D1608413

CARDIAC ARRHYTHMIA

MECHANISMS, DIAGNOSIS, AND MANAGEMENT

SECOND EDITION

CARDIAC ARRHYTHMIA

MECHANISMS, DIAGNOSIS, AND MANAGEMENT

SECOND EDITION

Editors

PHILIP J. PODRID, M.D.

Professor of Medicine
Associate Professor, Pharmacology and Experimental Therapeutics
Boston University School of Medicine
Boston, Massachusetts

PETER R. KOWEY, M.D.

Professor of Medicine
Jefferson Medical College
Philadelphia, Pennsylvania;
Chief, Division of Cardiovascular Diseases
Lankenau Hospital and Main Line Health System;
President, Main Line Health Heart Center
Wynnewood, Pennsylvania

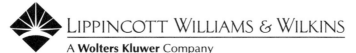

LIPPINCOTT WILLIAMS & WILKINS
A **Wolters Kluwer** Company
Philadelphia • Baltimore • New York • London
Buenos Aires • Hong Kong • Sydney • Tokyo

Acquisitions Editor: Ruth W. Weinberg
Developmental Editor: Ellen DiFrancesco
Production Manager: Toni Ann Scaramuzzo
Production Editor: Michael Mallard
Manufacturing Manager: Colin Warnock
Cover Designer: Mark Lerner
Compositor: Lippincott Williams & Wilkins Desktop Division
Printer: Maple Press

Library of Congress Cataloging-in-Publication Data
Cardiac arrhythmia : mechanisms, diagnosis, and management / editors, Philip J. Podrid, Peter R. Kowey.—2nd ed.
    p. ;   cm.
Includes bibliographical references and index.
ISBN 0-7817-2486-4
1. Arrhythmias.   I. Podrid, Philip J.   II. Kowey, Peter R.
[DNLM: 1. Arrhythmia—diagnosis.   2. Arrhythmia—therapy.
WG 330 C2649 2001]
RC685.A65 C24 2001
616.1′28—dc21   2001029293

Care has been taken to confirm the accuracy of the information presented and to describe generally accepted practices. However, the authors, editors, and publisher are not responsible for errors or omissions or for any consequences from application of the information in this book and make no warranty, expressed or implied, with respect to the currency, completeness, or accuracy of the contents of the publication. Application of this information in a particular situation remains the professional responsibility of the practitioner.

The authors, editors, and publisher have exerted every effort to ensure that drug selection and dosage set forth in this text are in accordance with current recommendations and practice at the time of publication. However, in view of ongoing research, changes in government regulations, and the constant flow of information relating to drug therapy and drug reactions, the reader is urged to check the package insert for each drug for any change in indications and dosage and for added warnings and precautions. This is particularly important when the recommended agent is a new or infrequently employed drug.

Some drugs and medical devices presented in this publication have Food and Drug Administration (FDA) clearance for limited use in restricted research settings. It is the responsibility of the health care provider to ascertain the FDA status of each drug or device planned for use in their clinical practice.

10 9 8 7 6 5 4 3 2 1

The first edition of this textbook was dedicated to our wives and children to whom we remain so very grateful for their unconditional love and patience. This edition is dedicated to our parents, Irving and Shirley Podrid and Peter and Edith Kowey who raised us to respect our fellow man and to appreciate the importance of hard work and perseverance. Without their support and encouragement, not only would this book not have been possible, but as doctors and people, we would be much diminished.

CONTENTS

Contributors ix
Foreword xiii
Preface xv
Acknowledgments xvii

SECTION I: BASIC SCIENCE

1. **Anatomy and Physiology of the Conduction System 3**
   Michael R. Lauer and Ruey J. Sung

2. **Basic Electrophysiology: Generation of the Cardiac Action Potential 37**
   Augustus O. Grant and Michael Carboni

3. **Mechanisms of Arrhythmogenesis 51**
   Charles Antzelevitch and Alexander Burashnikov

4.1. **Genetics of Arrhythmogenic Disorders 81**
   Silvia G. Priori, and Carlo Napolitano

4.2. **Influence of Autonomic Factors and Behavioral State on Vulnerability to Cardiac Arrhythmias 109**
   Richard L. Verrier, Julie A. Kovach, and Murray A. Mittleman

SECTION II: DIAGNOSTIC MODALITIES

5. **The Use of the Electrocardiogram in the Diagnosis of Arrhythmia 127**
   David B. Bharucha and Philip J. Podrid

6.1. **Role of Holter Monitoring and Exercise Testing for Arrhythmia Assessment and Management 165**
   Harold L. Kennedy and Philip J. Podrid

6.2. **Heart Rate Variability, Signal-Averaged Electrocardiography QT Dispersion and T Wave Alternans 195**
   Daniel Bloomfield, Anthony R. Magnano, and J. Thomas Bigger

7. **Electrophysiologic Testing and Cardiac Mapping 231**
   Hasan Garan and Brian McGovern

SECTION III: THERAPEUTIC MODALITIES

8. **Antiarrhythmic Drugs 265**
   Gerald V. Naccarelli, Philip T. Sager, and Bramah N. Singh

9. **Cardioversion and Defibrillation 303**
   Javier E. Sanchez, Andrew E. Epstein, and Raymond E. Ideker

10. **Cardiac Pacemakers 323**
    Amit Shanker and Sanjeev Saksena

11. **Implantable Cardioverter-Defibrillators 357**
    N. A. Mark Estes III and David S. Cannom

12. **Catheter and Surgical Ablation for Cardiac Arrhythmias 383**
    Ronald Berger, Michael D. Lesh, and Hugh Calkins

SECTION IV: SPECIFIC ARRHYTHMIAS

Tachyarrhythmia

13. **Sinoatrial/Atrial Tachyarrhythmias 411**
    Jeffrey J. Goldberger and Alan H. Kadish

14. **Atrioventricular Nodal Reentry 433**
    Richard I. Fogel and Eric N. Prystowsky

15. **Atrial Fibrillation 457**
    Arshad Jahangir, Thomas M. Munger, Douglas L. Packer, and Harry J.G.M. Crijns

16. **Atrial Flutter 501**
    Albert L. Waldo

17. **Tachycardias in Wolff-Parkinson-White Syndrome 517**
    Roger A. Marinchak and Seth J. Rials

18. **Ventricular Premature Depolarizations and Nonsustained Ventricular Tachycardia 549**
    Alfred E. Buxton and James Duc

19. **Sustained Monomorphic Ventricular Tachycardia 573**
    David Martin and J. Marcus Wharton

20. Polymorphous Ventricular Tachycardia, Including Torsade de Pointes 603
Stefan H. Hohnloser

21. Sudden Cardiac Death 621
Philip J. Podrid and Peter R. Kowey

Bradyarrhythmias

22. Sinus Node Function and Dysfunction 653
James A. Reiffel

23. Atrioventricular Nodal Conduction Abnormalities 671
Morton F. Arnsdorf and Ralph Verdino

24. His-Purkinje Disease 693
Pablo Denes

SECTION V: SPECIFIC SYNDROMES

25. Arrhythmias in Hypertrophic, Dilated, and Right Ventricular Cardiomyopathies 721
William J. McKenna, Joseph M. Galvin, and Shoaib Hamid

26. Arrhythmias in Congenital Heart Disease 749
Ronald J. Kanter and Arthur Garson

27. Arrhythmias and Conduction Disturbances Associated with Pregnancy 785
Samer R. Dibs and Leslie A. Saxon

28. Arrhythmia in Athletes 805
Michael A. Brodsky and Cyril Y. Leung

29. Arrhythmias After Cardiac and Noncardiac Surgery 831
Mina K. Chung, Craig R. Asher, David Yamada, and Kim A. Eagle

30. Periinfarction Arrhythmias 863
Azad V. Ghuran and A. John Camm

31. Arrhythmias in Mitral Valve Disease 889
Paul Kligfield and Richard B. Devereux

32. Arrhythmias in Cardiac Transplantation 907
Steven A. Rothman, Joyce Wald, and Howard J. Eisen

33. Syncope: Pathophysiology, Evaluation, and Treatment 925
David G. Benditt

Index 945

CONTRIBUTORS

Charles Antzelevitch, Ph.D. Executive Director, Masonic Medical Research Laboratory, Utica, New York 13501

Morton F. Arnsdorf, M.D. Professor, Department of Medicine, University of Chicago, Chicago, Illinois 60637

Craig R. Asher, M.D. Department of Cardiology, Section of Cardiac Electrophysiology, Cleveland Clinic Foundation, Cleveland, Ohio 44195

Ronald Berger, M.D. Arrhythmia Service and Electrophysiology Laboratory, Johns Hopkins Hospital, Baltimore, Maryland 21287

David G. Benditt, M.D. Professor of Medicine, Cardiac Arrhythmia Center, University of Minnesota Medical School, Minneapolis, Minnesota 55455

David B. Bharucha, M.D., Ph.D. Lankenau Hospital, Wynnewood, Pennsylvania 19096

J. Thomas Bigger, M.D. Professor, Department of Medicine, Columbia University, New York, New York 10032

Daniel Bloomfield, M.D. Division of Cardiology, Columbia University, New York, New York 10032

Michael A. Brodsky, M.D. Professor of Medicine, Division of Cardiology, University of California, Irvine, Irvine, California 92697; University of California, Irvine Medical Center, Orange, California 92868

Alexander Burashnikov, M.D. Masonic Medical Research Laboratory, Utica, New York 13501

Alfred E. Buxton, M.D. Professor of Medicine, Brown University School of Medicine, Director, Arrhythmia Services, Rhode Island Hospital, Providence, Rhode Island 02905

Hugh Calkins, M.D. Professor, Department of Medicine and Pediatrics, Johns Hopkins University; Chief, Arrhythmia Service and Clinical Electrophysiology Laboratory, Johns Hopkins Hospital, Baltimore, Maryland 21287

A. John Camm, M.D., F.R.C.P. Professor, Department of Cardiological Sciences, St. George's Hospital Medical School, London, SW17 0RE, United Kingdom

David S. Cannom, M.D. Clinical Professor of Medicine, University of California, Los Angeles School of Medicine, Los Angeles, California 90024; Medical Director of Cardiology, Good Samaritan Hospital, Los Angeles, California 90017

Michael Carboni, M.D. Departments of Medicine and Pediatrics, Duke University Medical Center, Durham, North Carolina 27710

Mina K. Chung, M.D. Department of Cardiology, Section of Cardiac Electrophysiology, Cleveland Clinic Foundation, Cleveland, Ohio 44195

Harry J.G.M. Crijns, M.D. Professor of Cardiology, University of Maastricht; Chair, Department of Cardiology, University Hospital Maastricht, 6200 Maastricht, The Netherlands

Pablo Denes, M.D. Professor, Department of Medicine, Northwestern University Memorial Hospital, Northwestern University, Chicago, Illinois 60611

Richard B. Devereux, M.D. Professor of Medicine, Division of Cardiology, Weill Medical College of Cornell University, The New York Presbyterian Hospital, New York, New York 10021

Samer R. Dibs, M.D. Assistant Professor, Division of Cardiology/Cardiac Electrophysiology, Northwestern University, Northwestern Memorial Hospital, Chicago, Illinois 60611

James Duc, M.D. Division of Cardiology, Brown University School of Medicine, Providence, Rhode Island 02912

Kim A. Eagle, M.D. Albion Walter Hewlett Professor of Internal Medicine, Department of Internal Medicine, University of Michigan; Chief, Clinical Cardiology, University of Michigan Medical Center, Ann Arbor, Michigan 48109

Howard J. Eisen, M.D. Professor of Medicine and Physiology, Department of Medicine, Section of Cardiology, Temple University School of Medicine; Medical Director, Advanced Heart Failure and Transplant Center, Temple University Hospital, Philadelphia, Pennsylvania 19140

Andrew E. Epstein, M.D. Department of Internal Medicine, Division of Cardiovascular Diseases, University of Alabama at Birmingham, Birmingham, Alabama 35294

N.A. Mark Estes, III, M.D. Professor of Medicine, Tufts University School of Medicine; Director, Cardiac Arrhythmia Service, New England Medical Center, Boston, Massachusetts 02111

Richard I. Fogel, M.D. Clinical Electrophysiologist, Department of Cardiology, St. Vincent Hospital/Indiana Heart Institute, Indianapolis, Indiana 46260

Joseph M. Galvin, M.D. Department of Cardiac Medicine, St. George's Hospital Medical School, London, SW17 0RE, United Kingdom

Hasan Garan, M.D. Professor, Department of Cardiology, University of Texas, Houston Medical School, Houston, Texas 77030

Arthur Garson, M.D., M.P.H. Senior Vice President and Dean for Academic Operations, Baylor College of Medicine; Vice President, Quality and Outcomes Management, Texas Children's Hospital, Houston, Texas 77030

Azad V. Ghuran, M.B.Ch.B., M.R.C.P.(UK) Cardiology Research Fellow, Department of Cardiological Sciences, St. George's Hospital Medical School, London, SW17 0RE, United Kingdom

Jeffrey J. Goldberger, M.D. Department of Cardiology, Northwestern University Medical School, Chicago, Illinois 60611

Augustus O. Grant, M.B., Ch.B., Ph.D. Professor of Medicine, Duke University, Duke University Medical Center, Durham, North Carolina 27710

Shoaib Hamid, M.D. Department of Cardiac Medicine, St. George's Hospital Medical School, London, SW17 0RE, United Kingdom

Stefan H. Hohnloser, M.D. Professor of Medicine, Division of Cardiology, J.W. Goethe University, 60590 Frankfurt, Germany

Raymond E. Ideker, M.D., Ph.D. Jeanne V. Marks Professor of Medicine, Department of Medicine, University of Alabama at Birmingham, Birmingham, Alabama 35294

Arshad Jahangir, M.D. Department of Cardiology, Mayo Foundation, Rochester, Minnesota 55902

Alan H. Kadish, M.D. Professor of Medicine, Northwestern University; Director, Cardiac Electrophysiology, Northwestern Memorial Hospital, Chicago, Illinois 60611

Ronald J. Kanter, M.D. Associate Professor, Department of Pediatrics, Duke University; Director, Pediatric Electrophysiology, Duke University Medical Center, Durham, North Carolina 27710

Harold L. Kennedy, M.D., M.P.H. Professor, Department of Medicine, University of Nevada, Veterans Administration Medical Center, Reno, Nevada 89502

Paul Kligfield, M.D., F.A.C.C. Professor, Department of Medicine, Weill Medical College of Cornell University; Director, Cardiac Graphics Laboratory, New York-Cornell Center of New York-Presbyterian Hospital, New York, New York 10021

Julie A. Kovach, M.D. Department of Cardiology, University of Michigan Health System, Ann Arbor, Michigan 48109

Peter R. Kowey, M.D. Professor of Medicine, Thomas Jefferson University, Philadelphia, Pennsylvania 19107; Chief, Division of Cardiovascular Diseases, Lankenau Hospital, Wynnewood, Pennsylvania 19096

Michael R. Lauer, M.D. Department of Medicine, Stanford University School of Medicine, San Jose, California 95119

Michael D. Lesh, M.D. Division of Cardiac Electrophysiology, University of California, San Francisco, San Francisco, California 94143

Cyril Y. Leung, M.D. Assistant Clinical Professor, Department of Medicine, Division of Cardiology, University of California-Irvine Medical Center, University of California-Irvine, Orange, California 92868

Anthony R. Magnano, M.D. Division of Cardiology, Columbia University, New York, New York 10032

Roger A. Marinchak, M.D. Clinical Associate Professor of Medicine, Thomas Jefferson University School of Medicine, Philadelphia, Pennsylvania 19107; Director, Arrhythmia Services, Main Line Health System, The Lankenau Hospital, Wynnewood, Pennsylvania 19096

David Martin, M.D. Department of Medicine, Duke University Medical Center, Durham, North Carolina 27710

Brian McGovern, M.D. Massachusetts General Hospital, Boston, Massachusetts 02114

William J. McKenna, M.D. Professor of Cardiac Medicine, St. George's Hospital Medical School, London, SW17 0RE, United Kingdom

Murray A. Mittleman, M.D. Department of Medicine, Harvard Medical School; Institute for Prevention of Cardiovascular Disease, Beth Israel Deaconess Medical Center, Boston, Massachusetts 02215

Thomas M. Munger, M.D. Department of Cardiology, Mayo Foundation, Rochester, Minnesota 55902

Gerald V. Naccarelli, M.D. Professor, Department of Medicine, Penn State University College of Medicine; Chief, Division of Cardiology, The Milton S. Hershey Medical Center, Hershey, Pennsylvania 17033

Carlo Napolitano, M.D. University of Pavia, 27100 Pavia, Italy

Douglas L. Packer, M.D. Professor of Medicine, Department of Electrophysiology, Mayo Foundation, St. Mary's Hospital, Rochester, Minnesota 55905

Philip J. Podrid, M.D. Professor of Medicine, Department of Medicine/Cardiology; Associate Professor of Pharmacology and Experimental Therapeutics, Boston University School of Medicine, Boston, Massachusetts 02118

Silvia G. Priori, M.D., Ph.D. Associate Professor of Cardiology, University of Pavia; Director, Molecular Cardiology Division, Fondazione Salvatore Maugeri, 27100 Pavia, Italy

Eric N. Prystowsky, M.D. Consulting Professor of Medicine, Duke University Medical Center, Durham, North Carolina 27710; Director, Clinical Electrophysiology Laboratory, St. Vincent's Hospital, Indianapolis, Indiana 46260

James A. Reiffel, M.D. Professor of Clinical Medicine, Division of Cardiology, Columbia University; Director, ECG Laboratory, The New York Presbyterian Hospital, New York, New York 10032

Seth J. Rials, M.D., Ph.D. Heart Care, Inc., Columbus, Ohio 43214

Steven A. Rothman, M.D. Department of Medicine, Division of Clinical Electrophysiology, Temple University School of Medicine, Philadelphia, Pennsylvania 19140

Philip T. Sager, M.D. Department of Cardiology, University of California, Los Angeles School of Medicine; Veterans Administration Medical Center West Los Angeles, Los Angeles, California 90073

Sanjeev Saksena, M.D. Cardiovascular Institute of the Atlantic Health System, Passaic, New Jersey 07055

Javier E. Sanchez, M.D. Department of Internal Medicine, Division of Cardiovascular Diseases, University of Alabama at Birmingham, Birmingham, Alabama 35294

Leslie A. Saxon, M.D. Associate Professor of Medicine, Department of Cardiac Electrophysiology; Director, Electrophysiology Laboratory and Implantable Device Service, University of California, San Francisco, California 94143

Amit Shanker, M.D. Department of Medicine, Robert Wood Johnson School of Medicine, New Brunswick, New Jersey 08903

Bramah N. Singh, M.D., Ph.D. Professor of Medicine, Department of Cardiology, University of California, Los Angeles School of Medicine; Veterans Administration Medical Center West Los Angeles, Los Angeles, California 90073

Ruey J. Sung, M.D. Professor of Medicine, Stanford University School of Medicine, Stanford University Medical Center, Stanford, California 94305

Ralph Verdino, M.D. Section of Cardiology, University of Chicago Hospital, Chicago, Illinois 60637

Richard L. Verrier, Ph.D. Department of Medicine, Harvard Medical School; Institute for Prevention of Cardiovascular Disease, Beth Israel Deaconess Medical Center, Boston, Massachusetts 02215

Joyce Wald, M.D. Department of Medicine, Temple University School of Medicine, Philadelphia, Pennsylvania 19140

Albert L. Waldo, M.D. The Walter H. Pritchard Professor of Cardiology and Professor of Medicine, Case Western Reserve University; Director, Cardiac Electrophysiology Program, University Hospital, Cleveland, Ohio 44106

J. Marcus Wharton, M.D. Associate Professor of Medicine, Division of Cardiology, Duke University; Director, Clinical Cardiac Electrophysiology, Duke University Medical Center, Durham, North Carolina 27710

David Yamada, M.D. Department of Cardiology, Section of Cardiac Electrophysiology, Cleveland Clinic Foundation, Cleveland, Ohio 44195

FOREWORD

It was a pleasant surprise to be reinvited by Drs. Podrid and Kowey to write once again some introductory words now for the second edition of their textbook. Having reviewed my foreword for the first edition, I believe the weathering of time's passage has not diminished the cogency of these comments nor my expressed high regard for their text.

The Bible declares "of making many books there is no end." This wise observation antedates Gutenberg. At present, 1000 books are published daily worldwide. The total of all printed knowledge doubles every 8 years. The deluge has not spared cardiology. On the contrary, we are in the very midst of the torrent. An especially popular cardiologic subject is arrhythmias, a topic that fills numerous texts, monographs, hardcover as well as softcover books, and endless throwaways. What then is the justification for still another book?

The answer is straightforward: there is always a place for a good book—and in no field more insistently than arrhythmology. The reasons are several. Existing books are largely skewed toward the experts and are filled with specialized jargon, not distinguishing the esoteric detail from the essential points. A number of these books are written for budding electrophysiologists or for those readying to hang a shingle announcing themselves as arrhythmologists, whatever that means. In these books the technologic tail wags the clinical dog, and the everyday problems of internists and practicing cardiologists, who encounter the majority of patients experiencing arrhythmias, are largely ignored. There is therefore a need for an authoritative book positing the significant scientific and technologic advances within a sound clinical framework.

A well-planned book is especially needed at present to help the clinician orient during a period of substantial medical advances and great leaps in the development of the therapeutic armamentarium. This is nowhere more in evidence than in arrhythmology. The extensive persuasive data recently accumulated pointing to the paradox that all antiarrhythmic drugs can cause dangerous and even life-threatening arrhythmias leaves the practitioner in a quandary. Too often and unnecessarily the recourse is to use technology to solve even simple problems.

The majority of arrhythmias are readily manageable by the internist and general cardiologist. More than 95% of such disorders consist of extrasystoles, either atrial or ventricular, sinus tachycardia or bradycardia, and atrial fibrilla-tion. These disorders are better identified by a careful history than by an invasive procedure. The classic, long-established methods of management continue to be relevant and, when fully understood, still carry the day.

For the difficult and at time intractable rhythm disorders, new techniques, some with substantial efficacy have emerged and continue to be refined. Implantable devices, ever more elegant in design, can keep the physician informed as to what is transpiring while protecting the patient from potentially lethal arrhythmias. Current advances have dramatically changed the approach for managing a number of tachyarrhythmias. The aim has shifted from palliation to total cure by eliminating the pathologic nidus with radiofrequency ablation. While the initial applications have proved effective for atrial tachyarrhythmias, ventricular rhythm derangements will not be left unattended, as computer-driven cardiac mapping techniques define site of origin or pathway of arrhythmia traverse for permanent abolition.

Clinicians need to be continually alerted to the latest breakthroughs. More important, they deserve sound information, enabling them to distinguish the experimental and promising from the therapeutically proven.

Cardiac Arrhythmia: Mechanisms, Diagnosis, and Management, Second edition, is a comprehensive text edited by two leaders in arrhythmia studies, both seasoned clinicians, who, in addition to contributing their own wealth of experience, have mobilized leaders in the field to provide a panoramic perspective. That both Drs. Kowey and Podrid have received their early indoctrination and arrhythmia tutelage in my experimental laboratory at the Harvard School of Public Health and in the clinics of the Brigham and Women's Hospital makes me especially partial to their efforts.

Sir William Osler once commented, "To study medicine without books is to sail an uncharted sea; whilst to study medicine only from books is to not to go to sea at all." This book offers a well-charted journey. It is conceived from a clinician's perspective and provides a balanced approach invaluable for the practitioner.

Bernard Lown, M.D.
Professor Emeritus
Harvard School of Public Health
Brigham and Women's Hospital
Boston, Massachusetts 02115

PREFACE

Editing the first edition of our textbook *Cardiac Arrhythmia: Mechanisms, Diagnosis, and Management,* published in 1995, was a daunting task, as an enormous amount of material needed to be pulled together and synthesized into a cohesive book, which would be useful for cardiologists and noncardiologists. We thought that editing the second edition would be an easier task, requiring only updating of the material. However, we grossly underestimated the amount of work involved and editing this second edition turned out to be a more extensive project than anticipated since over the past 5 years there has been an explosion of information in the field of arrhythmia. The rapid evolution in new approaches for the evaluation and management of patients with various rhythm disorders has been staggering, requiring extensive rewriting of all of the chapters.

The evaluation of patients with arrhythmia continues to evolve. Many techniques are no longer used; some are of less relevance, while others have become more important as clinical tools. Perhaps the most dramatic developments have occurred in the management of arrhythmias. The results from a number of large randomized trials have caused a major change in the primary method of treatment of many patients, with a marked expansion in the use of non-pharmacologic therapy, including ablative techniques and implantable devices. These therapies have offered patients important alternatives for management, with the potential for a "cure" in many cases; as a result there has been a marked shift in the primary approach to therapy. Non-pharmacologic therapy is now the preferred therapeutic approach for controlling most rhythm abnormalities, while in many cases pharmacologic therapy with antiarrhythmic drugs has been relegated to a secondary role, most frequently used as adjunctive rather than primary therapy to facilitate or modify device function or to improve on the results of a partially successful ablation. However, the use of parenteral forms of some of these agents has evolved with a growing interest in acute arrhythmia management.

The growing use of ablation as a first-line therapy has provided the impetus for many advances in the field of electrophysiologic mapping, with the development of impressive technology for precise localization of the arrhythmogenic focus. Today, almost all patients with supraventicular tachyarrhythmias, including atrial tachycardia, atrioventricular nodal reentrant tachycardia, atrioventricular reentrant tachycardia associated with a preexcitation syndrome, and atrial flutter as well as many with monomorphic ventricular tachycardia can be successfully treated with radiofrequency catheter ablation. Although drugs are still the mainstay of therapy for atrial fibrillation, there is a growing interest in and use of ablation. The primary approach to therapy of life-threatening ventricular tachyarrhythmias, including ventricular tachycardia and ventricular fibrillation, is an implantable device and there have been major advances in the ability of these devices to accurately identify these arrhythmia; they now have the capability to defibrillate, cardiovert, and provide dual chamber pacing for bradycardia.

While the established mechanisms for arrhythmogenesis have not changed, research has yielded many exciting insights into the etiology and basic electrophysiology of arrhythmia. In particular new studies have linked genetic abnormalities to a variety of conditions associated with arrhythmia and have provided a sound basis for understanding the etiology of specific arrhythmias on a cellular level.

As a result, the second edition had to be completely revised to reflect these developments in the field, prompting substantial changes in the chapters contained in this textbook. Additionally, the chapters had to be appropriately fashioned to avoid being too complex and unwieldy. The chapters about basic electrophysiology and methods for arrhythmia evaluation have been extensively updated. Chapters about device therapy (pacemakers and implantable defibrillators) and ablation and their application to therapy of various rhythm abnormalities have been entirely rewritten and expanded, while the sections on pharmacologic therapy have been appropriately trimmed. The chapters dealing with each of the specific arrhythmias and syndromes have been extensively rewritten to reflect the changes in management that have occurred over the past 5 years.

The second edition is substantially shorter than the first one to accommodate the needs of busy trainees and practitioners. With these major revisions, the second edition provides concise, yet complete information about the current state of the art of arrhythmia management, which can be used by both cardiologists and noncardiologists who see and treat patients with a wide range of rhythm disturbances. We hope that all who use this textbook will find it not only easy and enjoyable to read but also informative and useful for their clinical practice.

ACKNOWLEDGMENTS

The editors wish to thank our contributing authors who worked so hard to create an extraordinary and cohesive set of treatises that represents the state of knowledge in our field. Their clinical insight was especially important in crafting a useful textbook for practitioners. We very much appreciate their patience during our aggressive editing and in particular the difficult process of chapter consolidation. Ellen DiFrancesco, our developmental editor, and Ruth Weinberg, our acquisitions editor, are due special thanks for helping to launch this most ambitious project, for managing the logistics of chapter collection and distribution, and for chiding us to complete the project, and to get our book into production in a timely fashion. Our deep gratitude goes to Rose Marie Wells who provided unflagging secretarial support, toiling with characteristic good humor and without complaint, and to our administrative assistants and clerical staff who never balked at helping us with the seemingly endless task of paper shuffling and word processing. Our clinical partners and colleagues cheerfully shouldered an extra portion of work while we were occupied with the book's development and for that we are in their debt. We thank our mentors and teachers who showed us the way to their discipline and gave us the tools to understand its most important principles, and most importantly, helped us to understand what being a doctor really means. And most of all, we thank our wonderful patients who, by their courage and strength of character, inspire us to understand and conquer the afflictions that beset them.

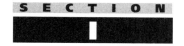

SECTION I

BASIC SCIENCE

1

ANATOMY AND PHYSIOLOGY OF THE CONDUCTION SYSTEM

MICHAEL R. LAUER
RUEY J. SUNG

Fundamentally, clinical cardiac electrophysiology is the study of the normal and abnormal functional properties of the electrically excitable tissues of the heart. Although an appreciation for the anatomy of the discrete components of the cardiac conduction system is important, cardiac electrophysiologists are generally less concerned with the precise anatomic details than the functional behavior of electrical conduction within and through these structures. The anatomic conduction system is best viewed as a physiologic continuum through which electrical current flows within three-dimensional structures. At different points along the course of the conduction system, there occur normal variations in conduction pattern, velocity, and direction. Clinically significant disruptions of cardiac rhythm may develop when altered anatomy (structure) leads to abnormal alterations of conduction pattern, velocity, and direction (function). The widespread use of ablation also necessitates knowledge of the conduction system.

FUNCTIONAL ANATOMY OF THE CONDUCTION SYSTEM

Most of the gross anatomic features of the heart and conduction system critical to the study of cardiac electrophysiology are presented in introductory or intermediate-level physiology courses. The histologic details and specifics of the cellular architecture of the normal and abnormal specialized conducting system continue to emerge and have been reviewed in detail elsewhere (1–18).

Figure 1-1 schematically depicts the normal conduction system. The heart's normal intrinsic pacemaker, called the sinoatrial (SA) node, lies within the sulcus terminalis

between the superior vena cava and the right atrial appendage. It is up to 2 cm long and 0.5 cm wide. Specialized cells within the SA node generate calcium (Ca^{2+})-dependent action potentials that spread through the transitional cells at the node's border to activate the atrial myocardium. This wavefront of depolarization conducts through the atria to the atrioventricular (AV) node, possibly by preferential internodal tracts composed of cells that are indistinguishable from working atrial myocardium. At least three such preferential approaches to the AV node have been proposed, including the superior, inferior, and middle pathways (15,16). However, other authorities have persuasively argued no such anatomically definable preferential pathways exist (19). The superior internodal tract proceeds from the cephalic portion of the SA node to the anterior portion of the atrial septum to merge with the anterior and superior approaches to the AV node. The middle pathway arises from the middle portion of the SA node and travels along the limbus fossa ovalis to also merge with the anterior atrial septal approaches to the AV node. The inferior tract runs from the caudal portion of the SA node along the lower part of the atrial septum near the opening of the inferior vena cava to reach the posterior approaches to the AV node near the ostium of the coronary sinus. Some authorities believe that an anterosuperiorly directed pathway runs through the atrial appendage to the anterior or superior approaches to the AV node. Bachmann's bundle may provide a preferential connection from the SA node to the left atrial septum with a left atrial extension connecting to the anterior approaches to the AV node.

In the absence of an accessory pathway, the AV node–His bundle axis provides the only electrical connection between the atria and ventricles. The gross and microscopic anatomy of the AV junction is complex, and the structural definition of the AV node has been the subject of controversy virtually since its original description (20–24). Based on histologic examination, three different areas of specialized tissues can be observed connecting the working atrial and ventricular myocardia at the AV junction: transi-

M. R. Lauer: Department of Medicine, Stanford University School of Medicine, San Jose, California 95119.

R. J. Sung: Department of Medicine, Stanford University School of Medicine, and Cardiac Electrophysiology Service, Stanford University Medical Center, Stanford, California 94305.

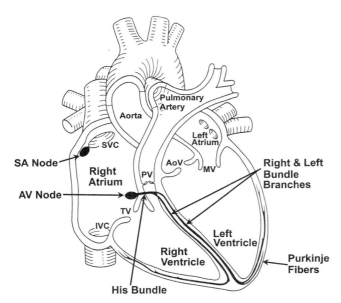

FIGURE 1-1. Cardiac specialized conduction system, including the sinoatrial node, atrioventricular node, His bundle, bundle branches, arborizing network of Purkinje fibers, right (RA) and left (LA) atria, and right (RV) and left (LV) ventricles.

tional cells (i.e., nodal approaches) positioned between the atrial myocardium and the compact node, the compact node proper, and the nonbranching part of the His bundle (3) (Fig. 1-2). The atrial components of these specialized tissues at the AV junction are contained within the triangle of Koch, an important landmark for AV nodal ablation. Two of its sides are formed by the tendon of Todaro and the tricuspid annulus, and its base is marked by the ostium of the coronary sinus (Fig. 1-3). In the adult human heart, the mean length of the triangle of Koch (measured from the central fibrous body to the nearest edge of the coronary sinus) is 17 ± 3 mm (range, 10 to 24 mm), and the mean width (measured from the tricuspid annulus to the nearest edge of the coronary sinus) is 13 ± 3 mm (range, 6 to 21 mm) (25). The compact node has a length of 5 to 7 mm and a width of 2 to 5 mm (26).

Lying at the apex of the triangle of Koch, the compact node penetrates the central fibrous body to become the His bundle. Transitional cells can be grouped into three zones: superficial, deep, and posterior. The superficial zone is continuous with the anterior and superior aspect of the compact node, the posterior zone joins the inferior and posterior part of the compact node, and the deep zone connects

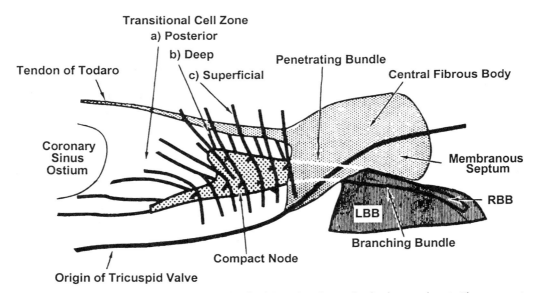

FIGURE 1-2. Diagram of the atrioventricular (AV) junctional area in the human heart. The compact node is composed of leftward- and rightward-going components and is continuous anteriorly with the penetrating AV bundle. The compact node is continuous with three groups of transitional cells: (1) superficial, passing superficial to the tendon of Todaro and partly extending over the compact node into the tricuspid valve base; (2) deep, connecting with the left side of the septum; and (3) posterior, connecting the atrial myocardium above and below the ostium of the coronary sinus. LBB, left bundle branch; RBB, right bundle branch. (From Becker AE, Anderson RH. Morphology of the human atrioventricular junctional area. In: Wellens HJJ, Lie KI, Janse MJ, eds. *The conduction system of the heart: structure, function and clinical implication.* Leiden, The Netherlands: Sterfest Kroese, 1976:263, with permission.)

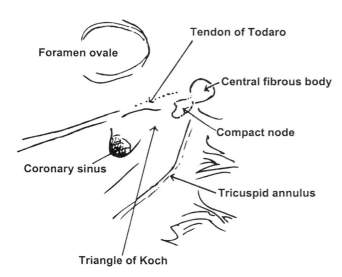

FIGURE 1-3. The central fibrous body at the apex, the tendon of Todaro and the tricuspid annulus at the sides, and the coronary sinus at the base demarcate the triangle of Koch. The compact atrioventricular (AV) node, which penetrates the central fibrous body to become the AV (His) bundle, is approximately 5 to 7 mm long and 2 to 5 mm wide. The triangle of Koch has a mean length (measured from the central fibrous body to the nearest edge of the coronary sinus) of approximately 17±3 mm and a mean height (measured from the tricuspid annulus to the nearest edge of the coronary sinus) of approximately 13±3 mm.

the left atrial septum to the deep part of the compact node (3) (Fig. 1-2). These transitional cell zones are also referred to as *nodal approaches* (22) or *atrionodal bundles* (13). In canine heart experiments, the transitional cell zones have been demonstrated to possess functional properties of specialized conduction tissues distinctly different from those of the working atrial myocardium (27).

In the rabbit heart, there is a dual input to the compact node during anterograde conduction (7, 28–32): an anterior input entering the node as a broad wavefront anterior to the coronary sinus ostium and a posterior input entering the node beneath the coronary sinus ostium through the crista terminalis. During retrograde conduction, the earliest exit to the atrium is in the interatrial septum, anterior to the coronary sinus ostium, at the same location of the anterior input during anterograde conduction; the crista terminalis is activated much later than the interatrial septum (Fig. 1-4).

Although not all investigators agree, the AV junction appears to consist of histologically distinct cell types, including P cells, and various types of transitional cells (33). P cells make up about 5% of the specialized cells in the AV junction, and transitional cells account for approximately 95%. Transitional cells vary in size and morphology, and they appear to have an intricate interwoven arrangement displaying various connections, including end-to-end, side-to-side, end-to-side, and combinations of these forms. Con-

nections appear not to be by conventional intercalated disks or gap junctions (i.e., containing mainly connexin 45 and 40 with little or no connexin 43) (34–37). The highest concentration of P cells is at the distal junction of the AV node and His bundle, and the cells are often associated with nerve endings.

Based on cellular electrophysiologic properties, the AV node has been divided into AN, N, and NH cell zones and into even smaller subdivisions (7,28–31) (Fig. 1-4). The AN region consists of large Purkinje-like cells comprising the internodal pathways with a large portion of the slender transitional cells. The N region corresponds primarily to the mass of interweaving and interconnected transitional cells of all types, and the NH region appears to be where P cells and some transitional cells connect with large Purkinje-type cells of the His bundle (33). The disparity in cell types and arrangements accounts for anisotropic conduction demonstrated at the AV junction (38).

The His or AV bundle begins as the AV node penetrates the central fibrous body, arising from the penetrating portion of the His bundle and soon arises as the major branching fascicles of the specialized conducting tissue in the ventricles called the His-Purkinje system. The main left bundle branch arborizes into fan-shaped posterior and anterior radiations. Further divisions from the larger posterior fascicle combine with contributions from the anterior fascicle to produce a septal branch of the left bundle branch. The large right bundle branch bifurcates from the continuation of the penetrating segment of the His bundle and ends with a trifurcation supplying the anterolateral papillary muscle, parietal band, and lower septal aspect of the right ventricle. Conduction in the atrial and ventricular muscle and the His-Purkinje system occurs relatively rapidly because of fast sodium (Na^+)-dependent action potentials. Rapid activation of the working ventricular muscle through the His-Purkinje system triggers ventricular contraction.

The complex regional endocardial anatomy of the right atrium also plays a crucial role in a number of tachyarrhythmias, including atrial tachycardias and atrial flutter. Orifices of superior and inferior vena cava lie in the superior and inferior aspects of the right atrium, respectively. The tricuspid annulus lies anterior to the cavity of the right atrium. The endocardium of the right atrium is divided into an anterior trabeculated portion (the true embryonic right atrium) and a posterior, smooth-walled segment that is derived from the embryonic sinus venosus. Separating these distinct anatomic regions laterally is the crista terminalis and, inferiorly, the eustachian ridge. The crista terminalis extends from the high interatrial septum anteriorly and superiorly to the orifice of the superior vena cava and radiates caudally along the posterolateral wall. At its inferior extent, it courses anterior to the orifice of the inferior vena cava. The eustachian ridge is the remnant of the embryonic sinus venosus valve and extends from the orifice of the infe-

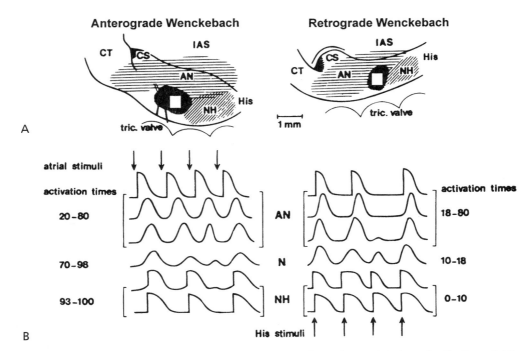

FIGURE 1-4. Representations of action potential configuration and timing of activation of AN, N, and NH cell regions during antegrade and retrograde Wenckebach phenomenon in the rabbit heart. The AN region consists of large Purkinje-like cells comprising the internodal pathways with a large portion of the slender transitional cells. The N region corresponds to the mass of interweaving and interconnected transitional cells of all types, and the NH region is where P cells and some transitional cells connect with large Purkinje-type cells of the His bundle. **A:** The location of the atrioventricular junctional regions (AN, N, and NH zones) in which action potentials are recorded. Notice the central position of the relatively small N zone. **B:** Resting potential configuration in the various zones during anterograde stimulation *(left)* and during retrograde stimulation *(right)*. Activation times are pooled from different experiments and are expressed as a percentage of total A-H or H-A conduction time. (From Janse MJ, van Capelle FJL, Anderson RH, et al. Electrophysiology and structure of the atrioventricular node of the isolated rabbit heart. In: Wellens HJJ, Lie KI, Janse MJ, eds. *The conduction system of the heart: structure, function and clinical implication.* Leiden, The Netherlands: Sterfest Kroese, 1976:296, with permission.)

rior vena cava along the floor of the right atrium to the ostium of the coronary sinus. A 1- to 2-cm-wide isthmus resides between the inferior aspect of the tricuspid valve annulus and the eustachian ridge. The ostium of the coronary sinus lies medial to the orifice of the inferior vena cava, where the floor of the right atrium rises to become the atrial septum.

Vascular Supply

The vascular supply to the SA node originates from the right coronary artery in 55% of patients and the left coronary artery in 45%. In approximately 90% of individuals, the AV node receives its blood supply from a branch of the right coronary artery. In 10%, an additional or the sole vascular supply comes from the left coronary artery. In 90% of patients, the His bundle vascular supply comes from branches of the left anterior descending artery. In the remaining 10% of patients, the His bundle receives its blood supply from the right coronary artery. The right and main left bundle branches receive their blood from perforating branches of the anterior and posterior descending arteries (i.e., mixed right and left coronary contribution). The left bundle anterior radiation generally receives its vascular supply from anterior perforating branches, and the posterior radiation is supplied by posterior perforating branches.

Autonomic Innervation and Nervous Control

There is extensive sympathetic and parasympathetic innervation of the SA and AV nodes (39). The cardiac plexus, formed by sympathetic nerves originating from the upper thoracic spinal cord and parasympathetic nerves from the medulla, surrounds the aortic arch and is the source of the cardiac autonomic innervation. The rate of depolarization and generation of action potentials in the SA node is exquisitely sensitive to the level of sympathetic and parasympathetic tone. Enhanced parasympathetic activity or decreased sympathetic activity results in a decrease in the rate of depolarization in the SA node, decreasing the rate of action potential generation, as well as increased conduction time through the AV node. However, enhanced sympathetic and reduced parasympathetic tone increases the rate of depolarization and action potential generation and decreases conduction time through the AV node. Although the SA and AV node regions receive extensive autonomic innervation, there is sparse innervation distal to the AV node, including the His bundle and bundle branches.

ARRHYTHMOGENIC ANATOMY

The three major mechanisms for clinical cardiac arrhythmias include reentry, automaticity, and triggered activity. A number of normal and abnormal anatomic structures (Fig.

1-5) have been implicated in the genesis of cardiac arrhythmias (Table 1-1). SA reentrant tachycardia may result from reentry within the SA node or the SA node and adjacent atrial myocardium. There is still debate whether the anatomic substrate for AV node reentry lies entirely within the confines of the AV node proper or may also involve adjacent atrial tissue, possibly atrial myocardium or transitional cells.

In the fully developed human heart, fibrous AV rings (i.e., annulus fibrosus) almost completely electrically insulate the atrial and ventricular myocardia from each other. Only at the AV node–His bundle region is electrical continuity established, permitting cardiac impulse conduction from the atria to the ventricles. As long as the insulation of the annulus fibrosus is not breached, atrial impulses are conducted to the ventricle only by way of the AV node-His-Purkinje system (40,41).

Because of its decremental conduction properties, the AV node functions as a protective barrier (42), delaying AV conduction and preventing an excessive number of

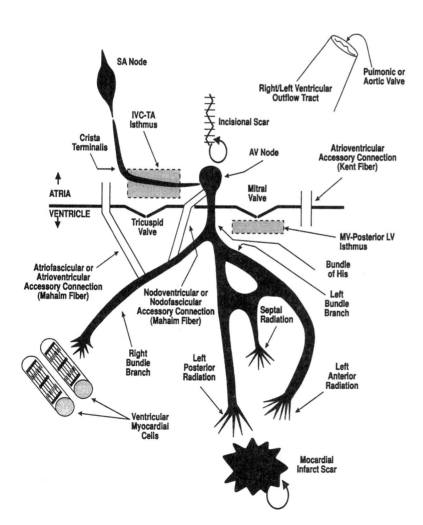

FIGURE 1-5. Locations of many of the anatomic substrates associated with the development of cardiac arrhythmias.

TABLE 1-1. ANATOMIC SUBSTRATES ASSOCIATED WITH THE DEVELOPMENT OF CARDIAC ARRHYTHMIAS

Anatomic Structure	Type of Arrhythmia	Mechanism of Arrhythmia
SA node ± adjacent tissues	SART	Microreentry
AV node ± adjacent tissues	AVNRT	Microreentry
Accessory connection (Kent fiber)	Orthodromic & antidromic AVRT	Macroreentry
Accessory connection (PJRT type)	Orthodromic AVRT with long RP′ interval	Macroreentry
Accessory connection (Mahaim fiber)	Antidromic AVRT	Macroreentry
Crista terminalis	AT	Reentry/automaticity/triggered activity?
Atrial isthmus: IVC-TV annulus and crista terminalis	AFL	Macroreentry
Bundle branches (with IVCD)	Bundle branch reentrant VT or fascicular tachycardia	Macroreentry
Myocardial scar (± isthmus) associated with infarct or cardiomyopathy	AT, AF, VT, VF	Macroreentry or microreentry
Ventricular isthmus: MV annulus–posterior basilar left ventricular MI scar	VT	Macroreentry or microreentry
Subvalvular right or left ventricular outflow tracts	VT	Reentry/automaticity/triggered activity?
Right or left ventricular dysplasia	VT	Macroreentry or microreentry
Pulmonary vein	AF, AFL, AT	Reentry/automaticity/triggered activity?
"Remodeled" atria	AF	Reentry (multiple wavefronts?)
Healed atrial myocardial surgical incision	AT, AFL	Macroreentry or microreentry

AF, atrial fibrillation; AFL, atrial flutter; AT, atrial tachycardia; AV, atrioventricular, AVNRT, atrioventricular node reentrant tachycardia; AVRT, atrioventricular reciprocating tachycardia; IVC, inferior vena cava; IVCD, intraventricular conduction delay; MI, myocardial infarction; MV, mitral valve; PJRT, permanent form of junctional reciprocating tachycardia; SA, sinoatrial; SART, sinoatrial reentrant tachycardia; TV, tricuspid valve; VF, ventricular fibrillation; VT, ventricular tachycardia.

atrial impulses from reaching the ventricles. When the annulus fibrosus insulation is disrupted or the normal AV node-His-Purkinje pathway is short-circuited by an accessory AV connection, the ventricle can be excited earlier than would normally be expected. This phenomenon is referred to as *ventricular preexcitation* (43,44). Based on findings of anatomic and electrophysiologic studies, accessory connections can be classified as accessory AV muscle bundles, accessory nodoventricular muscle bundles, atriofascicular bypass tracts, intranodal bypass tracts, nodal malformations, and fasciculoventricular accessory connections (43). Some of these accessory connections exist only anatomically or electrophysiologically, a few exist anatomically and electrophysiologically, but others are only hypothetical and remain very much debatable. The tachyarrhythmias associated with the ventricular preexcitation syndromes are the best studied examples of reentry (i.e., circus movement) and are discussed in other chapters of this book.

The crista terminalis (45–48) is a ridge of tissue that runs posteriorly from the "tail" of the SA node along the lateral right atrial wall and then medially to merge with the eustachian ridge, which ends near the ostium of the coronary sinus. During their routes, the crista and eustachian ridge provide the posterior border of the isthmus of atrial tissue forming the floor of the right atrium lying between the inferior vena cava and tricuspid valve annulus (IVC-

TV isthmus). Typical clockwise and counterclockwise atrial flutter traverse this isthmus as part of their macroreentry circuit, and this isthmus therefore has become the anatomic target for curative catheter ablation of atrial flutter (Fig. 1-6). Along its course, the crista terminalis appears to provide fertile ground for the origin of atrial tachycardia (45–48) because of automaticity, triggered activity, or reentry. Atrial tachycardia related to a healed atrial scar from a past surgical incision for repair of an atrial septal defect, other congenital heart disease, or valvular heart disease has also been described (49,50). The ostia of the pulmonary veins have been recognized as a frequent source of atrial premature depolarizations and rapid atrial tachycardias that can trigger atrial fibrillation and atrial flutter. Ablation of these triggering foci may provide a curative treatment for selected patients with atrial fibrillation and atrial flutter (51,52). Electrical and structural "remodeling" of the atria due to dilation, enlargement, and stretch resulting from atrial fibrillation may predispose to more atrial fibrillation (53–58).

Various forms of ventricular tachycardia have been associated with specific anatomic structures. Ventricular tachycardias originating in the right ventricular outflow and left ventricular outflow tracts have been identified (59–68). In each case, the tachycardia focus appears to be located immediately proximal to the pulmonic valve or aortic valve, respectively. The mechanism of these tachycardias is

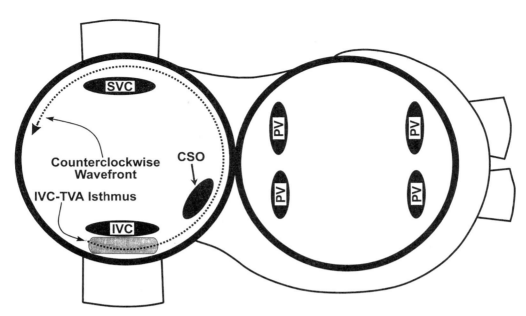

FIGURE 1-6. Cross-sectional view through the atrioventricular groove at the level of the mitral and tricuspid valve annulae as seen from the cardiac apex. The reentrant wavefront in patients with the typical clockwise and counterclockwise (shown here) forms of atrial flutter conducts through the isthmus bordered by the inferior vena cava (IVC) and the tricuspid valve annulus (TVA). The IVC-TVA isthmus is the anatomic target during ablation of typical atrial flutter. CSO, ostium of the coronary sinus; PV, pulmonary vein; SVC, superior vena cava.

still open to debate and may have characteristics consistent with automaticity, reentry, triggered activity, or possibly all three. Data from magnetic resonance imaging studies suggest that the ventricular location of the foci of tachycardia in some of these patients may not be entirely structurally normal (69,70). Bundle branch reentrant ventricular tachycardia using the main right and left bundle branches along with a poorly defined transseptal myocardial pathway for macroreentry has been described (71–74). Fascicular tachycardias that exclusively use the His-Purkinje system for macroreentry have also been observed (75–81). Ventricular tachycardia related to right or left ventricular dysplasia involving replacement of normal myocardium with fat and fibrous tissue has also been reported (59,82–90).

The most common and most dangerous cause of ventricular tachycardia is myocardial reentrant ventricular tachycardia related to an old myocardial infarct scar (91–100). Classically, this form of tachycardia is related to residual viable myocardium, possibly at the border zone of the infarct scar, which contains a zone of slow conduction and unidirectional conduction block. However, the concept of a viable isthmus region lying between two areas of nonconducting tissue has been proposed as a substrate for this form of ventricular tachycardia, in a fashion analogous to atrial flutter in the right atrium. In some patients with a posterior basilar and left ventricular myocardial infarct scar,

a viable isthmus between the scar and the posterior aspect of the mitral valve annulus may be responsible for macroreentry in these patients (101,102).

CLINICAL ELECTROPHYSIOLOGY OF THE CARDIAC CONDUCTION SYSTEM

Intracardiac Electrograms

Performance of a diagnostic electrophysiology procedure involves electrical stimulation of various cardiac chambers and recording of local cardiac electrical activity, called electrograms, using temporary electrode catheters placed percutaneously into the atria, ventricles, or lumens of epicardial vessels. An electrogram represents a recording of a voltage or electrical potential difference. A unipolar electrogram is the potential difference recorded between an intracardiac electrode in close association with cardiac tissue and a distant indifferent electrode. Recording of bipolar electrograms involves recording a potential difference between a pair of closely spaced electrodes. Bipolar electrodes primarily record local voltage signals and limit the recording of far-field signals and noise. Consequently, the signal-to-noise ratio of a bipolar recording is generally greater than that with unipolar recording, making bipolar recording the preferred method of electrogram recording in clinical cardiac electrophysiology. Clinically useful electrode pairs usually are 1 to 5 mm apart. Bipolar signals are normally filtered below 30 to 40 Hz and above 400 to 500 Hz. The eliminated low-frequency signals generally represent far-field voltages, and the high-frequency signals usually are noise.

Figure 1-7 shows intracardiac bipolar electrograms recorded from the high right atrium near the SA node, His bundle region, and right ventricular apex using quadripolar catheters. Not unexpectedly, during sinus rhythm, the electrogram recorded from the high right atrium precedes the inscription of the atrial electrogram recorded from the electrode catheter in the low septal right atrium. Because the catheter positioned near the His bundle is located at the junction of the right atrium and right ventricle, it records a local atrial electrogram and a right ventricular electrogram resulting from local activation of the right ventricular septum. Between these two signals is inscribed the His bundle electrogram. This deflection represents electrical activation

of the His bundle as the wavefront passes the pair of electrodes on the His bundle catheter.

Pacing Protocols and Programmed Electrical Stimulation

Atrial or ventricular muscle tissue consists of single cells with a negative resting potential of about −80 to −90 mV. Activation of single heart cells requires application of an electrical current that moves the cell's resting potential to the threshold potential. After the cell reaches its threshold potential, ion channels open, and a self-regenerating all-or-none action potential conducts to adjacent cells spreading throughout the conduction system. The minimum amount of electrical current that must be applied to heart tissue to produce a regenerating wavefront of depolarization is called the *threshold current* (or simply threshold).

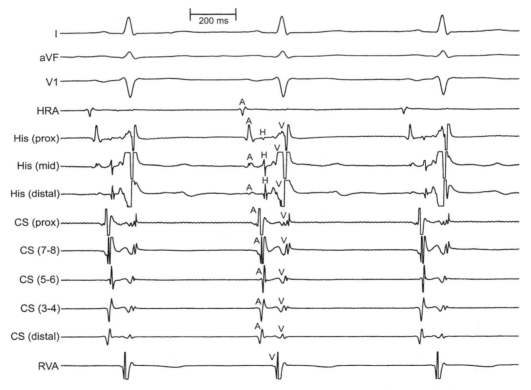

FIGURE 1-7. Basic 13-channel recording during a cardiac electrophysiology study of a patient with documented or presumed supraventricular tachycardia. From top to bottom, recordings taken from surface electrocardiographic leads I, aVF, and V₁, along with intracardiac electrograms recorded from the high right atrium (HRA); from the proximal (prox), middle (mid), and distal (dist) electrode pairs of a quadripolar electrode catheter positioned at the His bundle region; from a coronary sinus (CS) catheter positioned within the great cardiac vein along the posterior and lateral atrioventricular (AV) groove between the left atrium and left ventricle; and from the right ventricular apex (RVA). Arterial blood pressure (not shown) is often also recorded. For patients undergoing electrophysiology testing for presumed ventricular tachycardia, the coronary sinus catheter generally is not used. Some electrophysiologists only record from two, or rarely from one, bipolar electrode pairs in the His bundle region. A, atrial electrogram; H, His bundle electrogram; V, ventricular electrogram.

The electrical conduction properties of cardiac tissues, including the atria, ventricles, and specialized conducting system, are investigated using programmed electrical stimulation (PES). PES involves electrical stimulation of heart tissue using one of a number of pacing protocols. The atria or ventricles can be stimulated during electrical pacing. During pacing protocols, electrical stimulation is performed at a particular cycle length. The cycle length represents the time between any two successive stimuli. The relationship between pacing rate (PR) and cycle length (CL) is easily described (e.g., PR = 60,000/CL), with the pacing rate expressed as pulses or stimuli per minute and the cycle length measured in milliseconds. Pacing at a cycle length of 600 ms corresponds to a pacing rate of 100 pulses/min.

The first type of pacing used in electrophysiologic studies is called fixed-rate or fixed-cycle-length pacing (Fig. 1-8). In this type of pacing, the cycle length (pacing rate) of all the stimuli in the pacing train is the same and fixed. For example, fixed-cycle-length pacing of the right atrium may be performed at a cycle length of 600 ms, which means that the time interval between any two stimuli in the pacing train is 600 ms and the rate is 100 bpm. The length of the pacing train may range from only a few stimuli to many stimuli. A common length for a pacing train is 9 pr 10 stimuli. Pacing for this duration allows stabilization of the refractory period, which is discussed later in this chapter. Each of the pacing events in a pacing train is referred to as S_1. If the pacing is performed in the atrium, capture and conduction of the S_1 stimulus through the atria results in an atrial depolarization, called A_1. If the ventricle is being paced, capture and conduction of the S_1 in the ventricle results in a ventricular depolarization, called V_1.

The second common type of pacing protocol performed involves fixed-cycle-length (fixed-rate) pacing with extrastimuli. In this type of pacing, a fixed pacing train is followed by the introduction of one or more premature extrastimuli at the end of a fixed pacing train (Fig. 1-8). For example, if the cycle length of the eight stimuli in the drive train is 600 ms, a ninth stimulus may be added with the time between the last drive stimulus and the premature stimulus being 350 ms instead of 600 ms. This ninth premature stimulus is called S_2, which can cause premature atrial (A_2) or ventricular (V_2) depolarization. In this example, the S_1-S_2 coupling interval or coupling cycle length is 350 ms. The reason for introducing premature stimuli is to determine a refractory period or attempt to induce an arrhythmia. It is common to introduce multiple premature stimuli at the end of a fixed cycle pacing train; often up to three extra stimuli are used. The first extrastimulus is S_2, the second is called S_3, the third is referred to as S_4, and so on, with A_2, A_3, and A_4 or V_2, V_3, and V_4 corresponding to the resultant atrial or ventricular depolarizations, respectively.

A variant of this second type of pacing is fixed-cycle-length pacing with long-short extrastimuli (Fig. 1-8). This type of pacing is often useful for inducing some types of

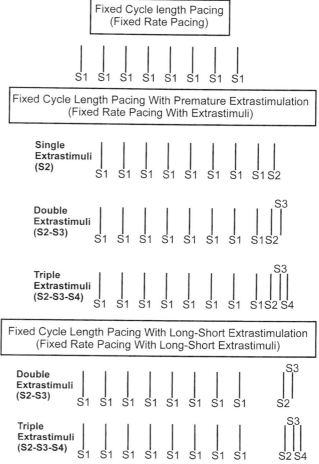

FIGURE 1-8. Two pacing protocols commonly used in electrophysiology studies. During fixed-cycle-length (fixed-rate) pacing, a train of electrical stimuli (S_1) is delivered in which the time between successive stimuli in the train is a fixed time interval (i.e., cycle length). During fixed-cycle-length pacing with premature extrastimuli, the cardiac tissue is stimulated as previously described, but at the end of the fixed pacing train, one or more premature stimuli are delivered earlier than the previous fixed cycle length. In practice, this premature extrastimulus is delivered earlier and earlier during subsequent pacing trains until it fails to depolarize the tissue. This type of pacing is used to determine the refractory periods of the atrium, ventricle, and specialized conduction system and to induce reentrant arrhythmias. The long-short extrastimuli pacing protocol is often used to induce reentrant ventricular tachycardia, especially bundle branch reentrant ventricular tachycardia.

ventricular tachycardia, especially bundle branch reentrant ventricular tachycardia.

Although a complete diagnostic electrophysiologic evaluation may entail the use of a variety of pacing protocols in different cardiac chambers before and after the administration of a variety of pharmacologic agents, at a minimum, the basic diagnostic study has the following main goals: an analysis of baseline rhythm, evaluation of baseline conduction properties, assessment of pacemaker function, pro-

TABLE 1-2. STANDARD COMPONENTS OF BASIC DIAGNOSTIC ELECTROPHYSIOLOGY STUDY

Component	Items of Phenomenon Evaluated	Parameters Measured and Examples
Baseline rhythm	Surface ECG and intracardiac electrograms	Sinus, AFL, AF, and others
Baseline conduction intervals	Surface ECG intervals	V-V, PR, QT intervals, QRS duration
	Intracardiac intervals	AH, HV intervals
Pacemaker function	SA node function	SNRT, corrected SNRT, SACT, CSM
Anterograde refractoriness and conduction patterns	Atrial and AV refractory periods	AERP, AVN ERP/FRP, WBCL, HP ERT/FRP, anterograde AP ERP/BCL
	AV conduction patterns	NP or AP; AVN FP or AVN SP
	Arrhythmia induction	Mode of induction, QRS axis and morphology, arrhythmia CL
Retrograde refractoriness and conduction patterns	Ventricular and VA refractory periods	VERP, retrograde NP ERP/BCL, retrograde AP ERP/BCL
	VA conduction patterns	NP or AP; AVN FP or AVN SP
	Arrhythmia induction	Mode of induction, QRS axis and morphology, arrhythmia CL
Arrhythmia induction and mechanism	Various pacing techniques and procedures; IV drugs	SART, AVNRT, AFL, AT, VT, AVRT, and others

A, atrial electrogram; AERP, atrial effective refractory period; AF, atrial fibrillation; AFL, atrial flutter; AP, accessory pathway; AV, atrioventricular; AT, atrial tachycardia; AVN, atrioventricular node; AVNRT, atrioventricular node reentrant tachycardia; AVRT, atrioventricular reciprocating tachycardia; BCL, block cycle; CSM, carotid sinus massage; ERP, effective refractory period; FP, fast conduction pathway of the atrioventricular node; FRP, functional refractory period; H, His bundle electrogram; HP, HisPurkinje; IV, intravenous; NP, normal pathway (atrioventricular node and HisPurkinje system); PES, programmed electrical stimulation; SA, sinoatrial; SACT, sinoatrial conduction time; SART, sinoatrial reentrant tachycardia; SNRT, sinus node recovery time; SP, slow conduction pathway of the atrioventricular node; V, ventricular electrogram; VERP, ventricular effective refractory period; VA, ventriculoatrial; VT, ventricular tachycardia; WBCL, Wenckebach block cycle length.

grammed electrical stimulation of the atria and ventricles to quantify the refractoriness of the anterograde and retrograde conduction pathways and to assess atrioventricular and ventriculoatrial conduction patterns, attempts to provoke a clinical arrhythmia, and determination of the mechanism of any induced tachyarrhythmias or bradyarrhythmias (Table 1-2).

Baseline Conduction Intervals

Baseline conduction intervals are measured from the surface electrocardiogram (ECG) and the intracardiac electrograms (Fig. 1-9). The PR, QRS, QT, P-P (A-A), and R-R (V-V) intervals are measured in the usual fashion. The time between the onset of the atrial spike in the His bundle recording and the onset of the His bundle electrogram is called the A-H interval (Fig. 1-9). The A-H interval represents the conduction time from the low septal right atrium through the AV node to the His bundle. Because a major component of the A-H interval is AV node conduction and because AV node conduction is significantly effected by autonomic nervous system tone, the A-H interval can be widely variable. In general, the normal range is 50 to 150 ms (103–113). Prolongation of the A-H interval may indicate high vagal tone but may also signify AV node disease or the effect of drugs. With enhanced sympathetic tone or the

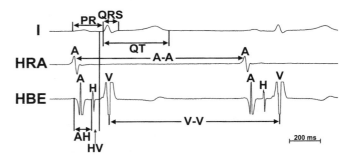

FIGURE 1-9. Measurement of baseline conduction intervals using surface electrocardiograms (ECG) and intracardiac electrograms. Surface ECG lead I is shown. Surface intervals (PR, QRS, QT) are measured in the usual ways. The A-A (P-P) interval is the cycle length of atrial depolarization recorded from the surface ECG or intracardiac electrograms. The V-V (R-R) interval is the cycle length of ventricular depolarization recorded from the surface ECG or intracardiac electrograms. During sinus rhythm, the high right atrial (HRA) electrogram occurs earliest. The atrial electrogram (A) recorded at the low septal right atrium by the His bundle (HBE) catheter occurs later. The A-H interval represents the conduction time between the low septal right atrium and the proximal His bundle region (measured in the HBE recording). The His bundle (H) deflection represents the depolarization wavefront traveling through the His bundle as it conducts to the bundle branches and ventricles. The H-V interval represents the time required for the wavefront to conduct from the proximal His bundle to earliest ventricular activation as measured from HBE recording or any surface ECG lead. In this case, the earliest ventricular activation is recorded in the His bundle region.

administration of catecholamines, the A-H interval shortens. The AV node exhibits decremental conduction properties, meaning that, with very rapid atrial pacing rates or with premature atrial stimuli, the AV node conduction time increases, and the A-H interval prolongs.

The time between the onset of the His spike and the earliest activation of the ventricle, as measured from the surface ECG or the ventricular electrogram in the His bundle recording, is called the H-V interval (Fig. 1-9). The H-V interval represents the time required for the electrical impulse to conduct from the proximal His bundle until it first activates any portion of the ventricle. This is normally much less than the A-H interval, and the normal range for the H-V interval is 30 to 55 ms (103–113). An apparent H-V interval of less than 30 ms may result from mistakenly recording the right bundle branch depolarization instead of the His bundle depolarization. However, a short H-V interval can also be seen in patients with accessory AV connections and ventricular preexcitation. Significant prolongation of the H-V interval can occur with drugs, or it may indicate fixed His bundle disease that may lead to complete heart block. Unlike the AV node, the His bundle normally is not affected by levels of autonomic tone and does not exhibit decremental conduction. The His-Purkinje system, however, may exhibit decremental conduction properties when it is exposed to antiarrhythmic drugs, becomes ischemic, or otherwise becomes diseased.

Evaluation of Sinoatrial Node Function

Evaluation of the native pacemaker function—the SA node—is often the first component of the invasive study performed during the basic diagnostic electrophysiology study (although in diagnostic studies for supraventricular tachycardia, the study generally begins in the ventricle with an analysis of ventriculoatrial conduction). The sinoatrial conduction time (SACT) is occasionally evaluated. Carotid

sinus massage is an easy method to test for the presence of carotid sinus hypersensitivity in patients with syncope. However, the most common invasive assessment of sinus node function involves measurement of the sinus node recovery time (SNRT), which is normally corrected for sinus rate (i.e., corrected sinus node recovery time [$SNRT_C$]).

Measurement of the SNRT involves fixed-cycle-length pacing of the high right atrium near the SA node at progressively shorter cycle lengths, beginning with a cycle length just below the sinus cycle length. Each drive train lasts for 60 seconds. One minute is allowed for full SA node recovery between drive trains. The interval between the last atrial-paced event and the appearance of the first sinus-derived atrial depolarization is the uncorrected SNRT (Fig. 1-10). Care must be taken to ensure that the escape depolarizations at the termination of overdrive pacing originate from the SA node. This can be done by comparing the P-wave morphology of these beats with the P waves generated during sinus rhythm or by having a second electrode catheter in the low right atrium to record the morphology, origin, and timing of electrograms during sinus rhythm and at the termination of the rapid pacing.

In normal persons, the longest SNRT is generally obtained in response to overdrive pacing at a cycle length of 400 to 450 ms. In patients in which abnormal SA node function is highly suspected, overdrive pacing can be performed at various cycle lengths (less than the sinus cycle length) down to 300 to 350 ms, generating SNRT and $SNRT_C$ values at each cycle length. Because patients with significant SA node dysfunction may have SA node entrance block, especially at short pacing cycle lengths, not all atrial pacing is necessarily effective at overdrive suppression of the SA node pacemaker activity. The examiner may find the largest SNRT or $SNRT_C$ is measured in response to overdrive pacing at 500 to 600 ms rather than at 400 to 500 ms. In general, a $SNRT_C$ of less than 500 to 550 ms is considered normal.

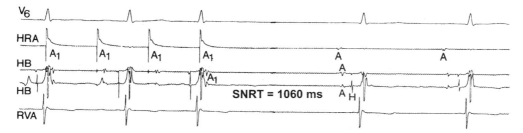

FIGURE 1-10. Surface electrocardiogram (ECG) and intracardiac recording during determination of sinus node recovery time (SNRT). Shown are the surface ECG lead V_6 and intracardiac electrograms from the high right atrium (HRA), His bundle region (HB), and right ventricular apex (RVA). Fixed-cycle-length pacing of the HRA is performed for 1 minute (A_1-A_1 = 400 ms); the last four atrial stimuli are shown here. The interval between the last atrial-paced event (A_1) and the appearance of the first sinus-derived atrial depolarization (A) is the uncorrected SNRT (1,060 ms). H, His bundle electrogram.

Assessment of Anterograde Refractoriness and Patterns of Conduction

Refractory Periods

In general, when a premature stimuli, S_2, is introduced at the end of a fixed pacing train, S_1, the S_2 may or may not generate a self-sustaining depolarizing wavefront in the cardiac tissue depending on the degree of prematurity of S_2. The S_1-S_2, A_1-A_2, H_1-H_2, or V_1-V_2 coupling intervals are used to determine the refractory periods of various cardiac tissues. For example, as the S_1-S_2 coupling interval is made shorter, an S_1-S_2 interval eventually is reached where S_2 fails to capture the heart tissue. Refractory periods are the "fundamental currency" of intracardiac electrophysiology and the means by which the electrical properties of cardiac tissues are described and compared (Tables 1-3 and 1-4).

The relative refractory period of a cardiac tissue is defined as the longest premature coupling interval that results in prolonged conduction of the premature impulse compared with the conduction of the stimulus delivered during the basic drive train (Figs. 1-11 and 1-12). For example, if atrial pacing is being performed, the atrial relative refractory period is the longest S_1-S_2 that results in an S_2-A_2 interval longer than the S_1-A_1 interval.

The *effective refractory period* of a cardiac tissue is defined as the longest premature coupling interval that fails to conduct through a tissue (Figs. 1-11 and 1-12). The atrial effective refractory period is the longest S_1-S_2 coupling interval that fails to depolarize the atria (S_2 without A_2), and the AV node effective refractory period is the longest A_1-A_2 interval that fails to conduct through the AV node to the His bundle.

The *relative refractory period* is generally slightly longer than the effective refractory period by an amount called the *latency period* (Figs. 1-11 and 1-12). Although the tissue remains excitable during the latency period, conduction may be slower or even decremental if activation occurs during this period. When the S_2 stimulus is delivered sufficiently close to the preceding S_1 (i.e., S_1-S_2 interval between atrial relative refractory period and atrial effective refractory period) in the high right atrium, a relatively isoelectric period of delay is seen in the high right atrial recording, and the A_1-A_2 interval recorded at the low septal right atrium near the His bundle is much longer than the S_1-S_2 interval recorded by the high right atrial catheter; the atrial activation (A_2) resulting from S_2 conducts slowly from the high right atrium to the His bundle region.

The *functional refractory period* is the shortest interval between two consecutively conducted impulses out of a cardiac tissue resulting from any two consecutive input impulses into that tissue (Figs. 1-12 and 1-13). The functional refractory period is a measure of output of a tissue and, unlike the relative refractory period or effective refractory period, is a "shortest" interval rather than a "longest" interval. In a sense, it is the shortest output interval that can occur in response to any input interval in a particular tissue. For example, the atrial functional refractory period is the shortest A_1-A_2 interval in response to any S_1-S_2 interval (Fig. 1-12), and the functional refractory period of the AV node is the shortest H_1-H_2 interval resulting from any A_1-A_2 interval (Fig. 1-13).

The effective refractory period is not an absolute value but varies depending on the stimulus intensity of the extrastimulus and on the cycle length between the fixed stimuli making up the pacing train. The effective refractory

TABLE 1-3. DEFINITION OF ANTEROGRADE PERIODS

Conduction System Component	Effective Refractory Period	Relative Refractory Period	Functional Refractory Period
Atrium	Longest S_1-S_2 that fails to produce an atrial depolarization	Longest S_1-S_2 at which S_2-A_2 is > S_1-A_1	Shortest A_1-A_2 resulting from any S_1-S_2
AV node	Longest A_1-A_2 (measured at the His bundle region) that fails to produce a His bundle depolarization	Longest A_1-A_2 at which A_2-H_2 is > A_1-H_1	Shortest H_1-H_2 resulting from any A_1-A_2
Accessory AV connection	Longest A_1-A_2 interval that fails to depolarize any portion of the ventricles through the accessory connection	Not normally measured	Shortest preexcited V_1-V_2 resulting from any A_1-A_2
His-Purkinje system	Longest H_1-H_2 that fails to result in ventricular depolarization[a]	Longest H_1-H_2 at which H_2-V_2 is > H_1-V_1 or generates an aberrant QRS complex	Shortest V_1-V_2 resulting from any H_1-H_2

S_1, A_1, H_1, V_1: stimulus artifact, atrial, His bundle, and ventricular electrograms during fixed cyclelength pacing train; S_2, A_2, H_2, V_2: stimulus artifact, atrial, His bundle, and ventricular electrograms of premature depolarization.
[a]Normally not measurable because the effective refractory period of the AV node is generally greater than for the His bundle or His Purkinje system.

TABLE 1-4. DEFINITION OF RETROGRADE REFRACTORY PERIODS

Conduction System Component	Effective Refractory Period	Relative Refractory Period	Functional Refractory Period
Ventricle	Longest S_1-S_2 that fails to produce a ventricular depolarization	Longest S_1-S_2 at which S_2-V_2 is > S_1-V_1[a]	Shortest V_1-V_2 resulting from any S_1-S_2
AV node	Longest H_1-H_2 (or S_1-H_2) that fails to produce an atrial depolarization near the His bundle region[b]	Not normally measurable	Shortest A_1-A_2 resulting from any H_1-H_2[b]
Accessory AV connection	Longest V_1-V_2 interval that fails to depolarize any portion of the atria through the accessory connection	Not normally measurable	Shortest A_1-A_2 resulting from any V_1-V_2[c]
His-Purkinje system	Longest V_1-V_2 (or S_1-S_2) interval that fails to produce His bundle depolarization[b]	Not normally measurable	Shortest H_1-H_2 (or S_1-H_2) resulting from any V_1-V_2[b]

S_1, A_1, H_1, V_1: stimulus artifact, atrial, His bundle, and ventricular electrograms during fixed cyclelength pacing train; S_2, A_2, H_2, V_2: stimulus artifact, atrial, His bundle, and ventricular electrograms of premature depolarization.
[a]Earliest V measured on the surface electrocardiogram or intracardiac assessment.
[b]Assumes that the examiner can clearly record retrograde His bundle activation resulting from premature stimulation.
[c]Measured near the site of the atrial input of accessory connection, assuming all retrograde normal pathway conduction is blocked.

period of atrial, ventricular, and His-Purkinje systems decreases with decreasing cycle length of the pacing train (i.e., rate-related refractoriness), whereas the AV nodal effective refractory period increases with decreasing cycle length (114–116). In the case of atrial, ventricular, and His-Purkinje tissue, the shortening of effective refractory period with increased pacing rate is called *peeling back of refractoriness*. It results from the fact that rapid pacing in these tissues causes shortening of the action potential duration. Under normal physiologic conditions, the effective refractory period in these tissues is regulated by and usually less than the action potential duration. Shortening the action potential duration with rapid pacing decreases the effective refrac-

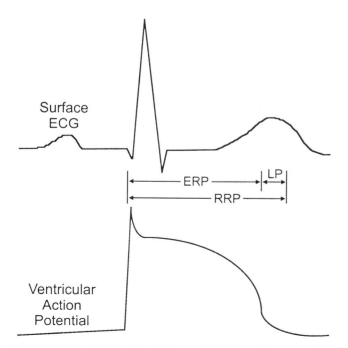

FIGURE 1-11. Relationship between effective refractory period (ERP), relative refractory period (RRP), latency period (LP), and the surface electrocardiogram (ECG) and the ventricular muscle cell action potential.

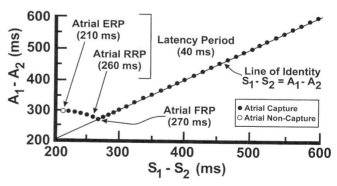

FIGURE 1-12. Determination of atrial functional, relative, and effective refractory periods and of the latency period by plotting A_1-A_2 versus S_1-S_2. A line of identity corresponds to the condition where S_1-S_2 = A_1-A_2. As S_1-S_2 shortens to 270 ms, the atrial functional refractory period (FRP) is reached. As S_1-S_2 shortens to less than 270 ms, the resultant A_1-A_2 deviates from the line of identity as the relative refractory period (RRP) is reached and the latency period is entered. During this period, the A_1-A_2 interval increases despite further decreases in S_1-S_2. Eventually, with further shortening of S_1-S_2, the atrial effective refractory period (ERP) is reached. Pacing stimulus intensity is at twice the diastolic threshold.

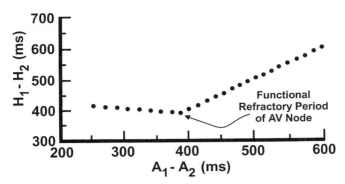

FIGURE 1-13. Plot of H_1-H_2 versus A_1-A_2 to determine functional refractory period of the atrioventricular node.

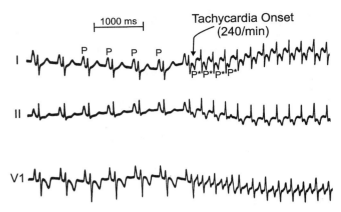

FIGURE 1-14. Change in the P-wave axis with a change in the direction of atrial activation. Surface electrocardiographic leads I, II, and V_1 were simultaneously recorded immediately before and after the onset of atrioventricular (AV) reciprocating tachycardia. Prominent positive P waves are seen in each of these leads during sinus rhythm, indicative of atrial activation proceeding from the high right atrium to the low right atrium. After the onset of tachycardia, the P waves become negative (P*) in leads I and II and biphasic in lead V_1. This tachycardia involves retrograde conduction from the ventricles to the atria through an accessory AV connection, and the retrograde atrial depolarization wavefront proceeds away from the positive poles of leads I and II and is perpendicular to lead V_1. The high right atrium is activated after the lower portions of the atria.

tory period. This rate-related shortening of action potential duration appears to result from a pacing-induced increase of one component of the delayed rectifier potassium (K^+) current (117–119).

The AV node displays post-repolarization refractoriness. AV node cells exhibiting slow, Ca^{2+}-dependent action potentials may not become reexcitable until after repolarization is complete, even though they exhibit very short action potential duration (120–123). The ionic mechanisms responsible for these differences are in dispute.

Intraatrial Conduction and Atrial Activation

Endocardial mapping indicates that normal atrial activation begins in the high or middle lateral right atrium, with the former more likely to occur at sinus rates of more than 100 bpm and the latter more likely at rates of less than 60 bpm. These different activation patterns may reflect different exit routes from a single sinus node or a sinus node consisting of multiple pacemaker regions (124). Spread of the atrial impulse to the right AV junction requires about one half of the time required to reach the left atrial free wall. Whether specific interatrial tracts exist between the SA and AV nodes is the subject of debate (125).

When normal atrial activation spreads from the high right atrium to the low right atrium, the surface ECG displays upright P waves in inferior leads II, III, and aVF because the depolarization wavefront is moving toward the positive poles of these leads. If, however, atrial activation proceeds in the opposite direction, as occurs with the usual form of atrial flutter or low right atrial tachycardias, the P wave is inverted in these leads because the depolarization wavefront is moving toward the negative poles of the inferior leads (Fig. 1-14). The morphology of a P wave produced by a premature atrial depolarization depends on the location of its origin. Its morphology is usually different from the P wave produced by the normal SA node depolarization.

Atrial Vulnerability

The period of atrial vulnerability roughly corresponds to the interval between the atrial relative refractory period and effective refractory period (i.e., latency period). The normal atrial effective refractory period ranges from 150 to 260 ms (116,126–129), and the atrial relative refractory period is normally 10 to 30 ms greater than the atrial effective refractory period. Atrial extrastimuli delivered during the period of atrial vulnerability are often followed by repetitive atrial activity that can become sustained, resulting in atrial flutter or fibrillation (130–138) (Fig. 1-15). Atrial extrastimuli with progressively shorter coupling intervals less than the relative refractory period and ever closer to the effective refractory period increase the incidence of repetitive responses and the risk of atrial flutter or fibrillation. In normal atria, the atrial vulnerable period is very brief, usually 10 to 30 ms. However, the vulnerable interval increases as the fixed drive cycle length is made shorter because of a drive cycle length–dependent decrease in the effective refractory period without any reduction in the relative refractory period (139). The repetitive atrial responses result from reentry of a premature atrial extrastimulus conducting through tissues that are relatively refractory. The conduction velocity is reduced, and in the presence of regions of unidirectional block, sustained reentrant atrial arrhythmias can result.

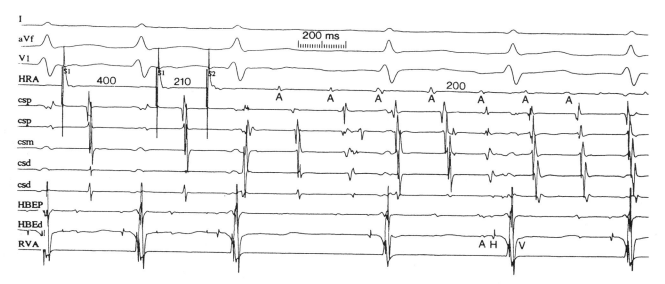

FIGURE 1-15. Atrial extrastimulus delivered during the period of atrial vulnerability results in repetitive atrial responses and sustained atrial flutter. From top to bottom, recordings from surface electrocardiographic leads I, aVF, and V₁, along with intracardiac electrograms from the high right atrium (HRA), five coronary sinus leads (proximal [csp], middle [csm], and distal [csd]), proximal His bundle (HBEP), distal His bundle (HBEd), and right ventricular apex (RVA). After fixed atrial pacing at a cycle length (S_1-S_1) of 400 ms, introduction of an atrial premature stimulus (S_1-S_2 = 210 ms) results in repetitive atrial depolarizations (A-A = 220 ms) and sustained atrial flutter with 3 : 1 atrioventricular conduction. A, atrial electrogram; H, His bundle electrogram; V, ventricular electrogram.

Anterograde Atrioventricular Conduction Pathways

When the high right atrium is electrically stimulated with a suprathreshold stimulus, capture occurs with spread of the wavefront of depolarization throughout both atria. Normally, the wavefront conducts from the atria to the ventricles through the AV node-His-Purkinje pathway, called the *normal pathway.* In patients with a normal conduction system, this results in a normal PR, A-H, and H-V intervals with a short QRS duration because of rapid conduction within the His-Purkinje system.

In the fully developed human heart, the fibrous AV ring (annulus fibrosis) almost completely electrically insulates the atrial and ventricular myocardium from each other. In most people, the normal pathway is the only conduction pathway from the atria to the ventricles because only at the AV node–His bundle region is the annulus fibrosis breached and electrical continuity established, permitting cardiac impulse conduction from the atria to the ventricles. As long as the insulation of the annulus fibrosis is not disrupted anywhere else, atrial impulses are conducted to the ventricle only by way of the AV node-His-Purkinje system. Because of its decremental conduction properties, the AV node functions as a protective barrier, delaying AV conduction and preventing one-to-one conduction to the ventricles of rapid impulses generated in the atria.

Whereas the AV nodal pathway normally behaves as a one-way street connecting the atria to the ventricles, in some patients, the normal AV nodal pathway behaves as if it allows two-way traffic with dual AV conduction pathways. In many patients, this has no functional significance, but in some individuals, this provides the substrate for the most common type of supraventricular tachycardia, called AV nodal reentrant tachycardia.

In rare patients, the annulus fibrosis insulation is breached at one or more locations by conductive muscle bundles, allowing an alternative conduction pathway from the atria to the ventricles. These accessory connections or accessory pathways are the cause of ventricular preexcitation (i.e., ventricular activation through the accessory pathway occurs earlier than by the normal AV node-His-Purkinje pathway), and by creating a high-speed bypass from the atria to the ventricles, they may permit rapid one-to-one AV conduction, with possible life-threatening consequences. These accessory connections are also critical anatomic components necessary for the development of one of the most common forms of supraventricular tachycardia, called orthodromic AV reciprocating tachycardia.

Atrial Pacing and Decremental Atrioventricular Nodal Conduction

The AV node exhibits decremental conduction properties; with very rapid atrial pacing or with premature atrial stimuli, the AV node conduction time (A-H interval) increases (Fig. 1-16). On a plot of the A_2-H_2 interval versus the A_1>-A_2 interval (Fig. 1-17), a gradual increase in the A_2-H_2 interval is observed with reductions in A^1-A^2 coupling interval until the AV node or atrial effective refractory period is reached (Fig. 1-16). Similarly, pacing at a critical A_1-A_1 interval results in progressive prolongation of the A-H interval until eventually there is atrial capture without conduction to the His bun-

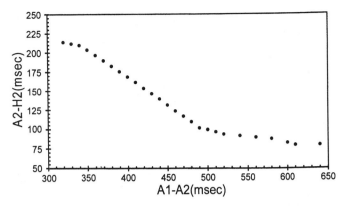

FIGURE 1-17. Plot of the A_2-H_2 interval versus the A_1-A_2 interval, illustrating normal decremental conduction properties of the atrioventricular (AV) node. Fixed-cycle-length pacing of the high right atrium (A_1-A_1 = 650 ms) is followed by the introduction of a premature atrial extrastimulus (A_2). As the duration of the premature coupling interval (A_1-A_2) is reduced, the conduction through the AV node is prolonged (i.e., increased duration of the A_2-H_2 interval). This increase in AV node conduction time is gradual, without any abrupt changes or discontinuities.

dle or ventricles. In normal hearts, the conduction block almost always occurs within the AV node, not the His bundle. The AV node Wenckebach cycle length is the longest A_1-A_1 interval that fails to result in one-to-one conduction through the AV node to the His bundle.

Certain individuals may have AV nodes exhibiting multiple transnodal conduction pathways. In these patients, the curve relating A_2-H_2 to A_1-A_2 often fails to show a smooth increase in A_2-H_2 with reductions in A_1-A_2 and instead

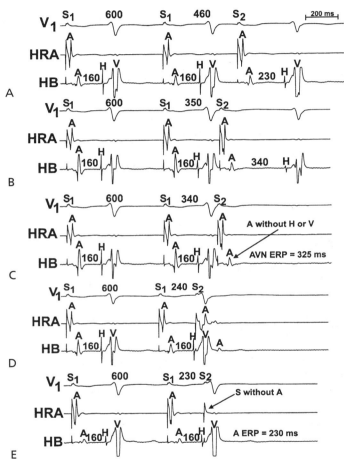

FIGURE 1-16. Demonstration of anterograde atrioventricular (AV) nodal decremental conduction, AV node effective refractory period, and atrial effective refractory period. In each panel, electrocardiographic lead V_1 is shown along with intracardiac electrograms from the high right atrium (HRA) and His bundle region. An eight-pulse fixed-rate drive train (S_1-S_1) (only last two stimuli shown) is delivered in the HRA, followed by increasingly premature extrastimulus (S_2) at coupling intervals (S_1-S_2) of 460 ms **(A)**, 350 ms **(B)**, 340 ms **(C)**, 240 ms **(D)**, and 230 ms **(E)**. The A-H interval during the drive train is significantly shorter than that seen with an extrastimulus, and A-H prolongs as the coupling interval of the extrastimulus decreases (i.e., decremental conduction). The AV node effective refractory is reached at the longest A_1-A_2, which fails to conduct to the His bundle **(C)**, while the atrial effective refractory period is the longest S_1-S_2, which fails to capture the atria **(E)**. A, atrial electrogram; A ERP, atrial effective refractory period; AVN ERP, atrioventricular node effective refractory period; H, His bundle electrogram; V, ventricular electrogram; S, stimulus artifact.

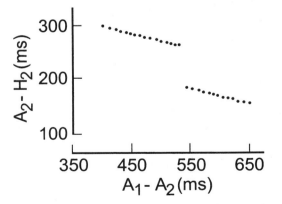

FIGURE 1-18. Plot of the A_2-H_2 interval versus the A_1-A_2 interval in a patient with dual atrioventricular (AV) node physiology. Fixed-cycle-length pacing of the high right atrium (HRA) (A_1-A_1 = 650 ms) is followed by the introduction of a premature atrial depolarization (A_2). As the premature coupling interval (A_1-A_2) is reduced from 540 to 530 ms, there is an abrupt increase in the duration of the A_2-H_2 interval (compare with Fig. 1-17). This abrupt increase in AV node conduction time at a discrete premature coupling interval indicates the presence of sudden block in the fast AV nodal pathway, with anterograde conduction continuing by means of the slow AV nodal pathway.

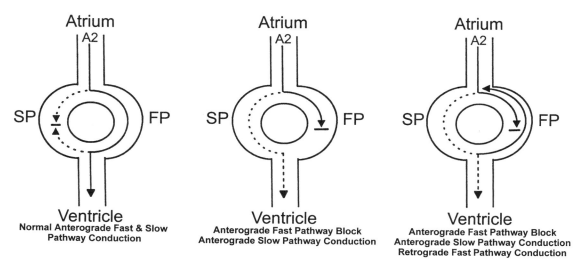

FIGURE 1-19. Schematic diagram of the atrioventricular node with fast and slow pathways.

exhibits an abrupt discontinuity at a critical A_1-A_2 coupling interval (Fig. 1-18). The explanation for this finding is that many normal AV nodes contain a fast conducting pathway and a slow conducting pathway (Fig. 1-19). Normally, conduction occurs preferentially down the fast pathway to activate the His bundle and ventricle. However, because the effective refractory period of the fast pathway usually is longer than that of the slow pathway, as the A_1-A_2 coupling interval is decreased, the effective refractory period of the

fast pathway is reached, and conduction blocks in that pathway. Conduction, however, continues down the nonrefractory slow pathway even as the A_1-A_2 coupling interval is shortened further. When the impulse conduction changes from the fast pathway to slow pathway, the A-H interval dramatically prolongs because conduction through this AV node pathway is much slower. This change from fast pathway to slow pathway conduction is marked by an A-H interval "jump" (Fig. 1-20). An A-H interval jump is

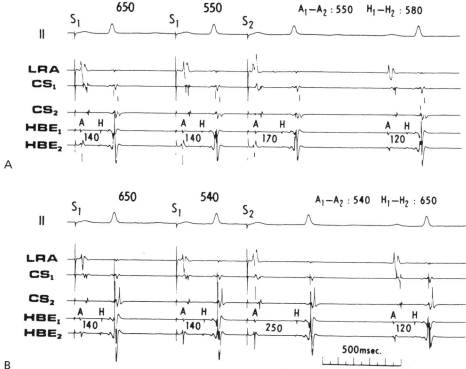

FIGURE 1-20. Intracardiac recording showing jump in the A-H interval. From top to bottom in each panel are the surface electrocardiographic recordings from lead II and endocardial recordings from the low right atrium (LRA), proximal and distal epicardial recordings from the coronary sinus catheter (CS$_1$ and CS$_2$, respectively), and proximal and distal endocardial His bundle recordings (HBE$_1$ and HBE$_2$, respectively). **A:** Fixed-cycle-length pacing of the right atrium is performed at a cycle length (S$_1$-S$_1$) of 650 ms, followed by the introduction of a premature stimulus at a coupling interval (S$_1$-S$_2$) of 550 ms (A_1-A_2 = 550 ms). The resultant A-H interval increases from 140 to 170 ms (i.e., normal decremental AV node conduction). **B:** After reducing the S$_1$-S$_2$ coupling interval to 540 ms (A_1-A_2 = 540), the A-H interval dramatically increases to 250 ms, indicating conduction block in the fast AV nodal pathway, although with continued anterograde conduction in the slow AV nodal pathway. A, atrial electrogram; H, His bundle electrogram; S, stimulus artifact.

defined as a 50-ms or greater increase in the A-H interval in response to a 10-ms reduction in the A_1-A_2 coupling interval. Because of the prolonged conduction time in the anterograde slow pathway, by the time the impulse reaches the lower junction of the slow and fast pathways, the retrograde fast pathway may no longer be refractory and may conduct the impulse retrogradely to reexcite the atria. Meanwhile, if the anterograde slow pathway has recovered, the wavefront of depolarization may reenter this anterograde pathway, possibly leading to a sustained circus movement tachyarrhythmia called the slow/fast form of AV node reentrant tachycardia (Fig. 1-19). However, many individuals with dual AV node physiology never develop a clinical tachycardia.

Accessory Atrioventricular Connections and the Concept of Preexcitation

Most people only have AV conduction within the normal AV conduction pathway (i.e., AV node-His-Purkinje system). Rare patients also exhibit AV conduction occurring over an accessory pathway. Functionally, there are three distinct varieties of accessory connections: those that conduct only in the anterograde direction (from atrium to ventricle), called manifest pathways; those that conduct only in the retrograde direction (from ventricle to atrium), called concealed pathways; and those that conduct in both directions, also called manifest pathways. Within each of theses types, accessory pathways exhibit rapid all-or-none conduction (i.e., similar to atrial or ventricular muscle) or decremental conduction (i.e., similar to the AV node), with the former much more common than the latter.

When the annulus fibrosis insulation is disrupted by a rapidly conducting manifest accessory AV connection, the normal AV node-His-Purkinje pathway is short-circuited, and the ventricle may be excited earlier (i.e., ventricular preexcitation) than would have otherwise occurred. Some areas of ventricular myocardium are activated through the accessory pathway, and other regions continue to be activated through the normal pathway. When viewed with surface ECG mapping, this multipathway activation of the ventricle manifests characteristic ECG changes (hence the term *manifest* accessory connection), including a shortened PR interval, slurring of the QRS complex upstroke (delta wave), increased duration of the QRS complex, and often an atypical QRS complex axis. Fast conduction over the AV connection bypassing the AV node accounts for the short P-R (P-delta wave) interval duration. This abnormal, multipathway activation of the ventricle results in ventricular fusion, generating a hybrid QRS complex that is different from that resulting from exclusive conduction over the normal or accessory pathway. Different degrees of ventricular preexcitation with dynamic variations in the QRS complex configuration can be observed in the same patient at different times. The greater the contribution of ventricular activation through the normal pathway (relative to the accessory connection), the less ventricular preexcitation is evident. The greater the contribution to ventricular depolarization through the accessory connection (relative to the normal pathway), the greater is the degree of ventricular preexcitation that occurs (Fig. 1-21).

Ventricular preexcitation during sinus rhythm is often more pronounced with right-sided than with left-sided accessory AV connections, because right-sided accessory connections are relatively closer to the sinus node. As a result, more ventricular activation has already occurred by way of the nearby accessory pathway (i.e., more ventricular preexcitation) before the impulse has had a chance to activate the ventricle through the slower conducting and more distant normal pathway. A shift in location of the atrial pacemaker or atrial pacing site can also change the degree of ventricular preexcitation. The closer the site of the ectopic pacemaker to the accessory AV connection, the greater is the degree of preexcitation. A change in the cardiac cycle length may also cause variation in the degree of ventricular preexcitation. Before reaching the anterograde effective refractory period of an accessory AV connection, atrial pacing at faster rates and atrial premature stimulation with progressively shorter coupling intervals increase the degree of ventricular preexcitation (Fig. 1-21). This happens because progressive lengthening of AV nodal conduction time associated with shortening of the cardiac

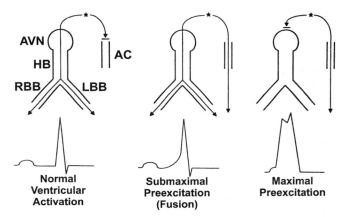

FIGURE 1-21. Differential contributions to ventricular depolarization through the normal atrioventricular (AV) conduction pathway and an accessory AV connection result in different degrees of preexcitation (i.e., fusion). If all the ventricular activation is through the normal AV nodal (AVN) pathway, normal ventricular activation occurs through the bundle branches, and there is no preexcitation. If all the ventricular activation occurs through the accessory connection (AC), maximal preexcitation occurs. Between these two extremes, ventricular depolarization is the result of variable contributions to ventricular activation (i.e., ventricular fusion) through the normal and accessory connections. HB, His bundle; LBB, left bundle branch; RBB, right bundle branch.

cycle length (i.e., decremental conduction) permits more ventricular excitation to occur through the accessory pathway. Despite the increasing degree of ventricular preexcitation, the atrial stimulus artifact-to-delta wave (P-delta wave interval) remains constant in nondecrementally conducting accessory pathways. Vagal stimulation may also be expected to increase the degree of preexcitation by prolonging AV nodal conduction time, thereby promoting the contribution of accessory pathway conduction to ventricular excitation.

Normalization of the QRS complex morphology with disappearance of ventricular preexcitation may also occur under a variety of situations. For example, a reduction in vagal tone during exercise or by blocking vagal effects with atropine facilitates normal pathway conduction, thereby lessening or possibly eliminating preexcitation, with normalization of the QRS complex. Other situations associated with the disappearance of preexcitation and normalization of ventricular activation include late activation of the accessory AV connection relative to the normal AV conduction pathway, ineffective atrial conduction at the entrance of the accessory AV connection, enhanced AV nodal conduction, and rate-dependent conduction block within the accessory pathway at critical cardiac cycle lengths.

Rarely, an atrial impulse conducted simultaneously over the normal and accessory pathways may produce a double ventricular response (i.e., 1 : 2 AV conduction). This phenomenon may also occur in patients with dual AV nodal pathways. This pattern can occur because of the marked difference in conduction time between the two AV conduction pathways, with an atrial impulse first activating the ventricle through an accessory pathway and then reactivating the ventricle through the normal pathway. The difference in conduction time between the two AV conduction pathways therefore must be longer than the effective refractory period of the His-Purkinje system and ventricle. Slow conduction in the AV node, a minimal degree of retrograde concealed conduction within the His-Purkinje system, and a short effective refractory period of the ventricle favor the development of this phenomenon. Repetition of double ventricular responses during sinus rhythm or an atrial arrhythmia may theoretically generate a nonreentrant form of supraventricular tachycardia.

In patients with the common variety of manifest accessory connection (i.e., Kent bundle), fixed atrial pacing at slow rates (i.e., slightly faster than the patient's sinus rate) results in conduction over the anterograde normal and accessory pathways. With increasing pacing rate, the anterograde block cycle length of the normal pathway and the accessory pathway will be reached. In each case, this is defined as the slowest fixed rate of atrial pacing (i.e., longest fixed cycle length) at which 1 : 1 AV conduction over the accessory pathway or normal pathway cannot be maintained. Which block cycle length is reached first depends on which pathway—normal or accessory—has the longest effective refractory period (with the longest effective refractory period within the normal pathway usually residing within the AV node). If the block cycle length of the normal pathway is reached first (i.e., block cycle length of normal pathway is greater than that of the accessory pathway), all AV conduction at faster rates will be within the accessory connection, and maximal preexcitation will be present (with no ventricular fusion). If the block cycle length of the accessory pathway is reached first (i.e., block cycle length of the accessory pathway is greater than that of the normal pathway), all AV conduction at faster rates will be within the normal pathway, and no preexcitation will be evident (with no ventricular fusion). When pacing at cycle lengths longer than the accessory and normal pathway block cycle lengths, anterograde conduction will proceed over the accessory and normal pathways, resulting in various degrees of ventricular fusion occurring and submaximal preexcitation evident. With continued more rapid atrial pacing, a cycle length eventually will be reached at which anterograde block occurs in both pathways; the refractory period of the atrial tissue is reached with a loss of atrial capture.

Most accessory connections exhibit all-or-none conduction, meaning that over a wide range of extrastimulus coupling intervals conduction time within the accessory pathway of the extrastimulus (i.e., Kent fibers) is unchanged. However, in response to a premature atrial extrastimulus, some accessory connections with anterograde conduction exhibit decremental conduction properties, similar to that seen in the AV node. Included in this group are classic Mahaim fibers (nodoventricular), as well as some right atriofascicular and rare right and left atrioventricular fibers. From a functional standpoint, the main distinguishing characteristic between these two types of accessory connections during extrastimulus pacing is that the P-to-delta wave interval (or stimulus artifact-to-delta wave interval) remains constant in the case of the Kent fiber because conduction time of an extrastimulus within the accessory connection does not change, whereas the P-to-delta wave interval does increase in the case of the Mahaim fiber because the conduction time of an extrastimulus within the accessory connection increases (Fig. 1-22).

Assessment of Retrograde Refractoriness and Patterns of Conduction

In general, anterograde AV conduction is more robust than retrograde ventriculoatrial conduction, with AV conduction block occurring in normal individuals at very short A_1-A_1 or A_1-A_2 coupling intervals that are usually shorter than the corresponding V_1-V_1 and V_1-V_2 intervals at which ventriculoatrial conduction is blocked. As in the case of anterograde conduction, retrograde ventriculoatrial conduction may occur

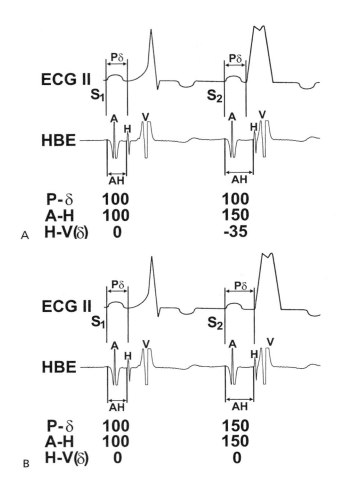

P-δ	100	100
A-H	100	150
H-V(δ)	0	-35

A

P-δ	100	150
A-H	100	150
H-V(δ)	0	0

B

FIGURE 1-22. The diagram illustrates the differences between anterograde conduction patterns in accessory connections exhibiting all-or-none conduction **(A)** and decremental conduction **(B)** in response to an atrial extrastimulus. In the basal state with fixed-rate pacing (S_1), there is minimal preexcitation. In both cases, the P-delta wave interval is 100 ms. With the introduction of a premature extrastimulus (S_2) in the atria, the conduction time from the atria to the His bundle through the atrioventricular (AV) node prolongs from 100 ms to 150 ms. In the case of the accessory connection with nondecremental conduction **(A)**, this increased conduction time allows a greater degree of preexcitation (i.e., greater proportion of the ventricles activated through the accessory connection) as seen in the QRS complex of the surface electrocardiogram and the H-V interval changing from zero to –35 ms (i.e., anterograde His bundle activation occurs 35 ms after the earliest ventricular activation through the accessory connection). However, because the conduction time within the accessory connection does not change in response to the extrastimulus, the P-delta wave interval does not change and is still measured at 100 ms. In the case of the accessory connection with decremental conduction properties **(B)**, the extrastimulus is associated with an increase of conduction time in the AV node and the accessory connection. Because conduction time increases in the accessory connection, the P-delta wave interval must increase (in this case, from 100 to 150 ms). Even with this increase in anterograde conduction time within the accessory connection, preexcitation can still increase (as evidenced by the increased QRS duration) so long as conduction time within the normal AV nodal pathway increases even more. Many accessory connections exhibiting decremental conduction are atriofascicular (i.e., running from the right atrium to a branch of the right bundle branch). In this case, the H-V interval may be largely unchanged because His bundle activation results from an impulse traveling in the retrograde direction within right bundle branch back to the proximal His bundle. This retrograde His bundle activation also can occur in cases of accessory connections lacking decremental conduction, especially if the anterograde conduction is very prolonged, as in the case of conduction within a slow AV nodal pathway. Whether His bundle activation is the result of anterograde AV nodal conduction or retrograde right bundle branch conduction often can be determined only if right bundle and His bundle electrograms are simultaneously recorded.

within the normal pathway (i.e., His-Purkinje-AV nodal pathway), an accessory pathway (i.e., an accessory ventriculoatrial connection), or the normal and accessory pathways. As with anterograde AV conduction, several retrograde refractory periods are routinely measured during the ventricular pacing portion of an electrophysiology study (Table 1-4).

Normal Retrograde Ventriculoatrial Conduction

Fixed-rate pacing in the ventricles with or without extrastimuli results in characteristic conduction patterns in a manner analogous to atrial pacing. Conduction may proceed unimpeded from its ventricular origin all the way to the atria. Retrograde conduction block may develop anywhere along the ventriculoatrial conduction pathway (Fig. 1-23). However, evaluating retrograde conduction, particularly the site of ventriculoatrial block, is more difficult than evaluating conduction in the anterograde direction (Fig. 1-23). The reason for this is that, during anterograde AV conduction, His bundle activation reliably occurs well before ventricular activation (except in the case of preexcitation), and the His bundle electrogram is predictably found clearly

delineated 30 to 60 ms before local ventricular activation. During retrograde conduction, the ventricular myocardium near the His bundle or proximal bundle branches may be activated before or nearly simultaneous with the His bundle or proximal right and left bundle branches (Fig. 1-24). Consequently, the retrograde His bundle, right bundle, or left bundle electrograms may not be recorded because they are hidden within the much larger local ventricular depolarization recorded by the electrode catheter positioned to record those electrograms, because a conduction block has occurred below the level of the His bundle or proximal bundle branches, or because it could merely indicate that the catheter is malpositioned. However, because conduction is rapid within the bundle branches (relative to ventricular muscle), rapid retrograde conduction within the right bundle branch block often results in the retrograde His bundle inscription before local activation of the ventricle in the His bundle region. Only by recording immediately proximal and distal to a particular site (and verifying correct catheter position) can conduction block be said to occur at that particular site.

Conduction in the His-Purkinje system after right apical endocardial activation may proceed within the right or left

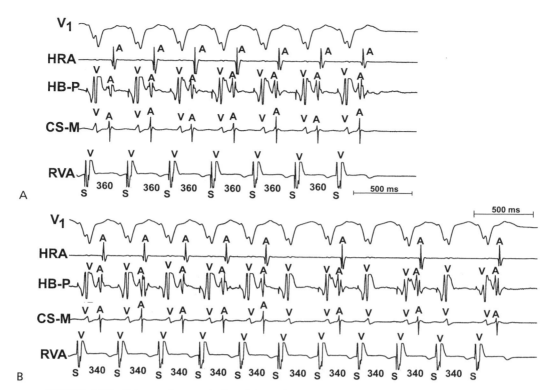

FIGURE 1-23. Retrograde ventriculoatrial conduction within the normal pathway and demonstration of the retrograde normal pathway block cycle length. Displayed from top to bottom are electrocardiographic lead V1 and intracardiac recordings from the high right atrium (HRA), proximal (HB-P) and distal (HB-D) His bundle (HB) region, middle coronary sinus (CS-M), and right ventricular apex (RVA). **A:** Fixed-rate right ventricular pacing is performed at a cycle length of 360 ms resulting in 1 : 1 ventriculoatrial conduction with retrograde earliest atrial activation in the His bundle region, which is consistent with retrograde conduction through the normal His bundle–atrioventricular (AV) nodal pathway. **B:** The pacing cycle length is reduced to 340 ms, and 1 : 1 ventriculoatrial conduction changes to 2 : 1 conduction *(right half of panel)*. The exact level of the conduction block cannot be determined because the retrograde His bundle electrogram cannot be seen. Although this is often called the retrograde Wenckebach block cycle length, the designation is inappropriate. The term Wenckebach block should be reserved for a conduction block that can be verified to occur within the AV node. Because, in the example shown, it cannot be said with certainty that the conduction block is within the AV node (it is probably in the His-Purkinje system), it is more correct to call this the retrograde normal pathway block cycle length.

bundle branch (Fig. 1-24). Not uncommonly, conduction proceeds through the right bundle branch at long coupling intervals. At shorter coupling intervals, retrograde conduction block may develop in the right bundle branch. Retrograde conduction, however, may continue within the left bundle branch after a delay resulting from right-to-left transseptal intramyocardial conduction ADDIN ENRfu (140, 141) (Fig. 1-24).

The most common site of retrograde conduction delay or block during ventriculoatrial conduction is in the His-Purkinje system (141–143) (Fig. 1-25). Right ventricular stimulation using fixed-cycle ventricular pacing with a single ventricular extrastimulus (V_1-V_2) can be used to study the behavior of the His-Purkinje system as long as a retrograde His bundle deflection can be recorded. Progressive prolongation of His-Purkinje conduction (V_2-H_2) occurs

with increasing prematurity of the ventricular extrastimulus (V_1-V_2) in a relatively constant fashion (Fig. 1-26). At any given V_1-V_2 interval, the V_2-H_2 interval is shorter at shorter drive cycle lengths (V_1-V_1). Eventually, with increasing prematurity, the ventricular effective refractory period is reached (Fig. 1-27).

Before reaching the ventricular effective refractory period, the introduction of a ventricular extrastimulus may result in repetitive ventricular responses even in individuals with normal hearts. The most common type of response is bundle branch reentry (144–148) (Figs. 1-27 through 1-29). In a significant percentage of patients, fixed right ventricular pacing with ventricular extrastimulation results in retrograde conduction of V_2 through the right bundle branch. This can be proved by observing a retrograde right bundle or His bundle deflection before the ventricular

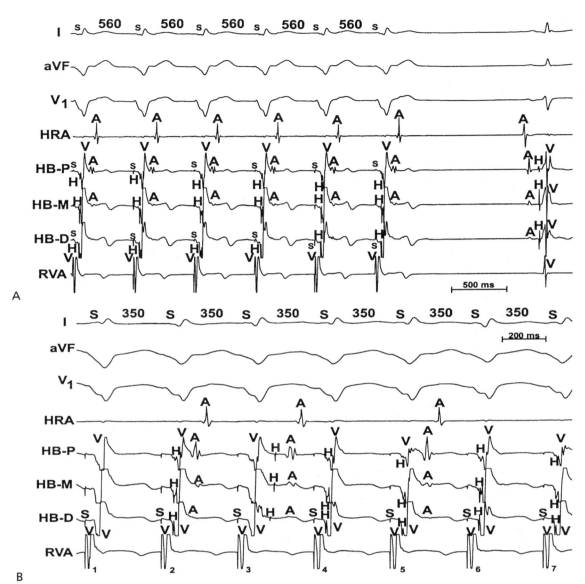

FIGURE 1-24. Fixed-cycle-length pacing at the right ventricular apex at two different drive cycle lengths shows 1 : 1 ventriculoatrial conduction **(A)** and conduction block at various levels within the retrograde normal pathway **(B)**. Displayed in each panel are electrocardiographic leads I, aVF, V_1 and intracardiac electrograms recorded from the high right atrium (HRA); proximal (HB-P), middle (HB-M), and distal (HB-D) His bundle regions; and right ventricular apex (RVA). **A:** The S_1–S_1 drive of 500 ms results in 1 : 1 ventriculoatrial conduction with the retrograde His bundle electrogram (H), which is inscribed as the sharp deflection recorded in the early portion of the local ventricular electrogram in each of the HB leads. **B:** The S_1–S_1 coupling interval was reduced to 350 ms. At this pacing rate, there is no longer 1 : 1 ventriculoatrial conduction. Ventricular depolarization 1 (numbers are at the bottom of **B**) captures the ventricle, but there is conduction block in the His-Purkinje system because no retrograde His bundle electrogram is recorded. Ventricular depolarizations 2 and 5 conduct to the atrium with inscription of the His bundle electrogram in the early portion of the local ventricular electrogram after rapid retrograde conduction within the right bundle branch. Ventricular depolarization 3 blocks retrogradely in the right bundle branch, conducts transseptally, and then proceeds up the left bundle branch to activate the His bundle, which is inscribed well after the local ventricular electrogram is recorded in the His bundle region. Retrograde conduction thereafter continues through the atrioventricular (AV) node to depolarize the atrium. Ventricular depolarizations 4, 6, and 7 all conduct retrograde by means of the right bundle branch to activate the His bundle, without continuing onward through the AV node to activate the atrium (i.e., conduction block within the AV node). A, atrial electrogram; H, His bundle electrogram; S, stimulus artifact ; V, ventricular electrogram.

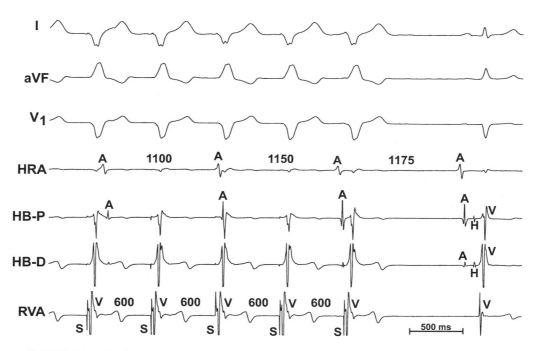

FIGURE 1-25. Fixed rate ventricular pacing with no ventriculoatrial conduction and retrograde conduction block within the His-Purkinje system (below the His bundle). Displayed from top to bottom are the electrocardiographic leads I, aVF, and V_1 and the intracardiac electrograms recorded from the high right atrium (HRA); proximal (HB-P), middle (HB-M), and distal (HB-D) His bundle regions; and right ventricular apex (RVA). Ventricular pacing is performed at a fixed-cycle-length (S_1-S_1) of 600 ms. The atrial activation occurs by the normal sinus mechanism with a "high to low" intraatrial activation sequence (i.e., high right atrium is activated before the low septal right atrium at the His bundle recording site). Atrial activation is dissociated from the retrograde ventricular depolarizations that block below the His bundle (i.e., no retrograde His bundle activation) in the His-Purkinje system. A, atrial electrogram; H, His bundle electrogram; S, stimulus artifact ; V, ventricular electrogram.

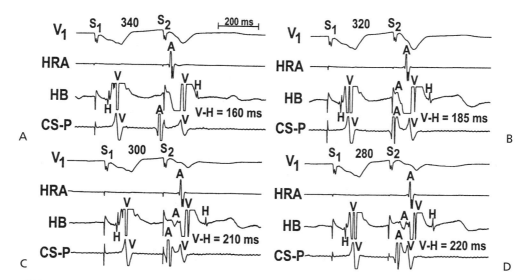

FIGURE 1-26. Decremental conduction within the retrograde His-Purkinje system. Displayed are electrocardiographic lead V_1 and intracardiac electrograms recorded from the high right atrium (HRA), His bundle (HB) region, and proximal coronary sinus (CS-P) region. After a fixed drive train (S_1-S_1 = 600 ms, not shown), a premature ventricular extrastimulus is introduced at the right ventricular apex at a cycle length (S_1-S_2) of 340 ms **(A)**, 320 ms **(B)**, 300 ms **(C)**, or 280 ms **(D)**. A, atrial electrogram; H, His bundle electrogram; S, stimulus artifact ; V, ventricular electrogram.

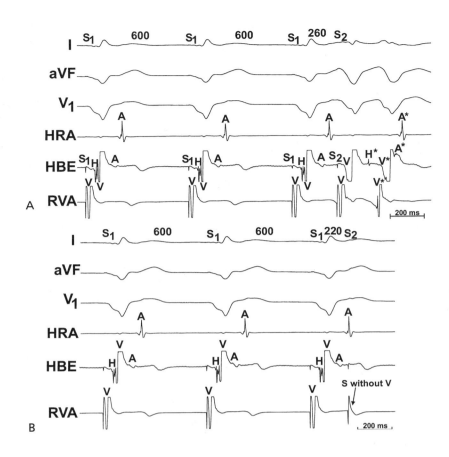

FIGURE 1-27. Retrograde conduction patterns resulting from ventricular extrastimulus pacing. Electrocardiographic leads I, aVF, V_1 and intracardiac electrograms from the high right atrium (HRA), His bundle region (HBE), and right ventricular apex (RVA) are displayed. Fixed-rate drive pacing (S_1-S_1) at the right ventricular apex at a cycle length of 600 ms is followed by a premature extrastimulus with a coupling interval (S_1-S_2) of 260 ms **(A)** or 220 ms **(B)**. **A:** There is 1 : 1 retrograde ventriculoatrial conduction during the fixed drive, with the retrograde His bundle electrogram (H) inscribed as the sharp deflection recorded in the early portion of the local ventricular electrogram in the HBE lead. The premature ventricular depolarization blocks in the retrograde right bundle, conducts transseptally, and then proceeds up the left bundle to activate the His bundle (H*), which is plainly visible after the large ventricular electrogram recorded by the HBE lead. Retrograde decremental conduction continues through the atrioventricular (AV) node to activate the atrium (A*). After activating the His bundle (H*), the wavefront conducts anterogradely within the previously refractory right bundle branch (i.e., bundle branch reentry) to reexcite the ventricle (V*). The S_1-S_2 coupling interval is further reduced (not shown) until eventually failure to capture the ventricle occurs at an S_1-S_2 coupling interval of 220 ms **(B)**. This is the ventricular effective refractory period. A, atrial electrogram; V, ventricular electrogram.

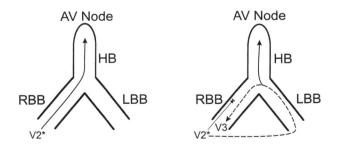

FIGURE 1-28. Circuit of bundle branch reentry. A premature right ventricular depolarization (V_2*) normally conducts retrogradely in the right bundle branch (RBB), through the His bundle (HB), to the atrioventricular (AV) node. With greater prematurity, retrograde V_2* conduction is blocked in the RBB and instead continues transseptally and proceeds retrogradely through the left bundle branch (LBB) to the HB. At the junction of the HB, RBB, and LBB, conduction can continue retrogradely to the AV node but also may proceed anterogradely within the RBB to reexcite the ventricle (V_3). Reentrant anterograde conduction in the RBB occurs because the delay resulting from transseptal and LBB conduction allows recovery of RBB excitability.

electrogram in the His bundle recording. As the premature coupling interval (V_1-V_2) is reduced, progressive retrograde conduction delay (prolongation of V_2-H_2 or S_2-H_2) occurs in the right bundle branch until block occurs. At this point, the retrograde conduction continues by means of the left bundle branch after transseptal activation, and the retrograde His potential is then observed after the local ventricular electrogram in the His recording. As the V_1-V_2 interval is further decreased, the V_2-H_2 (or S_2-H_2) further prolongs. When a critical degree of retrograde conduction delay has occurred, excitability can recover in the previously refractory right bundle branch. This allows V_2 to reenter the right bundle branch and conduct anterogradely, reexciting the ventricle as V_3 with a left bundle branch block QRS morphology pattern, similar to the QRS complex resulting from right ventricular apex stimulation (144–148). In the case of bundle branch reentry, the retrograde His bundle potential (H_2) precedes the anterograde right bundle deflection (RB_2), and the H-V interval preceding the extra beat (H_2-V_3) is equal to or greater than the H-V interval in sinus rhythm. For patients with normal hearts without a fixed bundle branch conduction delay, bundle branch reentry is rarely sustained and self-terminates after one or two beats.

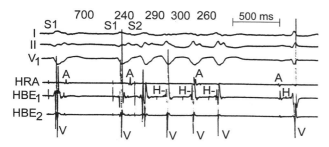

FIGURE 1-29. Surface electrocardiographic (ECG) and intracardiac recording of bundle branch reentry. Recordings top to bottom are from ECG leads I, II, and V_1, along with intracardiac recordings from the high right atrium (HRA) and proximal (HBE_1) and distal (HBE_2) His bundle regions. Right ventricular pacing is performed at a cycle length (S_1-S_1) of 700 ms, followed by the introduction of an extrastimulus at a premature coupling interval (S_1-S_2) of 240 ms. During the S_1-S_1 drive train, there is 1 : 1 ventriculoatrial conduction with the retrograde His bundle depolarization resulting from rapid conduction in the right bundle branch (RBB) is buried in the much larger ventricular depolarization recorded at the His bundle region. The paced premature ventricular depolarization is followed by a series of three spontaneous ventricular depolarizations with left bundle branch block (LBBB) morphology. The extrastimulus fails to conduct retrogradely in the RBB and instead proceeds transseptally and travels retrogradely in the left bundle branch (LBB). After this depolarization reaches the junction of the RBB and His bundle, the RBB is no longer refractory, allowing anterograde conduction again to proceed within the RBB. The ventricles are again activated from this reentrant depolarization wavefront with LBBB morphology. The long V-H- interval results because, with the RBB refractory, the His bundle is activated only after the impulse travels the long pathway from the right ventricle to the left ventricle and then retrogradely in the LBB. A, atrial depolarization; H, anterograde His bundle depolarization. H-, retrograde His bundle depolarization. (From Sung RJ, Juma Z, Saksena S. Electrophysiologic properties and antiarrhythmic mechanisms of intravenous *N*-acetylprocainamide in patients with ventricular dysrhythmias. *Am Heart J* 1983;105:811, with permission.)

Retrograde Conduction Using Accessory Ventriculoatrial Connections

Despite the fact that it is often difficult to record the retrograde His bundle activation, the hallmark of retrograde normal pathway (i.e., His-Purkinje-AV node) conduction is that it is decremental (Fig. 1-30) and that the earliest retrograde atrial activation occurs at the anterior right atrial septum at the site where the maximal His bundle electrogram is recorded during sinus rhythm (Fig. 1-30). However, if retrograde AV nodal conduction is through the slow AV nodal pathway and not the fast pathway, the earliest retrograde atrial activation is recorded more posterior than the site at which the maximal His bundle is recorded (i.e., closer to the ostium of the coronary sinus) (149).

If ventriculoatrial conduction occurs within an accessory connection, the retrograde pattern of conduction is different than that seen in Figure 1-30, unless the accessory connection lies immediately adjacent to the normal AV node–His bundle and exhibits decremental conduction. The most common type of accessory connection is a concealed (i.e., conducts only from the ventricle to atrium), left-sided pathway running between the left ventricle and the left atrium. If fixed-cycle-length ventricular pacing is performed in such a patient with ventriculoatrial conduction proceeding exclusively within the accessory connection, the earliest retrograde atrial activation is recorded by an electrode positioned adjacent to the location of the accessory connection in the distal coronary sinus/great cardiac vein (Fig. 1-31).

If fixed-rate ventricular pacing is performed in a patient with normal and accessory connections capable of retrograde conduction, various patterns of conduction may occur. Pacing at slow rates (i.e., just slightly faster than the

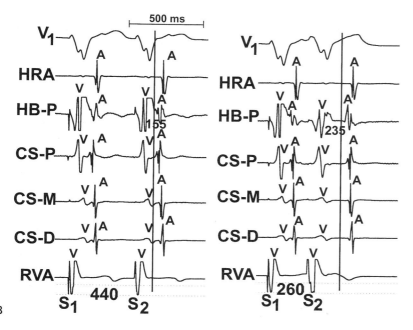

FIGURE 1-30. Decremental conduction properties of the retrograde normal pathway. Displayed are electrocardiographic lead V_1 and intracardiac electrograms recorded from the high right atrium (HRA); proximal His bundle region (HB-P); proximal (CS-P), middle (CS-M), and distal (CS-D) coronary sinus regions; and right ventricular apex (RVA). After a fixed drive train (S_1-S_1 = 600 ms, not shown), a premature ventricular extrastimulus is introduced at the RVA at a coupling interval (S_1-S_2) of 440 ms **(A)** or 260 ms **(B)**. As the extrastimulus coupling interval decreases from 440 to 260 ms, the ventriculoatrial conduction interval (measured as the local ventriculoatrial conduction time in the His bundle recording) increases from 155 to 235 ms. The retrograde atrial activation sequence remains unchanged, with the earliest atrial activation occurring in the proximal His bundle (HB-P) region and the latest activation in the distal coronary sinus (CS-D). Although the prolongation of conduction time is obvious, the sites of conduction delay cannot be identified because the His bundle electrogram is hidden within the ventricular depolarization recorded by the His bundle leads. A, atrial electrogram; H, His bundle electrogram; S, stimulus artifact ; V, ventricular electrogram.

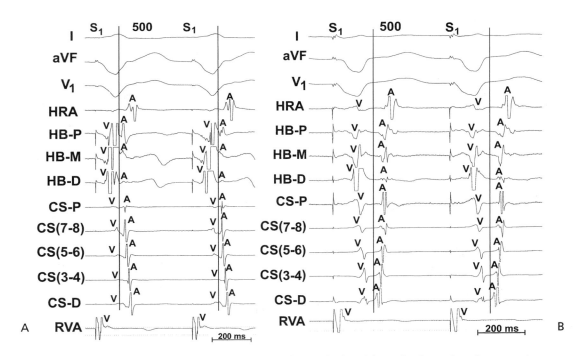

FIGURE 1-31. Fixed-rate ventricular pacing with ventriculoatrial conduction using the normal pathway **(A)** and a left lateral accessory connection **(B)**. From top to bottom are displayed surface electrocardiographic leads I, aVF, and V_1 and intracardiac electrograms from the high right atrium (HRA); proximal (HB-P), middle (HB-M), and distal (HB-D) His bundle regions; proximal (CS-P), middle (CS[3-4], CS[5-6], CS[7-8]), and distal (CS-D) coronary sinus or great cardiac vein; and right ventricular apex (RVA). The tip of the coronary sinus catheter (CS-D) is located at the far left lateral mitral annulus within the great cardiac vein, far from the interatrial septum and the His bundle region. **A:** Fixed-rate pacing (S_1-S_1) at 500 ms at the RVA results in ventriculoatrial conduction, with the earliest retrograde atrial activation recorded in the His bundle region and progressively later atrial activations recorded as assessment proceeds from the right anterior interatrial septum to the lateral coronary sinus region (CS-D). **B:** Fixed-rate pacing (S_1-S_1) at 500 ms at the RVA results in ventriculoatrial conduction, with the earliest retrograde atrial activation recorded in the distal coronary sinus and progressively later atrial activations recorded as assessment proceeds from the lateral coronary sinus region to the ostium of the coronary sinus (CS-P) and then to the anterior interatrial septum (HB-P). A, atrial electrogram; V, ventricular electrogram.

patient's sinus rate) may result in conduction over the retrograde normal and accessory pathways. At these cycle lengths, there is fusion activation of the atria, with some portions of the atria being activated using the accessory connection and other portions activated through the normal pathway. With increasing pacing rate, the retrograde block cycle length of the accessory pathway and the normal pathway will be reached. In each case, this is defined as the slowest fixed rate of ventricular pacing (i.e., longest fixed cycle length) at which 1 : 1 ventriculoatrial conduction over the accessory pathway or normal pathway, respectively, cannot be maintained (i.e., conduction block occurs at any faster pacing rate). Which block cycle length is reached first depends on which pathway—normal or accessory—has the longest effective refractory period. If the retrograde block cycle length of the normal pathway is reached first (i.e., block cycle length of normal pathway is greater than that of the accessory pathway), all ventriculoatrial conduction at faster rates will be within the accessory connection (with no atrial fusion). If the block cycle length of the accessory

pathway is reached first (i.e., block cycle length of the accessory pathway is greater than that of the normal pathway), all ventriculoatrial conduction at faster rates will be within the normal pathway (with no atrial fusion). When pacing at cycle lengths that are greater than the accessory and normal pathway retrograde block cycle lengths, ventriculoatrial conduction will proceed over the accessory and normal pathways, resulting in various degrees of ventricular fusion.

Concealed Conduction

Concealed conduction refers to incompletely penetrating electrical (nonpropagated) impulses in the heart that are themselves electrically silent on the surface ECG but that alter the conduction of subsequent propagated impulses. For example, incomplete penetration of the AV node by premature atrial or ventricular depolarizations can result in the unexpected prolongation of conduction or unexpected failure of propagation of an impulse (32,150–152). Figures 1-15, 1-32, and 1-33 illustrate examples of concealed con-

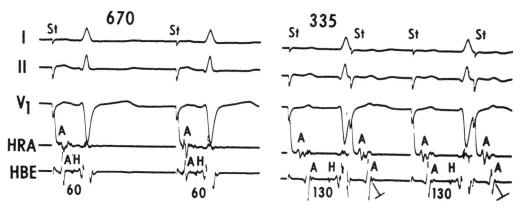

FIGURE 1-32. Demonstration of concealed conduction into the atrioventricular (AV) node with prolongation of AV nodal conduction time. Recordings from top to bottom are surface electrocardiographic leads I, II, and V_1 and endocardial electrograms from the high right atrium (HRA) and His bundle region (HBE). **A:** Electrical stimulation (St) of the HRA at an St-St cycle length of 670 ms results in 1 : 1 intraatrial and AV conduction with an A-H interval of 60 ms. **B:** The rate of atrial stimulation is increased (St-St = 335) resulting in 2 : 1 AV conduction (A-A cycle length = 335 ms, V-V cycle length = 670 ms) with an A-H interval of 130 ms. Despite the fact that the ventricular rate is identical in **A** and **B**, the A-H interval during AV conduction increases from 60 to 130 ms when the atrial depolarization rate is doubled. This result indicates that the atrial depolarization not conducted to the His bundle or ventricles nevertheless incompletely penetrates the AV node, thereby prolonging AV nodal conduction (i.e., A-H interval) during the subsequent AV-conducted impulse (i.e., concealed conduction). A, electrogram; H, His bundle electrogram; St, stimulus artifact.

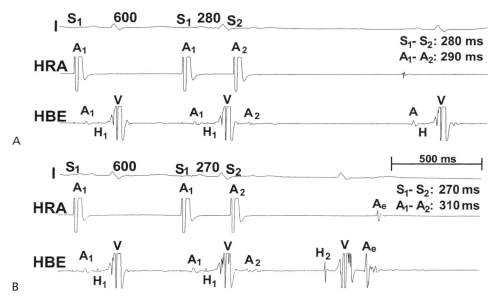

FIGURE 1-33. Intracardiac recordings of type 4 gap phenomenon. Surface electrocardiographic lead I is shown at the top of each panel. Fixed-rate pacing (S_1-S_1) at 600 ms is performed in the high right atrium (HRA), followed by the introduction of an extrastimulus at a coupling interval (S_1-S_2) of 280 ms **(A)** or 270 ms **(B)**. **A:** The extrastimulus results in an A_1-A_2 interval of 290 ms recorded in the His bundle region (HBE), with the atrial premature depolarization (A_2) failing to conduct through the atrioventricular (AV) node (i.e., A_2 not followed by H_2). **B:** With a further reduction in S_1-S_2 to 270 ms, the intraatrial conduction interval (A_1-A_2) recorded at the His bundle region increases to 310 ms. This intraatrial conduction delay of 20 ms between the HRA and the AV junction (i.e., A_1-A_2 increases from 290 ms to 310 ms) occurs despite a 10-ms decline in the extrastimulus coupling interval (S_1-S_2) from 280 to 270 ms. Because of this intraatrial conduction delay, the AV node has time to recover excitability, allowing the atrial extrastimulus (A_2) to conduct to the His bundle (H_2) and ventricle. This phenomenon, whereby AV nodal conduction that occurs at long extrastimulus coupling intervals (not shown) is blocked at shorter coupling intervals **(A)** but resumes despite a further reduction in the extrastimulus coupling interval **(B)**, is called the gap phenomenon. In general, a conduction gap can occur when conduction delay in a proximal tissue (in this case, the right atrium) allows previously blocked conduction to resume through a distal tissue (in this case, the AV node). The atrial electrogram (Ae) is an atrial echo beat resulting from retrograde activation of the atrium using the retrograde fast AV nodal conduction pathway after anterograde conduction of A_2 within the slow conduction pathway. A, atrial electrogram; H, His bundle electrogram; S, stimulus artifact; V, ventricular electrogram.

duction involving slowing or blocking of AV nodal or intraatrial conduction by premature impulses or during atrial flutter. In the situation depicted in Figure 1-32, right atrial premature depolarizations that fail to conduct to the His bundle or ventricles nevertheless delay subsequent conduction of impulses in the AV node. Nonpropagated atrial stimuli can increase the intraatrial conduction time of subsequent propagated atrial stimuli.

During atrial flutter, many of the rapid atrial depolarizations penetrate into, but do not conduct through, the AV node to the His bundle; notice that the atrial depolarizations are not followed by His depolarizations in Figure 1-15. Under normal conditions, this concealed conduction functions to prevent rapid 1:1 AV conduction during atrial tachycardias. However, exercise, with its reduction in parasympathetic and increase in sympathetic tone, can alter the effects of concealed conduction and enhance AV conduction during atrial flutter. The concealed AV nodal conduction is markedly diminished by the high adrenergic tone of exercise, resulting in a increase in the ventricular rate to the atrial flutter rate of 215 bpm.

Gap Phenomenon

The gap phenomenon refers to an unusual situation whereby atrial premature depolarizations of greater prematurity are more likely to conduct to the ventricles than less premature atrial depolarizations. The resumption of conduction at shorter coupling intervals was originally interpreted as a manifestation of supernormal conduction; however, it is now clear that this phenomenon has a simple physiologic basis.

In general, the gap phenomenon requires a distal region of the conduction system to have an effective refractory period longer than the functional refractory period of a more proximal region. In this case, premature atrial depolarizations block first in the distal location, but with continued prematurity, delay develops in the proximal site permitting time for the distal tissue to recover excitability, allowing resumption of distal conduction (143,153–158) (Fig. 1-33). Although numerous types of gap phenomenon have been demonstrated in human hearts, the most common gaps involve the AV node as the proximal region and various components of the His-Purkinje system as the distal site (143,153–158) (Table 1-5).

An unusual example of the gap phenomenon involves a right-sided accessory AV connection. Anterograde conduction through an accessory connection results in a wide QRS complex morphology on the surface ECG because of the depolarization wavefront proceeding independent of the His-Purkinje system. In this case, ventricular depolarization must conduct from myocardial cell to myocardial cell without the benefit of the arborizing specialized conduction system. Activation of the ventricle through the AV node-His-Purkinje axis results in a rapid, almost simultaneous

TABLE 1-5. CLASSIFICATION OF GAP PHENOMENON

Type	Distal (Initial) Site of Block	Proximal (Delayed) Site of Block
Anterograde		
1	HPS	AV node
2	HPS (distal)	HPS (proximal)
3	HPS	His bundle
4	HPS or AV node	Atrium
5	AV node (distal)	AV node (proximal)
6	HPS	Supernormal conduction
Retrograde		
1	AV node	HPS
2	HPS (proximal)	HPS (distal)

AV, atrioventricular; HPS, HisPurkinje system. Adapted from (156). Adapted from Damato AN, Akhtar M, Ruskin J, et al. Gap phenomena: antegrade and retrograde. In: Wellens HJJ, Lie KI, Janse MJ, eds. *The conduction system of the heart: structure, function and clinical implications.* Philadelphia: Lea & Febiger, 1976, with permission.

depolarization of all regions of the ventricles, eliciting a narrow QRS complex morphology. There is exclusive AV conduction through an accessory AV connection and not the AV node–His bundle axis, during fixed atrial pacing at a rate of 150 bpm. However, a gap exists allowing atrial premature depolarizations delivered at a specific coupling interval to conduct through the AV node, whereas earlier or later premature atrial depolarizations conduct through the accessory connection. The accessory AV connection (i.e., distal tissue) has an effective refractory period that is longer than the functional refractory period of the atrium (i.e., proximal tissue).

Supernormal and Pseudo-supernormal Conduction

In clinical electrophysiology, *supernormal conduction* has been classically used to describe situations in which conduction is better than anticipated or occurs when block was expected (159,160). It is in dispute whether true supernormal conduction occurs in human hearts, and many phenomena that have been attributed to supernormal conduction can be explained by concealed conduction, the gap phenomenon, facilitation, rate-related changes in refractoriness, summation and reflection, and dual AV node physiology (161–163). These examples of supernormal phenomena have been more correctly classified as *pseudo-supernormal conduction* (150,161–163).

Figure 1-34 shows a series of intracardiac recordings that are difficult to explain without invoking supernormal conduction. In this case, AV conduction and ventricular activation occurs such that the 12-lead ECG exhibits a right bundle branch block pattern. Premature atrial depolarizations delivered after the fixed drive train are conducted

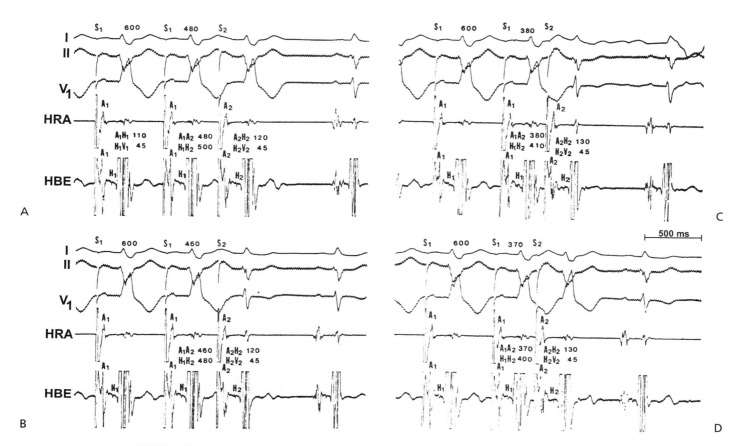

FIGURE 1-34. Evidence of supernormal conduction in the right bundle branch. Recordings from top to bottom in each panel include surface electrocardiographic leads I, II, and V_1 and intracardiac electrograms from the high right atrium (HRA) and His bundle region (HBE). Fixed-cycle-length pacing (S_1-S_1 = 600 ms) is performed in the HRA, followed by the introduction of increasingly premature extrastimulus (S_2). During the fixed pacing train, atrioventricular (AV) conduction occurs with a right bundle branch block (RBBB) QRS complex morphology (detected through the surface leads). **A to C:** With reductions in the S_1-S_2 (and A_1-A_2) coupling interval from 480 to 380 ms, the QRS complex morphology of the premature beat (V_2) changes from the RBBB pattern to a normal pattern. Associated with this change is the finding that the input coupling interval into the RBB (H_1-H_2) decreases from 500 to 480 ms, with only slight or no changes in the AV nodal (A_1-H_2) and His-Purkinje (H_2-V_2) conduction times. Despite the increase in prematurity of the input impulse to the RBB (and the absence of any delay in conduction in other portions of the conduction system), conduction within the RBB improves, contrary to expectations (i.e., supernormal conduction). **D:** With continued prematurity of S_2 and further reductions of the H_1-H_2 interval to 400 ms, conduction blocks in the RBB result again in the RBBB QRS morphology. Consequently, there is a 90-ms window of H_1-H_2 intervals ranging from 500 to 410 ms, within which conduction is enhanced in the RBB.

without right bundle branch block. With increasing prematurity, the input coupling interval into the right bundle branch (H_1-H_2) actually decreases, with only a minor or no change in AV nodal and His-Purkinje conduction times. Contrary to expectations, despite the increase in prematurity of the input impulse to the right bundle branch and the absence of any delay in conduction in other portions of the conduction system, conduction within the right bundle branch recovers and results in normal His-Purkinje conduction (i.e., narrow QRS complex).

REFERENCES

1. Anderson RH, Janse MJ, van Capelle FJ, et al. A combined morphological and electrophysiological study of the atrioventricular node of the rabbit heart. *Circ Res* 1974;35:909.
2. Anderson RH, Becker AE, Tranum-Jensen J, et al. Anatomic-electrophysiological correlations in the conduction system—a review. *Br Heart J* 1981;45:67.
3. Becker AE, Anderson RH. Morphology of the human atrioventricular junctional area. In: Wellens HJJ, Lie KI, Janse MJ, eds. *The conduction system of the heart: structure, function and clinical*

implication. Leiden, The Netherlands: Sterfest Kroese, 1976: 263.

4. Becker AE, Anderson RH, Durrer D, et al. The anatomical substrates of Wolff-Parkinson-White syndrome: a clinicopathologic correlation in seven patients. *Circulation* 1978;57:870.
5. Bharati S, Rosen KM, Towne WD, et al. The conduction system in the baboon heart. *Chest* 1979;75:62.
6. Bharati S, Nordenberg A, Bauernfiend R, et al. The anatomic substrate for the sick sinus syndrome in adolescence. *Am J Cardiol* 1980;46:163.
7. Janse MJ, Capelle FJV, Anderson RH, et al. Correlation between electrophysiologic recordings and morphologic findings in the rabbit atrioventricular node. *Arch Int Physiol Biochim* 1974;82:331.
8. Inoue S, Becker AE. Posterior extensions of the human compact atrioventricular node: a neglected anatomic feature of potential clinical significance. *Circulation* 1998;97:188.
9. Lev M, Unger PN, Rosen KM, et al. The anatomic substrate of complete left bundle branch block. *Circulation* 1974;50:479.
10. Lev M, Fox SMD, Bharati S, et al. Mahaim and James fibers as a basis for a unique variety of ventricular preexcitation. *Am J Cardiol* 1975;36:880.
11. Lev M, Unger PN, Rosen KM, et al. The anatomic base of the electrocardiographic abnormality left bundle branch block. *Adv Cardiol* 1975;14:16.
12. McGuire MA, de Bakker JM, Vermeulen JT, et al. Atrioventricular junctional tissue. Discrepancy between histological and electrophysiological characteristics. *Circulation* 1996;94:571.
13. Racker DK. Atrioventricular node and input pathways: a correlated gross anatomical and histological study of the canine atrioventricular junctional region. *Anat Rec* 1989;224:336.
14. Davies MJ, Anderson RH, Becker AE. *The conduction system of the heart.* London: Butterworth, 1983.
15. Bharati S, Lev M. The anatomy and pathology of the conduction system. In: Samet P, El-Sherif N, eds. *Cardiac pacing.* Orlando, FL: Grune & Stratton, 1980.
16. Becker AE. *Atrioventricular nodal anatomy revisited.* : Learning Center, 1994:17.
17. Fitzgerald D, Lazzara R. Functional anatomy of the conduction system. *Hosp Pract (Off Ed)* 1988;23:81.
18. Sealy WC, Gallagher JJ, Pritchett EL. The surgical anatomy of Kent bundles based on electrophysiological mapping and surgical exploration. *J Thorac Cardiovasc Surg* 1978;76:804.
19. Rossi L. Interatrial, internodal and dual reentrant atrioventricular nodal pathways: an anatomical update of arrhythmogenic substrates. *Cardiologia* 1996;41:129.
20. Keith A, Flack M. The form and nature of the muscular connections between the primary divisions of the vertebrate heart. *J Anat Physiol* 1907;41:172.
21. James TN. Morphology of the human atrioventricular node, with remarks pertinent to its electrophysiology. *Am Heart J* 1961;62:756.
22. Hecht HH, Kossmann CE, Childers RW, et al. Atrioventricular and intraventricular conduction. Revised nomenclature and concepts. *Am J Cardiol* 1973;31:232.
23. Tawara S. *Das Reizleitungssystem des Saugetierherzens.* Jena: Gustav Fisher, 1906.
24. Truex RC, Smythe MO. Reconstruction of the human atrioventricular node. *Anat Rec* 1967;158:11.
25. McGuire MA, Johnson DC, Robotin M, et al. Dimensions of the triangle of Koch in humans. *Am J Cardiol* 1992;70:829.
26. Widran J, Lev M. The dissection of the atrioventricular node, bundle and bundle branches in the human heart. *Circulation* 1951;4:863.
27. Racker DK. Sinoventricular transmission in 10 M K$^+$ by canine atrioventricular nodal inputs: superior atrionodal bundle and proximal atrioventricular bundle. *Circulation* 1991;83:1738.
28. Janse MJ, van Capelle FJL, Anderson RH, et al. Electrophysiology and structure of the atrioventricular node of the isolated rabbit heart. In: Wellens HJJ, Lie KI, Janse MJ, eds. *The conduction system of the heart: structure, function and clinical implication.* Leiden, The Netherlands: Sterfest Kroese, 1976:296.
29. Janse MK, Anderson RH, van Capelle FJ, et al. A combined electrophysiological and anatomical study of the human fetal heart. *Am Heart J* 1976;91:556.
30. Janse MJ. Influence of the direction of the atrial wave front on A-V nodal transmission in isolated hearts of rabbits. *Circ Res* 1969;25:439.
31. Meijler FL, Janse MJ. Morphology and electrophysiology of the mammalian atrioventricular node. *Physiol Rev* 1988;68:608.
32. Zipes DP, Mendez C, Moe GK. Evidence for summation and voltage dependency in rabbit atrioventricular nodal fibers. *Circ Res* 1973;32:170.
33. Sherf L, James TN, Woods WT. Function of the atrioventricular node considered on the basis of observed histology and fine structure. *J Am Coll Cardiol* 1985;5:770.
34. Oosthoek PW, Viragh S, Lamers WH, et al. Immunohistochemical delineation of the conduction system. II: The atrioventricular node and Purkinje fibers. *Circ Res* 1993;73:482.
35. Oosthoek PW, Viragh S, Mayen AE, et al. Immunohistochemical delineation of the conduction system. I: The sinoatrial node. *Circ Res* 1993;73:473.
36. Sugi Y, Hirakaw R. Freeze-fracture studies of the sinoatrial and atrioventricular nodes of the caprine heart, with special reference to the nexus. *Cell Tissue Res* 1986;245:273.
37. Davis LM, Rodefeld ME, Green K, et al. Gap junction protein phenotypes of the human heart and conduction system. *J Cardiovasc Electrophysiol* 1995;6[Pt 1]:813.
38. Spach MS, Josephson ME. Initiating reentry: the role of nonuniform anisotropy in small circuits. *J Cardiovasc Electrophysiol* 1994;5:182.
39. Randall WC. Differential autonomic control of SAN and AVN regions of the canine heart: structure and function . In: Mazgalev T, Dreifus LS, Michelson EL, eds. *Progress in clinical biological research: electrophysiology of the sinoatrial and atrioventricular nodes,* vol 275. New York: Alan R Liss, 1988:15.
40. Lev M. Anatomic basis for atrioventricular block. *Am J Med* 1964;37:742.
41. Truex RC, Bishof JK, Hoffman EL. Accessory atrioventricular bundles of the developing human heart. *Anat Rec* 1958;135:45.
42. Childers R. The AV node: normal and abnormal physiology. *Prog Cardiovasc Dis* 1977;13:361.
43. Anderson RH, Becker AE, Brechenmacher C, et al. Ventricular preexcitation: A proposed nomenclature for its substrates. *Eur J Cardiol* 1975;3:27.
44. Gallagher JJ, Gilbert M, Svenson RH, et al. Wolff-Parkinson-White syndrome: the problem, evaluation, and surgical correction. *Circulation* 1975;51:767.
45. Kalman JM, Olgin JE, Saxon LA, et al. Activation and entrainment mapping defines the tricuspid annulus as the anterior barrier in typical atrial flutter. *Circulation* 1996;94:398.
46. Olgin JE, Kalman JM, Fitzpatrick AP, et al. Role of right atrial endocardial structures as barriers to conduction during human type I atrial flutter: activation and entrainment mapping guided by intracardiac echocardiography. *Circulation* 1995;92:1839.
47. Olgin JE, Kalman JM, Lesh MD. Conduction barriers in human atrial flutter: correlation of electrophysiology and anatomy. *J Cardiovasc Electrophysiol* 1996;7:1112.
48. Kalman JM, Olgin JE, Karch MR, et al. "Cristal tachycardias": origin of right atrial tachycardias from the crista terminalis iden-

tified by intracardiac echocardiography. *J Am Coll Cardiol* 1998;
31:451.

49. Kalman JM, VanHare GF, Olgin JE, et al. Ablation of "incisional" reentrant atrial tachycardia complicating surgery for congenital heart disease: use of entrainment to define a critical isthmus of conduction. *Circulation* 1996;93:502.

50. Lesh MD, Kalman JM, Saxon LA, et al. Electrophysiology of "incisional" reentrant atrial tachycardia complicating surgery for congenital heart disease. *Pacing Clin Electrophysiol* 1997;20 [Pt 2]:2107.

51. Haissaguerre M, Jais P, Shah DC, et al. Spontaneous initiation of atrial fibrillation by ectopic beats originating in the pulmonary veins. *N Engl J Med* 1998;339:659.

52. Haissaguerre M, Shah DC, Jais P, et al. Role of catheter ablation for atrial fibrillation. *Curr Opin Cardiol* 1997;12:18.

53. Elvan A, Wylie K, Zipes DP. Pacing-induced chronic atrial fibrillation impairs sinus node function in dogs: electrophysiological remodeling. *Circulation* 1996;94:2953.

54. Daoud EG, Knight BP, Weiss R, et al. Effect of verapamil and procainamide on atrial fibrillation-induced electrical remodeling in humans. *Circulation* 1997;96:1542.

55. Goette A, Honeycutt C, Langberg JJ. Electrical remodeling in atrial fibrillation: time course and mechanisms. *Circulation* 1996;94:2968.

56. Tieleman RG, Van Gelder IC, Crijns HJ, et al. Early recurrences of atrial fibrillation after electrical cardioversion: a result of fibrillation-induced electrical remodeling of the atria? *J Am Coll Cardiol* 1998;31:167.

57. Wijffels MC, Kirchhof CJ, Dorland R, et al. Electrical remodeling due to atrial fibrillation in chronically instrumented conscious goats: roles of neurohumoral changes, ischemia, atrial stretch, and high rate of electrical activation. *Circulation* 1997;96:3710.

58. Yue L, Feng J, Gaspo R, et al. Ionic remodeling underlying action potential changes in a dog model of atrial fibrillation. *Circ Res* 1997;81:512.

59. Nibley C, Wharton JM. Ventricular tachycardias with left bundle branch block morphology. *Pacing Clin Electrophysiol* 1995; 18:334.

60. Ng KS, Wen MS, Yeh SJ, et al. The effects of adenosine on idiopathic ventricular tachycardia. *Am J Cardiol* 1994;74:195.

61. Lokhandwala YY, Smeets JL, Rodriguez LM, et al. Idiopathic ventricular tachycardia—characterisation and radiofrequency ablation. *Indian Heart J* 1994;46:281.

62. Merliss AD, Seifert MJ, Collins RF, et al. Catheter ablation of idiopathic left ventricular tachycardia associated with a false tendon. *Pacing Clin Electrophysiol* 1996;19[Pt 1]:2144.

63. Mont L, Seixas T, Brugada P, et al. The electrocardiographic, clinical, and electrophysiologic spectrum of idiopathic monomorphic ventricular tachycardia. *Am Heart J* 1992;124: 746.

64. Okumura K, Yamabe H, Tsuchiya T, et al. Characteristics of slow conduction zone demonstrated during entrainment of idiopathic ventricular tachycardia of left ventricular origin. *Am J Cardiol* 1996;77:379.

65. Nishizaki M, Arita M, Sakurada H, et al. Demonstration of Purkinje potential during idiopathic left ventricular tachycardia: a marker for ablation site by transient entrainment. *Pacing Clin Electrophysiol* 1997;20[Pt 1]:3004.

66. Vora AM, Tang AS, Green MS. Idiopathic left ventricular tachycardia: what is the mechanism? *Pacing Clin Electrophysiol* 1997;20:2855.

67. Wen MS, Yeh SJ, Wang CC, et al. Radiofrequency ablation therapy in idiopathic left ventricular tachycardia with no obvious structural heart disease. *Circulation* 1994;89:1690.

68. Zardini M, Thakur RK, Klein GJ, et al. Catheter ablation of idiopathic left ventricular tachycardia. *Pacing Clin Electrophysiol* 1995;18:1255.

69. Markowitz SM, Litvak BL, Ramirez de Arellano EA, et al. Adenosine-sensitive ventricular tachycardia: right ventricular abnormalities delineated by magnetic resonance imaging. *Circulation* 1997;96:1192.

70. Carlson MD, White RD, Trohman RG, et al. Right ventricular outflow tract ventricular tachycardia: detection of previously unrecognized anatomic abnormalities using cine magnetic resonance imaging. *J Am Coll Cardiol* 1994;24:720.

71. Blanck Z, Dhala A, Deshpande S, et al. Bundle branch reentrant ventricular tachycardia: cumulative experience in 48 patients. *J Cardiovasc Electrophysiol* 1993;4:253.

72. Blanck Z, Deshpande S, Jazayeri MR, et al. Catheter ablation of the left bundle branch for the treatment of sustained bundle branch reentrant ventricular tachycardia. *J Cardiovasc Electrophysiol* 1995;6:40.

73. Cohen TJ, Chien WW, Lurie KG, et al. Radiofrequency catheter ablation for treatment of bundle branch reentrant ventricular tachycardia: results and long-term follow-up. *J Am Coll Cardiol* 1991;18:1767.

74. De Lima GG, Dubuc M, Roy D, et al. Radiofrequency ablation of bundle branch reentrant tachycardia in a patient with atrial septal defect. *Can J Cardiol* 1997;13:403.

75. Bogun F, El-Atassi R, Daoud E, et al. Radiofrequency ablation of idiopathic left anterior fascicular tachycardia. *J Cardiovasc Electrophysiol* 1995;6:1113.

76. Gonzalez RP, Scheinman MM, Lesh MD, et al. Clinical and electrophysiologic spectrum of fascicular tachycardias. *Am Heart J* 1994;128:147.

77. Katritsis D, Heald S, Ahsan A, et al. Catheter ablation for successful management of left posterior fascicular tachycardia: an approach guided by recording of fascicular potentials. *Heart* 1996;75:384.

78. Wieland JM, Marchlinski FE. Electrocardiographic response of digoxin-toxic fascicular tachycardia to Fab fragments: implications for tachycardia mechanism. *Pacing Clin Electrophysiol* 1986;9:727.

79. Vergara I, Wharton JM. Ventricular tachycardia and fibrillation in normal hearts. *Curr Opin Cardiol* 1998;13:9.

80. Kim SS, Gallastegui J, Welch WJ, et al. Paroxysmal fascicular tachycardia and ventricular tachycardia due to mechanical stimulation by a mitral valve prosthesis. *J Am Coll Cardiol* 1986;7: 176.

81. Crijns HJ, Smeets JL, Rodriguez LM, et al. Cure of interfascicular reentrant ventricular tachycardia by ablation of the anterior fascicle of the left bundle branch. *J Cardiovasc Electrophysiol* 1995;6:486.

82. Berder V, Vauthier M, Mabo P, et al. Characteristics and outcome in arrhythmogenic right ventricular dysplasia. *Am J Cardiol* 1995;75:411.

83. Blake LM, Scheinman MM, Higgins CB. MR features of arrhythmogenic right ventricular dysplasia. *AJR Am J Roentgenol* 1994;162:809.

84. Leclercq JF, Coumel P. Characteristics, prognosis and treatment of the ventricular arrhythmias of right ventricular dysplasia. *Eur Heart J* 1989;10[Suppl D]:61.

85. Leclercq JF, Coumel P. Late potentials in arrhythmogenic right ventricular dysplasia. Prevalence, diagnostic and prognostic values. *Eur Heart J* 1993;14[Suppl E]:80.

86. Leclercq JF, Potenza S, Maison-Blanche P, et al. Determinants of spontaneous occurrence of sustained monomorphic ventricular tachycardia in right ventricular dysplasia. *J Am Coll Cardiol* 1996;28:720.

87. Manyari DE, Klein GJ, Gulamhusein S, et al. Arrhythmogenic right ventricular dysplasia: a generalized cardiomyopathy? *Circulation* 1983;68:251.

88. Furlanello F, Bertoldi A, Dallago M, et al. Cardiac arrest and sudden death in competitive athletes with arrhythmogenic right ventricular dysplasia. *Pacing Clin Electrophysiol* 1998;21[Pt 2]:331.

89. Peters S. Right ventricular cardiomyopathy: diffuse dilatation, focal dysplasia or biventricular disease. *Int J Cardiol* 1997;62:63.

90. Proclemer A, Crani R, Feruglio GA. Right ventricular tachycardia with ventricular dysplasia: clinical features, diagnostic techniques and current management. *Am Heart J* 1989;103:415.

91. Horowitz LN, Vetter VL, Harken AH, et al. Electrophysiologic characteristics of sustained ventricular tachycardia occurring after repair of tetralogy of Fallot. *Am J Cardiol* 1980;46:446.

92. Horowitz LN, Josephson ME, Farshidi A, et al. Recurrent sustained ventricular tachycardia. 3. Role of the electrophysiologic study in selection of antiarrhythmic regimens. *Circulation* 1978;58:986.

93. Horowitz LN, Josephson ME, Harken AH. Epicardial and endocardial activation during sustained ventricular tachycardia in man. *Circulation* 1980;61:1227.

94. Horowitz LN, Spielman SR, Greenspan AM, et al. Mechanisms in the genesis of recurrent ventricular tachyarrhythmias as revealed by clinical electrophysiologic studies. *Ann N Y Acad Sci* 1982;382:116.

95. Horowitz LN, Spielman SR, Greenspan AM, et al. Role of programmed stimulation in assessing vulnerability to ventricular arrhythmias. *Am Heart J* 1982;103[Pt 2]:604.

96. Josephson ME, Horowitz LN. Recurrent ventricular tachycardia: an electrophysiologic approach. *Med Clin North Am* 1979;63:53.

97. Josephson ME, Horowitz LN, Spielman SR, et al. Electrophysiologic and hemodynamic studies in patients resuscitated from cardiac arrest. *Am J Cardiol* 1980;46:948.

98. Josephson ME. Treatment of ventricular arrhythmias after myocardial infarction. *Circulation* 1986;74:653.

99. Josephson ME, Wit AL. Fractionated electrical activity and continuous electrical activity: fact or artifact? *Circulation* 1984;70:529.

100. Josephson ME, Almendral JM, Buxton AE, et al. Mechanisms of ventricular tachycardia. *Circulation* 1987;75[Pt 2]:III-41.

101. Wilber DJ, Kopp DE, Glascock DN, et al. Catheter ablation of the mitral isthmus for ventricular tachycardia associated with inferior infarction. *Circulation* 1995;92:3481.

102. Hadjis TA, Stevenson WG, Harada T, et al. Preferential locations for critical reentry circuit sites causing ventricular tachycardia after inferior wall myocardial infarction. *J Cardiovasc Electrophysiol* 1997;8:363.

103. Bekheit S, Murtagh JG, Morton P, et al. Measurements of sinus impulse conduction from electrogram of bundle of His. *Br Heart J* 1971;33:719.

104. Castellanos A, Castillo C, Agha A. Contribution of the His bundle recording to the understanding of clinical arrhythmias. *Am J Cardiol* 1971;28:499.

105. Castellanos A Jr, Castillo CA, Agha AS, et al. His bundle electrograms in patients with short P-R intervals, narrow QRS complexes, and paroxysmal tachycardias. *Circulation* 1971;43:667.

106. Damato AN, Lau SH, Berkowitz WD, et al. Recording of specialized conducting fibers (A-V nodal, His bundle, and right bundle branch) in man using an electrode catheter technic. *Circulation* 1969;39:435.

107. Damato AN, Lau SH, Helfant RH, et al. Study of atrioventricular conduction in man using electrode catheter recordings of His bundle activity. *Circulation* 1969;39:287.

108. Damato AN, Lau SH. Clinical value of the electrogram of the conduction system. *Prog Cardiovasc Dis* 1970;13:119.

109. Narula OS, Cohen LS, Samet P, et al. Localization of A-V conduction defects in man by recording of the His bundle electrogram. *Am J Cardiol* 1970;25:288.

110. Narula OS, Scherlag BJ, Samet P, et al. Atrioventricular block: localization and classification by His bundle recordings. *Am J Med* 1971;50:146.

111. Rosen KM. Evaluation of cardiac conduction in the cardiac catheterization laboratory. *Am J Cardiol* 1972;30:701.

112. Rosen KM, Scherlag BJ, Samet P, et al. His bundle electrogram. *Circulation* 1972;46:831.

113. Bekheit S, Murtagh JG, Morton P, et al. Studies of heart block with His bundle recordings. *Br Heart J* 1972;34:717.

114. Batsford WP, Akhtar M, Caracta AR, et al. Effect of atrial stimulation site on the electrophysiological properties of the atrioventricular node in man. *Circulation* 1974;50:283.

115. Cagin NA, Kunstadt D, Wolfish P, et al. The influence of heart rate on the refractory period of the atrium and the A-V conducting system. *Am Heart J* 1973;85:358.

116. Denes P, Wu D, Dhingra R, et al. The effects of cycle length on cardiac refractory periods in man. *Circulation* 1974;49:32.

117. Jurkiewicz NK, Sanguinetti MC. Rate-dependent prolongation of cardiac action potentials by a methane sulfonalide class III antiarrhythmic agent: specific block of rapidly activating delayed rectifier K+ current by dofetilide. *Circ Res* 1993;72:75.

118. Sanguinetti MC, Jurkiewicz NK. Two components of cardiac delayed rectifier K+ current: Differential sensitivity to block by class III antiarrhythmic agents. *J Gen Physiol* 1990;96:194.

119. Sanguinetti MC, Jurkiewicz NK. Delayed rectifier outward K+ current is composed of two currents in guinea pig atrial cells. *Am J Physiol* 1991;260:H393.

120. Hoffman BF, Paes de Carvalho A, De Mello WC. Transmembrane potentials of single fibres of the atrio-ventricular node. *Nature* 1958;181:66.

121. Hoffman BF, Paes de Carvalho A, De Mello WC, et al. Electrical activity of single fibers of the atrio-ventricular node. *Circ Res* 1959;7:11.

122. Jalife J. The sucrose gap preparation as a model of AV nodal transmission: are dual pathways necessary for reciprocation or AV nodal echoes? *Pacing Clin Electrophysiol* 1983;6:1106.

123. Simson MB, Spear JF, Moore EN. Electrophysiologic studies on atrioventricular nodal Wenckebach cycles. *Am J Cardiol* 1978;41:244.

124. Josephson ME (Ed.). Electrophysiologic investigation: general concepts. In: *Clinical cardiac electrophysiology: techniques and interpretations*. Philadelphia: Lea & Febiger, 1993:28.

125. Sherf L. The atrial conduction system: clinical implications. *Am J Cardiol* 1976;37:814.

126. Schuilenburg RM, Durrer D. Conduction disturbances located within the His bundle. *Circulation* 1972;45:612.

127. Josephson ME (Ed.). Atrial flutter and fibrillation. In: *Clinical cardiac electrophysiology: techniques and interpretations*. Philadelphia: Lea & Febiger, 1993.

128. Akhtar M, Caracta AR, Lau SH, et al. Demonstration of intra-atrial conduction delay, block, gap and reentry: a report of two cases. *Circulation* 1978;58:947.

129. Akhtar M, Damato AN, Batsford WP, et al. A comparative analysis of antegrade and retrograde conduction patterns in man. *Circulation* 1975;52:766.

130. Allessie MA, Bonke FI, Schopman FJ. Circus movement in rabbit atrial muscle as a mechanism of tachycardia. *Circ Res* 1973;33:54.

131. Allessie MA, Bonke FI, Schopman FJ. Circus movement in rabbit atrial muscle as a mechanism of tachycardia. II. The role of nonuniform recovery of excitability in the occurrence of unidirectional block, as studied with multiple microelectrodes. *Circ Res* 1976;39:168.

132. Allessie MA, Bonke FI, Schopman FJ. Circus movement in rabbit atrial muscle as a mechanism of tachycardia. III. The "leading circle" concept: a new model of circus movement in cardiac tissue without the involvement of an anatomical obstacle. *Circ Res* 1977;41:9.

133. Allessie MA, Lammers WJ, Bonke IM, et al. Intra-atrial reentry as a mechanism for atrial flutter induced by acetylcholine and rapid pacing in the dog. *Circulation* 1984;70:123.

134. Boineau JP, Schuessler RB, Mooney CR, et al. Natural and evoked atrial flutter due to circus movement in dogs. *Am J Cardiol* 1980;45:1167.

135. Bennett MA, Pentecost BL. The pattern of onset and spontaneous cessation of atrial fibrillation in man. *Circulation* 1970;41:981.

136. Frame LH, Page RL, Hoffman BF. Atrial reentry around an anatomic barrier with a partially refractory excitable gap: a canine model of atrial flutter. *Circ Res* 1986;58:495.

137. Haft JI, Lau SH, Stein E, et al. Atrial fibrillation produced by atrial stimulation. *Circulation* 1968;37:70.

138. Killip T, Gault JH. Mode of onset of atrial fibrillation in man. *Am Heart J* 1965;70:172.

139. Buxton AE, Marchlinski FE, Miller JM, et al. The human atrial strength-interval relationship: influence of cycle length and procainamide. *Circulation* 1989;79:271.

140. Akhtar M, Gilbert CJ, Wolf FG, et al. Retrograde conduction in the His-Purkinje system. Analysis of the routes of impulse propagation using His and right bundle branch recordings. *Circulation* 1979;59:1252.

141. Akhtar M. Retrograde conduction in man. *Pacing Clin Electrophysiol* 1981;4:548.

142. Akhtar M, Damato AN, Caracta AR, et al. The gap phenomena during retrograde conduction in man. *Circulation* 1974;49:811.

143. Akhtar M, Damato AN, Caracta AR, et al. The gap phenomenon during retrograde conduction in man. *Circulation* 1974;49:811.

144. Akhtar M, Damato AN, Ruskin JN, et al. Characteristics and coexistence of two forms of ventricular echo phenomena. *Am Heart J* 1976;92:174.

145. Akhtar M, Denker S, Lehmann MH, et al. Macro-reentry within the His-Purkinje system. *Pacing Clin Electrophysiol* 1983;6:1010.

146. Akhtar M, Damato AN, Batsford WP, et al. Demonstration of re-entry within the His-Purkinje system in man. *Circulation* 1974;50:1150.

147. Farshidi A, Michelson EL, Greenspan AM, et al. Repetitive responses to ventricular extrastimuli: incidence, mechanism, and significance. *Am Heart J* 1980;100:59.

148. Roy D, Brugada P, Bar FWHM, et al. Repetitive responses to ventricular extrastimuli: incidence and significance in patients without organic heart disease. *Eur Heart J* 1983;4:79.

149. Sung RJ, Waxman HL, Saksena S, et al. Sequence of retrograde atrial activation in patients with dual atrioventricular nodal pathways. *Circulation* 1981;64:1059.

150. Josephson ME (Ed.). Miscellaneous phenomena related to atrioventricular conduction. In: *Clinical cardiac electrophysiology: techniques and interpretations.* Philadelphia: Lea & Febiger, 1993.

151. Knoebel SB, Fisch C. Concealed conduction. *Cardiovasc Clin* 1973;5:21.

152. Moore EN, Knoebel SB, Spear JF. Concealed conduction. *Am J Cardiol* 1971;28:406.

153. Agha AS, Castellanos A, Wells D, et al. Type II and type III gaps in bundle branch conduction. *Circulation* 1973;47:325.

154. Agha AS, Castellanos A Jr, Wells D, et al. Type I, type II, and type 3 gaps in bundle-branch conduction. *Circulation* 1973;47:325.

155. Akhtar M, Damato AN, Batsford WP, et al. Unmasking and conversion of gap phenomenon in the human heart. *Circulation* 1974;49:624.

156. Damato AN, Akhtar M, Ruskin J, et al. Gap phenomena: antegrade and retrograde. In: Wellens HJJ, Lie KI, Janse MJ, eds. *The conduction system of the heart: structure, function and clinical implications.* Philadelphia: Lea & Febiger, 1976.

157. Moe GK, Mendez C, Han J. Aberrant A-V impulse propagation in the dog heart: a study of functional bundle branch block. *Circ Res* 1965;16:261.

158. Wu D, Denes P, Dhingra R, et al. Nature of the gap phenomenon in man. *Circ Res* 1974;34:682.

159. Childers RW. Supernormality. *Cardiovasc Clin* 1973;5:135.

160. Pick A, Langendorf R, Katz LN. The supernormal phase of atrioventricular conduction. *Circulation* 1962;26:322.

161. Gallagher JJ, Damato AN, Caracta AR, et al. Gap in A-V conduction in man; types I and II. Am Heart J 1973;85:78.

162. Gallagher JJ, Damato AN, Varghese PJ, et al. Alternative mechanisms of apparent supernormal atrioventricular conduction. *Am J Cardiol* 1973;31:362.

163. Moe GK, Childers RW, Merideth J. An appraisal of "supernormal" A-V conduction. *Circulation* 1968;38:5.

164. Greenspan AM, Camardo JS, Horowitz LN, et al. Human ventricular refractoriness: effects of increasing current. *Am J Cardiol* 1981;47:244.

165. Sung RJ, Juma Z, Saksena S. Electrophysiologic properties and antiarrhythmic mechanisms of intravenous *N*-acetylprocainamide in patients with ventricular dysrhythmias. *Am Heart J* 1983;105:811.

166. Sung RJ, Myerburg RJ, Castellanos A. Electrophysiological demonstration of concealed conduction in the human atrium. *Circulation* 1978;58:940.

167. Nguyen NX, Yang PT, Huycke EC, et al. Effects of beta-adrenergic stimulation on atrial latency and atrial vulnerability in patients with paroxysmal supraventricular tachycardia. *Am J Cardiol* 1988;61:1031.

2

BASIC ELECTROPHYSIOLOGY: GENERATION OF THE CARDIAC ACTION POTENTIAL

AUGUSTUS O. GRANT
MICHAEL CARBONI

The action potential (AP) describes the time course of membrane voltage during the cardiac cycle. It plays a central role in the normal function of the heart. The myogenic origin of the heartbeat is established and reflects the first important function of the AP, autorhythmicity. Normal cardiac function requires the ordered coordinate contraction of the cell in each region of the heart. The myocardial cells contract in a cephalad to caudal direction in the atria and from apex to base in the ventricles. Competence of the AV valves requires the appropriately timed contraction of the papillary muscles. The AP is the signal between cells that coordinates the contraction. In contrast to nerve and skeletal muscle, in which the AP last tens of milliseconds, the cardiac AP last hundreds of milliseconds. Emptying of the cardiac chambers is effected by sustained contractions. The control of the AP must be sufficiently dynamic that excitability and contractility can respond to changes in cycle length on a beat to beat basis. This chapter provides a description of the prototype AP in a ventricular cell and an analysis of variations within and between the various chambers. This is followed by a critical analysis of the membrane ion channels that play major roles in the generation of the various phases of the AP.

GENERATION OF THE ACTION POTENTIAL

Ventricular Myocyte Action Potential

The AP recorded from a normal ventricular myocyte has five phases, 0 through 4 (1) (Fig. 2-1). Phase 0 defines the period of rapid depolarization during which the membrane potential moves from its resting value of approximately −90 mV to +40 mV. It is the result of an increase membrane per-

meability to sodium ions (Na⁺), leading to a rapid influx of Na⁺. As depolarization increases the opening kinetics of the Na channels, the process is regenerative. The rate of depolarization of the membrane during phase 0, dV/dt_{max}, is an indirect measure of the current carried by Na⁺ (2).

Three processes contribute to the transition from phase 0 to the early period of repolarization called phase 1:

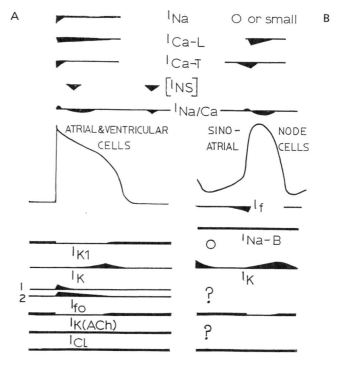

FIGURE 2-1. Cardiac action potential (AP) and underlying membrane currents. **A:** The AP and currents underlying the ventricular AP. **B:** The AP and currents underlying the sinoatrial node AP. Inward currents are shown above and outward currents below the panels.

A. O. Grant and M. Carboni: Departments of Medicine and Pediatrics, Duke University Medical Center, Durham, North Carolina 27710.

1. Depolarization moves the membrane potential close to the reversal potential for Na⁺. The decrease in the driving force for Na⁺ movement reduces I_{Na}.
2. Inactivation of the Na channels reduces their permeability to zero. The membrane must undergo repolarization before Na⁺ channels revert to a state in which they can undergo a further increase in conductance.
3. Activation of transient outward potassium ion (K⁺) current.

The amplitude of the outward current during phase 1 sets the voltage of the plateau phase (3) of the AP. A large outward current results in a plateau voltage in the negative range of membrane potential. The resulting AP has a "spike and dome configuration," as is seen in epicardial myocytes. With a small outward current, the plateau voltage is in the positive range of membrane potential. AP with small transient outward current has a square AP configuration, as is seen in guinea pig ventricular myocytes. Because the level of the plateau voltage sets the amplitude of the delayed rectifier K⁺ currents that are critical determinants of phases 2 and 3, the phase 1 outward currents are important determinants of AP shape. The marked regional and species variations in the phase 1 outward currents play important roles in the variation of AP configuration (Fig. 2-2). Multiple K⁺ channels contribute to phase 1 in each region of the heart and in various species. The major phase 1 outward current is the transient outward K-selective current, I_{to1}, which is analogous to the neuronal A-type current. A calcium (Ca²⁺)-activated outward current, I_{to2}, also contributes to phase 1. Ventricular myocytes have a c-AMP activated chloride (Cl⁻) current. It reverses potential at −45 to −65 mV and contributes to AP phase 1 current during sympathetic stimulation.

Phase 2, or the plateau, is the longest phase of the cardiac AP. The small net membrane current is the result of a delicate balance between inward and outward currents. The high membrane resistance during phase 2 means that small currents can result in large changes in membrane potential. This permits an energetically efficient basis for regulation of the AP duration. The L-type Ca current and a late component of Na current are the major sources of depolarizing current. At least four subtypes of K current contribute outward current during the plateau. Ultra-rapid, rapid, and slow components of delayed rectifier K⁺ current (I_{ur}, I_{Kr}, I_{Ks}) have been identified during phase 2. They were identified based on their kinetics and sensitivity to block by specific drugs. Molecular genetic studies have defined the molecular basis of at least two components of the delayed rectifier (I_{Kr} and I_{Ks}). A sustained outward K⁺ current, I_{Kp}, that is distinct from the delayed rectifiers has been identified in the plateau range of membrane potential in the guinea pig AP.

Phase 3 is the rapid phase of terminal repolarization of the AP. Outward currents predominate during phase 3. In addition to the outward currents activated during phase 2, the inward rectifier potassium current, I_{K1}, also makes significant contributions to repolarization. The property of refractoriness defines the ability of an excited cell to respond to a second stimulus. Cardiac cells do not respond to a premature stimulus during phase 2 of the AP, regardless of the size of the stimulus. This period defines the absolute refractory period. Excitability recovers slowly during phase 3. Initially, the threshold stimulus strength far exceeds that during phase 4. There is a brief period in late phase 3 called the *supernormal period* in which the threshold stimulus strength is less than that in phase 4. Full recovery of excitability occurs early during phase 4. The requirements for excitability during phase 3 include the application of sufficient charge to shift the membrane trajectory from the repolarizing (outward) to the depolarizing (inward) direction. It is the charge ($\int idt$) that determines the effectiveness of the applied stimulus. However, brief stimuli of large amplitude are more effective than prolonged stimuli of low amplitude. In the case of the ventricular cell, a third of the Na current must recover from inactivation before a regenerative depolarization can be elicited. There is a time lag between membrane repolarization to a given potential and the recovery of the Na channels from inactivation at that potential. The relationship between available Na conductance and membrane potential during phase 3 is called the *membrane responsiveness curve*. Agents such as antiarrhythmic drugs that slow apparent recovery from inactivation prolong the effective refractory period (ERP) of cardiac muscle. The magnitude of the outward K currents is an important determinant of refractoriness during phase 3.

Phase 4 defines the resting or diastolic phase of membrane potential. In contractile atrial and ventricular cells, the resting membrane potential is maintained at a steady level of −85 to −90 mV, which is primarily determined by

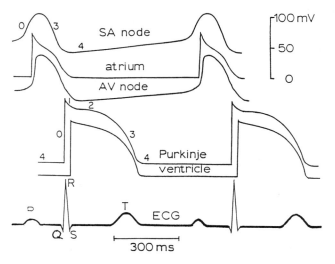

FIGURE 2-2. Variation of the action potential (AP) in various regions of the heart and the relation of AP timing to the surface electrocarediogram.

the ratio of internal to external K^+ concentrations and maintained by an influx of K^+ and outflux of Na^+ by means of an ATPase Na^+-K^+ pump. The cell membrane is primarily permeable to K^+ during this phase. The inward rectifier K channel dominates the resting membrane conductance. The resting membrane potential is slightly positive to the K equilibrium potential, E_K. The relationship between the external and internal K^+ concentrations ($[K^+]_o$ and $[K^+]_i$), and E_K is given by the Nernst equation:

$$E_K = RT/F \ln [K^+]_o/[K^+]_I$$

in which R is the gas constant, T is the absolute temperature, and F is the Faraday constant. Elevation of $[K^+]_o$ reduces E_K and the resting potential.

The AP acts as a current source for the propagation of information between neighboring cells. The neighboring cells that are connected by low resistance gap junctions function as current sinks. The effectiveness of the AP as a propagating signal depends on the size of the inward Na current during phase 0; large currents are effective stimuli for rapid conduction. The conduction velocity is proportional to the inverse square root of the internal resistance (Ω). The gap junctions are the sites of the low resistance connection between cardiac cells. Gap junction density is highest along the length of the cells and lower in the transverse direction . Conduction velocity is rapid in the direction of fiber orientation and slower in the transverse direction, which results in anisotropic conduction. Abnormalities of propagation during pathologic states such as myocardial ischemia are discussed in Chapter 3.

Sinoatrial and Atrioventricular Nodal Cells

Cells in the sinoatrial (SA) and atrioventricular (AV) nodes form the primary and subsidiary cardiac pacemakers. These cells have a very high input resistance (about $10^9 \Omega$). Small currents can result in substantial changes in membrane potential. SA and AV nodal cells have a maximum diastolic potential of approximately -60 mV during the early part of phase 4. The membrane potential undergoes spontaneous slow diastolic depolarization of 0.02 to 0.1 V/sec during the remainder of phase 4. This slow spontaneous diastolic depolarization is the hallmark of the AP in pacemaker cells. Multiple membrane ion channels and electrogenic transporters contribute to phase 4 depolarization:

1. Delayed rectifier K current activated during the preceding AP: time-dependent outward I
2. Background Na current I_B: time-independent inward I
3. Hyperpolarization activated current, I_f: time-dependent inward I
4. L-type Ca^{2+} current: late-phase-4, time-dependent inward I

5. Electrogenic Na-Ca exchanger current (coupling ratio, r = 3 : 1)
6. Electrogenic Na-K pump current (coupling ratio, r = 3 : 2): outward I

The delayed rectifier K current activated during the preceding AP deactivates during early phase 4. Its hyperpolarizing influence is reduced and allows the depolarizing influence of the inward currents to cause progressive depolarization. The extent to which I_f contributes to pacemaker activity during phase 4 is uncertain. Pacemaker activity persists when I_f is blocked by external cesium (Cs^+). Large-scale mutagenesis in zebra fish yielded mutants with slow heart rates associated with defects in I_f. The L-type Ca^{2+} channel is activated in the last one third of phase 4 and accelerates membrane depolarization to threshold. The Na-Ca exchanger and the Na-K pump play relatively minor roles in cardiac pacemaking.

There is a smooth transition between the terminal portion of phase 4 and phase 0 of the pacemaker AP. The L- and T-type Ca^{2+} channels are the major charge carriers during phase 0. The membrane current density during phase 0 of the nodal AP is substantially lower than that in atrial, ventricular, and Purkinje cells. The lowest AP propagation rates in the heart (0.1 to 0.2 m/sec) are observed in the SA and AV nodes. The central role of the L-type calcium channels makes conduction over the SA and AV nodes especially susceptible to calcium channel blocking drugs. Repolarization is effected by inactivation of the calcium currents and activation of outward K^+ currents.

The effective discharge rate of pacemaker cells is modulated by the three AP parameters: the maximum diastolic potential, the slow diastolic depolarization during phase 4, and the threshold potential. Drugs and the autonomic neurotransmitters may alter one or more of the AP parameters.

The neurohormonal regulation of heart rate is the result of neurotransmitter action on the sinus node pacemaker cells. Vagal stimulation releases acetylcholine from postganglionic parasympathetic nerve terminals. Acetylcholine activates the muscarinic M_2 receptor, initiating a series of events that slow the heart rate. Sympathetic stimulation releases norepinephrine and epinephrine. These sympathetic neurotransmitters increase the rate of sinus node pacemaker discharge. Much controversy surrounds the mechanisms involved in these autonomic responses. The analysis of the responses is complicated by the observation that vagal stimulation activates a different subset of receptors compared with application of acetylcholine (4). Differences have also been suggested between sympathetic stimulation and application of norepinephrine and epinephrine. The sequence of events after receptor activation appears to be similar for the parasympathetic and sympathetic neurotransmitters. Agonist binding activates a guanine nucleotide–binding, heterotrimeric (e.g., alpha, beta, gamma) G protein. The released G protein subunits, G_α and $G_{\beta\gamma}$, may then act as direct effectors through a membrane-delineated pathway. Alternatively, they may act as stimulators or inhibitors of enzymes, including adenylyl cyclase (AC), guanine 3′,5′-cyclic monophosphate phosphodiesterase (cGMP-PDE), and phospholipase C. These enzymes then interact with ion channel proteins to produce an effect of heart rate or conduction.

The initial effect of vagal stimulation is a reduction in the slope of phase 4 depolarization, with little change in the AP characteristics. Strong vagal stimulation or the application of acetylcholine also causes hyperpolarization of the maximum diastolic potential and abbreviation of the AP. Because of the relationships among all the currents that contribute to the AP in pacemaker cells, the current resulting from one channel alters the AP and the contribution of all the other membrane channels (5). The following changes in ionic current have been identified as consequences of parasympathetic stimulation:

1. Reduction of the background current I_b, identified even at low levels of vagal stimulation
2. Activation of an inward rectifying K channel, I_{KACh} (This is the best-studied response to vagal stimulation. Direct [$G_{I\alpha}$ or $G_{I\beta\gamma}$] and indirect pathways [phospholipase C] may be involved in the channel activation. Activation of I_{KACh} abbreviates the AP duration [APD] and increases the maximum diastolic potential.)
3. Reduction of I_{Ca} as a result of inhibition of adenylyl cyclase

Computer modeling is the best strategy to analyze the potential contribution of each of these factors to the slowing of pacemaker rate.

Sympathetic stimulation increases the slope of diastolic depolarization but does not increase the amplitude of the pacemaker AP. Multiple ionic currents are affected. The activation kinetics of the hyperpolarization-activated current, I_f, is shifted to more positive potentials. The magnitude of the inward Ca current is increased. Both current changes can contribute to the increase of phase 4 diastolic slope.

The characteristics of the AP are not uniform across the SA node. Cells in the center of the node have the lowest maximum diastolic potential and the steepest phase 4 slope. Toward the atrial margins of the node, the maximum diastolic potential increases, the phase 4 slope decreases, and the phase 0 slope increases. The fast Na current contributes to phase 4 in the cell at the SA node–crista terminalis junction. There is a difference in sensitivity of the pacemaker cells to parasympathetic and sympathetic stimulation. Increase in activity of either system is accompanied by a shift in the site of origin of the earliest pacemaker activity.

Anatomic-electrophysiologic correlative studies show that there are no discrete AV nodal cells with distinct characteristics. At the atrial margins of the node, there is a gradual transition of AP characteristics from the true atrial cells to the cells at the middle of the node. Similarly, there is a gradual transition of AP characteristics distally from the AV node to the proximal His bundle. For descriptive purposes, the AV junctional region is described as consisting of AN, N, and NH regions (6). The site of greatest conduction delay occurs in the N region. The cells in the N region have a low maximum diastolic potential. Phase 4 depolarization is present. The ionic basis of this depolarization has not been analyzed in as much detail as the SA nodal AP. The slope of phase 0 is slow and, in multicellular preparations, may show one or more notches. This is consistent with the contribution of Na and Ca channels to phase 0. Electrotonic interactions may also contribute to the notches. Reversal of the membrane potential at the peak of phase 0 is minimal or absent, and the peak of the AP is rounded, with no discrete phase 1.

Atrial Myocyte

Typical atrial myocytes have a stable membrane potential of −80 to −90 mV during phase 4. The rate of depolarization during phase 0 is about 100 V/sec, somewhat less than that observed in the ventricle. Phase 1 is well developed, reducing the membrane potential below 0 mV. The phase 2 plateau is usually not prominent and passes almost imperceptibly into phase 3. Terminal phase 3 repolarization is usually more prolonged than in ventricular myocytes. Overall, AP duration is 100 to 200 ms. There is some regional variation in AP characteristics within the atrium. Fibers around and within the AV valve have AP characteristics reminiscent of the SA node AP with phase 4 depolarization.

His-Purkinje System

The resting potential of cells in the His-Purkinje system is usually a few millivolts more negative than that observed in ventricular myocytes. The upstroke velocity during phase 0 is in the range of 500 to 1,000 V/sec and is the fastest recorded in the heart. The large dV/dt$_{max}$ is the result of a high density of Na channels. The high dV/dt$_{max}$ and large fiber diameter are responsible for the rapid conduction of the AP in the His-Purkinje system. A prominent phase 1 reduces the membrane potential below zero during phase 2. There is typically a secondary depolarization during phase 2, giving the AP a spike and dome characteristic. A maintained plateau phase is followed by rapid repolarization during phase 3. The APD of 300 to 500 msec is among the longest recorded in the heart. There is a gradation of APD along the His-Purkinje system such that the longest APD is recorded at the Purkinje-myocardial (PM) junction. The long APD at the PM junction is believed to form an electrical "gate," controlling the rate of excitation of the ventricle. The typical AP in a His-Purkinje cell shows minimal phase 4 depolarization. However, the slope of phase 4 can be readily increased by reduction of $[K^+]_o$, epinephrine, stretch, or membrane depolarization.

Transmural Variation of the Action Potential in the Ventricle and Atrium

Studies by Antzelovitch and colleagues documented important differences in the characteristics of the AP recorded from the epicardium, mid-myocardium, and endocardial regions of the ventricle (7) (Fig. 2-3). Transmural variations in AP characteristics have also been documented in the atria. Epicardial myocytes have a prominent phase 1 and a spike and dome AP configuration. Phase 1 is also prominent in the mid-myocardial (M) cells. The APD is much longer in M cells, particularly at slow heart rates or during exposure to class III drugs. Phase 1 is not very prominent in endocardial myocytes, and the APD is brief. These differences in APD characteristics are primarily the result of a graded density of I_{to1} across the myocardial wall. I_{to1} is well developed in epicardial myocytes, is less prominent in M cells, and may be absent in endocardial myocytes.

A variable distribution of the slow component of the delayed rectifier K current across the myocardial wall is also present, with the M cells having the lowest density. The differences in AP configuration and underlying current density in the epicardial, M, and endocardial myocytes may result in transmural differences in the response to neurotransmitters and drugs. A reduction in the I_{Na}, such as by drug blockade or an increase in the rate of inactivation, or an increase in I_{to1} shifts the membrane domain IV relationship in the outward direction. This may result in all-or-none repolarization and marked abbreviation of the AP. The differences in AP shape and duration result in significant transmural potential gradients during phases 2 and 3 of the AP and account for many electrocardiographic (ECG) abnormalities in pathologic states. Some of the consequences of the AP differences and their relationship to the ECG are summarized in Table 2-1. The role of the AP differences in the genesis of arrhythmias in the long QT and Brugada syndromes are discussed in Chapter 3.

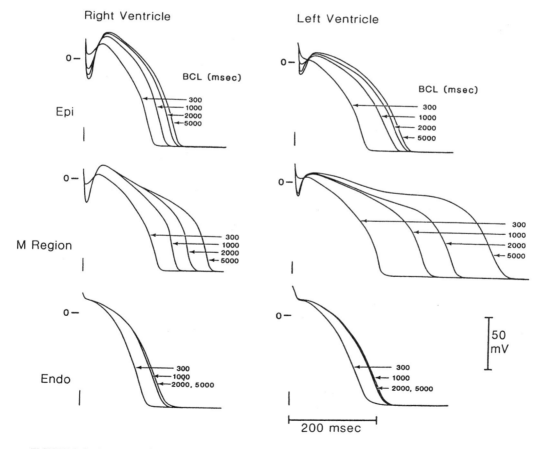

FIGURE 2-3. Transmural variation of the action potential (AP) characteristics in the right and left ventricles. The AP is recorded from the epicardium, mid-myocardium, and endocardium as a function of cycle length.

TABLE 2-1. CONSEQUENCES OF THE DIFFERENCES IN ACTION POTENTIAL CONFIGURATION AND UNDERLYING CURRENTS BETWEEN ENDOCARDIAL AND EPICARDIAL MYOCYTES

J wave, particularly during hypothermia
Differential sensitivity to ischemia
Differential sensitivity to neurotransmitters and drugs
   Isoproterenol and acetylcholine
   I_{TO} I_{CaL} I_{Na} I_K blockers
Rate dependence of the action potential duration more
   prominent in the epicardium
Epicardium more sensitive to $[K^+]_o$
Supernormal conduction observed in epicardial but not in
   endocardium

MEMBRANE CURRENT UNDERLYING THE CARDIAC ACTION POTENTIAL

Sodium Current

Membrane ion channels are integral membrane proteins that reduce the energy barrier for ion movement between the extracellular and intracellular fluid compartments. The fundamental properties of ion conduction and gating describe the behavior of the Na channel. Ion conduction or permeability is the process by which Na^+ crosses the lipid bilayer. Gating describes the opening and closing transitions of the channel. A quantitative analysis of the properties of the Na channel was first performed in nerves (8). The geometric complexity of naturally occurring cardiac preparations prevented a similar analysis in the heart for more than 25 years. However, the preparation of Ca-tolerant enzyme-dissociated single myocytes and the development of the patch clamp technique permitted a similar analysis in cardiac myocytes (9,10,11). Similar ion conduction and gating are observed in the cardiac and neuronal Na channels. The cloning and functional expression of the cardiac, neuronal, and skeletal muscle Na channel indicated that structure and function is relatively conserved among tissues and species.

Permeability of the Na channel for Na^+ exceeds that of other alkali metal cations such as K^+ and Cs^+ by a ratio of 25 : 1 or more. The transit rate for Na^+ exceeds 10^8 ions/sec. Na channels are blocked by divalent cations such as Ca^{2+}, Cd^{2+}, and Zn^{2+}. Sensitivity is greatest to the transition metal cation Cd^{2+} that has a K_d of 270 μM (12). Several studies have suggested that the Na^+ channel can be converted to a channel primarily permeable to Ca^{2+} by treatment with atrial natruretic peptide or β-adrenergic stimulation (13,14). However, none of these studies has been confirmed. The specific requirement for Na^+ versus Ca^{2+} permeability of membrane ion channel makes any such interconversion unlikely (15,16,17).

At the normal resting membrane potential of about −90 mV, Na channels are closed. They markedly increase their permeability in response to membrane depolarization. Even if the depolarization is maintained, the channels close. Closure at depolarized potential changes the channel to a refractory or inactivated state. To undergo another cycle of increased permeability, repolarization must occur. About 50 years ago, Hodgkin and Huxley proposed a physical model for the gating processes that result in the transient permeability increase of the Na channel. They proposed that Na channels exist in three states: closed, open, and inactivated:

$$\text{Closed} \rightleftharpoons \text{Open} \rightleftharpoons \text{Inactivated}$$

Channel state is determined by the relative position of activation (*m*) and inactivation (*h*) particles or gates in the membrane. To account for the lag in the rise in conductance, they proposed the presence of at least three *m* particles. In the resting state, *m* particles are in a nonconducting location, and *h* particles are in a conducting locus. During early depolarization, the *m* particles move outward and the channel assumes a conducting configuration. However, this is soon followed by movement of the *h* particle to a nonconducting configuration. Strong support for the physical model was provided by Armstrong and Bezanillia who measured small "gating currents" that precede the ionic current and reflect the movement of the gating particles (18). The structural studies discussed later have identified highly charged regions of the protein that are the likely source of the gating current.

The basic Hodgkin-Huxley model has proved enduring. However certain features of the model have had to be modified in the light of later studies. Hodgkin and Huxley proposed that both activation and inactivation were voltage dependent, but the processes were independent of each other. Subsequent studies have shown that activation and inactivation are coupled processes (3,19,20). Inactivation of closed channels is slow and voltage dependent. Inactivation of open channels is very rapid and relatively voltage independent.

Na channel function can be related to structure. Before reviewing the structural basis for ion conduction, the overall structure of the Na channel is reviewed (Fig. 2-4). The channel consists of a large α subunit and two auxiliary β subunits. Ion permeation and gating resides in the β subunit. The three-dimensional structure of ion channels has only been resolved for the K channel of *Streptomyces lividans* (21). However, the membrane organization of other membrane proteins such as the Na^+ channel β subunit can be inferred from hydropathy plot of the constituent amino acids. The α subunit is made up of four homologous domains, DI through DIV. The amino and carboxyl termini and the interdomain loops are intracellular. Each domain consists of six transmembrane segments, S1 through S6. The fourth transmembrane segment (S4) has a positively charged amino acid at every third or fourth posi-

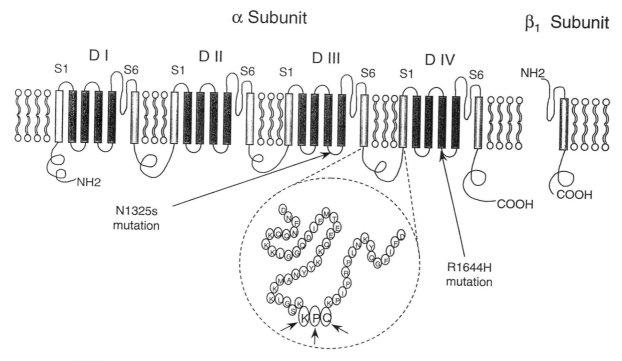

FIGURE 2-4. Structural organization of the β₁ and α subunits of the cardiac sodium (Na) channel. The transmembrane organization of the Na channel has been inferred from the constituent amino acids. DI through DIV are the four homologous domains, each containing six membrane-spanning segments (S1 through S6). Mutations associated with long QT syndrome (e.g., *LQT3*) have been highlighted.

tion. S4 acts as the voltage sensor that responds to activating transmembrane voltages. The loops between the transmembrane segments alternate between the intracellular and extracellular sides of the membrane. The extracellular loop between the fifth and sixth transmembrane segments dips deeply into the membrane and forms the ion channel pore or P loop. The sequence of ten amino acids in the P loops of DI through DIV are summarized in Figure 2-5. In each P loop, an amino acid triplet forms the critical selectivity filter residues. In DI through DIII, the middle residue has a free carboxyl group. The oxygen atom of the carboxyl group coordinates with Na^+, stripping it of its water at hydration as it crosses the membrane. The structure of the Ca channel selectivity filter is similar, with the exception that all four domains contribute glutamate residues (E) to the critical selectivity region. In the cardiac Na channel isoform, the third selectivity filter residue of DI, cysteine, confers Cd^{2+} sensitivity and tetrodotoxin (TTX) resistances. Mutation of this residue to tyrosine or phenylalanine converts the channel to a TTX-sensitive, Cd^{2+}-resistant subtype.

The loop between the third and fourth Na channel domains, $ID_{III/IV}$, is highly conserved between Na channel isoforms. Antibodies directed against epitopes in this region slow inactivation (22). Chain interruption in the middle of this region yields channels that fail to inactivate (23). A series of 10-amino deletions narrowed the location of the residues critical to inactivation (24). Mutation of a three–amino acid sequence in one segment of IFM to QQQ produced Na channels that fail to inactivate (25). West and colleagues proposed a hinged-lid model of channel inactivation in which the $ID_{III/IV}$ loop swings into the inner vestibule of the channel to effect inactivation (25). The hydrophobic IFM triplet acts as the latch for the hinged-lid mechanism. Actual movement of the inactivation gate has been tentatively identified by the technique of cysteine scanning. Accessibility of the cysteinyl residue in the mutant ICM to modification is reduced when the channel inactivates (26). Cytoplasmic regions of DIII and DIV act as the "docking site" for the $ID_{III/IV}$ linker during the process of inactivation. Inactivation depends on a precise channel structure. Naturally occurring mutation over a widespread area of the channel protein disrupts inactivation and is responsible for cardiac arrhythmias in the long QT syndrome (LQT3, now designated as SCN5A).

Auxiliary β-Subunit Modulation

In contrast to brain, the β₁ subunit is the only auxiliary Na channel subunit expressed in heart. The β₁ subunit in heart,

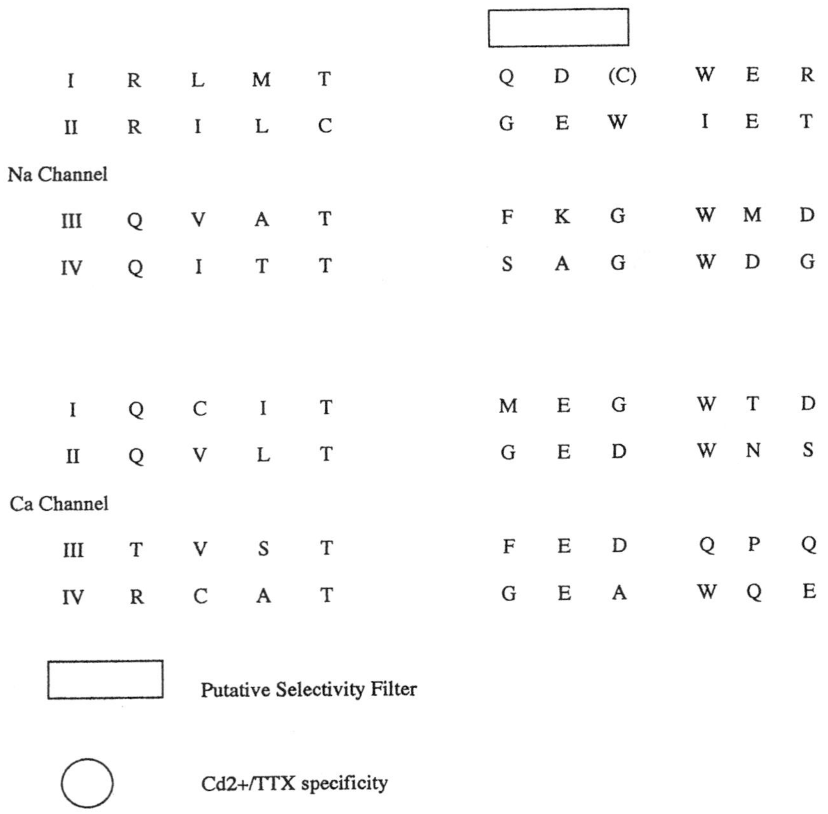

						☐				
I	R	L	M	T		Q	D	(C)	W	E	R
II	R	I	L	C		G	E	W	I	E	T

Na Channel

III	Q	V	A	T		F	K	G	W	M	D
IV	Q	I	T	T		S	A	G	W	D	G

I	Q	C	I	T		M	E	G	W	T	D
II	Q	V	L	T		G	E	D	W	N	S

Ca Channel

III	T	V	S	T		F	E	D	Q	P	Q
IV	R	C	A	T		G	E	A	W	Q	E

☐ Putative Selectivity Filter

◯ Cd2+/TTX specificity

FIGURE 2-5. The amino acids, designated by standard codes, are associated with the pore of the sodium and calcium channels. The rectangle identifies the selectivity filter. The cysteine bracketed in Na channel domain 1 confers tetrodotoxin resistance and cadmium sensitivity.

brain, and skeletal muscle is encoded by a single gene. The β_1 subunit consists of a small cytoplasmic domain, a single transmembrane segment, and a large extracellular amino terminus with multiple *N*-linked glycosylation sites and immunoglobulin-like folds. The β_1-subunit coexpression influences channel density and gating. Current density is increased. In oocytes, β-subunit coexpression has no effect or shifts the inactivation curve in a hyperpolarization direction (27). In HEK-293 cells, shifts in a depolarizing direction have been reported (28). The basis for the differences in the oocyte and mammalian expression system is uncertain. One possibility is that other proteins are involved in the α-β_1-subunit interaction and that these are differentially expressed in oocytes and mammalian cells. Use dependence for lidocaine in oocytes is attenuated by β-subunit coexpression (29).

Site-directed mutagenesis and spontaneous mutations have provided clues to the sites of α-β_1-subunit interactions. Deletion of the carboxyl terminus of the β_1 subunit results in loss of function (i.e., oocyte expression system). However, the mutation of the β_1-subunit carboxyl terminus eliminates the β_1-subunit–induced shift in inactivation in HEK-293 cells. Studies in oocytes suggest that the amino terminus interacts with the S5-S6 loop of domains I and IV.

Sodium Channel Regulation by Second Messengers

Na channel function is modulated through direct and indirect mechanisms by adrenergic stimulation. Modulation of channel development, level of expression, gating, and ion conduction has been reported with β-adrenergic stimulation. Na currents recorded from neonatal myocytes have reduced density and slow macroscopic inactivation. Coculture with sympathetic neurons or membrane-permeable cAMP analogues increases channel density and promotes adult phenotype gating (30). A similar developmental change has been described with AT1 cells (31). Despite extensive studies, the effects of β-adrenergic stimulation on current density, gating, and conductance remain controversial. Most upstroke velocity determinations in multicellular preparations show a reduction in dV/dt_{max} at depolarized membrane potentials (32,33). This finding is supported by Na current measurements in single myocytes (34,35,36). At hyperpolarized potentials, an increase in current density has been reported (37). The disparate results can be reconciled by a hyperpolarizing shift in the steady-state inactivation curve and an increase in maximum conductance (37,38). A few studies stand alone in showing no shift in gating and an increase in conductance.

Calcium Channels

Two classes of calcium channels, L- and T-type channels, are expressed in the heart (39). The two types are selectively permeable to Ca^{2+} but are the products of distinct genes. The L-type Ca channel is activated at low membrane potentials (about −50 mV) and undergoes relatively slow voltage and $[Ca_i^{2+}]$-dependent inactivation. The T-type channel inactivates at relatively high membrane potentials and undergoes more rapid inactivation. The two types of Ca channels also differ in their susceptibility to drugs. They appear to fulfill different roles. The L-type channel is primarily expressed in contractile myocytes of the atrium and ventricle and are a source of Ca^{2+} to trigger sarcoplasmic reticulum release and fill its stores. The T-type channel is expressed primarily in conduction system myocytes but may be upregulated in ventricular myocytes during development and hypertrophy. In conduction system myocytes, the T-type Ca channels may play a role in pacemaker activity. The properties of the two of Ca channels are compared in Table 2-2.

Regulation of the amplitude of the Ca channel is an important mechanism for varying cardiac inotropy. The β-adrenergic receptor stimulation activates adenylyl cyclase and a cAMP-dependent protein kinase that phosphorylates the Ca channel. Multiple mechanisms contribute to the changes in I_{Ca} during β-adrenergic stimulation. The voltage dependence of activation and inactivation is shifted to more negative potentials. Single-channel conductance is unchanged, but mean open time is increased, and the fraction of depolarization *without* channel openings (nulls) is reduced. Interactions with other G-protein receptor pathways occur at the level of adenylyl cyclase or cGMP-inhibited phosphodiesterase. Acetylcholine has no direct effect on I_{Ca}. However, activation of G_i by acetylcholine inhibits adenylyl cyclase and β-adrenergic–stimulated I_{Ca}. Nitric oxide stimulates cGMP production and can reduce stimulated I_{Ca} by inhibition of adenylyl cyclase. Physiologic increases in heart rate result in a positive I_{Ca} staircase. This increase in I_{Ca} depends on $[Ca^{2+}]_i$ and is mediated by CAMK II-dependent phosphorylation. Facilitation of I_{Ca} also occurs in response to marked membrane depolarization. This facilitation is apparently mediated by cAMP dependent protein kinase.

Calcium channels are multisubunit complexes consisting of α_{IC}, $\alpha_2\delta$, and β subunits. The α_{IC} is sufficient to form the ion conducting pore and to bind dihydropyridine. The α_{IC} subunit has been cloned from a cardiac cDNA library. It is structurally homologous to the Na channel β subunit, consisting of four homologous domains each containing six membrane-spanning segments. The major structural difference between voltage-gated cardiac Na and Ca channels is in the region of their selectivity filter. Glutamate residues on the ascending limb of the P loop of all four repeats (I through IV) form the Ca binding site. The structural basis of Ca_i-dependent inactivation is believed to involve a site 3′ to DIV-S6. However, a precise location is yet to be defined.

The $\alpha_2\beta$ subunit is the product of a single gene, and δ is apparently a proteolytic fragment. The cardiac-specific isoform of $\alpha_2\beta$ is produced by alternative splicing. Coexpression of the $\alpha_2\beta$ with the α_{IC} subunit increases channel expression twofold and increases activation and inactivation rates. Dihydropyridine binding is increased almost fourfold.

Multiple Ca channel β subunits (β_1 through β_3) are expressed in the heart. However, β_2 is the major subunit. Coexpression of α_{IC} and β_2 result in a 10-fold increase in current and dihydropyridine binding. Phosphorylation of the β_2 subunit may also be responsible for the β-receptor–mediated increase in I_{Ca}.

Fewer data are available on the molecular basis of the T-type Ca channel. Two α_1 subunits have been cloned, and both are expressed in the heart. The T-channel α subunit has the same basic structure as that of the L-type channel: four homologous domains, each with six membrane-spanning segments. However, the sequence homology between the two types of subunits is low (<15%).

TABLE 2-2. COMPARISON OF CALCIUM CURRENTS IN CARDIAC MUSCLE

Characteristic	L Type	T Type
Activation voltage V_{fi} (mV)	−50	+5
Inactivation voltage V_{fi} (mV)	−30 to −20	−60
Inactivation kinetics	Slow	Fast
Single channel conductance (pS)	15–25	8
Blockers		
Organic	Dihydropyridines	Mebefridil
Inorganic	Cd^{2+}	Ni^{2+}
β-adrenergic stimulation	Marks increase	Neutral
Tissue distribution	Contractile myocytes	Conduction system myocytes
	Atrium, ventricle	Sinoatrial and atrioventricular nodes
		Purkinje cells

Potassium Channels

Diversity of cardiac ion channels is greatest among K channels (40). No fewer that 10 types of K channels have been identified in cardiac myocytes. They fall into two broad categories: voltage-gated channels and inward rectifier channels. Each group has specific functions in the control of the AP. All channel subgroups are highly selective for K over other monovalent cations. Figure 2-6 contrasts the kinetic properties of the voltage-gated K channels. The transient outward current (I_{to}) in Figure 2-6A activates rapidly to a peak and then undergoes rapid voltage-dependent inactivation. The kinetics of recovery from inactivation varies between species. Slow recovery from inactivation contributes to the loss of the spike and dome configuration of the AP as heart rate increases. I_{to} is blocked by 4-aminopyridine, quinidine, and flecainide. Three classes of delayed rectifier K channels, the ultrarapid (I_{ur}), rapid (I_{Kr}), and slow (I_{Ks}) are present in heart muscle. The current illustrated in Figure 2-6B is representative of the class. They undergo little inactivation during maintained depolarization and close by deactivation on repolarization. The rapid and slow delayed rectifiers have been well characterized and can be separated based on their susceptibility to organic and inorganic blockers (41) (Table 2-3).

The other major category of cardiac K channels are the inward rectifiers. These channels can carry substantial current at negative membrane potentials because of their high membrane density and conductance. However, they carry very little current at the depolarized potentials of the AP plateau because of inward rectification. Block by cytoplasmic magnesium ions (Mg^{2+}) and polyamines are responsible for the inward rectification. The inward rectifier I_{K1} maintains the resting membrane potential. It is present in all cardiac myocytes. I_{K1} is blocked by Ba^{2+} and Cs^+. The channel activated by acetylcholine, I_{ACh}, belongs to the class of inwardly rectifying K channels. It is present in atrial and conduction system myocytes such as the SA and AV nodes.

TABLE 2-3. COMPARISON OF THE PROPERTIES OF DELAYED RECTIFIER CURRENTS I_K AND I_{Ks}

Characteristic	I_{Kr}	I_{Ks}
Conductance (pS)	10	3
Current density (pA/pF)	1	12
Rectification	Inward	None
Activation curve $V_{1/2}$	−21	+16
β-adrenergic stimulation	Neutral	Increase
Blockers		
Organic	Dofetilide E4031 Azimilide	Azimilide
Inorganic	La^{3+}	

I_{KACh} is activated by $G_{βγ}$. The ATP-sensitive K channel, I_{KATP}, is a heteromeric complex consisting of an inwardly rectifying K^+ channel and an ATP-binding cassette, the sulfonylurea receptor, SUR1. I_{KATP} is blocked by glibenclamide and other sulfonylureas. It is activated by vasodilators such as nicorandil. The density of the I_{KATP} channel is among the highest in the heart.

Molecular Basis of the Wide Array of Cardiac Potassium Channels

The application of the techniques of molecular genetics and of whole-cell and single-channel recordings has shed considerable light on the molecular basis of the various K currents identified by classic electrophysiologic techniques. The analysis of the molecular basis of the long QT syndromes (LQTS) has served as a catalyst for defining the substrate of the various cardiac K^+ channels. Results of the human genome project will identify multiple signature ion channel sequences. The relationship between such clones of the native channel in cardiac muscle can be an informative exercise. Snyders outlined criteria for assigning cloned K^+ channels to the underlying endogenous currents (40). These include agreement in the biophysical properties of conductance, ion selectivity, and voltage-dependent kinetics; correspondence in pharmacologic susceptibility to known blockers; and localization by immunohistochemistry and *in situ* hybridization.

There are two corresponding subgroups of structures for voltage-gated and inward rectifying K channels. The voltage-gate K channels have a structure similar to one of the four domains of the voltage-gated Na channels. The α-subunit structure consists of six putative transmembrane segments (S1 through S6), with intracellular amino and carboxyl termini. S4 has a charged amino acid at every third position. The regular array of five to seven charges acts as the voltage sensor for gating. During activation, S4 moves outward as a part of the sequence of events that lead to channel opening. The loop between S5 and S6 curves back into the membrane

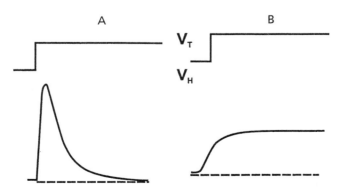

FIGURE 2-6. Characteristics of voltage-gated potassium (K) channels. **A:** Response of a transient K channel to step depolarization (e.g., I_{To1}). The current undergoes inactivation during the sustained pulse. **B:** Response of a delayed rectifier to depolarization. The current is sustained for the duration of the depolarizing pulse.

to form the pore, or P loop. The amino acid sequence GYG is the signature K-selective sequence found in a wide range of K channels. For the K channels that undergo rapid voltage-dependent inactivation, the amino terminus acts as a tethered ball that swings into position to occlude the cytoplasmic end of the channel pore. Four α subunits coassemble to form the functional channel. An early view that subunit coassembly is promiscuous, resulting in a wide array of heteromeric K channel complexes, is now known to be incorrect. There is a very limited range of coassembly between α-subunit subtypes. The subunit structure of the voltage-gated K channels is summarized in Figure 2-7.

The inward rectifier K channels have the simplest structure of the membrane ion channels. They are complexes of four subunits, each consisting of two membrane-spanning segments and an intervening P loop. They retain the GYG selectivity sequence characteristic of K⁺-selective ion channels. The crystal structure of a homologous channel, the membrane K channel of *S. lividans*, has been resolved to 3.2 angstroms (42). The analysis revealed a structure of four homologous subunits in the form of an inverted teepee. The selectivity filter is a narrow region about 12 by 6 angstroms. It is lined by the carbonyl oxygen atoms of the K channel selectivity filter signature sequence. The carbonyl atoms coordinate the K⁺ and stabilize it as it loses water or undergoes hydration during transition through the selectivity filter. The remainder of the channel pore is a large water-filled cavity lined by hydrophobic amino acids. Two ions occupy the pore, and their electrostatic repulsion promotes ion transit. Doyle and coworkers suggested that Na and Ca channel pore regions may have a similar structure (42).

Potassium Channel β Subunits

The single membrane-spanning protein, MinK (now designated KCNE1), was cloned from brain. When expressed in frog oocytes, MinK yielded a delayed rectifier K-selective channel. However, there was always the concern that a single membrane-spanning peptide of about 120 amino acids could form an ion-conducting channel. The analysis of a subgroup of patients with the congenital long QT syndrome helped to resolve the issue. The largest subgroup of LQTS patients had mutations in a putative K-channel protein KvLQT1 (now designated KCNQ1). However, when expressed in frog oocytes, KvLQT1 had kinetics that corresponded to no known native K channel. It was only when KvLQT1 was coexpressed with minK that channel current characteristic of the slow component of the delayed rectifier I_{Ks} was observed (43,44). The delayed activation characteristic of I_{Ks} was recapitulated by the KvLQT1-MinK complex, with MinK functioning as an auxiliary subunit to KvLQT1. The results with the isolated expression of MinK in oocytes can be reconciled with the fact that oocytes express an endogenous homologue of LQTS1.

Voltage Gated K⁺ Channels

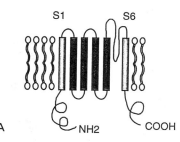

	Mammalian Classes	Native Currents
	KvΔ.x	I_{to}
	herg	I_{Kr}
	KvLQT1 + minK	I_{Ks}
	Kv1.x	I_{ur}

Inward Rectifier K⁺ Channels

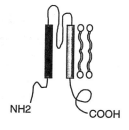

	Mammalian Classes	Native Currents
	$K_{ir}2.1$	I_{K1}
	$K_{ir}3.1 + K_{ir}3.4$	I_{ACh}
	$K_{ir}2.1$ + Sur1	I_{KATP}

FIGURE 2-7. Structure of cardiac potassium (K) channels. The structures of voltage-gated **(A)** and inward rectifier **(B)** K channels are shown. The middle column denotes the channel class, and the right column provides the native channels.

MinK is a member of a family of small K channel subunits. Four members of the family have been identified: KCNE1 through KCNE4. *KCNE1* encodes MinK. *KCNE2* encodes the MinK-related peptide MiRP1. It coassembles with HERG to reproduce the rapid component of the delayed rectifier I_{Kr}. The subunits exert multiple effects on the pore-forming α subunits (45). When coassembled with KvLQT1, MinK increases single-channel conductance and the rate of activation and deactivation. Coassembly of MiRP1 with HERG reduces single-channel conductance and slows the rate of channel deactivation. The effects of the auxiliary subunits is essential for normal function of I_{Ks} and I_{Kr} in the *in situ* heart. Mutations in the subunits are a cause for LQTS, including the Jervell-Lange-Neilsen syndrome. Mutations and polymorphisms in *KCNE1* and *KCNE2* predispose to drug-induced LQTS.

Hyperpolarization-Activated Action Channel

Conduction system myocytes express a cation channel with the unique property of activation on hyperpolarization. The half-potential for activation is about -100 mV. With $[K^+]$ of 5.4 mV, it reverses at about -30 mV, indicating mixed Na^+-K^+ selectivity. cAMP and cGMP shift the voltage dependence of activation in the depolarizing direction. The modulation does not involve channel phosphorylation as it persists in the presence of the nonspecific inhibitor, H-89. A channel, HAC1, that shares these characteristics has been cloned from brain and expression in the heart demonstrated by *in situ* hybridization (46). The channel belongs to the superfamily of voltage channels, with a six transmembrane segment–single pore subunit. The usual pattern of a charged amino acid in every third position of S4 is interrupted by a single serine in register. Despite the weak cation selectivity, the pore region has the K selectivity sequence, GYG. The cyclic nucleotide binding cassette is present in the carboxyl terminus.

Chloride Channels

Three distinct Cl^- channels have been detected in the heart: a cAMP-dependent current, a Ca-activated current, and a swelling-induced current (47). The cAMP-dependent Cl^- current is reduced by Cl^- removal and blocked by anthracene-9-carboxylic acid (A9C). Agents that inhibit adenylyl cyclase, such as acetylcholine, attenuate the isoproterenol-stimulated current. The cAMP-dependent Cl^- current is carried by a spliced variant of CFTR that lacks exon 5. Data supporting the presence of CFTR in the human heart are controversial. If present, it is likely to play only a minor role in the generation of the cardiac AP. Gating of the Ca-activated Cl^- current is correlated with the release of Ca^{2+} from the sarcoplasmic reticulum. It is abol-ished by drugs such as ryanodine and caffeine that interfere with the release of Ca from the sarcoplasmic reticulum or by the removal of external calcium.

The swelling-induced Cl^- current is activated by an increase in cell volume or by tyrosine phosphorylation. The current is time independent in the physiologic range of the membrane potential. The current is blocked by tamoxifen, A9C, and glibenclamide. The molecular identity of the current is unknown. The channel is widely distributed in the heart. The swelling-induced current plays little role in the generation of the AP in the basal state, but it may be important in states such as myocardial ischemia.

CARDIAC ACTION POTENTIAL IN DISEASE STATES

Arrhythmias may arise as primary disorders or as a complication of structural heart disease. Most arrhythmias arise from disturbances in the function of the ion channels that generate the normal AP. One subgroup of arrhythmias is the result of inherited defects of cardiac Na and K channels or the regulatory subunits. Other ion channel defects are acquired. The changes in the AP and the underlying membrane channels that occur in myocardial ischemia, cardiac hypertrophy, and atrial fibrillation are briefly reviewed.

Acute ischemia reduces the resting membrane potential, the maximum upstroke velocity of phase 0, and the AP duration. K^+ moves out of ischemic cardiac cells as a counter ion with lactate. The pH_i and pH_o values fall. The increase in $[K^+]_o$ and the fall in pH decrease the resting membrane potential. The reduced membrane potential inactivates the Na channels, and this results in a decrease in phase 0 depolarization rate. The is no evidence that elevated $[K^+]_o$ has a membrane potential–independent effect on the Na current (48). A reduction of [ATP] and an increase in the ADP : ATP ratio activate I_{KATP} and abbreviate the AP. I_{KATP} channels are present in abundance, and the activation of only a small fraction of the available channels can cause marked abbreviation of the APD.

The basis of the increased susceptibility to ventricular arrhythmias in cardiac hypertrophy and heart failure has been investigated extensively at the cellular level. The most consistent change in the AP is prolongation of the APD. Prolongation is the result of decreased expression of the transient outward K current I_{to}.

Sustained increases in heart rate such as in atrial fibrillation result in marked shortening of the ERP over a period of hours (49,50). The reduction of the ERP favors the persistence of atrial fibrillation. The ionic basis of the reduction of the ERP has been examined in human atrial specimens obtained at surgery and in rapid-pacing models of atrial fibrillation. In human atrial fibrillation, outward K current was reduced compared with control hearts. The reduction was surprising because it would be predicted to prolong the APD and the ERP. In the rapid-pacing model, I_{Ca} and I_{Na} were reduced; the major K currents were unchanged.

CONCLUSIONS

The AP is the signal for information transmission and initiation of contraction in cardiac cells. It is the result of an ordered sequence of changes in membrane permeability to specific ions. Most cardiac ion channels have been cloned and sequenced, and we are in the process of defining the molecular identity of the channels previously described by their biophysical and pharmacologic properties. Arrhythmias may arise from inherited defects of membrane ion channels. Acquired diseases may change membrane ion channel function by altering the milieu in which channels operate or reducing their number. Membrane ion channels are the targets for antiarrhythmic drugs, and their precise molecular definition should lead to more effective therapies.

REFERENCES

1. Hoffman BF, Cranefield PF. The atrium. In: *Electrophysiology of the heart.* New York: McGraw-Hill, 1960:19–74.
2. Cohen CJ, Bean BP, Tsien RW. Maximum upstroke velocity as an index of available sodium conductance. *Circ Res* 1984;54:636–651.
3. Aldrich RW, Stevens CF. Inactivation of open and closed sodium channels determined separately. *Symp Quant Biol* 1983;47:147–153.
4. Hirst GDS, Edwards FR, Bramich NJ, Klemm MF. Neural control of cardiac pacemaker potentials. *NIPS* 1991;6:185–190.
5. Campbell DL, Rasmusson RL, Strauss HC. Ionic current mechanisms generating vertebrate primary cardiac pacemaker activity at the single cell level: an integrative view. *Annu Rev Physiol* 1992;54:279–302.
6. Meijler FL, Janse MJ. Morphology and electrophysiology of the mammalian atrioventricular node. *Physiol Rev* 1988;68:608–647.
7. Litovsky SH, Antzelevitch C. Transient outward current prominent in canine ventricular epicardium but not endocardium. *Circ Res* 1988;62:116–126.
8. Hodgkin AL, Huxley AF. A quantitative description of membrane current and its application to conduction and excitation in nerve. *J Physiol* 1952;117:500–544.
9. Colquhoun D, Hawkes AG. The principles of the stochastic interpretation of ion-channel mechanisms. In: Sakmann B, Neher E, eds. *Single channel recordings.* New York: Plenum Press, 1993:135–175.
10. Grant AO, Wendt DJ, Zilberter Y, Starmer CF. Kinetics of interaction of disopyramide with the cardiac sodium channel: fast dissociation from open channels at normal rest potentials. *J Membrane Biol* 1993;136:199–214.
11. Powell T, Twist VW. A rapid technique for the isolation and purification of adult cardiac muscle cells having respiratory control and a tolerance to calcium. *Biochem Biophys Res Commun* 1976;72:327–333.
12. Sheets MF, Hanck DA. Mechanisms of extracellular divalent and trivalent cation block of the sodium current in canine cardiac Purkinje cells. *J Physiol* 1992;454:299–320.
13. Santana LF, Gomez AM, Lederer WJ. Ca^{2+} flux through promiscuous cardiac Na^+ channels: slip-mode conductance. *Science* 1998;279:1027–1033.
14. Sorbera LA, Morad M. Atrionaturitic peptide transforms cardiac sodium channels into calcium-conducting channels. *Science* 1990;247:969–973.
15. Chandra R, Chauhan VS, Starmer CF, Grant AO. Modulation of wild-type and ΔKPQ mutant human cardiac Na channels by β-adrenergic stimulation: shifts in gating but no change in Ca^{2+}/Na^+ selectivity. *Circulation* 1998;98:I-55.
16. Heinemann SH, Terlau H, Stuhmer W, et al. Calcium channel characteristics conferred on the sodium channel by single mutations. *Nature* 1992;356:441–443.
17. Nuss HB, Marban E. Whether "slip-mode conductance" occurs. *Science* 1999;284: 711A.
18. Armstrong CM, Bezanilla F. Inactivation of the sodium channel. II. Gating current experiments. *J Gen Physiol* 1977;70:567–590.
19. Aldrich RW, Stevens CF. Voltage-dependent gating of single sodium channels from mammalian neuroblastoma cells. *J Neurosci* 1987;7:418–431.
20. Nattel S, Mittleman M. Treatment of ventricular tachyarrhythmias resulting from amitriptyline toxicity in dogs. *J Pharmacol Exp Ther* 1984;231:430–435.
21. Doyle DA, Cabral JM, Pfuetzner RA, et al. The structure of the potassium channel: molecular basis of K^+ conduction and selectivity. *Science* 1998;280:69–77.
22. Vassilev P, Scheuer T, Catterall WA. Inhibition of single sodium channels by a site-directed antibody. *Proc Natl Acad Sci U S A* 1989;86:8147–8151.
23. Stuehmer W, Conti F, Suzuki H, et al. Structural parts involved in activation and inactivation of the sodium channel. *Nature* 1993;339:597–603.
24. Patton DE, West JW, Catterall WA, Goldin AL. Amino acid residues required for fast Na^+-channel inactivation: charge neutralizations and deletions in the III-IV linker. *Proc Natl Acad Sci U S A* 1992;89:10905–10909.
25. West JW, Patton DE, Scheuer T, et al. A cluster of hydrophobic aminoacid residues required for fast Na^+-channel inactivation. *Proc Natl Acad Sci U S A* 1992;89:10910–10914.
26. Kellenberger S, West JW, Scheuer T, Catterall WA. Molecular analysis of the Na^+ channel inactivation gate. *Biophysical J* 1996;70:A318.
27. Makita N Jr, Bennett PB, George AL Jr. Voltage-gated Na^+ channel $β_1$ subunit mRNA expressed in adult human skeletal muscle, heart and brain is encoded by a single gene. *J Biol Chem* 1994;269:7571–7578.
28. An RH, Wang XL, Kerem B, et al. Novel LQT-3 mutations affects Na^+ channel activity through interactions between α- and $β_1$-subunits. *Circ Res* 1998;83:141–146.
29. Makielski JC, Limberis JT, Chang SY, et al. Coexpression of beta 1 with cardiac sodium channel alpha subunits in oocytes decreases lidocaine block. *Mol Pharmacol* 1996;49:30–39.
30. Zhang J-F, Robinson RB, Siegelbaum SA. Sympathetic neurons mediate developmental change in cardiac sodium channel gating through long-term neurotransmitter action. *Neuron* 1992;9:97–103.
31. Yang T, Roden DM. Regulation of sodium current development in atrial tumor myocytes (AT-1 cells). *Am J Physiol* 1996;271:H541–H547.
32. Histome I, Kiyosue T, Imanishi S, Arita M. Isoproterenol inhibits residual fast channel via stimulation of β-adrenoceptors in guinea-pig ventricular muscle. *J Mol Cell Cardiol* 1985;17:657–665.
33. Windisch H, Tritthart HA. Isoproterenol, norepinephrine and phosphodiesterase inhibitors are blockers of the depressed fast Na^+-system in ventricular muscle fibers. *J Mol Cell Cardiol* 1982;14:431–434.
34. Ono K, Kiyosue T, Arita M. Isoproterenol, DBcAMP and forskolin inhibit cardiac sodium current. *Am J Physiol* 1989;256:C1131–C1137.

35. Schubert B, VanDongen AMJ, Kirsh GE, Brown AM. Inhibition of cardiac Na+ currents by isoproterenol. *Am J Physiol* 1990;258: H977–H982.

36. Schubert B, VanDongen AMJ, Kirsh GE, Brown AM. β-adrenergic inhibition of cardiac sodium channels by dual G-protein pathways. *Science* 1989;245:516–519.

37. Kirstein M, Eickhorn R, Langfeld H, et al. Influence of β-adrenergic stimulation of the fast sodium current in the intact rat papillary muscle. *Basic Res Cardiol* 1991;86:441–448.

38. Ono K, Fozzard HA, Hanck D. On the mechanism of cAMP-dependent modulation of cardiac sodium channel current kinetics. *Circ Res* 1993;72:807–815.

39. Bers DM, Perez-Reyes E. Ca channels in cardiac myocytes: structure and function in Ca influx and intracellular Ca release. *Cardiovasc Res* 1999;42:339–360.

40. Snyders DJ. Structure and function of cardiac potassium channels. *Cardiovasc Res* 1999;42:377–390.

41. Sanguinetti MC, Jurkiewicz NK. Two components of cardiac delayed rectifier K+ current. *J Gen Physiol* 1990;96:195–215.

42. Doyle DA, Cabral JM, Pfuetzner RA, et al. The structure of the potassium channel: molecular basis of K+ conduction and selectivity. *Science* 1998;280:69–77.

43. Barhanin J, Lesage F, Guillemare E, et al. K$_v$LQT1 and IsK (minK) proteins associate to form the I$_{Ks}$ cardiac potassium current. *Nature* 1996;384:78–80.

44. Sanguinetti MC, Curran ME, Zou A, et al Coassembly of K$_v$LQT1 and minK (IsK) proteins to form cardiac I$_{Ks}$ potassium channel. *Nature* 1996;384:80–83.

45. Abbott GW, Goldstein SA. A superfamily of small potassium channel subunits: form and function of the MinK-related peptides (MiRPs). *Q Rev Biophys* 1998;31:357–398.

46. Ludwig A, Zong X, Jeglitsch M, et al. A family of hyperpolarization-activated mammalian cation channels. *Nature* 1998;393: 587–591.

47. Sorota S. Insights into the structure, distribution and function of the cardiac chloride channels. *Cardiovasc Res* 1999;42:361–376.

48. Whalley DW, Wendt DJ, Starmer CF, Grant AO. Cardiac sodium channel kinetics are not influenced by external potassium. *Biophys J* 1993;64:A396.

49. Wijffels MCEF, Kirchhof CJHJ, Dorland R, Allessie MA. Atrial fibrillation begets atrial fibrillation. *Circulation* 1995;92: 1954–1968.

50. Wijiffels MCEF, Kirchof CJHJ, Darland R, Allessie MA. Electrical remodeling due to atrial fibrillation. In: Allessie MA, Fromer M, eds. *Atrial and ventricular fibrillation: mechanisms and device therapy.* Armonk, NY: Futura Publishing, 1996:215–234.

3

MECHANISMS OF ARRHYTHMOGENESIS

CHARLES ANTZELEVITCH
ALEXANDER BURASHNIKOV

Active cardiac arrhythmias are generally divided into two major categories: enhanced or abnormal impulse formation and reentry (Fig. 3-1). Reentry occurs when a propagating impulse fails to die out after normal activation of the heart and persists to reexcite the heart after expiration of the refractory period. Evidence implicating reentry as a mechanism of cardiac arrhythmias goes back to the turn of the century (1–16). Among the mechanisms responsible for abnormal impulse formation are enhanced automaticity and triggered activity. Automaticity is further divided into normal and abnormal, and triggered activity which further divided into two subcategories: early afterdepolarizations (EADs) and delayed afterdepolarizations (DADs). This chapter provides an overview of the cellular mechanisms underlying these cardiac arrhythmias.

REENTRY

Circus Movement Reentry

The circuitous propagation of an impulse around an anatomic or functional obstacle leading to reexcitation of the heart is referred to as *circus movement reentry*. Four distinct models have been described: the ring model, the leading circle model, the figure-of -eight model, and the spiral wave model. The ring model of reentry differs from the other three in that an anatomic obstacle is required. The leading circle, figure-of-eight, and spiral wave models of reentry require only a functional obstacle.

Ring Model

The simplest form of reentry, the ring model, first emerged as a concept shortly after the turn of the 19th century, when A. G. Mayer reported the results of experiments involving the subumbrella tissue of a jellyfish, the scychomedusa *Cas-*

siopeia (1,2). The muscular disk did not contract until ring-like cuts were made and pressure and a stimulus applied. This caused the disk to "spring into rapid rhythmical pulsation so regular and sustained as to recall the movement of clockwork" (1).

Mayer also demonstrated similar circus movement excitation in rings cut from the ventricles of turtle hearts, but he did not consider this to be a plausible mechanism for the development of cardiac arrhythmias. His experiments proved valuable in identifying two fundamental conditions necessary for the initiation and maintenance of circus movement excitation: unidirectional block, which is the impulse initiating the circulating wave must travel in one direction only, and in order for the circus movement to continue, the circuit must be long enough to allow each site in the circuit to recover before the return of the circulating wave.

Several years later, Mines (3) developed the concept of circus movement reentry as a mechanism responsible for cardiac arrhythmias (4). Mines confirmed Mayer's observations and suggested that the recirculating wave could be responsible for clinical cases of tachycardia (3). This concept was reinforced (4) after Kent discovered an extra accessory pathway connecting the atrium and ventricle of a human heart (17). The criteria developed by Mines for the identification of circus movement reentry is still in use today: an area of unidirectional block must exist; the excitatory wave progresses along a distinct pathway, returning to its point of origin and then following the same path again; and interruption of the reentrant circuit at any point along its path should terminate the circus movement.

Fourteen years later, Schmitt and Erlanger (18) suggested that coupled ventricular extrasystoles in mammalian hearts could arise as a consequence of circus movement reentry within loops composed of terminal Purkinje fibers and ventricular muscle. Using a theoretical model consisting of a Purkinje bundle that divides into two branches that insert distally into ventricular muscle (Fig. 3-2), they suggested that a region of depression within one of the terminal Purkinje branches could provide for unidirectional

C. Antzelevitch and A. Burashnikov: Masonic Medical Research Laboratory, Utica, New York 13501.

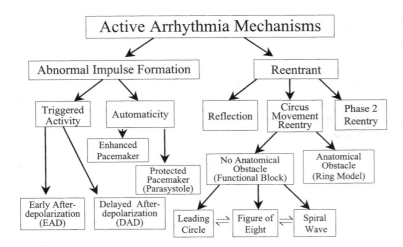

FIGURE 3-1. Classification of active cardiac arrhythmias.

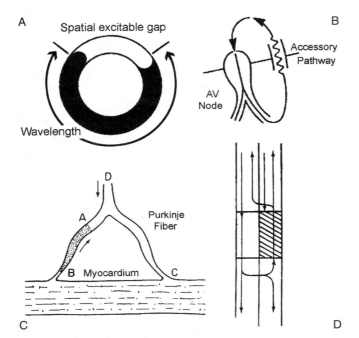

FIGURE 3-2. Ring models of reentry. **A:** Schematic of a ring model of reentry. **B:** Mechanism of reentry in the Wolf-Parkinson-White syndrome involving the atrioventricular (AV) node and an AV accessory pathway (AP). **C:** A mechanism for reentry in a Purkinje-muscle loop proposed by Schmitt and Erlanger. The diagram shows a Purkinje bundle (D) that divides into two branches, both connected distally to ventricular muscle. Circus movement was considered possible if the stippled segment, A → B, showed unidirectional block. An impulse advancing from D would reach and be blocked at A but would reach and stimulate the ventricular muscle at C by way of the other terminal branch. The wavefront would then reenter the Purkinje system at B, traversing the depressed region slowly so as to arrive at A after expiration of refractoriness. **D:** Schematic representation of circus movement reentry in a linear bundle of tissue as proposed by Schmitt and Erlanger. The upper pathway contains a depressed zone *(shaded)* that serves as a site of unidirectional block and slow conduction. Anterograde conduction of the impulse is blocked in the upper pathway but succeeds along the lower pathway. Beyond the zone of depression, the impulse crosses over through lateral connections and reenters through the upper pathway. (**C** and **D** from Schmitt FO, Erlanger J. Directional differences in the conduction of the impulse through heart muscle and their possible relation to extrasystolic and fibrillary contractions. *Am J Physiol* 1928;87:326–347, with permission.)

block and conduction slow enough to permit successful reexcitation within a loop of limited size (10 to 30 mm).

The early investigators recognized that successful reentry could occur only when the impulse was sufficiently delayed in an alternate pathway to allow for expiration of the refractory period in the tissue proximal to the site of unidirectional block. Both conduction velocity and refractoriness determine the success or failure of reentry and the general rule is that the length of the circuit (*pathlength*) must exceed or equal that of the *wavelength*, with the wavelength defined as the product of the conduction velocity and the refractory period or that part of the pathlength occupied by the impulse and refractory to reexcitation. The theoretical minimum pathlength required for development of reentry was initially thought to be quite long. In the early 1970s, microreentry within narrowly circumscribed loops was suggested to be within the realm of possibility. Cranefield, Hoffman, and coworkers (19,20) demonstrated that segments of canine Purkinje fibers that normally display impulse conduction velocities of 2 to 4 m/sec can conduct impulses with apparent velocities of 0.01 to 0.1 m/sec when encased in high-potassium (K⁺) agar. This finding and the demonstration by Sasyniuk and Mendez (21) of a marked abbreviation of action potential duration and refractoriness in terminal Purkinje fibers just proximal to the site of block greatly reduced the theoretical limit of the pathlength required for the development of reentry.

Several years later, single and repetitive reentry was reported by Wit and coworkers (22) in small loops of canine and bovine conducting tissues bathed in a high-K⁺ solution containing catecholamines, demonstrating reentry over a relatively small path. In some experiments, they used linear unbranched bundles of Purkinje tissue to demonstrate a phenomenon similar to that observed by Schmitt and Erlanger in which slow anterograde conduction of the impulse was sometimes followed by a retrograde wavefront that produced a "return extrasystole" (23). They proposed that the nonstimulated impulse was caused by a circus movement reentry made possible by longitudinal dissociation of the bundle, as in the Schmitt and Erlanger model (Fig. 3-2). Noting that in many of their experiments "the rapid upstroke within the depressed segment arises after the rapid upstroke of the normal fiber," Wit and coworkers (23,24) also considered the possibility that "the reflected impulse that travels slowly backward through the depressed segment is evoked by retrograde depolarization of the cells within the depressed segment by the rapid upstrokes of the cells beyond" (24). From this information, the idea arose that reexcitation could occur in a single fiber through a mechanism other than circus movement, namely reflection. Although both explanations appeared plausible, proof for either was lacking at the time. Proof for reflection as a mechanism of reentrant activity did not come until the early 1980s.

These pioneering studies led to our understanding of how anatomic obstacles such as the openings of the venae cava in the right atrium, an aneurysm in the ventricles, or the presence of a bypass tract between atria and ventricles can form a ringlike path for the development of extrasystoles, tachycardia, and flutter.

Leading Circle Model

The suggestion that reentry could be initiated without the involvement of anatomic obstacles and that "natural rings are not essential for the maintenance of circus contractions" was first made by Garrey in 1924 (25). Allessie and coworkers (26–28) were the first to provide support for this hypothesis in experiments in which they induced a tachycardia in isolated preparations of rabbit left atria by applying properly timed premature extrastimuli. Using multiple intracellular electrodes, they showed that, although the basic beats elicited by stimuli applied near the center of the tissue spread normally throughout the preparation, premature impulses propagate only in the direction of shorter refractory periods. An arc of block develops around which the impulse is able to circulate and reexcite the tissue. Recordings near the center of the circus movement showed only subthreshold responses, giving rise to the concept of the leading circle (28), a form of circus movement reentry occurring in structurally uniform myocardium requiring no anatomic obstacle (Fig. 3-3). The functionally refractory region that develops at the vortex of the circulating wave-

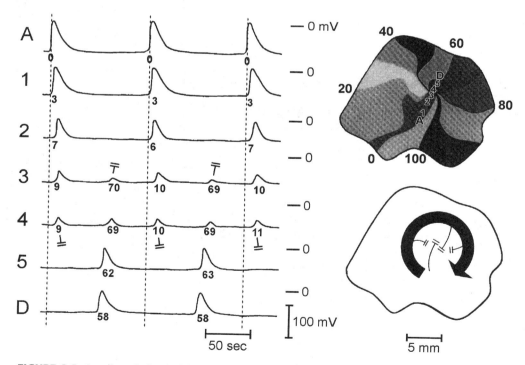

FIGURE 3-3. Leading circle model of reentry. Activation maps during steady-state tachycardia induced by a premature stimulus in an isolated rabbit atrium *(upper right)*. On the left are transmembrane potentials recorded from seven fibers located on a straight line through the center of the circus movement. The central area is activated by centripetal wavelets, and the fibers in the central area show double responses of subnormal amplitude. Both responses are unable to propagate beyond the center, preventing the impulse from short-cutting the circuit. The activation pattern *(lower right)* is schematically represented, showing the leading circuit and the converging centripetal wavelets. The block is indicated by double bars. (From Allessie MA, Bonke FIM, Schopman JG. Circus movement in rabbit atrial muscle as a mechanism of tachycardia. III. The "leading circle" concept: a new model of circus movement in cardiac tissue without the involvement of an anatomic obstacle. *Circ Res* 1977;41:9–18, with permission.)

front prevents the centripetal waves from short-circuiting the circus movement and maintains the reentry. Because the head of the circulating wavefront usually travels on relatively refractory tissue, a fully excitable gap of tissue may not be present; unlike other forms of reentry, the leading circle model may not be readily influenced by extraneous impulses initiated in areas outside the reentrant circuit and may not be easily entrained.

Kamiyama and coworkers (29) later showed that the leading circle mechanism could mediate tachycardia induced in isolated ventricular tissues. Allessie and coworkers (30) also described the development of circus movement reentry without the involvement of an anatomic obstacle in a two-dimensional model of ventricular epicardium created by freezing the endocardial layers of a Langendorff method–perfused rabbit heart.

Functional arcs or lines of block attending the development of a circus movement reentry were shown to develop in *in vivo* models of canine infarction in which a thin surviving epicardial rim overlies the infarcted ventricle (9,31–36). The lines of block observed during tachycardia are usually oriented parallel to the direction of the myocardial fibers, suggesting that anisotropic conduction properties (faster conduction in the direction parallel to the long axis of the myocardial cells) also play an important role in defining the functionally refractory zone (37–39). Dillon and coworkers (36) presented evidence that the long lines of functional block that sustain reentry in the epicardial rim overlying canine infarction may represent zones of very slow conduction, implying that the dimensions of the area of functional block may be relatively small and may even approach that of the vortex of functional block described by Allessie and coworkers.

Figure-of-Eight Model

El-Sherif and coworkers first described the figure-of-eight model of reentry in the surviving epicardial layer overlying infarction produced by occlusion of the left anterior descending artery in canine hearts (14,31–33,40). In the figure-of-eight model, the reentrant beat produces a wavefront that circulates in both directions around a long line of functional conduction block (Fig. 3-4) and rejoins on the distal side of the block. The wavefront then breaks through the arc of block to reexcite the tissue proximal to the block. The single arc of block is divided into two, and the reentrant activation continues as two circulating wavefronts that travel in clockwise and counterclockwise directions around the two arcs in a pretzel-like configuration. The diameter of the reentrant circuit in the ventricle may be as small as a few millimeters or as large as several centimeters. Lin and coworkers (41) described a novel quatrefoil-shaped reentry induced by delivering long stimuli during the vulnerable phase in rabbit ventricular myocardium. This pattern, a variant of figure-of-eight reentry, consists of two

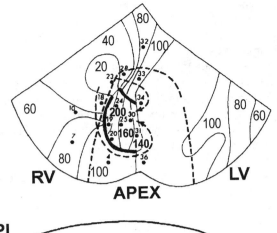

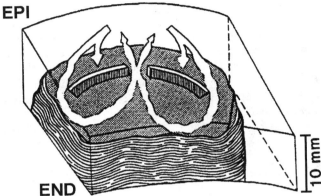

FIGURE 3-4. Figure-of eight model of reentry: isochronal activation map during monomorphic reentrant ventricular tachycardia occurring in the surviving epicardial layer overlying an infarction. Recordings were obtained from the epicardial surface of a canine heart 4 days after ligation of the left anterior descending coronary artery. Activation isochrones are drawn at 20-ms intervals. The reentrant circuit has a characteristic figure-of-eight activation pattern. Two circulating wavefronts advance in clockwise and counterclockwise directions, respectively, around two zones (arcs) of conduction block *(heavy solid lines)*. The epicardial surface is depicted as if the ventricles were unfolded after a cut from the crux to the apex. A three-dimensional diagrammatic illustration of the ventricular activation pattern during the reentrant tachycardia is shown in the lower panel. END, endocardium; EPI, epicardium; LV, left ventricle; RV, right ventricle. (From El-Sherif N. Reentry revisited. *Pacing Clin Electrophysiol* 1988;11:1358–1368, with permission.)

pairs of opposing rotors with all four circuits converging in the center.

Spiral Waves and Rotors

Originally used to describe reentry around an anatomic obstacle (42), the term spiral wave reentry was later adopted to describe circulating waves in the absence of an anatomic obstacle (43,44), similar to the circulating waves of the leading circle mechanism described by Allessie and colleagues (26,28). The spiral wave theory has advanced our understanding of the mechanisms responsible for the functional form of reentry. Although leading circle and spiral wave reentry are considered by some to be nearly identical, several distinctions have been suggested (28,45–47).

The curvature of the spiral wave is the key to the formation of the core (47). The curvature of the waveforms a region of high impedance mismatch (i.e., sink-source mismatch), where the current provided by the reentering wavefront (i.e., source) is insufficient to charge the capacity and excite the much larger volume of tissue ahead (i.e., sink). A prominent curvature of the spiral wave is generally encountered after a wave break, a situation in which a planar wave encounters an obstacle and breaks into two or more daughter waves. Because it has the greatest curvature, the broken end of the wave moves most slowly. As curvature decreases along the more distal parts of the spiral, propagation speed increases.

The term *spiral wave* typically is used to describe reentrant activity in two dimensions. The center of the spiral wave is called the *core*, and the distribution of the core in three dimensions is referred to as the *filament* (Fig. 3-5). The three-dimensional form of the spiral wave is called a *scroll wave* (48). In its simplest form, the scroll wave has a straight filament spanning the ventricular wall (i.e., from epicardium to endocardium). Theoretical studies have described three major scroll wave configurations with curved (L-, U-, and O-shaped) filaments (48), although numerous variations of these three-dimensional filaments in space and time are assumed to exist during cardiac arrhythmias (48). Anisotropy and anatomic obstacles can substantially modify the characteristics and spatiotemporal behavior of the vortex-like reentries. As anatomic obstacles are introduced, approaching a ring model of reentry, the

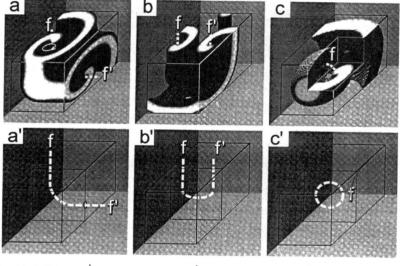

Underlying Mechanism	Spatial Dynamics	ECG	Clinical Presentation
stable spiral wave			monomorphic VT
quasiperiodically meandering spiral wave			torsade de pointes
chaotically meandering spiral wave			polymorphic VT
spiral wave breakup			VF

FIGURE 3-5. Basic scroll-type reentry in three-dimensional and spiral wave phenotypes with their possible clinical manifestations. **A:** Basic configurations of vortex-like reentry in three dimensions; a and a' are the L-shaped scroll wave and filament, respectively. The scroll rotates in a clockwise direction *(top)* about the L-shaped filament (f, f') shown in a'. The b and b' indicate the U-shaped scroll wave and filament, respectively. The c and c' indicate the O-shaped wave and filament, respectively. (From Pertsov AM, Jalife J. Three-dimensional vortex-like reentry. In: Zipes DP, Jalife J, eds. *Cardiac electrophysiology: from cell to bedside.* Philadelphia: WB Saunders, 1995:403–410, with permission.). **B:** Four types of spiral wave phenotypes and associated clinical manifestations. A stable spiral wave mechanism gives rise to monomorphic ventricular tachycardia (VT) on the electrocardiogram. A quasi-periodic meandering spiral wave is responsible for torsade de pointes, whereas a chaotically meandering spiral wave is revealed as polymorphic VT. A ventricular fibrillation (VF) pattern is caused by spiral wave breakup. In the second column, spiral waves are shown in gray, and the paths of their tips are shown as solid lines. (From Garfinkel A, Qu Z. Nonlinear dynamics of excitation and propagation in cardiac muscle. In: Zipes DP, Jalife J, eds. *Cardiac electrophysiology: from cell to bedside.* Philadelphia: WB Saunders, 1999:515–520, with permission.)

curvature of the wave becomes less of a determinant of the characteristics of the arrhythmia.

Spiral wave activity has been used to explain the electrocardiographic patterns observed during monomorphic and polymorphic cardiac arrhythmias, as well as during fibrillation (44,49,50). Monomorphic ventricular tachycardia (VT) results when the spiral wave is anchored and not able to drift within the ventricular myocardium. In contrast, a polymorphic VT such as that encountered with long QT syndrome (LQTS)–induced torsade de pointes is caused by a meandering or drifting spiral wave. Ventricular fibrillation (VF) seems to be the most complex representation of rotating spiral waves in the heart. VF is often preceded by VT. VF develops when the single spiral wave responsible for VT breaks up, leading to the development of multiple spirals that are continuously extinguished and re-created. There are likely to be variations on this theme. For example, it has been suggested that a single, meandering spiral wave could underlie the mechanism of VF (51–53), as in the case of the Brugada syndrome (53). Studies suggest that a single, stable, high-frequency intramural reentrant source can underlie VF, causing fibrillatory patterns by propagating into electrically heterogeneous regions (54,55). Fibrillatory patterns in the atria may be caused by multiple wandering reentrant wavelets, as in VF (56,57), to a single stable reentry (58) or even a focal automatic mechanism firing at a high rate (59).

Reflection

The concept of reflection was first suggested by Cranefield, Wit, and coworkers based on their studies of the propagation characteristics of slow action potential responses in K+-depolarized Purkinje fibers (19,20,22,24). Using strands of Purkinje fiber, Wit and coworkers demonstrated a phenomenon similar to that observed by Schmitt and Erlanger in which slow anterograde conduction of the impulse was sometimes followed by a retrograde wavefront that produced a "return extrasystole" (23). They proposed that the nonstimulated impulse was caused by circuitous reentry at the level of the syncytial interconnections, made possible by longitudinal dissociation of the bundle, as the most likely explanation for the phenomenon but also suggested the possibility of reflection. Direct evidence in support of reflection as a mechanism of arrhythmogenesis was first provided by Antzelevitch and coworkers (60,61).

Several models of reflection have been developed (60–63). The first model involved use of "ion-free" isotonic sucrose solution to create a narrow (1.5- to 2-mm) central inexcitable zone (i.e., gap) in unbranched Purkinje fibers mounted in a three-chamber tissue bath (60) (Fig. 3-6). In this model, stimulation of the proximal (P) segment elicits an action potential that propagates to the proximal border of the sucrose gap. Active propagation across the gap is not possible because of the ion-depleted extracellular milieu, but local circuit current continues to flow through the intercellular low-resistance pathways (a Ag/AgCl extracellular shunt pathway is provided). This local circuit or electrotonic current, much reduced on emerging from the gap, slowly discharges the capacity of the distal (D) tissue, giving rise to a depolarization that manifests as a subthreshold response (i.e., the last distal response) or a foot-potential that brings the distal excitable element to its threshold potential (Fig. 3-7). Active impulse propagation stops and then resumes after a delay that can be as long as several hundred milliseconds. When anterograde (P → D) transmission time is sufficiently delayed to permit recovery of refractoriness at the proximal end, electrotonic transmission of the impulse in the retrograde direction reexcites the proximal tissue, generating a closely coupled reflected reentry.

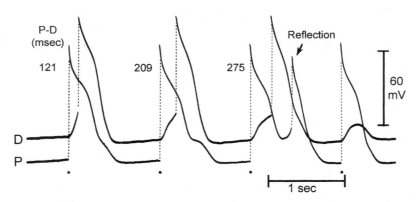

FIGURE 3-6. Delayed transmission and reflection across an inexcitable gap created by superfusion of the central segment of a Purkinje fiber with an "ion-free" isotonic sucrose solution. The two traces were recorded from proximal (P) and distal (D) active segments. P-D conduction time (indicated in milliseconds in the upper portion) increased progressively with a 4 : 3 Wenckebach periodicity. The third stimulated proximal response was followed by a reflection. (From Antzelevitch C. Clinical applications of new concepts of parasystole, reflection, and tachycardia. *Cardiol Clin* 1983;1:39–50, with permission.)

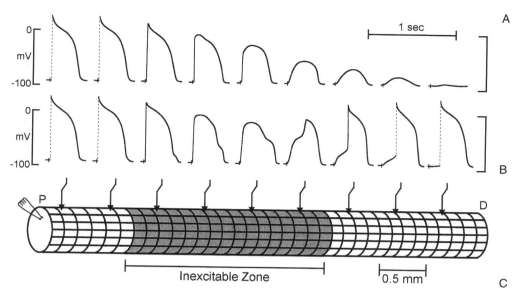

FIGURE 3-7. Discontinuous conduction **(B)** and conduction block **(A)** in a Purkinje strand with a central inexcitable zone **(C)**. The schematic illustration is based on transmembrane recordings obtained from canine Purkinje fiber–sucrose gap preparations. An action potential elicited by stimulation of the proximal (P) side of the preparation conducts normally up to the border of the inexcitable zone. Active propagation of the impulse stops at this point, but local circuit current generated by the proximal segment continues to flow through the preparation encountering a cumulative resistance (i.e., successive gap junctions). Transmembrane recordings from the first few inexcitable cells show a response not very different from the action potentials recorded in the neighboring excitable cells, despite the fact that no ions may be moving across the membrane of these cells. The responses recorded in the inexcitable region are the electrotonic images of activity generated in the proximal excitable segment. The resistive-capacitive properties of the tissue lead to an exponential decline in the amplitude of the transmembrane potential recorded along the length of the inexcitable segment and to a slowing of the rate of change of voltage as a function of time. If, as in B, the electrotonic current is sufficient to bring the distal excitable tissue to its threshold potential, an action potential is generated after a step delay imposed by the slow discharge of the capacity of the distal (D) membrane by the electrotonic current (i.e., foot-potential). Active conduction of the impulse therefore stops at the proximal border of the inexcitable zone and resumes at the distal border after a step delay that may range from a few to tens or hundreds of milliseconds. (Modified from Antzelevitch C. Electrotonus and reflection. In: Rosen MR, Janse MJ, Wit AL, eds. *Cardiac electrophysiology: a textbook.* Mount Kisco, NY: Futura Publishing, 1990:491–516, with permission.)

Reflection therefore results from the back and forth, electrotonically mediated transmission of the impulse across the same inexcitable segment; neither longitudinal dissociation nor circus movement need be invoked to explain the phenomenon.

A second model involves the creation of an inexcitable region permitting delayed conduction by superfusion of a central segment of a Purkinje bundle with a solution designed to mimic the extracellular milieu at a site of ischemia (61). With a K$^+$ concentration of between 15 and 20 mM, the "ischemic" solution induced major delays in conduction, which were as long as 500 ms across the 1.5-mm-wide ischemic central gap. The gap was shown to be largely composed of an inexcitable cable across which conduction of impulses was electrotonically mediated. The long delays of impulse conduction across the ischemic gap permit the development of reflection. When propagation across the gap is mediated by "slow responses," transmission is relatively prompt, and reflection does not occur (61).

Reflected reentry has been demonstrated in isolated atrial and ventricular myocardial tissues (63–65). Reflection has also been demonstrated in Purkinje fibers, in which a functionally inexcitable zone is created by focal depolarization of the preparation with long-duration constant current pulses (66). This phenomenon is also observed in isolated canine Purkinje fibers homogeneously depressed with high K$^+$ solution and in branched preparations of normal Purkinje fibers (67).

Success or failure of reflection depends critically on the degree to which conduction is delayed in both directions across the functionally inexcitable zone. These transit delays depend on the width of the blocked segment, the intracellular and extracellular impedance to the flow of local circuit current across the inexcitable zone, and the excitability of the distal active site (i.e., sink). Because the excitability of cardiac tissues continues to recover for hundreds of milliseconds after an action potential, impulse transmission across the inexcitable zone is a sensitive function of frequency (60,68–70). Consequently, the incidence and patterns of manifest ectopic activity encountered in models of reflection are highly rate dependent (62,65,69,71,72). Similar rate-dependent changes in extrasystolic activity have been reported in patients with frequent extrasystoles evaluated with Holter recordings (73) and in patients evaluated by atrial pacing (71,74).

Because reflection can occur within areas of tissue as small as 1 to 2 mm^2, it is likely to appear to be of focal origin. Its identification as a mechanism of arrhythmia may be difficult even with very high spatial resolution mapping of the electrical activity of discrete sites. The delineation of delayed impulse conduction mechanisms at discrete sites requires the use of intracellular microelectrode techniques in conjunction with high-resolution extracellular mapping techniques. These limitations considered, reflection has been suggested as the mechanism underlying reentrant extrasystolic activity in ventricular tissues excised from a 1-day-old infarcted canine heart (75) and in a clinical case of incessant ventricular bigeminy in a young patient with no evidence of organic heart disease (76).

Phase 2 Reentry

Phase 2 reentry is another example of a reentrant mechanism that may have a focal appearance. Phase 2 reentry occurs when the dome of the epicardial action potential propagates from sites at which it is maintained to sites at which it is abolished, causing local reexcitation of the epicardium and the generation of a closely coupled extrasystole. A more detailed description of this mechanism is described later in this chapter.

The Role of Heterogeneity

Several studies have shown that the ventricular myocardium is far from homogeneous, as previously thought, and that it is composed of at least three electrophysiologically and functionally distinct cell types: epicardial, mid-myocardial (M), and endocardial. These three ventricular myocardial cell types differ principally with respect to phase 1 and phase 3 repolarization characteristics (Fig. 3-8). Ventricular epicardial and M, but not endocardial, cells typically display a conspicuous phase 1 because of a prominent 4-aminopyridine (4-AP)–sensitive transient outward current (I_{to}), giving the action potential a spike and dome or notched configuration. These regional differences in I_{to}, first suggested on the basis of action potential data (77), have been demonstrated using whole-cell patch clamp techniques in canine (78), feline (79), rabbit (80), rat (81), and human (82,83) ventricular myocytes.

It is unknown whether I_{to2}, a calcium-activated component of the transient outward current, differs among the three ventricular myocardial cell types (84). I_{to2}, initially ascribed to a K$^+$ current, is thought to be primarily caused by the calcium-activated chloride current, $I_{Cl(Ca)}$ (84). Myocytes isolated from the epicardial region of the left ventricular wall of the rabbit show a higher density of cAMP-activated chloride current when compared with endocardial myocytes (85).

Major differences in the magnitude of the action potential notch and corresponding differences in I_{to} have been described between right and left ventricular epicardium (86). Similar interventricular differences in I_{to} have also been described for canine ventricular M cells (87). This distinction is thought to form the basis for why the Brugada syndrome, a channelopathy-mediated cause of sudden death, is a right ventricular disease.

FIGURE 3-8: Ionic distinctions among epicardial, M, and endocardial cells. **A:** Action potentials recorded from myocytes isolated from the epicardial, endocardial, and M regions of the canine left ventricle. **B:** I through V relations for I_{K1} in epicardial, endocardial, and M region myocytes. Values are given as the mean ± SD. **C:** Transient outward current (I_{to}) recorded from the three cell types. Current traces were recorded during depolarizing steps from a holding potential of –80 mV to test potentials ranging between –20 and +70 mV. **D:** The average peak current-voltage relationship for I_{to} for each of the three cell types. Values are given as the mean ± SD. **E:** Voltage-dependent activation of the slowly activating component of the delayed rectifier K$^+$ current (I_{Ks}). Currents were elicited by the voltage pulse protocol shown in the inset using a Na$^+$-, K$^+$-, and Ca^{2+}- free solution. **F:** Voltage dependence of I_{Ks} (current remaining after exposure to E-4031) and I_{Kr} (E-4031-sensitive current). Values are given as the mean ± SE. (*P < 0.05 compared with endocardial or epicardial). (Data from references 78, 91, and 93.) **G:** Reverse-mode sodium-calcium exchange currents recorded in potassium- and chloride-free solutions at a voltage of –80 mV. I_{Na-Ca} was maximally activated by switching to sodium-free external solution at the time indicated by the arrow. **H:** Mid-myocardial sodium-calcium exchanger density is 30% greater than endocardial density, calculated as the peak outward I_{Na-Ca} normalized by cell capacitance. Endocardial and epicardial densities were not significantly different. **I:** Tetrodotoxin (TTX)-sensitive late sodium current. Cells were held at –80 mV and briefly pulsed to –45 mV to inactivate fast sodium current before stepping to –10 mV. **J:** Normalized late sodium current measured 300 ms into the test pulse was plotted as a function of test pulse potential. (Adapted Zygmunt AC, Goodrow RJ, Antzelevitch C. I $_{Na-Ca}$ contributes to electrical heterogeneity within the canine ventricle. *Am J Physiol* 2000;278:H1671–H1678, with permission.)

The M cell is distinguished by the ability of its action potential to prolong disproportionately relative to the action potential of other ventricular myocardial cells in response to a slowing of rate or in response to action potential duration (APD)-prolonging agents (88–90) (Fig. 3-9). In the dog, the ionic basis for these features of the M cell include the presence of a smaller slowly activating delayed rectifier current (I_{Ks}) (91), a larger late sodium current (late I_{Na}) (92), and a larger Na-Ca exchange current (I_{Na-Ca}) (93). The rapidly activating delayed rectifier (I_{Kr}) and inward rectifier (I_{K1}) currents are similar in the three transmural cell types. Transmural and apicobasal differences in the density of I_{Kr} channels have been described in the ferret heart (94). I_{Kr} message and channel protein were shown to be much larger in the ferret epicardium. I_{Ks} is larger in M cells isolated from the right versus left ventricles of the dog (87).

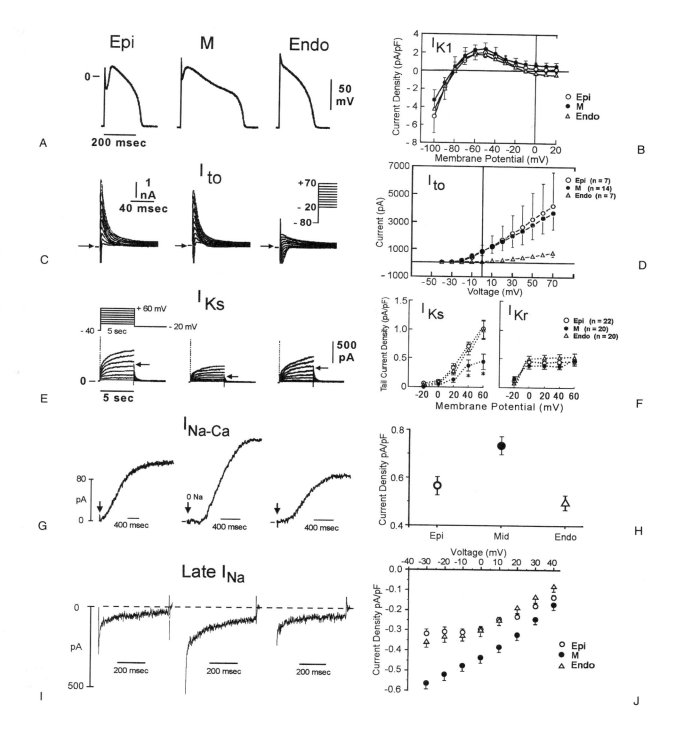

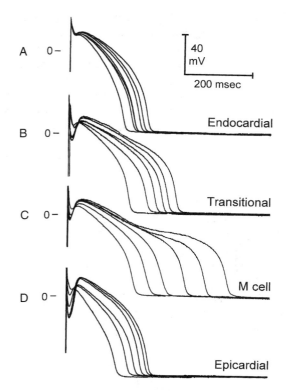

FIGURE 3-9. Transmembrane activity recorded from cells isolated from the epicardial (Epi), M, and endocardial (Endo) regions of the canine left ventricle at basic cycle lengths (BCLs) of 300 to 5,000 ms (i.e., steady-state conditions). The M and transitional cells were enzymatically dissociated from the midmyocardial region. Deceleration-induced prolongation of action potential duration in M cells is much greater than in epicardial and endocardial cells. The spike and dome morphology is also more accentuated in the epicardial cell.

Histologically, M cells are similar to epicardial and endocardial cells. Electrophysiologically and pharmacologically, they appear to be a hybrid between Purkinje and ventricular cells. Like Purkinje fibers, M cells show a prominent APD prolongation and develop EADs in response to I_{Kr} blockers, whereas epicardium and endocardium do not. Like Purkinje fibers, M cells develop DADs in response to agents that calcium load or overload the cardiac cell; epicardium and endocardium do not. Unlike Purkinje fibers, M cells display an APD prolongation in response to I_{Ks} blockers; epicardium and endocardium also have increased APDs in response to I_{Ks} blockers. Purkinje and M cells also respond differently to α-adrenergic agonists. $α_1$-Adrenoceptor stimulation produces APD prolongation in Purkinje fibers but abbreviation in M cells and little or no change in endocardium and epicardium (95).

The position of M cells within the ventricular wall has been investigated in greatest detail in the left ventricle of the canine heart. Although transitional cells are found throughout the wall in the canine left ventricle, M cells displaying the longest action potentials (basic cycle lengths ≥2,000 ms)

are often localized in the deep subendocardium to midmyocardium in the anterior wall, (96) deep subepicardium to mid-myocardium in the lateral wall (88), and throughout the wall in the region of the right ventricular outflow tracts (97). M cells are also present in the deep layers of endocardial structures, including papillary muscles, trabeculae, and the interventricular septum (98). Unlike Purkinje fibers, they are not found in discrete bundles or islets (98,99). Cells with the characteristics of M cells have been described in the canine, guinea pig, rabbit, pig, and human ventricles (78,88,90,91,96,98–117).

Amplification of transmural heterogeneities normally present in the early and late phases of the action potential can lead to the development of a variety of arrhythmias, including the Brugada syndrome and LQTS.

Brugada Syndrome

The Brugada syndrome, first described as a clinical entity by Brugada and Brugada in 1992 (118), is characterized by an ST segment elevation in the right precordial leads of V_1 to V_3 (unrelated to ischemia, electrolyte abnormalities, or structural heart disease) and by a high risk of sudden cardiac death (118–127). This topic is extensively reviewed elsewhere (128–130).

Most prevalent in males of Asian origin, the Brugada syndrome is familial, with an autosomal dominant mode of transmission (131). The age for the first arrhythmic event is between 2 and 77 years, with a mean age of approximately 40 years (120,127,129). Although Brugada syndrome patients generally have structurally normal hearts, small amounts of lipid infiltration into the deep subepicardium can be detected in some cases. The Brugada syndrome is unrelated to any chromosomal loci described for arrhythmogenic right ventricular cardiomyopathy (132).

The only gene mutations linked to the Brugada syndrome are in the cardiac sodium channel gene, *SCN5A* (133). Chen and associates described several mutations in *SCN5A* at sites other than those known to contribute to the LQT3 form of LQTS. Frame-shift and deletion mutations lead to failure of the channel to express, importantly reducing I_{Na} density (133,134). Missense mutations cause a shift in the voltage and time dependence of activation, inactivation, and reactivation. In the case of one missense mutation (T1620M), acceleration of the kinetics of inactivation of I_{Na} provides the substrate for the syndrome (135).

The Brugada syndrome is thought to be precipitated by an outward shift of the current active at the end of phase 1 of the right ventricular epicardial action potential (where I_{to} is most prominent) (128,136). Such a shift can cause all-or-none repolarization at the end of phase 1 and loss of the epicardial action potential dome, leading to marked abbreviation of the action potential. Pathophysiologic conditions (e.g., ischemia, metabolic inhibition, hypothermia) and some pharmacologic interventions cause loss of the dome and abbreviation of the action potential in canine and feline ventricular cells in which I_{to} is prominent. Under ischemic conditions and in response to agents that block I_{Na} or I_{Ca} or activate the ATP-sensitive potassium current (I_{K-ATP}), canine ventricular epicardium exhibits an all-or-none repolarization as a result of the rebalancing of currents flowing at the end of phase 1 of the action potential. Failure of the dome to develop occurs when outward currents (principally I_{to}) overwhelm the inward currents (chiefly I_{Ca}), resulting in a marked abbreviation of the action potential. This occurs when I_{to} remains strong, and inward current is reduced or outward current is augmented. In the case of the T1620M mutation of *SCN5A* that has been linked to the Brugada syndrome, the contribution of I_{Na} to the early part of the action potential is severely reduced because of an acceleration of the kinetics of inactivation of the current (135).

Loss of the action potential dome in epicardium but not endocardium creates a voltage gradient during phases 2 and 3 of the action potential that manifests as an ST segment elevation. Studies involving the arterially perfused right ventricular wedge preparation provide direct evidence in support of the hypothesis that loss or depression of the action potential dome in epicardium, but not endocardium, underlies the development of a prominent ST segment elevation in the Brugada syndrome and other syndromes associated with an ST segment elevation (136,137) (Fig. 3-10).

Loss of the action potential dome is usually not homogeneous. The action potential dome may be abolished at some epicardial sites but not others, causing a marked dispersion of repolarization within the epicardium. Conduction of the action potential dome from sites at which it is maintained to sites at which it is abolished can cause local reexcitation of the preparation. This mechanism, called phase 2 reentry, produces extrasystolic beats capable of initiating circus movement reentry (138–140) (Fig. 3-10). The arrhythmia often takes the form of a polymorphic VT, resembling a rapid torsade de pointes, which in some cases cannot be readily distinguished from VF. Investigators in the field have long appreciated the fact that circus movement reentry is more often than not precipitated by an extrasystole. This mechanism provides the substrate for the development of circus movement reentry in the form of epicardial and transmural dispersion of repolarization, as well as the phase 2 reentrant extrasystole that triggers the VT/VF episode.

A prominent I_{to} is a prerequisite for phase 2 reentry. Agents that inhibit I_{to}, including 4-aminopyridine and quinidine, are effective in restoring the action potential dome and electrical homogeneity and in aborting all arrhythmic activity in experimental models of this syndrome (136,139). Class Ia and Ic antiarrhythmic agents that block I_{Na}, but little to no I_{to} (i.e., flecainide, ajmaline, and procainamide), exacerbate or unmask the Brugada syndrome, whereas those with actions to block both I_{Na} and I_{to}

(i.e., quinidine and disopyramide) can exert an ameliorative effect (136). The anticholinergic effects of quinidine and disopyramide may also contribute to their effectiveness. However, the only therapeutic measure with proven effectiveness is the implantable cardioverter-defibrillator.

Long QT Syndrome

Amplification of intrinsic heterogeneities of ventricular repolarization also contribute to the development of LQTS. In this case, exaggeration of differences in final repolarization of the action potential of cells spanning the ventricular wall provide the arrhythmogenic substrate. The congenital and acquired (drug-induced) LQTS are characterized by the development of long QT intervals in the electrocardiographic (ECG) abnormal T waves and an atypical polymorphic tachycardia known as torsade de pointes (141–145). Genetic linkage studies have identified several forms of the congenital LQTS caused by mutations in ion channel genes located on chromosomes 3, 7, 11, and 21. Mutations in genes for KvLQT1 *(KCNQ1)* and minK *(KCNE1)* are responsible for defects in the I_{Ks} that underlies the LQT1 and LQT5 forms of LQTS, whereas mutations in *HERG* and *SCN5A* are responsible for defects in I_{Kr} and sodium current (I_{Na}) that underlie the LQT2 and LQT3 syndromes. Mutations in the gene *(KCNE2)* for minK-related protein, MiRP1, which associates with HERG to form the I_{Kr} channel, are responsible for the LQT6 form of LQTS (146).

The electrophysiologic, electrocardiographic, and pharmacologic characteristics of the LQT1, LQT2, and LQT3 syndromes have been studied in the arterially perfused canine left ventricular wedge preparation. Simultaneous recording of transmembrane activity from epicardial, M, and endocardial or Purkinje sites, together with a transmural ECG recorded along the same axis, permits correlation of transmembrane and electrocardiographic activity (96,108, 113–115,147). The wedge preparation is capable of developing and sustaining a variety of arrhythmias, including torsade de pointes. Pharmacologic models that mimic the clinical congenital syndromes with respect to prolongation of the QT interval, T-wave morphology, rate dependence of repolarization, and response to antiarrhythmic drugs have been developed (96,108,113–115) (Fig. 3-11).

The I_{Ks} blocker, chromanol 293B, was used to mimic LQT1 and the β-adrenergic agonist, isoproterenol, was used to assess β-adrenergic influence. I_{Ks} block alone produces a homogeneous prolongation of repolarization and refractoriness across the ventricular wall and does not induce arrhythmias. The addition of isoproterenol causes abbreviation of epicardial and endocardial APD but a prolongation or no change in the APD of the M cell, resulting in a marked augmentation of transmural dispersion of repolarization (TDR) and the development of spontaneous and stimulation-induced torsade de pointes (113). These changes give rise to a broad-based T wave and the long QT

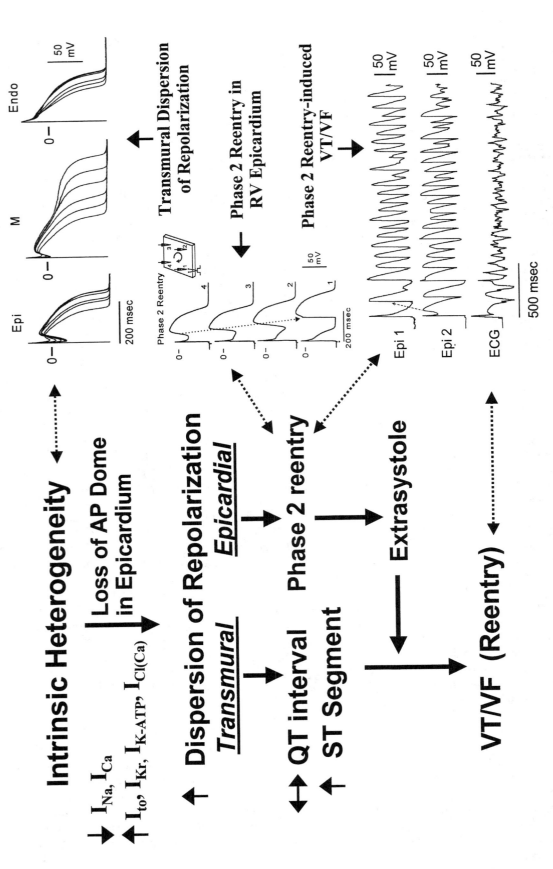

FIGURE 3-10. Proposed cellular and ionic mechanisms for the Brugada syndrome. (**Inset,** adapted from Lukas A, Antzelevitch C. Phase 2 reentry as a mechanism of initiation of circus movement reentry in canine epicardium exposed to simulated ischemia: the antiarrhythmic effects of 4-aminopyridine. *Cardiovasc Res* 1996;32:593–603, with permission.)

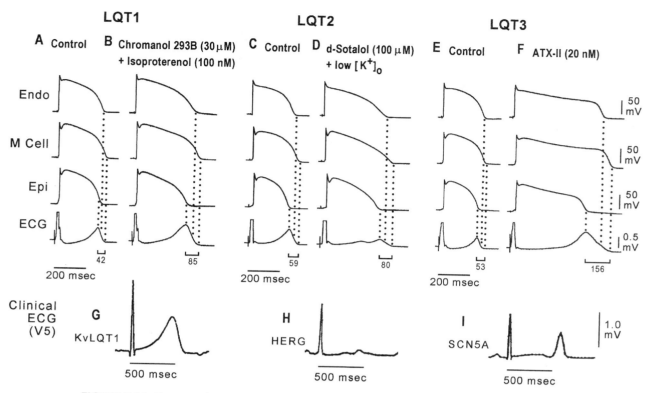

FIGURE 3-11. Transmembrane action potentials and transmural electrocardiograms (ECG) in the LQT1 (**A** and **B**), LQT2 (**C** and **D**), and LQT3 (**E** and **F**) models (arterially perfused canine left ventricular wedge preparations) and clinical ECG lead V₅ of patients with LQT1 (*KvLQT1* defect) (**G**), LQT2 (*HERG* defect) (**H**), and LQT3 (*SCN5A* defect) (**I**) syndromes. Isoproterenol + chromanol 293B (an I_{Ks} blocker), d-sotalol + low [K⁺]ₒ, and ATX-II (an agent that slows inactivation of late I_{Na}) are used to mimic the LQT1, LQT2, and LQT3 syndromes, respectively. **A** to **F**: Action potentials are simultaneously recorded from endocardial (Endo), M, and epicardial (Epi) sites together with a transmural ECG. The basic cyle length (BCL) = 2,000 ms. In all cases, the peak of the T wave in the ECG is coincident with the repolarization of the epicardial action potential, whereas the end of the T wave is coincident with the repolarization of the M cell action potential. Repolarization of the endocardial cell is intermediate between that of the M cell and epicardial cell. Transmural dispersion of repolarization across the ventricular wall, defined as the difference in the repolarization time between M and epicardial cells, is denoted below the ECG traces. **B**: Isoproterenol (100 nM) in the presence of chromanol 293B (30 μM) produced a preferential prolongation of the APD of the M, resulting in an accentuated transmural dispersion of repolarization and broad-based T waves as commonly seen in LQT1 patients (**G**). **D**: d-Sotalol (100 μM) in the presence of low potassium (2 mM) gives rise to low-amplitude T waves with a notched or bifurcated appearance caused by a significant slowing of repolarization as commonly seen in LQT2 patients (**H**). **F**: ATX-II (20 nM) markedly prolongs the QT interval, widens the T wave, and causes a sharp rise in the dispersion of repolarization. ATX-II also produces a marked delay in onset of the T wave because of relatively large effects of the drug on the action potential duration of epicardium and endocardium, consistent with the late-appearing T-wave pattern observed in LQT3 patients (**I**). (Adapted from references Shimizu W, Antzelevitch C. Sodium channel block with mexiletine is effective in reducing dispersion of repolarization and preventing torsade de pointes in LQT2 and LQT3 models of the long-QT syndrome. *Circulation* 1997;96:2038–2047 and from Shimizu W, Antzelevitch C. Cellular basis for the electrocardiographic features of the LQT1 form of the long QT syndrome: effects of β-adrenergic agonists, antagonists and sodium channel blockers on transmural dispersion of repolarization and torsade de pointes. *Circulation* 1998;98:2314–2322, with permission.)

interval characteristics of LQT1. The development of torsade de pointes in the model requires β-adrenergic stimulation, consistent with a high sensitivity of congenital LQTS (LQT1 in particular) to sympathetic stimulation (143, 148–151).

The I_{Kr} blocker, d-sotalol, was used to mimic LQT2 and the most common form of acquired (drug-induced) LQTS. A greater prolongation of the M cell action potential and slowing of phase 3 of the action potential of all three cell types results in a low-amplitude T wave, long QT interval, large TDR, and development of spontaneous and stimulation-induced torsade de pointes. The addition of hypokalemia gives rise to low-amplitude T waves with a deeply notched or bifurcated appearance, similar to those commonly seen in patients with the LQT2 syndrome (108,115). Isoproterenol further exaggerates transmural dispersion of repolarization, increasing the incidence of torsade de pointes (152).

ATXII, a sea anemone toxin that increases late I_{Na}, was used to mimic LQT3 (108). ATXII markedly prolongs the QT interval, delays the onset of the T wave (in some cases also widening it), and produces a sharp rise in TDR as a result of a greater prolongation of the APD of the M cell. The differential effect of ATXII to prolong the M cell action potential probably results from the presence of a larger late sodium current in the M cell (92). ATXII pro-

duces a marked delay in onset of the T wave because of a relatively large effect of the drug on epicardial and endocardial APD. This feature is consistent with the late-appearing T wave (long isoelectric ST segment) observed in patients with the LQT3 syndrome. In agreement with the clinical presentation of LQT3, the model displays a steep rate dependence of the QT interval and develops torsade de pointes at slow rates. β-Adrenergic influence in the form of isoproterenol reduces transmural dispersion of repolarization by abbreviating the APD of the M cell more than that of epicardium or endocardium and by reducing the incidence of torsade de pointes. Whereas the β-adrenergic blocker propranolol is protective in LQT1 and LQT2 wedge models, it has the opposite effects in LQT3, acting to amplify transmural dispersion and promoting torsade de pointes (152).

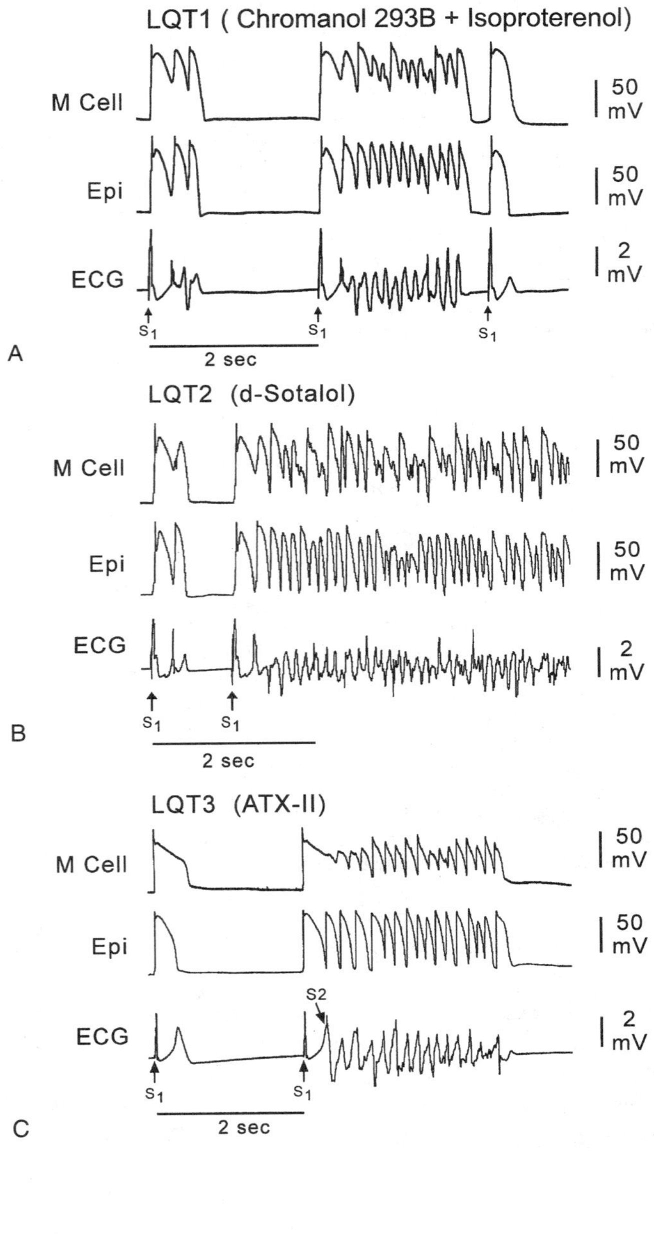

FIGURE 3-12. Polymorphic ventricular tachycardia displaying features of torsade de pointes (TdP) in the LQT1 (**A**), LQT2 (**B**), and LQT3 (**C**) models (arterially perfused canine left ventricular wedge preparations). Isoproterenol + chromanol 293B, d-sotalol, and ATX-II are used to mimic the three long QT syndromes, respectively. Each trace shows action potentials simultaneously recorded from M and epicardial (Epi) cells together with a transmural electrocardiogram. The preparation was paced from the endocardial surface at a basic cycle length (BCL) of 2,000 ms (S₁). **A** and **B:** Spontaneous torsade de pointes is induced in the LQT1 and LQT2 models, respectively. In both models, the first groupings show spontaneous ventricular premature beat (or couplets) that fail to induce torsade de pointes, and a second grouping shows spontaneous premature beats that succeed. The premature response appears to originate in the deep subendocardium (M or Purkinje). **C:** Programmed electrical stimulation-induces torsade de pointes in the LQT3 model. ATX-II produced significant dispersion of repolarization (first grouping). A single extrastimulus (S₂) applied to the epicardial surface at an S₁-S₂ interval of 320 ms initiates torsade de pointes (second grouping). (Adapted from references Shimizu W, Antzelevitch C. Sodium channel block with mexiletine is effective in reducing dispersion of repolarization and preventing torsade de pointes in LQT2 and LQT3 models of the long-QT syndrome. *Circulation* 1997;96:2038–2047 and from Shimizu W, Antzelevitch C. Cellular basis for the electrocardiographic features of the LQT1 form of the long QT syndrome: effects of β-adrenergic agonists, antagonists and sodium channel blockers on transmural dispersion of repolarization and torsade de pointes. *Circulation* 1998; 98:2314–2322, with permission.)

Torsade de pointes is a life-threatening, atypical, polymorphic VT commonly associated with LQTS. Torsade de pointes has been reported in patients receiving potassium channel blockers such as d-sotalol and quinidine, usually at slow heart rates or after long pauses. These conditions are similar to those under which these agents induce EADs and triggered activity in isolated Purkinje fibers and M cells, suggesting a role for EAD-induced triggered activity in the genesis of torsade de pointes. Although EADs may underlie the premature beat that initiates torsade de pointes, studies provide evidence in support of circus movement reentry as the mechanism responsible for the maintenance of the arrhythmia (97,100,108,109,113,115,144,147,153,154). In the wedge, torsade de pointes develops spontaneously in all three models and can be readily induced by introduction of a single premature beat to the epicardial surface (the site of earliest repolarization) (Fig. 3-12).

The available data support the hypothesis outlined in Figure 3-13. The hypothesis presumes the presence of electrical heterogeneity, principally in the form of TDR, under baseline conditions. The intrinsic heterogeneity is amplified by agents that decrease net repolarizing current by reducing I_{Kr} or I_{Ks} or augmenting late I_{Ca} or late I_{Na} or by ion channel mutations that affect these currents and are responsible for the various forms of LQTS. I_{Kr} blockers and LQT2 mutations or late I_{Na} promoters and LQT3 mutations produce a preferential prolongation of the M cell action potential. As a consequence, the QT interval prolongs and is accompanied by a dramatic increase in transmural dispersion of repolarization, which creates a vulnerable window for the development of reentry. The decrease in net repolarizing current can also give rise to EAD-induced triggered activity in M and Purkinje cells that is responsible for the extrasystole that triggers torsade de pointes. β-Adrenergic

agonists further amplify transmural heterogeneity (transiently) in the case of I_{Kr} and LQT2 but reduce it in the case of late I_{Na} enhancers or LQT3 (152). I_{Ks} blockers or LQT1 mutations cause a homogeneous prolongation of APD throughout the ventricular wall, leading to a prolongation of the QT interval but with no increase in transmural dispersion of repolarization. Under these conditions, torsade de pointes does not occur spontaneously, nor can it be induced by programmed stimulation until a β-adrenergic agonist is introduced. Isoproterenol dramatically increases transmural dispersion under these conditions by abbreviating the APD of epicardium and endocardium, creating a vulnerable window that an EAD- or DAD-induced triggered response can capture to generate torsade de pointes, a circus movement arrhythmia. Data from our laboratory suggest that DAD-induced triggered beats may be involved in the initiation of torsade de pointes in LQT1. I_{Ks} block, alone or in combination with β-adrenergic stimulation, did not induce EADs in epicardium, M cell, endocardium, or Purkinje fibers. However, the combination readily produces DAD and DAD-induced triggered activity in ventricular working myocardium (155).

Slow or Delayed Conduction

Slow or delayed impulse conduction can facilitate the development of reentrant arrhythmias by reducing the wavelength of the reentering wavefront so that it can be accommodated by the available pathlength. A number of factors determine the velocity at which an action potential propagates through cardiac tissue. Among these is the intensity of the fast inward sodium current that flows during the upstroke of the action potential and the axial resistance to the flow of local circuit current.

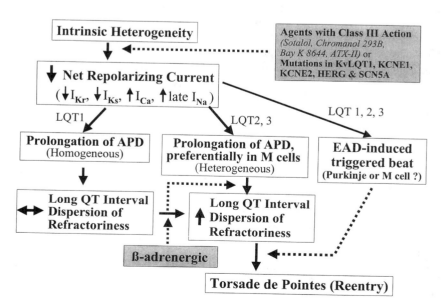

FIGURE 3-13. Proposed cellular and ionic mechanisms for the long QT syndrome.

Discontinuities in conduction can give rise to apparently very slow conduction and reentry in cardiac tissues by allowing for the development of prominent step delays in the transmission of impulses at discrete sites. Any agent or situation capable of suppressing the active generator properties of cardiac tissues may diminish excitability to the point of rendering a localized region functionally inexcitable and creating a discontinuity in the propagation of the advancing wavefront. Examples include an ion-free, ischemic, or high K^+ environment (60,61,63,68,69), as well as electrical blocking current (66,156,157), localized pressure (68,158), and localized cooling (158). Inhibition of the inward currents using sodium or calcium blockers (or both) can also create discontinuities in conduction when applied to localized segments (61).

Very slow conduction encountered under these conditions is caused by the development of major step delays caused by electrotonically mediated (saltatory) transmission of impulses across a functionally inexcitable zone (i.e., across a large cumulative axial resistance imposed between two excitable regions) rather than to a uniform or homogeneous slowing of impulse propagation (159) (Fig. 3-7). The functionally inexcitable zone effectively diminishes the electrical coupling between the excitable regions participating in the conduction of the impulse. The decay of the wavefront as it courses the inexcitable or refractory zone leads to slow activation of the tissue beyond and to a step delay in the conduction of the impulse. The resistive barriers created are not very different from those observed in anisotropy (160). With either condition, small changes in the effective impedance to the flow of local circuit current from one excitable element to the next can cause major delays in conduction. Conduction delays on the order of tens or hundreds of milliseconds occur when the electrotonic communication between the region already activated (i.e., source) and the region awaiting activation (i.e., sink) is weak. With progressive electrical uncoupling of the source and sink, conduction characteristics become progressively more sensitive to changes in the active and passive membrane properties of both the source and sink (70). Although the importance of the intensity of the source current, as reflected by the action potential amplitude, duration, or maximum rate of rise, $(dV/dt)_{max}$, is well appreciated (70,161–163), several studies suggest that under a variety of conditions the threshold current requirement of the sink (i.e. changes in excitability) (68,70,163) may be a more critical determinant of conduction delay or block.

Step delays of impulse conduction associated with electrotonic prepotentials have been observed in intracellular recordings obtained from human and animal infarcted myocardium (10,75,164,165). Extracellular mapping experiments also have uncovered step delays in the propagation of impulses in canine hearts subjected to acute regional myocardial ischemia (166). These studies lend support to an electrotonic interaction across a high impedance barrier as a mechanism responsible for apparently slow conduction.

Nonuniform recovery of refractoriness and geometric factors also play an important role in determining impulse conduction velocity and the success or failure of conduction. Disparity in the recovery of refractoriness has already been discussed as the basis for unidirectional block or the lines of block that develop in response to premature extrasystoles. Disparity of local refractoriness can also contribute to a major slowing of impulse propagation and to reentry (97,128,159,167).

The effect of geometry on impulse conduction has been the subject of considerable study. Regions at which the cross-sectional area of interconnected cells increases abruptly are potential sites for the development of unidirectional block or delayed conduction because of an impedance mismatch. Slowing or block of conduction occurs when the impulse propagates in the direction of increasing diameter because the local circuit current provided by the advancing wavefront is insufficient or barely sufficient to charge the capacity of the larger volume of tissue ahead and bring the larger mass to its threshold potential. The Purkinje-muscle junction is an example of a site at which unidirectional block and conduction delays are observed (168–170). The preexcitation (Wolff-Parkinson-White) syndrome is another example, in which a thin bundle of tissue, the Kent bundle, inserts into a larger ventricular mass.

ABNORMAL IMPULSE FORMATION

Normal Automaticity

Automaticity is defined as the ability of cardiac cells to generate spontaneous action potentials. Spontaneous activity is the result of diastolic depolarization caused by a net inward current flowing during phase 4 of the action potential that progressively brings the membrane potential to threshold. The sinoatrial (SA) node normally displays the highest intrinsic rate. All other pacemakers are referred to as subsidiary or latent pacemakers, because they take over the function of initiating excitation of the heart only when the SA node is compromised or when impulses of SA nodal origin fail to propagate.

The ionic mechanisms underlying normal SA node and Purkinje fibers automaticity include a hyperpolarization-activated inward current (I_f) (171,172) and decay of outward potassium current (I_K) (173,174). The contribution of I_f and I_K differs in SA or atrioventricular (AV) nodes and Purkinje fiber because of the different potential ranges of these two pacemaker types (i.e., -70 to -35 mV and -90 to -65 mV, respectively). The contribution of other voltage-dependent currents may be different as well. For example, I_{Ca} participates in the late phase of diastolic depolarization in the SA and AV nodes but not in Purkinje fibers. The action potential upstroke is provided largely by the fast sodium current in His-Purkinje system and predominantly by the slow calcium current in SA and AV nodes.

Sympathetic and parasympathetic influences and extracellular potassium levels modulate the rate of diastolic depolarization. In general, β-adrenergic receptor stimulation increases but muscarinic receptor stimulation reduces the rate of phase 4 depolarization. In the His-Purkinje system, parasympathetic effects are less apparent than those of the sympathetic system. Although acetylcholine produces little in the way of a direct effect, it can significantly reduce Purkinje automaticity by means of inhibition of the sympathetic influence, a phenomenon called *accentuated antagonism* (175). In all pacemaker cells, increased extracellular potassium concentration reduces the rate of diastolic depolarization, and decreased extracellular potassium has the opposite effect.

Abnormal Automaticity

Abnormal automaticity or depolarization-induced automaticity is observed under conditions of reduced resting membrane potential, such as ischemia, infarction, or other depolarizing influences (i.e., current injection) (Fig. 3-14). Abnormal automaticity is experimentally observed in tissues that normally develop diastolic depolarization (i.e., Purkinje fiber) and in those that normally do not display this feature (i.e., ventricular or atrial working myocardium). Compared with normal automaticity, abnormal automaticity in Purkinje fibers or ventricular and atrial myocardium is more readily suppressed by calcium channel blockers and shows little to no overdrive suppression (176,177). The ionic basis for diastolic depolarization in abnormal automaticity may be similar to that of normal automaticity in SA and AV nodes, consisting of a time-dependent decay of I_K with progressive activation of I_{Ca} (178,179).

The rate of abnormal automaticity is substantially higher than that of normal automaticity and is a sensitive function of resting membrane potential (i.e., the more depolarized the resting potential, the faster the rate). Similar to normal automaticity, abnormal automaticity is enhanced by β-

adrenergic agonists and by reduction of external potassium (176,178).

Automaticity as a Mechanism of Cardiac Arrhythmias

Enhanced normal automaticity can be the cause of some, usually benign, cardiac arrhythmias, including sinus tachycardia. Accelerated idioventricular rhythms have been attributed to enhanced normal automaticity in the His-Purkinje system (180). Although automaticity is not responsible for most rapid tachyarrhythmias, it can precipitate or trigger reentrant arrhythmias. The rate of automatic discharge recorded in isolated tissue under artificial experimental conditions may not be representative of the discharge rate to be expected *in vivo*, where endogenous factors such as catecholamines, histamine, and endothelin-1 and other factors such as stretch may accelerate automaticity.

Overall, the role of automaticity in experimental and clinical arrhythmias *in vivo* is not well defined. Although experimental and clinical three-dimensional mapping studies have shown that ventricular arrhythmias arising under conditions of acute ischemia, infarction, heart failure, and other cardiomyopathies can be ascribed to focal mechanisms (181–185), it is often difficult to discern between automatic and focal reentrant mechanisms such as reflection, phase 2 reentry, and microreentry.

Several experimental studies suggest a role for automaticity in cardiac arrhythmias. Haissaguerre and coworkers showed that atrial fibrillation can be triggered by rapid automaticity arising in the pulmonary veins (59). Myocytes isolated from failing and hypertrophied animal and human hearts have been shown to manifest diastolic depolarization (186,187) and to possess enhanced I_f pacemaker current (188,189), suggesting that these mechanisms contribute to extrasystolic and tachyarrhythmias arising with these pathologies. It is also noteworthy that atrial tissues isolated from patients with atrial fibrillation exhibit increased I_f mRNA levels (190).

Parasystole and Modulated Parasystole

Latent pacemakers throughout the heart are generally reset by the propagating wavefront initiated by the dominant pacemaker and are therefore unable to activate the heart. An exception to this rule occurs when the pacemaking tissue is somehow protected from the impulse of sinus origin. A region of entrance block arises when cells exhibiting automaticity are surrounded by ischemic, infarcted, or otherwise compromised cardiac tissues that prevent the propagating waveform invading the focus but that permit the spontaneous beat generated within the automatic focus to exit and activate the rest of the myocardium. A pacemaker region exhibiting entrance block and exit conduction defines a parasystolic focus (191).

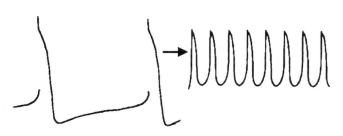

FIGURE 3-14. Transition of normal to abnormal automaticity (i.e., depolarization-induced low-voltage activity) in a Purkinje fiber.

The ectopic activity generated by a parasystolic focus is characterized by premature ventricular complexes with variable coupling intervals, fusion beats, and interectopic intervals that are multiples of a common denominator. This rhythm is relatively uncommon. Although it is usually considered benign, any premature ventricular activation can induce malignant ventricular rhythms in the ischemic myocardium or in the presence of a suitable myocardial substrate.

In the late 1970s and early 1980s, Moe and coworkers described a variant of classic parasystole, which they called *modulated parasystole* (192–194). This variant of the arrhythmia was suggested to result from incomplete entrance block of the parasystolic focus. Electrotonic influences arriving early in the pacemaker cycle delayed and those arriving late in the cycle accelerated the firing of the parasystolic pacemaker, so that ventricular activity could entrain the partially protected pacemaker (Fig. 3-15). As a consequence, at select heart rates, extrasystolic activity generated by the entrained parasystolic pacemaker would mimic reentry, generating extrasystolic activity with fixed coupling (60,62,71,192–200) (Figs. 3-16 and 3-17).

After depolarizations and Triggered Activity

Oscillations that attend or follow the cardiac action potential and depend on preceding transmembrane activity for their manifestation are referred to as *afterdepolarizations* (201). They are generally divided into early (EAD) and delayed (DAD) subclasses. EADs interrupt or retard repolarization during phase 2 or phase 3 (or both) of the cardiac action potential, whereas DADs arise after full repolarization. When an EAD or DAD amplitude suffices to bring the membrane to its threshold potential, a spontaneous action potential referred to as a *triggered response* is the result (202). These triggered events may be responsible for extrasystoles and tachyarrhythmias that develop under conditions predisposing to the development of afterdepolarizations.

Early Afterdepolarizations and Early Afterdepolarization-Induced Triggered Activity

Characteristics of Early Afterdepolarizations and Induced Beats

EADs are observed in isolated cardiac tissues exposed to injury (203), altered electrolytes, hypoxia, acidosis (204, 205), catecholamines (206,207), and pharmacologic agents (208), including antiarrhythmic drugs (209–213). Ventricular hypertrophy and heart failure also predispose to the development of EADs (187,214,215).

EAD characteristics vary as a function of animal species, tissue or cell type, and method by which the response is elicited. Although specific mechanisms of EAD may differ, a critical prolongation of repolarization accompanies most EADs. Figure 3-18 illustrates the two types of EADs generally encountered in Purkinje fiber. Oscillatory events appearing at potentials positive to −30 mV are generally referred to as phase 2 EADs. Those occurring at more negative potentials are called phase 3 EADs. Phase 2 and phase 3 EADs sometimes appear in the same preparation. The right panels show that triggered responses develop when the preparations are paced at slower rates (212). In contrast to Purkinje fibers, EAD activity recorded in ventricular preparations is always phase 2 EADs (100).

EAD-induced triggered activity is sensitive to changes in stimulation rate. Class III agents generally induce EAD activity at slow stimulation rates and totally suppress EADs at rapid rates (212,216). In contrast, β-adrenergic agonist-induced EADs are fast rate dependent (206,207). Studies have shown that, in the presence of I_{Kr} block, β-adrenergic agonists or acceleration from an initially slow rate transiently facilitates induction of EAD activity in ventricular

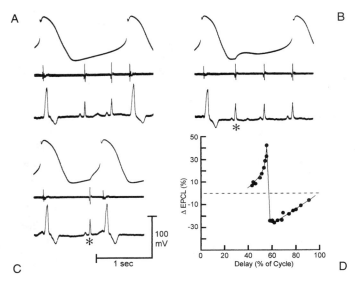

FIGURE 3-15. Electrotonic modulation of a parasystolic pacemaker. Traces were recorded from an experimental model consisting of a sucrose gap preparation *in vitro* coupled to the heart of an open-chest dog. Traces *(top to bottom)*: transmembrane potentials recorded from a distal segment of a Purkinje fiber–sucrose gap preparation and a right ventricular electrogram and electrocardiographic lead II from the *in vivo* preparation. **A:** The Purkinje pacemaker was allowed to beat free of any influence from ventricular activation. **B** and **C:** Pacemaker activity of the Purkinje area is electrotonically influenced by ventricular activation. An electrotonic influence arriving early in the pacemaker cycle delays the next discharge, whereas that arriving late accelerates the next discharge. **D:** The electrotonic modulation of pacemaker discharge is described in the form of a phase-response curve. The percentage change in ectopic pacemaker cycle length (EPCL) is plotted as a function of the temporal position of the electrotonic influence in the pacemaker cycle. (From Antzelevitch C, Bernstein MJ, Feldman HN, Moe GK. Parasystole, reentry, and tachycardia: a canine preparation of cardiac arrhythmias occurring across inexcitable segments of tissue. *Circulation* 1983;68:1101–1115, with permission.)

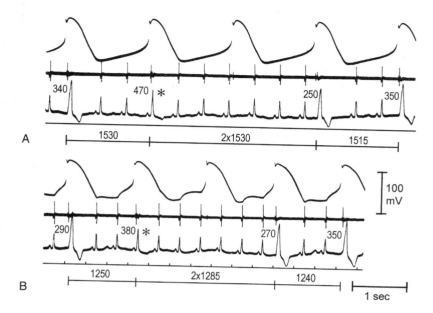

FIGURE 3-16. Patterns of classic parasystole generated by the experimental model described in Figure 3-15 in the absence **(A)** and presence **(B)** of modulating influence from the ventricles. The lowest trace is a stimulus marker. Numbers denote the coupling intervals of the ectopic responses to the preceding normal beats (in milliseconds). Asterisks denote fusion beats. Classic parasystolic features are apparent in both cases. (From Antzelevitch C, Bernstein MJ, Feldman HN, Moe GK. Parasystole, reentry, and tachycardia: a canine preparation of cardiac arrhythmias occurring across inexcitable segments of tissue. *Circulation* 1983;68:1101–1115, with permission.)

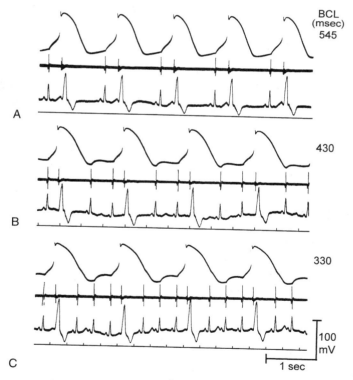

FIGURE 3-17. Records were obtained from the same preparation as in Figure 3-16 but at different cycle lengths. At the basic cycle lengths (BCL) shown, the activity generated was characteristic of reentry (i.e., fixed coupling of the premature beats to the basic beats). **A:** Bigeminy. **B:** Trigeminy. **C:** Quadrigeminy. (From Antzelevitch C, Bernstein MJ, Feldman HN, Moe GK. Parasystole, reentry, and tachycardia: a canine preparation of cardiac arrhythmias occurring across inexcitable segments of tissue. *Circulation* 1983;68:1101–1115, with permission.)

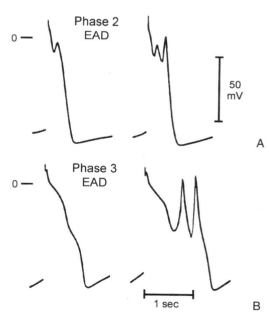

FIGURE 3-18. Early afterdepolarizations (EAD) and triggered activity. Each panel shows intracellular activity recorded from a Purkinje preparation pretreated with quinidine. Left panels depict responses displaying only EADs; right panels show responses manifesting triggered activity. **A:** EAD and triggered activity occurring at the plateau level (phase 2). **B:** EAD and triggered activity occurring during phase 3. (Adapted from Davidenko JM, Cohen L, Goodrow RJ, Antzelevitch C. Quinidine-induced action potential prolongation, early afterdepolarizations, and triggered activity in canine Purkinje fibers: effects of stimulation rate, potassium, and magnesium. *Circulation* 1989;79:674–686, with permission.)

M cells, although not in epicardium or endocardium and rarely in Purkinje fibers (111). This biphasic effect is thought to be caused by an initial priming of I_{Na-Ca}, which provides electrogenic inward current to sustain the action potential plateau, followed by recruitment of cAMP and Ca^{2+}-activated I_{Ks} that abbreviates APD.

Origin of Early Afterdepolarizations

Until about a decade ago, our understanding of the EAD was based largely on data obtained from studies involving Purkinje fiber preparations. With few exceptions (217,218), EADs were not observed in early experiments involving tissues isolated from the surface of the mammalian ventricle (219–222). Later studies showed that, although canine epicardial and endocardial tissues generally fail to develop EADs when exposed to APD-prolonging agents, mid-myocardial M cells readily develop EAD activity under these conditions (223). Failure of epicardial and endocardial tissues to develop EADs has been ascribed to the presence of a strong I_{Ks} in these cells (91). M cells have a weak I_{Ks} (91), predisposing them to the development of EADs in the presence of I_{Kr} block.

I_{Ks} block with chromanol 293B does not induce EAD in any of the four ventricular cell types (155). However, a combination of I_{Ks} and I_{Kr} block (i.e., chromanol 293B plus E-4031 or sotalol) induces EAD activity in canine isolated epicardial and endocardial tissues (224) and in perfused left ventricular wedge preparations. The predisposition of cardiac cells to the development of EADs depends principally on the reduced availability of I_{Kr} and I_{Ks}, as occurs in many forms of cardiomyopathy. Under these conditions, EADs can appear in any part of the ventricular myocardium.

Three-dimensional mapping of torsade de pointes arrhythmias in canine experimental models suggests that the extrasystole that initiates torsade de pointes can originate from subendocardial, mid-myocardium, or subepicardial regions of the left ventricle (109,225). These data point to Purkinje fibers and M cells as the principal sources of EAD-induced triggered activity *in vivo*. In the presence of combined I_{Kr} and I_{Ks} block, epicardium is often the first to develop an EAD.

Ionic Mechanisms Underlying Early Afterdepolarizations

EADs are usually associated with a prolongation of the repolarization phase because of a reduction of net outward current secondary to an increase in inward currents or decrease of outward currents. Most pharmacologic interventions associated with EADs can be grouped as acting predominantly through one of four different mechanisms:

1. A reduction of repolarizing potassium currents (e.g., I_{Kr}, class Ia and III antiarrhythmic agents; I_{Ks}, chromanol 293B)
2. An increase in the availability of calcium current (i.e., I_{Ca})
3. An increase in the sodium-calcium exchange current because of augmentation of intracellular calcium activity or upregulation of the exchanger (e.g., Bay K 8644, catecholamines)
4. An increase in late sodium current (i.e., late I_{Na}) (e.g., aconitine, anthopleurin-A, ATXII)

Combinations of these interventions (e.g., calcium loading plus I_{Kr} reduction) may act synergistically to facilitate the development of EADs (111,222,226,227).

The upstroke of the EAD usually is carried by calcium current. There is less agreement on the ionic basis for the critically important conditional phase of the EAD, defined as the period just before the EAD upstroke. Intracellular calcium levels and Na-Ca exchange current play a pivotal role in the conditional phase of isoproterenol-induced EADs (152,206,207). Data from several groups of investigators suggest that intracellular calcium levels do not influence the formation of this phase 2 EAD (218,228–230), whereas other groups have presented strong evidence in support of the influence of intracellular calcium levels in the formation of at least the conditional phase of the EAD (111,231). This discrepancy is in part caused by the type of tissues or cells studied.

There are major differences in the ionic mechanisms of EAD generation in canine Purkinje fibers and ventricular M cells. EADs induced in the canine M cells are exquisitely sensitive to change in intracellular calcium levels, whereas EADs elicited in Purkinje are largely insensitive (111,232). Ryanodine, an agent known to block calcium release from the sarcoplasmic reticulum (SR), abolishes EAD activity in canine M cells, but not in Purkinje fibers (232). These distinctions may reflect differences in intracellular calcium handling in M cells, in which the SR is well developed, compared with Purkinje fibers, in which the SR is poorly developed.

Early Afterdepolarizations-Induced Triggered Activity as a Cause of Arrhythmia

EAD-induced triggered activity is thought to be involved in precipitating torsade de pointes under conditions of congenital and acquired LQTSs (145,233). EAD-like deflections have been observed in ventricular MAP recordings immediately preceding torsade de pointes arrhythmias in the clinic and in experimental models of LQTS (220,234–237).

EAD activity may also be involved in the genesis of cardiac arrhythmias in cases of hypertrophy and heart failure. These syndromes are commonly associated with prolongation of the ventricular action potential, which predisposes to the development of EADs (186,187,214,215,238–240).

Delayed Afterdepolarization-Induced Triggered Activity

DADs are oscillations of transmembrane activity that occur after full repolarization of the action potential and depend on previous activation of the cell for their manifestation. DADs that reach the threshold potential give rise to spontaneous responses also referred to as triggered activity (202).

Causes and Origin of Delayed Afterdepolarization-Induced Triggered Activity

DADs and DAD-induced triggered activity are generally observed under conditions that cause large increases in intracellular calcium, $[Ca^{2+}]_i$, such as after high levels of cardiac glycosides (e.g., digitalis) (241–243) or catecholamines (206,244–246). This activity also occurs in hypertrophied and failing hearts (186,214) and in Purkinje fibers surviving myocardial infarction (161). In contrast to EADs, DADs are always induced at relatively rapid rates.

Digitalis-induced DADs and triggered activity have been well characterized in isolated Purkinje fibers (202). In the ventricular myocardium, they are rarely observed in epicardial or endocardial tissues, but they are readily induced in cells and tissues from the M region. However, DADs are frequently observed in myocytes enzymatically dissociated from ventricular myocardium (247–249). Digitalis, isoproterenol, high $[Ca^{2+}]_o$, or Bay K 8644, a calcium agonist,

have been shown to cause DADs and triggered activity in tissues isolated from the M region but not in epicardial or endocardial tissues (89,102,155,223) (Fig. 3-19). The failure of epicardial and endocardial cells to develop DADs has been ascribed to a high density of I_{Ks} in these tissues (91) compared with M cells, in which I_{Ks} is small (91). Reduction of I_{Ks} promoted isoproterenol-induced DAD activity in canine and guinea pig endocardium and epicardium (155,250).

Any intervention capable of altering intracellular calcium by modifying transsarcolemmal calcium current or by inhibiting sarcoplasmic reticulum storage or release of calcium can affect the DAD manifestation. DADs can also be modified by interventions capable of directly inhibiting or enhancing I_{ti}. DADs are modified by extracellular K^+, Ca^{2+}, lisophosphoglycerides, and metabolic factors such as ATP, hypoxia, and pH. Lowering extracellular K^+ (<4 mM) promotes DADs, and increasing K^+ attenuates or totally suppresses DADs (202,251). Lysophosphatidylcholine, in concentrations similar to those that accumulate in ischemic myocardium, have been shown to induce DAD activity (252). Elevating extracellular Ca^{2+} promotes DADs (202),

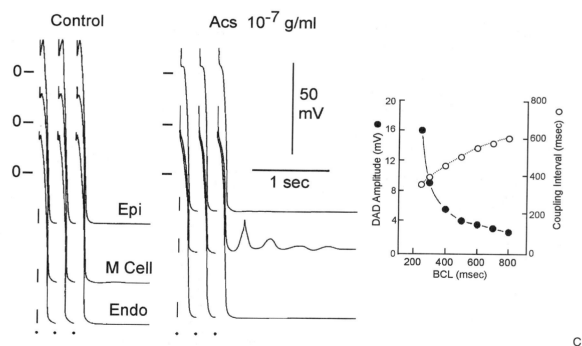

FIGURE 3-19. Digitalis-induced delayed afterdepolarizations in M cells but not epicardium or endocardium. Effects of acetylstrophanthidin (AcS) on transmembrane activity of epicardial (Epi), endocardial (Endo), and M cell preparations ($[K^+]_o = 4$ mM). **A:** Control. **B:** Recorded after 90 minutes of exposure to 10^{-7} g/mL of AcS. Each panel shows the last 3 beats of a train of 10 basic beats elicited at a basic cycle length (BCL) of 250 ms. Each train is followed by a 3-second pause. AcS induced prominent delayed afterdepolarizations (DADs) in the M cell preparation but not in epicardium or endocardium. **C:** Rate dependence of the coupling interval and amplitude of the AcS-induced DADs. Measured is the first DAD recorded from the M cell. (From Sicouri S, Antzelevitch C. Afterdepolarizations and triggered activity develop in a select population of cells (M cells) in canine ventricular myocardium: the effects of acetylstrophanthidin and Bay K 8644. *Pacing Clin Electrophysiol* 1991;14:1714–1720, with permission.)

and an increase of extracellular ATP potentiates isoproterenol-induced DAD (253).

Agents that prolong repolarization such as quinidine and clofilium facilitate the induction of DAD activity by augmenting calcium entry. Calcium calmodulin kinase can facilitate the induction of DADs by augmenting I_{Ca} (254).

Pharmacologic agents that affect the release and reuptake of calcium by the SR, including caffeine and ryanodine, also influence the manifestation of DADs and triggered activity. Low concentrations of caffeine facilitate Ca^{2+} release from the SR and contribute to the augmentation of DAD and triggered activity. High concentrations of caffeine prevent Ca^{2+} uptake by the SR and abolish I_{ti}, DADs, aftercontractions, and triggered activity. Doxorubicin, an anthracycline antibiotic, is effective in suppressing digitalis-induced DADs, possibly through inhibition of the Na-Ca exchange mechanism (255). Potassium channel activators such as pinacidil can also suppress DAD and triggered activity by activating ATP-regulated potassium current (I_{K-ATP}) (102,248).

Ionic Mechanisms Underlying Delayed Afterdepolarizations

DADs and accompanying aftercontractions are thought to be caused by oscillatory release of calcium from the SR under calcium overload conditions. The afterdepolarization is thought to be induced by a transient inward current (I_{ti}) generated by a nonselective cationic current (I_{ns}) (256,257), activation of an electrogenic Na-Ca exchanger (256,258–260), or calcium-activated Cl^- current (259,260). All occur after the release of Ca^{2+} from the overloaded SR.

Delayed Afterdepolarization-Induced Triggered Activity as a Cause of Arrhythmia

Although a wide variety of studies performed in isolated tissues and cells suggest an important role for DAD-induced triggered activity in the genesis of cardiac arrhythmias, especially bigeminal rhythms and tachyarrhythmias observed in the setting of digitalis toxicity (202), little direct evidence of DAD-induced triggered activity *in vivo* is available. Consequently, even when triggered activity appears a likely mechanism, it is often impossible to completely exclude other mechanisms such as reentry or enhanced automaticity.

Clinical arrhythmias that may be caused by DAD-induced triggered activity include *idiopathic ventricular tachyarrhythmias* (261–264) and *idioventricular rhythms*, which are accelerated AV junctional escape rhythms that occur as a result of digitalis toxicity or in a setting of myocardial infarction. Other possible DAD-mediated arrhythmias include exercise-induced, adenosine-sensitive VT, as described by Lerman and Belardinelli (265); repetitive monomorphic VT caused presumably cAMP-mediated triggered activity (266); supraventricular tachycardias, including arrhythmias originating in the coronary sinus (267); and some heart failure–related arrhythmias (185, 186,240).

ACKNOWLEDGMENTS

This work was supported by grants from the National Institutes of Health (HL 47678); the American Heart Association, New York State Affiliate; and the Masons of New York State and Florida.

REFERENCES

1. Mayer AG. *Rhythmical pulsations in scyphomedusae.* Publication 47. Pittsburg: Carnegie Institute, 1906:1–62.
2. Mayer AG. *Rhythmical pulsations in scyphomedusae. II.* Publication 102. Pittsburg: Carnegie Institute, 1908:115–131.
3. Mines GR. On dynamic equilibrium in the heart. *J Physiol* 1913;46:349–382.
4. Mines GR. On circulating excitations in heart muscles and their possible relation to tachycardia and fibrillation. *Trans R Soc Can* 1914;8:43–52.
5. Lewis T. The broad features and time-relations of the normal electrocardiogram: principles of interpretation. In: *The mechanism and graphic registration of the heart beat.* London: Shaw & Sons, 1925:44–77.
6. Moe GK. Evidence for reentry as a mechanism for cardiac arrhythmias. *Rev Physiol Biochem Pharmacol* 1975;72:55–81.
7. Kulbertus HE. .In: Kulbertus HE, ed. *Reentrant arrhythmias, mechanisms and treatment.* Baltimore: University Park Press, 1977.
8. Wit AL, Cranefield PF. Re-entrant excitation as a cause of cardiac arrhythmias. *Am J Physiol* 1978;235:H1–H17.
9. Wit AL, Allessie MA, Fenoglic JJ Jr, et al. Significance of the endocardial and epicardial border zones in the genesis of myocardial infarction arrhythmias. In: Harrison D, ed. *Cardiac arrhythmias: a decade of progress.* Boston: GK Hall, 1982:39–68.
10. Spear JF, Moore EN. Mechanisms of cardiac arrhythmias. *Annu Rev Physiol* 1982;44:485–497.
11. Janse MJ. Reentry rhythms. In: Fozzard HA, Haber E, Jennings RB, et al, eds. The heart and cardiovascular system. New York: Raven Press, 1986:1203–1238.
12. Hoffman BF, Dangman KH. Mechanisms for cardiac arrhythmias. *Experientia* 1987;43:1049–1056.
13. Antzelevitch C. Reflection as a mechanism of reentrant cardiac arrhythmias. *Prog Cardiol* 1988;1:3–16.
14. El-Sherif N. Reentry revisited. *Pacing Clin Electrophysiol* 1988;11:1358–1368.
15. Lazzara R, Scherlag BJ. Generation of arrhythmias in myocardial ischemia and infarction. *Am J Cardiol* 1988;61:20A-26A.
16. Rosen MR. The links between basic and clinical cardiac electrophysiology. *Circulation* 1988;77:251–63.
17. Kent AFS. Observation on the auriculo-ventricular junction of the mammalian heart. *Q J Exp Physiol* 1913;7:193–197.
18. Schmitt FO, Erlanger J. Directional differences in the conduction of the impulse through heart muscle and their possible relation to extrasystolic and fibrillary contractions. *Am J Physiol* 1928;87:326–347.
19. Cranefield PF, Hoffman BF. Conduction of the cardiac impulse. II. Summation and inhibition. *Circ Res* 1971;28:220–233.
20. Cranefield PF, Klein HO, Hoffman BF. Conduction of the car-

diac impulse. I. Delay, block and one-way block in depressed Purkinje fibers. *Circ Res* 1971;28:199–219.

21. Sasyniuk BI, Mendez C. A mechanism for reentry in canine ventricular tissue. *Circ Res* 1971;28:3–15.

22. Wit AL, Cranefield PF, Hoffman BF. Slow conduction and reentry in the ventricular conducting system. II. Single and sustained circus movement in networks of canine and bovine Purkinje fibers. *Circ Res* 1972;30:11–22.

23. Wit AL, Hoffman BF, Cranefield PF. Slow conduction and reentry in the ventricular conducting system. I. Return extrasystoles in canine Purkinje fibers. *Circ Res* 1972;30:1–10.

24. Cranefield PF. *The conduction of the cardiac impulse.* Mount Kisco, NY: Futura Publishing, 1975:153.

25. Garrey WE. Auricular fibrillation. *Physiol Rev* 1924; 4: 215–250.

26. Allessie MA, Bonke FIM, Schopman JG. Circus movement in rabbit atrial muscle as a mechanism of tachycardia. *Circ Res* 1973;33:54–62.

27. Allessie MA, Bonke FIM, Schopman JG. Circus movement in rabbit atrial muscle as a mechanism of tachycardia: II. The role of nonuniform recovery of excitability in the occurrence of unidirectional block as studied with multiple microelectrodes. *Circ Res* 1976;39:168–177.

28. Allessie MA, Bonke FIM, Schopman JG. Circus movement in rabbit atrial muscle as a mechanism of tachycardia. III. The "leading circle" concept: a new model of circus movement in cardiac tissue without the involvement of an anatomic obstacle. *Circ Res* 1977;41:9–18.

29. Kamiyama A, Eguchi K, Shibayama R. Circus movement tachycardia induced by a single premature stimulus on the ventricular sheet: evaluation of the leading circle hypothesis in the canine ventricular muscle. *Jpn Circ J* 1986;50:65–73.

30. Allessie MA, Schalij MJ, Kirchhof CJ, et al. Experimental electrophysiology and arrhythmogenicity: anisotropy and ventricular tachycardia. *Eur Heart J* 1989;10[Suppl E]:2–8.

31. El-Sherif N, Smith RA, Evans K. Canine ventricular arrhythmias in the late myocardial infarction period. 8. Epicardial mapping of reentrant circuits. *Circ Res* 1981; 49:255–265.

32. El-Sherif N, Mehra R, Gough WB, Zeiler RH. Ventricular activation pattern of spontaneous and induced ventricular rhythms in canine one-day-old myocardial infarction: evidence for focal and reentrant mechanisms. *Circ Res* 1982;51:152–166.

33. Mehra R, Zeiler RH, Gough WB, El-Sherif N. Reentrant ventricular arrhythmias in the late myocardial infarction period. 9. Electrophysiologic-anatomic correlation of reentrant circuits. *Circulation* 1983;67:11–24.

34. El-Sherif N, Mehra R, Gough WB, Zeiler RH. Reentrant ventricular arrhythmias in the late myocardial infarction period: interruption of reentrant circuits by cyrothermal techniques. *Circulation* 1983;68:644–656.

35. Wit AL, Allessie MA, Bonke FIM, et al. Electrophysiological mapping to determine the mechanisms of experimental ventricular tachycardia initiated by premature impulses: experimental approach and initial results demonstrating reentrant excitation. *Am J Cardiol* 1982;49:166–185.

36. Dillon SM, Allessie MA, Ursell PC, Wit AL. Influences of anisotropic tissue structure on reentrant circuits in the epicardial border zone of subacute canine infarcts. *Circ Res* 1988;63:182–206.

37. Clerc L. Directional differences of impulse spread in trabecular muscle from mammalian heart. *J Physiol (Lond)* 1976;255:335–346.

38. Harumi K, Burgess MJ, Abildskov JA. A theoretic model of the T wave. *Circulation* 1966;34:657–668.

39. Spach MS, Kootsey JM, Sloan JD. Active modulation of electrical coupling between cardiac cells of the dog: a mechanism

for transient and steady state variations in conduction velocity. *Circ Res* 1982;51:347–362.

40. El-Sherif N. The figure 8 model of reentrant excitation in the canine post-infarction heart. In: Zipes DP, Jalife J, eds. *Cardiac electrophysiology and arrhythmias.* New York: Grune & Stratton, 1985:363–378.

41. Lin SF, Roth BJ, Wikswo JP Jr. Quatrefoil reentry in myocardium: an optical imaging study of the induction mechanism. *J Cardiovasc Electrophysiol* 1999;10:574–586.

42. Weiner N, Rosenblueth A. The mathematical formulation of the problem of conduction of impulses in a network of connected excitable elements, specifically in cardiac muscle. *Arch Inst Cardiol Mex* 1946;16:205–265.

43. Davidenko JM, Kent PF, Chialvo DR, et al. Sustained vortex-like waves in normal isolated ventricular muscle. *Proc Natl Acad Sci U S A* 1990;87:8785–8789.

44. Pertsov AM, Davidenko JM, Salomonsz R, et al. Spiral waves of excitation underlie reentrant activity in isolated cardiac muscle. *Circ Res* 1993;72:631–650.

45. Jalife J, Davidenko JM, Michaels DC. A new perspective on the mechanisms of arrhythmias and sudden cardiac death: spiral wave of excitation in heart muscle. *J Cardiovasc Electrophysiol* 1991;2:S133–S152.

46. Athill CA, Ikeda T, Kim YH, et al. Transmembrane potential properties at the core of functional reentrant wave fronts in isolated canine right atria. *Circulation* 1998;98:1556–1567.

47. Jalife J, Delmar M, Davidenko JM, Anumonwo JMB. *Basic cardiac electrophysiology for the clinician.* Armonk, NY: Futura Publishing, 1999.

48. Pertsov AM, Jalife J. Three-dimensional vortex-like reentry. In: Zipes DP, Jalife J, eds. *Cardiac electrophysiology: from cell to bedside.* Philadelphia: WB Saunders, 1995:403–410.

49. Davidenko JM. Spiral wave activity: a possible common mechanism for polymorphic and monomorphic ventricular tachycardias. *J Cardiovasc Electrophysiol* 1993;4:730–746.

50. Garfinkel A, Qu Z. Nonlinear dynamics of excitation and propagation in cardiac muscle. In: Zipes DP, Jalife J, eds. *Cardiac electrophysiology: from cell to bedside.* Philadelphia: WB Saunders, 1999:515–520.

51. Gray RA, Jalife J, Panfilov AV, et al. Mechanisms of cardiac fibrillation [Letter; comment]. *Science* 1995;270:1222–1223.

52. Janse MJ, Wilms-Schopman FJG, Coronel R. Ventricular fibrillation is not always due to multiple wavelet reentry. *J Cardiovasc Electrophysiol* 1995;6:512–521.

53. Antzelevitch C. Ion channels and ventricular arrhythmias: cellular and ionic mechanisms underlying the Brugada syndrome. *Curr Opin Cardiol* 1999;14:274–279.

54. Chen J, Mandapati R, Berenfeld O, et al. High-frequency periodic sources underlie ventricular fibrillation in the isolated rabbit heart. *Circ Res* 2000;86:86–93.

55. Zaitsev AV, Berenfeld O, Mironov SF, et al. Distribution of excitation frequencies on the epicardial and endocardial surfaces of fibrillating ventricular wall of the sheep heart [See comments]. *Circ Res* 2000;86:408–417.

56. Moe GK, Rheinboldt WC, Abildskov JA. A computer model of atrial fibrillation. *Am Heart J* 1964;67:200–220.

57. Allessie MA, Lammers WJEP, Bonke FIM, Hollen J. Experimental evaluation of Moe's multiple wavelet hypothesis of atrial fibrillation. In: Zipes DP, Jalife J, eds. *Cardiac electrophysiology and arrhythmias.* New York: Grune & Stratton, 1985:265–276.

58. Schuessler RB, Grayson TM, Bromberg BI, et al. Cholinergically mediated tachyarrhythmias induced by a single extrastimulus in the isolated canine right atrium. *Circ Res* 1992;71:1254–1267.

59. Haissaguerre M, Jais P, Shah DC, et al. Spontaneous initiation of atrial fibrillation by ectopic beats originating in the pulmonary veins. *N Engl J Med* 1998;339:659–666.

60. Antzelevitch C, Jalife J, Moe GK. Characteristics of reflection as a mechanism of reentrant arrhythmias and its relationship to parasystole. *Circulation* 1980;61:182–191.

61. Antzelevitch C, Moe GK. Electrotonically mediated delayed conduction and reentry in relation to "slow responses" in mammalian ventricular conducting tissue. *Circ Res* 1981;49:1129–1139.

62. Antzelevitch C, Bernstein MJ, Feldman HN, Moe GK. Parasystole, reentry, and tachycardia: a canine preparation of cardiac arrhythmias occurring across inexcitable segments of tissue. *Circulation* 1983;68:1101–1115.

63. Rozanski GJ, Jalife J, Moe GK. Reflected reentry in nonhomogeneous ventricular muscle as a mechanism of cardiac arrhythmias. *Circulation* 1984;69:163–173.

64. Lukas A, Antzelevitch C. Reflected reentry, delayed conduction, and electrotonic inhibition in segmentally depressed atrial tissues. *Can J Physiol Pharmacol* 1989;67:757–764.

65. Davidenko JM, Antzelevitch C. The effects of milrinone on action potential characteristics, conduction, automaticity, and reflected reentry in isolated myocardial fibers. *J Cardiovasc Pharmacol* 1985;7:341–349.

66. Rosenthal JE, Ferrier GR. Contribution of variable entrance and exit block in protected foci to arrhythmogenesis in isolated ventricular tissues. *Circulation* 1983;67:1–8.

67. Antzelevitch C, Lukas A. Reflection and reentry in isolated ventricular tissue. In: Dangman KH, Miura DS, eds. *Basic and clinical electrophysiology of the heart.* New York: Marcel Dekker, 1991:251–257.

68. Antzelevitch C, Moe GK. Electrotonic inhibition and summation of impulse conduction in mammalian Purkinje fibers. *Am J Physiol* 1983;245:H42–H53.

69. Jalife J, Moe GK. Excitation, conduction, and reflection of impulses in isolated bovine and canine cardiac Purkinje fibers. *Circ Res* 1981;49:233–247.

70. Davidenko JM, Antzelevitch C. Electrophysiological mechanisms underlying rate-dependent changes of refractoriness in normal and segmentally depressed canine Purkinje fibers: the characteristics of post- repolarization refractoriness. *Circ Res* 1986;58:257–268.

71. Antzelevitch C. Clinical applications of new concepts of parasystole, reflection, and tachycardia. *Cardiol Clin* 1983;1:39–50.

72. Davidenko JM, Antzelevitch C. The effects of milrinone on conduction, reflection and automaticity in canine Purkinje fibers. *Circulation* 1984;69:1026–1035.

73. Winkle RA. The relationship between ventricular ectopic beat frequency and heart rate. *Circulation* 1982;66:439–446.

74. Nau GJ, Aldariz AE, Acunzo RS, et al. Clinical studies on the mechanism of ventricular arrhythmias. In: Rosenbaum MB, Elizari MV, eds. *Frontier of cardiac electrophysiology.* Amsterdam: Martinus Nijhoff, 1983:239–273.

75. Rosenthal JE. Reflected reentry in depolarized foci with variable conduction impairment in 1 day old infarcted canine cardiac tissue. *J Am Coll Cardiol* 1988;12:404–411.

76. Van Hemel NM, Swenne CA, De Bakker JMT, et al. Epicardial reflection as a cause of incessant ventricular bigeminy. *Pacing Clin Electrophysiol* 1988;11:1036–1044.

77. Litovsky SH, Antzelevitch C. Transient outward current prominent in canine ventricular epicardium but not endocardium. *Circ Res* 1988;62:116–126.

78. Liu DW, Gintant GA, Antzelevitch C. Ionic bases for electrophysiological distinctions among epicardial, midmyocardial, and endocardial myocytes from the free wall of the canine left ventricle. *Circ Res* 1993;72:67–87.

79. Furukawa T, Myerburg RJ, Furukawa N, et al. Differences in transient outward currents of feline endocardial and epicardial myocytes. *Circ Res* 1990;67:1287–1291.

80. Fedida D, Giles WR. Regional variations in action potentials and transient outward current in myocytes isolated from rabbit left ventricle. *J Physiol (Lond)* 1991;442:191–209.

81. Clark RB, Bouchard RA, Salinas-Stefanon E, et al Heterogeneity of action potential waveforms and potassium currents in rat ventricle. *Cardiovasc Res* 1993;27:1795–1799.

82. Wettwer E, Amos GJ, Posival H, Ravens U. Transient outward current in human ventricular myocytes of subepicardial and subendocardial origin. *Circ Res* 1994;75:473–482.

83. Nabauer M, Beuckelmann DJ, Überfuhr P, Steinbeck G. Regional differences in current density and rate-dependent properties of the transient outward current in subepicardial and subendocardial myocytes of human left ventricle. *Circulation* 1996;93:168–177.

84. Zygmunt AC. Intracellular calcium activates chloride current in canine ventricular myocytes. *Am J Physiol* 1994;267:H1984–H1995.

85. Takano M, Noma A. Distribution of the isoprenaline-induced chloride current in rabbit heart. *Pflugers Arch* 1992;420:223–226.

86. Di Diego JM, Sun ZQ, Antzelevitch C. I_{to} and action potential notch are smaller in left vs. right canine ventricular epicardium. *Am J Physiol* 1996;271:H548–H561.

87. Volders PG, Sipido KR, Carmeliet E, et al. Repolarizing K^+ currents I_{TO1} and I_{Ks} are larger in right than left canine ventricular midmyocardium. *Circulation* 1999;99:206–210.

88. Sicouri S, Antzelevitch C. A subpopulation of cells with unique electrophysiological properties in the deep subepicardium of the canine ventricle: the M cell. *Circ Res* 1991;68:1729–1741.

89. Antzelevitch C, Sicouri S, Litovsky SH, et al. Heterogeneity within the ventricular wall: Electrophysiology and pharmacology of epicardial, endocardial and M cells. *Circ Res* 1991;69:1427–1449.

90. Anyukhovsky EP, Sosunov EA, Rosen MR. Regional differences in electrophysiologic properties of epicardium, midmyocardium and endocardium: *in vitro* and *in vivo* correlations. *Circulation* 1996;94:1981–1988.

91. Liu DW, Antzelevitch C. Characteristics of the delayed rectifier current (I_{Kr} and I_{Ks}) in canine ventricular epicardial, midmyocardial and endocardial myocytes: a weaker I_{Ks} contributes to the longer action potential of the M cell. *Circ Res* 1995;76:351–365.

92. Eddlestone GT, Zygmunt AC, Antzelevitch C. Larger late sodium current contributes to the longer action potential of the M cell in canine ventricular myocardium. *Pacing Clin Electrophysiol* 1996;19:II-569(abst).

93. Zygmunt AC, Goodrow RJ, Antzelevitch C. I_{Na-Ca} contributes to electrical heterogeneity within the canine ventricle. *Am J Physiol* 2000;278:H1671–H1678.

94. Brahmajothi MV, Morales MJ, Reimer KA, Strauss HC. Regional localization of ERG, the channel protein responsible for the rapid component of the delayed rectifier, K^+ current in the ferret heart. *Circ Res* 1997;81:128–135.

95. Burashnikov A, Antzelevitch C. Differences in the electrophysiologic response of four canine ventricular cell types to $β_1$-adrenergic agonists. *Cardiovasc Res* 1999;43:901–908.

96. Yan GX, Shimizu W, Antzelevitch C. Characteristics and distribution of M cells in arterially perfused canine left ventricular wedge preparations. *Circulation* 1998;98:1921–1927.

97. Antzelevitch C, Shimizu W, Yan GX, et al. The M cell: its contribution to the ECG and to normal and abnormal electrical function of the heart. *J Cardiovasc Electrophysiol* 1999;10:1124–1152.

98. Sicouri S, Antzelevitch C. Electrophysiologic characteristics of M cells in the canine left ventricular free wall. *J Cardiovasc Electrophysiol* 1995;6:591–603.

99. Sicouri S, Fish J, Antzelevitch C. Distribution of M cells in the canine ventricle. *J Cardiovasc Electrophysiol* 1994;5:824–837.

100. Antzelevitch C, Sicouri S. Clinical relevance of cardiac arrhythmias generated by afterdepolarizations: the role of M cells in the generation of U waves, triggered activity and torsade de pointes. *J Am Coll Cardiol* 1994;23:259–277.

101. Stankovicova T, Szilard M, De Scheerder I, Sipido KR. M cells and transmural heterogeneity of action potential configuration in myocytes from the left ventricular wall of the pig heart. *Cardiovasc Res* 2000;45:952–960.

102. Sicouri S, Antzelevitch C. Drug-induced afterdepolarizations and triggered activity occur in a discrete subpopulation of ventricular muscle cell (M cells) in the canine heart: quinidine and Digitalis. *J Cardiovasc Electrophysiol* 1993;4:48–58.

103. Drouin E, Charpentier F, Gauthier C, et al. Electrophysiological characteristics of cells spanning the left ventricular wall of human heart: Evidence for the presence of M cells. *J Am Coll Cardiol* 1995;26:185–192.

104. Weissenburger J, Nesterenko VV, Antzelevitch C. Transmural heterogeneity of ventricular repolarization under baseline and long QT conditions in the canine heart *in vivo*. Torsades de pointes develops with halothane but not pentobarbital anesthesia. *J Cardiovasc Electrophysiol* 2000;11:290–304.

105. Sicouri S, Quist M, Antzelevitch C. Evidence for the presence of M cells in the guinea pig ventricle. *J Cardiovasc Electrophysiol* 1996;7:503–511.

106. Li GR, Feng J, Yue L, Carrier M. Transmural heterogeneity of action potentials and I_{to1} in myocytes isolated from the human right ventricle. *Am J Physiol* 1998;275:H369–H377.

107. Rodriguez-Sinovas A, Cinca J, Tapias A, et al. Lack of evidence of M-cells in porcine left ventricular myocardium. *Cardiovasc Res* 1997;33:307–313.

108. Shimizu W, Antzelevitch C. Sodium channel block with mexiletine is effective in reducing dispersion of repolarization and preventing torsade de pointes in LQT2 and LQT3 models of the long-QT syndrome. *Circulation* 1997;96:2038–2047.

109. El-Sherif N, Caref EB, Yin H, Restivo M. The electrophysiological mechanism of ventricular arrhythmias in the long QT syndrome: tridimensional mapping of activation and recovery patterns. *Circ Res* 1996;79:474–492.

110. Weirich J, Bernhardt R, Loewen N, et al. Regional- and species-dependent effects of K⁺-channel blocking agents on subendocardium and mid-wall slices of human, rabbit, and guinea pig myocardium. *Pflugers Arch* 1996;431:R-130(abst).

111. Burashnikov A, Antzelevitch C. Acceleration-induced action potential prolongation and early afterdepolarizations. *J Cardiovasc Electrophysiol* 1998;9:934–948.

112. Shimizu W, McMahon B, Antzelevitch C. Sodium pentobarbital reduces transmural dispersion of repolarization and prevents torsade de pointes in models of acquired and congenital long QT syndromes. *J Cardiovasc Electrophysiol* 1999;10:156–164.

113. Shimizu W, Antzelevitch C. Cellular basis for the electrocardiographic features of the LQT1 form of the long QT syndrome: effects of β-adrenergic agonists, antagonists and sodium channel blockers on transmural dispersion of repolarization and torsade de pointes. *Circulation* 1998;98:2314–2322.

114. Shimizu W, Antzelevitch C. Cellular and ionic basis for T wave alternans under long QT conditions. *Circulation* 1999;99:1499–1507.

115. Yan GX, Antzelevitch C. Cellular basis for the normal T wave and the electrocardiographic manifestations of the long QT syndrome. *Circulation* 1998;98:1928–1936.

116. Balati B, Varro A, Papp JG. Comparison of the cellular electrophysiological characteristics of canine left ventricular epicardium, M cells, endocardium and Purkinje fibres [In process citation]. *Acta Physiol Scand* 1998;164:181–190.

117. McIntosh MA, Cobbe SM, Smith GL. Heterogeneous changes in action potential and intracellular Ca^{2+} in left ventricular myocyte sub-types from rabbits with heart failure [In process citation]. *Cardiovasc Res* 2000;45:397–409.

118. Brugada P, Brugada J. Right bundle branch block, persistent ST segment elevation and sudden cardiac death: a distinct clinical and electrocardiographic syndrome: a multicenter report. *J Am Coll Cardiol* 1992;20:1391–1396.

119. Brugada J, Brugada P. Further characterization of the syndrome of right bundle branch block, ST segment elevation, and sudden cardiac death. *J Cardiovasc Electrophysiol* 1997;8:325–331.

120. Brugada J, Brugada R, Brugada P. Right bundle-branch block and ST-segment elevation in leads V_1 through V_3. A marker for sudden death in patients without demonstrable structural heart disease. *Circulation* 1998;97:457–460.

121. Aizawa Y, Tamura M, Chinushi M, et al. Idiopathic ventricular fibrillation and bradycardia-dependent intraventricular block. *Am Heart J* 1993;126:1473–1474.

122. Aizawa Y, Tamura M, Chinushi M, et al. An attempt at electrical catheter ablation of the arrhythmogenic area in idiopathic ventricular fibrillation. *Am Heart J* 1992;123:257–260.

123. Bjerregaard P, Gussak I, Kotar Sl, Gessler JE. Recurrent syncope in a patient with prominent J-wave. *Am Heart J* 1994;127:1426–1430.

124. Martini B, Nava A, Thiene G, et al. Ventricular fibrillation without apparent heart disease: description of six cases. *Am Heart J* 1989;118:1203–1209.

125. Miyazaki T, Mitamura H, Miyoshi S, et al. Autonomic and antiarrhythmic drug modulation of ST segment elevation in patients with Brugada syndrome. *J Am Coll Cardiol* 1996;27:1061–1070.

126. Kasanuki H, Ohnishi S, Ohtuka M, et al. Idiopathic ventricular fibrillation induced with vagal activity in patients without obvious heart disease. *Circulation* 1997; 95:2277–2285.

127. Nademanee K. Sudden unexplained death syndrome in southeast Asia. *Am J Cardiol* 1997;79:10–11.

128. Antzelevitch C, Brugada P, Brugada J, et al. The Brugada Syndrome. Armonk, NY: Futura Publishing, 1999:1.

129. Marcus FI. Idiopathic ventricular fibrillation. *J Cardiovasc Electrophysiol* 1997;8:1075–1083.

130. Gussak I, Antzelevitch C, Bjerregaard P, et al. The Brugada syndrome: clinical, electrophysiological and genetic aspects. *J Am Coll Cardiol* 1999;33:5–15.

131. Corrado D, Nava A, Buja G, et al. Familial cardiomyopathy underlies syndrome of right bundle branch block, ST segment elevation and sudden death [See comments]. *J Am Coll Cardiol* 1996;27:443–448.

132. Ahmed F, Li D, Karibe A, et al. Localization of a gene responsible for arrhythmogenic right ventricular dysplasia to chromosome 3p23. *Circulation* 1998;98:2791–2795.

133. Chen Q, Kirsch GE, Zhang D, et al. Genetic basis and molecular mechanisms for idiopathic ventricular fibrillation. *Nature* 1997;392:293–296.

134. Alings M, Wilde A. "Brugada" syndrome: clinical data and suggested pathophysiological mechanism. *Circulation* 1999;99:666–673.

135. Dumaine R, Towbin JA, Brugada P, et al. Ionic mechanisms responsible for the electrocardiographic phenotype of the Brugada syndrome are temperature dependent. *Circ Res* 1999;85:803–809.

136. Yan GX, Antzelevitch C. Cellular basis for the Brugada syndrome and other mechanisms of arrhythmogenesis associated with ST segment elevation. *Circulation* 1999;100:1660–1666.

137. Antzelevitch C. The Brugada syndrome. *J Cardiovasc Electrophysiol* 1998;9:513–516.

138. Lukas A, Antzelevitch C. Phase 2 reentry as a mechanism of ini-

tiation of circus movement reentry in canine epicardium exposed to simulated ischemia: the antiarrhythmic effects of 4-aminopyridine. *Cardiovasc Res* 1996;32:593–603.

139. Antzelevitch C, Yan GX, Shimizu W, Burashnikov A. Electrical heterogeneity, the ECG, and cardiac arrhythmias. In: Zipes DP, Jalife J, eds. *Cardiac electrophysiology: from cell to bedside.* Philadelphia: WB Saunders, 1999:222–238.

140. Antzelevitch C, Shimizu W, Yan GX, Sicouri S. Cellular basis for QT dispersion. *J Electrocardiol* 1998;30[Suppl]: 168–175.

141. Schwartz PJ, Periti M, Malliani A. The long QT syndrome. *Am Heart J* 1975;89:378–390.

142. Moss AJ, Schwartz PJ, Crampton RS, et al. The long QT syndrome: a prospective international study. *Circulation* 1985;71: 17–21.

143. Zipes DP. The long QT interval syndrome: a Rosetta stone for sympathetic related ventricular tachyarrhythmias. *Circulation* 1991;84:1414–1419.

144. Shimizu W, Ohe T, Kurita T. et al. Effects of verapamil and propranolol on early afterdepolarizations and ventricular arrhythmias induced by epinephrine in congenital long QT syndrome. *J Am Coll Cardiol* 1995;26:1299–1309.

145. Roden DM, Lazzara R, Rosen MR, et al. Multiple mechanisms in the long-QT syndrome: current knowledge, gaps, and future directions. *Circulation* 1996;94:1996–2012.

146. Abbott GW, Sesti F, Splawski I, et al. MiRP1 forms I_{Kr} potassium channels with HERG and is associated with cardiac arrhythmia. *Cell* 1999;97:175–187.

147. Antzelevitch C, Sun ZQ, Zhang ZQ, Yan GX. Cellular and ionic mechanisms underlying erythromycin-induced long QT and torsade de pointes. *J Am Coll Cardiol* 1996;28:1836–1848.

148. Schwartz PJ. The idiopathic long QT syndrome: progress and questions. *Am Heart J* 1985;109:399–411.

149. Moss AJ, Schwartz PJ, Crampton RS, et al. The long QT syndrome: prospective longitudinal study of 328 families. *Circulation* 1991;84:1136–1144.

150. Crampton RS. Preeminence of the left stellate ganglion in the long Q-T syndrome. *Circulation* 1979;59:769–778.

151. Ali RH, Zareba W, Moss AJ, et al. Clinical and genetic variables associated with acute arousal and nonarousal-related cardiac events among subjects with long QT syndrome. *Am J Cardiol* 2000;85:457–461.

152. Shimizu W, Antzelevitch C. Differential response to β-adrenergic agonists and antagonists in LQT1, LQT2, and LQT3 models of the long QT syndrome. *J Am Coll Cardiol* 2000;35: 778–786.

153. El-Sherif N, Chinushi M, Caref EB, Restivo M. Electrophysiological mechanism of the characteristic electrocardiographic morphology of torsade de pointes tachyarrhythmias in the long-QT syndrome: detailed analysis of ventricular tridimensional activation patterns. *Circulation* 1997;96:4392–4399.

154. Akar FG, Yan GX, Antzelevitch C, Rosenbaum DS. Optical maps reveal reentrant mechanism of torsade de pointes based on topography and electrophysiology of mid-myocardial cells. *Circulation* 1997;96:I-355(abst).

155. Burashnikov A, Antzelevitch C. Block of I_{Ks} does not induce early afterdepolarization activity but promotes β-adrenergic agonist-induced delayed afterdepolarization activity in canine ventricular myocardium. *J Cardiovasc Electrophysiol* 2000;11: 458–465.

156. Ferrier GR, Rosenthal JE. Automaticity and entrance block induced by focal depolarization of mammalian ventricular tissues. *Circ Res* 1980;47:238–248.

157. Wennemark JR, Ruesta VJ, Brody DA. Microelectrode study of delayed conduction in the canine right bundle branch. *Circ Res* 1968;23:753–769.

158. Downar E, Waxman MB. Depressed conduction and unidirec-

tional block in Purkinje fibers. In: Wellens HJ, Lie KI, Janse MJ, eds. *The conduction system of the heart.* Philadelphia: Lea & Febiger, 1976:393–409.

159. Antzelevitch C, Spach MS. Impulse conduction: continuous and discontinuous. In: Spooner PM, Rosen MR, eds. *Foundations of cardiac arrhythmias. Basic concepts: fundamental approaches.* New York: Marcel Dekker, 1999.

160. Spach MS, Miller WT, Geselowitz DB, et al. The discontinuous nature of propagation in normal canine cardiac muscle: evidence for recurrent discontinuities of intracellular resistance that affect the membrane currents. *Circ Res* 1981;48:39–54.

161. Lazzara R, El-Sherif N, Scherlag BJ. Electrophysiological properties of canine Purkinje cells in one-day-old myocardial infarction. *Circ Res* 1973;33:722–734.

162. Antzelevitch C, Jalife J, Moe GK. Frequency-dependent alternations of conduction in Purkinje fibers: a model of phase-4 facilitation and block. In: Rosenbaum MB, Elizari MV, eds. *Frontiers of cardiac electrophysiology.* Amsterdam: Martinus Nijhoff, 1983:397–415.

163. Gilmour RF Jr, Salata JJ, Zipes DP. Rate-related suppression and facilitation of conduction in isolated canine cardiac Purkinje fibers. *Circ Res* 1985;57:35–45.

164. Gilmour RF Jr, Heger JJ, Prystowsky EN, Zipes DP. Cellular electrophysiologic abnormalities of diseased human ventricular myocardium. *Am J Cardiol* 1983;51:137–144.

165. Gilmour RF Jr, Zipes DP. Cellular basis for cardiac arrhythmias. *Cardiol Clin* 1983;1:3–11.

166. Janse MJ, Van Capelle FJL. Electrotonic interactions across an inexcitable region as a cause of ectopic activity in acute regional myocardial ischemia: a study in intact porcine and canine hearts and computer models. *Circ Res* 1982;50:527–537.

167. Antzelevitch C, Shimizu W, Yan GX. Electrical heterogeneity and the development of arrhythmias. In: Olsson SB, ed. *Dispersion of ventricular repolarization.* Mount Kisco, NY: Futura Publishing, 2000.

168. Gilmour RF Jr. Phase resetting of circus movement reentry in cardiac tissue. In: Zipes DP, Jalife J, eds. *Cardiac electrophysiology: from cell to bedside.* New York: WB Saunders, 1989.

169. Matsuda K, Kamiyama A, Hoshi T. Configuration of the transmembrane action potential at the Purkinje-ventricular fiber junction and its analysis. In: Sano T, Mizuhira V, Matsuda K, eds. *Electrophysiology and ultrastructure of the heart.* New York: Grune & Stratton, 1967:177–187.

170. Overholt ED, Joyner RW, Veenstra RD, et al. Unidirectional block between Purkinje and ventricular layers of papillary muscles. *Am J Physiol* 1984;247:H-584–H-595.

171. DiFrancesco D. The cardiac hyperpolarizing-activated current, I_f: origins and developments. *Prog Biophys Mol Biol* 1985;46: 163–183.

172. DiFrancesco D. The pacemaker current (I(f)) plays an important role in regulating SA node pacemaker activity [See comments]. *Cardiovasc Res* 1995;30:307–308.

173. Vassalle M. Analysis of cardiac pacemaker potential using a "voltage clamp" technique. *Am J Physiol* 1966;210:1335–1341.

174. Vassalle M. The pacemaker current (I(f)) does not play an important role in regulating SA node pacemaker activity [Comment]. *Cardiovasc Res* 1995;30:309–310.

175. Levy MN. Sympathetic-parasympathetic interactions in the heart. *Circ Res* 1971;29:437–445.

176. Imanishi S, Surawicz B. Automatic activity in depolarized guinea pig ventricular myocardium: characteristics and mechanisms. *Circ Res* 1976;39:751–759.

177. Dangman KH, Hoffman BF. Studies on overdrive stimulation of canine cardiac Purkinje fibers: maximal diastolic potential as a determinant of the response. *J Am Coll Cardiol* 1983;2: 1183–1190.

178. Katzung BG, Morgenstern JA. Effects of extracellular potassium on ventricular automaticity and evidence for a pacemaker current in mammalian ventricular myocardium. *Circ Res* 1977;40:105–111.

179. Pappano AJ, Carmeliet EE. Epinephrine and the pacemaking mechanism at plateau potentials in sheep cardiac Purkinje fibers. *Pflugers Arch* 1979;382:17–26.

180. Katz LN, Pick A. The arrhythmias. In: Clinical electrocardiography. Philadelphia: Lea & Febiger, 1956:224, 225, 236.

181. Pogwizd SM, Hoyt RH, Saffitz JE, et al. Reentrant and focal mechanisms underlying ventricular tachycardia in the human heart. *Circulation* 1992;86:1872–1887.

182. Arnar DO, Bullinga JR, Martins JB. Role of the Purkinje system in spontaneous ventricular tachycardia during acute ischemia in a canine model. *Circulation* 1997;96:2421–2429.

183. Pogwizd SM. Focal mechanisms underlying ventricular tachycardia during prolonged ischemic cardiomyopathy. *Circulation* 1994;90:1441–1458.

184. Pogwizd SM. Nonreentrant mechanisms underlying spontaneous ventricular arrhythmias in a model of nonischemic heart failure in rabbits. *Circulation* 1995;92:1034–1048.

185. Pogwizd SM, McKenzie JP, Cain ME. Mechanisms underlying spontaneous and induced ventricular arrhythmias in patients with idiopathic dilated cardiomyopathy. *Circulation* 1998;98:2404–2414.

186. Vermeulen JT, McGuire MA, Opthof T, et al. Triggered activity and automaticity in ventricular trabeculae of failing human and rabbit hearts. *Cardiovasc Res* 1994;28:1547–1554.

187. Nuss HB, Kaab S, Kass DA, et al. Cellular basis of ventricular arrhythmias and abnormal automaticity in heart failure. *Am J Physiol* 1999;277:H80–H91.

188. Hoppe UC, Jansen E, Sudkamp M, Beuckelmann DJ. Hyperpolarization-activated inward current in ventricular myocytes from normal and failing human hearts. *Circulation* 1998;97:55–65.

189. Cerbai E, Barbieri M, Mugelli A. Occurrence and properties of the hyperpolarization-activated current I_f in ventricular myocytes from normotensive and hypertensive rats during aging. *Circulation* 1996;94:1674–1681.

190. Lai LP, Su MJ, Lin JL, et al. Measurement of funny current (I(f)) channel mRNA in human atrial tissue: correlation with left atrial filling pressure and atrial fibrillation. *J Cardiovasc Electrophysiol* 1999;10:947–953.

191. Scherf D, Boyd LJ. Three unusual cases of parasystole. *Am Heart J* 1950;39:650–663.

192. Jalife J, Moe GK. A biological model of parasystole. *Am J Cardiol* 1979;43:761–772.

193. Jalife J, Antzelevitch C, Moe GK. The case for modulated parasystole. *Pacing Clin Electrophysiol* 1982;5:911–926.

194. Moe GK, Jalife J, Mueller WJ, Moe B. A mathematical model of parasystole and its application to clinical arrhythmias. *Circulation* 1977;56:968–979.

195. Antzelevitch C, Jalife J, Moe GK. Electrotonic modulation of pacemaker activity: further biological and mathematical observations on the behavior of modulated parasystole. *Circulation* 1982;66:1225–1232.

196. Castellanos A, Melgarejo E, Dubois R, Luceri RM. Modulation of ventricular parasystole by extraneous depolarizations. *J Electrocardiol* 1984;17:195–198.

197. Jalife J, Moe GK. Effect of electrotonic potentials on pacemaker activity of canine Purkinje fibers in relation to parasystole. *Circ Res* 1976;39:801–808.

198. Moe GK, Jalife J, Antzelevitch C. Models of parasystole and reentry in isolated Purkinje fibers. *Mayo Clin Proc* 1982;57 [Suppl]:14–19.

199. Oreto G, Luzza F, Satullo G, Schamroth L. Modulated ventricular parasystole as a mechanism for concealed bigeminy. *Am J Cardiol* 1986;58:954–958.

200. Oreto G, Luzza F, Satullo G, et al. Sinus modulation of atrial parasystole. *Am J Cardiol* 1986;58:1097–1099.

201. Cranefield PF. Action potentials, afterpotentials and arrhythmias. *Circ Res* 1977;41:415–423.

202. Wit AL, Rosen MR. Afterdepolarizations and triggered activity: distinction from automaticity as an arrhythmogenic mechanism. In: Fozzard HA, et al., eds. *The heart and cardiovascular system.* New York: Raven Press, 1992:2113–2164.

203. Lab MJ. Contraction-excitation feedback in myocardium: physiologic basis and clinical relevance. *Circ Res* 1982;50:757–766.

204. Adamantidis MM, Caron JF, Dupuis BA. Triggered activity induced by combined mild hypoxia and acidosis in guinea pig Purkinje fibers. *J Mol Cell Cardiol* 1986;18:1287–1299.

205. Coraboeuf E, Deroubaix E, Coulombe A. Acidosis-induced abnormal repolarization and repetitive activity in isolated dog Purkinje fibers. *J Physiol (Paris)* 1980;76:97–106.

206. Priori SG, Corr PB. Mechanisms underlying early and delayed afterdepolarizations induced by catecholamines. *Am J Physiol* 1990;258:H1796–H1805.

207. Volders PGA, Kulcsar A, Vos MA, et al. Similarities between early and delayed afterdepolarizations induced by isoproterenol in canine ventricular myocytes. *Cardiovasc Res* 1997;34:348–359.

208. Brachmann J, Scherlag BJ, Rosenshtraukh LV, Lazzara R. Bradycardia-dependent triggered activity: Relevance to drug-induced multiform ventricular tachycardia. *Circulation* 1983;68:846–856.

209. Damiano BP, Rosen MR. Effects of pacing on triggered activity induced by early afterdepolarizations. *Circulation* 1984;69:1013–1025.

210. El-Sherif N, Zeiler RH, Craelius W, et al. QTU prolongation and polymorphic ventricular tachyarrhythmias due to bradycardia-dependent early afterdepolarizations: afterdepolarizations and ventricular arrhythmias. *Circ Res* 1988;63:286–305.

211. January CT, Riddle JM, Salata JJ. A model for early afterdepolarizations: induction with the Ca^{2+} channel agonist BAY K 8644. *Circ Res* 1988;62:563–571.

212. Davidenko JM, Cohen L, Goodrow RJ, Antzelevitch C. Quinidine-induced action potential prolongation, early afterdepolarizations, and triggered activity in canine Purkinje fibers: effects of stimulation rate, potassium, and magnesium. *Circulation* 1989;79:674–686.

213. Carmeliet E. Electrophysiologic and voltage clamp analysis of the effects of sotalol on isolated cardiac muscle and Purkinje fibers. *J Pharmacol Exp Ther* 1985;232:817–825.

214. Aronson RS. Afterpotentials and triggered activity in hypertrophied myocardium from rats with renal-hypertension. *Circ Res* 1981;48:720–727.

215. Volders PG, Sipido KR, Vos MA, et al. Cellular basis of biventricular hypertrophy and arrhythmogenesis in dogs with chronic complete atrioventricular block and acquired torsade de pointes. *Circulation* 1998;98:1136–1147.

216. Roden DM, Hoffman BF. Action potential prolongation and induction of abnormal automaticity by low quinidine concentrations in canine Purkinje fibers: relationship to potassium and cycle length. *Circ Res* 1986;56:857–867.

217. Bril A, Faivre JF, Forest MC, et al. Electrophysiological effect of BRL-32872, a novel antiarrhythmic agent with potassium and calcium channel blocking properties, in guinea pig cardiac isolated preparations. *J Pharmacol Exp Ther* 1995;273:1264–1272.

218. Marban E, Robinson SW, Wier WG. Mechanism of arrhythmogenic delayed and early afterdepolarizations in ferret muscle. *J Clin Invest* 1986;78:1185–1192.

219. Boutjdir M, El-Sherif N. Pharmacological evaluation of early

afterdepolarisations induced by sea anemone toxin (ATXII) in dog heart. *Cardiovasc Res* 1991;25:815–819.

220. Carlsson L, Abrahamsson C, Drews C, Duker GD. Antiarrhythmic effects of potassium channel openers in rhythm abnormalities related to delayed repolarization in the rabbit. *Circulation* 1992;85:1491–1500.

221. El-Sherif N, Zeiler RH, Craelius W, et al. QTU prolongation and polymorphic ventricular tachyarrhythmias due to bradycardia-dependent early afterdepolarizations. *Circ Res* 1988;63:286–305.

222. Nattel S, Quantz MA. Pharmacological response of quinidine induced early afterdepolarizations in canine cardiac Purkinje fibers: insights into underlying ionic mechanisms. *Cardiovasc Res* 1988;22:808–817.

223. Sicouri S, Antzelevitch C. Afterdepolarizations and triggered activity develop in a select population of cells (M cells) in canine ventricular myocardium: the effects of acetylstrophanthidin and Bay K 8644. *Pacing Clin Electrophysiol* 1991;14:1714–1720.

224. Burashnikov A, Antzelevitch C. Failure of canine ventricular epicardial and endocardial cells to develop early afterdepolarization activity is due to the presence of a prominent I_{Ks}. *Circulation* 1997;96:I-292(abst).

225. Murakawa Y, Sezaki K, Yamashita T, et al. Three-dimensional activation sequence of cesium-induced ventricular arrhythmias. *Am J Physiol* 1997;273:H1377–H1385.

226. Szabo B, Kovacs T, Lazzara R. Role of calcium loading in early afterdepolarizations generated by Cs in canine and guinea pig Purkinje fibers. *J Cardiovasc Electrophysiol* 1995;6:796–812.

227. Patterson E, Scherlag BJ, Szabo B, Lazzara R. Facilitation of epinephrine-induced afterdepolarizations by class III antiarrhythmic drugs. *J Electrocardiol* 1997;30:217–224.

228. January CT, Riddle JM. Early afterdepolarizations: mechanism of induction and block: a role for L-type Ca^{2+} current. *Circ Res* 1989;64:977–990.

229. Zeng J, Rudy Y. Early afterdepolarizations in cardiac myocytes: mechanism and rate dependence. *Biophys J* 1995;68:949–964.

230. Ming Z, Nordin C, Aronson MD. Role of L-type calcium channel window current in generating current-induced early afterpolarizations. *J Cardiovasc Electrophysiol* 1994;5:323–334.

231. Patterson E, Scherlag BJ, Lazzara R. Early afterdepolarizations produced by d,l-sotalol and clofilium. *J Cardiovasc Electrophysiol* 1997;8:667–678.

232. Burashnikov A, Antzelevitch C. Mechanisms underlying early afterdepolarization activity are different in canine Purkinje and M cell preparations: role of intracellular calcium. *Circulation* 1996;94:I-527(abst).

233. Antzelevitch C, Yan GX, Shimizu W, et al. Electrophysiologic characteristics of M cells and their role in arrhythmias. In: Franz MR, ed. *Monophasic action potentials: bridging cell and bedside.* Armonk, NY: Futura Publishing, 2000:583–604.

234. Ben-David J, Zipes DP. Differential response to right and left ansae subclaviae stimulation of early afterdepolarizations and ventricular tachycardia induced by cesium in dogs. *Circulation* 1988;78:1241–1250.

235. Jackman WM, Friday KJ, Anderson JL, et al. The long QT syndromes: a critical review, new clinical observations and a unifying hypothesis. *Prog Cardiovasc Dis* 1988;31:115–172.

236. Shimizu W, Ohe T, Kurita T, et al. Early afterdepolarizations induced by isoproterenol in patients with congenital long QT syndrome. *Circulation* 1991;84:1915–1923.

237. Asano Y, Davidenko JM, Baxter WT, et al. Optical mapping of drug-induced polymorphic arrhythmias and torsade de pointes in the isolated rabbit heart [See comments]. *J Am Coll Cardiol* 1997;29:831–842.

238. Ben-David J, Zipes DP, Ayers GM, Pride HP. Canine left ventricular hypertrophy predisposes to ventricular tachycardia induction by phase 2 early afterdepolarizations after administration of BAY K 8644. *J Am Coll Cardiol* 1992;20:1576–1584.

239. Beuckelmann DJ, Nabauer M, Erdmann E. Alterations of K^+ currents in isolated human ventricular myocytes from patients with terminal heart failure. *Circ Res* 1993;73:379–385.

240. Vermeulen JT. Mechanisms of arrhythmias in heart failure. *J Cardiovasc Electrophysiol* 1998;9:208–221.

241. Ferrier GR, Saunders JH, Mendez C. A cellular mechanism for the generation of ventricular arrhythmias by acetylstrophanthidin. *Circ Res* 1973;32:600–609.

242. Rosen MR, Gelband H, Merker C, Hoffman BF. Mechanisms of digitalis toxicity—effects of ouabain on phase four of canine Purkinje fiber transmembrane potentials. *Circulation* 1973;47:681–689.

243. Saunders JH, Ferrier GR, Moe GK. Conduction block associated with transient depolarizations induced by acetylstrophanthidin in isolated canine Purkinje fibers. *Circ Res* 1973;32:610–617.

244. Rozanski GJ, Lipsius SL. Electrophysiology of functional subsidiary pacemakers in canine right atrium. *Am J Physiol* 1985;249:H594–H603.

245. Marchi S, Szabo B, Lazzara R. Adrenergic induction of delayed afterdepolarizations in ventricular myocardial cells: beta-induction and alpha-modulation. *J Cardiovasc Electrophysiol* 1991;2:476–491.

246. Wit AL, Cranefield PF. Triggered and automatic activity in the canine coronary sinus. *Circ Res* 1977;41:435–445.

247. Matsuda H, Noma A, Kurachi Y, Irisawa H. Transient depolarizations and spontaneous voltage fluctuations in isolated single cells from guinea pig ventricles. *Circ Res* 1982;51:142–151.

248. Spinelli W, Sorota S, Siegel MB, Hoffman BF. Antiarrhythmic actions of the ATP-regulated K^+ current activated by pinacidil. *Circ Res* 1991;68:1127–1137.

249. Belardinelli LL, Isenberg G. Actions of adenosine and isoproterenol on isolated mammalian ventricular myocytes. *Circ Res* 1983;53:287–297.

250. Schreieck J, Wang YG, Gjini V, et al. Differential effect of beta-adrenergic stimulation on the frequency-dependent electrophysiologic actions of the new class III antiarrhythmics dofetilide, ambasilide, and chromanol 293B. *J Cardiovasc Electrophysiol* 1997;8:1420–1430.

251. Coetzee WA, Opie LH. Effects of components of ischemia and metabolic inhibition on delayed afterdepolarizations in guinea pig papillary muscle. *Circ Res* 1987;61:157–165.

252. Pogwizd SM, Onufer JR, Kramer JB, et al. Induction of delayed afterdepolarizations and triggered activity in canine Purkinje fibers by lysophosphoglycerides. *Circ Res* 1986;59:416–426.

253. Song Y, Belardinelli L. ATP promotes development of afterpolarizations and triggered activity in cardiac myocytes. *Am J Physiol* 1994;267:H2005–H2011.

254. Wu Y, Roden DM, Anderson ME. Calmodulin kinase inhibition prevents development of the arrhythmogenic transient inward current. *Circ Res* 1999;84:906–912.

255. Caroni P, Villani F, Carafoli E. The cardiotoxic antibiotic doxorubicin inhibits the Na^+/Ca^{2+} exchange of dog heart sarcolemmal vesicles. *FEBS Lett* 1981;130:184–186.

256. Kass RS, Tsien RW, Weingart R. Ionic basis of transient inward current induced by strophanthidin in cardiac Purkinje fibres. *J Physiol (Lond)* 1978;281:209–226.

257. Cannell MB, Lederer WJ. The arrhythmogenic current I_{TI} in the absence of electrogenic sodium-calcium exchange in sheep cardiac Purkinje fibres. *J Physiol (Lond)* 1986;374:201–219.

258. Fedida D, Noble D, Rankin AC, Spindler AJ. The arrhythmogenic transient inward current I_{ti} and related contraction in isolated guinea-pig ventricular myocytes. *J Physiol (Lond)* 1987;392:523–542.

259. Laflamme MA, Becker PL. Ca^{2+}-induced current oscillations in rabbit ventricular myocytes. *Circ Res* 1996;78:707–716.
260. Zygmunt AC, Goodrow RJ, Weigel CM. I$_{Na-Ca}$ and I$_{Cl(Ca)}$ contribute to isoproterenol-induced delayed afterdepolarizations in midmyocardial cells. *Am J Physiol* 1998;275:H1979–H1992.
261. Ritchie AH, Kerr CR, Qi A, et al. Nonsustained ventricular tachycardia arising from the right ventricular outflow tract. *Am J Cardiol* 1989;64:594–598.
262. Wilber DJ, Blakeman BM, Pifarre R, Scanlon PJ. Catecholamine sensitive right ventricular outflow tract tachycardia: intraoperative mapping and ablation of a free-wall focus. *Pacing Clin Electrophysiol* 1989;12:1851–1856.
263. Cardinal R, Scherlag BJ, Vermeulen M, Armour JA. Distinct activation patterns of idioventricular rhythms and sympathetically induced ventricular tachycardias in dogs with atrioventricular block. *Pacing Clin Electrophysiol* 1992;15:1300–1316.
264. Cardinal R, Savard P, Armour JA, et al. Mapping of ventricular tachycardia induced by thoracic neural stimulation in dogs. *Can J Physiol Pharmacol* 1986;64:411–418.
265. Lerman BB, Belardinelli LL, West GA, et al. Adenosine-sensitive ventricular tachycardia: evidence suggesting cyclic AMP-mediated triggered activity. *Circulation* 1986;74:270–280.
266. Lerman BB, Stein K, Engelstein ED, et al. Mechanism of repetitive monomorphic ventricular tachycardia. *Circulation* 1995;92:421–429.
267. Ter Keurs HE, Schouten VJA, Bucx JJ, et al. Excitation-contraction coupling in myocardium: implications of calcium release and Na^{+}-Ca^{2+} exchange. *Can J Physiol Pharmacol* 1987;65:619–626.
268. Antzelevitch C. Electrotonus and reflection. In: Rosen MR, Janse MJ, Wit AL, eds. *Cardiac electrophysiology: a textbook.* Mount Kisco, NY: Futura Publishing, 1990:491–516.

GENETICS OF ARRHYTHMOGENIC DISORDERS

SILVIA G. PRIORI
CARLO NAPOLITANO

The impressive developments that have occurred during the last 10 years in the field of human genetics have made an impact on cardiology (Fig. 4.1-1). After the identification of the genetic basis of monogenic diseases of the heart, cardiologists have become interested in molecular genetics. They have rapidly realized that genetic testing, gene-specific treatments, and gene-based risk stratification algorithms are entering clinical cardiology and are here to stay and will influence clinical practice during the next several years.

In this chapter, we review the current understanding of the molecular basis of "primary electrical disorders" and "structural heart diseases" predisposing to arrhythmias and sudden death (1).

Before dealing with individual diseases, we provide some general concepts about patterns of transmission of genetic diseases and nomenclature used when referring to genes and chromosomal regions. The concepts that are presented in this introduction are instrumental to the understanding of current knowledge about inherited arrhythmogenic diseases and are not intended to provide exhaustive coverage of the topic. The interested reader is directed to the specific literature reported in the Reference list.

MENDELIAN PATTERNS OF INHERITANCE

Most human disorders, with the exception of infectious diseases, are ultimately caused by genetic traits, although their genetic background is often very difficult to study because the clinical phenotype results from multiple genetic factors and from their interaction with the environment (polygenic diseases). It is much easier to study and identify the genetic substrate of the relatively rare monogenic disorders in which the phenotype is caused by a specific defect in one

major gene. The inheritance of monogenic diseases follows specific patterns that may be identified through the analysis of the family pedigree. Monogenic diseases may be inherited as dominant or recessive traits. The dominant traits are those causing the phenotype in the heterozygous state; recessive diseases are those that determine a phenotype only when a "double dose" (homozygosity) of the genetic defect is present. The heterozygous carriers of a recessive trait usually are normal or present with subclinical form of the disease. Because both autosomal and sexual chromosomes are present in the human genome, genetic traits are defined as autosomal or sex-linked.

Four different inheritance patterns may be described for the mendelian traits (Fig. 4.1-2).

- Autosomal dominant has a 50% chance of transmission to the offspring, and both men and women can be affected.

- Autosomal recessive means only the homozygous is clinically affected while the heterozygous is defined as a "healthy carrier." The inheritance chance of two defective alleles/genes in the same subject (one from the mother and one from the father) is 25%. Fifty percent of the offspring will receive only one defective allele (heterozygote) and 25% will receive two wild-type alleles.

- X-linked dominant is where both men and women can be affected, but no male-to-male transmission is possible and an affected male has a 100% chance to transmit the disease to daughters. Female-to-female transmission chance of the defective allele is 50%.

- X-linked recessive is where heterozygous women are healthy carriers of the genetic defect and all their sons are clinically affected. No female-to-female transmission of the disease is possible, but 50% of daughters are silent carriers (heterozygous for the defective allele). Affected man will generate unaffected men and heterozygous unaffected women (healthy carriers).

S. G. Priori: Department of Molecular Cardiology, Fondazione Salvatore Maugeri, Pavia, Italy 27100.
C. Napolitano: University of Pavia, Pavia, Italy, 27100.

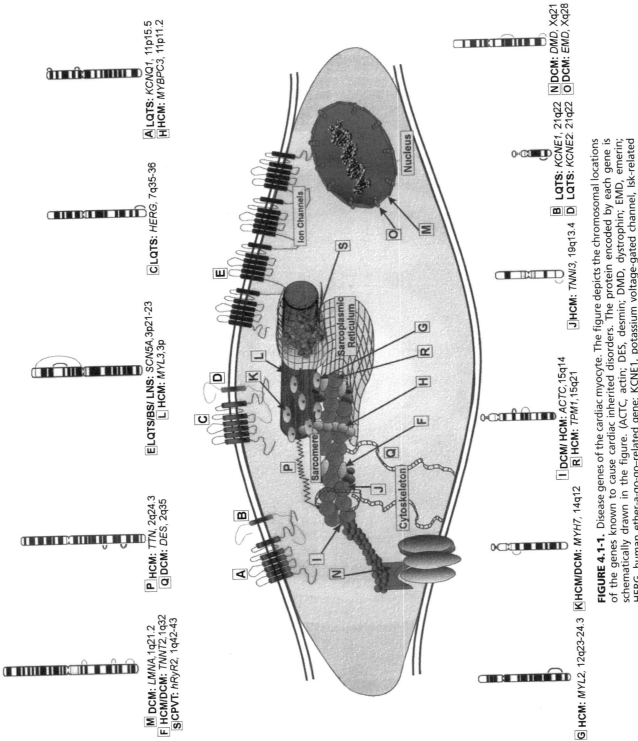

FIGURE 4.1-1. Disease genes of the cardiac myocyte. The figure depicts the chromosomal locations of the genes known to cause cardiac inherited disorders. The protein encoded by each gene is schematically drawn in the figure. (ACTC, actin; DES, desmin; DMD, dystrophin; EMD, emerin; HERG, human ether-a-go-go-related gene; KCNE1, potassium voltage-gated channel, Isk-related family, minK; KCNE2, potassium voltage-gated channel, Isk-related family, MiRP1; KCNQ1, potassium voltage-gated channel precursor, KQT-like subfamily, member 1; LMNA, lamin A/C; MYBPC3, myosin-binding protein C; MYH7, β-myosin heavy chain; MYL2, myosin regulatory light chain; MYL3, myosin essential light chain; hRyR2, human ryanodine receptor gene; SCN5A, voltage-gated cardiac sodium channel; TNNI3, troponin I; TNNT2, troponin T; TPM1, α-tropomyosin; TTN, titin.)

M DCM: *LMNA*, 1q21.2
F HCM/DCM: *TNNT2*, 1q32
S CPVT: *hRyR2*, 1q42-43

A LQTS: *KCNQ1*, 11p15.5
H HCM: *MYBPC3*, 11p11.2

C LQTS: *HERG*, 7q35-36

E LQTS/BS/ LNS: *SCN5A*, 3p21-23
L HCM: *MYL3*, 3p

P HCM: *TTN*, 2q24.3
Q DCM: *DES*, 2q35

B LQTS: *KCNE1*, 21q22
D LQTS: *KCNE2*, 21q22

N DCM: *DMD*, Xq21
O DCM: *EMD*, Xq28

J HCM: *TNNI3*, 19q13.4

I DCM/ HCM: *ACTC*, 15q14
R HCM: *TPM1*, 15q21

G HCM: *MYL2*, 12q23-24.3

K HCM/DCM: *MYH7*, 14q12

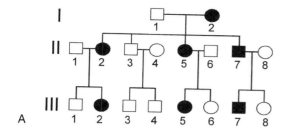

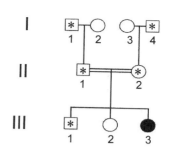

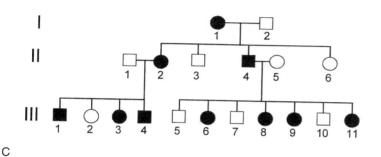

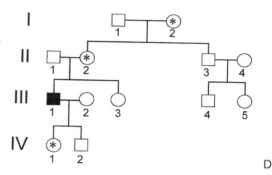

FIGURE 4.1-2. Patterns of familial transmission of mendelian inherited monogenic diseases. **A:** Autosomal dominant. **B:** Autosomal recessive. **C:** X-linked dominant. **D:** X-linked recessive.

In clinical practice, it is often arduous to identify the patterns of inheritance because low penetrance and variable expressivity may obscure the picture.

The penetrance of a genetic defect is defined as the ratio between the gene carriers and the individuals showing the diseased phenotype. In other words, a penetrance of 20% means that one gene carrier has one out of five chances to develop the disease. The variable expressivity is defined as the presence of different manifestations of the same genetic defect in different individuals. Low penetrance and variable expressivity may be caused by genetic and/or epigenetic (environmental) factors. For example, it has been shown (2) that some cases of drug-induced long QT syndrome (LQTS) and torsade de pointes may indeed be explained by the presence of low-penetrance mutations in cardiac ion channel proteins. These mutations behave like a predisposing substrate that manifests with arrhythmias only after exposure to a triggering factor.

Late-onset diseases are another example of variable penetrance. The penetrance of Huntington disease may be up to 100% if all the gene carriers in a family live long enough to manifest the phenotype, but the penetrance is much lower in young individuals. A similar example in cardiology is that of late-onset hypertrophic cardiomyopathy (HCM) (3).

NOMENCLATURE FOR GENES AND CHROMOSOMES

When dealing with the genetic bases of inherited arrhythmogenic conditions, one is presented with two scenarios (4). In the case of a few diseases, a lot of information is available: the gene causing a particular disease has been identified, the altered protein is known, and its function within cardiac cells is also well understood. In these cases, when most of the information is available, a major step can be accomplished in the understanding of the disease and in the definition of specific therapeutic approaches. It also becomes possible to screen genomic DNA of clinically affected individuals and their family members to search for specific mutations in the implicated gene (Fig. 4.1-3).

In the description of the diseases with known genetic aspects, we will report the name of the gene implicated in the disease and that of the related protein according to the international nomenclature. The name of the gene may be identical to the name of the protein; in these cases, there is common agreement to write the name of the gene in italics and that of the corresponding protein in normal characters. For example, the gene encoding the cardiac sodium channel is called *SCN5A* and the corresponding protein is SCN5A. In other instances, the name of the gene is different from

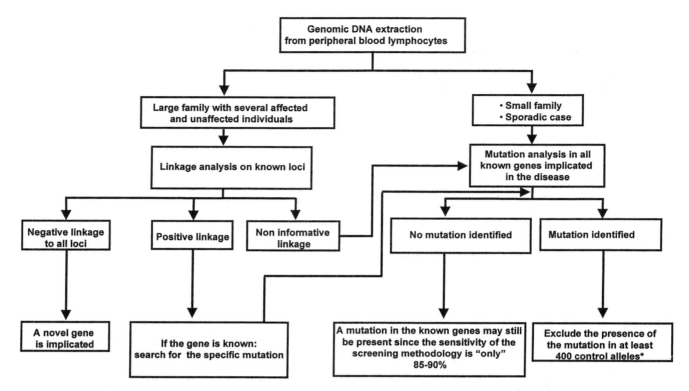

FIGURE 4.1-3. Clinical applications of genetic testing. The flow chart summarizes the main steps performed in the molecular biology laboratory to identify the DNA alterations causing the inherited arrhythmogenic disorders. This scheme is mainly applied to the identification of mutations in the known disease genes. The search for new genes requires different experimental procedures. The analysis of a panel of genomic DNA obtained from healthy individuals is needed to exclude the possibility of rare polymorphisms.

that of the peptide: In the case of the sarcomeric protein called "β-myosin heavy chain," the corresponding gene is called *MYH7*.

In the description of genotype-phenotype correlation, we will report the individual mutations that have been identified. In most cases, the defect is defined as a "point mutation," that is, a change of a single DNA base that results in the substitution of an amino acid with respect to the normal (wild-type) protein. Occasionally, more complex defects are associated with the disease such as deletions (absence of one or more amino acids), insertions (addition of one or more amino acids not present in the normal protein), or "splicing errors," which are alterations of the information leading to messenger RNA (mRNA) processing from genomic DNA (see the Glossary).

Point mutations are described with a sequence of letters and numbers, by which the first series of letters identifies the amino acid that is normally present and is followed by a number that identifies the position of that amino acid in the polypeptide chain. This sequence is then followed by letters that identify the amino acid that is present in the

mutated DNA (e.g., Ala234Val means that an alanine at position 234 is substituted by a valine).

For most diseases reviewed in this chapter, the genetic substrate is still unknown and genetic understanding is limited to the identification of a region of a specific chromosome in which the disease gene is most likely located (Table 4.1-1). This level of understanding is very preliminary, as it does not provide information concerning the gene involved or the type of defective protein implicated in the disease. The localization of the chromosomal region in which the disease gene is located is identified with a method called "linkage analysis." What is relevant here is to realize that for diseases such as arrhythmogenic right ventricular dysplasia, atrial fibrillation, and for several variants of dilated cardiomyopathy (DCM), we will present chromosomal locations using terms such as "the disease has been mapped to" followed by a sequence of letters and numbers (e.g., 14q23). For the novice to molecular biology, this code should be interpreted as follows: The first number ("14" in the example) indicates the chromosome in which it is expected that the gene for that

TABLE 4.1-1. GENE LOCI AND PROTEINS RELATED TO SPECIFIC DISEASES

Disease	Locus	Gene	Protein	Reference
XLDCM	Xq28	*EMD*	Emerin	Towbin et al. (41)
	Xp21.2	*DMD*	Dystrophin	Ortiz-Lopez et al. (44)
Barth	Xq28	*G.4.5*	Tafazzin	Bione et al. (63)
AD DCM	1q32	?	?	Durand et al. (73)
	2q35	*DES*	Desmin	Goldfarb (49), Li et al. (50)
	2p31	?	?	Siu et al. (76)
	3p22–p25	?	?	Olson et al. (74)
	6q23	?	?	Messina et al. (75)
	9q13–q21	?	?	Krajinovic et al. (71)
	10q21–q23	?	?	Bowles et al. (72)
	2q14–q22	?	?	Jung et al. (77)
	1q21.2	*LMNA*	Lamin A/C	Kass et al. (57), Fatkin et al. (58)
	14q12	*MYH7*	β-Myosin heavy chain	Kamisago et al. (40)
	1q32	*TNNT2*	Troponin T	Kamisago et al. (40)
HCM	1q32	*TNNT2*	Troponin T	Watkins et al. (17)
	3p	*MYL3*	Myosin essential light chain	Poetter et al. (15)
	7q3	?	?	MacRae et al. (25)
	11p11.2	*MYBPC3*	Myosin-binding protein C	Bonne et al. (21) Watkins et al. (22)
	12q23–q24.3	*MYL2*	Myosin regulatory light chain	Poetter et al. (15)
	14q12	*MYH7*	β-Myosin heavy chain	Geisterfer et al. (14)
	15q14	*ACTC*	Actin	Olson et al. (45)
	15q21	*TPM1*	α-Tropomyosin	Thierfelder et al. (18)
	15q14	*ACTC*	Actin	Mogensen et al. (23)
	2q24.3	*TTN*	Titin	Satoh et al. (24)
	19p13.2–q13.2	?	?	Kimura et al. (16)
FA.Fib	10q22–q24	?	?	Brugada et al. (207)
PFHB-I	19q13.2–q13.3	?	?	Brink et al. (221), De Meeus et al. (222)
Lenegre	3p21–p23	*SCN5A*	SCN5A	Schott et al. (223)
LQTS (R-W)	3p21–p23	*SCN5A*	SCN5A	Wang et al. (121)
	4q25–q27	?	?	Schott et al. (118)
	7q35–q36	*HERG*	HERG	Curran et al. (120)
	11p15.5	*KCNQ1*	KVLQT1	Wang et al. (119)
	21q22.1–p22.2	*KCNE1*	MinK	Splawski et al. (126)
	21q22.1–p22.2	*KCNE2*	MiRP1	Abbott et al. (141)
LQTS (JL-N)	11p15.5	*KCNQ1*	KVLQT1	Neyroud et al. (123)
	21q22.1–q22.2	*KCNE1*	MinK	Schultze-Bahr et al. (127)
ARVD	1q42–q43	?	?	Rampazzo et al. (89)
	14q12–q22	?	?	Severini et al. (90)
	14q23–q24	?	?	Rampazzo et al. (86)
	2q32.1–q32.2	?	?	Rampazzo et al. (91)
	3p23	?	?	Ahmad et al. (87)
	10q14–p12	?	?	Li et al. (88)
Naxos	17q21	PLK	PLK	McKoy et al. (84)
Brugada	3p21–p23	*SCN5A*	SCN5A	Chen et al. (183)
CPVT	1q42–q43	*hRyR2*	hRyR2	Priori et al. (197)

XLDCM, X-linked dilated cardiomyopathy; AD DCM, autosomal dominant dilated cardiomyopathy; Barth, Barth syndrome; FHCM, Familial hypertrophic cardiomyopathy; FA Fib, familial atrial fibrillation; PFHB-I, progressive familial heart block type I; LQTS (R-W), long QT syndrome Romano-Ward type; LQTS (JL-N), long QT syndrome Jervell and Lange-Nielsen type; ARVD, arrhythmogenic right ventricular cardiomyopathy; Naxos, Naxos disease; Brugada, Brugada syndrome; CPVT, catecholaminergic polymorphic ventricular tachycardia.

disease will be located, and the letter "p" or "q" indicates the arm of the chromosome ("p" represents the short arm, and "q" the long arm). The final sequences of numbers that follow indicate the *region* of the arm of the chromosome: Numbers are attributed according to international rules established by the Standing Committee of Human Cytogenetic Nomenclature. The example provided indicates that the gene is most likely located on the long arm of chromosome 14 in region 23 (read *two-three*, not *twenty-three*).

INHERITED STRUCTURAL ABNORMALITIES OF THE HEART

Hypertrophic Cardiomyopathy

Clinical Characteristics and Clinical Diagnosis

HCM is an inherited disease characterized by left ventricular hypertrophy developing in the absence of obvious causes such as hypertension or aortic stenosis. The degree of left ventricular hypertrophy is largely heterogeneous, frequently showing preferential involvement of the septum (asymmetric septal hypertrophy). Most patients have remarkable regional variations in the extent of hypertrophy. Although involvement of the septum is most common, patients do present with disproportionate involvement of the apex or left ventricular free wall and only a minority of patients present with concentric hypertrophy.

Based on the distribution of cardiac hypertrophy, four types of HCM have been described: type 1 with hypertrophy limited to the anterior segment of the ventricular septum; type 2 with hypertrophy of both the anterior and the posterior segments of the ventricular septum; type 3 with involvement of both the ventricular septum and the free wall of the left ventricle; and type 4 with involvement of the posterior segment of the septum, the anterolateral free wall, or the apical half of the septum (5,6). Although distribution of cardiac hypertrophy may vary, histological assessment has revealed that irregular arrangement of cardiac myocytes and disorganization of the myofibrillar architecture are constant findings. Similarly, diastolic dysfunction is present in most patients.

Initial reports described the presence of a dynamic left ventricular outflow tract pressure gradient, emphasized as a diagnostic feature of the disease. This gradient is caused by the narrowing of the subaortic area as a result of the midsystolic movement of the anterior mitral valve leaflet (systolic anterior motion) against the hypertrophic septum. It became evident later that only a few patients (less than 25%) present an outflow tract gradient. HCM is now described as a highly heterogeneous disease. The clinical phenotype may vary, presenting even among members of the same family with various amounts of hypertrophy, and the prognosis does not seem to correlate with the severity of the hypertrophy.

Clinical Management

Clinical management of HCM is complicated by the large heterogeneity of clinical manifestations. According to Spirito and colleagues (7), "The diverse clinical and genetic features of HCM make it impossible to define precise guidelines for management." Because the genetic defect leading to cardiac hypertrophy cannot be substantially modified, therapy is directed toward the treatment of symptoms to improve quality of life.

Sudden cardiac death is the most severe complication of HCM; major efforts have been devoted to the identification of prophylactic treatment for high-risk patients. Maron and colleagues (8) conducted a retrospective study that indicated that implantable defibrillators are highly effective in terminating life-threatening ventricular tachyarrhythmias in high-risk patients. In an accompanying editorial, Watkins (9) stated that adverse effects of an implantable device should be carefully weighed against the risk of sudden cardiac death. Medical therapy may be a plausible alternative according to the data presented in 1985 by McKenna and colleagues (10), who showed that patients treated with low-dose amiodarone had fewer arrhythmic events as compared to historical controls. β Blockers have also been suggested (11) as an effective prophylactic treatment. Lifestyle changes with reduction of physical activity and avoidance of competitive sports have also been recommended for affected individuals.

Prevalence and Inheritance

A positive family history compatible with autosomal dominant transmission is present only in 40% to 50% of cases. However, this figure might underestimate the actual number of familial forms, due to the large variability of clinical presentation among family members (incomplete penetrance).

The prevalence of HCM is currently estimated to be 1 in 500, suggesting that the disease is not as rare as was previously thought. Maron and colleagues (12) evaluated autopsy results performed in 158 sudden deaths that occurred in trained North American athletes. They concluded that the most common structural cardiovascular disease causing sudden death is HCM (48 athletes, 36%), which was disproportionately prevalent in black subjects compared with white athletes (48% versus 26% of deaths; $p = 0.01$).

Molecular Genetics

Nine genes have been associated with various forms of HCM and they all encode proteins of the *sarcomere*—the basic contractile unit of cardiac myocytes.

These sarcomeric proteins interact by following specific roles and stoichiometry to ensure appropriate contraction and relaxation of cardiac muscle. The schematic structure of the sarcomere comprises thin filaments and thick filaments (Fig. 4.1-1). Myosin is the major component of the thick filaments. Myosin consists of two heavy chains (β-myosin heavy chain) and four light chains (two myosin essential light chains and two myosin regulatory light chains). The light chains stabilize the long α helix neck of the myosin head; their precise role in cardiac muscle is only poorly understood. In skeletal muscle, the myosin regulatory light chain is thought to regulate myosin adenosine triphosphatase (ATPase) activity. Myosin light chains are located in the hinge region of the β-myosin heavy chain. The thin filaments of the sarcomere include actin, the troponin complex, and α-tropomyosin.

The troponin complex (troponin T, troponin I, and troponin C) binds α-tropomyosin and operates as a calcium-sensitive switch regulating actin-myosin interaction and force generation. Each of these three genes is subject to alternative splicing, resulting in the production of tissue-specific isoforms. For example, alternative splicing at the 5-prime region is responsible for the different isoforms of troponin T present in the human heart (13). The α-tropomyosin is a rod-shaped dimer of two α helices and lies within actin filaments where it works as a bridge connecting actin to troponin complex.

Another component of the sarcomere is cardiac myosin-binding protein C that is arrayed transversely and binds myosin heavy chain and titin; it appears to regulate contraction through a phosphorylation pathway. Actin is the major constituent of the thin filaments; it binds to the myosin heads to accomplish sarcomere contraction. There are several actin genes in human genomes. Although they show a high level of homology and probably derive from a single ancestor gene, they have distinguished into different polypeptides during evolution. Human platelet and human cardiac actin, for example, differ by a single amino acid. It is presently unknown whether there is a functional counterpart to account for this diversity.

Titin is a large and particularly abundant constituent of striated muscle. Its molecules are string-like and are likely to interact with myosin. One or both of the domain types are therefore likely to bind to myosin-binding protein C.

Most of the genes encoding for sarcomeric proteins have been identified and linked to HCM: β-myosin heavy chain (*MYH7* gene) on 14q12 (14), myosin essential light chain (*MYL3* gene) on 3p (15), myosin regulatory light chain (*MYL2* gene) on 12q23-q24.3 (15), troponin I (*TNNI3* gene) on 19q13.4 (16), troponin T (*TNNT2* gene) on 1q.32 (17), α-tropomyosin (*TPM1* gene) on 15q22.1 (18,19), myosin-binding protein C (*MYBPC3* gene) on 11p11.2 (20–22), actin (*ACTC* gene) on 15q14 (23), and titin (*TTN* gene) on 2q24.3 (24). MacRae and colleagues (25) described the existence of an additional locus on 7q3 to which familial HCM associated with Wolff-Parkinson-White (WPW) syndrome mapped; this gene has not been identified.

Genotype-Phenotype Correlation

β-Myosin Heavy Chain Mutations

A major focus of research has been directed toward the attempt to derive prognostic information based on the specific defect. Before reviewing the available data, we must review the following considerations. Most HCM patients with known genetic abnormalities carry mutations that are unique to their family. Few mutational hot spots have been

reported and data are available concerning the clinical outcome of families that share these mutations. However, these data should be handled as research information and the direct extrapolation to clinical management appears premature because the sample size is still limited.

The β-myosin heavy chain gene is the gene more frequently implicated in the genesis of HCM; it has been proposed that approximately 30% of patients with this disease carry defects in this gene.

A single mutation Arg403Gln appears to be relatively common, and it, as well as other mutations (e.g., Arg719Trp and Arg453Cys), has been associated with an adverse prognosis (26). Near-normal life expectancy was reported for mutations such as Val606Met, Leu908Val, and Gly256Gln (26,27).

Anan and colleagues (28) described a Phe513-to-Cys mutation in which affected family members had near-normal life expectancy; and an Arg719-to-Trp mutation with a high incidence of premature death and an average life expectancy in affected individuals of 38 years. The authors speculated that mutations that alter the charge of the encoded amino acid affects survival more significantly than those that produce a conservative amino acid substitution. This may occur because substitution of an amino acid with another with different chemical characteristics may lead to destabilization of the protein affecting its functional properties. The location of the substitution may also be of functional relevance and it might be expected that amino acid changes in regions of the protein that are involved in critical function, such as ATP hydrolysis and interaction with thin filaments, may be associated with more severe phenotypes. Even if these hypotheses are supported by observations made in some kindred, exceptions have also been identified, thus supporting words of caution for extrapolation to the clinical setting.

Interesting functional studies have been performed in the attempt to link functional consequences of some mutations to their implications on the natural history of the disease. Lankford and colleagues (29) compared the contractile properties of single muscle fibers from patients with three different mutations with those from normal controls. They reported large variability in the nature and extent of functional impairments in skeletal fibers affected by the different mutations and suggested that the observed variability may correlate with the severity and penetrance of the disease resulting from each mutation.

Interesting insights on functional consequences of β-myosin heavy chain mutations have emerged from several studies on transgenic animals. Geisterfer-Lowrance and colleagues (30) engineered the arg403-to-gln (R403Q) mutation into the mouse genome and observed premature death of homozygous mice and development of clinical signs of the disease in heterozygous mice. Interestingly, manifestation of the disease presented gender and developmental differences, with men being more severely affected and older animals presenting progressively more severe manifestations of the disease. Functional studies (29) initially demonstrated that the R403Q mutation resulted in a depressed mechanical state including diminished isometric force generation and lower shortening velocities, resulting in decreased power output and depressed force to stiffness ratios. In light of these functional consequences, the hypothesis has been raised that hypertrophy results as a compensatory mechanism in response to reduced sarcomeric function. Recently, however, a different interpretation of the functional consequences of the R403Q mutation has been provided. Tyska and colleagues (31) reported that a "gain of function" is responsible for an enhanced functional state that may result in excessive energetic requirements and functional hyperactivity of the mutated myosin that could be the origin of myocytes disarray seen in HCM. Thus, despite the hundreds of mutations that have been identified and transgenic models that have been developed, there is still inconsistency in the interpretation of the mechanisms by which mutations influence the clinical phenotype of HCM.

Cardiac Troponin T

Mutations of the cardiac Troponin T appear to be rather frequent among patients affected by HCM. Watkins and colleagues (32) suggested that *TNNT2* mutations might be present in 15% of patients with HCM. It has been suggested by these authors that *TNNT2* defects are associated with milder cardiac hypertrophy than other genetic variants of the disease, yet they may manifest with a high proportion of arrhythmic events and sudden cardiac death. Incomplete penetrance has also been reported in *TNNT2* genetic defects: Moolman and colleagues (33) reported a penetrance in adult individuals of 40% by echocardiography and 80% with the combination of echocardiography and electrocardiography.

In a transgenic model of TnT mutations, Tardiff and colleagues (34) observed the development of mild hypertrophy and mild systolic dysfunction, but a significant degree of diastolic dysfunction. Transfection of troponin T defects in quail myotubes demonstrated (35) a decrease of force production, leading the authors to speculate that the hypertrophic phenotype could reflect the augmented energetic load to the heart.

Myosin-Binding Protein C Mutations

Mutations in the gene encoding myosin-binding protein C were initially considered an uncommon cause of HCM. More recent data, however, suggested that the *MYBPC3* gene most likely involved in 15% of cases of HCM. This variant of the disease is characterized by late onset and severe prognosis (3). These authors demonstrated that penetrance of the disease remained incomplete until the sixth decade of life. Despite presenting a relatively low lethality, *MYPBC3* defects caused a high proportion of sudden cardiac deaths.

Epidemiologic data collected in patients with this variant of the disease emphasize the need to continue tight monitoring of individuals in families affected by HCM because delayed onset may unexpectedly pose a risk of sudden death for adults and middle-aged individuals who had been defined as unaffected at an early age.

α-Tropomyosin Gene

Mutations of the α-tropomyosin gene are a relatively infrequent cause of HCM, representing approximately 3% to 5% of the genotyped individuals (26,36). The phenotype is considered intermediately severe with heterogeneous cardiac hypertrophy, although it should be always remembered that only few observations have been made and that in individual patients, the possibility of developing marked ventricular hypertrophy and severe clinical manifestations cannot be ruled out. Dissimilar levels of cardiac hypertrophy have been reported among carriers of α-tropomyosin mutations (37). An unusual manifestation of α-tropomyosin mutations has been reported by Yamauchi-Takihara and colleagues (36), who reported cardiac dilation and heart failure in members of families with Ala63Val, Lys70Thr, and Asp175Asn mutations.

Myosin Essential Light Chain, Myosin Regulatory Light Chain, Actin, and Titin Mutations

Together, these rare forms account for about 5% to 8% of HCM cases. The limited number of families with these specific defects has made it impossible to derive specific genotype-phenotype correlation.

Dilated Cardiomyopathy

DCM represents the outcome of a heterogeneous group of disorders including myocarditis, coronary artery disease, and systemic diseases. In approximately half of the cases, however, DCM is defined as " idiopathic" because no etiologic factor is identified.

The prevalence of idiopathic DCM is estimated to be about 36.5 per 100,000; it accounts for more than 10,000 deaths per year in North America and is the leading indication for cardiac transplantation. Familial occurrence accounts for 20% to 25% and is mainly characterized by an autosomal dominant pattern of inheritance, with the exception of rare cases associated with X-linked diseases and of a few that are caused by defects of mitochondrial DNA that present matrilineal transmission.

The first familial forms of DCM to be genetically defined were those associated with skeletal muscle abnormalities such as the X-linked Duchenne and Becker muscular dystrophy and the X-linked and autosomal dominant forms of Emery-Dreifuss muscular dystrophy (38,39). Although these diseases are quite rare and their diagnosis is in most instances handled by the neurologist, their understanding has brought novel information relevant to the cardiologist. Identification of candidate genes implicated in DCM is frequently based on analogy observed with skeletal muscle disorders. At least two groups of heterogeneous proteins have been implicated in the genesis of DCM. The first group includes cytoskeletal proteins such as dystrophin (that is a gene on chromosome X and is responsible for Duchenne and Becker muscular dystrophy), actin, and desmin. The second group of proteins includes the so-called proteins of the "nuclear envelope" (such as lamin A/C) and proteins of the "nuclear lamina" (such as emerin). Their role in cardiac muscle is still debated (Fig. 4.1-1).

Although only few DCM genes are known, many loci have been identified, thus pointing to a large genetic heterogeneity in DCM. Interestingly, several inherited forms of DCM are associated with extracardiac involvement (skeletal myopathy) and with intracardiac conduction defects. It is fascinating to realize that "pure" skeletal muscle myopathies and "pure cardiomyopathies" may share the same genes (lamin A/C, desmin, dystrophin) and that transitional forms may present with mixed phenotype and large variability of clinical manifestations even among members of the same family.

Recently, Kamisago and colleagues (40) demonstrated that mutations in the genes encoding for the sarcomeric proteins β-myosin heavy chain and cardiac troponin T, which have been associated with HCM (see the Hypertrophic Cardiomyopathy section), may also cause familial DCM (Fig. 4.1-1), thus suggesting that the two diseases are, in some of their genetic variants, allelic diseases.

Genetic variants of DCM are outlined according to the following scheme: (a) DCM associated with defects of the cytoskeletal proteins, which include X-linked dystrophin DCM, actin-related autosomal dominant DCM, desmin-related autosomal dominant DCM, and β-myosin heavy chain and troponin T–related autosomal dominant DCM; (b) DCM associated with defects of the proteins of the nuclear lamina and nuclear envelope, which includes X-linked Emery-Dreifuss, autosomal dominant Emery-Dreifuss, and autosomal dominant cardiomyopathy with conduction defects; (c) tafazzin-related X-linked Barth syndrome and X-linked DCM; (d) mitochondrial DCM; and (e) loci associated with DCM.

Dilated Cardiomyopathy Associated with Defects of the Cytoskeletal Proteins

A genetic defect of the cytoskeletal protein dystrophin is the cause for muscular dystrophy of the Duchenne and Becker type and of one form of X-linked DCM.

Dystrophin acts as a "functional link" between the cytoskeleton and extracellular matrix through the activity of the so-called "dystrophin-associated glycoproteins." The sarcomere is attached to the cellular wall by nonsarcomeric actin and by other cytoskeletal proteins; therefore, these proteins ensure that when the sarcomere generates contraction, the entire cell shortens.

The intermediate filaments, along with microfilaments (actins) and microtubules (tubulins), represent a third class of well-characterized cytoskeletal elements. The subunits of the intermediate filaments display a tissue-specific pattern of expression. Desmin is the muscle-specific subunit. This gene has been associated with skeletal muscle disease and only recently, mutations in this gene have been associated with a novel form of DCM.

Based on the identification of genetic defects on dystrophin, actin, and desmin genes, it has been initially suggested that DCM is a disease of cytoskeletal proteins. The picture has already changed, as novel classes of proteins have been associated with DCM. Now let's review the three variants of DCM associated with dystrophin, actin, and desmin.

X-Linked Dystrophin Dilated Cardiomyopathy

The identification of dystrophin as a gene (Xp21.2) responsible for a form of X-linked DCM was provided for the first time by Towbin and colleagues (41), who used antidystrophin antibody and demonstrated paucity of cardiac dystrophin but normal skeletal muscle dystrophin in patients with X-linked cardiomyopathy. The same group performed linkage studies in the large family originally reported by Berko and Swift (42) and in a smaller new pedigree. Linkage of X-linked cardiomyopathy to the centromeric portion of the dystrophin locus was demonstrated and abnormalities of cardiac dystrophin were shown in experiments with antidystrophin antibodies. These observations demonstrated that a *DMD* gene exists that manifests with cardiac phenotype and normal skeletal muscle function.

Along the same line of research, Muntoni and colleagues (43) demonstrated a deletion in the promoter region and first exon of the *DMD* gene in a family with X-linked DCM. Ortiz-Lopez and colleagues (44) found a causative mutation in exon 9 of the *DMD* gene in the large North American kindred described by Towbin and colleagues (41).

Actin-Related Autosomal Dominant Dilated Cardiomyopathy

α-Actin is a protein of the sarcomere that has been implicated in familial HCM (23). Unexpectedly, it has recently been shown that actin not only is present in the sarcomere and involved in force generation, but also functions as a cytoskeletal protein being involved in force transmission. Olson and colleagues (45) tested the hypothesis that genetic defects in the gene encoding for cardiac "actin" could be responsible for DCM. They screened unrelated families and were able to identify single amino acid substitutions in two families; both mutations affected universally conserved amino acids in domains of actin that attached to Z bands and intercalated disks. (A G-to-A substitution in codon 312 in exon 5 and a GAG (glu)-to-GGG (gly) mutation in codon 361 in exon 6.) Other studies have attempted to define the prevalence of actin defects in families with history of DCM but failed to find other kindred with actin-related disease.

Takai and colleagues (46) studied 136 Japanese cases and concluded that mutation in the *ACTC* gene is a rare cause of DCM in Japanese patients. Mayosi and colleagues (47) studied 57 South African patients with DCM (56% of black African origin) and failed to identify mutations in skeletal or cardiac actin genes.

Desmin-Related Autosomal Dominant Dilated Cardiomyopathy

Desmin-related myopathy is a familial disorder character-ized by skeletal muscle weakness associated with cardiac conduction blocks, arrhythmias, and restrictive heart fail-ure, as well as by intracytoplasmic accumulation of desmin-reactive deposits in cardiac and skeletal muscle cells (48). Goldfarb and colleagues (49) reported a family with desmin-related cardioskeletal myopathy associated with mutations in the highly conserved C-terminal portion of the desmin rod domain. Li and colleagues (50) identified in 1 out of 44 unrelated probands with autosomal dominant DCM a heterozygous ile451-to-met substitution in the *DES* gene. This mutation was not present in more than 900 control chromosomes. The reports of Goldfarb and coworkers (49) and Li and associates (50) suggest a distinct cardiac genotype-phenotype correlation for mutations in the *DES* gene.

β-Myosin Heavy Chain and Troponin T–Related Autosomal Dominant Dilated Cardiomyopathy

The association of mutations in the β-myosin heavy chain gene and in the troponin-T gene to DCM is very recent; therefore, only three mutations have been identified in four families reported in a single study (40). Kamisago and col-leagues (40) speculated that 10% of dilated cardiomy-opathies might be caused by defects in these genes, but because data are not available, this figure should be regarded as an educated guess. The study by Kamisago and associates (40) reports two β-myosin heavy chain point mutations (Ser532Pro and Phe764Leu) identified in two relatively large families with HCM and a single amino acid deletion (δLys210) in the troponin T gene identified in two appar-ently unrelated families.

No functional studies are yet available to explain how these mutations cause the clinical phenotype of DCM and the differences between the mutations on the same gene that causes HCM. The authors advance the hypothesis that the sarcomere mutations identified in families with DCM are likely to diminish the mechanical function of cardiac myocytes at variance with mutations identified in patients with HCM that would increase contractility. Evidence that at least one β-myosin heavy chain mutation associated with HCM causes enhanced contractile function (31) supports their hypothesis. The interpretation that gain of function versus loss of function determines the type of cardiomyopa-thy associated with mutations of sarcomeric proteins is appealing. However, as discussed in the section on HCM, several authors described loss of function as a consequence of mutations causing the HCM phenotype; therefore, more data are required to clarify the issue.

Dilated Cardiomyopathy Associated with Defects of the Proteins of the Nuclear Lamina and Nuclear Envelope

Two genes implicated in DCM cases encode for proteins called emerin (*EMD*) and lamin A/C (*LMNA*). Emerin is a member of the family of the so-called "nuclear lamina–asso-ciated proteins." Cartegni and colleagues (51) proposed that emerin accounts for a membrane's anchorage to the cytoskeleton. In the heart, *emerin* has been identified in desmosomes and fasciae adherents, and it is believed that its role could contribute to cell-to-cell communication and tight adhesion between cells; this function could explain the cardiac phenotype of emerin-related DCM that manifests with conduction defects.

The second gene implicated in DCM is called lamin A/C, which is a filamentous protein contained in the nuclear matrix and is attached to the inner nuclear mem-brane. It is currently unknown whether emerin and lamin A/C interact, although it is suggested that they are found in the nuclear matrix.

X-Linked Emery-Dreifuss

Emery-Dreifuss muscular dystrophy is an X-linked inher-ited degenerative myopathy characterized by (a) slowly progressive muscle wasting and weakness with humero-peroneal distribution in the early stages; (b) early contrac-tures of the elbows, Achilles tendons, and postcervical muscles; and (c) cardiomyopathy. Emery (38) suggested that this disorder could also be inherited as an autosomal dominant trait.

It is important that cardiologists become aware of this disorder because even if Emery-Dreifuss' most obvious phe-notype involves skeletal muscles, the most serious and life-threatening clinical manifestation reflects cardiac involve-ment. Interestingly, cardiac manifestations, such as conduction disturbances, may be present also in the female carriers (38), who never show the full-blown disease. Initial cardiac manifestations are subtle, presenting with pro-longed PR intervals that may progress over a variable amount of time to complete heart block with bradycardic idioventricular rhythms that frequently require pacemaker implantation. Patients may need a pacemaker even before manifesting muscular weakness (52). At least 70 different mutations in the emerin gene have been identified in indi-viduals affected by X-linked Emery-Dreifuss muscular dys-trophy. Remarkably different levels of severity for clinical manifestations have been reported among individuals with the same mutation, suggesting that environmental or

genetic factors may be pivotal in the definition of the phenotype.

Autosomal Dominant Emery-Dreifuss

Fenichel and colleagues (53) and Miller and colleagues (54)
described families affected by an autosomal dominant muscular dystrophy with cardiac involvement that closely
resembled Emery-Dreifuss muscular dystrophy. Affected
individuals (men and women) had contractures of posterior
cervical muscles, elbows, and ankles associated with cardiac
involvement showing atrial arrhythmias and slow ventricular rate. Other descriptions of similar cases followed (55)
and confirmed the phenotypical similarities with Emery-
Dreifuss muscular dystrophy, leading to the acceptance of
the existence of two patterns of inheritance for the disease.
The search for the gene responsible for the autosomal dominant Emery-Dreifuss muscular dystropy was initiated
based on the evidence that "emerin" is normal in the autosomal dominant form. To explain the phenotypical similarity of the two forms (X-linked and autosomal dominant),
one might suggest that a protein that has functional interactions with emerin would be an ideal candidate gene for
the autosomal dominant form of the disease. It wasn't until
1999, with the work of Bonne and colleagues (56), that the
locus for autosomal dominant Emery-Dreifuss muscular
dystrophy was mapped to chromosome 1 (1q11-q23). This
region contains the lamin A/C gene that encodes two proteins of the nuclear lamina: lamins A and C that are produced by alternative splicing. Laminae form dimers
through their rod domain and interact with the chromatin
and with key proteins of the inner nuclear membrane.
Bonne and coworkers (56) confirmed that lamin A/C is the
gene responsible for autosomal dominant Emery-Dreifuss
and identified mutations that co-segregate with the disease
phenotype. This finding by Bonne and associates (56) is
important not only because the authors identified the disease gene, but also because their data implicate for the first
time components of the nuclear lamina in the genesis of a
muscle disease.

Autosomal Dominant Cardiomyopathy with Conduction Defects

Having discussed DCM associated with skeletal muscle
myopathy, it will be surprising to realize that one of the
few known genes responsible for a "pure" cardiac variant of
autosomal dominant DCM has been mapped to 1p1-q21
(57), the same region where the lamin A/C gene is located.
As we discussed, mutations in the head or tail domain of
this gene cause autosomal dominant Emery-Dreifuss muscular dystrophy. Recently, Fatkin and colleagues (58)
demonstrated genetic defects on the *LMNA* gene in families with autosomal dominant DCM and conduction system defects. Five novel missense mutations were identified
in the heterozygous state: four in the α-helical rod domain
of the *LMNA* gene, and one in the lamin C tail domain.

Each mutation caused heritable, progressive conduction
system disease (sinus bradycardia, atrioventricular [AV]
conduction block, or atrial arrhythmias) and DCM. Heart
failure and sudden death occurred frequently in these families. No family members with mutations had joint contractures or skeletal myopathy. Furthermore, serum creatine kinase levels were within the normal range in family
members with mutations in the lamin rod domain, but
mildly elevated in family members with a defect in the tail
domain of lamin C. These findings indicate that lamin A
and lamin C play an important role in cardiac conduction
and contractility. These data demonstrate that autosomal
dominant Emery-Dreifuss muscular dystrophy and DCM
with conduction disturbances are allelic diseases. This evidence points to the existence of variants of the disease
combining cardiac and muscle phenotypes. This interpretation blurs the distinction between two diseases that not
only are unrelated, but also fall in the area of competence
of different medical specialists, namely the neurologist and
the cardiologist.

Tafazzin-Related Barth Syndrome and X-Linked Dilated Cardiomyopathy

Barth and colleagues (59,60) described a large family
affected by an X-linked disorder characterized by DCM,
neutropenia, skeletal myopathy, and abnormal mitochondria. In this family, premature mortality was observed in
three generations caused by sepsis due to agranulocytosis or
cardiac failure. Weakness of skeletal muscles was also present in some (but not all) affected individuals. Subsequent
reports presented cases of X-linked diseases that included all
or some of the features of Barth syndrome. Neustein and
associates (61) reported a family that may have had the
same disorder. They demonstrated abnormal mitochondria
and cardiac endocardial fibroelastosis but apparently no
neutropenia in four men who died of DCM. Hodgson and
coworkers (62) described a family with multiple cases of
men who died of cardiac failure within the first 8 months
of life and presented with endocardial fibroelastosis and
abnormality of mitochondria. Kelley and colleagues (63)
reported increased levels of urinary 3-methylglutaconic acid
and 2-ethylhydracrylic acid and referred to the disorder as
Barth syndrome. The clinical course of the syndrome
includes severe cardiac dysfunction and recurrent infections
during infancy and early childhood. The disease may manifest as DCM or as isolated neutropenia without clinical
evidence of heart disease.

Linkage studies demonstrated that the gene of Barth
syndrome is located in Xq28. Bione and colleagues (64)
identified mutations in a gene called *G4.5* that is highly
expressed in cardiac and skeletal muscle. Different mRNAs
were produced by alternative splicing of the primary *G4.5*
transcript, encoding proteins called tafazzin, whose function is yet unknown.

As with other genetic defects that can have phenotypic heterogeneity, it has been shown that Barth syndrome may manifest in some individuals as an infantile cardiomyopathy. For example, D'Adamo and colleagues (65) demonstrated that the affected members of the family with DCM, which was reported by Gedeon and associates (66), had a mutation in the *G4.5* gene, supporting the evidence that the disease may present with the isolated feature of X-linked DCM.

Mitochondrial Dilated Cardiomyopathy

Evidence of a mitochondrial form of DCM was initially provided by Suomalainen and colleagues (67), when they described a mother and son who died of idiopathic DCM at ages 37 and 22 years, respectively. These authors demonstrated the presence of mitochondrial DNA, with multiple large deletions in muscle of both victims in this family with DCM, which was associated with severe muscle fatigue and weakness. Other reports followed (68–70), although conclusive demonstration that mutations of mitochondrial DNA were the only cause of DCM in these cases is missing.

Loci Associated with Dilated Cardiomyopathy

In the last section in this chapter, which is dedicated to DCM, we briefly review loci where one or few families have been linked, but here we give a short clinical description aimed at highlighting other phenotypes that are associated with DCM. The letters indicate the name given in the online database *Mendelian Inheritance in Man* (OMIM) database to each genetic variant of the DCM, and it is followed by the chromosomal locus (available at: http://www3.ncbi.nlm.nih.gov/omim/).

Gene Map Locus: 9q13 *CMD1B*

In one large six-generation family with autosomal dominant DCM, Krajinovic and colleagues (71) demonstrated linkage to 9q13-q22.

Gene Map Locus: 10q21-q23 *CMD1C*

Bowles and colleagues (72) found linkage between familial autosomal dominant DCM and markers at 10q21-q23 in a family in which 12 of 26 members were affected.

Gene Map Locus: 1q32 *CMD1D*

Durand and colleagues (73) studied a family residing in California and Utah with DCM in multiple members of three generations and by implication a fourth. Linkage analysis indicated the locus to be on 1q32.

3p25-p22 *CMD1E*

Olson and Keating (74) studied a family with DCM associated with sinus node dysfunction, supraventricular tachyarrhythmias, conduction delay, and stroke.

Gene Map Locus: 6q23 *CMD1F*

Messina and colleagues (75) observed DCM with conduction defect and adult-onset limb-girdle muscular dystrophy in an extensively affected four-generation family.

Gene Map Locus: 2q31 *CMD1G*

Siu and colleagues (76) clinically evaluated three generations of a Native American family with autosomal dominant transmission of DCM. Nine surviving affected individuals had early-onset disease (ventricular chamber dilation during the teenage years and congestive heart failure during the third decade of life). The disease was nonpenetrant in two obligate carriers.

Gene Map Locus: 2q14-q22 *CMD1H*

Jung and colleagues (77) studied a German family with 12 individuals affected by autosomal dominant DCM characterized by ventricular dilation, impaired systolic function, and conduction disease. After exclusion of the known loci for DCM, they performed a whole-genome screen and detected linkage to 2q14-q22.

Right Ventricular Cardiomyopathy

Arrhythmogenic right ventricular cardiomyopathy (also called dysplasia; ARVD) is a disease characterized by fibrofatty infiltration of the right ventricle (occasionally the left ventricle may be involved) (78). More frequently, the degenerative changes involve the free wall of the right ventricle, the subtricuspid region, and the outflow tract (79).

As with LQTS, two forms are described: the most common one being inherited as autosomal dominant (80) and one rare variant characterized by combined cardiac and extracardiac involvement (palmar keratosis and kinky hair) inherited as a recessive trait (81,82). The recessive trait has been described in the island of Naxos and is called Naxos disease. In a study on the population of Ecuador, Carvajal-Huerta (83) described 18 patients with an epidermolytic palmoplantar keratoderma, woolly hair, associated with cardiac left ventricular DCM. It remains unclear whether these patients have a different clinical disease or they may represent the same disorder as "Naxos disease" with biventricular involvement.

Naxos disease was first mapped to the long arm of chromosome 17 (17q21) by Coonar and colleagues in 1998 (81). Subsequently, a deletion in the human plakoglobin gene (*PLK*) in families with Naxos disease was demonstrated (84). This is the first gene that is associated with ARVD, indicating that this cardiomyopathy is caused by a cytoskeleton abnormality involving the cell-to-cell junction. Plakoglobin, a member of the armadillo protein gene family, is a constituent protein in adherens and desmosomal junctions with adhesive and signaling function. It is an important component of the cell-cell and cell-adhesion complex.

Arrhythmias represent the most important clinical manifestation of ARVD and may lead to sudden cardiac death. Ventricular extrasystoles show a left bundle branch block pattern; frequently arrhythmias are precipitated by intense physical activity. Diagnosis (79) is based on the identification of right ventricular dilation, adipose tissue infiltration and kinetic abnormalities with cardiac imaging techniques (echocardiography/cineangiography and magnetic resonance imaging [MRI]). Electrocardiographic (ECG) abnormalities are also important diagnostic criteria (T-wave inversion in leads V_1 through V_3). The most important ECG abnormalities are T-wave inversion in the right precordial leads and the presence of late potentials on signal averaged ECG. The diagnosis of right ventricular cardiomyopathy is based on echocardiographic and angiographic documentation of localized or widespread structural and dynamic abnormalities involving mainly or exclusively the right ventricle, in the absence of valve disease, shunts, active myocarditis, and coronary disease. Endomyocardial biopsy (85) may be useful in the differential diagnosis.

Rampazzo and colleagues (86) estimated that the prevalence of ARVD ranges from 6 per 10,000 in the general population to 4.4 per 1,000 in some areas with higher prevalence. For example, the Veneto region of northern Italy seems to present an unusually high prevalence of the disease; in this country, several large families have been identified and studied. Linkage has been established to several loci, but no gene has been identified. Two linkage studies performed in North American families, mapped on different and novel loci (87,88). Overall, six loci have been reported for the autosomal dominant form that correspond to six variants of the disease: *ARVD1* on 14q23-q24 (86), *ARVD2* on 1q42-q43 (89), *ARVD3* on 14q12-q22 (90), *ARVD4* on 2q32.1-q32.3 (91), *ARVD5* on 3p23 (87), and *ARVD6* on 10p14-p12 (88). The autosomal recessive form has been mapped to a novel locus (82) on chromosome 17.

An important observation concerning the physiopathologic basis of ARVD was made by Mallat and colleagues (92), who reported evidence of apoptosis in six out of seven patients with the disease and in none of four control individuals. These authors proposed that apoptosis might contribute to loss of myocardial tissue in the disease. Along the same line of research, Valente and colleagues (93) examined right ventricular endomyocardial biopsies from 20 subjects with the disease and demonstrated evidence of apoptotic myocytes with ARVD by electron microscopy and revealed the presence of apoptotic myocytes in 7 of 20. The authors concluded that myocardial destruction might occur intermittently with replacement by fat and might be episodic, rather than progressive. The role of viral infections in triggering destructive phases has been suggested (78).

Mitral Valve Prolapse

Idiopathic prolapse of the mitral valve leaflets into the left atrium is a highly prevalent condition, occurring in 5% to 10% of young adults, and this abnormality is more commonly observed in women than in men (94,95). Diagnosis is suspected at cardiac auscultation (midsystolic, nonejection click) and established at echocardiogram.

This abnormality is called *idiopathic* when it does not occur as a result of a structural heart disease or a connective tissue disorder (such as Marfan syndrome).

Idiopathic mitral valve prolapse may be associated with symptoms such as chest pain, dyspnea (96), and dysrhythmia (97). It has been suggested that symptoms may be the consequence of abnormal stretch of the mitral annulus (98). Familial occurrence of mitral valve prolapse was reported already in the seventies (99,100) and autosomal dominant inheritance was suggested (101).

The condition is usually benign; predisposition to bacterial endocarditis may be present in these patients. It has been reported that sudden cardiac death may be associated (102), particularly in those subjects with myxomatous degeneration of the valve leaflets.

Disse and colleagues (103) identified four pedigrees with autosomal dominant inheritance, linkage analysis of the largest pedigree (24 individuals in 3 generations) identified the locus for mitral valve prolapse at 16p12.1-p11.2

PRIMARY ELECTRICAL DISORDERS ASSOCIATED WITH VENTRICULAR ARRHYTHMIAS

Long QT Syndrome

In the early 1960s, Romano and colleagues (104) and Ward (105) independently described a disease characterized by QT prolongation, abnormal T-wave morphology, and high incidence of lethal cardiac arrhythmias transmitted as an autosomal dominant trait (Romano-Ward syndrome). A similar cardiac phenotype associated with neurosensorial deafness and an autosomal recessive pattern of inheritance had been described a few years earlier by Jervell and Lange-Nielsen (Jervell and Lange-Nielsen syndrome) (106). Throughout the years, an increasing number of families with congenital QT prolongation and ventricular arrhythmias have been collected in a Prospective Registry created by Moss and coworkers (107). Data obtained by this collaborative project have allowed the definition of the main clinical features of the disease (108), which is generally defined as LQTS.

Clinical Manifestations

In most cases, patients with LQTS are first referred to a physician because of the occurrence of a syncopal episode or cardiac arrest in a young individual (child or teenager). Syncope and fainting are the typical symptoms of LQTS and their occurrence is often associated with conditions of physical or emotional stress (e.g., fear, anger, loud noises, and sudden awakening). Auditory stimuli (e.g., alarm clock and thunder) and swimming may be specific triggers of syncope for some patients. Overall, an increased sympathetic activity is often associated with the onset of cardiac events in patients with LQTS, although in a smaller subset of individuals, cardiac events typically occur during rest or sleep (108). Clinical manifestations of LQTS may be highly variable, ranging from full-blown disease with markedly prolonged QT interval and recurrent syncope to subclinical forms with borderline QT-interval prolongation.

Clinical Management of Long QT Syndrome

The relevant role of the sympathetic nervous system in triggering the onset of cardiac events in many patients with LQTS provided the rationale for the use of antiadrenergic interventions (109). β Blockers were considered an effective therapy (110,111), based on the evidence of a significantly lower mortality rate among patients treated with beta blockade and left-sided cardiac sympathetic denervation compared with that for patients treated with nonantiadrenergic interventions (111). Left-sided cardiac sympathetic denervation has been proposed for patients who are unresponsive to or do not tolerate β-blocking therapy (112).

Although β blockers are considered a first-line treatment, a randomized, double-blind, placebo-controlled trial has never been performed. Recently, the investigators of the International Registry of Long QT Syndrome database analyzed the efficacy of beta blockade in patients with LQTS and showed a significant residual risk of sudden death (113). Patients that appear to be at higher risk despite treatment are those who survived aborted cardiac arrest; prophylactic implantable cardioverter-defibrillator (ICD) device should be considered for these patients. Permanent pacemaker implantation is indicated in selected patients who have LQTS with AV block and whenever there is evidence of bradycardia-dependent or pause-dependent malignant arrhythmias, but these devices should always be used in combination with β-blocker therapy (114,115).

Genetic Basis of Long QT Syndrome

As of today, five genes and six loci have been implicated in the genesis of LQTS (1). Linkage analysis was applied to large kindred, which allowed the mapping of four LQTS loci on chromosome 11 (116), 3 and 7 (117), and 4 (118). The gene on chromosome 11 (LQT1) *KCNQ1* was identified by Wang and colleagues (119) using positional cloning. Candidate gene approach allowed the identification of the genes corresponding to chromosome 7 (LQT2) and 3 (LQT3), *HERG* and *SCN5A*, respectively (120,121). All

these genes encode for ion-channel subunits critical for the physiologic excitability of cardiac myocytes.

KVLQT1 (LQT1) and *KCNE1* (LQT5).

The cardiac delayed rectifier current (I_K) is one of the major determinants of the phase 3 repolarization of the cardiac action potential and has been found to be the result of two independent components in isolated cardiac myocytes: a rapid (I_{Kr}) and a slow catecholamine-sensitive component (I_{Ks}) (122). *KCNQ1* (LQT1) constitutes the alpha subunit of the channel conducting the slow component of the cardiac delayed rectifier current I_{Ks}. *KCNQ1* mutations are the most prevalent genetic defect of LQTS. Approximately half of genotyped patients carry a mutation on this gene.

More than 70 different *KCNQ1* mutations (mainly single amino acid substitutions) have been described. Homozygous or compound heterozygous mutations of *KCNQ1* have been associated with the recessive Jervell and Lange-Nielsen form of LQTS (JLN1) (123). The beta subunit of the I_{Ks} channel (124,125) is encoded by the *KCNE1* gene (on chromosome arm 21q22.1-q22.2), which has been shown, in analogy with *KCNQ1,* to cause Romano-Ward (LQT5) and Jervell and Lange-Nielsen (JLN2) syndromes (126,127).

Expression studies of *KCNQ1* and *KCNE1* mutated proteins suggested multiple mechanisms of functional failure. Defective proteins may coassemble with wild-type proteins and act as a "poison peptide" that alters in a dominant negative fashion a channel's function. Other mutations do not assemble with wild-type peptides, causing a loss of function by haploinsufficiency (128–130). Defective peptides may alter intracellular protein trafficking (131). Overall, it is assumed that LQTS-related defects in *KCNQ1* and *KCNE1* reduce the repolarizing current I_{Ks}, thus prolonging action potential duration and QT interval.

HERG (LQT2) and *KCNE2* (LQT6)

The LQT2 variant of LQTS is caused by mutations in the *HERG* gene on chromosome arm 7q35-q36. *HERG* (human ether-a-go-go–related gene) was originally cloned by Warmke and Ganetzky (132) in 1994 and identified as a disease gene for LQTS one year later by Curran and colleagues (120). HERG protein is responsible for the fast component of the delayed rectifier current I_{Kr} (133).

Many *HERG* mutations have been reported in the last 5 years (134–139), suggesting that this is the second most common variant of LQTS accounting for 30% to 35% of mutations in LQTS-genotyped patients. One family with a homozygous mutation has been described (140). Compared with *KCNQ1*, *HERG* coassembles with a beta subunit to form a functionally intact channel. This beta subunit is called Mirp1 (minK-related peptide) and is encoded by a small intron-free gene on chromosome arm 21q22.1-q22.2 contiguous to the *KCNE1* gene (141). Only one third of *KCNE2* mutations identified so far were associated with the clinical phenotype of QT prolongation. In our series, only 1 of 250 LQTS probands has been found to be a carrier of a *KCNE2* mutation, a 9–base pairs deletion truncating the protein at the central portion of the transmembrane segment of the predicted topology. Thus, LQT6 appears to be a rare variant of LQTS.

Functional expression studies have demonstrated that *HERG* mutations cause a reduction of the I_{Kr} current (142). Compared with *KVLQT1* genetic defects, *HERG*-mutated subunits reduce repolarizing current through dominant negative (poison peptide) and nondominant negative (haploinsufficiency) (142). Recently detailed evaluation mutations have been associated with changes in the gating kinetics and defects in the intracellular protein trafficking (143,144).

SCN5A (LQT3)

The cardiac sodium channel gene was cloned by Gellens and coworkers in 1992 (145) and mapped to chromosome 3p21 by George and colleagues in 1995 (146). The structure of the SCN5A protein is quite different from most of the other voltage-dependent cardiac ion channels, which coassemble to form homomultimers or heteromultimers in the membrane. The Na^+ channel protein is a relatively large molecule that folds onto itself to surround the channel's pore (145). When linkage was established to the region 3p21-p23, SCN5A was immediately considered a most likely candidate for LQTS.

The first mutations, identified by Wang and colleagues (121,147), were clustered in the regions functionally relevant to the channel inactivation (delKPQ, R1623Q, N1325S). Functional studies demonstrated that these mutations cause an increased late inward sodium current (I_{Na}) (148,149). It was concluded that Na^+ channel mutations originate the LQTS phenotype by inducing a gain of function of the protein with an enhanced inward current, which prolongs action potential duration.

Few SCN5A mutations have been reported in the literature (121,147–152) and the relative prevalence of LQT3 among LQTS patients is estimated to be 10% to 15% (153).

LQT4 on Chromosome 4 (4q25-q27)

The gene associated with the LQTS locus on chromosome 4 is still unknown. Only one family linked to this locus (4q25-q27) has been reported (118). Of note, the phenotype of the LQT4 patients differs from that of the typical LQTS. Most of the affected individuals, besides QT-interval prolongation, also present with severe sinus bradycardia, paroxysmal atrial fibrillation (detected in more than 50% of the patients), and polyphasic T waves (118). Recent experimental data based on ankyrin(b) knock-out mice suggested that this protein is pivotal in the regulation of the Na^+ channel function, suggesting that the ankyrin(b) gene that maps to chromosome arm 4q25-q27 may be a candidate gene for LQT4 (154).

Genotype-Phenotype Correlation

Recently a number of genotype-phenotype correlation studies have been performed in the attempt to provide novel indicators for risk stratification.

The analysis of the ECG patterns revealed gene-specific alterations of the ST-T segment (155,156) and a different behavior of QT-interval adaptation to changes in heart rate, with an increased shortening at high frequency among LQT3 patients (157) and a reduced adaptation among LQT1 (158,159).

Schwartz and colleagues (160) have recently provided evidence that *KCNQ1* mutations increase the risk of cardiac events during physical or emotional stress. Carriers experience 97% of cardiac events in this setting, compared with LQT2 and LQT3 patients who have 50% of their events at rest. Along the same line, it has been proposed that auditory stimuli are a relatively specific trigger for LQT2 patients (161,162) and swimming is predominantly associated with cardiac events in LQT1 patients (162,163).

The analysis of the event-free survival performed by the investigators of the International Registry of Long QT Syndrome (164) shows that the lethality of cardiac events is influenced by the genetic substrate. LQT3 patients have fewer events that are characterized by high lethality (164).

Prediction of the severity of clinical manifestation from *in vitro* studies is not possible (165), as even the same mutation may cause variable severity of clinical manifestations (136); however, it has been suggested that the position of a mutation may allow some level of prediction of the phenotype. For example, mutations located in the carboxy terminus of *KCNQ1* (166) are mostly benign and are associated with a mild clinical phenotype. Napolitano and colleagues (2) and Neyroud and coworkers (167) showed that mutations occurring in functionally critical regions of the KCNQ1 protein might remain subclinical until a provocative factor unmasks the unstable electrical substrate.

These observations are extremely interesting but caution should be used in their extrapolation to clinical practice. For example, when larger groups of LQT3 patients carrying mutations other than the few originally reported have been studied, the presence of variable ST-T ECG patterns has been demonstrated (156). The variable penetrance of LQTS mutations (136,168) and the evidence that up to 6% of genotyped LQTS probands may indeed carry two independently inherited genetic defects (169,170) introduce additional complexity and limit the possibility to predict prognosis in the individual patient.

Gene-Specific Therapy

Gene-specific therapies are therapeutic strategies targeted to counteract the consequences of a specific genetic defect, as opposed to gene therapy, which is the attempt to correct the mutation, restoring a wild-type gene. Given the major technical limitations still existing for an effective gene therapy, gene-specific treatment may represent a feasible and targeted therapeutic approach for a genetic disease.

The understanding of the molecular basis of LQTS has suggested attempting to counteract the consequences of the genetic defect. Based on the evidence that LQT3 is caused by an increased late I_{Na} (148) and that LQT2 is caused by a reduction in I_{Kr} (120), we developed an experimental preparation mimicking LQT3 and LQT2, respectively (171). In this model, we demonstrated the Na$^+$ channel blocker mexiletine significantly reduced the action potential duration in the LQT3 model while it did not modify action potential duration in the LQT2 model. We later attempted to test the feasibility of this pharmacologic intervention in a small group of LQT3 patients (157), confirming that sodium-channel blockade shortened the QT interval among LQT3 patients, but not among LQT2 patients. Benhorin and colleagues (172) reported that flecainide may also shorten QT interval in LQT3 patients; however, the safety of flecainide in LQT3 has been subsequently questioned (173).

A similar approach was devised by Compton and colleagues (174) for the management of LQT2 patients. As previously discussed, LQT2 is caused by mutations in the *HERG* gene encoding the I_{Kr} potassium channel. I_{Kr} current is augmented by increases in the extracellular potassium levels. These authors hypothesized that I_{Kr} function could be improved by exogenous administration of potassium and potassium sparing diuretics. This gene-specific approach was tested in seven LQT2 patients obtaining a significant QT shortening.

A word of caution is required because there are no data proving that gene-specific therapy, besides shortening QT interval, is able to prevent life-threatening events.

Brugada Syndrome

In 1992, Brugada and colleagues (175) described a novel clinical entity characterized by ST-segment elevation in right precordial leads (V_1 through V_3), incomplete or complete right bundle branch block, and susceptibility to the development of ventricular tachyarrhythmias. This disease is now frequently called *Brugada syndrome*. Familial occurrence has been described with an autosomal dominant pattern of inheritance. The prevalence of Brugada syndrome is not known, although high prevalence has been reported in eastern countries (176).

The age of onset of clinical manifestations is the third or fourth decade of life and the cardiac events typically occur during sleep or at rest (177). Malignant forms with earlier onset and even with neonatal manifestations have been reported (178).

The diagnostic ECG pattern is intermittently present in affected individuals. It has been suggested that the autonomic nervous system may modify the ECG phenotype as intravenous administration of isoproterenol attenuates or acetylcholine accentuates the ECG abnormalities in affected individuals (179). Pharmacologic challenge with some class I antiarrhythmic drugs, namely, ajmaline, flecainide, and procainamide, may unmask the typical ECG pattern in affected patients and it has been proposed as a diagnostic test in patients with borderline ECG readings (180).

In a recent report from Brugada and colleagues (181), it has been shown that the risk of sudden death at a 3-year follow-up after diagnosis is 27% to 34% in asymptomatic and symptomatic patients, respectively (181). Because no pharmacologic treatment is associated with reduction of cardiac events, the treatment of choice is the ICD. Implantation of an ICD has been recommended for symptomatic individuals and for patients with inducible ventricular tachyarrhythmias at programmed electrical stimulation. This approach is still debated and data have been provided (182) showing a lower incidence of cardiac events among asymptomatic patients and a lower than expected predictive accuracy of programmed electrical stimulation.

Genetic Basis of Brugada Syndrome

In 1998, the molecular basis of Brugada syndrome had been identified and the disease had been demonstrated to be allelic to the LQTS (LQT3) (183). The first three *SCN5A* mutations identified by SSCP and DNA sequencing are two truncations (one frame-shift and one splice-donor mutation), resulting in a premature termination of the amino acid sequence, and one missense mutation in the fourth domain of the predicted transmembrane topology of *SCN5A* (183). Additional mutations have been reported in the literature (152,178,182,184). Data from our laboratories suggest that no more than 30% of patients with Brugada syndrome carry *SCN5A* mutations, pointing to the evidence that the disease is genetically heterogeneous.

In vitro functional characterization of *SCN5A* mutations showed that the missense mutation (T1620M) resulted in a faster recovery of inactivation of the mutated channels and a shift of voltage dependence of steady-state inactivation toward more positive potentials (183). Mutations in the *SCN5A* gene may modify the interaction with the sodium channel beta subunit, thereby leading to channel dysfunction (185,186).

An overlapping phenotype of LQTS 3 (LQT3) and Brugada syndrome has been reported by Bezzina and colleagues (152), who described the simultaneous presence of QT prolongation and ST-segment elevation in a family in which an *SCN5A* mutation (InsD1795) was present. Subsequently, we demonstrated that ST-segment elevation may be induced in LQT3 patients by administration of intravenous flecainide (173), suggesting that the response to this drug is similar in the two diseases and supporting the existence of clinical overlap.

It has been proposed that the ST-segment elevation phenotype is a feature of a novel type of cardiomyopathy (187,188). Few reports support this view: (a) a typical ARVD pattern at the cardiac MRI scan was identified in 1 of 35 patients with ST-segment elevation and right bundle branch block (189) and (b) "Brugada-like" ECG modifications were elicited in response to class Ic drugs and autonomic modulations in a patient with a clinical diagnosis of ARVD (190).

Catecholaminergic Polymorphic Ventricular Tachycardia

In 1983 and more extensively in 1995, Coumel and coworkers (191) and Leenhardt and colleagues (192) described a typical pattern of ventricular arrhythmias manifesting in children and young adults, characterized by polymorphic tachyarrhythmias often presenting a typical bidirectional pattern. In these patients, arrhythmias are precipitated by stress or emotion. Patients have a normal ECG reading and a normal QT-interval and lack structural abnormalities of the right and the left ventricle. A familiar occurrence of the disease occurred in approximately 30% of cases described by Leenhardt and colleagues (192) and an autosomal dominant pattern of inheritance was suggested. The condition has since then referred to as *catecholaminergic polymorphic ventricular tachycardia* (CPVT). The bidirectional pattern of CPVTs closely resembles the arrhythmias observed during digitalis intoxication, for example, or arrhythmias caused by triggered activity (193) due to delayed afterdepolarizations. Delayed afterdepolarizations are caused by abnormal calcium release from the sarcoplasmic reticulum, are enhanced by β-adrenergic stimulation (delayed afterdepolarization *in vivo*), and are suppressed by administration of ryanodine, a specific blocker of the sarcoplasmic reticulum channel responsible for intracellular calcium release. These pathophysiologic facts pointed to triggered activity as a likely mechanism for CPVT and suggested that genes encoding proteins responsible for intracellular calcium handling were likely candidates for this genetic disorder.

In 1999, Swan and colleagues (194) mapped the locus of CPVT to the chromosomal locus 1q42-q43 in two families. This region contains the gene encoding for the human cardiac ryanodine receptor (hRyR2) (195), the key protein involved in Ca^{2+} release from the sarcoplasmic reticulum (196). In December 2000, Priori and coworkers identified hRyR2 mutations in four families with the typical pattern of CPVT and a history of sudden cardiac death, thus demonstrating that hRyR2 is the gene for catecholaminergic ventricular tachycardia (197).

Idiopathic Ventricular Tachycardia and Fibrillation

Idiopathic ventricular tachycardia and fibrillation may present with familial clustering even in individuals with a structurally normal heart and in the absence of ECG signs of primary electrical diseases such as Brugada syndrome and LQTS (see specific sections). Several possibilities may account for this evidence. Genes encoding for cardiac ion channels may be potential candidates for these unclassified forms of familial idiopathic arrhythmias. Genes encoding for gap junctions, ion exchangers (such as the Na^+-Ca^{2+} exchanger) or ion pumps (such as the Na^+-K^+ pump) may be among other candidates. It is also possible that "idiopathic" ventricular arrhythmias are "formes frustes" of Brugada syndrome and LQTS (LQTS with normal QT interval). We recently (178) reported a family with five cases of sudden cardiac death and apparently no clinical phenotype that was subsequently characterized as genetically affected by Brugada syndrome.

Among the possible explanations for "idiopathic ventricular tachycardia and fibrillation" we hypothesize that in some families atypical variants of cardiomyopathies may cause electrical instability without manifesting a clinically overt cardiomyopathy (cases such as HCM without hypertrophy described, for example, with troponin T mutations). Among the forms of ventricular tachycardia that may occur in families but are not classified as "inherited" conditions, there are right ventricular outflow tract tachycardia, catecholaminergic ventricular tachycardia, and short coupled torsade de pointes.

Rubin and colleagues (198) reported a four-generation family with affected individuals presenting with paroxysmal ventricular tachycardia (right bundle branch block, with left axis deviation morphology) and sudden cardiac death in the absence of structural heart disease and repolarization abnormalities. No genetic studies were reported for this family.

An interesting observation that may open a new direction in the understanding of the genetic bases of ventricular arrhythmias was reported by Lerman and colleagues (199). They studied a patient with adrenergically mediated idiopathic right ventricular outflow tract tachycardia unresponsive to adenosine and vagal maneuvers. The authors performed genetic analysis on a biopsy sample obtained from the arrhythmogenic focus. In DNA extracted from the tissue (but not in genomic DNA or in DNA extracted from cardiac cells distant from the site of origin of the arrhythmias), they identified a "somatic" point mutation in the *GNAI2* gene (guanine nucleotide–binding protein, alpha-inhibiting activity polypeptide), which upon expression studies was proven to increase the level of cAMP.

This finding suggests that somatic cell mutations in the cAMP-dependent signal transduction pathway occurring during myocardial development may be responsible for some forms of idiopathic ventricular tachycardia. So far no other reports from the same group or other groups have confirmed this finding in other subjects.

SUPRAVENTRICULAR ARRHYTHMIAS

Sick Sinus Syndrome and Atrial Fibrillation

Familial clusters of atrial arrhythmias have been reported in the literature. However, at variance with inherited diseases associated with ventricular arrhythmias that are clearly inherited with autosomal dominant and recessive patterns and represent "pure" electrical disorders, the genetic transmission of "pure" atrial electrical abnormalities is less well defined. Structural abnormalities are frequently combined with atrial arrhythmias, particularly bradyarrhythmias. It is frequently hypothesized that these forms are actually electrical manifestations of regional cardiomyopathies or are even associated with extracardiac familial manifestations. Families have been reported with atrial arrhythmias associated with mental retardation (200) or with limb abnormalities. In some families, abnormalities of the sinus node are associated with tachyarrhythmias such as atrial fibrillation. The families described by Bacos and colleagues (201), Spellberg (202), Surawicz and Hariman (203), and Beyer and colleagues (204) presented with variable atrial arrhythmias including junctional rhythms, paroxysms of atrial fibrillation, and occasionally sudden death. It is extremely difficult to establish whether these familial "clusters" are different phenotypes that belong to a single inherited disease. For example, the observation of the existence of genetic factors in AV conduction time raises the issue whether cases reported as clusters of "short" or clusters of "long" PR interval are the 'tail' of the distribution for a multifactorial trait.

A familial disorder of the sinoatrial node was also described by Nordenberg and colleagues (205) and Mackintosh and Chamberlain (206). Frequently, sinus node dysfunction is combined with various types of conduction defects (AV block or intraventricular conduction delay). Although the pattern of inheritance may not be obvious in most cases, the frequency of multiple familial cases led Lehmann and Klein (200) to propose that 2% to 6% of cases of "sick sinus syndrome" are inherited.

The only hard finding supporting the concept of atrial arrhythmias as the manifestation of monogenic disorders comes from the study by Brugada and colleagues (207), who identified linkage for familial atrial fibrillation (logarithm of odds score of 3.60) to the region 10q22-q24 in Spanish families. Most patients included in the study had chronic atrial fibrillation, and the age of onset of the arrhythmias ranged from 2 to 50 years. In the last 3 years, Brugada and coworkers have actively worked to reduce the region of interest on chromosome 10 and have excluded several candidate genes such as β-adrenergic receptor (*ADRB1*) and α-adrenergic receptor (*ADRA2*) and a gene for G-protein–coupled receptor kinase (*GPRK5*), which interacts with adrenergic receptors. It is known that families with atrial fibrillation exist that do not link to the locus on chromosome 10, suggesting genetic heterogeneity of familial atrial fibrillation.

Wolff-Parkinson-White and Preexcitation Syndromes

WPW syndrome is characterized by a short PR interval, prolonged QRS, with a slurred upstroke of the R wave called a *delta wave,* and predisposition to manifest paroxysmal supraventricular tachycardia. The incidence of WPW is not known and figures ranging from 0.1 to 3 per 1,000 ECGs have been reported (1,208). Although the syndrome occurs most frequently as an isolated abnormality, the familial occurrence of WPW syndrome has been reported (209,210). Vidaillet (211) studied first-degree relatives of 383 patients with electrophysiologically proved accessory AV pathways. Thirteen of 383 patients (3.4%) had at least one first-degree relative with accessory pathways. Patients with family history of preexcitation had a higher incidence of multiple accessory pathways and an increased risk of sudden cardiac death. It was hypothesized that WPW may be transmitted as an autosomal dominant trait.

Occasionally, familial preexcitation has been associated with familial cardiomyopathy (212,213). MacRae and colleagues (25) described a large family with 25 surviving individuals in which WPW and familial HCM were segregated and the disorder was linked to DNA markers on band 7q3. An association between WPW and familial HCM had been reported already in the early descriptions of HCM, and Braunwald and coworkers (214) proposed that abnormal ventricular activation might lead to regional myocardial hypertrophy or that localized hypertrophy might disrupt normal cardiac electrical discontinuity at the AV junction.

Kimura and colleagues (16) presented data indicating that WPW syndrome can be associated with more than one type of HCM. Approximately 5% to 10% of patients with HCM also present with WPW. The issue relevant to the genetic understanding of these diseases is whether the association of WPW represents a genetically distinct variant of HCM. Data reported by Kimura and colleagues (16) in 1997 supports the evidence that more than one genetic form of HCM may be associated with WPW. These authors reported combined WPW and HCM in three individuals with a mutation in the cardiac troponin I gene and one with a deletion at a codon in the cardiac myosin-binding protein C gene. The latter mutation had been identified also in subjects with HCM not associated with WPW syndrome.

Progressive Cardiac Conduction Defect

Progressive cardiac conduction defect, also called Lenègre-Lev disease (215,216), is a common cardiac conduction defect characterized by progressive impairment of intracardiac conduction. In the early stages, the diagnosis of the disease is mainly based on ECG findings, and when complete

AV block develops, patients manifest syncope and even sudden death. Lenègre-Lev disease is considered a degenerative disorder of the conduction system, histologically characterized by focal sclerosis, and it is one of the major causes of pacemaker implantation.

Familial occurrence of conduction disturbances of the heart leading to complete AV block have been described in medical literature since the 1950s. It was the work by Brink and Torrington (217) that provided a complete description of the disease. These authors described the existence of two distinct forms (type I heart block and type II heart block). They described as typical of type I heart block the presence of a right bundle branch block with or without left anterior hemiblock that may progress to complete AV block; Adams-Stokes events occur more frequently in the neonatal period, during adolescence, or toward middle age. Presentation among family members may vary. Type II heart block is described as manifesting with sinus bradycardia and left posterior hemiblock that progresses to complete AV block.

One of the largest families reported presenting with multigenerational evidence of conduction defects is the Lebanese kindred studied by Stephan and colleagues (218–220). Of the 209 family members examined, 32 of them showed abnormalities of the conduction system (complete right bundle branch block, incomplete right bundle branch block, right bundle branch block with left axis deviation, right bundle branch block with right axis deviation, and complete heart block).

Given the heterogeneous clinical manifestation and the variable penetrance, it is difficult to assess whether the families reported by different authors have a single disease (caused by a single genetic abnormality) or whether they represent a heterogeneous group of conduction disturbances.

The first step toward the identification of a genetic substrate for familial heart block came when Brink and colleagues (221) performed linkage analysis in the family on which they originally reported (217) and found an association of progressive familial heart block, type I (PFHB1) to 19q13.2-q13.3. They pointed out that these kindred descended from an ancestor who emigrated from Portugal in 1696. de Meeus and colleagues (222) confirmed linkage to the same locus also in the Lebanese family described by Stephan and colleagues (220). No gene for PFHBI has been identified so far.

In 1999, Schott and colleagues (223) described two families with conduction defects and identified in both a mutation in the *SCN5A* gene; this gene has been previously implicated in LQTS (LQT3) and Brugada syndrome (see specific sections). Thus, according to Schott and colleagues, progressive conduction defect is allelic to LQT3 and Brugada syndrome. This finding is puzzling and stimulating at the same time. It is unclear from the description of the two families described by Schott extent to which the presence of phenotypic characteristics of LQT3 and Brugada syndrome were excluded. More specifically, because Brugada syndrome is frequently associated with a prolonged HV interval at electrophysiologic evaluation, it is intriguing to speculate that the two families presented with a form of Brugada syndrome. No data on provocative ajmaline challenge were reported to conclusively dismiss the diagnosis of Brugada syndrome.

GENETIC TESTING AND CLINICAL PRACTICE: PROSPECTIVE AND IMPLICATIONS

Genetic testing for arrhythmogenic disorders is not yet routinely available even though the number of laboratories performing these analyses worldwide is increasing. In light of the wider availability of molecular screening, it is important to discuss value and implications of genetic screening. In most diseases, molecular diagnosis has a diagnostic value but is not yet useful to guide clinical management and to predict clinical outcome (risk stratification).

Molecular diagnosis can be applied in two groups of patients: (a) the clinically affected individuals and (b) the apparently healthy family members of an affected patient. The value and impact of genetic screening in the two settings is profoundly different.

Molecular Diagnosis in Clinically Affected Individuals

In a subject that is seeking medical attention because he or she has a clinical problem, molecular diagnosis may help the clinician achieve the correct diagnosis in patients with borderline or unclear clinical manifestations of a disease. Even in a subject with a definitive clinical diagnosis, molecular analysis is valuable, as it may define the subtype of the disease carried by the individual patient (and in some of the diseases, this may have implications for clinical management) and it allows screening of family members. The identification of a genetic defect in a clinically affected individual allows access to prenatal and preimplant diagnosis. There is little doubt that in clinically affected patients, availability of genetic screening is going to be beneficial.

Molecular Diagnosis in Clinically Unaffected Individuals

Because most of the diseases discussed in this chapter are characterized by incomplete penetrance and variable expression, only genetic analysis may rule out the presence of the disease in an asymptomatic family member. Accordingly, during clinical evaluation of members of families affected by genetic diseases, unaffected individuals should be informed that although they are apparently healthy, they may still carry a genetic defect that may remain "silent" or may suddenly manifest later in life.

In families in which the genetic diagnosis has been established in the proband, the issue is raised whether family members should be tested.

Presymptomatic diagnosis prompts considerations that should be addressed before offering testing. The pros and cons of presymptomatic diagnosis vary with different diseases and should be tailored to the individual, so there is no single answer to the question "when should we offer genetic testing to asymptomatic individuals?"

Learning to be a "gene carrier" exposes asymptomatic subjects to the unexpected evidence that they carry and may transmit a potentially fatal disease. Counseling these patients is very difficult. Before undergoing genetic testing, these individuals should be educated about the implication of a positive result and they should always be offered the opportunity to refuse testing.

These subjects will ask about the "benefits" of knowing that they carry the genetic defect, and once more the answer will vary in the different diseases. In diseases such as the LQTS and CPVT, for example, in which prophylactic pharmacologic treatment is available (β blockers) and "lifestyle precautions" could be adopted to reduce events (e.g., the avoidance of competitive sport and drugs known to prolong repolarization), there may be a clear benefit in knowing who is at risk. For other diseases such as Brugada syndrome, HCM, or DCM, in which the clinical manifestations are frequently delayed in life and treatment to prevent symptoms is not yet available, the need for presymptomatic diagnosis is debatable. Commenting on the role of presymptomatic molecular diagnosis of HCM, Clarke and Harper (224) suggested that "the parallels between this cardiomyopathy and Huntington disease (a late-onset disease) are sufficiently striking that we would be very cautious about testing for it in childhood. The emotional consequences of being brought up under a cloud of doom may be damaging, and the lack of any uncertainty in identifying gene carriers by mutation analysis might paradoxically make this worse." A profoundly different prospective was that of Watkins and colleagues (225), who countered this view by saying that children with the condition face a 4% to 6% risk of sudden death each year. Genetic diagnosis will allow evaluation of prophylactic use of antiarrhythmic agents or implantable defibrillator devices. We support the latter view, but we strongly believe that genetic counseling should always accompany genetic testing to allow individuals to decide for themselves (right of "not knowing") after having received appropriate information on the value and limitation of genetic analysis in the specific case.

GLOSSARY

allele   alternative forms (i.e., differences in the nucleotide sequence) of a gene in a specific locus on the genome.

α helix   frequently found secondary structure of a protein. This structure is particularly stable because it allows the highest possible number of hydrogen bonds. One turn of the helix encompasses approximately 3.5 amino acid residues.

alternative splicing   process producing different proteins from the same gene. Most of the human genes are made up of coding DNA sequences (exons) and noncoding DNA sequences (introns), which are removed by the splicing process leading to mRNA production. Single exons may be skipped during splicing to generate different isoforms of the same protein. Alternative splicing may be tissue specific.

amino acid sequence   the linear order of amino acids constituting a protein.

autosome   all chromosomes except the sexual chromosomes. The autosomal genes follow the distribution of the autosomal chromosome during meiosis (autosomal inheritance) while the genes on sexual chromosomes (X or Y) follow the sex-linked pattern of inheritance. Human genome comprises 22 autosomal chromosomes.

band designation   classification of the typical bands of the human chromosomes stained with Giemsa quinacrine method. The short (p) and the long (q) arms of the chromosomes are divided into two or more regions to localize the genes or other genetic markers.

base pair   the bond between two complementary nucleotides, such as adenine (A) with thymine (T) or cytosine with guanine. In the DNA molecule, complementary bases are held together by hydrogen bonds.

base pair substitution   a DNA mutation resulting in the change of a single base pair. Two types of substitution are possible: (a) transition, in which a purine (adenine and guanine) is substituted by the other purine (the same for pyrimidine thymine and cytosine), and (b) transversion, a substitution of a purine with a pyrimidine, and vice versa.

bases of the DNA   single molecules constituting the base of genetic code. There are four bases: two purines (adenine and guanine) and two pyrimidines (thymine and cytosine). In the RNA molecule, uracil substitutes thymine.

centimorgans (cM)   unit of measure of the genetic distance between two markers on a chromosome. It is widely used in linkage analysis. The cM distance is calculated (by statistical linkage analysis) as genetic distance (as opposed to physical distance) that is measured in nucleotides. One cM is approximately 1 million base pairs.

chromatin   nucleotide molecules (DNA and RNA). DNA associated proteins present in the nucleus of the eukaryotic cells.

chromosome   in the eukaryotic cells is the chromatin material organized in a linear sequence, carrying the genetic information. Chromosomes are visible only in dividing cells during metaphase.

chromosome bands   bands generated from the staining of chromosomes and used to study chromosomal abnormalities. Four main procedures for staining of the human chromosomes produce four different sets of chromosomal bands: G bands, C bands, Q bands, and R bands. These different staining techniques allow the identification of different chromosomal characteristics. For instance, C-banding is useful to study the centromeres while Q bands are useful to identify the Y chromosome.

clone   two genetically identical organisms descending from the same genome (e.g., homozygous twins). For a single DNA sequence, a clone is an identical copy obtained by genetic engineering.

cloning   DNA manipulation (often done by the insertion of a DNA sequence into a plasmid vector with subsequent replication in bacterial strains) resulting in the generation of one or usually many identical copies of the same original DNA sequence.

coding region   the DNA sequences containing the code to generate RNA. The coding region of a gene results from the sum of the exons.

codon   a group of three nucleotides coding for a single amino acid. Every protein starts with the specific codon "ATG" coding for a methionine. The end of coding region is marked by three possible codons: TAG, TAA, or TGA.

congenital   a phenotypic trait existing at birth. Congenital traits may or may not be genetically determined.

cytogenetic map   the map localizing the genes on a chromosome.

cytoskeleton   the protein array allowing the cells to assume a specific shape, determining the matrix fixing intracellular organelles in the cell.

deletion   a DNA mutation resulting in the loss of genetic material. The size of the deletion may vary from a few nucleotides to large chromosomal segments.

deoxyribonucleic acid (DNA)   molecule formed by the linear sequence of purine and pyrimidine bases bonded to deoxyribose sugar and constituting the molecular structure of the genes.

dominant inheritance   a genetic trait that phenotypically manifests in the heterozygous state.

exons   DNA sequences containing the information for (a) transcription start and signaling to direct mRNA to ribosomes; (b) genetic information to translate DNA into proteins; (c) transcription and translation end and the polyadenylation signal (the adenine tail added to mRNA molecule).

frame shift   DNA mutations resulting from the addition or loss of genetic material (one or more nucleotides), which determines a change in the message during the DNA translation into proteins, that is, change of the triplet's sequence.

frame (or reading frame)   the DNA triplet's sequence coding for the amino acids of a protein.

gene   the DNA sequence containing all the information for the synthesis of a specific protein including the upstream regulatory sequences, the exons, and the introns.

genetic linkage   two or more chromosomal loci lying close enough to be inherited together with no recombination (e.g., a chromosomal marker and a disease gene). Crossing over during meiosis leads to random distribution of chromosomal segments (recombination). Recombination between two loci is more likely to happen when their genetic distance is longer.

genomic DNA   the entire DNA contained in the nucleus (as opposed to mitochondrial DNA).

genotype   the genetic asset of an individual at a specific locus or loci.

hot spot   a DNA site that is subject to mutation with a significantly higher frequency in respect to the mean mutation rate of the DNA molecule.

incomplete dominance   partial expression of a dominant trait or disease.

insertion   a DNA mutation consisting in an addition of genetic material (one or more base pairs).

intron-exon boundaries   DNA sequence that marks the start and the end of the introns, therefore determining the exons' limits.

locus   the position of a gene in a chromosome.

lod (logarithm of odds) score   a measure of the statistical power of the linkage analysis to determine the association between a genetic marker and a phenotype. A lod score of more than 3 (1 chance out of 1,000 of a casual relationship) is considered significant to establish a linkage to a locus while a lod score of less than 2 excludes the linkage.

marker   a gene or a DNA sequence with a known chromosomal location used to map other genes on the chromosome.

missense mutation   a DNA mutation resulting in a single amino acid substitution.

penetrance   the proportion of the gene carriers showing the clinical phenotype.

phenotype   detectable character of an individual due to a specific genetic setting interacting with the environment.

point mutation a DNA mutation consisting in a single nucleotide substitution.

polymerase chain reaction (PCR) a widely used molecular biology tool allowing the production of thousands of copies of a specific DNA sequence (usually ranging from 100 to 5,000 base pairs) by means of an enzymatic reaction with DNA polymerase. Bacterially derived DNA polymerases are generally used to perform a PCR reaction (e.g., Taq polymerase from thermophilus aquaticus).

polymorphism a DNA sequence variant frequently observed in a population.

regulatory sequence a DNA sequence controlling the gene expression (e.g., the promoter of a gene). Both inhibiting and enhancing regulatory sequences are present in the human genome.

wild type the most frequently observed phenotype. Term may be a synonym of "normal."

REFERENCES

1. Priori SG, Barhanin J, Hauer RNW, et al. Genetic and molecular basis of cardiac arrhythmias: impact on clinical management. Part I and II. *Circulation* 1999;99:518–528, and *Eur Heart J* 1999;20:174–195.
2. Napolitano C, Schwartz PJ, Brown AM, et al. Evidence for cardiac ion-channel mutation underlying drug-induced torsades de pointes. *J Cardiovasc Electrophysiol* 2000;11:691–696.
3. Niimura H,. Bachinski LL, Sangwatanaroj S, et al. Mutations in the gene for cardiac myosin-binding protein C and late-onset familial hypertrophic cardiomyopathy. *N Engl J Med* 1998;338:1248–1257.
4. Priori SG. Long QT and Brugada syndromes: from genetics to clinical managements. *J Cardiovasc Electrophysiol* 2000;11:1174–1178.
5. Ciro E, Nichols PF, Maron BJ. Heterogeneous morphologic expression of genetically transmitted hypertrophic cardiomyopathy: two-dimensional echocardiographic analysis. *Circulation* 1983;67:1227–1233.
6. Maron BJ, Bonow RO, Seshagiri T, et al. Hypertrophic cardiomyopathy with ventricular septal hypertrophy localized to the apical region of the left ventricle (apical hypertrophic cardiomyopathy). *Am J Cardiol* 1982;49:1838–1848.
7. Spirito P, Seidman CE, McKenna WJ, Maron BJ. The management of hypertrophic cardiomyopathy. *N Engl J Med* 1997;336:775–785.
8. Maron BJ, Shen WK, Link MS, et al. Efficacy of implantable cardioverter-defibrillators for the prevention of sudden death in patients with hypertrophic cardiomyopathy. *N Engl J Med* 2000;342:365–373.
9. Watkins H. Sudden death in hypertrophic cardiomyopathy [Editorial]. *N Engl J Med* 2000;342:422–424.
10. McKenna WJ, Oakley CM, Krikler DM, Goodwin JF. Improved survival with amiodarone in patients with hypertrophic cardiomyopathy and ventricular tachycardia. *Br Heart J* 1985;53:412–416.
11. Ostman Smith I, Wettrell G, Riesenfeld TA. A cohort study of childhood hypertrophic cardiomyopathy: improved survival following high-dose beta-adrenoceptor antagonist treatment. *J Am Coll Cardiol* 1999;34:1813–1822.
12. Maron BJ, Shirani J, Poliac LC, et al. Sudden death in young competitive athletes: clinical, demographic, and pathological profiles. *JAMA* 1996;276:199–204.
13. Townsend PJ, Farza H, MacGeoch C, et al. Human cardiac troponin T: identification of fetal isoforms and assignment of the TNNT2 locus to chromosome 1q. *Genomics* 1994;21:311–316.
14. Geisterfer-Lowrance AAT, Kass S, Tanigawa G, et al. A molecular basis for familial hypertrophic cardiomyopathy: a beta cardiac myosin heavy chain gene missense mutation. *Cell* 1990;62:999–1006.
15. Poetter K, Jiang H, Hassanzadeh S, et al. Mutations in either the essential or regulatory light chains of myosin are associated with a rare myopathy in human heart and skeletal muscle. *Nat Genetics* 1996;13:63–69.
16. Kimura A, Harada H, Park JE, et al. Mutations in the cardiac troponin I gene associated with hypertrophic cardiomyopathy. *Nat Genetics* 1997;16:379–382.
17. Watkins H, MacRae C, Thierfelder L, et al. A disease locus for familial hypertrophic cardiomyopathy maps to chromosome 1q3. *Nat Genetics* 1993;3:333–337.
18. Thierfelder L, MacRae C, Watkins H, et al. A familial hypertrophic cardiomyopathy locus maps to chromosome 15q2. *Proc Natl Acad Sci U S A* 1993;90:6270–6274.
19. Thierfelder L, Watkins H, MacRae C, et al. Alpha-tropomyosin and cardiac troponin T mutations cause familial hypertrophic cardiomyopathy: a disease of the sarcomere. *Cell* 1994;77:701–712.
20. Carrier L, Hengstenberg C, Beckmann JS, et al. Mapping of a novel gene for familial hypertrophic cardiomyopathy to chromosome 11. *Nat Genetics* 1993;4:311–313.
21. Bonne G, Carrier L, Bercovici J, et al. Cardiac myosin binding protein-C gene splice acceptor site mutation is associated with familial hypertrophic cardiomyopathy. *Nat Genetics* 1995;11:438–440.
22. Watkins H, Conner D, Thierfelder L, et al. Mutations in the cardiac myosin binding protein-C gene on chromosome 11 cause familial hypertrophic cardiomyopathy. *Nat Genetics* 1995;11:434–437.
23. Mogensen J, Klausen IC, Pedersen AK, et al. Alpha-cardiac actin is a novel disease gene in familial hypertrophic cardiomyopathy. *J Clin Invest* 1999;103:R39–R43.
24. Satoh M, Takahashi M, Sakamoto T, et al. Structural analysis of the titin gene in hypertrophic cardiomyopathy: identification of a novel disease gene. *Biochem Biophys Res Commun* 1999;262:411–417.
25. MacRae CA, Ghaisas N, Kass S, et al. Familial hypertrophic cardiomyopathy with Wolff-Parkinson-White syndrome maps to a locus on chromosome 7q3. *J Clin Invest* 1995;96:1216–1220.
26. Watkins H, Rosenzweig A, Hwang DS, et al. Characteristics and prognostic implications of myosin missense mutations in familial hypetrophic cardiomyopathy. *N Engl J Med* 1992;326:1108–1114
27. Epstein ND, Cohn GM, Cyran F, Fananapazir L. Differences in clinical expression of hypertrophic cardiomyopathy associated with two distinct mutations in the beta-myosin heavy chain gene. *Circulation* 1992;86:345–352.
28. Anan R, Greve G, Thierfelder L, et al. Prognostic implications of novel beta-cardiac myosin heavy chain gene mutations that cause familial hypertrophic cardiomyopathy. *J Clin Invest* 1994;93:280–285.
29. Lankford EB, Epstein ND, Fananapazir L, Sweeney HL. Abnormal contractile properties of muscle fibers expressing beta-myosin heavy chain gene mutations in patients with hypertrophic cardiomyopathy. *J Clin Invest* 1995;95:1409–1414.
30. Geisterfer-Lowrance AA, Christe M, Conner DA, et al. A

mouse model of familial hypertrophic cardiomyopathy. *Science* 1996;272:731–734.

31. Tyska MJ, Hayes E, Giewat M, et al. Single-molecule mechanics of R403Q cardiac myosin isolated from the mouse model of familial hypertrophic cardiomyopathy. *Circ Res* 2000;86: 737–744.

32. Watkins H, McKenna WJ, Thierfelder L, et al. Mutations in the genes for cardiac troponin T and alpha-tropomyosin in hypertrophic cardiomyopathy. *N Engl J Med* 1995;332:1058–1064.

33. Moolman JC, Corfield VA, Posen B, et al. Sudden death due to troponin T mutations. *J Am Coll Cardiol* 1997;29:549–555.

34. Tardiff JC, Factor SM, Tompkins BD, et al. A truncated cardiac troponin T molecule in transgenic mice suggests multiple cellular mechanisms for familial hypertrophic cardiomyopathy. *J Clin Invest* 1998;101:2800–2811.

35. Sweeney HL, Feng HS, Yang Z, Watkins H. Functional analyses of troponin T mutations that cause hypertrophic cardiomyopathy: insights into disease pathogenesis and troponin function. *Proc Nat Acad Sci* 1998;95:14406–14410.

36. Yamauchi-Takihara K, Nakajima-Taniguchi C, Matsui H, et al. Clinical implications of hypertrophic cardiomyopathy associated with mutations in the alpha-tropomyosin gene. *Heart* 1996;76:63–65

37. Coviello DA, Maron BJ, Spirito P, et al. Clinical features of hypertrophic cardiomyopathy caused by mutation of a "hot spot" in the alpha-tropomyosin gene. *J Am Coll Cardiol* 1997; 29:635–640

38. Emery AEH. Emery-Dreifuss syndrome. *J Med Genetics* 1989; 26:637–641.

39. Emery AEH. X-linked muscular dystrophy with early contractures and cardiomyopathy (Emery-Dreifuss type). *Clin Genetics* 1987;32:360–367.

40. Kamisago M, Sharma SD, DePalma SR, et al. Mutations in sarcomere protein genes as a cause of dilated cardiomyopathy. *N Engl J Med* 2000;343:1688–1696.

41. Towbin JA, Hejtmancik JF, Brink P, et al. X-linked dilated cardiomyopathy: molecular genetic evidence of linkage to the Duchenne muscular dystrophy (dystrophin) gene at the Xp21 locus. *Circulation* 1993;87:1854–1865.

42. Berko BA, Swift M. X-linked dilated cardiomyopathy. *N Engl J Med* 1987;316:1186–1191.

43. Muntoni F, Cau M, Ganau A, et al. Deletion of the dystrophin muscle-promoter region associated with X-linked dilated cardiomyopathy. *N Engl J Med* 1993;329:921–925.

44. Ortiz-Lopez R, Li H, Su J, et al. Evidence for a dystrophin missense mutation as a cause of X-linked dilated cardiomyopathy. *Circulation* 1997;95:2434–2440.

45. Olson TM, Michels VV, Thibodeau SN, et al. Actin mutations in dilated cardiomyopathy, a heritable form of heart failure. *Science* 1998;280:750–752.

46. Takai E, Akita H, Shiga N, et al. Mutational analysis of the cardiac actin gene in familial and sporadic dilated cardiomyopathy. *Am J Med Genetics* 1999;86:325–327.

47. Mayosi BM, Khogali SS, Zhang B, Watkins H. Cardiac and skeletal actin gene mutations are not a common cause of dilated cardiomyopathy. *J Med Genetics* 1999;36:796–797.

48. Dalakas MC, Park KY, Semino-Mora C, et al. Desmin Myopathy, a skeletal myopathy with cardiomyopathy caused by mutations in the desmin gene. *N Engl J Med* 2000; 342:770–780.

49. Goldfarb LG, Park KY, Cervenakova L, et al. Missense mutations in desmin associated with familial cardiac and skeletal myopathy. *Nat Genetics* 1998;19:402–403.

50. Li D, Tapscoft T, Gonzalez O,et al. Desmin mutation responsible for idiopathic dilated cardiomyopathy. *Circulation* 1999; 100:461–464.

51. Cartegni L, Raffaele di Barletta M, Barresi R, et al. Heart-spe-

cific localization of emerin: new insights into Emery-Dreifuss muscular dystrophy. *Hum Mol Genetics* 1997;6:2257–2264.

52. Takahashi K. Neurogenic scapuloperoneal amyotrophy associated with dystrophic changes. *Clin Neurol* 1971;11:650–658.

53. Fenichel GM, Sul YC, Kilroy AW, Blouin R. An autosomal dominant dystrophy with humeropelvic distribution and cardiomyopathy. *Neurology* 1982;32:1399–1401.

54. Miller RG, Layzer RB, Mellenthin MA, et al. Emery-Dreifuss muscular dystrophy with autosomal dominant transmission. *Neurology* 1985;35:1230–1233.

55. Orstavik KH, Kloster R, Lippestad C, et al. Emery-Dreifuss syndrome in three generations of females, including identical twins. *Clin Genetics* 1990;38:447–451.

56. Bonne G, Di Barletta MR, Varnous S, et al. Mutations in the gene encoding lamin A/C cause autosomal dominant Emery-Dreifuss muscular dystrophy. *Nat Genetics* 1999;21:285–288.

57. Kass S, MacRae C, Graber HL, et al. A gene defect that causes conduction system disease and dilated cardiomyopathy maps to chromosome 1p1-1q1. *Nat Genetics* 1994;7:546–551.

58. Fatkin D, MacRae C, Sasaki T, et al. Missense mutations in the rod domain of the lamin A/C gene as causes of dilated cardiomyopathy and conduction-system disease. *N Engl J Med* 1999;341:1715–1724.

59. Barth PG, Van't Veer-Korthof ET, Van Delden L, et al. An X-linked mitochondrial disease affecting cardiac muscle, skeletal muscle and neutrophil leukocytes. In: Busch HFM, Jennekens FGI, Schotte HR, eds. *Mitochondria and muscular diseases.* Beetsterzwaag, The Netherlands: Mefar Publishing, 1981: 161–164.

60. Barth PG, Scholte JA, Berden JA, et al. An X-linked mitochondrial disease affecting cardiac muscle, skeletal muscle and neutrophil leucocytes. *J Neurol Sci* 1983;62:327–355.

61. Neustein HB, Lurie PR, Fugita M. Endocardial fibroelastosis found on transvascular endomyocardial biopsy in children. *Arch Pathol Lab Med* 1979;103:214–219.

62. Hodgson S, Child A, Dyson M. Endocardial fibroelastosis: possible X linked inheritance. *J Med Genetics* 1987;24:210–214.

63. Kelley RI, Clark BJ, Morton DH, Sherwood WG. X-linked cardiomyopathy, neutropenia, and increased urinary levels of 3-methylglutaconic and 2-ethylhydracrylic acids. *Am J Hum Genetics* 1989;45[Suppl]:A7(abst).

64. Bione S, D'Adamo P, Maestrini E, et al. A novel X-linked gene, G4.5. [sic] is responsible for Barth syndrome. *Nat Genetics* 1996;12:385–389.

65. D'Adamo P, Fassone L, Gedeon A, et al. The X-linked gene G4.5 is responsible for different infantile dilated cardiomyopathies. *Am J Hum Genetics* 1997;61:862–867.

66. Gedeon AK, Wilson MJ, Colley AC, et al. X linked fatal infantile cardiomyopathy maps to Xq28 and is possibly allelic to Barth syndrome. *J Med Genetics* 1995;32:383–388.

67. Suomalainen A, Paetau A, Leinonen H, et al. Inherited idiopathic dilated cardiomyopathy with multiple deletions of mitochondrial DNA. *Lancet* 1992;340:1319–1320.

68. Tanaka M, Ino H, Ohno K, et al. Mitochondrial mutation in fatal infantile cardiomyopathy [Letter]. *Lancet* 1990;336:1452.

69. Zeviani M, Sevidei S, Gellera C, et al. An autosomal dominant disorder with multiple deletions of mitochondrial DNA starting at the D-loop region. *Nature* 1989;339:309–311.

70. Taniike M, Fukushima H, Yanagihara I, et al. Mitochondrial tRNA(ile) mutation in fatal cardiomyopathy. *Biochem Biophys Res Commun* 1992;186:47–53.

71. Krajinovic M, Pinamonti B, Sinagra G, et al, and the Heart Muscle Disease Study Group. Linkage of familial dilated cardiomyopathy to chromosome 9. *Am J Hum Genetics* 1995;57: 846–852.

72. Bowles KR, Gajarski R, Porter P, et al. Gene mapping of famil-

ial autosomal dominant dilated cardiomyopathy to chromosome 10q21-23. *J Clin Invest* 1996;98:1355–1360.

73. Durand JB, Bachinski LL, Bieling LC, et al. Localization of a gene responsible for familial dilated cardiomyopathy to chromosome 1q32. *Circulation* 1995;92:3387–3389.

74. Olson TM, Keating MT. Mapping a cardiomyopathy locus to chromosome 3p22-p25. *J Clin Invest* 1996;78:528–532.

75. Messina DN, Speer MC, Pericak-Vance MA, McNally EM. Linkage of familial dilated cardiomyopathy with conduction defect and muscular dystrophy to chromosome 6q23. *Am J Hum Genetics* 1997;61:909–917.

76. Siu BL, Niimura H, Osborne JA, et al. Familial dilated cardiomyopathy locus maps to chromosome 2q31. *Circulation* 1999;99:1022–1026.

77. Jung M, Poepping I, Perrot A, et al. Investigation of a family with autosomal dominant dilated cardiomyopathy defines a novel locus on chromosome 2q14-q22. *Am J Hum Genetics* 1999;65:1068–1077.

78. Fontaine G, Fontaliran F, Hebert JL, et al. Arrhythmogenic right ventricular dysplasia. *Annu Rev Med* 1999;50:17–35.

79. McKenna WJ, Thiene G, Nava A, et al. Diagnosis of arrhythmogenic right ventricular dysplasia/cardiomyopathy. *Br Heart J* 1994;71:215–218.

80. Corrado D, Nava A, Buja G, et al. Familial cardiomyopathy underlies syndrome of right bundle branch block, ST segment elevation and sudden death. *J Am Coll Cardiol* 1996;27:443–448.

81. Protonotarios N, Tsatsopoulou A, Patsourakos P, et al. Cardiac abnormalities in familial palmoplantar keratosis. *Br Heart J* 1986;56:321–326.

82. Coonar AS, Protonotarios N, Tsatsopoulou A, et al. Gene for arrhythmogenic right ventricular cardiomyopathy with diffuse nonepidermolytic palmoplantar keratoderma and woolly hair (Naxos disease) maps to 17q21. *Circulation* 1998;97:2049–2058.

83. Carvajal-Huerta L. Epidermolytic palmoplantar keratoderma with woolly hair and dilated cardiomyopathy. *J Am Acad Dermatol* 1998;39: 418–421.

84. McKoy G, Protonotarios N, Crosby A, et al. Identification of a deletion in plakoglobin in arrhythmogenic right ventricular cardiomyopathy with palmoplantar keratoderma and woolly hair (Naxos disease). *Lancet* 2000;355:2119–2124

85. Angelini A, Thiene G, Boffa GM, et al. Endomyocardial biopsy in right ventricular cardiomyopathy. *Int J Cardiol* 1993;40:273–282.

86. Rampazzo A, Nava A, Danieli GA, et al. The gene for arrhythmogenic right ventricular cardiomyopathy maps to chromosome 14q23-q24. *Hum Mol Genetics* 1994;3:959–962.

87. Ahmad F, Li D, Karibe A, et al. Localization of a gene responsible for arrhythmogenic right ventricular dysplasia to chromosome 3p23. *Circulation* 1998;98:2791–2795.

88. Li D, Ahmad F, Gardner MJ, et al. The locus of a novel gene responsible for arrhythmogenic right-ventricular dysplasia characterized by early onset and high penetrance maps to chromosome 10p12-p14. *Am J Hum Genetics* 2000;66:148–156.

89. Rampazzo A, Nava A, Erne P, et al. A new locus for arrhythmogenic right ventricular cardiomyopathy (ARVD2) maps to chromosome 1q42-q43. *Hum Mol Genetics* 1995;4:2151–2154.

90. Severini GM, Krajinovic M, Pinamonti B, et al, and the Heart Muscle Disease Study Group. A new locus for the arrhythmogenic right ventricular dysplasia on the long arm of chromosome 14. *Genomics* 1996;31:193–200.

91. Rampazzo A, Nava A, Miorin M, et al. ARVD4, a new locus for arrhythmogenic right ventricular cardiomyopathy, maps to chromosome 2 long arm. *Genomics* 1997;45:259–263.

92. Mallat Z, Tedgui A, Fontaliran F, et al. Evidence of apoptosis in arrhythmogenic right ventricular dysplasia. *N Engl J Med* 1996;335:1190–1196.

93. Valente M, Calabrese F, Thiene G, et al. *In vivo* evidence of apoptosis in arrhythmogenic right ventricular cardiomyopathy. *Am J Pathol* 1998;152:479–484.

94. Procacci PM, Savran SV, Schreiter SL, Bryson AL. Prevalence of clinical mitral valve prolapse in 1169 young women. *N Engl J Med* 1976;294:1086–1088.

95. Sbarbaro JA, Mehlman DJ, Wu L, Brooks HL. A prospective study of mitral valvular prolapse in young men. *Chest* 1979;75:555–559.

96. BonTempo CP, Ronan JA Jr, de Leon AC Jr, Twigg HL. Radiographic appearance of the thorax in systolic-click late systolic murmur syndrome. *Am J Cardiol* 1975;36:27–31.

97. Gooch AS, Vicencio F, Maranhao V, Goldberg H. Arrhythmias and left ventricular asynergy in the prolapsing mitral leaflet syndrome. *Am J Cardiol* 1972;29:611–620.

98. Hutchins GM, Moore GW, Skoog DK. The association of floppy mitral valve with disjunction of the mitral annulus fibrosus. *N Engl J Med* 1986;314:535–541.

99. Rizzon P, Biasco G, Brindicci G, Mauro F. Familial syndrome of midsystolic click and late systolic murmur. *Br Heart J* 1973; 35:245–259.

100. Hunt D, Sloman G. Prolapse of the posterior leaflet of the mitral valve occurring in eleven members of a family. *Am Heart J* 1969;78:149–153.

101. Weiss AN, Mimbs JW, Ludbrook PA, Sobel BE. Echocardiographic detection of mitral valve prolapse: exclusion of false positive diagnosis and determination of inheritance. *Circulation* 1975;52:1091–1096.

102. Shappell SD, Marshall CE, Brown RE, Bruce TA. Sudden death and the familial occurrence of mid-systolic click, late systolic murmur syndrome. *Circulation* 1973;48:1128–1134.

103. Disse S, Abergel E, Berrebi A, et al. Mapping of a first locus for autosomal dominant myxomatous mitral-valve prolapse to chromosome 16p11.2-p12.1. *Am J Hum Genetics* 1999;65:1242–1251.

104. Romano C, Gemme G, Pongiglione R. Aritmie cardiache rare in eta' pediatrica. *Clin Pediatr* 1963;45:656.

105. Ward OC. New familial cardiac syndrome in children. *J Ir Med Assoc* 1964;54:103.

106. Jervell A, Lange-Nielsen F. Congenital deaf mutism, functional heart disease with prolongation of the QT interval and sudden death. *Am Heart J* 1957;54:59.

107. Moss AJ, Schwartz PJ, Crampton RS, et al. The long QT syndrome: prospective longitudinal study of 328 families. *Circulation* 1991;84:1136.

108. Schwartz PJ, Priori SG, Napolitano C. Long QT syndrome. In: Zipes DP, Jalife J, eds. *Cardiac electrophysiology. From cell to bedside,* 3rd ed. Philadelphia: WB Saunders, 2000: 597–615.

109. Schwartz PJ, Periti M, Malliani A. The long Q-T syndrome. *Am Heart J* 1975;89:378.

110. Schwartz PJ. Idiopathic long QT syndrome: progress and questions. *Am Heart J* 1985;109:399.

111. Schwartz PJ, Locati E. The idiopathic long QT syndrome. Pathogenetic mechanisms and therapy. *Eur Heart J* 1985;6 [Suppl D]:103.

112. Schwartz PJ, Locati EH, Moss AJ, et al. Left cardiac sympathetic denervation in the therapy of the congenital long QT syndrome. A world-wide report. *Circulation* 1991;84:503.

113. Moss AJ, Zareba W, Hall WJ, et al. Effectiveness and limitations of beta-blocker therapy in congenital long-QT syndrome. *Circulation* 2000;101:616–623.

114. Eldar M, Griffin JC, Van Hare GF, et al. Combined use of beta-adrenergic blocking agents and long-term cardiac pacing for

patients with the long QT syndrome. *J Am Coll Cardiol* 1992; 20:830–837.

115. Cantù F, Priori SG, Napolitano C, et al. Ruolo del pace maker nella sindrome del QT lungo: dati dal registro internazionale. *Cardiologia* 1997;42[Suppl 4]:50.

116. Keating M, Atkinson D, Dunn C, et al. Linkage of a cardiac arrhythmia, the long QT syndrome, and the Harvey ras-1 gene. *Science* 1991;252:704–706.

117. Jiang C, Atkinson D, Towbin JA, et al. Two long QT syndrome loci map to chromosomes 3 and 7 with evidence for further heterogeneity. *Nat Genetics* 1994;8:141–147.

118. Schott JJ, Peltier S, Foley P, et al. Mapping of a new gene for the LQTS syndrome. *Am J Hum Genetics* 1995;57:1114–1122.

119. Wang Q, Curran ME, Splawski I, et al. Positional cloning of a novel potassium channel gene: KVLQT1 mutations cause cardiac arrhythmias. *Nat Genetics* 1996;12:17–23.

120. Curran ME, Splawski I, Timothy KW, et al. A molecular basis for cardiac arrhythmia: HERG mutations cause long QT syndrome. *Cell* 1995;80:795–803.

121. Wang Q, Shen J, Splawski I, et al. SCN5A mutations associated with an inherited cardiac arrhythmia, long QT syndrome. *Cell* 1995;80:805–811.

122. Sanguinetti MC, Jurkiewicz NK. Two components of cardiac delayed rectifier K^+ current. Differential sensitivity to block by class III antiarrhythmic agents. *J Genet Physiol* 1990;96: 195–215.

123. Neyroud N, Tesson F, Denjoy I, et al. A novel mutation in the potassium channel gene KVLQT1 causes the Jervell and Lange-Nielsen cardioauditory syndrome. *Nat Genetics* 1997;15:186–189.

124. Barhanin J, Lesage F, Guillemare E, et al. K(V)LQT1 and lsK (minK) proteins associate to form the I(Ks) cardiac potassium current. *Nature* 1996;384:78–80.

125. Sanguinetti MC, Curran ME, Zou A, et al. Coassembly of KvLQT1 and minK (IsK) proteins to form cardiac I(Ks) potassium channel. *Nature* 1996;384:80–83.

126. Splawski I, Tristani-Firouzi M, Lehmann MH, et al. Mutations in the hminK gene cause long-QT syndrome and suppress IKs function. *Nat Genetics* 1997;17:338–340.

127. Schulze-Bahr E, Wang Q, Wedekind H, et al. KCNE1 mutations cause Jervell and Lange-Nielsen syndrome. *Nat Genetics* 1997;17:267–268.

128. Chouabe C, Neyroud N, Guicheney P, et al. Properties of KvLQT1 K^+ channel mutations in Romano-Ward and Jervell and Lange-Nielsen inherited cardiac arrhythmias. *EMBO J* 1997;16:5472–5479.

129. Mitcheson JS, Sanguinetti MC. Biophysical properties and molecular basis of cardiac rapid and slow delayed rectifier potassium channels. *Cell Physiol Biochem* 1999;9:201–216.

130. Franqueza L, Lin M, Shen J, et al. Long QT syndrome-associated mutations in the S4-S5 linker of KvLQT1 potassium channels modify gating and interaction with minK subunits. *J Biol Chem* 1999;274:21063–21070.

131. Bianchi L, Shen Z, Dennis AT, et al. Cellular dysfunction of LQT5-minK mutants: abnormalities of IKs, IKr and trafficking in long QT syndrome. *Hum Mol Genetics* 1999;8:1499–1507.

132. Warmke JW, Ganetzky B. A family of potassium channel genes related to eag in *Drosophila* and mammals. *Proc Natl Acad Sci U S A* 1994;91:3438–3442.

133. Sanguinetti MC, Jiang C, Curran ME, Keating MT. A mechanistic link between an inherited and an acquired cardiac arrhythmia: HERG encodes the IKr potassium channel. *Cell* 1995;81:299–307.

134. Chen J, Zou A, Splawski I, et al. Long QT syndrome–associated mutations in the Per-Arnt-Sim (PAS) domain of HERG potassium channels accelerate channel deactivation. *J Biol Chem* 1999;274:10113–10118.

135. Tanaka T, Nagai R, Tomoike H, et al. Four novel KVLQT1 and four novel HERG mutations in familial long-QT syndrome. *Circulation* 1997;95:565–567.

136. Priori SG, Napolitano C, Schwartz PJ. Low penetrance in the long QT syndrome. Clinical impact. *Circulation* 1999;99:529–533.

137. Jongbloed RJ, Wilde AA, Geelen JL, et al. Novel KCNQ1 and HERG missense mutations in Dutch long-QT families. *Hum Mutat* 1999;13:301–310.

138. Satler CA, Vesely MR, Duggal P, et al. Multiple different missense mutations in the pore region of HERG in patients with long QT syndrome. *Hum Genetics* 1998;102:265–272.

139. Splawski I, Shen J, Timothy KW, et al. Genomic structure of three long QT syndrome genes: KVLQT1, HERG, and KCNE1. *Genomics* 1998;51:86–97.

140. Hoorntje T, Alders M, van Tintelen P, et al. Homozygous premature truncation of the HERG protein: the human HERG knockout. *Circulation* 1999;100:1264–1267.

141. Abbott GW, Sesti F, Splawski I, et al. MiRP1 forms IKr potassium channels with HERG and is associated with cardiac arrhythmia. *Cell* 1999;97:175–187.

142. Sanguinetti MC, Curran ME, Spector PS, Keating MT. Spectrum of HERG K^+-channel dysfunction in an inherited cardiac arrhythmia. *Proc Natl Acad Sci U S A* 1996;93:2208–2212.

143. Furutani M, Trudeau MC, Hagiwara N, et al. Novel mechanism associated with an inherited cardiac arrhythmia: defective protein trafficking by the mutant HERG (G601S) potassium channel. *Circulation* 1999;99:2290–2294.

144. Roden DM, Balser JR. A plethora of mechanisms in the HERG-related long QT syndrome. Genetics meets electrophysiology. *Cardiovasc Res* 1999;44:242–246.

145. Gellens ME, George AL Jr, Chen LQ, et al. Primary structure and functional expression of the human cardiac tetrodotoxin-insensitive voltage-dependent sodium channel. *Proc Natl Acad Sci U S A* 1992;89:554–558.

146. George AL Jr, Varkony TA, Drabkin HA, et al. Assignment of the human heart tetrodotoxin-resistant voltage-gated Na^+ channel alpha-subunit gene (SCN5A) to band 3p21. *Cytogenet Cell Genetics* 1995;68:67–70.

147. Wang Q, Shen J, Li Z, et al. Cardiac sodium channel mutations in patients with long QT syndrome, an inherited cardiac arrhythmia. *Hum Mol Genetics* 1995;4:1603–1607.

148. Bennett PB, Yazawa K, Makita N, George AJ. Molecular mechanism for an inherited cardiac arrhythmia. *Nature* 1995;376: 683–685

149. Dumaine R, Wang Q, Keating MT, et al. Multiple mechanisms of Na^+ channel-linked long-QT syndrome. *Circ Res* 1996;78: 916–924.

150. Wattanasirichaigoon D, Vesely MR, Duggal P, et al. Sodium channel abnormalities are infrequent in patients with long QT syndrome: identification of two novel SCN5A mutations. *Am J Med Genetics* 1999;86:470–476.

151. An RH, Wang XL, Kerem B, et al. Novel LQT-3 mutation affects Na^+ channel activity through interactions between alpha- and beta$_1$-subunits. *Circ Res* 1998;83:141–146.

152. Bezzina C, Veldkamp MW, van Den Berg MP, et al. A single $Na^{(+)}$ channel mutation causing both long-QT and Brugada syndromes. *Circ Res* 1999;85:1206–1213.

153. Napolitano C, Ronchetti E, Memmi M, et al. Molecular epidemiology of LQTS in a cohort of 267 probands. *J Am Coll Cardiol* 2001 *(in press)*.

154. Chauhan VS, Tuvia S, Buhusi M, et al. Abnormal cardiac $Na^{(+)}$ channel properties and QT heart rate adaptation in neonatal ankyrin(B) knockout mice. *Circ Res* 2000;86:441–447.

155. Moss AJ, Zareba W, Benhorin J, et al. ECG T-wave patterns in genetically distinct forms of the hereditary long QT syndrome. *Circulation* 1995;92:2929–2934.

156. Zhang L, Timothy KW, Vincent GM, et al. Spectrum of ST-T–wave patterns and repolarization parameters in congenital long-QT syndrome: ECG findings identify genotypes. *Circulation* 2000;102:2849–2855

157. Schwartz PJ, Priori SG, Locati EH, et al. Long QT syndrome patients with mutations on the SCN5A and HERG genes have differential responses to Na⁺ channel blockade and to increases in heart rate. Implications for gene-specific therapy. *Circulation* 1995;92:3381–3386.

158. Moretti P, Calcaterra P, Napolitano C, et al. High prevalence of concealed long QT syndrome among carriers of KVLQT1 defects. *Circulation* 2000;102:II584(abst).

159. Swan H, Viitasalo M, Piippo K, et al. Sinus node function and ventricular repolarization during exercise stress test in long QT syndrome patients with KvLQT1 and HERG potassium channel defects. *J Am Coll Cardiol* 1999;34:823–829.

160. Schwartz PJ, Priori SG, Spazzolini C, et al. Genotype-phenotype correlation in the long QT syndrome. Gene-specific triggers for life-threatening arrhythmias. *Circulation* 2001 *(in press)*.

161. Wilde AA, Jongbloed RJ, Doevendans PA, et al. Auditory stimuli as a trigger for arrhythmic events differentiate HERG-related (LQTS2) patients from KVLQT1-related patients (LQTS1). *J Am Coll Cardiol* 1999;33:327–332.

162. Moss AJ, Robinson JL, Gessman L, et al. Comparison of clinical and genetic variables of cardiac events associated with loud noise versus swimming among subjects with the long QT syndrome. *Am J Cardiol* 1999;84:876–879.

163. Ackerman MJ, Tester DJ, Porter CJ. Swimming, a gene-specific arrhythmogenic trigger for inherited long QT syndrome. *Mayo Clin Proc* 1999;74:1088–1094.

164. Zareba W, Moss AJ, Schwartz PJ, et al. Influence of the genotype on the clinical course of the long QT syndrome. *N Engl J Med* 1998;339:960–965.

165. Priori SG, Napolitano C, Brown AM, et al. The loss of function induced by HERG and KVLQT1 mutations does not correlate with the clinical severity of the long QT syndrome. *Circulation* 1998;98[Suppl 1]: I457.

166. Donger C, Denjoy I, Berthet M, et al. KVLQT1 C-terminal missense mutation causes a forme fruste long-QT syndrome. *Circulation* 1997;96:2778–2781.

167. Neyroud N, Denjoy I, Donger C, et al. Heterozygous mutation in the pore of potassium channel gene KvLQT1 causes an apparently normal phenotype in long QT syndrome. *Eur J Hum Genetics* 1998;6:129–133.

168. Priori SG, Schwartz PJ, Napolitano C, et al. A recessive variant of the Romano-Ward long QT syndrome? *Circulation* 1998; 97:2420–2425.

169. Napolitano C, Memmi M, Ronchetti E, et al. Silent mutation on cardiac ion channel genes and sudden death: a lesson from the long QT syndrome. *Circulation* 1999;Suppl 1:I8(abst).

170. Berthet M, Denjoy I, Donger C, et al. C-terminal HERG mutations. The role of hypokalemia and KCNQ1-associated mutation in cardiac event occurrence. *Circulation* 1999;99: 1464–1470.

171. Priori SG, Napolitano C, Cantù F, et al. Differential response to Na⁺ channel blockade, β-adrenergic stimulation, and rapid pacing in a cellular model mimicking the SCN5A and HERG defects present in the long QT syndrome. *Circ Res* 1996;78: 1009–1015.

172. Benhorin J, Taub R, Goldmit M, et al. Effects of flecainide in patients with new SCN5A mutation: mutation-specific therapy for long-QT syndrome? *Circulation* 2000;101:1698–1706.

173. Priori SG, Napolitano C, Schwartz PJ, et al. The elusive link between LQT3 and Brugada syndrome: the role of flecainide challenge. *Circulation* 2000;102:945–947.

174. Compton SJ, Lux RL, Ramsey MR, et al. Genetically defined therapy of inherited long-QT syndrome. Correction of abnormal repolarization by potassium. *Circulation* 1996;94: 1018–1022.

175. Brugada P, Brugada J. Right bundle-branch block, persistent ST segment elevation and sudden cardiac death: a distinct clinical and electrocardiographic syndrome. *J Am Coll Cardiol* 1992; 20:1391–1396.

176. Nademanee K, Veerakul G, Nimmannit S, et al. Arrhythmogenic marker for the sudden unexplained death syndrome in Thai men. *Circulation* 1997;96:2595–2600.

177. Brugada J, Brugada P, Brugada R. The syndrome of right bundle branch block and ST segment elevation in V₁ to V₃ and sudden death—the Brugada syndrome. *Europace* 1999;1:156–166.

178. Priori SG, Napolitano C, Giordano U, et al. Brugada syndrome and sudden cardiac death in children. *Lancet* 2000;355: 808–809.

179. Miyazaki T, Mitamura H, Miyoshi S, et al. Autonomic and antiarrhythmic drug modulation of ST segment elevation in patients with Brugada syndrome. *J Am Coll Cardiol* 1996;27: 1061–1070.

180. Brugada R, Brugada J, Antzelevitch C, et al. Sodium channel blockers identify risk for sudden death in patients with ST-segment elevation and right bundle branch block but structurally normal hearts. *Circulation* 2000;101:510–515.

181. Brugada J, Brugada R, Brugada P. Right bundle-branch block and ST segment elevation in leads V₁–V₃: a marker of sudden death in patients with no demonstrable structural heart disease. *Circulation* 1998;97:457–460.

182. Priori SG, Napolitano C, Gasparini M, et al. Clinical and genetic heterogeneity of the right bundle branch block and ST segment elevation syndrome. A prospective evaluation of 52 families. *Circulation* 2000;102:2509–2515.

183. Chen Q, Kirsch GE, Zhang D, et al. Genetic basis and molecular mechanism for idiopathic ventricular fibrillation. *Nature* 1998;392:293–296.

184. Rook MB, Alshinawi CB, Groenewegen WA, et al. Human SCN5A gene mutations alter cardiac sodium channel kinetics and are associated with the Brugada syndrome. *Cardiovasc Res* 1999;44:507–517.

185. Wehrens XH, Wattanasirichaigoon D, Memmi M, et al. Mutation-dependent regulation of human cardiac Na⁺ channels by sympathetic stimulation in long QT and Brugada syndromes. *Circulation* 1999;99[Suppl 1]:I496(abst).

186. Makita N, Shirai N, Wang DW, et al. Cardiac Na(⁺) channel dysfunction in Brugada syndrome is aggravated by beta(₁)-subunit. *Circulation* 2000;101:54–60.

187. Martini B, Nava A, Thiene G, et al. Ventricular fibrillation without apparent heart disease: description of six cases. *Am Heart J* 1989;118:1203–1209.

188. Martini B, Nava A, Canciani B, Thiene G. Right bundle branch block, persistent ST segment elevation and sudden cardiac death. *J Am Coll Cardiol* 1993;22:633.

189. D'Onofrio A, Cuomo S, Musto B, Boccalatte A. Right bundle branch block, persistent ST-segment elevation in V₁–V₃ and sudden cardiac death: always a distinct syndrome? *G Ital Cardiol* 1995;25:1171–1175.

190. Izumi T, Ajiki K, Nozaki A, et al. Right ventricular cardiomyopathy showing right bundle branch block and right precordial ST segment elevation. *Intern Med* 2000;39:28–33.

191. Coumel P, Fidelle J, Lucet V, et al. Catecholaminergic-induced severe ventricular arrhythmias with Adams-Stokes syndrome in children: report of four cases. *Br Heart J* 1978;40[Suppl]: 28–37.

192. Leenhardt A, Lucet V, Denjoy I, et al. Catecholaminergic polymorphic ventricular tachycardia in children. A 7-year follow-up of 21 patients. *Circulation* 1995;91:1512–1519.

193. Rosen MR, Danilo P Jr. Effects of tetrodotoxin, lidocaine, verapamil and AHR-2666 on oubain-induced delayed after depolarizations in canine Purkinje fibers. *Circ Res* 1980;46:117–124.

194. Swan H, Piippo K, Viitasalo M, et al. Arrhythmic disorder mapped to chromosome 1q42-q43 causes malignant polymorphic ventricular tachycardia in structurally normal hearts. *J Am Coll Cardiol* 1999;34:2035–2042.

195. Otsu K, Fujii J, Periasamy M, et al. Chromosome mapping of five human cardiac and skeletal muscle sarcoplasmic reticulum protein genes. *Genomics* 1993;17:507–509.

196. Tunwell RE, Wickenden C, Bertrand BM, et al. The human cardiac muscle ryanodine receptor-calcium release channel: identification, primary structure and topological analysis. *Biochem J* 1996;318:477–487.

197. Priori SG, Napolitano C, Tiso N, et al. Mutations in the cardiac ryanodine receptor gene (hRyR2) underlie catecholaminergic polymorphic ventricular tachycardia. *Circulation* 2000;102:r49–r53.

198. Rubin DA, O'Keefe A, Kay RH, et al. Autosomal dominant inherited ventricular tachycardia. *Am Heart J* 1992;123:1082–1084.

199. Lerman BB, Dong B, Stein KM, et al. Right ventricular outflow tract tachycardia due to a somatic cell mutation in G protein subunit-alpha-i2. *J Clin Invest* 1998;101:2862–2868.

200. Lehmann H, Klein UE. Familial sinus node dysfunction with autosomal dominant inheritance. *Br Heart J* 1978;40:1314–1316.

201. Bacos JM, Eagan JT, Orgain ES. Congenital familial nodal rhythm. *Circulation* 1960;22:887–895.

202. Spellberg RD. Familial sinus node disease. *Chest* 1971;60:246–251.

203. Surawicz B, Hariman RJ. Follow-up of the family with congenital absence of sinus rhythm. *Am J Cardiol* 1988;61:467–469.

204. Beyer F, Paul T, Luhmer I, et al. Familiaeres idiopathisches Vorhofflimmern mit bradyarrhythmie. *Z Kardiol* 1993;82:674–677.

205. Nordenberg A, Varghese PJ, Nugent EW. Spectrum of sinus node dysfunction in two siblings. *Am Heart J* 1976;91:507–512.

206. Mackintosh AF, Chamberlain DA. Sinus node disease affecting both parents and both children. *Eur J Cardiol* 1979;10:117–122.

207. Brugada R, Tapscott T, Czernuszewicz GZ, et al. Identification of a genetic locus for familial atrial fibrillation. *N Engl J Med* 1997;336:905–911.

208. Wellens HJJ, Farre J, Bar FW. The Wolff-Parkinson-White syndrome. In: Mandel WJ, ed. *Cardiac arrhythmias. Their mechanisms, diagnosis and management.* Philadelphia: JP Lippincott Co, 1987:274–296.

209. Harnischfeger WW. Hereditary occurrence of the pre-excitation (Wolff-Parkinson-White) syndrome with re-entry mechanism and concealed conduction. *Circulation* 1959;19:28–40.

210. Chia BL, Yew FC, Chay SO, Tan ATH. Familial Wolff-Parkinson-White syndrome. *J Electrocardiol* 1982;15:195–198.

211. Vidaillet HJ Jr, Pressley JC, Henke E, et al. Familial occurrence of accessory atrioventricular pathways (preexcitation syndrome). *N Engl J Med* 1987;317:65–69.

212. Massumi RA. Familial Wolff-Parkinson-White syndrome with cardiomyopathy. *Am J Med* 1967;43:951–955.

213. Schneider RG. Familial occurrence of Wolff-Parkinson-White syndrome. *Am Heart J* 1969;78:34–36.

214. Braunwald E, Morrow AG, Cornell WP, et al. Idiopathic hypertrophic subaortic stenosis: clinical, hemodynamic and angiographic manifestations. *Am J Med* 1960;29:924–945.

215. Lenegre J. Etiology and pathology of bilateral bundle branch block in relation to complete heart block. *Prog Cardiovasc Dis* 1964;6:409–444.

216. Lev M, Kinare SG, Pick A. The pathogenesis of atrioventricular block in coronary disease. *Circulation* 1970;42:409–425

217. Brink AJ, Torrington M. Progressive familial heart block—two types. *S Afr Med J* 1977;52:53–59.

218. Stephan E. Hereditary bundle branch system defect: survey of a family with four affected generations. *Am Heart J* 1978;95:89–95.

219. Stephan E, Aftimos G, Allam C. Familial fascicular block: histologic features of Lev's disease. *Am Heart J* 1985;109:1399–1401.

220. Stephan E, de Meeus A, Bouvagnet P. Hereditary bundle branch defect: right bundle branch blocks of different causes have different morphologic characteristics. *Am Heart J* 1997;133:249–256.

221. Brink PA, Ferreira A, Moolman JC, et al. Gene for progressive familial heart block type I maps to chromosome 19q13. *Circulation* 1995;91:1633–1640.

222. de Meeus A, Stephan E, Debrus S, et al. An isolated cardiac conduction disease maps to chromosome 19q. *Circ Res* 1995;77:735–740.

223. Schott JJ, Alshinawi C, Kyndt F, et al. Cardiac conduction defects associate with mutations in SCN5A [Letter]. *Nat Genetics* 1999;23:20–21.

224. Clarke A, Harper P. Genetic testing for hypertrophic cardiomyopathy. *N Engl J Med* 1992;327:1175–1176.

225. Watkins H, Seidman JG, Seidman CE. Genetic testing for hypertrophic cardiomyopathy. *N Engl J Med* 1992;327:1176.

INFLUENCES OF AUTONOMIC FACTORS AND BEHAVIORAL STATE ON VULNERABILITY TO CARDIAC ARRHYTHMIAS

RICHARD L. VERRIER
JULIE A. KOVACH
MURRAY A. MITTLEMAN

Neural and behavioral factors have been widely implicated in the genesis of life-threatening arrhythmias in animals and humans. In the experimental laboratory, it has been shown that activation of the sympathetic nerve by stimulation of central (1–4) and peripheral adrenergic structures (5), infusion of catecholamines (6), and imposition of behavioral stress (7–11) can increase cardiac vulnerability in the healthy and ischemic heart. These arrhythmogenic effects are substantially blunted by β-adrenergic receptor blockade (12). Various supraventricular arrhythmias can also be elicited by activation of the autonomic nervous system (13,14). Vagus nerve activation is generally effective against arrhythmias involving the atrioventricular node but has the potential for precipitating fibrillation in atria damaged by disease and even in the healthy atrium (14–15). In humans, arrhythmogenesis attributable to sympathetic nerve activity has been demonstrated in the context of acute myocardial ischemia and infarction (16–18), in the long QT syndrome (19), and during behavioral stress (20–22).

The most compelling evidence for a pivotal role of sympathetic nerve activity in the genesis of malignant arrhythmias clinically derives from multicenter trials of β-adrenergic blocking agents (23–27). Overall, it has been shown that this class of compounds is capable of reducing reinfarction and sudden cardiac death by 30% or more. Although the mechanisms whereby these agents exert their salutary influence is a matter of considerable debate, there is general agreement that their ability to reduce myocardial ischemia is a critical factor (27a).

The goal of this chapter is to discuss the mechanisms whereby neural and behavioral factors conduce to life-threatening arrhythmias. This includes a discussion of the effects of enhanced autonomic nervous system activity on excitable properties of the heart and its specialized conducting system, an impairment in myocardial perfusion, and changes in platelet aggregability (Fig. 4.2-1). The clinical significance of the latter effect is underscored by the circadian pattern of sudden cardiac death, which is most prevalent in the early morning hours coincident with upregulation of platelets and proaggregatory surges in sympathetic nerve discharge (28–30). There is evidence that increased adrenergic discharge can predispose to disruption of ather-

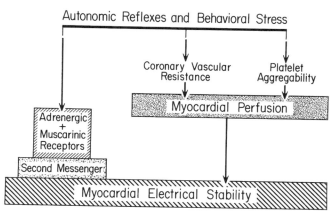

FIGURE 4.2-1. Summary of mechanisms mediating the effects of the autonomic nervous system on ventricular electrical stability. These modes of action provide the strategic loci for reduction of arrhythmogenesis by blockade of adrenergic receptors. (From Verrier RL. Central nervous system modulation of cardiac rhythm. In: Rosen MR, Palti Y, eds. *Lethal arrhythmias resulting from myocardial ischemia and infarction.* Boston: Kluwer Academic Publishers, 1988:149–164, with permission.)

R. L. Verrier and M. A. Mittleman: Department of Medicine, Harvard Medical School, and Institute for Prevention of Cardiovascular Disease, Beth Israel Deaconess Medical Center, Boston, Massachusetts 02215.

J. A. Kovach: Department of Cardiology, University of Michigan Health System, Ann Arbor, Michigan 48109.

osclerotic plaques and lead to coronary thrombosis (31). The reduction in the morning peak in myocardial infarction incidence by β-adrenergic blockade or aspirin lends further support for these putative mechanisms (32–35).

T-WAVE ALTERNANS AS A MARKER OF CARDIAC VULNERABILITY

Assessment of cardiac vulnerability is made more challenging by the transitory nature of neural triggers and the dynamic changes in cardiac substrate that occur during acute ischemia and reperfusion. The traditional method has been the ventricular fibrillation threshold technique, which involves determining the minimum current required to elicit the arrhythmia during the vulnerable phase of the cardiac cycle (6,36,37). The major disadvantage of the technique is the disruptive effects of repeated inductions of ventricular fibrillation and the attendant resuscitative procedures.

Considerable evidence has been accrued that suggests that quantification of T-wave alternans, defined as a consistent 2 : 1 variation in T-wave morphology, may provide a robust way to assess the dynamic changes in vulnerability. In addition, this index circumvents problems associated with cardiac electrical testing. Adam and coworkers (38) and Smith and colleagues (39) demonstrated a significant correlation between fluctuations in overall energy of the T wave and the ventricular fibrillation threshold during coronary artery occlusion and hypothermia in dogs. We demonstrated that the magnitude of T-wave alternans provides a continuous measure of vulnerability to fibrillation during both occlusion and reperfusion (Fig. 4.2-2) (40,41). In a study involving 61 chloralose-anesthetized dogs during 122 ten-minute left anterior descending coronary occlusions followed by abrupt reperfusion, a close temporal linear ($r^2 = 0.98$, $p < 0.01$) relationship

between the spontaneous occurrence of ventricular tachycardia and fibrillation and the magnitude of T-wave alternans was observed (Fig. 4.2-3) (41).

There is growing evidence that T-wave alternans testing may be useful clinically, as has been recently reviewed (42). Among the most salient observations are that it can be employed to detect changes in repolarization in patients with cardiac disease during angioplasty (41), ambulatory ischemia (43), and exercise stress testing (44–44b) and to delineate the degree of vulnerability to lethal arrhythmias in patients referred for programmed electrical stimulation (45) or implantable cardioverter-defibrillators (46). Rosenbaum and coworkers (45) found that repolarization alternans was a significant and independent predictor of inducible arrhythmias in 83 patients referred for electrophysiologic testing. The sensitivity and specificity of alternans to predict the results of electrophysiologic testing in their study was 81% and 84%, respectively, with a relative risk of 5.2. The presence of T-wave alternans in the microvolt range and arrhythmia inducibility were found to be significant and essentially equivalent predictors of arrhythmia-free survival ($p < 0.001$). In a prospective study (46), T-wave alternans was compared with the other current noninvasive markers of risk for ventricular arrhythmias (namely, invasive electrophysiologic testing, left ventricular ejection fraction, baroreceptor sensitivity, heart rate variability, signal-average electrocardiogram, the presence of nonsustained ventricular tachycardia on Holter monitoring, and QT dispersion) in patients who had received implantable cardioverter-defibrillators because of high risk for ventricular arrhythmias. On multivariate analysis, T-wave alternans was the only significant independent predictor of event-free survival during an 18-month follow-up. The available clinical data are summarized in Table 4.2-1. Collectively, these experimental and clinical observations carry important implications because they suggest that assessment of T-wave alternans may

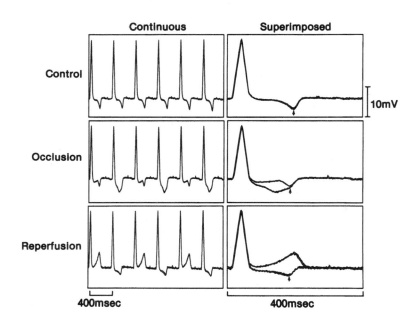

FIGURE 4.2-2. Electrocardiogram recorded within the left ventricle before, during, and after coronary artery occlusion in a single representative animal. Right panels show superimposition of six successive beats. Before occlusion *(top tracing)*, the T waves of each succeeding beat are uniform (arrow designates apex of T wave). After 4 minutes of coronary artery occlusion *(middle tracing)*, there is marked alternation of the first half of the T wave, coinciding with the vulnerable period of the cardiac cycle. The second half of the T wave remains uniform. After release of the occlusion *(bottom tracing)*, alternans is bidirectional, with T waves alternately inscribed above and below the isoelectric line. (From Nearing BD, Huang AH, Verrier RL. Dynamic tracking of cardiac vulnerability by complex demodulation of the T-wave. *Science* 1991;252: 437–440, with permission.)

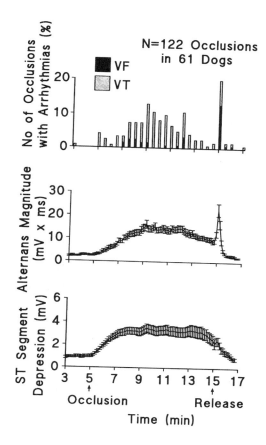

FIGURE 4.2-3. Simultaneous time course of spontaneous ventricular fibrillation (VF) and tachycardia (VT), T-wave alternans, and ST-segment depression during 10 minutes of left anterior descending coronary artery occlusion and reperfusion in 61 chloralose-anesthetized dogs monitored with a left ventricular electrocardiographic catheter. Two occlusion-release sequences were performed in each dog. Incidence of spontaneous VT and VF was summed for each 30-second period. T-wave alternans and ST-segment changes were summed for each 10-ms interval. The waxing and waning of T-wave alternans magnitude closely parallels the spontaneous occurrence of malignant ventricular arrhythmias during occlusion and reperfusion. By contrast, the ST-segment changes were dissociated from arrhythmogenesis during the initial and latter minutes of the occlusion and upon reperfusion. The alternans and ST-segment values are means ± standard error of the mean. VT was defined as four or more successive ventricular ectopic beats. (From Nearing BD, Oesterle SN, Verrier RL. Quantification of ischaemia-induced vulnerability by precordial T-wave alternans analysis in dog and human. *Cardiovasc Res* 1994:28:1440–1449, with permission.)

TABLE 4.2-1. CLINICAL STUDIES ON PREDICTIVE POWER OF T-WAVE ALTERNANS IN HIGHRISK PATIENTS

Patient Group	No. of Patients	End Point	Findings	Investigators
Electrophysiologic patients (64% CAD, 75% of whom had MI; 8% dilated cardiomyopathy; 24% no organic heart disease)	83	Inducible during PES	Sensitivity = 81%, specificity = 84%, PPV = 76%, NPV = 88%, RR = 5.2	Rosenbaum and colleagues (45)
Electrophysiologic patients	45	Inducible during PES	Sensitivity = 85%, specificity = 68%	Kavesh and colleagues (121)
Electrophysiologic patients (64% CAD, 75% of whom had MI; 8% dilated cardiomyopathy; 24% no organic heart disease)	66	Ventricular tachyarrhythmia events	Sensitivity = 89%, specificity = 89%, PPV = 80%, NPV = 94%, RR = 13.3	Rosenbaum and colleagues (45)
Consecutive ICD patients with ventricular arrhythmia (75% CAD, 17% dilated-cardiomyopathy)	95	Ventricular tachyarrhythmic events	Sensitivity = 78%, specificity = 61%, PPV = 67%, NPV = 73%, RR = 2.5	Hohnloser and colleagues (46)
Consecutive ICD patients with ventricular arrhythmia and CAD	71	Ventricular tachyarrhythmic events	Sensitivity = 85%, specificity = 68%, PPV = 73%, NPV = 81%, RR = 3.9	Hohnloser and colleagues 1998 (46)

ICD, implantable cardioverter-defibrillator; CAD, coronary artery disease; MI, myocardial infarction; PES, programmed electrical stimulation; PPV, positive predictive value; NPV, negative predictive value; RR, relative risk.
Source: Verrier RL, Cohen RJ. Risk identification and markers of susceptibility. In: Spooner P, Rosen MR, eds. *Foundations of cardiac arrhythmias.* New York: Marcel Dekker 2001:745–777, with permission.

provide a useful means of predicting risk for sudden cardiac death. This possibility is particularly attractive in light of the ubiquity of the phenomenon of T-wave alternans, which is evident with cardiac disease patients with ischemia or infarction (43–45,47–51) or primary arrhythmia (46), as well as the long QT syndrome (19,52–55) and Prinzmetal angina (56–62).

ADRENERGICALLY INDUCED CARDIAC VULNERABILITY

Experimentally, we have shown that within a few minutes of left anterior descending coronary artery occlusion, there is a striking surge in sympathetic nerve activity. This has been documented by direct nerve recording measurements (63) and by complex demodulation of heart rate variability (64). The enhancement in sympathetic nerve activity is associated with a marked increase in susceptibility to ventricular fibrillation as evidenced by the spontaneous occurrence of the arrhythmia (41), a fall in ventricular fibrillation threshold (63) (Fig. 4.2-4), and increased T-wave alternans magnitude (40,41,65) (Fig. 4.2-3). Upon reperfusion, a second peak in vulnerability occurs, probably due to washout products of cellular ischemia (63,66,67). Stellectomy significantly blunts the surge in vulnerability to ventricular fibrillation during occlusion but enhances its magnitude during reperfusion (63). These findings are consistent with the facts that adrenergic factors play a key role during ischemia (68) and that stellectomy increases the reactive hyperemic response to "release reperfusion" (63), which in turn probably leads to greater liberation of ischemic by-products.

Sympathetic-Parasympathetic Nerve Interactions

Enhanced cardiac vagus nerve activity can reduce susceptibility to ventricular fibrillation (69). The antifibrillatory action derives mainly through an antagonism of the deleterious effects of sympathetic nerve activity. The molecular and cellular bases for this accentuated antagonism appear to be presynaptic inhibition of norepinephrine release and stimulation of muscarinic receptors, which inhibit second messenger formation by catecholamines (70). The vagus nerve is not effective in preventing reperfusion-induced ventricular fibrillation during fixed-rate pacing. However, during spontaneous rhythm, the rate-reducing effect of vagus nerve excitation decreases susceptibility to fibrillation by increasing diastolic perfusion time and reducing myocardial oxygen deficit, thereby lessening the release of ischemic by-products.

Today there is no direct evidence for an antiarrhythmic effect of vagus nerve activation at the ventricular level in human subjects. However, there are inferential data that

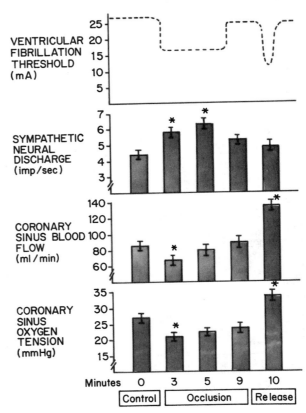

FIGURE 4.2-4. Effects of a 10-minute period of left anterior descending coronary artery occlusion and release on neural sympathetic activity, coronary sinus blood flow, and oxygen tension. A schematic representation of the time course of changes in ventricular fibrillation threshold is also displayed. Left anterior descending coronary artery occlusion results in a consistent activation of sympathetic preganglionic fibers, which corresponds with the period of maximal increase in vulnerability to ventricular fibrillation. The concomitant changes in coronary sinus blood flow and reperfusion are also displayed (*, *p* < 0.05 compared to control period). (From Lombardi F, Verrier RL, Lown B. Relationship between sympathetic neural activity, coronary dynamics, and vulnerability to ventricular fibrillation during myocardial ischemia and reperfusion. *Am Heart J* 1983;105:958–965, with permission.)

suggest that some of the mechanisms described in experimental animals may operate in the clinical setting. In particular, it has been shown that impairment of or a decrease in either vagal tone, as assessed by heart rate variability, or reflex activation of the nerve, as assessed by baroreceptor sensitivity to phenylephrine infusion, are both associated with increased mortality rates and incidence of sudden death among post–myocardial infarction patients (69, 71,72) (Fig. 4.2-5).

Mechanisms Responsible for Arrhythmogenesis during β-Adrenergic Receptor Activation

The mechanisms whereby enhanced sympathetic nerve activity increases cardiac vulnerability in the healthy and

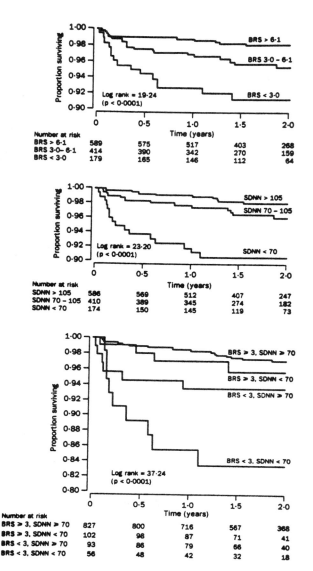

FIGURE 4.2-5. Kaplan-Meier survival curves for total cardiac mortality in post–myocardial infarction patients according to baroreceptor sensitivity (*BRS*) in the Autonomic Tone and Reflexes After Myocardial Infarction Study (*p* value refers to differences in event rates among subgroups). (From La Rovere MT, Bigger JT Jr, Marcus FI, et al. Baroreflex sensitivity and heart-rate variability in prediction of total cardiac mortality after myocardial infarction. ATRAMI [Autonomic Tone and Reflexes After Myocardial Infarction] investigators. *Lancet* 1998;351:478–484, with permission.)

ischemic heart are complex (14). The major indirect effects include impairment of oxygen supply-demand ratio resulting from increased cardiac metabolic activity, coronary vasoconstriction, particularly in vessels with damaged endothelium, and changes in preload and afterload (73). The direct effects on cardiac electrophysiologic function include derangements in impulse formation, conduction, or both (14,74). Increased levels of catecholamines stimulate β-adrenergic receptors, which in turn alter adenylate cyclase activity and intracellular calcium flux (Fig. 4.2-6). These effects are probably mediated by the cyclic nucleotide and protein kinase regulatory cascade, which can alter spatial heterogeneity of calcium transients and consequently increase dispersion of repolarization. The net effect is an increase in vulnerability to ventricular fibrillation (75,76). The converse is also true: reduction of cardiac sympathetic neural drive by stellectomy provides an antifibrillatory influence in animals and humans.

Effectiveness of β₁- and β₂-Adrenergic Receptor Blockade in Preventing Ischemia-Induced Vulnerability

Clinical trials in the postinfarction phase support the effectiveness of β-adrenergic receptor blockade in reducing the risk of sudden death and reinfarction (23–26,31). Although the mechanisms whereby these agents exert their salutary influence is a matter of considerable debate, there is general agreement that their ability to reduce myocardial ischemia is a critical factor. Central and peripheral sites of action (23) have been proposed for the effectiveness of β-adrenergic receptor blockade in reducing susceptibility to ventricular fibrillation during acute myocardial ischemia. Propranolol and metoprolol are the most extensively studied and have been found to reduce mortality rates by 30% or more in long-term studies (23–26,31). Although the Cardiac Arrhythmia Suppression Trial (CAST) had failed to show improved survival with agents designed to suppress ventricular premature beats, a subset of the CAST supported the secondary preventive benefit of beta-blockade therapy in high-risk post–myocardial infarction patients (ejection fraction ≤ 40%) (24). It was determined that beta-blockade therapy was independently associated with one-third reduction in arrhythmia-related death or cardiac arrest, with enhanced survival at 30 days, as well as with suppression of all-cause and arrhythmic death or nonfatal cardiac arrest at 1 and 2 years of follow-up. Metoprolol also reduced all-cause mortality rates and overall mortality rates of patients with acute myocardial infarction who were enrolled in the Goteborg Metoprolol Trial (25). The Beta-Blocker Heart Attack Trial determined that propranolol had its greatest beneficial effect in post–myocardial infarction patients with persistent ST-segment depression, in whom the drug significantly reduced mortality rates, including sudden death (26).

The Acebutolol et Prevention Secondaire de l'Infarctus (APSI) Trial, a randomized, double-blind, placebo-controlled trial involving more than 600 post–myocardial infarction patients, demonstrated that the drug reduced cardiovascular mortality rates by 58% (*p* = 0.006) (77). This significant finding challenges the widely held view that drugs with intrinsic sympathomimetic activity are not suitable for secondary prevention after acute myocardial infarction. The APSI investigators suggested that part of the dif-

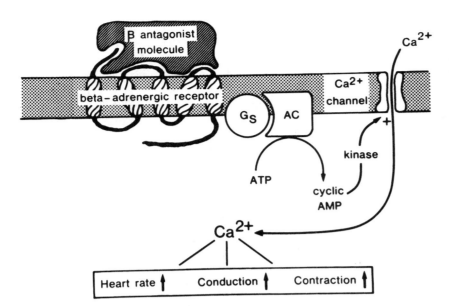

FIGURE 4.2-6. The cardiac β-adrenoceptor and signaling system. The β-antagonist molecule interacts with the β receptor, whose molecular structure has been revealed and the amino acid sequence characterized. In the presence of the stimulatory form of the G protein (Gs), adenylate cyclase (AC) converts adenosine 5′-triphosphate (ATP) to cyclic adenosine 5′-monophosphate (AMP), which acting by means of a protein kinase, enhances phosphorylation of the calcium channel and permits more calcium to enter through the calcium channel during voltage-induced depolarization. Such calcium releases much more from the sarcoplasmic reticulum (calcium-induced calcium release) to increase cytosolic calcium, heart rate, conduction, and contraction, as well as the rate of relaxation (the latter by phosphorylation of the protein phospholamban in the sarcoplasmic reticulum). (From Opie LH. *Drugs for the heart,* 3rd ed. Philadelphia: WB Saunders, 1991, with permission.)

ference in the findings may be attributed to the fact that a rather low acebutolol dosage, 200 mg twice daily, was administered and that the drug has only moderate intrinsic sympathomimetic activity.

More recently, the effectiveness of beta blockade in the setting of congestive heart failure has been examined. Treatment with metoprolol in heart failure patients in New York Heart Association classes II, III, and IV, in addition to optimum standard therapy, was associated with a more than 30% decrease in all-cause mortality rates, cardiovascular morality rates, sudden deaths, and deaths resulting from progressive heart failure (27). In a subset of the Goteborg Metoprolol Trial involving patients with suspected acute myocardial infarction and indirect signs of congestive heart failure, it was determined that the β blocker markedly improved survival at 3 months and 1 year (78). Furthermore, in the CAST patients with congestive heart failure, beta-blockade therapy was associated with longer time to occurrence of new or worsened congestive heart failure (24).

Peripheral Sites of Action

There is considerable evidence indicating that β-adrenergic receptor blockade reduces arrhythmogenesis by an action at the neurocardiac effector junction. In particular, β-adrenergic receptor blockade by drugs such as propranolol and metoprolol afford significant protection against ventricular fibrillation (67,79) and reduce T-wave alternans (80) during acute coronary artery occlusion in the experimental animal. The salutary influence of these agents appears to be a result of their β-adrenergic receptor blocking properties, rather than their membrane-stabilizing actions (16). Opie (81) suggested that part of the beneficial effects of β-adren-

ergic receptor blockade by the noncardioselective agent propranolol may be negated by its potential vasoconstrictor effect, which is a result of its inhibition of coronary β2-adrenergic receptor–mediated vascular smooth muscle relaxation. Indeed, in a number of patients with Prinzmetal variant angina, propranolol has exacerbated symptoms (82), presumably by unopposed α-receptor–mediated coronary vasoconstriction. Such an effect would not be anticipated from cardioselective agents.

Cardiac β2-adrenergic receptors do not appear to play a significant role in modulating ventricular excitable properties. Hohnloser and coworkers (83) have studied the effects of the selective β2-adrenergic receptor agonist salbutamol and the antagonist ICI 118,551 on excitability, refractoriness, and ventricular fibrillation threshold in the canine heart. These agents, even in relatively high doses, failed to alter any of the electrophysiologic end points that were investigated. These results and those of others seem to suggest no significant involvement of β2-adrenergic receptors in altering cardiac excitable properties, at least in the canine heart. It is unknown whether this receptor subtype plays a role in modulating electrophysiologic properties of the human ventricle.

Central Effects of β-Adrenergic Receptor Blockade

There is evidence indicating that the antifibrillatory influence of β-adrenergic receptor blockade may result in part from blockade of central β-adrenergic receptors (84–86). Parker and coworkers (85) have shown that intracerebroventricular administration of subsystemic doses of l-propranolol but not d-propranolol was capable of significantly reducing the incidence of ventricular fibrillation during combined left anterior descending coronary artery occlusion and behavioral stress in the pig. Surprisingly, intravenous administration of even a relatively high dose of l-propranolol did not exhibit antifibrillatory action. The latter effect may relate in part to a species dependence, because unlike canines, pigs do not show a suppression of ischemia-induced arrhythmias in response to beta blockade (86). Parker and coworkers proposed that the centrally mediated protective effect of beta blockade is due to a decrease in sympathetic nerve activity and in plasma norepinephrine concentration (87,88). Eckberg (84) suggested that β-blocking agents with lipophilic properties may protect against ventricular fibrillation, not only by decreasing sympathetic neural tone but also by increasing cardiac vagal drive. It is important to point out that in the long term, penetration of cerebrospinal fluid is achieved even by lipid-insoluble β-blocking agents (81).

Whereas central actions of β-adrenergic receptor blockade may be a contributing factor to reducing susceptibility to ventricular fibrillation during acute myocardial ischemia, these are unlikely to be the sole mechanisms. This conclusion is drawn from the fact that administration of β-blocking agents is capable of negating the profibrillatory effect of direct sympathetic nerve stimulation (4,5). It is interesting to note that the prominent β-blocking agents, which have demonstrated long-term effects on mortality rates, namely, propranolol and metoprolol, are all lipophilic. It remains to be determined whether the long-term protective effects are different for the less lipophilic compounds. It is possible that with time, the differences between effectiveness of agents based on lipophilicity are offset by diffusion of the agent across the blood-brain barrier.

EXPERIMENTAL STUDIES OF BEHAVIORAL STRESS AND ARRHYTHMOGENESIS

Several behavioral models have been developed to define the impact of behavioral state on cardiac electrical stability (7,11,89,90). These have included aversive behavioral conditioning paradigms and models eliciting natural emotions, notably anger and fear (7,11,89). Quantification of changes in cardiac electrical stability in the healthy and ischemic heart was achieved by means of the repetitive extrasystole threshold technique (7,91). Aversive conditioning of dogs in a pavlovian sling with mild chest shock on 3 consecutive days showed that subsequent exposure to the environment without shock elicited a reduction in the repetitive extrasystole threshold of more than 30% (7,10). The same paradigm elicited a threefold increase in the occurrence of spontaneous ventricular fibrillation when occlusion was carried out in the aversive sling, compared with the nonaversive cage environment. In dogs recovering from myocardial infarction, exposure to the aversive environment consistently elicited ventricular tachycardia for several days during the healing process (Fig. 4.2-7) (8). After this time, the animals continued to exhibit signs of behavioral stress in the aversive environment but no longer experienced ventricular arrhythmias, indicating that the arousal state required a substrate of cardiac electrical instability for the induction of rhythm disturbances. The stress-induced changes in cardiac excitable properties are largely obtunded by β-adrenergic receptor blockade with propranolol or the cardioselective drugs tolamolol and metoprolol (92,93).

Using the precordial V5 electrocardiogram, it was demonstrated in canines that a standardized protocol for

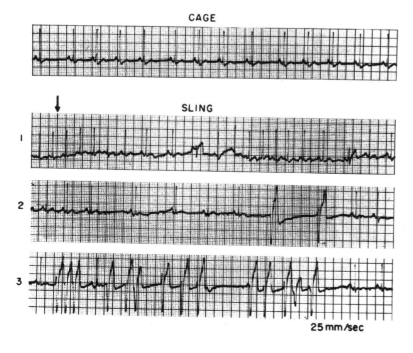

FIGURE 4.2-7. Provocation of ventricular arrhythmias by psychologic stress during myocardial infarction. In the nonstressful environment (*cage, upper tracing*), the animal exhibited normal sinus rhythm at a rate of 90 beats per minute. In comparison, when the animals were placed in the stressful environment (*sling, lower three continuous tracings*), ventricular arrhythmias were evoked. *(1)* Upon presentation of stressful stimuli (*arrow*), a brief period of sinus tachycardia (160 beats per minute) was followed by *(2)* sinus bradycardia (72 beats per minute). *(3)* Normal rhythm was interrupted by ventricular premature beats, culminating in ventricular tachycardia with bouts of R-on-T phenomenon. The observations were made 48 hours after myocardial infarction. (From Corbalan R, Verrier RL, Lown B. Psychological stress and ventricular arrhythmias during myocardial infarction in the conscious dog. *Am J Cardiol* 1974;34:692–696, with permission.)

induction of anger (11) induced a sizable increase in T-wave alternans before occlusion and increased by twofold the magnitude of alternation produced by 3 minutes of occlusion alone. The stress-related effects were significantly lessened by metoprolol (1.5 mg/kg intravenously) (80) (Fig. 4.2-8), further implicating a major role of β_1-adrenergic receptors in sympathetic nerve induction of cardiac vulnerability and T-wave alternans. Gang and colleagues (94) found that timolol and propranolol were protective against inducible sustained ventricular tachyarrhythmias in dogs with subacute myocardial infarction. Kaplan and colleagues (95,96) observed in socially dominant male monkeys that social disruption induced increased sympathetic nerve activity and endothelial injury in the coronary arteries and aorta. These effects were prevented in similarly aggressive monkeys by β-adrenergic blockade.

The net effect of neural activation on heart rhythm during infarction may be further complicated by functional or anatomic changes due to necrosis of afferent and efferent sympathetic and vagus nerve fibers within the ventricles. In an extensive series of experiments, Zipes and coworkers showed that sympathetic efferent nerve fibers en route to the ventricle cross at the atrioventricular groove travel within the superficial subepicardium in a base-to-apex direction and penetrate the myocardium to innervate the endocardium (97). They have suggested that myocardial infarction can produce functionally denervated areas within the ventricle. These investigators have shown that zones apical to the infarction fail to exhibit afferent reflexes in response to bradykinin or nicotine. Moreover, refractoriness of the affected areas is not altered by stimulation of the vagus nerve or the stellate ganglion. There is a significant reduction of norepinephrine levels in myocardial tissue. The affected zone is supersensitive to infused norepinephrine or isoproterenol (98). Thus, these investigators suggest that selective myocardial damage to the epicardium or endocardium may preferentially interrupt one or the other limb of the autonomic nervous system and this interruption in turn may predispose subjects to some ventricular arrhythmias. In addition, the functional denervation of sympathetic nerve fibers can lead to arrhythmogenic supersensitivity to catecholamines in areas distal to the zone of infarction.

Clinical Evidence of the Role of Behavioral Stress in Cardiovascular Events

The contribution of behavioral stress to triggering major cardiovascular events, including myocardial ischemia and infarction, arrhythmias, and sudden cardiac death, is gaining greater appreciation through controlled behavioral studies, standardized clinical stress testing, and experimental models of stress-induced cardiac sympathetic nerve activity.

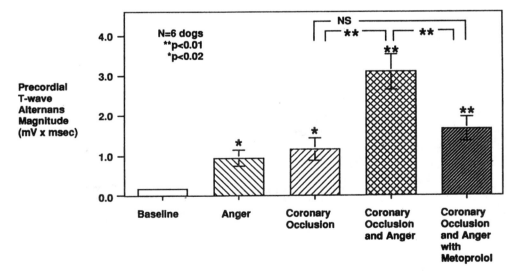

FIGURE 4.2-8. The effects of inducing anger in canines on T-wave alternans before and during a 3-minute period of left anterior descending coronary artery occlusion. The behavioral paradigm consisted of a confrontation over access to food (12). The precordial V$_5$ electrocardiographic lead demonstrates that even in the absence of coronary occlusion, aggressive arousal elicits a significant degree of T-wave alternans (0.92 ± 0.2 μV·ms, as quantified by complex demodulation). When aggressive arousal was superimposed on coronary occlusion, the magnitude in alternans was nearly twice that observed with occlusion alone. The stress-related effects were significantly lessened by intravenous administration of metoprolol (1.5 mg/kg). The results were obtained during spontaneous rhythm. (From Kovach JA, Nearing BD, Verrier RL. Effect of aggressive arousal on precordial T-wave alternans magnitude in the normal and ischemic canine heart with and without beta $_1$-adrenergic blockade with metoprolol. *J Am Coll Cardiol* 1994;23:329A[abst], with permission.)

In the United States alone, there are 1 million nonfatal infarctions and 250,000 sudden cardiac deaths annually, resulting in the classification of cardiac events as the leading cause of death in men and women in the industrially developed world. Descriptive studies indicate that emotional stress, particularly anger, fear, anxiety, bereavement, and depression, precedes fatal and nonfatal myocardial infarction in approximately 210,000 to 270,000 (14% to 18%) cases annually (99).

Controlled Behavioral Studies of Behavioral Stress and Myocardial Infarction

The role of anger as an acute precipitant of nonfatal myocardial infarction was identified in the large, controlled ONSET study (100). Among the 1,623 patients with acute infarction interviewed an average of 4 days after onset of cardiac symptoms, 2.4% reported that they had been "very angry" during the 2-hour period before myocardial infarction. Specific, frequent triggers of anger were arguments with family members (25%), conflicts at work (22%), and legal problems (8%). The case-crossover method (101,102) was employed. The elevated risk of myocardial infarction was found to be confined to the first 2 hours after an outburst of anger, as computed by using each patient's usual exposure during the prior year as the control information (100). The risk of infarction onset was estimated to be elevated by 2.3 times during the 2-hour period immediately after "very angry" (95% confidence interval [CI], 1.7–3.2), compared with control information based on each patient's usual frequency of anger (Fig. 4.2-9). Similar results were obtained from control information based on the frequency of anger episodes during the day before infarction. These data indicated that risk was increased fourfold (95% CI, 1.9–9.4). Analyses that employed the anger subscale of the State-Trait Personality Inventory indicated the increased risk of myocardial infarction at 1.9 times the normal (95% CI, 1.3–2.7), and state anxiety was calculated at a transient 1.6-fold (95% CI, 1.1–2.2) increase in risk of myocardial infarction onset. The relative risk of myocardial infarction attributable to anger was nearly half of the 5.9-fold increased risk associated with heavy physical exertion previously identified by the same authors (99). Among the possible explanations for this difference is the persistence of the affective state as the individual ruminates over the events precipitating the episode. Accordingly, the period of increased risk resulting from heavy exertion is transient, lasting less than 1 hour, whereas that of anger persists for up to 2 hours. A second possibility is that anger-induced ischemia may result from delayed constriction of the large coronary arteries, as found in studies in experimental animals (11).

The Normative Aging Study, a prospective study that enrolled men diagnosed free of coronary disease and followed them for 7 years, spawned several investigations that

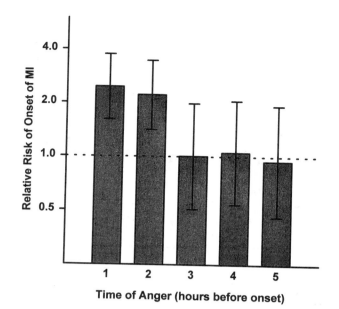

FIGURE 4.2-9. Bar graph shows the time of onset of myocardial infarction (MI) after an outburst of anger (induction time). Each of the 5 hours before MI onset was assessed as an independent hazard period, and anger in each hour was compared with that of the control intervals. Only the two 1-hour periods immediately before MI onset were associated with an increased risk, suggesting that the induction time for MI is less than 2 hours. Error bars indicate 95% confidence intervals. Dotted line represents baseline risk. (From Mittleman MA, Maclure M, Sherwood JB, et al. Triggering of acute myocardial infarction onset by episodes of anger. *Circulation* 1995;92:1720–1725, with permission.)

yielded valuable evidence of a causal role for anger in the increased incidence of coronary heart disease. The 1,305 study subjects completed the revised Minnesota Multiphasic Personality Inventory 2 (MMPI 2) and were grouped according to their responses to the MMPI 2 Anger Content scale. During the 7 years of follow-up, 30 nonfatal myocardial infarctions and 20 fatal coronary events were observed. None of the 20 fatal coronary events occurred in men reporting the lowest level of anger. Kawachi and colleagues (103) calculated the risk of a fatal or nonfatal coronary event to be 3.2 (95% CI, 0.9–10.5) times higher among the men reporting the highest compared with the lowest level of anger on the MMPI 2 Anger Content scale.

Standardized Clinical Stress Testing of Ischemia

Because myocardial ischemia during daily life activities is associated with an increased risk of acute cardiac events, standardized provocative stress testing has been employed as a tool for identifying individuals at risk for stress-induced ischemia and cardiac arrhythmias, and on a population level, to probe the association between emotional or mental arousal and the development of ischemia (104–116). Gottdiener and colleagues (111) determined that daily life

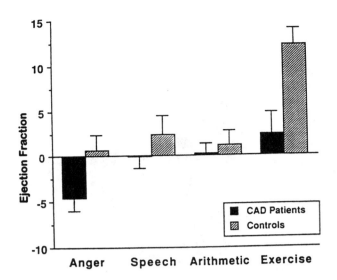

FIGURE 4.2-10. Change in ejection fraction (with standard deviation) from baseline for the anger, speech, and arithmetic tasks and the bicycle exercise test for patients with coronary artery disease *(CAD)* and control subjects. (From Ironson G, Taylor CB, Boltwood M, et al. Effects of anger on left ventricular ejection fraction in coronary artery disease. *Am J Cardiol* 1992;70:281–285, with permission.)

stresses provoked silent ischemia at lower heart rates and blood pressure measurements than exercise. These findings suggest that ischemia in response to mental stress results not only from increased myocardial oxygen demand, but also from decreased coronary flow, probably as a result of transient coronary vasoconstriction. Exercise stress testing did not adequately identify individuals susceptible to triggers of ischemia during sedentary activities, whereas left ventricular wall motion response to mental arithmetic and a simulated public speech task on a personal topic did predict susceptibility.

A new behavioral stress paradigm, "anger recall," has been employed by several investigators to test whether the mere act of describing a recent episode of anger might reproduce the impact of the emotion itself on myocardial perfusion and cardiac mechanical function. Ironson and coworkers (108) demonstrated that anger recall was the most potent behavioral stress paradigm tested for eliciting myocardial ischemia and left ventricular dysfunction in patients with single-vessel coronary artery disease. "Anger recall" produced a greater reduction in ejection fraction than did exercise stress testing (Fig. 4.2-10). Boltwood and coworkers (109) documented that coronary artery segments narrowed by atherosclerosis constricted while normal segments dilated in response to anger recall. They attributed this response to intact endothelial function in normal segments despite the vasoconstrictor effects of circulating plasma catecholamines. Current knowledge regarding elevations in risk of fatal and nonfatal cardiac events resulting from behavioral stress are summarized in Table 4.2-2 (117).

TABLE 4.2-2. BEHAVIORAL STUDIES AND RISK OF FATAL OR NONFATAL CARDIAC EVENTS

Behavior	Outcome	Risk Ratio	Investigator
Anger	Nonfatal MI	2.3 for 2 hours	Mittleman and colleagues (100)
Anger	Fatal or nonfatal MI	3.2	Kawachi and colleagues (103)
Anxiety	Nonfatal MI	1.6	Mittleman and colleagues (100)
Anxiety	Fatal MI	1.9	Kawachi and colleagues (122)
Anxiety	Sudden death (within 24 h)	4.5	Kawachi and colleagues (122)
Phobic anxiety	Fatal MI	3.0	Kawachi and colleagues (123)
Phobic anxiety	Sudden death (within 24 h)	6.1	Kawachi and colleagues (123)
Worry	Nonfatal MI	2.4	Kubzansky and colleagues (124)
Daily life stresses (tension, sadness, frustration)	Silent myocardial ischemia in patients with coronary disease	2–3 for 1 h	Gullette and colleagues (125)
Major depression in early survivors of MI	Cardiac death	3.64 for 18 mo	Frasure-Smith and colleagues (126)
Depressive symptomatology in early survivors of MI	Cardiac death	7.82	Frasure-Smith and colleagues (126)
Depressive symptomatology in early survivors of MI	Cardiac death in patients with ≥10 premature ventricular contractions	29.1	Frasure-Smith and colleagues (126)
Vital exhaustion	Nonfatal MI	2.28	Appels and Mulder (127)
Vital exhaustion	Recurrent MI	2.7	Kop and colleagues (128)

MI, myocardial infarction.
Source: Verrier RL, Mittleman MA. The impact of emotions on the heart. In: Mayer EA, Saper CB, eds.
The biologic basis for mind body interactions. Amsterdam: Elsevier Science, with permission.

SLEEP-RELATED CARDIAC RISK

Healthy people find sleep to be generally salutary and restorative. Ironically, during sleep in patients with respiratory or heart disease, the brain can precipitate breathing disorders, myocardial ischemia, arrhythmias, and even death. An estimated 250,000 nocturnal myocardial infarctions and 38,000 nocturnal sudden deaths occur annually in the U.S. population, based on our recent observation that 20% of myocardial infarctions and 15% of sudden deaths occur during the period from 12:00 A.M. to 6:00 A.M. (118). This event rate is equivalent to 91% of the number of fatalities resulting from automobile accidents and 20% more than the number of deaths caused by HIV infection. Thus, sleep is not a protected state. The distribution of deaths and myocardial infarctions during nighttime is nonuniform, a pattern consistent with provocation by pathophysiologic triggers. Precise characterization of the precipitating factors for nocturnal cardiac events is incomplete. Although death during sleep may be presumed to be painless, in many cases,

it is premature, as it occurs in infants and adolescents and in adults with ischemic heart disease, for whom the median age is 59 years. High-risk populations for nocturnal cardiorespiratory events include a number of sizable patient groups (Table 4.2-3).

The two main factors that have been implicated in nocturnal cardiac events are sleep-state–dependent surges in autonomic nervous system activity and depression of respiratory control mechanisms, which have an impact on a vulnerable cardiac substrate. The brain, in subserving its needs for periodic reexcitation during rapid eye movement (REM) sleep and dreaming, imposes significant demands on the heart by inducing bursts in sympathetic nerve activity, which reaches levels higher than those during wakefulness. In susceptible individuals, this degree of sympathetic nerve activity may compromise coronary artery blood flow, as metabolic demand outstrips supply, and may trigger sympathetically mediated life-threatening arrhythmias. Obstructive sleep apnea, which impairs ventilation during sleep and can generate reductions in arterial oxygen satura-

TABLE 4.2-3. PATIENT GROUPS AT POTENTIALLY INCREASED RISK FOR NOCTURNAL CARDIAC EVENTS

Indication (US Patients/y)	Possible Mechanism
Angina, myocardial infarction, arrhythmias, ischemia, or cardiac arrest at night	The nocturnal pattern suggests a sleep-state–dependent autonomic trigger or respiratory distress; 20% of myocardial infarctions (~250,000 cases/y) and 15% of sudden deaths (~38,000 cases/y) occur between midnight and 6:00 A.M.
Unstable angina, non–Q-wave infarction, Prinzmetal angina	Non-demand ischemia and angina and non–Q-wave infarction peak between midnight and 6:00 A.M.
Acute myocardial infarction (1.5 million)	
Disturbances in sleep, respiration, and autonomic balance may be factors in nocturnal arrhythmogenesis. Spousal or family report of highly irregular breathing, excessive snoring, or apnea in patients with coronary disease (5 to 10 million US patients with apnea)	Patients with hypertension or coronary artery disease should be screened for the presence of sleep apnea, which conduces to hypertension, ischemia, arrhythmia, and atrial fibrillation, and is a risk factor for lethal daytime cardiac events, including myocardial infarction.
Heart failure (4.6 million)	20% of sudden deaths in heart failure patients occur between midnight and 6:00 A.M.
Long QT syndrome	The profound cycle-length changes associated with sleep may trigger pause-dependent torsade de pointes in these patients.
Nearmiss or siblings of sudden infant death syndrome victims	Crib death commonly occurs during sleep with characteristic cardiorespiratory symptoms.
Asians with warning signs of sudden unexplained nocturnal death (SUNDS)	SUNDS is attributable to sleeprelated arrhythmia.
Atrial fibrillation (2.5 million)	29% of episodes occur between midnight and 6:00 A.M. Respiratory and autonomic mechanisms are suspected.
Patients on cardiac medications (13.5 million US patients with cardiovascular disease)	β–Blockers and calcium channel blockers that cross the bloodbrain barrier may increase nighttime risk, as poor sleep and violent dreams may be triggered. Medications that increase the QT interval may conduce to pause-dependent torsade de pointes during the profound cycle-length changes of sleep. Because arterial blood pressure is decreased during nonrapid eye movement sleep, additional lowering by antihypertensive agents may induce a risk of ischemia and infarction because of lowered coronary perfusion.

Source: Verrier RL, Mittleman MA. Sleep-related cardiac risk. In: Kryger MH, Roth T, Dement WC, eds. *Principles and practice of sleep medicine,* 3rd ed. Philadelphia: WB Saunders, 2000, with permission.

tion, afflicts 5 to 10 million Americans, or 2% to 4% of the population (119). This condition has been strongly implicated, when severe, in the cause of hypertension, ischemia, arrhythmias, myocardial infarction, and sudden death in individuals with coexisting ischemic heart disease. Autonomic or respiratory disturbances during sleep may trigger atrial fibrillation in certain patient populations. A challenge is also presented by non-REM sleep, when malperfusion of the heart and brain may result from hypotension and decreased blood flow in stenosed vessels. These conditions may be confounded by medications that cross the blood-brain barrier, alter sleep structure, and provoke nightmares with severe cardiac autonomic discharge. Finally, an insidious component of the problem of nocturnal risk results from the fact that many individuals are unaware of their respiratory or cardiac distress at night and take no corrective action. Thus, sleep presents unique autonomic, hemodynamic, and respiratory challenges to the diseased myocardium, which cannot be monitored by daytime diagnostic tests. The importance of monitoring nocturnal arrhythmias extends beyond identifying sleep-state–dependent triggers of cardiac events, as nighttime ischemia, arrhythmias, autonomic activity, and respiratory disturbances carry predictive value for daytime events. The evidence supporting these comments has recently been reviewed (120).

SUMMARY

An impressive body of information underscores the importance of neural and behavioral factors in the genesis of cardiac arrhythmias in the healthy and ischemic heart. The main intermediary mechanisms of autonomic influences include direct effects on myocardial excitable properties and indirect actions resulting from alterations in coronary vasomotor tone and platelet aggregability. There is growing evidence that changes in behavioral state, as occur during intense arousal and dreaming, exert a major impact on myocardial perfusion and vulnerability to cardiac arrhythmias. Particularly underappreciated has been the importance of disturbed respiratory function during sleep in patients with underlying cardiac ailments including ischemic heart disease, heart failure, and atrial fibrillation. The availability of new tools from the disciplines of epidemiology, cardiovascular pathophysiology, behavioral medicine, and noninvasive cardiac risk assessment are likely to accelerate our understanding of the triggers of life-threatening arrhythmias and the development of effective therapeutic modalities.

ACKNOWLEDGMENTS

This work was supported by grant no. P01 ES008129 and P01 ES09825-01 from the National Heart, Lung, and Blood Institute of the National Institutes of Health and grant no. 9630115N from the American Heart Association. The authors thank Sandra S. Verrier for her editorial contributions.

REFERENCES

1. Hockman CH, Mauck HP, Hoff EC. ECG changes resulting from cerebral stimulation: II. A spectrum of ventricular arrhythmias of sympathetic origin. *Am Heart J* 1966;71:695–700.
2. Manning JW, Cotten M de V. Mechanism of cardiac arrhythmias induced by diencephalic stimulation. *Am J Physiol* 1962;203:1120–1124.
3. Korteweg GCJ, Boeles JTF, Ten Cate J. Influence of stimulation of some subcortical areas on electrocardiogram. *J Neurophysiol* 1957;20:100–107.
4. Verrier RL, Calvert A, Lown B. Effect of posterior hypothalamic stimulation on the ventricular fibrillation threshold. *Am J Physiol* 1975;228:923–927.
5. Verrier RL, Thompson PL, Lown B. Ventricular vulnerability during sympathetic stimulation: role of heart rate and blood pressure. *Cardiovasc Res* 1974;8:602–610.
6. Han J, Moe GK. Nonuniform recovery of excitability in ventricular muscle. *Circ Res* 1964;14:44–60.
7. Lown B, Verrier RL, Corbalan R. Psychologic stress and threshold for repetitive ventricular response. *Science* 1973;182:834–836.
8. Corbalan R, Verrier RL, Lown B. Psychological stress and ventricular arrhythmias during myocardial infarction in the conscious dog. *Am J Cardiol* 1974;34:692–696.
9. Lown B, Verrier RL. Neural activity and ventricular fibrillation. *N Engl J Med* 1976;294:1165–1170.
10. Verrier RL, Lown B. Behavioral stress and cardiac arrhythmias. *Annu Rev Physiol* 1984;46:155–176.
11. Verrier RL, Hagestad EL, Lown B. Delayed myocardial ischemia induced by anger. *Circulation* 1987;75:249–254.
12. Verrier RL, Lown B. Adrenergic blockade and the prevention of behaviourally-induced cardiac arrhythmias. In: Zanchetti A, ed. *Advances in beta-blocker therapy II*. Amsterdam: Excerpta Medica, 1982:130–146.
13. Coumel P. Autonomic influences in atrial tachyarrhythmias. *J Cardiovasc Electrophysiol* 1996;7:999.
14. Jayachandran JV, Sih HJ, Winkle W, et al. Atrial fibrillation produced by prolonged rapid atrial pacing is associated with heterogeneous changes in atrial sympathetic. *Circulation* 2000;101:1185.
14a. Geddes LA, Hinds M, Babbs CF, et al. Maintenance of atrial fibrillation in anesthetized and unanesthetized sheep using cholinergic drive. *Pacing Clin Electrophysiol* 1996;19:165.
14b. Liu L, Nattel S. Differing sympathetic and vagal effects on atrial fibrillation in dogs: role of refractoriness heterogeneity. *Am J Physiol* 1997;273:H805.
15. Allessie MA, Bonke FIM. Atrial arrhythmias: basic concepts. In: Mandel WJ, ed. *Cardiac arrhythmias: their mechanisms, diagnosis, and management*. Philadelphia: JB Lippincott Co, 1987:186–207.
16. Fitzgerald JD. The role of beta-adrenergic blockade in acute myocardial ischemia. In: Oliver MF, Julian DG, Donald KW, eds. *Effect of acute ischemia on myocardial function*. Baltimore: Williams & Wilkins, 1972:321–351.
17. Webb SW, Adgey AAJ, Pantridge JF. Autonomic disturbance at onset of acute myocardial infarction. *BMJ* 1972;3:89–92.
18. Schwartz PJ, La Rovere MT, Vanoli E. Autonomic nervous sys-

tem and sudden cardiac death: experimental basis and clinical observations for post-myocardial infarction risk stratification. *Circulation* 1992;85[Suppl I]:I77–I91.

19. Schwartz PJ, Zaza A, Locati E, et al. Stress and sudden death: the case of the long QT syndrome. *Circulation* 1991;83[Suppl II]:II71–II80.

20. Taggart P, Carruthers M, Somerville W. Electrocardiogram, plasma catecholamines and lipids, and their modification by oxprenolol when speaking before an audience. *Lancet* 1973;2: 341–346.

21. Taggart P, Gibbons D, Somerville W. Some effects of motor-car driving on the normal and abnormal heart. *BMJ* 1969;4: 130–134.

22. Lown B. Sudden cardiac death: biobehavioral perspective. *Circulation* 1987;76[Suppl I]:I186–I196.

23. Yusuf S, Peto R, Lewis J, et al. Beta blockade during and after myocardial infarction: an overview of the randomized trials. *Prog Cardiovasc Dis* 1985;27:335–371.

24. Kennedy HL, Brooks MM, Barker AH, et al. Beta-blocker therapy in the Cardiac Arrhythmia Suppression Trial. CAST Investigators. *Am J Cardiol* 1994;74:674–680.

25. Herlitz J, Elmfeldt D, Holmberg S, et al. Goteborg Metoprolol Trial: mortality and causes of death. *Am J Cardiol* 1984;53: 9D–14D.

25a. Shivkumar K, Schultz L, Goldstein S, et al. Effects of propranolol in patients entered in the Beta-Blocker Heart Attack Trial with their first myocardial infarction and persistent electrocardiographic ST-segment depression. *Am Heart J* 1998;135[Suppl 2, Pt 1]:261–267.

26. Effect of metoprolol CR/XL in chronic heart failure: Metoprolol CR/XL Randomised Intervention Trial in Congestive Heart Failure (MERIT-HF). *Lancet* 1999;353:2001–2007.

27. CIBIS-II Investigators and Committees. The Cardiac Insufficiency Bisoprolol Study II (CIBIS-II): A randomised trial. *Lancet* 1999;353:9.

27a. Nagatsu, M, Spinale, FG, Koide M, et al. Bradycardia and the role of beta-blockade in the amelioration of left ventricular dysfunction. *Circulation* 2000;101:653.

28. Muller JE, Stone PH, Turi ZG, et al. Circadian variation in the frequency of onset of acute myocardial infarction. *N Engl J Med* 1985;313:1315–1322.

29. Tofler GH, Brezinski D, Schafer AI, et al. Concurrent morning increase in platelet aggregability and the risk of myocardial infarction and sudden cardiac death. *N Engl J Med* 1987; 316:1514–1518.

30. ISIS-2 (Second International Study of Infarct Survival) Collaborative Group. Morning peak in the incidence of myocardial infarction: experience in the ISIS-2 trial. *Eur Heart J* 1992;13:594–598.

31. Frishman WH, Lazar EJ. Reduction of mortality, sudden death and non-fatal reinfarction with beta-adrenergic blockers in survivors of acute myocardial infarction: a new hypothesis regarding the cardioprotective action of beta-adrenergic blockade. *Am J Cardiol* 1990;66:66G–70G.

32. Willich SN, Linderer T, Wegscheider K, et al. Increased morning incidence of myocardial infarction in the ISAM Study: Absence with prior beta-adrenergic blockade. *Circulation* 1989; 80:853–858.

33. Ridker PM, Manson JE, Buring JE, et al. Circadian variation of acute myocardial infarction and the effect of low-dose aspirin in a randomized trial of physicians. *Circulation* 1990;82:897–902.

34. Peters RW. Propranolol and the morning increase in sudden cardiac death: (The Beta-Blocker Heart Attack Trial experience). *Am J Cardiol* 1990;66:57G–59G.

35. McCall NT, Tofler GH, Schafer AI, et al. The effect of enteric-coated aspirin on the morning increase in platelet activity. *Am Heart J* 1991;121:1382–1388.

36. Moore EN, Spear JF. Ventricular fibrillation threshold. Its physiological and pharmacological importance. *Arch Intern Med* 1975;135:446–453.

37. Verrier RL, Brooks WW, Lown B. Protective zone and the determination of vulnerability to ventricular fibrillation. *Am J Physiol* 1978;234:H592–H596.

38. Adam DR, Smith JM, Akselrod S, et al. Fluctuations in T-wave morphology and susceptibility to ventricular fibrillation. *J Electrocardiol* 1984;17:209–218.

39. Smith JM, Clancy EA, Valeri CR, et al. Electrical alternans and cardiac electrical instability. *Circulation* 1988;77:110–121.

40. Nearing BD, Huang AH, Verrier RL. Dynamic tracking of cardiac vulnerability by complex demodulation of the T-wave. *Science* 1991;252:437–440.

41. Nearing BD, Oesterle SN, Verrier RL. Quantification of ischaemia-induced vulnerability by precordial T-wave alternans analysis in dog and human. *Cardiovasc Res* 1994;28: 1440–1449.

42. Verrier RL, Cohen RJ. Risk identification and markers of susceptibility. In: Spooner P, Rosen MR, eds. *Foundations of cardiac arrhythmias.* New York: Marcel Dekker Inc. 2001:745–777.

43. Verrier RL, Nearing BD, MacCallum G, et al. T-wave alternans during ambulatory ischemia in patients with coronary heart disease. *Ann Noninvasive Electrocardiol* 1996;1:113–20.

44. Nearing BD, Stone PH, MacCallum G, et al, for the Vascular Basis Study Group. New median beat analysis method for T-wave alternans detection in standard treadmill testing of patients with stable coronary disease. *Pace* (abst) *(in press).*

44a. Hohnloser SH, Klingenheben T, Zabel M, et al. T wave alternans during exercise and atrial pacing in humans. *J Cardiovasc Electrophysiol* 1997;8:987.

44b. Estes NA III, Michaud G, Zipes DP, et al. Electrical alternans during rest and exercise as predictors of vulnerability to ventricular arrhythmias. *Am J Cardiol* 1997;80:1314.

45. Rosenbaum DS, Jackson LE, Smith JM, et al. Electrical alternans and vulnerability to ventricular arrhythmia. *N Engl J Med* 1994;330:235–241.

46. Hohnloser SH, Klingenheben T, Li YG, et al. T-wave alternans as a predictor of recurrent ventricular tachyarrhythmias in ICD recipients: prospective comparison with conventional risk markers. *J Cardiovasc Electrophysiol* 1998;9:1258–1268.

47. Salerno JA, Previtali M, Panciroli C, et al. Ventricular arrhythmias during acute myocardial ischaemia in man. The role and significance of R-ST-T alternans and the prevention of ischaemic sudden death by medical treatment. *Eur Heart J* 1986;7:63–75.

48. Sutton PMI, Taggart P, Lab M, et al. Alternans of epicardial repolarization as a localized phenomenon in man. *Eur Heart J* 1991;12:70–78.

49. Pantridge JF. Autonomic disturbance at the onset of acute myocardial infarction. In: Schwartz PJ, Brown AM, Malliani A, Zanchetti A, eds. *Neural mechanisms in cardiac arrhythmias.* New York: Raven Press, 1978:7–17.

50. Puletti M, Curione M, Righetti G, et al. Alternans of the ST-segment and T-wave in acute myocardial infarction. *J Electrocardiol* 1980;13:297–300.

51. Cinca J, Janse MJ, Morena H, et al. Mechanisms and time course of the early electrical changes during acute coronary artery occlusion. An attempt to correlate the early ECG changes in man to cellular electrophysiology in the pig. *Chest* 1980; 77:499–505.

52. Schwartz PJ, Malliani A. Electrical alternation of the T-wave: clinical and experimental evidence of its relationship with the sympathetic nervous system and with the long Q-T syndrome. *Am Heart J* 1975;89:45–50.

53. Schwartz PJ. Idiopathic long QT syndrome: progress and questions. *Am Heart J* 1985;109:399–411.

54. Rosenbaum MB, Acunzo RS. Pseudo 2:1 atrioventricular block and T wave alternans in the long QT syndromes. *J Am Coll Cardiol* 1991;18:1363–1366.

55. Surawicz B, Fisch C. Cardiac alternans: diverse mechanisms and clinical manifestations. *J Am Coll Cardiol* 1992;20:483–499.

56. Turitto G, El-Sherif N. Alternans of the ST segment in variant angina. *Chest* 1988;93:587–591.

57. Williams RR, Wagner GS, Peter RH. ST-segment alternans in Prinzmetal's angina. A report of two cases. *Ann Intern Med* 1974;81:51–54.

58. Kleinfeld MJ, Rozanski JJ. Alternans of the ST segment in Prinzmetal's angina. *Circulation* 1977;55:574–577.

59. Rozanski JJ, Meller J, Kleinfeld M, et al. Nonmechanical ST-segment alternans in Prinzmetal's angina. *Ann Intern Med* 1978; 89:76–77.

60. Rozanski JJ, Kleinfeld M. Alternans of the ST segment and T wave. A sign of electrical instability in Prinzmetal's angina. *Pacing Cardiac Electrophysiol* 1982;5:359–365.

61. Miller DD, Waters DD, Szlachcic J, et al. Clinical characteristics associated with sudden death in patients with variant angina. *Circulation* 1982;66:588–592.

62. Cheng TC. Electrical alternans: an association with coronary artery spasm. *Arch Intern Med* 1983;143:1052–1053.

63. Lombardi F, Verrier RL, Lown B. Relationship between sympathetic neural activity, coronary dynamics, and vulnerability to ventricular fibrillation during myocardial ischemia and reperfusion. *Am Heart J* 1983;105:958–965.

64. Nearing BD, Verrier RL. Simultaneous assessment of autonomic regulation and cardiac vulnerability during coronary occlusion and reperfusion by complex demodulation of heart rate variability and T-wave alternans. *Circulation* 1992;86:I639 (abst).

65. Verrier RL, Nearing BD. Electrophysiologic basis for T-wave alternans as an index of vulnerability to ventricular fibrillation. *J Cardiovasc Electrophysiol* 1994;5:445–461.

66. Verrier RL, Hagestad EL. Mechanisms involved in reperfusion arrhythmias. *Eur Heart J* 1986;7[Suppl A]:13–22.

67. Corbalan R, Verrier RL, Lown B. Differing mechanisms for ventricular vulnerability during coronary artery occlusion and release. *Am Heart J* 1976;92:223–230.

68. Elharrar V, Zipes DP. Cardiac electrophysiologic alterations during myocardial ischemia. *Am J Physiol* 1977;233:H329–H345.

69. DeFerrari GM, Vanoli E, Schwartz PJ. Vagal activity and ventricular fibrillation. In: Levy MN, Schwartz PJ, eds. *Vagal control of the heart.* Mt. Kisco, NY: Futura Publishing, 1994: 613–636.

70. Levy MN, Warner MR. Autonomic interactions in cardiac control: role of neuropeptides. In: Zipes DP, Jalife J, eds. *Cardiac electrophysiology and arrhythmias.* Orlando: Grune & Stratton, 1985:305.

71. Kleiger RE, Miller JP, Bigger JT Jr, et al, and the Multicenter Post-Infarction Research Group. Decreased heart rate variability and its association with increased mortality after acute myocardial infarction. *Am J Cardiol* 1987;59:256–262.

72. La Rovere MT, Bigger JT Jr, Marcus FI, et al. Baroreflex sensitivity and heart-rate variability in prediction of total cardiac mortality after myocardial infarction. ATRAMI (Autonomic Tone and Reflexes After Myocardial Infarction) investigators. *Lancet* 1998;351:478–484.

73. Verrier RL. Autonomic modulation of arrhythmias in animal models. In: Rosen MR, Wit AL, Janse MJ, eds. *Cardiac electrophysiology: a textbook in honor of Brian Hoffman.* New York: Futura Publishing, 1990:933–949.

74. Corr PB, Yamada KA, Witkowski FX. Mechanisms controlling cardiac autonomic function and their relation to arrhythmoge-nesis. In: Fozzard HA, Haber H, Jennings RB, et al, eds. *The heart and cardiovascular system.* New York: Raven Press, 1986: 1343–1403.

75. Levy MN. Role of calcium in arrhythmogenesis. *Circulation* 1989;80[Suppl IV]:IV23–IV30.

76. Billman GE. The antiarrhythmic and antifibrillatory effects of calcium antagonists. *J Cardiovasc Pharmacol* 1991;18[Suppl 10]:S107–S117.

77. Boissel JP, Leizorovicz A, Picolet H, et al, and the APSI investigators. Efficacy of acebutolol after acute myocardial infarction (the APSI Trial). *Am J Cardiol* 1990;66:24C–31C.

78. Herlitz J, Waagstein F, Lindqvist J, et al. Effect of metoprolol on the prognosis for patients with suspected acute myocardial infarction and indirect signs of congestive heart failure (a subgroup analysis of the Goteborg Metoprolol Trial). *Am J Cardiol* 1997;80:40J–44J.

79. Anderson JL, Rodier HE, Green LS. Comparative effects of beta-adrenergic blocking drugs on experimental ventricular fibrillation threshold. *Am J Cardiol* 1983;51:1196–1202.

80. Kovach JA, Nearing BD, Verrier RL. Effect of aggressive arousal on precordial T-wave alternans magnitude in the normal and ischemic canine heart with and without beta 1-adrenergic blockade with metoprolol. *J Am Coll Cardiol* 1994;23:329A(abst).

81. Opie LH. *Drugs for the heart,* 3rd ed. Philadelphia: WB Saunders, 1991.

82. Yasue H. Beta-adrenergic blockade and coronary arterial spasm. In: Sandφe E, Julian DG, Bell JW, eds. Management of Ventricular Tachycardia: Role of Mexiletine. Amsterdam: Excerpta Medica, 1978:305–313.

83. Hohnloser SH, Verrier RL, Lown B. Influence of beta-adrenoceptor stimulation and blockade on cardiac electrophysiologic properties and serum potassium concentration in the anesthetized dog. *Am Heart J* 1987;113:1066–1070.

84. Eckberg DL. Beta-adrenergic blockade may prolong life in post-infarction patients in part by increasing vagal cardiac inhibition. *Med Hypoth* 1984;15:421–432.

85. Parker GW, Michael LH, Hartley CJ, et al. Central beta-adrenergic mechanisms may modulate ischemic ventricular fibrillation in pigs. *Circ Res* 1990;66:259–270.

86. Benfey BG, Elfellah MS, Ogilvie RI, et al. Antiarrhythmic effects of prazosin and propranolol during coronary artery occlusion and reperfusion in dogs and pigs. *Br J Pharmacol* 1984;82:717–725.

87. Lewis PJ, Haeusler G. Reduction in sympathetic nervous activity as a mechanism for the hypotensive action of propranolol. *Nature* 1975;256:440.

88. Privitera PJ, Webb JG, Walle T. Effect of centrally administered propranolol on plasma renin activity, plasma norepinephrine, and arterial pressure. *Eur J Pharmacol* 1979;54:51–60.

89. Verrier RL, Dickerson LW. Autonomic nervous system and coronary blood flow changes related to emotional activation and sleep. *Circulation* 1991;83[Suppl II]:II81–II89.

90. Skinner JE. Regulation of cardiac vulnerability by the cerebral defense system. *J Am Coll Cardiol* 1985;5:88B–94B.

91. Matta RJ, Verrier RL, Lown B. Repetitive extrasystole as an index of vulnerability to ventricular fibrillation. *Am J Physiol* 1976;230:1469–1473.

92. Matta RJ, Lawler JE, Lown B. Ventricular electrical instability in the conscious dog. Effects of psychological stress and beta adrenergic blockade. *Am J Cardiol* 1976;38:594–598.

93. Verrier RL, Lown B. Influence of neural activity on ventricular electrical stability during acute myocardial ischemia and infarction. In: Sandoe E, Julian DC, Bell JW, eds. *Management of ventricular tachycardia: role of mexiletine.* Amsterdam: Excerpta Medica, 1978:133–150. International Congress Series, No 458.

94. Gang ES, Bigger JT Jr, Uhl EW. Effects of timolol and propra-

nolol on inducible sustained ventricular tachyarrhythmias in dogs with subacute myocardial infarction. *Am J Cardiol* 1984; 53:275–281.

95. Kaplan JR, Manuck SB, Adams MR, et al. The effects of beta-adrenergic blocking agents on atherosclerosis and its complications. *Eur Heart J* 1987;8:928–944.

96. Kaplan JR, Pettersson K, Manuck SB, et al. Role of sympathoadrenal medullary activation in the initiation and progression of atherosclerosis. *Circulation* 1991;84[Suppl VI]: VI23–VI32.

97. Zipes DP, Barber MJ, Takahashi N, et al. Recent observations on autonomic innervation of the heart. In: Zipes DP, Jalife J, eds. *Cardiac electrophysiology and arrhythmias.* Orlando: Grune & Stratton, 1985.

98. Inoue H, Zipes DP. Results of sympathetic denervation in the canine heart: supersensitivity that may be arrhythmogenic. *Circulation* 1987;75:877–887.

99. Verrier RL, Mittleman MA. Life-threatening cardiovascular consequences of anger in patients with coronary heart disease. In: Deedwania PC, Tofler GH, eds. *Triggers and timing of cardiac events.*

100. Mittleman MA, Maclure M, Sherwood JB, et al. Triggering of acute myocardial infarction onset by episodes of anger. *Circulation* 1995;92:1720–1725.

101. Maclure M. The case-crossover design: a method for studying transient effects on the risk of acute events. *Am J Epidemiol* 1991;133:144–153.

102. Mittleman MA, Maclure M, Robins JM. Control sampling strategies for case-crossover studies: An assessment of relative efficiency. *Am J Epidemiol* 1995;142:91–98.

103. Kawachi I, Sparrow D, Spiro A III, et al. A prospective study of anger and coronary heart disease. The Normative Aging Study. *Circulation* 1996;94:2090–2095.

104. Deanfield JE, Shea M, Kennett M, et al. Silent myocardial ischaemia due to mental stress. *Lancet* 1984;2:1001–1005.

105. Barry J, Selwyn AP, Nabel EG, et al. Frequency of ST-segment depression produced by mental stress in stable angina pectoris from coronary artery disease. *Am J Cardiol* 1988;61: 989–993.

106. Rozanski A, Bairey CN, Krantz DS, et al. Mental stress and the induction of silent myocardial ischemia in patients with coronary artery disease. *N Engl J Med* 1988;318:1005–1012.

107. Bairey CN, Krantz DS, Rozanski A. Mental stress as an acute trigger of ischemic left ventricular dysfunction and blood pressure elevation in coronary artery disease. *Am J Cardiol* 1990; 66:28G–31G.

108. Ironson G, Taylor CB, Boltwood M, et al. Effects of anger on left ventricular ejection fraction in coronary artery disease. *Am J Cardiol* 1992;70:281–285.

109. Boltwood MD, Taylor CB, Burke MB, et al. Anger report predicts coronary artery vasomotor response to mental stress in atherosclerotic segments. *Am J Cardiol* 1993;72:1361–1365.

110. Burg MM, Jian D, Soufer R, et al. Role of behavioral and psychological factors in mental stress-induced silent left ventricular dysfunction in coronary artery disease. *J Am Coll Cardiol* 1993; 22:440–448.

111. Gottdiener JS, Krantz DS, Howell RH, et al. Induction of silent myocardial ischemia with mental stress testing: relation to the

triggers of ischemia during daily life activity and to ischemic functional severity.*J Am Coll Cardiol* 1994;24:1645–1651.

112. Blumenthal JA, Jiang W, Waugh RA, et al. Mental stress-induced ischemia in the laboratory and ambulatory ischemia during daily life. Association and hemodynamic features. *Circulation* 1995;92:2102–2108.

113. Gabbay FH, Krantz DS, Kop WJ, et al. Triggers of myocardial ischemia during daily life in patients with coronary artery disease: physical and mental activities, anger and smoking. *J Am Coll Cardiol* 1996;27:585–592.

114. Jiang W, Babyak M, Krantz DS, et al. Mental stress-induced myocardial ischemia and cardiac events. *JAMA* 1996;275: 1651–1656.

115. Krantz DS, Kop WJ, Santiago HT, et al. Mental stress as a trigger of myocardial ischemia and infarction. In: Deedwania PC, Tofler GH, eds. *Triggers and timing of cardiac events.*

116. Papademetriou V, Gottdiener JS, Kop WJ, et al. Transient coronary occlusion with mental stress. *Am Heart J* 1996;132: 1299–1301.

117. Verrier RL, Mittleman MA. The impact of emotions on the heart. In: Mayer EA, Saper CB, eds. *The biological basis for mind body interactions.* Amsterdam: Elsevier Science.

118. Lavery CE, Mittleman MA, Verrier RL, et al. Nonuniform nighttime distribution of acute cardiac events: a possible effect of sleep states. *Circulation* 1997;96:3321–3327.

119. Young T, Palta M, Dempsey J, et al. The occurrence of sleep-disordered breathing among middle-aged adults. *N Engl J Med* 1993;328:1230–1235.

120. Verrier RL, Mittleman MA. Sleep-related cardiac risk. In: Kryger MH, Roth T, Dement WC, eds. *Principles and practice of sleep medicine,* 3rd ed. Philadelphia: WB Saunders, 2000.

121. Kavesh NG, Shorofsky SR, Gold MR, et al. The effect of heart rate on T-wave alternans. *J Cardiovasc Electrophysiol* 1998;9: 703–708.

122. Kawachi I, Sparrow D, Vokonas PS, et al. Symptoms of anxiety and risk for coronary heart disease: The Normative Aging Study. *Circulation* 1994;90:2225–2229.

123. Kawachi I, Colditz GA, Ascherio A, et al. Prospective study of phobic anxiety and risk of coronary heart disease in men. *Circulation* 1994;89:1992–1997.

124. Kubzansky LD, Kawachi I, Spiro A, et al. Is worrying bad for your heart? *Circulation* 1997;95:818–824.

125. Gullette ECD, Blumenthal JA, Babyak M, et al. Effects of mental stress on myocardial ischemia during daily life. *N Engl J Med* 1997;277:1521–1526.

126. Frasure-Smith N, Lesperance F, Talajic M. Depression and 18 month prognosis after myocardial infarction. *Circulation* 1995; 91:999–1005.

127. Appels A, Mulder P. Fatigue and heart disease. The association between 'vital exhaustion' and past, present and future coronary heart disease. *J Psychosom Res* 1989;33:727–738.

128. Kop WJ, Appels AP, Mendes de Leon CF, et al. Vital exhaustion predicts new cardiac events after successful coronary angioplasty. *Psychosom Med* 1994;56:281–287.

129. Verrier RL. Central nervous system modulation of cardiac rhythm. In: Rosen MR, Palti Y, eds. *Lethal arrhythmias resulting from myocardial ischemia and infarction.* Boston: Kluwer Academic Publishers, 1988:149–164.

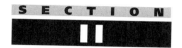

SECTION II

DIAGNOSTIC MODALITIES

USE OF THE ELECTROCARDIOGRAM IN THE DIAGNOSIS OF ARRHYTHMIA

DAVID B. BHARUCHA
PHILIP J. PODRID

Electrocardiography is the most commonly used laboratory procedure in medicine and the role of the electrocardiogram (ECG) in the diagnosis and therapy of arrhythmias is unique because it is the most practical method of recording cardiac arrhythmias (1–3). A task force of the American College of Cardiology, 10th Bethesda Conference on Optimal Electrocardiography, stated that "careful assessment of the surface ECG eliminates need for intracardiac electrocardiography in many instances" (4). The ECG reflects the voltage generated by the atrial and ventricular myocardium, whereas an arrhythmia is often the result of abnormalities of impulse formation or conduction (or both) of the specialized conduction tissue. Because the activity of the specialized tissue is not recorded on the ECG, its function must be deduced from the temporal relations of the waveforms generated by the myocardium. Such deductive analysis is facilitated by the recognition of electrophysiologic ECG concepts, including rate-related and non–rate-related aberration and the Ashman phenomenon, electrical alternans, ventricular fusion, retrograde conduction, reciprocation, parasystole, exit block, supernormality, and concealed conduction.

LIMITATIONS OF THE ELECTROCARDIOGRAM IN THE INTERPRETATION OF ARRHYTHMIAS

Despite the high sensitivity and specificity of the ECG for the diagnosis of arrhythmias, there are limitations (5,6).

D. B. Bharucha: Cardiovascular Division, Lankenau Hospital, Wynnewood, Pennsylvania 19096.

P. J. Podrid: Department of Medicine, Boston University School of Medicine, Boston, Massachusetts 02118.

When a diagnosis and recognition of the mechanism of an arrhythmia depends on analysis of an altered behavior of the specialized tissue and has to be extrapolated from the behavior of the atrial and ventricular myocardium, a single or even a correct diagnosis or mechanism may not always be possible. Multiple diagnoses and mechanisms are possible because of the inability to record the activity of the specialized conduction tissue and the necessity to rely on deductive analysis. Because the ECG lacks sensitivity for small but physiologically significant interval changes, an interval change should be assumed when the ECG pattern changes, even if the interval change is not recognizable in the surface tracing. Such an assumption is supported by intracardiac studies demonstrating that small changes in cycle length, often in the order of only a few milliseconds, may slow or block conduction.

ELECTROCARDIOGRAPHIC CLUES TO THE ELECTROPHYSIOLOGIC MECHANISMS OF ARRHYTHMIAS

Although extrapolation from the cell, tissue, or animal to the human is often difficult or impossible, ECG clues may allow recognition of the underlying mechanism with some degree of reliability. ECG manifestations suggesting automaticity include gradual acceleration of an arrhythmia, long coupling intervals, variable coupling of uniform complexes, gradual emergence of an arrhythmia, and fusion as the first complex of an emerging arrhythmia (Figs. 5-1 and 5-2). Examples of some of the more common automatic arrhythmias include escape rhythms, parasystole, some forms of atrial tachycardia, nonparoxysmal junctional tachycardia, fascicular ventricular tachycardia (VT), accelerated idioventricular rhythm, and parasystolic tachycardia.

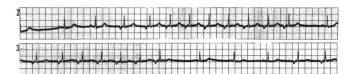

FIGURE 5-1. Repetitive junctional tachycardia. Automatic mechanisms are suggested by the long coupling and gradual coupling and gradual acceleration of the rate.

The ECG features that favor reentry include fixed and relatively short coupling interval of the ectopic impulses, onset of the arrhythmia accompanied by prolongation of conduction, evidence of dual atrioventricular (AV) nodal conduction, an accessory pathway, and abrupt cessation of a tachycardia, especially when terminated by an ectopic impulse (Figs. 5-3 and 5-4). Some of the reentrant arrhythmias include isolated atrial, junctional, and ventricular premature beats; atrial tachycardia; sinus node reentry, which is a form of atrial tachycardia that uses sinus node as part of the reentrant tachycardia; AV nodal reentrant tachycardia (AVNRT); permanent or incessant junctional reentrant tachycardia; VT; and AV reentrant tachycardia (AVRT) (7–10).

Although triggered activity can be evoked in a wide variety of cardiac tissues, there are only isolated references to clinical arrhythmias as possibly caused by afterdepolarizations (11–16). The problem in identifying afterdepolarization as a mechanism of clinical arrhythmias is a lack of specific ECG criteria. Many of the ECG features of reentry and triggered automaticity are common to both, making a differential diagnosis difficult. Some criteria may be helpful in separating triggered arrhythmias from those due to automaticity or reentry (17,18):

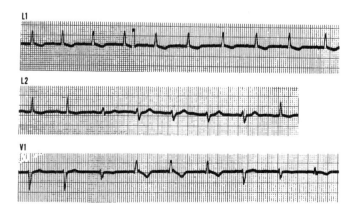

FIGURE 5-2. Accelerated idioventricular rhythm. The automatic mechanism is suggested by long coupling and ventricular fusions. (From Fisch C. *Electrocardiography of arrhythmias.* Philadelphia: Lea & Febiger, 1989:150, with permission)

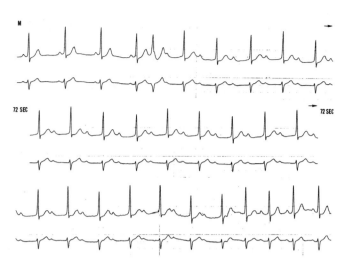

FIGURE 5-3. Long and short PR reflect dual atrioventricular nodal conduction, which is further supported by atrial and ventricular reentry. (From Fisch C. *Electrocardiography of arrhythmias.* Philadelphia: Lea & Febiger, 1989:388, with permission.)

1. Induction of the arrhythmia by multiple extrastimuli
2. Induction by overdrive pacing and failure to recur
3. Induction of arrhythmias favored by a rapid sinus rate or pacing rather than by relatively slow spontaneous or pacing rates
4. Decrease of the cycle length of the induced arrhythmia paralleling the decrease of the cycle length of the dominant rhythm
5. Dependence of initiation of the triggered rhythm on the number of preceding stimuli

The most helpful criterion for diagnosis of a triggered rhythm is the response to overdrive pacing. Although automaticity is suppressed and reset by overdrive pacing and resumes after pacing ceases, triggered activity is

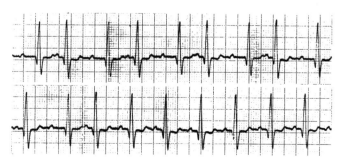

FIGURE 5-4. Alternans of atrioventricular (AV) conduction due to dual AV nodal conduction. (From Surawitz B, Fisch C. Cardiac alternans: diverse mechanisms and clinical manifestations. *J Am Coll Cardiol* 1992;20:483–499, with permission.)

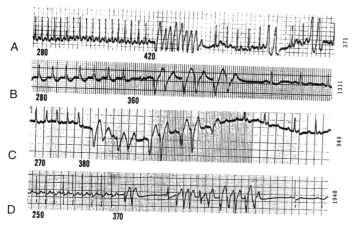

FIGURE 5-5. Supraventricular tachycardia triggering biventricular tachycardia. (From Fisch C, Knoebel SB. Accelerated junctional escape. In: Zipes, DP, Jalife J, eds. *Cardiac electrophysiology.* Orlando: Grune & Stratton, 1985:469, with permission.)

induced by overdrive pacing and does not resume after the arrhythmia and pacing stop. Evidence suggests that some of the early arrhythmias of myocardial infarction, accelerated junctional escapes and tachycardias, certain exercise- or adrenergic-induced VTs, and supraventricular tachycardias (SVTs), including arrhythmias originating in the coronary sinus, may be triggered (19). A phenomenon observed many years ago—the appearance of VT with termination of SVT —may well represent triggered activity (20,21) (Fig. 5-5). The fact that the arrhythmias were observed almost exclusively in patients given large doses of digitalis in an effort to terminate the arrhythmia supports this idea.

ELECTROCARDIOGRAPHIC FEATURES OF NARROW-COMPLEX TACHYCARDIAS

A regular narrow-complex tachycardia is almost always supraventricular in origin; the etiology may be an atrial flutter or an SVT, including atrial tachycardia, junctional tachycardia, typical or atypical AVNRT, or an orthodromic atrioventricular reentrant tachycardia (OAVRT) (22–24) (Fig. 5-6). Issues regarding the ECG diagnosis of an SVT are summarized in Table 5-1. Algorithms for the ECG differentiation of these arrhythmias are presented in Figures 5-7 and 5-8.

An antidromic AVRT (AAVRT) presents with wide QRS complexes, and its diagnosis is discussed later in the sections on wide-complex tachycardias. A narrow-complex VT is uncommon, and it is usually established by the same crite-

ria used for diagnosing VT, as is also discussed in the sections on wide-complex tachycardia (25).

Atrial Activity

The presence of atrial activity, its timing related to ventricular activity, and its morphology comprise the cornerstone of ECG evaluation of SVT (26,27) (Table 5-2 and Figs. 5-7 and 5-9). These criteria have been described in ECG texts as *cherchez le P* and *who's married to whom?* and described in the correlation of ECG findings with electrophysiologic observations (26). There are, however, important cautions in using this approach. P-wave activity often cannot be identified with certainty, and the position of the P wave does not indicate whether atrial activation is responsible for ventricular activation or whether it is itself the result of retrograde or eccentric activation from a remote site.

Absence of Atrial Activity

Determining the presence or absence of atrial activity (i.e., P waves) is the first important step for establishing the mechanism. However, atrial activity can be difficult to ascertain if there are a limited number of ECG leads available. A 12-lead ECG should be obtained whenever possible. If P waves are still not obvious, the use of Lewis leads may be valuable; the arm electrodes are brought onto the precordium, thereby creating a neo-limb lead I that, by accentuating the atrial electrical signal, may provide evidence of a P wave.

After careful examination of all available ECG leads, the absence of clear atrial activity in an SVT that has QRS complexes with regular R-R intervals suggests a junctional focus or AV junctional substrate for the tachycardia (Fig. 5-8D). Most commonly, this is a typical AVNRT (slow/fast type) in which ventricular activation occurs through the slow pathway and retrograde atrial activation occurs through the fast pathway; as a result, there is simultaneous atrial and ventricular activation, and the QRS complex obscures atrial electrical activity, because the P wave is inscribed simultaneously with or buried within the QRS complex (Figs 5-9 through 5-11). Occasionally, the atrial activity in typical AVNRT is slightly delayed, occurring shortly after the QRS complex; the P wave occurs at the very end of the QRS complex and manifests by alteration in the terminal portion of the QRS complex: a pseudo-S wave in the inferior leads and a pseudo-R deflection in lead V_1 (Fig. 5-12). Often, these subtle alterations in the QRS complex can only be appreciated after comparison with an ECG tracing obtained during sinus rhythm. Atrial activity that occurs distinctly after a narrow QRS complex can become inapparent, buried with in the QRS complex, with the development of bundle branch

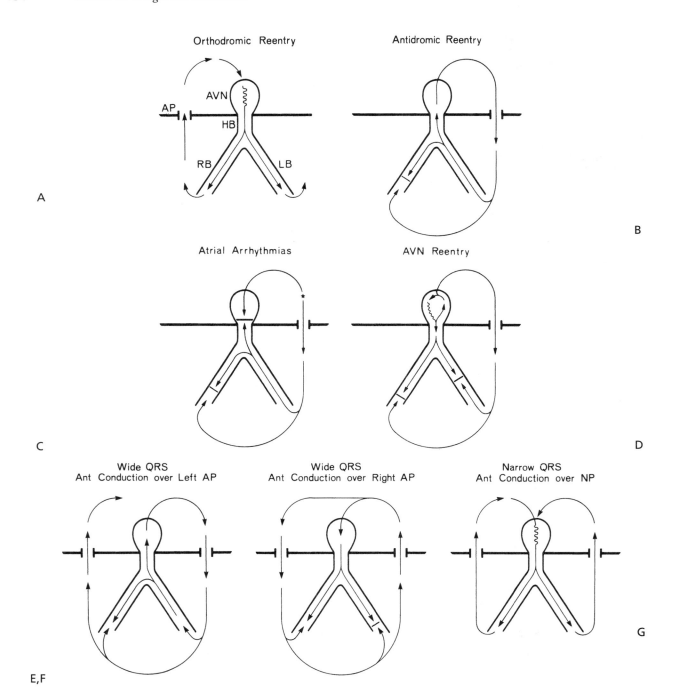

FIGURE 5-6. Schematic representation of some of the possible tachycardia circuits in patients with the Wolff-Parkinson-White syndrome. **A:** In orthodromic reentry, the antegrade limb of the reentry circuit is the atrioventricular (AV) node-His-Purkinje system and the retrograde limb is the accessory pathway. **B:** In true antidromic tachycardia, the reverse is seen, with antegrade conduction through the accessory pathway and retrograde conduction through the His-Purkinje-AV node. **C** and **D:** In atrial and atrioventricular nodal reentrant tachycardia (AVNRT), the accessory pathway is not a part of the reentry circuit. Nonetheless, ventricular preexcitation may occur because of antegrade conduction through the accessory pathway. **E** to **G:** These panels depict some of the possible reentry circuits in patients with multiple accessory pathways. In these patients, at least three (AV node-His-Purkinje and two more accessory pathways) conduits exist for antegrade or retrograde conduction between the atria and ventricles, and multiple reentry circuits are therefore possible. AP, accessory pathway; HB, His bundle; RB, right bundle; LB, left bundle; NP, AV node-His-Purkinje. (Adapted from Akhtar M. Electrophysiologic basis for wide QRS tachycardia. *Pacing Clin Electrophysiol* 1983;6:81, with permission.)

TABLE 5-1. NARROW COMPLEX SUPRAVENTRICULAR TACHCYARDIA: POSITION OF ATRIAL ACTIVITY WITHIN THE CARDIAC CYCLE

No Clear Atrial Activity
Typical AVNRT
JT
AT, ST, SNRT (with prolonged and fortuitously timed
  conduction)
Short RP–Long PR
Typical AVNRT
AVRT with relatively rapid retrogade conduction
AT, ST, SNRT (with relatively prolonged AV conduction)

Long RP–Short PR
Atypical AVRT
O-AVRT with slow retrograde conduction
PJRT
AT, ST, SNRT
RP = PR
Typical AVNRT with 2:1 AV block
Atrial flutter with 2:1 AV block
AT, ST, SNRT (with fortuitously timed AV conduction)

AT, atrial tachycardia; AV, atrioventricular; AVNRT, atrioventricular nodal reentrant tachycardia; AVRT, atrioventricular reentrant tachycardia; JT, junctional tachycardia; O-AVRT, orthodromic atrioventricular reentrant tachycardia; PJRT, permamnent form of junctional reciprocating tachycardia; SNRT, sinus node reentrant tachycardia; ST, sinus tachycardia.

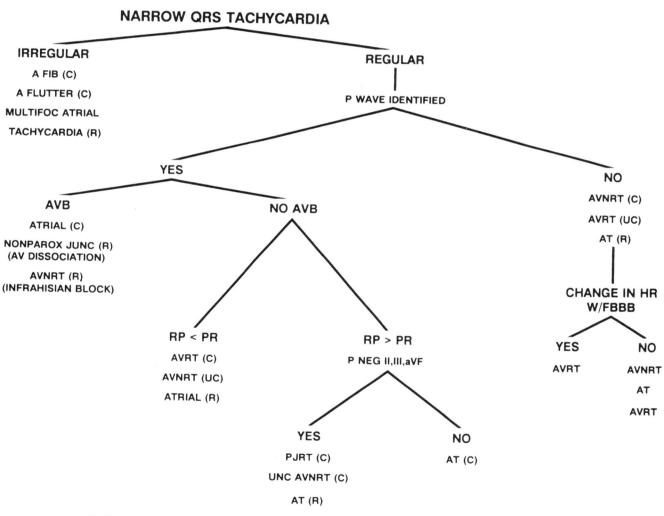

FIGURE 5-7. A simple algorithm for the differential diagnosis of narrow QRS tachycardia assessed by surface electrocardiography. Differentiation is based on regularity, identification of P waves, presence of a concomitant atrioventricular (AV) block, location of the P waves, and effect of functional bundle branch block. The frequency with which a specific feature is given within parentheses. AT, atrial tachycardia; AVNRT, atrioventricular nodal reentrant tachycardia; AVRT, atrioventricular reentrant tachycardia; C, common; FBBB, functional bundle branch block; PJRT, permanent form of junctional reciprocating tachycardia; R, rare; UC, uncommon.

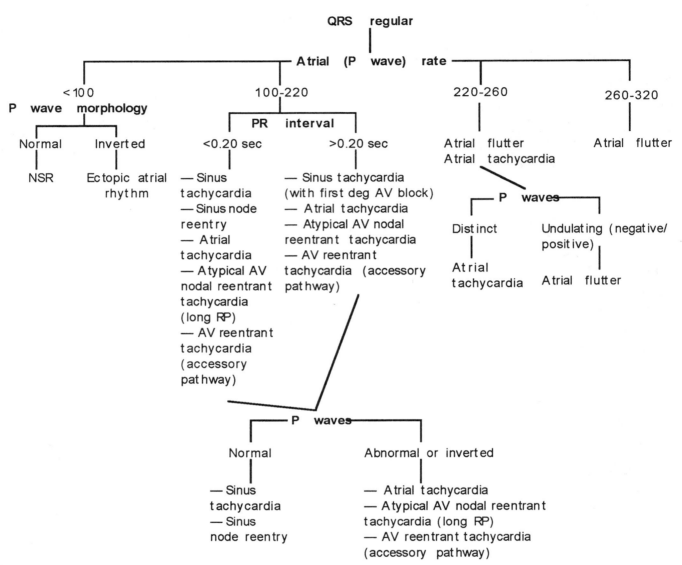

FIGURE 5-8. Algorithms for establishing etiology of various tachyarrhythmias. AV, atrioventricular.

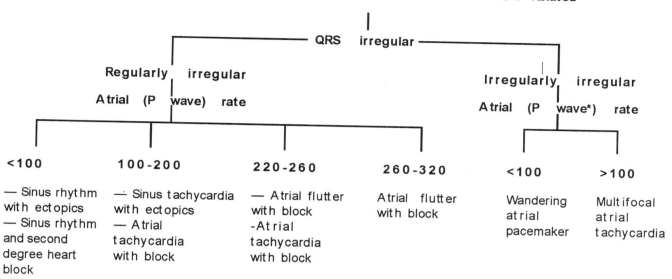

B   *P wave morphology and PR interval variable

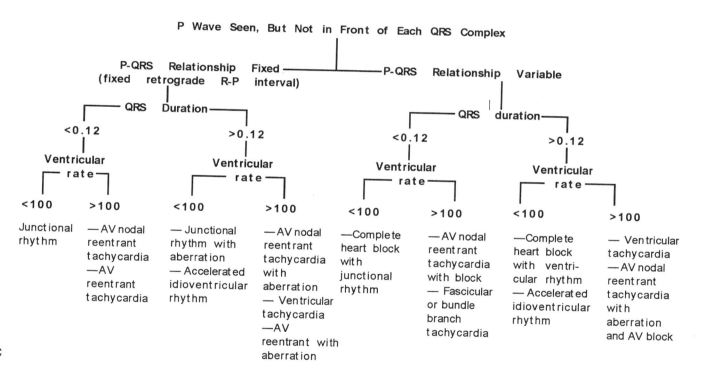

C

FIGURE 5-8. *(continued)*

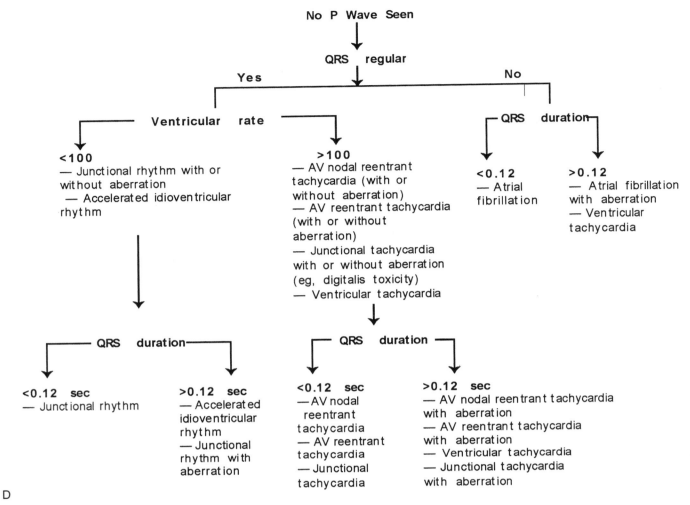

FIGURE 5-8. *(continued)*

TABLE 5-2. ELECTROCARDIOGRAPHIC AND MECHANISTIC CHARACTERISTICS OF SUPRAVENTRICULAR TACHYCARDIA

Rhythm	Site of Origin or of Crucial Substrate	Subtypes of Related Tachycardias	RP/PR Relationship	QRS Morphology and Response to BBB	Presence of AV Block and SVT Termination	Rate Considerations
AVNRT	AV nodal related pathways	Typical, atypical, "other" atypical	RP < PR (RP > PR)[a] (RP = PR)	Variable	Often but not always terminated	Sudden halving or doubling of rate can occur because of 2:1 AV nodal block
AVRT	Atrioventricular accessory connection	Orthodromic, antidromic	RP < PR (RP > PR)	Alternans; BBB ipsilateral to BPT should increase rate or VA interval for orthodromic AVRT	Terminating	—
AT	Atrial myocardium, sometimes at structural abnormality	SA reentry, inappropriate ST, MAT	RP > PR (RP < PR) If MAT, PR will vary beat to beat	Variable	Does not terminate	MAT—by definition will be irregular
Atrial flutter	Atrial myocardium, sometimes at structural abnormality. For some atrial flutters: tricuspid valvular isthmus	Typical vs atypical; isthmus-dependent vs independent	Often RP = PR	Variable	Does not terminate	A ventricular rate of 150 bpm suggests typical atrial flutter
Atrial fibrillation	Atrial myocardium	If initiated by reproducible PAC: "focal AF"	—	Variable	Does not terminate	*NB*: If regular, consider digoxin excess
PJRT	Retrogradely conducting pathway with decremental properties	Permanent, paroxysmal	RP > PR	—	Terminates	—
JT	Automatic junctional focus	—	Variable; AV dissociation often present	—	Variable	—
Mahaim fiber tachycardia	Atriofascicular or atrioventricular decrementally conducting connections	—	RP < PR	LBBB morphology	Terminates	—

AF, atrial fibrillation; AT, atrial tachycardia; AVNRT, atrioventricular nodal reentrant tachycardia; AVRT, atrioventricular reentrant tachycardia; BPT, bypass tract; JT, junctional tachycardia; LBBB, left bundle branch block; MAT, multifocal atrial tachycardia; PAC, premature atrial contraction; PJRT, permanent or paroxysmal junctional reciprocating tachycardia; SA, sinoatrial; VA, ventriculoatrial.
[a]Parenthetic notes indicate a less frequent occurrence.

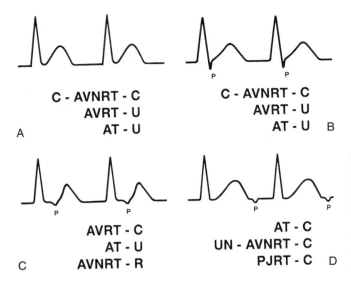

A

C - AVNRT - C
AVRT - U
AT - U

B

C - AVNRT - C
AVRT - U
AT - U

C

AVRT - C
AT - U
AVNRT - R

D

AT - C
UN - AVNRT - C
PJRT - C

FIGURE 5-9. Relationship of P to QRS in supraventricular tachyarrhythmias (SVTs). **A:** SVTs in P waves are not identified. This situation typically is seen in common atrioventricular nodal reentrant tachycardia (AVNRT). When the P wave can be seen in AVNRT, it immediately follows the QRS or may deform it as shown in **B. C:** The typical location of the P wave in atrioventricular (AV) reentrant tachycardia is depicted. When the P wave precedes the QRS **(D)**, the permanent form of junctional ectopic tachycardia, reentrant tachycardia, exists. AT, atrial tachycardia; C, common; PJRT, permanent junctional reciprocating tachycardia; R, rare; U, common.

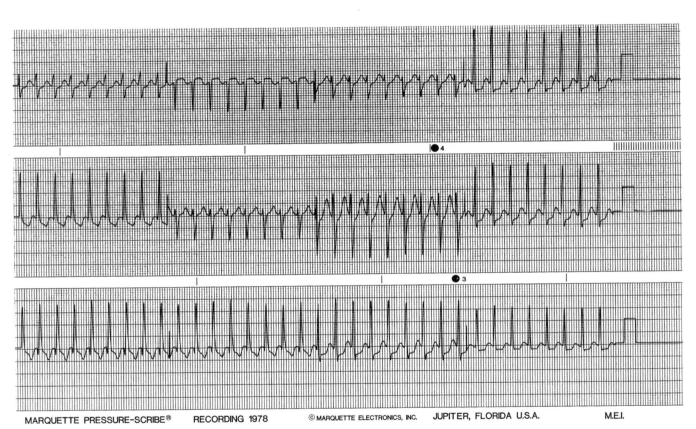

MARQUETTE PRESSURE-SCRIBE®   RECORDING 1978   © MARQUETTE ELECTRONICS, INC.   JUPITER, FLORIDA U.S.A.   M.E.I.

FIGURE 5-10. Twelve-lead electrocardiogram of atrioventricular nodal reentrant tachycardia (AVNRT) of the common type. A typical electrocardiographic appearance of the common type of AVNRT is shown. P waves are infrequently identified in this type of tachycardia because the timing of atrial activation is often simultaneous with that of the QRS. In the uncommon type of AVNRT, P waves with a negative polarity in leads II, III, and aVF are seen preceding the QRS, similar to that seen in Figures 5-9 and 5-17.

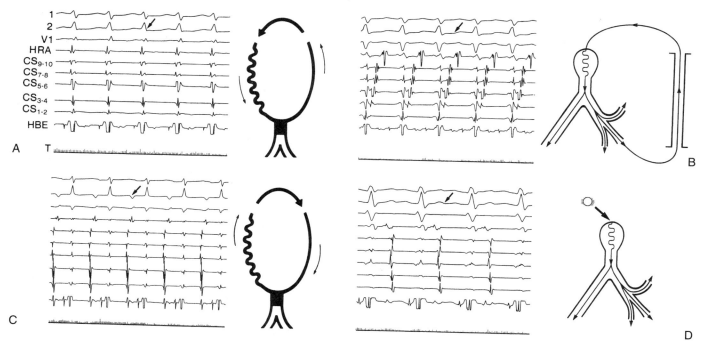

FIGURE 5-11. Schema of reentry circuits and appearance of intracardiac electrograms in atrioventricular (AV) nodal, orthodromic, and atrial tachycardias. Surface electrocardiographic (ECG) leads I, II, and V_1; high right atrial (HRA), coronary sinus (CS), and His bundle electrograms (HBE); and time lines (T) are shown *(right)* along with a schema for the reentry circuits. The arrows indicate the location of the P wave on the surface ECG. **A:** The common variety of atrioventricular nodal reentrant tachycardia (AVNRT), with a long A-H and short H-A time reflecting conduction through the slow and fast pathways, respectively. **B:** The uncommon AVNRT circuit is shown with conduction down the fast pathway and up the slow pathway, resulting in short A-H and long H-A intervals. **C:** An orthodromic tachycardia circuit uses a left free wall accessory pathway. The ventriculoatrial conduction time is greater than 60 ms, with the earliest atrial activation occurring at the site of insertion of the accessory pathway. Antegrade conduction occurs by means of the AV node. **D:** In atrial tachycardias, the atrial activation sequence reflects the site of origin of the tachycardia in the atria. The location of the P wave relative to the QRS on the surface level ECG depends solely on AV conduction times.

block (BBB) during the SVT, resulting in slowed, antegrade ventricular activation.

Atrial activity may also be absent during an atrial tachycardia in which the P wave is embedded in the T wave, often because of prolonged PR interval from slowed AV nodal conduction. This situation can be clarified by comparison of the ECG during the tachycardia with a tracing during sinus rhythm. However, rate-related changes in the repolarization phase of the ECG signal, or

the T wave, may make this challenging. Atrial activity may become obvious with maneuvers that may alter the rate of the tachycardia or the rate of conduction through the AV node, such as carotid sinus pressure or a Valsalva maneuver, and during the pause that follows a premature ventricular contraction (PVC). The timing and positioning of atrial activity in an SVT and the implications for establishing the causes of the SVT are summarized in Table 5-2.

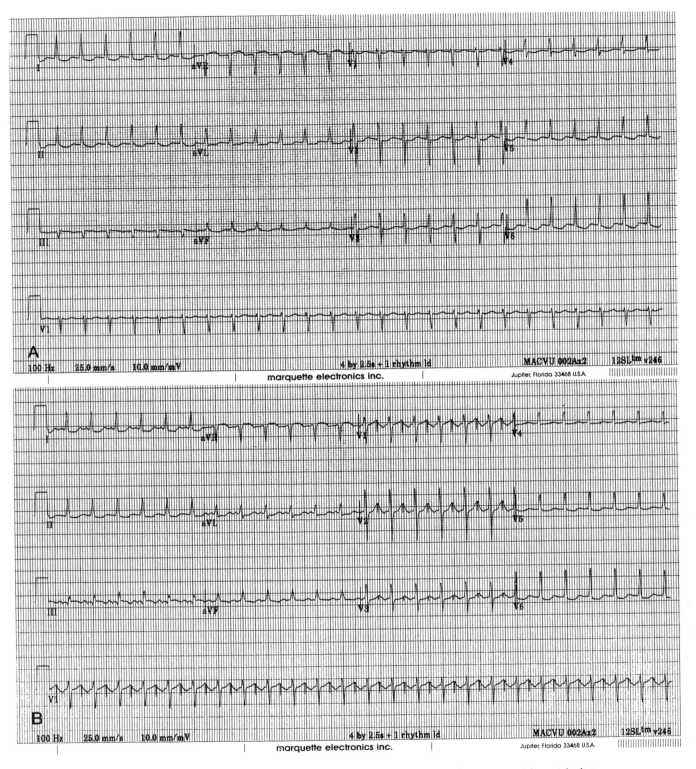

FIGURE 5-12. Twelve-lead electrocardiogram (ECG) of a patient with common atrioventricular nodal reentrant tachycardia (AVNRT) demonstrates a pseudo-R' in V₁. **A:** A narrow QRS tachycardia at a rate of 150 bpm without discernible P waves is seen. **B:** When compared with a 12-lead ECG during atrial pacing at a similar rate, it can be appreciated that V₁ during tachycardia has a terminal R'. This occurs because of inscription of the P wave, whose timing in AVNRT may coincide with the terminal part of the QRS.

Short RP–Long PR Relationships in Tachycardias

Several mechanisms causing SVT result in a tachycardia in which the RP interval is shorter than the PR interval, including OAVRT occurring in the Wolff-Parkinson-White syndrome, in which there is antegrade ventricular activation through the His-Purkinje system and retrograde atrial activation through the accessory pathway (Figs. 5-9 and 5-13); some cases of atypical AVNRT in which there is fast antegrade ventricular activation and slow retrograde atrial activation (fast-slow type); and a slow/slow atypical AVNRT (Fig. 5-14). Atrial tachycardia (AT), sinus node reentrant tachycardia (SNRT), or inappropriate sinus tachycardia can result in a short RP–long PR pattern if intrinsic AV conduction is slow or the rate of the atrial focus impinges on AV nodal refractoriness, resulting in decremental and slow conduction.

Long RP–Short PR Relationships

Several tachycardias can present with a long RP interval, in which ventricular activation occurs through the fast pathway and retrograde atrial conduction occurs through the slow pathway. They include OAVRT, which uses a slowly conducting bypass tract as the retrograde limb; the permanent form of junctional reciprocating tachycardia, which is most often an OAVRT using a concealed bypass tract (usually but not exclusively posteroseptally located) with slowly conducting and decremental properties (28); an atypical or uncommon AVNRT (Figs. 5-15 and 5-16); AT (Fig. 5-17); and a sinus node–based tachycardia. In approximately 2% of cases, typical AVNRT exhibits a long RP–short PR pattern, with a resultant pseudo-Q wave in the inferior leads (22,23).

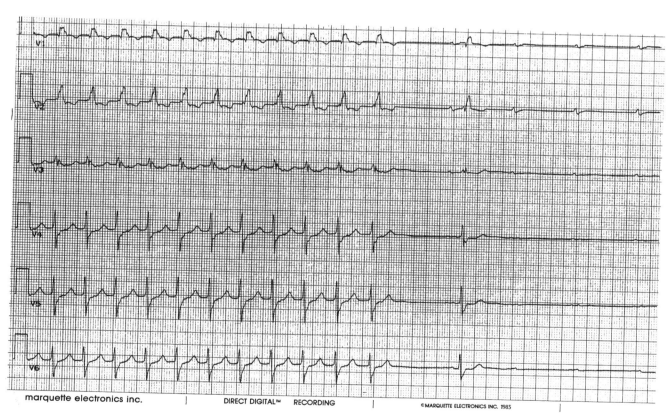

marquette electronics inc. | DIRECT DIGITAL™ RECORDING | ©MARQUETTE ELECTRONICS INC. 1985 |

FIGURE 5-13. Diagnostic value of atrioventricular (AV) nodal blockade on supraventricular tachyarrhythmia (SVT). Tracings are shown for the precordial electrocardiographic leads in a patient with orthodromic reciprocating tachycardia with right bundle branch aberration. The typical location of the P wave in the ST segment resulting in a short RP and long PR can be appreciated, especially in leads V₃, V₄, and V₅. After administration of adenosine, termination of tachycardia is seen with a P wave not followed by a QRS, suggesting that the tachycardia circuit involves the AV node in the antegrade direction.

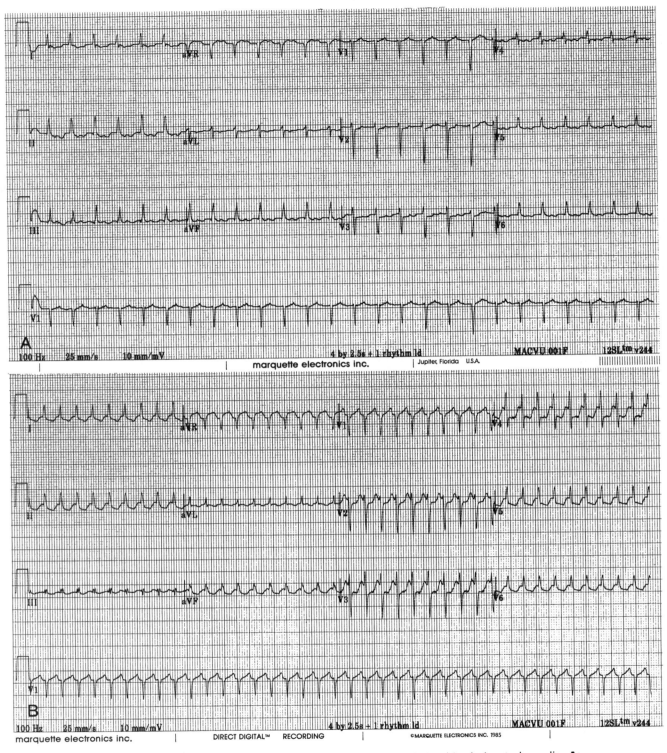

FIGURE 5-14. Electrophysiologic significance of the PR-RP relationship during tachycardia. **A:** Twelve-lead electrocardiographic and V₁ rhythm strip for a patient with orthodromic tachycardia. The P wave is identified in the upstroke of the T wave such that the PR interval is greater than the RP interval. This occurs because of the relatively shorter conduction time through the accessory pathway (RP interval) compared with the atrioventricular (AV) node (PR interval). **B:** Twelve-lead electrocardiogram for the same patient. The RP interval remains unchanged. The significant shortening of the tachycardia cycle length primarily is caused by shortening of the PR interval, resulting in a RP : PR ratio of almost 1. The change in PR interval in this particular patient resulted from the presence of dual AV nodal pathways with antegrade conduction through the slow pathway and retrograde conduction through the accessory pathway in **A**. In B, although retrograde conduction remains unchanged, antegrade conduction occurs through the fast pathway.

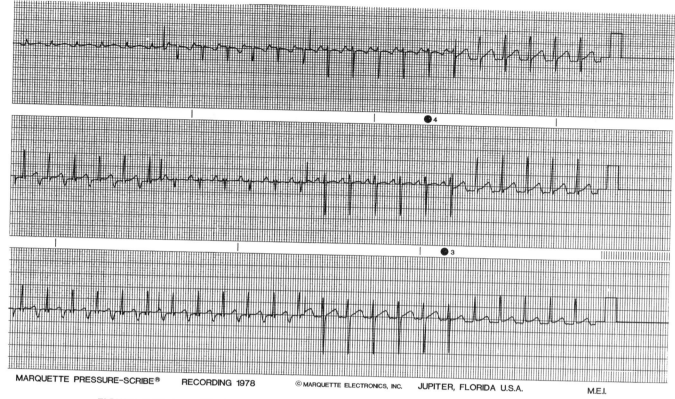

FIGURE 5-15. Long RP–short PR tachycardia. Twelve-lead electrocardiogram of the permanent form of junctional reciprocating tachycardia is shown. In this tachycardia, ventricular activation occurs by means of the atrioventricular (AV) node-His-Purkinje rhythm and retrograde conduction through a posteroseptal accessory pathway with decremental conduction properties. The typical electrocardiographic pattern is that of an incessant tachycardia with a long RP–short PR interval and negative P waves in II, III, and aVF leads.

Other Concerns about Atrial Activity in Tachycardia

The observation of atrial activity precisely halfway across the R-R interval suggests an SVT in the presence of 2 : 1 AV block (Fig. 5-18). In this situation, alternate signals of atrial activity are obscured by the QRS. Examples of this relationship include atrial flutter, AT, or typical AVNRT with 2 : 1 AV block; the presence of 2 : 1 AV block during an SVT excludes OAVRT, in which there is a macroreentrant circuit using an accessory pathway and atrial and ventricular tissue that requires the presence of 1 : 1 AV conduction for arrhythmia generation and continuation.

AV conduction can be profoundly influenced by disease state, drugs, and autonomic tone. The RP-PR relationship of an SVT, especially an AT, can vary depending on the state of the AV node.

A constant RP interval, regardless of the SVT cycle length, strongly suggests an OAVRT using a rapidly retrogradely conducting bypass tract (Fig. 5-14). Such a tract has no decremental properties; there is no relationship between rate and conduction velocity within it, and oscillations in the R-R interval, which cause variations in AV conduction, do not alter the RP interval. The opposite observation is made in ATs as changes in the R-R interval result in changes in the RP interval.

P-Wave Morphology and Axis

The morphology and axis of atrial activity can be diagnostic of the type of SVT and the location of an accessory connection in OAVRT (Fig. 5-8A). For example, a negative P wave in limb lead I suggests a left-to-right direction of atrial activation; a negative P wave in lead aVF would suggest atrial activation from inferior to superior.

In the case of typical AVNRT, even when most atrial activity occurs during ventricular activation and the P wave is buried within the QRS complex in some leads, the P wave may be obvious in other leads, providing directional

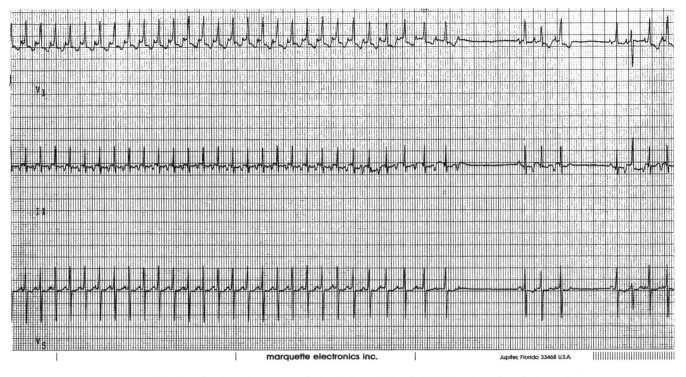

FIGURE 5-16. Termination of supraventricular tachyarrhythmia (SVT) by adenosine. Surface electrocardiographic leads V₁, II, and V₅ are shown during administration of an intravenous bolus of adenosine. This patient has a long RP and short PR tachycardia, with an inverted P wave in lead II (and in III and aVF [not shown]), suggesting the permanent form of atrioventricular (AV) junctional tachycardia or the uncommon form of atrioventricular nodal reentrant tachycardia (AVNRT). After administration of adenosine, progressive prolongation of the PR interval is seen because of the AV nodal conduction delay until AV block and termination of the tachycardia occurs. With resumption of sinus rhythm, the effect of adenosine on the retrograde limb of the tachycardia circuit is seen with progressive prolongation of the RP interval until ventriculoatrial block occurs. This behavior is most consistent with the permanent form of junctional reciprocating tachycardia.

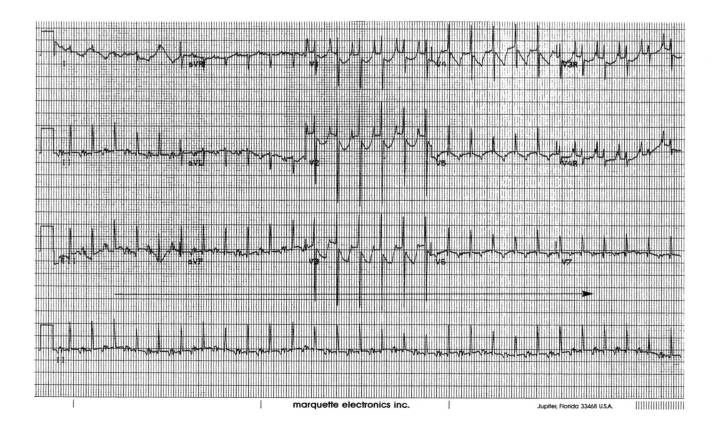

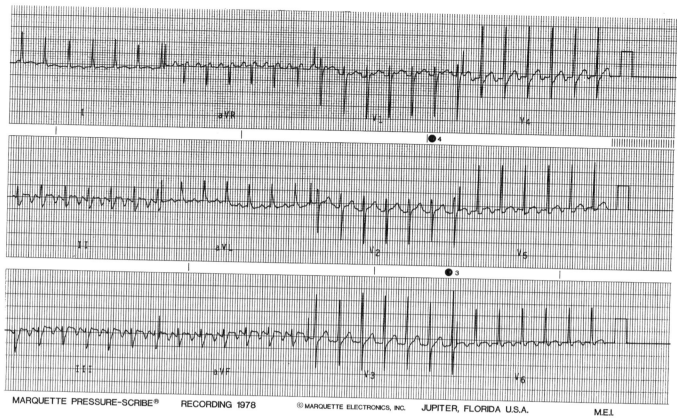

FIGURE 5-18. A 2:1 block during supraventricular tachyarrhythmia (SVT). A 12-lead electrocardiogram of atrial flutter with 2:1 atrioventricular (AV) block is shown. A similar 12-lead configuration is used in all subsequent electrocardiograms. Because every alternate flutter wave falls on the terminal part of the QRS, it may be difficult to identify, especially if a single lead recording such as V₁ alone is available. However, with the aid of multiple electrocardiographic lead recordings (best seen in lead aVR in this example), atrial flutter with 2:1 AV conduction is identified.

information. The presence of a pseudo-S wave in inferior leads, representing inverted P waves, implies inferior-to-superior activation of the atria; the absence of atrial activity in lead I and equal atrial activity in aVR and aVL suggest midline activation of the atria from the AV junction region (24–28). This retrograde atrial activation pattern is also seen with an OAVRT using a paraseptal connection, except that atrial activity is more obvious because of the longer RP interval observed with this AVRT; the atrial activity in the

lateral precordial leads can be negative, especially if the posteroseptal tract is slowly conducting.

OAVRT using a left free wall accessory connection frequently has a negative P wave in lead I as a consequence of left-to-right retrograde atrial activation, and OAVRT using a right-sided free wall bypass tract has a positive P wave in the lateral leads (29). For posterior, left-sided bypass tracts, the positivity of retrograde P waves in aVR is greater than in aVL, particularly when the tract is

FIGURE 5-17. Twelve-lead electrocardiogram of a patient with automatic atrial tachycardia. The location of the P waves in atrial tachycardias depends entirely on atrioventricular (AV) conduction, and therefore the usual appearance in the absence of concomitant AV conduction delay is that of a long RP–short PR tachycardia. Although not shown in this example, AV block is not infrequent, especially when the vagal tone is increased. The prolonged and bizarre morphology of the P waves is also typical of automatic atrial tachycardias.

located leftward of the septum; for posterior, right-sided tracts, the positivity of retrograde atrial activity in aVL is greater than in aVR, especially for tracts more rightward of the septum.

Atrial activity that is identical to the sinus P wave in multiple leads raises the possibility of SNRT or sinus tachycardia; the former mechanism is characterized by an abrupt increase and decrease in rate on the initiation and termination of the SVT, and in the latter case, there are gradual changes in rate with arrhythmia onset and offset. SNRT can be induced by a premature atrial contraction (Fig. 5-19).

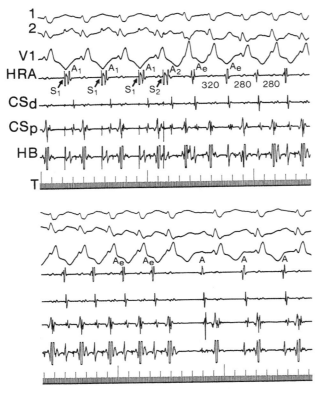

FIGURE 5-19. Electrophysiologic features of sinoatrial reentrant tachycardia. Tracings from top to bottom are for surface electrocardiograph leads (I, II, V₁), the high right atrial (HRA) electrogram, the proximal (CSp) and distal (CSd) coronary sinus electrograms, His bundle (HB) electrogram, and time lines (T). At a drive cycle length of 350 ms, an atrial premature beat (A₂) initiates a tachycardia. Several features suggest sinoatrial reentry as the mechanism of the tachycardia. The sequence of atrial activation is similar to that during sinus rhythm; no consistent ventriculoatrial relationship is seen, especially at the initiation of the tachycardia, and the tachycardia terminates with an A followed by a V. The latter finding is less likely to be seen in atrioventricular nodal reentrant tachycardia (AVNRT) and orthodromic tachycardia in which the tachycardia usually terminates with atrioventricular (AV) nodal block and A is not followed by a V. A, atrial; Ae, atrial echo; S, sinus.

QRS Morphology

Several QRS morphologies may be helpful in establishing the cause of the tachyarrhythmia.

QRS Alternans

QRS alternans describes a beat-to-beat oscillation in the amplitude of the QRS complex and can be observed in several types of SVT. The underlying mechanism for alternans may involve subtle beat-to-beat variation in His-Purkinje system refractoriness, resulting in a small degree of beat-to-beat aberration in the QRS complex.

Alternans has been most frequently observed with OAVRT and infrequently with other forms of SVT associated with very rapid rates. Green and colleagues observed that the finding of QRS alternans in an SVT had a 96% specificity and a 92% predictive accuracy for identifying an OAVRT with retrograde atrial activation through an accessory tract (30). The absence of alternans, however, does not have predictive value for excluding the involvement of an accessory tract. QRS alternans has been reported to occur in one third of AVRTs, 12% of ATs, and 2% of AVNRTs.

Pseudo-alterations in the QRS Complex

Atrial activity during an SVT can be partially embedded in and therefore deform the QRS. This pattern is most characteristically seen in typical AVNRT.

Bundle Branch Block and Supraventricular Tachyarrhythmia

Functional or rate-related BBB can be observed for several beats at the initiation of SVT if the refractory period of one fascicle or bundle fails to adapt to the abrupt increase in rate, resulting in conduction delay or block within the fascicle or bundle. This aberration may resolve as the rate-related shortening of the refractory period of the His-Purkinje system accommodates during sustained SVT. This phenomenon occurs less frequently at the initiation of typical slow/fast AVNRT compared with OAVRT because initial, prolonged slow pathway input into the His-Purkinje system during AVNRT is less likely to encroach on His-Purkinje system refractoriness (23).

Induced PVCs occurring during AVNRT have caused transient left bundle branch block (LBBB) rather than right bundle branch block (RBBB) aberration, most likely because of the use of a right ventricular catheter for PVC introduction and results in earlier recovery of the right bundle after earlier activation.

Bundle Branch Block and Atrioventricular Reentrant Tachycardia

BBB ipsilateral to a bypass tract may produce a critical delay, a condition that may promote the initiation of an OAVRT. A BBB that occurs ipsilateral to an accessory connection in OAVRT can prolong the cycle length of the SVT because of the fact that the reentrant impulse, which is conducted antegradely through the contralateral bundle, is delayed or slowed because of muscle-to-muscle conduction from the bundle to the bypass tract (31–33) (Fig. 5-20), or to be more precise, the prolongation in OAVRT cycle length with BBB can be accounted for by an increase in the ventriculoatrial (VA) interval (i.e., time from earliest ventricular activation in SVT to earliest atrial activation) (34,35). Because longer VA times may occasionally cause AV times to shorten as a result of less decremental conduction through the AV node because of the slower rate of the AVRT, the overall AVRT cycle length can remain the same or even shorten (32). Free wall bypass tracts ipsilateral to BBB during OAVRT are more likely than paraseptal bypass tracts to result in discernible differences in VA times and the SVT cycle length; this occurs because of the longer distance the impulse must travel from muscle to muscle before reaching the bypass tract (34–36). In one study of 95 patients, an increase in the VA time interval by ≥40 ms in the absence of fascicular block had a sensitivity and specificity of 95% and 100%, respectively, for the presence of a free wall bypass tract

(37). In contrast, BBB occurring contralateral to a free wall AV accessory pathway has no effect on the VA interval and the tachycardia cycle length.

Wide QRS Complex Supraventricular Tachyarrhythmia Not Related to a Bundle Branch Block

Two types of SVT may be associated with a wide QRS complex during the tachycardia, but the QRS aberration is not the result of a rate-related or functional BBB. The first is AAVRT, which uses an accessory pathway, such as an AV, nodoventricular, or atriofascicular connection, as its antegrade limb for ventricular activation and the AV node-His-Purkinje system as the retrograde limb for atrial activation; the AAVRT results in a tachycardia with a wide QRS complex that is not rate related but caused by direct myocardial conduction through the accessory pathway, which results in aberrant conduction (Fig. 5-21). In this situation, the QRS complex during the AVRT resembles the preexcited QRS complex that is recorded during sinus rhythm. Differentiation of AAVRT from SVT with bundle branch aberrancy or VT is discussed in the sections on wide-complex tachycardias.

The second type is Mahaim fiber tachycardia. Mahaim fibers are atriofascicular or AV connections that conduct the impulse decrementally; they are often the antegrade limb for macroreentrant, wide-complex, preexcited tachycardia. As a result of decremental or slowed conduction during the tachycardia, the QRS complexes are widened. The ECG appearance typically has a LBBB-morphology QRS because the insertion of the atriofascicular-type connection is near the distal right bundle branch in the region of the right ventricular apex and that of the AV-type connection is near the tricuspid annulus of the right ventricle. ECG characteristics of a Mahaim fiber–based SVT include the following (38) (Fig. 5-22):

1. QRS with a LBBB or LBBB-like morphology
2. QRS axis between 0 and +75 degrees
3. QRS duration of 0.15 seconds or less
4. R wave in lead I
5. rS complex in lead V_1
6. Precordial transition in lead V_4 or later
7. Heart rate of 130 to 270 bpm

Although there may be ventricular preexcitation, there is no delta wave on the ECG during sinus rhythm in patients with Mahaim fibers because impulse conduction and ventricular activation preferentially occur through the AV node; however, conduction by these pathways can become more apparent or revealed in situations in which conduction through the AV node is slowed or blocked, as may occur with high vagal tone, adenosine, or atrial pacing.

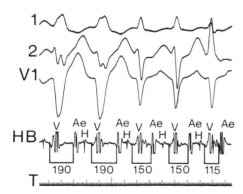

FIGURE 5-20. Effect of ipsilateral functional bundle branch block on VA conduction time during atrioventricular (AV) reentrant (orthodromic) tachycardia. Tracings from top to bottom are for the electrocardiographic leads (I, II, and V₁), His bundle (HB) electrograms, and time line (T). During orthodromic tachycardia, the atrial (Ae) His deflection (H) and ventricular electrograms (V) are shown. Complete functional left bundle branch block (first and second beats), left anterior fascicular block (third and fourth beats), and narrow QRS complex (fifth beat) are shown. Prolongation of ventriculoatrial conduction time with functional left bundle branch block suggests that it is part of the tachycardia circuit and is therefore presumptive evidence of a left-sided accessory pathway.

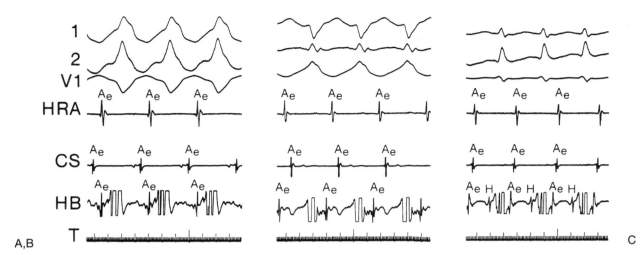

FIGURE 5-21. Preexcited tachycardia in the presence of multiple accessory pathways. Tracings from top to bottom are for the surface electrocardiographic leads (I, II, V₁) and the high right atrial (HRA), coronary sinus (CS), and His bundle (HB) electrograms, followed by the time lines (T). These tracings are obtained from a patient with two accessory pathways located in the left free wall and right anteroseptal regions. **A:** A preexcited tachycardia uses the right anteroseptal pathway antegradely and the left free wall pathway retrogradely. **B:** A preexcited tachycardia in which the left free wall and the right anteroseptal pathways are the antegrade and retrograde reentrant limbs, respectively. **C:** A narrow QRS complex tachycardia (orthodromic) in which the normal pathway is activated antegradely, and both accessory pathways are activated retrogradely. Ae, atrial echo; H, His deflection. (From Jazayeri MR, Sra JS, Akhtar M. Wide QRS complexes: electrophysiologic basis of a common electrocardiographic diagnosis. *J Cardiovasc Electrophysiol* 1992;3:378, with permission.)

Atrioventricular Block during Supraventricular Tachyarrhythmia

The presence of AV block during SVT effectively excludes any macroreentrant rhythm requiring the ventricular myocardium as a part of its circuit, especially an AVRT.

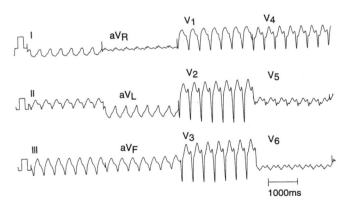

FIGURE 5-22. Twelve-lead electrocardiogram taken during reciprocating atrioventricular tachycardia in a patient with a Mahaim-type connection demonstrated the left bundle branch block (LBBB) and left axis deviation characteristic of this condition.

The *2:1 Atrioventricular Block*

The 2:1 AV block often results in an ECG pattern in which one P wave is seen halfway between QRS complexes, and the second one is buried within the QRS complex. The most common cause for 2:1 AV block is atrial flutter, and flutter most often initially presents with 2:1 AV block (Fig. 5-18). Exceptions include the use of drugs or the presence of a disease that slows AV conduction, resulting in higher degrees of AV block; drugs or atrial disease that slow the atrial rate in flutter, thereby decreasing the degree of decremental AV nodal conduction, possibly allowing for 1:1 AV conduction; drugs that accelerate AV nodal conduction, resulting in 1:1 AV conduction; and the presence of an antegradely conducting accessory bypass tract with properties that allow rapid antegrade AV conduction.

Other causes of 2:1 AV block include AT and, infrequently, AVNRT. In the case of typical AVNRT, the location of the 2:1 AV block is most frequently infra-Hisian rather than intranodal.. However, in this situation, infra-Hisian block does not imply His-Purkinje system pathology and most often is evident at the start of SVT before accommodation of rate-related His-Purkinje refractoriness. Often, 1:1 conduction resumes with a sudden period of aberration as a consequence of recovery of conduction eccentrically, improving in one, but not all, parts of the His-Purkinje system. The presence of 2:1 AV block in typical AVNRT can be a useful characteristic in distinguishing this SVT from OAVRT using a posteroseptal bypass tract, which may have a similar ECG pattern; 1 : 1 AV conduction always exists with an OAVRT because this arrhythmia cannot persist in the presence of any block.

Atypical AVNRT with 2 : 1 AV block rarely has been reported (39). The persistence of AVNRT with any AV block, but particularly high-grade or complete AV block, has been used as evidence to suggest that infranodal structures are not required for the occurrence of this arrhythmia.

Variable Atrioventricular Block

Variable AV block, producing a regularly irregular or irregularly irregular ventricular response, can be observed with a variety of SVTs, most often with tachyarrhythmias originating in the atrium, such as automatic AT, atrial flutter, sinus node reentry, or atrial fibrillation. Typical AVNRT with second-degree Wenckebach AV block is infrequently observed but results in a regularly irregular QRS pattern. Multifocal atrial tachycardia, by definition, has a varying PR interval.

Atrioventricular Dissociation

AV dissociation can be observed in a variety of circumstances; any SVT not dependent on a bypass tract for maintenance can be associated with complete heart block and AV dissociation. AV dissociation can occur with the non-paroxysmal form of AV junctional tachycardia (40) (Fig. 5-23) or conditions provoking accelerated AV junctional automaticity, including after valvular cardiac surgery, after radiofrequency ablation of the AV junctional region, after acute infarction, or with digitalis toxicity.

Initiation or Termination of the Supraventricular Tachyarrhythmia

The recording of an ECG during the initiation or termination of an SVT can provide critical information about the mechanism of the tachycardia.

Arrhythmia Initiation

SVTs due to a microreentrant or macroreentrant mechanism frequently are initiated by a premature beat, most often a premature atrial contraction (PAC) (Fig. 5-24). A premature beat, which is likely to conduct slowly through cardiac tissue and a potential reentrant circuit, can result in a critical delay, conduction recovery, and unidirectional block, resulting in a tachycardia. When the SVT is initiated by a PAC with a prolonged PR interval, the presence of dual AV nodal physiology is suggested, and the arrhythmia is most likely an AVNRT or OAVRT using a slow AV nodal pathway as the antegrade limb. SNRT can be discriminated from sinus tachycardia by virtue of its initiation with a PAC or its abrupt termination by a PAC or a vagal maneuver.

Initiation of an SVT by a PVC, particularly when it has a long coupling cycle, makes the SVT more likely to be an AVRT associated with a bypass pathway that conducts slowly in a retrograde direction. Although initiation of an SVT with a gradual acceleration (i.e., warm up) is sometimes ascribed to an automatic mechanism, it is seen in a variety of circumstances. For example, SVTs using slowly

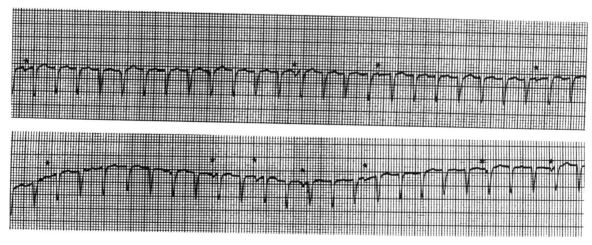

FIGURE 5-23. Example of a junctional tachycardia with atrioventricular (AV) dissociation in a patient with an underlying cardiomyopathy. The narrow-complex junctional tachycardia has a rate of 180. Intermittently seen are P waves *(asterisks)*. Although not always clearly seen, the P waves that are obvious have a variable relationship to the QRS complexes and are therefore dissociated.

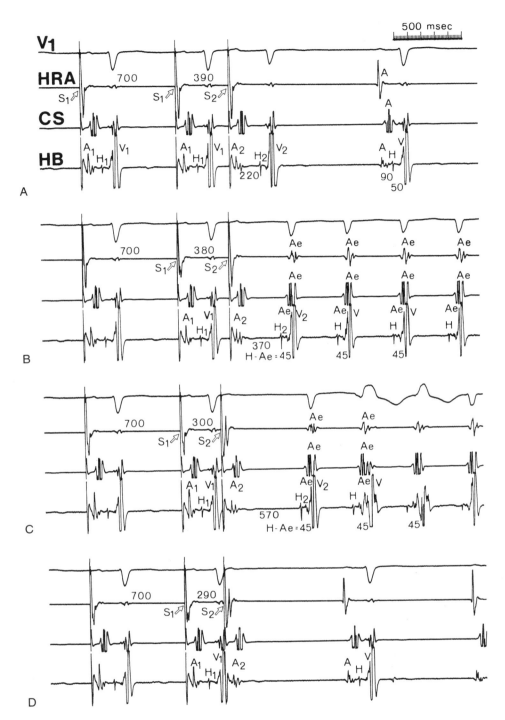

FIGURE 5-24. Initiation of common atrioventricular (AV) node reentry. **A:** At a basic cycle length of 700 ms, an atrial premature beat with an A_1-A_2 interval of 390 ms (A_2) conducts with an A_1-H_2 interval of 220 ms. **B:** With a shorter A_1-A_2 interval of 380 ms, a sudden jump in AV nodal conduction time (A_2-H_2) coincides with the onset of tachycardia, during which the H-Ae interval is 45 ms. **C:** The shortest A_1-A_2 interval is associated with the onset of tachycardia. **D:** With a block in the AV node, the arrhythmia could not be induced, suggesting that propagation beyond the atria is important for induction. This finding also argues against intraatrial reentry as the mechanism. Ae, atrial echo; H-Ae, His bundle deflection to atrial echo; HRA, high right atrial electrogram; CS, coronary sinus; HB, His bundle electrogram. (From Akhtar M, Tchou P, Jazayeri M: Supraventricular tachycardias: clinical characteristics, diagnosis, and management. In: El-Sherif N, Samet P, eds. *Cardiac pacing and electrophysiology,* 3rd ed. Philadelphia: WB Saunders, 1991:173, with permission.)

conducting bypass tracts can be associated with rate acceleration (41).

Termination of the Arrhythmia

The termination of an SVT may provide clues to its mechanism. Termination of the SVT with AV block (i.e., atrial activity not followed by a QRS) suggests, but does not prove, that the mechanism of the SVT is not an AT or another arrhythmia originating in the atrium and that the AV node is a part of the reentrant circuit, with block occurring in the antegrade limb of the AV node (Figs. 5-13 and 5-16).

Diagnostic Interventions

Diagnostic interventions during SVT can provide valuable information about the mechanism of the tachycardia. Transient AV block can be caused by vagal maneuvers, such as carotid sinus massage, or pharmacologically with intravenous adenosine or verapamil (42–44). During AV block, the atrial activity (P wave) of tachycardias originating in the atria (e.g., atrial tachycardias, atrial flutter, SNRT, sinus tachycardia) should become apparent and is independent of QRS complexes (Fig. 5-25). The development of AV block results in the termination of an arrhythmia, which requires the AV node as one limb of the reentrant circuit, such as AVNRT or OAVRT (Figs. 5-13 and 5-16).

There are, however, several cautionary notes on the use of intravenous agents during tachycardias. Some atrial tachycardias and bypass tracts are sensitive to adenosine.

The presence of continued atrial tachycardic activity during adenosine-induced AV block helps to include an AT, but the absence of that finding does not exclude AT. It is not completely certain that termination of an SVT, which relies on a bypass tract, occurs because of block in the AV node.

Intravenous adenosine is useful in the diagnosis of dual AV nodal physiology, even when administered during sinus rhythm (49). Findings with adenosine that suggest a dual AV node includes at least a 50-ms increase in the PR interval between two successive beats and the presence of an AV nodal echo beat; however, an increase in PR interval may be difficult to appreciate if AV nodal block is induced by adenosine.

Administration of intravenous agents can be medically risky in several circumstances. In the presence of a bypass tract that can conduct antegradely and that has a short refractory period, the administration of an AV nodal blocking agent in the presence of atrial fibrillation can lead to exclusive conduction down the bypass tract and possibly to ventricular arrhythmias (45); ventricular arrhythmias, including torsade des pointes, have been observed in patients without preexcitation but who may have bradycardic-dependent arrhythmias (46). Intravenous verapamil can cause peripheral vasodilation and hypotension, a compensatory surge in catecholamines, and a resultant increase in bypass tract conduction times and decrease in refractory periods. Intravenous adenosine has induced atrial fibrillation in a variety of SVTs or after long-short sequences of atrial rhythms (47,48). Intravenous adenosine can have a markedly prolonged effect in patients who are concurrently taking Persantine, resulting in malignant bradyarrhythmias.

Rate and Regularity on the Electrocardiogram

The rate of the tachycardia and the regularity of the P-P and R-R intervals can provide some aid in establishing the etiology.

Regularity of the Supraventricular Tachyarrhythmia

Most SVTs have R-R and P-P intervals that are completely regular. Irregularity of the R-R intervals during an SVT raises the possibility of atrial fibrillation, multifocal atrial tachycardia, AT or atrial flutter with variable conduction, or AVNRT with Mobitz type I (Wenckebach) second-degree AV block, although this is rare. When the underlying rhythm is atrial fibrillation, but the R-R intervals are perfectly regular, digitalis toxicity is suggested.

Rate of the Supraventricular Tachyarrhythmia

The rate of the SVT usually provides little help in establishing the cause of the tachycardia because there is much

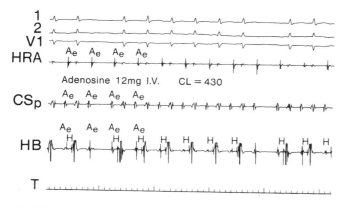

FIGURE 5-25. Continuation of tachycardia despite an atrioventricular (AV) block. Tracings from top to bottom are for the electrocardiographic leads (I, II, and V₁), high right atrial (HRA) electrogram, proximal coronary sinus (CSp) electrogram, His bundle (HB) electrogram, and time lines (T). Recordings obtained after administration of adenosine reveal a continuation of tachycardia, with a cycle length (CL) of 430 ms, despite the presence of AV nodal block. This finding excludes the diagnosis of AV reentrant tachycardia and virtually excludes the diagnosis of atrioventricular nodal reentrant tachycardia (AVNRT) as well.

overlap; the rate of AT or sinus node reentry is often 120 to 180 bpm, the rate of AVNRT is often 140 to 220 bpm, and the rate of AVRT is 140 to 240 bpm (Fig. 5-8A, B). However, an SVT at rate of 150 bpm strongly suggests the possibility of atrial flutter with 2 : 1 AV block. An SVT whose rate is suddenly observed to double or to halve raises the possibility of AVNRT with 1 : 1 conduction alternating with 2 : 1 AV conduction. When the rate of the SVT is very rapid, QRS alternans may occur; the presence of QRS alternans generally suggests an OAVRT as the mechanism, but this abnormality can be seen with any rapid SVT.

Incessant Supraventricular Tachyarrhythmia

An SVT is defined as incessant if it is present for at least 90% of a monitoring period (50). An incessant SVT can result in a tachycardia-associated cardiomyopathy. The causes of an incessant SVT include nonparoxysmal junctional tachycardia, atypical fast/slow AVNRT, SNRT, and atrial tachycardias, particularly those with evidence for abnormal automaticity and triggered activity (51).

Premature Ventricular Contraction during Supraventricular Tachyarrhythmia

A PVC during SVT can be valuable for elucidating mechanism, especially when atrial activity is visible during SVT. A late-coupled PVC that resets (or advances) atrial activity of the SVT without terminating the SVT suggests an OAVRT using a paraseptal bypass tract or a bypass tract ipsilateral to the origin of the PVC; however, the absence of tachycardia reset does not exclude this or any other cause.

A PVC during SVT can also be useful for establishing the cause when it results in a compensatory pause and reveals atrial activity (52). A PVC can result in the narrowing of a previously wide QRS by allowing for a recovery of bundle branch refractoriness or because of a disruption in concealed penetration into a bundle branch; narrowing of the QRS can also result in evidence of atrial activity.

Effect of Bundle Branch Block

A change in SVT rate with the development of a BBB suggests that the mechanism is an OAVRT with a bypass tract ipsilateral to the block; the BBB causes the impulse to travel farther, crossing the septum to reach the contralateral bundle, increasing the time for retrograde atrial activation, and slowing the rate of the AVRT (Fig. 5-20).

DIAGNOSIS AND EVALUATION OF A WIDE QRS COMPLEX TACHYCARDIA

The differential diagnosis of a wide QRS complex tachycardia is clinically relevant for several reasons. In the pres-

ence of underlying heart disease, the prognosis of a patient with VT is worse than the prognosis of a patient with SVT. Intravenous administration of drugs, such as verapamil, often used in the treatment of SVT can cause severe hemodynamic deterioration in patients with VT, resulting in hypotension and ischemia and rendering the arrhythmia impossible to cardiovert and possibly precipitating ventricular fibrillation (53,54).

Causes of a Wide-Complex Tachycardia

Tachycardias with a wide QRS complex (QRS width ≥0.12 seconds) may be supraventricular or ventricular in origin (Table 5-3). Causes include AVRT due to a preexcitation syndrome with antegrade conduction to the ventricle over an accessory pathway and retrograde conduction back to the AV node and atrium through the normal His-Purkinje pathway (i.e., AAVRT); any SVT, such as sinus tachycardia, atrial flutter, or AVNRT, associated with a functional or rate-related BBB; a functional rate-related BBB as a result of therapy with class Ia or Ic antiarrhythmic drugs that possesses the property of use dependency (i.e., slowing of conduction is more pronounced at higher heart rates) (55); preexistent intraventricular conduction delay or BBB that is present during sinus rhythm and that persists during the tachycardia; and VT (56).

General Clinical Approach to the Diagnosis of Wide-Complex Tachycardia

The initial approach to establishing the cause of a wide-complex tachycardia involves evaluation of information obtained from the history, physical examination, response to certain maneuvers, and careful inspection of the ECG, including a rhythm strip and a 12-lead tracing (57,58) (Table 5-4). Comparison of the ECG during the tachycardia with that recorded during sinus rhythm is important.

History

The history is an important first step for establishing the cause of the arrhythmia. Patients who have VT tend to be

---

TABLE 5-3. CAUSES OF WIDE QRS COMPLEX TACHYCARDIA

Ventricular tachycardia
Antidromic atrioventricular reentrant tachycardia (A-AVRT) in Wolff-Parkinson-White syndrome
Any supraventricular tachycardia (e.g., sinus tachycardia, atrial flutter, atrial tachycardia, atrioventricular nodal reentrant tachycardia [AVNRT] with bundle branch block):
    Preexistent bundle branch block
    Functional (rate-related) bundle branch block as from a class IA or IC antiarrhythmic drug or underlying conduction abnormality.

TABLE 5-4. WIDE COMPLEX TACHYCARDIA: VENTRICULAR TACHYCARDIA VERSUS SUPRAVENTRICULAR TACHYCARDIA WITH ABERRANCY

Diagnostic Aids	Usefulness
Presenting symptom	Unhelpful
History	
CAD and previous MI	VT
First arrhythmia after MI	VT
Physical examination	
Evidence of AV dissociation	VT
Blood pressure	Unhelpful
Heart rate	Unhelpful
Electrocardiogram	
Rate	Unhelpful
QRS width >0.16	VT
QRS width <0.16	Unhelpful
Axis shift	VT
Left axis	Suggests VT
Right or normal axis	Unhelpful
QRS morphology	Usually unhelpful
Positive QRS concordance	VT
Negative QRS concordance	Unhelpful
AV dissociation	VT
No AV dissociation	Unhelpful
Response to lidocaine	Suggests VT
Response to verapamil	Suggests SVT

AV, atrioventricular; CAD, coronary artery disease; MI, myocardial infarction; SVT, supraventricular tachycardia; VT, ventricular tachycardia.

older than those with an SVT, but extensive overlap makes this criterion unreliable. However, the younger the patient (especially if younger than 20 years old), the more likely is the diagnosis of an SVT, particularly that associated with an accessory pathway.

Perhaps the most important historical fact that strongly suggests VT as the cause is the presence of structural heart disease, especially coronary artery disease and a previous myocardial infarction (57,58). The first occurrence of the tachycardia after a myocardial infarction makes VT the most likely cause. In more than 98% of patients with a previous myocardial infarction, the cause of a wide-complex tachycardia is VT, but only 7% of those with SVT have a history of a prior infarction.

The duration of the tachycardia is helpful. When it has been present for more than 3 years, an SVT is the more likely cause.

It is important to establish the medication being taken by the patient, particularly antiarrhythmic drugs and other cardiac agents. The class I antiarrhythmic agents slow conduction and have a property of use dependency, and the slowing of impulse conduction is more pronounced at higher heart rates (59). Therapy with these agents may result in rate-related aberration during any supraventricular

arrhythmia (i.e., sinus tachycardia, atrial flutter or fibrillation, and SVT) (60).

The symptoms associated with a tachycardia are not related to the mechanism but are the result of the rapid heart rate, associated heart disease, and left ventricular function (57,58). Because SVT is more likely to occur in a younger patient without heart disease who has intact left ventricular function, there are often no associated symptoms that suggest hemodynamic instability. However, if the rate is extremely rapid or if there is underlying heart disease (especially valvular or congenital), hemodynamic instability and hypotension may be present.

In contrast, VT is not always associated with hypotension (57, 61). In addition to the factors previously mentioned, the hemodynamic effect of this arrhythmia is related to the development of AV asynchrony and the location of the VT focus, which affect the left ventricular activation sequence.

Physical Examination

The physical examination can provide important clues to the cause of the tachyarrhythmia. Although vital signs are obtained, the blood pressure and heart rate are not helpful.

Evidence of AV dissociation is of great importance. AV dissociation is present, although not always evident, in approximately 60% to 75% of patients with VT, but it is rarely seen in SVT (57,58). Evidence of AV dissociation usually establishes VT as the mechanism, but its absence is less helpful. The presence of AV dissociation may be established by close inspection of the ECG or with physical examination (Table 5-5). Because AV dissociation results in

TABLE 5-5. ESTABLISHING ATRIOVENTRICULAR DISSOCIATION

Physical examination
  Cannon "A" waves
  "Cacophony" of heart sounds
  Variability of first heart sound
  Variability of blood pressure
Electrocardiogram
  Dissociated P waves with rate slower than ventricular rate
  Irregular changes in ST-T waves
  Non–rate-related changes in QRS width and morphology
  Fusion beats
  Dressler beats (intermittent capture)
Esophageal lead (or nasogastric tube or central i.v. line)
  P wave and QRS complexes at different rates
Electrophysiologic techniques
  Dissociated atrial electrograms with cycle length greater than ventricular electrograms
  No His electrogram before the ventricular electrogram (none present or follows the ventricular electrogram)
  His potential preceding ventricular electrogram with short HV interval

AV asynchrony and variability in the relationship between atrial and ventricular contraction, examination of the jugular pulsation in the neck reveals cannon A waves, which are intermittent and irregular pulsation, due to ventricular contraction, which produces a transient increase in atrial and venous pressure as a result of atrial contraction against a closed AV valve. AV dissociation also produces fluctuation in blood pressure, reflecting variability in the degree of atrial contribution to left ventricular filling, stroke volume, and cardiac output. AV dissociation also produces variability in the occurrence and intensity of heart sounds, particularly S_1.

Responses to Interventions and to Drugs

Several interventions are helpful in establishing the cause of the tachycardia. Carotid sinus pressure enhances vagal tone and hence depresses sinus and AV nodal activity. The heart rate during sinus tachycardia gradually slows with carotid sinus pressure and then accelerates on release. The ventricular rate of atrial tachycardia and atrial flutter abruptly slows, the result of AV nodal blockade; the arrhythmia itself, which is generated within the atria, is unaffected. An SVT terminates or remains unaltered. In general, VT is unaffected, although carotid sinus pressure slows the atrial rate and in some cases exposes the presence of AV dissociation not otherwise obvious, establishing the diagnosis of VT. In rare cases, a VT may terminate with carotid sinus pressure.

Response to lidocaine suggests, but does not prove, that VT is the mechanism, whereas a response to digoxin, verapamil, or adenosine strongly suggests SVT, although very infrequently VT may terminate with these agents. However, unless the cause for the wide-complex tachycardia is definitely established, verapamil and adenosine should not be given, because they have been reported to cause hemodynamic collapse in patients with VT (53).

Analysis of the Electrocardiogram

Careful inspection of the ECG, including a 12-lead and rhythm strip, is of great importance. Comparison of the ECG obtained during the tachycardia with an ECG recorded during sinus rhythm is helpful (62,63). A significant shift in QRS axis and a marked change in QRS morphology, when compared with sinus rhythm, are of great help in establishing the diagnosis of VT. Their similarity to QRS complexes during sinus rhythm suggests SVT (Fig. 5-26).

VT is often associated with slight irregularity of R-R intervals, subtle or more marked variation of QRS morphology, and variability in ST-T waves (Fig. 5-27). These abnormalities result from changes in the direction of impulse conduction as it exits from the reentrant circuit and variability in the activation and repolarization pattern of the ventricular myocardium, which results in underlying heterogeneity of the ventricular myocardium and its response to depolarization and repolarization contribute to this variability.

Occasionally, there is evidence of AV dissociation manifested as obviously dissociated P waves, fusion beats, and intermittent captured (Dressler) beats (Figs. 5-28 through 5-30). In some cases, marked changes in the QRS morphology and in the ST and T waves are manifestations of AV dissociation.

In contrast, there is uniformity of the R-R intervals, QRS morphology, and ST and T waves with an SVT, because the activation of the ventricular myocardium always follows the same pathway, which involves the AV node and His-Purkinje system or an accessory bypass tract. Usually there is 1 : 1 atrial and ventricular activity.

The most diagnostic ECG finding associated with VT is the presence of AV dissociation. Although AV dissociation is not evident in all cases of VT, its presence establishes this arrhythmia as the likely cause. In the presence of AV dissociation, retrograde atrial activation is absent (i.e., there is no VA conduction because of retrograde AV nodal block). Atrial activity or the P wave is independent of the ventricular activity or QRS complex and is usually at a rate slower than the ventricular rate. Establishing AV dissociation therefore is of great importance for diagnosing VT (Table 5-5).

Dissociated P waves may be obvious on the ECG or rhythm strip or may be superimposed on the ST segment or T wave, altering their morphology (Fig. 5-28). The presence of a fusion beat, which has a morphology that is intermediate between a sinus beat and ventricular complex, results from simultaneous activation of the ventricular myocardium through the normal conduction system and from the ventricular focus. A Dressler beat represents intermittent ventricular capture, and the QRS complex is normalized and is identical to the sinus QRS complex (Fig. 5-30). It results from ventricular activation, which occurs as a result of impulse conduction that can occur by means of the normal conduction system (i.e., from the atrium through the AV node and His Purkinje system).

Fusion and Dressler beats are seen with AV dissociation and are more evident when the tachycardia rate is slower (Fig. 5-29). Fusion and capture do not alter the rate of the VT, although they may produce a change in R-R intervals.

If P waves are not obvious or suggested on the ECG, alternative methods for their identification may be useful:

1. Use of a modified chest lead placement (i.e., Lewis leads)
2. Carotid sinus pressure for altering the relationship between the P wave and QRS complex
3. Use of an esophageal lead (using an electrode wire or nasogastric tube)

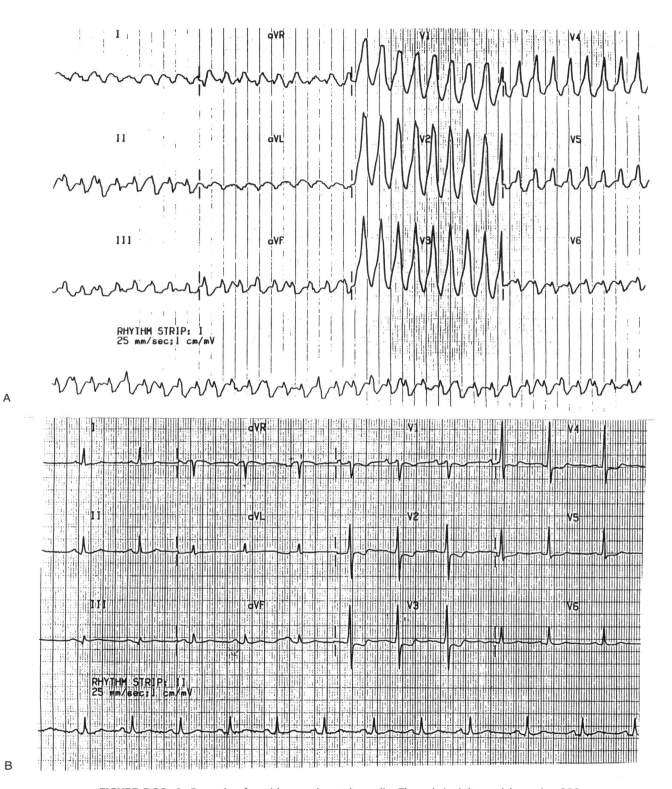

FIGURE 5-26. A: Example of a wide-complex tachycardia. The axis is rightward (negative QRS complexes in leads I and aVL), and there are tall, monophasic R-waves in leads V_1 through V_5 and a deep S-wave in V_6. These electrocardiographic findings favor ventricular tachycardia (VT). Most importantly, there is evidence of atrioventricular (AV) dissociation, which is best identified in leads II, III, and aVF. The lead II rhythm strip shows obviously dissociated P waves and marked changes in QRS morphology and of the ST segments and T waves. **B:** Recorded after sinus rhythm was restored, the electrocardiogram shows a normal axis and normal QRS morphology in the limb and precordial leads.

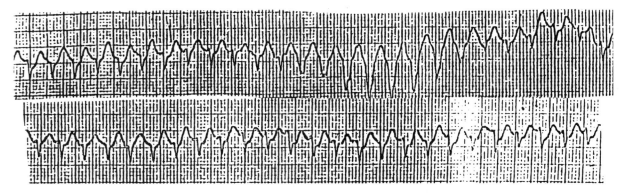

FIGURE 5-27. Continuous lead II rhythm strip of ventricular tachycardia (VT). Seen are subtle changes in the ST segments and T waves. There is a sudden change of QRS morphology, becoming widened, which is not rate related but occurs spontaneously.

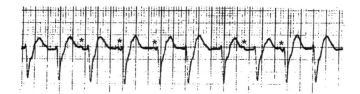

FIGURE 5-28. Example of ventricular tachycardia (VT) with obvious atrioventricular (AV) dissociation. The P waves *(asterisks)* are dissociated from the QRS complexes and occur at a rate slower than the ventricular rate.

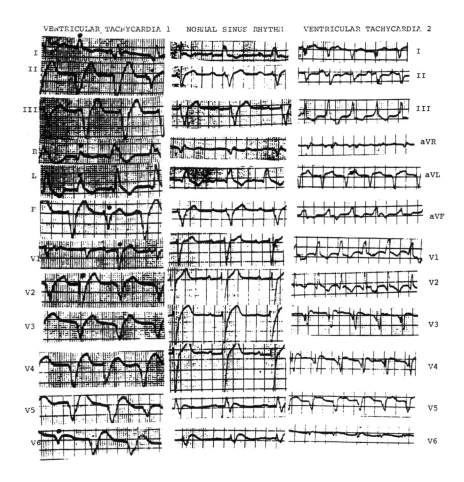

FIGURE 5-29. Patient with ventricular tachycardia (VT) of two different morphologies. VT1 has a QRS morphology that resembles that seen in sinus rhythm in all leads. However, the complexes are wider. Occasional QRS complexes *(solid circles)* are different in morphology from the others but are identical to the QRS morphology recorded during sinus rhythm. A P wave and constant PR can be seen before these "normal" QRS complexes, and the PR interval is the same as measured during sinus rhythm. These are Dressler beats (i.e., QRS complexes that are normalized because of intermittent capture). VT2 has a QRS morphology different from those of sinus rhythm and VT1. Although the QRS is narrowed, there has been a marked shift in the axis; there is a tall, monophasic R-wave in V_1; and most importantly, there is atrioventricular (AV) dissociation, best seen in the limb leads. Notice the marked changes in the ST segments and T waves and the occasional distinct P waves.

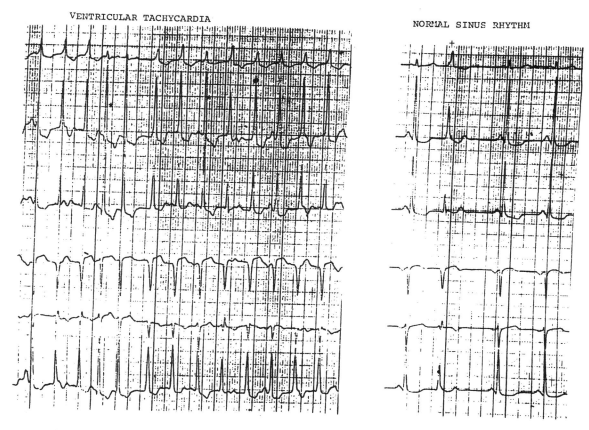

VENTRICULAR TACHYCARDIA

NORMAL SINUS RHYTHM

FIGURE 5-30. Example of ventricular tachycardia (VT) with the six limb leads recorded simultaneously. During VT, there are marked changes in QRS morphology that are best seen in leads I *(first line)* and aVL *(fifth line)*. In lead II *(second line)*, there are distinct P waves that are dissociated from the QRS complexes. Some of the P waves can be seen within the ST segment or T wave. Occasionally, there is a P wave that is followed by a normalized QRS complex, such as the fourth and eighth QRS *(asterisk)*. These are Dressler beats. Fusion complexes *(circle)* are occasionally seen. When compared with sinus rhythm, the captured beats are identical to the sinus QRS complexes. The QRS complexes during VT are identical in morphology to a spontaneous ventricular premature beat (+) seen during sinus rhythm.

4. Right atrial recording obtained by an electrode catheter in the right atrium or from a central intravenous line
5. Invasive electrophysiologic studies to expose AV dissociation if present, establishing the diagnosis (Fig. 5-31)

Classic Electrocardiographic Criteria for Distinguishing between Ventricular Tachyarrhythmias and Supraventricular Tachyarrhythmias with Aberrant Conduction

Several other features on the surface ECG are helpful for establishing the cause of a wide-complex tachycardia. Criteria in current use were defined from analysis of the 12-lead ECGs recorded during tachycardia in patients in whom the mechanism of the arrhythmia was determined during electrophysiologic investigation.

Four criteria seem particularly helpful in the differential diagnosis (62–66):

1. Morphologic features of the QRS
2. AV dissociation, fusion, or capture beats
3. Duration of the QRS complex
4. Axis of the QRS complex in the frontal plane

Classic criteria suggesting VT or SVT are summarized in Figure 5-32 and Table 5-4.

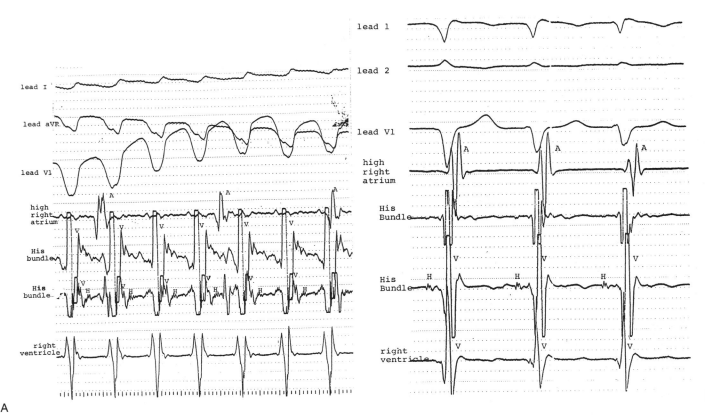

FIGURE 5-31. A: Example of an electrophysiologic study of a patient with ventricular tachycardia (VT). Atrioventricular (AV) dissociation is evidenced by the atrial activity (A) at a slower rate than the ventricular activity (V), and there is no relationship between A and V. His bundle activation (H spike on the His bundle electrogram) follows ventricular activity, indicating retrograde activation of His. **B:** Example of an electrophysiologic study during supraventricular tachyarrhythmia (SVT) with aberration. The 1:1 atrial (A) and ventricular (V) activations occur simultaneously, although the retrograde A electrogram occurs slightly after V activity. Before each V wave is a bundle of His spike (H), with a fixed H-V interval, indicating a supraventricular origin for the tachycardia.

QRS Morphology Pattern in the Precordial Leads

To make a diagnosis based on the morphology pattern of the QRS complex in the precordial leads, QRS polarity in lead V_1 or V_2 must be defined as positive (i.e., RBBB-like pattern) or negative (i.e., LBBB-like pattern). Lead V_6 can offer additional diagnostic clues (66–71) (Figs. 5-32 and 5-33).

V_1-Positive Wide QRS Tachycardia

RBBB aberrancy can be identified in lead V_1 from a triphasic rSR′ pattern and in lead V_6 from a triphasic qRS pattern with the R : S ratio greater than 1. The small initial waves (rV_1 and qV_6) reflect normal septal activation that is preserved in RBBB, whereas the tall terminal forces ($R′V_1$ and SV_6) indicate late activation of the right ventricle because of conduction delay in the right bundle (Fig. 5-33).

In VT, intraventricular conduction is bizarre and does not follow the rules that apply to functional or structural interruption of the normal conduction system. In contrast with the findings in SVT, a monophasic R or a biphasic qR pattern in lead V_1 and a deep S wave (R : S ratio <1) in lead V_6 suggest a ventricular origin of the tachycardia (Figs. 5-32 and 5-33).

When a double-peaked R wave is recorded in V_1, with a left peak taller than the right one (i.e., so-called rabbit ear sign), a ventricular origin is likely (67). However, a taller right rabbit ear does not help in distinguishing a ventricular from a supraventricular site of origin.

V_1-Negative Wide QRS Tachycardia

A ventricular origin of a V_1-negative (LBBB-like) wide QRS tachycardia is highly suspected in the presence of the following ECG findings (64,68,69) (Fig. 5-32):

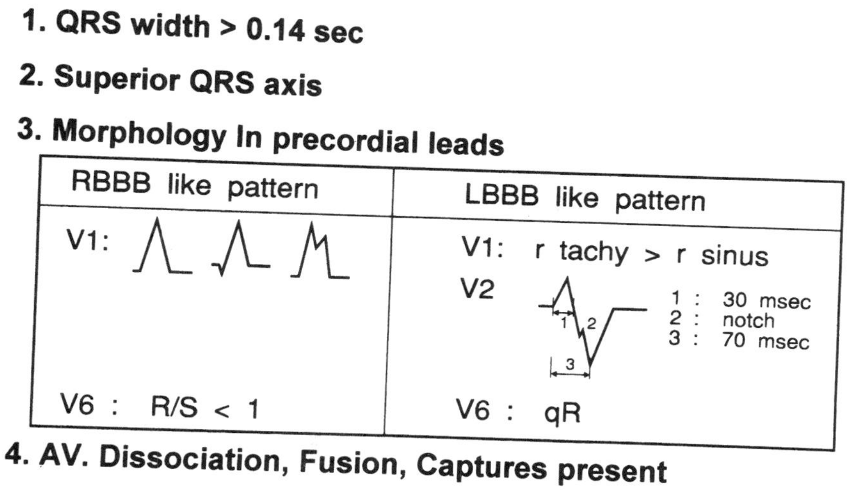

1. QRS width > 0.14 sec

2. Superior QRS axis

3. Morphology In precordial leads

RBBB like pattern	LBBB like pattern
V1: ⋀ ⋀ ⋈	V1: r tachy > r sinus V2: ⟍⟋⟍_ 1 : 30 msec ⟍⟍ 2 : notch 3 : 70 msec
V6 : R/S < 1	V6 : qR

4. AV. Dissociation, Fusion, Captures present

FIGURE 5-32. Criteria used in the differential diagnosis between supraventricular tachyarrhythmia (SVT) with intraventricular aberrant conduction and ventricular tachycardia (VT) that favor a diagnosis of VT.

1. A broad initial R wave of 30 ms or more in lead V_1 or V_2, with the initial R wave in V_1 that is often taller during tachycardia than during sinus rhythm
2. A slurred or notched downstroke of the S wave in lead V_1 or V_2
3. A duration of 70 ms or longer from the onset of the ventricular complex to the nadir of the QS or S wave in leads V_1 and V_2
4. The presence of any Q wave in lead V_6

SVT with LBBB can be recognized by several ECG markers, which are caused by the typical changes in ventricular activation pattern because of left bundle conduction delay. In a LBBB, the electrical activation of the septum, which normally occurs from left to right, is reversed. Ventricular activation begins in the right side of the interventricular septum and proceeds from right to left through the septum. This results in a small, narrow R wave in V_2 and often in the absence of any initial positive deflection in V_1. The right-to-left septal vector is directed toward V_6, causing initial positivity and absence of any Q wave in this lead. During LBBB

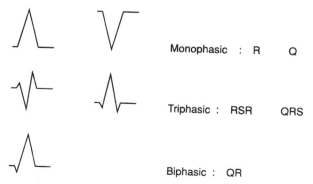

FIGURE 5-33. Examples of QRS complexes that are not RS complexes.

Monophasic : R   Q

Triphasic : RSR   QRS

Biphasic : QR

aberrancy, the downstroke of the S wave is clean, without any slurring or notch, and has a swift inscription.

Additional Information from V_6

After the diagnosis of VT has been established, the morphology of the QRS complex in V_6 yields information on the basal-apical vector of the tachycardia. A predominantly positive VT QRS complex in V_6 implies a basal-to-apical activation sequence. In contrast, a predominately negative VT QRS complex in V_6 implies an apical-to-basal activation sequence.

Atrioventricular Dissociation, Fusion, and Capture Beats

In the presence of AV dissociation, the atria and ventricles are activated independently of each other. AV dissociation, the hallmark of VT, can be recognized on the 12-lead ECG by the identification of independent P waves that have no relation to QRS complexes (i.e., they are dissociated) (Figs. 5-28 through 5-30). Identifying P waves is sometimes difficult because T waves and initial or terminal QRS portions can resemble atrial activity. Artifacts can be mistaken for P waves. When atrial fibrillation is the underlying supraventricular rhythm, the diagnosis of AV dissociation is impossible.

Occasionally, a fusion or captured beat (i.e., partially or completely normalized QRS) may be fortuitously observed during VT (Fig. 5-30). When a sinus impulse can be conducted to the ventricles during VT, it may activate the ventricles entirely (i.e., captured or Dressler beat) or activate the ventricles at the same time as activation from the ventricular impulse (i.e., fusion). In both circumstances, the resulting beat is narrower than the QRS complexes during the tachycardia. However, a narrower beat during a wide QRS tachycardia is not always a marker for VT, because it may occur in SVT with aberrancy when ventricular premature beats arise from the ventricle ipsilateral to the BBB. In

Wolff-Parkinson-White syndrome, atrial fibrillation occasionally can conduct over the AV node-His axis, resulting in narrower beats; in this situation, however, the rhythm is irregularly irregular.

QRS Complex Width and Axis

Other diagnostic criteria are related to the width and frontal plane axis of the QRS complex. A QRS duration of 0.14 second or more and a superior or indeterminate axis, which is extremely leftward (> −90) or extremely rightward (>180), favor the diagnosis of VT. A marked rightward or leftward shift in axis, primarily of the initial portion of the QRS complex, when compared with the axis during sinus rhythm strongly suggests VT.

Limitations of the Classic Electrocardiographic Criteria

The clinical accuracy of the classic criteria was assessed in a prospective analysis of 236 wide QRS tachycardias that were evaluated with electrophysiologic testing to localize the origin of the tachycardia (70). A superior axis deviation of the QRS complex in the frontal plane is far from an exclusive finding in VT because it occurs in 23% of SVTs, is even more common in the presence of LBBB, and becomes the rule when antegrade conduction occurs over an inferiorly located accessory pathway (i.e., septal, right-sided, or Mahaim).

A QRS width exceeding 140 ms was found in 23% of patients with SVT and may be even more common in patients treated with class Ia and Ic antiarrhythmic drugs (71,72). However, a relatively narrow QRS complex (<140 ms) was present in 21% of VTs, especially when the arrhythmia was idiopathic or fascicular in origin or when digitalis toxicity was the cause.

AV dissociation frequently is absent during VT, and it could be clearly demonstrated in only 21% of cases of VT; independent beating of atria and ventricles cannot be diagnosed if atrial fibrillation is the underlying supraventricular rhythm. In about one half of the patients with VT, some form of retrograde conduction to the atria is present; this may be 2:1 retrograde conduction or retrograde Wenckebach. A high incidence of discordance in the QRS morphology criteria was observed and was present equally in 40% of VTs and SVTs.

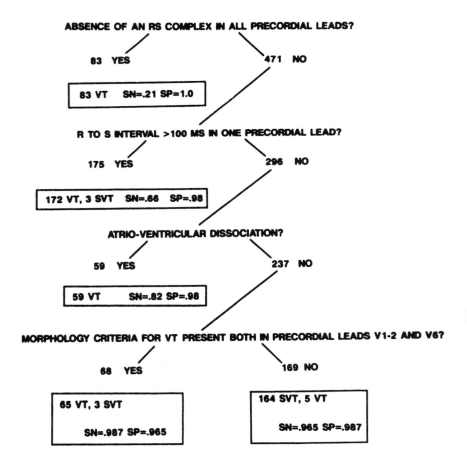

FIGURE 5-34. Algorithm of the diagnosis made by two observers of 554 tachycardias with widened QRS complexes. The number of tachycardias classified at each step is given. Sensitivities (SN) and specificities (SP) for the diagnosis of ventricular tachycardia (VT) are also shown at each step and for the diagnosis of supraventricular tachyarrhythmia (SVT) with aberrant conduction at the last step. The four consecutive criteria reached a sensitivity of 98.7% and a specificity of 96.5% for the diagnosis of SVT with aberrant conduction.

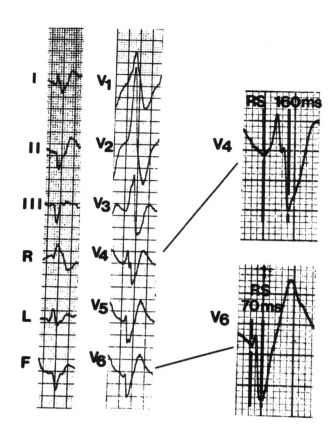

FIGURE 5-35. Tracings from the 12-lead electrocardiogram illustrate the measurements of the RS interval. A ventricular tachycardia (VT) with a right bundle branch block (RBBB)-like QRS complex is shown. An RS complex is observed in precordial leads V_3 through V_6. The S wave is, however, not sharp enough in lead V_3 to measure confidently an RS interval. The RS interval (enlarged in the right panel) measures 160 ms in lead V_4 and 70 ms in lead V_6. The longest RS interval is more than 100 ms and diagnostic of VT. Paper speed was 25 mm/sec.

Stepwise Approach to Wide QRS Tachycardias

Because patients with wide QRS tachycardias commonly are seen in emergency situations, there is a need for simple criteria that can be applied quickly and easily. Two algorithms have been developed by Brugada for establishing the cause of a wide-complex tachycardia: the first for differentiating VT from SVT with aberrant conduction and the second for differentiating VT from antidromic tachycardia (70). These two algorithms can be used sequentially but not in tandem.

Algorithm 1

Algorithm 1 allows the differential diagnosis between VT and SVT with aberrant conduction (Fig. 5-34). In the first step, all precordial leads are inspected to detect the presence or absence of an RS complex (Figs. 5-35 and 5-36). If an RS complex cannot be identified in any precordial lead, the diagnosis of VT can be made with 100% specificity, and further analysis is not needed. Monophasic R or Q complexes, triphasic RSR or QRS, and biphasic qR should not be labeled as RS (Fig. 5-33).

In the second step, if an RS complex is clearly distinguished in one or more precordial leads, the next step

involves careful measurement of the interval between the onset of the R wave and the deepest part of the S wave (i.e., RS interval). If the RS interval exceeds 100 ms, the diagnosis of VT can be made with a specificity of 98%; if RS complexes are present in multiple precordial leads, the one with the largest RS interval is considered (Fig. 5-35).

In the third step, if the RS interval is less than 100 ms, a ventricular or supraventricular site of origin of the tachycardia is possible, and the presence or absence of AV dissociation should be established. Clear-cut demonstration of AV dissociation is 100% specific for the diagnosis of VT.

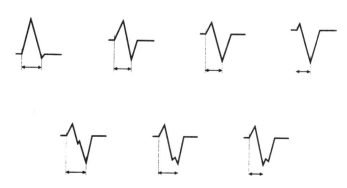

FIGURE 5-36. RS complexes and measurement of the RS interval.

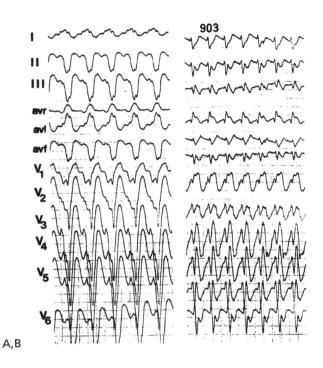

FIGURE 5-37. Twelve-lead electrocardiograms illustrate the value of the new criteria compared with old criteria in the differential diagnosis between ventricular tachycardia (VT) and supraventricular tachycardia (SVT) with aberrant conduction. **A:** VT in a patient with surgically corrected tetralogy of Fallot. The RS complex occurs in leads V_2 through V_6. The RS interval is clearly longer than 100 ms and is diagnostic for VT. **B:** SVT with right bundle branch block (RBBB) aberrant conduction from the same patient. The duration of the QRS complex is more than 200 ms. Atrioventricular dissociation is not visible, and the axis of the QRS complex in the frontal plane is of no help in the differential diagnosis. The QRS complex is triphasic in lead V_1, but the R : S wave ratio is less than 1 in lead V_6. Old criteria favor the diagnosis of VT in this case. With the new criteria, the correct diagnosis of SVT with RBBB aberrant conduction was made as follows: (a) Absence of an RS complex in precordial leads? An RS is observed in lead V_6. (b) RS interval greater than 100 ms in one precordial lead? RS interval is less than 100 ms. (c) Atrioventricular dissociation? Not recognizable. (d) Morphology criteria for VT present in precordial leads V_1 and V_6? No, because lead V_1 has a triphasic complex. By excluding VT with the four steps, the correct diagnosis of SVT was made.

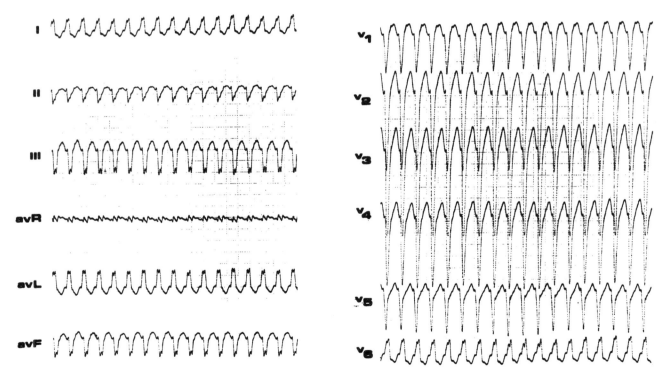

FIGURE 5-38. The diagnosis is made using **Algorithm 1:** *Step 1.* RS complex is present in V_2 through V_5. In V_1, there is a monophasic R, and in V_6, there is a QS complex. *Step 2.* The RS interval (200 ms) is longest in V_2 and clearly exceeds 100 ms, which is diagnostic for ventricular tachycardia (VT). Further analysis of algorithm 1 is not needed. **Algorithm 2:** *Step 1.* Dominantly negative QRS complexes occur in leads V_5 and V_6, excluding antidromic tachycardia. The diagnosis is VT.

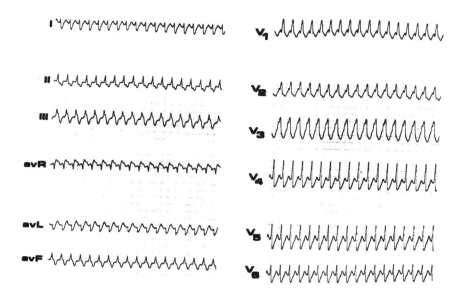

FIGURE 5-39. Using **Algorithm 1**: *Step 1.* RS complexes are present in leads V_4, V_5, and V_6. *Step 2.* In all these leads, the RS interval is less than 100 ms. *Step 3.* Atrioventricular (AV) dissociation is not evident. *Step 4.* The morphology criteria for V_1-positive ventricular tachycardia (VT) are not fulfilled in V_1 (triphasic QRS complex) or in V_6 (R : S > 1). The diagnosis is supraventricular tachycardia with right bundle branch block aberrancy.

In the fourth step, if the RS interval is less than 100 ms and AV dissociation cannot clearly be demonstrated, the classic morphology criteria for V_1-positive and V_1-negative wide QRS complex tachycardias are considered. For diagnosing VT, the classic morphologic criteria must be present in lead V_1 (V_2) and in lead V_6.

This algorithm is highly accurate in the differentiation of VT from SVT with aberrant conduction. The specificity is 97%, and sensitivity is 99% (Figs. 5-37 through 5-39).

Algorithm 2

Algorithm 2 allows the differential diagnosis between VT and antidromic tachycardia in Wolff-Parkinson-White syndrome (Fig. 5-40). This algorithm addresses two important problems in the differential diagnosis between VT and SVT with aberrant conduction: antidromic tachycardia and treatment with class Ia and Ic antiarrhythmic drugs. Several important concepts form the basis of this algorithm.

The first step is to define the polarity of the QRS complex in leads V_4 through V_6; they are predominantly positive or predominantly negative. Accessory pathways are located in the AV ring, and they activate the ventricles from the base to the apex, resulting in predominantly positive QRS complexes in the precordial leads V_4 through V_6 (Fig. 5-40). Predominantly negative complexes in these leads cannot be observed during a preexcited tachycardia and favor the diagnosis of VT with 100% specificity, and further analysis is unnecessary (Figs. 5-41 and 5-42). If the polarity of the QRS complex is predominantly positive in V_4 through V_6, the cardiologist should proceed to the second step.

The second step is to identify a qR complex. In the absence of structural heart disease, qR complexes in leads

V_2 through V_6 cannot be observed with an antidromic tachycardia; if a qR is present, VT can be diagnosed with a specificity of 100%, and further analysis is omitted (Fig. 5-41). If a qR wave in leads V_2 to V_6 is absent, the third step is necessary.

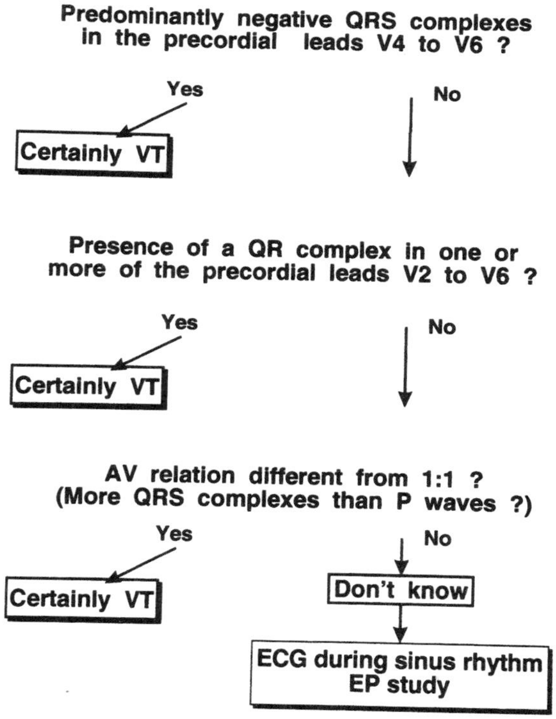

Predominantly negative QRS complexes in the precordial leads V4 to V6 ?

Yes → **Certainly VT**

No → ↓

Presence of a QR complex in one or more of the precordial leads V2 to V6 ?

Yes → **Certainly VT**

No → ↓

AV relation different from 1:1 ?
(More QRS complexes than P waves ?)

Yes → **Certainly VT**

No → **Don't know** → **ECG during sinus rhythm EP study**

FIGURE 5-40. Wide QRS complex tachycardia. Algorithm 2 is suggested for the differential diagnosis between ventricular and preexcited tachycardia.

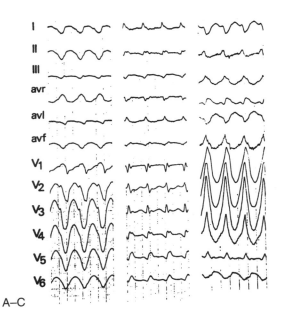

A–C

FIGURE 5-41. A: Example of ventricular tachycardia (VT) with predominantly negative QRS complexes in the precordial leads V_5 and V_6. **B:** VT with a QR complex in leads V_3 to V_6. **C:** Preexcited regular tachycardia using a left lateral accessory pathway.

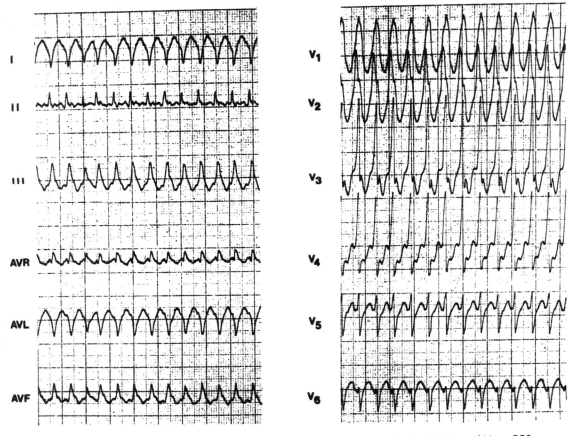

FIGURE 5-42. Case study 5. **Algorithm 1:** *Step 1.* There is a monophasic R in V_1 and V_2, a QRS complex in V_6, but an RS complex in V_3, V_4, and V_5. The S-wave in V_3 is the notch in the descending limb of the ventricular complex. *Step 2.* The RS interval does not exceed 100 ms. *Step 3.* Atrioventricular (AV) dissociation cannot be clearly demonstrated. *Step 4.* The morphology criteria for V_1-positive ventricular tachycardia (VT) are present in V_1 (monophasic R) and in V_6 (R : S < 1). **Algorithm 2:** *Step 1.* Predominantly negative QRS complexes in leads V_5 and V_6 exclude antidromic reentrant tachycardia. The diagnosis is VT.

The third step is to evaluate the AV relationship, especially whether AV dissociation is present. Antidromic tachycardia is always associated with 1 : 1 retrograde AV conduction, and AV dissociation is 100% specific for VT.

If all these steps are answered negatively, the diagnosis of preexcited (antidromic) tachycardia has to be considered. Algorithm 2 has a specificity of 100% for VT but a sensitivity of 75%. Comparison of the ECG in VT with that during sinus rhythm could further clarify the diagnosis.

REFERENCES

1. Fisch C. The clinical electrocardiogram: a classic. *Circulation* 1980;62[Suppl 111]:1–4.
2. Wellens HJI. The electrocardiogram 80 years after Einthoven. *J Am Coll Cardiol* 1986;7:484–491.
3. Krikler DM. Electrocardiography then and now: where next? *Br Heart J* 1987;57:113–117.
4. American College of Cardiology tenth Bethesda conference: optimal electrocardiography. *Am J Cardiol* 1978;41:111–191.
5. Fisch C. The electrocardiogram and arrhythmias: limitations of a technique. *Circulation* 1987;75[Suppl III]:48–52.
6. Fisch C. *Electrocardiography of arrhythmias.* Philadelphia: Lea & Febiger, 1989:197.
7. Narula OS. Sinus node reentry: a mechanism for supraventricular tachycardia. *Circulation* 1974;50:1114–1128.
8. Wellens HJJ. Unusual examples of supraventricular reentrant tachycardias. *Circulation* 1975;51:997–1002.
9. Wu D, Amat-Y-Leon F, Denes P, et al. Demonstration of sustained sinus and atrial reentry as a mechanism of paroxysmal supraventricular tachycardia. *Circulation* 1975;51:234–243.
10. Coumel P, Flammang D, Attuel P, Leclerc JF. Sustained intraatrial reentrant tachycardia electrophysiologic study of 20 cases. *Clin Cardiol* 1979;2:167–178.
11. Mendez C, Delmar M. Triggered activity: its possible role in cardiac arrhythmias. In: Zipes DP, Jalife J, eds. *Cardiac electrophysiology and arrhythmias.* Orlando: Grune & Stratton, 1985.
12. Wittenberg SM, Strevli F, Klocke FJ. Acceleration of ventricular pacemakers by transient increases in heart rate in dogs during Ouabain administration. *Circ Res* 1970;26:705–716.
13. Knoebel SB, Fisch C. Accelerated junctional escape: a clinical and electrocardiographic study. *Circulation* 1974;50:151–158.
14. Rosen MR, Fisch C, Hoffman BF, et al. Can accelerated atrioventricular escape rhythms be explained by delayed afterdepolarizations? *Am J Cardiol* 1980;45:1272–1284.
15. Zipes DP, Foster PR, Troup PJ, et al. Atrial induction of ventricular tachycardia: reentry versus triggered automaticity. *Am J Cardiol* 1979;44:1–8.
16. Wellens HJJ, Brugada P, Nanagt EJDM, et al. New studies with triggered automaticity. In: Harrison DC, ed. *Cardiac arrhythmias.* Boston: GK Hall, 1981;591–599.
17. Wellens HJJ, Brugada P. The role of triggered activity in clinical arrhythmias. In: Rosenbaum MB, Elizari MV, eds. *Frontiers of cardiac electrophysiology.* The Hague: Martinus Nijhoff, 1983: 195–216.
18. Castellanos A Jr, Lemberg L, Centurion MJ, et al. Concealed digitalis-induced arrhythmias unmasked by electrical stimulation of the heart. *Am Heart J* 1967;173:484–490.
19. Cranefield PF, Aronson RS. *Cardiac arrhythmias: the role of triggered activity and other mechanisms.* Mount Kisco, NY: Futura Publishing, 1988;135.
20. Cranefield PF, Aronson RS. Triggered activity sustained by delayed afterdepolarizations: initiation, persistence, and termination. In: *Cardiac arrhythmias: the role of triggered activity and other mechanisms.* Mount Kisco, NY: Futura, 1988;203–243.
21. Henning B, Wit AL. The time course of action potential repolarization affects delayed afterdepolarization amplitude in atrial fibers of the canine coronary sinus. *Circ Res* 1984;55:110–115.
22. Josephson ME, Wellens HJJ. Differential diagnosis of supraventricular tachycardia. *Cardiology Clinics* 1990;8:411–442.
23. Josephson ME. *Clinical cardiac electrophysiology: Techniques and interpretations.* Philadelphia: Lea & Febiger, 1993.
24. Akhtar M. Supraventricular tachycardia. Electrophysiologic mechanisms, diagnosis and pharmacologic therapy. In: Josephson ME, Wellens HJJ, eds. *Tachycardias: mechanisms, diagnosis, treatment.* Philadelphia: Lea & Febiger, 1984:137–169
25. Bar FW, Brugada P, Dassen WRM, et al. Differential diagnosis of tachycardia with narrow QRS complex (shorter than 0.12 second). *Am J Cardiol* 1984;54:555–560.
26. Marriott HJL. *Practical electrocardiography.* Baltimore: Williams & Wilkins, 1988.
27. Farre J, Wellens HJJ. The value of the electrocardiogram in diagnosing site of origin and mechanism of supraventricular tachycardia. In: Wellens HJJ, Kulbertus HE, eds. *What's new in electrocardiography.* The Hague, Martinus Nijhoff, 1981: 131–171.
28. Farshidi A, Josephson ME, Horowitz LN. Electrophysiologic characteristics of concealed bypass tracts: clinical and electrocardiographic correlates. *Am J Cardiol* 1978;41:1052.
29. Puech P, Grolleau R, Cinca J. Reciprocating tachycardia using a latent left-sided accessory pathway: diagnostic approach to conventional ECG. In: Kulbertus H, ed. *Re-entrant arrhythmias: mechanisms and treatment.* Lancaster, England: MTP, 1977: 117–131.
30. Green M, Heddle B, Dassen W, et al. Value of QRS alternation in determining the site of origin of narrow QRS supraventricular tachycardia. *Circulation* 1983;68:368–573.
31. Coumel P, Attuel P. Reciprocating tachycardia in overt and latent pre-excitation. Influence of functional bundle branch block on the rate of tachycardia. *Eur J Cardiol* 1974;1: 423–436.
32. Ross DL, Uther JB. Diagnosis of concealed accessory pathways in supraventricular tachycardia. *Pacing Clin Electrophysiol* 1984; 7:1069–1085.
33. Wellens HJJ, Durrer D. The role of an accessory atrioventricular pathway in reciprocal tachycardia. *Circulation* 1975;52:58–72.
34. Pritchett ELC, Tonkin AM, Dugan FA, et al. Ventriculo-atrial conduction time during reciprocating tachycardia with intermittent bundle-branch block in Wolff-Parkinson-White syndrome. *Br Heart J* 1976;38:1058–1064.
35. Kerr CR, Gallagher JJ, German LD. Changes in ventriculoatrial intervals with bundle branch block aberration during reciprocating tachycardia in patients with accessory atrioventricular pathways. *Circulation* 1982;66:196–201.
36. Tonkin AM, Gallagher JJ, Svenson RH, et al. Anterograde block in accessory pathways with retrograde conduction in reciprocating tachycardia. *Eur J Cardiol* 1975;3:143–152.
37. Yang, Y, Cheng, J, Glatter, K, et al. Quantitative effects of functional bundle branch block in patients with atrioventricular reentrant tachycardia. *Am J Cardiol* 2000; 85:826–831.
38. Bardy GH, Fedor JM, German LD, et al. Surface electrocardiographic clues suggesting presence of a nodofascicular Mahaim fibre. *J Am Coll Cardiol* 1984;3:1161–1168.
39. Vassallo JA, Cassidy DM, Josephson ME. Atrioventricular nodal supraventricular tachycardia. *Am J Cardiol* 1985;56:193–195.
40. Santinelli V, Chiariello M, Condorelli M. Nonparoxysmal atrioventricular junctional rhythm: a clinical and electrophysiologic study. *Eur Heart J* 1984;5:304–307.

41. Farre J, Ross D, Wiener I, et al. Reciprocal tachycardia using accessory pathways with long conduction times. *Am J Cardiol* 1979;44:1099–1109.

42. Glatter KA, Cheng J, Dorostkar P, et al. Electrophysiologic effects of adenosine in patients with supraventricular tachycardia. *Circulation* 1999;99:1034–1040.

43. Singh BN, Hecht HS, Nademanee K, Chew CYC. Electrophysiological and hemodynamic actions of slow-channel blocking compounds. *Prog Cardiovasc Dis* 1982; 25:103–132.

44. Singh BN, Nademanee K, Baky S. Calcium antagonists: clinical uses in treating arrhythmias. *Drugs* 1983; 25:125–153.

45. Kaplan IV, Kaplan AV, Fisher JD. Adenosine induced atrial fibrillation precipitating polymorphic ventricular tachycardia. *Pacing Clin Electrophysiol* 2000; 23:140–141.

46. Romer M, Candinas R. Adenosine-induced nonsustained polymorphic ventricular tachycardia. *Eur Heart J* 1994; 15:281–282.

47. Strickberger SA, Man KC, Daoud EG, et al. Adenosine-induced atrial arrhythmia: a prospective analysis. *Ann Intern Med* 1997; 127:417–422.

48. Glatter KA, Cheng J, Dorostkar P, et al. Electrophysiologic effects of adenosine in patients with supraventricular tachycardia. *Circulation* 1999;99:1034–1040.

49. Belhassen B, Fish R, Glikson M, et al. Noninvasive diagnosis of dual AV node physiology in patients with AV nodal reentrant tachycardia by administration of adenosine-5'-triphosphate during sinus rhythm. *Circulation* 1998;98:47–53.

50. Sung RJ. Incessant supraventricular tachycardia. *Pacing Clin Electrophysiol* 1983;6:1306–1326.

51. Moro C, Rufilanchas JJ, Tamargo J, et al. Evidence of abnormal automaticity and triggering activity in incessant ectopic atrial tachycardia. *Am Heart J* 1988;116:550–552.

52. Wang K, Hodges M. The premature ventricular complex as a diagnostic aid. *Ann Intern Med* 1992;117:766–770.

53. Buxton AE, Marchlinsky FE, Doherty JU, et al. Hazards of intravenous verapamil for sustained ventricular tachycardia. *Am J Cardiol* 1987;59:1107–1110.

53a. Rankin AC, Rae AP, Cobbe SM. Misuse of intravenous verapamil in patients with ventricular tachycardia. *Lancet* 1987;2: 472–474

54. Stewart RB, Bardy GH, Greene HL. Wide complex tachycardia: misdiagnosis and outcome after emergency therapy. *Ann Intern Med* 1986;104:766–771.

55. Wellens HJJ, Ross DL, Farre J, Brugada P. Functional bundle branch block during supraventricular tachycardia in man: observations on mechanisms and their incidence. In: Zipes D, and Jalife J, eds. *Cardiac electrophysiology and arrhythmias.* New York: Grune & Stratton 1985:435–441.

56. Dancy M, Camm AJ, Ward D. Misdiagnosis of chronic recurrent ventricular tachycardia. *Lancet* 1985;2:320–323.

57. Akhtar M, Shenasa M, Jazayeri M, et al. Wide complex tachycardia. reappraisal of a common clinical problem. *Ann Intern Med* 1988;109:905–912.

58. Tchou P, Young P, Mahmud R, Dinker S, et al. Useful clinical criteria for the diagnosis of ventricular tachycardia. *Am J Med* 1988;84:53–56.

59. Ranger S, Talajic M, Lemery R, et al. Kinetics of use-dependent ventricular conduction slowing by antiarrhythmic drugs in humans. *Circulation* 1991;83:1987–1992.

60. Ranger S, Talajic M, Lemery R, et al. Amplification of flecainide induced ventricular conduction slowing by exercise: a potentially significant consequence of use dependent sodium channel blockade. *Circulation* 1989;79:1000–1006.

61. Morady F, Baerman JM, DiCarlo LA, et al. A prevalent misconception regarding wide-complex tachycardias. *JAMA* 1985; 254:2790–2792.

62. Wellens HJJ, Bar FW, Lie KI. The value of the electrocardiogram in the differential diagnosis of a tachycardia with a widened QRS complex. *Am J Med* 1978;64:27–33.

63. Wellens HJJ, Bar FW, Vanagt EJ, et al. The differentiation between ventricular tachycardia and supraventricular tachycardia with aberrant conduction: the value of the 12-lead electrocardiogram. In: Wellens HJJ, Kulbertus HE, eds. *What's new in electrocardiography.* Boston: Martinus Nijhoff, 1981:184–192.

64. Kindwall KE, Brown J, Josephson ME. Electrocardiographic criteria for ventricular tachycardia in wide complex left bundle branch block morphology tachycardias. *Am J Cardiol* 1988;61: 1279–1283.

65. Marriot HJL. Differential diagnosis of supraventricular and ventricular tachycardia. *Geriatrics* 1970;25:91–94.

66. Sandler A, Marriott HJL. The differential morphology of anomalous ventricular complexes of RBBB type in ventricular ectopy versus aberration. *Circulation* 1965;31:551–556.

67. Gozensky C, Thorne D. Rabbit ear: an aid in distinguishing ventricular ectopy from aberration. *Heart Lung* 1974;3: 634–636.

68. Rosenbaum MB. Classification of ventricular extrasystoles according to form. *J Electrocardiol* 1969;2:289–298.

69. Swanick EJ, La Camera F, Marriott HJL. Morphologic features of right ventricular ectopic beats. *Am J Cardiol* 1972;30:888–891.

70. Brugada P, Brugada J, Mont L, et al. A new approach to the differential diagnosis of a regular tachycardia with a wide QRS complex. *Circulation* 1991;83:1649–1659.

71. Crijns HJ, van Gelder IC, Lie KI. Supraventricular tachycardia mimicking ventricular tachycardia during flecainide treatment. *Am J Cardiol* 1988;62:1303–1306.

72. Murdock CJ, Kyles AE, Yeung-Lai-Wah JA, et al. Atrial flutter in patients treated for atrial fibrillation with propafenone. *Am J Cardiol* 1990;66:755–757.

ROLE OF HOLTER MONITORING AND EXERCISE TESTING FOR ARRHYTHMIA ASSESSMENT AND MANAGEMENT

HAROLD L. KENNEDY
PHILIP J. PODRID

Ambulatory monitoring and exercise testing are the two most valuable noninvasive methods of assessing ventricular and supraventricular tachyarrhythmias and bradyarrhythmias in a wide range of patient groups.

ROLE OF AMBULATORY MONITORING

Ambulatory (Holter) electrocardiography (ECG) is a widely used noninvasive test to evaluate ECG abnormalities in patients with various cardiac disease states. The clinical utility of the ambulatory ECG recording lies in its ability to continuously examine the patient's rhythm over an extended time, permitting ambulatory activity and facilitating examination of the diurnal physical and psychologic changes. In contrast to the standard ECG, which provides a fixed picture of 12 leads that demonstrate cardiac electrical events over a brief period (less than 30 seconds), the 24-hour ambulatory ECG provides a more narrow view of 2 or 3 leads of ECG data but has the strength of recording changing dynamic cardiac electrical phenomena that often are transient and of brief duration. More recent technology has applied 12 leads to the ambulatory ECG to capture more adjunctive ECG parameters. Ambulatory monitoring provides a record of past events, permitting detailed analysis of dynamic and transient ECG changes, although today's technology permits online continuous monitoring (1). The increased sensitivity of the ambulatory ECG, compared with other ECG tests (which have great inherent variability), for detecting spontaneous cardiac arrhythmias has been clearly demonstrated in various clinical studies (2,3).

H. L. Kennedy: Department of Medicine, University of Nevada, Reno, Nevada 89502.

P. J. Podrid: Department of Medicine, Boston University School of Medicine, Boston, Massachusetts 02118.

Although ambulatory ECG is an important clinical diagnostic test for the recording of cardiac tachyarrhythmias and bradyarrhythmias (including conduction disturbances), it also can evaluate ST-segment changes (for myocardial ischemia), R-R–interval changes (for heart rate variability), QRS-complex measurements (for specific intervals, e.g., QT-interval and T-wave changes), and the high-resolution signal-average ECG (for electrical fragmentation, e.g., late potentials) (4). These latter parameters provide additional adjunctive ECG data that may help in the analysis of arrhythmogenesis, mechanism of drug action, or the prediction of a specific cardiac arrhythmia.

Clinical experience has shown ambulatory ECG to be one of the most cost-effective clinical tools in the diagnosis and assessment of symptomatic or asymptomatic cardiac arrhythmias, prognostic assessment or risk stratification of various cardiac populations, and the evaluation of arrhythmia management modalities.

Pathophysiology of Cardiac Arrhythmias and the Rationale for the Use of Ambulatory Monitoring

The physiology of cardiac arrhythmias classically involves concepts of abnormal impulse generation and propagation that account for the genesis of both bradyarrhythmias and tachyarrhythmias (5,6). These concepts recognize that the electrical genesis of cardiac arrhythmias commonly encompasses three important determinants (Fig. 6.1-1).

1. Cardiac substrate is most commonly a structural abnormality of the ventricular myocardium that may be the result of some disease state or abnormal genetic ion channel disorders (7,8).
2. Electrical triggers, such as spontaneous ventricular arrhythmias, were initially thought to be the major

provocateur of fatal cardiac arrhythmias but are now recognized as only one pathophysiologic component of the mechanism and not always required.

3. Physiologic or pathophysiologic modulating factors are arrhythmogenic triggers or events thought to initiate electric instability within an underlying myocardial abnormality at any given point in time.

These latter modulating factors may be ischemia, electrolyte abnormalities, acidosis, hypoxia, toxic or proarrhythmic medications, or other systemic factors; however, the most important are those that result from changes in sympathetic and parasympathetic tone (5) (Fig. 6.1-2). Current understanding of the importance of the autonomic nervous system in this regard has truly taken place only in the last decade but nonetheless focuses attention on methods to assess an ever-changing autonomic milieu in a manner widely applicable to patients.

The concept that "triggers" (i.e., premature ventricular ectopic beats) were the predominant mechanism of cardiac arrhythmias emerged in the 1960s and 1970s and led to the wide popularity of the ambulatory ECG. Ambulatory ECG observations from patients who experienced sudden death during examination led to the recognition that most instantaneous cardiovascular sudden deaths were caused by ventricular tachyarrhythmias, which culminated in ventricular fibrillation and death (9).

Although two decades of investigation have employed invasive electrophysiologic studies to substantiate the role and importance of the myocardial substrate in the mecha-

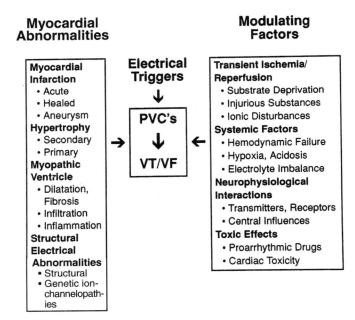

FIGURE 6.1-2. Clinical profile of pathophysiologic determinants. (PVC, premature ventricular contraction; VT/VF, ventricular tachycardia fibrillation.)

nisms of arrhythmia, the ambulatory ECG has experienced an "off again/on again" romance with investigators studying arrhythmic mechanisms. During this time, many investigators became disenchanted with ambulatory ECG because data obtained from monitoring concerning triggers were not found to be highly predictive of a cardiac event in an individual patient. Additionally, there was the observation about late proarrhythmia and the realization from the Cardiac Arrhythmia Suppression Trial that successful treatment and suppression of spontaneous premature ventricular contractions (VPCs) ectopic beats (triggers) did not necessarily decrease the risk of arrhythmic death (10,11). The dilemma of how to direct clinical antiarrhythmic intervention in an individual patient was heightened. There emerged the confrontation of what evaluation process (and the treatment guided by such methods) was most efficacious for various subsets of patients, ambulatory ECG or invasive electrophysiologic studies.

From this controversy came the Electrophysiologic Study Versus Electrocardiographic Monitoring (ESVEM) Study. ESVEM was the first large prospective, randomized trial designed to determine whether ambulatory ECG monitoring or electrophysiologic study–guided drug therapy was superior in predicting long-term outcome in patients with malignant ventricular tachyarrhythmias or syncope who manifested both spontaneous frequent ventricular arrhythmias and inducible ventricular tachycardia (12,13). Despite the criticisms that the trial was conducted in a highly selective group of patients (14), ESVEM demonstrated that the ambulatory ECG (augmented by exercise testing) resulted in a larger yield of predicted drug efficacy

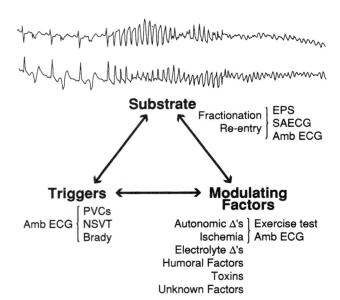

FIGURE 6.1-1. Pathophysiologic determinants of arrhythmia genesis. (EPS, electrophysiologic studies; SAECG, signal-average electrocardiogram; Amb ECG, ambulatory electrocardiogram; PVCs, premature ventricular contractions; NSVT, nonsustained ventricular tachycardia; Brady, bradyarrhythmia; Δ's, changes.)

and was obtained more readily at less cost (13). Moreover, the predictive accuracy of ambulatory ECG was equivalent to that of electrophysiologic studies (13). The noninvasive methods of ambulatory ECG and exercise testing were attested to again as effective and cost-effective methodology of managing patients with malignant ventricular arrhythmias (Fig. 6.1-3) (15).

It has now become apparent that the presence of an abnormal myocardial substrate alone, as detected by electrophysiologic studies, does not account for all the inciting factors of most cardiac arrhythmias and that the ambulatory ECG is useful and cost-effective in assessing patients with malignant ventricular tachyarrhythmias. Attention has focused on the ambulatory ECG to explore various cardiac modulators that could initiate and affect cardiac arrhythmias, including ST-segment changes associated with ischemia, heart rate variability, QT-interval changes (T wave alternans), or QT alternans.

Information Derived from Ambulatory Monitoring

Role for Arrhythmia Assessment

Interest has shifted back to the ambulatory ECG to define the high-risk post–myocardial infarction patients with frequent and complex ventricular arrhythmias who might benefit from amiodarone therapy (16,17). The Canadian Amiodarone Myocardial Infarction Arrhythmia Trial (CAMIAT) randomized 1,202 patients with frequent (mean of more than 10 PVCs per hour) and complex (more

than one run of nonsustained ventricular tachyarrhythmias) ventricular arrhythmias detected by 24-hour ambulatory ECG to placebo or amiodarone therapy 6 to 45 days after myocardial infarction (16). Clinical follow-up for a mean of 1.8 years showed a 48.5% relative risk reduction of resuscitated ventricular fibrillation or arrhythmic death among amiodarone-treated patients as compared with placebo-treated patients (1.77% versus 3.38% per year). Surprisingly, all-cause mortality rates were not significantly improved (amiodarone 4.4% versus placebo 5.4%) (16). These findings were similar in outcome to those of the European Myocardial Infarction Amiodarone Trial (EMIAT) (17). EMIAT identified high-risk post–myocardial infarction patients based on a decreased left ventricular ejection fraction (≤40%). Although EMIAT also demonstrated that amiodarone decreased arrhythmic death incidences, it failed to show any overall benefit on all-cause mortality rates (17). Both CAMIAT and EMIAT showed a beneficial interaction between amiodarone and β-blocker therapy (18,19).

Role for Assessment of ST-Segment and QT-Interval Changes

Additional interest in the use of ambulatory ECG for evaluating ST-segment changes emerged with new knowledge of the vascular endothelium and the multiple processes of atherosclerosis. This spawned new investigations of silent myocardial ischemia and focused attention on new therapeutic agents whose actions modify endothelial mecha-

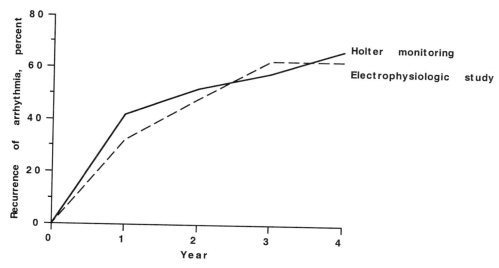

FIGURE 6.1-3. Results from the Electrophysiologic Study Versus Electrocardiographic Monitoring (ESVEM) Study in which the arrhythmia recurrence rate was assessed in patients with previous ventricular tachycardia or fibrillation who were treated with an antiarrhythmic drug, which was selected by a Holter monitor or electrophysiologic study. There was no difference between the two groups (*p* = 0.69). (From Mason JW, for the ESVEM Investigators. A comparison of electrophysiologic testing with Holter monitoring to predict antiarrhythmic drug efficacy for ventricular tachyarrhythmias. *N Engl J Med* 1993;329:445, with permission.)

nisms (20,21). Such studies have been accompanied by myriad investigations employing heart rate variability and QT-interval dynamic changes. Fatal cardiac arrhythmias in patients without structural cardiac disease that result from genetic abnormalities of ion channel disorders have also gained scientific interest. Definition of the long QT and Brugada syndromes and their characteristic phenotypic ECG pattern resulting from abnormal ion channel defects, which sometimes is only manifested by pharmacologic challenge, provides new insight to the enigma of primary electrical disorders (7,8,22). Whether or not ambulatory ECG can play a diagnostic role in the diagnosis of the latter group of patients awaits further investigations.

Role of Monitoring for Assessing Late Potentials

In addition to the time-honored clinical mainstay of documenting and identifying spontaneous ectopic triggers, such as ventricular or supraventricular tachyarrhythmias and bradyarrhythmias resulting from atrioventricular and intraventricular conduction disturbances, ambulatory ECG can also be a valuable adjunct in recognizing abnormal structural myocardial substrate as identified by fractionated late potentials (23). Whether it will prove valuable in detecting the heterogeneous abnormalities of ion channel disorders, which result in abnormal myocardial dispersion and fatal ventricular arrhythmias, remains to be determined.

Nevertheless, ambulatory monitoring remains one of the most specific sources of information for noninvasively evaluating the modulating factors of ischemia (through ST-seg-

ment changes), repolarization abnormalities (QT- or TU-wave changes), or autonomic changes (R-R changes of heart rate variability) (4).

Ambulatory ECG Methodology and Technology

The continuous ambulatory ECG is obtained technologically by (a) conventional tape or solid-state storage (Holter) recording and appropriate playback instrumentation systems and (b) solid-state technology using a real-time analysis microcomputer and memory storage.

Other technologies often used to complement the ambulatory ECG in the study of cardiac arrhythmias include (a) in-hospital long-term ambulatory ECG, (b) transtelephonic monitoring, and (c) implantable loop recorders.

Conventional Ambulatory ECG

The conventional ambulatory ECG system includes a continuous tape or solid-state storage recording of all ECG data for a minimum of 24 or 48 hours and playback analysis. The technology uses a small, lightweight, battery-operated electromagnetic tape or solid-state storage recorder that records from bipolar leads either two or three channels (although 12 leads are possible) of ECG data on reel to reel, magnetic tape cassette, microcassette, compact disc, or more recently on Flash card storage (24) (Figs. 6.1-4 and 6.1-5). State-of-the-art recorders have patient-activated event markers and encoded time or time markers and range from the size of a small book to that of a cigarette package.

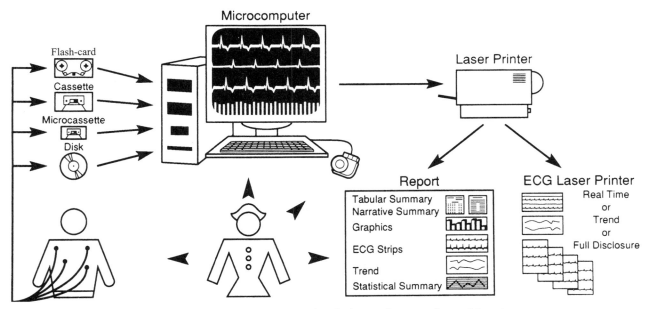

FIGURE 6.1-4. Modern conventional ambulatory electrocardiographic system.

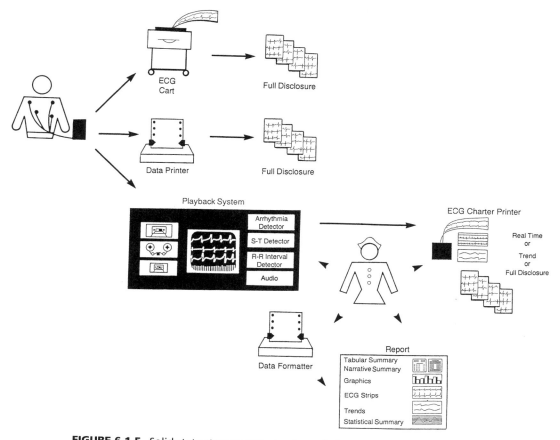

FIGURE 6.1-5. Solid-state storage recorder for ambulatory electrocardiography.

The recorded data are digitized (if not already so recorded) and analyzed with a playback instrument system that demands operator interaction with an arrhythmia analyzer, ST-segment detector, R-R–interval analysis, signal-averaging computer, and various audiovisual detection and review displays, as well as a printer for generating printouts of ECG recordings, trends, or statistical summaries (Figs. 6.1-4 through 6.1-6). Solid-state storage recorders using 11 to 160 megabytes of storage space (disc or Flash card) have been interfaced with a manufacturer's standard ECG cart or a data printer to provide continuous "full-disclosure" hourly printouts for all the data recorded, permitting total visual interpretation. Alternatively, these data can be submitted in digital format for conventional playback analysis (Fig. 6.1-5).

Solid-State ECG Recording Systems

Solid-state ambulatory ECG systems originated from the capability of chip and microprocessor electronic memory storage and were initially introduced for ambulatory ECG as real-time analysis devices (1). These real-time ambulatory ECG instruments consist of (a) a small, lightweight, battery-operated microcomputer that analyzes data online and records the ambulatory ECG and (b) a report generator that receives the data from the real-time analysis recorder and permits editing, generation of analog and graphic hard copy results, and data storage and retrieval (Fig. 6.1-7). This instrumentation also typically continuously evaluates for 24 hours two or three channels of ECG data from bipolar leads. Some instruments purport to examine continuous long-term ECG data for extended periods (up to 5 days with battery changes) (1). This continuous technology examines ambulatory beat-by-beat ECG data during real time to determine various decision-analysis diagnoses within the capability of the algorithm of the specific microcomputer (Fig. 6.1-7). Modern solid-state real-time analysis instruments store a decision analysis in a computational summary data format in solid-state memory and have developed innovative data-compression techniques that are capable of storing all ECG complexes that occur during a continuous 24-hour examination. Whereas the major advantage of real-time analysis technology is cited to be the preprocessing of ECG data—making it immediately available on completion of the examination—major disadvantages are (a) the absence of continuous storage of all ECG data for subsequent analysis and verification in some instruments and (b) the recent documentation that regardless of excellent real-time analysis algorithm accuracy as judged by authoritative databases, artifact introduced during

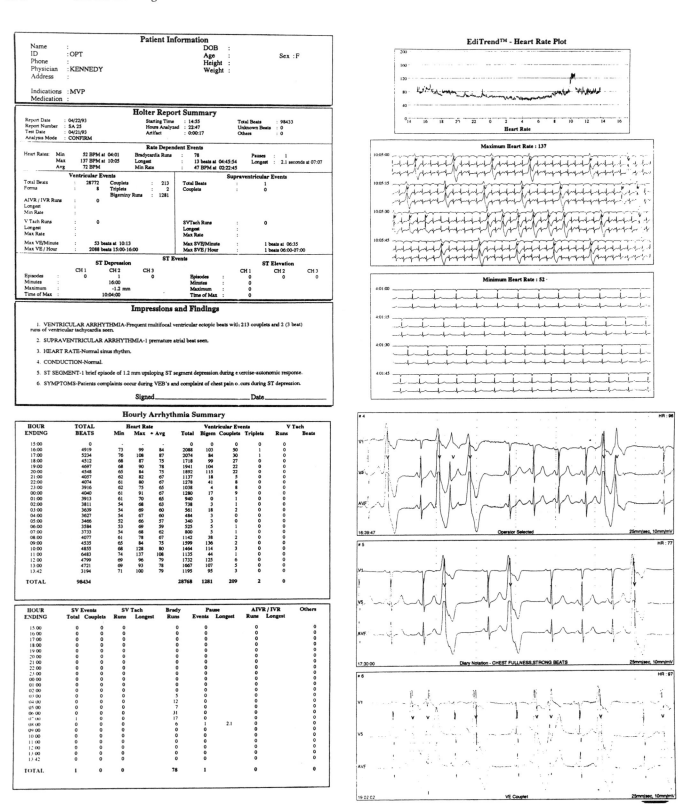

FIGURE 6.1-6. Printouts of trend, tabular data, full-disclosure, and real-time electrocardiographic data obtained from a laser printer.

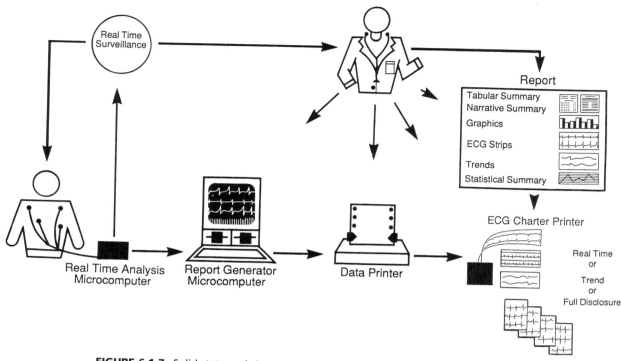

FIGURE 6.1-7. Solid-state real-time analysis ambulatory electrocardiographic system.

the 24-hour ambulatory ECG requires some form of limited operator interaction to attain optimum accuracy (25). Some early versions of real-time analysis instrument systems were equipped with various "warning" systems that were to alert the patient to specific ECG phenomena (e.g., sustained ventricular tachycardia) in an ongoing surveillance manner to permit early medical intervention (26).

In-Hospital Telemetry

Hospital telemetry provides continuous ECG monitoring within the setting of the coronary care unit or the intermediate care unit and continues to be the mainstay of surveillance monitoring of cardiac arrhythmia in patients who are seriously ill or have life-threatening cardiac arrhythmia disturbances. More recently, the improvement of telemetry systems has evolved to accommodate two channels of ECG data, permitting analysis of both cardiac arrhythmias and ST-segment changes (27). The most recent change of this technology was the introduction of solid-state storage of all online ECG data in a digitized format, permitting total reexamination and printout of stored "full-disclosure" continuous ECG data. This solid-state storage is accomplished with low-cost personal computer memory and presents the same options of a solid-state storage ambulatory ECG.

The continuously looping (12- to 24-hour) stored telemetry signal is presented in an hourly full-disclosure format to permit a review of all continuous events that occurred during the previous 12 to 24 hours. New applications of in-hospital long-term ECG telemetry continue to emerge with the addition of other sensors such as thoracic and abdominal respiratory movements, vascular oxygen or CO_2 monitoring, or body movements (28).

Transtelephonic Recording Devices

There are several types of transtelephonic ECG devices and transmitters, capable of direct transmission of an ECG by telephone as an audio signal. These ECG signals are most commonly received at a base station equipped with a demodulator and an ECG strip-chart recorder. The base station may be staffed by a cardiovascular technician or nurse on a 24-hour availability basis or may at times be interfaced to a microcomputer capable of receiving and storing the data for interpretation later. Although such devices most commonly provide limited noncontinuous sample ECG data, the type of examination required may necessitate noncontinuous or continuous application of the recording device.

Noncontinuously applied transtelephonic devices with and without memory are small (beeper size), lightweight instruments that are generally inexpensive. These devices are carried by the patient and can be applied with temporary contact to the precordial area or are attached by electrodes and worn continuously. Older versions of these devices (without memory) required immediate access to a telephone to perform transmission of the ECG data online to the base station. This technology was most widely used for routine pacemaker follow-up of a limited ECG sample (29) but also was used to provide a prolonged (5- to 7-minute) ECG sample in specific patient populations under surveillance (30–33). A modification of these devices was the development of noncontinuously applied transtelephonic or solid-state devices with limited solid-state memory (usually $1^1/_2$ to 5 minutes) whose major advantage is the capability of recording a sample of data without the necessity of immediate access to telephone transmission. Patients in the latter instance could apply the device to the precordial area, obtain a recording of ECG data into solid-state memory, and later (when telephonic transmission was available) transmit the ECG data for interpretation. These circumstances facilitated the examination of patients with intermittent or rare symptoms by recording ECG data during symptoms, although it required that the patient was not incapacitated during the symptom and had a reasonable amount of physical dexterity to apply the device.

More recently, continuously applied transtelephonic or solid-state devices are being used to take advantage of a memory loop circuitry through constant examination using applied conventional bipolar electrodes (34–39). Patients wearing such a continuously applied device with "loop" memory, therefore, can activate it, permitting recording of stored data before the event (typically 1 to 4 minutes) and after the event (30 to 60 seconds) (35–38). Later, the patient can send the ECG recording to the base station printout recorder by means of telephone transmission for interpretation or it may be printed on a standard ECG machine or automatically stored on a microcomputer for later review (24–26). Because such devices continuously have the ECG in memory before activation, they are excellent for documenting transient symptomatic or incapacitating events and displaying the antecedent onset and offset of a paroxysmal cardiac arrhythmic event. This technology seeks to limit the necessity of rapid manual dexterity, such as that required with applied precordial devices, and is more suitable for persons who are physically distraught or incapacitated by their symptoms or who have limited manual dexterity (Fig.6.1-8). Proponents of such technology indicate that 95% of calls for symptoms suspicious for transient cardiac rhythm disturbances occur within 4 weeks, with documentation of serious arrhythmias (52%) and the recurrence of symptoms (70%) most common in the first week of examination (39). Nevertheless, there are some practical limitations of the technology because of patient error or device malfunction (35). Whereas 25% of patients with recurrent syncope obtained diagnostic benefit, it was recognized that 20% of patients were noncompliant, and appreciable difficulties of cognitive implementation were present in some patients (particularly the elderly) (35).

The latest innovation of this technology uses a readily available wrist recorder, whose circuitry is completed by contact of the index finger and thumb or hand contact to the opposite wrist. This action results in the loop storage

(retrospective and prospective time) of a 4- to 5-minute ECG sample of lead I and permits direct printout or transtelephonic transmission (40). Another innovation of this technology is the ability to transmit the stored data by telephone directly to a facsimile machine. This avoids the necessity of a "base station" and provides the capability of telephone transfer to virtually any location. This important adaptation permits ready and direct access to responsible medical personnel or the managing physician.

It is important to appreciate that transtelephonic technology is also growing as a result of increasing interest from electrophysiologists who see patients for whom the cause of recurrent syncope remains unknown after electrophysiologic studies or tilt table testing (41). Current evidence indicates that intermittent loop ECG recorders are the examination of choice in patients with recurrent or unexplained syncope who have undergone previous clinical and ambulatory ECG examination without occurrence of symptoms or disclosure of an etiologic ECG abnormality (34–38) (Fig. 6.1-8). On the other hand, their use as a primary form of ambulatory ECG examination to replace the 24-hour continuous ambulatory ECG as the initial examination has not currently been established and is to be avoided (42).

Although there is one relatively small randomized clinical trial comparing the technologies of ambulatory ECG with transtelephonic monitoring in a specific population (43), several contrasts derived from the literature are apparent (Table 6.1-1). These technologies do not compete against each other but are complementary. When the history and physical examination, aided by a standard ECG, does not disclose the diagnosis of a suspected cardiac arrhythmia, a continuous 24-hour ambulatory ECG is obtained. Further diagnostic tests including transtelephonic loop recording or long-term surveillance may be indicated, depending on the nature and frequency of the complaint. Transtelephonic recording has a value in the follow-up of patients treated with antiarrhythmic drugs as a method for intermittent evaluation of drug efficacy during a long time.

Implantable Loop Recorders

A recent innovation in loop recorders for prolonged examination led to the development of a recorder, smaller than a pack of gum, which is inserted just beneath the skin in the upper chest area in a brief outpatient procedure (44). The device is capable of continuously recording the ECG for up to 14 months. The patient places a hand-held pager-like device over the loop recorder after any event (including syncope) and presses a button to retain the data in the hand-held device. The physician then analyzes this information, which is stored on a solid-state Flash card, by printout to real-time ECG. Early experience has been reported in 24 patients with recurrent unexplained syncope, negative tilt and electrophysiologic testing; 21 patients had recurrent syncope 5 months after device implantation and 18 had a

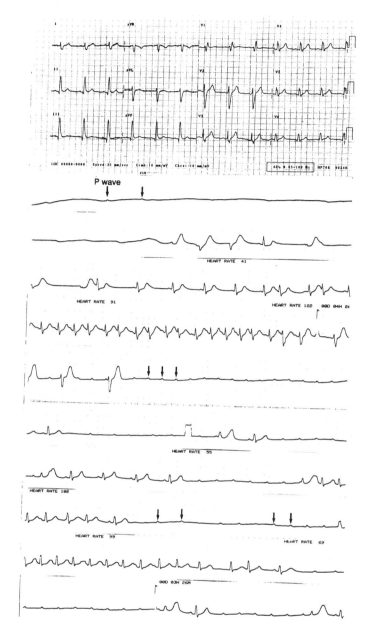

FIGURE 6.1-8. Recordings of a recently referred 67-year-old white man with 14 episodes of recurrent syncope during a 3-year period who had undergone cardiologic evaluation of echocardiography, exercise testing, and 24-hour ambulatory electrocardiography. During the initial 30 days of transtelephonic monitoring, the present episode was recorded. The patient received a DDD pacemaker.

treatable diagnosis (44). The long-term merit of this approach is yet to be determined.

Ambulatory ECG for Arrhythmia Diagnosis

Ambulatory ECG is the most widely employed technology to evaluate the patient with symptoms suggestive of a car-

diac arrhythmia. Although clinical experience has shown that cardiac ECG abnormalities are often associated with such complaints, it is imperative to correlate the ECG rhythm recorded simultaneously with the occurrence of such symptoms. Ambulatory (Holter) ECG is the most commonly used technology to evaluate such patient symptoms, often for extended periods of monitoring. The type of ambulatory ECG technology employed depends on the

TABLE 6.1-1. TECHNICAL AND CLINICAL DIFFERENCES OF AMBULATORY ECG AND TRANSTELEPHONIC LOOP RECORDER

	Ambulatory ECG	Transtelephonic Loop
Technical		
ECG data	24 or 48 h of two- or three- channel ECG Continuous ECG data	4–5 min of one-channel ECG Intermittent and patient-activated ECG data Transtelephonic loop recorder
Resources needed	Holter recorder Holter playback analysis system Operator interaction	Telephone communication with audio modem Base station printout recorder (24-h availability) Operator interaction 30-d surveillance—$200–300
Cost	24-h examination—$150–300	Moderate/substantial (sending and recording
Patient participation	Minimal (diary for symptoms)	ECG data)
Clinical		
Indications	To diagnose cardiac arrhythmias with qualitative/ quantitative assessment	To diagnose infrequent or rare cardiac arrhythmias qualitatively only
As first-line diagnostic test	Often	Never
As arrhythmic follow-up	Often	Rarely or special situation (e.g., sudden death cohorts or effects on QT interval)
As pacemaker follow-up	Often	Often

ECG, electrocardiography.

nature of the symptoms (disturbing versus incapacitating), the frequency and duration of the symptom, and the necessity to observe ECG data before and after the compliant (i.e., the onset and offset).

In most instances, all patients benefit from an initial examination with either 24 or 48 hours of continuous ambulatory ECG to examine the underlying cardiac rhythm and assess background arrhythmias or conduction disturbances that may be present. The symptoms that occur can then be readily correlated with the onset and offset of complaints and evaluated for their causal nature. Most often such examinations serve to exclude cardiac arrhythmias as a specific cause of a patient's complaint.

For less frequently occurring symptoms, transtelephonic monitoring (with or without loop memory) may be better suited and more cost-effective for the examination of an intermittent or sporadic complaint. However, if symptoms are severe and potentially life-threatening, such as syncope, presyncope, or sustained lightheadedness, it is probably more appropriate to admit the patient to the hospital for monitoring by telemetry or to use continuous 24- or 48-hour ambulatory ECG examination within the safety of the hospital environment. In these patients, tilt table testing, intracardiac electrophysiologic studies, and exercise testing are used adjunctively with ambulatory ECG and transtelephonic techniques (45–46). On rare occasions, the diagnostic dilemma may require the implantable loop recorder for prolonged chronic monitoring (44).

Many older studies have documented the clinical efficacy of ambulatory ECG in the examination of symptoms, including palpitations, dizziness, presyncope, or syncope (47–52). Approximately 25% to 50% of patients will experience a complaint during a 24-hour ambulatory ECG,

approximately 2% to 15% will have a causal cardiac arrhythmia, and 35% will have a complaint without ECG abnormality (51–53). When the recording is extended to 3 days, half of the patients have symptoms, and if it is extended to 5 to 21 days (mean of 9), 75% have symptoms (53).

Recent attention has been drawn to the differences in complaints between hospital inpatients and outpatients (54). Symptoms from ventricular arrhythmias in 6.3% of 306 hospitalized patients correlated with causal arrhythmias detected by 24-hour ambulatory ECG in 95% (19 of 20 patients); in contrast, complaints occurred in 55% of 278 outpatients and correlated in only 43.5% (67 of 154 patients) (54). Furthermore, Nwasokwa and Wenger (55) showed that in 1,010 hospitalized patients, age, gender, and presenting symptoms predicted the findings of ambulatory ECG. The presenting symptom was such a powerful predictor that patients being examined by ambulatory ECG should be considered in two broad categories: those with or those without syncope. The latter patient group has a consistently higher rate of diary maintenance, of reporting symptoms during ambulatory ECG, and of a conclusive examination (55). Age and gender were relatively unimportant predictors in this group but were quite important for those having syncope. Women younger than 60 years were most likely to maintain diaries and report nonsyncopal symptoms, whereas men older than 60 years being evaluated for syncope were four times less likely to report symptoms or maintain a diary (55).

These data are difficult to interpret because they include various population groups, examined for various durations of time, with varying definitions of ECG abnormalities that were being evaluated for temporal correlation of the symptom. Moreover, detected ECG abnormalities of sinus bradycardias, sinus pauses, supraventricular arrhythmias, and ventricular arrhythmias are known to occur in healthy asymptomatic populations. Therefore, the occurrence of such arrhythmias does not necessarily establish a causal mechanism for a transient disturbance in consciousness. If the presence of symptoms, cardiac arrhythmias, or both are accepted as clinically relevant, a 24-hour ambulatory ECG in all patients with complaints may be diagnostic in 76% (56). In contrast, if detection of temporal concordance of symptoms and cardiac arrhythmias is mandated, ambulatory monitoring is diagnostic in 16% (56).

Kapoor and colleagues reported that demanding temporal correlation between symptoms and ECG findings will underestimate the prevalence of important arrhythmias and will be demonstrated in only 2% to 3% of patients, although arrhythmias as a causal phenomenon during such complaints will be excluded in 20% to 35% of patients (57,58). Kapoor and colleagues (57) correlated detected arrhythmias to ultimate outcome: Patients with frequent and complex ventricular arrhythmias who had syncope experienced a higher incidence of sudden death. Thus, specific therapeutic intervention perhaps should be directed at patients with sustained syncope who have frequent and repetitive ventricular ectopy regardless of whether the ectopy produces symptoms.

Recent data support the value of ambulatory ECG in determining who benefits from electrophysiologic studies for unexplained syncope. Linzer and colleagues. (58) developed a model of clinical characteristics in predicting the outcome of electrophysiologic studies in such patients and validated it in 141 consecutive patients with unexplained syncope (59). A combination of clinical, ECG, and ambulatory ECG findings could predict the outcome of electrophysiologic testing in syncope. In particular, serious ventricular tachyarrhythmias were predicted by the presence of organic heart disease and nonsustained ventricular tachycardia on ambulatory ECG (sensitivity 100%), whereas sinus bradycardia, first-degree heart block, or bundle branch block by ECG were sensitive for bradyarrhythmic outcomes (sensitivity, 79%). Alternatively, bradyarrhythmic "medium-risk" patients could be evaluated noninvasively with long-term loop transtelephonic ambulatory ECG to document the causative event (35,59). Patients with none of the clinical predictors are at almost no risk for a serious ventricular arrhythmia and at very slight risk of a bradyarrhythmia.

Ambulatory ECG is ideally suited for characterizing the qualitative aspects of spontaneous cardiac arrhythmias; various QRS morphologies, "onset and offset" data of various tachyarrhythmias and bradyarrhythmias, coupling intervals, rate dependence, and changes in QT interval provide deductive information concerning site of origin of the arrhythmia or pathway of reentry (60,61). Additionally P-wave presence and axis often render clues to the specific electrophysiologic abnormality and may be particularly aided by a three-channel ambulatory ECG recording (61).

It has been recognized for some time that the 24-hour ambulatory ECG trend provides valuable heart rate data in atrial fibrillation to guide pharmacologic therapy for control of ventricular response or to assess the control of paroxysmal events.

Role of Ambulatory ECG for Risk Assessment

Ambulatory ECG is useful to assess risk associated with cardiac arrhythmias in specific asymptomatic populations, including patients with coronary heart disease, particularly after a myocardial infarction, those with hypertrophic and dilated cardiomyopathy, and apparently healthy persons without evidence of cardiac disease. Conventional 24-hour ambulatory ECG recording is also useful for risk assessment in symptomatic patients presenting with hemodynamically unstable ventricular tachycardia or ventricular fibrillation resulting in sudden death.

Coronary Heart Disease

The Coronary Drug Project and other studies called attention to the prognostic value of frequent and complex ventricular arrhythmias for identifying post–myocardial infarction patients at excess risk of death, including sudden death; complex forms of ventricular arrhythmia in men were associated with a twofold risk of death from all causes and threefold increased risk of sudden death (62–64). Another study found that after a 5-year follow-up, the age-adjusted risk for sudden coronary death in men with ventricular tachycardiac or early cycle beats was four to five times more than that in men without ventricular arrhythmias (65). Although some debate ensued over whether ventricular arrhythmias were an independent variable, further studies unequivocally demonstrated that the frequency and complexity of ventricular arrhythmias detected on ambulatory electrocardiography had independent prognostic risk, which was additive to increased risk of an adverse outcome associated with decreased left ventricular function (66). These data have also been confirmed in the postthrombolytic era (67).

Ambulatory ECG studies of post–myocardial infarction patients have shown that heart rate variability derived from ambulatory monitoring, as measured by the standard deviation of the R-R intervals in sinus rhythm, was a powerful predictor of prognosis, independent of ventricular arrhythmias or left ventricular function (68,69). Patients with decreased heart rate variability have reduced vagal or increased sympathetic tone and may have a higher risk of ventricular fibrillation. Decreased heart rate variability has been identified during ambulatory ECG in patients who experienced sudden death (70,71). A newly described parameter investigated from Holter recordings is heart rate turbulence; this methodology investigates sinus-rhythm cycle length after a single ventricular premature beat (VPB) and characterizes the fluctuations by turbulence onset and slope (72). Using multivariate analysis, heart rate turbulence was found to be in the most powerful stratifier of mortality in EMIAT and the second most powerful stratifier in Multicenter Post Infarction Trial (72). This methodology awaits further evaluation

Cardiomyopathy

Approximately two thirds of patients with hypertrophic cardiomyopathy have frequent and complex ventricular arrhythmias on ambulatory ECG; the presence of ventricular tachycardia, found in approximately 25% of patients, predicts those with subsequent occurrence of sudden death (73,74). There is evidence that amiodarone prevents sudden death in this subset of patients by abolishing ventricular tachycardia as assessed by 48-hour ambulatory ECG (75). However, other data cast doubt on the outcome with ventricular tachycardia suppression while continuing to acknowledge nonsustained ventricular tachycardia as an important risk factor for sudden death (76).

In ischemic or nonischemic dilated cardiomyopathy, complex and frequent ventricular arrhythmias are detected by ambulatory ECG in 80% to 90% of patients, and although some investigators have found that they do not predict prognosis (77), several small prospective follow-up studies have shown that complex or repetitive ventricular

arrhythmias are an independent predictor of sudden death in patients with a dilated cardiomyopathy (78,79). This association appears to be independent of hemodynamic or neuroendocrine variables (79), and sudden death may occur despite a seemingly favorable clinical response to medical therapy (80). These conclusions have been supported by several large clinical trials, which continue to identify repetitive ventricular arrhythmias and nonsustained ventricular tachycardia as independent risk factors of sudden death in this population (80,80a) (Fig. 6.1-9), while other trials have demonstrated only a trend (81). However, establishing a definite relationship is difficult because patients are receiving multiple secondary preventive therapies, which interact with the relationship of sudden death.

Healthy Persons without Heart Disease

As assessed by 24 to 48 hours of continuous ambulatory ECG, ventricular arrhythmias are found in 40% to 75% of normal persons (82–87). The incidence and frequency of ventricular ectopy increase with age, and even frequent and complex forms have been found in 1% to 4% of the general population (85,88); in the absence of structural heart disease, complex ventricular ectopy is not associated with an increased risk and subjects with this arrhythmia have a favorable long-term prognosis (89). This good prognosis was even true in the presence of asymptomatic coronary

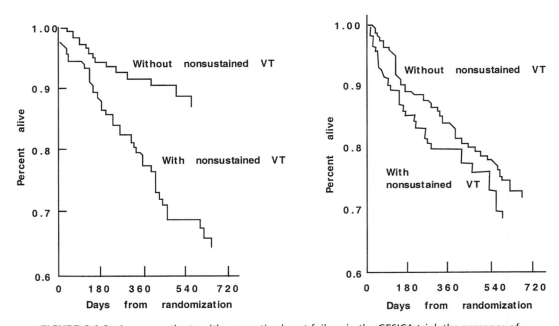

FIGURE 6.1-9. Among patients with congestive heart failure in the GESICA trial, the presence of nonsustained ventricular tachycardia was associated with an increased incidence of sudden cardiac death (*p* = 0.001) (*left panel*) but no change in death from progressive heart failure (*right panel*). (From Doval HC, Nul DR, Grancelli HO, et al, for the GESICA-GEMA Investigators. Nonsustained ventricular tachycardia in severe heart failure. Independent marker of increased mortality due to sudden death. *Circulation* 1996;94:3198, with permission.)

artery disease, but not when there was an unrecognized myocardial infarction (89).

Symptomatic Ventricular Tachycardia or Ventricular Fibrillation

An increasing number of patients have been resuscitated from sudden cardiac death from ventricular tachycardia or ventricular fibrillation; many have severe coronary artery disease that predisposes to recurrent symptomatic ventricular tachycardia and a decreased long-term survival rate when they are untreated or are treated empirically, (90,91). Studies have shown that when antiarrhythmic therapy abolishes repetitive ventricular activity on ambulatory ECG and exercise testing long-term survival is excellent, and there is a 2.3% annual mortality rate. In contrast, when advanced ventricular arrhythmias cannot be controlled, the annual mortality rate is 52.5% (15,92). Similar observations were noted by Hoffman and colleagues (93) in patients with chronic coronary artery disease and frequent and complex ventricular ectopy, but without malignant ventricular arrhythmias. In light of the findings of the ESVEM Study (12–14), ambulatory ECG appeared to be the first-line method of assessment in this population. However, today, patients with sustained symptomatic ventricular tachycardia or ventricular fibrillation are immediately identified as candidates for the internal cardioverter-defibrillator device. Thus, the use of ambulatory ECG in this population is no longer indicated.

Evaluation of Therapeutic Intervention

Ambulatory ECG has proven valuable for evaluating various therapies used to treat cardiac arrhythmias. Most commonly, an assessment of antiarrhythmic drug therapy and pacemaker function are the major indications for ambulatory ECG.

Antiarrhythmic Drug Therapy

When serious or potentially lethal ventricular arrhythmias are discovered on ambulatory monitoring in a patient with underlying organic heart disease, physicians may treat such arrhythmias with antiarrhythmic drugs in the hope of altering an adverse prognosis. However, several pitfalls developed in this approach.

It was observed that there is a great deal of spontaneous variability of arrhythmias within each individual. Early observations described spontaneous changes in ventricular arrhythmia frequency and complexity and found that arrhythmic efficacy had to be defined by a certain percentage reduction in spontaneous arrhythmia that would account for this variability (94,95). Further, it was discovered that 25% to 27% of patients with benign and potentially lethal ventricular arrhythmia would have spontaneous resolution of ventricular arrhythmias after 12 to 17 months

of antiarrhythmic therapy, therefore not requiring long-term therapy (96). This variability of ventricular arrhythmia was found to be time dependent and greater in patients with low-density ventricular arrhythmias, coronary artery disease, or frequent ventricular tachycardia runs (97,98).

Follow-up Holter monitoring of patients being treated with antiarrhythmic drug therapy showed that there were frequent episodes during which there was a transient loss of antiarrhythmic efficacy criteria, the development of late proarrhythmia, and the spontaneous resolution of ventricular arrhythmias during therapy (99–101). These factors have tempered the clinician's casualness in prescribing antiarrhythmic drug therapy.

More recently the multicenter Cardiac Arrhythmia Suppression Trial (CAST) (10,11) and the Survival With Oral d-Sotalol (SWORD) Trial (102) have cast doubt on the merit of the antiarrhythmic drug suppression of ventricular arrhythmia in post–myocardial infarction patients, as therapy with encainide, flecainide, moricizine, and d-sotalol was associated with an increased rate of cardiac and arrhythmic mortality compared with that of patients receiving placebo (Figs. 6.1-10 and 6.1-11). Other clinical trials employing amiodarone also failed to demonstrate the merit of suppressing ventricular arrhythmias in post–myocardial infarction patients (16,17). Nevertheless, the conventional 24- to 48-hour ambulatory ECG examination remains the mainstay of assessing the suppression of spontaneous arrhythmia, based on a reduction of the number of VPBs by 70% to 90% and elimination of all repetitive forms (runs and couplets).

In addition, transtelephonic monitoring has been used to evaluate antiarrhythmic therapy (102–105) and has been extended to provide "surveillance" of specific high-risk subgroups (106). Although studies exist that substantiate the value of transtelephonic monitoring in antiarrhythmic drug assessment programs, these trials were not directed at specific high-risk subgroups and the value of transtelephonic monitoring in such patients is uncertain (107,108).

Evaluation of Pacemakers

It is estimated that about 90% of pacemaker patients are followed by their private physician or pacemaker surveillance service (109). With the emergence of pacemaker and automatic implantable cardioverter-defibrillator (ICD) technology in recent years, the need for a dedicated cardiac pacemaker follow-up clinic has become apparent (110). Digital counters, exercise testing (for rate-response pacing), transtelephonic surveillance (111,112), and ambulatory ECG (113–115) proved valuable in the assessment of pacemaker function. Although special pacemaker and ICD interrogative devices, which use telemetry interrogation of software programs contained within the pacemaker, can assess myriad electrical parameters indicating proper pacemaker function, the use of ambulatory ECG does increase the diagnosis of pacemaker malfunction by

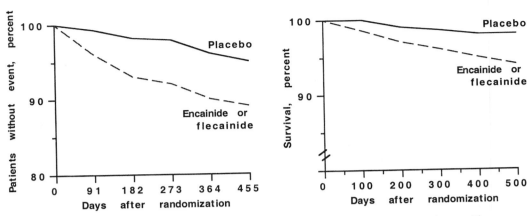

FIGURE 6.1-10. Results of the Cardiac Arrhythmia Suppression Trial (CAST) in patients with ventricular premature beats after myocardial infarction. When compared with patients receiving placebo, patients receiving encainide or flecainide had a significantly lower rate of avoiding a cardiac event (death or resuscitated cardiac arrest) (*left panel*) (p = 0.001) and a lower overall survival rate (*right panel*) p = 0.00006. The cause of death was arrhythmia or cardiac arrest. (From Echt DS, Liebson PR, Mitchell B, et al. *N Engl J Med* 1991;324:781, with permission.)

examining the patient for 24 hours or more during daily activities. Enhanced detection of pacemaker dysfunction by ambulatory ECG has proven valuable in the early postimplant period compared with in-hospital telemetry monitoring and has allowed therapeutic intervention before patient discharge (114). The increased diagnostic yield associated with ambulatory ECG is not simply related to the more prolonged time of examination but has been facilitated by Holter technology that permits detection and recognition of the pacing stimulus artifact with amplification and recording of it on a separate dedicated channel (116). Thus, information concerning failure to capture, failure to sense, failure of output, the number of

pacing stimuli, and the percentage of beats paced are all provided by the current ambulatory ECG assessment of pacemaker function.

Holter technology has proven to be a valuable aid in the visual interpretation of ECGs from dual-chamber pacemakers. To date, only the conventional continuous Holter recordings have enjoyed success in such applications. The use of routine transtelephonic transmissions is now part of the official recommendations of pacemaker follow-up, as indicated by the policy conference of the North American Society of Pacing and Electrophysiology (117). Such transtelephonic devices most commonly assess pacemaker rate but on modern programmable mod-

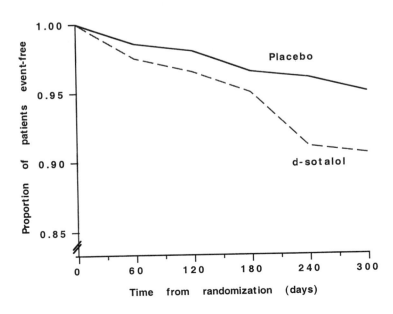

FIGURE 6.1-11. Results from the Survival With Oral d-Sotalol (SWORD) trial. The administration of d-sotalol to patients with an ejection fraction of 40% or less after either recent myocardial infarction (MI) or after symptomatic heart failure with a remote (less than 42 days) MI was associated with increased mortality rate, compared with placebo (5% versus 3.1%). The excess number of deaths was presumed to be primarily the result of arrhythmias. (From Waldo AL, Camm AJ, DeRuyter H, et al. *Lancet* 1996;348:7, with permission.)

els may allow varying forms of interrogation. Despite these advantages, Holter technology has lagged behind pacemaker technology.

ROLE OF EXERCISE TESTING IN ARRHYTHA MANAGEMENT

Exercise testing is a well-established technique that is valuable for the evaluation of patients with heart disease, providing important information about dynamic cardiac function. Although most often used in the evaluation of coronary artery disease, exercise testing produces a number of physiologic changes that have a role in arrhythmia management, particularly in the evaluation of antiarrhythmic drugs action (Table 6.1-2).

1. Exercise testing may be important and necessary for exposing the clinical arrhythmia, particularly in a small but important subset of patients with a history of a sustained tachyarrhythmia that cannot be induced in the electrophysiologic laboratory or documented on ambulatory monitoring.
2. It is an adjunctive technique used with ambulatory monitoring or electrophysiologic testing for evaluating and managing the patient with a history of supraventricular or ventricular arrhythmia, particularly in the selection of an antiarrhythmic drug. It has an important role in evaluating rate control in atrial fibrillation and for establishing the rate cutoff for an ICD by identifying the maximum sinus rate achieved during physical activity.
3. Exercise testing may have a role for aiding in the stratification of patients with heart disease in whom the risk of sudden cardiac death is increased, particularly those with a recent myocardial infarction.
4. Exercise testing may also be of use for those patients with transient symptoms, suggesting arrhythmia in whom other techniques fail to document a cause.
5. Perhaps the most important role for exercise testing is in the evaluation of both the beneficial and the possible harmful effects of antiarrhythmic drugs.

TABLE 6.1-2. USES OF EXERCISE TESTING IN ARRHYTHMIA EVALUATION AND MANAGEMENT

1. Provocation of arrhythmia
2. Evaluation of antiarrhythmic drug efficacy
3. Exposure of harmful drug effects
   a. Negative inotropy
   b. Conduction abnormalities
   c. Arrhythmia aggravation
4. Prognostication—establish risk of an arrhythmic event
5. Rate control in atrial fibrillation

Physiologic Effects of Exercise

Exercise results in a number of physiologic changes, particularly involving the autonomic nervous system. There is withdrawal of vagal tone and more importantly activation of the sympathetic nervous system and an increase in circulating catecholamines (118) (Fig. 6.1-12). This results in an increase in heart rate, systolic blood pressure, and myocardial contractility or inotropy, all of which cause an increase in myocardial oxygen demand, provoking myocardial ischemia in patients with coronary artery disease.

Biochemical Changes

Ischemia causes myocardial acidosis and electrolyte shifts, particularly the development of extracellular hyperkalemia. These pH and electrolyte abnormalities alter the electrophysiologic properties of the membrane:

1. The resting membrane potential becomes less negative, resulting in a slowing of action potential generation and impulse conduction velocity.
2. Refractoriness is decreased.
3. Automaticity is enhanced.

Changes in these parameters affect the basic mechanisms responsible for arrhythmogenesis, such as reentry, triggered automaticity, and enhanced automaticity (119). Moreover, because ischemia and the resulting changes are not uniform, electrophysiologic heterogeneity is increased, providing the appropriate milieu for arrhythmia.

Mechanical Effects

Sympathetic stimulation produces a direct positive inotropic effect, which can cause mechanical changes on the myocardium and an increase in myocardial wall stress

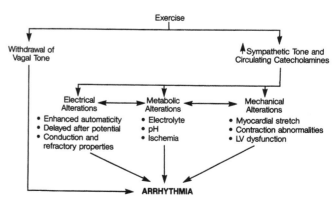

FIGURE 6.1-12. Scheme of physiologic changes produced by exercise. The primary effect is activation of the sympathetic nervous system and an increase in circulating catecholamines. This results in electrical, metabolic, and mechanical changes that are important in arrhythmogenesis.

and tension, changes that along with ischemia can provoke regional myocardial dysfunction and contraction abnormalities, as well as increase myocardial stretch; it has been well documented that there is a mechanoelectrical effect; that is, stretch results in an increased membrane automaticity and changes in myocardial refractoriness and conduction (120).

Hemodynamic Changes

Sympathetic stimulation may produce regional differences in blood flow and oxygen delivery, resulting in localized or regional shifts in electrolytes and changes in pH level, even in the absence of coronary artery disease (121). During exercise, there is the potential for enhancement of these differences of blood flow and possible ischemia, even in the healthy heart, although this is more pronounced in the presence of heart disease (122).

A decrease in coronary artery perfusion pressure produces a more profound reduction of blood flow and oxygen supply to the endocardial layer compared with that to the epicardium; therefore, differences in pH levels, electrolyte levels, and oxygen delivery may develop not only between ischemic and nonischemic tissue, but also between the endocardial and epicardial layers within an ischemic region (122,123). The heterogeneity between adjacent areas as well as nonuniformity between endocardial and epicardial layers could produce an appropriate precondition for reentry, the most important mechanism for arrhythmia.

Electrophysiologic Effects

Activation of the sympathetic nervous system and an increase in circulating catecholamine levels can directly affect the mechanisms responsible for arrhythmogenesis. Catecholamines shorten membrane refractory periods and increase myocardial conduction velocity. These changes are nonuniform when underlying heart disease is present, as normal and abnormal tissue respond differently and in the presence of regional ischemia and electrolyte and pH abnormalities, the nonuniform changes in these electrophysiologic parameters may be augmented, resulting in even greater myocardial electrophysiologic heterogeneity, an important precondition for reentry (119).

Sympathetic stimulation also causes an increase in spontaneous automaticity of the membrane by increasing the rate of phase 4 spontaneous depolarization. This enhanced automaticity may be particularly pronounced in diseased myocardial tissue that already exhibits underlying abnormal automaticity (124). Finally, sympathetic stimulation increases the influx of calcium ions, thereby increasing the amplitude of delayed afterpotentials, which may result in triggered automaticity (125).

Incidence of Arrhythmia during Exercise

Ventricular Arrhythmia

Ventricular arrhythmia, particularly VPBs, is commonly seen during exercise testing. The type and frequency of ventricular arrhythmia provoked by exercise are related to the presence and extent of underlying heart disease (126–134) (Table 6.1-3). Similar to the data obtained from ambulatory monitoring, the occurrence of ventricular arrhythmia is also directly related to age. The recognition of arrhythmia, particularly of repetitive forms including couplets and runs of nonsustained ventricular tachycardia, is enhanced with the use of continuous monitoring during the test (126).

TABLE 6.1-3. PREVALENCE OF VENTRICULAR ARRHYTHMIA DURING EXERCISE—PERCENTAGE WITH ARRHYTHMIA

Study	Simple VPBs		Repetitive VPBs	
	Normal	Heart Disease	Normal	Heart Disease
Beard and Owen (127)	8.0		0.3	
Master (128)	18.0		0.3	15.0
Whinnery (129)	5.0	50.0	0	22.0
McHenry and colleagues (130)	34.0	50.0	6.0	31.0
Poblete and colleagues (131)	7.0	62.0	0	20.0
Ryan and colleagues (133)		55.0		
Gaoch and McConnell (134)		45.0		
Califf and colleagues (137)	14.0	23.0	2.4	8.2
Weiner and colleagues (138)		19.0		
Detry and colleagues (141)				0.58[a]
Jelinek and Lown (132)	19.0	36.0	1.8	3.6

VPB, ventricular premature beats.
[a]Ventricular tachycardia or ventricular fibrillation.

Age and sex, independent of underlying heart disease, are also important factors associated with the prevalence of VPBs during exercise. In one study of 289 healthy men and women, the frequency of VPBs with exercise was 35% among men and 14% in women (135). In patients younger than 30 years, the incidence of exercise-induced ventricular arrhythmia was 18% while 50% of patients older than 50 had ventricular arrhythmia.

An additional factor related to the occurrence of VPBs during exercise is the extent or severity of underlying disease, similar to observations from ambulatory monitoring (136,137). One study, which retrospectively reviewed the data from the Coronary Artery Surgical Study (CASS) of 1,486 patients with coronary artery disease documented by cardiac catheterization, found that VPBs during exercise were observed in only 10% of patients; however, among the 245 patients with minimal coronary disease, only 6.5% had VPBs, and they were documented in 10.5% of 1,241 patients with significant coronary artery disease (136). There was also a relationship between left ventricular function and the presence of VPBs. Among those with minimal coronary artery disease, the average ejection fraction in those with VPBs was 50% versus 64% in patients without VPBs ($p < 0.05$), while in the group with significant coronary artery disease, the occurrence of VPBs was associated with a previous myocardial infarction, a reduced left ventricular ejection fraction, and more extensive coronary artery disease. Other studies have found that the incidence of VPBs is greater in patients with left main or three-vessel coronary disease, in those with more segmental wall motion abnormalities, a greater degree of ST-segment depression during exercise, or more severe defects on thallium imaging (138,139).

Of more concern are complex or repetitive arrhythmias; as with isolated VPBs, there is also an association between exercise-induced repetitive arrhythmia, particularly runs of nonsustained ventricular tachycardia, and age and the presence and extent of heart disease (137,140). Although ambulatory monitoring is a more sensitive method of documenting repetitive arrhythmia, exercise testing is an important adjunct method. The incidence of repetitive arrhythmia in healthy patients ranges from 1.5% to 6%. In contrast, exercise-induced repetitive VPBs, particularly nonsustained ventricular tachycardia, are more frequently seen in patients with heart disease, and the prevalence ranges from 15% to 31% (Table 6.1-3). There is also a relationship with the severity of the underlying disease: Patients with a prior myocardial infarction have more frequent repetitive arrhythmia compared with those patients without a prior infarction.

The occurrence of a serious sustained ventricular tachyarrhythmia during exercise testing is uncommon, even in those patients with underlying heart disease; the reported incidence is less than 1%. When it occurs, it is most often within the first few minutes of recovery (Fig. 6.1-13). One review of data from 7,500 consecutive exercise tests reported that only 6 patients had an episode of ventricular

fibrillation (0.08%) while 40 (0.55%) had ventricular tachyarrhythmia that was sustained in 13 (0.17%) and nonsustained in 27 (0.36%) (141).

In an attempt to establish differences between patients with and without exercise-induced ventricular tachyarrhythmia, one study evaluated clinical, angiographic, and electrophysiologic characteristics of 112 patients with a clinical history of a sustained ventricular arrhythmia, 13% of whom had ventricular tachyarrhythmia during exercise. Five of these patients (group A) had coronary artery disease and four had ventricular tachyarrhythmia induced during electrophysiologic study. No heart disease was documented in 10 patients (group B), and during electrophysiologic study 8 had ventricular tachyarrhythmia induced, but in 4 of these patients, isoproterenol was required (142). It was concluded that in contrast to exercise-induced ventricular tachyarrhythmia in patients with heart disease who have an abnormal substrate, the provocation of this arrhythmia with exercise in those without heart disease is primarily the result of catecholamines. In patients with coronary artery disease, there are no clinical, angiographic, or electrophysiologic

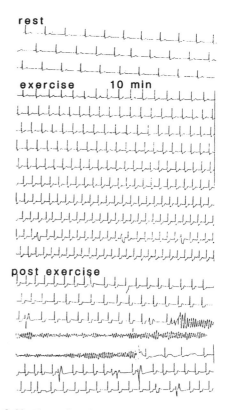

FIGURE 6.1-13. Example of ventricular fibrillation during exercise testing in an asymptomatic patient with coronary artery disease. The patient exercised for 10 minutes, at which time there was a 2-mm horizontal ST-segment depression. The patient was asymptomatic but stopped for leg fatigue. Within 3 minutes of recovery, spontaneous ventricular fibrillation occurred, requiring defibrillation.

differences between those with or without exercise-induced ventricular tachyarrhythmia.

All forms of exercise-induced ventricular arrhythmia are more common in patients who have experienced a clinical episode of a sustained ventricular tachyarrhythmia or sudden cardiac death. Each of these patients, regardless of the presence or extent of heart disease, will have VPBs during exercise testing, and approximately 50% to 75% will have repetitive forms (143,144). Although ambulatory monitoring is a more sensitive method for exposing repetitive ventricular arrhythmia, particularly nonsustained ventricular tachycardia, approximately 10% of patients with a clinical history of a spontaneous episode of serious sustained ventricular tachyarrhythmia will have sustained or nonsustained ventricular tachyarrhythmia exposed only during exercise testing, although no arrhythmia is documented on ambulatory monitoring (145). In some of these patients, arrhythmia cannot be induced with electrophysiologic testing and it is likely that in these patients, the arrhythmia is largely the result of enhanced sympathetic stimulation and elevated levels of circulating catecholamines. Often these patients have no heart disease present. A sustained ventricular tachyarrhythmia occurring during exercise is also more frequent in those patients with a clinical history of such arrhythmia.

Supraventricular Arrhythmia

Supraventricular arrhythmia during exercise is fairly common; most frequently observed are atrial or junctional premature beats and their frequency ranges from 3% to 27% (Table 6.1-4) (127–130,132,134). The occurrence of supraventricular premature beats is associated with the presence of heart disease and is 40% and 5% in those with or without heart disease, respectively. There is also an association with age and they are present in 6% of those 25 to 34 years of age and in 14% of those 45 to 54.

Although premature beats are commonly observed during exercise testing, a sustained supraventricular tachyarrhythmia is infrequent; in patients without heart disease, supraventricular tachycardia is provoked during exercise in up to 3% while atrial fibrillation is observed in up to 1%

(Table 6.1-4) (127,128,132,134). A sustained supraventricular arrhythmia is more commonly induced by exercise in patients with a history of such arrhythmia and up to 14% of such patients have a sustained arrhythmia with exercise (Fig. 6.1-14) (146).

Prognostic Significance of Ventricular Arrhythmia during Exercise Testing

Although most data regarding the prognostic significance of VPBs in patients with heart disease are based on studies using ambulatory monitoring to document their presence, there are some data about the prognostic importance of exercise-induced ventricular arrhythmia in patients with coronary artery disease, particularly those with a recent myocardial infarction; data in other groups of patients are lacking.

In patients with a recent myocardial infarction, the first-year mortality rate is 12% among patients with VPBs induced by exercise compared with a 4% incidence of death in those with VPBs present at rest but not during exercise; mortality rate was 16% among the group of patients with VPBs observed both at rest and with exercise (147). In a study of 667 patients with a recent myocardial infarction, the presence of any VPB during low-level exercise testing increased the first-year mortality rate from 3% to 7% ($p <$ 0.05), whereas exercise-induced couplets increased the mortality rate threefold, from 4% to 13% ($p <$ 0.05) (148). In another study of 163 patients with an uncomplicated myocardial infarction, the presence of VPBs during exercise was the only exercise-related variable associated with an increased risk of sudden death (149).

A similar relationship between arrhythmia during exercise and mortality has also been reported in patients with chronic coronary artery disease who have not had a myocardial infarction, although this association is uncertain (136,138) (Table 6.1-5). The prognostic importance of exercise-induced VPBs is primarily associated with evidence of ischemia, as indicated by ST-segment changes; in patients with coronary artery disease without ST-segment depression, the 1-year mortality rate was 2% in the absence of VPBs, 15% with simple VPBs, and 29% in the presence of repeti-

TABLE 6.1-4. PREVALENCE OF SUPRAVENTRICULAR ARRHYTHMIA DURING EXERCISE TESTING—PERCENTAGE WITH ARRHYTHMIA

Study	Simple	Supraventricular Tachycardia	Atrial fibrillation
Beard and Owen (127)	2.5	0.1	
Master (128)	4.8		0.3
Jelinek and Lown (132)	17.7	2.2	1.1
McHenry and colleagues (130)	10.0		
Whinnery (129)	27.0		
Gooch and McConnell (134)		2.8	0.3
Graboys and Wright (146)		0.8	0.1

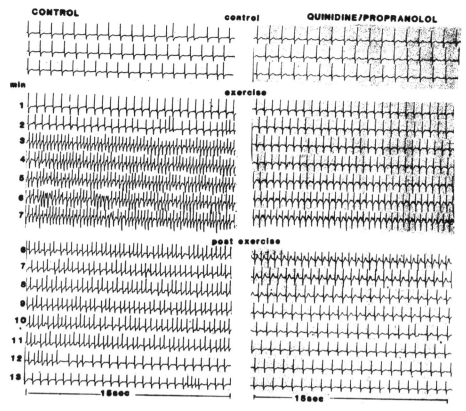

FIGURE 6.1-14. Use of exercise testing in the treatment of atrial fibrillation. During the base-line, the patient developed atrial fibrillation after 3 minutes of exercise. A second exercise test during therapy with quinidine and propranolol failed to induce atrial fibrillation.

TABLE 6.1-5. PROGNOSTIC SIGNIFICANCE OF EXERCISE-INDUCED VENTRICULAR PREMATURE BEATS

Study	Population	Followup (y)	No VPBs	Simple VPBs	Complex VPBs	Significant
Califf and colleagues (137)	Normal	3.0	0	0	0	No
Califf and colleagues	CAD	3.0	10	17	25	Yes
Weiner and colleagues (138)	Significant CAD	4.3	11	13	?	No
	Minimal CAD	5.0	2	9	?	No
Udall and Ellestad (150)	CAD (−ST)	1	2	15	29	Yes
	CAD(+ST)	1	10	33	42	Yes
Weld and colleagues (147)	PostMI	1	4	12	?	Yes
Krone and colleagues (148)	PostMI	1	3	7	13	Yes
Henry and colleagues (149)	PostMI	2	8	25	?	Yes
Graboys and colleagues (143)	SCD survivors	2.5	?	2.3	43.6	Yes

CAD, coronary artery disease; MI, myocardial infarction; SCD, sudden cardiac death; +ST, ST segment depression; −ST, no ST segment changes; VPBs, ventricular premature beats; ?, no data available.

tive or complex VPBs (150). In contrast, the 1-year mortality rate in those with coronary disease with ST-segment depression during exercise testing was 10% when VPBs were absent, 33% when simple VPBs were provoked, and 42% with complex VPBs. In another study of 620 patients with coronary artery disease who underwent cardiac catheterization, the annual mortality rate during a 3-year follow-up was 25% in those with repetitive arrhythmia provoked by exercise testing, compared with a 17% yearly mortality rate in patients with simple VPBs and 10% in those without exercise-induced arrhythmia (137). In contrast, there was no cardiac mortality among 673 patients without heart disease regardless of the presence, type, or frequency of ventricular arrhythmia induced during exercise testing.

Reproducibility of Exercise-Induced Arrhythmia

One of the major problems limiting the use of noninvasive methods for arrhythmia assessment and management is the lack of reproducibility in the occurrence, frequency, and type of VPBs. Although such spontaneous variability has most often been reported when ambulatory monitoring is used to document arrhythmia, some studies have found substantial random variability and a lack of reproducibility of VPBs during exercise testing (151–153). However, the reproducibility of exercise-induced VPBs tends to be greater in patients with underlying cardiovascular disease (154,155). Age may also be a factor related to reproducibility of arrhythmia during exercise.

It has been observed that all forms of VPBs, including repetitive forms, are more frequently induced during exercise testing in patients with a previous history of a sustained ventricular arrhythmia and that all forms of exercise-induced arrhythmia are highly reproducible; in one study, 78% of patients with a clinical history of sustained ventricular tachyarrhythmia or ventricular fibrillation had all forms of ventricular arrhythmia reproducibly induced (155).

There are no data regarding the reproducibility of supraventricular arrhythmia. Based on ambulatory monitoring, supraventricular premature beats are very variable, and their presence and frequency vary greatly from hour to hour and day to day. Likewise, the provocation of a sustained supraventricular tachyarrhythmia during exercise is not reproducible, which is not unexpected given the sporadic clinical occurrence of these arrhythmias.

Use of Exercise Testing for Management of Patients with Ventricular Arrhythmia

Exercise testing has an important adjunctive role in the management of patients with a ventricular tachyarrhythmia, regardless of whether noninvasive ambulatory monitoring or invasive electrophysiologic testing is used as the primary method for selecting an effective antiarrhythmic drug (Fig. 6.1-15). Exercise testing produces important physiologic changes that affect the myocardium and may alter or modulate the frequency and type of spontaneous VPBs (the triggers) or the properties and stability of the substrate (the reentrant circuit) (Fig. 6.1-1). These changes may play a role in the exposure of arrhythmia, but more importantly, exercise testing and the resulting physiologic electrical, mechanical, and metabolic effects have important implications with regard to antiarrhythmic drug therapy. The changes produced by exercise testing—particularly the increase in sympathetic tone, the elevated circulating catecholamine levels, and the metabolic changes of potassium, other electrolytes, pH, and oxygen supply—may interact with, negate, or enhance antiarrhythmic drug activity, possibly resulting in arrhythmia recurrence or aggravation.

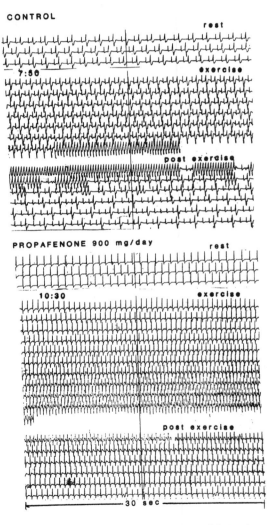

FIGURE 6.1-15. Use of exercise testing as a guide to drug selection. Before therapy, the rhythm was sinus with ventricular bigeminy. Exercise provoked runs of nonsustained ventricular tachycardia at rates of 220 beats per minute. With propafenone therapy, arrhythmia was abolished.

One group of patients for whom exercise testing is particularly important are those who have experienced a serious sustained ventricular tachyarrhythmia (ventricular tachycardia or ventricular fibrillation), as the selection of a drug that is effective under various conditions is critical. In one study of 123 patients presenting with a serious ventricular tachyarrhythmia who underwent noninvasive testing for the selection of an effective antiarrhythmic drug, the continued presence of runs of nonsustained ventricular tachycardia during exercise testing, even if absent on monitoring, was associated with a significantly higher annual mortality rate, compared with the mortality rate for patients in whom such forms were absent during exercise and monitoring after antiarrhythmic drug therapy (156).

Catecholamines and Antiarrhythmic Drugs

Exercise testing is an important adjunctive method, used along with either ambulatory monitoring or electrophysiologic study, as it provides important information about antiarrhythmic drug activity that is complementary to information derived from other tests. Activation of the sympathetic nervous system and an increase in circulating catecholamines during exercise are factors that may have an impact on antiarrhythmic drug action. Antiarrhythmic drugs produce a decrease in membrane conductivity, prolongation of membrane refractory period, a reduction in excitability, and a decrease in membrane automaticity (157). In contrast, administration of catecholamines results in a shortening of the refractory period, an increase in membrane excitability, an increase in membrane conductivity, and an augmentation in automaticity, changes that are in direct opposition to those caused by antiarrhythmic drugs (158) (Fig. 6.1-16). Therefore, catecholamines may interfere with and negate the action of antiarrhythmic drugs by reversing their beneficial effects.

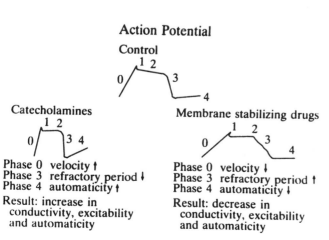

FIGURE 6.1-16. Electrophysiologic actions of antiarrhythmic drugs and catecholamines. The effects of catecholamines are in contrast to the depressive actions of the membrane active agents.

There are a number of studies evaluating the interaction between catecholamines and antiarrhythmic drugs in which electrophysiologic techniques were used to identify an effective drug that prevented the induction of a sustained ventricular tachyarrhythmia or supraventricular tachycardia (Table 6.1-6) (159–165). In approximately 50% of patients, the clinical arrhythmia was reinduced with electrophysiologic testing when catecholamines were infused, confirming that they negated or reversed antiarrhythmic drug action, resulting in drug inefficacy. During follow-up of patients in whom arrhythmia was reinduced during the catecholamine infusion, there was a significant recurrence rate of the clinical arrhythmia despite the use of an antiarrhythmic drug initially identified as being effective by electrophysiologic techniques. Because exercise testing is a physiologic way of activating the sympathetic nervous system and increasing circulating catecholamines, it is a logical and important method for providing a complete evaluation of antiarrhythmic drug action, yielding data that are complimentary to those derived from either monitoring or electrophysiologic testing (166).

Exercise Testing and Exposure of Drug-Related Toxicity

Exercise testing is of major importance for exposing potential toxic effects of antiarrhythmic agents. The degree of conduction slowing produced by these drugs varies among these agents and the reduction of impulse conduction is rate dependent; that is, the depressive effects on conduction are more pronounced at rapid heart rates (167,168). This property is known as *use dependency* (or rate dependency) and exercise testing is an important technique for establishing the degree of use dependency and may expose potentially harmful effects of these agents on atrioventricular or intraventricular conduction, presenting as a rate-related prolongation of PR or QRS intervals and, not infrequently, a new right or left bundle branch block (Fig. 6.1-17). In some cases, this rate-dependent slowing of conduction may cause complete blockade of impulse conduction through the atrioventricular node, resulting in complete heart block. The development of ventricular tachyarrhythmia with exercise is observed in patients with the greatest degree of rate-related increase in QRS duration.

In a drug-free state, the increase in heart rate occurring with exercise decreases the time for membrane repolarization and the QT interval usually shortens, a result of sympathetic stimulation and increased catecholamine levels. The effect of heart rate on the QT interval may be significantly blunted by antiarrhythmic drugs, and there may be a paradoxical prolongation in repolarization time and the QT interval; another factor that may be responsible for arrhythmogenesis or arrhythmia aggravation, specifically torsade de pointes. It has been observed that patients with a prolonged QT syndrome (Romano-Ward syndrome or Jervell and Lange-Nielsen syndrome) who have an abnormally prolonged time for mem-

TABLE 6.1-6. EFFECT OF CATECHOLAMINE INFUSION ON ANTIARRHYTHMIC DRUG EFFICACY

Study	N	Arrhythmia	Drug	Reinducible with Catecholamine		Recurrence in Follow-Up of Those Reducible	Recurrence in Follow-Up of Those not Reducible
						(%)	
Morady and colleagues (164)	21	VT	Quinidine	10	(48)	NR[a]	NR
Jozayeri and colleagues (160)	17	VT	1A, 1C	10	(59)	3 (30)	0/7
Niazi and colleagues (163)	16	SVT	Encainide	10	(63)	4 (40)	0/6
Brugada and colleagues (165)	10	SVT	Amiodarone	10	(100)	NR	NR
Helmy	10	SVT	Flecainide	5	(50)	3 (60)	0/5
Dubuc	37	SVT	1A, 1C	16	(43)	9 (56)	2/21 (10)
Akhtar and colleagues (162)	32	SVT	Encainide	20	(63)	8 (40)	0/12
Dongas and colleagues (161)	8	SVT	Procainamide	5	(63)	NR	NR
Cockrell and colleagues (159)	21	SVT	Flecainide	11	(52)	7 (64)	1/10 (10)
Overall	172			97	(56)	34 (47)[b]	3 (5)[c]

VT, ventricular tachyarrythmia; SVT, supraventricular tachycardia.
[a]NR, not reported.
[b]34/72 patients reported.
[c]3/61 patients reported.

brane repolarization at baseline do not have appropriate shortening of the QT interval with exercise (169). It has been suggested that patients with underlying, but not clinically obvious, abnormalities of repolarization and the QT interval may also be at an increased risk for this arrhythmic complication with class Ia drugs and that failure to appropriately shorten the QT interval during exercise may be a marker of patients at risk for this complication (170).

Aggravation of arrhythmia, a frequent and potentially serious complication of antiarrhythmic drugs, may often be exposed by exercise testing in patients with ventricular arrhythmia, even when ambulatory monitoring or electro-

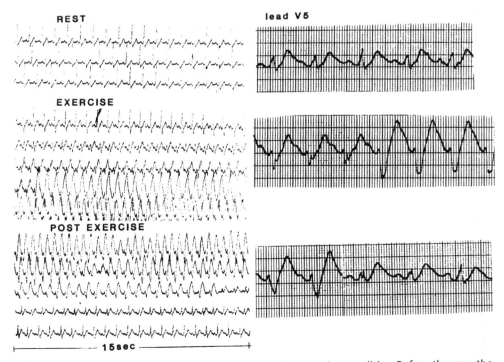

FIGURE 6.1-17. Use of exercise testing to expose conduction abnormalities. Before therapy, the electrocardiogram showed a normal QRS complex at rest and during exercise testing. During therapy with a class Ic antiarrhythmia drug, a rate-related left bundle branch block occurred during exercise.

physiologic testing demonstrate suppression of arrhythmia (Fig. 6.1-18) (171,172). Exercise testing may also be useful for exposing potentially serious ventricular arrhythmia in patients receiving antiarrhythmic drug therapy for suppression of an atrial arrhythmia (173,174).

As previously indicated, there is an increase in sympathetic neural activity and circulating catecholamines and the occurrence of ischemia with exercise; these situations produce changes of extracellular potassium and pH levels that may foster arrhythmia. More importantly, these changes can have an impact on antiarrhythmic drug action. The development of extracellular hyperkalemia and tissue acidosis causes a reduction in resting membrane potential and a slowing of impulse conduction velocity that may exaggerate the depressive effects of antiarrhythmic drugs on conduction, possibly resulting in localized intraventricular block. Ischemia and acidosis may also alter the tissue binding and hence the concentration of these agents, further modifying their electrophysiologic actions. In contrast, hypokalemia, which may be a result of circulating catecholamines and activation of β_2-mediated insulin secretion (175), causes a shortening of the refractory period and an increase in membrane excitability, hence reversing the prolongation of refractoriness and the reduction in excitability produced by antiarrhythmic drugs.

Each of the antiarrhythmic drugs is negatively inotropic and has the potential to depress left ventricular contractility and provoke congestive heart failure (176). Unfortunately, the left ventricular ejection fraction measured at rest may not demonstrate any significant drug-induced change; the resting ejection fraction is therefore an unreliable method for predicting whether the patient is at risk for this complication. However, it is possible that determination of the left ventricular ejection fraction during exercise will be more useful, as the effects of ischemia and catecholamines may exacerbate the negative inotropic effect of these agents (177).

Use of Exercise Testing for the Management of Supraventricular Arrhythmia

Supraventricular tachyarrhythmia is infrequently provoked by exercise, and its reproducibility during exercise is poor. However, if the tachyarrhythmia is reproducibly induced,

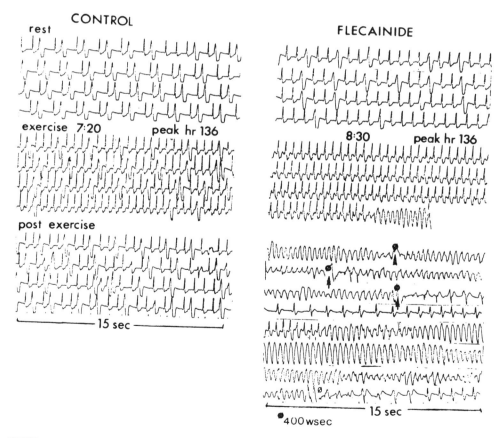

FIGURE 6.1-18. Arrhythmia aggravation exposed by exercise testing. Before therapy, there were brief episodes of nonsustained ventricular tachycardia. During therapy with flecainide, a class Ic antiarrhythmic agent, sustained ventricular tachycardia, and ventricular fibrillation resulting in collapse were provoked. Defibrillation was required.

exercise testing is a useful tool for its management (Fig. 6.1-14). Repetitive exercise testing during an antiarrhythmic drug administration is an effective method for determining drug effect and for establishing an effective program for control.

Role in Atrial Fibrillation

Exercise testing has an important role in the management of patients with chronic atrial fibrillation, primarily for establishing the ventricular rate during activity that is dependent on the state of the atrioventricular node and its electrophysiologic properties (178–180). An important element in the management of patients with chronic atrial fibrillation is slowing of the heart rate by impairing impulse conduction through the atrioventricular node. During any form of exercise, atrioventricular nodal conduction is enhanced and heart rate becomes increased, often to an excessively high level (181) (Fig. 6.1-19). Drugs that block atrioventricular nodal impulse conduction, including digoxin, calcium channel blockers, or β blockers, are useful for rate control during atrial fibrillation, and exercise testing is an important method for establishing their effectiveness (178,179,182). If heart rate is not well controlled with one agent, another atrioventricular nodal blocking agent is administered and its effect is assessed with a second exercise test. This is important because poor heart rate control can over time result in progressive cardiomegaly, a reduction in left ventricular ejection fraction, and ultimately congestive heart failure (183).

Use of Exercise Testing in Other Conditions

In addition to its important role in evaluating the beneficial or harmful effects of antiarrhythmic drugs, exercise testing has also been useful for the evaluation of other conditions associated with arrhythmia. As indicated previously, patients with the prolonged QT syndrome do not have the expected shortening of the QT interval during exercise (169,170) and many will develop serious arrhythmia with exercise, a result of increased sympathetic tone and further autonomic imbalance (184). It is possible that patients with an idiosyncratic reaction to the class Ia drugs, who develop substantial QT prolongation and the associated increased risk of torsade de pointes even with low serum concentrations of a drug, have a *forme fruste* of the QT syndrome. Exercise testing may help identify these patients, as the QT interval will not shorten appropriately.

Exercise testing has been used to identify patients with the Wolff-Parkinson-White syndrome who are at an increased risk for sudden death (185). The persistence of preexcited QRS complexes during exercise testing has a 17% specificity but a 90% sensitivity for identifying patients at risk for sudden death as determined by electrophysiologic testing, which is defined as the shortest R-R interval of ≤250 ms during induced atrial fibrillation.

Safety of Exercise Testing

A very important concern about the use of exercise testing for arrhythmia management, particularly in patients with far advanced heart disease, is safety. In several surveys involving thousands of patients with heart disease or varying causes and severity, mortality caused by the precipitation of a serious arrhythmia has been rare, with the incidence range from 0.2% to 0.5% (186,187).

The data about the safety of exercise testing are limited in patients who have a history of a ventricular tachyarrhythmia and usually have significant underlying heart disease and impaired left ventricular function. In one retrospective study of 263 patients with a history of a sustained ventricular tachyarrhythmia who underwent 1,377 tests, a serious

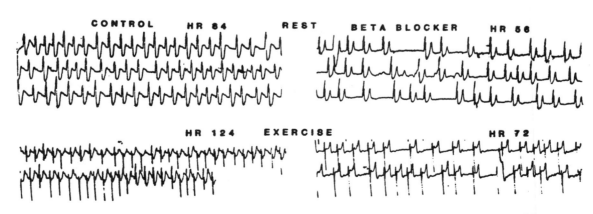

FIGURE 6.1-19. Use of exercise testing for rate control of atrial fibrillation. During therapy with digoxin alone, heart rate was moderately well controlled at rest, but with exercise on a bicycle ergometer, heart rate was excessively rapid. After the addition of a β blocker, heart rate at rest—but more importantly with exercise—was better controlled.

arrhythmia complication requiring an intervention (cardioversion, defibrillation, or intravenous drug administration) occurred in 32 tests (2.3%) involving 24 patients (9.1%) (188). It was also observed in this study that the risk of a sustained tachyarrhythmia during exercise was greater during antiarrhythmic drug therapy when compared with testing performed in a baseline state. Therefore, it appears that exercise testing in patients with far advanced heart disease who have a history of sustained ventricular tachyarrhythmia is a safe procedure. Although the risk of inducing a serious ventricular tachyarrhythmia during exercise testing is increased when compared with a population of patients with heart disease who have no clinical history of serious arrhythmia, most events occur during antiarrhythmic drug use when exercise is performed for an evaluation of efficacy, suggesting that the arrhythmia results from aggravation of arrhythmia caused by the antiarrhythmic drug.

REFERENCES

1. Kennedy HL, Wiens RD. Ambulatory (Holter) electrocardiography using real-time analysis. *Am J Cardiol* 1987;59:1190.
2. Boudalas H, Schaal SF, Lewis RP, et al. Superiority of 24 hour outpatient monitoring over multi-stage exercise testing for the evaluation of syncope. *J Electrocardiol* 1979;12:103.
3. Poblete PF, Kennedy HL, Caralis DG. Detection of ventricular ectopy in patients with coronary heart disease and normal subjects by exercise testing and ambulatory electrocardiography. *Chest* 1978;74:402.
4. Kennedy HL. Ambulatory (Holter) electrocardiography technology. *Cardiol Clin* 1992;10:341–359.
5. Coumel P, Leenhardt A. Mental activity, adrenergic modulation, and cardiac arrhythmias in patients with heart disease. *Circulation* 1991;83[Suppl II]:II58–II70.
6. Meyerburg RJ, Kessler KM, Bassett AL, et al. A biological approach to sudden cardiac death: structure, function and cause. *Am J Cardiol* 1989;63:1512–1516.
7. Shimizu W, Antzelevitch C. Cellular basis for long QT, transmural dispersion of repolarization and torsade de pointe long QT syndrome. *J Electrocardiol* 1999;32[Suppl]:177–184.
8. Yan GX, Antzelevitch C. Cellular basis for the Brugada syndrome and other mechanisms of arrhythmogenesis associated with ST-segment elevation. *Circulation* 1999;100:1660–1666.
9. Bayes de Luna A, Coumel P, Leclercq JF. Ambulatory sudden death: mechanisms of production of fatal arrhythmia on the basis of data from 157 cases. *Am Heart J* 1989;117:151–159.
10. The Cardiac Arrhythmia Suppression Trial (CAST) Investigators. Preliminary report: effect of encainide and flecainide on mortality in a randomized trial of arrhythmia suppression after myocardial infarction. *N Engl J Med* 1989;321:406–412.
11. The Cardiac Arrhythmia Suppression Trial II Investigators. The effect of the antiarrhythmic agent moricizine on survival after myocardial infarction. *N Engl J Med* 1992;327:227–233.
12. The ESVEM Investigators. The ESVEM Trial: electrophysiologic study versus electrocardiographic monitoring for selection of antiarrhythmic therapy of ventricular tachyarrhythmias. *Circulation* 1989;79:1354–1360.
13. Mason JW, for the ESVEM Investigators. A comparison of electrophysiologic testing with Holter monitoring to predict antiarrhythmic drug efficacy for ventricular tachyarrhythmias. *N Engl J Med* 1993;329:445–451.
14. Ward DE, Camm AJ. Dangerous ventricular arrhythmias; can we predict drug efficacy? *N Engl J Med* 1993;329:498–499.
15. Graboys TB, Lown B, Podrid PJ, DeSilva R. Long-term survival of patients with malignant ventricular arrhythmia treated with antiarrhythmic drugs. *Am J Cardiol* 1982;50:437–443.
16. Cairns JA, Connolly SJ, Roberts R, Gent M. Randomised trial of outcome after myocardial infarction in patients with frequent or repetitive ventricular premature depolarisations: CAMIAT. *Lancet* 1997;349:675–682.
17. Julian DG, Camm AJ, Frangin G, et al. Randomised trial of effect of amiodarone on mortality in patients with left ventricular dysfunction after recent myocardial infarction: EMIAT. *Lancet* 1997;349:667–674.
18. Kennedy HL. Beta-blocker prevention of proarrhythmia and proischemia. Clues from CAST, CAMIAT and EMIAT. *Am J Cardiol* 1997;80:1208–1211.
19. Boutitie F, Boissel JP, Connolly SJ, et al, and the EMIAT and CAMIAT Investigators. Amiodarone interaction with beta-blockers: analysis of the merged EMIAT (European Myocardial Infarction Amiodarone Trial) and CAMIAT (Canadian Amiodarone Myocardial Infarction Trial) databases. *Circulation* 1999;99:2268–2275.
20. Davies RF, Goldberg DA, Forman S, et al. Asymptomatic Cardiac Ischemia Pilot (ACIP) study two-year follow-up. *Circulation* 1997;95:2037–2043.
21. van Boven AJ, Jukema W, Zwinderman AH, et al, and the REGRESS study group. Reduction of transient myocardial ischemia with pravastatin in addition to the conventional treatment in patients with angina pectoris. *Circulation* 1996;94:1503–1505.
22. Brugada R, Brugada J, Antzelevitch C, et al. Sodium channel blockers identify risk for sudden death in patients with ST-segment elevation and right bundle branch block but structurally normal hearts. *Circulation* 2000;101:510–515.
23. Kennedy HL, Bavishi NS, Buckingham TA. Ambulatory (Holter) electrocardiography signal-averaging: a current prospective. *Am Heart J* 1992;124:1339–1346.
24. De Maso J, Myers S, Nels D, Sellers C. Ambulatory high-resolution ECG recorder using disk storage. *J Ambul Monit* 1992;5:317–322.
25. Kennedy HL, Smith SC, Mizera J, et al. Limitations of ambulatory ECG real-time analysis for ventricular and supraventricular arrhythmia accuracy detected by clinical evaluation. *Am J Noninvasive Cardiol* 1992;6:137–146.
26. Barry J, Campbell S, Nabel EG, et al. Ambulatory monitoring of the digitized electrocardiogram for detection and early warning of transient myocardial ischemia in angina pectoris. *Am J Cardiol* 1987;60:483–488.
27. Hassin Y, Frieman I, Gotsman MS. Two-channel ECG monitoring in the coronary care unit. *Clin Cardiol* 1984;7:102.
28. Aly AF, Afchine D, Esser P, et al. Telemetry as a new concept in long term monitoring of SIDS-risk infant. *Eur J Med Res* 2000;5:19–22.
29. Furman S, Escher DJW. Telephone pacemaker monitoring. *Ann Thorac Surg* 1975;20:326.
30. Antaman FM, Ludmer PI, McGowan N, et al. Transtelephonic electrocardiographic transmission for management of cardiac arrhythmias. *Am J Cardiol* 1986;58:1021.
31. Chadda KD, Harrington D, Kushnik H, et al. The impact of transtelephonic documentation of arrhythmia on morbidity and mortality rate in sudden death survivors. *Am Heart J* 1986;112:1159.
32. Folick MJ, Gorkin I, Capone RJ, et al. Psychological distress as a predictor of ventricular arrhythmias in a post-myocardial infarction population. *Am Heart J* 1988;116:32.
33. Pratt CM, Slyman DJ, Wierman AM, et al. Asymptomatic tele-

phone ECG transmission as an outpatient surveillance system of ventricular arrhythmias: relationship to quantitative ambulatory ECG recordings. *Am Heart J* 1987;113:1.

34. Brown AP, Dawkins KD, Davies JG. Detection of arrhythmias: use of a patient-activated ambulatory electrocardiogram device with a solid-state memory loop. *Br Heart J* 1987;58:251.

35. Linzer M, Pritchett ELC, Pontinen M, et al. Incremental diagnostic yield of loop electrocardiographic recorders in unexplained syncope. *Am J Cardiol* 1990;66:214–219.

36. Linzer M, Prystowsky EN, Brunetti LL, et al. Recurrent syncope of unknown origin diagnosed by ambulatory continuous loop recording. *Am Heart J* 1988;116:1632–1634.

37. Goldstein MA, Hesslein P, Dunnigan A. Efficacy of transtelephonic electrocardiographic monitoring in pediatric patients. *Am J Dis Child* 1990;144:178–182.

38. Linzer M, Comegno A. Long-term ambulatory ECG monitoring in syncope: the state of the art. *Cardiovasc Rev Rep* 1993; 14(June):11–21.

39. Reiffel JA, Schulhof E, Joseph B, et al. Optimum duration of transtelephonic ECG monitoring when used for transient symptomatic event detection. *J Electrocardiol* 1991;24:165–168.

40. Kamalvand K, Tan K, Kotsakis A, et al. Ambulatory patient-activated arrhythmia monitoring: comparison of a new wrist-applied monitor with a conventional precordial device. *J Electrocardiol* 1997;30:127–131.

41. Prystowsky EN, Knilans TK, Evans JJ. Diagnostic evaluation and treatment strategies for patients at risk for serious cardiac arrhythmias. Part 1: syncope of unknown origin. *Mod Conc Cardiovasc Dis* 1991;60:49–53.

42. Zimetbaum PJ, Josephson ME. The evolving role of ambulatory arrhythmia monitoring in general clinical practice. *Ann Intern Med* 1999;130:848–856.

43. Kinlay S, Leitch JW, Neil A, et al. Cardiac event recorders yield more diagnoses and are more cost-effective than 48-hour Holter monitoring in patients with palpitations. A controlled clinical trial. *Ann Intern Med* 1996;124:16–20.

44. Krahn AD, Klein GJ, Yee R, Norris C. Final results from a pilot study with an implantable loop recorder to determine the etiology of syncope in patients with negative noninvasive and invasive testing. *Am J Cardiol* 1998;82:117–119.

45. Boudoulas H, Geleris P, Schaal SF, et al. Comparison between electrophysiologic studies and ambulatory monitoring in patients with syncope. *J Electrocardiol* 1983;16:91–96.

46. Boudalas H, Schaal SF, Lewis RP, Robinson JL. Superiority of 24 hour outpatient monitoring over multi-stage exercise testing for the evaluation of syncope. *J Electrocardiol* 1979;12:103–109.

47. Lipski J, Cohen L, Espinoza J, et al. Value of Holter monitoring in assessing cardiac arrhythmias in symptomatic patients. *Am J Cardiol* 1976;37:102–107.

48. Hertzenau H, Yahini JH, Neufeld NH. Holter monitoring in dizziness and syncope. *Acta Cardiol (Brux)* 1979;34:375–383.

49. Goldberg AD, Raftery EB, Cashman PMM. Ambulatory electrocardiographic records in patients with transient cerebral attacks or palpitations. *BMJ* 1975;6:569–571.

50. Zeldis SM, Levine BJ, Michaelson El, Morganroth J. Cardiovascular complaint. Correlation with cardiac arrhythmias on 24 hour electrocardiographic monitoring. *Chest* 1980;78:456–462.

51. Gibson TC, Heitzman MR. Diagnostic efficacy of 24 hour electrocardiographic monitoring for syncope. *Am J Cardiol* 1984;53:1013–1017.

52. Shotan A, Ostrzega E, Mehra A, et al. Incidence of arrhythmias in normal pregnancy and relation to palpitations, dizziness, and syncope. *Am J Cardiol* 1997;79:1061–1064.

53. Johansson BW. Evaluation of alteration of consciousness and palpitations. In: Wenger NK, Mock MB, Ringquist I, eds. *Ambulatory electrocardiographic recording*. Chicago: Year Book, 1981:321–330.

54. Surawicz B, Pinto RP. Symptoms in hospital patients and outpatients with ventricular arrhythmias during ambulatory ECG monitoring. *J Ambul Monit* 1991;4:83–90.

55. Nwasokwa ON, Wenger NK. Diagnostic value of ambulatory electrocardiography: dependence on presenting symptom, age and sex. *Am J Noninvasive Cardiol* 1988;2:140–147.

56. Montague TJ, Bewick DJ, Spencer CA, Klassen GA. Clinical utility of a single 24 hour electrocardiogram in the investigation of patients with suspected cardiac dysrhythm. *Am J Noninvasive Cardiol* 1989;3:193–198.

57. Kapoor WN, Cha R, Peterson JR, et al. Prolonged electrocardiographic monitoring in patients with syncope. *Am J Med* 1987;82:20–28.

58. Linzer M, Prystowsky EN, Divine GW, et al. Predicting outcome of electrophysiologic studies in patients with unexplained syncope: preliminary validation of a derived model. *J Gen Intern Med* 1991;6:113–120.

59. Bachinsky WB, Linzer M, Weld L, Estes NAM. Usefulness of clinical characteristics in predicting the outcome of electrophysiologic studies in unexplained syncope. *Am J Cardiol* 1992;69:1044–1049.

60. Coumel P. Diagnostic and prognostic values and limitations of Holter monitoring. *Eur Heart J* 1989;10[Suppl E]:19–30.

61. Kennedy HL. Importance of the standard electrocardiogram in ambulatory (Holter) electrocardiography. *Am Heart J* 1992;123:1660–1677.

62. The Coronary Drug Project Research Group. Prognostic importance of premature beats following myocardial infarction. *JAMA* 1973;223:1116–1124.

63. Kotler MN, Tabatznik B, Mower MM, Tominaga S. Prognostic significance of ventricular ectopic beats with respect to sudden death in the late post-infarction period. *Circulation* 1973;7(5):959–966.

64. Ruberman W, Weinblatt E, Goldberg JD, et al.. Ventricular premature beats and mortality after myocardial infarction. *N Engl J Med* 1977;297:750–757.

65. Ruberman W, Weinblatt E, Goldberg JD, et al. Ventricular premature complexes and sudden death after myocardial infarction. *Circulation* 1981;64:297–305.

66. Bigger JT, Fleiss JL, Kleiger RE, et al. The relationships among ventricular arrhythmias, left ventricular dysfunction, and mortality in the 2 years after myocardial infarction. *Circulation* 1984;69:250–258.

67. Maggioni AP, Zuanetti G, Franzosi MG, et al. Prevalence and prognostic significance of ventricular arrhythmias after acute myocardial infarction in the fibrinolytic era. GISSI-II results. *Circulation* 1993;87:312–322.

68. Kleiger RE, Miller JP, Bigger JT, Moss AJ, and the Multicenter Post-Infarction Research Group. Decreased heart rate variability and its association with increased mortality after acute myocardial infarction. *Am J Cardiol* 1987;59:256–262.

69. Farrell TG, Bashir Y, Cripps T, et al. Risk stratification for arrhythmic events in post-infarction patients based on heart rate variability, ambulatory electrocardiographic variables and the signal-averaged electrocardiogram. *J Am Coll Cardiol* 1991;18:687–697.

70. Algra A, Tijssen JGP, Roelandt RTC, et al. Heart rate variability from 24 hour electrocardiography and the 2-year risk for sudden death. *Circulation* 1993;88:180–185.

71. Dougherty CM, Burr RL. Comparison of heart rate variability in survivors and nonsurvivors of sudden death cardiac arrest. *Am J Cardiol* 1992;70:441–448.

72. Schmidt G, Malik M, Barthel P, et al. Heart-rate turbulence after ventricular premature beats as a predictor of mortality after acute myocardial infarction. *Lancet* 1999;353:1390–1396.

73. Maron BJ, Savage DD, Wolfson JK, Epstein SE. Prognostic significance of 24 hour ambulatory electrocardiographic monitoring in patients with hypertrophic cardiomyopathy: a prospective study. *Am J Cardiol* 1981;48:252–257.

74. McKenna WJ, England D, Dio YL, et al. Arrhythmia in hypertrophic cardiomyopathy: influence on prognosis. *Br Heart J* 1981;46:168–172.

75. McKenna WJ, Oakley CM, Krikler DM, Goodwin JR. Improved survival with amiodarone in patients with hypertrophic cardiomyopathy and ventricular tachycardia. *Br Heart J* 1985;53:412–416.

76. Spirito P, Bellone P, Harris KM, et al. Magnitude of left ventricular hypertrophy and risk of sudden death in hypertrophic cardiomyopathy. *N Engl J Med* 2000;342:1778–1785.

77. Huang SK, Messer JV, Denes P. Significance of ventricular tachycardia in idiopathic dilated cardiomyopathy: observations in 35 patients. *Am J Cardiol* 1983;51:507–512.

78. Meinertz T, Hoffman T, Kasper W, et al. Significance of ventricular arrhythmias in idiopathic dilated cardiomyopathy. *Am J Cardiol* 1984;53:902–907.

79. Holmes J, Kubo SH, Cody RJ, Kligfield P. Arrhythmias in ischemic and nonischemic dilated cardiomyopathy: prediction of mortality by ambulatory electrocardiography. *Am J Cardiol* 1985;55:46–151.

80. Chakkao CS, Gheorghiade M. Ventricular arrhythmia in severe heart failure: incidence, significance, and effectiveness of antiarrhythmic therapy. *Am Heart J* 1985;109:497–504.

80a. Doval HC, Nul DR, Grancelli HO, et al, for the GESICA-GEMA Investigators. Nonsustained ventricular tachycardia in severe heart failure. Independent marker of increased mortality due to sudden death. *Circulation* 1996;94:3198–3203.

81. Singh SN, Fisher SG, Carson PE, Fletcher RD, and the Department of Veteran Affairs CHF STAT Investigators. Prevalence and significance of nonsustained ventricular tachycardia in patients with premature ventricular contractions and heart failure treated with vasodilator therapy. *J Am Coll Cardiol* 1998;32:942–947.

82. Brodsky M, Wu D, Denes P, et al. Arrhythmias documented by 24 hour continuous electrocardiographic monitoring in 50 male medical students without apparent heart disease. *Am J Cardiol* 1977;39:390–395.

83. Sobotka PA, Mayer JH, Bauernfeind RA, et al. Arrhythmias documented by 24 hour continuous ambulatory electrocardiographic monitoring in young women without apparent heart disease. *Am Heart J* 1981;101:753–759.

84. Raftery EB, Cashman PMM. Long-term recording of the electrocardiogram in a normal population. *Postgrad Med J* 1976;52 [Suppl 7]:32–37.

85. Bjerregaard P. Premature beats in healthy subjects 40-79 years of age. *Eur Heart J* 1982;3:493–503.

86. Fleg JL, Kennedy HL. Cardiac arrhythmias in a healthy elderly population: detection by 24 hour ambulatory electrocardiography. *Chest* 1982;81:302–307.

87. Kostis JB, McCrone K, Moreyra AE, et al. Premature ventricular complexes in the absence of identifiable heart disease. *Circulation* 1981;63:1351–1356.

88. Kennedy HL, Underhill SJ. Frequent and complex ventricular ectopy in apparently healthy subjects: a clinical study of 25 cases. *Am J Cardiol* 1976;38:141–148.

89. Kennedy HL, Whitlock JA, Sprague MK, et al. Long-term follow-up of asymptomatic healthy subjects with frequent and complex ventricular ectopy. *N Engl J Med* 1985;312:193–197.

90. Schaffer WA, Cobb LA. Recurrent ventricular fibrillation and modes of death in survivors of out-of-hospital ventricular fibrillation. *N Engl J Med* 1975;293:259–262.

91. Eisenberg MS, Hallstrom A, Bergner L. Long-term survival after out-of-hospital cardiac arrest. *N Engl J Med* 1982;306:1340–1343.

92. Hohnloser SH, Raeder EA, Podrid PJ, et al. Predictors of antiarrhythmic drug efficacy in patients with malignant ventricular tachyarrhythmias. *Am Heart J* 1987;114:1–7.

93. Hoffman A, Schultz E, White R, et al. Suppression of high-grade ventricular ectopic activity by antiarrhythmic drug treatment as a market for survival in patients with chronic coronary artery disease. *Am Heart J* 1984;107:1103–1108.

94. Winkle RA. Antiarrhythmic drug effect mimicked by spontaneous variability of ventricular ectopy. *Circulation* 1978;57:1116–1121.

95. Morganroth J, Michelson EL, Horowitz LN, et al. Limitations of routine long-term electrocardiographic monitoring to assess ventricular ectopy frequency. *Circulation* 1978;58:408–414.

96. Pratt CM, Delclos G, Wierman AM, et al. The changing baseline of complex ventricular arrhythmias. A new consideration in assessing long-term antiarrhythmic drug therapy. *N Engl J Med* 1985;313:1444–1449.

97. Pratt CM, Theroux P, Slymen D, et al. Spontaneous variability of ventricular arrhythmias in patients at increased risk for sudden death after acute myocardial infarction: consecutive ambulatory electrocardiographic recordings of 88 patients. *Am J Cardiol* 1987;59:278–283.

98. Anastasiou-Nana MI, Menlove RL, Nanas JN, Anderson JL. Changes in spontaneous variability of ventricular ectopic activity as a function of time in patients with chronic arrhythmias. *Circulation* 1988;78:286–295.

99. Kennedy HL, Sprague MK, Homan SM, et al. Natural history of potentially lethal ventricular arrhythmias in patients treated with long-term antiarrhythmic drug therapy. *Am J Cardiol* 1989;64:1289–1297.

100. Velebit V, Podrid PJ, Lown B, et al. Aggravation and provocation of ventricular arrhythmias by antiarrhythmic drugs. *Circulation* 1982;65:886–894.

101. Kennedy HL. Late proarrhythmia and understanding the time of occurrence of proarrhythmia. *Am J Cardiol* 1990;66:1139–1143.

102. Hasin Y, David D, Rogel S. Diagnostic and therapeutic assessment by telephone electrocardiographic monitoring of ambulatory patients. *BMJ* 1976;2:609–612.

103. Pritchett ELC, Zimmerman JM, Hammill K, et al. Electrocardiogram recording by telephone in antiarrhythmic drug trials. *Chest* 1982;81:473–476.

104. Antman EM, Ludmer PL, McGowan N, et al. Transtelephonic electrocardiographic transmission for management of cardiac arrhythmias. *Am J Cardiol* 1986;58:1021–1024.

105. Shen WK, Holmes DR, Hammill SC. Transtelephonic monitoring: documentation of transient cardiac rhythm disturbances. *Mayo Clin Proc* 1987;62:109–112.

106. Pratt CM, Slymen DJ, Wierman AM, et al. Asymptomatic telephone ECG transmission as an outpatient surveillance system of ventricular arrhythmias: relationship to quantitative ambulatory ECG recordings. *Am Heart J* 1987;113:1–7.

107. Capone RJ, Visco J, Curwen E, Van Every S. The effect of early prehospital transtelephonic coronary intervention on morbidity and mortality: experience with 284 post-myocardial infarction patients in a pilot program. *Am Heart J* 1984;107:1153–1160.

108. David D, Kaplinsky E. The role of outpatient transtelephonic monitoring and self-medication following acute myocardial infarction. In: Califf GM, Wagner GS, eds. *Acute coronary care: principles and practice.* Boston: Martinus Nijhoff, 1985:531–536.

109. Parsonnet V, Bernstein AD. Pacing in perspective: concepts and controversies. *Circulation* 1986;73:1087–1093.

110. Griffin JC, Schuenemeyer TD. Current concepts in pacemaker follow-up. *Intell Report in Cardiac Pacing Electrophysiol* 1984;2:1–5.

111. Griffin JC, Schuenemeyer TD. Pacemaker follow-up: an introduction and overview. *Clin Prog Pacing Electrophysiol* 1983;1:30.

112. Dreifus LS, Zinberg A, Hurzeler P, et al. Transtelephonic monitoring of 25,919 implanted pacemakers. *Pace* 1986;9:371–378.

113. Famularo MA, Kennedy HL. Ambulatory electrocardiography in the assessment of pacemaker function. *Am Heart J* 1982;104:1086–1094.

114. Janosik DL, Redd RM, Buckingham TA, et al. The utility of ambulatory electrocardiography in detecting pacemaker dysfunction in the early post-implant period. *Am J Cardiol* 1987;60:79F–82F.

115. Bethge KP, Brandes A, Gonska D. Diagnostic sensitivity of Holter monitoring in pacemaker patients. *J Ambul Monit* 1989;2:79–89.

116. Kelen GJ, Bloomfield DA, Hardage M, et al. A clinical evaluation of an improved Holter monitoring technique for artificial pacemaker function. *Pace* 1980;3:192–197.

117. Levine PA, Belott PH, Bilitch M, et al. Recommendations of the NASPE Policy Conference on Pacemaker Programmability and Follow-up. *Pace* 1983;6:1222–1223.

118. Bruce TA, Chapman CP, Baker O, Fisher JN. Role of autonomic and myocardial factors in cardiac control. *J Clin Invest* 1963;42:721.

119. Wit AL, Rosen MR. Pathophysiologic mechanisms of cardiac arrhythmias. *Am Heart J* 1983;106:798.

120. Dean JW, Lab MJ. Arrhythmia in heart failure: role of mechanically induced changes in electrophysiology. *Lancet* 1989;10:1309.

121. Marcus ML, Kerber RE, Erhardt JC, et al. Spatial and temporal heterogeneity of left ventricular perfusion in awake dogs. *Am Heart J* 1977;94:748.

122. Coggens DL, Flynn AE, Austin RE, et al. Nonuniform loss of regional flow reserve during myocardial ischemia in dogs. *Circ Res* 1990;67:253.

123. Kageyama Y, Hill JC, Gettes LS. Interaction of acidosis and increased intracellular potassium on action potential characteristics and conduction in guinea pig ventricular muscle. *Clin Res* 1982;51:614.

124. Hauswurth D, Noble D, Tsien RW. Adrenalin mechanism of action of the pacemaker potential in cardiac Purkinje fibers. *Science* 1968;162:916.

125. Wit AL, Cranfield PF. Triggered activities in cardiac muscle fibers of the simian mitral valve. *Circ Res* 1976;38:85.

126. Antman ES, Graboys TB, Lown B. Comparison of continuous intermittent electrocardiographic monitoring during exercise testing for exposure of cardiac arrhythmias. *JAMA* 1979;241:2802.

127. Beard EF, Owen CA. Cardiac arrhythmias during exercise stress testing in healthy men. *Aerospace Med* 1973;44:286.

128. Master AM. Cardiac arrhythmias elicited by the two-step exercise test. *Am J Cardiol* 1973;32:766.

129. Whinnery JE. Dysrhythmia comparison in apparently healthy males during and after treadmill and accelerated stress test. *Am Heart J* 1983;105:732.

130. McHenry PL, Fisch C, Jordan JW. Cardiac arrhythmia observed during maximal exercise testing in clinically normal men. *Am J Cardiol* 1978;39:311.

131. Poblete PF, Kennedy HL, Cavalis DG. Detection of ventricular ectopy in patients with coronary heart disease and normal subjects by exercise testing and ambulatory electrocardiography. *Chest* 1978;74:402.

132. Jelinek MV, Lown B. Exercise stress testing for exposure of cardiac arrhythmia. *Prog Cardiovasc Dis* 1974;16:497.

133. Ryan M, Lown B, Horn H. Comparison of ventricular ectopic activity during 24-hour monitoring and exercise testing in patients with coronary heart disease. *N Engl J Med* 1975;292:224.

134. Gaoch AS, McConnell D. Analysis of transient arrhythmia and conduction disturbances during submaximal treadmill exercise testing. *Prog Cardiovasc Dis* 1970;13:293.

135. Ekblum B, Hartley LH, Day WC. Occurrence and reproducibility of exercise-induced ventricular ectopy in normal subjects. *Am J Cardiol* 1979;43:35.

136. Sami M, Chaitman B, Fisher L, et al. Significance of exercise-induced ventricular arrhythmia in stable coronary artery disease. A Coronary Artery Surgery Study project. *Am J Cardiol* 1984;54:118.

137. Califf RM, McKinnis RA, McNeer F, et al. Prognostic value of ventricular arrhythmias associated with treadmill exercise testing in patients studied with cardiac catheterization for suspected ischemic heart disease. *J Am Coll Cardiol* 1983;2:1060.

138. Weiner DA, Levine PR, Klein MD, Ryan TJ. Ventricular arrhythmias during exercise testing: mechanism, response to coronary bypass surgery, and prognostic significance. *Am J Cardiol* 1984;53:1553.

139. Schweikert RA, Pashkow FJ, Snader CE, et al. Association of exercise-induced ventricular ectopic activity with thallium myocardial perfusion and angiographic coronary artery disease in stable, low-risk populations. *Am J Cardiol* 1999;83:530.

140. Yang JC, Wesley RC, Froelicher VF. Ventricular tachycardia during routine treadmill testing: risk and prognosis. *Arch Intern Med* 1991;51:349.

141. Detry JM, Abouantoun S, Wyms W. Incidence and prognostic implications of severe ventricular arrhythmias during maximal exercise testing. *Am J Cardiol* 1981;48:35.

142. Rodriguez LM, Weleffe A, Brugada P, et al. Exercise induced sustained symptomatic ventricular tachycardia. Incidence, clinical, angiographic and electrophysiologic characteristics. *Eur Heart J* 1990;11:225.

143. Graboys TB, Lampert S, Lown B. Yield of a ventricular arrhythmia during exercise testing in patients with prior cardiac arrest. *Circulation* 1980;66[Suppl II]:II27(abst).

144. Lown B, Podrid PJ, DeSilva RA, Graboys TB. Sudden cardiac death: management of the patient at risk. *Curr Probl Cardiol* 1980;4:1.

145. Graboys TB, Lown B, Podrid PJ, et al. Long-term survival of patients with malignant ventricular arrhythmia. *Am J Cardiol* 1982;50:437.

146. Graboys TB, Wright RF. Provocation of supraventricular tachycardia during exercise stress testing. *Cardiovasc Rev Rep* 1980;1:57–58.

147. Weld FM, Chu KL, Bigger JT, Rolnitzky LM. Risk stratification with low level exercise testing two weeks after myocardial infarction. *Circulation* 1981;64:306.

148. Krone RJ, Gillespie JA, Weld FM, et al, and the Multicenter Postinfarction Research Group. Low-level exercise testing after myocardial infarction usefulness in enhancing clinical risk stratification. *Circulation* 1985;71:80.

149. Henry RL, Kennedy GT, Crawford MH. Prognostic value of exercise-induced ventricular ectopy activity for mortality after acute myocardial infarction. *Am J Cardiol* 1987;59:1251.

150. Udall JA, Ellestad MJ. Prediction implications of ventricular premature contractions associated with treadmill stress testing. *Circulation* 1977;56:985.

151. Sheps DS, Ernst JC, Briese RF, et al. Decreased frequency of exercise-induced ectopic activity in the second of two consecutive treadmill tests. *Circulation* 1977;55:892.

152. Drory Y, Pines A, Fisman EZ, Kellerman JJ. Persistence of arrhythmia-exercise response in healthy young men. *Am J Cardiol* 1990;66:1092.

153. Handler CE, Sowton E. Stress testing predischarge and six weeks after myocardial infarction to compare submaximal and maximal exercise predischarge and to assess the reproducibility of induced abnormalities. *Int J Cardiol* 1985;9:173.

154. Faris JV, McHenry PC, Jordan JW, Morris SN. Prevalence and reproducibility of exercise-induced ventricular arrhythmias during maximal exercise testing in normal men. *Am J Cardiol* 1976;37:617.

155. Saini V, Graboys T, Towne V, Lown B. Reproducibility of exercise induced ventricular arrhythmia in patients undergoing evaluation for malignant ventricular arrhythmia. *Am J Cardiol* 1989;63:697.

156. Graboys TB, Lown B, Podrid PJ, DeSilva R. Long-term survival of patients with malignant ventricular arrhythmia. *Am J Cardiol* 1982;50:437.

157. Rosen MR, Wit AL. Electropharmacology of antiarrhythmic drugs. *Am Heart J* 1983;106:829.

158. Wit AL, Hoffman BF, Rosen MR. Electrophysiology and pharmacology of cardiac arrhythmias. IX. Cardiac electrophysiologic effects of beta adrenergic receptor stimulation and blockade. Part A. *Am Heart J* 1975;90:521.

159. Cockrell JL, Scheinman MM, Titus C, et al. Safety and efficacy of oral flecainide therapy in patients with atrioventricular re-entrant tachycardia. *Ann Intern Med* 1991;114:189.

160. Jazayeri MR, Wyhe G, Avitall B, et al. Isoproterenol reversal of antiarrhythmic effects in patients with inducible sustained ventricular tachyarrhythmias. *J Am Coll Cardiol* 1989;14:705.

161. Dongas J, Tchou P, Mahmud R, et al. Catecholamine mediated reversal of procainamide induced retrograde block in paroxysmal supraventricular tachycardias: possible cause of treatment failures. *Circulation* 1985;72[Suppl III]:III126(abst).

162. Akhtar M, Niazi I, Naccarelli G, et al. Role of adrenergic stimulation by isoproterenol in reversal of effects of encainide in supraventricular tachycardia. *Am J Cardiol* 1988;62:45L.

163. Niazi I, Naccarelli G, Dougherty A, et al. Treatment of atrioventricular nodal re-entrant tachycardia with encainide: reversal of drug effect with isoproterenol. *J Am Coll Cardiol* 1989;13:904.

164. Morady F, Kou WH, Kadish AH, et al. Antagonism of flecainide electrophysiologic effects by epinephrine in patients with ventricular tachycardia. *J Am Coll Cardiol* 1988;12:388.

165. Brugada P, Facchini M, Wellens HJJ. Effects of isoproterenol and amiodarone and the role of exercise in initiation of circus movement tachycardia in the accessory atrioventricular pathway. *Am J Cardiol* 1986;57:146.

166. Van Wijk LM, Crijns HJ, Kingma HJ, et al. Flecainide long-term effects in patients with sustained ventricular tachycardia or ventricular fibrillation. *J Cardiovasc Pharmacol* 1990;15:884.

167. Ranger S, Talajic M, Lemnery R, et al. Kinetics of use-dependent ventricular conduction slowing by antiarrhythmic drugs in humans. *Circulation* 1991;83:1987.

168. Ranger S, Talajic M, Lemery R, et al. Amplification of flecainide induced ventricular conduction slowing by exercise. A potentially significant clinical consequence use dependent sodium channel blockade. *Circulation* 1989;79:1000.

169. Vincent GM, Jaiswal D, Timothy KW. Effects of exercise on heart rate, QT, QTc and QT/QS2 in the Romano-Ward inherited long QT syndrome. *Am J Cardiol* 1991;68:498.

170. Kadish AH, Weisman HF, Veltri EP, et al. Paradoxic effects of exercise on the QT interval in patients with polymorphic ventricular tachycardia receiving type 1A antiarrhythmic agents. *Circulation* 1990;81:14.

171. Anastasiou-Nana MI, Anderson JL, Stewart JR, et al. Occurrence of exercise induced and spontaneous wide complex tachycardia during therapy with flecainide for complex ventricular arrhythmia. A possible proarrhythmic effect. *Am Heart J* 1987;113:1071–1072.

172. Slater W, Lampert SC, Podrid PJ, Lown B. Clinical predictors of arrhythmia worsening by antiarrhythmic drugs. *Am J Cardiol* 1988;61:349.

173. Falk RH. Flecainide induced ventricular tachycardia and fibrillation in patients treated for atrial fibrillation. *Ann Intern Med* 1989;111:107.

174. Feld GK, Chen PS, Nicod P, et al. Possible atrial proarrhythmic effects of class Ic antiarrhythmic agents. *Am J Cardiol* 1990;60:378–383.

175. Brown MJ, Brown DL, Murphy MN. Hypokalemia from beta-2 receptor stimulation by circulating catecholamines. *N Engl J Med* 1983;307:1414.

176. Ravid J, Podrid PJ, Lampert S, Lown B. Congestive heart failure induced by antiarrhythmic drugs. *J Am Coll Cardiol* 1989;14:1326.

177. Pratt CM, Podrid PJ, Scals A, et al. Effects of ethmozine (moricizine HCl) on ventricular function using echocardiographic, hemodynamic and radionuclide assessments. *Am J Cardiol* 1987;60:73F.

178. Roth A, Harrison E, Mitani G, et al. Efficacy of medium and high dose diltiazem alone and in combination with digoxin for control of heart rate at rest and during exercise in patients with chronic atrial fibrillation. *Circulation* 1986;73:316–324.

179. Lang R, Klein H, Segni E, et al. Verapamil improves exercise capacity in chronic atrial fibrillation: double-blind crossover study. *Am Heart J* 1983;105:820–824.

180. Gaffney TE, Kahn JB, Van Maanen EF, Acheson GH. A mechanism of the vagal effect of cardiac glycosides. *J Pharmacol Exp Ther* 1958;122:423–426.

181. Beasely R, Smith DA, McHaffie DJ. Exercise heart rates at different serum digoxin concentration in patients with atrial fibrillation. *BMJ* 1985;290:9–11.

182. Atwood JE, Sullivan M, Forbes S, et al. Effect of beta-adrenergic blockage on exercise performance in patients with chronic atrial fibrillation. *J Am Coll Cardiol* 1987;10:314–320.

183. Peters KG, Kienzle MG. Severe cardiomyopathy due to chronic rapid atrial fibrillation: complete recovery after reversion to sinus rhythm. *Am J Med* 1988;85:242–244.

184. Schwartz PJ, Periti M, Malliani A. The long QT syndrome. *Am Heart J* 1975;89:378.

185. Gaita F, Giustetto C, Riccardi RM, et al. Stress and pharmacologic tests as methods to identify patient with Wolf-Parkinson-White syndrome at risk of sudden death. *Am J Cardiol* 1989;64:487.

186. Atterhog J, Jonssen B, Samuels MC. Exercise testing: a preoperative study of complication rates. *Am Heart J* 1979;98:572.

187. Irving J, Bruce R. External hypertension and post-exertional ventricular fibrillation in stress testing. *Am J Cardiol* 1977;39:849.

188. Young, D, Lampert, S, Graboys, TB, et al. Safety of maximal exercise testing in patients at high risk for ventricular arrhythmia. *Circulation* 1984;70:184.

HEART RATE VARIABILITY, SIGNAL-AVERAGED ELECTROCARDIOGRAPHY QT DISPERSION AND T WAVE ALTERNANS

DANIEL BLOOMFIELD
ANTHONY R. MAGNANO
J. THOMAS BIGGER

The field of noninvasive electrocardiology has progressed steadily. The objectives of this field are to quantify abnormalities of cardiac depolarization and repolarization and determine their predictive values for cardiovascular events. A substantial effort is underway to use noninvasive electrophysiologic information to predict sudden cardiac death and to select patients for therapy that is proven to prevent this event, for example, β-adrenergic blocking drugs, amiodarone, and implantable cardioverter-defibrillators (ICDs). This chapter discusses the role of R-R variability, baroreceptor sensitivity, signal-average electrocardiogram (SAECG), QT variability, and microvolt T-wave alternans for assessing the status of the autonomic nervous system, cardiac depolarization, and cardiac repolarization. The predictive value of these measures and their role in the selection of therapy and prophylaxis are reviewed.

R-R–INTERVAL VARIABLITY

R-R variability has been used for many years as a laboratory tool to evaluate the autonomic nervous system in short-term experiments. During the past 15 years, cardiovascular uses of R-R variability have increased substantially to study cardiovascular physiology and pharmacology and to assess risk of death in patients with cardiac disease. The first paper about the prognostic significance of R-R variability was published in 1978 by Wolf and colleagues (1). Since that time, R-R variability has been established as an excellent predictor of death and nonfatal arrhythmic events after myocardial infarction.

D. Bloomfield, A. R. Magnano, and J. T. Bigger: Division of Cardiology, Columbia University, New York, New York 10032.

For prediction of death, time and frequency domain measures of R-R variability are equivalent. Frequency domain measures of R-R variability are more commonly used for mechanistic studies because they resolve parasympathetic and sympathetic influences better than time domain measures.

Physiologic Basis for the Use of Spectral Analysis of R-R Variability for Arrhythmia Assessment

Spectral analysis of R-R variability quantifies vagal modulation of R-R intervals. Under special circumstances, spectral analysis of R-R variability can provide insight into the activity of the sympathetic nervous system as well. There is a large body of evidence that indicates that the autonomic nervous system plays a significant role in the genesis of cardiac arrhythmias, including malignant ventricular arrhythmias such as sustained ventricular tachycardia (VT) and ventricular fibrillation (2–5).

The parasympathetic nervous system plays a protective role, decreasing the likelihood of malignant ventricular arrhythmias. Some of the most impressive studies on vagal protection from malignant ventricular arrhythmias were done by Schwartz and Vanoli (3), Schwartz and Stone (6), and Schwartz and colleagues (7) in a dog model of sudden cardiac death. Anterior myocardial infarction was produced in dogs by open-chest ligation of the anterior descending coronary artery and an occluder was placed around the circumflex coronary artery. After recovery, dogs were exercised on a treadmill to near maximal heart rates, about 200 beats per minute (bpm), at which time the circumflex coronary artery was occluded. The sudden coronary occlusion produced myocardial ischemia in the setting of decreased vagal activity and increased sympathetic activity. Under these circumstances, about 55% of the dogs repeatedly developed ventricular fibrillation (susceptible dogs). The binary response to exercise/ischemia was reproducible; some dogs fibrillated repeatedly (susceptible) while others did not (nonsusceptible).

Using this model, the response to exercise/ischemia was predicted by baroreflex sensitivity (BRS) quantified as the increase in R-R interval as a function of the increase in systolic blood pressure engendered by intravenous injection of phenylephrine (8). Dogs with low BRS were susceptible to ventricular fibrillation when faced with the exercise/ischemia challenge, whereas dogs with high BRS were not. BRS dropped substantially after myocardial infarction but maintained its rank order; that is, dogs with the lowest preinfarction BRS tended to have the lowest postinfarction BRS and thus tended to be susceptible to ventricular fibrillation. Thus, risk to ventricular fibrillation during myocardial ischemia was predicted by BRS measured in healthy dogs before experimental myocardial infarction was induced. After infarction, susceptible dogs could be converted to nonsusceptible by exercise training, which increased BRS (9) or by direct vagal stimulation (10). A smaller set of experiments in the same model of sudden death showed that R-R variability dropped after myocardial infarction in the dog and predicted ventricular fibrillation during the exercise/ischemia challenge (11). However, preinfarction values for R-R variability did not predict postinfarction values or response to the exercise/ischemia challenge (12).

Methodology

Most measures of R-R–interval variability are critically dependent on the quality of the input data. Often the sequence of R-R intervals is obtained from inherently noisy ambulatory ECG recordings. It is particularly important to correctly label QRS complexes when R-R variability is small because a few mislabeled QRS complexes may produce large errors in calculating R-R variability. Wow and flutter resulting from tape-transport errors can be avoided using Holter recorders that provide a phase-locked timing track or using digital recorders. VPCs and APCs must be accurately labeled. Missed QRS complexes must be corrected as well.

Time Domain Analysis of R-R–Interval Variability

A 24-hour continuous ECG recording is standard for calculating time domain measures of R-R variability (13,14). The total variance during the 24-hour interval, the square of standard deviation of the normal R-R intervals (SDNN), is divided into the variance within 5-minute intervals, ASDNN squared, and the variance between 5-minute intervals, SDANN squared (Table 6.2-1). In addition, several

TABLE 6.2-1. DEFINITIONS FOR TIME AND FREQUENCY DOMAIN MEASURES OF HEART PERIOD VARIABILITY

Variable	Domain	Units	Definition
Night-day difference	Time	ms	Difference between the average of all the normal R-R intervals at night (24:00–05:00) and the average of all the normal R-R intervals during the day (07:30–21:30).
SDNN	Time	ms	Standard deviation of all normal R-R intervals in the entire 24-h ECG recording.
SDANN index	Time	ms	Standard deviation of the average normal R-R intervals for all 5-min segments of a 24-h ECG recording (each average is weighted by the fraction of the 5 min that has normal R-R intervals).
SDNN index	Time	ms	Mean of the standard deviations of all normal R-R intervals for all 5-min segments of a 24-h ECG recording.
R-MSSD	Time	ms	Root-mean-square successive difference, the square root of the mean of the squared differences between adjacent normal R-R intervals over the entire 24-h ECG recording.
pNN50	Time	None	Percentage of differences between adjacent normal R-R intervals that are more than 50 ms computed over the entire 24-h ECG recording.
NN50	Time	%	Number of adjacent normal R-R intervals that are more than 50 ms counted over the entire 24-h ECG recording.
Total power	Frequency	ms^2	The energy in the heart period power spectrum up to 0.40 Hz.
Ultra low frequency power	Frequency	ms^2	The energy in the heart period power spectrum up to 0.0033 Hz.
Very low frequency power	Frequency	ms^2	The energy in the heart period power spectrum between 0.0033 and 0.04 Hz.
Low frequency power	Frequency	ms^2	The energy in the heart period power spectrum between 0.04 and 0.15 Hz.
High frequency power	Frequency	ms^2	The energy in the heart period power spectrum between 0.15 and 0.40 Hz.
Low frequency to high frequency ratio	Frequency	None	The ratio of low to high frequency power.

time domain measures have been used to quantify high-frequency (HF) R-R–interval fluctuations that are modulated by respiration, such as the root-mean-square successive difference (RMSSD) or the proportion of differences between adjacent R-R intervals that are more than 50 ms (i.e., pNN50) (13,14). The standard deviation of 100 or fewer R-R intervals reflects respiratory sinus arrhythmia but is influenced by fluctuations of R-R intervals with longer periods (14). The standard deviation of longer recordings is importantly influenced by fluctuations of R-R intervals with periods longer than respiratory sinus arrhythmia and thus is not specific for vagal modulation.

Spectral Analysis of R-R–Interval Variability

Spectral analysis of R-R intervals identifies periodic components and estimates their frequency and power. There are three important steps in spectral analysis. First, missing data and ectopic beats must be handled to generate a continuous sequence of normal-to-normal (NN) intervals. In patients with heart disease, the sequence of R-R intervals rarely will consist entirely of NN intervals, R-R variability calculations are only concerned with such intervals. In time domain analysis, non-NN intervals (and sometimes the subsequent NN interval) can just be excluded. However, for frequency analysis, this is not appropriate, because it is important to maintain the temporal ordering and spacing of the sequence of NN intervals. Typically, linear interpolation (splines) is used to fill in the R-R sequence when missing or ectopic beats are present (15). Second, a continuous function is derived from the discrete NN intervals. The function is then filtered and sampled to produce a time series suitable for spectral analyses (16). Third, the average NN interval is subtracted from the time series and

a fast Fourier transform is performed to resolve the frequency components of cyclic activity.

The fast Fourier transform is only one method of spectral analysis. Spectral estimation is an area of continuing active research in mathematics, statistics, and signal processing and proponents of various approaches sometimes advocate their positions with great zealotry. There is no "best" method of spectral estimation. In "classical spectral analysis," the Fourier transform is employed to represent the time series as a sum of periodic functions. This decomposition yields a specific energy or power for a discrete set of uniformly distributed frequencies. Total spectral power equals the variance of the original sequence. Thus, the Fourier transform decomposes the variance of the input data into the variance attributable to each specific frequency. Bartlett (17) suggested that by averaging sequential power spectra, statistically superior behavior can be obtained, and this approach is now widely used. Power-spectral data are inherently "spiky," and although this does not affect statistical validity, it is visually unattractive. Power spectra can be "smoothed" to overcome this drawback without affecting its statistical properties or substantially increasing the time necessary for its computation. Spectral analysis resulting from averaging more than 5-minute segments of R-R data from a 24-hour recording is illustrated in Figure 6.2-1. A peak in the "low-frequency (LF) range" can be appreciated near 0.13 Hz and a broader peak representing respiratory modulation is centered near 0.27 Hz.

A number of refinements and variations to classical spectral estimation have been proposed to improve the resolution or statistical properties of the resulting spectra (18). Yule approached spectral analysis with an alternative method, in which a linear predictive model is fitted to the time-series data (19). As applied to the analysis of R-R vari-

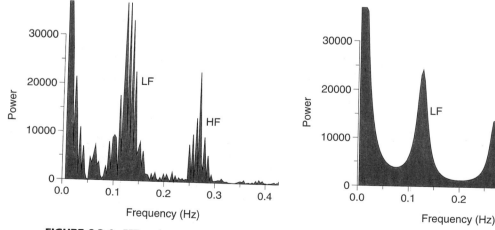

FIGURE 6.2-1. FFT and autoregressive power spectra. FFT analysis of a 5-minute recording of R-R intervals. The results of autoregression analysis (*right panel*) of the same 5-minute recording. The mathematical algorithm smooths the data but gives almost identical areas under the curves in the frequency bands of interest. In the supine recording, there is a peak at about 0.27 Hz (the high-frequency power band) and a peak at about 0.13 Hz (the low-frequency power band).

ability, these techniques typically use regression techniques to predict an R-R interval from a linear combination of the immediately prior R-R intervals. The popularity of these parametric identification techniques has expanded with the development of efficient computational algorithms. They do not make classical spectral analysis obsolete but provide another approach by which a signal can typically be represented as a sum of a smaller number of periodic components chosen at specific frequencies at which power is maximal. For analysis of R-R variability data, the ability to obtain a small number of discrete frequencies has been the primary advantage of these techniques, rather than the HF resolution required for many applications in geophysics or communications. This simpler frequency decomposition facilitates cross-spectral analysis of R-R–interval data with other physiologic time series such as blood pressure and respiration (20,21). Another alternative for spectral analysis of R-R–interval data is complex demodulation (18). In this technique, a continuous estimate of power in the vicinity of a small number of discrete frequencies is produced. Such an approach can be used, for example, to track the HF component representing vagal activity with various conditions (22,23).

Other analysis techniques being applied to the R-R–interval data come from the theory of nonlinear dynamics, or the "chaos theory" as it is popularly known (24–28). These techniques assume the data is aperiodic, but not random. Most of the nonlinear dynamic measures can be derived from 24-hour Holter ECG recordings digitized at 128 samples per second; Skinner's point estimate of the correlation dimension (PD2) has been calculated from ECG recordings digitized at 512 samples per second. Nonlinear dynamics is less intuitive in its interpretation, less understandable in direct terms, and its statistical theory less advanced. However, nonlinear dynamic measures quantify the complexity of the R-R–interval time series in a way that linear methods including conventional power-spectral analysis do not. A lack of complexity may not only characterize the effects of disease in a useful way but also may improve the prediction of outcomes of patients with cardiac diseases.

Despite the common use of the term "heart rate variability," most investigators actually perform power-spectral analysis on R-R intervals (thus our use of the term R-R–interval variability). Some investigators calculate a series of instantaneous heart rates from a sequence of R-R intervals and perform power-spectral analysis on the instantaneous heart rates. For physiologic or pharmacologic studies, such as effect of posture, breathing maneuvers, and drug effects, power spectra obtained from a series of R-R intervals (heart period or R-R variability) or from a series of instantaneous heart rates (heart rate variability) yield virtually identical results. However, in correlations and multivariate analyses, R-R variability and heart rate variability are not equivalent. For example, the standard deviation of instantaneous heart rate has almost no correlation with average heart rate while the

standard deviation of normal R-R intervals has a substantial correlation with average R-R interval ($r \sim 0.50$).

Physiologic Significance of Standard Frequency Bands

Power-spectral measures of the R-R time series delineate cyclic fluctuations in the R-R intervals in terms of their frequency and power. Table 6.2-1 lists the standard frequencies that are estimated for use in cardiac physiologic or epidemiologic studies. To estimate spectral, data should be collected for about 15 times the period of the fluctuations being estimated, that is, for HF power with a frequency of 0.25 Hz about 1.0 minutes (4-second period × 15) should be the minimum duration used for analysis. For LF power (0.04 to 0.15 Hz) centered on 0.10 Hz, data should be collected for about 2.5 minutes (10-second period × 15). Below 0.04 Hz, R-R–interval power spectra are log-linear and inversely related to the frequency; that is, the lower the frequency, the greater the power (so-called 1/f relationship) (29). Because of the 1/f relationship, power spectra done on 24-hours of R-R–interval data have more than 80% of their power in the frequency band less than 0.04 Hz.

Physiologic perturbations and pharmacologic interventions help to define physiologic systems responsible for cyclic fluctuations in the R-R intervals. HF power (0.15 to 0.40 Hz) represents a pure vagal efferent signal that is modulated by ventilation (respiratory sinus arrhythmia) (30–32). The HF peak varies with ventilatory frequency and usually is found at a frequency of about 0.25 Hz, corresponding to 15 breaths per minute. Breathing cued to several metronome rates shows that the peak of HF power moves to the frequency of breathing (32,33). HF power disappears almost totally after intravenous injection of atropine, indicating that the efferent neural signal travels on the vagus nerve (32,33). LF power (0.04 to 0.15 Hz) has contributions from vagal and sympathetic modulation of R-R intervals (32–34). LF power seems to modulate on the spontaneous cycling of arterial blood pressure, that is, the Mayer waves, at a frequency of about 0.10 Hz. The ratio of LF to HF power is a useful index of sympathetic-parasympathetic balance, particularly during postural changes. On standing, HF power decreases to about 25% of its supine value; LF power decreases slightly or increases. Thus, the LF : HF ratio increases very substantially due to an increase in Mayer waves upon standing up and the increased BRS in the upright posture (33). The LF power in the supine position is abolished by atropine; the increase in LF : HF ratio seen on standing or being tilted upright is attenuated markedly after β-adrenergic blockade (32,33). Although somewhat crude, HF and LF power in a power spectrum of the R-R time series can provide important information about the autonomic nervous system in intact humans during normal daily activities. Spectral analysis is readily available and inexpensive, which makes the test feasible to use in large-scale epidemiologic studies or clinical trials. Also, the methodology lends itself to physiologic or pharmacologic studies that measure autonomic nervous system activity before and after an intervention.

Strong correlations are found among time and frequency domain measures of R-R variability in healthy subjects and after myocardial infarction. Each frequency domain measure of R-R variability is so strongly correlated ($r \geq 0.90$) with a time domain variable that the variables are essentially equivalent (Table 6.2-2).

Day-to-Day Reproducibility of R-R Variability

Many Holter variables, such as ventricular arrhythmias or ischemic episodes, are quite variable from day to day. Although it might be anticipated that there would be considerable day-to-day instability in measures of R-R variability (particularly those components that reflect sympathetic or parasympathetic nervous activity), this is not the case.

Kleiger and colleagues (35) studied 14 healthy subjects, 20 to 55 years of age, to determine day-to-day stability of R-R variability. Time and frequency domain measures of R-R variability were measured on two 24-hour recordings made 3 to 65 days apart (median of 18 days): one under baseline conditions and the other during placebo treatment. The power-spectral measures of R-R variability were essentially constant from day to day during the range of the time studied (3 to 65 days) despite marked differences among the 5-minute intervals within a day. Day-to-day stability makes it easy to detect small differences in R-R variability resulting from disease or drug treatment. Although a significant "placebo effect" can be found for blood pressure or frequency of myocardial ischemic episodes, none was found for R-R variability (35).

Several studies show that the day-to-day stability of R-R variability is greater for patients with heart disease than for healthy persons (36). The sicker the patient group, the more stable R-R variability is from day-to-day (35,36). The stability of measures of R-R variability facilitates distinguishing real changes caused by progression or regression of cardiac disease or those caused by drug effects from apparent changes resulting from random variation.

Predictive Value of R-R Variability in Heart Disease

The prognostic value of R-R variability has been shown in several large samples of patients with coronary heart disease studied by several groups of investigators. R-R variability has substantial, independent predictive value in coronary heart disease when measured at various times after myocardial infarction—soon after admission, at hospital discharge, and after full recovery. The initial studies of R-R variability were done before thrombolysis became the standard of care for the treatment of acute myocardial infarction (37,38). More recently, a number of studies in the "thrombolytic era" have confirmed that R-R variability is still a potent predictor of mortality in post–myocardial infarction patients treated with thrombolytic agents (39–42). Also, R-R variability has predictive value in patients with chronic congestive heart failure (43,44).

R-R Variability to Assess Prognosis after Myocardial Infarction

R-R variability is an excellent predictor of risk after myocardial infarction. In 1978, Wolf and colleagues (1) first

TABLE 6.2-2. CORRELATIONS AMONG MEASURES OF HEART PERIOD VARIABILITY (N = 715)

	Night-Day Difference	SDNN	In Total Power	In ULF Power	SDANN Index	In VLF Power	SDNN Index	In LF Power	In R-MSSD	In pNN50	In HF Power	In LF/HF Power
Night-day difference	1.00											
SDNN	0.71	1.00										
In Total power	0.68	0.96	1.00									
In ULF power	0.71	0.95	0.99	1.00								
SDANN index	0.75	0.98	0.94	0.96	1.00							
In VLF power	0.43	0.78	0.82	0.75	0.68	1.00						
SDNN index	0.44	0.82	0.79	0.71	0.70	0.90	1.00					
In LF power	0.42	0.72	0.75	0.67	0.61	0.91	0.89	1.00				
In R-MSSD	0.28	0.62	0.58	0.52	0.51	0.60	0.78	0.65	1.00			
In pNN50	0.27	0.57	0.56	0.50	0.49	0.59	0.71	0.64	0.93	1.00		
In HF power	0.35	0.67	0.66	0.59	0.57	0.70	0.82	0.77	0.92	0.89	1.00	
In LF/HF power	0.17	0.20	0.26	0.23	0.17	0.45	0.25	0.49	-0.25	-0.22	-0.18	1.00

In = natural logarithm; SDNN, SD of 211 normal R-R intervals in the entire 24-h ECG recording; ULF, ultra low frequency; SDANN index, SD of the average normal R-R intervals for all 5-min segments of a 24-h ECG recording; VLF, very low frequency; SDNN index, mean of the SD of all normal R-R intervals for all 5-min segments of a 24-h ECG recording; R-MSSD, root-mean-square successive difference; pNN50, percentage of differences between adjacent normal R-R intervals that are more than 50 ms computed over the entire 24-h ECG recording; LF, low frequency; HF, high frequency.

reported an association between R-R variability and prognosis in patients with acute myocardial infarction. A 60-second ECG recording was made for 176 patients on admission to the coronary care unit. Short-term R-R variability was estimated as the variance of 30 consecutive R-R intervals from the 60-second strip. A variance for such a short time interval measures primarily respiratory sinus arrhythmia, that is, vagal activity modulated by breathing. They arbitrarily chose a variance value of 1,000 ms^2, which dichotomized their group into 103 patients (59%) without sinus arrhythmia (variance, <1,000 ms^2) and 73 patients (42%) with sinus arrhythmia. They found that patients with R-R variance of less than 1,000 ms^2 were more likely to have anterior myocardial infarction, a Norris index of more than or equal to 10, low values for average R-R interval, and later admission to hospital. The mean age in the two groups was almost the same (56 and 57 years). The hospital mortality rate of patients with R-R variance of less than 1,000 ms^2 was 15.5%, compared with 4.1% for patients with R-R variance of more than or equal to 1,000 ms^2, a relative risk of 3.8 (95% confidence interval [CI], 1.1–12.5). After adjusting for heart rate or location of the infarct, we found that low R-R variance was still significantly associated with higher mortality rates. Only 19 deaths occurred in the study group, so the strength of the association was not estimated precisely. Also, no account was taken of left ventricular function, ventricular arrhythmias, or myocardial ischemia as covariate, so the independent predictive value of R-R variability was not established. Nevertheless, this study was the first to call attention to the possible prognostic significance of R-R variability measured early after myocardial infarction.

In 1987, Kleiger and colleagues (37) reported that the standard deviation of the normal R-R intervals (SDNN), calculated during a 24-hour period, predicted death after myocardial infarction. This measure of R-R variability is correlated very strongly with total power in a 24-hour R-R power spectrum (45). This study included 808 patients and 127 deaths. The 24-hour Holter recordings were done 11 ± 3 days after infarction. An SDNN of 50 ms was chosen arbitrarily to dichotomize their group into 125 patients (16%) with low values and 683 patients (84%) with high values. During 2 to 4 years of follow-up, the mortality rate of patients with an SDNN of less than 50 ms was 34%, compared with a 12% mortality rate in patients with an SDNN of more than or equal to 50 ms, a relative risk of 2.8 (95% CI, 2.0–3.8) (Fig. 6.2-2). SDNN predicted mortality independent of previously known risk predictors such as left ventricular ejection fraction (EF) or ventricular arrhythmias. This study was the first to show the independent predictive value of R-R variability for all-cause mortality after myocardial infarction.

Bigger and colleagues (38) studied 715 patients 2 weeks after myocardial infarction to establish the associations between six power-spectral measures of R-R–period variability calculated from continuous 24-hour ECG recordings and mortality during 4 years of follow-up before and after adjust-

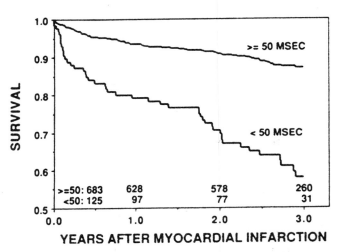

FIGURE 6.2-2. Survival curves of standard deviation of normal R-R intervals (SDNN). (From Kleiger RI, Miller JP, Bigger JT, et al. Decreased heart rate variability and its association with increased mortality after acute myocardial infarction. *Am J Cardiol* 1987;59:256–262, with permission.)

ing for five previously established risk predictors. The association between the six measures of R-R variability and three mortality end points were evaluated: death from all causes, cardiac death, and arrhythmic death by the Hinkle-Thaler definition (46). Each measure of R-R variability had a significant and at least moderately strong univariate association with all-cause mortality, cardiac death, and arrhythmic death (Fig. 6.2-3). Ultra LF and very LF power had stronger associations with all three mortality end points than HF power. The 24-hour total power (equivalent to SDNN) also had a strong association with all three mortality end points (38).

Power-spectral measures of R-R variability were significantly and strongly associated with subsequent all-cause mortality and arrhythmic death after adjusting for other postinfarction risk predictors, such as age, New York Heart Association (NYHA) functional class, rales in the coronary care unit, left ventricular EF, and ventricular arrhythmias detected in a 24-hour Holter ECG recording (38). Adding power-spectral measures of R-R variability, measured about 10 days after myocardial infarction, to previously known postinfarction risk predictors identified small subgroups with a 2.5-year mortality risk of approximately 50% (38).

Bigger and colleagues (47) also showed that power-law analysis of R-R–interval variability in 24-hour ECG recordings made soon after myocardial infarction was a better predictor of cardiac death than the usual power-spectral analyses of R-R variability (47). The slope and the intercept of the regression of log(power) on log(frequency) between 10^{-4} and 10^{-2} Hz were strongly associated with cardiac and arrhythmic death after myocardial infarction. Huikuri and colleagues (48) had very similar results in a study of 305 elderly (65 years or older) Finns who were living in the city of Turku. During 10 years of follow-up, 184 participants

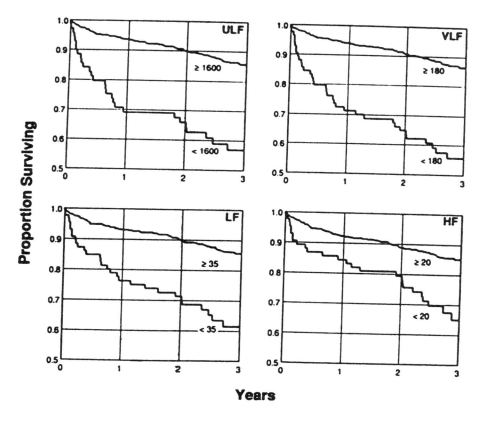

FIGURE 6.2-3. Survival curves of frequency domain measures. (From Bigger JT, Fleiss JL, Steinman RC, et al. Frequency domain measures of heart period variabiliy and mortality after myocardial infarction. *Circulation* 1992; 85:164–171, with permission.)

died; 74 died of cardiac disease. The slope of the regression of log(power) on log(frequency) between 10^{-4} and 10^{-2} Hz (called the β slope by this group) was strongly associated with total mortality and with cardiac and cerebrovascular deaths (relative risk, 2.0 and 2.8, respectively). The regression slope (β slope) was a significant and the strongest predictor of cardiac and cerebrovascular mortality after adjusting statistically for various cardiovascular risk factors. Huikuri and colleagues (49) conducted another study of R-R variability in a subgroup of 446 patients with acute myocardial infarction and a left ventricular EF of less than 0.36 selected from the Danish Investigations of Arrhythmia and Mortality on Dofetilide-Myocardial Infarction (DIAMOND-MI) study (49). A 24-hour ECG was done 5 to 10 days after infarction and the patients were followed for an average of 2 years. Time, frequency, and fractal measures of R-R–interval variability were calculated and related to death during follow-up. The fractal measures of R-R–interval variability included Poincaré plot analysis, power-law scaling analysis (the β slope between 10^{-4} and 10^{-2} Hz), and short (less than 11 R-R intervals) and intermediate (more than 11 R-R intervals) fractal scaling exponents (called α_1 and α_2 slopes, respectively) calculated by detrended fluctuation analysis. During follow-up, 114 patients died, 75 of arrhythmic deaths and 28 of nonarrhythmic cardiac deaths. Of the large number of measures of R-R variability performed in this study, reduced short-term fractal scaling exponent was a somewhat more power-

ful predictor of total mortality, arrhythmic deaths, and nonarrhythmic cardiac deaths (relative risk, 3.0; 95% CI, 2.5–4.2) than the other measures . The short-term scaling exponent, α_1, remained a significant predictor of death after statistical adjustment for age, NYHA functional class, EF, and use of cardiac medications.

Short-Term Measures of R-R Variability

Previous studies have shown that the activity of the sympathetic and parasympathetic nervous system can be characterized adequately by R-R variability from time periods as short as 2 to 15 minutes (32–34). Bigger and colleagues (50) compared short-term (from 2- to 15-minute) and long-term (24-hour) measures of R-R variability in their ability to predict mortality in the same sample of 715 patients post–myocardial infarction. Short segments of ECG recordings were selected from two time periods for analysis: 8:00 A.M. to 4:00 P.M. and 12:00 A.M. to 5:00 A.M. The former corresponds to the time interval during which short-term measures of R-R variability would most likely be obtained. The latter, during sleep, represents a period of increased vagal tone similar to the conditions that exist when a person is lying quietly in a laboratory. Frequency domain measures were calculated from spectral analysis of heart period data during a 24-hour interval and for 15-, 10-, 5-, and 2-minute segments during the day and at night. Mean power-spectral values from short periods during the day and night were similar to 24-hour values, and the correlations between short-segment values and 24-hour values were strong (many correlations were 0.75 or more). Using the optimal cutpoints determined previously for the 24-hour power-spectral values, we determined the predictive value of R-R variability measured from short segments of ECG recordings. Power spectral measures of R-R variability from short segments were excellent predictors of all-cause, cardiac, and arrhythmic mortality, as well as sudden death. Patients with low values were two to four times as likely to die during an average follow-up of 31 months, as were patients with high values. Power-spectral measures of R-R variability calculated from short (2 to 15 minutes) ECG recordings are remarkably similar to those calculated during 24 hours and are excellent predictors of all-cause mortality and sudden cardiac death. These data suggest that R-R variability can be measured from a short-term recording done in a laboratory or office setting and may not require a full 24-hour ambulatory ECG recording.

R-R Variability Predicts Arrhythmic Events

Farrell and colleagues (39) found that R-R variability predicted arrhythmic events (sustained ventricular arrhythmias or arrhythmic death) better than nonarrhythmic deaths or recurrent ischemic events after myocardial infarction. The study group of 416 patients experienced 24 arrhythmic events and 47 deaths during follow-up. A 24-hour ECG recording and an SAECG were performed 6 or 7 days after myocardial infarction. R-R variability was measured by triangular interpolation of the frequency distribution of R-R intervals (the R-R variability index). The mean value for the R-R variability index was 27 ± 11 ms (range, 3 to 81 ms). Their group was dichotomized using a R-R variability index of 20 ms; 113 patients (27%) had low values and 348 patients (73%) had high values. Risk of an arrhythmic event during 2 years of follow-up was 32 times higher in the group with a R-R variability index of less than 20 ms, compared with the group with a value of more than or equal to 20 ms and the risk of experiencing a cardiac death was about seven times as high. The R-R variability index was a stronger univariate predictor of arrhythmic events or cardiac death than ventricular arrhythmias, SAECG, left ventricular EF, exercise test, or coronary angiography. The R-R variability index did not predict recurrent myocardial infarction. The best combination to predict arrhythmic events was an R-R variability index value of less than 20 ms, a positive SAECG recording, and repetitive ventricular premature contractions present in a 24-hour Holter recording. Figure 6.2-4 shows how combinations of risk predictors improve positive predictive accuracy for arrhythmic events during long-term follow-up after myocardial infarction. Adding the SAECG to the R-R variability index doubled positive predictive accuracy, and adding repetitive ventricular premature contractions to the combination almost doubled positive predictive accuracy again. The combination of these

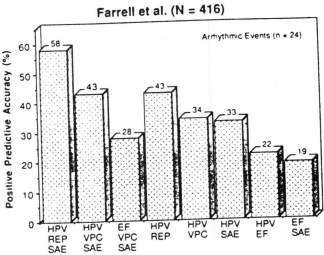

FIGURE 6.2-4. Bar graphs of mortality rates with combined risk factors. (From Farrell TG, Bashir Y, Cripps T, et al. Risk stratification for arrhythmic events in postinfarction patients based on heart rate variability, ambulatory electrocardiographic variables and the signal-averaged electrocardiogram. *J Am Coll Cardiol* 1991;18:687–697, with permission.)

three variables had a positive predictive accuracy of 58%. Skinner and colleagues (51) showed that a decrease in the PD2 of the R-R–interval time series occurred a few hours before ventricular fibrillation in Holter recordings of 11 patients, but not in recordings from 13 high-risk patients who did not develop ventricular fibrillation. These authors speculated that the ability of the PD2 to predict imminent sudden death was explained by its ability to measure deterministic chaos, unlike linear measures, such as standard deviation of R-R intervals, a measure of stochastic noise.

R-R Variability Predicts Death and Arrhythmic Events after Thrombolysis

Most original studies of R-R variability were done before the institution of thrombolytic therapy of acute myocardial infarction. Two more recent studies in which a significant number of patients received thrombolytic therapy demonstrated that R-R variability is still a strong predictor of mortality after myocardial infarction (40,42). Copie and colleagues (40) evaluated the predictive power of R-R variability, left ventricular EF, and mean R-R interval in 579 patients followed for 2 or more years after acute myocardial infarction. More than half of the patients received thrombolytic therapy. R-R variability was measured by triangular interpolation of the frequency distribution of R-R intervals (the R-R variability index). Both mean R-R interval and the R-R variability index were strong univariate predictors of cardiac mortality and all-cause mortality. Mean R-R interval dichotomized at 700 ms had a sensitivity of 45%, a specificity of 85%, and a positive predictive accuracy of 20%. R-R variability index dichotomized at 17 units had a sensitivity of 40%, a specificity of 86%, and a positive predictive accuracy of 20%. The association of low R-R variability and increased mortality was independent of mean R-R interval.

Role of R-R Variability and Baroreceptor Sensitivity

Autonomic Tone and Reflexes After Myocardial Infarction (ATRAMI) was a prospective, longitudinal epidemiologic study to delineate the role of autonomic nervous system markers for predicting cardiac death or nonfatal cardiac arrest after myocardial infarction (42). SDNN was used as the measure of R-R variability and BRS was determined using the phenylephrine method (52). Although both of these autonomic markers provide information about autonomic activity, they measure different aspects of physiology. R-R variability provides information about tonic autonomic modulation under ambulatory conditions, whereas BRS provides information about reflex autonomic activity in response to activation of the baroreceptor and can be viewed as a "vagal stress test." The main objective of ATRAMI was to determine whether BRS provided additional prognostic information for cardiac mortality independent of R-R variability, left ventricular EF, and ventricular arrhythmias. ATRAMI was a multicenter, international prospective study that enrolled 1,284 patients with a recent (less than 28 days) myocardial infarction; 63% of patients were treated with thrombolytic therapy, and 24-hour ECG recordings were done to quantify R-R variability and ventricular arrhythmias. During 21 months of follow-up, the primary end point occurred in only 49 patients (3.9%) and included 44 cardiac deaths and 5 nonfatal cardiac arrests. Low values of either R-R variability (SDNN of less than 70 ms) or BRS (less than 3.0 ms/mm Hg) carried a significant multivariate risk of cardiac mortality (3.2 [95% CI, 1.42–7.36] and 2.8 [95% CI, 1.24–6.16], respectively) (Fig. 6.2-5). The combination of low SDNN and low BRS further increased risk; the 2-year mortality rate was 17% when both were below the cutoffs and 2% (*p* < 0.0001) when both were well preserved (SDNN > 105 ms; BRS > 6.1 ms/mm Hg). Importantly, SDNN and BRS added significant prognostic value to left ventricular EF. The combination of low SDNN or BRS with a left ventricular EF of 0.35 carried a relative risk of 6.7 (3.1 to 14.6) or 8.7 (4.3 to 17.6), respectively, compared with patients with a left ventricular EF of more than or equal to 0.35 and less compromised SDNN (≥70 ms) and BRS (≥3 ms/mm Hg). Power-spectral measures of R-R variability also were demonstrated to be strong independent predictors of cardiac mortality after myocardial infarction (53). Each power-spectral measurement of R-R variability had a statistically significant and strong (relative risk, >3) univariate association with cardiac mortality. LF power was the strongest univariate predictor of the power-spectral measures of R-R variability. The independent prognostic information

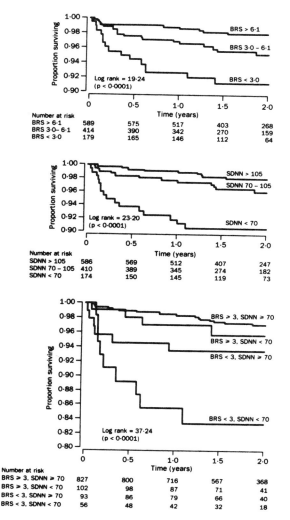

FIGURE 6.2-5. Kaplan-Meier survival curves for total cardiac mortality rate according to baroreflex sensitivity, standard deviation of normal R-R intervals (SDNN), and their combination. *p* Value refers to difference in event rate between subgroups. (From La Rovere MT, Bigger JT Jr, Marcus FI, et al. Baroreflex sensitivity and heart-rate variability in prediction of total cardiac mortality after myocardial infarction. ATRAMI [Autonomic Tone and Reflexes After Myocardial Infarction] investigators. *Lancet* 1998;351:480, with permission.)

provided by BRS and R-R variability provides compelling evidence for the hypothesis that altered autonomic balance contributes to cardiac mortality after myocardial infarction. The finding that R-R variability and BRS independently predict cardiac mortality suggests that tonic autonomic modulation and reflex autonomic activity identify different aspects of susceptibility to fatal ventricular arrhythmias.

Effect of Myocardial Infarction on R-R Variability

R-R variability is reduced to about 25% of normal 2 to 3 weeks after myocardial infarction (54). Several small studies have studied the recovery of R-R variability early and late after myocardial infarction.

Early Recovery of R-R Variability Varies with Location of Myocardial Infarction

Flapan and colleagues (55) studied the recovery of a time domain measure of HF power in 20 highly selected patients who experienced their first myocardial infarction. All patients were treated with streptokinase and aspirin acutely and continued to receive atenolol and aspirin during the 3-month follow-up. Continuous 24-hour ECG recordings were made at less than 1.5, 7, 42, and 140 days after myocardial infarction. Cardiac parasympathetic activity was measured using the counts of the number of times that successive R-R intervals differed by more than 50 ms (NN50) in a 24-hour period. For all 20 patients, NN50 doubled between 1.5 days and 6 weeks after infarction and tripled between 1.5 days and 3 months. There was a striking difference in the pattern of recovery of NN50 depending on the site of infarction. For the nine patients with inferior myocardial infarction, NN50 was within normal limits at 1.5 days after infarction and did not change significantly during the 3-month follow-up. For the 11 patients with anterior myocardial infarction, NN50 was 20% of normal at 1.5 days and recovered progressively to 67% of normal by 3 months. By 6 weeks after myocardial infarction, there was no significant difference in NN50 between patients with anterior infarcts and those with inferior infarcts. In anterior infarcts, there was a striking difference in the recovery of heart rate, which stabilized by day 7, and R-R variability, which continued to increase for 3 months. The patients in this study were highly selected and few in number. Therefore, the study needs to be confirmed. If confirmed, the mechanism for the difference between early vagal activity for inferior and anterior myocardial infarction needs further exploration. Flapan and colleagues (55) postulate that the infarct process, particularly prostaglandin release, causes increased vagal afferent nerve traffic, which is responsible for preserving efferent vagal activity. However, it is not clear why increased afferent vagal nerve traffic would not increase NN50 above normal values rather than just preserve normal values. Also, their explanation does not account for the marked decrease in cardiac vagal activity in anterior myocardial infarction. Bigger and colleagues (56) explained decreased cardiac vagal activity in anterior infarction by postulating an increase in afferent sympathetic nerve traffic, an effect that has been shown to decrease efferent vagal nerve traffic in experimental myocardial ischemia. Surely, we have much more to learn about the mechanisms accounting for changes in cardiac neural activity that occur during acute myocardial infarction.

Late Phase of Recovery

Long-term recovery of R-R variability after myocardial infarction was studied in the placebo cohort of the Cardiac Arrhythmia Pilot Study (CAPS) (54), that is, the 68 patients who had 24-hour ECG recordings at baseline, 3, 6, and 12 months. The 24-hour power-spectral density was computed using fast Fourier transforms. The baseline values (25 days after myocardial infarction) for R-R variability were similar in CAPS patients to those found in 715 patients who participated in the Multicenter Post Infarction Program (MPIP), indicating that the CAPS sample is generally representative of postinfarction patients with respect to these measures. The values for the five measures were one third to one half of those found in 95 healthy persons of similar age and gender. There was a substantial increase in all measures of R-R variability between the baseline 24-hour ECG recording and the 3-month recording ($p < 0.001$). Between 3 months and 12 months, the values were quite stable for the group as a whole and for individuals (intraclass correlation coefficients ≥ 0.66). Even at 12 months after infarction, full recovery values for the five measures of R-R variability were only one half to two thirds the values found in the sample of 95 healthy age- and sex-matched persons.

Predictive Value of Power-Spectral Measures of R-R Variability Late after Myocardial Infarction

To determine whether power-spectral measures of R-R variability predict death when measured late after infarction, Bigger and colleagues (57) studied the 331 patients in CAPS who survived for 1 year, had a 24-hour ECG recording made after the CAPS drug was washed out, and were discharged on no antiarrhythmic drug therapy. Thirty deaths occurred during an average of 788 days follow-up. Power-spectral measures of R-R variability were calculated using 24-hour continuous ECG recordings. Because of the increase in R-R variability that occurs after myocardial infarction, the optimum cutpoints in the 1-year recordings were substantially higher than those previously determined 2 weeks after infarction (Table 6.2-3). Each power-spectral

TABLE 6.2-3. OPTIMAL CUTPOINTS FOR PREDICTION OF ALL-CAUSE MORTALITY AFTER MYOCARDIAL INFARCTION BY FREQUENCY DOMAIN MEASURES OF HEART PERIOD VARIABILITY

	Optimal Cutpoints	
Variable	At Discharge 2 Weeks after MI	After Recovery From MI
Ultra-low-frequency power (ms²)	1600	5000
Very-low-frequency power (ms²)	180	600
Low-frequency power (m²)	35	120
High-frequency power < 35 (ms²)	20	35
Total power (ms²)	2000	6000
Low-frequency to high-frequency ratio	0.95	1.6

MI, myocardial infarction.

measure of R-R variability had a strong and significant univariate association with 2.5-year all-cause mortality; the relative risks ranged from 2.5 to 5.6 (Fig. 6.2-6). Prediction of death was not improved when measures of R-R variability made within a month of myocardial infarction were added to a survival model that contained measures of R-R variability made one year after myocardial infarction. After adjustment for age, NYHA functional class, rales in the cardiac care unit, left ventricular EF, and ventricular arrhythmias, measures of heart period variability made a year after infarction still had a strong and significant association with all-cause mortality. It is clear from this study that R-R variability, measured late after infarction, predicts death independent of other important postinfarction risk predictors. Some patients recover to normal values of R-R variability during the year after myocardial infarction. Others show very little recovery or actually decrease. The final recovery values for R-R variability are the best predictors of subsequent events; that is, knowledge of the recovery pattern does not improve prediction significantly.

The optimal cutpoints listed in Table 6.2-3 are derived from postinfarction samples in the prethrombolytic era. Post–myocardial infarction patients who receive thrombolytic therapy have higher values of R-R variability (42). Optimal cutpoints for the different measures of R-R variability in patients who have received thrombolytic therapy have not been formally analyzed, although they are likely to be near the optimal cutpoints for patients late after myocardial infarction in the prethrombolytic era (right-hand column of Table 6.2-3).

R-R Variability to Assess Prognosis in Patients with Heart Failure

Patients with heart failure have autonomic dysfunction. The United Kingdom Heart Failure Evaluation and Assessment of Risk Trial (UK-HEART) evaluated the prognostic value of R-R variability in a large prospective study of patients with heart failure (43). In this study, 433 patients with congestive heart failure (NYHA classes I to III) with a mean EF of 0.41 ± 0.17 were followed for 482 ± 161 days and the 54 deaths were classified as arrhythmic ($n = 18$), resulting from progressive heart failure ($n = 23$), or other ($n = 13$). SDNN was a strong predictor of mortality (Fig. 6.2-7); 6% of the patients had an SDNN of less than 50 ms with an annual mortality rate of 51.4%, 32% had an SDNN of 50 to 100 ms with an annual mortality rate of 12.7%, and 62% had an SDNN or more than 100 ms with an annual mortality rate of 5.5%. SDNN was only weakly related to left ventricular EF ($r = 0.12$). In a multivariate analysis, SDNN remained a significant predictor of mortality in a model that included cardiothoracic ratio, left ventricular end-systolic dimension, and serum sodium levels.

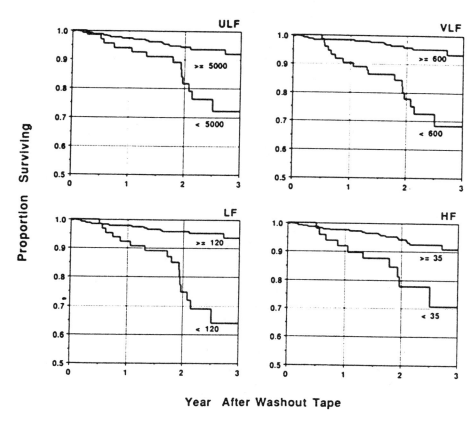

Year After Washout Tape

FIGURE 6.2-6. Survival curves of frequency domain measures from "late after myocardial infarction" data. (From Bigger JT Jr, Fleiss JL, Rolnitzky LM, Steinman RC. Frequency domain measures of heart period variability to assess risk late after myocardial infarction. *J Am Coll Cardiol* 1993;21:729–736, with permission.)

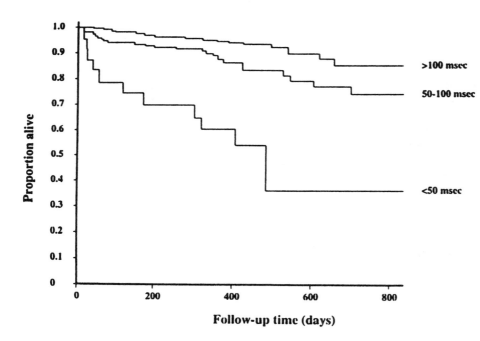

FIGURE 6.2-7. Kaplan-Meier survival curves in patients with heart failure categorized into standard deviation of normal R-R intervals (SDNN) subgroups. (From Nolan J, Batin PD, Andrews R, et al. Prospective study of heart rate variability and mortality in chronic heart failure: results of the United Kingdom Heart Failure Evaluation and Assessment of Risk Trial [UK-HEART]. *Circulation* 1998;98:1513, with permission.)

In the analysis of cause-specific mortality, 33% of the 54 deaths were classified as arrhythmic and 43% were classified as resulting from progressive heart failure. In multivariate analyses, predictors of arrhythmic death included cardiothoracic ratio, left ventricular end-diastolic dimension, the presence of unsustained VT, and serum potassium levels; SDNN was not a predictor of arrhythmic death. However, SDNN was the strongest predictor of death from progressive heart failure in a multivariate analysis that also included serum creatinine and serum sodium levels. A recent analysis of the Congestive Heart Failure–Survival Trial of Antiarrhythmic Therapy (CHF–STAT) heart failure group found that R-R variability was a strong predictor of total deaths and predicted arrhythmic deaths better than nonarrhythmic deaths (44).

The UK-HEART demonstrated that autonomic dysfunction measured by R-R variability was a strong predictor of death, particularly death from progressive heart failure, confirming the results of a number of smaller studies (58–61). The mechanisms of reduced R-R variability in heart failure are complex. Reduced values for R-R variability (particularly measures corresponding to rapid changes in R-R interval such as pNN50, RMSSD, and HF power) suggest that vagal modulation is reduced in heart failure and accompanies the well-known increases in sympathetic activation that occur in heart failure (43,62). Some investigators have suggested that abnormal breathing patterns and reduced physical activity in patients with heart failure may limit the prognostic utility of R-R variability in this group of patients (63,64). The data from the UK-HEART and CHF–STAT, however, demonstrate that R-R variability has prognostic significance in heart failure (43,44). Importantly, the UK-HEART and

CHF–STAT measured R-R variability from ambulatory 24-hour ECG recordings without measuring or controlling for breathing rate or physical activity.

R-R variability identifies patients with left ventricular dysfunction who benefit from amiodarone treatment. A substudy of the European Myocardial Infarct Amiodarone Trial (EMIAT) prospectively tested the hypothesis that patients with reduced R-R variability benefit from amiodarone treatment (65). EMIAT randomized 1,486 survivors of myocardial infarction with a left ventricular EF of less than or equal to 0.40 to amiodarone or placebo and followed them for 664 ± 107 days. EMIAT showed that amiodarone had no statistically significant effect on all-cause mortality rate but did reduce arrhythmic mortality. In the EMIAT substudy, 1,216 patients had 24-hour Holter recordings and two measures of R-R variability were calculated: R-R variability index of less than or equal to 20 units and SDNN of less than or equal to 50 ms. The Holter recordings were scanned at local centers and then analyzed centrally for R-R variability. This resulted in suboptimum identification of ectopic beats, which had a greater effect on SDNN (overestimating) than the R-R variability index. The substudy included 363 (29.9%) patients who had a heart rate variability index of less than or equal to 20 units. In the placebo arm of the study, patients with reduced R-R variability had a significantly higher mortality rate than patients with preserved R-R variability (22.8% versus 9.5%; *p* value not given).

In the prospectively defined subgroup of EMIAT with reduced R-R variability, there was a 23.2% reduction in all-cause mortality with amiodarone that did not meet statistical significance (22.8% versus 17.5%; *p* = 0.24) and a statistically significant 66% reduction in cardiac mortality

(12.8% versus 4.4%; *p* < 0.01). The efficacy of amiodarone in patients with reduced R-R variability was further evaluated in a number of patient categories (Fig. 6.2-8). The benefit of amiodarone was large in patients with reduced R-R variability and a resting heart rate more than or equal to 75 bpm; this subgroup had a 29.0% mortality rate when treated with placebo, compared with 19.3% when treated with amiodarone, a 33.7% reduction in mortality (*p* = 0.075). This important prospectively defined substudy is the first to demonstrate that R-R variability can select a group of patients with autonomic dysfunction who will benefit from prophylactic antiarrhythmic treatment. At least one randomized controlled trial is evaluating the use of prophylactic ICDs in patients with left ventricular dysfunction and reduced R-R variability (Defibrillator in Acute Myocardial Infarction Trial [DINAMIT]) (66). If this trial confirms a survival benefit for high-risk patients selected by low R-R variability and treated with an ICD, physicians will have a clear indication to use R-R variability to identify high-risk patients for prophylactic ICD therapy.

Conclusion

For many years, various short-term measures of R-R variability have been used to evaluate the status of the parasym-

pathetic nervous system in diseases such as diabetic neuropathy and for studying the responsiveness of the parasympathetic nervous system to laboratory protocols such as mental arithmetic. During the past 15 years, a number of large-scale epidemiologic studies have conclusively shown that measures of R-R variability predict death after myocardial infarction. Two studies demonstrated that R-R variability predicts mortality in patients with congestive heart failure. As univariate predictors, measures of R-R variability predict all-cause mortality, as well as left ventricular EF or unsustained ventricular arrhythmias. When measures of R-R variability are added to other risk predictors, such as left ventricular EF, unsustained ventricular arrhythmias, or SAECG, positive predictive accuracy is improved significantly. Measured early or late after infarction, R-R variability predicts death during long-term follow-up. R-R variability predicts arrhythmic events after myocardial infarction even better than all-cause mortality. Because R-R variability is a dynamic variable, it can be used to monitor physiologic or pharmacologic interventions or the progression of diseases. We have one example of R-R variability selecting patients who benefit from antiarrhythmic (amiodarone) therapy. Because R-R variability is useful, readily available, and inexpensive, we should see increasing use of this tool in the coming years.

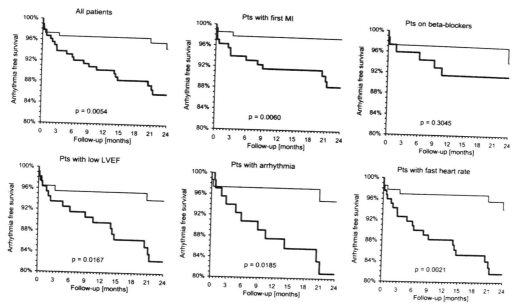

FIGURE 6.2-8. Curves of arrhythmia-free survival in patients in the European Myocardial Infarct Amiodarone Trial selected by a prospectively defined criterion: a heart rate variability index of ≤20 units. In each case, the *p* value corresponds to the log-rank statistics of the Kaplan-Meier survival model. Placebo arm (*bold line*) and the amiodarone arm (*fine line*) are both shown. Arrhythmia, ≥10 ventricular premature contractions per hour or 1 triplet; fast heart rate, baseline short-term heart rate of ≥75 beats per minute; low left ventricular ejection fraction, ≤0.30; MI, myocardial infarction. (From Malik M, Camm AJ, Janse MJ, et al. Depressed heart rate variability identifies postinfarction patients who might benefit from prophylactic treatment with amiodarone: a substudy of EMIAT [the European Myocardial Infarct Amiodarone Trial]. *J Am Coll Cardiol* 2000;35:1270, with permission.)

SIGNAL-AVERAGED ECG (SAECG)

The SAECG was developed 20 years ago to improve the signal to noise ratio of a surface ECG, thus permitting the identification of low-amplitude (microvolt level) signals at the end of the QRS complex that have been referred to as *late potentials*. Late potentials are thought to represent regional delayed activation and thus serve as a marker for the electrophysiologic substrate for reentrant ventricular tachyarrhythmias. As such, the SAECG has been used clinically to identify patients at high risk for developing sustained ventricular arrhythmias. Although a substantial amount of data demonstrate that patients with an abnormal SAECG are at high risk, the predictive accuracy of the SAECG is modest, 20% to 25%. The negative predictive accuracy of the SAECG, however, is extremely high, more than 90%. One of the most common uses of the SAECG today is to identify patients who are at low risk for having an arrhythmic event and who therefore do not need any further evaluation. In the following sections, the signal-processing techniques that are used to record the SAECG are discussed along with criteria for interpreting and classifying tracings. The pathophysiology of late potentials is briefly discussed, followed by a discussion of the clinical application of the SAECG.

Technical Aspects

An international task force of experts recommended standards for acquisition and analysis of the SAECG (67). The acquisition of the SAECG is most often done using a bipolar orthogonal lead system. The X lead should be positioned at the fourth intercostal space of the left and the right midaxillary lines. The Y lead should be positioned on the superior aspect of the manubrium sternum and on either the left iliac crest or the left upper leg. The Z lead should be positioned at the left parasternal fourth intercostal space (same as lead V_2 in the standard surface 12-lead ECG) and directly posterior on the left side of the vertebral column. Skin preparation is important. The skin should be cleansed and abraded to reduce impedance. Silver-silver chloride electrodes are recommended.

The primary signal-processing technique used to enhance the signal to noise ratio in the SAECG involves the temporal averaging of sequential QRS complexes (Fig. 6.2-9). This technique requires the detection and alignment of sequential QRS complexes. Random noise that is not synchronized to the QRS complex is ultimately "averaged out." As noise levels are reduced, low-amplitude signals that consistently appear on successive beats can be identified. Noise is reduced in proportion to the square root of the number of complexes that are averaged. If 400 beats are averaged, the noise levels are reduced 20-fold. The averaging technique requires that only QRS complexes with the same morphology be analyzed; premature ventricular beats or aberrantly conducted beats must be excluded. Selection of the correct QRS complexes is accomplished by an automated template-recognition algorithm, which first creates a template "normal beat" and then compares successive beats to the template. Only beats that are highly correlated with the template are averaged.

Digital filters are used in conjunction with averaging to reduce noise levels and enhance the identification of the

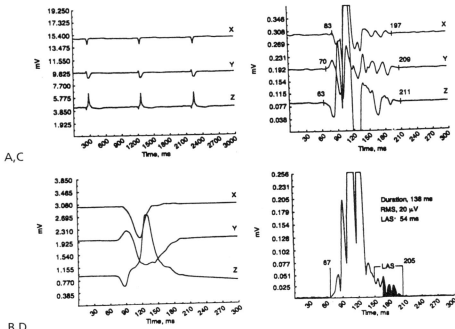

A,C

B,D

FIGURE 6.2-9. Example of signal-average electrocardiogram (SAECG). Sequence of processing an SAECG. **A:** The individual unfiltered orthogonal leads using time and amplitude scaling typical for an ECG. **B:** An averaged complex on an expanded timescale and increased gain, which allows detection of low-amplitude late potentials at the end of the QRS complex. **C:** Each lead at a higher gain after processing with a high-pass filter, which removes low-frequency components. **D:** The vector magnitude formed by a combination of the filtered orthogonal leads $(X^2 + Y^2 + Z^2)^{1/2}$. The duration (filtered QRS [*fQRS*]), the root mean square (*RMS*) listed as the RMS, and the low-amplitude signal are identified. (From Steinberg JS, Berbari EJ. *J Cardiovasc Electrophysiol* 1996;7: 974, with permission.)

onset and termination of the QRS complex. The most common filter used is a bidirectional filter (68), although other digital filters continue to be developed and evaluated. The high-pass component of a filter removes LF activity (usually less than 25 or 40 Hz) with only minimal attenuation of HF components. High-pass filters remove baseline drift of the ECG signal and the LF component of the ST segment and T wave, permitting better detection of QRS offset. Low-pass filters remove HF noise (usually more than 250 Hz) such as pectoral muscle potentials.

To optimize noise reduction, the acquisition of the SAECG should be done in a quiet room and after the patient has had a few minutes to relax. In most cases, the acquisition of the SAECG should continue until a sufficiently low noise level (for example, 0.3 to 0.5 μV) has been achieved (69). In most cases, this can be accomplished by averaging 200 to 300 beats (about 5 minutes), which should be sufficient to allow a recording of a signal with an acceptably low noise level. Acquisition can be considerably longer (10 to 20 minutes) in patients with atrial fibrillation or frequent ectopic beats.

Criteria for Interpretation and Classification

The criteria for interpreting the SAECG depend heavily on accurate recognition of the onset and offset of the QRS complex. Most studies use the vector magnitude of the filtered orthogonal leads $(X^2 + Y^2 + Z^2)^{1/2}$, also called *the filtered QRS,* to detect onset and offset of the QRS complex. The onset is relatively easy to identify, given the rapid deflection of the R wave. The offset of the QRS is more difficult to determine and by searching backward (from the T-wave region back toward the QRS) until the mean voltage exceeds three times the standard deviation of the baseline noise. The onset and offset of the QRS should be automatically determined but confirmed by a physician or adjusted manually when necessary.

Time domain analysis is most commonly used to interpret the SAECG. Three measurements are made: the duration of the filtered QRS (fQRS) duration, the root-mean-square (RMS) voltage of the terminal 40 ms of the filtered QRS (RMS40), and the duration of low-amplitude (less

than 40 μV) signal (Table 6.2-4 and Fig. 6.2-9). Different criteria for abnormality have been proposed and they are often based on using different filters. The criteria recommended by the Task Force are listed in Table 6.2-4 (67). The fQRS is the most important abnormality. Some investigators have required that two of three measurements should be abnormal to classify the SAECG as abnormal, although relatively few studies have compared different criteria. The Cardiac Arrhythmia Suppression Trial (CAST) SAECG substudy demonstrated that the fQRS had its optimum predictive accuracy (measured as the area under the receiver operating characteristic curve) when dichotomized at 120 ms rather than 114 ms (70). This study also demonstrated that the fQRS alone was the best predictor of arrhythmic events and the predictive accuracy was not improved by the addition of the RMS40 or the low-amplitude signal.

Other analytic techniques have been applied to the SAECG to improve the identification of late potentials or to improve the predictive accuracy of the SAECG. Spectral analysis of the SAECG takes advantage of differences in the frequency characteristics between late potentials and the QRS complex and ST segment. These techniques can identify the equivalent of "late potentials" within the QRS complex. Kelen and colleagues (71) first used spectral turbulence analysis of the SAECG to analyze abnormalities in the frequency content of overlapping narrow windows within the QRS complex. Recently, a combination of time domain and spectral turbulence analysis of the SAECG was shown to be better then either alone (72). Lander and colleagues (73) proposed another method of identifying intra-QRS "late potentials," which uses a parametric modeling of the SAECG to identify notches and slurs in the QRS complex in the time domain (73). In this study, the presence of abnormal intra-QRS potentials had a better predictive accuracy than standard time domain measures. Wavelet analysis has also been applied to the SAECG in an attempt to improve the temporal localization of abnormal frequency components within the QRS complex (74). The use of wavelet transformation has also been shown to improve the prognostic value of the SAECG after myocardial infarction (75). These new analytic tools are promising but need further validation.

TABLE 6.2-4. TIME DOMAIN MEASUREMENTS OF THE SIGNAL-AVERAGED ECG

Measurement	Abbreviation	Normal Values	Definition
Filtered QRS duration	fQRS	<114 ms	Duration of filtered QRS complex using a 40-Hz high-pass bidirectional filter
Root-mean square voltage in the terminal 40 ms	RMS	≥20 μV	Root-mean-square voltage in the terminal 40 ms of the filtered QRS complex
Late amplitude segment	LAS	≤38 ms	The amount of time that the terminal portion of filtered QRS complex is below 40 μV

See ref. 67.

Pathophysiology

Late potentials recorded using the SAECG from the body surface appear to be a manifestation of regional delayed activation of the myocardium. The delay in activation may be the result of a lengthened pathway of excitation, a decrease in conduction velocity, or both. Most myocardial infarctions do not result in complete transmural necrosis but leave behind a variable amount of surviving myocardium. Fibrosis not only creates barriers that lengthen the excitation pathway but also causes asynchronous and heterogeneous patterns of activation caused by disruption of the normal intercellular coupling and disruption of the parallel orientation of myocardial cell bundles (76,77). These heterogeneous patterns of activation are manifest as fragmented, low-amplitude local extracellular electrograms (Fig. 6.2-10).

The pathophysiologic link between late potentials detected on the SAECG and VT has been established from

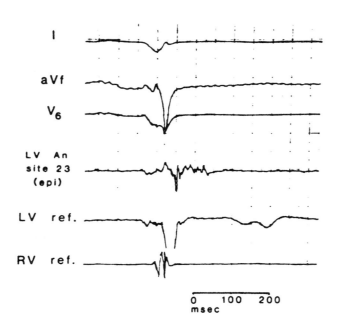

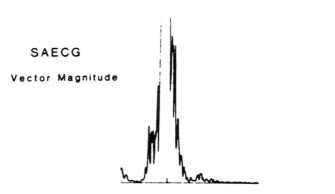

FIGURE 6.2-10. Correspondence of the signal-average electrocardiogram and fragmented intracardiac electrograms.

a number of experiments. In dogs and humans, late potentials recorded from the SAECG correspond in time to fragmented intracardiac electrograms that span diastole (78). This type of continuous diastolic electrical activity is associated with the initiation and perpetuation of reentrant VT (79). Late potentials from the SAECG or fragmented local intracardiac electrograms reflect a substrate for sustained VT. However, only a few patients with evidence of delayed myocardial activation develop ventricular arrhythmias, suggesting that additional triggers (such as ischemia, ventricular ectopic complexes, or autonomic nervous activity) are necessary to initiate sustained ventricular arrhythmias.

Clinical Applications of the Signal-Average Electrocardiogram

The initial relationship between late potentials on the SAECG and VT was established in cohort studies of patients with ischemic heart disease that compared patients with and without clinical or inducible sustained VT (68,80,81). The SAECG was abnormal in 70% to 80% of patients with sustained VT, in contrast to 10% to 15% of patients with ischemic heart disease but without VT, and only 6% of normal volunteers. One of the first applications of the SAECG was to identify the likelihood that patients with previous myocardial infarction and unsustained VT would have inducible sustained VT during an electrophysiologic test. Three small studies evaluated this use and found that the SAECG had a sensitivity of about 70% and a specificity of about 80% with a positive predictive accuracy of about 50% and a negative predictive accuracy of about 90% (82–84).

Risk Stratification after Myocardial Infarction

The initial studies of the prognostic significance of the SAECG after myocardial infarction were done in the 1980s before thrombolytic therapy was used. Breithardt and colleagues (80) published the first prospective study demonstrating that an abnormal SAECG predicted the occurrence of spontaneous arrhythmic events (sudden cardiac death and VT) after myocardial infarction. Subsequent studies confirmed the prognostic significance of an abnormal SAECG (39,85–87). These studies reported that late potentials were present in 20% to 50% of patients after myocardial infarction and were more common in patients with inferior wall myocardial infarction; the posterior wall normally depolarizes late in the cardiac cycle, so delayed activation in this region is more likely to give rise to late potentials. Delay in activation of the anterior wall may not give rise to late potentials. This identification of intra-QRS "late potentials" in anterior infarcts has been an area of active research (71,74,88). Although all of these early studies confirmed the prognostic significance of the SAECG after myocardial infarction, a low positive predictive accuracy, similar to other noninvasive tests, was consistently noted.

Use after Reperfusion

The impact of thrombolytic therapy on the SAECG has been evaluated in a number of studies. In an uncontrolled study of 106 patients, of whom 44 were treated with thrombolytic therapy, late potentials were less likely to be identified in patients who received thrombolytic therapy than those who did not (5% versus 23%) (89). Among the patients who received thrombolytic therapy, 2 of 6 patients with an occluded infarct–related artery had late potentials, whereas none of the 38 patients with a patent infarct–related artery had late potentials. Other investigators have confirmed a strong association between a closed infarct–related artery and the presence of late potentials (89–94).

A substudy of the CAST sought to determine whether the prognostic significance of an abnormal SAECG (defined as an fQRS duration of more than or equal to 120 ms) measured after myocardial infarction is influenced by coronary artery reperfusion (either thrombolytic therapy or angioplasty) in the acute myocardial infarction period (95). In this substudy, the predictive value of the SAECG was compared in patients with and without prior thrombolysis/angioplasty in 787 patients. The average follow-up was 10 ± 3 months

and arrhythmic events occurred in 33 patients (4.2%). The SAECG was less likely to be abnormal in patients with thrombolytic therapy/angioplasty (9.4%; 34 of 363 patients), compared with those who did not have either thrombolytic therapy or angioplasty (14.9%; 63 of 424 patients) (*p* < 0.02). The arrhythmic event rate for patients with abnormal SAECG, however, was similar for patients with and without thrombolysis/angioplasty (20.6% in both groups) (Fig. 6.2-11). The arrhythmic event rate for patients with normal SAECG with and without thrombolysis/angioplasty was 0.9% (3 of 329 patients) and 2.8% (10 of 361 patients), respectively. The authors concluded from this data that an abnormal SAECG is predictive of an increased incidence of arrhythmic events in all patients regardless of prior reperfusion therapy.

In a randomized, placebo-controlled trial of "late" thrombolytic therapy (given 6 to 24 hours after the onset of myocardial infarction) in 185 patients who presented with ST elevation, an abnormal SAECG (fQRS or more than 120 ms) was half as common in the group given thrombolytic therapy as in the group given placebo (11% versus 23%) (96). Other studies of the effect of late reperfusion on the SAECG had variable results (97).

After late reperfusion, a normal SAECG predicts improvement in wall motion in patients with a patent infarct–related artery (97). Despite a patent artery, patients with an abnormal

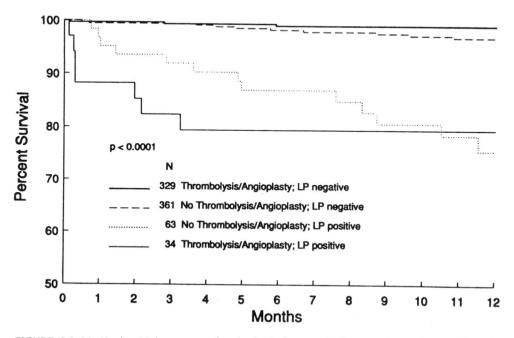

FIGURE 6.2-11. Kaplan-Meier curves of arrhythmia-free survival curves for patients with and without thrombolytic therapy/angioplasty. Patients with late potentials (LPs) had a worse outcome whether or not they received thrombolytic therapy/angioplasty. Patients who had no LPs had a low arrhythmic event rate. (From Denes P, El-Sherif N, Katz R, et al, and the Cardiac Arrhythmia Suppression Trial (CAST)/SAECG substudy Investigators. Prognostic significance of signal-averaged electrocardiogram after thrombolytic therapy and/or angioplasty during acute myocardial infarction [CAST substudy]. *Am J Cardiol* 1994;74:216–220, with permission.)

SAECG are less likely to have recovery of wall motion. A normal SAECG is a marker of myocardial viability and predicts improved EF after coronary artery bypass surgery (98,99).

Prospective studies of the SAECG after myocardial infarction in patients largely treated primarily with thrombolytic therapy have continued to demonstrate that the SAECG retains its prognostic significance with a positive predictive accuracy ranging from 11% to 25% (92,95,100–102). A number of investigators evaluated the use of the SAECG in combination with other noninvasive risk factors in an attempt to improve the predictive accuracy of identifying high-risk patients. Three early prethrombolytic post–myocardial infarction studies demonstrated that the association between an abnormal SAECG and cardiac death or arrhythmic events was independent of ventricular ectopy on a 24-hour Holter recording, left ventricular EF, and heart rate variability (39,86,103). The combination of these different risk markers left a relatively small group (10% to 15%) of extremely high-risk post–myocardial infarction patients with an estimated 50% chance of having an unfavorable outcome (cardiac death or an arrhythmic event) in the first 2 years after myocardial infarction.

A recent study of 575 patients after myocardial infarction compared these four major risk predictors—the SAECG, left ventricular EF, ventricular arrhythmias on a 24-hour Holter recording, and heart rate variability—for their ability to predict arrhythmic and nonarrhythmic death (104). In this study, 54% of the patients received thrombolytic therapy. All of the variables were univariate predictors of cardiac death and arrhythmic death. However, in multivariate analysis, only decreased heart rate variability and unsustained VT were independently associated with arrhythmic death; the SAECG did not provide independent prognostic information above that accounted for by these other variables.

The predictive accuracy of the SAECG regarding arrhythmic events after myocardial infarction can be improved by combining time domain and frequency domain methods (spectral turbulence) of analyzing the SAECG (72). Time domain methods of analyzing the SAECG have more false-positive results in inferior wall myocardial infarction, whereas spectral turbulence has more false-positive results in anterior wall myocardial infarction. The positive predictive accuracy of either of the two techniques alone was about 20%. However, when variables from the two methods were optimized and then entered into a stepwise discriminant model, a positive predictive accuracy of 36% was obtained. Moreover, positive predictive accuracy improved to 51% in patients with a left ventricular EF of less than 0.40.

Risk Stratification in Patients with Left Ventricular Dysfunction

The use of the SAECG to identify high-risk patients with left ventricular dysfunction was evaluated in the Multicenter Unsustained Tachycardia Trial (MUSTT) (105).

MUSTT enrolled 2,202 patients with ischemic heart disease, an EF of less than 0.40, and unsustained VT. All patients underwent electrophysiologic testing. Patients with inducible VT were then randomized to antiarrhythmic therapy (drugs or ICD) or to conventional therapy (such as angiotensin-converting enzyme inhibitors, β blockers, aspirin). In a substudy of MUSTT, the predictive accuracy of the SAECG was evaluated in 1,096 patients treated with conventional therapy. This sample included 207 patients with inducible VT who were randomized to conventional therapy and 889 patients without inducible VT who were being followed in the registry (106). In this substudy, patients with bundle branch block or intraventricular conduction delays were excluded. The SAECG was a significant predictor of arrhythmic death or cardiac death with a relative risk slightly less than 2. Moreover, the presence of inducible VT during electrophysiologic testing did not add prognostic value to the SAECG. In a separate study, these investigators demonstrated that the SAECG may not be a specific marker of arrhythmic death (107). Although a normal SAECG was associated with an excellent prognosis, an abnormal SAECG was more strongly associated with cardiac death than specifically arrhythmic death.

The CABG Patch trial used the SAECG to identify high-risk patients with left ventricular dysfunction (EF < 0.36) who were undergoing coronary artery bypass graft (CABG) surgery (108). In a preliminary study done in preparation for the CABG Patch trial, 258 patients with an abnormal SAECG were compared with 123 patients with a negative SAECG (109). The 3-year mortality rates were twice as high for patients with an abnormal SAECG (28% versus 14%). Subsequently, The CABG Patch trial was the only randomized ICD clinical trial that used the SAECG to identify high-risk patients. Nine hundred patients with left ventricular dysfunction and an abnormal SAECG who were undergoing CABG surgery were randomized to a prophylactic ICD or to no therapy (108). The CABG Patch trial found that ICD therapy did not reduce total mortality rates, although it did reduce the rate of arrhythmic death (110).

Results when the SAECG is used to identify high-risk patients with dilated nonischemic cardiomyopathy are inconsistent. Mancini and colleagues (111) evaluated 114 patients with nonischemic cardiomyopathy who were followed for about 1 year. The 20 patients with an abnormal SAECG had a significantly worse event-free survival than patients with a normal SAECG or patients with bundle branch block. The prognostic significance of the SAECG in patients with a nonischemic cardiomyopathy was also evaluated in two smaller studies (112,113). Silverman and colleagues (114) studied 200 patients with more severe heart failure than those in the study by Mancini and colleagues and found that an abnormal SAECG was not associated with a worse survival in the subgroup of 112 patients with a nonischemic cardiomyopathy. They also found that patients with nonischemic cardiomyopathy and either a bundle branch block or an intraventricular conduction defect had a significantly worse survival than patients with a normal QRS duration regardless of their SAECG results.

The SAECG may identify high-risk patients with amyloid cardiomyopathy, arrhythmogenic right ventricular dysfunction, or a hypertrophic cardiomyopathy (114a) and identify patients with arrhythmogenic right ventricular dysplasia and VT (114b,114c)

Unexplained Syncope

Syncope has multiple causes and often is a diagnostic challenge. Depending on the sample of patients, the cause of syncope is sustained VT in 15% to 35%. The SAECG has been recommended as a screening test for patients with unexplained syncope to determine which patients should have an electrophysiologic study. This use of the SAECG was evaluated in a multicenter study of 189 consecutive patients with unexplained syncope who all underwent electrophysiologic testing and had a 24-hour Holter recording (115). In this sample, 16% had previous myocardial infarction, 31% had left ventricular dysfunction (ischemic or nonischemic), and 31% had no demonstrable heart disease. The end point of the study was inducible VT during electrophysiologic testing. The SAECG had a sensitivity of 70% and a specificity of 55%. A history of myocardial infarction or left ventricular dysfunction was more specific but less sensitive. In multivariate analysis, only the SAECG and a history of myocardial infarction were independent predictors of inducible VT. The incremental clinical value of using the SAECG was evaluated in two groups classified as low or moderate risk based on clinical variables (age, gender, and history of myocardial infarction). In the moderate-risk group, the probability of VT was 28% to 42% and the risk doubled if the SAECG was abnormal. In the low-risk group, however, the SAECG provided no incremental predictive value. In the absence of clinical risk factors, an abnormal SAECG is likely to be a false-positive result. Based on these data, use of the SAECG is limited to patients with a history of myocardial infarction. Some clinicians refer all patients with a previous myocardial infarction and unexplained syncope for electrophysiologic testing while others use the SAECG to identify a lower risk group who do not need an electrophysiologic study. One important limitation of this study was the absence of follow-up, because the end point of this study was inducible VT. Limitations in the long-term predictive accuracy of an electrophysiologic study leaves open the question of whether patients with a history of myocardial infarction and a normal SAECG have a good long-term prognosis.

Summary

Despite improvements in signal processing, knowledge of the pathophysiologic link between the SAECG and reentrant ventricular tachyarrhythmias, and a number of studies demonstrating that the SAECG can identify high-risk patients in certain disease states, clinical applications of the SAECG have not gained widespread acceptance. With the exception of the CABG Patch trial, no other large randomized clinical trials have used the SAECG to select a high-risk population for evaluation of a specific treatment. Recent data from MUSTT, the CABG Patch trial, and other studies suggest that an abnormal SAECG may not be a specific marker of arrhythmic risk because it also identifies patients without myocardial viability who are also likely to die from pump failure. These limitations will be overcome only if large clinical treatment trials are performed to demonstrate that the SAECG can be used to select patients groups that will benefit from specific treatments.

QT Dispersion

Throughout the history of ECG, investigators have recognized that the QT interval differs amongst the 12 ECG standard leads (116). For much of this century, however, there has been a lack of consensus on the appropriate lead for QT-interval measurement. Lead II, lead aVL, or the lead showing the earliest Q wave, the most distinct T wave, or the longest QT interval have all been recommended (117). Implicit in this disagreement was the fact that interlead QT-interval differences exist on the 12-lead ECG. In 1985, Campbell and colleagues (118) performed a lead-by-lead comparison of QT-interval measurements in 32 patients after myocardial infarction, determining that the lead with the maximum QT interval was highly variable. Contemporaneously, body surface potential mapping studies using 150 unipolar torso electrodes confirmed that regional difference in ventricular repolarization time could be detected from the body surface (119). Increased attention to interlead differences in the QT interval during the latter half of the 1980s set the stage for the emergence of the current concept of QT dispersion (QTd). By convention, QTd has been defined as the difference (measured in milliseconds) between the minimum and maximum QT intervals on the standard 12-lead ECG. In 1988, Cowan and colleagues found that QTd was approximately 50 ms in a group of healthy subjects and more than 70 ms in patients with a history of myocardial infarction (117).

Since these initial observations, substantial interest has developed regarding QTd as a marker of arrhythmia risk. Unfortunately, a voluminous literature on QTd is plagued by methodological difficulties that contribute to conflicting results. At this time, it is unclear whether these methodological issues can be overcome. Therefore, QTd does not have a clear role in the identification of high-risk patients in clinical practice.

Physiologic Basis

It is well known that action potential duration (APD) differs, both transmurally and regionally (120). QTd has been proposed as a measure of regional differences in dispersion of APD, which may identify arrhythmogenic substrates (121). Thus, increased heterogeneity in ventricular repolarization time may be reflected in increased QTd.

Several studies using monophasic action potential recordings in human subjects support the validity of QTd as a surrogate for dispersion of APD. The first study compared QTd with monophasic action potential recordings from 12 epicardial sites in 10 patients undergoing open-chest cardiac surgery. During both sinus rhythm and ventricular pacing, a positive and significant correlation was found between QTd and regional APD (122). A second human study evaluated 17 patients using either epicardial or endocardial monophasic action potentials and reported that QTd, as measured on a 12-lead ECG from the same day, correlated well with APD dispersion (123). Two animal studies, however, were unable to find an association between QTd and activation recovery interval dispersion, a validated index of APD dispersion derived from epicardial unipolar electrodes. Wang (124) evaluated six anesthetized sheep wearing an epicardial elastic sock laced with 64 unipolar electrodes. Because intact animals were used, QTd could be measured from body surface electrodes, resembling the manner in which ECGs are recorded in humans. Nevertheless, no correlation was found between body surface QTd and regional dispersion of APD. Finally, Lux and colleagues (125) constructed a model in which a Langendorff-perfused isolated dog heart was suspended in a torso-shaped, electrolytic tank. In this experiment, a poor correlation was found between activation recovery interval and QTd.

Thus, the physiologic basis of QTd remains controversial and several important questions remain unanswered. Despite the data demonstrating a correlation between QTd and APD dispersion, a causal relationship is not established. In the isolated dog heart model of Lux and colleagues (125), QTd underestimated the true regional differences in APD. More importantly, QTd was insensitive to regional repolarization shortening in the presence of prolonged repolarization elsewhere. Several groups of investigators have suggested that QTd is simply a result of different projections of the heart's electrical activity onto varying lead axes and has little to do with regional dispersion of APD (126). The duration of the T wave in any given lead is dependent on the geometric orientation of repolarization to the lead axis (127). Thus, QTd could potentially arise for reasons not directly related to regional differences in action potential recovery time dispersion. Notably, QTd is not a unique ECG parameter in its ability to reflect action potential recovery time dispersion. Zabel and colleagues (123,128) have found that other T-wave indices such as late T-wave area, total T-wave area, and T peak–T end interval also show significant correlation with action potential recovery time dispersion. Whether these alternative ECG parameters, alone or com-

binations with QTd, are better correlated with ventricular repolarization dispersion is unsettled.

Methods of Measurement

QTd is generally defined as the difference between the maximum and minimum QT interval among the 12 standard ECG leads. The measurement of QTd requires identification of the beginning of the QRS deflection and end of the T wave in each ECG lead. In contrast to the HF and precise onset of the QRS complex, locating the end of the T wave is much more problematic given its low amplitude, variable morphology, and smooth return toward the isoelectric line (118,129). Indeed, accurate detection of the end of the T wave represents a major technical challenge in QTd methodology (130). Another important issue is the most appropriate approach to QTd measurement in the presence of U waves. Whether to include the U wave in QT-interval measurement is a subject of long-standing controversy. Because U waves are more pronounced in certain ECG leads (117), inclusion of U waves will increase the magnitude of QTd. Exclusion of U waves may lead to inaccuracies in determining the T-wave offset or loss of important information about repolarization processes (131) and produces variable effects on QTd measurement (132). At present, the most accepted convention is to exclude the U wave from QTd measurement (133). If the U wave cannot be separated from the T wave in a given ECG lead, then it is reasonable to exclude that ECG lead from QTd analysis.

Initial reports of QTd were based on manual measurements with calipers, frequently using paper speed of 50 mm per second and digitizing tablets to facilitate measurement. However, manual measurement is tedious, time-consuming, subject to human error, and difficult to employ in large-scale clinical studies (129,134,135). In an effort to overcome the difficulties inherent in manual measurement of QTd, several computerized algorithms have been developed (Fig. 6.2-12) (136). The threshold method marks the end of the T wave at the point where its amplitude decreases below a predefined threshold level (usually defined as a percentage of the peak T-wave amplitude). The differential threshold method is analogous but uses the first derivative (slope) of the T wave instead of the T wave itself. According to the slope intercept method, a tangent is drawn from the maximum slope of the terminal T wave to the isoelectric level; the intersection between the tangent and the isoelectric level is designated the end of the T wave. Finally, the peak slope intercept method identifies the point of maximal terminal T-wave slope. A line is drawn, which includes both the peak of the T wave and the point of maximal terminal T-wave slope; the end of T wave is defined by the intersection between this line and the isoelectric level.

Comparative studies of these automated methods have found that QTd values are highly dependent on the auto-

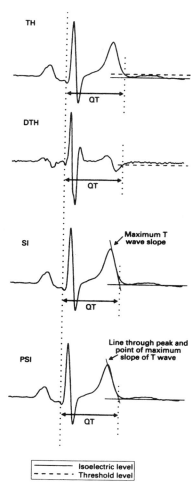

FIGURE 6.2-12. Four techniques used to automatically determine the end of the T wave. Three of the methods use the measurements from the actual electrocardiogram (ECG) signal to determine the end of the T wave: threshold (*TH*) method, slope-intercept (*SI*) method, and peak slope-intercept (*PSI*) method. The differential threshold (*DTH*) method uses the first derivative of the ECG signal to determine the end of the T wave. (From McLaughlin, et al. *BMJ* 1995;74:86, with permission.)

mated method used. In addition, the choice of parameters such as filtering bandwidth and definition of the isoelectric voltage level can significantly affect QTd. The slope intercept method appears to be the most reproducible and robust technique; however, multiple studies have found that this method consistently underestimates the manually measured QTd by approximately 20 ms (129,136,137). This systematic "underestimation" highlights the fact that the normal range for QTd will differ substantially by technique and that careful attention should be directed at the methodology used in research studies. Regardless of the technique chosen, it appears that reproducibility of QTd measurement is substantially lower than for other conventional ECG parameters, such as the PR, R-R, QRS, and QT intervals (138).

Another potential source of variability in the measurement of QTd is interlead differences in QRS onset. The relative contribution of QRS onset to QTd can be substantial, often exceeding 20 ms (117,139). Some investigators have evaluated the JT interval as a measure of repolarization time that is less confounded by ventricular activation (140,141). Accordingly, JT dispersion may be a useful alternative to QTd as a surrogate for ventricular repolarization time dispersion (123,128,142). Most computerized algorithms for measuring QTd use a common QRS onset point in all leads (143).

Several methods are used for determining which leads to exclude from estimation of QTd. Leads in which the QT interval cannot be measured reliably are typically designated "invalid leads" and excluded from analysis. Common causes for this problem include low-amplitude T waves, biphasic T waves, U waves (or P waves at fast heart rates) obscuring the end of the T wave, baseline artifact, and electrical noise (118,130). No standard criteria exist for the minimum number of leads required to measure a valid QTd and no standard algorithm exists for correcting QTd when leads are excluded (132).

Several automated software packages have been designed for QTd measurement, including the modular ECG analysis system (MEANS) (144), the Glasgow program (139), and the QT Guard program (137). QT Guard is a commercially available software package for QTd analysis (GE/Marquette Medical Systems, Milwaukee, WI) that can analyze standard 12-lead ECGs that have been digitally recorded using a GE/Marquette ECG acquisition unit. The program superimposes all normal QRS complexes in each lead to derive a "median beat," a method akin to signal averaging. QT Guard uses a common QRS onset point for all 12 leads, so the QTd calculated reflects only dispersion of the T-wave offset. Its default QTd measurement algorithm is a slope intercept method; however, the program can be modified to use the threshold method or differential threshold method. If threshold methods are used, the operator may choose the threshold level. Leads with low T-wave amplitude, complex T-wave morphology, and excessive noise are excluded; however, the operator can override computer decisions regarding which leads are valid. The operator also can override choices of both the peak and end of the T wave in each lead. QTd is provided as the difference between the maximum and minimum QT intervals and the standard deviation of all QT intervals (143,145).

Finally, some have questioned whether QTd is the optimal method to measure action potentia recovery time dispersion. Many other parameters have been proposed, including JT-interval dispersion, total T-wave area, late T-wave area and the T peak–T end interval. The correlation between each of these parameters and action potential dispersion was similar to the correlation between QTd and action potential dispersion in isolated rabbit hearts (123). Human studies also demonstrate that these measures add important information to QTd in multivariate models predicting action potential recovery time dispersion (128). These data suggest that QTd may not be unique in its ability to detect regional heterogeneity in repolarization. In addition, several studies showed a striking relationship between QTd and properties of the ventricular repolarization loop on the vectorcardiogram, demonstrating that similar information may be derived from an evaluation of the T-wave vector loop (126,127). It is uncertain whether these alternative ECG parameters will ultimately provide additional useful prognostic information, either instead of or in conjunction with QTd.

Predictive Value of QT Dispersion

A growing number of studies evaluates QTd as a predictor of mortality in various patient populations. Although two large population-based studies have found that increased QTd predicted sudden cardiac death, available data on the prognostic value of QTd within specific patient populations are variable. Most of these studies include few patients and use manual QTd measurement methodologies.

Prediction of Inducible Ventricular Tachycardia

Two studies have evaluated QTd in patients referred for electrophysiologic testing. In one study, QTd was longer in 56 patients with inducible VT, compared with 106 noninducible patients (85 ± 62 versus 66 ± 48 ms); both groups of patients had longer QTd than the 144 healthy controls (38 ± 21 ms) (146). Among several QTd indices studied, QT-apex (the interval from the QRS onset to the apex of the T wave) dispersion was found to be the best predictor of inducibility during electrophysiologic study. Although late potentials on SAECG and reduced EF were stronger predictors, QT-apex dispersion remained a significant parameter in a logistic regression model including all three measures (146). A second study of 66 patients reported that increased QTd (more than 60 ms) predicted inducible VT with a sensitivity of 67% and a specificity of 94% (147). However, this analysis did not adjust for significant differences in EF or history of myocardial infarction between the inducible and uninducible groups. Based on limited evidence, it appears that QTd measurement is a relatively weak predictor of inducibility at electrophysiologic study.

Congestive Heart Failure

Several studies have evaluated the relationship between QTd and outcome in patients with congestive heart failure. One prospective study of 104 patients with NYHA class II to IV heart failure found that a QTd of more than 90 ms was associated with a 2.8-fold higher death rate (95% CI, 1.2–6.4). In multivariate analysis, NYHA functional class and QTd were the only predictors of cardiac mortality. Although EF and average QRS duration were significant univariate predictors of mortality, they did not improve the

fit of the multivariate model (148). Pinsky and colleagues (149) evaluated the ability of QTd to predict all-cause mortality in 80 consecutive patients listed for cardiac transplantation. A QTd of more than 140 ms was associated with a 4.1-fold increased risk of death before transplantation. The unusually high QTd cutpoint used in this study likely reflects the severity of underlying structural and electrical cardiac dysfunction among patients in need of cardiac transplantation. Interestingly, QTd was the only variable associated with risk of death; functional class, QRS duration, QT/corrected QT (QTc) interval, heart rate, cause of heart failure, history of antiarrhythmic therapy, and history of ventricular arrhythmias were not statistically significant in either univariate or multivariate analyses (149).

In a third series of 200 patients with congestive heart failure followed for 24 ± 16 months, a QTd of more than 80 ms predicted arrhythmic events (sudden cardiac death, symptomatic sustained VT, or ventricular fibrillation) with a relative risk of 2.22 (95% CI, 1.01–4.89) (150). In a multivariate model, increased QTd was the only independent predictor of arrhythmic events; the model did not select unsustained VT or ventricular late potentials. However, QTd was not a significant predictor of other individual end points including all-cause mortality, cardiac mortality, or sudden cardiac death. Subgroup analysis of the 116 patients with nonischemic cardiomyopathy showed QTd to be an independent predictor of all-cause mortality (relative risk, 2.17; 95% CI, 1.00–4.78), cardiac mortality (relative risk, 2.28; 95% CI, 1.00–5.29), sudden cardiac death (relative risk, 4.48; 95% CI, 1.41–16.86), and arrhythmic events (relative risk, 4.49; 95% CI, 1.49–13.56) (150). In contrast, a smaller prospective series of 60 patients with nonischemic cardiomyopathy found no significant difference in QTd between survivors and 17 patients who died or who underwent transplantation (151).

Although QTd did not predict events in the ischemic cardiomyopathy subgroup from the Galinier and colleagues series, other investigators have reported increased QTd in those dying suddenly (150). Barr and colleagues (152) studied 44 subjects who were followed for an average of 36 months. The mean rate corrected QTd was 99 ms in 7 patients dying suddenly, 67 ms in 12 patients dying of progressive heart failure, and 53 ms in the 21 survivors (all differences were significant) (152).

In summary, it appears that QTd may have prognostic value for patients with congestive heart failure; however, further large prospective investigations of patients with ischemic and nonischemic cardiomyopathy are needed to substantiate this possibility.

QT Dispersion to Assess Prognosis after Myocardial Infarction

Evidence for the prognostic value of QTd for patients after myocardial infarction is lacking. A prospective study of 280 myocardial infarction survivors failed to show a difference in QTd for patients with cardiovascular events (153). Another prospective study of 936 patients with chronic coronary artery disease found that JT dispersion was significantly greater in 17 patients who died from arrhythmic death than in 51 matched survivors. In this study, QTd showed a trend toward being greater in patients who died but was not statistically significant (142). In contrast, one report of 30 patients with a recent myocardial infarction and recurrent ventricular arrhythmias found a QTd of 104 ms, which was significantly prolonged compared with the value in 40 patients with a recent infarct and no arrhythmia (65 ms) and with healthy patients (38 ms) (153a). Similar findings were noted in another series in which increased QTd was associated with VT but not ventricular fibrillation (153b). In a trial of 603 patients with a myocardial infarction and clinical evidence of heart failure, QTd was a predictor of all-cause mortality; an increase of 10 ms added a 5% to 7% relative risk of death (153c).

Successful thrombolytic therapy reduces the amount of QTd and, as with the improvement in baroreceptor sensitivity, may indicate enhanced vagal tone and reduced sympathetic activity (153d). The reduction in QTd may also reflect a greater amount of viable myocardium in the infarct region (153e).

Despite these observations, there is currently no compelling evidence for QTd as a useful index of arrhythmia risk in patients after myocardial infarction.

Long QT Syndrome

Patients with long QT syndrome are known to have increased QTd. However, only one small series of 10 patients with long QT syndrome has suggested that increased QTd may be a predictor of ventricular arrhythmias (121). There are some data supporting the use of QTd as a marker of therapeutic efficacy. Patients who were asymptomatic on β-adrenergic blocking medications (mean follow-up of 7 ± 4 years, minimum follow-up of 1 year) were found to have less QTd than untreated patients or those with recurrent syncope despite full-dose β blockers. Another study of 28 patients with long QT syndrome on β-blocking medications showed that increased QTd identified those with recurrent episodes of syncope despite therapy (154). In this study, a QTd of more than 100 ms while on β blockers identified those with recurrent syncopal episodes with 80% sensitivity and 82% specificity. Interestingly, 11 patients in this study who had recurrent syncope on β blockers underwent left cardiac sympathetic denervation and subsequently had no syncope during a mean follow-up of 5 ± 4 years. In these 11 patients, left-sided cardiac sympathetic denervation was associated with a significant reduction in QTd (154). Thus, limited evidence suggests that QTd may predict arrhythmia risk in patients with long

QT syndrome. However, the small number of patients studied makes these findings inconclusive.

Use of QT Dispersion to Predict Mortality in Population-Based Studies

Because QTd is measured from the standard 12-lead ECG, assessment of the prognostic value of QTd in large-scale population-based studies has been possible. Two prospective population-based studies using different computerized measurement techniques have found QTd to be an independent predictor of mortality. De Bruyne and colleagues (155) studied 5,812 men and women aged 55 or older in the Rotterdam Study using MEANS. During a mean follow-up of 4 years, cardiac death, sudden cardiac death, and total mortality rates were increased in the highest QTc dispersion tertile compared with the lowest tertile. A QTc dispersion of more than 66 ms was associated with a twofold increased risk of cardiac death, which remained significant after adjustment for age, hypertension, diabetes, and previous myocardial infarction (144). It is important to recognize that no adjustments were made for other ECG variables, such as heart rate, corrected QT interval, or QRS duration. Interestingly, T-wave axis, T-wave vector loop, and QTc were reported elsewhere as significant predictors of mortality in the same elderly population (155–157). This observation suggests that ECG parameters aside from QTd may also provide prognostically important information about abnormalities of repolarization in the context of a relatively unselected elderly population.

A second large-scale population-based study of 1,839 Native American Indians enrolled in the Strong Heart Study also demonstrated that QTd predicts mortality. QTd (measured using QT Guard) was found to be a significant predictor of all-cause mortality and cardiovascular mortality during a mean follow-up of 3.7 years. After multivariate adjustment for 13 possible confounding variables, a QTd of more than 58 ms was associated with a threefold increase in risk of cardiovascular death (Fig. 6.2-13). Both QTc and QTd remained significant independent predictors of cardiovascular mortality in a Cox multivariate model; however, ECG variables such as heart rate and QRS duration were not included in the analysis (158). Nevertheless, data from two separate sources suggest that QTd can predict sudden cardiac death in large heterogeneous community-based populations.

Summary

Despite voluminous literature, QTd does not currently have a clear role in clinical practice. The complexity surrounding the measurement of the end of the T wave has given rise to numerous methodological difficulties in the measurement of QTd. A number of recent automated computer algorithms for measuring QTd have been developed, although there is still no consensus on how to measure QTd. Without a consensus on how to measure QTd, there can be no consensus

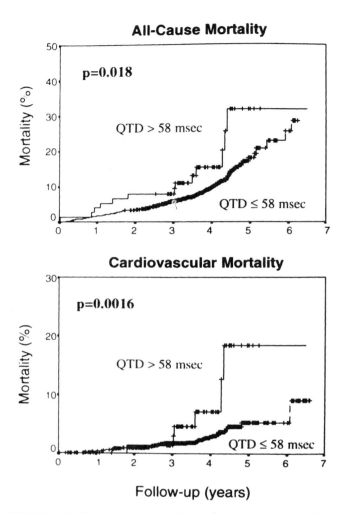

All-Cause Mortality

p=0.018

QTD > 58 msec

QTD ≤ 58 msec

Cardiovascular Mortality

p=0.0016

QTD > 58 msec

QTD ≤ 58 msec

Follow-up (years)

FIGURE 6.2-13. Kaplan-Meier plots of cumulative mortality resulting from all causes **(top)** and cardiovascular causes only **(bottom)** in participants from the Strong Heart Study grouped according to QT dispersion partitioned at 58 ms. (From Okin PM, Devereux RB, Howard BV, et al. Assessment of QT interval and QT dispersion for prediction of all-cause and cardiovascular mortality in American Indians: the Strong Heart Study. *Circulation* 2000;101[Jan 4]:64, with permission.)

on an optimal cutpoint above which QTd is considered abnormal. At this point, it is unclear whether these methodological issues can be overcome. A number of studies on the ability of QTd to predict mortality have yielded conflicting results. Because QTd is critically dependent on the way in which it is measured, it is impossible to reconcile divergent results from studies that use different measurement techniques. Although two large population-based studies demonstrated that QTd measured with computerized algorithms was a potent predictor of sudden cardiac death, the clinical utility of this finding in the evaluation of individual patients remains uncertain. Small sample sizes and inconsistent results limit the interpretation of available data from specific patient subgroups. Even if the methodological issues of QTd measurement are resolved, a number of large-scale studies will be needed to determine the role of QTd in clinical practice.

T-Wave Alternans

T-wave alternans is a 2:1 fluctuation in the amplitude or shape of T waves. Macroscopic T-wave alternans has been recognized as a harbinger of malignant ventricular arrhythmias (159) when found in long QT syndrome (160,161) and various electrolyte abnormalities (162,163). However, electrical alternans is a very rare ECG finding. Only 46 cases of macroscopic T-wave alternans have been reported and the mortality rate associated with these cases was 61% (164).

During the past 10 years, methods have been developed to quantify microvolt-level T-wave alternans (not visible with the naked eye) and the genesis of ventricular arrhythmias (165,166). The measurement of microvolt-level T-wave alternans required sophisticated noise-reduction techniques and analytic methods that are now commercially available (165,167). Even though this technology is new, the available data suggest that T-wave alternans is a potent predictor of arrhythmia risk in diverse disease states (165,166). Based on these data, the measurement of stress-induced microvolt-level T-wave alternans has been approved by the United States Food and Drug Administration for the following indication:

> The presence of T-wave alternans in patients with known, suspected or at risk of ventricular tachyarrhythmia predicts increased risk of a cardiac event (ventricular tachyarrhythmia or sudden death). T-wave alternans should be used only as an adjunct to clinical history and the results of other noninvasive and/or invasive tests.

Cellular Electrophysiologic Mechanisms Underlying T-Wave Alternans

Macroscopic T-wave alternans is associated with long QT syndrome (congenital or acquired) and with polymorphous VT or torsade de pointes. Recently, the mechanism responsible for generating T-wave alternans has been clarified, generalized, and linked to arrhythmogenesis in other forms of heart disease (168). In an experimental model using Langendorff-perfused guinea pig hearts, T-wave alternans elicited on the surface ECG during fixed-rate pacing was linked to localized action potential alternans recorded simultaneously from 128 epicardial sites with voltage-sensitive dyes (168). Localized action potential alternans is a rate-dependent property of myocytes and importantly varies in different regions of the heart and often occurs as a result of electrophysiologic uncoupling between cells. This type of uncoupling can occur with any myocardial disease process that leads to the development of interstitial fibrosis, such as the diffuse interstitial fibrosis that occurs in nonischemic cardiomyopathies, and does not require a discrete myocardial infarction.

Regional inhomogeneities in the phase and amplitude of action potential alternans in neighboring regions of cells result in discordant alternans; in one region, the action potential duration is short while in another region, the action potential duration is long. Discordant alternans is associated with the development of steep spatial electrotonic gradients that can cause marked dispersion of repolarization, unidirectional block, and reentry. Interestingly, the arrhythmia that resulted from discordant alternans was polymorphous VT when the layer of myocardial cells in the model was healthy and monomorphic VT when a lesion (scar) was introduced into the layer of cells. The reentrant arrhythmia used a circuit that encircled the lesion (169). This finding links the development of T-wave alternans to both polymorphous and monomorphic VT depending on the substrate. In long QT syndrome when the myocardium is otherwise structurally healthy, polymorphous VT is the most common ventricular arrhythmia (170,171). After myocardial infarction, the development of T-wave alternans may be associated with monomorphic VT (172). In either case, the development of T-wave alternans is indicative of electrophysiologic properties of the myocardium that are associated with arrhythmogenesis.

Animal Models Linking T-Wave Alternans and Vulnerability to Ventricular Arrhythmias

The relationship between the vulnerability of the myocardium to ventricular arrhythmias and the presence and magnitude of microvolt-level T-wave alternans were demonstrated in a series of intact animal studies (165,173). Under various conditions that increase susceptibility to ventricular

arrhythmias including hypothermia, ischemia, and rapid pacing, the magnitude of T-wave alternans was inversely related to the magnitude of the ventricular fibrillation threshold, a measure of cardiac electrical stability. One important characteristic of T-wave alternans was identified from these studies: T-wave alternans often was not present until the heart rate was more than 90 bpm. The magnitude of T-wave alternans then increased dramatically as heart rate was increased further above that threshold heart rate. This finding suggested that alternans needs to be measured at heart rates between 90 and 110 bpm, although the exact heart rate threshold is not known and may vary from subject to subject.

Measurement

The measurement of microvolt T-wave alternans combines sophisticated noise-reduction techniques with a spectral method for identifying any systematic oscillation in the morphologic pattern of the T-wave amplitude(165,167). Using the spectral method, beat-to-beat fluctuations in the T wave are measured from each sample point of the T wave from 128 time-aligned ECG complexes (Fig. 6.2-14). Each point from the T wave is measured at the same time relative to the QRS complex. Power spectra are calculated for each point within the T wave. The power spectrum depicts the

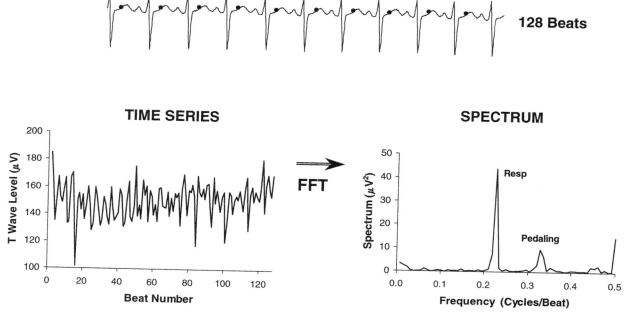

FIGURE 6.2-14. Spectral method of measuring T-wave alternans. The amplitudes of corresponding points on the T wave are measured for 128 beats. A time series consisting of these 128 amplitudes is created. The power spectrum of this time series is computed using fast Fourier transform methods. In the power spectrum obtained from recordings during bicycle exercise, peaks corresponding to frequencies of respiration, pedaling, and alternans are illustrated. (From Cohen RJ. T-wave alternans and Laplacian imaging. In: Zipes DP, Jalife J, eds. *Cardiac electrophysiology: from cell to bedside.* Philadelphia: WB Saunders, 1999:781–789, with permission.)

frequencies at which beat-to-beat fluctuations in the amplitude of the T wave occur. Because this spectrum is created by measurements taken once per beat, its frequencies are in the units of cycles per beat (instead of cycles per second). The point on the spectrum corresponding to exactly 0.5 cycles per beat indicates the magnitude of the alternation of the T wave. Spectra are generated from each point on the T wave and are then averaged to produce a composite spectrum. This composite spectrum has the characteristic that it is sensitive to any change in the morphology of the T wave even if the peak amplitude does not change.

The alternans power (μV^2) is defined as the difference between the power at the alternans frequency (0.5 cycles per beat) and the power at the noise frequency band (calculated over the frequency between 0.44 and 0.49 cycles per beat). This is a measure of the true physiologic alternans level. The alternans voltage (V_{alt} measured in μV) is simply the square root of alternans power and corresponds to the difference in the voltage (averaged over the T wave) between the overall mean beat and either the even-numbered or odd-numbered mean beats (i.e., is half the difference between the even mean and the odd mean). A measure of the statistical significance of the alternans is defined as the alternans ratio (*k* score) calculated as the ratio of the alternans power divided by the standard deviation of the noise (this statistic is similar to the *z* score based on the normal distribution). Alternans is considered significant if the *k* score is more than or equal to 3.

The spectral method has a number of features that provide for a robust measurement of T-wave alternans. The use of a 128-beat spectrum provides for a very accurate measurement of frequency in the beat frequency domain. This allows for differentiation of true physiologic alternans, which occurs at exactly one half of the beat frequency, from movement or other repetitive artifact that may cause peaks at close to half the beat frequency. The use of a reference noise band (close to the alternans frequency of 0.44 to 0.49 cycles per beat) and the subtraction of the mean noise level from the alternans power makes the alternans level relatively independent of mean noise levels. An increase in white noise raises the noise levels of the entire spectrum; this is corrected by subtracting the mean noise level from the power at the alternans frequency (0.5 cycles per beat). In addition, the use of the alternans ratio takes into account the variation of noise in the spectrum and requires that the magnitude of alternans power is greater than 3 standard deviations of the noise levels, indicating that alternans is statistically unlikely to be an artifact. Finally, the measurements of many points over the T wave make the alternans measurement sensitive to all T-wave morphology changes.

T-Wave Alternans Is Highly Dependent on Heart Rate

Therefore, it is necessary to elevate the heart rate to measure T-wave alternans with adequate sensitivity (165). In the initial clinical studies, heart rate was increased by atrial pacing (174). Subsequently, noninvasive measurement of T-wave alternans during exercise testing became possible after the development of multicontact electrodes in combination with sophisticated signal-processing techniques, which significantly reduced noise levels (167). In most patients with T-wave alternans, the magnitude of alternans is on the order of several microvolts (roughly one fiftieth of a millimeter in standard ECG tracings). The measurement of T-wave alternans therefore requires careful preparation of the skin (including shaving hair and moderate skin abrasion) to minimize electrode-to-skin impedance. The electrode-to-skin impedance should be measured before exercise to ensure proper lead placement and preparation. Placing ECG electrodes away from the pectoral muscles can reduce muscle artifact. Specialized multicontact electrodes have been developed (Hi-Res Electrodes, Cambridge Heart, Inc, Bedford, MA), which record and process ECG signals and a measurement of impedance from multiple segments of an electrode. The multicontact electrodes increase the signal to noise ratio by taking advantage of the fact that the ECG signal detected by each contact of an electrode should be nearly identical because the contacts are located in proximity to each other. In contrast, the local muscle noise and motion artifact recorded by each electrode may be quite different depending, in part, on the impedance of the contact-skin connection. The use of multicontact electrodes allows a noise-reduction process through an adaptive averaging method that cancels the noise. The electrode enhancement method forms a linear combination of the impedance signal and electrode segment that produces a composite ECG signal that has the same morphology but has lower noise than an ECG signal taken from the center segment of the electrode alone. Thus, the signals from each of the electrodes can be combined to increase the signal and reduce the noise. By using advanced signal processing in combination with multicontact electrodes, one can routinely measure T-wave alternans during bicycle or treadmill exercise stress with commercially available equipment (CH2000 system, Cambridge Heart, Inc, Bedford, MA). The method for increasing heart rate appears to be unimportant. A number of investigators have demonstrated high concordance between T-wave alternans measured during atrial pacing, exercise, and during pharmacologic testing with dobutamine and atropine (175–177).

Interpretation

The interpretation of the T-wave alternans test must consider the dynamic variation of heart rate with exercise. Patients susceptible to ventricular tachyarrhythmias tend to develop sustained alternans during exercise stress at heart rates of about 100 bpm). Ultimately, the interpretation of a T-wave alternans study will require answers to two sets of questions: (a) Is T-wave alternans present and is it sustained above a threshold heart rate? If it is present, is the alternans real or artifactual? (b) If alternans is not present, are there artifacts present that could obscure or mask true alternans? The definition of sustained alternans is alternans that is consistently present above a patient-specific onset heart rate. Alternans that occurs episodically and does bear a consistent relationship to heart rate has not been associated with increased arrhythmic risk.

T-wave alternans test results are classified as positive, negative, or indeterminate. The usual criterion used to define a positive T-wave alternans test result indicative of arrhythmic risk is the presence of sustained alternans with onset either at the resting heart rate or at a heart rate of less than or equal to 110 bpm (heart rates here refer to a 128-beat averaged heart rate). The alternans must have an amplitude of more than or equal to 1.9 μV, with a *k* score of at least 3.0, and must last for more than 1 minute and include some period of artifact-free data. Alternans can be identified in a single orthogonal (vector) lead or in two adjacent precordial leads. A test result is usually negative if it does not meet the criteria for a positive test result and if there is at least 1 minute of data at or above a heart rate of 105 bpm without significant alternans, with a noise level of less than or equal to 1.8 μV, and with fewer than 10% ectopic beats. An indeterminate test result is a result that does not meet the criteria for being classified as positive or negative. To optimize the interpretation of T-wave alternans tests, an exercise protocol should be used, which results in a gradual increase in heart rate from 90 to 110 bpm during a 3- to 5-minute period. For the purposes of measuring T-wave alternans, patients need only exercise to a heart rate of about 120 bpm; T-wave alternans is not significant at higher heart rates and can occur in healthy subjects.

An example of a T-wave alternans tracing is shown in Figure 6.2-15. In the left panel, the upper tracing represents heart rate and the lower tracing represents the alternans voltage in the vector magnitude lead. One box represents 2 μV of T-wave alternans. The x axis represents the time in minutes. The patient begins to exercise at minute 26:00 at a heart rate of 80 bpm. During the next 12 minutes, the patient exercises against increasing workloads and his heart rate increases from 80 bpm to a maximum of 120 bpm. Alternans begins to appear during exercise at 28:50 when the heart rate is 94 bpm (referred to as the "onset heart rate"). As the patient continues to exercise and his heart rate increases, the alternans voltage increases to approximately 6 μV. In this test, T-wave alternans persists for about 9 minutes and is consistently present above a threshold heart rate of 94 bpm. The power spectrum from the vector magnitude (displayed on the right) is illustrated from 128 beats at a point corresponding to a heart rate of 120 bpm (at 36:52). The power spectrum demonstrates a clear peak at 0.5 cycles per beat (the alternans frequency of every other beat).

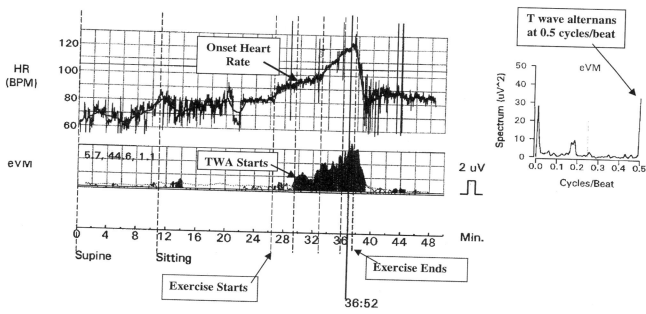

FIGURE 6.2-15. Example of T-wave alternans. **Left:** A portion of a T-wave alternans report from the CH2000 system (Cambridge Heart, Inc., Bedford, MA) and includes **(top)** a plot of heart rate and **(bottom)** a plot of the magnitude of T-wave alternans over the course of the exercise study. The magnitude of T-wave alternans reaches the threshold value of 1.9 μV at minute 28:45 and the magnitude increases as heart rate increases. **Right:** The power spectrum from 128 beats centered at minute 36:52 (the time at which magnitude of alternans has peaked). T-wave alternans is measured at 0.5 cycles per beat and the magnitude corresponds to the square root of the power in the power spectrum. (See text for details.)

Clinical Studies

The initial clinical studies of T-wave alternans are encouraging. In healthy subjects (age matched for patients with a heart disease), exercise-induced T-wave alternans is very rare (about 1%) (178). The presence of microvolt-level T-wave alternans is associated with an increased risk of future arrhythmic events. Equally important is the consistent finding that the absence of T-wave alternans is associated with an excellent prognosis. Many of these early studies are small and include patients already identified as being high risk (such as patients with VT referred for electrophysiologic testing). Large-scale epidemiologic studies are currently underway that will provide unbiased and accurate estimates of the magnitude of the increased risk associated with T-wave alternans.

T-Wave Alternans Measured during Atrial Pacing in Patients Referred for Electrophysiologic Testing

In 1994, Rosenbaum and colleagues (174) published the first prospective human study demonstrating a strong relationship between the presence of T-wave alternans and the inducibility of ventricular arrhythmias during electrophysiologic testing and 20-month arrhythmia-free survival. In this study, 83 patients undergoing an electrophysiologic test were evaluated for T-wave alternans during atrial pacing at 100 bpm. T-wave alternans was detected in 36 patients (43%) and 39 patients (47%) had inducible ventricular arrhythmias during programmed electrical stimulation. The sensitivity of T-wave alternans for predicting the inducibility of ventricular arrhythmias was 81% and the specificity was 84%. Patients who had T-wave alternans were 5.2 times more likely to have inducible ventricular arrhythmias than those patients who did not. Moreover, in a multivariate analysis, the increased risk of developing ventricular arrhythmias associated with T-wave alternans was independent of the presence of organic heart disease. Furthermore, the presence of T-wave alternans was associated with a markedly decreased arrhythmia-free survival during a 20-month follow-up: 19% of patients with T-wave alternans versus 94% without it had a 20-month arrhythmia-free survival. This landmark study clearly established a strong association between T-wave alternans and the risk of developing potentially fatal ventricular arrhythmias.

T-Wave Alternans Measured during Exercise in Patients Referred for Electrophysiologic Testing

A subsequent multicenter study evaluated the prognostic significance of T-wave alternans in patients referred for electrophysiologic testing measured during bicycle exercise (rather than atrial pacing) (178a,179). In this study, 337 patients referred for an electrophysiologic test underwent an SAECG and a T-wave alternans test using bicycle ergometry before their electrophysiologic test. Of the 313 patients who completed the study, 64% were men with a mean age of 56 ± 15 years. Nearly half of the patients had coronary artery disease and a reduced EF (≤0.40) was present in 46% of patients. The indication for the electrophysiologic test varied: syncope, 41%; evaluation of monomorphic VT, 16%; cardiac arrest, 5%; unsustained VT, 4%; and other indications (e.g., family history of sudden death, hypertrophic cardiomyopathy, or right ventricular dysplasia), 5%. The remaining 29% were referred for evaluation of supraventricular tachycardia and served as a control group.

In this study, T-wave alternans was strongly associated with the inducibility of monomorphic VT during the electrophysiologic test (180). The odds of having inducible VT if T-wave alternans was present were 5.7 ($p < 0.001$). The sensitivity of T-wave alternans for the induction of sustained monomorphic VT was 78% and the specificity was 73%. This comparison assumes that an electrophysiologic test is the gold standard, although it is possible that T-wave alternans predicts arrhythmic events better than electrophysiologic testing.

To compare the predictive value of T-wave alternans with that of the SAECG and electrophysiologic testing, 290 patients were followed for a mean of 9.9 months. There were 22 ventricular tachyarrhythmic events, which included 5 patients with sudden death and 17 nonfatal arrhythmias, most of which occurred in patients with ICDs. The Kaplan-Meier curves of event-free survival are shown in Figure 6.2-16. All three tests predicted the ventricular tachyarrhythmic events. Patients with T-wave alternans had an almost 11-fold increased risk of experiencing an event compared with patients without T-wave alternans ($p < 0.002$). The ventricular tachyarrhythmia event-free survival curves for SAECG (panel B) and electrophysiologic testing (panel C) also demonstrate an early and persistent separation between low-risk and high-risk subgroups. The results of electrophysiologic testing had a relative risk of 7.1 ($p < 0.001$) while the relative risk for the SAECG was 4.5 ($p < 0.002$). In this direct comparison of two noninvasive risk markers, T-wave alternans had a stronger association with arrhythmic events than the SAECG.

Multivariate models including other variables were used to evaluate the independent association of T-wave alternans (179). T-wave alternans had a 7.7-fold increased risk of having an arrhythmic event or death after accounting for EF (dichotomized at 0.40). With T-wave alternans in the model, EF was no longer predictive of having an arrhythmic event or death. In addition, the association between T-wave alternans and spontaneous arrhythmic events and death was independent of the cause of heart disease: The relative risk (after adjusting for a history of coronary artery disease) was 11.0 ($p < 0.005$).

Risk Stratification after Myocardial Infarction

Hohnloser and colleagues (175) evaluated T-wave alternans in 448 patients 5 to 21 days after acute myocardial infarction. The mean left ventricular EF of this sample was 0.48

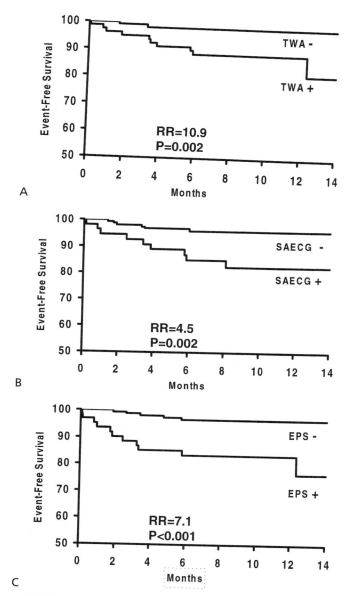

FIGURE 6.2-16. T-wave alternans **(A)**, signal-average ECG **(B)**, and the results for inducible tachycardia during electrophysiologic testing **(C)** in relation to arrhythmia-free survival among 290 patients. All three tests significantly discriminated patients for events. (From Gold MR, Bloomfield DM, Anderson KP, et al. A comparison of T-wave alternans, signal averaged electrocardiography and programmed ventricular stimulation for arrhythmia risk stratification. *J Am Coll Cardiol* 2000;36:2247–2253, with permission.)

in 102 patients after acute myocardial infarction. This study excluded patients with an EF of less than 0.20, although there was still an unusually sick sample of postinfarction patients: 27% had an EF of less than 0.40 and 15% had an arrhythmic event defined as sustained VT or ventricular fibrillation during 13 ± 6 months of follow-up. In this study, 49% of patients had T-wave alternans and 28% had an abnormal SAECG. T-wave alternans was highly associated with the development of arrhythmic events (relative risk, 16.8; *p* < 0.01) and had a sensitivity of 93% and an extremely high negative predictive accuracy of 98% (Fig. 6.2-17). The positive predictive accuracy of T-wave alternans was 28%. The SAECG was a weaker univariate predictor of arrhythmic events (relative risk, 5.7; *p* < 0.001) and had a sensitivity of 53%, a positive predictive accuracy of 38%, and a negative predictive accuracy of 91%. When T-wave alternans and the SAECG were combined, the positive predictive accuracy improved to 50%, although this was associated with a decrease in sensitivity to 53%.

Risk Stratification in Heart Failure

The prognostic significance of T-wave alternans in patients with congestive heart failure has been evaluated in a small German study (182). In this study, 107 patients with NYHA class II and III congestive heart failure without a history of arrhythmic events underwent T-wave alternans testing. The primary end point was a spontaneous arrhythmic event (including VT/ventricular fibrillation, nonfatal cardiac arrest, and arrhythmic death). The mean age was 55 ± 10 years, and 80% were men. The average EF was 0.28 ± 0.07. The cause of left ventricular dysfunction was ischemic in 58% and nonischemic in 42%. T-wave alternans had a strong association with arrhythmic events. None of the patients who had a negative T-wave alternans test had an arrhythmic event, compared with a 2-year arrhythmic event rate of 23% in patients with a positive T-wave alternans test.

Two small studies evaluated the prognostic significance of T-wave alternans in patients with a nonischemic dilated cardiomyopathy. Klingenheben and colleagues (183) evaluated 56 patients with nonischemic dilated cardiomyopathy, including 16 patients who had a history of arrhythmic events and had previously undergone ICD implantation. The prevalence of T-wave alternans in this sample was 29/56 (52%) and T-wave alternans was associated with arrhythmic events. There were six arrhythmic events in 6 months of follow-up and all of the events occurred in patients who had a positive T-wave alternans test. A second study of patients with dilated cardiomyopathy found that the percentage of patients with VT (predominantly unsustained) was significantly higher in patients with T-wave alternans than those without it (61% versus 8%) (184).

± 0.11. The prevalence of T-wave alternans early after myocardial infarction was 18%. The authors reported that T-wave alternans evolves during several weeks after infarction and suggested that risk stratification for late arrhythmic events should be performed 4 to 6 weeks after infarction. No follow-up data were available.

Ikeda and colleagues (181) evaluated the prognostic significance of T-wave alternans and an abnormal SAECG

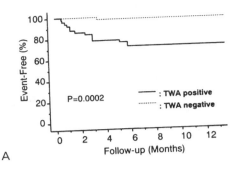

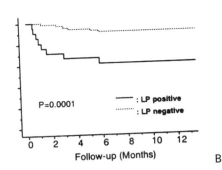

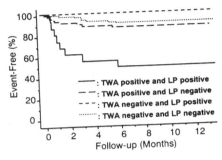

FIGURE 6.2-17. Kaplan-Meier actuarial curves for arrhythmia-free follow-up for groups with positive or negative **(A)** T-wave alternans, **(B)** late potentials, and **(C)** the combination of the two noninvasive tests after acute myocardial infarction. The combination of a positive T-wave alternans and a positive signal-average electrocardiogram predicted arrhythmic events better than either test alone. (From Ikeda T, Sakata T, Takami M, et al. Combined assessment of T-wave alternans and late potentials used to predict arrhythmic events after myocardial infarction. A prospective study. *J Am Coll Cardiol* 2000;35:729, with permission.)

Predicting ICD Shocks

In another study of high-risk patients, Hohnloser and colleagues (185) tested T-wave alternans as a predictor of appropriate discharge of an ICD during an 18-month follow-up in 95 patients who received ICDs for standard clinical indications. In addition to T-wave alternans testing, patients had a number of other noninvasive tests to evaluate arrhythmia risk, including VT induced during electrophysiologic test, left ventricular EF, baroreceptor sensitivity, SAECG, QTd, and the following variables from a 24-hour Holter recording: unsustained VT, mean R-R interval, and SDNN. The only univariate predictors of appropriate ICD shocks were T-wave alternans (relative risk, 2.5; $p < 0.01$), and left ventricular EF (relative risk, 1.4; $p < 0.05$). In a multivariate analysis, T-wave alternans was the only statistically significant independent predictor of ICD discharge.

Summary

These early data not only suggest that T-wave alternans is strongly associated with inducible monomorphic VT during an electrophysiologic test but also suggest that the test identifies patients who are at increased risk for dying or having spontaneous arrhythmic events. T-wave alternans appears to have a stronger association with the risk of developing spontaneous arrhythmic events than electrophysiologic tests or SAECG. The association between T-wave alternans and the risk of dying or having spontaneous arrhythmic events appears to be independent of EF and equally strong in patients with an ischemic and a nonischemic cardiomyopathy.

It is important to note, however, that many of the studies have included extremely high-risk patients (who have already had sustained ventricular arrhythmias) and low-risk patients (patients without structural heart disease), which tends to overestimate the magnitude of risk associated with the presence of T-wave alternans. Larger prospective epidemiologic studies are necessary to better estimate the magnitude of the increase in risk associated with T-wave alternans and to define the optimal combination of noninvasive tests for identifying patients at increased risk of developing arrhythmic events.

INTEGRATING INFORMATION FROM MULTIPLE RISK FACTORS: COMPARISONS AND COMBINATIONS

The optimal way to use noninvasive tests to predict arrhythmic events depends in part on the goals of screening. Most tests perform better at identifying low-risk patients (high negative predictive accuracy) than at identifying high-risk patients. Based on the available epidemiologic data, most of these noninvasive tests, when used individually, have a positive predictive accuracy that is on the order of 10% to 25%. When the goal of screening patients is to identify high-risk patients for prophylactic treatment, a higher positive predictive accuracy is needed. This has motivated investigators to combine risk factors to identify patients at high enough risk to warrant aggressive prophylactic antiarrhythmic therapy.

A number of studies have compared the ability of these diverse noninvasive risk factors to identify patients at high risk for sudden death and/or have used multiple risk factors in combination, attempting to enhance predictive accuracy. Three of these noninvasive risk factors, the SAECG, R-R variability, and T-wave alternans, have been shown to provide independent prognostic information above and beyond the information available from routine clinical care including the measurement of left ventricular EF (37,38,186,187). SAECG and R-R variability also have been shown to provide prognostic information that is independent of the amount of ventricular ectopy measured from a 24-hour Holter recording. This is important because R-R variability can be measured from 24-hour Holter recordings and suggests that both types of information from 24-hour Holter recordings provide independent prognostic information. When either R-R variability or the SAECG is combined with these other routinely available measurements (EF and ventricular arrhythmias measured from a 24-hour Holter recording), a small group of extremely high-risk patients can be identified. A number of early prethrombolytic post–myocardial infarction studies demonstrated that the association between an abnormal SAECG and cardiac death or arrhythmic events was independent of ventricular ectopy on a 24-hour Holter recording, left ventricular EF, and heart rate variability (39,86,103). Combining these different risk markers selected a relatively small group (10% to 15%) of extremely high-risk post–myocardial infarction patients with about a 50% chance of having an unfavorable outcome (cardiac death or an arrhythmic event) in the first 2 years after their myocardial infarction.

A recent study of 575 patients after myocardial infarction compared these four major risk predictors—the SAECG, left ventricular EF, ventricular arrhythmias on a 24-hour Holter recording, and R-R interval variability—for their ability to predict arrhythmic and nonarrhythmic death (104). In this study, 54% of the patients received thrombolytic therapy. All of the variables were univariate predictors of cardiac mortality and arrhythmic death. However, in multivariate analysis, only decreased R-R variability and unsustained VT were independently associated with arrhythmic death. The SAECG did not provide independent prognostic information above that accounted for by these other variables.

The combination of SAECG and T-wave alternans is theoretically attractive because it combines abnormalities detected during depolarization and repolarization. The predictive value of combining T-wave alternans and the SAECG was evaluated in two studies. In a study of patients referred for electrophysiologic testing, both T-wave alternans and the SAECG were independent predictors of inducible sustained VT during an electrophysiology study (172a,179). T-wave alternans was a stronger univariate predictor (relative risk, 10.9) than the SAECG (relative risk, 4.5) for the prediction of spontaneous ventricular arrhythmias during 1 year of follow-up. In a post–myocardial infarction study, the combination of an abnormal T-wave alternans test and an abnormal SAECG had a higher predictive accuracy than either test alone (181). When used together, T-wave alternans and the SAECG had a sensitivity of 53%, a specificity of 91%, and a positive predictive accuracy of 50%. In a multivariate Cox model, this combination had a hazard ratio of 19.9 (95% CI, 3.2–125.3). No studies have directly compared or evaluated a combination of T-wave alternans and R-R variability.

The optimum use of these three risk factors—R-R variability, the SAECG, and T-wave alternans—in combination with other readily available clinical markers of risk such as EF and ventricular arrhythmias on a 24-hour Holter recording, remains to be defined. A large epidemiologic study that includes all of these risk factors is needed.

CONCLUSION

Individually, R-R variability, SAECG, QTd, and microvolt-level T-wave alternans are useful for assessing the status of the autonomic nervous system, cardiac depolarization, or cardiac repolarization. R-R variability and SAECG already have proven useful for predicting cardiovascular death in general and sudden cardiac death in particular. Microvolt-level T-wave alternans shows great promise as a predictor of sudden cardiac death, but definitive studies have yet to be done. QTd seems to have less predictive value and it is not yet clear whether technical improvements will lead to better performance or whether this technique will ultimately prove inadequate for predicting sudden cardiac death.

REFERENCES

1. Wolf MM, Varigos GA, Hunt D, Sloman JG. Sinus arrhythmia in acute myocardial infarction. *Med J Aust* 1978;2:52–53.
2. Lown B, Verrier RL. Neural activity and ventricular fibrillation. *N Engl J Med* 1976;294:1165–1170.
3. Schwartz PJ, Vanoli E. Cardiac arrhythmias elicited by interaction between acute myocardial ischemia and sympathetic hyperactivity: a new experimental model for the study of antiarrhythmic drugs. *J Cardiovasc Pharmacol* 1981;3:1251–1259.
4. Schwartz PJ, Brown AM, Malliani A, Zanchetti A. *Neural mechanisms in cardiac arrhythmias.* New York: Raven Press, 1978.
5. Corr PB, Yamada KA, Witkowski FX. Mechanisms controlling cardiac autonomic function and their relation to arrhythmogenesis. In: *The heart and cardiovascular system.* New York: Raven Press, 1986:1343–1403.
6. Schwartz PJ, Stone HL. The role of the autonomic nervous system in sudden coronary death. *Ann N Y Acad Sci* 1982;382:162–180.
7. Schwartz PJ, Billman GE, Stone HL. Autonomic mechanisms in ventricular fibrillation induced by myocardial ischemia during exercise in dogs with healed myocardial infarction: an experimental preparation for sudden cardiac death. *Circulation* 1984; 69:790–800.
8. Billman GE, Schwartz PJ, Stone L. Baroreceptor reflex control of heart rate: a predictor of sudden cardiac death . *Circulation* 1982;66:874–880.

9. Billman GE, Schwartz PJ, Stone HL. The effects of daily exercise on susceptibility to sudden cardiac death. *Circulation* 1984; 69:1182–1189.

10. Vanoli E, De Ferrari GM, Stramba Badiale M, et al. Vagal stimulation and prevention of sudden death in conscious dogs with a healed myocardial infarction. *Circ Res* 1991;68:1471–1481.

11. Billman GE, Hoskins RS. Time-series analysis of heart rate variability during submaximal exercise. Evidence for reduced cardiac vagal tone in animals susceptible to ventricular fibrillation. *Circulation* 1989;80:146–157.

12. Hull SS Jr, Evans AR, Vanoli E, et al. Heart rate variability before and after myocardial infarction in conscious dogs at high and low risk of sudden death. *J Am Coll Cardiol* 1990;16:978–985.

13. Bigger JT, Fleiss JL. Methods for assessment of vagal tone and reflexes: time domain measures. In: Levy MN, Schwartz PJ, eds. *Vagal control of the heart: experimental basis and clinical implications.* Mt. Kisco, NY: Futura Publishing, 1994:419–432.

14. Kleiger RE, Stein PK, Bosner MS, Rottman JN. Time domain measurements of heart rate variability. *Cardiol Clin* 1992;10: 487–498.

15. Albrecht P, Cohen RJ. Estimation of heart rate power spectrum bands from real world data: dealing with ectopic beats and noise data. *Comput Cardiol* 1988;15:311–314.

16. Berger RD, Akselrod S, Gordon D, Cohen RJ. An efficient algorithm for spectral analysis of heart rate variability. *IEEE Trans Biomed Eng* 1986;9:900–904.

17. Bartlett MS. Smoothing periodograms from time series with contiguous spectra. *Nature (London)* 1948;161:686–687.

18. Bloomfield P. *Fourier analysis of time series: an introduction.* New York: John Wiley and Sons, 1975.

19. Oppenheim AV, Schafer RW. *Digital signal processing.* Englewood Cliffs, NJ: Prentice-Hall, 1975.

20. Mullen TJ, Appel ML, Mukkamala R, et al. System identification of closed-loop cardiovascular control: effects of posture and autonomic blockade. *Am J Physiol* 1997;272:H448–H461.

21. Baselli G, Cerutti S, Civardi S, et al. Spectral and cross-spectral analysis of heart rate and arterial blood pressure variability signals. *Comput Biomed Res* 1986;19:520–534.

22. Kiauta T, Jager F, Tapp WN. Complex demodulation of heart rate changes during orthostatic testing. *Comput Cardiol* 1990; 159–162.

23. Shin SJ, Reisman SS, Tapp WN, Atelson BH. Assessment of autonomic regulation of heart rate variability by the method of complex demodulation. *IEEE Trans Biomed Eng* 1989;36: 277–283.

24. Gleick J. *Chaos. Making a new science.* New York: Viking, 1987.

25. Saul JP, Albrecht P, Berger RD, Cohen RJ. Analysis of long term heart rate variability: methods, 1/f scaling and implications. *Comput Cardiol* 1987;14:419–422.

26. Peng CK, Havlin S, Stanley HE, Goldberger AL. Quantification of scaling exponents and crossover phenomena in nonstationary heart beat time series. *Chaos* 1995;5:82–87.

27. Skinner JE, Carpeggiani C, Landisman CE, Fulton KW. Correlation dimension of heartbeat intervals is reduced in conscious pigs by myocardial ischemia. *Circ Res* 1991;68:966–976.

28. Goldberger AL, West BJ. Applications of nonlinear dynamics to clinical cardiology. *Ann N Y Acad Sci* 1987;504:195–213.

29. Kobayashi M, Musha T. 1/f fluctuation of heartbeat period . *IEEE Trans Biomed Eng* 1982;29:456–457.

30. Katona PG, Jih F. Respiratory sinus arrhythmia: noninvasive measure of parasympathetic cardiac control. *J Appl Physiol* 1975; 39:801–805.

31. Fouad FM, Tarazi RC, Ferrario CM, et al. Assessment of parasympathetic control of heart rate by a noninvasive method. *Am J Physiol* 1984;246:H838–H842.

32. Pagani M, Lombardi F, Guzzetti S. Power spectral analysis of heart rate and arterial pressure variabilities as a marker of sympatho-vagal interaction in man and conscious dog. *Circ Res* 1986;59:178–193.

33. Pomeranz B, Macaulay RJB, Caudill MA, et al. Assessment of autonomic function in humans by heart rate spectral analysis. *Am J Physiol* 1985;248:H151–H153.

34. Akselrod S, Gordon D, Ubel FA, et al. Power spectrum analysis of heart rate fluctuations: a quantitative probe of beat-to-beat cardiovascular control. *Science* 1981;213:220–222.

35. Kleiger RE, Bigger JT Jr, Bosner MS, et al. Stability over time of variables measuring heart rate variability in normal subjects. *Am J Cardiol* 1991;68:626–630.

36. Bigger JT Jr, Fleiss JL, Rolnitzky LM, Steinman RC. Stability over time of heart period variability in patients with previous myocardial infarction and ventricular arrhythmias. The CAPS and ESVEM investigators. *Am J Cardiol* 1992;69:718–723.

37. Kleiger RE, Miller JP, Bigger JT, Moss AJ, and the Multicenter Post-Infarction Research Group. Decreased heart rate variability and its association with increased mortality after acute myocardial infarction. *Am J Cardiol* 1987;59:256–262.

38. Bigger JT, Fleiss JL, Steinman RC, et al. Frequency domain measures of heart period variability and mortality after myocardial infarction. *Circulation* 1992;85:164–171.

39. Farrell TG, Bashir Y, Cripps T, et al. Risk stratification for arrhythmic events in postinfarction patients based on heart rate variability, ambulatory electrocardiographic variables and the signal-averaged electrocardiogram . *J Am Coll Cardiol* 1991;18:687–697.

40. Copie X, Hnatkova K, Staunton A, et al. Predictive power of increased heart rate versus depressed left ventricular ejection fraction and heart rate variability for risk stratification after myocardial infarction. *J Am Coll Cardiol* 1996;27:270–276.

41. Zuanetti G, Mantini L, Hernandez-Bernal F, et al. Relevance of heart rate as a prognostic factor in patients with acute myocardial infarction: insights from the GISSI-2 study. *Eur Heart J* 1998;19[Suppl F]:F19–F26.

42. La Rovere MT, Bigger JT Jr, Marcus FI, et al. Baroreflex sensitivity and heart-rate variability in prediction of total cardiac mortality after myocardial infarction. ATRAMI (Autonomic Tone and Reflexes After Myocardial Infarction) investigators. *Lancet* 1998;351:478–484.

43. Nolan J, Batin PD, Andrews R, et al. Prospective study of heart rate variability and mortality in chronic heart failure: results of the United Kingdom Heart Failure Evaluation and Assessment of Risk Trial (UK-HEART). *Circulation* 1998;98:1510–1516.

44. Bilchick KC, Fetics B, Fischer SG, et al. The prognostic value of heart rate variability in congestive heart failure: a substudy of the Veterans Affairs' survival trial of antiarrhythmic therapy in congestive heart failure. *Circulation* 2000 *(in press)*.

45. Bigger JT Jr, Fleiss JL, Steinman RC, et al. Correlations among time and frequency domain measures of heart period variability two weeks after acute myocardial infarction. *Am J Cardiol* 1992;69:891–898.

46. Hinkle LE, Thaler JT. Clinical classification of cardiac deaths. *Circulation* 1982;65:457–464.

47. Bigger JT Jr, Steinman RC, Rolnitzky LM, et al. Power law behavior of RR-interval variability in healthy middle-aged persons, patients with recent acute myocardial infarction, and patients with heart transplants. *Circulation* 1996;93:2142–2151.

48. Huikuri HV, Makikallio TH, Airaksinen KE, et al. Power-law relationship of heart rate variability as a predictor of mortality in the elderly. *Circulation* 1998;97:2031–2036.

49. Huikuri HV, Makikallio TH, Peng CK, et al. Fractal correlation properties of R-R interval dynamics and mortality in patients with depressed left ventricular function after an acute myocardial infarction . *Circulation* 2000;101:47–53.

50. Bigger JT Jr, Fleiss JL, Rolnitzky LM, Steinman RC. The ability

of several short-term measures of RR variability to predict mortality after myocardial infarction. *Circulation* 1993;88:927–934.

51. Skinner JE, Pratt CM, Vybiral T. A reduction in the correlation dimension of heartbeat intervals precedes imminent ventricular fibrillation in human subjects. *Am Heart J* 1993;125:731–743.

52. Smyth HS, Sleight P, Pickering GW. Reflex regulation of arterial pressure during sleep in man: a quantitative method of assessing baroreflex sensitivity. *Circ Res* 1969;24:109–121.

53. Bigger JT Jr, Bloomfield DM, Steinman RC, Rolnitzky LM, and the ATRAMI Investigators. Frequency domain measures of RR variability predict cardiac mortality in the thrombolytic era. *Circulation* 1996;94:1–27.

54. Bigger JT Jr, Fleiss JL, Rolnitzky LM, et al. Time course of recovery of heart period variability after myocardial infarction. *J Am Coll Cardiol* 1991;18:1643–1649.

55. Flapan AD, Wright RA, Nolan J, et al. Differing patterns of cardiac parasympathetic activity and their evolution in selected patients with a first myocardial infarction. *J Am Coll Cardiol* 1993;21:926–931.

56. Bigger JT Jr, La Rovere MT, Steinman RC, et al. Comparison of baroreflex sensitivity and heart period variability after myocardial infarction. *J Am Coll Cardiol* 1989;14:1511–1518.

57. Bigger JT Jr, Fleiss JL, Rolnitzky LM, Steinman RC. Frequency domain measures of heart period variability to assess risk late after myocardial infarction. *J Am Coll Cardiol* 1993;21:729–736.

58. Szabo BM, van Veldhuisen DJ, van der Veer N, et al. Prognostic value of heart rate variability in chronic congestive heart failure secondary to idiopathic or ischemic dilated cardiomyopathy. *Am J Cardiol* 1997;79:978–980.

59. Brouwer J, van Veldhuisen DJ, Man in't Veld AJ, et al. Prognostic value of heart rate variability during long-term follow-up in patients with mild to moderate heart failure. The Dutch Ibopamine Multicenter Trial Study Group. *J Am Coll Cardiol* 1996;28:1183–1189.

60. Ponikowski P, Anker SD, Chua TP, et al. Depressed heart rate variability as an independent predictor of death in chronic congestive heart failure secondary to ischemic or idiopathic dilated cardiomyopathy. *Am J Cardiol* 1997;79:1645–1650.

61. Binder T, Frey B, Porenta G, et al. Prognostic value of heart rate variability in patients awaiting cardiac transplantation. *Pacing Clin Electrophysiol* 1992;15:2215–2220.

62. Saul JP, Arai Y, Berger RD, et al. Assessment of autonomic regulation in chronic congestive heart failure by heart rate spectral analysis. *Am J Cardiol* 1988;61:1292–1299.

63. Mortara A, Sleight P, Pinna GD, et al. Abnormal awake respiratory patterns are common in chronic heart failure and may prevent evaluation of autonomic tone by measures of heart rate variability. *Circulation* 1997;96:246–252.

64. Bernardi L, Valle F, Coco M, et al. Physical activity influences heart rate variability and very-low-frequency components in Holter electrocardiograms. *Cardiovasc Res* 1996;32:234–237.

65. Malik M, Camm AJ, Janse MJ, et al. Depressed heart rate variability identifies postinfarction patients who might benefit from prophylactic treatment with amiodarone: a substudy of EMIAT (the European Myocardial Infarct Amiodarone Trial). *J Am Coll Cardiol* 2000;35:1263–1275.

66. Pratt CM, Camm AJ, Bigger JT Jr, et al. Evaluation of antiarrhythmic drug efficacy in patients with an ICD: unlimited potential or replete with complexity and problems? *J Cardiovasc Electrophysiol* 1999;10:1534–1549.

67. Breithardt G, Cain ME, El-Sherif N, et al. Standards for analysis of ventricular late potentials using high-resolution or signal-averaged electrocardiography. A statement by a Task Force Committee of the European Society of Cardiology, the American Heart Association, and the American College of Cardiology. *Circulation* 1991;83:1481–1488.

68. Simson MB. Use of signals in the terminal QRS complex to identify patients with ventricular tachycardia after myocardial infarction. *Circulation* 1981;64:235–242.

69. Steinberg JS, Bigger JT Jr. Importance of the endpoint of noise reduction in analysis of the signal-averaged electrocardiogram. *Am J Cardiol* 1989;63:556–560.

70. El-Sherif N, Denes P, Katz R, et al. Definition of the best prediction criteria of the time domain signal-averaged electrocardiogram for serious arrhythmic events in the postinfarction period. The Cardiac Arrhythmia Suppression Trial/Signal-Averaged Electrocardiogram (CAST/SAECG) substudy investigators. *J Am Coll Cardiol* 1995;25:908–914.

71. Kelen GJ, Henkin R, Starr AM, et al. Spectral turbulence analysis of the signal-averaged electrocardiogram and its predictive accuracy for inducible sustained monomorphic ventricular tachycardia. *Am J Cardiol* 1991;67:965–975.

72. Vazquez R, Caref EB, Torres F, et al. Improved diagnostic value of combined time and frequency domain analysis of the signal-averaged electrocardiogram after myocardial infarction. *J Am Coll Cardiol* 1999;33:385–394.

73. Lander P, Gomis P, Caminal P, et al. Pathophysiological insights into abnormal intra-QRS signals in the high resolution ECG. In: *Computers in cardiology.* Los Alamitos, CA: IEEE, 1995: 273–275.

74. Meste O, Rix H, Caminal P, Thakor NV. Ventricular late potentials characterization in time-frequency domain by means of a wavelet transform. *IEEE Trans Biomed Eng* 1994;41:625–634.

75. Reinhardt L, Makijarvi M, Fetsch T, et al. Predictive value of wavelet correlation functions of signal-averaged electrocardiogram in patients after anterior versus inferior myocardial infarction. *J Am Coll Cardiol* 1996;27:53–59.

76. Gardner PI, Ursell PC, Fenoglio JJ Jr, Wit AL. Electrophysiologic and anatomic basis for fractionated electrograms recorded from healed myocardial infarcts. *Circulation* 1985;72:596–611.

77. Richards DA, Blake GJ, Spear JF, Moore EN. Electrophysiologic substrate for ventricular tachycardia: correlation of properties *in vivo* and *in vitro. Circulation* 1984;69:369–381.

78. Simson MB, Untereker WJ, Spielman SR. Relation between late potentials on the body surface and directly recorded fragmented electrograms in patients with ventricular tachycardia. *Am J Cardiol* 1983;51:105–112.

79. Josephson ME, Horowitz LN, Farshidi A. Continuous local electrical activity: a mechanism of recurrent ventricular tachycardia. *Circulation* 1978;57:658.

80. Breithardt G, Schwarzmaier J, Borggrefe M, et al. Prognostic significance of late ventricular potentials after acute myocardial infarction. *Eur Heart J* 1983;4:487–495.

81. Denes P, Santarelli P, Hauser RG. Quantitative analysis of the HF components of the terminal portion of the body surface QRS in normal subjects and in patients with ventricular tachycardia. *Circulation* 1983;67:1129–1138.

82. Buxton AE, Simson MB, Falcone RA, et al. Results of signal-averaged electrocardiography and electrophysiologic study in patients with nonsustained ventricular tachycardia after healing of acute myocardial infarction. *Am J Cardiol* 1987;60:80–85.

83. Winters SL, Ip J, Deshmukh P, et al. Determinants of induction of ventricular tachycardia in nonsustained ventricular tachycardia after myocardial infarction and the usefulness of the signal-averaged electrocardiogram. *Am J Cardiol* 1993;72:1281–1285.

84. Turitto G, Fontaine JM, Ursell SN, et al. Value of the signal-averaged electrocardiogram as a predictor of the results of programmed stimulation in nonsustained ventricular tachycardia. *Am J Cardiol* 1988;61:1272–1278.

85. Denniss AR, Richards DA, Cody DV. Prognostic significance of ventricular tachycardia and fibrillation induced at programmed stimulation and delayed potentials detected on the signal-aver-

aged electrocardiograms of survivors of acute myocardial infarction. *Circulation* 1986;74:731–745.

86. Kuchar DL, Thorburn CW, Sammel NL. Prediction of serious arrhythmic events after myocardial infarction: signal-averaged electrocardiogram, Holter monitoring, and radionuclide ventriculography. *J Am Coll Cardiol* 1987;9:531–538.

87. Gomes JA, Winters SL, Stewart D, et al. A new noninvasive index to predict sustained ventricular tachycardia and sudden death in the first year after myocardial infarction: based on signal-averaged electrocardiogram, radionuclide ejection fraction, and Holter monitoring. *J Am Coll Cardiol* 1987;10:349–357.

88. Lander P, Gomis P, Goyal R, et al. Analysis of abnormal intra-QRS potentials: improved predictive value for predicting arrhythmic events using the signal-averaged electrocardiogram. *Circulation* 1997;95:1386–1393.

89. Gang ES, Lew AS, Hong M, et al. Decreased incidence of ventricular late potentials after successful thrombolytic therapy for acute myocardial infarction. *N Engl J Med* 1989;321:712–716.

90. Vatterott PJ, Hammill SC, Bailey KR, et al. Late potentials on signal-averaged electrocardiograms and patency of the infarct-related artery in survivors of acute myocardial infarction. *J Am Coll Cardiol* 1991;17:330–337.

91. Zimmermann M, Adamec R, Ciaroni S. Reduction in the frequency of ventricular late potentials after acute myocardial infarction by early thrombolytic therapy. *Am J Cardiol* 1991;67:697–703.

92. Pedretti R, Laporta A, Etro MD, et al. Influence of thrombolysis on signal-averaged electrocardiogram and late arrhythmic events after acute myocardial infarction. *Am J Cardiol* 1992;69:866–872.

93. Lange RA, Cigarroa RG, Wells PJ, et al. Influence of anterograde flow in the infarct artery on the incidence of late potentials after acute myocardial infarction. *Am J Cardiol* 1990;65:554–558.

94. de Chillou C, Doevendans P, Cheriex E, et al. Echocardiographic wall motion abnormalities and the signal averaged electrocardiogram in the acute phase of a first myocardial infarction. *Eur Heart J* 1993;14:795–798.

95. Denes P, El-Sherif N, Katz R, et al, and the Cardiac Arrhythmia Suppression Trial (CAST)/SAECG substudy Investigators. Prognostic significance of signal-averaged electrocardiogram after thrombolytic therapy and/or angioplasty during acute myocardial infarction (CAST substudy). *Am J Cardiol* 1994;74:216–220.

96. Steinberg JS, Hochman JS, Morgan CD, et al, and the Late Assessment of Thrombolytic Efficacy (LATE) Ancillary Study Investigators. Effects of thrombolytic therapy administered 6 to 24 hours after myocardial infarction on the signal-averaged ECG. Results of a multicenter randomized trial. *Circulation* 1994;90:746–752.

97. Ragosta M, Sabia PJ, Kaul S, et al. Effects of late (1 to 30 days) reperfusion after acute myocardial infarction on the signal-averaged electrocardiogram. *Am J Cardiol* 1993;71:19–23.

98. Cook JR, Flack JE, Gregory CA, et al. Influence of the preoperative signal-averaged electrocardiogram on left ventricular function after coronary artery bypass graft surgery in patients with left ventricular dysfunction. The CABG Patch trial. *Am J Cardiol* 1998;82:285–289.

99. Ragosta M, Pagley PR, DiMarco JP, Beller GA. Relation between myocardial viability and abnormalities on the signal-averaged electrocardiogram in patients with low (<40%) ejection fraction and coronary artery disease. *Am J Cardiol* 2000 Feb15;85:405–410.

100. Malik M, Kulakowski P, Odemuyiwa O, et al. Effect of thrombolytic therapy on the predictive value of signal-averaged electrocardiography after acute myocardial infarction. *Am J Cardiol* 1992;70:21–25.

101. McClements BM, Adgey AA. Value of signal-averaged electrocardiography, radionuclide ventriculography, Holter monitoring and clinical variables for prediction of arrhythmic events in survivors of acute myocardial infarction in the thrombolytic era. *J Am Coll Cardiol* 1993;21:1419–1427.

102. Hohnloser SH, Franck P, Klingenheben T, et al. Open infarct artery, late potentials, and other prognostic factors in patients after acute myocardial infarction in the thrombolytic era. A prospective trial. *Circulation* 1994;90:1747–1756.

103. Freedman RA, Gillis AM, Keren A. Signal-averaged electrocardiographic late potentials in patients with ventricular fibrillation or ventricular tachycardia: correlation with clinical arrhythmia and electrophysiologic study. *Am J Cardiol* 1985;55:1350–1353.

104. Hartikainen JE, Malik M, Staunton A, et al. Distinction between arrhythmic and nonarrhythmic death after acute myocardial infarction based on heart rate variability, signal-averaged electrocardiogram, ventricular arrhythmias and left ventricular ejection fraction. *J Am Coll Cardiol* 1996;28:296–304.

105. Buxton AE, Lee KL, Fisher JD, et al. A randomized study of the prevention of sudden death in patients with coronary artery disease. *N Engl J Med* 1999;341:1882–1890.

106. Cain ME, Gomes JA, Hafley G, et al. Performance of the signal-averaged ECG and electrophysiologic testing in identifying patients vulnerable to arrhythmic or cardiac death. *Circulation* 1999;100:1267.

107. Gomes JA, Cain ME, Buxton AE, et al. The signal-averaged ECG is a powerful predictor of outcome in the Multicenter Unsustained Tachycardia Trial. *Circulation* 1999;100:1267.

108. Bigger JT Jr. Prophylactic use of implanted cardiac defibrillators in patients at high risk for ventricular arrhythmias after coronary-artery bypass graft surgery. *N Engl J Med* 1997;337:1569–1575.

109. Gottlieb CD, Bigger JT Jr, Steinman RC, Rolnitzky LM, for the CABG Patch Investigators. Signal-averaged ECG predicts death after CABG surgery. *Circulation* 1995;92:I406.

110. Bigger JT Jr, Whang W, Rottman JN, et al. Mechanisms of death in the CABG Patch trial: a randomized trial of implantable cardiac defibrillator prophylaxis in patients at high risk of death after coronary artery bypass graft surgery. *Circulation* 1999;99:1416–1421.

111. Mancini DM, Wong KL, Simson MB. Prognostic value of an abnormal signal-averaged electrocardiogram in patients with nonischemic congestive cardiomyopathy. *Circulation* 1993;87:1083–1092.

112. Denereaz D, Zimmermann M, Adamec R. Significance of ventricular late potentials in non-ischaemic dilated cardiomyopathy. *Eur Heart J* 1992;13:895–901.

113. Bloomfield DM, Hickey K, Sciacca RR, et al. Abnormal Signal-averaged electrocardiogram predicts mortality in patients with non-ischemic cardiomyopathy and severe congestive heart failure. *J Am Coll Cardiol* 1995;25:215A.

114. Silverman ME, Pressel MD, Brackett JC, et al. Prognostic value of the signal-averaged electrocardiogram and a prolonged QRS in ischemic and nonischemic cardiomyopathy. *Am J Cardiol* 1995;75:460–464.

114a. Dubrey SW, Bilazarian S, LaValley M, et al. Signal-averaged electrocardiography in patients with AL (primary) amyloidosis. *Am Heart J* 1997;134:994.

114b. Turrini P, Angelini A, Thiene G, et al. Late potentials and ventricular arrhythmia in arrhythmogenic right ventricular cardiomyopathy. *Am J Cardiol* 1999;83:1214.

114c. Hermida JS, Minassian A, Jarry G, et al. Familial incidence of late ventricular potentials and electrocardiographic abnormalities in arrhythmogenic right ventricular dysplasia. *Am J Cardiol* 1997;79:1375.

115. Steinberg JS, Prystowsky E, Freedman RA, et al. Use of the signal-averaged electrocardiogram for predicting inducible ventric-

ular tachycardia in patients with unexplained syncope: relation to clinical variables in a multivariate analysis. *J Am Coll Cardiol* 1994;23:99–106.

116. Wilson FN, MacLeod AG, Barker PS, Johnston FD. The determination and the significance of the areas of the ventricular deflections of the electrocardiogram. *Am Heart J* 1934;46–61.

117. Cowan JC, Yusoff K, Moore M, et al. Importance of lead selection in QT interval measurement. *Am J Cardiol* 1988;61:83–87.

118. Campbell RW, Gardiner P, Amos PA, et al. Measurement of the QT interval. *Eur Heart J* 1985;6[Suppl D]:81–83.

119. Mirvis DM. Spatial variation of QT intervals in normal persons and patients with acute myocardial infarction. *J Am Coll Cardiol* 1985;5:625–631.

120. Antzelevitch C, Shimizu W, Yan GX, Sicouri S. Cellular basis for QT dispersion. *J Electrocardiol* 1998;30[Suppl]:168–175.

121. Day CP, McComb JM, Campbell RW. QT dispersion: an indication of arrhythmia risk in patients with long QT intervals. *Br Heart J* 1990;63:342–344.

122. Hingham PD, Hilton CJ, Aitcheson JD, et al. Does QT dispersion reflect dispersion of ventricular recovery? *Circulation* 1992;86:I392(abst).

123. Zabel M, Lichten PR, Haverich A, Franz MR. Comparison of ECG variables of dispersion of ventricular repolarization with direct myocardial repolarization measurements in the human heart. *J Cardiovasc Electrophysiol* 1998;9:1279–1284.

124. Wang L. QT dispersion from body surface ECG does not reflect the spatial dispersion of ventricular repolarization in sheep. *Pacing Clin Electrophysiol* 2000;23(Mar):359–364.

125. Lux RL, Fuller MS, MacLeod RS, et al. QT interval dispersion: dispersion of ventricular repolarization or dispersion of QT interval? *J Electrocardiol* 1998;30[Suppl]:176–180.

126. Lee KW, Kligfield P, Okin PM, Dower GE. Determinants of precordial QT dispersion in normal subjects. *J Electrocardiol* 1998;31[Suppl]:128–133.

127. Kors JA, van Herpen G, van Bemmel JH. QT dispersion as an attribute of T-loop morphology. *Circulation* 1999;99:1458–1463.

128. Zabel M, Portnoy S, Franz MR. Electrocardiographic indexes of dispersion of ventricular repolarization: an isolated heart validation study. *J Am Coll Cardiol* 1995;25:746–752.

129. Xue Q, Reddy S. New algorithms for QT dispersion analysis. *IEEE Comput Cardiol* 1996;293–296.

130. McLaughlin NB, Campbell RWF, Murray A. Influence of T wave amplitude on automatic QT measurement. *IEEE Comput Cardiol* 1995;777–780.

131. Antzelevitch C, Nesterenko VV, Yan GX. Role of M cells in acquired long QT syndrome, U waves, and torsade de pointes. *J Electrocardiol* 1995;28[Suppl]:131–138.

132. Hnatkova K, Malik M, Kautzner J, et al. Adjustment of QT dispersion assessed from 12 lead electrocardiograms for different numbers of analysed electrocardiographic leads: comparison of stability of different methods. *Br Heart J* 1994;72:390–396.

133. Batchvarov V, Malik M. Measurement and interpretation of QT dispersion. *Prog Cardiovasc Dis* 2000;42(Mar/Apr):325–344.

134. Ahnve S. Errors in the visual determination of corrected QT (QTc) interval during acute myocardial infarction. *J Am Coll Cardiol* 1985;5:699–702.

135. Savelieva I, Yi G, Guo X, et al. Agreement and reproducibility of automatic versus manual measurement of QT interval and QT dispersion. *Am J Cardiol* 1998;81:471–477.

136. McLaughlin NB, Campbell RW, Murray A. Comparison of automatic QT measurement techniques in the normal 12 lead electrocardiogram. *Br Heart J* 1995;74:84–89.

137. Savelieva I, Yi G, Guo X, et al. Agreement and reproducibility of automatic versus manual measurement of QT interval and QT dispersion. *Am J Cardiol* 1998;81:471–477.

138. Gang Y, Guo XH, Crook R, et al. Computerised measurements of QT dispersion in healthy subjects. *Heart* 1998;80:459–466.

139. Macfarlane PW, McLaughlin SC, Rodger JC. Influence of lead selection and population on automated measurement of QT dispersion. *Circulation* 1998;98:2160–2167.

140. Spodick DH. Reduction of QT-interval imprecision and variance by measuring the JT interval [Editorial]. *Am J Cardiol* 1992;70:103.

141. Banker J, Dizon J, Reiffel J. Effects of the ventricular activation sequence on the JT interval. *Am J Cardiol* 1997;79:816–819.

142. Zareba W, Moss AJ, le Cessie S. Dispersion of ventricular repolarization and arrhythmic cardiac death in coronary artery disease. *Am J Cardiol* 1994;74:550–553.

143. Savelieva I, Yap YG, Yi G, et al. Comparative reproducibility of QT, QT peak, and T peak–T end intervals and dispersion in normal subjects, patients with myocardial infarction, and patients with hypertrophic cardiomyopathy. *Pacing Clin Electrophysiol* 1998;21:2376–2381.

144. de Bruyne MC, Hoes AW, Kors JA, et al. QTc dispersion predicts cardiac mortality in the elderly: the Rotterdam Study. *Circulation* 1998;97:467–472.

145. Batchvarov V, Yi G, Guo X, et al. QT interval and QT dispersion measured with the threshold method depend on threshold level. *Pacing Clin Electrophysiol* 1998;21:2372–2375.

146. Lee KW, Okin PM, Kligfield P, et al. Precordial QT dispersion and inducible ventricular tachycardia. *Am Heart J* 1997;134:1005–1013.

147. Stoletniy LN, Pai SM, Platt ML, et al. QT dispersion as a noninvasive predictor of inducible ventricular tachycardia. *J Electrocardiol* 1999;32:173–177.

148. Anastasiou-Nana MI, Nanas JN, Karagounis LA, et al. Relation of dispersion of QRS and QT in patients with advanced congestive heart failure to cardiac and sudden death mortality. *Am J Cardiol* 2000;85(May 15):1212–1217.

149. Pinsky DJ, Sciacca RR, Steinberg JS. QT dispersion as a marker of risk in patients awaiting heart transplantation. *J Am Coll Cardiol* 1997;29:1576–1584.

150. Galinier M, Vialette JC, Fourcade J, et al. QT interval dispersion as a predictor of arrhythmic events in congestive heart failure. Importance of aetiology. *Eur Heart J* 1998;19:1054–1062.

151. Fei L, Goldman JH, Prasad K, et al. QT dispersion and RR variations on 12-lead ECGs in patients with congestive heart failure secondary to idiopathic dilated cardiomyopathy. *Eur Heart J* 1996;17:258–263.

152. Barr CS, Naas A, Freeman M, et al. QT dispersion and sudden unexpected death in chronic heart failure. *Lancet* 1994;343:327–329.

153. Zabel M, Klingenheben T, Franz MR, Hohnloser SH. Assessment of QT dispersion for prediction of mortality or arrhythmic events after myocardial infarction: results of a prospective, long-term follow-up study. *Circulation* 1998;97:2543–2550.

153a. Perkiomaki JS, Koistinen MJ, Yli-Mayry S, et al. Dispersion of QT intervals in patients with and without susceptibility to ventricular tachyarrhythmias after previous myocardial infarction. *J Am Coll Cardiol* 1995;26:174.

153b. Oikarinen L, Viitasalo M, Toivonen L. Dispersion of the QT interval in postmyocardial infarction patients presenting with ventricular tachycardia or with ventricular fibrillation. *Am J Cardiol* 1998;81:694.

153c. Spargias KS, Lindsay SJ, Kawar GI, et al. QT dispersion as a predictor of long-term mortality in patients with acute myocardial infarction and clinical evidence of heart failure. *Eur Heart J* 1999;20:1158.

153d. Moreno FL, Villanueva MT, Karagounis LA, et al, for the Team-2 Study Investigators. Reduction in QT interval dispersion by successful thrombolytic therapy in acute myocardial infarction. *Circulation* 1994;90:94.

153e. Schneider CA, Voth E, Baer FM, et al. QT dispersion is determined by the extent of viable myocardium in patients with chronic Q-wave myocardial infarction. *Circulation* 1997;96: 3913.

154. Priori SG, Napolitano C, Diehl L, Schwartz PJ. Dispersion of the QT interval. A marker of therapeutic efficacy in the idiopathic long QT syndrome. *Circulation* 1994;89:1681–1689.

155. de Bruyne MC, Hoes AW, Kors JA, et al. Prolonged QT interval predicts cardiac and all-cause mortality in the elderly. The Rotterdam Study . *Eur Heart J* 1999;20:278–284.

156. Kors JA, de Bruyne MC, Hoes AW, et al. T axis as an indicator of risk of cardiac events in elderly people. *Lancet* 1998;352: 601–605.

157. Kors JA, de Bruyne MC, Hoes AW, et al. T-loop morphology as a marker of cardiac events in the elderly. *J Electrocardiol* 1998;31 [Suppl]:54–59.

158. Okin PM, Devereux RB, Howard BV, et al. Assessment of QT interval and QT dispersion for prediction of all-cause and cardiovascular mortality in American Indians: the Strong Heart Study. *Circulation* 2000;101(Jan 4):61–66.

159. Raeder EA, Rosenbaum DS, Bhasin R, Cohen RJ. Alternating morphology of the QRST complex preceding sudden death. *N Engl J Med* 1992;326:271–272.

160. Schwartz PJ, Malliani A. Electrical alternation of the T-wave: clinical and experimental evidence of its relationship with the sympathetic nervous system and with the long Q-T syndrome. *Am Heart J* 1975;89:45–50.

161. Hiejima K, Sano T. Electrical alternans of TU wave in Romano-Ward syndrome. *Br Heart J* 1976;38:767–700.

162. Reddy CV, Kiok JP, Khan RG, El-Sherif N. Repolarization alternans associated with alcoholism and hypomagnesemia. *Am J Cardiol* 1999;84:390–391.

163. Shimoni Z, Flatau E, Schiller D, et al. Electrical alternans of giant U waves with multiple electrolyte deficits. *Am J Cardiol* 1984;54:920–921.

164. Kalter HH, Schwartz ML. Electrical alternans. *N Y State J Med* 1948;1:1164–1166.

165. Smith JM, Clancy EA, Valeri CR, et al. Electrical alternans and cardiac electrical instability. *Circulation* 1988;77:110–121.

166. Nearing BD, Oesterle SN, Verrier RL. Complex demodulation of T-wave alternans in the precordial leads for noninvasive assessment of cardiac vulnerability in animals and man. *Circulation* 1992;86[Suppl I]:I300.

167. Rosenbaum DS, Albrecht P, Cohen RJ. Predicting sudden cardiac death from T wave alternans of the surface electrocardiogram: promise and pitfalls. *J Cardiovasc Electrophys* 1996;7:1095–1111.

168. Pastore JM, Girouard SD, Laurita KR, et al. Mechanism linking T-wave alternans to the genesis of cardiac fibrillation. *Circulation* 1999;99:1385–1394.

169. Pastore JM, Shah MH, Rosenbaum DS. Role of structural barriers in the mechanism of alternans-induced reentry. *Pace* 1999; 22:537.

170. Chinushi M, Restivo M, Caref EB, El-Sherif N. Electrophysiological basis of arrhythmogenicity of QT/T alternans in the long-QT syndrome: tridimensional analysis of the kinetics of cardiac repolarization. *Circ Res* 1998;83:614–628.

171. Platt SB, Vijgen JM, Albrecht P, et al. Occult T wave alternans in long QT syndrome. *J Cardiovasc Electrophysiol* 1996;7:144–148.

172. Gold MR, Kavesh NG, Bloomfield DM, et al. Correlation of T-wave alternans during exercise with the induction of ventricular tachycardia. *Pace* 1998;21.

172a. Gold MR, Bloomfield DM, Anderson KP, et al. A comparison of T-wave alternans, signal averaged electrocardiography and programmed ventricular stimulation for arrhythmia risk stratification. *J Am Coll Cardiol* 2000;36:2247–2253.

173. Adam DR, Smith JM, Akselrod S, et al. Fluctuations in T-wave morphology and susceptibility to ventricular fibrillation. *J Electrocardiol* 1984;17:209–218.

174. Rosenbaum DS, Jackson LE, Smith JM, et al. Electrical alternans and vulnerability to ventricular arrhythmias. *N Engl J Med* 1994;330:235–241.

175. Hohnloser SH, Klingenheben T, Zabel M, et al. T wave alternans during exercise and atrial pacing in humans. *J Cardiovasc Electrophysiol* 1997;8:987–993.

176. Coch M, Weber S, Buck L, Waldecker B. Assessment of T wave alternans using atropine. *Circulation* 1998;98:I442.

177. Ritvo BS, Magnano AR, Bloomfield DM. Comparison of exercise and pharmacologic methods of measuring T wave alternans. *Pace* 2000;23:688.

178. Caref EB, Stoyanovsky V, Cohen RJ, El-Sherif N. Incidence of T wave alternans in normal subjects and effects of heart rate on onset. *Circulation* 1987;96:I582.

179. Bloomfield DM, Gold MR, Anderson KP, et al. A comparison of T wave alternans and signal-averaged electrocardiography in predicting outcome of electrophysiology testing. *Pace* 1999;22:751.

180. Gold MR, Bloomfield DM, Anderson KP, et al. T wave alternans predicts arrhythmia vulnerability in patients undergoing electrophysiology study. *Circulation* 1998;98:I647.

181. Ikeda T, Sakata T, Takami M, et al. Combined assessment of T-wave alternans and late potentials used to predict arrhythmic events after myocardial infarction. A prospective study. *J Am Coll Cardiol* 2000;35:722–730.

182. Klingenheben T, Cohen RJ, Peetermans J, Hohnloser SH. Predictive value of T-wave alternans in patients with congestive heart failure. *Circulation* 1998;98:I864.

183. Klingenheben T, Credner SC, Bender B, et al. Exercise induced microvolt level T wave alternans identifies patients with non-ischemic dilated cardiomyopathy at high risk of ventricular tachyarrhythmic events. *Pace* 1999;22:860.

184. Adachi K, Ohnishi Y, Shima T, et al. Determinant of microvolt-level T-wave alternans in patients with dilated cardiomyopathy. *J Am Coll Cardiol* 1999;34:374–380.

185. Hohnloser SH, Klingenheben T, Li YG, et al. T wave alternans as a predictor of recurrent ventricular tachyarrhythmias in ICD recipients: prospective comparison with conventional risk markers. *J Cardiovasc Electrophysiol* 1998;9:1258–1268.

186. Steinberg JS, Regan A, Sciacca RR, et al. Predicting arrhythmic events after acute myocardial infarction using the signal-averaged electrocardiogram. *Am J Cardiol* 1992;69:13–21.

187. Bloomfield DM, Gold MR, Anderson KP, et al. T wave alternans predicts events independent of ejection fraction and etiology of heart disease in patients undergoing electrophysiologic testing for known or suspected ventricular arrhythmias. *Pace* 2000;23:593.

7

ELECTROPHYSIOLOGIC TESTING AND CARDIAC MAPPING

HARAN GARAN
BRIAN MCGOVERN

Invasive cardiac electrophysiology has evolved rapidly from a research tool to an established clinical technique for investigating and treating cardiac rhythm disorders (1,2). Detailed analysis of cardiac tachyarrhythmias or bradyarrhythmias with the use of an intracardiac electrophysiologic study may help the clinician make an accurate diagnosis of the underlying mechanism; evaluate prognosis in certain cases; acquire data regarding indications for specific forms of therapy, such as permanent pacemaker implantation; and evaluate the feasibility of nonpharmacologic drug therapy such as transcatheter radiofrequency (RF) ablation, antiarrhythmic surgery, or implantable cardioverter-defibrillator (ICD) therapy. Since the publication of the Electrophysiologic Study Versus Electrocardiographic Monitoring (ESVEM) and Cardiac Arrest in Seattle: Conventional versus Amiodarone Drug Evaluation (CASCADE) trials (3,4), programmed electrical stimulation (PES) has been used little for serial testing of the efficacy of antiarrhythmic drugs. PES is still used to assess the electrophysiologic effect of major nonpharmacologic interventions, such as surgical coronary revascularization and antiarrhythmic surgery. The emergence of transcatheter RF ablation as a highly effective and relatively safe technique for treatment of supraventricular (5–7) and ventricular (8–10) tachyarrhythmias has resulted in a resurgence of interest in arrhythmia mechanisms. In this context, invasive cardiac electrophysiologic studies with arrhythmia induction and intracardiac mapping play a pivotal role in the precise definition of the underlying mechanism, in the localization of the site of origin of the arrhythmia, and in providing appropriate targets for transcatheter ablation. Two multicenter, primary prevention cardiac arrhythmia trials, the first Multicenter Automatic Defibrillator Implantation Trial (MADIT I) and Multicenter Unsustained Tachycardia Trial (MUSTT) (11,12), which incorporated PES into their protocols, have resulted in new indications for cardiac electrophysiologic studies. Common indications for a cardiac electrophysiologic study and PES are listed in Table 7-1.

TABLE 7-1. INDICATIONS FOR CARDIAC ELECTROPHYSIOLOGY STUDIES

Diagnosis and Management of Bradyarrhythmias
  To acquire corroborative data in symptomatic patients with episodic bradyarrhythmia
  To define the level of AV conduction abnormality
Diagnosis and Management of Tachyarrhythmias
  To define the mechanism of narrow-complex tachycardia
  To define the mechanism of wide-complex tachycardia
  To reproduce the clinically documented narrow- or wide-complex tachycardia for mapping and transcatheter ablation
Syncope of Unknown Origin
  To assess the sinus node function and AV conduction and to search for inducible sustained ventricular tachyarrhythmias in patients with syncope and organic heart disease
Primary Prevention Protocols
  To search for PES-induced VT/VF in patients with coronary disease, depressed ventricular function, and nonsustained VT for ICD therapy
Miscellaneous Individualized Uses
  To select optimal ICD parameters for ICD therapy
  To assess the effect of cardiac surgery (e.g., coronary revascularization, endocardial resection)
  To assess the modifying (suppressing) effect of an antiarrhythmic drug (rare)

AF, atrial fibrillation; AV, atrioventricular; ICD, implantable cardioverter-defibrillator; PES, programmed electrical stimulation; VF, ventricular fibrillation; VT, ventricular tachycardia.

H. Garan: Department of Cardiology, University of Texas at Houston Medical School, Houston, Texas 77030.

B. McGovern: Massachusetts General Hospital, Boston, Massachusetts 02114.

METHODOLOGY OF CARDIAC ELECTROPHYSIOLOGY STUDIES

Basic Equipment and Personnel

Central components of a cardiac electrophysiologic study are a programmable, constant-current-source stimulator and a multichannel data acquisition system. The stimulator must be electrically isolated and have synchronous pacing capability with a cycle length range of 150 to 1,500 ms and a capability of incrementing or decrementing coupling intervals by 10 ms or less and of delivering a minimum of three programmable premature extrastimuli and burst pacing with an interstimulus accuracy of 1 ms. Based on experience with strength-interval curves, the stimulus strength is usually set at twice the diastolic threshold (i.e., threshold should ideally be less than 1mA) and the pulse width at 2 ms to limit induction of nonspecific rhythms occurring with higher currents during programmed stimulation (13) and to maintain uniformity among different laboratories. Typically, the surface electrocardiographic (ECG) leads I, aVF, and V_1 (approximating the mutually orthogonal Frank leads X, Y, Z) are recorded. Bipolar intracardiac signals are filtered below 30 to 40 Hz and above 400 to 500 Hz, and unipolar intracardiac recordings are typically left unfiltered because of the low-frequency nature of their signal content. The signals are then amplified, displayed in real time on an oscilloscope, and recorded continuously during the study with multichannel magnetic or optical disk recorders for later retrieval and analysis.

Ideally, biplane fluoroscopy is used to guide catheter placement. The frequently used, three-dimensional electroanatomic mapping technique has the potential to decrease the duration of fluoroscopy needed substantially. Induction of potentially lethal arrhythmias during the course of an electrophysiologic study typically occurs in 20% to 50% of patients (14), and the permanent presence and maintenance of cardiopulmonary resuscitation equipment, including a primary and a backup (second) external defibrillator, in the laboratory is mandatory.

Approach to the Patient

Preparation of the patient for the cardiac electrophysiologic study should begin with a clear explanation of the primary reason for the study and what to expect during the procedure. Informed consent specifically stating the possible risks and anticipated benefits must be obtained. Heart failure, myocardial ischemia, and electrolyte abnormalities need to be treated and under control before any invasive electrophysiologic study is undertaken. For baseline studies, a period of antiarrhythmic drug washout of at least five half-lives is required unless there is a specific reason to perform the procedure during drug therapy. The studies are performed in the postabsorptive, fasting state for aspiration prophylaxis in case of cardioversion or endotracheal intubation. Sedation is often achieved with benzodiazepines, which have relatively few and only mild to moderate electrophysiologic effects at the doses routinely employed (15). Intravenous midazolam is commonly used and usually provides adequate sedation and amnesia. Intravenous analgesia with opioids (e.g., fentanyl) is also commonly used.

In routine diagnostic studies, standard access is through the femoral veins using a percutaneous, modified Seldinger technique. An internal jugular or subclavian vein approach facilitates entry into the coronary sinus when it is required for diagnostic supraventricular tachycardia (SVT) studies. When access to the left heart is needed, such as for left ventricular mapping, it may be achieved retrogradely through the femoral artery or using the transseptal catheterization technique through the right femoral vein. Lidocaine for local anesthesia should be limited at a total dose of less than 2.5 mg/kg because larger subcutaneous doses may result in therapeutic serum levels that may interfere with the electrophysiologic findings (16). Systemic heparin is not routinely employed but is mandatory when left heart catheterization is required retrogradely or through the transseptal technique. It should also be used judiciously in individual cases even if the electrode catheters are confined to the venous circulation, especially for long procedures using a large number of catheters.

Baseline Cardiac Recordings and Analysis

A comprehensive diagnostic baseline study typically requires a minimum of four electrode catheters: in the right atrium close to the superior vena cava and right atrial junction; across the septal tricuspid leaflet to record a His bundle electrogram; at the right ventricular apex; and in the coronary sinus for left atrial recordings and stimulation. For most routine diagnostic electrophysiologic studies, quadripolar electrode catheters are sufficient. This configuration allows bipolar pacing with the distal pair and simultaneous bipolar recording with the proximal pair. Generally, bipolar pacing and recording are preferred. Bipolar waveforms often are complex and manifest multiple components and more than one rapid deflection. Under these circumstances, it is not possible to assign a local activation time to the electrogram with high precision. It is more difficult to time local events with unipolar recordings, but they provide directionality, which is not available with bipolar recordings. An activation wavefront moving toward the electrode results in a positive deflection, and one moving away produces a negative deflection. In a unipolar tracing, the rapid deflection that corresponds to the change of polarity and represents the pas-

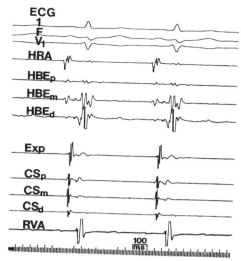

FIGURE 7-1. During a typical cardiac electrophysiologic study, local electrograms are recorded from the high right atrium (HRA), His bundle (HB), right ventricular apex (RVA), and coronary sinus (CS). When mapping is required, one or several more recording channels are dedicated to exploring (Exp) electrodes. p, proximal; m, middle; d, distal.

sage of the activation wavefront under the electrode, the intrinsicoid deflection, was historically taken to be the marker for local activation time (17). Laboratory studies have shown excellent correlation between bipolar and unipolar recordings and local activation times registered with intracellular recordings (18).

Figure 7-1 shows the baseline intracardiac recordings obtained during a typical diagnostic electrophysiologic study. These intracardiac tracings usually include the recording from the high right atrium, the His bundle electrogram, and the coronary sinus recordings, followed by the recording from the right ventricular apex. Depending on the particular study, other required recordings may include the right bundle electrogram, left ventricular recordings, transseptal left atrial recordings, pulmonary vein recordings, and atrial or ventricular exploring catheter tracings for mapping. Special multipolar catheters such as a halo catheter or a crista terminalis catheter are used for recording the activation sequence of the right atrium during atrial tachyarrhythmias. As more complex arrhythmias are mapped, other multipole special catheters, such as the basket catheters and noncontact mapping catheters, are deployed in different cardiac chambers.

The electrophysiologic analysis begins with the measurement of the basic intervals that reflect the integrity of the conduction system under rest conditions. The P-A interval is measured from the onset of the earliest regis-

tered surface P wave or intracardiac atrial activation to the onset of the septal atrial deflection recorded on the His bundle catheter. There is no general consensus about what constitutes a normal range, although values from 20 to 60 ms have been reported (19). Prolonged P-A interval times suggest abnormal atrial conduction and can be a clue to the presence of the cause of first-degree atrioventricular block (20).

The A-H interval is measured from the earliest rapid deflection of the septal atrial recording to the earliest onset of the His bundle deflection on the His bundle electrogram. This interval is taken to represent AV nodal conduction, although more correctly, it is the sum of conduction through the low right atrial inputs into the AV node, the AV node proper, and the proximal His bundle. The range of this interval in normal subjects is wide, 50 to 120 ms (19). Short A-H intervals may be seen with increased sympathetic tone, enhanced AV node conduction, preferential left atrial input into the AV node, and in unusual forms of preexcitation such as atrio-Hisian connections (21). Long A-H intervals are most commonly the result of negative dromotropic drugs such as β-receptor antagonists and calcium channel blockers, enhanced vagal tone, or intrinsic disease of the AV node. Care is needed to distinguish true A-H prolongation from artifactually prolonged A-H resulting from recording a right bundle branch potential instead of a proper His bundle potential. The His bundle electrogram duration reflects conduction through the short length of the compact His bundle, penetrating the membranous septum. Normally, it is of short duration (15 to 25 ms) and composed of high-frequency deflections (19,22). Fractionation, prolongation, or splitting of the His bundle potential is seen with disease of the His bundle (23,24) (Fig. 7-2).

The H-V interval, measured from the earliest onset of the His bundle deflection to the earliest registered surface or intracardiac ventricular activation recorded anywhere, reflects conduction time through the distal His-Purkinje tissue. Unlike the AV node, the His-Purkinje system is far less influenced by the autonomic nervous system, and the range in normal subjects is narrow, 33 to 55 ms (25). The most reliable method of validating the His potential is His bundle pacing through the His bundle recording bipole. A prolonged H-V interval is consistent with diseased distal conduction in all fascicles (26), although an artifactually prolonged H-V interval may be registered if the earliest ventricular activation is missed on the surface electrocardiogram and standard intracardiac recordings such as may occur in septal infarction.

After acquisition of baseline measurements, PES is carried out. The algorithms for programmed atrial and ventricular stimulation that are used for specific dysrhythmias and for different clinical presentations are reviewed subsequently (Table 7-2).

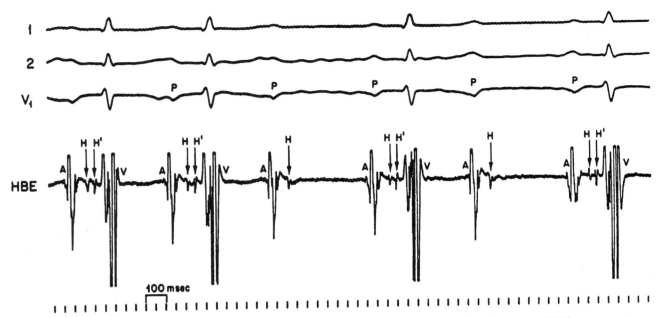

FIGURE 7-2. Advanced conduction disease in the His bundle. The His bundle electrogram (HBE) manifests two components (H and H') during conducted beats. The proximal component is present after a nonconducted P wave, but the distal His bundle is not activated. The level of atrioventricular block is sharply defined as intra-His during the cardiac electrophysiologic study.

TABLE 7-2. COMMONLY USED PROTOCOLS FOR PROGRAMMED CARDIAC STIMULATION FOR DIFFERENT SYNDROMES

	Site of Stimulation	Drive CL (ms)	Numbner of Programmed Extrastimuli	Use of Isoproterenol
Out-of-Hospital cardiac arrest	RVA RVOT	400,600	1,2,3	–
Recurrent sustained VT (ischemic disease)	RVA RVOT (LV)	400,600	1,2,3	–
Recurrent sustained VT (nonischemic disease)	RVA	400,600	1,2,3[a]	+
Idiopathic VT	RVA RVOT	400,600	1,2,3	++
No SHD Syncope[b]	RVA (RVOT ?)	400,600	1,2 (?3)	+
Nonsustained VT[b]	RVA (RVOT ?)	400,600	1,2 (?3)	±
Workup of VT for nonpharmacologic treatment[c]	RVA Multiple LV sites RVOT	400,600 and as needed	1,2,3	–

CL, cycle length; LV, left ventricle; RVA, right ventricular apex; RVOT, right ventricular outflow tract; SHD, structural heart disease; VT, ventricular tachycardia.

[a]Unusual coupling interval sequences (e.g., short-long-short) may be used to initiate suspected bundle branch reentry.

[b]The extent of the protocol in syncope and nonsustained VT may vary as concerns for sensitivity (reproducing sustained VT) or specificity (induction of a clinically irrelevant arrhythmia) predominate.

[c]Recordings, resetting, and entrainment from multiple RV and LV sites of stimulation are frequently needed.

SAFETY ISSUES: COMPLICATION OF INVASIVE CARDIAC ELECTROPHYSIOLOGIC STUDIES

Complications of invasive cardiac electrophysiologic studies are rare provided that high-risk patients such as those with critical aortic stenosis, severe hypertrophic obstructive cardiomyopathy, left main or severe three-vessel coronary artery disease, acute coronary syndromes, and uncompensated congestive heart failure are excluded. Appropriate patient selection is a crucial aspect of maintaining safety. Sustained tachyarrhythmias should not be induced in patients with left main coronary artery stenosis or critical left ventricular outflow tract obstruction. Assessment of the presence and the severity of structural heart disease and biventricular systolic function should be done in all patients before an invasive electrophysiologic study. This may be achieved by an echocardiogram alone in most cases. Coronary angiography may be required in certain cases to exclude critical coronary artery disease but is usually not needed in otherwise healthy patients with no ischemic symptoms or structural heart disease who are undergoing mapping and transcatheter ablation. The echocardiogram may also alert the operator to the presence of a patent foramen ovale, which requires special precautions to avoid paradoxical thromboembolism. When a right-to-left communication is suspected, intravenous injection of agitated saline should be performed. In special cases, a transesophageal echocardiogram may be used to exclude left atrial thrombus before transseptal catheterization and mapping of the left atrium.

Serious complications of diagnostic invasive electrophysiologic studies include vascular injury, deep vein thrombosis and subsequent pulmonary embolism, hemorrhage requiring transfusion therapy, cardiac chamber perforation resulting in pericardial tamponade, complete heart block, pneumothorax, sepsis, abscess at the catheterization site, myocardial infarction, stroke, and death (Table 7-3). In 359 patients undergoing 1,062 diagnostic procedures between 1977 and 1981 at the Massachusetts General Hospital, DiMarco and colleagues reported no deaths and a morbidity rate per procedure of 1.9% provided that the exclusion criteria mentioned previously were observed (27). All complications (e.g., thromboembolism, infections, pneumothorax, cardiac chamber perforation) were related to the catheterization process rather than to PES. In a series of approximately 6,500 procedures performed at the Hospital of the University of Pennsylvania, Josephson and coworkers reported one death and a less than 2% complication rate (28).

During the past decade, there has been a steady rise in the use of intracardiac mapping and transcatheter RF ablation for the treatment of supraventricular and ventricular arrhythmias. Compared with the mostly diagnostic

TABLE 7-3. COMPLICATIONS OF INVASIVE CARDIAC ELECTROPHYSIOLOGIC STUDIES

Associated with Percutaneous Catheterization of Veins and Arteries
Pain
Adverse drug reaction
Infection or abscess at the catheterization site
Sepsis
Bleeding or hematoma
Thrombophlebitis
Pulmonary thromboembolism
Arterial tean or aortic dissection
Systemic thromboembolism
Transient ischemic attack or stroke
Associated with Intracardiac Catheters and Programmed Cardiac Stimulation
Cardiac chamber or coronary sinus perforation
Hemopericardium or cardiac tamponade
Atrial fibrillation or ventricular fibrillation
Myocardial ischemia or myocardial infarction
Bundle branch block
Associated with Transcatheter Ablation
Complete heart block
Valvar injury or new-onset valvar insufficiency
Acute coronary artery thrombosis and chronic coronary stenosis
Proarrhythmia
Cardiac chamber, coronary sinus, or venae cavae perforation
Pericarditis
Myocardial necrosis, heart failure, or cardiogenic shock
Pulmonary vein stenosis
Phrenic nerve paralysis
Radiation skin burns

studies of the earlier series, ablation procedures are much longer, involve administration of higher doses of sedative and analgesic agents, and require more frequent catheterization of the left heart, longer periods of radiation exposure, and more frequent changes of catheters. The length of some of the RF ablation procedures may increase morbidity from vascular or thromboembolic complications. Catheter ablation procedures carry additional risks such as inadvertent complete heart block, valvar injury, aortic puncture during transseptal catheterization, left ventricular rupture, and systemic thromboembolism (29,30). Other complications unique to transcatheter RF ablation include phrenic nerve injury resulting in hemidiaphragmatic paralysis, RF-induced coronary thrombosis (31,32), and pulmonary vein stenosis (33) (Table 7-3). The overall incidence of life-threatening or disabling complications of RF ablation is low (1% to 2%) in most laboratories. A detailed list of multiple minor and major complications for catheter ablation of individual arrhythmias (4.4% total) has been published by the Multicenter European RF survey (34), and an overall 3.1% incidence of complications has been reported in a large series reporting 3,966 consecutive procedures (35).

ROLE OF INVASIVE CARDIAC ELECTROPHYSIOLOGY STUDIES IN THE DIAGNOSIS AND MANAGEMENT OF BRADYARRHYTHMIAS

Various measurements are made in the cardiac electrophysiology laboratory to evaluate sinus node function and the conduction system of the heart. Bradyarrhythmias may be broadly categorized into disorders of impulse initiation in the sinus node, such as sinus arrest or failure of a subsidiary focus to provide an adequate escape rhythm, and disorders of the cardiac conduction system, such as complete heart block. Both disorders may coexist in a patient. The problem is often episodic, and ambulatory ECG monitoring techniques have poor sensitivity. In these cases, findings from an electrophysiologic study may complement other clinical data by unmasking suspected but previously undocumented abnormal sinus impulse formation or AV conduction (Table 7-1).

Evaluation of Sinus Node Dysfunction

The methods of assessing sinus node function are indirect. Direct recordings of sinus node potentials have been reported and appear to correlate reasonably well with indirect measurements (36). However, this technique has not gained wide clinical application and presently is regarded as an investigational method. Sinus node recovery time (SNRT) as a measure of sinus node automaticity and the sinoatrial conduction time (SACT) as an estimate of conduction through sinoatrial tissue are the methods commonly employed in the electrophysiology laboratory (37,38).

The SNRT is estimated by pacing for at least 1 minute from a high right atrial site close to the sinus node and measuring the interval from the last paced atrial beat to the first spontaneous sinus beat; this is repeated with decreasing cycle lengths, noting the longest recovery. Pacing rates up to 200 bpm may be employed for improved sensitivity (39). The normal response is a postpacing pause not exceeding 1,400 ms, with gradual return to the baseline cycle length over the ensuing five to six beats. Because the absolute recovery time is a function of the spontaneous basic cycle length (BCL), adjusted parameters such as the corrected sinus recovery time ($SNRT_C = SNRT - BCL$) and normalized recovery time (SNRT/BCL), which are less than 550 ms and 150%, respectively, in normal subjects, are more reliable parameters (37,39). These corrections are less accurate at lower spontaneous rates (39).

As with corrected sinus node recovery times, the sinoatrial conduction is assessed indirectly in the electrophysiology laboratory by analyzing the response of the sinus node to atrial extrastimuli. Most commonly used is the Strauss technique (40), in which a single atrial extrastimulus (A_2) is initially introduced at a coupling interval just shorter than the basic cycle length and repeated every 8 to 10 sinus beats

(A_1-A_1) and the coupling interval decremented by 10 to 20 ms. The return intervals (A_2-A_3) are measured to identify the zone of reset to ensure penetration into the sinoatrial node. The return interval (A_2-A_3) in the reset zone is estimated to be the sum of sinoatrial conduction into the sinus node (SACT retrograde), the basic cycle length (A_1-A_1), and conduction of the reset impulse from the sinus node to the atrial tissue (SACT antegrade). With the assumption that antegrade and retrograde SACTs are equal (which is not strictly correct), one-way SACT is calculated as $[(A_2-A_3) - (A_1-A_1)]/2$. Normal SACT times range from 40 to 60 ms up to 70 to 150 ms, depending on the laboratory (40,41). The limitations of this technique result from the similar assumptions made as in measuring SNRT. This technique is rarely used for clinical decision making.

The techniques of assessing sinus node function in the electrophysiology laboratory are flawed with assumptions that limit the validity of the techniques used and hence their clinical utility. Although abnormal measurements correlate in general with the severity of clinical abnormality, this correlation may break down in individual cases, and neither the $SNRT_C$ nor the SACT measurement can be taken as a gold standard for assessment of sinus node function; rather, they must be interpreted in the setting of the clinical presentation and in the light of other findings, including documented spontaneous bradyarrhythmias, the rate response to exercise, and response to pharmacologic agents such as atropine and β-adrenergic blockers before clinical decisions are made.

Evaluation of Atrioventricular Block and Conduction Disturbances

An invasive electrophysiologic study has little to add to the diagnosis or management if spontaneous third-degree heart block, Mobitz type II second-degree heart block, or trifascicular block is documented electrocardiographically in the symptomatic patient. It may yield useful diagnostic information when symptomatic AV block is suspected, but because of its episodic nature, it cannot be documented by electrocardiography. In these circumstances, His bundle recording and programmed atrial stimulation may unmask severe latent conduction system disease and, more importantly, define the level of AV conduction disturbance.

The baseline His bundle electrogram recording provides information about the AV nodal (A-H), both proximal and distal Hisian, and His-Purkinje (H-V) conduction. Failure of an atrial depolarization to conduct to the ventricles associated with the absence of a His bundle depolarization after the local atrial electrogram on the corresponding intracardiac His bundle recording localizes the block to the AV node. Presence of a His bundle signal fragmented into separate proximal and distal components, the so-called split His potential (Fig. 7-2), or a single His potential with no ensuing ventricular depolarization localizes the conduction disturbance at the His bundle or distal to the His bundle, respectively. If there is complete AV dissociation and the surface QRS complex is narrow, the His bundle recording almost always demonstrates a His deflection before each ventricular depolarization. If QRS is wide, demonstration of a local His bundle electrogram preceding each ventricular complex, with a normal or borderline prolonged H-V interval, indicates an escape rhythm originating in the distal AV node or in the His bundle with aberrant conduction, which is more stable and reliable compared with a ventricular escape rhythm originating from a more distal His-Purkinje site. This distinction usually cannot be made electrocardiographically.

The combination of the electrocardiographic documentation of high-grade AV block and symptoms usually dictates the therapy, and invasive electrophysiologic studies have limited or no diagnostic roles. They may be helpful in situations such as 2 : 1 AV block, in which case, insight into the precise site of block may influence therapy. If the block is intra- or infra-Hisian, pacemaker therapy, even in the absence of symptoms or with mild symptoms, may be indicated. Intra-His block may be observed during an atrial premature stimulus in the setting of a split His potential recorded at baseline (i.e., proximal component present with no recorded distal component and no ventricular depolarization). This is a rare but extremely specific finding that warrants pacemaker therapy (42). Perhaps equally rarely, His bundle recordings can diagnose pseudo-AV block where spontaneous His depolarizations, not apparent on the surface ECG, may fail to conduct to the ventricle and prevent the proper conduction of the subsequent sinus impulse through the AV node because of retrograde concealment, masquerading as type II AV block (43).

Patients who show true evidence of trifascicular disease on the surface ECG do not need electrophysiologic evaluation of the His-Purkinje conduction system because they already have clear evidence of diffuse disease in the His-Purkinje system. His bundle recordings may be of use for patients with chronic bifascicular block in predicting the risk of developing complete heart block. Finding a prolonged H-V interval in such patients signifies conduction disease in all three fascicles. An H-V interval longer than 100 ms has been a useful predictor of clinical high-grade AV block over a mean follow-up period of 2 years (44). If there is first-degree AV block in addition to chronic bifascicular block, a His bundle recording determines whether the delay is in the AV node or in the His-Purkinje system. However, it is not clear that cardiovascular mortality can be substantially lowered by permanent pacing in this population even if the electrophysiologic study shows extensive distal disease, because mortality in this group of patients results mostly from other events, such as ventricular tachyarrhythmias, heart failure, and recurrent ischemic events, which are related to the presence and severity of underlying heart disease.

The AV conduction system can be stressed to reveal its functional reserve during an electrophysiologic study. Atrial pacing with gradually decreasing cycle lengths (not abrupt onset), which results in distal infra-His conduction block during 1-1 AV nodal conduction, has been shown to have prognostic importance for subsequent AV block in patients with bundle branch block, although this finding occurs with a low frequency (45). Administration of atropine to decrease the functional refractory period of the AV node allows more strenuous testing of the His-Purkinje system by allowing 1-1 conduction through the AV node at shorter cycle lengths. Another method used to stress the AV conduction system is rapid infusion of antiarrhythmic drugs such as procainamide, which increases conduction time in the His-Purkinje system. Infusion of up to 10 mg/kg of procainamide while in sinus rhythm may induce second- or third-degree distal AV block in patients with bifascicular block suspected of having intermittent advanced AV block (46,47).

Cardiac electrophysiologic testing is limited in its clinical utility in asymptomatic patients even when the techniques used during the electrophysiologic evaluation include atropine and procainamide administration. In contrast to the asymptomatic patients, those presenting with syncope or presyncopal episodes and whose electrocardiograms manifest bifascicular block but no other abnormality should have an electrophysiologic study (48). A markedly prolonged H-V interval at rest or demonstration of intra- or infra-His block during atrial pacing enhances the specificity of the electrocardiographic intraventricular conduction disturbance and becomes an indication for permanent pacemaker therapy.

CARDIAC ELECTROPHYSIOLOGY STUDIES IN THE DIAGNOSIS AND MANAGEMENT OF TACHYARRHYTHMIAS

The following sections describe the common techniques used in the cardiac electrophysiologic laboratory as part of a general approach for the diagnosis and mapping of cardiac tachyarrhythmia.

Narrow QRS Complex Tachycardia

Narrow QRS complex tachycardia is almost always supraventricular in origin and, when there is no structural heart disease, is only rarely life threatening. An invasive electrophysiologic study for a documented narrow-complex tachycardia is needed for its precise diagnosis, mapping, and treatment by transcatheter RF ablation. Even if the clinician's inclination is toward pharmacologic therapy, there is often a benefit to be gained from understanding the underlying mechanism with precision to optimize treatment. Multiple mechanisms may be present in the same patient, and the distinction between separate forms may not be possible electrocardiographically.

One study showed that the mechanism of a regular, narrow-complex tachycardia could be correctly predicted from the 12-lead electrocardiogram taken during the tachycardia in 85% of the patients (49). Although most narrow-complex tachycardias can be diagnosed correctly provided that a 12-lead ECG can be obtained during the SVT, the incidence of correct diagnosis becomes nearly 100% after an invasive cardiac electrophysiologic study. In reality, when transcatheter ablative treatment is being contemplated, invasive electrophysiologic studies are performed to confirm the underlying mechanism of the tachycardia with certainty, to exclude other mechanisms, and to define the targets for RF current application. In modern practice, the diagnostic electrophysiologic study and transcatheter ablation are typically performed during the same session.

Techniques for Investigating Supraventricular Tachycardia Mechanisms

The atrial and ventricular activation sequence during SVT, pacing maneuvers such as resetting with critically timed extrastimuli, entrainment mapping, and observation of the responses to pharmacologic agents during pacing or spontaneous tachycardia allow the diagnosis of the SVT mechanism in most cases. An intracardiac electrophysiologic study is especially indicated in patients when SVT is associated with severe symptoms such as syncope or pulmonary edema. An invasive electrophysiologic study in such a markedly symptomatic patient is mandatory when the resting ECG manifests the pattern of preexcitation. Similarly, in patients with underlying organic heart disease who develop angina or heart failure during their arrhythmia or when SVT is incessant, resulting in tachycardia-related cardiomyopathy, there is an urgency to define the precise

mechanism and implement definitive and curative treatment rather than palliative management.

Diagnosis and treatment (i.e., transcatheter ablation) of SVT have become the most common indications for cardiac electrophysiologic study. Electrode catheters placed at the high right atrium, close to the sinus node, at the His bundle position, at the right ventricular apex, and within the coronary sinus usually suffice to make the diagnosis of SVT with certainty in most cases. In more complex SVT mechanisms and in patients undergoing mapping and transcatheter ablation, additional special mapping catheters such as the multipolar halo catheter or additional exploring catheters recording special signals such as accessory pathway potentials, right or left bundle potential, left ventricular endocardial or epicardial (recorded from coronary sinus branches) electrograms, potentials recorded from the crista terminalis, and pulmonary vein electrograms may be desirable (Fig. 7-3).

Programmed atrial stimulation is usually performed from the high right atrium, and a second atrial site, such as the coronary sinus, is also commonly employed. One and two atrial extrastimuli with progressively shorter coupling intervals are delivered after a train of eight or more drive beats at several cycle lengths until atrial refractoriness is encountered. Incremental atrial pacing in steps of 10 ms is also performed until second-degree AV block develops. Atrial extrastimulus technique and incremental atrial pacing may uncover ventricular preexcitation with wide QRS complex and shortened H-V interval. Ventricular preexcitation in the presence of an unchanging AV interval suggests an AV connection, whereas preexcitation (i.e., shortening H-V interval) occurring in association with progressive AV delay suggests a decrementally conducting atriofascicular connection (50). Localization of the site of critical delay required for the initiation of SVT may help identify the mechanism and the site

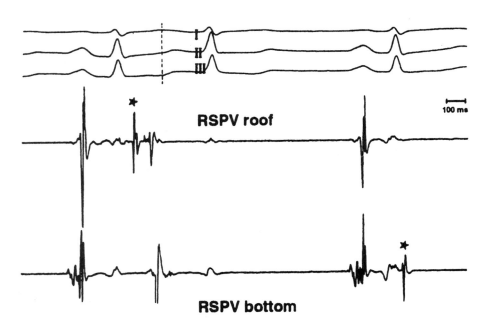

RSPV roof

RSPV bottom

100 ms

FIGURE 7-3. Pulmonary vein (PV) potentials (i.e., high-frequency spikes) are recorded from an electrode catheter positioned with the right superior pulmonary vein (RSVP). During the atrial premature beats that originate within the RSVP, PV potential (star) precedes the atrial electrogram. The second ectopic beat does not conduct to the atrium (concealed). (From Haissaguerre M, Jais P, Shah DC, et al. *Circulation* 2000;101:1410, with permission.)

of the tachycardia. Critical intraatrial delay suggests intraatrial reentry. Critical prolongation of the A-H interval, especially a sudden increment in A-H duration of more than 50 ms in response to 10- to 20-ms shortening of the coupling interval (the so-called jump followed by an atrial echo beat) indicates the presence of dual-pathway AV nodal physiology and suggests AV nodal reentry as the mechanism. AV reciprocating tachycardia also requires critical delay, but this may be intraatrial, in the AV node, in the His-Purkinje system, intraventricular, or in all of them.

When tachycardia is induced by atrial stimulation (Fig. 7-4), several important observations and maneuvers could be used to diagnose the mechanism with certainty. AV reentrant tachycardia (AVRT) requires an obligatory 1:1 atrial-ventricular ratio and cannot sustain in the presence of AV or ventriculoatrial (VA) dissociation. AV nodal reentry also manifests 1:1 AV ratio in most cases, although atria or ventricles at the infra-His level rarely may be dissociated from the tachycardia circuit (51). Frequently, simultaneous or nearly simultaneous atrial and ventricular activation are seen with typical slow-fast AV nodal reentrant tachycardia (AVNRT). In AVRT and in certain forms of AVNRT (slow/slow), the retrograde P wave follows the QRS and is usually within the first half of the R-R interval. In atypical AVNRT (fast/slow) and rarely in AVRT with a decrementally conducting retrograde pathway, the H-A interval may be substantially longer than the A-H interval in the His bundle recording. With this finding, the differential diagnosis also includes atrial tachycardia (AT).

Recording of the atrial activation sequence during the tachycardia is critical in making the diagnosis. In slow node reentrant tachycardia, a high-to-low and right-to-left atrial activation pattern is seen, and the interatrial septum depolarizes in an anterocranial to posterocaudal direction as during a sinus beat. In typical AVNRT, the atrial activation sequence is concentric, and the interatrial septal activation is caudal to cranial with the site of earliest atrial activation at the anterior septum adjacent to the site of His bundle recording. In fast/slow AVNRT, the atrial activation is also low to high, but with the site of earliest atrial activation usually observed close to or within the coronary sinus os or at posterocaudal interatrial septum. In orthodromic AVRT, the retrograde atrial activation is eccentric, reflecting the site of atrial insertion for right or left free wall AV connections, but concentric for septal accessory pathways. In antidromic AVRT, the retrograde atrial activation is low to high and concentric, exactly like typical AVNRT because VA conduction is usually, but not always (e.g., a second accessory pathway), through the His-Purkinje and AV nodal tissue. The electrophysiologic study also reveals the presence of a second accessory pathway if the proper observations are carried out. These include changing preexcitation morphology in manifest cases or a changing site of the earliest atrial activation during VA conduction. The appearance of bundle branch block or fascicular block during SVT

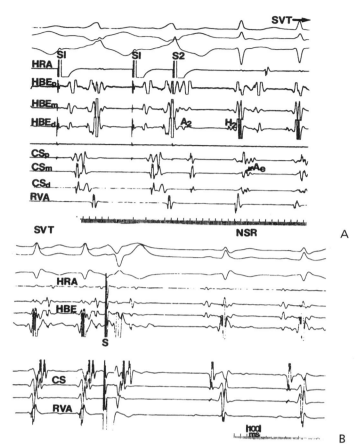

FIGURE 7-4. A: This tracing shows the initiation of orthodromic atrioventricular (AV) reciprocating tachycardia by a programmed atrial premature stimulus (S₂) in a patient with Wolff-Parkinson-White syndrome. The premature stimulus blocks anterogradely in the accessory pathway and conducts through the AV node slow pathway, generating the necessary delay for the recovery of the accessory pathway excitability. The mechanism of the tachycardia (i.e., AV reciprocating, incorporating a left-sided accessory pathway) is immediately suggested from the atrial activation sequence (i.e., earliest in the mid-coronary sinus [CSₘ]) during the first echo (Aₑ) beat. **B:** Termination of the supraventricular tachycardia (SVT) by a programmed ventricular extrastimulus. The mechanism is AV reciprocating tachycardia incorporating a left posterolateral accessory pathway. The ventricular extrastimulus conducts to the left atrium but encounters the refractory period of the AV node. There is no AV conduction, and SVT is interrupted by a block in the anterograde limb.

with an associated increase in the tachycardia cycle length and in the VA interval is diagnostic of an ipsilateral, retrogradely conducting accessory pathway (52).

Introduction of synchronized atrial or ventricular extrastimuli may further confirm the mechanism and the site of the arrhythmia. When properly timed, such extrastimuli encounter the reentrant circuit within the excitable gap and advance (reset) the tachycardia. For example, during narrow-complex tachycardia, if a ventricular extrastimulus, delivered at a time when His bundle is refractory, advances the following atrial electrogram, the presence of an extranodal AV connection is confirmed. If in addition the extrastimulus resets the SVT cycle and does not alter the atrial electrogram morphology and activation sequence seen during SVT, it is confirmed that the extranodal connection is part of the circuit (Fig. 7-5). Similarly, during a wide-complex tachycardia, advancing the ventricular activation by an atrial extrastimulus synchronized with the septal atrial electrogram, which is not captured by the extrastimulus, favors antidromic AVRT.

When the atrial activation sequence during SVT is eccentric (e.g., a left atrial site earlier than the septal atrium), the differential diagnosis includes AVRT and AT. Reproducible termination of the tachycardia by a ventricular extrastimulus that does not capture the atrium strongly favors AVRT. Advancing the timing of atrial depolarization by a ventricular extrastimulus delivered during the refractory period of His bundle shows the presence of an extranodal connection but does not exclude AT. Beat-by-beat changes in cycle length of a magnitude ≥40 ms without the appearance of bundle branch block favors AT, especially when the A-A' interval predicts the corresponding H-H' interval, rather than the H-H' predicting the A-A' interval. Failure to advance the atrial depolarization by a slightly premature ventricular extrastimulus delivered to the base of the left or the right ventricle, immediately adjacent to the site of the earliest atrial electrogram, strongly argues against an accessory pathway and suggests AT.

If the atrial activation sequence is concentric during SVT and during ventricular pacing, the differential diagnosis includes septal AT, AVNRT, and AVRT incorporating a septal accessory pathway. A ventricular extrastimulus (or

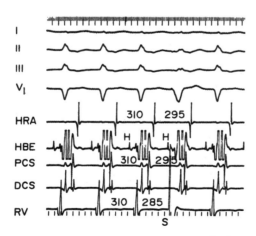

FIGURE 7-5. A critically timed right ventricular (RV) extrastimulus, delivered at a time when the His bundle is refractory, advances the atrial electrogram using a left posterior (extranodal) atrioventricular (AV) connection and resets the tachycardia, demonstrating participation of the AV connection in the mechanism of the tachycardia. During the premature beat, the atrial activation sequence does not change. DCS, distal coronary sinus; HBE, His bundle electrogram; HRA, high right atrium; PCS, proximal coronary sinus; RV, right ventricle. (From Tchou P, Lehmann MH, Jazayeri M, Akhtar M. Atriofascicular connection or a nodoventricular Mahaim fiber? Electrophysiologic elucidation of the pathway and associated reentrant circuit. *Circulation.* 1988;77(4):837–48, with permission.)

extrastimuli) that advances the His electrogram convincingly without changing the timing of atrial depolarization argues against slow/fast AVNRT and in favor of septal AT. As in the case of eccentric atrial activation, critically timed ventricular extrastimuli, delivered close to the basal-septal right ventricle, play a critical role in making the correct diagnosis. Comparing the atrial activation sequence, the VA and His-to-atrium intervals during His and ventricular (simultaneous) pacing from the His bundle catheter versus basoseptal ventricular pacing but without capturing the His bundle can help differentiate between a concealed anteroseptal accessory pathway and an AV nodal fast pathway (53).

Assessment of VA conduction at baseline by ventricular extrastimulus technique and incremental pacing reveals useful information. Absence of VA conduction excludes AVRT but not AVNRT, because VA conduction in the fast pathway often recovers with atropine or isoproterenol, and the absence of baseline conduction may reflect high resting vagal tone or withdrawn sympathetic tone with prolonged refractoriness. Retrograde atrial activation during ventricular pacing may suggest the presence of an accessory pathway if eccentric activation is identified (e.g., left atrial activation before septal-atrial activation). The observation of concentric and decremental VA conduction with shortening of coupling intervals argues against the presence of a concealed accessory pathway except in rare cases of decremental posteroseptal connections. However, sudden onset of 2:1 VA block without prior decrement does not exclude an accessory pathway.

Administration of pharmacologic agents is frequently helpful. Selectively blocking conduction in the AV node with adenosine may unmask latent accessory pathway conduction. Adenosine is particularly useful in the diagnosis of AT if it blocks AV nodal conduction without terminating the AT mechanism. Atropine or isoproterenol may be used to facilitate the induction of AVNRT, AVRT, or AT, which then may be mapped to define the precise mechanism.

Differential Diagnosis of Wide-Complex Tachycardia

The differential diagnosis of wide-complex tachycardia with a constant cycle length includes any SVT mechanism with aberrant conduction; SVT with "innocent bystander" accessory pathway that results in preexcitation during AVNRT, AT, or atrial flutter (AFL) without participating in the actual mechanism; antidromic AVRT (including atriofascicular pathways); ventricular tachycardia (VT); and bundle branch reentry. In a prospective study, Wellens and colleagues evaluated 62 consecutive patients with regular wide QRS complex tachycardia with 12-lead ECG and subsequently with invasive electrophysiologic studies (54). In their study, five SVTs were misdiagnosed as VT, demonstrating that, even in a specialized center serving as a tertiary referral institution, the ECG alone may be misleading. Because of the prognostic implications of sustained VT or an anterogradely conducting accessory pathway with a markedly short functional refractory period, the mechanism underlying the wide-complex tachycardia must be clearly identified. The underlying heart disease and a 12-lead ECG may sometimes be enough to make the diagnosis of VT. However, as reported by Akhtar and coworkers, the most reliable electrocardiographic marker, VA dissociation, was present and discernible on the surface ECG in only one half of the cases in a group of nonselected patients with wide-complex tachycardia presenting to the emergency room, and the sensitivity and the specificity of the other morphologic electrocardiographic markers favoring VT over aberration were not high enough for a certain diagnosis (55). A diagnostic electrophysiologic study may be important and becomes imperative if in addition the (undiagnosed) wide-complex tachycardia is associated with severe symptoms such as syncope or hemodynamic collapse (Table 7-1).

The clinical utility of the electrophysiologic study is limited by the inducibility of the clinical wide-complex arrhythmia by PES. The reproducibility is high if the mechanism is reentry in the scarred myocardium, bundle branch reentry, idiopathic left VT, or arrhythmogenic right ventricular dysplasia (ARVD) or if the arrhythmia is supraventricular with aberration or preexcitation. In advanced organic nonischemic heart disease, the sensitivity of PES, as defined by induction of any sustained VT or ventricular fibrillation (VF) as an end point, may be high, but its capability to reproduce the clinically documented wide-complex tachycardia is lower than in ischemic heart disease (56). It is important to record a 12-lead ECG during each episode of electrically induced sustained arrhythmia and to compare these ECGs to the tracing recorded during the clinical tachycardia. The reproducible induction by PES of idiopathic right ventricular or left ventricular outflow tract tachycardia is lower than the rate of induction of idiopathic interfascicular or septal left VT (57).

If the clinical arrhythmia cannot be reproduced by the PES protocol, administration of atropine or isoproterenol, provided that precipitation of clinical myocardial ischemia is not a concern, may facilitate tachycardia induction. To the extent that it is safe, it may be necessary to continue the antiarrhythmic drugs that the patient is taking at the time of the spontaneous wide-complex tachycardia, because these drugs may have promoted the arrhythmia or its modification (e.g., aberrant conduction), and PES may be able to reproduce the clinical wide-complex tachycardia only under these circumstances.

In the absence of any tachycardia induction, the electrophysiologic study may provide useful indirect information such as unmasking preexcitation or aberrant conduction, similar to the surface QRS morphology of the clinical arrhythmia, during atrial pacing at clinically observed cycle lengths (favoring an SVT mechanism) or demonstrating the absence of one-to-one AV and VA conduction at cycle lengths observed during the clinical episode (favoring VT). It is important to underscore that, especially in view of the

role played by uncontrollable factors such as the autonomic nervous system, this type of inferential information is no substitute for reproducing the clinically documented tachycardia, and caution must be exercised before any clinical decisions are based on such indirect evidence.

THE ROLE OF CARDIAC ELECTROPHYSIOLOGIC STUDIES IN THE MANAGEMENT OF VENTRICULAR TACHYARRHYTHMIAS

Application and Protocols

In the early days of clinical cardiac electrophysiology, PES was widely used to guide antiarrhythmic drug therapy in patients presenting with cardiac arrest or sustained VT (58). Later, clinical trials such as CASCADE (4) and ESVEM (3) raised doubts about the reliability of PES in selecting effective antiarrhythmic drugs for patients with organic heart disease and documented sustained ventricular tachyarrhythmias. Although the PES protocol used to assess drug efficacy in ESVEM differed from that commonly employed in most clinical electrophysiology laboratories (3), the results of this trial nevertheless increased awareness of the limitations of serial electrophysiologic testing for evaluating drug efficacy.

The role of cardiac electrophysiologic testing in patients presenting with cardiac arrest or hemodynamically unstable VT further diminished after the publication of the multicenter secondary prevention arrhythmia trials—Antiarrhythmics Versus Implantable Defibrillators (AVID), Cardiac Arrest Study Hamburg (CASH), and Canadian Implantable Defibrillator Study (CIDS)—which showed the superiority of ICD over empirically chosen or PES-guided antiarrhythmic drug therapy, at least for patients with poor ventricular systolic function (left ventricular ejection fraction [LVEF] <0.35) (59–61). These patients do not need PES for diagnosis or for guiding therapy. Cardiac electrophysiologic testing in patients with documented VT is mostly reserved for candidates for nonpharmacologic treatment such as transcatheter RF ablation. These are patients with idiopathic VT or bundle branch reentry and patients with advanced organic heart disease, already protected with an ICD, in whom transcatheter RF ablation is used as a palliative intervention to decrease the frequency of VT and ICD therapies (62).

Several protocols exist for programmed ventricular stimulation. They differ in the basic drive cycle, number of premature ventricular extrastimuli, and sites of stimulation (63–69). Examples of adequate protocols (90% sensitivity) for VT induction, as outlined by the North American Society of Pacing and Electrophysiology (NASPE), are those that use a basic drive train of at least eight captured beats immediately followed by single, double, and if necessary, triple ventricular extrastimuli that scan the electrical diastole (66) (Fig. 7-5). At least two drive trains that differ by at least 20 bpm are recommended for stimulation at the right ventricular apex, followed by stimulation at the right ventricular outflow tract. Maintaining the coupling intervals at 180 ms or longer during ventricular stimulation is a commonly accepted precaution to minimize the probability of inducing polymorphic VT or VF, which are undesirable outcomes during attempts to induce and map monomorphic VT. Depending on the clinical circumstances, left ventricular stimulation is an option and is more commonly used if the intention is to reproduce a clinical left VT for mapping and catheter ablation.

Isoproterenol infusion during ventricular stimulation has been reported to increase the yield of VT induction and thereby the sensitivity of the technique (70). Isoproterenol is more commonly used for induction of "idiopathic" VT and may be necessary for successfully inducing VT based on triggered activity as its mechanism. Isoproterenol may be contraindicated if the patient has advanced coronary artery disease. Other intravenous agents used to facilitate tachycardia induction in the electrophysiology laboratory include epinephrine, phenylephrine, atropine, and methylxanthines. In triggered idiopathic VT of right ventricular outflow tract and rarely in reentrant VT, atrial pacing has also been effective in VT induction (71).

Generally, the short- and long-term reproducibility of the response to PES is high if two or three ventricular extrastimuli are used and the patient has structural heart disease caused by coronary artery disease. One study reported a 91% success rate in immediate reproduction of a second induced, sustained VT episode after the first induction and a 100% success rate of initiating a third episode after two previous inductions in patients with sustained monomorphic VT (72). The reproducibility rate of the induction technique itself was 81% after one induction and 88% after two inductions. These figures apply to induction of any sustained monomorphic VT and not necessarily the same electrocardiographic VT morphology. Especially in the setting of advanced organic heart disease, it is common to induce several sustained monomorphic VTs with distinct surface ECG morphologies in the same patient (i.e., pleomorphism). Although pleomorphism of recurrent spontaneous VT is also a clinically observed phenomenon (73), the relationship between multiple clinical and multiple induced ECG morphologies still needs further clarification.

PES protocols for VT must not be rigid and should be selected and modified depending primarily on the clinical presentation (e.g., documented monomorphic VT versus syncope of unknown origin), underlying heart disease (e.g., ischemic heart disease versus no structural heart disease), and the indication for the study (e.g., testing the efficacy of a prior intervention versus VT induction for intracardiac mapping).

Ventricular Tachycardia in Ischemic Heart Disease

The multicenter clinical trial ESVEM showed that PES-guided drug therapy was not superior to pharmacologic therapy guided by electrocardiographic monitoring. However, PES-guided therapy can still be used in patients without frequent ectopy in whom ECG monitoring is not practical (3). Another way to interpret the findings from this study is to conclude that both are poor techniques for guiding therapy, because recurrence rates were unacceptably high in both arms (3). Because ESVEM was not a controlled study, it is difficult to know whether the high VT recurrence, strictly defined, was caused by the proarrhythmic effect of the drugs used. It is of interest that, unlike VT recurrence, the incidence of sudden death and cardiac arrest was low in both arms of the trial (3), a potentially hypothesis-generating observation.

In patients with ischemic heart disease, the presence of inducible VT that continues to be inducible in the presence of antiarrhythmic drugs is thought to be a poor prognostic sign. Data from the MUSTT registry shed light on this issue. Cardiac mortality at 2 and 5 years was lower in patients with no inducible VT/VF (i.e., registry patients) than that observed in patients in inducible VT/VF randomized to no antiarrhythmic therapy. All of these patients had ischemic heart disease (LVEF ≤0.40) and nonsustained VT (12). However, in absolute terms, cardiac mortality was still high (24% at 5 years) in patients meeting the clinical criteria for inclusion who were not randomized because they had no inducible VT. In a group with even more advanced ischemic heart disease, the mortality rate may be higher still, further diminishing the discriminating role of VT/VF induction by PES.

PES is often used to guide antiarrhythmic protection in patients with coronary artery disease in several other settings, but its role in this area needs clarification. One such setting is the case of the patient who presents with a ventricular tachyarrhythmia (sustained VT/VF) not associated with an acute myocardial infarction is discovered to have extensive coronary artery disease, undergoes coronary revascularization, and retains relatively well preserved, but not necessarily completely normal left ventricular function (LVEF of 0.40 to 0.50). Surgical coronary revascularization alone may render previously inducible VF no longer inducible after surgery, especially if overall left ventricular function is relatively well preserved (74). The response to PES is frequently used to decide whether ICD therapy should also be used in addition to coronary revascularization in these patients. However, reliable data on this issue do not exist. In contrast, induced monomorphic VT in a heart with depressed function is rarely, if ever, suppressed by coronary revascularization alone (74). Map-guided endocardial resection may be curative in eliminating recurrent VT by itself in some patients. Persistently inducible VT during postsurgical PES is commonly used to justify implantation of an ICD, because this finding appears to predict clinical recurrence (75).

Cardiac electrophysiologic studies with PES may also provide practical information regarding the choice of a particular device in patients undergoing ICD therapy. All of the available devices have tiered-therapy capabilities, and the efficacy of specific responses such as low-energy cardioversion or various antitachycardia pacing algorithms may be investigated during cardiac electrophysiologic studies. Similarly, the finding of coincident conduction disease may prompt implantation of a dual-chamber ICD. However, the most clear-cut indication for cardiac electrophysiologic studies in patients with ischemic VT is for testing the feasibility of transcatheter RF ablation as a palliative intervention. These patients are usually found among those previously treated with ICD or amiodarone and experience highly frequent or incessant VT (76). The mapping techniques used in these patients are described subsequently.

Ventricular Tachyarrhythmias in Nonischemic Cardiac Disease

Patients with hypertrophic cardiomyopathy are at risk for sudden cardiac death (77–79). However, estimation of the precise rate of sudden cardiac death is limited by referral bias and ever-changing clinical practices. A 2% to 4% incidence of sudden cardiac death for adults and a 4% to 6% incidence for children and adolescents have been reported (77–79) and are a sensitive function of the particular genetic mutations (80). VT is thought to be the major cause of sudden cardiac death and has been documented on rare occasions by ambulatory ECG recording (78,79). However the positive predictive value of clinical findings such as non-sustained VT or even syncope remains low.

The role of PES in the management of hypertrophic cardiomyopathy has been investigated in terms of its utility in diagnosis, prognosis, and therapy (81–83), but to this day, it remains controversial. One such study found a 43% induction rate of sustained ventricular tachyarrhythmia using a stimulation protocol with up to three right or left ventricular extrastimuli in 155 consecutive hypertrophic cardiomyopathy patients, already known to be at high risk for sudden cardiac death (83). A history of prehospital cardiac arrest or syncope was associated with an increased likelihood of ventricular tachyarrhythmia induction by PES. A potpourri of electrophysiologic abnormalities such as prolonged sinus node recovery times, prolonged sinoatrial conduction times, increased H-V interval, infra-Hisian block during rapid atrial pacing, accessory pathways, and inducible AF or AFL have been identified (83).

Despite the good correlation between VT induction and the presenting symptoms of syncope or prehospital cardiac arrest, the positive predictive accuracy of the response to PES is low, and more importantly, there is no conclusive evidence supported by controlled data that suppression by antiarrhythmic drugs of inducible VT or VF in this group improves prognosis (84). The available data do not support the routine use of PES in patients with hypertrophic cardiomyopathy, and invasive cardiac electrophysiologic studies should be reserved

for patients with specifically treatable arrhythmias such as AFL or SVT that depend on an accessory pathway.

Dilated Cardiomyopathy

Electrophysiologic testing plays a relatively limited role in the management of ventricular arrhythmias associated with idiopathic dilated cardiomyopathy (IDCM). It is of particular importance in establishing the diagnosis of VT based on bundle branch reentry, which can be permanently abolished by catheter ablation of the right bundle branch (85). The incidence of bundle branch reentry has been proposed to be as high as one third of all monomorphic VT in the IDCM population. A stimulation protocol, which includes an abrupt cycle length prolongation in the basic drive cycle just before the introduction of ventricular extrastimuli, may be used in patients suspected of having sustained bundle branch reentry. This technique exploits the immediate changes in His-Purkinje system refractoriness in response to changes in diastolic interval and has been reported to enhance the induction of sustained bundle branch reentry (86,87).

Cardiac electrophysiologic studies, however, have not been very useful in the management of the more commonly encountered ventricular tachyarrhythmias that are thought to result from myocardial reentry in patients with IDCM. Electrophysiologic evaluation of IDCM patients has shown that the clinical presentation is a major determinant of the response to PES; those who present with sustained monomorphic VT have the highest likelihood of developing sustained monomorphic VT in response to PES. The absence of induced sustained monomorphic VT has not been a reliable negative predictor for subsequent arrhythmic events (88,89). Analysis of pooled data shows that a satisfactory event-free course is not the observed outcome during follow-up among those few whose ventricular arrhythmias were suppressed with an antiarrhythmic agent at the time of electrophysiologic testing (90–92). An important limitation of PES-guided therapy in patients with IDCM is the low reproducibility of the response to PES. In studies performed in our laboratory, this reproducibility of response to PES, at baseline or after drug therapy, is lower compared with the reproducibility observed in patients with ischemic heart disease.

Arrhythmogenic Right Ventricular Dysplasia

The response to PES in patients with ARVD is similar to that observed in patients with ischemic heart disease: if there is a history of spontaneous VT, the rate of induction of sustained monomorphic VT is high, except the site of origin in ARVD is most commonly right ventricular (93). The invasive studies are usually reserved for patients who are candidates for intracardiac mapping and transcatheter ablation. Electrophysiologic testing does not play any role in evaluation of patients with congenital long QT syndromes. This is not true for all genetically determined "channelopathies," and PES, at baseline or after infusion of a sodium channel blocking drug, may have a role in the workup of patients with the Brugada syndrome (94).

Idiopathic Ventricular Tachycardia

Idiopathic left VT commonly presents with right bundle branch block mimicry and left axis deviation on the surface 12-lead ECG and can be terminated with verapamil but not adenosine or vagal maneuvers (95,96). Atrial or ventricular pacing or ventricular extrastimuli commonly induce the tachycardia (97). Endocardial mapping during VT has localized the site of origin to the inferoapical portion of the left ventricle in patients with right bundle branch block mimicry associated with left axis deviation and to the apical anteroseptal site in a few patients with right bundle branch block mimicry associated with right axis deviation. The tachycardias have been shown to be entrainable, and high-frequency local electrogram components have been recorded close to the site of origin, suggesting involvement of the His-Purkinje system (98). The role of invasive cardiac electrophysiologic studies in this form of VT is mostly for non-pharmacologic treatment with catheter ablation (99).

Catecholamine-mediated VT is usually seen in young patients and is frequently precipitated by exercise (100). The mechanism is thought to be triggered activity. This VT typically manifests with left bundle branch block mimicry and an inferiorly directed frontal axis on the surface ECG, reflecting its usual site of origin in the right or left ventricular outflow tract. As with other forms of idiopathic VT, the role of cardiac electrophysiologic studies is related less to the need for accurate diagnosis and more to the feasibility of potentially curable ablative therapy (101–103). This VT can be reproduced in the electrophysiology laboratory, but the rate of induction, particularly without catecholamines, is low. Isoproterenol infusion alone may initiate VT or transform nonsustained to sustained episodes, although programmed stimulation can also succeed in tachycardia induction by rapid atrial stimulation, rapid ventricular stimulation, or ventricular extrastimuli (101,102). The site of origin is determined by activation sequence mapping or by pace mapping and may be at the right ventricular or left ventricular outflow tract, is usually endocardial, and rarely is epicardial (104).

THE ROLE OF CARDIAC ELECTROPHYSIOLOGY STUDY IN SYNCOPE OF UNKNOWN ORIGIN

The cardiac causes of syncope may be structural (e.g., calcific aortic stenosis, dynamic outflow tract gradient in hypertrophic cardiomyopathy, left atrial myxoma, pulmonary hypertension), but are more commonly arrhythmic and related to a tachycardia or a bradycardia (105). If the correlation between an arrhythmia and syncope has been documented, an invasive cardiac electrophysiologic study is not needed for further diagnosis except in rare cases of documented syncopal wide-complex tachycardia for which the underlying mechanism is uncertain. When the cause of syncope is unknown, cardiac electrophysiologic testing may be indicated in certain settings (105–107). It is usually considered after the history, physical examination, blood tests, and the appropriate noninvasive studies, such as 24-hour ambulatory monitoring, carotid sinus massage, echocardiography, event recorders, loop recorders, and tilt-table studies, have not revealed a specific cause.

Cardiac electrophysiologic studies are performed to collect inferential data, searching for markedly abnormal electrophysiologic findings commonly associated with high specificity and for inducible arrhythmias that reproduce presyncope or syncope in patients with structural, especially ischemic, heart disease with evidence of prior myocardial infarction. The findings usually accepted as specific enough to single out bradycardia or conduction disturbance as a cause for syncope are a SNRT of more than 3 seconds, markedly long secondary pauses during sinus node recovery, a baseline H-V interval of $\geq$100 ms, and intra-His or infra-His conduction block (except during abrupt shortening in basic cycle length, which may be a normal finding). However, normal results may be found in patients previously documented to have syncope resulting from sinus arrest or high-grade AV conduction disturbances, and the sensitivity of the test is not high; the specificity of these findings, except perhaps for intra-His block, is also low. The predictive value of marked H-V prolongation (>100 ms) in response to rapid intravenous infusion of procainamide is controversial (47). VT may be the cause of syncope in patients with surface ECG evidence of conduction system disease, and consequently, programmed ventricular stimulation should be part of the cardiac electrophysiologic evaluation of these patients, especially when there is advanced organic heart disease (108,109).

Unless there is a convincing history of palpitations preceding syncope or a suspicion of SVT or idiopathic VT as the underlying cause, as in a patient with previously documented tachycardia, there is almost no yield for PES in patients with structurally normal hearts presenting with syncope. In contrast, VT is usually the most common arrhythmia induced during PES in the patients with syncope and organic heart disease. In a compilation of 11 studies reporting the results of electrophysiologic testing in a total of 844 patients with history of syncope of unknown cause, Kapoor found a 45% incidence of VT induction, a 22% incidence of SVT induction, a 28% incidence of conduction disturbances, and 5% incidence of other causes (107). The diagnostic yield of invasive cardiac electrophysiologic testing depends highly on the selection process, especially on the presence or absence of structural heart disease in the syncope patient (110). In a study of 104 patients in which 22 had VT and 2 had SVT induced, a negative study result was associated with LVEF of more than 0.40, absence of structural heart disease, a normal electrocardiogram, and a normal ambulatory ECG monitor recording (111). In another series of 141 patients with unexplained syncope selected to undergo cardiac electrophysiologic studies, those who had no organic heart disease, no unsustained VT on ambulatory monitoring, and no first-degree AV block or bundle branch block recorded during a resting electrocardiogram were at almost no risk for induction of arrhythmia and at very slight risk for a conduction system abnormality (112). In another report of 86 patients with syncope, among the patients with structural heart disease, 71 had abnormal cardiac electrophysiologic studies, with induced sustained monomorphic VT being the most common abnormality, whereas among the patients without detectable structural heart disease, only 13% had abnormal findings, with induced SVT being the most common.

Induction by PES of a previously undocumented ventricular arrhythmia during syncope workup should always be evaluated critically regarding its specificity. There is no commonly accepted standard stimulation protocol for syncope, but in most of the laboratories, up to three extrastimuli are applied to two right ventricular stimulation sites when there is underlying organic heart disease. What stimulation protocol, if any, should be used in syncope with no structural heart disease is controversial, and it is difficult to know the clinical significance of VF induced by an aggressive PES protocol in a syncope patient with no structural heart disease, except perhaps in the setting of certain channelopathies (94). There is general agreement that induced nonsustained VT lacks the specificity necessary for a clinically important end point. Induced VT in a patient presenting with syncope must be interpreted in the setting of clinical presentation, the underlying heart disease, and the symptoms reproduced. The largest secondary prevention trial, AVID, did include patients presenting with syncope who later had sustained VT/VF induced by PES (59). This particular patient subgroup was not large enough for a conclusive subgroup analysis; nevertheless, it appeared that ICD benefit was independent of clinical presentation. The specificity of induced VT or VF in a patient presenting with syncope is still problematic, but acceptance rate of this finding as a clinical end point requiring attention and treatment in patients with advanced organic heart disease has increased greatly. With the availability of stored electrogram recordings in ICDs, the prognostic significance of PES-induced VT/VF should be further classified.

THE ROLE OF CARDIAC ELECTROPHYSIOLOGY STUDIES IN EVALUATING THE HIGH-RISK PATIENT

Patients with advanced organic heart disease who have already survived a prehospital cardiac arrest have the greatest risk of sudden cardiac death. Invasive cardiac electrophysiologic stud-

ies are playing an ever-decreasing role in the management of such patients and are usually not used for risk stratification any more. However, in other patient populations with somewhat lower risk of sudden cardiac death, there is still a need for clinical tools capable of defining this risk reliably.

The mortality in the year after acute myocardial infarction, which was approximately 10% until a decade ago (113), has decreased with aggressive early management. Much of this early mortality is attributed to sudden death from ventricular arrhythmias. Two studies prospectively evaluating the role of PES in predicting sudden cardiac death after acute myocardial infarction in small groups of patients arrived at sharply disparate results (114,115). A larger study investigated the utility of a system of risk stratification for 230 patients with recent myocardial infarction and at risk for sudden death who were followed prospectively for more than 2 years (116). In this select group, the annual event rate was 1.8% with a total of 17 cardiac events, defined as sudden death, out-of-hospital cardiac arrest, or syncope associated with an ICD countershock. Eighty-two percent (14 of 17) of the cardiac events occurred in patients who had sustained VT induced by PES (116). In the asymptomatic group, the excess event rate—13% in those with inducible VT versus 0% in those with no induced VT ($p = 0.01$)—was even more significant if VT had been induced with two or fewer ventricular extrastimuli: 20% versus 0% ($p = 0.001$). However, the positive predictive value of PES in this setting is low. In general, PES alone has not led to consistent conclusions about its clinical utility in screening for the high-risk patients among those with an uncomplicated acute infarction, and its routine use for this purpose is not recommended.

The largest population at an increased risk of sudden cardiac death comprises patients with depressed ventricular function due to advanced ischemic heart disease and nonsustained VT. Two large, multicenter, primary prevention trials, MADIT I and MUSTT, have evaluated the role of preventive therapy prospectively in such patients using a randomized design (11,12). Programmed cardiac stimulation was included in the protocol of both of these studies. The findings changed substantially how clinicians approach these patients, and the studies themselves resulted in new indications for PES, at least until future data from other large, prospective clinical studies further change the current practice.

MADIT I recruited patients with prior Q-wave myocardial infarction, asymptomatic nonsustained VT, and LVEF of ≤0.35 (11). Patients meeting these criteria underwent PES, and those with electrically induced sustained VT underwent repeat PES after intravenous procainamide. Only patients in whom sustained inducible VT persisted after intravenous procainamide were randomized to ICD therapy versus conventional therapy, primarily antiarrhythmic drug therapy with sotalol or amiodarone. Even though it included a small number of patients, MADIT I was the first randomized study that convincingly demonstrated the

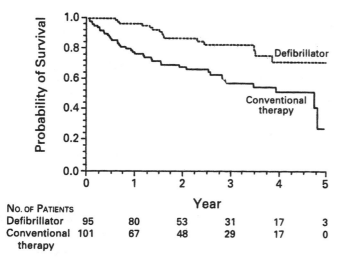

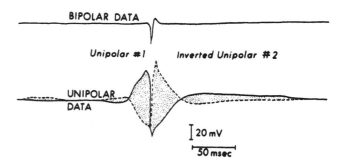

FIGURE 7-6. Intention-to-treat Kaplan-Meier survival curves of the patients randomized to receive an implantable cardioverter-defibrillator (ICD) versus those who were randomized to other (antiarrhythmic drug) therapies in the MADIT I Trial. (From Moss AJ, Hall WT, Cannon DS, et al. *N Engl J Med* 1996;335:1939, with permission.)

FIGURE 7-7. Generation of a bipolar electrogram from the unipolar recordings from the bipoles. The upper trace is the bipolar recording. The lower trace shows overlapping, simultaneous unipolar recordings from the two poles comprising the bipole. The solid line is from unipolar 1, and the dashed line is from the inverted trace from unipolar 2. The unipolar 2 trace is inverted to correspond to the recording vector it serves in the bipolar recording. In the unipolar recordings, notice the gradual up-sloping and down-sloping potentials generated by far-field activation. The stippled area between the two unipolar traces represents the portion of the signal subtracted by the bipolar recording. (From Gallagher JJ, Kasell JH, Cox JL, et al. Techniques of intraoperative electrophysiologic mapping. *Am J Cardiol* 1982; 49:221–240, with permission.)

superiority of ICD as an effective primary prevention therapy (Fig. 7-6). It also defined a new clinical role for PES in identifying candidates for ICD treatment among the high-risk patients with ischemic heart disease and nonsustained VT. It is important to emphasize that MADIT I was not a controlled study, and the long-term registry data on patients with no inducible sustained VT/VF are not available. The higher use of β blockers in the ICD group may have played a role in the better outcome of this group. The absence of PES-induced sustained ventricular arrhythmia should not be equated with favorable long-term outcome for patients fitting the clinical profile required by the MADIT inclusion criteria.

The population of patients targeted by MUSTT, another primary prevention trial, was similar: ischemic heart disease, LVEF of less than 0.40, and documented asymptomatic nonsustained VT. This was a larger trial that took nearly 10 years to finish (12). The patients who, in addition to meeting the inclusion criteria, had inducible sustained VT or VF in response to PES were randomized to no antiarrhythmic therapy or to electrophysiologically guided antiarrhythmic therapy. The latter group did better, but the survival benefit was limited entirely to those treated with ICD, whereas the patients given antiarrhythmic drugs did at least as poorly as or worse than the untreated patients. Another important detail was the outcome of patients in whom sustained polymorphic VT or VF was induced using three extrastimuli. According to the protocol, these patients were considered as having no inducible sustained ventricular arrhythmia (because VT/VF was not induced by two extrastimuli) and were followed in the registry. The event rate for this group was almost as high as that observed for patients with VT induced with two extrastimuli, who were

subsequently randomized to no treatment. This observation suggests that basing "clinical relevance" of the induced arrhythmia on whether two or three extrastimuli are used to induce it may not be justified in this particular patient population (12).

Other findings from MUSTT regarding the role of PES are noteworthy. Patients who had no inducible VT/VF and who were followed in the registry had a lower rate of sudden cardiac death compared with those with no inducible VT/VF. These patients, however, still had a relatively high event rate, and their mortality rate was higher than for the patients treated with ICDs, and much is consistent with the MADIT I results. The absence of PES-induced VT does not necessarily predict a favorable outcome for this group of high-risk patients. Several large, multicenter clinical trials evaluating the role of ICD in primary prevention in patients at high risk for sudden cardiac death, such as MADIT II, Defibrillators in Non-Ischemic Cardiomyopathy Treatment Evaluation (DEFINITE), and Sudden Cardiac Death–Heart Failure Trial (SCD-HeFT) (117–119), are bypassing the PES step altogether, and their results may further modify the ever-evolving role of PES in the management of such patients.

CARDIAC MAPPING

Cardiac mapping is the process of identifying the temporal and spatial distributions of electrical potential generated by myocardium during normal or abnormal rhythms. This process allows description of the spread of activation from its initiation to its completion within a region of interest, and in its usual application, it focuses on the identification of the site of origin or a critical site of conduction for an arrhythmia. Although traditionally aimed at detecting myocardial activation, advances have expanded cardiac mapping applications to measuring repolarization and potential amplitudes in so-called voltage mapping.

The development of techniques for intraoperative mapping allowed the first successful surgical division of an accessory pathway (120). By the late 1970s, mapping techniques allowed the successful surgical ablation of VT (121). Further refinements in mapping techniques over the past 10 years have enabled the development of highly effective transcatheter techniques for ablation of most types of SVT and various VTs (5–10). These transcatheter mapping techniques, including nonfluoroscopic electroanatomic mapping (122) and noncontact endocardial mapping (123), have all but replaced intraoperative mapping, which is now rarely performed.

The amplitude of the extracellular potential generated by myocardial depolarization depends on a number of factors, principally the magnitude of the currents generated by each cell, the number of cells simultaneously generating this current, the proximity of the recording electrode to these cells, and the resistance to current flow between the source in the myocardium and the recording site (124). Recorded electrograms can yield two important pieces of information: the local activation time (i.e., the time of activation of myocardium immediately adjacent to the recording electrode relative to a reference) and the complexity of myocardial activation within the "field of view" of the recording electrode.

Recording electrodes may be unipolar or bipolar; in actuality, both so-called unipolar and bipolar recordings are bipolar, except that the bipoles are much more widely spaced in the former than the in the latter. The more the interelectrode spacing is increased on a conventional bipolar electrode, the more the recorded electrogram resembles a "unipolar" recording. Because extracellular potential decreases inversely by the square of the distance from a point source (124), far-field events generate relatively low-amplitude signals compared with electrogram components generated by near-field sources in unipolar recordings. The major component of the unipolar electrogram allows determination of the local activation time, although exceptions have been observed. If a recording electrode is at the source from which all wavefronts propagate, the recorded potential is an entirely negative, or QS, deflection (125–127). Unlike unipolar recordings, bipolar electrodes with short interpolar distances are relatively unaffected by far-field events. The bipolar electrogram is the sum of the two unipolar electrograms recorded at the bipoles (Fig. 7-7). The shape and the amplitude of the bipolar electrograms are determined by the orientation of the bipolar recording axis to the direction of propagation of the activation wavefront.

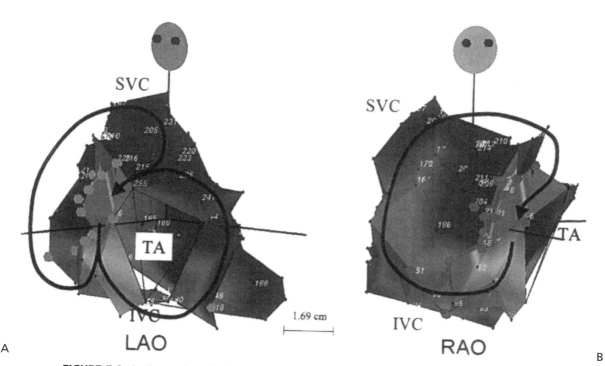

FIGURE 7-8. A: Grayscale activation isochrones generated during focal right atrial tachycardia. The earliest activation, relative to a remote fiducial point, is represented. The spread of activation is centrifugal from a focal point located along distal crista terminalis. **B:** Figure-of-eight atrial tachycardia circuit results from macroreentry around atrial scar tissue. (From Shah, et al. *Circulation* 2000;101:635, with permission.)

Establishing electrogram criteria that allow accurate determination of the moment of myocardial activation at the recording electrode is critical for construction of an area map of the activation sequence. Most studies have suggested that the local activation is best determined in the unipolar electrogram by the point with maximum slope (i.e., maximum change in potential, or dV/dt) (128). Using this fiducial point, errors in determining the local activation time compared with intracellular recordings typically have been less than 1 ms (129). Algorithms for detecting local activation time from bipolar electrograms have been more problematic, in part because of the fact that the bipolar electrogram is generated by two spatially separated recording poles. Among several options, the absolute maximum electrogram amplitude appears to most consistently correlate with local activation time determined by other means (129). For complex multicomponent bipolar electrograms, such as those with marked fractionation and prolonged duration seen in regions with complex conduction patterns (e.g., in regions of slow conduction in cases of AFL or VT), determination of local activation time becomes problematic, and the decision of which activation time is most appropriate needs to be made in the context of the particular rhythm being mapped (128,130).

Methodology

A large variety of multipolar electrode catheters has been developed to facilitate placement of the catheter in the desired place and to fulfill various recording requirements. These include multipolar recording electrode-catheters placed within the coronary sinus and along the crista terminalis in the right atrium, the halo catheter used to map the reentrant electrical activity around the tricuspid annulus during right atrial macroreentry, special catheters used to record left atrial and left ventricular epicardial activity from the coronary sinus branches, electrodes to record electrical activity from the pulmonary veins, basket electrodes capable of conforming to the chamber size and shape, and "noncontact" composite electrodes for simultaneous acquisition of a high number of electrograms. Steerable or deflectable catheters allow precise and detailed mapping and catheter ablation of many different types of tachyarrhythmias.

To ensure high-quality recordings, direct cardiac electrograms should be recorded with amplifiers with high-input impedances to decrease unwanted electrical interference (131). For most of the digital systems used today, after amplification of the data at each channel, the data undergo analog to digital (A/D) conversion. Amplifiers are also used to filter the low- and high-frequency content of the signal. The range of frequencies not filtered out is frequently called the *bandpass*. The high-pass filter allows frequencies above a limit to remain in the signal (i.e., it filters out lower frequencies), and the low-pass filter filters out frequencies above a certain limit. Typical bandpass for intracardiac

bipolar electrograms is 30 to 300 Hz. The high-pass filter is set at 30 Hz to filter out low-frequency repolarization events and limit baseline drift. Because most of the signal content is less than 300 Hz, the low-pass filter is set from 300 Hz to eliminate high-frequency noise. Unipolar electrograms are typically filtered across a wider bandpass, typically 0.05 to 300 Hz. For digital systems, the sampling rate should be at least twice as fast as the highest frequency component of the signal to avoid aliasing (i.e., the Nyquist limit) (132). For practical purposes of activation mapping, sampling rates of 1,000 Hz are generally adequate (133).

Single-Catheter Mapping

The simplest form of mapping is achieved by moving the single electrode sequentially to various points of interest to measure local activation. Local activation times must be measured relative to some external fiducial marker, such as the onset of the P wave or QRS complex on the surface ECG or a reference electrode in the heart. However, the success of roving-point mapping is predicated on the sequential beat-by-beat stability of the activation sequence being mapped and the ability of the patient to tolerate the sustained arrhythmia. However, these assumptions do not always apply, as in the mapping of polymorphic VT. Similarly, monomorphic VT may have a repetitive sequence of endocardial activation but can be hemodynamically too unstable to allow time for complete roving endocavitary catheter mapping in the electrophysiology laboratory. The more sites that are simultaneously mapped, the less roving of a single point is required. In the electrophysiology laboratory, additional data are obtained by placing a limited number of catheters within the heart (i.e., right ventricular apex, His bundle region, high right atrium, and coronary sinus) in addition to the mapping electrodes. During initial arrhythmia evaluation, recording from these limited number of sites allows rough estimation of the site of interest.

Mapping simultaneously from as many sites as possible greatly enhances the precision, detail, and speed of identifying regions of interest. Unfortunately, transcatheter endocardial mapping as performed in the electrophysiology laboratory is limited by the number, size, and type of electrodes that can be placed within the heart. Development of high-density electrode arrays that can be deployed from a catheter and computerized multichannel mapping systems (56 to 256 channels) may change this in the near future. These systems allow high-speed data acquisition from various electrode arrays, depending on the clinical application.

Nonfluoroscopic Electroanatomic Mapping

The technique of nonfluoroscopic electroanatomic mapping, widely used in many of the cardiac electrophysiologic laboratories worldwide, is based on the use of a special catheter with a locatable tip connected to a mapping and navigation system

(134.). An external magnetic field is created by a very low magnetic field emitter. A miniature magnetic field sensor at the tip of the catheter can determine the location (x, y, and z coordinates) and the orientation (roll, pitch, and yaw) of the catheter. The catheter generates an accurate and individualized three-dimensional reconstruction of the chamber size and local geometry in addition to the usual local electrograms. The accuracy and the reproducibility of the three-dimensional localization have been validated (134).

The system can generate isochrones of electrical activity as color-coded static maps or animated dynamic maps of activation wavefront. These pictures can define reentrant circuits and the site of origin or breakthrough of an ectopic activity with centrifugal, monoregional, or asymmetric spread of electrical activity. An additional advantage is local electrogram voltage mapping during sinus, paced, or any other rhythm that defines anatomically correct regions of no voltage (presumed scar), low voltage, and normal voltage, although the true range of normal is often difficult to define, especially with bipolar recordings, and when different criteria have been used.

Since the introduction of three-dimensional electroanatomic mapping, many reports have been published describing its use in mapping of accessory pathways (135), typical AFL (136), focal ATs (137), and idiopathic VTs (138). Other reports have described its utility in defining activation patterns of more complex atrial and ventricular tachyarrhythmias with the use of propagation maps to identify slowly conducting critical pathways (139) and substrate mapping to identify the geometry of scars and their relationship to pathways in ischemic VT or postsurgical atrial tachyarrhythmias (140) (Fig. 7-8). The technique can also differentiate markedly slow conduction from complete conduction block when effective linear lesions are essential for the success of catheter ablation (141).

A major advantage of this technique is its ability to allow the catheter to anatomically and accurately "revisit" a critically important recording site identified previously during the study, even if the tachycardia is no longer present or inducible and therefore map-guided catheter navigation is no longer possible. This accurate repositioning can allow pace mapping from or further application of RF current to critically important sites that otherwise cannot be performed with a high degree of accuracy and reproducibility. Although fluoroscopy is always needed for initial orientation, an experienced operator can usually generate an extensive endocardial activation map with substantially reduced radiation for the practitioner and the patient.

Noncontact Endocardial Activation Mapping

Historically, mathematical methods based on the inverse solution to Laplace's equation have been applied to describe the cardiac epicardial activation from the changing distribution of the isopotential regions on the skin of chest wall during the cardiac cycle (142). Similar mathematical techniques lie behind the generation of endocardial activation maps based on the electrical field detected by a composite electrode placed in the blood pool in the center of the cardiac chamber of interest (143).

The noncontact catheter is a multielectrode array mounted on a balloon-tipped catheter. This balloon can be filled with contrast dye and visualized fluoroscopically (144). The location of any conventional mapping catheter with respect to this multielectrode array can be determined by passing a high-frequency, low-current locator signal by means of a process described and validated previously (144).

Clinically, the multielectrode array has been deployed in the right atrium, in the left atrium, through the transseptal approach, and in the left ventricle through the retrograde, transaortic approach to map right and the left atrial tachyarrhythmias and VT (145–147). Systemic anticoagulation is critical to avoid thromboembolic complications. An intravenous bolus of heparin usually is given at an initial dose of 10,000 IU, and additional supplements are needed during the course of the study to maintain the activated clotting time between 350 and 400 seconds.

The system generates isopotential maps of the endocardial surface at successive cross sections of time, and when these are animated, the spread of the depolarization wave is visualized. The maps are particularly useful for identifying slowly conducting pathways such as the critical slow pathways in ischemic VT (147) and rapid breakthrough points (Fig. 7-9). In macroreentrant tachycardias such as typical or atypical AFL, the reentry circuit may be fully identifiable along with other aspects, such as slowing of the activation wavefront in the isthmus (148).

It has been argued that the biggest advantage of noncontact endocardial mapping is its ability to recreate the endocardial activation sequence from simultaneously acquired multiple data points over a very few (theoretically one) tachycardia beats, obviating the need for prolonged tachycardia that may be poorly tolerated. Although in theory this sounds logical, more investigation is needed to define its clinical benefits and its precise range of applicability.

Mapping of Specific Tachyarrhythmias

Detailed descriptions of the mapping techniques used for specific supraventricular and ventricular arrhythmias and their treatment are given in later chapters of this book. A brief discussion is presented here, emphasizing the aspects relevant to transcatheter mapping.

Preexcitation Syndromes

Several parameters can be used to identify an accessory pathway location during catheter-based mapping. To determine the atrial insertion site, the earliest site of retrograde atrial activation during orthodromic AV reciprocating tachycardia or ventricular pacing must be identified (149,150). The

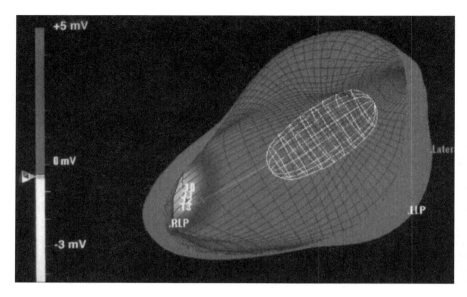

FIGURE 7-9. Three-dimensional isopotential half-open map of the left atrium generated by the noncontact system being used to map focal atrial fibrillation. The ectopic activity (i.e., depolarization) spreads centrifugally from the ostium of the left upper pulmonary (LUP) vein. (From Schneider MA, Ndrepepa G, Zrenner B, et al. Noncontact mapping-guided catheter ablation of atrial fibrillation associated with left atrial ectopy. *J Cardiovasc Electrophysiol* 2000;11: 477, with permission.)

assumption is that the local VA interval on the recording electrode is shortest at the atrial insertion site. For ventricular pacing, rates rapid enough to prolong retrograde AV nodal conduction should be used to allow identification of eccentric retrograde atrial activation and avoid fusion activation of the atria. This may not be possible with rapidly (retrogradely)

conducting AV nodes and may require pharmacologic block. With left-sided accessory pathways, the multiple recording electrodes on the coronary sinus catheter demonstrate eccentric retrograde atrial activation arising earliest on one pole of the coronary sinus catheter (Fig. 7-9). Ideally, the earliest site should be flanked on either side by electrodes recording

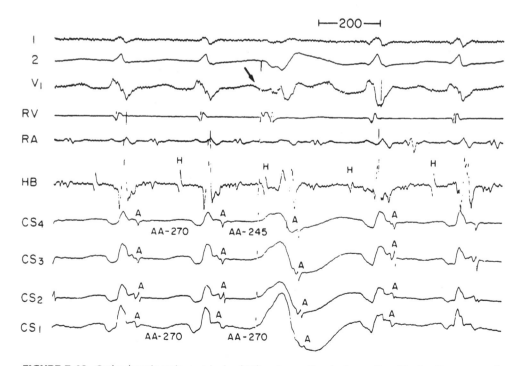

FIGURE 7-10. Orthodromic atrioventricular (AV) reciprocating tachycardia with simultaneous activation of proximal and distal coronary sinus (CS) recording sites because of fusion activation of the left atrium. A ventricular extrastimulus (*arrow*) delivered when the His bundle is refractory advances the atrial activation by the posteroseptal pathway but blocks in the lateral pathway, thereby unmasking the presence of two accessory pathways. (From Yee R, et al. In: Zipes, Jalife, eds. *Cardiac electrophysiology from cell to bedside.* St. Louis: W.B. Saunders, 1999:467, with permsission.)

slightly later atrial activation, which is referred to as bracketing of the earliest site. If the distal (or proximal) pole of the coronary sinus catheter records the earliest atrial activation, advancing or withdrawing the coronary sinus catheter by a few centimeters should allow bracketing of the retrograde atrial activation sequence. The earliest activation occurring simultaneously at two adjacent coronary sinus recording sites may result from a single pathway located between the two recording electrodes or two pathways with atrial insertions at the two recording electrodes (Fig. 7-10). Advancing or withdrawing the coronary sinus catheter by a few millimeters to determine the absolute earliest sites of activation can help distinguish the two possibilities (150).

Recording electrodes placed within the right coronary artery have been used to allow precise localization of right free wall pathways using a pull-back technique, in a fashion analogous to the coronary sinus pull-back technique for left-sided accessory pathways (151). However, careful attention to mapping the tricuspid annulus aided by specialized preformed guiding sheaths to keep the deflectable catheters at the valve annulus generally circumvents the need for right coronary artery mapping and avoids its potential complications.

Anteroseptal, posteroseptal, and intermediate septal accessory pathways result in "concentric" retrograde atrial activation during orthodromic AVRT or ventricular pacing because of their proximity to the AV node. If the recording poles of the coronary sinus catheter are pulled back to the coronary sinus ostium, activation at this site can be seen to precede atrial activation on the His bundle catheter for a posteroseptal accessory pathway. More precise mapping of septal accessory pathways depends on detailed mapping with a roving catheter (152). To avoid confusing retrograde AV nodal conduction from septal accessory pathway conduction, mapping during orthodromic AVRT is preferred over ventricular pacing. Pacing near the atrial insertion of the accessory pathway creates a greater degree of preexcitation with a shorter delay between the stimulus and the onset of the delta wave than pacing at sites more remote from the accessory pathway (153). By pacing at various right and left atrial sites and measuring the degree of preexcitation and the stimulus-delta wave onset interval (so-called differential pacing), the site of the accessory pathway can be approximated. More precise localization of the ventricular insertion site is obtained by mapping along the AV groove in sinus rhythm to determine the site of earliest ventricular activation during preexcited beats. Local ventricular activation at the ventricular insertion site frequently precedes the onset of the delta wave on the surface ECG by 10 to 40 ms (154,155). If preexcitation is minimal in sinus rhythm, atrial pacing at decremental cycle lengths can be performed to facilitate ventricular preexcitation by delaying AV nodal conduction.

In the anterograde or retrograde directions, discrete potentials can be seen bridging the atrial and ventricular

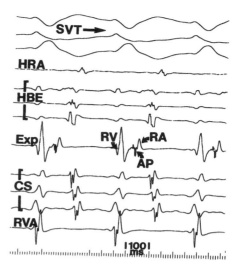

FIGURE 7-11. The tracings show a right-sided accessory pathway potential recorded during orthodromic atrioventricular reciprocating tachycardia with right bundle branch block aberration in a patient with preexcitation syndrome. The pathway potential is a high-frequency component, juxtaposed between the ventricular (V) and atrial (A) electrograms. Application of radiofrequency current at this site successfully eliminated the pathway.

electrograms at the site of the accessory pathway (150, 155–159) (Fig. 7-11). Such potentials are thought to be generated by the accessory pathways, and their identity can be validated by showing that they dynamically follow atrial and ventricular premature activation in a fashion parallel to accessory pathway function. Recording of accessory pathway potentials has proven a reliable means of directing RF catheter ablation of the accessory pathway (155–159). This is also true for atriofascicular connections (160).

For anterogradely functioning accessory pathways, the presence of accessory pathway potentials, a local ventricular activation preceding onset of the surface delta wave by 30 to 40 ms, and a short interval between the accessory pathway potential and the ventricular electrogram predict successful ablation and indicate the greatest proximity of the catheter to the accessory pathway (155). For retrogradely functioning pathways, the presence of accessory pathway potentials, continuous electrical activity between the local ventricular and atrial electrograms, and the shortest local VA interval during reciprocating tachycardia are most predictive (155). Some investigators have shown that additional information can be gained from recording unipolar electrograms (144). If the unipolar electrode is situated at the site of ventricular insertion of an accessory pathway, all ventricular activation conducts away from the electrode to generate a QS-pattern ventricular electrogram after a fused or very short PQ deflection, given the short accessory pathway activation time (159). Identification of a QS complex may be even more important in localizing the ventricular insertion of accessory pathways that insert remotely from the AV groove, such as an atriofascicular or a nodofascicular pathway inserting into the His-Purkinje fibers (160).

Atrioventricular Nodal Reentry

In the typical form of slow/fast AVNRT, retrograde conduction occurs across the fast pathway and anterograde conduction across the slow pathway. Identification of the fast pathway rests on localization of the earliest site of retrograde atrial activation during AVNRT in an anteroseptal region near the His bundle (161,162). Because atrial activation in the anterior septal region occurs concomitantly with or slightly before the local ventricular activation, it is sometimes difficult to differentiate the atrial from the ventricular activation complex on the His bundle recording. Atrial mapping of the His bundle region can be facilitated by placing a relatively early premature ventricular activation during tachycardia to advance local ventricular septal activation, allowing distinction of the local atrial electrogram. The VA interval at the His bundle electrogram, ordinarily −20 to 0 ms during typical AVNRT, may be slightly positive at the site closest to the fast pathway (162).

During the fast/slow AVNRT or during ventricular pacing with retrograde conduction across the slow pathway, earliest retrograde atrial activation occurs at the coronary sinus ostial area (i.e., posteroseptal region). Mapping of the slow pathway of the AV node rests on its spatial proximity to the coronary sinus ostium. During sinus or atrially paced rhythm, complex atrial electrograms are seen in the posteroseptal space, with discrete potentials perhaps representing an activation potential from a discrete slow pathway or perhaps representing complexities of anisotropic conduction in the posterior AV nodal complex in a region critical for AV nodal reentry (163,164) (Fig. 7-12). The observation that such "slow pathway potentials" occur in patients without AVNRT or dual AV nodal physiology further suggests that such complex electrograms in the posteroseptal space represent the normal conduction characteristics of this area (165). Regardless of its origin, the slow pathway potential designates an area critical for the maintenance of AVNRT because ablation of this site prevents initiation of tachycardia, although dual AV nodal physiology may persist (163,164). In some variants of AVNRT, retrograde activation may occur in intermediate septal regions or within the os of coronary sinus.

Atrial Tachycardia

AT due to reentry or focal mechanisms (i.e., ectopic or triggered) is a relatively uncommon form of SVT, except in patients who have had prior cardiac surgery. For tachycardias without an obvious macroreentrant circuit, mapping is performed by identifying the site of earliest atrial activation during tachycardia and confirming that there is centrifugal activation away from this site. Detailed mapping of the

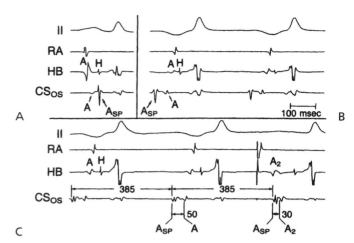

FIGURE 7-12. Tracings recorded from the posterior margin of the coronary sinus ostium (CSos). **A:** During sinus rhythm, a large, so-called slow pathway potential (Asp), followed by a smaller, far-field atrial (A) electrogram, is recorded. **B:** The order is reversed during atypical (i.e., fast-slow) atrioventricular (AV) nodal reentrant tachycardia. **C:** An atrial extrastimulus during atrioventricular nodal reentrant tachycardia (AVNRT) advances the atrial activation timing while altering neither the timing nor the morphology of Asp. (From Jackman WM, Beckman KJ, McClelland JH, et al. Treatment of supraventricular tachycardia due to atrioventricular nodal reentry by radiofrequency catheter ablation of slow-pathway conduction. *N Engl J Med* 1992;327: 314, with permission.)

atrial activation sequence during tachycardia is performed using one or more mapping catheters (7,166–168). The older technique of two-catheter mapping (i.e., dueling catheters technique) has been replaced by the three-dimensional electroanatomic mapping method (134,137). Magnetic electroanatomic mapping has facilitated the mapping of focal tachycardias. This technique generates isochrones of activation that show a centrifugal spread from a source. For mapping and ablation of left AT, a transseptal approach to the left atrium is usually needed (166). Most ATs arise within the right atrium (167,168). Local electrograms are frequently fractionated, low amplitude, and prolonged at the site of origin of AT in adults (7,167,168) (Fig. 7-13), although this finding may not be as common in children (166).

The use of pace mapping for comparison of P-wave morphology and the intraatrial activation sequence during AT and during pacing from the mapping catheter has been described elsewhere (168). However, pace mapping of the atria is complicated by the frequent difficulties of precise 12-lead ECG identification of P-wave morphology during tachycardia because of overlap of the P wave with the preceding QRST segment. Relative to activation mapping during tachycardia, pace mapping of the atria seems to add little additional benefit except when the AT is not inducible or not sustained long enough to allow activation mapping.

Some patients with AT, especially those with structural heart disease or prior cardiac surgery, have reentrant cir-

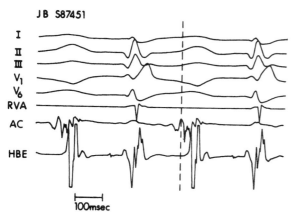

FIGURE 7-13. Intracardiac recordings during right atrial tachycardia. The ablation catheter (AC) is located at the site of earliest atrial activity during the tachycardia. The onset of the atrial electrogram on the ablation catheter precedes the onset of the tachycardia P wave by 35 ms, and the local atrial electrogram is fractionated and prolonged. Radiofrequency ablation was successful at this site.

cuits in which the diastolic limb can be fully or partially mapped over one to several centimeters of myocardium. These macroreentrant tachycardias require mapping of the entire reentrant circuit using roving-catheter techniques or special electrode catheters capable of simultaneous recordings from multiple sites. Activation times are recorded at each site and the points registered on a display of the atria for graphic registration of the circuit. Pacing within the diastolic limb of the circuit may result in entrainment of the tachycardia without evidence of fusion activation of the P wave, which is called *entrainment with concealed fusion.* The amount of latency between the stimulus and the onset of the P wave during concealed entrainment is inversely proportioned to the distance from the exit site. Identification of sites that allow concealed entrainment and confirmation that they lie within the circuit by measurement of postpacing intervals may allow a higher rate of successful ablation. Dynamic isochronous activation maps generated by electroanatomic mapping and isopotential maps generated by composite noncontact mapping electrodes may greatly aid the definition of the circuit underlying a macroreentrant AT.

Voltage mapping during sinus rhythm and tachycardia by the electroanatomic mapping technique has been used to delineate the scarred areas that serve as the anatomic barriers and the corridors and isthmuses between these barriers, which are the critical pathways, to better define the geometry of the circuits involved (140).

Atrial Flutter

The typical form of AFL is a macroreentrant tachyarrhythmia with the circuit revolving around an area of

functional block located in the posterolateral right atrium along the crista terminalis (169–173). During AFL, systole is defined by the onset of the negative saw-toothed flutter wave in the inferior electrocardiographic leads. Earliest presystolic activity occurs in the region of the coronary sinus ostium, and activation proceeds counterclockwise around the area of block. Electrograms obtained from the region of block occur throughout much of diastole and are markedly prolonged and fractionated (172–174). Endocardial mapping in the electrophysiology laboratory is generally performed with right atrial special multipolar catheters, such as the halo catheter. Feld and coworkers (172) showed that a site of successful ablation of AFL was near the coronary sinus ostium, pacing from which demonstrated concealed entrainment of the AFL associated with minimal latency (<40 ms) between the stimulus and the local atrial activation. Others have advocated ablation across the diastolic limb of the circuit between the tricuspid annulus and inferior vena cava ostium (174). Atypical forms of AFL have also been mapped in the electrophysiology laboratory and similarly represent macroreentrant circuits around large areas of presumed functional block similar to that in typical AFL (175). The macroreentrant circuit may be a clockwise variant of typical AFL or may be the result of smaller macroreentrant circuits located in the right atrium and still using the isthmus between the inferior vena cava and the tricuspid annulus, such as the lower loop reentry (lower half of the typical AFL circuit) (176) (Fig. 7-14). Alternatively, the circuit may be around a core of functional block in the crista terminalis area in the free lateral wall of the right atrium (177). Atypical AFL arising in the left atrium is uncommon (178) and usually occurs in patients with left heart disease or prior cardiac surgery. Unlike the typical flutter, which can be ablated by an anatomic approach targeting the right atrial isthmus, the tissue between the inferior vena cava and the tricuspid annulus, these atypical forms must be mapped individually in detail using activation sequence and entrainment techniques. The presence of isthmus conduction as a critical component (i.e., isthmus dependence) must be demonstrated before the anatomic approach can be used.

Ventricular Tachycardia

Mapping of VT in the electrophysiology laboratory uses the same steerable mapping catheters as used for the mapping and ablation of SVT. Several means of localizing the origin of a VT have been developed and include pace mapping, activation sequence mapping during VT, entrainment mapping during tachycardia, identification of areas of fractionated conduction and low-voltage electrograms during sinus or atrially paced rhythm, and identification of slowly conducting regions during "electrical diastole" by noncontact isopotential mapping.

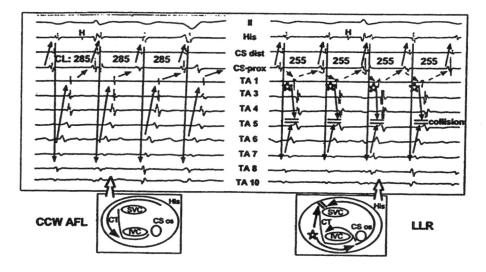

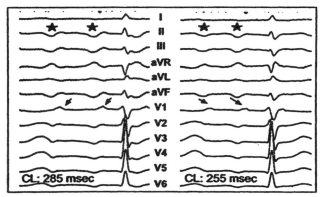

FIGURE 7-14. The tracing shows the halo catheter activation sequences during counterclockwise atrial flutter and its spontaneous transformation into sustained lower loop reentry with corresponding changes in cycle length (CL) and the activation sequence. CS_{os}, coronary sinus ostium; CT, crista terminalis; IVC, inferior vena cava; SVC, superior vena cava. (From Cheng J, Cabeen WR, Scheinman MM. Right atrial flutter due to lower loop reentry. *Circulation* 1999; 99:1700, with permission.)

Pace Mapping

Pace mapping involves manipulation of the mapping catheter to the region of origin of VT. Pacing at this site using the same cycle length as the tachycardia should generate QRS complexes resembling those during VT (179–181) (Fig. 7-15). The greater the degree of concordance between QRS morphology during pacing and tachycardia, the closer the catheter is to the site of origin of the tachycardia. Concordance should occur in 12 of 12 leads on the surface ECG; however, this is frequently not achievable. Kadish and colleagues (180) showed that, if only major QRS configuration changes were evaluated on the 12-lead ECG, sites as disparate as 15 mm could be similar; if only minor configuration changes were allowed, this measurement decreased to 5 mm. However, 83% of patients had some QRS configuration change with pacing 5 mm from the index site, and all patients had changes with pacing 10 mm from the index site. These data suggest that detailed pace mapping with allowance of only minor QRS configuration changes would allow identification of the site of origin of a tachycardia. Pace mapping has advantages over activation mapping in that induction of VT is not required, and it allows identification of the site of origin when the

induced tachycardia is poorly tolerated or when the VT is not inducible by PES but 12-lead QRS morphology is available. However, pace mapping only identifies the site of breakthrough into the myocardial tissue that generates surface vectors. This may be adequate for certain forms of idiopathic VT. However, if the circuit geometry is complex as it usually is in postinfarction VT, the essential sites are not accurately identified by pace mapping.

Activation Sequence Mapping

The most commonly used method of identifying the site of origin of a VT is mapping to find the site of earliest endocardial activation during tachycardia (182). Such early activation sites precede the inscription of the QRS during tachycardia and presumably reflect the site from which electrical systole emanates. This assumption holds whether the mechanism of tachycardia is focal (i.e., triggered or automatic) or reentrant. In reentrant VT, a zone of slow conduction over a pathway of possibly quite complex geometry (e.g. nonlinear, nonhomogeneously anisotropic) provides the diastolic limb of the reentrant circuit. After emerging from the zone of slow conduction, the wave front propagates rapidly throughout the ventricles to generate the QRS complex. Early or

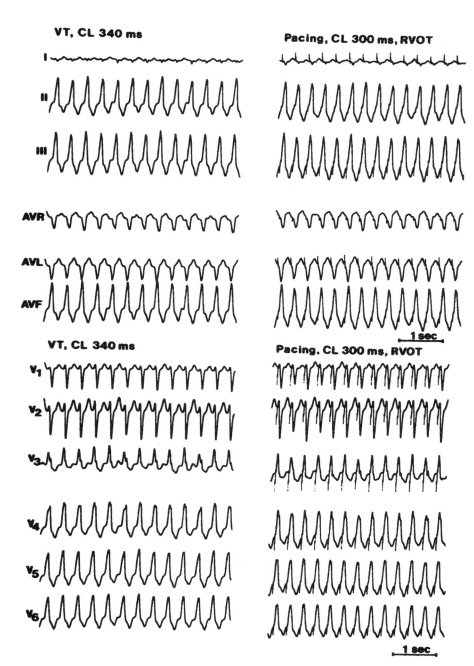

FIGURE 7-15. Twelve-lead electrocardiograms of sustained idiopathic right ventricular tachycardia during infusion of isoproterenol and during pacing at the site of successful ablation at a similar cycle length (i.e., pace mapping). Notice the similarity in QRS morphologies in all of the 12 electrocardiographic leads. (From Morady F, Kadish A, Dicarlo L, et al. Long term results of catheter ablation of idiopathic right ventricular tachycardia. *Circulation* 1990;82:2093–2099, with permission.)

presystolic activation occurs in close proximity to the exit region from the zone of slow conduction.

Electrograms in the region of presystolic activation are often complex, with long prepotentials preceding the major deflection on the electrogram that coincides with the onset of the QRS complex (183–185). Such prepotentials merge into the major deflection, typically without an intervening isoelectric segment. If an intervening isoelectric segment exists, the prepotentials are called mid-diastolic potentials (186) (Fig. 7-16). They identify a region of functional or anatomic conduction block adjacent to the recording

catheter. These prepotentials may precede the major ventricular deflection by tens to hundreds of milliseconds. It is important to demonstrate that, during initiation and resetting of the tachycardia, the mid-diastolic potential always precedes all complexes of the tachycardia in a parallel manner and that loss of the mid-diastolic potential is associated with termination of the tachycardia (187). Those that do not dynamically precede the QRS of tachycardia may represent blind-end alleys (187) of late activation or motion artifact (188). Brugada and colleagues (183) demonstrated that near continuous electrical activity spanning the dias-

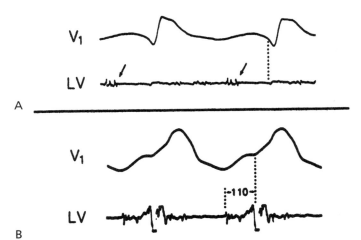

FIGURE 7-16. A: Mid-diastolic potentials during left ventricular (LV) endocardial mapping of ventricular tachycardia. The dotted vertical line marks the onset of the QRS complex during ventricular tachycardia. The mid-diastolic fractionated electrogram *(arrow)* is followed by an isoelectric baseline that precedes the onset of the QRS during tachycardia. **B:** Typical presystolic fractionated activity with an onset 110 ms before the QRS complex in tachycardia. However, unlike the mid-diastolic potentials in **A**, the presystolic component of the electrogram is continuous with the major component of the electrogram and the onset of the QRS complex. Such mid-diastolic activity probably represents a zone of conduction block with surrounding tissue activated by different wavefronts. (From Fritzgerald DM, Friday KJ, Yeung Lai Wah JA, et al. Electrogram patterns predicting successful catheter ablation of ventricular tachycardia. *Circulation* 1988;77:806–814, with permission.)

tolic segment may be seen in patients with VT in the setting of ischemic heart disease or right ventricular dysplasia; however, in 17 of the 20 episodes of continuous electrical activity, the activity was dissociated from the VT. Such behavior presumably results from slow and fractionated conduction into nonessential areas of diseased myocardium.

Entrainment Mapping

Another technique that has been proposed for identification of the zone of slow conduction in patients with macroreentrant VT is entrainment mapping (189,190). If pacing is performed within the zone of slow conduction during VT at a pacing cycle length slightly shorter than the tachycardia cycle length, the tachycardia circuit may be entrained. Because retrograde activation of the zone of slow conduction does not occur fast enough to provide antidromic activation of the ventricles but does propagate antegradely to activate the ventricles orthodromically, there is no evidence of fusion of the QRS complex on the surface ECG—hence the term *entrainment with concealed fusion*. The tachycardia accelerates to the rate of pacing without a change in the VT QRS morphology (Fig. 7-17). This phenomenon can be demonstrated in at least 50% of patients with ischemic heart disease undergoing mapping for ablation (190,191). It has been argued that the postpacing

interval at the pacing site should be comparable (within 20 to 30 ms) to the tachycardia cycle length to ensure that the site is not a blind-end alley within the zone of slow conduction (190). There is typically latency between the stimulus delivery and the recording of the onset of the QRS or local electrogram at the exit site, suggesting stimulation directly into a zone of slow conduction with delay before activating the ventricles. Morady and associates published data obtained during ischemic VT mapping that showed postpacing intervals were not useful in discriminating between sites of concealed entrainment that were within or outside the VT circuit (192). The optimal endocardial mapping technique for postinfarction VT needs to be refined further.

Fractionated Local Electrograms and Voltage Mapping

During sinus rhythm in patients with prior myocardial infarction, endocardial electrograms in and adjacent to the area of infarction frequently have complex morphologic patterns, including fractionation, split potentials, decreased amplitude, and prolonged duration (186) (Fig. 7-17). Similar fractionated electrograms have been seen for patients with right ventricular dysplasia and scleroderma (193), but they occur less often for patients with nonischemic dilated cardiomyopathies. Endocardial mapping for these fractionated, prolonged, and late electrograms in sinus rhythm has been suggested as a means for localizing the site of origin of VT in patients with ischemic heart disease (194,195). However, one problem is the overlap in amplitude and duration measurements between the sites of VT origin and other recording sites. Several studies have shown that fractionated, low-amplitude, and late electrograms can occur in other areas, particularly within the infarct zone, but do not participate in tachycardia (196). The predictive accuracy of fractionated endocardial activity for localizing the site of origin of VT is limited, and the other methods listed previously provide more direct approaches to mapping. With the electroanatomic mapping technique that uses a location sensor incorporated into a mapping catheter, a more complete and global endocardial voltage map of the ventricles may be generated during sinus rhythm. The low-voltage areas may be helpful in defining the circuits and slowly conducting pathways underlying the VT mechanism, especially when the activation maps are superimposed (197).

Role of Epicardial Mapping

The site of origin of the tachycardia may not be accessible from the endocardial approach. Animal and human studies have shown that approximately one third of VTs in the setting of ischemic heart disease depend on mid-myocardial, subepicardial, or intraseptal regions (198–201). Although

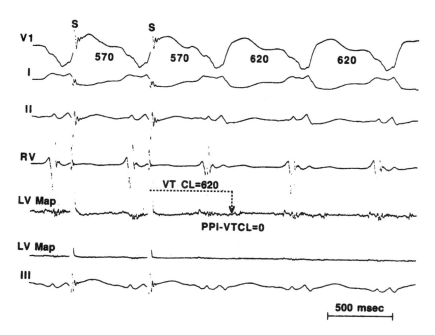

FIGURE 7-17. The tracing shows surface and local electrograms recorded during entrainment with concealed fusion of sustained, monomorphic ventricular tachycardia (VT) in a patient with chronic myocardial infraction. The postpacing interval (PPI) is considered to be zero because the point after the last stimulus at an interval equal to the VT cycle length (CL) falls within a wide fractionated electrogram. The surface QRS morphology remains unrelated during entrainment with concealed fusion. (From Bogun F, Knight B, Goyal R, et al. Clinical value of the postpacing interval for mapping of ventricular tachycardia in patients with prior myocardial infarction. *J Cardiovasc Electrophysiol* 1999;10:47, with permission.)

the general vicinity may be definable with endocardial mapping in these situations, precise localization is impossible. Epicardial ventricular mapping is possible using special recording catheters that may be manipulated into the branches of the coronary sinus. Epicardial mapping using this technique has been used for mapping ischemic VT and for mapping idiopathic VT of outflow tract origin and VT seen in nonischemic cardiomyopathy (202). This technique may be particularly important in identifying the outflow tract VTs that may be difficult to ablate with the endocardial approach only.

Another epicardial mapping technique using a subxiphoid percutaneous approach for accessing the epicardial surface has been used to map VT in the setting of Chagas disease (203). A wider application of this technique may be possible, but it is currently investigational (204).

CONCLUSIONS

Cardiac electrophysiologic studies, PES, and intracardiac mapping have become indispensable techniques in the diagnosis and nonpharmacologic treatment of supraventricular and VTs. They continue to be helpful clinically in the management of the patients with bradyarrhythmias, conduction disturbances, and syncope. Programmed cardiac stimulation is widely used in clinical decision making and risk stratification for selected patients with a high-risk profile for potentially lethal ventricular tachyarrhythmias. In some areas of clinical cardiac electrophysiology, the clinical utility of PES remains uncertain and needs to be defined clearly by prospective, randomized studies.

REFERENCES

1. Zipes D, Rahimtoola S. State-of-the-art consensus conference on electrophysiologic testing in the diagnosis and treatment of patients with cardiac arrhythmia. *Circulation* 1987;75[Suppl III]:1–199.
2. Zipes DP, DiMarco JP, Gillette PC, et al. Guidelines for clinical intracardiac electrophysiologic and catheter ablation procedures. *Circulation* 1995;92:673–691.
3. Mason JW, for the ESVEM Investigators. A comparison of electrophysiologic testing with Holter monitoring to predict antiarrhythmic efficacy for ventricular tachyarrhythmias. *N Engl J Med* 1993;329:445–451.
4. The CASCADE Investigators. Randomized antiarrhythmic drug therapy in survivors of cardiac arrest. *Am J Cardiol* 1993; 72:280–287.
5. Jackman WM, Wang XZ, Friday KJ, et al. Catheter ablation of accessory and atrioventricular pathways (Wolff-Parkinson-White syndrome) by radiofrequency current. *N Engl J Med* 1991;324:1618–1662.
6. Calkins H, Sousa J, El-Atassi R, et al. Diagnosis and cure of the Wolff-Parkinson-White syndrome or paroxysmal supraventricular tachycardias during a single electrophysiologic test. *N Engl J Med* 1991;324:1612–1618.
7. Lesh MD, Van Hare GF, Epstein LM, et al. Radiofrequency catheter ablation of atrial arrhythmias: results and mechanism. *Circulation* 1994;89:1074–1089.
8. Morady F, Harvey M, Kalfleisch SJ, et al. Radiofrequency catheter ablation of ventricular tachycardia in patients with coronary artery disease. *Circulation* 1993;87:363–372.
9. Kim Y, Sosa-Suarez G, Trouton TG, et al. Treatment of ventricular tachycardia by transcatheter radiofrequency ablation in patients with ischemic heart disease. *Circulation* 1994;89: 1094–1102.
10. Coggins DL, Lee RL, Sweeney J. Radiofrequency catheter ablation as a cure for idiopathic tachycardia of both left and right ventricular origin. *J Am Coll Cardiol* 1994;23:1333–1341.
11. Moss AJ, Hall WJ, Cannom DS. Improved survival with an

implanted defibrillator in patients with coronary disease at high risk for ventricular arrhythmia. *N Engl J Med* 1996;335: 1933–1940.

12. Buxton AE, Kee KL, Fisher JD, et al. A randomized study of the prevention of sudden death in patients with coronary artery disease. *N Engl J Med* 1999;341:1882–1890.

13. Kennedy EE, Rosenfeld LE, McPherson CA, et al. Mechanisms and relevance of arrhythmias induced by high-current programmed ventricular stimulation. *Am J Cardiol* 1986;57: 598–603.

14. Brugada P, Green M, Abdollah H, Wellens HJJ. Significance of ventricular arrhythmias initiated by programmed ventricular stimulation: the importance of the type of ventricular arrhythmia induced and the number of premature stimuli required. *Circulation* 1984:69–87.

15. Ruskin JN, Caracta A, Batsford W, et al. Electrophysiologic effects of diazepam in man. *Clin Res* 1974;22:302A.

16. Nattel S, Rickenberger R, Lehrman L, Zipes D. Therapeutic blood lidocaine concentrations after local anesthesia for cardiac electrophysiologic studies. *N Engl J Med* 1979;30:415–420.

17. Durrer D, van der Tweel LH. The spread of activation in the left ventricular wall of the dog. *Am Heart J* 1953;46:683–691.

18. Steinhaus BM. Estimating cardiac trans-membrane activation and recovery times from unipolar and bipolar extracellular electrograms: a stimulation study. *Circ Res* 1989;64:449–462.

19. Castellanos A Jr, Castillo C, Agha A. Contribution of His bundle recording to the understanding of clinical arrhythmias. *Am J Cardiol* 1971; 28:499.

20. Sherron P, Torres-Arraut E, Tamer D, et al. Site of conduction delay and electrophysiologic significance of first-degree atrioventricular block in children with heart disease. *Am J Cardiol* 1985;55:1323–1327.

21. Benditt DG, Klein GJ, Kriett JM, Dunnigan A, Benson DW Jr. Enhanced atrioventricular nodal conduction in man: electrophysiologic effects of pharmacologic autonomic blockade. *Circulation* 1984;68:1088–1095.

22. Damato AN, Lau SH. Clinical value of the electrogram of the conduction system. *Prog Cardiovasc Dis* 1970; 13(2):119–40.

23. Amat-y-Leon F, Dhingra R, Denes P, et al The clinical spectrum of chronic His bundle block. *Chest* 1976;70:747.

24. Bharati S, Lev M, Wu D, et al. Pathophysiologic correlates in two cases of split His bundle potentials. *Circulation* 1974;47: 776.

25. Kupersmith J, Krongrad E, Waldo A. Conduction intervals and conduction velocity in the human cardiac conduction system. *Circulation* 1973;47:776.

26. Dhingra RC, Palileo E, Strasberg B, et al. Significance of the HV interval in 517 patients with chronic bifascicular block. *Circulation* 1981;64:1265.

27. DiMarco JP, Garan H, Ruskin JN. Complications in patients undergoing cardiac electrophysiologic procedures. *Ann Intern Med* 1982;97:490.

28. Horowitz LN. Safety of electrophysiologic studies. *Circulation* 1986;73:11–28.

29. Epstein MR, Knapp LD, Martindill M, et al. Embolic complications associated with radiofrequency catheter ablation. Atakr Investigator Group. *Am J Cardiol* 1996;77:655–658.

30. Thakur RK, Klein GJ, Yee R, Zardini M. Embolic complications after radiofrequency catheter ablation. *Am J Cardiol* 1994;74:278–279.

31. Hope EJ, Haigney MC, Calkins H, Resar JR. Left main coronary thrombosis after radiofrequency ablation: Successful treatment with percutaneous transluminal angioplasty. *Am Heart J* 1995;129:1217–1219.

32. Pons M, Beck L, Leclercq F, et al. Chronic left main coronary artery occlusion: a complication of radiofrequency ablation of

idiopathic left ventricular tachycardia. *Pacing Clin Electrophysiol* 1997;20:1874–1876.

33. Robbins IM, Colvin EV, Doyle TP, et al. Pulmonary vein stenosis after catheter ablation of atrial fibrillation. *Circulation* 1998; 98:1769–1775.

34. Hindricks G. The Multicenter European Radiofrequency Survey (MERFS): complications of radiofrequency catheter ablation of arrhythmias. *Eur Heart J* 1993;14:1644–1653.

35. Chen SA, Chiang CE, Tai CT, et al. Complications of diagnostic electrophysiologic studies and radiofrequency catheter ablation in patients with tachyarrhythmias: an eight-year survey of 3966 consecutive procedures in a tertiary referral center. *Am J Cardiol* 1996;77:41–46.

36. Reiffel JA, Gang E, Gliklich J, et al. The human sinus node electrogram: a transvenous catheter technique and a comparison of directly measured and indirectly estimated sinoatrial conduction time in adults. *Circulation* 1980;62:1324.

37. Narula OS, Samel P, Javier RP. Significance of the sinus node recovery time. *Circulation* 1972;45:140.

38. Narula OS, Shanto N, Vasquez M, et al. A new method for measurement of sinoatrial conduction time. *Circulation* 1978; 58:706.

39. Heddle WF, Dorveaux LD, Tonkin AM. Use of rapid atrial pacing to assess sinus node function. *Clin Prog Electrophysiol Pacing* 1985;3:299.

40. Strauss HC, Saroff AL, Bigger JT Jr, Giardina EGV. Premature atrial stimulation as a key to the understanding of sinoatrial conduction in man. *Circulation* 1973;47:86.

41. Dhingra RC, Wyndham C, Amat-y-Leon F, et al. Sinus nodal response to atrial extrastimuli in patients without apparent sinus node disease. *Am J Cardiol* 1975;36:445.

42. Guimond C, Puech P. Intra-His bundle blocks (102 cases). *Eur J Cardiol* 1976;4:481.

43. Rosen KM, Rahimtoola SH, Gunnar RM. Pseudo AV block secondary to premature non-propaged His bundle depolarization. *Circulation* 1970;42:367.

44. Scheinman MM, Peters RW, Sauve MJ, et al. Value of the H-Q interval in patients with bundle branch block and the role of prophylactic permanent pacing. *Am J Cardiol* 1982;50:1316.

45. Dhingra RC, Wyndham C, Bauernfeind R, et al. Significance of block distal to the His bundle induced by atrial pacing in patients with chronic bifascicular block. *Circulation* 1979;60: 1455.

46. Scheinman MM, Weiss AN, Shaffar E, et al. Electrophysiologic effects of procainamide in patients with interventricular conduction delay. *Circulation* 1974;49:422.

47. Tonkin AM, Heddle WF, Tornos P. Intermittent atrioventricular block: procainamide administration as a provocative test. *Aust N Z J Med* 1978;8:594.

48. Fujimura O, Yee R, Klein GJ, et al. The diagnostic sensitivity of electrophysiologic testing in patients with syncope caused by a transient bradycardia. *N Engl J Med* 1989;321:1703–1707.

49. Wellens HJJ, Brugada P, Bar FW. Indications for the use of intracardiac electrophysiologic studies for the diagnosis of site of origin and mechanism of tachycardias. *Circulation* 1987;75 [Suppl III]:III-110–III-115.

50. Gallagher JJ, Smith WM, Kasell JH, et al. Role of Mahain fibers in cardiac arrhythmias in man. *Circulation* 1981;64:176.

51. Akhtar M, Damato AN, Ruskin JN, et al. Antegrade and retrograde conduction characteristics in three patterns of paroxysmal atrioventricular junctional reentrant tachycardia. *Am Heart J* 1978;95:22.

52. Coumel P, Attuel P. Reciprocating tachycardia in overt and latent pre-excitation: influence of functional bundle branch block on the rate of the tachycardia. *Eur J Cardiol* 1974;1: 423–431.

53. Hirao K, Otomo K, Wang X, et al. Para-Hisian pacing. A new method for differentiating retrograde conduction over an accessory AV pathway from conduction over the AV node. *Circulation* 1996;94:1027–1035.

54. Wellens HJJ, Bar FWHM, Lie KI. The value of the electrocardiogram in the differential diagnosis of a tachycardia with a widened QRS complex. *Am J Med* 1978;64:27–33.

55. Akhtar M, Shenasa M, Jazayeri M, et al. Wide QRS tachycardia: reappraisal of a common clinical problem. *Ann Intern Med* 1988;109:905–912.

56. Poll DS, Marchlinski FE, Buxton AE, Josephson ME. Sustained ventricular tachycardia in patients with idiopathic dilated cardiomyopathy: electrophysiologic testing and lack of response to antiarrhythmic drug therapy. *Circulation* 1984;70:451–456.

57. Buxton A, Waxman H, Marchlinski F, et al. Right ventricular tachycardia: clinical and electrophysiologic characteristics. *Circulation* 1983;68:917–927.

58. Ruskin JN, DiMarco JP, Garan H. Antiarrhythmic drugs. Out-of-hospital cardiac arrest: electrophysiologic observations and selection of long-term antiarrhythmic therapy. *N Engl J Med* 1980;303:607–613.

59. The Antiarrhythmics Versus Implantable Defibrillators (AVID) Investigators. A comparison of antiarrhythmic drug therapy with implantable defibrillators in patients resuscitated from near-fatal ventricular arrhythmias. *N Engl J Med* 1997;337:1576–1583.

60. Siebels J, Cappato R, Ruppel R, and the CASH Investigators. Preliminary results of the Cardiac Arrest Study Hamburg (CASH). *Am J Cardiol* 1993;72:109F–113F.

61. Connolly SJ, Gent M, Roberts RS, et al. Canadian implantable defibrillator study (CIDS): a randomized trial of the implantable cardioverter defibrillator against amiodarone. *Circulation* 2000;101:1297–1302.

62. Strickberger SA, Man KC, Daoud EG, et al. A prospective evaluation of catheter ablation of ventricular tachycardia as adjuvant therapy in patients with coronary artery disease and an implantable cardioverter-defibrillator. *Circulation* 1997;96:1525–1531.

63. Herre JM, Mann DE, Luck JC, et al. Effect of increased current, multiple pacing sites and number of extrastimuli on induction of ventricular tachycardia. *Am J Cardiol* 1986;57:102–107.

64. Stevenson WG, Wiener I, Weiss JN. Comparison of bipolar and unipolar programmed electrical stimulation for the initiation of ventricular arrhythmias: significance of a nodal excitation during bipolar stimulation. *Circulation* 1986;73:693.

65. Morady F, Kadish A, de Buitlier M, et al. Prospective comparison of a conventional and an accelerated protocol for programmed ventricular stimulation in patients with coronary artery disease. *Circulation* 1991;83:764–773.

66. Estes NAM, Garan H, McGovern B, Ruskin JN. Influence of drive cycle length during programmed stimulation on induction of ventricular arrhythmias: analysis of 403 patients. *Am J Cardiol* 1986;57:108–112.

67. Simonson JS, Gang E, Mandel W, Peter T. Increasing the yield of ventricular tachycardia induction: a prospective, randomized comparative study of the standard ventricular stimulation protocol to a short-to-long protocol and a new two-site protocol. *Am Heart J* 1991;121:68–76.

68. Artoul SG, Fisher JD, Kim SG, et al. Stimulation hierarchy: optimal sequence for double and triple extrastimuli during electrophysiologic studies. *Pacing Clin Electrophysiol* 1992;15:790–800.

69. Cain ME, Martin TC, Marchlinski FE, Josephson ME. Changes in ventricular refractoriness after an extrastimulus: effects of prematurity, cycle length, and procainamide. *Am J Cardiol* 1983;52:996–1002.

70. Freedman R, Swerdlow C, Echt D, et al. Facilitation of ventricular tachyarrhythmia induction by isoproterenol. *Am J Cardiol* 1984;54:765–770.

71. German L, Packer D, Bardy G, Gallagher J. Ventricular tachycardia induced by atrial stimulation in patients without symptomatic cardiac disease. *Am J Cardiol* 1983;52:1202–1207.

72. DeBuitleir M, Morady F, DiCarlo LA, et al. Immediate reproducibility of clinical and nonclinical forms of induced ventricular tachycardia. *Am J Cardiol* 1986;58:279–282.

73. Wilber DJ, Davis MJ, Rosenbaum M, et al. Incidence and determinants of multiple morphologically distinct sustained ventricular tachycardias. *J Am Coll Cardiol* 1987;10:583–591.

74. Kelly P, Ruskin JN, Vlahakes GJ, et al. Surgical coronary revascularization in survivors of prehospital cardiac arrest: its effect on inducible ventricular arrhythmias and long-term survival. *J Am Coll Cardiol* 1990;16:267–273.

75. Miller JM, Kienzle MG, Harken AH, Josephson ME. Subendocardial resection for ventricular tachycardia: predictors of surgical success. *Circulation* 1984;70:624–631.

76. Cao K, Gonska BD. Catheter ablation of incessant ventricular tachycardia: acute and long-term results. *Eur Heart J* 1996;17:756–763.

77. Maron B, Fannapazir L. Sudden cardiac death in hypertrophic cardiomyopathy. *Circulation* 1992;85[Suppl I];I-57–I-63.

78. McKenna W, Camm A. Sudden death in hypertrophic cardiomyopathy: assessment of patients at high risk. *Circulation* 1989;80:1489–1492.

79. Nicod P, Polikar R, Peterson KL. Hypertrophic cardiomyopathy and sudden cardiac death. *N Engl J Med* 1988;318:1255–1257.

80. Watkins H, McKenna WJ, Thierfelder L, et al. Mutations in the genes for cardiac troponin T and alpha-tropomyosin in hypertrophic cardiomyopathy. *N Engl J Med* 1995;332:1058–1064.

81. Watson R, Schwartz J, Maron B, et al. Inducible polymorphic ventricular tachycardia in a subgroup of patients with hypertrophic cardiomyopathy at high risk for sudden death. *J Am Coll Cardiol* 1987;10:761–774.

82. Kuck K, Kunze K, Schluter M, et al. Programmed electrical stimulation in hypertrophic cardiomyopathy: results in patients with and without cardiac arrest or syncope. *Eur Heart J* 1988;9:177–185.

83. Fananapazir L, Tracy C, Leon M, et al. Electrophysiologic abnormalities in patients with hypertrophic cardiomyopathy: a consecutive analysis in 155 patients. *Circulation* 1989;80:1259–1268.

84. Fananapazir L, Change A, Epstein S, McAreavey D. Prognostic determinants in hypertrophic cardiomyopathy: prospective evaluation of a therapeutic strategy based on clinical Holter hemodynamic and electrophysiologic findings. *Circulation* 1992;86:730–740.

85. Tchou P, Jazayeri M, Denker S, et al. Transcatheter electrical ablation of right bundle branch: a method of treating macroreentrant ventricular tachycardia due to bundle branch reentry. *Circulation* 1988;8:246–257.

86. Denker S, Lehman M, Mahmud R, et al. Facilitation of ventricular tachycardia induction with abrupt changes in ventricular cycle length. *Am J Cardiol* 1984;53:508–515.

87. Caceres J, Jazayeri M, McKinnie J, et al. Sustained bundle branch reentry as a mechanism of clinical tachycardia. *Circulation* 1989;79:256–270

88. Brembilla-Perrot B, Donetti J, Terrier de la Chaise A, et al. Diagnostic value of ventricular stimulation in patients with idiopathic dilated cardiomyopathy. *Am Heart J* 1991;121:1124–1131.

89. Liem BL, Swerdlow CD. Value of electrophysiologic testing in idiopathic dilated cardiomyopathy and sustained ventricular tachyarrhythmias. *Am J Cardiol* 1988;62:611–616.

90. Constantin L, Martins JB, Kienzle MG, et al. Induced sustained ventricular tachycardia in nonischemic dilated cardiomyopathy: dependence on clinical presentation and response to antiarrhythmic agents. *Pacing Clin Electrophysiol* 1989;12:776–783.

91. Poll DS, Marchlinski FE, Buxton AE, Josephson ME. Usefulness of programmed stimulation in idiopathic dilated cardiomyopathy. *Am J Cardiol* 1986;58:992–997.

92. Rae AP, Spielman SR, Kutalek S, et al. Electrophysiologic assessment of antiarrhythmic drug efficacy for ventricular tachyarrhythmias associated with dilated cardiomyopathy. *Am J Cardiol* 1987;59:291–295.

93. Leclercq JF, Chouty F, Cauchemez B, et al. Results of electrical fulguration in arrhythmogenic right ventricular disease. *Am J Cardiol* 1988;62:220–224.

94. Brugada J, Brugada P. Right bundle branch block, persistent ST segment elevation and sudden cardiac death: a distinct clinical and electrocardiographic syndrome: a multicenter report. *J Am Coll Cardiol* 1992;20:1391–1396.

95. Belhassen B, Shapira I, Pelleg A, et al. Idiopathic recurrent sustained ventricular tachycardia responsive to verapamil: an ECG-electrophysiologic entity. *Am Heart J* 1984;108:1034–1037.

96. Ohe T, Shimomura K, Aihara N, et al. Idiopathic sustained left ventricular tachycardia: clinical and electrophysiologic characteristics. *Circulation* 1988;77:560–568.

97. German L, Packer D, Bardy G, Gallagher J. Ventricular tachycardia induced by atrial stimulation in patients without symptomatic cardiac disease. *Am J Cardiol* 1983;52:1202–1207.

98. Okumura K, Matsuyama K, Miyagi H, et al. Entrainment of idiopathic ventricular tachycardia of left ventricular origin with evidence for reentry with an area of slow conduction and effect of verapamil. *Am J Cardiol* 1988;62:727–732.

99. Klein L, Shih H, Hackett FK, et al. Radiofrequency catheter ablation of ventricular tachycardia in patients without structural heart disease. *Circulation* 1992;85:1666–1674.

100. Lerman BB, Stein K, Engelstein ED. Mechanism of repetitive monomorphic ventricular tachycardia. *Circulation* 1995;92:421–429.

101. Morady F, Kadish A, Dicarlo L, et al. Long term results of catheter ablation of idiopathic right ventricular tachycardia. *Circulation* 1990;82:2093–2099.

102. Breithardt G, Borggrefe M, Wichter T. Catheter ablation of idiopathic right ventricular tachycardia. *Circulation* 1990;82:2273–2276.

103. Wilber D, Baerman J, Olshansky B, et al. Adenosine-sensitive ventricular tachycardia: clinical characteristics and response to catheter ablation. *Circulation* 1993;87:126–134.

104. Calkins H, Kalbfleish SJ, El-Atassi R, et al. Relation between efficacy of radiofrequency catheter ablation and the site of origin of idiopathic ventricular tachycardia. *Am J Cardiol* 1993;71:827–833.

105. DiMarco JP. Electrophysiologic studies in patients with unexplained syncope. *Circulation* 1987;75[Suppl III]:III-140–III-143.

106. McAnulty JH. Syncope of unknown origin: the role of the electrophysiologic studies. *Circulation* 1987;75[Suppl III]:III-144–III-145.

107. Kapoor WM, Hammill SC, Gersh BJ. Diagnosis and natural history of syncope and the role of invasive electrophysiologic testing. *Am J Med* 1989;63:730–734.

108. Fizri M, Lerman BB, Marchlinski PE, et al. Electrophysiologic evaluation of syncope in patients with bifascicular block. *Am Heart J* 1983;106:693–697.

109. Morady F, Higgins J, Peters RW, et al. Electrophysiologic testing in bundle branch block and unexplained syncope. *Am J Cardiol* 1984;54:587–591.

110. Denes P, Uretz E, Ezri MD, Borbola J. Clinical predictors of electrophysiologic findings in patients with syncope of unknown origin. *Arch Intern Med* 1988;148:1922–1928.

111. Krol RB, Morady F, Flaker GC, et al. Electrophysiologic testing in patients with unexplained syncope: clinical and noninvasive predictors of outcome. *J Am Coll Cardiol* 1987;10:358–363.

112. Bachinsky WB, Linzer M, Weld L, Estes NAM. Usefulness of clinical characteristics in predicting the outcome of electrophysiologic studies in unexplained syncope. *Am J Cardiol* 1992;69:1044–1049.

113. Gomes J, Winters S, Stewart D, et al. A new noninvasive index to predict sustained ventricular tachycardia and sudden death in the first year after myocardial infarction based on signal averaged electrocardiogram, radionuclide ejection fraction and Holter monitoring. *J Am Coll Cardiol* 1987;10:349–357.

114. DeBelder M, Camm A. Use of electrophysiologic studies in patients after myocardial infarction. *J Cardiovasc Electrophysiol* 1991;2:53–64.

115. Bhandari AK, Hong R, Kotlewski A, et al. Prognostic significance of programmed ventricular stimulation in survivors of acute myocardial infarction. *Br Heart J* 1989;61:410–416.

116. Cripps T, Bennett D, Camm A, Ward D. Inducibility of sustained monomorphic ventricular tachycardia as a prognostic indicator in survivors of recent myocardial infarction: a prospective evaluation in relation to other prognostic variables. *J Am Coll Cardiol* 1989;14:289–296.

117. Klein H, Auricchio A, Reek S, Geller C. New primary prevention trials of sudden cardiac death in patients with left ventricular dysfunction: SCD-HEFT and MADIT II. *Am J Cardiol* 1999;83:91D–97D.

118. Kadish A, Quigg R, Schaechter A, et al. Defibrillators in nonischemic cardiomyopathy treatment evaluation. *Pacing Clin Electrophysiol* 2000;23:338–343.

119. Cannom DS. Other primary prevention trials—what is clinically and economically necessary? *J Interv Card Electrophysiol* 2000;4:109–115.

120. Cobb FR, Blumenschein SD, Sealy WC, et al. Successful surgical interruption of the bundle of Kent in a patient with Wolff-Parkinson-White syndrome. *Circulation* 1968;38:1018–1029.

121. Wittig JH, Boineau JP. Surgical treatment of ventricular arrhythmias using epicardial, transmural, and endocardial mapping. *Ann Thorac Surg* 1975;20:117–126.

122. Gepstein L, Hayam G, Ben-Haim SA. A novel method for nonfluoroscopic catheter-based electroanatomical mapping of the heart. *Circulation* 1997;95:1611–1622.

123. Khoury DS, Taccardi B, Lux RL, *Ershler PR, Rudy Y*. Reconstruction of endocardial potentials and activation sequences from intracavitary probe measurements: localization of pacing sites and effects of myocardial structure. *Circulation* 1995;91:845–863.

124. Plonsey R. *Bioelectric phenomenon*. New York: McGraw-Hill, 1969.

125. Spach MS, Miller WT, Geselowitz DB, et al. The discontinuous nature of propagation in normal canine cardiac muscle: evidence for recurrent discontinuities of intracellular resistance that affect the membrane currents. *Circ Res* 1981;48:39–54.

126. Gallagher JJ, Kasell J, Sealy WC, et al. Epicardial mapping in the Wolff-Parkinson-White syndrome. *Circulation* 1978;57:854–866.

127. Haissaguerre M, Warin JF, LeMetayer P, et al. Catheter ablation of Mahaim fibers with preservation of atrioventricular nodal conduction. *Circulation* 1990;82:418–427.

128. Biermann M, Shenasa M, Borggrefe M, et al. The interpretation of cardiac electrograms. In: Shenasa M, Borggrefe M, Breithardt G, eds. *Cardiac mapping*. Mount Kisco, NY: Futura Publishing, 1993:11–34.

129. Anderson KP, Walker R, Fuller M, et al. Criteria for local electrical activation: effects of electrogram characteristics. *IEEE Trans Biomed Eng* 1993;40:169–181.

130. Damiano RJ Jr, Blanchard SM, Asano T, et al. The effects of distant potentials on unipolar electrograms in an animal model utilizing the right ventricular isolation procedure. *J Am Coll Cardiol* 1988;11:1100–1109.

131. Claydon RJ III, Pilkington TC, Ideker RE. Classification of heart tissue from bipolar and unipolar intramural potentials. *IEEE Trans Biomed Eng* 1985;32:513–520.

132. Ziemer RE, Tranter WH. *Principles of communications: systems, modulation, and noise.* Boston: Houghton Mifflin, 1976:68–70.

133. Barr RC, Spach MS. Sampling rates required for digital recording of intracellular and extracellular cardiac potentials. *Circulation* 1977;55:40–48.

134. Ben-Haim SA, Osadchy D, Schuster I. Nonfluoroscopic, in vivo navigation and mapping technology. *Nat Med* 1996;2: 1393–1395.

135. Hindricks G, Kottkamp H, Brunn J. A new three dimensional electromagnetic mapping technology for non-fluoroscopic catheter ablation of left-sided accessory pathways. *Eur Heart J* 1997;18:205.

136. Shah DC, Jais P, Haissaguerre M, Chouairi S, et al. Three dimensional mapping of the common atrial flutter in the right atrium. *Circulation* 1997;96:3901–3912.

137. Hoffmann E, Nimmermann P, Reithmann C, et al. New mapping technology for atrial tachycardias. *J Interv Card Electrophysiol* 2000;4:117–120.

138. Friedman PA, Packer DL, Hammill SC. Catheter ablation of mitral isthmus ventricular tachycardia using electroanatomically guided linear lesions. *J Cardiovasc Electrophysiol* 2000;11: 466–471.

139. Delacretaz E, Stevenson WG, Ganz LI, et al. Entrainment mapping combined with 3D electroanatomic mapping for ablation of multiple atrial macroreentry circuits in adults with repaired congenital heart disease. *Pacing Clin Electrophysiol* 1999;22:892.

140. Dorostkar PC, Cheng JIE, Scheinman MM. Electroanatomical mapping and ablation of the substrate supporting intraatrial reentrant tachycardia after palliation for complex congenital heart disease. *Pacing Clin Electrophysiol* 1998;21:1810–1819.

141. Shah DC, Haissaguerre M, Jais P, et al. High-density mapping of activation through an incomplete isthmus ablation line. *Circulation* 1999;99:211–215.

142. Rudy Y, Messinger-Rapport BJ. The inverse problem in electrocardiography: solutions in terms of epicardial potentials. *Crit Rev Biomed Eng* 1988;16:214–268.

143. Khoury DS, Rudy Y. A model study of volume conductor effects on endocardial and intracavitary potentials. *Circ Res* 1992;71:511–525.

144. Schilling RJ, Peters NS, Davies DW. Noncontact mapping of cardiac arrhythmias. *J Electrocardiol* 1999;32:13–15

145. Schneider MA, Ndrepepa G, Zrenner B, et al. Noncontact mapping-guided catheter ablation of atrial fibrillation associated with left atrial ectopy. *J Cardiovasc Electrophysiol* 2000;11: 475–479.

146. Kadish A, Schilling RC, Peters NS. Endocardial mapping of human atrial fibrillation using a novel non-contact mapping system. *Pacing Clin Electrophysiol* 1997;20:1063.

147. Schilling RC, Peters NS, Davies DW. Feasibility of a noncontact catheter for endocardial mapping of human ventricular tachycardia. *Circulation* 1999;99:2543–2552.

148. Strickberger SA, Knight BP, Michaud GF, et al. Mapping and ablation of ventricular tachycardia guided by virtual electrograms using a noncontact computerized mapping system. *J Am Coll Cardiol* 2000;35:414–421.

149. Crossen KJ, Lindsay BD, Cain ME. Reliability of retrograde atrial activation patterns during ventricular pacing for localizing accessory pathways. *J Am Coll Cardiol* 1987;9:1279–1287.

150. Jackman WM, Friday KJ, Yeung-Lai-Wah JA, et al. New

catheter technique for recording left free-wall accessory atrioventricular pathway activation: identification of pathway fiber orientation. *Circulation* 1988;78:598–610.

151. Lesh MD, Van Hare GF, Schamp DJ, et al. Curative percutaneous catheter ablation using radiofrequency energy for accessory pathways in all locations: results in 100 consecutive patients. *J Am Coll Cardiol* 1992;19:1303–1309.

152. Epstein AE, Kirklin JK, Holman WL, et al. Intermediate septal accessory pathways: electrocardiographic characteristics, electrophysiologic observations and their surgical implications. *J Am Coll Cardiol* 1991;17:1570–1578.

153. Denes P, Wyndham CR, Amat-Y-Leon F, et al. Atrial pacing at multiple sites in the Wolff-Parkinson-White syndrome. *Br Heart J* 1977;39:506–514.

154. Mitchell LB, Mason JW, Scheinman MM, et al. Recordings of basal ventricular preexcitation from electrode catheters in patients with accessory atrioventricular connections. *Circulation* 1984;69:233–241.

155. Chen A, Broggrefe M, Shenasa M, et al. Characteristics of local electrogram predicting successful radiofrequency ablation of left-sided accessory pathways. *J Am Coll Cardiol* 1992;20: 656–665.

156. Calkins H, Kim Y-N, Schmaltz S, et al. Electrogram criteria for identification of appropriate target sites for radiofrequency catheter ablation of accessory atrioventricular connections. *Circulation* 1992;85:565–573.

157. Jackman WM, Friday KJ, Scherlag BJ, et al. Direct endocardial recording from an accessory atrioventricular pathway: localization of the site of block, effect of antiarrhythmic drugs, and attempt at nonsurgical ablation. *Circulation* 1983;69:906–915.

158. Kuck KH, Schluter M. Single-catheter approach to radiofrequency current ablation of left-sided accessory pathways in patients with Wolff-Parkinson-White syndrome. *Circulation* 1991;84:2366–2375.

159. Haissaguerre M, Dartigues JF, Warin JF, et al. Electrogram patterns predictive of successful catheter ablation of accessory pathways: value of unipolar recording. *Circulation* 1991;84:188–202.

160. Kottkamp H, Hindricks G, Shenasa H, et al. Variants of preexcitation: specialized atriofascicular pathways, nodofascicular pathways, and fasciculoventricular pathways: electrophysiologic findings and target sites for radiofrequency catheter ablation. *J Cardiovasc Electrophysiol* 1996;7:916–930.

161. Sung RJ, Waxman HL, Saksena S, Juma Z. Sequence of retrograde atrial activation in patients with dual atrioventricular nodal pathways. *Circulation* 1981;64:1059–1067.

162. Haissaguerre M, Warin JF, Lemetayer P, et al. Closed-chest ablation of retrograde conduction in patients with atrioventricular nodal reentrant tachycardia. *N Engl J Med* 1989;320:426–433.

163. Jackman WM, Beckman KJ, McClelland JH, et al. Treatment of supraventricular tachycardia due to atrioventricular nodal reentry by radiofrequency catheter ablation of slow-pathway conduction. *N Engl J Med* 1992;327:313–318.

164. Haissaguerre M, Gaita F, Fischer B, et al. Elimination of atrioventricular nodal reentrant tachycardia using discrete slow potentials to guide application of radiofrequency energy. *Circulation* 1992;85:2162–2175.

165. Hazlitt HA, Beckman KJ, McClelland JH, et al. Prevalence of slow AV nodal pathway potentials in patients without AV nodal reentrant tachycardia. *J Am Coll Cardiol* 1993;21[Suppl II]: 281A.

166. Walsh EP, Saul P, Hulse JE, et al. Transcatheter ablation of ectopic atrial tachycardia in young patients using radiofrequency current. *Circulation* 1992;86:1138–1146.

167. Kay GN, Chong F, Epstein AE, et al. Radiofrequency ablation for treatment of primary atrial tachycardias. *J Am Coll Cardiol* 1993;21:901–909.

168. Tracy CM, Swartz JF, Fletcher RD, et al. Radiofrequency catheter ablation of ectopic atrial tachycardia using paced activation sequence mapping. *J Am Coll Cardiol* 1993;21:910–917.

169. Disertori M, Inama G, Vergara G, et al. Evidence of a reentry circuit in the common type of atrial flutter in man. *Circulation* 1983;67:434–440.

170. Cosio FG, Arribas F, Barbero JM, et al. Validation of double-spike electrograms as markers of conduction delay or block in atrial flutter. *Am J Cardiol* 1988;61:775–780.

171. Olshansky B, Okumura K, Hess PG, Waldo AL. Demonstration of an area of slow conduction in human atrial flutter. *J Am Coll Cardiol* 1990;16:1639–1648.

172. Feld GK, Fleck RP, Shen P-S, et al. Radiofrequency catheter ablation for the treatment of human type I atrial flutter: identification of a critical zone in the reentrant circuit by endocardial mapping techniques. *Circulation* 1992;86:1233–1240.

173. Cosio FG, Arribas F, Palacios J, et al. Fragmented electrograms and continuous electrical activity in atrial flutter. *Am J Cardiol* 1986;57:1309–1314.

174. Cosio FG, Lopez-Gil M, Goicolea A, et al. Radiofrequency ablation of the inferior vena cava-tricuspid valve isthmus in common atrial flutter. *Am J Cardiol* 1993;71:705–709.

175. Cosio FG, Goicolea A, Lopez-Gil M, et al. Atrial endocardial mapping in the rare form of atrial flutter. *Am J Cardiol* 1990;66:715–720.

176. Cheng J, Cabeen WR, Scheinman MM. Right atrial flutter due to lower loop reentry. *Circulation* 1999;99:1700–1705.

177. Kall JG, Rubenstein DS, Kopp DE, et al. Atypical flutter originating in the right atrial free wall. *Circulation* 2000;101:270–279.

178. Jais P, Shah DC, Haissaguerre M, et al. Mapping and ablation of left atrial flutters. *Circulation* 2000;101:2928–2934.

179. Kuchar DL, Ruskin JN, Garan H. Electrocardiographic localization of the site of origin of ventricular tachycardia in patients with prior myocardial infarction. *J Am Coll Cardiol* 1989;13:893–900.

180. Kadish AH, Childs K, Schmaltz S, Morady F. Differences in QRS configuration during unipolar pacing from adjacent sites: implications for the spatial resolution of pace-mapping. *J Am Coll Cardiol* 1991;17:143–151.

181. Sippens-Groenewegen A, Spekhorst H, van Hemel NM, et al. Localization of the site of origin of postinfarction ventricular tachycardia by endocardial pace mapping. *Circulation* 1993;88:2290–2306.

182. Josephson ME, Horowitz LN, Spielman SR, et al. Comparison of endocardial catheter mapping with intraoperative mapping of ventricular tachycardia. *Circulation* 1980;61:395–404.

183. Brugada P, Abdollah H, Wellens HJJ. Continuous electrical activity during sustained monomorphic ventricular tachycardia. *Am J Cardiol* 1985;55:402–411.

184. Fitzgeral DM, Friday KJ, Yeung Lai Wah JA, et al. Electrogram patterns predicting successful catheter ablation of ventricular tachycardia. *Circulation* 1988;77:806–814.

185. Josephson ME, Horowitz LN, Farshidi A. Continuous local electrical activity. *Circulation* 1978;57:659–665.

186. Morady F, Frank R, Kou WH, et al. Identification and catheter ablation of a zone of slow conduction in the reentrant circuit of ventricular tachycardia in humans. *J Am Coll Cardiol* 1988;11:775–782.

187. Stevenson WG, Weiss JN, Wiener I, et al. Resetting of ventricular tachycardia: implications for localizing the area of slow conduction. *J Am Coll Cardiol* 1988;11:522–529.

188. Ideker RE, Lofland GK, Bardy GH, et al. Late fractionated potentials and continuous electrical activity caused by electrode motion. *Pacing Clin Electrophysiol* 1983;6:908–914.

189. Morady F, Kadish A, Rosenheck S, et al. Concealed entrainment as a guide for catheter ablation of ventricular tachycardia in patients with prior myocardial infarction. *J Am Coll Cardiol* 1991;17:678–689.

190. Stevenson WG, Sager PT, Friedman PL. Entrainment techniques for mapping atrial and ventricular tachycardias. *J Cardiovasc Electrophysiol* 1995;6:201–206.

191. Hadjis TA, Hasada T, Stevenson WG, et al. Effects of recording site on postpacing interval measurement during catheter mapping and entrainment of postinfarction ventricular tachycardia. *J Cardiolvasc Electrophysiol* 1997;8:398–404.

192. Bogun F, Knight B, Goyal R, et al. Clinical value of the postpacing interval for mapping of ventricular tachycardia in patients with prior myocardial infarction. *J Cardiovasc Electrophysiol* 1999;10:43–51.

193. Rankin AC, Osswald S, McGovern BA, et al. Mechanism of sustained monomorphic ventricular tachycardia in systemic sclerosis. *Am J Cardiol* 1999;83:633–636.

194. Cassidy DM, Vassallo JA, Buxton AE, et al. The value of catheter mapping during sinus rhythm to localize site of origin of ventricular tachycardia. *Circulation* 1984;69:1103–1110.

195. Cassidy DM, Vasallo JA, Miller JM. Endocardial catheter mapping in patients in sinus rhythm: relationship to underlying heart disease and ventricular arrhythmias. *Circulation* 1986;73:645–652.

196. Kienzle MG, Miller J, Falcone RA, Harken A, Josephson ME. Intraoperative endocardial mapping during sinus rhythm: relationship to site of origin of ventricular tachycardia. *Circulation* 1984;70:957–965.

197. Marchlinski FE, Callans DJ, Gottlieb CD, Zado E. Linear ablation lesions for control of unmappable ventricular tachycardia in patients with ischemic and nonischemic cardiomyopathy. *Circulation* 2000;101:1288–1296.

198. Downar E, Harris L, Mickleborough LL, et al. Endocardial mapping of ventricular tachycardia in the intact human ventricle: evidence for reentrant mechanisms. *J Am Coll Cardiol* 1988;11:783–791.

199. Downar E, Kimber S, Harris L, et al. Endocardial mapping of ventricular tachycardia in the intact human heart: evidence for multiuse reentry in a functional sheet of surviving myocardium. *J Am Coll Cardiol* 1992;20:869–878.

200. Kramer JB, Saffitz JE, Witkowski FX, Corr PB. Intramural reentry as a mechanism of ventricular tachycardia during evolving canine myocardial infarction. *Circ Res* 1985;56:736–754.

201. Garan H, Fallon JT, Rosenthal S, Ruskin JN. Endocardial, intramural, and epicardial activation patterns during sustained monomorphic ventricular tachycardia in late canine myocardial infarction. *Circ Res* 1987;60:879–896.

202. Littman L, Svenson RH, Gallagher JJ, et al. Functional role of the epicardium in postinfarction ventricular tachycardia: observations derived from computerized epicardial activation mapping, entrainment, and epicardial laser photoablation. *Circulation* 1991;83:1577–1591.

203. Sosa E, Scanavacca M, D'Avila A, et al. Radiofrequency catheter ablation of ventricular tachycardia guided by nonsurgical epicardial mapping in chronic Chagasic heart disease. *Pacing Clin Electrophysiol* 1999;22:128–130.

204. Tomassoni G, Stanton M, Richey M, et al. Epicardial mapping and radiofrequency ablation of ischemic ventricular tachycardia using a three-dimensional nonfluoroscopic mapping system. *J Cardiovasc Electrophysiol* 1999;10:1643–1648.

SECTION

III

THERAPEUTIC MODALITIES

8

ANTIARRHYTHMIC AGENTS

GERALD V. NACCARELLI
PHILIP T. SAGER
BRAMAH N. SINGH

PHARMACOKINETIC AND PHARMACODYNAMIC PRINCIPLES OF ANTIARRHYTHMIC AGENTS

Antiarrhythmic agents have a relatively narrow window between therapeutic and toxic effects: Small decreases in plasma concentration can result in arrhythmia recurrence while increases in plasma concentrations can cause toxicity. By understanding a drug's pharmacokinetics, the clinician can optimize proper dosing to maximize benefits and reduce risks. Plasma concentrations of an antiarrhythmic drug will be affected by absorption, distribution, metabolism, and excretion. Several factors may affect the plasma drug concentration in an individual patient.

1. Disease states can affect the rate or extent of absorption.
2. Distribution is often affected by alterations in protein binding.
3. Changes in renal and hepatic function may prolong the time it takes to remove a drug from the body.
4. Absorption, distribution, metabolism, and excretion can be affected by other drugs that the patient is taking (i.e., drug-drug interactions).

Absorption

Most absorption occurs in the small intestine and this process is relatively rapid after drug ingestion with a half-life of approximately 20 to 40 minutes. Absorption can range from less than 50% to more than 90% and can be altered by concomitant food or drug ingestion, pH level, bowel motility, malabsorption syndromes, and other factors. Absorption can also be modulated by certain disease

states (e.g., congestive heart failure [CHF] can cause bowel edema, which can substantially reduce drug absorption). Different preparations of the same drug can have marked variability in the rates of absorption because of the capsule or tablet properties, which may be of major clinical significance if the patient changes antiarrhythmic drug brands (1). Slow-release forms of agents (e.g., procainamide and disopyramide) have been developed using a nonabsorbable matrix to slow the rates of intestinal absorption. Drug absorption is usually a fairly rapid process; however, the rate and extent of absorption may be affected by gastric and bowel pH level, bowel bacterial flora, concomitant food intake, bowel motility, or other drugs.

Bioavailability

Bioavailability is the percentage of drug that reaches the systemic circulation after absorption and first-pass metabolism, predominantly in the liver and to a lesser extent in the intestinal wall. Drugs that undergo extensive "first-pass" metabolism, such as propranolol and verapamil, need to be administered in much greater quantities when given orally, compared with intravenous administration.

The systemic circulation distributes the drug to the various compartments. The volume of distribution indicates the extent a drug distributes into body fluids and tissues. Once a drug reaches the systemic circulation, it will be distributed extravascularly and intracellularly, usually consistent with a two-compartment model (2–4). The degree to which a drug enters cells and tissues depends on its lipid solubility and the extent to which the agent is bound to proteins within the systemic circulation and the cellular surface (2). After drug administration, agents that functionally have two-compartment distribution exhibit an initial phase of rapid reduction in drug levels (the alpha phase) secondary to distribution to the peripheral compartment followed by a more gradual reduction in plasma concentration resulting from elimination (the beta phase) (4). The volume

G. V. Naccarelli: Division of Cardiology, Penn State University, College of Medicine, Hershey, Pennsylvania 17033.
P. T. Sager and B. N. Singh: UCLA School of Medicine, and VA Greater Los Angeles Healthcare System, Los Angeles, California 90073.

of distribution is a measure of the extent of a drug's extravascular distribution and represents the volume by which the drug would have to be diluted to obtain the plasma concentration observed before the drug has undergone any elimination.

Many drugs bind to plasma proteins, which reduce the availability of the drug to interact with cardiac channels or receptors. Drug assays usually measure the bound and unbound drug concentration and do not reflect the amount of drug available to cardiac targets. In most cases, this is not a problem because the percentage of a drug bound to plasma proteins is relatively constant. However, concomitant drug administration can alter plasma protein binding. In the case of disopyramide, propafenone, and lidocaine, protein binding can become saturated, and increases in drug dosing will result in significantly greater augmentation of the plasma-free drug concentration available to interact with cardiac targets.

Another important pharmacokinetic parameter is clearance, which is the ability of the body to remove drugs from the blood. Clearance represents the volume of blood from which the drug is removed during a specific period. A drug's clearance and volume of distribution determine the rate of removal from the body. Clearance represents the sum of the different processes by which a drug is eliminated and is a function of the half-life (clearance = [volume distribution] × [0.693/half-life]). First-pass clearance may be affected by CHF with decreased perfusion of the liver, cirrhosis, inherited metabolism phenotype, and drug interactions altering metabolism.

Metabolism

Enzymatic metabolism of a drug is genetically determined (2–4). Several antiarrhythmic drugs undergo biotransformation by hepatic oxidative metabolism through the cytochrome P450 system. Cimetidine and amiodarone inhibit the cytochrome P450 enzymes (CYP), causing an increased concentration of certain drugs when used concomitantly. Phenytoin and phenobarbital induce the P450 system, resulting in an increased metabolism of some antiarrhythmics. CYP D6 is the major enzyme system for biotransforming propafenone, flecainide, acebutolol, metoprolol, and propranolol. Most patients are "extensive metabolizers," and the remaining 5% to 10% of the population, who have reduced amounts of the CYP D6, are labeled "poor metabolizers." Many serotonin uptake inhibitors (including paroxetine [Paxil] and fluoxetine [Prozac]) and quinidine inhibit this enzyme (4). CYP A4 is the most prevalent enzyme in the liver and metabolizes many drugs including quinidine, lidocaine, and mexiletine, as well as many calcium channel blockers, terfenadine, and cyclosporine. The enzyme is inhibited by cimetidine, erythromycin, ketoconazole, and grapefruit juice, and its activity is augmented by rifampin and phenytoin. In patients

taking terfenadine, the concomitant administration of erythromycin or drinking grapefruit juice has been associated with the development of torsade de pointes, probably secondary to reductions in CYP A4 activity and increased terfenadine-induced prolongation of repolarization (5,6).

Drugs such as procainamide are metabolized by *N*-acetyltransferase. About 50% of blacks and whites and 90% of Asians are rapid acetylators. Many drugs have active metabolites. The time to reach steady state will be determined by the half-life of the active metabolite if it has a longer half-life than that of the parent compound. This is typical for drugs such as propafenone and acebutolol. Although loading doses of antiarrhythmic agents are often used to treat patients with clinical cardiac arrhythmias, this approach may not decrease the amount of time it takes to reach pharmacologic steady state.

Elimination

Most drugs follow a first-order elimination process. First-order elimination kinetics refers to a process in which the amount of drug in the body diminishes logarithmically over time. This means that the fraction of a drug in the body eliminated during a period of time remains constant. The time it takes to get one half, or 50%, of the drug eliminated from this initial compartment is referred to as the β half-life. One would expect the serum drug concentration to decline by one half during the period known as *the elimination half-life*. After a drug is discontinued, it will take approximately four to five half-lives before it is almost completely removed (93% to 97%) from the body. With drugs that follow first-order elimination, if the dose given is doubled, the serum drug concentrations will also double. Some drugs, such as disopyramide and propafenone, follow nonlinear or dose-dependent pharmacokinetics; in this situation, doubling the dose may increase serum concentrations by more than a factor of two, leading to toxicity.

In CHF, the volume of distribution may be decreased by as much as 40% and drug clearances may be diminished because of decreased renal or hepatic blood flow and reduced hepatic enzyme activity (2). These changes may prolong elimination half-life and require a reduction of the dose to avoid toxicity.

RECEPTOR PHYSIOLOGY

The interaction of antiarrhythmic agents with cardiac ionic substrates results in modulation of refractoriness, conduction, and cable properties of cardiac cells. As an overview, antiarrhythmic agents appear to prevent or terminate reentrant arrhythmias by prolonging the wavelength (by prolonging the refractory period, usually by increasing the action potential duration [APD]) to such a degree that the advancing wavefront encounters refractory tissue. Conduction slowing, by shortening the wavelength (wavelength = [refractory period] × [conduction velocity]), can result in stabilization of reentry and is thought to be the major mechanism for proarrhythmia seen in patients receiving some antiarrhythmic drugs, such as propafenone or flecainide. There is an important interplay between a drug's actions on refractoriness and conduction, affecting the antiarrhythmic and proarrhythmic properties of an agent. When flecainide was studied in canine investigations of atrial fibrillation, arrhythmia termination was related to the degree that flecainide increased the atrial APD and refractory period, compared with slowing conduction. In addition, recent mapping studies show a significant source-sink mismatch where the reentrant circuit turns (i.e., the pivot point) that is associated with conduction slowing and alterations in cardiac action potential characteristics (7). Further drug-induced increases in this mismatch may result in prevention or termination of reentry.

Antiarrhythmic agents bind to specific cell membrane channels, receptors, and cellular pumps, resulting in alterations in the flow of ions across the cell membrane and subsequent changes in the action potential characteristics, causing modulation of cardiac conduction, refractoriness, excitability, and impulse formation (8,9,10). The autonomic nervous system plays an important role in the genesis of cardiac arrhythmias and β-adrenergic, α-adrenergic, muscarinic, and purinergic receptors modulate the actions of ionic channels and pumps. Drugs usually reduce ionic currents, but in some instances, drugs may increase ion flow through channels, possibly by interfering with channel closing. For example, ibutilide increases the slow inward sodium current (I_{Na}) (11–13), and adenosine triphosphate (ATP)–sensitive potassium channel activators (e.g., pinacidil) increase repolarizing potassium currents (14). Some agents work entirely (β blockers) or in part (e.g., d,l-sotalol, which blocks potassium channels and is a β receptor blocker) by interaction with cellular receptors to modify membrane ionic fluxes. Cardiac receptors are coupled to G proteins, which modulate physiologic responses by activation of a protein kinase with subsequent phosphorylation of proteins altering the function of an ionic channel or by linking receptors to second messenger systems or directly to pumps.

Antiarrhythmic drug actions are usually the summation of the effects of the agent on multiple channels or receptors. For example, amiodarone has a complex pharmacologic profile. It inhibits the fast inward sodium current, repolarizing potassium currents, inward calcium currents, and exerts antiadrenergic actions and alters thyroid homeostasis. d,l-Sotalol blocks β receptors at lower doses than those that result in significant effects on repolarization, resulting from potassium channel blockade.

Antiarrhythmic drugs can only bind to the channel during specific phases of the cardiac action potential, corresponding to specific conformational states of the channel (8–10). In the resting state, ionic current is not being passed through the channel, and in the open state, the channel has undergone conformational changes so ions can pass through the channel. The inactivated state follows the open state as an intermediate stage during which ions can no longer traverse the channel because the gates that modulate ionic flow have closed (Fig. 8-1). Most antiarrhythmic agents appear to bind to channels during only one or two of the states and disassociate from the channel during the other state(s). For example, quinidine largely binds during the open states and dissociates during the resting state. The effects of pharmacologic agents on cardiac electrophysiology are modulated by factors that influence the access to channel-binding sites. Many channels have rectification, which means they largely permit ions to pass in only one direction.

Drugs bind to channels with certain onset-offset kinetics and this has been worked out for blockers of the fast inward sodium current, I_{Na} (8). Agents with slow kinetics (class Ic drugs such as flecainide and propafenone) have the most potent sodium channel-blocking activity and this action will be augmented to the greatest degree during rapid heart rates (see discussion of frequency dependence). Class Ia

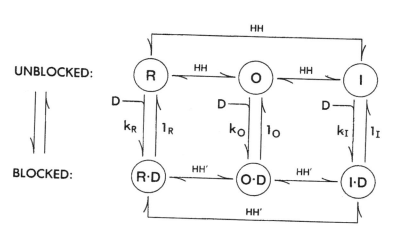

FIGURE 8-1. Schematic diagram of a simplified state-dependent drug-receptor mechanism for channel blockade. Unblocked ion channels, such as sodium channels, are assumed to cycle through three states: rested *(R)*, open *(0)*, and inactivated *(I)*, according to Hodgkin-Huxley kinetics *(HH)*. A channel-blocking drug *(D)* can combine with the channel receptor in any of the three states, resulting in drug-complexed channels such as R.D, O.D, and I.D, which are incapable of conducting ionic current (blocked). The drug-receptor interaction is governed by association and dissociation rate constants (k and l) that are different for each state. The blocked channels can cycle between states and may recover with modified Hodgkin-Huxley kinetics *(HH')*. Recovery from the I.D to the R.D state is made difficult by an apparent shift of the normal recovery curve to more negative potentials. (From Naccarelli G. Antiarrhythmic drugs. In: Willerson JT, Cohn J, eds. *Cardiovascular medicine,* 2nd ed. Philadelphia: WB Saunders, 2000:1632–1649, with permission.)

agents (such as quinidine, procainamide, and disopyramide) have moderate onset-offset kinetics while class Ib agents (such as lidocaine, tocainide, and mexiletine) have rapid kinetics producing the least degree of sodium channel blockade. This difference in the kinetics of drug channel binding and dissociation can result in remarkable differences in drug action as a function of heart rate (i.e., frequency dependence).

Antiarrhythmic agents may exert different electrophysiologic actions in the atria and the ventricles because of differences in cellular ionic currents and action potential characteristics. For example, flecainide prolongs the atrial APD but has little effect on this parameter in the ventricle, probably because of differences in ionic currents. Mexiletine largely binds to ionic channels during the APD plateau, and because phase 2 is abbreviated in atrial cells, compared with ventricular cells, this agent exerts little electrophysiologic effects in the atria.

Frequency Dependence

Drug binding to the sodium channel occurs during the open state (phase 0) and during the action potential plateau (phase 2) and dissociation occurs during diastole (phase 4) (8–10). During tachycardia, the diastolic internal (phase 4) is reduced to a greater degree than the action potential plateau (phase 2), and the number of depolarizations and phase 0 states are increased per unit of time. Subsequently, during rapid heart rates, there is less time for dissociation during phase 4 and more opportunity for phase 0 binding, and cells spend proportionally less time in phase 4, which is when dissociation usually occurs (Fig. 8-2). Tachycardia results in enhanced conduction slowing and a widened QRS complex during treatment with sodium channel blockers secondary to enhanced drug channel binding (Fig. 8-3). Therefore, the effects of a drug on cardiac cells are dependent on processes that directly effect drug binding and dissociation. Rate-related conduction slowing is seen to

a greater degree with class Ic agents, compared with class Ia or class Ib agents, because of the slower dissociation kinetics of class Ic drugs. Frequency dependence of sodium channel blockade may be observed clinically during pacing (15–17) or exercise (18), and sinus tachycardia–induced conduction slowing has been associated with the development of sustained monomorphic ventricular tachycardia (VT) in patients receiving class Ic agents (18). Drug binding may also be voltage-dependent, which means that binding is influenced by the resting membrane voltage of the action potential. Thus, certain situations, such as ischemia-induced increases in the resting membrane potential, can have significant effects on drug binding and the pharmacologic actions of antiarrhythmic agents (19,20). For example, lidocaine slows conduction to a greater degree in partially depolarized cells versus normal cells, such as occurs during ischemia (9).

Drug-induced prolongation of repolarization by blocking potassium channels usually results in a substantially different frequency-dependent profile than that of sodium channel blockers (21–23). Most class III agents, such as dofetilide (24), sematilide (21), and sotalol (25), prolong repolarization to a greater degree during bradycardia than during tachycardia (reverse frequency dependence; Fig. 8-4). Enhanced repolarization and APD prolongation during bradycardia can lead to torsade de pointes while attenuation in drug-induced prolongation of repolarization during the rapid heart rates commonly associated with clinical tachycardias may result in drug inefficacy to terminate or prevent tachycardia initiation (22–23).

There are significant differences between the individual class III agents in their proclivity to exhibit reverse frequency-dependent effects. Agents that work primarily by blocking I_{Kr} have the greatest degree of reverse frequency dependence (e.g., dofetilide [24] and sematilide [21]) while agents that also block I_{Ks} (e.g., azimilide [26] or ambasilide [27,28]) appear to have limited frequency dependence. Amiodarone (which blocks I_{Ks}, I_{Kr}, I_{K1}, and I_{CA}) is devoid

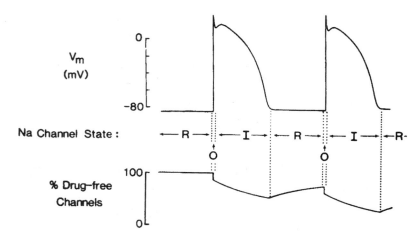

FIGURE 8-2. Schematic illustration of the time-dependent changes in sodium *(Na)* channel states, rested *(R)*, open *(0)*, and inactivated *(I)*, associated with cardiac action potentials **(top)** and the resulting changing level of block **(bottom)** by a local anesthetic–type antiarrhythmic drug. Note that this drug causes some block during the open channel state (upstroke of the action potential) and additional block during the inactivated state (plateau). During diastole, partial recovery from block occurs because the affinity of the drug for rested channels is low. (From Clarkson CW, Hondeghem LM. Mechanism for bupivacaine depression of cardiac conduction: fast block of sodium channels during the action potential with slow recovery from block. *Anesthesiology* 1985;62:396, with permission.)

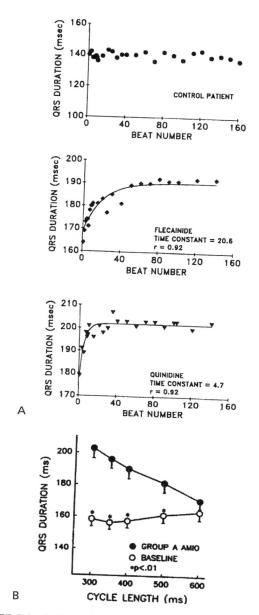

FIGURE 8-3. A: Plots of the kinetics of QRS duration prolongation during the initiation of ventricular pacing (400 ms) in patients in the antiarrhythmic drug-free state **(top)**, in patients receiving flecainide **(middle)**, and in patients receiving quinidine **(bottom).** Onset-time kinetics for the best-fit nonlinear regression line (*shown*) are in number of beats. (From Villemaire C, Talajic M, Nattel S. Mechanisms by which sotalol prevents atrial fibrillation at doses that fail to terminate the arrhythmia. *Circulation* 1997;96(8)[Suppl]:I236(abst), with permission.) **B:** Graph shows the frequency-dependent effects of amiodarone on the QRS duration during ventricular pacing, demonstrating significant frequency-dependent prolongation of this parameter during rapid pacing. (From Buchanan LV, Le MR, Walters RR, et al. Antiarrhythmic and electrophysiologic effects of intravenous ibutilide and sotalol in the canine sterile pericarditis model. *J Cardiovasc Electrophysiol* 1996;7:113–119, with permission.)

of reverse frequency dependence (15,29) and this property may explain, in part, the agent's low incidence of proarrhythmia and high degree of efficacy. Compared with other agents, in the atrium, flecainide and propafenone exhibit positive frequency-dependent effects on repolarization, increasing the APD to a greater degree during tachycardia than during bradycardia (30), and this may play a significant mechanistic role in their ability to terminate recent-onset atrial fibrillation. Frequency dependence may be important regarding the risks associated with prolongation of repolarization (torsade de pointes) and may explain differences between a drug's ability to prevent an arrhythmia (when repolarization is significantly prolonged during normal resting heart rates) and its ability to terminate a reentrant tachycardia (when the drug's electrophysiologic actions on repolarization may be markedly attenuated). In an experimental study, azimilide did not exhibit frequency-dependent effects on repolarization and was significantly more effective in terminating atrial fibrillation than sotalol, whose actions to prolong repolarization were attenuated at rapid heart rates (31). When ibutilide was compared with d,l-sotalol in a multicenter trial examining the ability of these agents to terminate atrial fibrillation, ibutilide was significantly more efficacious than d,l-sotalol (32). This finding may be related to the observation that ibutilide is devoid of frequency-dependent effects whereas d,l-sotalol–induced prolongation of the atrial APD is markedly reduced during rapid heart rates (33–35). However, the presence of reverse frequency-dependent effects on repolarization does not indicate that an agent will be clinically ineffective. Dofetilide has reverse frequency dependence and has been shown to be a clinically effective therapy to terminate and prevent atrial fibrillation (36,37).

In contrast to sodium channel blockade, the mechanisms responsible for reverse frequency dependence of potassium channel blockers on repolarization do not appear to be secondary to drug channel binding. Many of these agents prolong repolarization by blocking the rapidly activating component of the delayed rectifier potassium current, I_{Kr}, during rapid heart rates. However, at fast rates, because of the kinetics of inactivation of the slowly activating component of the delayed rectifier potassium current (I_{Ks}), there is insufficient time for I_{Ks} to fully deactivate and there is a buildup of repolarizing potassium current (38). This results in APD shortening that overwhelms the APD-prolonging effects of I_{Kr} blockade. In addition, a buildup of potassium in the intracellular clefts may enhance potassium repolarizing currents

Proarrhythmia

Ventricular Proarrhythmia

Proarrhythmic effects of antiarrhythmic agents have been variously defined as an increase in ventricular ectopy, runs

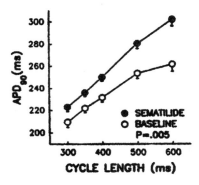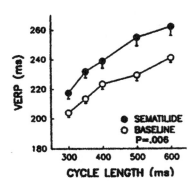

FIGURE 8-4. Graphs showing the frequency-dependent effects of sematilide on the action potential duration (APD_{90}) and the right ventricular effective refractory period *(RVERP)*. Sematilide significantly increased the APD_{90} and the RVERP to a greater extent at longer cycle lengths than at shorter paced cycle lengths ($p \le 0.05$, repeated measures analysis of variance). (From Velebit V, Podrid PJ, Cohen B, et al. Aggravation and provocation of ventricular arrhythmia by antiarrhythmic drugs. *Circulation* 1982;65: 886, with permission.)

of nonsustained VT, new sustained monomorphic VT, ventricular fibrillation (VF), or torsade de pointes (39,40). It has been hypothesized that sustained monomorphic VT observed during treatment with class Ic or class Ia agents is secondary to the effects of sodium channel blockade–induced conduction slowing and stabilization of reentrant circuits, whereas torsade de pointes is usually secondary to action potential prolongation and calcium-induced afterdepolarizations (41). Irrespective of the mechanism, drug-induced proarrhythmia is markedly increased in patients with CHF, significant structural heart disease, and clinical sustained ventricular tachyarrhythmias (42–46). Additionally, changes in pharmacokinetics, such as decreased clearance of a drug, resulting in increased plasma concentrations can cause proarrhythmia while alterations in underlying cardiac substrate (e.g., development of CHF) may increase the proarrhythmic risks of antiarrhythmic therapy.

Monomorphic Ventricular Tachycardia

The development of new monomorphic VT can be observed with any antiarrhythmic agent but is most common during administration of sodium channel blockers. It is thought that drug-induced slowing of conduction within diseased areas of the myocardium causes wavelength shortening, heightening the likelihood of reentry because circulating wavefronts will not encounter refractory tissue (47–50). The risk of development of this type of proarrhythmia appears to be greatest with class Ic agents, probably because they exhibit the most potent sodium channel blockade. The proarrhythmic risk with class Ic agents is most marked in patients with depressed left ventricular function and CHF (41,43,51) but is only rarely observed in patients with structurally normal hearts without ischemia (43). Ischemia can result in further slowing of conduction and an increased likelihood of developing proarrhythmia during class Ic drug administration (48). Similarly, enhanced conduction slowing during sinus tachycardia in patients receiving flecainide has also been correlated with the development of sustained monomorphic VT (18). Clinically, such arrhythmias may be very difficult to treat because they can be incessant, despite multiple defibrillations. Hypertonic saline (3% NaCl; possi-

bly effective by increasing the rapid inward sodium current) and β blockers may be helpful in such patients. In contrast to many studies of proarrhythmia, the increased mortality rate observed in the Cardiac Arrhythmia Suppression Trial (CAST), which evaluated flecainide and encainide after myocardial infarction, was not an early event but continued at a fairly constant rate during the study, suggesting an interaction with acute precipitating events such as ischemia (52). The previous discussion has focused on reentrant arrhythmias. In the case of an automatic focus, a drug could be beneficial by decreasing the automaticity of the focus. Alternatively, an automatic focus could be clinically silent because of a high degree of exit block, but drug-induced slowing of the firing rate could be proarrhythmic by permitting the focus to locally activate myocardial tissue causing clinical tachycardia (53).

The effects of left ventricular function on proarrhythmia were highlighted by a retrospective analysis of the Stroke Prevention in Atrial Fibrillation study (42). Survival was examined based on whether patients with atrial fibrillation were receiving antiarrhythmic agents (predominantly quinidine or procainamide). Administration of these drugs did not affect mortality in patients without CHF but significantly reduced survival in patients with CHF. Metaanalysis of studies examining the effects of antiarrhythmic agents on post–myocardial infarction mortality have shown a worsened survival with class I agents but not class III agents (54). When amiodarone (55–57), dofetilide (36,58), and d,l-sotalol (59) were examined in patients after myocardial infarction or who had significant CHF, there were no negative effects on survival. Thus, it is not recommended that class I agents be used in patients with CHF or marked left ventricular dysfunction. In addition, class Ic agents are usually only used in patients without significant structural heart disease.

Torsade de Pointes

Torsade de pointes is closely associated with drugs that prolong repolarization and the action potential (class I and class III agents) and it is thought to result from reactivation of calcium channels during phase 3 of the APD, with resulting increases in calcium currents and afterdepolarizations (60).

Thus, although torsade de pointes can be caused by blockade of potassium channels, it is not potassium channel blockade itself that causes the proarrhythmia, but secondary ionic currents resulting from APD prolongation. Alternatively, marked dispersion of APD in various areas of the ventricle ("dispersion of repolarization") may be the mechanism for this arrhythmia in some individuals. Although usually associated with pronounced QT-interval prolongation, in some patients, the QT interval is not markedly increased or prolongation is observed only after a preceding pause.

Clinical studies have demonstrated that the development of torsade de pointes is most common in women, patients with increased baseline QT intervals or marked QT-interval prolongation during drug therapy, CHF, bradycardia, left ventricular hypertrophy, and hypokalemia (44,60). Torsade de pointes is usually an early event occurring within the first several days of drug initiation, but in some patients, it occurs after changes in dosing regimen, alterations in drug clearance, or with the development of precipitating factors such as hypokalemia. Recent genetic analysis has demonstrated that some patients who develop drug-induced torsade de pointes have a "forme fruste" of long QT syndrome (61–63). Such patients have normal QT intervals at baseline but have a defect in the gene that codes for a sodium or potassium channel, resulting in enhanced susceptibility to drug-induced prolongation of repolarization and torsade de pointes. Torsade de pointes appears to be directly related to drug concentrations in patients receiving the I_K blockers d,l-sotalol (0.5% at 160 mg per day and 4.4% at 480 mg per day [64]) or dofetilide (36,65) but occurs at low concentrations in patients receiving quinidine (60,66,67), possibly related to quinidine-induced blockade of potassium currents at low concentrations and sodium channels at only higher plasma levels. Overall, the incidence of torsade de pointes appears to be the lowest with amiodarone (56–68). This is possibly a result of the agent' s complex pharmacology and multiple ionic actions, as well as the absence of excessive APD prolongation during bradycardia (15). Drug-induced torsade de pointes is usually treated by removing the offending agent and the rapid administration of intravenous and magnesium sulfate (69).

Atrial Proarrhythmia

In some patients receiving sodium channel blockers (most commonly, flecainide or propafenone) for treatment of supraventricular tachycardias, particularly atrial fibrillation, the atrial conduction slowing properties of these compounds can result in the development of atrial flutter, often with a long flutter cycle length or slow rate (70). Such slowing can result in a 1 : 1 atrioventricular (AV) conduction of atrial depolarization, resulting in marked tachycardia (e.g., 150 to 200 beats per minute). The vagolytic properties of class Ia agents can, in some patients, facilitate conduction through the AV node. In some patients, the fast ventricular rates may be associated with marked QRS prolongation (as a result of use-dependent effects of the drug or drug-induced ventricular conduction slowing and the development of a bundle branch block), mimicking VT. Concomitant administration of an AV nodal blocking agent with a sodium channel blocker in patients with atrial fibrillation or flutter can prevent such rapid AV nodal conduction. The conduction slowing effects of these agents may facilitate reentry and the development of atrial flutter in some patients by slowing conduction within the right atrium. If these drugs control a patient's atrial fibrillation but atrial flutter is a recurrent problem, the flutter can be ablated (71–73).

Hemodynamic Effects

Class Ia and class III antiarrhythmic agents can have significant hemodynamic effects that may be different with oral and intravenous administration. Oral flecainide and disopyramide are the most potent negative inotropic agents and they can exacerbate CHF (74). The β-blocking properties of d,l-sotalol can exacerbate CHF, which may be offset in some patients by possible positive inotropic effects from sotalol-induced APD prolongation and increased inward calcium flux. Quinidine, procainamide, lidocaine, mexiletine, and tocainide have mild negative inotropic effects. Dofetilide appears to be well tolerated hemodynamically in patients with significant CHF (36), and in human hemodynamic investigations, dofetilide did not significantly affect cardiac output or left ventricular filling pressures in patients with low ejection fractions (75). Amiodarone has been said to have mild negative inotropic effects, but in two large investigations of patients with significant CHF (57,76), amiodarone was well tolerated without CHF exacerbation. Intravenous procainamide, bretylium, and amiodarone (77) are potent vasodilators and administration can result in significant hypotension that may require concomitant saline or inotropic administration. In a multicenter randomized study (78), amiodarone was associated with less hypotension compared with bretylium. The hypotension associated with intravenous amiodarone may be a result of the polysorbate 80 dilutor and an aqueous preparation of this pharmacologic agent is currently in clinical trials. Intravenous ibutilide has been shown to be without significant hemodynamic effects (79).

β-Adrenergic blockers are negative inotropic agents and the use of these agents in patients with CHF, when initiated in low doses in stable patients, has been shown to reduce symptoms of heart failure and improve survival. Verapamil and to a lesser extent diltiazem are negative inotropic agents that should be used cautiously in patients with CHF. Newer dihydropyridine agents, such as amlodipine, do not exert negative inotropic effects but do not have clinically useful electrophysiologic actions. Digoxin exerts positive inotropic effects and has been shown to result in a reduction of symptoms in patients with CHF.

COMBINATION THERAPY

Class I and III agents have been combined in patients with cardiac arrhythmias and there is substantially more experience using combination therapy to treat ventricular tachyarrhythmias than there is to treat supraventricular tachycardias. However, with the increased use of the implantable cardioverter-defibrillator, the interest in combination antiarrhythmic therapy has been significantly reduced. Class Ib agents, usually mexiletine, have been combined with class I agents or amiodarone to suppress VT (80). The combination of mexiletine with quinidine or procainamide has not been highly efficacious in suppressing inducible VT (81,82) and has not shown clinical benefit. The combination of class I agents and amiodarone has been shown to result in significant slowing of the VT cycle length elicited during electrophysiologic testing (83), but the absence of long-term studies with clinical follow-up precludes drawing firm conclusions about the clinical significance of this finding. The combination of sotalol and quinidine or procainamide has been examined and resulted in a low incidence of proarrhythmia or recurrent ventricular tachyarrhythmias during follow-up (84). Suppression of inducible VT was related to significant prolongation of refractoriness, and combination therapy eliminated the frequency-dependent effects on refractoriness usually observed with sotalol (85).

There are substantial data demonstrating that β-adrenergic sympathetic stimulation can significantly attenuate or reverse the electrophysiologic actions of antiarrhythmic drugs (17,86–89). Studies have demonstrated that low-dose sympathetic stimulation can fully reverse the electrophysiologic actions of sematilide (87) (a pure class III agent) and quinidine (17) and partially attenuate the actions of amiodarone (87,89) to prolong ventricular repolarization. In contrast, the effects of d,l-sotalol on repolarization were not significant during isoproterenol infusion, likely because of its β-blocking activity (17). The addition of β blockers to class I and III drugs might be useful to prevent reversal of pharmacologic actions during increases in sympathetic stimulation. Patients receiving a β blocker and a class I antiarrhythmic agent in the Electrophysiological Study Versus Electrocardiographic Monitoring (ESVEM) Study had an improved survival rate compared with those treated with class I agents alone (90). Concomitant β-blocker therapy in the CAST study was associated with an amelioration of the mortality-inducing effects of encainide or flecainide (91). An examination of the European Myocardial Infarction Amiodarone Trial (EMIAT) and the Canadian Amiodarone Myocardial Infarction Trial (CAMIAT) demonstrates that in these post–myocardial infarction studies, there was a synergistic interaction between β blockers and amiodarone, with a significant reduction in arrhythmic mortality in patients receiving combination therapy (92).

Drugs that exhibit negative chronotropic effects on the AV node are frequently used in combination to slow the ventricular response during atrial fibrillation. The negative chronotropic effects of digoxin are easily reversed by sympathetic stimulation, and using a β blocker with digoxin can prevent this.

Antiarrhythmic Classification

The classification of antiarrhythmic drugs according to the modified Vaughan Williams classification assumes that individual drugs have a predominant mechanism of action (93). Although this classification has limited clinical utility and does not account for the complicated electrophysiologic and autonomic interactions that may occur, it does highlight the major mode of action of these agents, particularly the ionic channels that are altered.

1. The class I drugs act by modulating or closing the sodium channels, thereby inhibiting phase 0 depolarization. Three different subgroups have been identified because their mechanism or duration of action is somewhat different because of variable rates of drug binding to and dissociation from the channel receptor. (a) The class Ic agents (flecainide, propafenone), which are the most potent sodium channel blockers, have the slowest binding and dissociation from the receptor. (b) The class Ib agents (mexiletine, tocainide, and lidocaine) are the weakest sodium channel blockers and have the most rapid binding and dissociation. (c) The class Ia agents (quinidine, procainamide, and disopyramide) are intermediate. These agents also possess potassium channel-blocking activity and prolong repolarization.
2. The class II drugs (β blockers) act by inhibiting sympathetic activity, primarily by causing beta blockade.
3. The class III drugs (amiodarone, ibutilide, dofetilide, and sotalol) block the potassium channels, thereby prolonging repolarization and the duration of the action potential and the refractory period. Some of these drugs also have other antiarrhythmic effects. Sotalol has β-blocking activity while amiodarone can block the sodium channel in depolarized tissues and may block the calcium channel.
4. The class IV drugs are calcium channel blockers. Verapamil has a more pronounced inhibitory effect on the slow response sinoatrial and AV nodes than diltiazem. In comparison, the dihydropyridines, such as nifedipine, have little electrophysiologic effect.

Table 8-1 lists a classification of antiarrhythmic drugs as proposed by Vaughan Williams (84). This classification has been modified over the years. In addition, autonomic and unique features of these drugs are not used as part of this classification. These characteristics, as listed in the paper describing the Sicilian Gambit (9), are listed in Table 8-2. These classification schema are limited in usefulness because they do not characterize drugs by basic electrophysiologic differences such as onset-offset kinetics (9,94),

TABLE 8-1. VAUGHAN WILLIAMS ANTIARRHYTHMIC DRUG CLASSIFICATION

Class	Action	Drug
I	Sodium channel blockers	
Ia	Moderate phase 0 depression	Quinidine
	Moderate conduction slowing	Procainamide
	Prolongs repolarization	Disopyramide
Ib	Minimal phase 0 depression	Lidocaine
	Shortens repolarization	Tocainide
		Mexiletine
Ic	Marked phase 0 depression	Flecainide
	Marked conduction slowing	Propafenone
	Slight effect on repolarization	Moricizine
II	β blockers	Propranol
		Acebutolol
		Esmolol
III	Prolongs repolarization	Bretylium
		Amiodarone
		Sotalol
		Ibutilide
		Dofetilide
IV	Calcium channel blockers	Verapamil
		Diltiazem
	Purine agonist	Adenosine
	Digitalis glycosides	Digoxin
		Digitoxin

use dependency, and whether drugs block open or inactivated states. In addition to macroscopic changes in cardiac substrate, disease states can also alter the number or function of ionic channels. CHF is associated with reductions in the transient inward current (I_{to}) and alterations in intracellular calcium handling (95–97). The development of left

ventricular hypertrophy in rabbits has been shown to result in decreases in the inward rectifier potassium current and increases in the transient outward current, as well as reductions in the VF threshold (98,99), which resolved during captopril therapy.

Quinidine (Quinidex, Quinaglute, Cardioquin)

Quinidine is a class Ia antiarrhythmic agent. It is manufactured as a sulfate salt with long-acting trade name formulations (Quinidex) and as the polygalacturonate (Cardioquin) and gluconate salts (Quinaglute).

Electrophysiology

Basic experiments demonstrate that quinidine reduces automaticity by raising threshold potential and decreasing the rate of rise of phase 4 depolarization. Quinidine decreases the rate of rise of phase 0 of the action potential by blocking sodium influx predominantly in the activated state, thus slowing conduction. This action of quinidine is frequency-dependent with depression of V_{max} being greater at faster heart rates (94). Rate-dependent block occurs at an intermediate rate. Quinidine prolongs APD, primarily by blocking the potassium channel (I_{Kr}) (100). Quinidine also prolongs the effective refractory period (ERP) and the ERP to APD ratio.

Quinidine has vagolytic effects, which can increase sinus heart rate, enhance AV nodal conduction and shorten AV node refractory periods. Quinidine mildly blocks α_2 and muscarinic subtype 2 receptors (9). Because of conduction slowing and competitive vagolytic properties, the PR and A-H intervals may not increase. Quinidine increases the

TABLE 8-2. REPOLARIZATION-PROLONGING ANTIARRHYTHMIC DRUGS: NEW AND OLD[a]

Antiarrhythmic Drug	Cardiomyocyte Membrane Effects	Possible Antiadrenergic Action	Route of Administration	Likely Major Indications
Ibutilide	Activates I_{Na-s}, blocks I_{Kr}	—	IV	AF (FL)
Azimilide[b]	Blocks I_{Kr} and I_{Ks}	—	PO	AF (FL)/PSVT/VA/SCD proph.
Tedisamil[b]	Blocks I_{Kr} and I_{to}	+ (?)	IV and PO	AF
Ersentilide[b]	Blocks I_{Kr} and β_1 receptors	Beta blockade	IV and PO	AF (FL)/PSVT/VA/SCD proph
Dofetilide	Blocks I_{Kr}	—	IV and PO	AF (FL)/PSVT
Trecetilide[b]	Probably similar to ibutilide	—	IV and PO	AF (FL)
Dronedarone[b]	Multiple actions, but same as those for amiodarone for ion channel block	Noncompetitive	IV and PO	AF (FL)/PSVT/VA/SCD proph; ICD combination
Amiodarone	Multiple actions but predominantly blocks I_{to}, I_{Kr}, I_{Ca}, and I_{Na}	Noncompetitive	IV and PO	AF (FL)/PSVT/VA/SCD proph; ICD combination
Sotalol	Blocks I_{Kr} and β_1 and β_2 receptors	Beta blockade	PO	AF (FL)/PSVT/VA/SCD proph; ICD combination

AF (FL), atrial fibrillation (flutter); PSVT, paroxysmal supraventricular tachycardia; SCD proph, prophylaxis against sudden cardiac death; VA, sustained ventricular arrhythmia; —, no; +, yes; ICD, implantable cardioverter-defibrillator
[a]In the United States, amiodarone and sotalol are approved for ventricular arrhythmia; sotalol and dofetilide have been approved for atrial fibrillation.
[b]Under investigation.

ERP of the atria, His-Purkinje system, ventricles, and accessory pathways (101). Quinidine will increase the H-V, QT, and QRS intervals (102,103).

Pharmacokinetics

Because quinidine has various preparations, pharmacokinetics varies. With quinidine sulfate, 95% is absorbed orally and bioavailability is about 70% to 80% and peak levels occur 1 to 3 hours after ingestion (Table 8-3). From 20% to 50% is excreted unchanged by the kidneys. Otherwise, quinidine is metabolized by hydroxylation in the liver. 3-Hydroxyquinidine and 2′-oxoquinidine have minimal antiarrhythmic activity. The half-life of quinidine sulfate is 5 to 7 hours and thus takes about 24 to 36 hours to reach steady state. Therapeutic plasma levels are 2 to 7 μg/mL. Extended-release preparations release about one third of the dose immediately with the remainder time-released for 6 to 10 hours.

Dosing

The dosage of the quinidine sulfate is usually 200 to 600 mg four times a day, depending on levels, efficacy, and intolerance. Quinidex is given at the same total daily dosage using a twice-daily or a three-times-a-day schedule. Quinaglute dosages range from 324 to 972 mg twice daily or three times a day.

Efficacy

Quinidine is effective in suppressing premature atrial contractions and ectopic atrial tachycardias. Quinidine has been useful in the chemical cardioversion and maintenance of patients with atrial flutter and fibrillation. About 50% of atrial fibrillation patients treated with quinidine remain in sinus rhythm 1-year postcardioversion (104).

By suppressing premature atrial contractions and premature ventricular contractions and by slowing conduction and prolonging refractoriness of accessory pathways and the retrograde limb of the AV node, quinidine has been effective in treating premature supraventricular tachycardia secondary to AV nodal reentrant tachycardia and AV reentrant tachycardia. Like procainamide, quinidine rarely completely blocks conduction in accessory pathways with refractory periods of less than 270 ms (101).

Quinidine is effective for the chronic suppression of ventricular ectopic activity. Based on Holter monitoring, quinidine will effectively suppress premature ventricular contractions, ventricular couplets, and nonsustained VT in about 60% of patients (105). In patients with sustained VT or VF, efficacy rates, as determined by programmed stimulation, range from 16% in the ESVEM Study (105) to 20% to 25% in uncontrolled trials (102). Combination therapy with tocainide or mexiletine, using lower maintenance doses of both drugs, achieves added efficacy and lower toxicity (106).

Adverse Effects

Subjective toxicity with quinidine is common. From 10% to 35% of patients will develop nausea, vomiting, anorexia, or diarrhea. In ESVEM (105), 32% of patients discontinued quinidine because of adverse effects. Some of these adverse reactions are dose-related. Fever, rash, and tinnitus can rarely occur. End-organ toxicity includes the occurrence of a rare drug-induced thrombocytopenia and granulomatous hepatitis.

Quinidine has mild negative inotropic activity, but its overall effect on cardiac output appears to be minimal. Its peripheral vasodilatory effects, mediated partially by alpha blockade, may counterbalance some of its direct negative inotropic activity. Rarely, the vasodilatory properties of quinidine can lead to orthostatic hypotension.

Quinidine can be used with amiodarone, although because of a drug-drug interaction, quinidine doses need to be lowered by about one third (107).

Importantly, quinidine interacts with digoxin, increasing digoxin levels by a factor of two (108). This occurs secondary to quinidine displacing digoxin from the tissues and by reducing renal clearance rates of digoxin. When used in combination, digoxin doses should be halved. Quinidine by inhibiting the CYP D6 enzyme system also can increase the levels of antiarrhythmic agents such as propafenone metabolized by this enzyme system when used concomitantly (109).

Because of its vagolytic effects, quinidine may cause an increase in ventricular response when used to treat patients for atrial fibrillation or flutter. Also, by slowing the atrial

TABLE 8-3. PHARMACOKINETIC PROPERTIES OF CLASS IA ANTIARRHYTHMICS

Variable	Quinidine	Procainamide	Disopyramide
Bioavailability	70–80%	75–95%	70–85%
Elimination	Hepatic (50–70%)/renal	Hepatic (30–60%)/renal	Renal/hepatic
Elimination half-life	6–7	3–6	4–10
Therapeutic range	2–7	4–10	2–5 (μg/mL)
Renal/hepatic	50–70	30–60	None
Active metabolite	None	N-acetylprocainamide	Mono-N-dealkylated disopyramide
Protein binding	80%	20%	30% nonlinear
Drug interactions	Amiodarone, digoxin, propafenone	Amiodarone	Amiodarone

rate and decreasing concealed AV nodal block in the AV node, atrial flutter with a 1 : 1 conduction ratio can occur.

Quinidine may worsen infranodal block. By slowing conduction, quinidine can be proarrhythmic with the development of new-onset monomorphic VT. Of more concern, quinidine may prolong the QT interval and cause torsade de pointes in up to 5% of patients (110,111). Because of this, in-hospital initiation under telemetry conditions is recommended. There is no QT-interval cutoff to predict torsade de pointes with quinidine. However, if the corrected QT interval (QTc) becomes longer than 525 ms, caution should be used in further titrating the dose of this drug. Also, it is recommended that quinidine should not be used in patients with a baseline prolonged QT interval. There are no large controlled trials defining the safety of using quinidine in post–myocardial infarction or CHF patients. One small study (42) suggests that quinidine and other class I agents increase mortality rates in patients with atrial fibrillation who also have a history of CHF. Quinidine can raise the defibrillation and pacing threshold when used with implantable cardioverter-defibrillators or pacemakers.

Procainamide (Procan-SR, Pronestyl-SR, Procanbid)

Procainamide is a class Ia antiarrhythmic agent useful in both atrial and ventricular arrhythmias. It is available intravenously and in oral shorter-acting and sustained-release preparations. Procan-SR is delivered via an early-release wax matrix and Pronestyl-SR as an early-release inner core. Procanbid is a longer-acting formulation that can be given on a twice-daily dosing schedule.

Electrophysiology

Procainamide has electrophysiologic properties similar to those of quinidine but has less vagolytic effects.

Pharmacokinetics

Procainamide is 95% absorbed in the small intestine, with peak levels occurring 15 minutes to 2 hours after oral administration (Table 8-3). Bioavailability is about 85%. Procainamide is acetylated in the liver by N-acetyltransferase to an active metabolite, N-acetylprocainamide (NAPA), which possesses class III antiarrhythmic activity and probably accounts for the prolongation of the QT interval seen with procainamide therapy (112). The rate of acetylation depends on a genetically determined acetylation phenotype. In rapid acetylators, NAPA levels usually exceed that of the parent compound. NAPA is an active metabolite with 70% of the antiarrhythmic activity of the parent compound. From 30% to 60% of the drug is excreted unchanged in the urine and the remainder is excreted as NAPA. Orally, the half-life of procainamide is only 3 to 4 hours, so steady state is achieved within 24 hours. NAPA has a half-life of 6 hours. Therapeutic procainamide levels

are in the 4- to 8-μg/mL ranges with NAPA levels of 8 to 16, and combined levels of more than 16 to 20 μg/mL are commonly associated with toxicity.

Dosing

Procainamide is usually initiated at about 50 mg/kg per day; the average dosage is thus 1,500 to 4,000 mg per day, administered in 2 to 4 doses. Doses are titrated to efficacy, toxicity, and blood levels. Intravenous procainamide requires loading doses of 10 to 15 mg/kg given at 25 to 50 mg per minute depending on blood pressure. This can be followed by a 1- to 4-mg per minute intravenous drip.

Efficacy

Both intravenous and oral procainamide may be used to chemically convert and treat patients with ectopic atrial tachycardia, atrial flutter, atrial fibrillation, and premature supraventricular tachycardia. In hemodynamically tolerated atrial fibrillation with overt preexcitation, intravenous procainamide is the treatment of choice to slow antegrade accessory pathway conduction and thus the ventricular response. Procainamide is about 60% effective in suppressing premature ventricular contractions, ventricular couplets, and nonsustained VT as assessed by Holter monitoring (105). In sustained VT, procainamide is effective in about 20% to 25% as assessed by programmed stimulation (105). Added efficacy is achieved when procainamide is used with mexiletine. The response to intravenous procainamide in the electrophysiology laboratory appears to predict an acceptable electrophysiologic response to oral procainamide and other antiarrhythmic agents, although this is controversial (113). Intravenous procainamide is one of the parenteral treatments of choice for ventricular tachyarrhythmias and is more likely to terminate VT than lidocaine (114).

Adverse Effects

Procainamide may cause nausea, anorexia, vomiting, and rash. End-organ toxicity of concern is a rare agranulocytosis that usually occurs during the first 3 months of treatment.

The major limiting adverse reaction with procainamide has been the development of a systemic lupus-like reaction in 10% to 20% of patients. This is more likely to occur in slow acetylators, in whom procainamide levels are high and NAPA levels are low. Although 70% of patients will develop a positive antinuclear antibody titer within a year, this laboratory abnormality alone does not warrant discontinuation of therapy. Overall, 31% of patients treated with procainamide in the ESVEM Study discontinued therapy secondary to adverse effects (105).

Procainamide has a negative inotropic effect that is mild (115). Procainamide can cause high-degree AV block and ventricular proarrhythmia including the new onset of sustained, monomorphic VT or torsade de pointes; the torsade is likely related to NAPA and its class III activity (112). In renal failure, patients may develop significantly increased levels of both procainamide and NAPA with the development of torsade de pointes. Like quinidine, procainamide has been associated with increased mortality rates when used in CHF patients (42). No safety data exist in the post–myocardial infarction setting. Procainamide, because of its mixed class I/III activity, has neutral effects on defibrillation thresholds.

Although there are no known teratogenic effects, procainamide does cross the placenta and can be used for the treatment of fetal tachycardias.

Disopyramide (Norpace, Norpace CR)

Disopyramide is a type Ia antiarrhythmic agent approved by the Food and Drug Administration (FDA) for the treatment of ventricular arrhythmias. Disopyramide also has efficacy in the treatment of atrial fibrillation and neurocardiogenic syncope.

Electrophysiology

In basic animal and human experiments, disopyramide has similar electrophysiologic and more anticholinergic effects than quinidine and procainamide.

Pharmacokinetics

Ninety percent of an oral dose of disopyramide is absorbed and its bioavailability is 70% to 85% (Table 8-3). Peak levels occur in 2 hours. Fifty-five percent of a dose is recovered after renal excretion unchanged in the urine while 25% is recovered as the active *N*-monodealkylated metabolite. Disopyramide has nonlinear pharmacokinetics with decreasing plasma protein binding as serum concentrations increase (116).

The half-life varies from 4 to 10 hours (averages 6 to 7 hours) and steady state is achieved within 40 hours. In patients with renal failure and CHF, elimination half-life is significantly increased. Usually therapeutic levels are in the 2- to 5-µg/mL range.

Dosing

Dosage ranges from 400 to 800 mg four times a day with the short-acting form or twice daily when the controlled-release formulation is used.

Efficacy

Disopyramide is very effective in treating patients with ectopic atrial tachycardia, atrial flutter, atrial fibrillation, and premature supraventricular tachycardia (117,118). Disopyramide is as effective as procainamide and quinidine in suppressing premature ventricular contractions, ventricular couplets, and nonsustained runs of VT as assessed by Holter monitoring, and suppressing sustained VT as assessed by programmed stimulation (119). Because of the anticholinergic properties of disopyramide, it is often used to treat patients with neurocardiogenic syncope (120).

Adverse Effects

Disopyramide's subjective toxicity is primarily secondary to its anticholinergic activity and includes dry mouth, blurred vision, urinary retention, constipation, and worsening of glaucoma. These reactions require discontinuation in about 10% of patients. If needed, long-acting pyridostigmine can be given with disopyramide to minimize anticholinergic adverse effects. No significant end-organ toxicity has been noted with disopyramide (121).

Disopyramide's most important adverse reaction is worsening of CHF secondary to its significant negative inotropic activity and increase of peripheral vascular resistance. CHF occurs in 50% of patients with a prior history of CHF and only 5% of other patients (122). No well-controlled data exist to determine the safety of using disopyramide in CHF or post–myocardial infarction patients.

Disopyramide by slowing conduction can cause complete AV block and bundle branch block. Slowing of conduction and prolongation of QT interval can cause proarrhythmias such as monomorphic sustained VT and torsade de pointes.

Lidocaine Hydrochloride (Xylocaine)

Lidocaine hydrochloride is a short-acting intravenous, type Ib antiarrhythmic agent that is useful in the acute treatment of ventricular arrhythmias.

Electrophysiology

Electrophysiologically, lidocaine minimally blocks the sodium channels predominantly in the inactivated state and thus minimally slows conduction in the His-Purkinje system and myocardium. Rate-dependent block develops rapidly with lidocaine. Lidocaine has more conduction-slowing properties in ischemic tissue. Lidocaine has little to no effect on atrial, AV nodal, or accessory pathway tissue; thus, it is ineffective in treating supraventricular arrhythmias. Lidocaine depresses automaticity in Purkinje fibers and thus would be predicted to be efficacious in suppressing irritable ventricular foci. Its ability to slow conduction in cardiac tissue and a net increase in the ERP-APD ratio may help prevent reentrant ventricular arrhythmias.

Pharmacokinetics

Lidocaine has poor oral absorption and 90% of an administered dose is rapidly metabolized in the liver into two major metabolites: monoethylglycinexylidide (MEG) and glycinexylidide (GX) (123). MEG is 80% and GX 10% as potent as the parent compound. Because of its rapid first-pass metabolism; lidocaine is not useful orally and must be administered parenterally to achieve therapeutic blood levels.

Lidocaine administered as an intravenous bolus is distributed rapidly into the intravascular compartment (half-life = 8 minutes) and then diffuses quickly into the peripheral compartment. Lidocaine has a half-life of 1.5 to 2 hours in the second pass of redistribution, with extensive metabolism occurring hepatically. Because of this, if an infusion is started without a bolus loading dose, it takes 20 to 60 minutes to attain therapeutic levels.

Dosing

Recommended dosing includes a loading bolus infusion of 75 to 200 mg intravenously followed by a 1- to 4-mg per minute maintenance infusion. Within 15 minutes of the first bolus, a second bolus of 100 mg can be given to maintain levels. If maintenance infusions at higher doses are needed, patients should receive a 50- to 75-mg intravenous bolus before increasing the rate of the maintenance infusion to avoid delays in attaining higher blood levels (124).

In patients with severe heart failure, there is decreased hepatic blood flow and metabolism of lidocaine. In this situation, lower doses need to be used to avoid toxicity (125). Elderly patients are more sensitive to the toxic effects of lidocaine. In older patients, lower loading and maintenance doses should be used.

Efficacy

Lidocaine is used as a drug of choice for the rapid suppression of premature ventricular contractions, warning arrhythmias, and prophylaxis in the post–myocardial infarction setting (126). A metaanalysis suggests that lidocaine should not be routinely used as a post–myocardial infarction prophylactic antiarrhythmic against the occurrence of VT or VF (127). It is not as effective as procainamide for slowing or terminating sustained VT (114).

Adverse Effects

Lidocaine has dose-related neurologic and gastrointestinal adverse effects. Neurologic side effects include numbness, tingling, seizures, tremors, paresthesias, disorientation, dulled sensorium, tinnitus, and drowsiness. Gastrointestinal side effects include nausea and vomiting. Lidocaine causes a dose-related increase in defibrillation thresholds (128). Lidocaine is well tolerated hemodynamically. Lidocaine only minimally slows conduction in the His-Purkinje system. Therapeutic blood levels are in the 1- to 5-μ/mL range.

Tocainide (Tonocard)

Tocainide (oral lidocaine) is an orally useful primary amine analogue of lidocaine with class Ib effects.

Electrophysiology

Its electrophysiologic effects *in vitro* are similar to those of lidocaine and mexiletine.

Pharmacokinetics

Tocainide has excellent oral absorption and bioavailability, exceeding 95% (Table 8-4). The renal and hepatic routes eliminate tocainide. No major active metabolites exist. Its onset of action is 1.5 hours and its half-life averages 11 to

TABLE 8-4. PHARMACOKINETIC PROPERTIES OF MEXILETINE AND TOCAINIDE

	Mexiletine	Tocainide
Bioavailability	>90%	>95%
Elimination	Hepatic	Hepatic/renal (40%)
Elimination half-life	10–15 h	9–40 h
Mean	12 h	14 h
Therapeutic range	1–2 μg/mL	4–10 μg/mL
Protein binding	60–70%	4–20%
Active metabolite	None	None
Drug interactions	None	None

19 hours. Therapeutic levels of tocainide are between 4 and 10 μg/mL (129).

Dosing

Oral dosing with tocainide is usually initiated at 300 to 400 mg two to three times a day. Rarely, a dosage as high as 600 mg three times a day is required.

Efficacy

Tocainide has been found to be an effective suppresser of premature ventricular beats. An effective response to lidocaine may be predictive of a tocainide response. Using programmed stimulation as a measure of efficacy; tocainide is effective in less than 15% of patients with sustained ventricular tachyarrhythmias (129–131). Combination of tocainide with a type Ia agent has demonstrated an added efficacy of 15% to 35% in patients with ventricular arrhythmias, compared with either agent alone.

Adverse Effects

Like lidocaine and mexiletine, side effects of tocainide are primarily gastrointestinal and neurologic. Gastrointestinal side effects include anorexia, nausea, vomiting, abdominal pain, and constipation. Neurologic side effects include tremors, nervousness, dizziness, paresthesias, and confusion. Because of subjective intolerance, which is often dose-related, tocainide has to be discontinued in 15% to 30% of patients. Lowering the dose or taking the medication after meals can often minimize subjective side effects. Up to 8% of patients who take tocainide get a drug-induced rash, which resolves after discontinuing the drug. Rare occurrences of pulmonary fibrosis or agranulocytosis (0.2%) with tocainide have limited the use of this drug. From a cardiac viewpoint, tocainide is well tolerated. The incidence of drug-aggravated heart failure or arrhythmia is less than 4%. No major drug interaction problems have been reported. No post–myocardial infarction or CHF safety data exist for tocainide.

Mexiletine (Mexitil)

Mexiletine is a class Ib oral agent that resembles lidocaine and tocainide in structure.

Electrophysiology

Its electrophysiologic and electrocardiographic effects are like those of lidocaine and tocainide.

Pharmacokinetics

Mexiletine is well absorbed orally with more than 90% bioavailability (Table 8-4). Hepatic metabolism is the major route of elimination and only 10% to 15% of the parent drug is excreted unchanged in the urine. The onset of action occurs within 1 to 2 hours and the elimination half-life averages 10 to 12 hours. Mexiletine is 70% protein bound. No important drug interactions have been identified with mexiletine (132).

Dosing

The dosage of mexiletine is usually initiated at 200 mg three times a day. Maintenance dosages vary from 150 to 300 mg three times a day. In some patients, twice-daily dosing may be effective.

Efficacy

Like tocainide, mexiletine has been effective in approximately 50% of patients with potentially lethal ventricular arrhythmias studied by a Holter monitor model. In the ESVEM Study, 67% of patients had suppression of their ventricular arrhythmia as assessed by Holter monitoring (105). Mexiletine has been shown to be comparable to quinidine in suppressing ventricular ectopic activity. Adding a type Ia antiarrhythmic agent to mexiletine is associated with added efficacy and decreased toxicity (106,133). Mexiletine was not found to reduce mortality in a post–myocardial infarction population (IMPACT study), although it significantly reduced the frequency of premature ventricular contractions (134). Mexiletine's effects on survival in CHF patients have not been studied. In patients with recurrent sustained VT studied in the electrophysiology laboratory, mexiletine appears to be effective in 10% to 15% of patients. Efficacy rates between 20% and 30% have been demonstrated in patients with VF who survived an out-of-hospital cardiac arrest (135,136). Combination therapy with type Ia agents in patients with sustained ventricular tachyarrhythmias may increase the efficacy rates by an additional 15% to 30% (106,133). Mexiletine is very effective in treating pediatric patients who have ventricular arrhythmias after surgery for tetralogy of Fallot. Mexiletine, by shortening the QT interval, is effective in treating some patients with prolonged QT syndrome who have an abnormal amino acid substitution in the sodium channel (137).

Adverse Effects

Like lidocaine and tocainide, mexiletine has dose-related central nervous system and gastrointestinal side effects. Central nervous system toxicity includes tremors, dizziness, blurred vision, and confusion. The primary gastrointestinal side effect is nausea, although vomiting and heartburn are also seen. Taking the drug with meals or antacids can minimize subjective side effects.

Mexiletine is relatively free of end-organ toxicity, although rare cases of drug-induced hepatitis have been reported.

Hemodynamically, mexiletine is well tolerated. No change in left ventricular ejection fraction has been noted during mexiletine therapy when compared with baseline (138). Mexiletine has minimal proarrhythmic effects. Because mexiletine shortens the QT interval, torsade de pointes does not occur. Mexiletine can cause an elevation in defibrillation thresholds if used in patients with an implantable cardioverter-defibrillator.

Flecainide (Tambocor)

Flecainide is a class Ic antiarrhythmic agent, approved by the FDA, that is used to treat ventricular arrhythmias and atrial fibrillation.

Electrophysiology

Flecainide prolongs refractoriness and slows conduction in the atria, AV node, His-Purkinje system, ventricles, and accessory pathways (139,140). It predominantly blocks sodium channels in the activated state with rate-dependent block occurring slowly.

Pharmacokinetics

Flecainide's bioavailability is 90% to 95% (Table 8-5). Its half-life averages between 12 and 27 hours (mean, 20 hours). Although flecainide is mostly metabolized (70%) in the liver, 30% is excreted by the kidney. Peak blood levels are achieved in 2 to 4 hours (139). Because of its long half-life, flecainide is effective using a twice-daily dosing schedule.

Dosing

Flecainide is available as 100-mg tablets. We usually initiate therapy at 100 mg twice daily. After steady state has been achieved, we increase the dosage to 150 mg twice daily as necessary. Rarely, higher dosages (200 mg twice daily) are required. Therapeutic levels are 0.2 to 1.0 μg/mL. Prolongation of the PR and QRS intervals occur when therapeutic plasma levels are achieved.

Efficacy

Flecainide has been shown to be extremely effective (more than 70%) in decreasing the frequency of premature ventricular contractions in patients with frequent ventricular ectopy (141,142). In comparative trials with quinidine and disopyramide, flecainide has been shown to be statistically superior in the suppression of premature ventricular contractions, ventricular couplets, and runs of nonsustained VT. In patients with symptomatic ventricular arrhythmias in the post–myocardial infarction period, the CAST study demonstrated that both encainide and flecainide enhanced

TABLE 8-5. CLINICAL PHARMACOLOGY OF PROPAFENONE, FLECAINIDE, AND MORICIZINE

	Propafenone	Flecainide	Moricizine
Bioavailability	Dose-related 13–55% (first-pass hepatic clearance)	95%	30–40% (first-pass hepatic metabolism)
Elimination	Hepatic (99%) (rapid extensive metabolizers, 90% of patients)	Hepatic (70%)/renal	Hepatic (>99%)
Elimination half-life	6 h (3–12 h) in extensive metabolizers	20 h (11–30 h)	2-4 h (10–13 h in patients with heart disease)
Therapeutic range	Variable	0.2–1.0 µg/mL	Variable
Protein binding	90–95%	40%	95%
Active metabolites	5-hydroxypropafenone	None	None
Drug interactions	Quinidine	Amiodarone	Cimetidine, theophylline

mortality compared with placebo, despite effective premature ventricular contraction suppression (52). In patients with sustained VT, the efficacy of flecainide (20%) has been comparable to that of type Ia antiarrhythmic agents (143,144). Efficacy rates are higher in patients with preserved left ventricular function and ejection fractions of more than 0.30 (144). Recent data suggest that flecainide may be useful in treating some patients with prolonged QT syndromes (145).

Flecainide has been demonstrated to be a very effective agent in the treatment of reentrant supraventricular arrhythmias (140), atrial origin arrhythmias (140), and atrial fibrillation (146). A prospective study demonstrated that flecainide was equally effective as quinidine in treating atrial fibrillation and was associated with less toxicity (146). Flecainide is predominantly used for the treatment of supraventricular tachyarrhythmias without concomitant organic heart disease. Bolus oral doses (300 mg) expedite the medical conversion of recent-onset atrial fibrillation to sinus rhythm (147).

Adverse Effects
Subjectively, flecainide is very well tolerated. Noncardiac side effects, which are dose-related, include dizziness, visual disturbances, and headache. Cardiovascular adverse reactions of concern include depression of left ventricular function and aggravation of CHF in some patients (139,140).

Of major concern is flecainide's proarrhythmic potential. In patients with premature ventricular contractions and nonsustained VT that is not in the post–myocardial infarction period, the incidence of ventricular proarrhythmia appears to be less than 3%. In the CAST study, mortality rates were increased compared with placebo in patients treated for asymptomatic ventricular arrhythmias post–myocardial infarction (52). In patients without significant structural heart disease and supraventricular tachycardia, there is no risk of worsening survival (148). In patients with sustained ventricular tachyarrhythmias, the incidence of proarrhythmia, including the development of incessant VT, averages between 7% and 17% (45,144), with severe organic heart disease and left ventricular dysfunction. Fle-

cainide may worsen preexisting sinus node dysfunction, and because of its potent effects on slowing His-Purkinje conduction, it may aggravate preexisting conduction disturbances and precipitate the development of advanced AV block. Flecainide has caused acute and chronic elevation of permanent pacemaker thresholds and defibrillator thresholds. Flecainide may slightly increase digoxin levels. When used with amiodarone, flecainide levels may increase 15% to 30%.

Propafenone (Rythmol)

Propafenone, another class Ic antiarrhythmic agent, also has weak associated β-blocking characteristics (149,150). It is useful in the treatment of ventricular and supraventricular arrhythmias.

Electrophysiology
The drug has type Ic electrophysiologic effects like those of flecainide. However, it differs from flecainide in several ways. Propafenone has weak β-blocking effects (structure similar to that of propranolol); its onset-offset kinetics is more similar to that of disopyramide than that of flecainide (8); and it blocks sodium channels in both the activated and the inactivated state.

Pharmacokinetics
Propafenone is totally absorbed then undergoes first-pass hepatic elimination by way of a storable oxidative pathway (Table 8-5). Metabolism of propafenone is genetically determined using the CYP 2D6 enzyme system (109,151). Ten percent of patients are "poor metabolizers" with a prolonged half-life of parent compound. The half-life of the parent compound ranges from 2 to 12 hours, with a mean of 6 hours. Poor metabolizers often have half-lives in the 10- to 12-hour range. The major metabolites of propafenone are 5-hydroxypropafenone (active) and N-debutyl propafenone. Although the half-life of the parent compound is only 6 hours, steady state is not usually reached for 72 hours because of the active metabolite's half-life. At higher doses, propafenone demonstrates nonlinear

pharmacokinetics with decreasing plasma protein binding as serum concentrations increase.

Dosing

The recommended starting dosage of propafenone is 150 mg three times a day. The dosage may be increased to 225 to 300 mg three times a day if necessary.

Efficacy

In patients with potentially lethal ventricular arrhythmias, propafenone has been effective in controlling premature ventricular contractions, ventricular couplets, and nonsustained VT in 48% to 65% of patients (149,150). Studies have demonstrated at least equal and in some cases more efficacy than quinidine, mexiletine, and disopyramide (152). In patients with a history of sustained VT or VF, programmed stimulation studies have demonstrated propafenone to be effective in suppressing inducible VT in about 14% to 20% of patients (153,154). In the Cardiac Arrest Study Hamburg (CASH) trial (154), propafenone decreased survival rates of sudden death survivors compared with an implantable cardioverter-defibrillator.

Propafenone prolongs refractoriness and slows conduction in the atria, AV node, and accessory AV connections (155). Propafenone is effective in treating more than 50% of patients with reentrant supraventricular tachycardia and paroxysmal atrial fibrillation (156). Like flecainide, propafenone is primarily used as a front-line agent for the suppression of atrial fibrillation in patients with no to minimal structural heart disease. Oral bolus doses of propafenone (600 mg) expedite medical conversion of atrial fibrillation to sinus rhythm (147).

Adverse Effects

Subjective adverse effects with propafenone include a bitter metallic taste, nausea, vomiting, constipation, and dizziness. A drug-induced rash has been induced in about 3% of patients. End-organ toxicity such as neutropenia and a positive antinuclear antibody titer with a drug-induced lupus syndrome is rarely caused by propafenone. Because of its β-blocking activity, it can accentuate AV nodal block. Because of its type Ic effects, it can aggravate His-Purkinje block. Propafenone has some negative inotropic activity and should be used cautiously in patients with left ventricular dysfunction (74). Proarrhythmia occurs in about 3% of patients treated for benign or potentially lethal ventricular arrhythmias and 10% of patients with a prior history of sustained VT or VF. Propafenone can cause an elevation in pacing thresholds but at low doses seems to have minimal effects on defibrillation thresholds.

Propafenone interacts with digoxin and can raise digoxin levels by 40% to 60%. Propafenone also appears to increase the plasma concentration of warfarin and can cause significant increases in prothrombin times. No post–myocardial infarction or CHF safety data exist for propafenone.

Moricizine (Ethmozine)

Moricizine hydrochloride is a phenothiazine derivative developed in the Soviet Union that is useful in the treatment of ventricular arrhythmias (157,158).

Electrophysiology

Moricizine has membrane-stabilizing activity and local anesthetic activity, and it moderately inhibits the sodium channels in phase 0 of the action potential. It primarily blocks the fast sodium channel in the inactivated state. The electrophysiologic effects of moricizine do not clearly define this agent into any of the subclasses defined by Vaughan Williams. Its electrophysiologic actions are similar to those of a mild class Ic agent, but in isolated Purkinje fibers of dogs, moricizine shortens phase 2 and 3 repolarization, similar to class Ib agent, along with a dose-related decrease in V_{max}. In the canine model, no significant effects have been observed in the sinus node or atria. In man, moricizine decreases conduction velocity through the AV node with an increase in the A-H interval. It also slows conduction in the ventricular myocardium with prolongation of the H-V, PR, and QRS intervals. There is little change in the J-T interval, suggesting that the drug does not prolong ventricular repolarization or block potassium channels. Intracardiac studies have shown that moricizine slows AV node conduction without prolonging ventricular ERP (159). Retrograde AV node and accessory pathway conduction are also slowed.

Pharmacokinetics

Moricizine is the ethyl ester hydrochloride of 10-(3-morpholinoproprinonyl) phenothiazine-2-carbonic acid. It is well absorbed by the gastrointestinal tract (Table 8-4). However, because of significant first-pass metabolism, bioavailability is only 38%. Peak blood levels are reached 0.5 to 2 hours after oral administration. Moricizine is highly plasma bound to protein (95%). The mean elimination half-life is 6 hours. With chronic dosing, the half-life may increase to 12 hours. Moricizine is extensively metabolized (at least 26 metabolites) with significant first-pass metabolism occurring. Two active metabolites probably have little importance because they represent less than 1% of the administered parent drug dose. About 56% of moricizine is excreted in the feces and 39% in the urine.

Dosing

Moricizine is available as 200-, 250-, and 300-mg tablets. The typical daily oral dosage is 200 to 400 mg three times a day. We usually initiate therapy at 200 mg three times a day then increase by 150 mg per day at 3-day intervals.

Efficacy

In non–life-threatening ventricular arrhythmias, moricizine is usually effective in 50% to 65% of patients as assessed by Holter monitoring regardless of ejection fraction (160). In comparative studies, moricizine has been demonstrated to be equally effective as propranolol, quinidine, and disopyramide (161). In the Cardiac Arrhythmia Suppression Trial II (CAST II), moricizine was shown to have an early (first 14 days) enhanced mortality rate (p = 0.02) when compared with placebo in post–myocardial infarction ventricular arrhythmia patients (162). During chronic follow-up, no statistical difference in mortality rates was noted. These results have limited the use of this drug. In refractory sustained VT, as assessed by programmed stimulation, the response rate is less than 20%, although moricizine usually slows the VT rate in patients who remain inducible (163,164). The efficacy of moricizine in treating various supraventricular tachyarrhythmias has not been well established. It has been shown to suppress retrograde AV nodal and accessory pathway conduction and have some efficacy in suppressing atrial fibrillation.

Adverse Effects

Moricizine causes proarrhythmia in about 3% to 4% of patients with potentially lethal ventricular arrhythmias (45,46). In CAST II, some early post–myocardial infarction mortality cases secondary to moricizine were felt to result from enhanced proarrhythmic potential in the ischemic setting (162). In patients with depressed ejection fractions and lethal arrhythmias, the proarrhythmic rate exceeds 10%. The most common adverse reactions include dry mouth, paresthesias, vertigo, dizziness (15%), nausea, headache, fatigue, dyspnea, palpitations, dyspepsia, diarrhea, vomiting, and sweating. Dizziness appears to be dose-related. Rarely, moricizine can cause a fever and elevation of liver function test scores. No other significant end-organ toxicity has been reported. Moricizine has minimal negative inotropic activity. Moricizine worsened heart failure in 2.8% of 374 patients with a prior history of heart failure and only 0.1% of 545 patients without a history of heart failure (165). There is no known significant interaction with digoxin or warfarin. Cimetidine raises moricizine levels by 40% and moricizine improves the clearance and shortens the half-life of theophylline derivatives.

Propranolol (Inderal, Inderal-LA)

Propranolol is a β blocker that has had FDA approval for treating supraventricular and ventricular arrhythmias since 1973. Propranolol is noncardioselective, has no intrinsic sympathomimetic activity, but does have membrane-stabilizing activity. It is available as a short-acting and long-acting (Inderal-LA) oral preparation and also parenterally.

Pharmacokinetics

Propranolol is almost completely absorbed orally, but bioavailability is markedly reduced as a result of first-pass metabolic breakdown by way of the CYP D6 enzyme system in the liver. With chronic administration, there is saturation of the hepatic system with an increase in bioavailability from 10% or 20% to 50%. The major metabolite is 4-OH-propranolol. The half-life of propranolol is 3 to 6 hours with steady state being achieved within 30 hours. Inderal-LA has a duration of action exceeding 24 hours. Intravenously, propranolol has an initial α half-life of 10 minutes followed by a β half-life of 2 to 3 hours. Therefore, after intravenous propranolol, systemic effects may last for hours.

Dosing

Oral dosage varies from 40 to 640 mg daily. Because of first-pass metabolism, only about 10% is given as an intravenous dose (1 to 10 mg). Complete sympathetic blockade requires 0.15 to 0.2 mg/kg of intravenous propranolol.

Electrophysiology

Propranolol has membrane-stabilizing effects with mild sodium channel blocking effects. Propranolol inhibits many of the effects of β-receptor stimulation such as blocking enhanced automaticity and adrenergic improvement in conduction velocities and shortening of refractory periods. Propranolol also blocks adrenergic activation of calcium channels. Propranolol decreases resting heart rate, prolongs sinus node recovery times, increases PR and A-H intervals and may decrease the QT interval. Propranolol prolongs refractoriness in the AV node with little effect on refractoriness of other cardiac tissues.

Efficacy

Propranolol is effective in slowing the ventricular response (particularly during exercise) but rarely terminates or prevents the occurrence of atrial flutter and fibrillation or paroxysmal supraventricular tachycardia. Propranolol is also effective in slowing sinus heart rate in patients with inappropriate symptomatic sinus tachycardia. With ventricular arrhythmias, propranolol will suppress premature ventricular contractions, ventricular couplets, and nonsustained VT in 45% to 50% of patients. In the electrophysiology laboratory, propranolol is effective in less than 5% of patients with inducible sustained VT. Propranolol is the drug of choice in exercise-aggravated or exercise-induced arrhythmias and in patients with prolonged QT syndrome. Propranolol is effective as adjunct therapy with a sodium channel blocker for supraventricular tachycardia and VT. Adrenergic reversal of sodium channel blockers can be blunted by propranolol. Intravenously, propranolol can be used to acutely slow the ventricular response or treat arrhythmia patients in the critical care setting. Like timolol, metoprolol, and acebutolol, propranolol has been shown to significantly reduce mortality rates in the post–myocardial infarction period (166,167). Carvedilol, bisoprolol, and long-acting metoprolol have also been shown to prolong survival in CHF patients (168–170).

Adverse Effects

Propranolol can aggravate sinus node dysfunction and AV block as well as slow heart rate. Because propranolol is not cardioselective, it can cause bronchospasm or mask the sympathetic-mediated warning signs of hypoglycemia in insulin-dependent diabetics. Because of its significant negative inotropic effects, dose-related worsening of CHF is common. Subjective side effects include fatigue and mental blunting.

Acebutolol (Sectral)

Acebutolol is a β blocker that has been approved for the management of ventricular arrhythmias. Acebutolol differs from propranolol in that it is more cardioselective, has intrinsic sympathomimetic activity, and is more hydrophilic. Like propranolol, it has membrane-stabilizing activity at higher doses.

Electrophysiology
Acebutolol has electrophysiologic effects that are like those of other β blockers, except that its intrinsic sympathomimetic activity causes less reduction in heart rate than propranolol.

Pharmacokinetics
Acebutolol is well absorbed from the gastrointestinal tract and is subject to extensive first-pass hepatic metabolism by way of the CYP D6 enzyme system into the pharmacologically active *N*-acetylmetabolite, diacetolol. Although the half-life of acebutolol is only 3 to 4 hours, the half-life of diacetolol is longer (8 to 13 hours), making twice-daily dosing an option. The drug is partially excreted in the urine.

Dosing
Drug therapy is initiated with 200 mg twice daily and increased to 400 mg twice daily if necessary.

Efficacy
Acebutolol has efficacy rates like those of propranolol in suppressing ventricular ectopic activity (171). Acebutolol is effective in controlling about 45% to 50% of patients with benign and potentially lethal ventricular arrhythmias as defined by Holter monitoring (172). In one study, efficacy rates of acebutolol were like those of quinidine. In patients with sustained VT, acebutolol has been effective in less than 5% of patients. Acebutolol reduced mortality rate by 48% in one high-risk post–myocardial infarction study (173) with long-term maintenance of this protective effect.

Adverse Effects
The most frequent adverse reactions from acebutolol are those typically associated with β blockers, such as depression and fatigue. Because of its intrinsic sympathomimetic activity, symptomatic bradycardia is less common with acebutolol than with propranolol. Although acebutolol is relatively cardioselective, asthma and other bronchospastic lung disease can be exacerbated. Worsening of AV block and aggravation of heart failure can result from its negative inotropic activity. Rare cases of reversible hepatic toxicity represent the only known end-organ toxicity.

Esmolol Hydrochloride (Brevibloc)

Esmolol is an intravenous β-blocking agent that is relatively cardioselective, has no intrinsic sympathomimetic or membrane-stabilizing activity, and is weakly lipid soluble (174).

Electrophysiology
After an intravenous infusion of esmolol, electrophysiologic effects, as determined by a slowing in sinus cycle length and prolongation of sinus node recover times, occur within 5 minutes. Esmolol also slows AV nodal conduction. No direct effect on atrial or ventricular refractoriness or H-V interval has been noted.

Pharmacokinetics
Esmolol is an ultrashort-acting intravenous β blocker (about one fortieth the blocking potency of propranolol) (175). Within 24 hours of termination, up to 88% of the drug is accounted for in the urine, as the clinically inactive acid metabolites. Esmolol given intravenously has a distribution half-life of 2 minutes and an elimination half-life of 9 minutes. After a loading infusion, steady-state blood levels can be reached in 5 minutes. After discontinuation, blood levels deplete rapidly within 10 minutes and are negligibly present within 30 minutes.

Dosing
Esmolol is usually given as a 500 mcg/kg loading dose intravenously for 1 minute. This is usually followed by a 4-minute infusion at 50 μg/kg per minute. The infusion can be increased up to 300 μg/kg per minute if necessary.

Efficacy
In patients with supraventricular tachycardia and atrial fibrillation, a slowing of mean ventricular rate quickly occurs. In a 63-patient study, esmolol produced a therapeutic response in 72% of patients with various supraventricular tachycardias, compared with 6% on placebo. In a comparative study, a therapeutic response was noted in 72% of patients receiving esmolol compared with 69% of those receiving intravenous propranolol (176).

Adverse Effects
Esmolol exhibits equal effects on heart rate slowing as those of propranolol with more rapid reversal of beta blockade on discontinuation. Esmolol, like other β blockers, has significant negative inotropic activity. Decreases in hemodynamics are similar to those seen after administration of 4 mg of intravenous propranolol. Dose-related hypotension is the most common adverse effect.

Amiodarone (Cordarone)

Amiodarone is an iodinated benzofuran derivative that is commercially available intravenously and orally. It is a coronary vasodilator with antiischemic effects.

Electrophysiology

Amiodarone has been subclassified as a class III antiarrhythmic agent. However, amiodarone has class I, II, III, and IV (l-type calcium channel) actions (9,177,178). Because the sodium channels are depressed in phase 0 in a use-dependent fashion, the effects of amiodarone become more pronounced at faster heart rates. Amiodarone also has some sympatholytic properties, although catecholamine-reversal studies suggest these effects are weak. *In vivo*, amiodarone prolongs refractoriness and slows conduction in the atria AV node, His-Purkinje system, ventricles, and accessory pathways. *In vitro* and *in vivo*, amiodarone slows sinus node automaticity and thus heart rate. Prolongation of APD, without reverse use dependency, is secondary to potassium channel-blocking effects, both I_{Kr} and I_{Ks}. Some of the electrophysiologic and antiarrhythmic effects of amiodarone may be secondary to impairing the peripheral conversion of thyroxine to $3,5,3'$-triiodothyronine.

Intravenously, amiodarone slows heart rate and prolongs AV nodal refractoriness. Intravenous amiodarone has little acute effect on atrial or ventricular refractoriness (179). Intravenous amiodarone is not associated with any significant prolongation of APD of use-dependent sodium channel blockade. Its acute effects may be partially explained by its sympatholytic and calcium channel-blocking effects.

Pharmacokinetics

The clinical pharmacology of oral amiodarone is not well understood, although it is best represented by a three-compartment model (180) (Table 8-6). Amiodarone has a large volume of distribution (500 L) and a long half-life (average of 53 days) requiring months for blood levels to reach equilibrium. The bioavailability of amiodarone averages 30% to 50%. Serum levels are higher when amiodarone is taken with food. Excretion is minimal by both hepatic and fecal routes. It is not dialyzable. Because of its high lipophilicity, amiodarone and its metabolites are extensively distributed into fat, muscle, liver, lung, and spleen. Amiodarone is extensively metabolized to desethylamiodarone. Amiodarone has biphasic elimination with a decrease in levels during the first 3 to 10 days after cessation of therapy, fol-

lowed by an increased drug concentration rebound that is thought to be a result of elimination of parent compound from poorly perfused tissues. Because of the drug's long half-life, plasma levels of amiodarone and desethylamiodarone can be measured as long as 9 months after cessation of therapy with clinically significant plasma levels lasting 3 months or more. Myocardial concentrations are 10 to 50 times those of plasma.

Intravenous amiodarone has complex pharmacokinetics. Peak serum concentrations range from 5 to 41 mg/L after a 15-minute infusion. Because of the rapid distribution of the drug, serum concentrations decrease to 19% of peak values within 30 to 45 minutes of discontinuing an infusion (181). Although parent-compound plasma levels are high with intravenous use, desethylamiodarone levels are quite low.

Dosing

Amiodarone requires an oral loading dosage of 800 to 1,400 mg a day for several weeks. By 4 weeks of therapy, dosages average about 600 mg a day. By 4 months, most of our patients are taking 400 mg a day. In an attempt to minimize toxicity, maintenance dosages ranging from 200 mg every other day to 400 mg a day are preferred. Therapeutic blood levels are in the l.0- to 2.5-μg/mL range. Blood levels, along with a clinical judgment of efficacy and toxicity, are used to titrate the dose downward. Low dosages of 200 mg four times a week to every day can be used in patients with atrial fibrillation.

Intravenous dosing starts with a 150-mg bolus injection given during 10 minutes, followed by a slow loading infusion of 360 mg given during 6 hours at 1 mg per minute and 540 mg given at 0.5 mg per minute during the remaining 18 hours (181). Supplemental infusions of 150 mg given during 10 minutes can be given for breakthrough arrhythmias (181).

Efficacy

Amiodarone has been approved for the treatment of life-threatening ventricular arrhythmias. Amiodarone is effective in more than 60% of patients with refractory sustained VT or VF (182,183), although noninducibility may only be demonstrated in 20% of patients. Its long half-life and delayed effects, or asymptomatic recurrences of self-terminating, slower VT may explain low recurrence rates despite noninducibility. Although empiric therapy with amiodarone has been demonstrated to be more effective than guided therapy with most conventional antiarrhythmics (184), several trials have demonstrated that the implantable cardioverter-defibrillator is more effective in improving survival in patients with sustained ventricular tachyarrhythmias (154,185,186) (Table 8-7). In the Antiarrhythmics Versus Implantable Defibrillators trial, the implantable-cardioverter defibrillator decreased the total mortality rate by 39% ($p <$ 0.02) compared with empiric amiodarone-guided sotalol therapy (185). In CASH, 2-year efficacy rates of amiodarone

TABLE 8-6. PHARMACOKINETIC PROPERTIES OF AMIODARONE

Bioavailability	Variable (22–86%)
Elimination	Hepatic and intestinal
Elimination half-life	
Acute	3–21 h
Chronic	52.6 d
Therapeutic range	1.0–2.5 μg/mL
Protein binding	96%
Active metabolites	Mono-*N*-desethylamiodarone
Drug interactions	Warfarin, digoxin, quinidine, procainamide, flecainide

TABLE 8-7. AMIODARONE/ICD TRIALS IN SUSTAINED VT/VF

	AVID	CIDS	CASH
N	1,016	659	349
Therapy	ICD vs empiric amiodarone or guided sotalol	ICD vs empiric amiodarone	ICD vs empiric amiodarone, metoprolol or propafenone
Primary End point	Total mortality	Total mortality	Total mortality
Drug event rate	17.7%	8.3%	9.8%
Principal finding	ICD decreased TM by 39% ($p < 0.02$) compared with amiodarone or sotalol group	ICD decreased TM by 19.6% ($p = 0.072$) compared with amiodarone group	ICD group decreased TM by 30% ($p = 0.047$) compared with metoprolol plus amiodarone group

ICD, implantable cardioverterdefibrillator; VT, ventricular tachycardia; VF, ventricular fibrillation; TM, total mortality; AVID, Antiarrythmia Versus Implantable Defibrillators; CIDS, Canadian Implantable Defibrillators Study; CASH, Cardiac Arrest Study Hamburg.

were no higher than those of metoprolol (187). In the Cardiac Arrest in Seattle: Conventional versus Amiodarone Drug Evaluation (CASCADE) study (184), event-free survival of survivors of cardiac arrest was statistically better ($p = 0.001$) for empiric amiodarone than guided conventional therapy. However, 4-year amiodarone treated recurrent cardiac arrest/arrhythmic death rates were still high (52%), suggesting a benefit of concomitant implantable cardioverter-defibrillator therapy in such patients.

Although not approved for use in patients with potentially lethal ventricular arrhythmias, amiodarone is a very effective (more than 70%) suppresser of ventricular ectopic activity as assessed by Holter monitoring. Although the Grupo de Estudio de la Sobrevida en la Insuficiencia Cardiac en Argentina (GESICA) trial (76) demonstrated an improvement in survival in amiodarone patients with CHF (most with concomitant ventricular arrhythmias), the Congestive Heart Failure–Survival Trial of Antiarrhythmic Therapy (CHF–STAT) study (57) demonstrated a neutral effect on survival even in patients whose ventricular arrhythmias were suppressed (Table 8-8). In CAMIAT (55), post–myocardial infarction patients with concomitant ventricular arrhythmias had decreased arrhythmic death but no statistical improvement in total survival when treated with amiodarone. In EMIAT (56), amiodarone was used to treat post–myocardial infarction patients with depressed ejection fractions. In EMIAT, as in CAMIAT, arrhythmic death was statistically reduced, but there was no statistical improvement in overall survival (Table 8-9). In both EMIAT and CAMIAT, the addition of a β blocker to amiodarone improved survival (92). In the Multicenter Automatic Implantable Defibrillator Implantation Trial (188), there was a 54% improvement in survival using an implantable cardioverter-defibrillator instead of amiodarone (or other antiarrhythmics) in post–myocardial infarction populations with a depressed ejection fraction, nonsustained VT, and inducible sustained VT not suppressed by intravenous procainamide. Similar results were reported in the Multicenter Unsustained Tachycardia Trial (189) with implantable cardioverter-defibrillator superiority over amiodarone and other antiarrhythmic drugs.

Oral amiodarone, even at low doses, can be effective in controlling two thirds of the patients with otherwise drug-refractory atrial fibrillation or paroxysmal supraventricular tachycardia. Because of its AV node effects, amiodarone is effective in slowing the ventricular response in chronic or recurrent episodes of atrial fibrillation. Gosselink and colleagues (190) noted that amiodarone maintained normal sinus rhythm in 61% (1 year) and 56% (2 years) after spontaneous or electrical conversion. Recent data from the Canadian Trial of Atrial Fibrillation (191) suggest amiodarone is more effective than sotalol or propafenone in maintaining sinus rhythm.

Intravenous amiodarone controls life-threatening ventricular tachyarrhythmias with an efficacy comparable to bretylium but with better tolerance (77,78,181). An amiodarone resus-

TABLE 8-8. SELECTED FEATURES OF GESICA AND CHF–STAT

	GESICA	CHF–STAT
No. of patients	516	674
LVEF	<35%	≤40%
Ischemic cardiomyopathy	39%	70%
NYHA III/IV	79%	43%
Mean heart rate (bpm)	90	80
Atrial fibrillation	29%	15%
>1 PVC/h	71%	100%
Nonsustained VT	33%	77%
Primary end point	Total mortality	Total mortality
Placebo event rate	21.0%	9.4%
Follow-up (median)	13 mo	45 mo
Treatment withdrawal	3%	41%
Principal finding	Amiodarone reduced TM ($p = 0.024$)	TM (pNS) TM in nonischemic patients trended ($p = 0.07$) favorably

GESICA, Grupo de Estudio de la Sobrevida en la Insuficiencia Cardiac en Argentina; CHF–STAT, Congestine Heart Failure-Survival Trial of Antiarrythmic Therapy; TM, total mortality; LVEF, left ventricular ejection fraction; PVC, premature ventricular contractions; VT, ventricular tachycardia.

TABLE 8-9. SELECTED FEATURES OF EMIAT AND CAMIAT

	EMIAT	CAMIAT
Entry criteria		
Days post-myocardial infarction	5–21	6–45
LVEF	<40%	No requirement
Ectopy	Not required	≥10 PVCs/h or ≥1 run
n	1,486	1,202
Double-blind Rx	Amiodarone-placebo	Amiodarone-placebo
Primary End point		Total mortality AD/recuscitated VF
Secondary End point	Resuscitated CA	CD, AD, AD + AD, CD, TM
Placebo event rate	7.8%	4.2%
Amiodarone dosing after loading	200 mg/d	1 g/wk–300 mg/d
Follow-up	≥1 y	2 y
Patients on β blocker	44% (amiodarone)	60% (amiodarone, placebo)
	45% (placebo)	
Principal finding	Amiodarone reduced (p = 0.05)AD by 35%; no effect on TM	Amiodarone reduced AD/resuscitated (p = 0.029) no effect on TM

AD, arrhythmic death; CD, cardiac death; TM, total mortality; LVEF, left ventricular ejection fraction; CA, cardiac arrythmia; VF, ventricular fibrillation; PVC, premature ventricular contractions; EMIAT, European Myocardial Infarct Amiodarone Trial; CAMIAT, Canadian Amiodarone Myocardial Infarction Trial.

citation study demonstrated that patients treated with intravenous amiodarone out-of-hospital had a better chance of survival to hospital admission than those treated with placebo (192). Intravenous amiodarone is also effective in slowing AV nodal conduction in patients with rapid atrial tachyarrhythmias in the critical care setting (193). Because it has little acute effect on the atrial ERP, intravenous amiodarone is no more effective than placebo in terminating atrial fibrillation (194). If larger doses of intravenous amiodarone are used, some effects on atrial fibrillation conversion have been reported.

Adverse Effects

Adverse effects during amiodarone therapy are common (195–197). However, CASH, and Canadian Implantable Defibrillator Study (CIDS) demonstrated only a 3% to 4% per year amiodarone drug discontinuation rate resulting from adverse effects. Minor side effects that seldom require drug discontinuation include corneal microdeposits, asymptomatic transient elevation of hepatic enzymes, photosensitivity of the skin, blue-gray skin discoloration, and subjective gastrointestinal side effects. Very few cases of optic neuritis causing blindness have been reported. Amiodarone-induced hypothyroidism occurs in about 8% of our patients and requires the addition of thyroid replacement. Drug-induced hyperthyroidism (2%) may require discontinuation of therapy. Liver and thyroid function tests are recommended two times a year (198). The most serious adverse effect requiring discontinuation of amiodarone is interstitial pneumonitis (3% to 7%). Kudenchuk and colleagues (199) reported that patients with baseline abnormal chest x-rays or pulmonary function tests have a higher incidence of developing pulmonary fibrosis. This adverse effect is dose-related and occurs rarely if less than 400 mg per day is used as the maintenance dosage. Annual

chest x-rays and measurements of diffusion capacity can screen for this abnormality. Neurologic side effects, including a peripheral neuropathy and myopathy, usually resolve on lowering the dose. Drug-induced bradycardia may require backup permanent pacing in up to 2% of patients. Low-dose amiodarone may minimize the frequency of these adverse effects (195). Amiodarone increases the defibrillation threshold in patients who have implantable cardioverter-defibrillators (200). Amiodarone may also increase pacing thresholds. The safety of amiodarone in pregnant women has not been established. Amiodarone crosses the placenta and is present in breast milk. Venous sclerosis can be minimized if intravenous amiodarone is given through a central venous line.

Amiodarone is well tolerated hemodynamically with minimal negative inotropic effects. Fewer than 4% of orally treated patients will have worsening of CHF. The vasodilating properties of amiodarone partially compensate for its negative inotropic effects. The predominant adverse effect of intravenous amiodarone is drug-induced hypotension (181).

Although amiodarone prolongs APD, amiodarone-induced torsade de pointes is rare and the development of incessant sustained VT occurs in less than 4% of patients.

Amiodarone has been shown to interact with digoxin, warfarin, quinidine, procainamide, and flecainide (196,198). Digoxin levels will double, type I antiarrhythmic levels will increase 15% to 35% and prothrombin times will double or triple. Concomitant use of these drugs requires lower doses and close monitoring.

Bretylium (Bretylol)

Bretylium is an intravenous, class III agent useful in the acute treatment of sustained ventricular tachyarrhythmias.

Electrophysiology

Bretylium affects the heart through direct action on the membrane and indirectly through sympathetic denervation of the heart. Bretylium prolongs the APD and the ERP of Purkinje fibers in ventricular muscle through a direct effect without altering the ERP-APD ratio. However, this prolongation seems to be more significant in healthy tissue than ischemic tissue. Thus, bretylium may raise the VF threshold by reducing the disparity of ventricular refractoriness between ischemic and nonischemic tissue.

The electrophysiologic effects of bretylium are time-dependent and complex, a net result of its indirect and direct actions (201,202). Direct activity, which dominates later electrophysiologic effects including lengthening of APD and refractory period, becomes evident in the setting of the bretylium's antiadrenergic actions. These latter effects are important to chronic antiarrhythmic activity. However, both the direct (electrophysiologic actions on the cardiac membrane) and the indirect effects (sympatholytic) of the drug are clinically relevant, as is the absence of sodium channel-blocking or class I effects of the drug.

Bretylium characteristically lengthens the APD and the ERP proportionately in ventricular tissue and Purkinje fibers (201,202) primarily by lengthening the plateau (phase 2) of the action potential, a consequence of blockade of cardiac membrane potassium channels (203). The favorable electrophysiologic effects of bretylium in the ischemic tissue are accompanied by a reduction in the dispersion of myocardial refractoriness between nonischemic and ischemic zones. Unlike other class III compounds, bretylium does not induce torsade de pointes. From this, it may be inferred that the drug does not act predominantly by blocking I_{Kr} in myocardial muscle and it may not unduly prolong the APD in the M cells of the ventricle. The observation that bretylium can dramatically increase the electrical threshold for induction of VF in experimental studies of nonischemic and ischemic myocardium has served as a primary stimulus for its development as an antiarrhythmic-antifibrillatory agent (204).

Antiadrenergic Effects

Bretylium is an adrenergic neuron-blocking drug with complex pharmacologic properties. These include indirect effects that stem from its interactions with adrenergic neurons, as well as direct (cardiac membrane) ones on the myocardial membranes. Interaction with adrenergic neurons includes early sympathomimetic activity, caused by norepinephrine release, and subsequent adrenergic neuronal blockade. These actions are a consequence of selective accumulation of bretylium in sympathetic ganglionic and postganglionic adrenergic neurons, with uptake leading to initial norepinephrine release. This is followed by subsequent inhibition of norepinephrine release caused by depression of adrenergic neuronal excitability, leading to chemical sympathectomy, which *per se* may exert an antifibrillatory effect. The direct effects of the compound on cardiac membranes include the proportionate lengthening of action potential and of the refractory period, a class III effect, related to blockade of potassium-carrying ion channels (203).

Pharmacokinetics

Intravenous bretylium has a rapid onset of action that occurs within minutes. An intravenous injection of bretylium in human volunteers produces serum concentrations that are more than 10-fold greater than those observed after equivalent oral doses. Calculated oral bioavailability is variable, averaging only 20% to 25%. Elimination by both routes follows a biexponential decay, accounted for entirely by renal clearance. Similar kinetics have been shown to apply to cardiac patients given intravenous bretylium (205). Disposition was entirely accounted for by renal elimination, which averaged 400 mL per minute. Terminal elimination half-life of bretylium averages 13.5 hours. Apparent volumes of distribution of bretylium average 3 to 7 L/kg (205). Bretylium is negligibly bound to plasma proteins, has no known metabolites, and does not interact directly with other drugs. Therapeutic blood levels are in the range of 1 µg/mL.

Dosing

The initial recommended dose of bretylium is 5 to 10 mg/kg given intravenously. The maintenance dosage schedule is 1 to 2 mg per minute as a continuous intravenous infusion. Bretylium should be administered in a monitored, critical care setting. For VF and hemodynamically unstable VT, an initial dose of 5 mg/kg is given undiluted by rapid intravenous injection. If VF persists, the dose may be increased to 10 mg/kg and repeated, together with other measures. There is relatively little experience or rationale for using doses of more than 30 mg/kg.

When hemodynamically stable ventricular tachyarrhythmias are treated, the dosage is 5 to 10 mg/kg during at least 8 minutes (preferably, 15 to 30 minutes) to prevent nausea and vomiting. Subsequent doses may be given at 1- to 2-hour intervals if arrhythmia persists or recurs. For maintenance therapy, a diluted solution of bretylium is administered as a constant infusion, generally at a rate of 1 to 2 mg per minute. Alternatively, a dose of 5 to 10 mg/kg may be administered by slow injection (i.e., 10 to 30 minutes) every 6 hours. Intramuscular therapy may be given, if necessary, but intravenous administration is preferred.

Accumulation of bretylium may occur in patients with advanced renal failure (particularly when creatinine clearance is less than 25 mL per minute). Dialysis increases bretylium clearance twofold. Hepatic dysfunction and heart failure are not known to change the pharmacokinetics of bretylium, except to the extent that renal clearance has changed.

Efficacy

Bretylium is a unique antiarrhythmic agent. In addition to its antiarrhythmic properties, the drug has excellent antifibrillatory properties. Several studies have shown that defibrillation is possible with bretylium alone or with bretylium and cardioversion when lidocaine alone or cardioversion alone have failed to revert the patient to sinus rhythm (206). Overall, a beneficial effect of bretylium has been reported in 60% to 70% of patients, with antifibrillatory effects occurring within 10 to 15 minutes (207–210). In contrast, maximal antiarrhythmic activity (suppression of ventricular ectopy or tachycardia) has generally not been observed for several hours (211). In an important observational study, 27 consecutive patients with resistant VF attended by a hospital cardiac arrest team were given bretylium (212). Successful termination of VF was achieved in 20 (74%) within 9 to 12 minutes, and 12 (44%) survived to discharge. In a controlled emergency ward study of 59 patients with cardiopulmonary arrest, bretylium was associated with a 35% survival rate, compared with a 6% rate in patients treated with resuscitative measures and other therapies (including lidocaine) alone (213). The outcome of bretylium treatment, however, was adversely affected by increasing times from cardiac arrest to therapy in another study (214).

Bretylium was compared with lidocaine in a controlled study of 146 patients experiencing out-of-hospital VF (215). In this Seattle Heart Watch Study, no significant difference was observed in the percentage of patients converting to an organized rhythm (about 90%), the proportion of patients successfully resuscitated (about 60%), and the percentage surviving to hospital discharge. A similarly designed, randomized Milwaukee Paramedic Study involving 91 patients with refractory VF reported a similar pattern of response (216).

Adverse Effects

Adverse effects of bretylium are primarily related to its modification of adrenergic function. Injections of bretylium cause a biphasic cardiovascular response (217). Initially, increases in heart rate and blood pressure are observed, a result of norepinephrine release from adrenergic nerve endings. This is followed within 15 to 30 minutes by reductions in vascular resistance, blood pressure, and heart rate, which are manifestations of sympathetic neuronal blockade, a result of interference with release but not of depletion of norepinephrine stores. Studies have shown that bretylium may improve myocardial function directly by increasing the amount of calcium available for myocardial contraction from intracellular stores, and indirectly by its effect on the sympathetic nervous system. Because of the release of norepinephrine caused by bretylium, there may be a transient increase in blood pressure and heart rate, and premature ventricular contractions during the initial 20 minutes. Anxiety, excitement, flushing, substernal pressure, headache, and angina pectoris are other manifestations that may be associated with the initial catecholamine release. Within 15 minutes, as a result of some antiadrenergic effects after a dose, postural hypotension and less frequently supine hypotension may be seen. Hypotension has required

drug discontinuation in about 10% of patients. Rarely, some nausea and vomiting occur during administration of bretylium. Because bretylium is primarily excreted by way of the kidney, accumulation may occur in those with advanced renal failure. In these patients, when maintenance therapy is given, infusion doses should be reduced and intervals for injections increased.

Sotalol (Betapace)

Sotalol is a unique, noncardioselective β blocker with type III properties (218) (Table 8-10).

The commercially available drug is a racemic mixture of d,l-sotalol. Sotalol has one third the β-blocking potency of propranolol. It exhibits no intrinsic sympathomimetic or local anesthetic activity.

Electrophysiology

Sotalol prolongs repolarization in a concentration-dependent fashion resulting in increases in the QT interval and the APD as determined by basic electrophysiologic measurements and monophasic action potential recordings in people. Action potential lengthening is predominantly secondary to a reduction in the delayed rectifier potassium current in addition to a decrease in the inward rectifier current. In high concentrations, sotalol inhibits the inward sodium current, but not calcium currents. Sotalol slows the sinus node cycle length and lengthens AV nodal conduction time (A-H interval) and the ERPs of the atria, AV node, ventricle, and accessory pathway. Sotalol demonstrates reverse use dependence in the atria with less electrophysiologic effects at faster heart rates (25). No effect on the H-V interval has been noted. Electrocardiographically, sotalol

TABLE 8-10. PHARMACOKINETIC PROPERTIES OF SOTALOL

Absorption rate	T$_{max}$ 2–3 h
Extent of absorption	>90% of dose
Extent of bioavailability	~100% of dose
Binding to plasma protein	0%
Approximate volume of distribution	1.6–2.4 L/kg
Elimination	
Renal (unchanged)	~90%
Biotransformation	0%
Approximate plasma half-life	15 (7–18) h
Pattern of elimination kinetics	First order
Kinetic model applicable	Open two compartment
Metabolites	None detected
Steady state to dose ratio	Two-fold variation
Special features	Accumulation in renal failure, kinetics not affected by liver function

Source: Sundquist H. Basic review and comparison of β-blocker pharmacokinetics. *Curr Ther Res* 1980;28:385, with permission.

prolongs the PR and corrected J-T intervals with no significant change in the QRS duration (Table 8-10). Sotalol's β-blocking properties predominate at lower doses and its type III effects predominate at higher doses (218).

Pharmacokinetics

Sotalol is nearly completely absorbed (more than 90%) and excreted by the kidney with minimal metabolic breakdown (219). Bioavailability approaches 100%. Peak blood levels are noted 2 hours after a dose and the elimination half-life varies from 7 to 15 hours. The β-adrenergic antagonism effects of sotalol are longer than the elimination half-life.

Dosing

Oral sotalol is initiated at 80 mg twice daily. Dosages are increased to 120 mg to 160 mg twice daily as needed.

Efficacy

Because of its effects on atrial, AV node, and accessory pathway refractoriness, sotalol is effective in converting and maintaining sinus rhythm in patients with atrial fibrillation; however, it is less effective than class Ia and Ic drugs for atrial fibrillation reversion (220). Rate control at the level of the AV node is also achieved in these patients. Sotalol is also effective in the treatment of paroxysmal supraventricular tachycardia and atrial fibrillation, with efficacy rates like those of quinidine and propafenone (221,222).

Sotalol appears to be effective in suppressing ventricular ectopic activity as assessed by a Holter monitoring in 50% to 60% of patients. In the ESVEM Study, sotalol was equally effective as quinidine, procainamide, mexiletine, and propafenone in achieving suppression of ventricular arrhythmias as assessed by serial Holter monitoring (105). In a post–myocardial infarction study, sotalol reduced the mortality rate by 18% (no difference compared with placebo) and reduced reinfarction rate by 41% ($p < 0.05$) during the year after infarction (58).

In sustained VT, as assessed by programmed stimulation, sotalol has been demonstrated to be effective in suppressing VT induction in almost 40% of patients in multiple trials including ESVEM (105,223). It has also been effective when used as an adjunct to an implantable cardioverter-defibrillator, reducing the incidence of total mortality or a first appropriate shock and total mortality or a first inappropriate shock by 44% and 64%, respectively (224).

Adverse Effects

Because of its β-blocking properties, sotalol has some negative inotropic potential; however, this is minimal compared with that of other β-blocking agents because lengthening of APD may enhance cardiac contractility. Noncardiac side effects are those typically noted for the other β blockers. Cardiac side effects of sotalol include hypotension, symptomatic bradycardia, or AV nodal conduction abnormalities. Torsade de pointes is the most common proarrhythmia caused by sotalol with a frequency similar to that associated with quinidine. This side effect is minimized to less than 2% if the total daily dose is no more than 320 mg per day and the QTc is less than or equal to 525 ms. Given its post–myocardial infarction safety, sotalol is commonly used to treat symptomatic arrhythmias in this setting.

Ibutilide (Corvert)

Ibutilide is a class III intravenous, antiarrhythmic agent with a novel mechanism of action. It is useful for the pharmacologic conversion of atrial fibrillation and atrial flutter (225).

Electrophysiology

Ibutilide prolongs APD and thus the QT interval by its property of blocking the rapid component of the delayed rectifier current (I_{Kr}); at much lower concentrations, the drug also activates a slow inward current carried largely by sodium ions, a current that is not blocked by I_{Kr} blockers (11–13). These effects have been demonstrated in isolated cardiac myocytes. In isolated atrial and ventricular muscle preparations, ibutilide increases the APD and the ERP, effects on both of which are attenuated at increasing rates (225). In people, the drug produces a concentration-related increase in the QT and QTc intervals (13,225). In the appropriate experimental models, the drug has the propensity to generate early afterdepolarizations, which in the *in vivo* setting may be the basis of the drug's proclivity to induce torsade de pointes (225–227). Thus, ibutilide, like most other class III compounds, is likely to produce antifibrillatory and profibrillatory actions (227).

Although ibutilide does produce a mild slowing of the sinus rate and slows AV nodal conduction in healthy volunteers and patients, there is no significant effect on heart rate, PR interval, or the QRS interval, and the drug does not lower blood pressure or worsen heart failure, as it does not exert a negative inotropic effect in the atria or the ventricles (13). It exhibits no significant interaction with the autonomic nervous system. The property that is critical for its therapeutic utility is the significant and acute prolongation of the atrial ERP, which leads to rapid termination of atrial fibrillation and flutter, and the lowering of the energy for electrical defibrillation when these arrhythmias are not amenable to electrical conversion (228). Some of its effects may be secondary to blocking the delayed rectifier potassium channel. Ibutilide prolongs atrial refractoriness. It has no evidence of reverse use dependence with equal effects on atrial refractoriness at both slow and fast heart rates. It has negligible effects on heart rate or AV nodal conduction and refractoriness. Ibutilide prolongs ventricular ERPs and lowers the defibrillation threshold (13,225).

Pharmacokinetics

Ibutilide is available only as an intravenous formulation, as the drug is rapidly metabolized in the liver as a first-pass phenomenon. For this reason, the oral formulation is unlikely to be effective. The plasma concentration of the drug decreases in a multiexponential manner, with a high initial level followed by a rapid systemic clearance by the hepatic route (13). The drug's pharmacokinetic properties (Table 8-11) are linear with the dose; there is a large volume of distribution, with 40% protein binding. The elimination half-life is variable (2 to 12 hours, with a mean of 6 hours). The drug is extensively metabolized to eight inactive metabolites (13,225) and excreted largely by the kidney; however, intravenous dosing does not require dose adjustments relative to changes in renal and hepatic function. Coadministration of ibutilide with digoxin, calcium channel blockers, or β blockers exerts no effect on the pharmacokinetics, safety, or the efficacy of the drug for the conversion of atrial fibrillation or flutter. Similarly, the age or gender of the patient or the nature of the arrhythmia being treated has no effect on the drug's pharmacokinetics.

Dosing
The usual dose is 1 mg intravenously during 10 minutes followed by a second dose of 1 mg if ineffective.

Efficacy
Ibutilide is effective in terminating atrial fibrillation in about 35% to 40% of patients within 1 hour compared with 3% efficacy in placebo-treated patients, 18% efficacy with intravenous procainamide, and 11% for sotalol (32,226,229–231). It is even more effective in terminating atrial flutter with efficacy rates averaging 60%. Similar efficacy rates for atrial fibrillation and flutter have been reported in the post–coronary artery bypass graft setting (232). The major issues regarding the use of pure class III agents in the acute conversion of atrial fibrillation and atrial flutter have been summarized and critically discussed by Singh (233) and Roden (234).

Adverse Effects
Ibutilide's main toxicity is secondary to its ability to prolong APD and thus the QT interval. Nonsustained drug-induced torsade de pointes occurs in about 2% of patients with sustained polymorphic VT requiring cardioversion

occurring in an additional 2% of patients (44). All drug-induced proarrhythmia has occurred within 40 minutes of drug administration. Noncardiac side effects were indistinguishable from those of placebo, as were hypotension, conduction block, or bradycardia.

Dofetilide (Tikosyn)
Dofetilide is a class III antiarrhythmic that has been approved by the FDA for the treatment of atrial fibrillation.

Electrophysiology
Dofetilide is a methanesulfonanilide derivative with a similar structure to the non–β-blocking moiety of sotalol. The drug is a highly selective agent that delays repolarization and prolongs the APD in the atria, ventricles, and Purkinje fibers by I_{Kr} blockade, which is the sole identifiable action of the drug (235–237). The compound exerts no effects on sodium and calcium channels and therefore has minimal effects on conduction velocity and does not alter the PR interval or the QRS duration of the surface electrocardiogram. Its sole measurable electrophysiologic action is the lengthening of cardiac repolarization, as reflected in the QT-QTc interval, an effect that correlates directly with the lengthening of the refractory period. Dofetilide prolongs the atrial and ventricular ERP and the QT interval without affecting other conduction parameters; reverse use dependence of these changes has been reported. Dofetilide displays little affinity for adrenergic, adenosine, dopamine, or muscarinic receptors.

Pharmacokinetics
Dofetilide is well absorbed with a systemic bioavailability of more than 90% (Table 8-12). Peak plasma concentrations are achieved at about 2 hours, and the elimination half-life averages 9.5 hours. Steady state is achieved in about 2 days. More than 60% of the drug is excreted unchanged in the urine, with the remainder metabolized in the liver; dose adjustment is necessary in patients with impaired renal function.

Dosing
Dosing under telemetry conditions is based on baseline creatinine clearance resulting from the drug's predominant

TABLE 8-11. PHARMACOKINETIC PROPERTIES OF IBUTILIDE

- Linear pharmacokinetics
- Rapid, extensive extravascular distribution (V_{ds} range 6.6–13.4 L)
- High systemic clearance
- Elimination half-life 3–6 h
- Plasma protein bindings 41% bound
- Extensively hepatically metabolized—eight inactive metabolites

V_{ds}, Apparent volume of distribution.

TABLE 8-12. PHARMACOKINETIC PROPERTIES OF DOFETILIDE

Bioavailability	Absorbed >90% after oral ingestion, not affected by food
Elimination half-life	10 h
T_{max} (oral)	2–3 h
Elimination	80% by renal excretion, <20% by hepatic metabolism, no clinically active metabolites
Drug plasma concentration	Linear relationship
Increased plasma concentration	Directly related to increases in QTc

renal excretion. In patients with normal renal function, the dosage is 500 μg twice daily, and if abnormal renal function 250 μg twice daily. A reduction in the dose of the drug is also recommended if the QT-QTc interval increases by more than 15% or prolongs beyond 500 ms. These precautions have been shown to markedly reduce the incidence of torsade de pointes.

Efficacy

Dofetilide (Tikosyn) is the prototype of a pure or simple class III antiarrhythmic agent, the oral formulation of which was recently approved for the maintenance of sinus rhythm in patients with paroxysmal and persistent atrial fibrillation and flutter. Like ibutilide, the drug is effective in terminating recent-onset atrial fibrillation and flutter (238), although this indication is not approved for clinical use. In a placebo-controlled blinded study of 91 patients, Falk and colleagues (239) found a conversion rate of 13% and 31% in atrial fibrillation patients given 4 or 8 μg/kg of dofetilide intravenously; there were no conversions on placebo. In atrial flutter, the conversion rate was 54%.

Although effective in suppressing ventricular ectopy, dofetilide has been primarily studied in the prevention of atrial fibrillation and it is now approved for this indication. In the European and Australian Multicenter Evaluative Research on Atrial Fibrillation Dofetilide Study, the drug converted atrial fibrillation to sinus rhythm in about 29% of patients; at the end of the first year, 66% remained in sinus rhythm at the highest dosage (500 μg twice daily) compared with 26% on placebo ($p = 0.001$) (37). The median time to relapse of atrial fibrillation or flutter at the two higher dosages (250 and 500 μg twice daily) of the drug was more than 365 days compared with 34 for placebo. In a second study, Symptomatic Atrial Fibrillation Investigation and Randomized Evaluation of Dofetilide (240), involving 325 patients, 30% of patients converted on the 500 μg twice-daily dosage schedule, 70% of such conversions occurring during the first 24 hours. The 250 patients who achieved sinus rhythm only at the highest dosage (500 μg twice daily) showed significant efficacy when compared with placebo; the probability of the patients on 500 μg twice daily remaining in sinus rhythm at the end of 12 months was 58% in the case of dofetilide compared with 25% on placebo ($p = 0.001$). The median time for the patients to relapse to atrial fibrillation or flutter was more than 365 days on the active drug, compared with 27 days on placebo.

In the Danish Investigations of Arrhythmia and Mortality-Congestive Heart Failure (DIAMOND-CHF) study of 1,518 patients with heart failure and in the DIAMOND-Myocardial Infarction trial of 1,510 patients with a myocardial infarction, the drug had no effect on mortality rate (36). However, these studies have shown that the safety of the compound is critically dependent on the use of appropriate doses of the drug relative to renal function, therapy

initiation in hospital, and subsequent monitoring of the patient by following the changes in the QT-QTc intervals with adjustment of drug dose.

Adverse Effects

Subjectively, dofetilide is well tolerated. Its predominant concerning adverse effect is a 1.3% to 4% incidence of symptomatic torsade de pointes. The drug has no effect on myocardial contractility or on systemic hemodynamics. It does not depress systemic blood pressure. Hemodynamically, the drug is well tolerated and by prolonging APD is a positive inotropic agent. Dofetilide has been used safely in post–myocardial infarction and CHF patients in the DIAMOND trials (36) with neutral effects on overall survival. No known drug interactions with dofetilide exist.

The concomitant use of certain drugs during dofetilide therapy is contraindicated, particularly those that may substantially increase the plasma concentrations of dofetilide. These include verapamil, ketoconazole, cimetidine, trimethoprim/sulfamethoxazole, prochlorperazine, and magesterol. The drug is also contraindicated in patients with severe renal impairment and in those with acquired or congenital long QT syndrome. A previous history of torsade de pointes either on dofetilide or with any other QT-prolonging compounds is also a contraindication to the use of the drug for the treatment of atrial fibrillation or flutter.

New Class III Antiarrhythmic Drugs under Development

Some of the new class III antiarrhythmia drugs are listed in Table 8-2 (241).

Azimilide

Azimilide blocks multiple myocardial ion channels and the available data on the compound suggest that the compound may have a lower arrhythmogenic potential. The compound prolongs repolarization by predominantly blocking the slow component of the delayed rectifier current (I_{Ks}) with presumably somewhat lesser effects on the rapid component (242,243). In human isolated atrial and ventricular myocytes, azimilide produces a concentration-dependent inhibition of both the I_{Ks} and I_{Kr} (244). Such a property may not be associated with reverse use and rate dependency of action on repolarization; like amiodarone, azimilide maintains its class III action at high heart rates. It may therefore be less likely than other specific I_{Kr} blockers to produce torsade des pointes (243,244).

In healthy volunteers, oral azimilide in dosages of up to 200 mg per day (usual therapeutic dosages are 75, 100, and 125 mg per day) were well tolerated (245). It produced maximum increments in the QT interval, between 24% and 28%, although individual values ranged from 4% to 42% (246). The QT increases were dose-dependent without significant increases in the PR or QRS intervals or in heart rate or blood pressure, suggesting that the drug does not have sodium or calcium channel-blocking actions or significant influence on the sympathetic or parasympathetic nervous systems (241). Its effectiveness in maintaining stability in atrial fibrillation and flutter has been documented in large clinical trials (246). A mortality trial in the survivors of myocardial infarction with reduced left ventricular function is in progress (247).

Tedisamil

Tedisamil was developed for its antiischemic rather than its antiarrhythmic or antifibrillatory properties. Tedisamil blocks a complex aggregate of repolarizing myocardial ionic currents, has antiischemic properties, and slows the heart rate (248–250). The drug has been reported to block the delayed rectifier potassium channel (I_{Kr}) and the transient outward current, I_{to}. Tedisamil also modifies the responses of the K-channel (ATP-dependent or K_{ATP}) opener, pinacidil. Electrophysiologically, tedisamil has been found to prolong the APD in the atrial rather than in ventricular myocardium with corresponding increases in the ERP. It is in early stages for the development of its role in atrial fibrillation and flutter in regard to arrhythmia and maintenance of sinus rhythm.

Ersentilide

Ersentilide is a sotalol-like drug that is being investigated for the control of atrial fibrillation and flutter and ventricular arrhythmias, particularly in combination with the implantable cardioverter-defibrillator. It is an I_{Kr} blocker with the associated property of selectively blocking β_1 adrenoreceptor, in contrast to d,l-sotalol, which blocks both β_1 and β_2 adrenoreceptors. However, its pharmacodynamic and electrophysiologic properties (251) and its overall spectrum of clinical activity is likely to be similar to that of d,l-sotalol.

Trecetilide

Trecetilide exerts a similar mode of action on cardiac myocyte to that of ibutilide, but it is active orally and parenterally, with a high oral bioavailability.

Dronedarone

Dronedarone is a deiodinated derivative of amiodarone; it is in the early stages of development. This compound was developed with the expectation that the deletion of the iodine atoms from the aromatic ring, the substitution of the ethyl by butyl group in the terminal side chain, combined with the addition of methanesulfonyl to the benzofuran moiety will eliminate the well-recognized serious side effects of amiodarone. In the experimental setting, these expectations appear to have been met, but there is still paucity of clinical data with respect to the precise efficacy and the side effect profile of dronedarone. In contrast to amiodarone, dronedarone has a shorter elimination half-life, although the drug is metabolized in the liver; its electrophysiologic and pharmacologic time

course of action, particularly with respect to repolarization, is less time-dependent than that of amiodarone. In early human studies, it appears that much larger amounts of the drug may be needed to induce changes in heart rate and in the lengthening of the QT-QTc intervals of the surface electrocardiogram that are similar to those produced with amiodarone. The acute superfusion studies in isolated myocardial tissues revealed that like amiodarone, dronedarone shortened the APD and reduced the V_{max} of the upstroke velocity of the APD. In contrast, in tissues taken from animals pretreated with dronedarone for 3 weeks, there were marked and significant increases in the APD_{50} and APD_{90} and lengthening of the APD in the sinus node while slowing automaticity. In these respects, the drug appeared to be more potent than the parent compound in animals in which the drug also decreased heart rate and lengthened the QT-QTc intervals of the surface electrocardiogram. The available data indicate that the electrophysiologic properties including the influence on myocardial ion channels of dronedarone are similar to those of amiodarone, despite the absence of iodine in the molecular structure of the compound.

Verapamil (Calan, Isoptin)

Verapamil is a papaverine derivative that blocks the calcium channel and is classified as a type IV antiarrhythmic agent. Intravenous verapamil is available for the acute treatment of supraventricular tachycardia. Oral verapamil is available in a short-acting and controlled-release formulation and is useful in controlling the ventricular response in atrial fibrillation and preventing reentrant paroxysmal supraventricular tachycardia.

Electrophysiology

As a calcium l-channel antagonist, verapamil inhibits the slow channels by blocking the inward calcium current (252,253). Verapamil slows the sinus rate, although this direct suppressant effect may be counteracted by its vasodilatory properties, and slows AV nodal conduction, prolonging the A-H interval and the AV node effective and functional refractory periods. Verapamil has been noted to shorten the refractory period of accessory pathway tissue.

Pharmacokinetics

Although more than 90% of verapamil is absorbed, only 10% to 20% is bioavailable because of first-pass hepatic metabolism (252). Only 7% of the drug is excreted unchanged in the urine. Orally, peak levels occur in 2 hours and the half-life is 3 to 7 hours.

Dosing

When administered intravenously, verapamil effects occur in 3 to 5 minutes and last 20 to 30 minutes. The intravenous dose is 0.1 mg/kg (generally 5 to 10 mg) as a bolus; a second bolus can be given 15 minutes later if arrhythmia continues. If continuous infusions are needed, 0.005 mg/kg per minute is administered. Orally, the total daily dosage ranges from 160 to 720 mg per day; the short-acting form of the drug is administered three times daily while the long-acting form is a once-a-day drug.

Efficacy

Intravenous verapamil has been the drug of choice for the acute termination of reentrant premature supraventricular tachycardia using the AV node (254). Efficacy rates of 80% to 95% for reversion to sinus rhythm are comparable to those of intravenous adenosine. Intravenous verapamil can also be used to acutely slow the ventricular response in patients with atrial fibrillation and flutter (254–256). Intravenous verapamil should not be used in wide QRS tachycardias of undetermined origin because many of these tachycardias are VTs and verapamil may cause further hemodynamic compromise, including the precipitation of VF (257). The drug may also be hazardous in patients with atrial fibrillation with a wide complex in patients with the Wolff-Parkinson-White syndrome (258). Continuous infusions (0.1 mg/kg per hour) of verapamil may be useful for temporary rate control of multifocal atrial tachycardia and atrial fibrillation in the critical care setting.

Oral verapamil is useful in the control of the ventricular response in patients with atrial fibrillation and flutter; it may be used as a sole agent or in combination with digoxin or a β blocker (259,260). Oral verapamil may rarely be effective in preventing the recurrence of premature supraventricular tachycardia. Rarely, verapamil is effective in treating certain types of VT in patients with healthy hearts (261).

Adverse Effects

Verapamil can cause symptomatic bradycardia and sinus arrest and can worsen AV nodal block. Because of its significant negative inotropic effects, verapamil can depress left ventricular function and cause or worsen CHF. Intravenous verapamil can accelerate the preexcited ventricular response and potentially provoke VF in patients with atrial fibrillation and Wolff-Parkinson-White syndrome (258). Subjective toxicity includes nausea, dizziness, and constipation. Verapamil may increase the serum digoxin level during concomitant administration; this results from a reduction in digoxin clearance (262). Data suggest that verapamil may have beneficial effects on outcome in patients with a myocardial infarction who do not have heart failure (21% reduction in mortality rate) while it does not affect survival in those with heart failure (263).

Diltiazem (Cardizem)

Diltiazem is an l-channel calcium blocker with electrophysiologic effects similar to those of verapamil. Orally, it is approved for the treatment of angina and hypertension, although it is frequently used as adjunct therapy in rate control of atrial fibrillation. Intravenously, diltiazem has proven to be an effective drug for acutely terminating paroxysmal supraventricular tachycardia (264) with efficacy rates similar to those of verapamil and is approved for controlling the ventricular response with rapid atrial arrhythmias (265).

Dosing

Oral diltiazem is used at total daily dosages of 90 to 360 mg per day; it can be given once or twice per day. Intravenously, the dose is 0.25 mg/kg (average of 20 mg); a second dose of 25 mg may be given thereafter if necessary. Continuous intravenous infusions can be used at a dose of 10 to 15 mg per hour.

Electrophysiology

Diltiazem has electrophysiologic effects similar to those of verapamil. Because of less peripheral vasodilation, reflex changes are not as common; because of this, diltiazem more consistently slows heart rate. Diltiazem slows conduction (A-H interval) in the AV node and prolongs antegrade AV nodal refractoriness. It has no effect on accessory pathway tissue.

Efficacy

After an intravenous bolus, diltiazem will slow the ventricular response by about 25% within 3 to 7 minutes in patients with atrial tachyarrhythmias and a rapid ventricular response. Continuous intravenous infusion of diltiazem maintains a more than 20% decrease in heart rate in patients in atrial flutter and fibrillation and 76% will have adequate heart rate control for at least 10 hours (265). Intravenous diltiazem has been effective in terminating supraventricular tachycardia in more than 80% of cases within 3 minutes (264). Oral diltiazem is very effective in controlling the ventricular response in patients with rapid atrial fibrillation and flutter (266).

Adverse Effects

Intravenous diltiazem may cause substantial heart rate slowing, AV block, and hypotension. Compared with verapamil, hemodynamic compromise with diltiazem is less likely to occur. Oral diltiazem does not alter mortality in patients with a recent myocardial infarction and no heart failure, including those who receive a thrombolytic agent (267–269). However, the drug is associated with an increased mortality rate in post–myocardial infarction patients who have pulmonary congestion and heart failure (267,268).

Adenosine (Adenocard)

Adenosine is a purine agonist that is effective in terminating premature supraventricular tachycardia. The effects of adenosine are mediated by extracellular purinergic receptors.

Electrophysiology

Adenosine interacts with α_1 receptors on the extracellular surface of cardiac cells, activating potassium channels. The ensuing increase in potassium conductance is the predominant mechanism responsible for the action of adenosine on atrial myocardium, AV node, and sinus node cells (270,271). Enhanced potassium conductance shortens the duration of the atrial APD, hyperpolarizes the membrane potential, and reduces atrial contractility. The shortening of the atrial APD is probably responsible for the negative inotropic effect of adenosine in atrial myocardium, because it indirectly reduces calcium influx into the cells. Activation of the potassium conductance is also thought to be the major mechanism by which adenosine induces AV block; however, a decrease in calcium influx may also contribute. In contrast to atrial tissue, adenosine has no direct effect on the ventricular myocardium. As a result, adenosine has negative chronotropic and dromotropic effects on the sinoatrial and AV nodes. No effects on His-Purkinje conduction or ventricular refractoriness have been noted.

Pharmacokinetics

After injection, adenosine is rapidly cleared from the circulation by cellular uptake and metabolism. Adenosine enters the blood pool and metabolizes to inosine and adenosine monophosphate with an elimination half-life of less than 10 seconds. Onset of action is about 15 to 30 seconds after injection. Aminophylline counteracts the effects of adenosine. Dipyridamole, which is a potent adenosine uptake inhibitor, may potentiate the effect of adenosine (272,273).

Dosing

The dose of adenosine is 6 mg by bolus; an additional 6 to 12 mg can be given after 2 minutes if necessary. More than 90% of patients with premature supraventricular tachycardia will revert to sinus rhythm with a dose of less than 10 mg.

Efficacy

Adenosine at doses of 12 mg intravenously is effective in terminating supraventricular tachycardia in 91% of cases; this includes supraventricular tachycardia in the Wolff-Parkinson-White syndrome (272,273). Conversion to sinus rhythm usually occurs in less than 1 minute. Adenosine terminates supraventricular tachycardia quicker than verapamil (median of 30 versus 170 seconds). Adenosine is not effective for terminating other supraventricular tachyarrhythmias, including atrial fibrillation, atrial flutter, or atrial tachycardia. It has been found to be effective in terminating certain types of sustained VT, which occur in healthy hearts, are mediated by triggered activity resulting from calcium influxes, and are catecholamine sensitive (274). Because adenosine rarely affects VT and has a short half-life, it has been used as a diagnostic test in wide QRS tachycardia of undetermined origin (275). However, in patients with structural heart disease and hypotensive wide QRS tachycardia, adenosine should be avoided.

Adverse Effects

Dyspnea and flushing are the most common adverse effects that may occur transiently. Cardiac side effects include transient but significant sinus bradycardia, sinus tachycardia, sinus pauses, and AV block. More serious arrhythmias can occur, including prolonged ventricular asystole, VT, nonsustained polymorphic VT, or VF; torsade de pointes has been observed in patients at risk for bradycardia-dependent arrhythmias, particularly those with a prolonged QT interval (276,277). Atrial fibrillation after adenosine injection has been observed in up to 12% of patients; it is associated with a long-short atrial sequence, that is, an atrial premature beat with a short coupling cycle. At high doses, a transient decrease in blood pressure has been noted.

Digoxin (Lanoxin, Lanoxicaps) and Digitoxin (Crystodigin)

Digoxin and digitoxin are cardiac glycosides, often grouped in the digitalis glycoside family. These drugs are useful in controlling the ventricular response in atrial tachyarrhythmias and terminating and preventing supraventricular tachycardia; they also have positive inotropic effects in patients with systolic dysfunction (278).

Pharmacokinetics

Digoxin can be administered intravenously or orally. When administered orally, digoxin is 60% to 80% absorbed. After drug administration, a 6- to 8-hour distribution phase occurs. The volume of distribution is large. From 20% to 25% of digoxin is bound to protein. The time-to-onset effect is 0.5 to 2 hours and peak effect is 2 to 6 hours. Elimination of digoxin follows first-order kinetics. Because digoxin is primarily renally excreted, excretion may be diminished in patients with abnormal renal function. The elimination half-life in patients with normal renal function is l.5 to 2 days. This may be extended to 6 days in patients with significant renal dysfunction.

Digitoxin differs from digoxin in that it has a longer elimination half-life of 7 to 9 days and is primarily metabolized in the liver.

Electrophysiology

The major antiarrhythmic effect of digitalis glycosides is by way of an indirect action mediated by the autonomic nervous system; digoxin produces an enhancement of vagal activity. Thus, digitalis may slow sinus node automaticity and slow AV node conduction, prolonging AV node refractoriness. The direct effect of digoxin is to increase the force of myocardial contraction.

Dosing

The usual maintenance dosage of digoxin is 0.125 to 0.25 mg per day. As a result of drug-drug interaction, the dose of digoxin should be decreased in patients who are on concomitant quinidine, propafenone, verapamil, or amiodarone. It also should be decreased in patients with renal dysfunction. Because of the long elimination half-life, it may take more than a week for digoxin to reach steady state. Regardless of oral or intravenous administration, patients could be more rapidly digitalized using loading doses of 8 to 12 µg/kg (or 0.75 to 1.5 mg).

For digitoxin, digitalization can occur using 0.2 mg twice daily for 4 days after maintenance dosages of 0.05 to 0.3 mg daily, with the most common dosage being 0.1, 0.15, or 0.2 mg daily. In patients who develop life-threatening digitalis toxicity, Digibind can be given in an attempt to reverse some direct effects of digoxin acutely.

Efficacy

There is little proof in the literature that digoxin has a significant benefit in treating ventricular arrhythmias. However, there are some minimal reports and indirect evidence that in patients with systolic dysfunction, optimizing hemodynamics may have a beneficial antiarrhythmic effect (279). Digoxin is primarily used to control the ventricular rate in patients with atrial fibrillation, atrial flutter, and atrial tachycardia. Although digitalis is a useful drug for slowing conduction through the AV node and prolonging AV node refractoriness by way of its vagotonic effect, β blocker and calcium blockers are more effective; moreover, it is less likely to control the ventricular rate during exercise (when vagal tone is low and sympathetic tone is high). Although rapid digitalization is often used in patients who present with new-onset atrial fibrillation in an attempt to restore sinus rhythm, placebo-controlled studies have demonstrated that the conversion rates are similar to placebo (280–282). In patients with vagally induced atrial fibrillation, digitalis may make atrial fibrillation more likely to recur. Digitalis, by slowing conduction antegrade in the AV node, may be useful in slowing the ventricular response of patients with reentrant paroxysmal supraventricular tachycardias. In rare circumstances, this effect on AV nodal conduction may be beneficial in preventing recurrence of paroxysmal supraventricular tachycardia.

Adverse Effects

Noncardiac toxic manifestations of digitalis excess include anorexia, nausea, vomiting, headache, visual scotomas, and changes in color perception. Cardiac toxicity includes AV junctional escape rhythms, ventricular ectopic beats and bigeminy, VT, nonparoxysmal functional tachycardias, atrial tachycardia with block, and Mobitz type I AV block (283,284). In patients with heart failure, digitalis has not been shown to have any effects on long-term survival (285).

REFERENCES

1. Reiffel JA, Kowey PR. Generic antiarrhythmics are not therapeutically equivalent for the treatment of tachyarrhythmias. *Am J Cardiol* 2000;85(May 1):1151–1153.

2. Naccarelli G. Antiarrhythmic drugs. In: Willerson JT, Cohn J, eds. *Cardiovascular medicine,* 2nd ed. Philadelphia: WB Saunders, 2000:632–1649.

3. Buchert E, Woosley RL. Clinical implications of variable antiarrhythmic drug metabolism. *Pharmacogenetics* 1992;2:2–11.

4. Roden DM, Kim RB. Pharmacokinetics, pharmacodynamics, pharmacogenetics, and drug interactions. In: Zipes DP, Jalife J, eds. *Cardiac electrophysiology.* Philadelphia: WB Saunders, 2000:882–889.

5. Woosley RL, Chen Y, Freiman JP, Gillis RA. Mechanism of the cardiotoxic actions of terfenadine. *JAMA* 1993;269:1532–1536.

6. Honig PK, Woosley RL, Zamani K, et al. Changes in the pharmacokinetics and electrocardiographic pharmacodynamics of terfenadine with concomitant administration of erythromycin. *Clin Pharmacol Ther.* 1992;52:231–238.

7. Grant AO, Wendt DJ. Blockade of ion channels by antiarrhythmic drugs. *J Cardiovasc Electrophysiol* 1991;2:5153–5158.

8. Girouard SD, Pastore JM, Laurita KR, et al. Optical mapping in a new guinea pig model of ventricular tachycardia reveals mechanisms for multiple wavelengths in a single reentrant circuit. *Circulation* 1996;93:603–613.

9. Task Force of the Working Group on Arrhythmias of the European Society of Cardiology. The Sicilian gambit. A new approach to the classification of antiarrhythmic drugs based on their actions on arrhythmogenic mechanisms. *Circulation* 1991;84:1831–1851.

10. Katzung BG. New concept of antiarrhythmic drug action. In: Yu P, Goodwin J, eds. *Progress in cardiology.* Philadelphia: Lea & Febiger, 1987:5–16.

11. Lee KS, Gibson JK. Unique ionic mechanism of action of ibutilide on freshly isolated heart cells. *Circulation* 1995;92:2755–2757.

12. Lee KS. Ibutilide, a new compound with potent class III antiarrhythmic activity, activates a slow inward Na^+ current in guinea pig ventricular cells. *J Pharmacol Exp Ther* 1992;262:99–108.

13. Naccarelli GV, Lee KS, Gibson JK, VanderLugt J. Electrophysiology and pharmacology of ibutilide. *Am J Cardiol* 1996;78:12–16.

14. Schwanstecher M, Sieverding C, Dorschner H, et al. Potassium channel openers require ATP to bind to and act through sulfonylurea receptors. *EMBO J* 1998;17:5529–5535.

15. Sager PT, Uppal P, Follmer C, et al. Frequency-dependent electrophysiologic effects of amiodarone in humans. *Circulation* 1993;88:1063–1071.

16. Ranger S, Talajic M, Lemery R, et al. Kinetics of use-dependent ventricular conduction slowing by antiarrhythmic drugs in humans. *Circulation* 1991;83:1987–1994.

17. Sager PT, Behboodikhah M. Frequency-dependent electrophysiologic effects of d,l-sotalol and quinidine and modulation by beta-adrenergic stimulation. *J Cardiovasc Electrophysiol* 1996;7:102–112.

18. Ranger S, Talajic M, Lemery R, et al. Amplification of flecainide-induced ventricular conduction slowing by exercise. A potentially significant clinical consequence of use-dependent sodium channel blockade. *Circulation* 1989;79:1000–1006.

19. Montero M, Beyer T, Schmitt C, et al. Differential effects of quinidine on transmembrane action potentials of normal and infarcted canine Purkinje fibers. *J Cardiovasc Pharmacol* 1992;20:304–310.

20. Schmitt C, Kadish AH, Balke WC, et al. Cycle length-dependent effects on normal and abnormal intraventricular electrograms: effect of procainamide. *J Am Coll Cardiol* 1988;12:395–403.

21. Sager PT, Nademanee K, Antimisiaris M, et al. Antiarrhythmic effects of selective prolongation of refractoriness. Electrophysiologic actions of sematilide HCl in humans. *Circulation* 1993;88:1072–1082.

22. Hondeghem LM, Snyders DJ. Class III antiarrhythmic agents have a lot of potential but a long way to go. Reduced effectiveness and dangers of reverse use dependence. *Circulation* 1990; 81:686–690.
23. Nattel S, Zeng FD. Frequency-dependent effects of antiarrhythmic drugs on action potential duration and refractoriness of canine cardiac Purkinje fibers. *J Pharmacol Exp Ther* 1984; 229:283–291.
24. Sager PT. The frequency-dependent effects of dofetilide in humans. *Circulation* 1995;92:1I–774(abst).
25. Schmitt C, Brachmann J, Karch M, et al. Reverse use-dependent effects of sotalol demonstrated by recording monophasic action potentials of the right ventricle. *Am J Cardiol* 1991;68: 1183–1187.
26. Groh WJ, Gibson KJ, Maylie JG. Comparison of the rate-dependent properties of the class III antiarrhythmic agents azimilide (NE-10064) and E-4031: considerations on the mechanism of reverse rate-dependent action potential prolongation. *J Cardiovasc Electrophysiol* 1997;8:529–536.
27. Weyerbrock S, Schreieck J, Karch M, et al. Rate-independent effects of the new class III antiarrhythmic agent ambasilide on transmembrane action potentials in human ventricular endomyocardium. *J Cardiovasc Pharmacol* 1997;30:571–575.
28. Wang J, Feng J, Nattel S. Class III antiarrhythmic drug action in experimental atrial fibrillation. Differences in reverse use dependence and effectiveness between d-sotalol and the new antiarrhythmic drug ambasilide. *Circulation* 1994;90:2032–2040.
29. Anderson KP, Walker R, Dustman T, et al. Rate-related electrophysiologic effects of long-term administration of amiodarone on canine ventricular myocardium *in vivo*. *Circulation* 1989;79: 948–958.
30. Wang ZG, Pelletier LC, Talajic M, Nattel S. Effects of flecainide and quinidine on human atrial action potentials. Role of rate-dependence and comparison with guinea pig, rabbit, and dog tissues. *Circulation* 1990;82:274–283.
31. Nattel S, Liu L, St-Georges D. Effects of the novel antiarrhythmic agent azimilide on experimental atrial fibrillation and atrial electrophysiologic properties. *Cardiovasc Res* 1998;37:627–635.
32. Vos MA, Golitsyn SR, Stangl K, et al, for the Ibutilide/Sotalol Comparator Study Group. Superiority of ibutilide (a new class III agent) over d,l-sotalol in converting atrial flutter and atrial fibrillation. *Heart* 1998; 79:568.
33. Buchanan LV, Le MR, Walters RR, et al. Antiarrhythmic and electrophysiologic effects of intravenous ibutilide and sotalol in the canine sterile pericarditis model. *J Cardiovasc Electrophysiol* 1996;7:113–119.
34. Villemaire C, Talajic M, Nattel S. Mechanisms by which sotalol prevents atrial fibrillation at doses that fail to terminate the arrhythmia. *Circulation* 1997;96(8)[Suppl]:I236(abst).
35. Wang J, Bourne GW, Wang Z, et al. Comparative mechanisms of antiarrhythmic drug action in experimental atrial fibrillation. Importance of use-dependent effects on refractoriness. *Circulation* 1993;88:1030–1044.
36. Torp-Pedersen C, Moller M, Bloch-Thomsen PE, et al. Dofetilide in patients with congestive heart failure and left ventricular dysfunction. Danish Investigations of Arrhythmia and Mortality on Dofetilide Study. *N Engl J Med* 1999;341: 857–865.
37. Greenbaum RCT, Channer K, Dalrymple H, et al. Conversion of atrial fibrillation and maintenance of sinus rhythm by dofetilide: The EMERALD (European and Australian Multicenter Evaluative Research on Atrial Fibrillation Dofetilide) Study. *Circulation* 1998;98:I633(abst).
38. Jurkiewicz NK, Sanguinetti MC. Rate-dependent prolongation of cardiac action potentials by a methanesulfonanilide class III antiarrhythmic agent. Specific block of rapidly activating

39. Velebit V, Podrid PJ, Cohen B, et al. Aggravation and provocation of ventricular arrhythmia by antiarrhythmic drugs. *Circulation* 1982;65:886.
40. Zipes DP. Proarrhythmic effects of antiarrhythmic drugs. *Am J Cardiol* 1987;59:26E.
41. Levine JH, Morganroth J, Kadish AH. Mechanisms and risk factors for proarrhythmia with type Ia compared with Ic antiarrhythmic drug therapy. *Circulation* 1989;80:1063–1069.
42. Flaker GC, Blackshear JL, McBride R, et al. Antiarrhythmic drug therapy and cardiac mortality in atrial fibrillation. The Stroke Prevention in Atrial Fibrillation Investigators. *J Am Coll Cardiol* 1992;20:527–532.
43. Morganroth J. Risk factors for the development of proarrhythmic events. *Am J Cardiol* 1987;59:32E–37E.
44. Kowey PR, Vander LJ, Luderer JR. Safety and risk/benefit analysis of ibutilide for acute conversion of atrial fibrillation/flutter. *Am J Cardiol* 1996;78:46–52.
45. Podrid PJ, Lambert S, Graboys TB, et al. Aggravation of arrhythmia by antiarrhythmic drugs: incidence and predictors. *Am J Cardiol* 1987;59:38E.
46. Slater WS, Lampert S, Podrid PJ, Lown B. Clinical predictors of arrhythmia worsening by antiarrhythmic drugs. *Am J Coll Cardiol* 1988;61:349.
47. Brugada J, Boersma L, Kirchhof C, Allessie M. Proarrhythmic effects of flecainide. Experimental evidence for increased susceptibility to reentrant arrhythmias. *Circulation* 1991;84:1808–1818.
48. Wallace AA, Stupienski RF, Kothstein T, et al. Demonstration of proarrhythmic activity with the class Ic antiarrhythmic agent encainide in a canine model of previous myocardial infarction. *J Cardiovasc Pharmacol* 1993;21:397–404.
49. Ranger S, Nattel S. Determinants and mechanisms of flecainide-induced promotion of ventricular tachycardia in anesthetized dogs. *Circulation* 1995;92:1300–1311.
50. Coromilas J, Saltman AE, Waldecker B, et al. Electrophysiological effects of flecainide on anisotropic conduction and reentry in infarcted canine hearts. *Circulation* 1995;91:2245–2263.
51. Herre JM, Titus C, Oeff M, et al. Inefficacy and proarrhythmic effects of flecainide and encainide for sustained ventricular tachycardia and ventricular fibrillation. *Ann Intern Med* 1990; 113:671–676.
52. The Cardiac Arrhythmia Suppression Trial Investigators. Preliminary report: effect of encainide and flecainide on mortality in a randomized trial of arrhythmia suppression after myocardial infarction. *N Engl J Med* 1989;321:406–412.
53. Friedman PL, Stevenson WG. Proarrhythmia. *Am J Cardiol* 1998;82:50N–58N.
54. Teo KK, Yusuf S, Furberg CD. Effects of prophylactic antiarrhythmic drug therapy in acute myocardial infarction. An overview of results from randomized controlled trials. *JAMA* 1993;270:1589–1595.
55. Cairns JA, Connolly SJ, Roberts R, Gent M, for the Canadian Amiodarone Myocardial Infarction Arrhythmia Trial Investigators. Randomised trial of outcome after myocardial infarction in patients with frequent or repetitive ventricular premature depolarisations. CAMIAT. Canadian Amiodarone Myocardial Infarction Arrhythmia Trial. *Lancet* 1997;349:675–682.
56. Julian DG, Camm AJ, Frangin G, et al, for the European Myocardial Infarct Amiodarone Trial Investigators. Randomised trial of effect of amiodarone on mortality in patients with left-ventricular dysfunction after recent myocardial infarction: EMIAT. European Myocardial Infarct Amiodarone Trial Investigators. *Lancet* 1997;349:667–674.
57. Singh SN, Fletcher RD, Fisher SG, et al, for the Congestive Heart Failure–Survival Trial of the Antiarrhythmic Therapy

(CHF–STAT). Amiodarone in patients with congestive heart failure and asymptomatic ventricular arrhythmia (CHF–STAT). *N Engl J Med* 1995;333:77–82.

58. Anonymous. Dofetilide. UK 68, UK 68798, Tikosyn, Xelide. *Drugs R.D.* 1999;1:304–311.

59. Julian DG, Jackson FS, Szekely P, Prescott RJ. A controlled trial of sotalol for 1 year after myocardial infarction. *Circulation* 1983;67:I61–I62.

60. Jackman WM, Friday KJ, Anderson JL, et al. The long QT syndromes: a critical review, new clinical observations and a unifying hypothesis. *Prog Cardiovasc Dis* 1988;31:115–172.

61. Viskin S. Long QT syndromes and torsade de pointes. *Lancet* 1999;354:1625–1633.

62. Schultz-Bahr E, Haverkamp W, Hordt M. Do mutations in cardiac ion channel genes predispose to drug-induced long QT syndrome? *Circulation* 1997;96:I211(abst).

63. Napolitano C, Priori SG, Schwartz PJ. Identification of a long QT syndrome molecular defect in drug-induced torsade de pontes. *Circulation* 1997;I211:(abst).

64. Sotalol prescribing information [Pamphlet]. *Physicians' Desk Reference.* 2000.

65. Sager PT. New advances in class III antiarrhythmic drug therapy. *Curr Opin Cardiol* 1999;14:15–23.

66. Roden DM. Taking the "idio" out of "idiosyncratic": predicting torsade de pointes. *Pacing Clin Electrophysiol* 1998;21:1029.

67. Roden DM, Woosley RL, Primm K. Incidence of clinical features of the quinidine associated long QT syndrome. Implications for patient care. *Am Heart J* 1986;111:1088.

68. Hohnloser SH, Klingenheben T, Singh BN. Amiodarone-associated proarrhythmic effects. A review with special reference to torsade de pointes tachycardia. *Ann Intern Med* 1994;121:529–535.

69. Tzivoni D, Keren A, Cohen AM, et al. Magnesium therapy for torsade de points. *Am J Cardiol* 1984;53:528.

70. Feld GK, Chen PS, Nicod P, et al. Possible atrial proarrhythmic effects of class 1C antiarrhythmic drugs. *Am J Cardiol* 1990;66:378–383.

71. Nabar A, Rodriguez LM, Timmermans C, et al. Radiofrequency ablation of "class Ic atrial flutter" in patients with resistant atrial fibrillation. *Am J Cardiol* 1999;83:785–787.

72. Schumacher B, Jung W, Lewalter T, et al. Radiofrequency ablation of atrial flutter due to administration of class Ic antiarrhythmic drugs for atrial fibrillation. *Am J Cardiol* 1999;83:710–713.

73. Huang DT, Monahan KM, Zimetbaum P, et al. Hybrid pharmacologic and ablative therapy: a novel and effective approach for the management of atrial fibrillation. *J Cardiovasc Electrophysiol* 1998;9:462–469.

74. Ravid S, Podrid PJ, Lampert S, Lown B. Congestive heart failure induced by six of the newer antiarrhythmic drugs. *J Am Coll Cardiol* 1989;14:1326.

75. Nademanee K, Bailey W, O'Neill G, et al. Electrophysiologic and hemodynamic effects of dofetilide in patients with left ventricular function: a randomized, double-blind, placebo-controlled study. *Pace* 1998;21:867(abst).

76. Doval HC, Nul DR, Grancelli HO, et al. Randomised trial of low-dose amiodarone in severe congestive heart failure. Grupo de Estudio de la Sobrevida en la Insuficiencia Cardiac en Argentina (GESICA). *Lancet* 1994;344:493–498.

77. Kowey PR, Marinchak RA, Rials SJ, Filart RA. Intravenous amiodarone. *J Am Coll Cardiol* 1997;29:1190–1198.

78. Kowey PR, Levine JH, Herre JM, et al. Randomized, double-blind comparison of intravenous amiodarone and bretylium in the treatment of patients with recurrent, hemodynamically destabilizing ventricular tachycardia or fibrillation. The Intravenous Amiodarone Multicenter Investigators Group. *Circulation* 1995;92:3255–3263.

79. Stambler BS, Beckman KJ, Kadish AH, et al. Acute hemodynamic effects of intravenous ibutilide in patients with or without reduced left ventricular function. *Am J Cardiol* 1997;80:458–463.

80. Mendes L, Podrid PJ, Fuchs T, Franklin S. The role of combination therapy with a class Ic antiarrhythmic agent and mexiletine for ventricular tachycardia. *J Am Coll Cardiol* 1991;17:1396–1402.

81. Widerhorn J, Sager PT, Rahimtoola SH, Bhandari AK. The role of combination therapy with mexiletine and procainamide in patients with inducible sustained ventricular tachycardia refractory to intravenous procainamide. *Pace* 1991;14:420–426.

82. Bonavita GJ, Pires LA, Wagshal AB, et al. Usefulness of oral quinidine-mexiletine combination therapy for sustained ventricular tachyarrhythmias as assessed by programmed electrical stimulation when quinidine monotherapy has failed. *Am Heart J* 1994;127:847–851.

83. Toivonen L, Kadish A, Morady F. A prospective comparison of class Ia, Ib, and Ic antiarrhythmic agents in combination with amiodarone in patients with inducible, sustained ventricular tachycardia. *Circulation* 1991;84:101–108.

84. Dorian P, Newman D, Berman N, et al. Sotalol and type Ia drugs in combination prevent recurrence of sustained ventricular tachycardia. *J Am Coll Cardiol* 1993;22:106–113.

85. Lee SD, Newman D, Ham M, Dorian P. Electrophysiologic mechanisms of antiarrhythmic efficacy of a sotalol and class Ia drug combination: elimination of reverse use dependence. *J Am Coll Cardiol* 1997;29:100–105.

86. Sanguinetti MC, Jurkiewicz NK, Scott A, Siegl PK. Isoproterenol antagonizes prolongation of refractory period by the class III antiarrhythmic agent E-4031 in guinea pig myocytes. Mechanism of action. *Circ Res* 1991;68:77–84.

87. Sager PT, Follmer C, Uppal P, et al. The effects of beta-adrenergic stimulation on the frequency-dependent electrophysiologic actions of amiodarone and sematilide. *Circulation* 1994;90:1811–1819.

88. Groh WJ, Gibson KJ, McAnulty JH, Maylie JG. Beta-adrenergic blocking property of dl-sotalol maintains class III efficacy in guinea pig ventricular muscle after isoproterenol. *Circulation* 1995;91:262–264.

89. Calkins H, Sousa J, el-Atassi R, et al. Reversal of antiarrhythmic drug effects by epinephrine: quinidine versus amiodarone. *J Am Coll Cardiol* 1992;19:347–352.

90. Reiffel JA, Hahn E, Hartz V, Reiter MJ. Sotalol for ventricular tachyarrhythmias: beta-blocking and class III contributions, and relative efficacy versus class I drugs after prior drug failure. ESVEM Investigators. Electrophysiologic Study Versus Electrocardiographic Monitoring. *Am J Cardiol* 1997;79:1048–1053.

91. Kennedy HL, Brooks MM, Barker AH, et al. Beta-blocker therapy in the Cardiac Arrhythmia Suppression Trial. CAST Investigators. *Am J Cardiol* 1994;74:674–680.

92. Boutitie F, Boissel JP, Connolly SJ, et al. Amiodarone interaction with beta-blockers: analysis of the merged EMIAT (European Myocardial Infarct Amiodarone Trial) and CAMIAT (Canadian Amiodarone Myocardial Infarction Trial) databases. The EMIAT and CAMIAT Investigators. *Circulation* 1999;99:2268–2275.

93. Vaughan-Williams EM. A classification of antiarrhythmic action reassessed after a decade of new drugs. *J Clin Pharmacol* 1984;24:129.

94. Campbell TJ. Kinetics of onset of rate-dependent effects of class I antiarrhythmic drugs are important in determining effects on refractoriness in guinea pig ventricle, and provide a theoretical basis for their subclassification. *Cardiovasc Res* 1983;17:344–352.

95. Kaab S, Dixon J, Duc J, et al. Molecular basis of transient out-

ward potassium current downregulation in human heart failure: a decrease inKv4.3 mRNA correlated with a reduction in current density. *Circulation* 1998;98:1383–1393.

96. O'Rouke B, Kass DA, Tomaselli GF, et al. Mechanisms of altered excitation-contraction coupling in canine tachycardia-induced heart failure, I: experimental studies. *Circ Res* 1999;84: 562–570.

97. Schroder F, Handrock R, Beuckelmann DJ, et al. Increased availability and open probability of single l-type calcium channels from failing compared with nonfailing human ventricle. *Circulation* 1998;98:969–976.

98. Rials SJ, Xu X, Wu Y, et al. Regression of LV hypertrophy with captopril normalizes membrane currents in rabbits. *Am J Physiol* 1998;275:H1216–H1224.

99. Rials SJ, Wu Y, Xu X, et al. Regression of left ventricular hypertrophy with captopril restores normal ventricular action potential duration, dispersion of refractoriness, and vulnerability to inducible ventricular fibrillation. *Circulation* 1997;96:1130–1336.

100. Roden DM, Bennett PB, Snyders Dj, et al. Quinidine delays I_k activation in guinea pig ventricular myocytes. *Circ Res* 1988;62:1055–1058.

101. Wellens HJJ, Bar F, Dassen WRM, et al. Effect of drugs in the Wolff-Parkinson-White syndrome. Importance of initial length of the effective refractory period of the accessory pathway. *Am J Cardiol* 1980;46:665–669.

102. DiMarco JP, Garan H, Ruskin JN. Quinidine for ventricular arrhythmias. Value of electrophysiologic testing. *Am J Cardiol* 1983;51:90–95.

103. Josephson ME, Seides SF, Batsford WP, et al. The electrophysiological effects of intramuscular quinidine on the atrioventricular conducting system in man. *Am Heart J* 1974;87:55–64.

104. Coplen SE, Antman EM, Berlin JA, et al. Efficacy and safety of quinidine therapy for maintenance of sinus rhythm after cardioversion. A meta-analysis of randomized control trials. *Circulation* 1990;82:1106–1116.

105. Mason JW, and the ESVEM Investigators. A comparison of seven antiarrhythmic drugs in patients with ventricular tachyarrhythmias. *N Engl J Med* 1993;329:452–458.

106. Duff HJ, Mitchell LB, Manuari D, Wyse DG. Mexiletine-quinidine combination: Electrophysiologic correlates of a favorable antiarrhythmic interaction in humans. *J Am Coll Cardiol* 1987;10:1149–1156.

107. Naccarelli GV, Rinkenberger RL, Dougherty AH, Giebel RA. Amiodarone: Pharmacology and antiarrhythmic and adverse effects. *Pharmacotherapy* 1985;5:298–313.

108. Mungall DR, Robichaux RP, Perry W, et al. Effects of quinidine on serum digoxin concentration. A prospective study. *Ann Intern Med* 1980;93:689–693.

109. Siddoway LA, Thompson EA, McAllister CB, et al. Polymorphism propafenone metabolism and disposition in man: clinical and pharmacokinetic consequences. *Circulation* 1987;75: 785–791.

110. Selzer A, Wray HW. Quinidine syncope. Paroxysmal ventricular fibrillation occurring during treatment of chronic atrial arrhythmias. *Circulation* 1964;30:17.

111. Roden DM, Woosley RL, Primm K. Incidence and clinical features of the quinidine-associated long QT syndrome: implications for patient care. *Am Heart J* 1986;111:1088–1093.

112. Winkle RA, Jaillon P, Kates RE, Peters F. Clinical pharmacology and antiarrhythmic efficacy of *N*-acetylprocainamide. *Am J Cardiol* 1981;47:123.

113. Waxman HL, Buxton AE, Sadowski LM, Josephson ME. Response to procainamide during electrophysiologic study for sustained ventricular tachycardia predicts response to other drugs. *Circulation* 1982;67:30–37.

114. Gorgels APM, van den Dool A, Hofs A, et al. Comparison of

115. Gottlieb SS, Kukin ML, Medina N, et al. Comparative hemodynamic effects of procainamide, tocainide and encainide in severe chronic heart failure. *Circulation* 1991;81:860–864.

116. Karim A, Nissen C, Azarnoff DL. Clinical pharmacokinetics of disopyramide. *J Pharmacokinet Bipharm* 1982;10:465–494.

117. Arif M, Laidlaw JC, Oshrain C, et al. A randomized double-blind parallel group comparison of disopyramide phosphate and quinidine in patients with cardiac arrhythmias. *Angiology* 1983;34:393.

118. Karlson BW, Torstensson I, Abjorn C, et al. Disopyramide in the maintenance of sinus rhythm after electrocardioversion of atrial fibrillation: a placebo controlled one-year follow-up study. *Eur Heart J* 1988;9:284.

119. Lermann BB, Waxman HL, Buxton AE, Josephson ME. Disopyramide: evaluation of electrophysiologic effects and clinical efficacy in patients with sustained ventricular tachycardia or ventricular fibrillation. *Am J Cardiol* 1983;51:759–764.

120. Sra JS, Anderson AJ, Sheikh SH, et al. Unexplained syncope evaluated by electrophysiologic studies and head-up tilt testing. *Ann Intern Med* 1991;114:1013–1019.

121. Teichman SL, Ferrick A, Kim SG, et al. Disopyramide-pyridostigmine interaction: selective reversal of anticholinergic symptoms with preservation of antiarrhythmic effect. *J Am Coll Cardiol* 1987;10:633.

122. Podrid PJ, Schoeneberger A, Lown B. Congestive heart failure caused by oral disopyramide. *N Engl J Med* 1980;302:614–617.

123. Collingsworth KA, Kalman SN, Harrison DC. The clinical pharmacology of lidocaine as an antiarrhythmic drug. *Circulation* 1974;50:1217–1230.

124. Harrison DC. Practical guidelines for the use of lidocaine. Prevention and treatment of cardiac arrhythmias. *JAMA* 1975;233: 1202–1204.

125. Thompson PD, et al. Lidocaine pharmacokinetics in advanced heart failure, liver disease and renal failure in humans. *Ann Intern Med* 1973;78:499–508.

126. Lie KI, Wellens HJJ, VanCapelle FJ, Durrer D. Lidocaine in the prevention of ventricular fibrillation. *N Engl J Med* 1974;291: 1324–1326.

127. Hine LK, Laird N, Hewitt P, et al. Meta-analytic evidence against prophylactic use of lidocaine in acute myocardial infarction. *Arch Intern Med* 1989;149:2694–2698.

128. Dorian P, Fain ED, Davy JM, Winkle RA. Lidocaine causes a reversible concentration-dependent increase in fibrillation energy requirements. *J Am Coll Cardiol* 1986;8:327–332.

129. Kutalek SP, Morganroth J, Horowitz LN. Tocainide: a new oral antiarrhythmic agent. *Ann Intern Med* 1985;103:387–391.

130. Morganroth J, Nestico FF, Horowitz LN. A review of the uses and limitations of tocainide—a class Ib antiarrhythmic agent. *Am Heart J* 1985;110:856–863.

131. Podrid PJ, Lown B. Tocainide for refractory symptomatic ventricular arrhythmias. *Am J Cardiol* 1982;49:1279.

132. Campbell RWF. Mexiletine. *N Engl J Med* 1987;316:29–34.

133. Duff HJ, Kolodgie FD, Roden DM, Woosley RL. Electropharmacologic synergism with mexiletine and quinidine. *J Cardiovasc Pharmacol* 1986;8:840–846.

134. Impact Research Group. International mexiletine and placebo antiarrhythmic coronary trial. I. Report on arrhythmia and other findings. *J Am Coll Cardiol* 1984;4:1148–1163.

135. DiMarco JP, Garan H, Ruskin JN. Mexiletine for refractory ventricular arrhythmias: results using serial electrophysiologic testing. *Am J Cardiol* 1981;47:131.

136. Berns E, Naccarelli GV, Dougherty AH, et al. Mexiletine: lack of predictors of clinical response in patients treated for life-threatening tachyarrhythmias. *J Electrophysiol* 1988;2:201–206.

137. Shimizu W, Antzelvitch C. Cellular basis for the ECG features of the LQT1 form of the long-QT syndrome: effects of β-adrenergic agonists and antagonists and sodium channel blockers on transmural dispersion of repolarization and torsade de pointes. *Circulation* 1998;98:2314–2322.

138. Stein J, Podrid P, Lown B. Effects of oral mexiletine on left and right ventricular function. *Am J Cardiol* 1984;54:575.

139. Roden DM, Woosley RL. Drug therapy: flecainide. *N Engl J Med* 1986;315:36.

140. Anderson JL, Pritchett ELC, eds. International symposium on supraventricular arrhythmias; focus on flecainide. *Am J Cardiol* 1988;62:1D–67D.

141. Lal R, Chapman PD, Naccarelli GV, et al. Flecainide in the treatment of nonsustained ventricular tachycardia. *Ann Intern Med* 1986;105:493–498.

142. The Cardiac Arrhythmia Pilot Study (CAPS) Investigators. Effects of encainide, flecainide, imipramine and moricizine on ventricular arrhythmias during the year after myocardial infarction. The CAPS. *Am J Cardiol* 1988;61:501–509.

143. Lal R, Chapman PD, Naccarelli GV, et al. Short- and long-term experience with flecainide acetate in the management of refractory life-threatening ventricular arrhythmias. *J Am Coll Cardiol* 1985;6:772.

144. Flecainide Ventricular Tachycardia Study Group. Treatment of resistant ventricular tachycardia with flecainide acetate. *Am J Cardiol* 1986;57:1299–1304.

145. Benhorin J, Taub R, Golmit M, et al. Effects of flecainide in patients with new SCN5A mutation: mutation-specific therapy for long-QT syndrome? *Circulation* 2000;101:1698–1706.

146. Naccarelli GV, Dorian P, Hohnloser SH, Coumel P, for the Flecainide Multicenter Atrial Fibrillation Group. Prospective comparison of flecainide versus quinidine for the treatment of paroxysmal atrial fibrillation/flutter. *Am J Cardiol* 1996;77:53A–59A.

147. Capucci A, Boriani G, Botto GL, et al. Conversion of recent-onset atrial fibrillation by a single oral loading dose of propafenone or flecainide. *Am J Cardiol* 1994;74:503–505.

148. Pritchett ELC, Wilkinson WE, Clair WK, et al. Comparison of mortality in patients treated with flecainide to those treated with a variety of antiarrhythmic drugs for supraventricular arrhythmias. *Am J Cardiol* 1993;72:108–110.

149. Podrid PJ, Lown B. Propafenone: a new agent for ventricular arrhythmia. *J Am Coll Cardiol* 1984;4:117–125.

150. Podrid PJ, ed. Symposium on propafenone. *J Electrophysiol* 1989;1:517–590.

151. Connally SJ, Kates RE, Lebsack CS, et al. Clinical pharmacology of propafenone. *Circulation* 1983;68:589–596.

152. Naccarella F, Bracchetti D, Palmieri M, et al. Comparison of propafenone and disopyramide for treatment of chronic ventricular arrhythmias: placebo-controlled, double-blind, randomized crossover study. *Am Heart J* 1985;109:833–839.

153. Chilson DA, Heger JJ, Zipes DP, et al. Electrophysiologic effects and clinical efficacy of oral propafenone therapy in patients with ventricular tachycardia. *J Am Coll Cardiol* 1985;5:1407.

154. Siebels J, Cappato R, Ruppel R, et al, and the CASH Investigators. Preliminary results of the Cardiac Arrest Study Hamburg (CASH). *Am J Cardiol* 1993;72:109F–113F.

155. Ludmer PL, McGowan NE, Antman EM, Friedman PL. Efficacy of propafenone in Wolff-Parkinson-White syndrome: electrophysiologic findings and long-term followup. *J Am Coll Cardiol* 1987;9:1357–1363.

156. Reimold SC, Cantillon CO, Friedman PL, Antman EM. Propafenone versus sotalol for suppression of recurrent symptomatic atrial fibrillation. *Am J Cardiol* 1993;71:558–563.

157. Podrid PJ, Lyakishev A, Lown B, et al. Ethmozine, a new antiarrhythmic drug for suppressing ventricular premature complexes. *Circulation* 1980;61:450–457.

158. Ruggio JM, Somberg JC. New therapy focus: Ethmozine. *Cardiovasc Rev Rep* 1984;5:738–741.

159. Mann DE, Luck JC, Herre JM, et al. Electrophysiologic effects of Ethmozine in patients with ventricular tachycardia. *Am Heart J* 1984;107:674.

160. Hession MJ, Lampert S, Podrid PJ, Lown B. Ethmozine (moricizine HCl) therapy for complex ventricular arrhythmias. *Am J Cardiol* 1987;60:59F.

161. Pratt, CM, Butman, SM, Young, JB, et al. Antiarrhythmic efficacy of Ethmozine (moricizine HCl) compared with disopyramide and propranolol. *Am J Cardiol* 1987;60:52F.

162. The Cardiac Arrhythmia Suppression Trial II Investigators. Effect of the antiarrhythmic agent moricizine on survival after myocardial infarction. *N Engl J Med* 1992;327:227–233.

163. Horowitz LN. Efficacy of moricizine in malignant ventricular arrhythmias. *Am J Cardiol* 1990;65:41D.

164. Powell AC, Gold MR, Brooks R, et al. Electrophysiologic response to moricizine in patients with sustained ventricular arrhythmias. *Ann Intern Med* 1992;116:382.

165. Pratt CM, Podrid P, Greatrix B, et al. Efficacy and safety of moricizine in patients with congestive heart failure: a summary of the experience in the United States. *Am Heart J* 1990;119:1.

166. Beta-Blocker Heart Attack Trial Research Group:. A randomized trial of propranolol in patients with acute myocardial infarction. I: mortality results. *JAMA* 1982;247:1707–1714.

167. Naccarelli GV, Wolbrette Dl, Dell'Orfano JT, et al. A decade of clinical trial developments in postmyocardial infarction, congestive heart failure, and sustained ventricular tachyarrhythmias patients from CAST to AVID and beyond. *J Cardiovasc Electrophysiol* 1998;9:864–891.

168. MERIT-HF Study Group. Effect of metoprolol CR/XL in chronic heart failure: metoprolol CR/XL randomized interventional trial in congestive heart failure (MERIT-HF). *Lancet* 1999;353:2001–2007.

169. CIBIS II Investigators. The cardiac insufficiency bisoprolol study II (CIBIS II): a randomized trial. *Lancet* 1999;353:9–13.

170. Packer M, Bristow MR, Cohn JN, et al, for the U.S. Carvedilol Heart Failure Study Group. The effect of carvedilol on morbidity and mortality in patients with chronic heart failure. *N Engl J Med* 1996;334:1349–1355.

171. Singh SN, DiBianco R, Davidson ME, et al. Comparison of acebutolol and propranolol for treatment of chronic ventricular arrhythmia: a placebo-controlled, double-blind, randomized crossover study. *Circulation* 1982;65:1356–1364.

172. DeSoyza N, Shapiro W, Chandraratna PAN, et al. Acebutolol therapy for ventricular arrhythmias: a randomized, placebo-controlled double-blind multicenter study. *Circulation* 1982;65:1129–1133.

173. Boissel JP, Leizorovicz A, Picolet H, et al, and the APSI Investigators. Efficacy of acebutolol after acute myocardial infarction (the APSI trial). *Am J Cardiol* 1990;66:24C–31C.

174. Angaran DM, Schultz NJ, Tschida VH. Esmolol hydrochloride: an ultrashort-acting, beta-adrenergic blocking agent. *Clin Pharm* 1986;5(4):288–303.

175. Gorczynski RJ. Basic pharmacology of esmolol. *Am J Cardiol* 1985;56(11):3F–13F.

176. Anderson S, Blanski L, Byrd RC, et al. Comparison of the efficacy and safety of esmolol, a short-acting beta blocker with placebo in the treatment of supraventricular arrhythmias. *Am Heart J* 1986;111:429–438.

177. Zipes DP, Prystowsky EN, Heger JJ. Amiodarone: electrophysiologic actions, pharmacokinetics and clinical effects. *J Am Coll Cardiol* 1984;3:1059.

178. Mason JW. Amiodarone. *N Engl J Med* 1987;316:455.

179. Desai AD, Chun S, Sung RJ. The role of intravenous amio-

darone in the management of cardiac arrhythmias. *Ann Intern Med* 1997;127:294–303.

180. Holt DW, Tucker GT, Jackson PR, Storey GCA. Amiodarone pharmacokinetics. *Am Heart J* 1983;106:840–846.

181. Naccarelli GV, Jalal S. Intravenous amiodarone: another option in the acute management of sustained ventricular tachyarrhythmias. *Circulation* 1995;92:3154–3155.

182. Heger JJ, Prystowsky EN, Jackmn WM, et al. Amiodarone: clinical efficacy and electrophysiology during long-term therapy for recurrent ventricular tachycardia or ventricular fibrillation. *N Engl J Med* 1981;305:539–545.

183. Herre JM, Sauve MJ, Malone P, et al. Long-term results of amiodarone therapy in patients with recurrent sustained ventricular tachycardia or ventricular fibrillation. *J Am Coll Cardiol* 1989;13:442–449.

184. The CASCADE Investigators. Randomized antiarrhythmic drug therapy in survivors of cardiac arrest (the CASCADE study). *Am J Cardiol* 1993;72:280–287.

185. The Antiarrhythmics Versus Implantable Defibrillators (AVID) Investigators. A comparison of antiarrhythmic drug therapy with implantable defibrillators in patients resuscitated from near fatal ventricular arrhythmias. *N Engl J Med* 1997;337: 1576–1583.

186. Connolly S, Gent M, Roberts R, et al. Canadian Implantable Defibrillator Study (CIDS): a randomized trial of the implantable cardioverter defibrillator against amiodarone. *Circulation* 2000;101:1297–1302.

187. Kuck KH, Cappato R, Siebels J, Ruppel R, for the CASH Investigators. Randomized comparison of antiarrhythmic drug therapy with implantable defibrillators in patients resuscitated from cardiac arrest. The Cardiac Arrest Study Hamburg (CASH). *Circulation* 2000;102:748.

188. Moss AJ, Hall WJ, Cannom DS, et al, for the Multicenter Automatic Defibrillator Implantation Trial Investigators. Improved survival with an implanted defibrillator in patients with coronary disease at high risk for ventricular arrhythmia. *N Engl J Med* 1996;335:1933–1940.

189. Buxton AE, Lee KL, Fisher JD, et al, for the Multicenter Unsustained Tachycardia Trial Investigators. A randomized study of the prevention of sudden death patients with coronary artery disease. *N Engl J Med* 1999;341:1882–1890.

190. Gosselink AT, Crijns HJ, VanGelder IC, et al. Low-dose amiodarone for maintenance of sinus rhythm after cardioversion of atrial fibrillation or flutter. *JAMA* 1992;267:3289–3293.

191. Roy D, Talajic M, Dorian P, et al, for the Canadian Trial of Atrial Fibrillation Investigators. *N Engl J Med* 2000;342: 913–920.

192. Kudenchuk PJ, Cobb LA, Copass MK, et al. Amiodarone for resuscitation after out-of-hospital cardiac arrest due to ventricular fibrillation. *N Engl J Med* 1999;341:821–878.

193. Clemo HF, Wood MA, Gilligan DM, Ellenbogen KA. Intravenous amiodarone for acute heart rate control in the critically ill patient with atrial tachyarrhythmias. *Am J Cardiol* 1998;81: 594–598.

194. Galve E, Rius T, Ballester R, et al. Intravenous amiodarone in treatment of recent-onset atrial fibrillation: results of a randomized, controlled study. *J Am Coll Cardiol* 1996;27:1079–1082.

195. Vorperian VR, Havighurst TC, Milleer S, January CT. Adverse effects of low dose amiodarone: a meta-analysis. *J Am Coll Cardiol* 1997;30:791–798.

196. Podrid PJ. Amiodarone: reevaluation of an old drug. *Ann Intern Med* 1995;122:689–700.

197. Naccarelli GV, Rinkenberger RL, Dougherty AH, Fitzgerald DM. Adverse effects of amiodarone. *Med Toxicol Adverse Drug Exp* 189;4:246–253.

198. Goldschlager N, Epstein A, Naccarelli GV, et al, for the Practice Guidelines Subcommittee, North American Society of Pacing and Electrophysiology. Practice guidelines for clinicians who treat patients with amiodarone. *Arch Intern Med* 2000:160; 1741–1746.

199. Kudenchuk PJ, Pierson DJ, Greene HL, et al. Prospective evaluation of amiodarone pulmonary toxicity. *Chest* 1984;86: 541–548.

200. Jung W, Manz M, Pizzulli L, et al. Effects of chronic amiodarone therapy on defibrillation threshold. *Am J Cardiol* 1992;70:1023–1027.

201. Bigger JT Jr, Jaffe CC. The effect of bretylium tosylate on the electrophysiologic properties of ventricular muscle and Purkinje fibers. *Am J Cardiol* 1971;27:82–95.

202. Wit AL, Steiner C, Damato AN. Electrophysiologic effects of bretylium tosylate on single fibers of the canine specialized conducting system and ventricle. *J Pharmacol Exp Ther* 1970;173: 344–352.

203. Bacaner MB, Clay JR, Shrier A, et al. Potassium channel blockade: a mechanism for suppressing ventricular fibrillation. *Proc Natl Acad Sci U S A* 1986;83:2223–2231.

204. Anderson JL, Patterson E, Conlon M, et al. Kinetics of antifibrillatory effects of bretylium: correlation with myocardial drug concentrations. *Am J Cardiol* 1980;46:583–590.

205. Anderson JL, Patterson E, Wagner JG, et al. Clinical pharmacokinetics of intravenous and oral bretylium tosylate in survivors of ventricular tachycardia or fibrillation. *J Cardiovasc Pharmacol* 1981;3:485–592.

206. Fujimoto T, Hamamoto H, Peter T, et al. Electrophysiologic effects of bretylium on canine ventricular muscle during acute ischemia and reperfusion. *Am Heart J* 1983;105:966–975.

207. Chow MS, Kluger J, DiPersio DM, et al. Antifibrillatory effects of lidocaine and bretylium immediately postcardiopulmonary resuscitation. *Am Heart J* 1985;110:938–947.

208. Anderson JL, Brodine WN, Patterson E, et al. Electrophysiologic effects of bretylium in man. Correlation with plasma bretylium concentrations. *J Cardiovasc Pharmacol* 1982;4:871–880.

209. Heissenbuttel RH, Bigger JT. Bretylium tosylate: a newly available antiarrhythmic drug for ventricular arrhythmias. *Ann Intern Med* 1979;91:229–240.

210. Koch-Weser J. Drug therapy: bretylium. *N Engl J Med* 1979; 300:473–482.

211. Romhilt DW, Bloomfield SS, Lipicky RJ, et al. Evaluation of bretylium tosylate for the treatment of premature ventricular contractions. *Circulation* 1972;45:800–809.

212. Holder DA, Sniderman AD, Fraser G, et al. Experience with bretylium tosylate by a hospital cardiac arrest team. *Circulation* 1977;55:541–550.

213. Nowak RM, Bodnar TJ, Dronen S, et al. Bretylium tosylate as initial treatment for cardiopulmonary arrest: randomized comparison with placebo. *Ann Emerg Med* 1981;10:8–16.

214. Harrison BE, Amey BD. The use of bretylium in prehospital ventricular fibrillation. *Am J Emerg Med* 1983;1:1–8.

215. Haynes RE, Chinn RL, Copass MK, et al. Comparison of bretylium tosylate and lidocaine in management of out-of-hospital ventricular fibrillation: a randomized clinical trial. *Am J Cardiol* 1981;48:353–362.

216. Olson DW, Thompson BM, Darin JC, et al. A randomized comparison study of bretylium tosylate and lidocaine in resuscitation of patients from out-of-hospital ventricular fibrillation in a paramedic system. *Ann Emerg Med* 1984;13:807–816.

217. Boura ALA, Green AF. The actions of bretylium: adrenergic neurone blocking and other effects. *Br J Pharmacol* 1959;14: 536–540.

218. Singh BN, ed. Control cardiac arrhythmias with sotalol, a broad-spectrum anti-arrhythmic with beta-blocking effects and class III activity. *Am J Cardiol* 1990;765:1A–84A.

219. Hanyok JJ. Clinical pharmacokinetics of sotalol. *Am J Cardiol* 1993;72:19A–26A.

220. Ferreira E, Sunderji R, Gin K. Is oral sotalol effective in converting atrial fibrillation to sinus rhythm? *Pharmacotherapy* 1997;17:1233.

221. Benditt DG, Williams JH, Jin J, et al. Maintenance of sinus rhythm with oral d,l-sotalol therapy in patients with symptomatic atrial fibrillation and/or atrial flutter. d,l-Sotalol Atrial Fibrillation/Flutter Study Group. *Am J Cardiol* 1999;84:270.

222. Juul-Möller S, Edvardsson N, Rehnqvist-Ahlberg N. Sotalol versus quinidine for the maintenance of sinus rhythm after direct current conversion of atrial fibrillation. *Circulation* 1990; 82:1932.

223. Haverkamp W, Martinez-Rubio A, Hief C, et al. Efficacy and safety of d,l-sotalol in patients with ventricular tachycardia and in survivors of cardiac arrest. *J Am Coll Cardiol* 1997;30:487.

224. Pacifico A, Hohnloser SH, Williams JH, et al, for the d,l-Sotalol Implantable Cardioverter-Defibrillator Study Group. Prevention of implantable-defibrillator shocks by pretreatment with sotalol. *N Engl J Med* 1999;340:1855.

225. Murray KT. Ibutilide. *Circulation* 1998;97:493–497.

226. Volgman AS, Carberry PA, Stambler B, et al. Conversion efficacy and safety of intravenous ibutilide compared with intravenous procainamide in patients with atrial flutter or fibrillation. *J Am Coll Cardiol* 1998;31:1414–1419.

227. Buchanan LV, Kabell G, Brunden MN, et al. Comparative assessment of ibutilide, d-sotalol, clofilium, E-4031, and UK-68,798 in a rabbit model of proarrhythmia. *J Cardiovasc Pharmacol* 1993;22:540–549.

228. Oral H, Souza HJ, Michaud GF, et al. Facilitating transthoracic cardioversion of atrial fibrillation with ibutilide treatment. *N Engl J Med* 1999;340:1849–1854.

229. Stambler BS, Wood MA, Ellenbogen KA, et al, and the Ibutilide Repeat Dose Study Investigators. Efficacy and safety of repeated intravenous doses of ibutilide for rapid conversion of atrial flutter or fibrillation. *Circulation* 1996;94:1613.

230. Abi-Mansour P, Carberry PA, McCowan RJ, et al, and the Study Investigators. Conversion efficacy and safety of repeated doses of ibutilide in patients with atrial flutter and atrial fibrillation. *Am Heart J* 1998;136:632.

231. Ellenbogan KA, Clemo HF, Stambler BS, et al. Efficacy of ibutilide for termination of atrial fibrillation and flutter. *Am J Cardiol* 1996;78:42–45.

232. Mattioni T, Denker S, Riggio D, et al. Efficacy and safety of intravenous ibutilide in the treatment of atrial flutter and atrial fibrillation following valvular or coronary artery bypass surgery. *Pacing Clin Electrophysiol* 1997;20:1059(abst).

233. Singh BN. Acute conversion of atrial flutter and fibrillation: direct current cardioversion versus intravenously administered pure class III agents. *J Am Coll Cardiol* 1997;29:391–393.

234. Roden DM. Ibutilide and the treatment of atrial arrhythmias. A new drug almost unheralded is now available to US physicians. *Circulation* 1996;94:1499–1502.

235. Ward KJ, Gill JS. Dofetilide: first of new generation of class III agents. *Exp Opin Invest Drugs* 1997;6:1269–1281.

236. Sedgewisk ML, Dalrymple I, Rae AP. Effects of the new class III antiarrhythmic drug dofetilide on the atrial and ventricular intracardiac monophasic action potential in patients with angina pectoris. *Eur Heart J* 1992;69:513–517.

237. Tham TCK, MacLennan BA, Burke MT, et al. Pharmacodynamics and pharmacokinetics of the class III antiarrhythmic agent dofetilide(UK,68,798) in humans. *J Cardiovasc Pharmacol* 1993;21:507–512.

238. Rasmussen HS, Allen MJ, Blackburn KJ, et al. Dofetilide, a novel class II antiarrhythmic agent. *J Cardiovasc Pharmacol* 1992;20[Suppl 2]:S96–S105.

239. Falk RH, Pollak A, Singh SN, Friederich T, for Dofetilide Investigators. Intravenous dofetilide, a class III antiarrhythmic agent, for the termination of sustained atrial fibrillation or flutter. *J Am Coll Cardiol* 1997;29:385–90.

240. Singh S, Berk M, Yellon L, et al. Efficacy and safety of dofetilide in maintaining normal sinus rhythm in patients with atrial fibrillation/flutter: a multicenter study (abstract). *Eur Heart J* 1998;19(Suppl):363.

241. Camm AJ. What should we expect from the next generation of antiarrhythmic drugs? *J Cardiovasc Electrophysiol* 1999;10: 308–318.

242. Fermini B, Jurkiewicz NK, Jow B. Use dependent effect of the class III antiarrhythmic agent NE-10064(azimilide) on cardiac repolarization block or delayed rectifier potassium and l-type calcium currents. *J Cardiovasc Pharmacol* 1995;26:259–267.

243. Salata JJ, Brooks RR. Pharmacology of azimilide dihydrochloride (NE-10064), a class III antiarrhythmic agent. *Cardiovasc Drug Rev* 1997;15:137–156.

244. Lamorgese M, Kirian M, Van Wagoner DR. Azimilide (NE-10064) blocks outward K currents in human atrial and ventricular myocytes. *Circulation* 1997;92(8)[Suppl]:I1575.

245. Corey AE, Al-Khalidi H, Brezovic C, et al. Azimilide pharmacokinetics and pharmacodynamics upon multiple oral dosing. *Clin Pharmacol Ther* 1997;61:205–212.

246. Pritchett E, Connolly S, Marcello S. Azimilide treatment of atrial fibrillation. *Circulation* 1998;98[Suppl]7:1–633(abst).

247. Camm AJ, Karam R, Pratt CM. The azimilide post-infarct survival evaluation (ALIVE) trial. *Am J Cardiol* 1998;81:35D–39D.

248. Tsuchihashi K, Curtis MJ. Tedisamil possesses direct defibrillatory activity during myocardial ischemia and during reperfusion. *Br J Pharmacol* 1990;99:231P.

249. Tsuchihashi K, Curtis MJ. Chemical defibrillation in ischemia and reperfusion by selective blockade of the transient outward current (I_{to}). *Circulation* 1991;82[Suppl III]:III452.

250. Dukes ID, Morad M. Tedisamil inactivates transient outward K^+ channels in rat and guinea pig ventricular myocytes. *Am J Physiol* 1989;257:H1746–H174.

251. Argentieri TM, Troy HH, Carroll MS, et al. Electrophysiologic activity and antiarrhythmic efficacy of CK-3579, a new antiarrhythmic agent with beta-adrenergic blocking properties. *J Cardiovasc Pharmacol* 1992;21:647–655.

252. Singh BN, Ellrodt G, Peter CT. Verapamil: a review of its pharmacological properties and therapeutic use. *Drugs* 1978;15:169.

253. Singh BN, Hecht HS, Nademanee K, Chew CYC. Electrophysiological and hemodynamic actions of slow-channel blocking compounds. *Prog Cardiovasc Dis* 1982;25:103.

254. Rinkenberger RL, Prystowsky EN, Heger JJ, et al. Effects of intravenous and chronic oral verapamil administration in patients with supraventricular tachyarrhythmias. *Circulation* 1980;62:996–1010.

255. Sung RJ, Elser B, McAllister RG Jr. Intravenous verapamil for termination of reentrant supraventricular tachycardias. Intracardiac studies correlated with plasma verapamil concentrations. *Ann Intern Med* 1980;93:682–689.

256. Waxman HL, Myerburg RJ, Appel R, Sung RJ. Verapamil for control of ventricular rate in paroxysmal supraventricular tachycardia and atrial fibrillation or flutter. A double-blind randomized cross-over study. *Ann Intern Med* 1981;94:1–6.

257. Buxton AE, Marchlinski FE, Doherty JW, et al. Hazards of intravenous verapamil for sustained ventricular tachycardia. *Am J Cardiol* 1987;59:1107–1110.

258. Gulamhusein S, Ko P, Carruthers SG, Klein GJ. Acceleration of the ventricular response during atrial fibrillation in the Wolff-Parkinson-White syndrome after verapamil. *Circulation* 1982; 65:348–354.

259. Lundstrom T, Ryden L. Ventricular rate control and exercise

performance in chronic atrial fibrillation: Effects of diltiazem and verapamil. *J Am Coll Cardiol* 1990;16:86.

260. Waxman HL, Myerburg RJ, Appel R, Sung RJ. Verapamil for control of ventricular rate in paroxysmal supraventricular tachycardia and atrial fibrillation or flutter: A double blind randomized cross-over study. *Ann Intern Med* 1981;94:1.

261. Gill JS, Blaszyk K, Ward DE, et al. Verapamil for suppression of idiopathic ventricular tachycardia of left bundle branch–like morphology. *Am Heart J* 1993;126:1126.

262. Kirch W, Kleinbloesem CH, Belz GG. Drug interactions with calcium antagonists. *Pharmacol Ther* 1990;45:109.

263. The Danish Study Group on Verapamil in Myocardial Infarction. Effect of verapamil on mortality and major events after acute myocardial infarction (the Danish Verapamil Infarction Trial II–DAVIT II). *Am J Cardiol* 1990;66:779–785.

264. Dougherty AH, Jackman WM, Naccarelli GV, et al, and the IV Diltiazem Study Group. Acute conversion of paroxysmal supraventricular tachycardia with intravenous diltiazem: A multicenter dose response study. *Am J Cardiol* 1992;70:587–592.

265. Salerno DM, Dias VC, Kleiger RE, et al. Efficacy and safety of intravenous diltiazem for treatment of atrial fibrillation and atrial flutter. *Am J Cardiol* 1989;63:1046–1051.

266. Steinberg JS, Katz RJ, Bren GB, et al. Efficacy of oral diltiazem to control ventricular response in chronic atrial fibrillation at rest and during exercise. *J Am Coll Cardiol* 1987;9:405.

267. The Multicenter Diltiazem Post-Infarction Trial Research Group. The effect of diltiazem on mortality and reinfarction after myocardial infarction. *N Engl J Med* 1988;319:385–392.

268. Gibson RS, Boden WE, Theroux P, et al. Diltiazem and reinfarction in patients with non Q-wave infarction. *N Engl J Med* 1986;315:423–429.

269. Boden WE, van Gilst WH, Scheldewaert RG, et al. Diltiazem in acute myocardial infarction treated with thrombolytic agents: a randomised placebo-controlled trial. Incomplete Infarction Trial of European Research Collaborators Evaluating Prognosis post-Thrombolysis (INTERCEPT). *Lancet* 2000;355:1751.

270. Hollander BP, Webb JL. Effects of adenine nucleotide on the contractility and membrane potentials of rat atrium. *Circ Res* 1957;5:349.

271. Belardinelli L, Lerman BB. Adenosine: cardiac electrophysiology. *Pacing Clin Electrophysiol* 1991;14:1672.

272. DiMarco JP, Sellers TD, Lerman BB, et al. Diagnostic and therapeutic use of adenosine in patients with supraventricular tachyarrhythmias. *J Am Coll Cardiol* 1985;6:417–425.

273. DiMarco, Sellers TD, Berne RM, et al. Adenosine: electrophysiologic effects and therapeutic use for terminating paroxysmal supraventricular tachycardia. *Circulation* 1983;68:1254–1263.

274. Lerman BB, Belardinelli L, West GA, et al. Adenosine-sensitive ventricular tachycardia: evidence suggesting cyclic AMP–mediated triggered activity. *Circulation* 1986;74:270.

275. Griffith MJ, Linker NJ, Ward DE, Camm A. Adenosine in the diagnosis of broad complex tachycardia. *Lancet* 1988;I:672–675.

276. Romer M, Candinas R. Adenosine-induced non-sustained polymorphic ventricular tachycardia. *Eur Heart J* 1994;15:281.

277. Wesley RC Jr, Turnquest P. Torsades de pointes after intravenous adenosine in the presence of prolonged QT syndrome. *Am Heart J* 1992;123:794.

278. Smith TW. Digitalis. Mechanisms of action and clinical use. *N Engl J Med* 1988;318:358–36.

279. Lown B, Graboys TB, Podrid PJ, et al. Effect of a digitalis drug on ventricular premature beats. *N Engl J Med* 1977;296:301–306.

280. Falk RH, Knowlton AA, Bernard SA, et al. Digoxin for converting recent-onset atrial fibrillation to sinus rhythm. A randomized, double-blind trial. *Ann Intern Med* 1987;106:503–506.

281. The Digitalis in Acute Atrial Fibrillation (DAAF) Trial Group. Intravenous digoxin in acute atrial fibrillation. Results of a randomized, placebo-controlled multicentre trial in 239 patients. *Eur Heart J* 1997;18:649–654.

282. Jordaens L, Trouerbach J, Calle P, et al. Conversion of atrial fibrillation to sinus rhythm and rate control by digoxin in comparison to placebo. *Eur Heart J* 1997;18:643.

283. Pick A. Digitalis and the electrocardiogram. *Circulation* 1957;15:603–608.

284. Kelly RA, Smith TW. Recognition and management of digitalis toxicity. *Am J Cardiol* 1992;69:108.

285. Garg R, Gorlin R, Smith T, Yusuf S, for the Digitalis Investigation Group. The effect of digoxin on mortality and morbidity in patients with heart failure. *N Engl J Med* 1997;336:525–533.

9

CARDIOVERSION AND DEFIBRILLATION

JAVIER E. SANCHEZ
ANDREW E. EPSTEIN
RAYMOND E. IDEKER

Electrical energy has been used to treat cardiac rhythm disturbances for more than a century (1). Ventricular fibrillation was first treated with alternating current (AC) (2,3) and later with capacitor discharge shocks (4). Further refinements in the techniques of cardioversion and defibrillation have allowed the development of portable and implantable defibrillators for the treatment of atrial and ventricular fibrillation. In this chapter, the electrophysiology of cardioversion and defibrillation and general considerations in the clinical application of these forms of therapy are discussed.

Electrical cardioversion refers to the delivery of energy synchronized with the QRS complex. It can be used for the treatment of any tachyarrhythmia during which well-defined QRS complexes can be reliably identified. On the other hand, defibrillation refers to the delivery of unsynchronized energy. It is the only mode of electrical shock currently used for ventricular defibrillation and the mode of choice for the treatment of pulseless ventricular tachycardia and other ventricular tachycardias during which QRS complexes are difficult to identify.

ELECTROPHYSIOLOGY OF CARDIOVERSION AND DEFIBRILLATION

Ventricular fibrillation was early described as the uncoordinated electrical activity of the heart that renders it unable to pump blood effectively (5,6). In the 1930s, Carl Wiggers (7–10) systematically studied ventricular fibrillation and described the evolution of induced ventricular fibrillation in dogs. After carefully studying cinematographic recordings of the canine heart, he described four general stages in terms of decreasing degrees of observed ventricular contraction. These stages spanned from the onset of induced ventricular fibrillation to the cessation of all mechanical activity. His

careful observations remain influential in today's ideas about fibrillation. He described the *undulatory stage* as the initial period during which the fibrillation started with one extrasystole followed by three to six coordinated beats involving most of the ventricles. Although these were not electrical mapping studies, he was aware of Mines' experimental work (11) and proposed that these contractions were secondary to reentrant waves that used slightly different routes. During the second stage, *convulsive incoordination,* he noted that the heart seemed to be swept by progressively smaller and dissociated waves. These smaller wavefronts were described as still capable of inducing relatively vigorous, albeit uncoordinated, contractions of the ventricle. The *tremulous incoordination* stage, lasting up to 3 minutes, was characterized by reduction in the areas of visibly contracting myocardium. Finally, during the fourth (*atonic fibrillation*) stage, no contraction of the myocardium was visible despite the continued electrical activity recorded on the surface electrocardiogram (ECG). Detailed mapping studies of electrically induced ventricular fibrillation have expanded Wiggers' description about how the fibrillation process evolves over time. Recently, mapping studies using computerized algorithms have further characterized the breakdown in organization during ventricular fibrillation, quantifying how reentrant wavefronts increase in number, how the area swept by each wavefront decreases in size, and how the pathways used by each reentrant wavefront become more complex (12).

Based on limited ECG recordings, some authors (13–15) proposed that the stages described by Wiggers were the result of multiple reentrant waves that progressively decreased in size while others (16,17) suggested that the initiation and maintenance of fibrillation required rapidly firing ectopic foci. The views of Moe deserve particular attention. He advocated the concept of multiple wandering reentrant wavelets as the mechanism for the maintenance of fibrillation (18,19). He developed a computer model representing the heart as a two-dimensional sheet of cells (20) having different degrees of excitability and refractoriness, qualities that in those days were already known to be asso-

J. E. Sanchez, A. E. Epstein, and R. E. Ideker: Department of Internal Medicine, Division of Cardiovascular Diseases, University of Alabama at Birmingham, Birmingham, Alabama 35294.

ciated with the maintenance of fibrillation. His computer model behaved in several ways similar to atrial fibrillation. For instance, the "fibrillatory" activity could be initiated by premature excitation and maintained after the original stimulus was withdrawn. He also noted that the simulated electrical activity began with periodic waves that progressively decreased in size but increased in number. Furthermore, as in true fibrillation, prolongation of the refractory period led to increased organization of the turbulent activity until it ceased. Moe's computer model strongly supported the multiple-wavelet hypothesis as the mechanism for fibrillation in the heart.

Moe's hypothesis was experimentally verified by Allessie and colleagues (21) in a series of experiments using Langendorff-perfused canine hearts. They recorded the electrical activity of both atria with the use of two recording plaques, each containing 480 electrodes. Multiple wandering wavelets were present during sustained fibrillation and characterized as intraatrial reentrant circuits of the leading circle type (21). Subsequent mapping and computer-modeling studies by multiple laboratories studying atrial and ventricular fibrillation are consistent with the main principles of Moe's multiple-wavelet hypothesis. Modern mathematical predictions about how these electrical waves may evolve with time and interact with each other have been proposed (22), experimentally verified, and described in terms of spiral waves and drifting rotors (23–26). A recent review of these concepts in nonmathematical terms is presented in Gray (27).

Both Allessie and Moe suggested that the presence of multiple wavelets did not exclude the possibilities that ectopic foci were present and that they may be required for the initiation and maintenance of atrial fibrillation. Recent studies have shown that in some patients with frequent, paroxysmal atrial fibrillation, ectopic foci are responsible for the initiation of this arrhythmia (28).

Our current understanding of fibrillation and defibrillation is based on observations that are widely recognized. Chiefly among these is the observation that ventricular defibrillation is a probabilistic process (29,30). Figure 9-1 shows the expected response to shocks of increasing strength delivered to fibrillating myocardium. Defibrillation is accomplished over a range of delivered energies (29). There is no dividing line under which defibrillation is never achieved and over which defibrillation is always achieved. Shocks of equal energy are not observed to always have the same outcome. This probabilistic nature of defibrillation holds true for ventricular and atrial defibrillation regardless of whether the energy is applied externally or internally or whether the energy source is an alternating or a direct current (DC). For practical purposes, authors commonly refer to energy values associated with successful defibrillation as the defibrillation threshold (DFT) or effective dose (ED) and acknowledge the probabilistic nature of these values by stating the likelihood of successful defibrillation that is

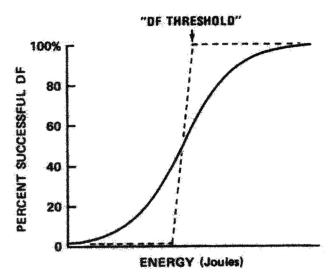

FIGURE 9-1. In contrast to the concept of a single "defibrillation (DF) threshold" (*dashed line*), the dose-response curve (*solid line*) reflects the probabilistic nature of defibrillation. As the shock strength is increased, successful defibrillation becomes more likely. (From Davy JM, Fain ES, Dorian P, et al. The relationship between successful defibrillation and delivered energy in open chest dogs: reappraisal of the "defibrillation threshold" concept. *Am Heart J* 1987;113:77–84, with permission.)

expected with the given energy shock. In this way, the shock energy associated with a 50% probability of successful defibrillation is referred to as the DFT_{50} or ED_{50}, and that value associated with more than or equal to 90% probability of success is referred to as the DFT_{90} or ED_{90}. It is also recognized that although shocks of increasing energy are associated with a higher likelihood of defibrillation, increasing up to nearly 100% success (31), further increases in energy are associated with a declining probability of success. This decrease in the efficacy is a result of the proarrhythmic effects of very high energy shocks (32,33).

The induction of ventricular fibrillation with electrical shocks is also a probabilistic process. The induction of fibrillation by electrical shocks is particularly efficient when shocks are delivered near the T wave of the cardiac cycle (8). Even when delivered during this period of ventricular vulnerability, shocks above a certain energy consistently fail to induce ventricular fibrillation (34). This phenomenon is referred to as the upper limit of vulnerability (ULV) for the electrical induction of ventricular fibrillation. As will be discussed later in this chapter, this ULV correlates with the DFT. These observations, namely, the probabilistic nature of defibrillation, the existence of a ULV, and the correlation between the ULV and the DFT, are the fundamental features of fibrillation and defibrillation that current hypotheses about fibrillation and defibrillation mechanisms attempt to explain. We discuss the two major hypotheses about the nature of defibrillation: the critical mass hypothesis and the ULV hypothesis. These hypotheses describe the process of ventricular and atrial fibrillation in a similar manner. Some differences between atrial and ventricular fibrillation exist, but these are envisioned to be related to the different anatomy and geometry of the cardiac chambers (35,36).

The concept that a critical mass of myocardium is necessary to sustain fibrillation originated when it was recognized that ventricular fibrillation was more difficult to induce and maintain in smaller hearts (6). In 1914, Garrey proposed a relation between the total mass required to sustain the fibrillatory process (37). He noted that up to three fourths of the ventricular mass had to be removed from a fibrillating canine heart for the fibrillation to stop. In 1975, Zipes and colleagues (38) defined *critical mass* as the minimal total amount of myocardium that must be present and excitable for ventricular fibrillation to continue spontaneously.

Zipes and colleagues (38) studied electrically induced ventricular fibrillation in canine hearts supported by cardiopulmonary bypass while recording electrical activity using epicardial electrodes positioned to record from the

vascular beds of each of the coronary arteries. By selectively infusing a hyperkalemic solution into the coronary arteries, they correlated the probability of successful defibrillation with the total mass of ventricular myocardium depolarized and rendered unexcitable by the hyperkalemic solution. As the total amount of depolarized myocardium increased, the probability of successful defibrillation also rose. The investigators also noted that although the electrical activity recorded from the areas infused with the hyperkalemic solution ceased, electrical activity consistent with ventricular fibrillation continued briefly in the remaining myocardium, even during episodes in which pharmacologic defibrillation was achieved (Fig. 9-2). They concluded that when a critical mass of myocardium was depolarized by the hyperkalemic infusion, ventricular fibrillation would eventually cease. In the same study, the authors also investigated the probability of successful electrical defibrillation as a function of the location of the shocking electrodes. Defibrillation could be accomplished more effectively by electrode

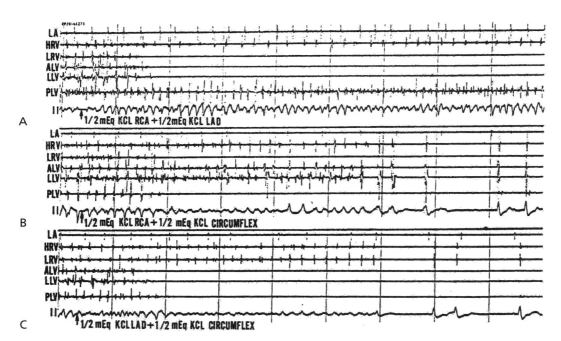

FIGURE 9-2. Termination of ventricular fibrillation by selective potassium chloride infusion. Electrograms recorded epicardially from the left atrium *(LA)*, high right ventricle near the outflow tract *(HRV)*, low right ventricle *(LRV)* along the inferior border, posterobasal left ventricle *(PLV)*, free wall of the left ventricle adjacent to the interventricular septum *(LLV)*, the apex of the left ventricle *(ALV)*, and lead II from the surface electrocardiogram. The epicardial electrodes record from the distributions of the right coronary artery (HRV and LRV), the left anterior descending (LAD) coronary artery (ALV and LLV), and the circumflex artery (PLV). **A:** Potassium chloride is injected simultaneously in the right coronary artery *(RCA)* and the LAD coronary arteries. Electrical activity in LRV, ALV, and LLV is suppressed but ventricular fibrillation continues in the PLV and is reflected on surface lead II. **B:** Potassium chloride is injected simultaneously in the RCA and circumflex arteries. Electrical activity recorded from the LRV and PLV were suppressed first. Other areas of the heart continued to fibrillate transiently until ventricular fibrillation terminated. **C:** Potassium chloride is injected simultaneously in the LAD and circumflex arteries. Electrical activity in the ALV, LLV, and PLV is suppressed and shortly after ventricular fibrillation terminates. (From Zipes DP, Fischer J, King RM, et al. Termination of ventricular fibrillation in dogs by depolarizing a critical amount of myocardium. *Am J Cardiol* 1975;36:37–44, with permission.)

systems that encompassed the left ventricle, rather than the right ventricle. This finding also was consistent and supportive of the critical mass concept.

The ULV concept was introduced by Fabiato and colleagues (34). Studying dogs, they noted that the induction of ventricular fibrillation by delivering shocks during the T wave of the cardiac cycle became increasingly difficult as the energy was increased to a certain shock strength, above which fibrillation could no longer be induced. Above this upper limit, shocks delivered at any point during the cardiac cycle, including the vulnerable period, fail to induce ventricular fibrillation. Furthermore, Fabiato and colleagues recognized that the strength of the upper limit shocks was similar to the DFT. In other words, the energy required to reliably defibrillate a fibrillating ventricle was approximately the same that would reliably fail to induce fibrillation when delivered to the ventricle in sinus rhythm. Expanding on these early observations, recent investigations have led to the following conclusions. First, a numerical correlation exists between the ULV and the DFT (39–41). Second, this correlation can be very strong when the location of the shocking electrodes and the timing of the ULV shocks are carefully controlled (42–44). Third, factors that influence the ULV affect the DFT similarly (45,46)

The concept of the ULV evolved into a hypothesis unifying the processes of fibrillation induction and defibrillation (47,48) after the observation in electrical mapping studies that after failed defibrillation shocks, a period of electrical quiescence was present (49–55). Figure 9-3 (51) shows epicardial recordings demonstrating a pause after a failed defibrillation shock followed by the regeneration of ventricular fibrillation. Because the critical mass hypothesis postulated that defibrillation shocks allowed ventricular fibrillation to continue in some areas of the heart, the observation that unsuccessful defibrillation shocks were able to transiently halt all fibrillatory activity was incongruent with the critical mass concept. Thus, a new hypothesis was required. The ULV hypothesis proposed that unsuccessful defibrillation shocks halt all activation wavefronts but a new process of ventricular fibrillation is induced by the shock. Thus, according to the ULV hypothesis, for a shock to be successful it not only has to halt all activation wavefronts but also must not induce new wavefronts that can refibrillate the heart.

Critical point reentry was proposed as a mechanism through which a shock can induce ventricular fibrillation after failed defibrillation shocks and after shocks delivered during the vulnerable period of ventricular depolarization. To understand critical point reentry, one must consider how the potential gradient field created by the shock is distributed throughout the ventricles.

Figure 9-4 shows the potential field distribution after a monophasic 500-V shock delivered between an electrode positioned in the right ventricular apex (cathode) and a cutaneous patch over the left lower thorax (anode) (56). As shown in Figure 9-4, the potential gradient distribution cre-

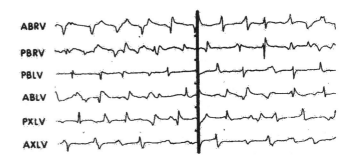

A

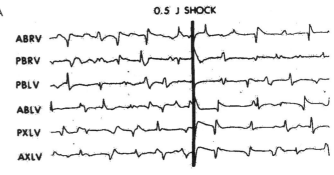

B

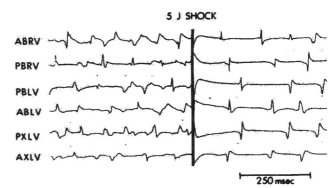

C

FIGURE 9-3. Electrical activity before and immediately after unsuccessful shocks to fibrillating myocardium. Electrodes were placed over the anterior and posterior aspects of the base of the right (*ABRV* and *PBRV*) and left ventricle (PBLV and ABLV), and apex (*AXLV* and *PXLV*). **A:** After a 0.01-J shock, ventricular fibrillation continues. **B:** After a 0.5-J shock, a brief pause in the electrical activity is recorded in all leads. **C:** After a 5-J shock, a longer pause is recorded in all leads. After the pause, ventricular fibrillation is reinitiated. (From Shibata N, Chen PS, Dixon EG, et al. Epicardial activation after unsuccessful defibrillation shocks in dogs. *Am J Physiol* 1988;255:H902–H909, with permission.)

ated by a shock varies throughout the heart as a function of the electrode location and the conductivity of the tissues. Areas of the heart that are distant from the current pathway have lower potential gradients.

The distribution of the potential gradient field is important because the response of the myocardium exposed to high-energy shocks is not an all-or-none response but is a function of local field strength. As shown in Figure 9-5 (57), the response of the myocardium to a stimulus greater than a critical value is graded, varying proportionally with

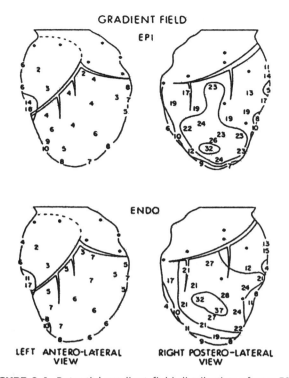

GRADIENT FIELD
EPI

ENDO

LEFT ANTERO-LATERAL VIEW   RIGHT POSTERO-LATERAL VIEW

FIGURE 9-4. Potential gradient field distribution after a 500-V monophasic shock delivered between the right ventricle apex (*cathode*) and a cutaneous patch over the left lower thorax. Gradients are shown in volts per centimeter for the epicardial (*epi*) and endocardial (*endo*) surfaces of the heart. The highest gradients were obtained near the shocking electrode at the apex. Significantly lower gradients were recorded far from the shocking electrodes, toward the base of the heart. (From Tang AS, Wolf PD, Claydon FJ, et al. Measurement of defibrillation shock potential distributions and activation sequences of the heart in three dimensions. *Proc IEEE* 1988;76:1176–1186, with permission.)

the stimulus strength and inversely with the degree of prematurity of the stimulus. The local response after a shock can vary from an all-or-none response, as observed for the 1.6-V/cm shock field, to a gradation of extension of the action potential and refractory period, as observed in Figure 9-5 for an 8.4-V/cm shock field. Critical point reentry occurs when the critical value shock strength intersects with a critical level of refractoriness leading to the formation of a reentrant circuit (22,47,58). Figure 9-6 (58) demonstrates an episode of ventricular fibrillation induction after the delivery of an electrical shock. In this study, a mapping plaque was positioned over the right ventricle, and the myocardium was paced from a linear electrode positioned along the right side of the plaque. Figure 9-6A shows the activation times after the last S1 stimulus. S2 shocks, delivered from a linear electrode positioned perpendicular to the pacing electrode at the bottom of the plaque, created a potential gradient field that decreased as a function of the distance from the S2 electrode, as shown in Figure 9-6B. S2 shocks were delivered at progressively shorter coupling intervals, scanning the vulnerable period after the S1 stimulus. As shown in Figure 9-6C, after a certain S_1-S_2 coupling interval a reentrant circuit was formed that eventually degenerated into ventricular fibrillation. This reentrant circuit circled around a "critical point" where the tissue was just past its refractory period and the local potential gradient was at the critical value of 5 to 6 V/cm. Myocardium to the right and below the critical point had a long period to recover from the last S1 stimulus and was exposed to a stimulus field larger than the critical value. Myocardium above and to the right of the critical point was exposed to a weaker stimulus field; therefore, only the tissue close to the S1 pac-

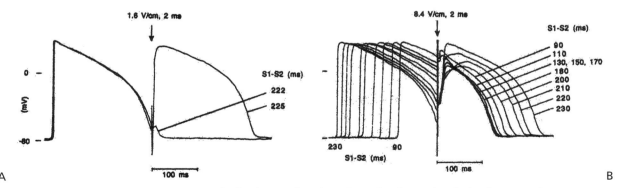

FIGURE 9-5. Response to an S2 stimulus as a function of coupling interval and stimulus strength. **A:** A 1.6-V/cm stimulus delivered with a 225-ms coupling interval causes a new action potential. Decreasing the coupling interval to 222 ms causes the stimulus with the same strength to elicit almost no response. **B:** An 8.4 V/cm stimulus delivered at increasing coupling intervals causes a range of responses in the action potential. The longer the S_1-S_2 coupling interval, the larger the extension of the action potential caused by the shock. The different tracings are time-aligned to the stimulus. (From Knisley SB, Smith WS, Ideker RE. Effect of field stimulation on cellular repolarization in rabbit myocardium—implications for reentry induction. *Circ Res* 1992;70:707–715, with permission.)

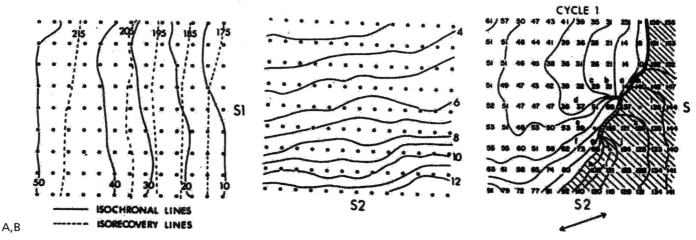

FIGURE 9-6. Induction of ventricular fibrillation caused by critical point reentry. **A:** Distribution of activation times and recovery times after the last S1 stimulus. The activation wavefront (*solid lines* with activation times in milliseconds at the bottom of the figure) advances from the right side of the plaque toward the left side, away from the pacing electrode. The recovery times (*dashed lines*) to a local 2 mA stimulus are shown in the upper part of the figure. The areas closer to the pacing electrode (on the right side of the figure) are activated first and therefore recover excitability sooner after the S1 stimulus. **B:** The S2 stimulus is delivered from the lower portion of the plaque, perpendicular to the pacing stimuli. The potential gradient field in volts per centimeter (*solid lines*) decreases as the distance from the S2 electrode is increased. **C:** Activation pattern of the first cycle after an S2 stimulus. The response to the S2 stimulus varied throughout the plaque as a function of distance away from the S2 stimulus and the degree of refractoriness of the tissue. A critical point occurred where the potential gradient field of 5 to 6 V/cm intersected tissue that was just passing out of its refractory period to a 2-ms local stimulus. The shock field was thought to have stimulated a new action potential in the tissue in the hatched area. (From Frazier DW, Wolf PD, Wharton JM, et al. Stimulus-induced critical point reentry: mechanism for electrical initiation of reentry in normal canine myocardium. *J Clin Inves* 1989;83:1030–1052, with permission.)

ing electrode was directly excited by the S2 stimulus. Myocardium to the left and above the critical point was still refractory and was not directly excited by the shock field because it was less than the critical value, so no graded response was elicited. The myocardium to the left and below the critical point experienced varying degrees of refractory period extension. Therefore, the activation wavefront starts in the area above and to the right of the critical point and circles around the critical point.

When a critical point occurs, after a shock delivered during the vulnerable period of an organized rhythm or immediately after a failed defibrillation attempt, a reentrant wavefront starts, which could progress to ventricular fibrillation. As the shock strength is increased, the regions with a potential gradient below the critical value become smaller and occur farther away from the shocking electrodes. Therefore, for shocks above the DFT and the ULV, critical points are unlikely to occur within the ventricles; hence, ventricular fibrillation is unlikely to be induced. Critical point reentry was postulated as one of the possible mechanisms by which the process of defibrillation and fibrillation reinduction could be related. Other mechanisms that could link the process of defibrillation and fibrillation induction still remain to be identified.

Other views regarding the mechanism of fibrillation and defibrillation have been proposed. Some authors emphasize the prolongation of the refractory period caused by the shock within the context of the critical mass (59,60) or the ULV (61) hypothesis. Others have emphasized shock-induced "virtual electrode" polarization patterns observed after failed defibrillation shocks (62). These "virtual electrode patterns" may cause postshock initiation of new wavefronts or dispersion of repolarization and provide the substrate for postshock reentrant arrhythmias. Further studies are required to more clearly understand the process of fibrillation induction, maintenance, and termination.

FACTORS ASSOCIATED WITH DEFIBRILLATION SUCCESS

Waveforms

The pioneering work on human transthoracic defibrillation by Zoll and others relied on a 60-Hz AC delivered during 20 to 150 ms. This allowed up to 10 cycles of the sinusoidal waveform to be delivered to the patient. Although undoubtedly able to defibrillate, these early waveforms were associated with a high incidence of fibrillation induction in the ventricle and in the atria (4). They also posed a health hazard to medical personnel, exposing the operator of the defibrillator to currents capable of inducing ventricular fibrillation (63). In addition, these early defibrillators required an AC energy source and were bulky and heavy, which made them difficult to transport during emergency situations. For these reasons AC shocks are no longer used in clinical practice. Instead, capacitor discharge pulses are favored. Because defibrillation efficacy depends on shock waveform, even when comparing shocks of similar strength, the clinician must become familiar with how the different waveforms compare.

Damped sinusoidal waveforms are generated by modifying a capacitor discharge with an inductor. The inductor smoothes the sharp leading edge of the capacitor discharge creating a waveform with gradual onset, as shown in Figure 9-7A. Early defibrillation studies in animals demonstrated that the efficacy and safety of capacitor discharge shocks were improved with the use of inductors (64,65). Thus, defibrillators for clinical use in humans were designed and manufactured using inductors (4). However, it is now recognized that with present technology, the incremental value added by the inductor (66) comes at the expense of a more than 50% increase in the weight, size, and cost of the device (67). Thus, for practical reasons, newer external defibrillators are commonly designed to use waveforms generated without the use of an inductor.

When a capacitor is allowed to discharge directly against a resistance (without the use of an inductor), a waveform

with a sharp leading edge followed by an exponential decay is created (Fig. 9-7B). After a capacitor discharge, most of the current flow occurs early after the leading edge of the pulse. The low-energy tail of the discharge does not contribute to the defibrillation efficacy of the waveform. Furthermore, the tail of certain waveforms can refibrillate the heart (68). Thus, waveforms are commonly truncated as shown in Figure 9-7C. Waveforms are monophasic when the polarity delivered to the electrodes remains unchanged during the shock, and biphasic (Fig. 9-7D) when the polarity is reversed once during the shock.

Figure 9-7C, D includes examples of truncated exponential waveforms. These waveforms, also referred to as trapezoidal waveforms, have a leading edge and a trailing edge. Trapezoidal waveforms are described in terms of their tilt and time constants. The tilt of the waveform is defined as the percentage of the leading edge voltage that is present in the trailing edge while the time constant is defined as the time required for the leading edge voltage to decrease by 63%. The time constant is a function of the capacitance and the resistance of the circuit and numerically equals their product. The tilt of the waveform is determined by the pulse duration and the time constant of the waveform. Increasing the pulse duration of a waveform will increase its tilt, and increasing the time constant of the waveform will decrease its tilt. The duration, tilt, and time constants of an exponentially decaying waveform are important determinants of its efficacy for defibrillation.

For biphasic waveforms, the efficacy is dependent not only on the duration, tilt, and time constants of each of the phases, but also on the interaction between the first and the second phase. Biphasic waveforms that deliver most of the charge during the first phase tend to have lower DFTs. Figure 9-8 (69) was constructed after determining the DFT using pulses with a fixed 10-ms duration. For this study, shocks were delivered from epicardial electrodes positioned on the right and left ventricle. As the duration of the second phase was increased from 2.5 ms to 5.0 ms, no significant change in the DFT voltage was noted, but as the duration of the second phase was further increased, the DFT voltage increased. The detrimental effect of prolonging the second phase longer than the first phase is more clearly revealed in Figure 9-9 (70). This graph was constructed after determining the DFTs for internal defibrillation shocks using a biphasic waveform with a fixed first-phase duration of 3.5 ms. Figure 9-9 shows how increasing the duration of the second phase up to 2.0 ms decreased the DFT current. Further increases in the duration of the second phase did not help decrease the DFT. When the second phase was 7.0 ms long, the DFT was more than that for the monophasic 3.5-ms shock alone.

Figures 9-8 and 9-9 show examples of biphasic waveforms that are more effective for defibrillation than monophasic waveforms. Other studies in animals and humans undergoing ventricular and atrial defibrillation also

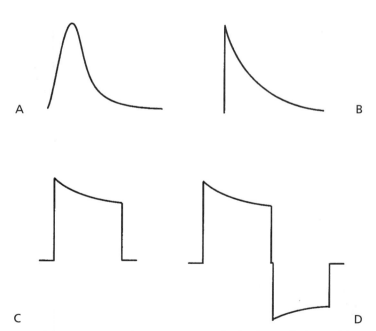

FIGURE 9-7. Waveforms. **A:** Monophasic damped sinusoidal waveform. **B:** Exponential decay observed after a capacitor discharge against a resistance. Notice the low amplitude tail of this waveform. **C:** Monophasic, truncated exponential waveform. **D:** Biphasic, truncated exponential waveform. See text.

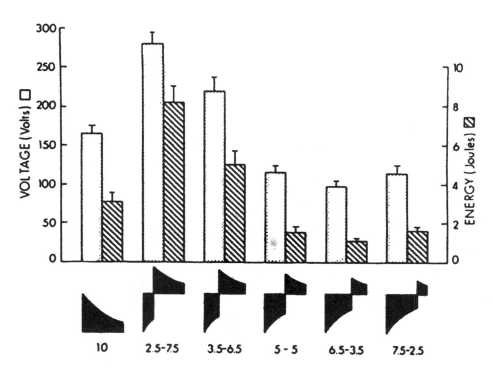

FIGURE 9-8. Defibrillation threshold voltage and energy values for six waveforms of the same total duration (10 ms). Diagrams of the waveforms are shown below the bar graphs. Biphasic waveforms with a second phase equal to or shorter than the first phase have the lowest defibrillation thresholds. (From Dixon EG, Tang ASL, Kavanagh KM, et al. Improved defibrillation thresholds with large contoured epicardial electrodes and biphasic waveforms. *Circulation*1987;76:1176–1184, with permission.)

demonstrated lower DFTs for biphasic shocks than for monophasic shocks (69–76). Despite the usual superiority of biphasic shocks over monophasic shocks, there are circumstances under which a biphasic shock can be less effective than a monophasic shock. As already discussed, Figure 9-9 shows an example of a biphasic waveform rendered less effective than the monophasic waveform by extending the duration of the second phase to more than the duration of the first phase. The mechanisms for explaining the superiority of biphasic over monophasic waveforms are not completely understood (76).

Investigations are in progress for the development of more effective waveforms. The results with internal defib-

rillation systems using a triphasic waveform have been mixed. Although some have found them less effective than biphasic waveforms (69–92), others (93,94) reported that at least one form of triphasic waveform can provide an advantage over a standard biphasic waveform. Another approach to increase the efficacy of defibrillation waveforms has been to use two separate, high-tilt capacitors for the delivery of each of the phases of the biphasic waveform (95). Finally, animal studies suggest that timing of the shock to the morphology electrogram (96), or delivering the shock very soon after the onset of fibrillation (97), may also improve the outcome of internal defibrillation shocks.

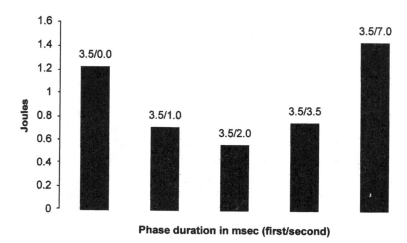

FIGURE 9-9. Defibrillation threshold energy for shocks with a 3.5-ms first phase. As the duration of the second phase was increased from 0.0 ms (a monophasic shock) to 2.0 ms, the defibrillation threshold improved. Further increases in the duration of the second phase were associated with an increase in the defibrillation threshold. (From Feeser SA, Tang ASL, Kavanagh KM, et al. Strength-duration and probability of success curves for defibrillation with biphasic waveforms. *Circulation* 1990; 82:2128–2141, with permission.)

Electrode Position

The performance of either monophasic or biphasic waveforms can be improved by choosing electrode positions that increase the minimal potential gradient across the heart.

For transthoracic shocks, the electrodes are commonly placed in the anteroapical or anteroposterior positions. For the anteroapical configuration, one electrode is placed toward the right side of the upper sternum below the clavicle and the other electrode is placed slightly lateral to the cardiac apex (98). For the anteroposterior configuration, one electrode is positioned anteriorly, to the left of the sternum, overlying the right ventricle, and the other electrode is placed posteriorly, to the left of the spine. When using either configuration in women, placement of an electrode over breast tissue should be avoided because in this location impedance is high (99). In this situation, it is preferable to place the electrode just lateral to or under the breast. For practical reasons, the anteroapical configuration is used during emergency situations, and for some elective procedures, the anteroposterior position is more convenient. Neither of these standard positions has been shown to be consistently superior in all patients (100), but individual patients may respond better to one electrode configuration over the other. Again, the use of an electrical coupler and the application of firm pressure on the electrodes may, in many situations, improve the outcome without the need for switching to a different electrode position.

For internal ventricular defibrillation, one of the electrodes is positioned at the right ventricular apex. The other electrode is commonly the can of the pulse generator, often linked to a second coiled electrode in the superior vena cava or the subclavian vein. Using the pulse generator, as with an active electrode, improves the shock vector and thus is associated with a decrease in the DFTs (77,78). Similarly, for internal atrial defibrillation, the lowest thresholds are obtained with configurations that encompass as much of the atria as possible (75,79–82).

Electrode Polarity

Electrode polarity can affect the DFT obtained with monophasic and biphasic waveforms. For internal ventricular defibrillation, the use of the right ventricular apex electrode as the anode has been shown to decrease the DFT of monophasic waveforms in animals (83,84) and humans (85). For biphasic waveforms, the use of the right ventricular electrode as the anode for the first phase has also been shown to decrease DFTs for some electrode configurations (84), although not for others (83). Despite these generalizations about optimal polarity, the optimal polarity for each patient can vary (86–88). Therefore, it is advised to reverse the polarity of the shock electrodes whenever a patient with a high DFT is encountered during implantation of a defibrillator. The effects of polarity on the DFT are less prominent when the electrodes are farther from the heart. Thus, for external defibrillation, the polarity of the shock does not seem to have a large effect on the DFT (89).

Transthoracic Impedance

The current flow across the myocardium is only a small fraction, perhaps as low as 4%, of the total current delivered by a transthoracic shock (101,102). The rest of the current is shunted across other structures such as the thoracic musculature and the mediastinum. Current flow across the heart is determined by the distribution of the transthoracic impedance. It has been documented that the total transthoracic impedance among different patients can range from 20 to 150 Ω (103). This variation can be explained by several factors, which are listed in Table 9-1. Electrode size is an important consideration. Diameters between 8 and 12 cm are optimal for use in adults (104,105). The use of smaller electrodes is discouraged except with infants weighing less than 10 kg (106). Electrical conduction at the electrode-skin interface is significantly improved by the use of an electrical coupler (i.e., conductive pads or gel). Attention must be paid when applying a conductive gel, particularly between subsequent shocks. If the gel is inadvertently smeared over the chest wall between the electrodes, a low-resistance electrical pathway is created. This pathway can effectively shunt the current between the electrodes, thus decreasing the energy delivered to the heart. Applying firm pressure over the electrodes will also improve conduction across the electrode-skin interface (105,107,108).

Transthoracic impedance decreases after repetitive shocks (109,110). This decrease may be a result of the tissue edema that follows a transthoracic shock (111). Consistent with this mechanism is the observation that the timing of successive shocks affects the decrease in the transthoracic impedance (109,110). Based on these observations, some authors advocate waiting 3 minutes before delivering another shock after a failed attempt during an elective cardioversion procedure (112). Finally, the delivery of the shock during expiration has been noted to marginally decrease the atrial DFT when compared with shocks delivered during inspiration (113).

TABLE 9-1. FACTORS AFFECTING TRANSTHORACIC IMPEDANCE

Electrode size, position, and distance
Electrode-skin interface
Contact pressure
Shock strength
Previous shocks
Interval between shocks
Phase of ventilation
Previous sternotomy
Patient size and body habitus

Other Factors

Other factors that affect transthoracic impedance such as morbid obesity, thick upper torso, and marked chronic hyperinflation of the lungs cannot be changed before delivery of a shock. The presence of these factors imposes on the clinician the need to be particularly attentive to the other considerations to improve the probability of successful defibrillation.

CLINICAL CONSIDERATIONS

Elective cardioversion should be performed by trained personnel familiar with airway management and resuscitation techniques. The procedure is performed in a medical facility equipped with resuscitation equipment. The supplies necessary for suction, airway management, and an oxygen source are required. Continuous rhythm and hemodynamic monitoring are mandatory, as is a supply of pharmacologic agents to use as an adjunct to therapy or in the event of complications.

The proper use of an anesthetic agent is extremely important. Patients not adequately anesthetized and sedated will experience pain secondary to the tetanic contraction of the chest wall musculature. They may also suffer excessive fear and apprehension about future necessary treatments or procedures. A single short-acting barbiturate such as methohexital or the combined use of a benzodiazepine and an opioid analgesic (e.g., midazolam and fentanyl) is useful in achieving transient sedation and amnesia. Sedation should be initiated in the patient in the fasting state to decrease the risk of aspiration of gastric contents. Manual ventilation with supplemental oxygen is required during the period of deepest sedation. Endotracheal intubation is not routinely required for the fasting patient, but the supplies and personnel for endotracheal ventilation should be readily available. Only ventricular fibrillation or other tachyarrhythmias associated with loss of consciousness justify shock therapy without sedation.

The electrode paddles should be used with a conductive material, a conductive pad or a gel, to decrease transthoracic impedance and avoid skin trauma. The electrodes are positioned firmly in the anteroapical or anteroposterior position as described above. The use of self-adhesive (114) electrode patches is convenient and allows for rescue shocks or pacing to be delivered promptly. However, the use of these electrodes can be associated with lower success rates because the firm contact achieved with handheld electrodes is not achieved (115). Cohen and colleagues (105) found that four of five patients with atrial fibrillation undergoing elective cardioversion that had failed at least one 360-J shock using self-adhesive skin electrodes could be successfully cardioverted by applying manual compression of the skin patches with defibrillator paddles. Therefore, when using self-adhesive skin electrodes, it is required to either switch to handheld electrodes or apply manual pressure (using disconnected paddles) before declaring that an arrhythmia is not responsive to electrical therapy.

For cardioversion, the physician must ensure adequate synchronization of the defibrillator output with the QRS complex. Visual inspection of the synchronization markers in the defibrillator ECG monitor is required to avoid shocking on the T wave. Most commercially available defibrillators default to the unsynchronized mode after the delivery of each shock; therefore, it is incumbent on the physician to resynchronize the output after each shock. For pulseless ventricular tachycardia and ventricular tachycardia with QRS and T waves of similar appearance, unsynchronized 200-J shocks are recommended (116).

The use of electrical therapy needs to be considered within the context of the clinical situation. Sustained tachyarrhythmias associated with angina, acute onset or worsening of congestive heart failure, or hypotension with signs or symptoms of poor end organ perfusion should be treated aggressively. If prompt reversion or improvement is not obtained with medical management, electrical therapy is indicated. Tachyarrhythmias that occur in a repetitive fashion, with episodes of spontaneous termination followed by resumption of the tachycardia, are unlikely to be resolved with electrical therapy. In these circumstances, successful electrical therapy is expected to be followed by rapid reinitiation of the arrhythmia.

Arrhythmias in the setting of digitalis intoxication do not respond well to electrical therapy. Furthermore, electrical interventions during digitalis intoxication can actually precipitate ventricular fibrillation refractory to any treatment (117). It is therefore advisable to avoid cardioversion of arrhythmias resulting from digitalis toxicity. When electrical therapy in this setting is unavoidable, pretreatment with lidocaine or phenytoin has been advocated and correction of potassium abnormalities is essential. It is prudent to start with low-energy shocks because the induction of arrhythmias in these patients may be dose-related. For elective cardioversion procedures in patients on chronic digoxin therapy, cardioversion can be easily and safely done as long as digoxin toxicity is absent and potassium abnormalities have been corrected (118).

ROLE OF CARDIOVERSION AND DEFIBRILLATION IN SPECIFIC ARRHYTHMIAS

Cardiac Arrest

The most effective therapy for ventricular fibrillation and a cardiac arrest resulting from pulseless ventricular tachycardia is prompt electrical defibrillation (119–122). Patients with ventricular fibrillation soon develop hypoxia, acidosis, and irreversible end organ damage. After 10 minutes of ventricular fibrillation, the probability of survival is dismal, even when basic cardiopulmonary resuscitation (CPR) is instituted. The need for early defibrillation and the interplay between bystander CPR and electrical defibrillation is demonstrated in Figure 9-10. This graph was generated by Valenzuela and colleagues (123) after analyzing two large retrospective series of witnessed cardiac arrest with documented ventricular fibrillation. As shown in the graph, survival to hospital discharge is a function of the time intervals from collapse to CPR and from collapse to defibrillation. For every minute that CPR and defibrillation are postponed, chance of survival decreases by 10%. The use of CPR is negated when defibrillation is delayed for more than 10 minutes. Similarly, the effectiveness of defibrillation is significantly improved by the institution of CPR immediately after collapse. The rapid delivery of CPR and early defibrillation are also important to maximize survival of inhospital cardiac arrest victims (124).

Factors other than the timing of CPR and defibrillation affect outcome after a resuscitation attempt (125). Preexisting medical conditions such as pulmonary, cerebrovascular, renal, and hepatic disease decrease the probability of a positive outcome (126,127). Some studies have also suggested that patients with high transthoracic impedance and ventricular fibrillation with an amplitude of less than 0.5 mV in the initial recorded rhythm ("fine" ventricular fibrillation) are less likely to respond to treatment (128).

The ideal first shock would be of sufficient energy to ensure a high success rate without causing undue myocardial and transthoracic damage. Studies have found that initial shock strengths of less than or equal to 200 J are associated with success rates similar to those for shocks of more than or equal to 300 J (129,130). Therefore, current guidelines (116) suggest that at least when using monophasic waveforms, the initial shock strength should be 200 J, followed by successive 300-J and 360-J shocks until successful

defibrillation. Some have advocated the adjustment of the shock energy based on the patient's transthoracic impedance (100), and at least one manufacturer has adopted this strategy. Studies in humans undergoing transthoracic shocks for the treatment of induced ventricular fibrillation have shown that lower energy biphasic shocks have the same efficacy as higher energy monophasic shocks. For instance, investigators in a single-center (131) and in a multicenter study (67) found that 115- to 130-J biphasic shocks were as successful as 200-J monophasic shocks. It is estimated that a 360-J shock from a standard commercially available defibrillator using a damped sinusoidal waveform is equivalent to a 200- to 220-J shock from a defibrillator using a biphasic, truncated exponential waveform. The finding that trapezoidal biphasic waveforms allow similar defibrillation success as standard monophasic waveforms (damped sinusoidal) with lower energy is of practical importance. Defibrillators able to deliver lower energy shocks using a biphasic waveform are smaller, lighter, and potentially more affordable than older defibrillators using the monophasic, damped sinusoidal waveform. Public initiatives to improve the survival of out-of-hospital cardiac arrest victims by making these devices available to the public (132) will significantly benefit from these advances (67).

Ventricular Tachycardia

Electrical cardioversion is indicated for the treatment of monomorphic ventricular tachycardia that fails to respond to drug therapy. As already discussed, it is important to properly sedate these patients. A properly delivered, synchronized 100-J shock is associated with nearly 100% efficacy and no significant increased risk of complications when compared with lower energy shocks. Therefore, an initial shock of 100 J is recommended for ventricular tachycardia that requires cardioversion. For polymorphic ventric-

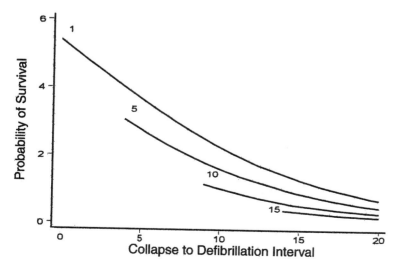

FIGURE 9-10. Relation of time interval from collapse to cardiopulmonary resuscitation (CPR) and defibrillation to survival. Each curve represents the probability of survival as a function of the collapse-defibrillation interval when CPR is started 1, 5, 10, and 15 minutes after collapse. As the interval from collapse to defibrillation increases, the probability of survival decreases. (From Valenzuela TD, Roe DJ, Cretin S, et al. Estimating effectiveness of cardiac arrest interventions: a logistic regression survival model. *Circulation* 1997;96:3308–3313, with permission.)

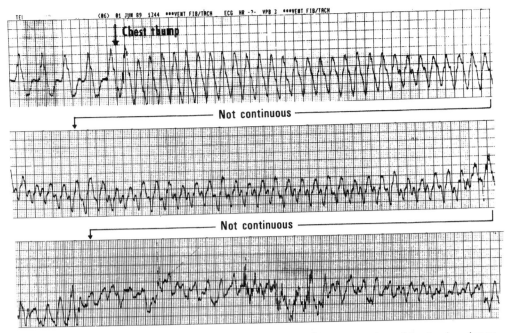

FIGURE 9-11. Ventricular fibrillation after precordial thump. Initial portion of the tracing shows monomorphic ventricular tachycardia. After the precordial thump, incidentally delivered during the T wave, the tachycardia accelerates and converts to ventricular fibrillation.

ular tachycardias or monomorphic tachycardias with T waves indistinguishable from the QRS, an unsynchronized shock of 200 J is used, followed successively by 300-J and 360-J shocks if needed. Some reports show that when no defibrillator is immediately available, a precordial thump (133), or even vigorous cough (134), can be used to terminate ventricular tachycardia. These strategies are unreliable and can accelerate the ventricular rate or induce ventricular fibrillation (135,136) (Fig. 9-11), so their use is usually limited to situations in which other therapies are not available.

Implantable Cardioverter-Defibrillator

In certain populations at high risk of life-threatening ventricular arrhythmias the implantable cardioverter-defibrillator (ICD) can improve survival (137,138). In these patients, effective defibrillation is delivered within seconds of the onset of the ventricular tachyarrhythmia. Further discussion about the role of the ICD can be found in Chapter 11.

Atrial Fibrillation

Electrical cardioversion for the treatment of atrial fibrillation plays a significant role in the management of symptomatic patients (139). Patients with atrial fibrillation commonly experience palpitations, malaise, and fatigue. Some may develop congestive heart failure. When patients do not respond to pharmacologic intervention, or when adverse drug effects occur, electrical cardioversion for selected

patients is indicated. Factors that affect the likelihood of successful maintenance of sinus rhythm after cardioversion are listed in Table 9-2.

Except in rare circumstances, atrial fibrillation patients can be stabilized medically to allow for elective or semielective electrical cardioversion. This allows the physician to have a discussion with the patient about the options for treatment. It is necessary to discuss with the patient the risk for thromboembolic events and the likelihood of immediate and long-term success after the cardioversion procedure. Every effort should be employed to reverse any treatable precipitating factor (e.g., hyperthyroidism) and to optimize the medical therapy, particularly in patients with signs and symptoms of volume overload. Although some patients have an excellent chance of long-term success, those who experience an episode of atrial fibrillation have a high risk of experiencing atrial fibrillation again. It is necessary to recognize that the relative value of a strategy of long-term maintenance of sinus rhythm versus rate control has not been established. The ongoing Atrial Fibrillation Follow-up Investigation of Rhythm Management (AFFIRM) Trial, sponsored by the National Heart, Lung, and Blood Institute, is addressing this important clinical question (140).

Once the decision for rhythm control with electrical cardioversion has been made, the timing of the procedure needs to be addressed. For patients with atrial fibrillation for longer than 48 hours or atrial fibrillation of unknown duration, anticoagulation with warfarin for 3 to 4 weeks is considered the accepted standard of care (139). Some

TABLE 9-2. DETERMINANTS OF SUCCESS AFTER ATRIAL DEFIBRILLATION

Duration of the atrial fibrillation
Patient age
Atrial diameter
Cause of heart disease
Volume status
Antiarrhythmic therapy
Presence of coexisting medical problems
History of prior cardioversion followed by atrial fibrillation
  recurrence

authors suggest that a thorough transesophageal echocardiographic (TEE) evaluation documenting the absence of atrial thrombus can obviate the need for the 3 weeks of anticoagulation before cardioversion (141). Patients with atrial fibrillation for less than 48 hours are considered at a lesser risk for the presence of intracardiac thrombi; therefore, current guidelines suggest that these patients can be cardioverted without preprocedure oral anticoagulation (139). Regardless of the precardioversion strategy, postcardioversion oral anticoagulation for at least 4 weeks is advisable for all patients, even when sinus rhythm has been restored (142–144). Postcardioversion anticoagulation is necessary because atrial transport function may not recover for up to several weeks after conversion (145,146), and in the absence of efficient transport, atrial thrombi may still develop, even during sinus rhythm.

The energy selection for the initial shock for the treatment of atrial fibrillation with conventional (monophasic) defibrillators remains a matter of controversy. Based on anecdotal reports and nonrandomized studies, it has long been advocated to start with a 100-J shock and to increase the energy for successive shocks (147). Recently, a preliminary report (148) from a randomized trial suggests that initial energies of 200 and 360 J are as safe as 100-J shocks with no increase in the incidence of significant sinus bradycardia, atrioventricular block, or troponin I enzyme elevation. Furthermore, the success rate with the higher energy initial shocks was significantly improved.

If the initial shock fails to terminate the atrial fibrillation, the energy of the subsequent shocks is commonly increased in a stepwise manner up to 360 J. For patients that have failed 360-J transthoracic shocks, higher energy shocks have been used. A shock energy of up to 720 J can be delivered by applying two sets of self-adhesive patches and connecting each pair of electrodes to a separate external defibrillator and delivering both synchronized shocks simultaneously (149,150). This approach can lead to effective and safe cardioversion of patients that have failed to cardiovert after receiving 360-J transthoracic shocks.

Biphasic waveforms may be more effective than monophasic waveforms because they use less delivered energy, which may result in less postshock myocardial dys-

function. This was evaluated in one study that randomized 174 patients with atrial fibrillation to cardioversion with monophasic waveform, using sequential shocks of 100 to 360 J, or biphasic waveform with energies of 70 to 170 J (150a). First-shock efficacy was greater with a biphasic waveform (68% versus 21%) and delivered energy was 50% less; the overall cardioversion rate was higher with the biphasic waveform (94% versus 79%).

The use of some antiarrhythmic agents before cardioversion is associated with improved outcomes. One study found that the use of ibutilide before elective cardioversion was associated with lower defibrillation energies and a high success rate (151). In this study, sustained polymorphic ventricular tachycardia occurred in 2 out of 64 patients and both of these patients had a left ventricular ejection fraction of less than 0.20. All the patients who were nonresponsive to up to a 360-J transthoracic shock were successfully cardioverted electrically after the administration of ibutilide. Other class III or class I agents can be used chronically to increase the likelihood of maintaining sinus rhythm after a successful cardioversion.

Atrial Flutter

Advances in the treatment of atrial flutter, including the widespread application of ablation therapy, have decreased the role of electrical cardioversion for this arrhythmia. When cardioversion is required, the initial shock energy can be 10 to 50 J, but a 100-J shock is preferred because it has a nearly 100% success rate without an increase in complications. Anticoagulation before cardioversion in patients with atrial flutter of recent onset and no other indication for anticoagulation is not required. The need to anticoagulate patients with chronic atrial flutter and the use of anticoagulation after cardioversion are a matter of debate. Some studies seem to suggest that chronic atrial flutter is associated with an increased risk of thromboembolic events that warrants anticoagulation (152,153). Other authors have shown an acute decrease in atrial transport function, with the development of spontaneous echo contrast and occasional thrombus formation, after the acute termination of the arrhythmia (154, 155). Whether these findings justify the use of anticoagulation with its attendant risk for bleeding complications will be difficult to settle without further studies.

Supraventricular Tachycardia

Reentrant supraventricular tachycardias, such as atrioventricular nodal reentrant tachycardia and atrioventricular reciprocating tachycardia, may be acutely terminated with vagal maneuvers or pharmacologic therapy in close to 100% of patients. Rarely, when significant hemodynamic compromise is present, electrical cardioversion is indicated. Like atrial flutter, these arrhythmias may respond to low-energy synchronized shocks in the range of 50 J, but a 100-

J shock is associated with a higher success rate without an increase in complications. The efficacy of electrical shocks for the treatment of atrial arrhythmias caused by increased automaticity of a single focus is less predictable and higher energy shocks are required. Multifocal atrial tachycardia responds poorly to electrical shocks and should be managed with rate control and treatment of the underlying medical conditions.

INTERNAL CARDIOVERSION AND DEFIBRILLATION

Transthoracic shocks are usually successful in stabilizing the patient with ventricular arrhythmias until reversible factors are corrected or more definitive therapy can be offered. Reports in the literature document occasional situations in which patients requiring frequent transthoracic shocks have been stabilized with the use of temporary endocardial defibrillation electrodes (156). The emergency use of internal defibrillation has also been documented for patients that have failed high-energy transthoracic shocks (157). However, in current clinical practice, the use of endocardial electrodes for the treatment of ventricular arrhythmias is mostly limited to the use of the ICD. Elsewhere in this book the use of ICDs is discussed in detail.

Internal cardioversion of atrial fibrillation can be offered to patients in whom transthoracic shocks have failed. Early procedures were performed with a single intracardiac electrode positioned in the right atrium and the use of an external paddle positioned posteriorly as the second electrode. The energy delivered was between 200 and 300 J and the success rates were marginally better than those with external 300- to 360-J shocks (79). More recently, the procedure has been performed with temporary catheter electrodes positioned in the distal coronary sinus and the right atrial appendage or right atrial lateral wall (75,80,81). With the use of intracardiac electrodes and a biphasic waveform (158), low-energy shocks (less than or equal to 5 J) can terminate atrial fibrillation reliably, particularly in patients with an atrial fibrillation duration of less than 1 year (82). The DFTs obtained with intracardiac electrodes can be further decreased with the use of intravenous agents (159).

Although internal atrial defibrillation is effective and safe for the treatment of acute episodes, it is an invasive form of therapy that should be reserved for patients in whom adequate attempts of chemical and transthoracic shock therapy have failed. With the advent of safe and efficient adjuvant pharmacologic treatment (151), few patients are likely to require this form of therapy.

The high acute success rate and safety of endocardial defibrillation have favored the development of the implantable atrial defibrillator. This device has been tested in a limited number of highly symptomatic patients with frequent episodes of paroxysmal atrial fibrillation (160).

The internal atrial defibrillator can reliably and safely terminate episodes of atrial fibrillation. However, the treatments are commonly distressing to the patient and continuation of antiarrhythmic drug therapy is usually required. The role of the implantable atrial defibrillator as a stand-alone treatment or as an adjunct to other forms of therapy remains to be determined (161).

A unique opportunity for internal defibrillation is presented by the patient with postoperative atrial fibrillation. In this setting, it is common to have temporary epicardial wires left by the surgeon at the time of surgery to facilitate the diagnosis and management of postoperative rhythm disturbances (162,163). Traditionally, these epicardial electrodes are used to pace-terminate reentrant arrhythmias or to temporarily pace the patient with postoperative bradycardia. Recently, epicardial electrodes placed at the time of cardiac surgery were used for the treatment of postoperative atrial fibrillation using cardioversion (164). In this study, atrial fibrillation was terminated with shocks averaging 5 J without significant complications from the shock or from the extraction of the electrodes.

COMPLICATIONS
Bradyarrhythmias

Bradyarrhythmias are common after successful defibrillation shocks. In patients with induced ventricular arrhythmias, Eysmann and colleagues (165) noted that 17 out of 64 transthoracic shocks were followed by early bradycardia, defined by the authors as any rhythm with a cycle length of more than or equal to 1,200 ms for the first 5 seconds after the shock. In this study, bradycardia was still present 10 seconds after the shock in nine (12%) episodes. The occurrence of bradycardia correlated with the need for multiple shocks and the presence of previous inferior myocardial infarction. Waldecker and colleagues (166) evaluated the interval after a successful shock before the first spontaneous activity after transthoracic shocks for the treatment of induced ventricular arrhythmias or atrial fibrillation. An escape rhythm after ventricular defibrillation appeared after a mean of 1,900 ± 960 ms (range, 700 to 7,500 ms) while after successful cardioversion of atrial fibrillation, the escape rhythm occurred after 1,150 ± 470 ms. The pauses were followed by conduction disturbances or bradycardia in nearly half the patients, but pacing was required only after 13% (13 of 99) of the shocks. The occurrence of bradycardia was more common in patients with ischemic cardiomyopathies, but unlike in the report by Eysmann and colleagues, it was not related to the total number of DC shocks. Out-of-hospital ventricular defibrillation is also associated with bradyarrhythmic complications and their incidence may be related to the shock strength. In a study of cardiac arrest victims, significant bradycardia, atrioventricular block, and asystole were reported in 24% of patients after receiving 320-J shocks, but only in 9% of patients who received 175-J shocks (130). Persistent bradyarrhythmias can also occur after cardioversion of atrial arrhythmias. Patients with sick sinus syndrome and those with unknown sinus node function (e.g., patients with chronic atrial fibrillation or flutter) may be at increased risk of this complication.

Tachyarrhythmias

Unsustained tachyarrhythmias have also been reported after successful internal (161) and transthoracic shocks (130,165,166). In a study of patients undergoing ICD testing, the incidence of these arrhythmias after internal defibrillation shocks was not related to the shock strength (167). However, the shock strength did influence the cycle length of these arrhythmias (168). For shocks with energy levels of at least 10 J above the defibrillation energy requirement, arrhythmias with a cycle length of more than 300 ms occurred after 32% of the shocks. When the shock strength was below the defibrillation energy requirement, only 7.1% of the shocks were followed by arrhythmias with a cycle length of more than 300 ms ($p < 0.05$). Conversely, successful low-energy shocks were followed by arrhythmias with a cycle length of less than or equal to 300 ms more frequently than after high-energy shocks (19% versus 1.5%; $p < 0.05$). The mechanisms explaining the results of this study were not explored, but the authors speculated that these differences may have been related to the deleterious effects of excessive shock energy on the integrity of the cell membrane.

Shocks for the treatment of atrial fibrillation, atrial flutter, or other supraventricular tachycardias rarely are complicated by the occurrence of sustained ventricular arrhythmias. When this occurs, it is usually a result of lack of synchronization of the shock, although ventricular fibrillation can occur after synchronized shocks (169).

ST-Segment Changes

ECG changes, particularly of the ST segment, are common after defibrillation and cardioversion shocks. In the study of Eysmann and colleagues (165), continuous three-lead monitoring and serial 12-lead ECGs were recorded after DC shocks for the treatment of induced ventricular arrhythmias. Transient ST-segment elevation or depression was noted in nearly 40% of patients. These ST changes resolved within 15 minutes in all patients. In this study, the ST-segment elevations occurred almost exclusively in the ECG and anatomic distributions where a myocardial scar was known to be present. Another study evaluated the relation between shock waveform and energy and the incidence of ST-segment changes (67). The authors compared the degree of ST-segment depression 10 seconds after a transthoracic shock for the treatment of induced ventricular arrhythmias. They reported a trend to greater ST-segment depressions after shocks of 115, 130, 200, and 360 J. An example from their study is shown in Figure 9-12. Although the observed trend was statistically significant, the clinical implications of these findings are not known. ECG changes have also been documented after the implantation and testing of ICDs (170).

Embolism

We have already discussed the use of anticoagulation in patients with atrial fibrillation to decrease the incidence of thromboembolic complications. Even patients with no thrombus evident on precardioversion transesophageal echocardiographic evaluation can develop embolic complications (170), possibly related to the atrial stunning commonly observed after DC cardioversion (142). Patients treated for ventricular arrhythmias can also suffer from embolic complications. These complications are more common in patients with left ventricular dysfunction and in patients with a history of anterior myocardial infarction.

Hemodynamic Complications

Hemodynamic complications such as acute pulmonary edema (171) and hypotension (172) occur rarely after DC shocks. It is important to recognize when these complications are secondary to other events such as pulmonary embolism to initiate adequate therapy. Transient decreases in cardiac output in the range of 10% to 15% after shocks have been documented to occur in humans possibly as a function of shock strength (173).

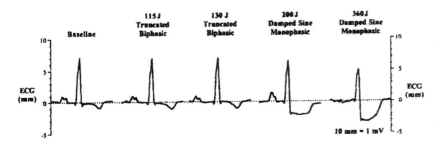

FIGURE 9-12. ST-segment changes after transthoracic shocks. Baseline and postshock electrocardiograms 10 seconds after shock delivery in a patient who received transthoracic shocks with monophasic and biphasic waveforms. Note how shock energy and waveform influence the degree of postshock ST-segment depression. (From Bardy GH, Marchilinski FE, Sharma AD, et al. Multicenter comparison of truncated biphasic shocks and standard damped sine wave monophasic shocks for transthoracic ventricular defibrillation. *Circulation* 1998;94:2507–2514, with permission.)

Myocardial Damage

Myocardial necrosis after defibrillation shocks can be documented with creatine kinase, creatine kinase-MB, or troponin elevations in a small percentage of patients. These elevations are usually mild and not associated with other manifestations of myocardial ischemia (174). Areas of local necrosis and fibrosis have been documented in patients with epicardial (175) and transvenous (176) defibrillation systems.

Myocardial Dysfunction

Global left ventricular dysfunction resulting from myocardial stunning may be seen in patients with cardiac arrest who have undergone successful CPR. This is related in part to defibrillation but is also a result of the arrhythmia itself and to the absence of cardiac output and coronary blood flow during the period of arrest with resultant ischemia. Thus, baseline evaluation of left ventricular function in such patients should be delayed for at least 48 hours after resuscitation (176a). In animals, the severity of postresuscitation myocardial dysfunction is related partly to the energy used for defibrillation (176b).

Pacemaker Dysfunction

Complications of pacemaker function after transthoracic shocks have been reported. Transient elevation of the pacing threshold is common immediately after transthoracic (177) and internal defibrillation shocks (178). Although these changes usually resolve within minutes, pacemaker-dependent patients may experience asystole after the shock, particularly if their chronic pacing threshold is relatively high or if their device is near end of life. After internal defibrillation shocks, the increase in pacing thresholds is more significant after monophasic than biphasic shocks, at least in patients with dedicated bipolar pacing electrodes (179,180). The incidence of pacing system malfunction after transthoracic shocks may be decreased by positioning the shocking electrodes away from the pulse generator.

Other Complications

A number of other complications can occur after cardioversion or defibrillation including painful skin burns from improper technique and placement of electrodes. A rare complication is physical trauma resulting from vigorous body movements during the delivery of the electric shock.

ACKNOWLEDGMENT

This work was supported in part by research grant no. T32HL07703 and HL42760 from the National Institutes of Health research grants.

REFERENCES

1. Prevost JL, Battelli F. Sur quelques effets des décharges électriques sur le coeur des Mammifères. *Comptes Rendus Hebdomadaires des Seances de l'academie des Sciences* 1899;129:1267–1268.
2. Zoll PM. Resuscitation of the heart in ventricular standstill by external electric stimulation. *N Engl J Med* 1952;13:768–771.
3. Zoll PM, Linenthal AJ, Gibson W, et al. Termination of ventricular fibrillation in man by externally applied electric countershock. *N Engl J Med* 1956;254:727–732.
4. Lown B, Amarasingham R, Neuman J. New method for terminating cardiac arrhythmias. *JAMA* 1962;182:548–555.
5. Hoffa M, Ludwig C. Einige neue versuche über herzebewegung. *Z Rationelle Med* 1850;9:107–144.
6. MacWilliam JA. Cardiac failure and sudden death. *BMJ* 1889;1:6–8.
7. Wiggers CJ. Studies of ventricular fibrillation caused by electric shock: cinematographic and electrocardiographic observations of the natural process in the dog's heart: its inhibition by potassium and the revival of coordinated beats by calcium. *Am Heart J* 1930;5:351–365.
8. Wiggers CJ, Wégria R. Ventricular fibrillation due to single, localized induction and condenser shocks applied during the vulnerable phase of ventricular systole. *Am J Physiol* 1940;128:500–505.
9. Wiggers CJ. The mechanism and nature of ventricular fibrillation. *Am Heart J* 1940;20:399–412.
10. Wiggers CJ. The physiologic basis for cardiac resuscitation from ventricular fibrillation: method for serial defibrillation. *Am Heart J* 1940;20:413–422.
11. Mines GR. On circulating excitations in heart muscles and their possible relation to tachycardia and fibrillation. *Proc Trans Royal Soc Can* 1914;4:43–52.
12. Huang J, Rogers JM, KenKnight BH, et al. Evolution of the organization of epicardial activation patterns during ventricular fibrillation. *J Cardiovasc Electrophysiol* 1998;9:1291–1304.
13. Moe GK, Harris AS, Wiggers CJ. Analysis of the initiation of fibrillation by electrographic studies. *Am J Physiol* 1941;134:473–492.
14. Harris AS, Rojas AG. The initiation of ventricular fibrillation due to coronary occlusion. *Exp Med Surg* 1943;1:105–122.
15. Surawicz B. Ventricular fibrillation. *Am J Cardiol* 1971;28:268–287.
16. Scherf D, Schott A. The localization of the site of origin and the spread of extrasystoles. *Extrasystoles and allied arrhythmias.* London: William Heinemann Medical Books Limited, 1973:529–559.
17. Sano T, Sawanobori T. Mechanism initiating ventricular fibrillation demonstrated in cultured ventricular muscle tissue. *Circ Res* 1970;26:201–210.
18. Moe GK, Abildskov JA. Experimental and laboratory reports. *Am Heart J* 1959;58:59–70.
19. Moe GK. On the multiple wavelet hypothesis of atrial fibrillation. *Arch Intern Pharmacodyn* 1962;140:183–187.
20. Moe GK, Rheinboldt WC, Abildskov JA. A computer model of atrial fibrillation. *Am Heart J* 1964;67:200–220.
21. Allessie MA, Bonke FIM, Schopman FJG. Circus movement in rabbit atrial muscle as a mechanism of tachycardia: III. the "leading circle" concept: a new model of circus movement in cardiac tissue without the involvement of an anatomical obstacle. *Circ Res* 1977;41:9–18.
22. Winfree AT. *When time breaks down: the three-dimensional dynamics of electrochemical waves and cardiac arrhythmias.* Princeton, NJ: Princeton University Press, 1987.
23. Jalife J, Davidenko JM, Michaels DC. A new perspective on the

mechanisms of arrhythmias and sudden cardiac death: spiral waves of excitation in heart muscle. *J Cardiovasc Electrophysiol* 1991;2:S133–S152.

24. Gray RA, Jalife J, Panfilov AV, et al. Mechanisms of cardiac fibrillation: drifting rotors as a mechanism of cardiac fibrillation. *Science* 1995;270:1222–1225.
25. Gray RA, Pertsov AM, Jalife J. Incomplete reentry and epicardial breakthrough patterns during atrial fibrillation in the sheep heart. *Circulation* 1996;94:2649–2661.
26. Gray RA, Pertsov AM, Jalife J. Spatial and temporal organization during cardiac fibrillation. *Nature* 1998;392:675–678.
27. Gray RA. Mechanisms of cardiac fibrillation: a basic scientist's report. *Cardiovasc Rev Rep* 1999;April:206–215.
28. Haïssaguerre M, Jaïs P, Shah DC, et al. Spontaneous initiation of atrial fibrillation by ectopic beats originating in the pulmonary veins. *N Engl J Med* 1998;339:659–666.
29. Davy JM, Fain ES, Dorian P, et al. The relationship between successful defibrillation and delivered energy in open-chest dogs: reappraisal of the "defibrillation threshold" concept. *Am Heart J* 1987;113:77–84.
30. Gliner BE, Murakawa Y, Thakor NV. The defibrillation success rate versus energy relationship: part I—curve fitting and the most efficient defibrillation energy. *Pace* 1990;13:326–338.
31. Schuder J. The role of an engineering oriented medical research group in developing improved methods and devices for achieving ventricular defibrillation: the University of Missouri experience. *Pace* 1993;16:95–124.
32. Ideker RE, Hillsley RE, Wharton JM. Shock strength for the implantable defibrillator: can you have too much of a good thing? *Pace* 1992;15:841–844.
33. Cates AW, Wolf PD, Hillsley RE, et al. The probability of defibrillation success and the incidence of postshock arrhythmia as a function of shock strength. *Pace* 1994;17:1208–1217.
34. Fabiato A, Coumel P, Gourgon R, et al. Le seuil de réponse synchrone des fibres myocardiques. Application è la comparaison expérimentale de l'efficacité des différentes formes de chocs électriques de défibrillation. *Arch Mal Coeur* 1967;60:527–544.
35. Ideker RE, Cooper RAS, Walcott KT. Comparison of atrial and ventricular fibrillation and defibrillation. *Pace* 1994;17:1034–1042.
36. Gray RA, Jalife J. Ventricular fibrillation and atrial fibrillation are two different beasts. *Chaos* 1998;8:65–78.
37. Garrey WE. The nature of fibrillatory contractions of the heart—its relation to tissue mass and form. *Am J Physiol* 1914;33:397–414.
38. Zipes DP, Fischer J, King RM, et al. Termination of ventricular fibrillation in dogs by depolarizing a critical amount of myocardium. *Am J Cardiol* 1975;36:37–44.
39. Chen P-S, Shibata N, Dixon EG, et al. Comparison of the defibrillation threshold and the upper limit of ventricular vulnerability. *Circulation* 1986;73:1022–1028.
40. Souza JJ, Malkin RA, Ideker RE. Comparison of upper limit of vulnerability and defibrillation probability of success curves using a nonthoracotomy lead system. *Circulation* 1995;91:1247–1252.
41. Chen P-S, Feld GK, Kriett JM, et al. Relation between upper limit of vulnerability and defibrillation threshold in humans. *Circulation* 1993;88:186–192.
42. Swerdlow CD, Ahern T, Kass RM, et al. Upper limit of vulnerability is a good estimator of shock strength associated with 90% probability of successful defibrillation in humans with transvenous implantable cardioverter-defibrillators. *J Am Coll Cardiol* 1996;27:1112–1118.
43. Swerdlow CD, Martin DJ, Kass RM, et al. The zone of vulnerability to T wave shocks in humans. *J Cardiovasc Electrophysiol* 1997;8:145–154.
44. Behrens S, Li C, Franz MR. Timing the upper limit of vulner-

45. ability is different for monophasic and biphasic shocks: implications for the determination of the defibrillation threshold. *Pace* 1997;20:2179–2187.
45. Idriss SF, Anstadt MP, Anstadt GL, et al. The effect of cardiac compression on defibrillation efficacy and the upper limit of vulnerability. *J Cardiovasc Electrophysiol* 1995;6:368–378.
46. Huang J, KenKnight BH, Walcott GP, et al. Effects of transvenous electrode polarity and waveform duration on the relationship between defibrillation threshold and upper limit of vulnerability. *Circulation* 1997;96:1351–1359.
47. Walcott GP, Walcott KT, Ideker RE. Mechanisms of defibrillation. *J Electrocardiol* 1995;28:1–6.
48. Walcott GP, Knisley SB, Zhou X, et al. On the mechanism of ventricular defibrillation. *Pace* 1997;20:422–431.
49. Chen P-S, Shibata N, Dixon EG, et al. Activation during ventricular defibrillation in open-chest dogs: evidence of complete cessation and regeneration of ventricular fibrillation after unsuccessful shocks. *J Clin Invest* 1986;77:810–823.
50. Chen P-S, Wolf PD, Claydon FJ III, et al. The potential gradient field created by epicardial defibrillation electrodes in dogs. *Circulation* 1986;74:626–636.
51. Shibata N, Chen P-S, Dixon EG, et al. Epicardial activation following unsuccessful defibrillation shocks in dogs. *Am J Physiol* 1988;255:H902–H909.
52. Chen P-S, Wolf PD, Melnick SD, et al. Comparison of activation during ventricular fibrillation and following unsuccessful defibrillation shocks in open chest dogs. *Circ Res* 1990;66:1544–1560.
53. Zhou X, Daubert JP, Wolf PD, et al. Epicardial mapping of ventricular defibrillation with monophasic and biphasic shocks in dogs. *Circ Res* 1993;72:145–160.
54. Cha Y-M, Peters BB, Chen P-S. The effects of lidocaine on the vulnerable period during ventricular fibrillation. *J Cardiovasc Electrophysiol* 1994;5:571–580.
55. Usui M, Callihan RL, Walker RG, et al. Epicardial shock mapping following monophasic and biphasic shocks of equal voltage with an endocardial lead system. *J Cardiovasc Electrophysiol* 1996;7:322–334.
56. Tang ASL, Wolf PD, Claydon FJ, et al. Measurement of defibrillation shock potential distributions and activation sequences of the heart in three-dimensions. *Proc IEEE* 1988;76:1176–1186.
57. Knisley SB, Smith WM, Ideker RE. Effect of field stimulation on cellular repolarization in rabbit myocardium: Implications for reentry induction. *Circ Res* 1992;70:707–715.
58. Frazier DW, Wolf PD, Wharton JM, et al. Stimulus-induced critical point: Mechanism for electrical initiation of reentry in normal canine myocardium. *J Clin Invest* 1989;83:1039–1052.
59. Tovar OH, Jones JL. Relationship between "extension of refractoriness" and probability of successful defibrillation. *Am J Physiol* 1997;272:H1011–H1019.
60. Dillon SM, Kwaku KF. Progressive depolarization: a unified hypothesis for defibrillation and fibrillation induction by shocks. *J Cardiovasc Electrophysiol* 1998;9:529–552.
61. Sweeney RJ, Gill RM, Reid PR. Refractory interval after transcardiac shocks during ventricular fibrillation. *Circulation* 1996;94:2947–2952.
62. Efimov IR, Cheng Y, Van Wagoner DR, et al. Virtual electrode-induced phase singularity: a basic mechanism of defibrillation failure. *Circ Res* 1998;82:918–925.
63. Tacker WA Jr, Geddes LA. *Electrical defibrillation.* Boca Raton, FL: CRC Press, 1980.
64. Edmark KW, Thomas G, Jones TW. DC pulse defibrillation. *J Thorac Cardiovasc Surg* 1966;3:326–333.
65. Mackay RS, Leeds SE. Physiological effects of condenser discharges with application to tissue stimulation and ventricular defibrillation. *J Appl Physiol* 1953;6:67–75.
66. Walcott GP, Melnick SB, Chapman FW, et al. Relative efficacy

of monophasic and biphasic waveforms for transthoracic defibrillation after short and long durations of ventricular fibrillation. *Circulation* 1998;98:2210–2215.

67. Bardy GH, Marchlinski FE, Sharma AD, et al. Multicenter comparison of truncated biphasic shocks and standard damped sine wave monophasic shocks for transthoracic ventricular defibrillation. Transthoracic Investigators. *Circulation* 1996;94:2507–2514.

68. Irnich W. Optimal truncation of defibrillation pulses. *Pace* 1995;18:673–688.

69. Dixon EG, Tang ASL, Wolf PD, et al. Improved defibrillation thresholds with large contoured epicardial electrodes and biphasic waveforms. *Circulation* 1987;76:1176–1184.

70. Feeser SA, Tang ASL, Kavanagh KM, et al. Strength-duration and probability of success curves for defibrillation with biphasic waveforms. *Circulation* 1990;82:2128–2141.

71. Chapman PD, Wetherbee JN, Vetter JW, et al. Strength-duration curves of fixed pulse width variable tilt truncated exponential waveforms for nonthoracotomy internal defibrillation in dogs. *Pace* 1988;11:1045–1050.

72. Bardy GH, Ivey TD, Allen MD, et al. A prospective randomized evaluation of biphasic versus monophasic waveform pulses on defibrillation efficacy in humans. *J Am Coll Cardiol* 1989;14:728–733.

73. Kavanagh KM, Tang ASL, Rollins DL, et al. Comparison of the internal defibrillation thresholds for monophasic and double and single capacitor biphasic waveforms. *J Am Coll Cardiol* 1989;14:1343–1349.

74. Saksena S, An H, Mehra R, et al. Prospective comparison of biphasic and monophasic shocks for implantable cardioverter-defibrillators using endocardial leads. *Am J Cardiol* 1992;70:304–310.

75. Cooper RAS, Alferness CA, Smith WM, Ideker RE. Internal cardioversion of atrial fibrillation in sheep. *Circulation* 1993;87:1673–1686.

76. Walcott GP, Walcott KT, Knisley SB, et al. Mechanisms of defibrillation for monophasic and biphasic waveforms. *Pace* 1994;17:478–498.

77. Mouchawar GA, Wolsleger WK, Doan PD, et al. Does an SVC electrode further reduce DFT in a hot-can ICD system? *Pace* 1997;20:163–167.

78. Bardy GH, Johnson G, Poole JE, et al. A simplified, single-lead unipolar transvenous cardioversion-defibrillation system. *Circulation* 1993;88:543–547.

79. Lévy S, Lauribe P, Dolla E, et al. A randomized comparison of external and internal cardioversion of chronic atrial fibrillation. *Circulation* 1992;86:1415–1420.

80. Murgatroyd FD, Slade AK, Sopher SM, et al. Efficacy and tolerability of transvenous low energy cardioversion of paroxysmal atrial fibrillation in humans. *J Am Coll Cardiol* 1995;25:1347–1353.

81. Alt E, Schmitt C, Ammer R, et al. Effect of electrode position on outcome of low-energy intracardiac cardioversion of atrial fibrillation. *Am J Cardiol* 1997;79:621–625.

82. Lévy S, Ricard P, Lau C, et al. Multicenter low energy Transvenous Atrial Defibrillation (XAD) trial. *J Am Coll Cardiol* 1997;29:750–755.

83. Usui M, Walcott GP, Strickberger SA, et al. Effects of polarity for monophasic and biphasic shocks on defibrillation efficacy with an endocardial system. *Pace* 1996;19:65–71.

84. Thakur R, Souza J, Chapman P, et al. Electrode polarity is an important determinant of defibrillation efficacy using a nonthoracotomy system. *Pace* 1994;17:919–923.

85. Strickberger SA, Hummel JD, Horwood LE, et al. Effect of shock polarity on ventricular defibrillation threshold using a transvenous lead system. *J Am Coll Cardiol* 1994;24:1069–1072.

86. Bardy GH, Ivey TD, Allen MD, et al. Evaluation of electrode polarity on defibrillation efficacy. *Am J Cardiol* 1989;63:433–437.

87. Tang W, Weil MH, Sun S, et al. Epinephrine increases the severity of postresuscitation myocardial dysfunction. *Circulation* 1995;92:3089–3093.

88. Troup P, Wetherbee JN, Chapman PD, et al. Does electrode polarity affect defibrillation efficacy? *Pace* 1990;13:528.

89. Weaver WD, Martin JS, Wirkus MJ, et al. Influence of external defibrillator electrode polarity on cardiac resuscitation. *Pace* 1993;16:285–291.

90. Chapman PD, Wetherbee JN, Vetter JW, et al. Comparison of monophasic, biphasic, and triphasic truncated pulses for nonthoracotomy internal defibrillation. *J Am Coll Cardiol* 1988;11:57A(abst).

91. Manz M, Jung W, Wolpert C, et al. Can triphasic shock waveforms improve ICD therapy in man? *Circulation* 1993;88:I593(abst).

92. Jung W, Manz M, Moosdorf R, et al. Comparative defibrillation efficacy of biphasic and triphasic waveforms. *New Trends Arrhyth* 1993;9:765.

93. Huang J, KenKnight BH, Rollins DL, et al. Defibrillation with triphasic waveforms. *Pace* 1997;20:1056(abst).

94. Huang J, KenKnight BH, Walcott GP, et al. Effect of electrode polarity on internal defibrillation with monophasic and biphasic waveforms using an endocardial lead system. *J Cardiovasc Electrophysiol* 1997;8:161–171.

95. Yamanouchi Y, Brewer JE, Olson KF, et al. Fully discharging phases. A new approach to biphasic waveforms for external defibrillation. *Circulation* 1999;100:826–831.

96. Hsu W, Lin Y, Lang DJ, et al. Improved internal defibrillation success with shocks timed to the morphology electrogram. *Circulation* 1998;98:808–812.

97. Strobel JS, Kenknight BH, Rollins DL, et al. The effects of ventricular fibrillation duration and site of initiation on the defibrillation threshold during early ventricular fibrillation. *J Am Coll Cardiol* 1998;32:521–527.

98. Kerber RE, Robertson CE. Transthoracic defibrillation. In: Paradis NA, Halperin HR, Nowak RM, eds. *Cardiac arrest: the science and practice of resuscitation medicine.* Baltimore, MD: Williams & Wilkins, 1996:370–381.

99. Pagan-Carlo LA, Spencer KT, Robertson CE, et al. Transthoracic defibrillation: importance of avoiding electrode placement directly on the female breast. *J Am Coll Cardiol* 1996;27:449–452.

100. Kerber RE, Jensen SR, Grayzel J, et al. Elective cardioversion: influence of paddle-electrode location and size on success rates and energy requirements. *N Engl J Med* 1981;305:658–662.

101. Lerman BB, Deale OC. Relation between transcardiac and transthoracic current during defibrillation in humans. *Circ Res* 1990;67:1420–1426.

102. Deale OC, Lerman BB. Intrathoracic current flow during transthoracic defibrillation in dogs: transcardiac current fraction. *Circ Res* 1990;67:1405–1419.

103. Kerber RE, Martins JB, Kienzle MG, et al. Energy, current, and success in defibrillation and cardioversion: clinical studies using an automated impedance-based method of energy adjustment. *Circulation* 1988;77:1038–1046.

104. Ewy GA, Horan WJ. Effectiveness of direct current defibrillation: role of paddle electrode size: II. *Am Heart J* 1977;93:674–675.

105. Kerber WJ, Grayzel J, Hoyt R, et al. Transthoracic resistance in human defibrillation: influence of body weight, chest size serial shocks, paddle size and paddle contact pressure. *Circulation* 1981;3:676–682.

106. Atkins DL. Pediatric defibrillation: Optimal techniques. In: Tacker WA Jr, ed. *Defibrillation of the heart: ICDs, AEDs, and manual.* St. Louis: Mosby–Year Book, 1994:169–181.

107. Cohen TJ, Noubani H, Goldner BG, et al. Active compression-decompression defibrillation provides effective defibrillation during cardiopulmonary resuscitation. *Am Heart J* 1995;130: 186–187.

108. Cohen TJ, Ibrahim B, Denier D, et al. Active compression cardioversion for refractory atrial fibrillation. *Am J Cardiol* 1997; 80:354–355.

109. Geddes LA, Tacker WA Jr, Cabler P, et al. The decrease in transthoracic impedance during successive ventricular defibrillation trials. *Med Instrum* 1975;4:179–180.

110. Dahl CF, Ewy GA, Thomas ED. Transthoracic impedance to direct current discharge—effect of repeated countershocks. *Med Instrum* 1976;3:151–154.

111. Sirna SJ, Kieso RA, Fox-Eastham KJ, et al. Mechanisms responsible for decline in transthoracic impedance to DC shocks. *Am J Physiol* 1989;257:H1180–H1183.

112. Ewy GA. Optimal technique for electrical cardioversion of atrial fibrillation. *Circulation* 1992;86:1645–1647.

113. Ewy GA, Hellman DA, McClung S, et al. Influence of ventilation phase on transthoracic impedance and defibrillation effectiveness. *Crit Care Med* 1980;8:164–166.

114. Kerber RE, Martins JB, Kelly KJ, et al. Self-adhesive preapplied electrode pads for defibrillation and cardioversion. *J Am Coll Cardiol* 1984;3:815–820.

115. Smith TW, Zimetbaum PJ, Korley V, et al. Adhesive pad electrodes versus hand-held electrodes for elective cardioversion of atrial fibrillation. *Pace* 1999;22:826(abst).

116. Kloeck W, Cummins RO, Chamberlain D, et al. The universal advanced life support algorithm: an advisory statement from the Advanced Life Support Working Group of the International Liaison Committee on Resuscitation. *Circulation* 1997;95: 2180–2182.

117. Kleiger R, Lown B. Cardioversion and digitalis. II. Clinical studies. *Circulation* 1966;33:878–887.

118. Mann DL, Maisel AS, Atwood JE, et al. Absence of cardioversion-induced ventricular arrhythmias in patients with therapeutic digoxin levels. *J Am Coll Cardiol* 1985;5:882–890.

119. Eisenberg MS, Copass MK, Hallstrom AP, et al. Treatment of out-of-hospital cardiac arrests with rapid defibrillation by emergency medical technicians. *N Engl J Med* 1980;302:1379–1383.

120. Stults KR, Brown DD, Schug VL, et al. Prehospital defibrillation performed by emergency medical technicians in rural communities. *N Engl J Med* 1984;310:219–223.

121. Weaver WD, Copass MK, Bufi D, et al. Improved neurologic recovery and survival after early defibrillation. *Circulation* 1984; 69:943–948.

122. Kloeck W, Cummins RO, Chamberlain D, et al. Early defibrillation: an advisory statement from the Advanced Life Support Working Group of the International Liaison Committee on Resuscitation. *Circulation* 1997;95:2183–2184.

123. Valenzuela TD, Roe DJ, Cretin S, et al. Estimating effectiveness of cardiac arrest intervention: a logistic regression survival model. *Circulation* 1997;96:3308–3313.

124. Cummins RO, Sanders A, Mancini E, et al. In-hospital resuscitation: a statement for healthcare professionals from the American Heart Association Emergency Cardiac Care Committee and the Advanced Cardiac Life Support, Basic Life Support, Pediatric Resuscitation, and Program Administration Subcommittees. *Circulation* 1997;95:2211–2212.

125. Gascho JA, Crampton RS, Cherwek ML, et al. Determinants of ventricular defibrillation in adults. *Circulation* 1979;60:231–240.

126. Hallstrom A, Cobb L, Yu BH. Influence of comorbidity on the outcome of patients treated for out-of-hospital ventricular fibrillation. *Circulation* 1996;93:2019–2022.

127. Epstein AE, Powell J, Yao Q, et al. In-hospital versus out-of-hospital presentation of life-threatening ventricular arrhythmias

128. Dalzell GW, Adgey AA. Determinants of successful transthoracic defibrillation and outcome in ventricular fibrillation. *Br Heart J* 1991;65:311–316.

129. Weaver WD, Cobb LA, Copass MK, et al. Ventricular defibrillation—a comparative trial using 175-J and 320-J shocks. *N Engl J Med* 1982;307:1101–1106.

130. Kerber RE, Jensen SR, Gascho JA, et al. Determinants of defibrillation: prospective analysis of 183 patients. *Am J Cardiol* 1983;52:739–745.

131. Bardy GH, Gliner BE, Kudenchuk PJ, et al. Truncated biphasic pulses for transthoracic defibrillation. *Circulation* 1995;91: 1768–1774.

132. Nichol G, Hallstrom AP, Kerber R, et al. American Heart Association report on the second public access defibrillation conference, April 17–19, 1997. *Circulation* 1998;97:1309–1314.

133. Pennington JE, Taylor J, Lown B. Chest thump for reverting ventricular tachycardia. *N Engl J Med* 1970;283:1192–1195.

134. Caldwell G, Millar G, Quinn E, et al. Simple mechanical methods for cardioversion: defence of the precordial thump and cough version. *BMJ* 1985;291:627–630.

135. Sclarovsky S, Kracoff O, Arditi A, et al. Ventricular tachycardia "pleomorphism" induced by chest thump. *Chest* 1982;81:97–98.

136. Krijne R. Rate acceleration of ventricular tachycardia after a precordial chest thump. *Am J Cardiol* 1984;53:964–965.

137. The AVID Investigators. A comparison of antiarrhythmic-drug therapy with implantable defibrillators in patients resuscitated from near-fatal ventricular arrhythmias. *N Engl J Med* 1997; 337:1576–1583.

138. Moss AJ, Hill WJ, Cannom DS, et al. Improved survival with an implanted defibrillator in patients with coronary disease at high risk for ventricular arrhythmia. *N Engl J Med* 1996;335: 1933–1940.

139. Prystowsky EN, Benson DW Jr, Fuster V, et al. Management of patients with atrial fibrillation. A statement for healthcare professionals. From the Subcommittee on Electrocardiography and Electrophysiology, American Heart Association. *Circulation* 1996;93:1262–1277.

140. The Planning and Steering Committees of the AFFIRM Study for the NHLBI AFFIRM Investigators. Atrial fibrillation follow-up investigation of rhythm management—the AFFIRM Study design. *Am J Cardiol* 1997;79:1198–1202

141. Steering and Publications Committees of the ACUTE Study. Design of a clinical trial for the assessment of cardioversion using transesophageal echocardiography (the ACUTE Multicenter Study). *Am J Cardiol* 1998;81:877–883.

142. Fatkin D, Kuchar DL, Thorburn CW, et al. Transesophageal echocardiography before and during direct current cardioversion of atrial fibrillation: evidence for "atrial stunning" as a mechanism of thromboembolic complications. *J Am Coll Cardiol* 1994;23:307–316.

143. Harjai KJ, Mobarek SK, Cheirif J, et al. Clinical variables affecting recovery of left atrial mechanical function after cardioversion from atrial fibrillation. *J Am Coll Cardiol* 1997;30:481–486.

144. Berger M, Schweitzer P. Timing of thromboembolic events after electrical cardioversion of atrial fibrillation or flutter: a retrospective analysis. *Am J Cardiol* 1998;82:1545–1547.

145. Manning WJ, Silverman DI, Katz SA, et al. Impaired left atrial mechanical function after cardioversion: relation to the duration of atrial fibrillation. *J Am Coll Cardiol* 1994;23: 1535–1540.

146. Maciera-Coelho E. Left atrial mechanical function after cardioversion. *Am J Cardiol* 1996;77:326.

147. Lown B. Electrical reversion of cardiac arrhythmias. *Br Heart J* 1967;29:469–489.

148. Joglar JA, Hamdan MH, Zagrodzky JD, et al. Initial energy for external cardioversion of atrial fibrillation. *Pace* 1999;22:898 (abst).

149. Bjerragaard P, El-Shafei A, Janosic D, et al. Double external direct-current shocks for refractory atrial fibrillation. *Am J Cardiol* 1999;83:972–974.

150. DeLurgio DB, Hanson KJ, Mera F, et al. Simultaneous transthoracic shocks from two defibrillators for conversion of refractory atrial fibrillation. *Circulation* 1998:98:I425(abst).

150a. Mittal S, Ayati S, Stein KM, et al. Transthoracic cardioversion of atrial fibrillation. Comparison of rectilinear versus damped sine wave monophasic shocks. *Circulation* 2000;101:1282.

151. Oral H, Souza JJ, Michaud GF, et al. Facilitating transthoracic cardioversion of atrial fibrillation with ibutilide pretreatment. *N Engl J Med* 1999;340:1849–1854.

152. Lanzarotti CJ, Olshansky B. Thromboembolism in chronic atrial flutter: is the risk underestimated? *J Am Coll Cardiol* 1997; 30:1506–1511.

153. Seidl K, Hauer B, Schwick NG, et al. Risk of thromboembolic events in patients with atrial flutter. *Am J Cardiol* 1998;82: 580–583.

154. Welch PJ, Afridi I, Joglar JA, et al. Effect of radiofrequency ablation on atrial mechanical function in patients with atrial flutter. *Am J Cardiol* 1999;84:420–425.

155. Jordaens L, Missault L, Germonpré E, et al. Delayed restoration of atrial function after conversion of atrial flutter by pacing or electrical cardioversion. *Am J Cardiol* 1993;71:63–67.

156. Zipes DP, Jackman WM, Heger JJ, et al. Clinical transvenous cardioversion of recurrent life-threatening ventricular tachyarrhythmias: low energy synchronized cardioversion of ventricular tachycardia and termination of ventricular fibrillation in patients using a catheter electrode. *Am Heart J* 1982;103:789–794.

157. Cohen TJ, Scheinman MM, Pullen BT, et al. Emergency intracardiac defibrillation for refractory ventricular fibrillation during routine electrophysiologic study. *J Am Coll Cardiol* 1991;18: 1280–1284.

158. Cooper RAS, Johnson EE, Wharton M. Internal atrial defibrillation in humans. Improved efficacy of biphasic waveforms and the importance of phase duration. *Circulation* 1997;95: 1487–1496.

159. Boriani G, Biffi M, Capucci A, et al. Favorable effects of flecainide in transvenous internal cardioversion of atrial fibrillation. *J Am Coll Cardiol* 1999;33:333–341.

160. Wellens HJ, Lau CP, Luderitz B, et al. Atrioverter: an implantable device for the treatment of atrial fibrillation. *Circulation* 1998;98:1651–1656.

161. Josephson ME. New approaches to the management of atrial fibrillation. The role of the atrial defibrillator. *Circulation* 1998; 98:1594–1596.

162. Harris PD, Malm JR, Bowman FO, et al. Epicardial pacing to control arrhythmias following cardiac surgery. *Circulation* 1968; 37:II178–II183.

163. Waldo AL, MacLean WA, Cooper TB, et al. Use of temporarily placed epicardial atrial wire electrodes for the diagnosis and treatment of cardiac arrhythmias following open-heart surgery. *J Thorac Cardiovasc Surg* 1978;76:500–505.

164. Liebold A, Wahba A, Birnbaum DE. Low-energy cardioversion with epicardial wire electrodes: new treatment of atrial fibrillation after open heart surgery. *Circulation* 1998;98:883–886.

165. Eysmann SB, Marchlinski FE, Buxton AE, et al. Electrocardiographic changes after cardioversion of ventricular arrhythmias. *Circulation* 1986;73:73–81.

166. Waldecker B, Brugada P, Zehender M, et al. Dysrhythmias after direct-current cardioversion. *Am J Cardiol* 1986;57:120–123.

167. Mower MM, Mirowski M, Spear JF, et al. Patterns of ventricular activity during catheter defibrillation. *Circulation* 1974;49: 858–861.

168. Zivin A, Souza J, Pelosi F, et al. Relationship between shock energy and postdefibrillation ventricular arrhythmias in patients with implantable defibrillators. *J Cardiovasc Electrophysiol* 1999; 10:370–377.

169. Zipes DP. Electrical therapy of cardiac arrhythmias. In: Braunwald E, ed. *Heart disease: a textbook of cardiovascular medicine,* 5th ed. Philadelphia: WB Saunders, 1997:619–639.

170. Osswald S, Roelke M, O'Nunain, et al. Electrocardiographic pseudo-infarct patterns after implantation of cardioverter-defibrillators. *Am Heart J* 1995;129:265–272.

171. Black IW, Fatkin D, Sagar KB, et al. Exclusion of atrial thrombus by transesophageal echocardiography does not preclude embolism after cardioversion of atrial fibrillation. A multicenter study. *Circulation* 1994;89:2509–2513.

172. Lindsay J Jr. Pulmonary edema following cardioversion. *Am Heart J* 1967;74:434–435.

173. Resnekov L, McDonald L. Complications in 220 patients with cardiac dysrhythmias treated by phased direct current shock, and indications for electroconversion. *Br Heart J* 1967;29:926–936.

174. Tokano T, Bach D, Chang J, et al. Effect of ventricular shock strength on cardiac hemodynamics. *J Cardiovasc Electrophysiol* 1998;9:791–797.

175. Joglar JA, Kessler DJ, Welch PJ, et al. Effects of repeated electrical defibrillations on cardiac troponin I levels. *Am J Cardiol* 1999;83:270–272.

176. Singer I, Hutchins GM, Mirowski M, et al. Pathologic findings related to the lead system and repeated defibrillations in patients with the automatic implantable cardioverter-defibrillator. *J Am Coll Cardiol* 1987;10:382–388.

176a. Kern KB, Hilwig RW, Rhee KH, et al. Myocardial dysfunction following resuscitation from cardiac arrest: an example of global myocardial stunning. *J Am Coll Cardiol* 1996; 28:232.

176b. Xie J, Weil MH, Sun S, et al. High-energy defibrillation increases the severity of postresuscitation myocardial dysfunction. *Circulation* 1997;96:683.

177. Epstein AE, Kay GN, Plumb VJ, et al. Gross and microscopic pathological changes associated with nonthoracotomy implantable defibrillator leads. *Circulation* 1998;98:1517–1524.

178. Altamura G, Bianconi L, Bianco FL, et al. Transthoracic DC shock may represent a serious hazard in pacemaker dependent patients. *Pace* 1995;18:194–198.

179. Yee R, Jones DL, Jarvis E, et al. Changes in pacing threshold and R wave amplitude after transvenous catheter countershock. *J Am Coll Cardiol* 1984;4:543–549.

180. Kudenchuk PJ, Poole JE, Dolack GL, et al. Prospective evaluation of the effect of biphasic waveform defibrillation on ventricular pacing thresholds. *J Cardiovasc Electrophysiol* 1997;8:485–495.

10

CARDIAC PACEMAKERS

AMIT SHANKER
SANJEEV SAKSENA

Modern pacemaker technology has improved the duration and quality of life for individuals with bradyarrhythmias. Since the introduction of the first temporary transcutaneous pacemaker in 1952, the use of temporary and permanent cardiac pacemakers markedly expanded after 1958, when temporary transvenous pacing and permanent implantation techniques were developed. Indications for cardiac pacing have expanded. Once relegated as a standby device for bradycardic patients requiring rate support, pacemakers are used for the treatment of hemodynamic abnormalities, conduction system defects, and tachyarrhythmias. Cardiac pacemaker function has become more complex, with physiologic electrical stimulation attempting to meet the metabolic and circulatory demands of the body.

This chapter reviews the principles and practice of cardiac pacing. A summary of the indications and assessment of pacemaker function and malfunction is included.

PRINCIPLES AND FUNCTIONAL ELEMENTS OF PULSE GENERATORS AND LEADS FOR CARDIAC PACING

A thorough understanding of applied scientific and engineering principles is essential in the management of technical problems that may arise in cardiac pacing (1). A cardiac pacemaker system consists of a pulse generator that is connected to the heart by means of catheter electrodes, referred to as *leads*. The titanium or stainless steel case of the pulse generator contains the power supply and the hardware and software required for sensing the natural cardiac rhythm and initiating stimulated cardiac depolarizations. The transceiver circuitry of the pulse generator allows for noninvasive external interrogation and programming of the pacemaker system. The catheter electrodes provide a conduit for bidi-

rectional exchange of current to and from the pulse generator and the myocardium.

Pulse Generator

A conventional, single-chamber pacemaker pulse generator consists of several important functional elements, including the power source, output circuit, sensing circuit, timing circuit, transceiver circuit, and the microprocessor.

The power source is a reservoir of electric charge performing two functions. It provides power to perform essential functions using the electric circuits in the pulse generator, and it delivers current to the myocardial tissue to stimulate cardiac depolarization. Lithium-iodine batteries are typically used with an estimated survival of approximately 10 to 12 years (with average current drain). Device sophistication and activation of these features increase current drain and shorten generator longevity. Most pulse generators internally monitor battery voltage and impedance to provide advance warning when the battery approaches its end of life.

An adequate stimulus current density (i.e., current per unit of cross-sectional area) and stimulus duration by the output circuit of the pulse generator are required to achieve threshold for myocardial stimulation (i.e., *capture*) to ensure impulse propagation as seen with spontaneous cardiac depolarizations. This is accomplished by applying the voltage across the lead electrodes in contact with the endocardium. Electrical configurations of leads vary with the number of catheter electrodes in the circuit (e.g., unipolar, bipolar, tripolar).

Most output circuits of pulse generators perform voltage-source pacing. The stimulus voltage and stimulus current decay during the stimulus as the charged capacitor discharges through the cardiac impedance. If current leaks develop in the insulation of the lead, the coil, or both, the voltage and current decay more rapidly. If the only parameter monitored during patient follow-up is the peak amplitude of the stimulus, the existence of an insulation failure may go unnoticed before capture is lost. A few pulse generators still perform

A. Shanker: Department of Medicine, Robert Wood Johnson School of Medicine, New Brunswick, New Jersey 08903.
S. Saksena: Cardiovascular Institute of the Atlantic Health System, Passaic, New Jersey 07055.

current-source pacing. In this form of pacing, the current is constant for the duration of the stimulus through the combination of the coupling capacitor and the myocardial impedance. In the event of insulation leakage, the peak stimulus voltage and current are significantly reduced, aiding in detection of battery depletion at follow-up.

The sensing circuit in the pulse generator detects spontaneous cardiac depolarizations. A conventional sensing circuit includes a sensing amplifier, a bandpass filter, and the threshold comparator. These functional elements have been implemented to prevent the pulse generator from interpreting extraneous electrical signals as spontaneous cardiac depolarizations. The sensing amplifier magnifies the voltage difference that appears across the electrodes and avoids undue corruption by the low-voltage electrical noise. To avoid having the amplifier affected by an anticipated high-amplitude input signal (e.g., electrical stimulus delivered in the atrium by a dual-chamber pacemaker as "seen" by the ventricular chamber sensing circuit), the sense amplifier can be deliberately disabled for a short period, referred to as the *blanking period.*

A bandpass filter screens and isolates the components of the amplified input signal that clearly signify cardiac depolarization. The bandpass filter rejects relatively slow-moving signal components and very rapidly moving signal components, such as skeletal muscle myopotentials from the chest wall and ambient electrical noise. The bandpass filter isolates components of rapid deflection with spontaneous cardiac depolarizations. An intrinsic or rapid deflection (duration of about 10 ms) with depolarization and subsequent slow deflection with repolarization are initially demonstrated in recently injured myocardium. The amplitude of the slow deflection decreases as the electrode-tissue interface matures with time.

The threshold comparator performs the actual detection of the signal. By comparing the instantaneous voltage at the filtered output with a fixed reference voltage (i.e., *sensing threshold*), the comparator produces a logic signal (i.e., *voltage pulse*). This logic signal is commonly used to reset the pacemaker's escape timing. A minimum interval between sensed events is established during which a logic signal produced by a sensed event is ignored by the timing circuitry. This is referred to as the *refractory period.*

With the three components of the sensing circuit, the pulse generator may be adjusted to increase or decrease its sensitivity to spontaneous depolarizations. An adjustment in the sensitivity of the pulse generator entails changing of the gain of the sensing amplifier with the threshold-detection reference voltage being held constant.

Certain basic intervals are tracked by the pulse generator's electronic timing circuitry. In single-chamber atrial and ventricular pacing, the spontaneous AA (i.e., successive atrial depolarizations) and VV (i.e., successive ventricular depolarization) intervals between successive atrial and ventricular stimuli are tracked. In dual-chamber pacing, the atrioventricular (AV) and ventriculoatrial interstimulus intervals are also tracked. These signals can be used to trigger the output circuit for anticipated depolarization or to control the blanking and refractory periods of the sensing circuit.

A transceiver circuit permits bidirectional communication between a pacemaker programming device and the pulse generator using pulsed radiofrequency signals or magnetic coupling, allowing noninvasive reprogramming of the pacemaker after implantation. With interrogation of the pulse generator, the electrophysiologist may also be able to obtain real-time intracardiac electrograms, marker channels reflecting logic pulses from cardiac chambers individually, lead and battery impedance, rate histograms of spontaneous cardiac activity, and delivered stimulus pulse energy parameters. Microprocessor-based functions also provide the capability for data gathering, storage, analysis, and display. The microprocessor allows for evaluation of device and cardiac function as detected by the pacemaker. Pacemaker clinic visits are devoted to review and response to such accumulated information in the period between visits.

Lead Electrode

The pacemaker lead is the connecting link between the myocardium and the pulse generator. It consists of an electrode (i.e., cathodal tip electrode only in unipolar leads and an anodal ring electrode in bipolar leads), a conductor coil, a distal lead anchoring mechanism, and a proximal terminal pin for connection with the pulse generator. The entire lead is encased in insulating material to ensure efficient transfer of energy from the pulse generator to the myocardium. The electrical configuration of a lead may be unipolar or bipolar. In both configurations, the cathode is the electrode tip. In a unipolar configuration, the anode is the metal housing of the pulse generator. In a bipolar configuration, the anode is an indifferent ring electrode proximal to the cathode. Among the important differences in these lead configurations is that of sensing, which is discussed later. With the arrival of coaxial conductors, bipolar leads are nearly the same diameter as unipolar leads.

The minimal amount of energy required for consistent depolarization to occur is called the *stimulation threshold.* This threshold depends on the mean stimulus amplitude (voltage or current) and the stimulus duration as demonstrated by the strength-duration curve for myocardial stimulation. Shortening the duration of the stimulus increases the required voltage or current threshold. In the initial steep portion of the strength-duration curve, a minor change in the pulse duration can have a major impact on the required stimulation threshold.

The stimulation threshold is affected by intrinsic and extrinsic factors. The endocardial stimulation threshold changes in a variety of physiologic states. Sleeping and eating typically increase the threshold, whereas exercise and postural changes decrease the threshold. These events mediate their effects through changes in sympathetic tone. Hyperglycemia, acidosis, and hyperkalemia may increase the required stimulation threshold. Endocrinologic abnormalities, such as hypothyroidism, increase threshold, and exogenous adrenocortical hormones and endogenous catecholamines lower the threshold. Use of antiarrhythmic medications can affect pacing thresholds. Type I and some type III drugs such as amiodarone that block cardiac sodium channels can raise the threshold by inhibiting the excitability of cardiac tissue.

The pathophysiologic mechanisms of inflammation explain the characteristic alterations seen in the endomyocardial stimulation threshold after lead implantation. Immediately after implantation, injury alters membrane permeability to sodium and potassium transfer, resulting in a diminished stimulation threshold. In the subacute period, inflammation, fibrin deposition, and capsule formation contribute to an increase in threshold. The eventual reduction in the inflammatory response by the fourth week results in the diminution of the stimulation threshold. Steroid-eluting electrodes reduce the degree of the inflammatory response, attenuating the bell-shaped rise and fall seen in threshold maturation with conventional leads.

To optimize pacemaker longevity, routine use of low-voltage stimulation is recommended. Electrode design is used to accomplish this goal. Electrodes' efficiency depends on metallurgic composition, macrostructure, and microstructure. They use platinum, platinum-iridium, activated carbon, titanium, or Elgiloy, which is an alloy of cobalt, iron, chromium, molybdenum, nickel, and manganese. The small surface area reduces the energy required for stimulation. Current density is maximal at the points of greatest curvature of an electrode. However, the small surface area may compromise sensing because of a higher source impedance. Newer lead tips are more porous to maximize the sensing surface area without affecting stimulation energy. Elution of dexamethasone from the porous lead electrode tip significantly reduces early postoperative and chronic peak stimulation thresholds. This effectively lowers the energy requirements from the pulse generator.

The incorporation of active- or passive-fixation devices has reduced the incidence of lead dislodgment. Active-fixation devices employ the use of springs, deployable radiating pins or needles, or endocardial claws or screws. Endocardial screw-in electrodes have received considerable attention because of their proven efficacy in patients with dilated ventricles, difficult atrial placements, and atrial appendectomies. Passive-fixation devices are designed to permit tissue ingrowth for improved anchoring. Tine leads have become the most commonly used passive-fixation device.

PACEMAKER CODES

Numerous coding systems have been developed to define the operational function of antiarrhythmic devices (2,3). The latest revision requires four positions to incorporate newer functions and a fifth position for antitachycardia devices (Table 10-1). Fewer than four positions is considered incomplete. The use of the letter O (denoting the absence of any such function) helps to ensure that each letter is in its proper position:

Position I designates the chambers paced (A, atrium; V, ventricle; D, dual).
Position II designates the chambers sensed (A, atrium; V, ventricle; D, dual).
Position III designates the response to a sensed signal (I, inhibited; T, triggered; D, dual).
Position IV describes the degree of programmability and the presence or absence of a rate modulation mechanism (M, multiprogrammable; C, communicating; R, rate response; O, no pacemaker settings can be altered).
Position V indicates the presence of antitachycardia functions by means of pacing modalities or shocking to terminate the tachyarrhythmia.

TABLE 10-1. NASPE/BPEG PACEMAKER CODE

Position I	Position II	Position III	Position IV	Position V
Chamber Paced	Chamber Sensed	Response to Sensing	Programmability, Rate Modulation	Antitachyarrhythmia Functions
O, none	O, none	O, none	O, none	O, none
A, atrium	A, atrium	T, triggered	P, simple programmable	P, Pacing (antitachyarrhythmia)
V, ventricle	V, ventricle	I, inhibited	M, multiprogrammable	S, shock
D, dual (A + V)[a]	D, dual (A + V)[a]	D, dual (D + I)[b]	C, communicating (telemetry)	D, dual (P + S)[c]
S, single chamber[d]	S, single chamber[d]		R, Rate modulation	

NASPE/BPEG, North American Society for Pacing and Electrophysiology/British Pacing and Electrophysiology Group.
[a]Atrial and ventricular.
[b]Dual (atrial/ventricular) and inhibited.
[c]Pacing and shock.
[d]Manufacturer's designation only.

The increasing complexity of dual-chamber devices has prompted the development of the North American Society of Pacing and Electrophysiology (NASPE) code (3). This code more specifically addresses the complexities and enhances the description of pacemaker function in the management of tachyarrhythmias and bradyarrhythmias. Because of the code's degree of detail, its practical clinical use is limited and is relegated as an adjunct to the NASPE/British Pacing and Electrophysiology Group Generic Code (NBG code).

TEMPORARY CARDIAC PACING

There are various methods for temporary cardiac pacing, including with an intracardiac electrode, external electrodes, an esophageal electrode, or epicardial electrodes (4–6). A number of pacing modes are available for temporary use; pacing can be atrial (AOO, AAI), ventricular (VVI, VOO), or dual chamber (DDI, DDD, VDD, or DVI). Pacing can be asynchronous or demand although with dual-chamber pacing, atrial sensing can trigger ventricular pacing.

Temporary Intracardiac Pacing

Temporary intracardiac pacing is performed by temporary transvenous electrode catheter insertion through a jugular or subclavian venous access; these approaches are preferred for catheter electrode introduction because they provide optimal electrode stability and a reduced likelihood of complications. Although antecubital and femoral venous cannulation may be used, there is significant likelihood of infection and phlebitis by these routes. To ensure appropriate positioning in the atrium or ventricle, the electrode tip is fluoroscopically guided into the right atrial appendage or the right ventricular apex. In the absence of fluoroscopy, balloon-tipped floatation electrodes can be used in emergent situations with sensed electrogram timing and morphology or with pacing electrograms used to guide positioning. A pacing threshold of less than 1 V is usually considered satisfactory.

With transvenous pacing, patients seldom complain of discomfort, making it ideal for prolonged use when necessary. However, because of its invasive nature, some complications may occur and include ventricular arrhythmias, particularly in patients with an acute myocardial infarction; pericarditis; ventricular perforation; bleeding; pulmonary and air embolism; pneumothorax with subclavian vein puncture; and infection.

External Cardiac Pacing

Gel patches are applied to the anterior chest and the lower left scapula. High-output pacing is required for ventricular

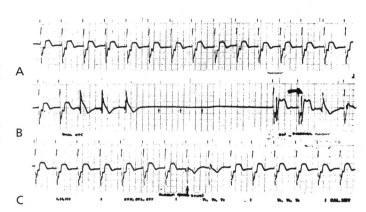

FIGURE 10-1. Recording from a patient undergoing external pacing. **A:** Successful pacing with 100% ventricular capture. **B:** The energy output of the device is reduced to below threshold, and there is no ventricular capture (beats 3 through 5). When the external pacemaker is turned off, there is no spontaneous ventricular activity, although small P waves (*arrows*) are seen. **C:** Pacing is reinstituted thereafter (bottom panel). (From Falk RH. Noninvasive external cardiac pacing. In: El Sherif NA, Samit P, eds. *Cardiac pacing and electrophysiology*, 3rd ed. Philadelphia: WB Saunders, 1991:675–684, with permission.)

capture. Unfortunately, this form of pacing causes significant patient discomfort and should be used only in the urgent treatment of asystole, symptomatic bradycardia due to heart block, or sinus node dysfunction (7,8). The external pacemaker is also important for prophylaxis in patients at high risk for heart block or during transport of acutely ill cardiac arrhythmia patients.

When used emergently during a cardiac arrest due to primary asystole, it can provide life-saving support to maintain cardiac rhythm until a stable temporary transvenous pacing system is inserted (Fig. 10-1). The external pacemaker is of little value in patients with a prolonged cardiac arrest in whom asystole develops as a result of prolonged ventricular fibrillation.

External cardiac pacing has also been used to overdrive and pace terminate a supraventricular or, less frequently, ventricular tachyarrhythmia (Figs. 10-2 and 10-3).

Transesophageal Pacing

The pacing electrode used for transesophageal pacing is enclosed in a soluble capsule and is swallowed by the patient. It is positioned so that consistent atrial capture is obtained. A special pulse generator is used for esophageal pacing because a longer pulse width and amplitude are required for capture. This method allows an easy and noninvasive approach for atrial pacing. Selective ventricular capture may occur in only 5% of cases. This method is not recommended for patients with AV block.

Transesophageal pacing is used in pediatric and other populations for the diagnosis and treatment of cardiac

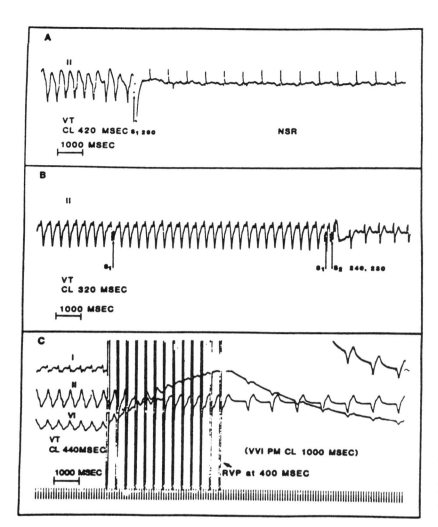

FIGURE 10-2. Example of external pacemaker used for termination of ventricular tachycardia. **A:** Ventricular tachycardia (VT) with a cycle length of 420 ms is terminated by a single extrastimulus. **B:** VT at a cycle length of 360 ms. The first stimulus (S$_1$) fails to capture the ventricle, and the VT is unaffected. Double extrastimuli (S$_1$, S$_2$) result in VT termination. **C:** VT with a cycle length of 440 ms is recorded on three surface electrocardiographic leads (I, II, V$_1$). Using the external pacemakers, rapid ventricular pacing (RVP) at a cycle length of 400 ms terminates the VT, and a paced rhythm is restored. (From Estes NAM, Deering TF, Manolis AS, et al. External cardiac programmed stimulation for noninvasive termination of sustained supraventricular and ventricular tachycardia. *Am J Cardiol* 1989;63:177–182, with permission.)

arrhythmias. It has been of some use for pace termination of atrial tachycardia or atrial flutter and for establishing the presence of P waves if they are not obvious on the electrocardiogram (ECG) (Fig. 10-4). Although complications are uncommon, most patients do experience some epigastric and substernal discomfort with pacing.

Epicardial Pacing

Epicardial pacing is used primarily during and after cardiac surgery and can be used for temporary pacing if bradycardia occurs or for overdrive pacing of a postoperative atrial tachyarrhythmia, especially atrial flutter. Teflon-coated stainless steel wires or tape electrodes with bared tips are sutured to the epicardium; there are unipolar or bipolar types, and the leads may be located in the atrium, ventricle, or both chambers. In the postoperative period, they can be removed by gentle traction. The use of atrial electrodes in addition to ventricular wires has been increasingly stressed to diagnose and treat ventricular and

atrial arrhythmias. Tape electrodes permit epicardial pacing and low-energy defibrillation. These leads can also be used for tachycardia termination and postoperative electrophysiologic testing.

Temporary Atrial and Dual-Chamber Cardiac Pacing

In most instances, temporary cardiac pacing is performed in the right ventricle. However, certain situations may warrant the use of temporary atrial and dual-chamber pacing. In these systems, the atrial lead may be placed in the right atrial appendage or as a secondary option in the lateral right atrium. Temporary, preformed atrial J electrodes and wire electrodes have been developed for this use. They may be inserted through a single venous sheath with two ports or using separate venous entry sheaths from the subclavian vein. Careful fixation of catheter and sheath to the skin helps prevent dislodgment. Atrial pacing may be appropriate in sinus node dysfunction without AV block, for over-

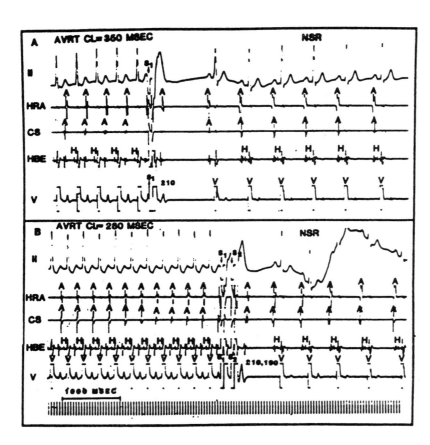

FIGURE 10-3. Example of supraventricular tachycardia (SVT) termination with the external pacemaker. **A:** An atrioventricular reentrant tachycardia (AVRT) with a cycle length of 350 ms is recorded on a surface electrocardiographic lead (II), in the high right atrium (HRA), coronary sinus (CS), at the His bundle (HBE), and in the ventricle (V). A single extrastimulus (S_1) captures the ventricle and terminates the SVT. This occurs because of retrograde conduction through a bypass tract with an antegrade block in the AV node. **B:** The AVRT is more rapid as a result of an isoproterenol infusion. Double extrastimuli terminate the tachycardia. A, atrial electrogram; H, His bundle electrogram; V, ventricular electrogram. (From Estes NAM, Deering TF, Manolis AS, et al. External cardiac programmed stimulation for noninvasive termination of sustained supraventricular and ventricular tachycardia. *Am J Cardiol* 1989;63:177–182, with permission.)

drive or underdrive pacing in atrial and junctional tachycardias such as AV nodal reentrant tachycardias or typical atrial flutter, or diagnostically for differentiation of an atrial or ventricular origin in patients with wide complex tachycardias.

Dual-chamber pacing is more appropriate for sinus node dysfunction with first-, second-, or third-degree AV block in a patient with noncompliant, poor left ventricular function or in patients with large myocardial infarctions, particularly associated with right ventricular infarction, who have sinoatrial nodal involvement and heart block. It is also used in assessment of hemodynamic efficacy in anticipated dual-chamber pacemaker implantation or in patients with a relative bradycardia who are hemodynamically unstable in the immediate postoperative period.

Indications for Temporary Cardiac Pacing

Temporary cardiac pacing is an integral approach to ensure a stable cardiac rhythm and maximize cardiac output in patients with symptomatic bradyarrhythmias. Temporary pacing is indicated in several clinical circumstances (9,10): acute myocardial infarction, drug-induced bradyarrhythmias, cardiac catheterization in specific subpopulations, uncontrolled tachyarrhythmias, reversible conditions, and permanent pacemaker or lead failure.

Acute Myocardial Infarction

The need for temporary cardiac pacing in patients with acute myocardial infarction is best understood when the impact of ischemia of the conduction system is considered. The sinoatrial node, located near the junction of the right atrium and the superior vena cava, is supplied by the sinoatrial nodal artery, a branch of the right coronary artery in 55% or the left circumflex artery in the remaining individuals. The AV node is supplied by the nodal branch of the right coronary artery in 90% of individuals and by the left circumflex artery in the remaining 10%. There is very little collateral blood supply for these structures. In contrast, the His bundle and proximal portions of the left and right bundles have a dual blood supply from the AV nodal artery and the septal branches of the left anterior descending artery. The right bundle branch and left anterior fascicle have blood supplied from branches of the left anterior descending artery. The left posterior fascicle is anatomically less discrete and has a dual blood supply from the AV nodal and posterior descending arteries.

Conduction disturbances in myocardial infarction depend on the site of arterial occlusion (11–14). Occlusion proximal to the sinoatrial artery can result in sinus node dysfunction. More distal occlusion can result in AV block at the AV node. AV block resulting from occlusion of the AV

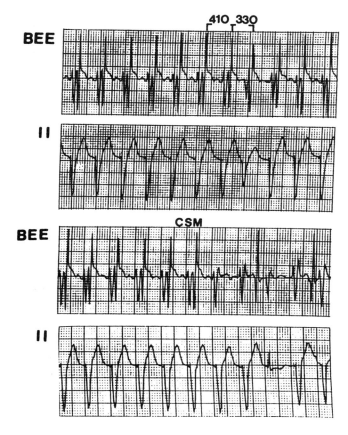

FIGURE 10-4. The wide QRS tachycardia at 150 bpm has atrial deflections on the bipolar esophageal electrograms after each QRS. A 1 : 1 retrograde ventriculoatrial association is strongly suggested when a premature ventricular beat shortens the P-P interval from 410 to 330 ms. Ventricular tachycardia is confirmed on the lower tracing when carotid sinus massage (CSM) creates retrograde block with no interruption of the ventricular rate. The dissociated atrium captures the ventricular with a premature QRS more normal than the QRS of the wide QRS tachycardia.

nodal branch may not necessarily be associated with extensive infarction. Because the bundle branches are anatomically more diffuse, bundle branch block is usually associated with an extensive, often anterior myocardial infarction. These rules can vary with patients with multivessel disease or prior occluded coronary arteries. The decision to insert a temporary pacemaker in patients with acute myocardial infarction depends on the location of the conduction disturbance, the extent of newly infarcted myocardium, and the presence of prior conduction system disease.

Inferior infarction is usually associated with conduction system disturbances proximal to the His bundle. Escape rhythms in this situation usually have a stable and narrow QRS complex, with rates greater than 40 bpm tending to be atropine responsive. AV block is usually but not invariably transient. Indications for temporary pacing in this group include a ventricular rate less than 40 bpm and

symptomatic bradycardia associated with angina or ventricular arrhythmias that are bradycardia dependent.

New conduction disorders located distal to the AV node are usually seen with an anterior myocardial infarction. High-degree AV block or bundle branch blocks can be observed. The escape rhythm is associated with an unstable and wide QRS complex with rates less than 45 bpm, often not atropine responsive. Frequently, this progresses to high-degree AV block, contributing to hemodynamic instability. Because progression to complete heart block contributes independently to morbidity and mortality in myocardial infarction, temporary cardiac pacing is immediately indicated. Patients at risk for third-degree or complete heart block include type II second-degree AV block, new bifascicular block, complete left or right bundle branch block with first- or second-degree AV block, alternating left and right bundle branch block, and preexisting right bundle branch block with new left fascicular block or first-degree AV block. The subsequent need for permanent pacing in a particular patient is based on whether the rhythm disturbance is temporary or permanent and on the severity of associated symptoms.

The American Heart Association and American College of Cardiology have published guidelines for the use of temporary bradycardia pacing in patients with acute myocardial infarction (15) (Tables 10-2 and 10-3). As with all the guidelines for the use of pacemakers, the following definitions apply:

Class I: conditions for which there is evidence or general agreement that a given procedure or treatment is useful and effective

Class II: conditions for which there is conflicting evidence or a divergence of opinion about the usefulness or efficacy of a procedure or treatment

Class IIa: weight of evidence or opinion favors usefulness or efficacy

Class IIb: usefulness or efficacy less well established by evidence or opinion

Class III: conditions for which there is evidence or general agreement that the procedure or treatment is not useful or may be harmful

Drug-Induced Bradyarrhythmias

Use of antiarrhythmic agents, including digoxin, at normal or toxic doses can result in sinus node dysfunction and AV nodal block. These arrhythmias may occur even at low or therapeutic levels as a consequence of underlying conduction system disease or an idiosyncratic predisposition due to undiagnosed gene mutations. Temporary cardiac pacing is indicated in these conditions for the duration of drug washout. If long-term therapy is considered, as in the case for some antiarrhythmic agents for ventricular arrhythmias, permanent pacing with backup defibrillation is indicated.

TABLE 10-2. RECOMMENDATIONS FOR PLACEMENT OF TRANSCUTANEOUS PATCHES AND ACTIVE (DEMAND) TRANSCUTANEOUS PACING IN MYOCARDIAL INFARCTION

Class I
1. Sinus bradycardia (rate <50 bpm) with symptoms of hypotension (systolic blood pressure <80 mm Hg) unresponsive to drug therapy[a]
2. Mobitz type II second-degree atrioventricular (AV) block[a]
3. Third-degree heart block[a]
4. Bilateral bundle branch block (BBB) (alternating BBB or RBBB and alternating left anterior fascicular block [LAFB], left posterior fascicular block [LPFB]) (irrespective of time of onset)[b]
5. Newly acquired or age-indeterminate LBBB, LBBB and LAFB, or RBBB and LPFB[b]
6. RBBB or LBBB and first-degree AV block[b]

Class IIa
1. Stable bradycardia (systolic blood pressure >90 mm Hg, no hemodynamic compromise, or compromise responsive to initial drug therapy)[b]
2. Newly acquired or age-indeterminate RBBB[b]

Class IIb
1. Newly acquired or age-indeterminate first-degree AV block[b]

Class III
1. Uncomplicated acute myocardial infarction without evidence of conduction system disease

---

[a]Transcutaneous patches applied; system may be attached and activated within a brief time if needed. Transcutaneous pacing may help as an urgent expedient. Because it is associated with significant pain, high-risk patients likely to require pacing should receive a temporary pacemaker.
[b]Apply patches and attach system; system is in active or standby mode to allow immediate use on demand as required. In facilities in which transvenous pacing or expertise are not available to place an intravenous system, consideration should be given to transporting the patient to one equipped and competent in placing transvenous systems.

Temporary cardiac pacing is indicated for the acute management of polymorphic ventricular tachycardia (i.e., torsade de pointes or other ventricular arrhythmias) with a prolonged QT interval (16,17). Temporary overdrive pacing should be employed until all reversible factors have been corrected or a permanent pacing system has been implanted.

During Cardiac Catheterization

Prophylactic temporary cardiac pacing is performed in the cardiac catheterization laboratory when there is a risk of complete AV block during this intervention. In patients with a preexisting left bundle branch block, right heart catheterization can result in transient or prolonged complete AV block. Prophylactic temporary pacemaker placement is also appropriate when pulmonary artery catheter (Swan-Ganz) insertion is required in a patient with a preexisting complete left bundle branch block. Significant bradycardia and asystole can also occur during injection of radiopaque dye into the right coronary artery but rarely requires cardiac pacing unless this precludes completion of coronary angiography.

TABLE 10-3. RECOMMENDATIONS FOR TEMPORARY TRANSVENOUS PACING IN ACUTE MYOCARDIAL INFARCTION

Class I
1. Asystole
2. Symptomatic bradycardia (includes sinus bradycardia with hypotension and type I second-degree atrioventricular [AV] block with hypotension not responsive to atropine)
3. Bilateral bundle branch block (BBB) (alternating BBB or RBBB with alternating left anterior or left posterior fascicular block [LAFB/LPFB]) (any age)
4. New or indeterminate age bifascicular block (RBBB with LAFB or LPFB, or LBBB) with first-degree AV block
5. Mobitz type II second-degree AV block

Class IIa
1. RBBB and LAFB or LPFB (new or indeterminate)
2. RBBB with first-degree AV block
3. LBBB, new or indeterminate
4. Incessant ventricular tachycardia, for atrial or ventricular overdrive pacing
5. Recurrent sinus pauses (>3 seconds) not responsive to atropine

Class IIb
1. Bifascicular block of indeterminate age
2. New or age-indeterminate isolated RBBB

Class III
1. First-degree heart block
2. Type I second-degree AV block with normal hemodynamics
3. Accelerated idioventricular rhythm
4. BBB or fascicular block known to exist before acute myocardial infarction

---

In choosing an intravenous pacemaker system, patients with substantially depressed ventricular performance, including right ventricular infarction, may respond better to atrial or atrioventricular sequential pacing than ventricular pacing.

Management of Tachycardias

Temporary cardiac pacing in patients with tachyarrhythmias can be used for diagnostic or therapeutic purposes. Simultaneous recording of the surface ECG during the tachycardia and the atrial electrogram using a temporary pacing electrode is useful in studying AV relationships. These recordings are useful in differentiating an atrial or ventricular origin of wide-complex tachycardias. Ventriculoatrial dissociation suggests the diagnosis of ventricular tachycardia, whereas one-to-one ventriculoatrial relationships may be seen in supraventricular tachycardias with aberrancy or preexcitation or ventricular tachycardia with 1:1 retrograde conduction. Further examination of the atrial electrograms may help in the diagnosis of atrial fibrillation or atrial flutter or a dual supraventricular and ventricular tachycardia.

Electrical stimulation with temporary electrodes is helpful in terminating many forms of reentrant regular supraventricular and ventricular tachycardias. Investigational pacing modes are being applied in type II atrial flutter and atrial fibrillation. Pacing should be employed if pharmacologic therapy is ineffective and recurrent cardioversion is required.

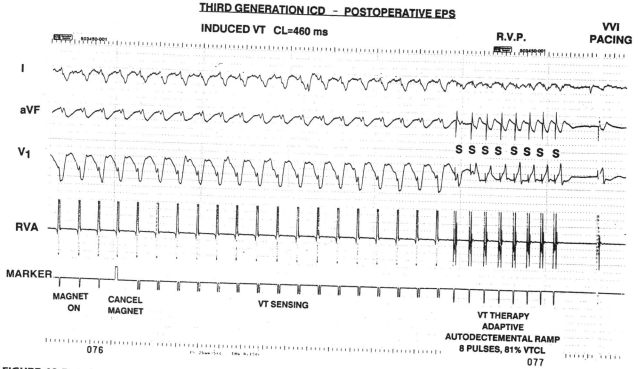

FIGURE 10-5. Induced ventricular tachycardia (VT) during an electrophysiologic study using the programmed electrical stimulation feature in the Medtronic 7216A implantable cardioverter-defibrillator. Readings for three surface electrocardiographic leads (I, aVF, V₁), the right ventricular apical electrogram, and the telemetric marker channel *(bottom)* are shown. The device is activated at the cancel magnet command shown on the marker channel at the bottom after VT induction. Sensing of the tachycardia in the programmed VT zone is shown by the double markers. Sixteen beats are sensed in this zone, and a rate-adaptive rapid ventricular pacing burst is delivered. This is an autodecremental ramp starting at 81% of the VT cycle length for eight pulses. After VT termination, demand ventricular pacing is observed. CL, cycle length; EPS, electrophysiologic study; ICD, implantable cardioverter-defibrillator; RVA, right ventricular apical electrogram; RVP, rapid ventricular pacing; S, pacing stimulus; VVI, command ventricular pacing; (From Saksena S. Implantable cardioverter: defibrillator devices for the future. In: Fisch C, Surawicz B, eds. *Cardiac electrophysiology and arrhythmias.* New York: Elsevier, 1991:449, with permission.)

Overdrive pacing can terminate atrial flutter, AV reentry tachycardia, and ventricular tachycardia; high-frequency pacing may be effective in atypical atrial flutter (Figs. 10-5 and 10-6). Timed premature beats or underdrive pacing can terminate reciprocating AV reentrant and ventricular tachycardias. Defibrillation capability should be available when pacing techniques are employed for tachycardia termination.

Pacing can prevent the onset of tachyarrhythmias that are bradycardia or conduction delay dependent or associated with a prolonged QT interval. Atrial pacing can be used to convert hemodynamically unstable atrial flutter to a hemodynamically more favorable atrial arrhythmia (i.e., atrial fibrillation), which has a slower ventricular response because of concealed AV nodal conduction. Multisite pacing methods are being used for prevention of atrial fibrillation in the postoperative cardiac surgery patient; its role, however, remains uncertain (18–21). In this approach, simultaneous dual-site pacing at the right and left atrium is performed with temporary wires for the immediate postoperative period, usually in combination with drug therapy such as β-blocking agents.

Temporary Pacing for a Reversible Condition

Temporary pacing is indicated for bradycardia that results from an acute and reversible cause that probably will not require permanent pacing, such as injury to the sinus or AV node or His-Purkinje system after heart surgery, Lyme disease, or heart transplantation associated with transient sinus node injury and dysfunction. Cardiac trauma, as occurs after a motor vehicle accident with associated chest trauma, can require temporary bradycardia pacing for transient asystole resulting from AV block. Temporary pacing is indicated for subacute bacterial endocarditis with an aortic valve abscess that damages the His-Purkinje system and causes AV block.

Catheter ablation of the AV node to slow the heart rate in atrial fibrillation usually results in complete heart block and requires permanent pacing. Temporary pacing is necessary until a permanent pacemaker can be placed.

Temporary pacing (i.e., single-chamber pacing in the atrium or ventricle or dual-chamber AV sequential pacing) has been used to establish the potential benefit of permanent pacemakers in patients with sinus bradycardia, first-degree

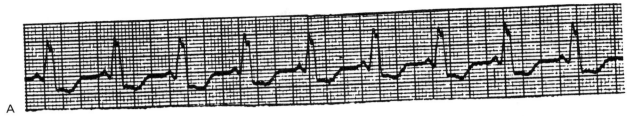

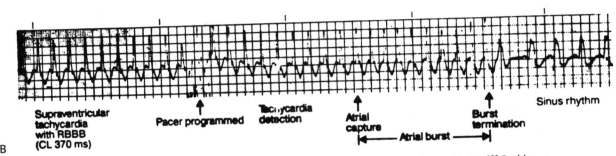

FIGURE 10-6. Management of supraventricular tachycardia in a patient with Wolff-Parkinson-White syndrome using a dual-chamber antitachycardia pacemaker. **A:** In this patient with incessant supraventricular tachycardia, a Medtronic model 7008 Symbios pacemaker was inserted, and bipolar stimulation was used to achieve permanent paced preexcitation. Atrioventricular (AV) sequential pacing was established in the DVI mode with an AV interval of 100 ms, which resulted in a marked decrease in the frequency of supraventricular tachycardia episodes. **B:** Recurrent paroxysmal supraventricular tachycardia was occasionally observed, and the same antitachycardia device as shown in **A** was programmed to the automatic mode using atrial burst pacing for tachycardia termination. Supraventricular tachycardia with a right bundle branch block configuration and with a cycle length of 370 ms occurred spontaneously. The pacemaker was programmed to the predetermined antitachycardia device termination mode. Automatic tachycardia detection ensued within the 2 seconds, followed by delivery of an atrial burst that reset the tachycardia, which results in antegrade AV nodal block with penetration of the accessory pathway antegradely and failure of maintenance of the tachycardia wavefront. The patient subsequently reverted to sinus rhythm with antegrade preexcitation. (From Saksena S, et al. Electrophysiologic mechanisms underlying management of supraventricular tachycardia by electrical stimulation. In: Saksena S, Goldschlager N, eds. *Electrical therapy for cardiac arrhythmias.* Philadelphia: WB Saunders, 1990:384, with permission.)

AV block, second-degree AV block, and hypertrophic cardiomyopathy when the cause of symptoms is unclear.

TECHNIQUE AND INDICATIONS FOR PERMANENT PACEMAKER IMPLANTATION

Permanent Pacemaker Insertion

The standard technique for permanent transvenous pacemaker insertion employs venous access from the subclavian or cephalic veins. The prepectoral region contralateral to the patient's dominant arm responsible for most activity is shaved and prepped before local anesthesia. Local anesthesia with 1% to 2% Xylocaine, with or without conscious sedation, is usually employed. Using a standard prepectoral incision curved along the deltopectoral groove, the cephalic vein is isolated; the subclavian vein is cannulated percutaneously if there is failure to achieve cephalic vein availability or additional access

for lead number or dimension is needed. Using fluoroscopy, bipolar or unipolar leads are placed in the right ventricular apex, high right atrium (usually in the appendage if feasible), and rarely in the coronary sinus for novel pacing methods (Figs. 10-7 and 10-8). The leads are fixed at the venous entry point with nonabsorbable sutures and a prepectoral pocket fashioned anterior to the pectoralis major fascial sheath for generator placement. The leads are tested for adequate sensing (sinus P wave >1.5 mV) , ventricular R wave >5 mV), and pacing (atrium or ventricle <1 V at 0.5-ms pulse width). The generator pocket is closed after adequate lead fixation, placing lead system below the generator and confirming lead position, providing available length for motion or postural changes, and checking stability radiographically (Fig. 10-9).

After implantation, the pocket should be checked for bleeding, collection, or drainage before hospital discharge. Postoperatively, a chest radiograph in the posteroanterior and lateral views is obtained to confirm lead position before

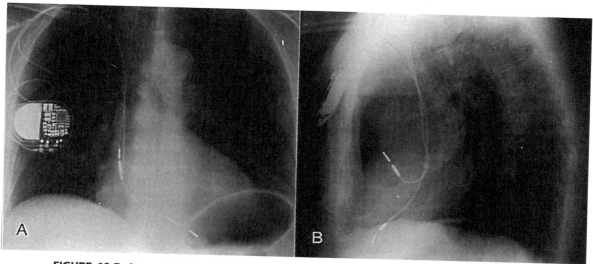

FIGURE 10-7. Posteroanterior **(A)** and lateral **(B)** radiographic views of a DDD dual-chamber pacemaker in a patient. The atrial lead is in the right atrial appendage, which on the lateral view is seen to be in an anterior position. The ventricular lead is in the right ventricular apex. The lateral view confirms the anterior position of the lead, excluding inadvertent placement of the lead into the coronary sinus or left ventricle.

discharge, and a paced ECG is examined to document device function. Postoperative antibiotics are used in many centers for reducing risk of infection.

Indications for Permanent Pacing

Pacing for Sinus Node Dysfunction

Sinus node dysfunction is defined by abnormal sinus node behavior at rest or during stimulation and includes a constellation of electrocardiographic findings such as sinus bradycardia, sinus arrest, sinus node exit block, or the bradycardia-tachycardia syndrome. Wandering atrial pacemaker characterized by pacemaker shift or atrial fibrillation may coexist in this disorder. Sinus bradycardia, sinus pauses, and type I second-degree AV block may be normal physical findings in the trained athlete who has an elevated basal vagal tone. Indications for pacing in sinus node dysfunction are listed in Table 10-4 (15).

Sick sinus syndrome refers to ECG findings with symptoms attributed to a diseased sinoatrial node. These symptoms can include those caused by a low cardiac output from fatigue or frank syncope. An electrocardiographic correlation of the symptoms with the bradyarrhythmia is essential for the diagnosis of sick sinus syndrome. Sick sinus syndrome occurs most often as a chronic disorder but rarely can occur during an acute myocardial infarction. In the latter instance, it should be treated only when a transient nature has been excluded.

The sick sinus syndrome accounts for more than one half of pacemakers implanted (22) (Table 10-4). Permanent pacing can alleviate symptoms in sick sinus syndrome (23,24). Atrial pacing and ventricular pacing have been employed. Single-chamber atrial pacemakers are appropriate only in those individuals with no evidence of AV block or conduction system disease; In contrast, patients with conduction system abnormalities are generally treated with a dual-chamber pacing, dual-chamber sensing, atrial-triggered, and ventricular-inhibited (DDD) pacemaker. Nevertheless, the use of a DDD pacemaker obviates the need for additional electrophysiologic evaluation of conduction system disease and anticipates the possible subsequent development of conducting system dysfunction. Rate-adaptive pacing in patients with symptomatic sinus node dysfunction restores a physiologically appropriate heart rate.

Studies comparing rate-responsive atrial-based (atrial or dual-chamber) pacemakers with ventricular pacing have been reported (25–28). Available data suggest that, in patients with a sick sinus syndrome, those with long-term atrial and dual-chamber pacing are less likely to develop chronic atrial fibrillation or cerebrovascular accidents and to have better survival than those treated with ventricular based pacing. The Pacemaker Selection in the Elderly (PASE) trial prospectively randomized 407 elderly patients (average age, 76 years) with sick sinus syndrome or complete AV block to rate-responsive VVI or DDD pacing (27). At 30 months, no difference was observed in the end points of total mortality (17% versus 16%); stroke or death; stroke, hospitalization for heart failure, or death (27% versus 22%); or atrial fibrillation (19% versus 17%). Nevertheless, in the subset of patients with a sick sinus syndrome, DDD pacing was associated with a nonsignificant trend toward a lower mortality (12% versus 20%); lower incidence of stroke; hospitalization for heart failure, or death (20% versus 31%); and less atrial fibrillation (19% versus 28%). Quality of life and functional status were moder-

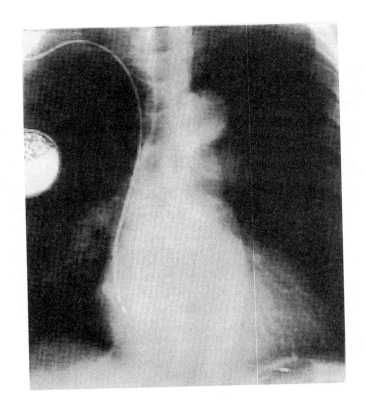

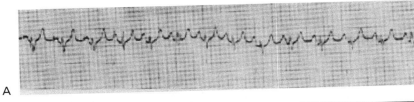

A

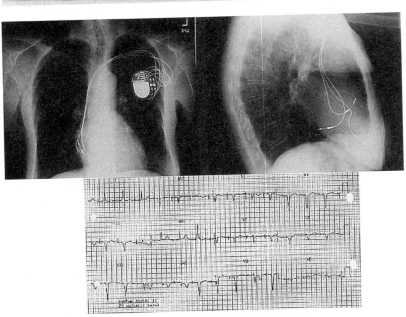

B

FIGURE 10-8. New developments of single- and dual-chamber pacing systems. **A:** Single-lead tripolar pacing system with ventricular sensing and pacing and with atrial sensing leads to permit atrial-triggered ventricular pacing *(bottom)*. (From Saksena S, et al. Electrophysiologic mechanisms underlying management of supraventricular tachycardia by electrical stimulation. In: Saksena S, Goldschlager N, eds. *Electrical therapy for cardiac arrhythmias.* Philadelphia: WB Saunders, 1990, with permission.) **B:** Dual-site right atrial pacing system used for atrial fibrillation and flutter prevention with electrocardiographic tracing of paced rhythm. (Adapted from Saksena S, Prakash A, Hill M, et al. Prevention of recurrent atrial fibrillation with chronic dual-site right atrial pacing. *J Am Coll Cardiol* 1996; 28:687, with permission.

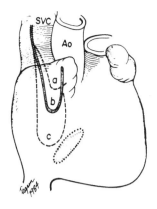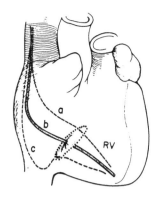

Atrial Lead Position   Ventricular Lead Position

FIGURE 10-9. Schematic diagram of appropriate lead positioning during dual-chamber pacemaker implantation. For the atrial and ventricular leads, position b is correct. Position a is too taut, and in position c, there is excessive lead. With deep inspiration, both leads should approximate position a.

ately better with DDD pacing in patients with sick sinus syndrome, but there was no difference in patients with AV block.

The Canadian Study on Physiologic Pacing found that the primary end point, cardiovascular death or stroke, was identical for ventricular and physiologic pacing (5.5 versus

4.9 events per year); there was no difference in the annual rate of all-cause mortality (6.6% versus 6.3%), incidence of stroke (1.09 versus 1.02 per year), or congestive heart failure (3.5 versus 3.1 events per year), and functional capacity, as assessed with a 6-minute walk, was identical (25). However, the incidence of atrial fibrillation was reduced by 18% with physiologic pacing (6.6 versus 5.3 events per year); this benefit was not apparent until 2 years after implantation. Improved survival is seen in patients with high-degree AV block and continuous pacing.

Physiologic atrial pacing can prevent or reduce atrial fibrillation recurrences, usually in combination with drug or ablation therapy in a "hybrid" therapy algorithm for patients with symptomatic recurrent or even permanent atrial fibrillation. Further studies are investigating the benefits of rate-responsive dual-chamber pacing over dual-chamber pacing alone and single-chamber atrial pacing versus dual-chamber AV pacing.

Pacing for Atrioventricular Block

The indications for permanent pacing in patients with an AV block due to myocardial infarction largely depend on persistence of the disorder after the acute phase of myocardial injury and the patient's symptoms (Table 10-5). Second- or third-degree degree AV block is more likely to result in symptoms and to require intervention. Rarely, first-degree AV block may result in a low-output state and left

TABLE 10-4. INDICATIONS FOR PERMANENT PACING IN SINUS NODE DYSFUNCTION

Class I
1. Sinus node dysfunction with documented symptomatic bradycardia, including frequent sinus pauses that produce symptoms. In some patients, bradycardia is iatrogenic and occurs as a consequence of essential long-term drug therapy of a type and dose for which there are no acceptable alternatives.
2. Symptomatic chronotropic incompetence

Class IIa
1. Sinus node dysfunction occurring spontaneously or as a result of necessary drug therapy with heart rate <40 bpm when a clear association between significant symptoms consistent with bradycardia and the actual presence of bradycardia has not been documented

Class IIb
1. In minimally symptomatic patients, chronic heart rate <30 bpm while awake

Class III
1. Sinus node dysfunction in asymptomatic patients, including those in whom substantial sinus bradycardia (heart rate <40 bpm) is a consequence of long-term drug treatment
2. Sinus node dysfunction in patients with symptoms suggestive of bradycardia that are clearly documented as not associated with a slow heart rate
3. Sinus node dysfunction with symptomatic bradycardia due to nonessential drug therapy

Adapted from Gregoratos G, Cheitlin M, Conill A, et al. *Circulation* 1998;97:1325, with permission.

TABLE 10-5. INDICATIONS FOR PERMANENT PACING AFTER THE ACUTE PHASE OF MYOCARDIAL INFARCTION

Class I
1. Persistent second-degree atrioventricular (AV) block in the His-Purkinje system with bilateral bundle branch block or third-degree AV block within or below the His-Purkinje system after acute myocardial infarction
2. Transient advanced (second- or third-degree) infranodal AV block and associated bundle branch block. If the site of block is uncertain, an eletrophysiologic study may be necessary
3. Persistent and symptomatic second or third-degree AV block

Class IIa
None

Class IIb
1. Persistent second- or third-degree AV block at the AV node level

Class III
1. Transient AV block in the absence of intraventricular conduction defects
2. Transient AV block in the presence of isolated left anterior fascicular block
3. Acquired left anterior fascicular block in the absence of AV block
4. Persistent first-degree AV block in the presence of bundle branch block that is old or age indeterminate

Adapted from Gregoratos G, Cheitlin M, Conill A, et al. *Circulation* 1998;97:1325, with permission.

heart failure. Pacing can theoretically improve survival and alleviate symptoms in this clinical scenario. Prior studies have demonstrated that the long-term survival of these patients is related primarily to the extent of myocardial damage and the character of intraventricular conduction disturbances (11). Although permanent pacing may have some survival impact, sudden death and myocardial failure are more frequent comorbidities impairing survival. Symptomatic patients with second- and third-degree AV block after the acute phase of infarction should be carefully considered for pacing and electrophysiologic evaluation may be helpful in predicting likelihood of long-term AV block.

The location of the infarction (e.g., anterior) and the timing and type of intraventricular conduction defect are significant factors in determining the need for permanent pacing in post–myocardial infarction patients with an acquired AV block. Patients with an acute inferior myocardial infarction often have transient first-, second-, or third-degree AV block and should not be candidates for permanent pacemaker implantation. However, the development of a new intraventricular conduction defect with an acquired AV block during acute myocardial infarction is likely to herald a more ominous prognosis with respect to persistent AV block. Accordingly, patients with new-onset bifascicular block (i.e., complete left bundle branch block or a right bundle branch block combined with left anterior or posterior fascicular block) and advanced second- or third-degree AV block deserve earlier consideration for permanent pacemaker implantation (12,13).

Thrombolytic therapy has reduced the incidence of these disturbances, such as AV block (29–32). However, these abnormalities in the presence of a partially or fully reperfused artery is still of concern and continues to predict a high mortality as seen in the second Thrombolysis in Myocardial Infarction (TIMI II) study (29). However, final assessment of the need for permanent pacing should await completion of the revascularization procedures contemplated, because progressive improvement can be anticipated. Electrophysiologic testing may be warranted when doubt exists regarding the need for permanent cardiac pacing.

In patients with abnormal AV conduction not associated with acute myocardial infarction, permanent pacemaker implantation is strongly influenced by the presence or absence of symptoms directly attributable to the bradycardia (33) (Table 10-6). Reversible causes of AV block should be sought out; these include electrolyte abnormalities, infectious conditions (i.e., Lyme disease), neurally mediated mechanisms, and physiologic AV block (i.e., exercise induced or tachycardia dependent). If these have been excluded, permanent pacing is considered in symptomatic patients or in patients with advanced AV block likely to develop symptoms or have increased arrhythmic mortality. These latter groups can include asymptomatic congenital heart block with unstable or subnormal escape rhythm during activity (34,35).

TABLE 10-6. INDICATIONS FOR PERMANENT PACING IN ACQUIRED ATRIOVENTRICULAR BLOCK IN ADULTS

Class I
1. Third-degree atrioventricular (AV) block at any anatomic level associated with any one of the following conditions:
    a. Bradycardia with symptoms presumed to be caused by AV block
    b. Arrhythmias and other medical conditions that require drugs that result in symptomatic bradycardia
    c. Documented periods of asystole ≥3.0 seconds or any escape rate <40 bpm in awake, symptom-free patients
    d. After catheter ablation of the AV junction. There are no trials to assess outcome without pacing, and pacing is virtually always planned in this situation unless the operative procedure is AV junction modification
    e. Postoperative AV block that is not expected to resolve
    f. Neuromuscular diseases with AV block such as myotonic muscular dystrophy, Kearns-Sayre syndrome, Erbs dystrophy (limb-girdle), and peroneal muscular atrophy
2. Second-degree AV block regardless of type or site of block, with associated symptomatic bradycardia

Class IIa
1. Asymptomatic third-degree AV block at any anatomic site with average awake ventricular rates of 40 bpm or faster
2. Asymptomatic type II second-degree AV block
3. Asymptomatic type I second-degree AV block at intra-His or infra-His levels found incidentally at electrophysiologic study performed for other indications
4. First-degree AV block with symptoms suggesting pacemaker syndrome and documented alleviation of symptoms with temporary AV pacing

Class IIb
1. Marked first-degree AV block (>0.30 second) in patients with left ventricular dysfunction and symptoms of congestive heart failure in whom a shorter AV interval results in hemodynamic improvement, presumably by decreasing left atrial filling pressure

Class III
1. Asymptomatic first-degree AV block
2. Asymptomatic type I second-degree AV block at the supra-His (AV node) level or not known to be intra-His or infra-Hisian
3. AV block expected to resolve and unlikely to recur (e.g., drug toxicity, Lyme disease)

Adapted from Gregoratos G, Cheitlin M, Conill A, et al. *Circulation* 1998;97:1325, with permission.

Some conditions may justify pacemaker implantation because of anticipated disease progression (e.g., sarcoidosis, amyloidosis, neuromuscular diseases) or adverse consequences (e.g., valvular repair or replacement). However, in most patients, pacing is reserved for symptomatic patients with second- or third-degree AV block, usually below the AV node (15). Studies have strongly suggested that permanent pacing confers a survival benefit in patients with transient or permanent, symptomatic, third-degree AV block regardless of the results of electrophysiologic study. Because progression to advanced or third-degree AV block is uncommon in patients with type I second-degree AV block, pacemaker implantation is not indicated. However, the incidental finding at electrophysiologic study of an intra-His or infra-His type I second-degree block is a class IIa indication for pacemaker placement. Accordingly, patients with type II second-degree AV block should be strongly considered for permanent pacemaker implantation.

Marked first-degree AV delay (>0.30 second) may result in a pseudo-pacemaker syndrome, in which AV dyssynchrony culminates in hemodynamic consequences similar to ventriculoatrial conduction (36). Decompensated heart failure may manifest in patients with left ventricular dysfunction. Pacing with a shorter AV delay may result in hemodynamic and symptomatic improvement. Echocardiographic or invasive documentation of hemodynamic improvement with pacing is recommended before permanent pacemaker implantation. The breadth of evidence does not support a survival benefit with pacing in patients with an isolated first-degree AV block.

Pacing for Chronic Fascicular Disease

Considerations in pacemaker placement in patients with symptomatic (i.e., syncope) fascicular disease depends on the presence or absence of associated advanced AV block (15). (Table 10-7). Third-degree AV block is most commonly preceded by bifascicular disease. Symptomatic fascicular disease in the presence of transient or permanent third-degree AV block is associated with an increased incidence of sudden cardiac death (37–45). Pacing in these patients relieves symptoms and probably confers a mortality benefit. If the cause of syncope in patients with fascicular disease cannot be determined or if pharmacologic treatment precipitates AV block,

consideration for permanent pacemaker implantation is warranted. Electrophysiologic testing is important to exclude a culprit ventricular arrhythmia as the mechanism of syncope (42,43). Recurrent syncope in a patient with significant cardiac disease, particularly with left ventricular dysfunction, should prompt such evaluation.

Cardiovascular mortality among patients with inducible ventricular tachycardia and syncope with this substrate may rival or even exceed that among patients with a history of recurrent ventricular tachycardia or cardiac arrest (46). Inducible ventricular tachycardia may be present with patients with bifascicular and trifascicular block and increased risk of sudden death.

In certain circumstances, permanent pacemaker implantation is indicated in patients with asymptomatic fascicular disease (47,48). These situations include incidental findings at electrophysiologic study of prolonged H-V interval of more than 100 ms and a pacing-induced nonphysiologic infra-His block. Some investigators have observed progression to high-degree AV block in both circumstances, but this may be best related to progression of the underlying cardiac disease with subsequent nonarrhythmic death. Pacing may not effectively prevent mortality in this situation.

Pacing for Hypersensitive Carotid

Hypersensitive carotid syndrome is a cause of syncope. It is characterized by a hyperactive response to carotid stimulation: minimal carotid pressure inducing asystole of more than 3 seconds, symptomatic decrease in systolic blood pressure in the absence of medications, or both conditions. There are two components to the reflex: a cardioinhibitory response with resultant negative chronotropic or dromotropic properties and a vasodepressor response with reduced sympathetic outflow and loss of vascular tone independent of heart rate changes. Indications for pacing are listed in Table 10-8 (15). It is important to establish that a hyperactive response with carotid stimulation is truly the cause of the patient's symptoms and discern the relative contribution of both components, which frequently coexist (i.e., mixed response) in a given patient. In a long-term follow-up of these patients, syncope recurred in 27% of patients with a mean follow-up of 44 months (49). Patients receiving AV pacemakers for pure cardioinhibitory response were free of recurrent syncope. Permanent pacing is effective and indicated in patients with a cardioinhibitory component alone or sometimes in the mixed form.

Pacing for Neurally Mediated Syncope

Neurally mediated syndromes refer to scenarios that trigger a neural reflex, culminating in self-limited episodes of hypotension or bradycardia. This form of syncope accounts for 10% to 40% of syncopal events. The role of permanent pacemaker implantation is evolving with the recognition of

TABLE 10-7. INDICATIONS FOR PERMANENT PACING IN CHRONIC BIFASCICULAR AND TRIFASCICULAR BLOCK

Class I
1. Intermittent third-degree atrioventricular (AV) block
2. Type II second-degree AV block

Class IIa
1. Syncope not proved to be caused by AV block when other likely causes have been excluded, specifically ventricular tachycardia
2. Incidental finding at electrophysiologic study of markedly prolonged H-V interval (≥100 ms) in asymptomatic patients
3. Incidental finding at electrophysiologic study of pacing-induced infa-His block that is not physiologic

Class IIb
None

Class III
1. Fascicular block without AV block or symptoms
2. Fascicular block with first-degree AV block without symptoms

Adapted from Gregoratos G, Cheitlin M, Conill A, et al. *Circulation* 1998;97:1325, with permission.

TABLE 10-8. INDICATIONS FOR PERMANENT PACING IN HYPERSENSITIVE CAROTID SINUS SYNDROME AND NEURALLY MEDIATED SYNCOPE

Class I
1. Recurrent syncope caused by carotid sinus stimulation; minimal carotid sinus pressure induces ventricular asystole of >3 seconds' duration in the absence of any medication that depresses the sinus node or atrioventricular (AV) conduction.

Class IIa
1. Recurrent syncope without clear, provocative events and with a hypersensitive cardioinhibtory response
2. Syncope of unexplained origin when major abnormalities of sinus node function or AV conduction are discovered or provoked in electrophysiologic studies

Class IIb
1. Neurally mediated syncope with significant bradycardia reproduced by a head-up tilt, with or without isoproterenol or other provocative maneuvers

Class III
1. A hyperactive cardioinhibitory response to carotid sinus stimulation in the absence of symptoms
2. A hyperactive cardioinhibitory response to carotid sinus stimulation in the presence of vague symptoms such as dizziness, light-headedness, or both
3. Recurrent syncope, light-headedness, or dizziness in the absence of a hyperactive cardioinhibitory response
4. Situational vasovagal syncope in which avoidance behavior is effective

Adapted from Gregoratos G, Cheitlin M, Conill A, et al. *Circulation* 1998;97:1325, with permission.

a frequently coexisting or predominant vasodepressor component without significant bradycardia or cardioinhibitory component (15) (Table 10-8). Even in patients with a primarily vasodepressor component, a slowing of the heart rate is often observed after the fall in blood pressure.

Several trials have examined the role of permanent pacing in these patients (50–53). Two randomized trials enrolling symptomatic patients with evidence of a cardioinhibitory component demonstrated that pacing can increase the time to recurrence of syncopal events. In the North American Vasovagal Pacemaker Study of 54 patients who had evidence of a cardioinhibitory response with tilt-table testing, there was an unexpectedly large treatment effect, with a relative risk reduction of 85% in the incidence of syncope with a dual-chamber compared with no pacemaker (22% versus 70%) (50). This effect was large enough to terminate the study after pilot enrollment only.

The Vasovagal Syncope International Study (VASIS) randomized 42 patients with cardioinhibitory, tilt-positive, neurally mediated syncope to a DDI pacemaker with hysteresis or no pacemaker (51). After a mean follow-up of 3.7 years, there was a significant reduction in the incidence of recurrent syncope with pacing (5% versus 61% without a pacemaker). In those without a pacemaker, the median time to recurrent syncope was 5 months, with a rate of 0.44 per

year. There was no difference in the incidence of a positive response to repeated tilt-table testing among those with or without a pacemaker (59% versus 61%). Some investigators have concluded that patients with syncope of undetermined origin in whom a bradycardic cause is strongly suspected (or provoked at electrophysiologic study) may benefit from empiric pacing.

Pacing for Tachyarrhythmias

Pacing therapies have been developed to terminate and prevent symptomatic ventricular and supraventricular tachycardias (15,54) (Tables 10-9 and 10-10). Major advantages of these electrical therapies are their painless nature and rapid application. However, pacing therapies are not universally effective in all types of tachycardia or for each episode in a specific patient. Each attempt at pacing-mediated termination has the potential risk of tachycardia acceleration into another, more symptomatic tachycardia or fibrillation.

Antitachycardia pacing is effective in terminating a variety of reentrant supraventricular tachycardias (i.e., AV reentry, AV nodal reentry, intraatrial reentry, or typical atrial flutter) and reentrant sustained monomorphic ventricular tachycardias due to anatomic or functional reentry. Tachycardia termination by electrical stimulation requires critically timed pacemaker impulses to arrive at an access site to the circuit when the tissue is excitable, referred to as the *excitable gap*. A larger excitable gap within the circuit allows stimuli to more easily penetrate the circuit. The use of multiple stimuli at progressively rapid rates and the use of multiple stimulating sites increase the likelihood of penetration of the excitable gap. Proximity of the stimulation site to the reentrant circuit may also facilitate penetration of the

TABLE 10-9. PACING INDICATIONS TO PREVENT TACHYCARDIA

Class I
1. Sustained pause-dependent ventricular tachycardia (VT), with or without prolonged QT, in which the efficacy of pacing is thoroughly documented

Class IIa
1. High-risk patients with congenital long QT syndrome

Class IIb
1. Atrioventricular (AV) reentrant or AV node reentrant supraventricular tachycardia not responsive to medical or ablative therapy
2. Prevention of symptomatic, drug-refractory, recurrent atrial fibrillation

Class III
1. Frequent or complex ventricular ectopic activity without sustained VT in the absence of the long QT syndrome
2. Long QT syndrome due to reversible causes

Adapted from Gregoratos G, Cheitlin M, Conill A, et al. *Circulation* 1998;97:1325, with permission.

TABLE 10-10. INDICATIONS FOR PERMANENT PACEMAKERS THAT AUTOMATICALLY DETECT AND PACE TO TERMINATE TACHYCARDIAS

Class I

1. Symptomatic recurrent supraventricular tachycardia that is reproducibly terminated by pacing after drugs and catheter ablation fail to control the arrythmia or produce intolerable side effects
2. Symptomatic recurrent sustained ventricular tachycardia as part of an automatic defibrillator system

Class IIa

None

Class IIb

1. Recurrent supraventricular tachycardia or atrial flutter that is reproducibly terminated by pacing as an alternative to drug therapy or ablation

Class III

1. Tachycardias frequently accelerated or converted to fibrillation by pacing
2. The presence of accesory pathways with the capacity for rapid anterograde conduction whether or not the pathways participate in the mechanism of the tachycardia

Adapted from Gregoratos G, Cheitlin M, Conill A, et al. *Circulation* 1998;97:1325, with permission.

excitable gap by reducing the probability of intervening anatomic or functional boundaries.

Three forms of electrical stimulation can interrupt a reentrant circuit and terminate tachycardias: underdrive pacing, overdrive pacing, and extrastimulus methods. Underdrive pacing employs electrical stimulation at interstimulus intervals that are longer than the tachycardia cycle length. This form of stimulation requires a relatively wide excitable gap (as seen in slower tachycardias with longer revolution times), limiting its use to tachycardias with rates less than 160 bpm. This approach is seldom used because of its limited efficacy. Its utility may be seen when converting a demand pacemaker to an asynchronous mode in a patient who develops a slow reentrant tachycardia where a stimulus may incidentally terminate the arrhythmia.

Programmed extrastimuli can be introduced into the cardiac cycle at intervals during diastole previously determined to be successful at electrophysiologic testing. If initial attempts are unsuccessful, multiple extrastimuli with progressive prematurity during diastole may be required.

The most common form of antitachycardia pacing is overdrive pacing, which employs electrical stimulation at interstimulus intervals that are shorter than tachycardia cycle length. The interval between these successive pacing pulses is referred to as the burst cycle length. The coupling interval defines the time between the last sensed event that fulfills the detection criteria and delivery of the first paced pulse. The coupling interval and the burst cycle length can be programmed as adaptive (with stimulus timing specified as a predetermined fraction of the tachycardia cycle length) or as a fixed interval.

A burst scheme introduces a series of stimuli with a constant burst cycle length. More aggressive therapy, referred to as *tiered therapy*, may be required to terminate the tachycardia. Two modes may be programmed to allow for the adjustment of the burst cycle length: ramp decrement and scan decrement burst pacing. With ramp decrement burst pacing, each successive burst cycle length is shortened. In a scan decrement scheme, the burst cycle length of each burst sequence is shortened with successive bursts.

Combination of the ramp and scan schema is possible when the first burst sequence follows a ramp scheme with successive bursts after a scan scheme in which each burst is a ramp. Occasionally, the burst cycle lengths within a single ramp sequence may be programmed to accelerate and decelerate, which is referred to as a *changing ramp*.

Pacing may prevent or terminate intraatrial, AV, and AV nodal reentrant tachycardias that are refractory to ablative or drug therapy (Figs. 10-6 and 10-10). In some patients with sick sinus syndrome and bradycardia-dependent atrial fibrillation, atrial-based pacing may reduce the frequency of atrial fibrillation recurrences (55–58).

Some investigations have provided the electrophysiologic basis for pacing applications for prevention of symptomatic drug-refractory atrial fibrillation. Atrial fibrillation is initiated by an ectopic atrial premature beat resulting from enhanced automaticity or triggered activity from either atrium. Maintenance of atrial fibrillation requires perpetuation of one or multiple microreentrant circuits triggering multiple atrial wavelets. The rationale for pacing in prevention of atrial fibrillation lies in one or a combination of the following mechanisms: overdrive suppression of triggers, electrophysiologic modification of atrial activation patterns preventing initiation of atrial fibrillation, or pacing-induced electrical remodeling preventing onset and maintenance of atrial fibrillation.

Dual-site atrial pacing may be more effective with respect to atrial fibrillation prevention than single-site pac-

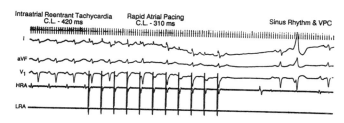

FIGURE 10-10. Termination of intraatrial reentrant tachycardia by rapid atrial pacing bursts. Atrial tachycardia is interrupted by a pacing train of 11 beats at 73% of tachycardia cycle length. This was reproducibly demonstrated in this patient. CL, cycle length; HRA, high right atrium; LRA, low right atrium; VPC, ventricular premature contraction. (From Saksena S, et al. Electrophysiologic mechanisms underlying management of supraventricular tachycardia by electrical stimulation. In: Saksena S, Goldschlager N, eds. *Electrical therapy for cardiac arrhythmias.* Philadelphia: WB Saunders, 1990:384. with permission.)

ing (59–62) (Fig. 10-8B). By altering the atrial activation sequence, dual-site atrial pacing can more effectively alter the hemodynamics of atrial contraction and the electrical properties of the atrial substrate. Daubert and associates demonstrated that, in patients with significant interatrial conduction delays, biatrial pacing significantly reduced pulmonary capillary wedge pressure compared with right atrial pacing (58). Alteration of the atrial activation sequence may explain the failure of atrial premature beats to trigger atrial fibrillation with dual-site rather than with single-site atrial pacing. If the site of abnormal substrate is unknown, pacing from two sites may increase the probability of preexciting the substrate of the reentrant circuit. Clinical studies examining the use of dual-site right atrial pacing in patients with symptomatic drug-refractory atrial fibrillation with and without concomitant bradyarrhythmias suggested an increase in arrhythmia-free intervals compared with the results of single-site atrial pacing.

Pacing for Hypertrophic Obstructive Cardiomyopathy

Pacing indications for hypertrophic obstructive cardiomyopathy are limited (15) (Table 10-11). Initial studies with permanent DDD pacing showed impressive reductions in the dynamic left ventricular outflow tract gradients with selection of an individualized optimal AV delay (63–67). Later studies demonstrated a more modest reduction in the left ventricular outflow tract gradient. The precise mechanisms by which pacing decreases the gradient are not completely understood but are most often ascribed to altered ventricular depolarization decreasing septal obstruction at the outflow tract. With conflicting results from many studies, the correlations for gradient reduction, subjective assessment, and objective end points remain uncertain for a given patient. The multicenter European Pacing in Cardiomyopa-

thy (PIC) study found that approximately 60% of patients improved with pacing at 12 weeks; these benefits persisted for 1 year (65). In the Multicenter Pacing Therapy for Hypertrophic Cardiomyopathy (M-PATHY) trial, which undertook a prospective crossover comparison of DDD pacing with no pacing in 48 patients, there was a symptomatic improvement in many patients; however, there was a substantial placebo effect (66). Improvement was not accompanied by concomitant improvement in peak oxygen consumption despite a 40% decrease in the left ventricular outflow tract gradient occurring in 57% of these patients. At 12 months, only 12% of patients were judged to have had a therapeutic response; these patients were significantly older than those without a response (69 versus 51 years, $p < 0.005$). As a consequence, DDD pacing should be considered a treatment option only for patients with medically refractory, symptomatic hypertrophic obstructive cardiomyopathy or those who do not wish to undergo surgical or ablative intervention or are poor candidate for such procedures.

Pacemaker in Dilated Cardiomyopathy

Several studies have suggested that dual-chamber pacing might minimally improve subjective end points in symptomatic patients with drug-refractory dilated cardiomyopathy and a prolonged PR interval or QRS duration; this has been called *resynchronization therapy* (15,68–74) (Table 10-12). Acute hemodynamic benefit with temporary pacing may be demonstrated before permanent pacemaker implantation but does not invariably predict the long-term results of pacing. However, the mechanisms through which dual-chamber pacing may benefit these patients remain poorly understood, although results of several studies have suggested that the most important mechanisms are increases in filling time, optimization of left heart mechanical AV delay, and normalization of intraventricular activation, which results

---

TABLE 10-11. PACING INDICATIONS FOR HYPERTROPHIC CARDIOMYOPATHY

Class I
1. Class I indications for sinus node dysfunction or atrioventricular block as previously described

Class IIA
None

Class IIb
1. Medically refractory, symptomatic hypertrophic cardiomyopathy with significant resting or provoked left ventricular (LV) outflow obstruction

Class III
1. Patients who are asymptomatic or medically controlled
2. Symptomatic patients without evidence of LV outflow obstruction

Adapted from Gregoratos G, Cheitlin M, Conill A, et al. *Circulation* 1998;97:1325, with permission.

TABLE 10-12. PACING INDICATIONS FOR DILATED CARDIOMYOPATHY

Class I
1. Class I indications for sinus node dysfunction or AV block as previously described

Class IIa
None

Class IIb
1. Symptomatic, drug-refractory, dilated cardiomyopathy with prolonged PR interval when acute hemodynamic studies have demonstrated hemodynamic benefit of pacing

Class III
1. Asymptomatic dilated cardiomyopathy
2. Symptomatic dilated cardiomyopathy when patients are rendered asymptomatic by drug therapy
3. Symptomatic ischemic cardiomyopathy

Adapted from Gregoratos G, Cheitlin M, Conill A, et al. *Circulation* 1998;97:1325, with permission.

in a more coordinated ventricular contraction pattern and an improvement in left ventricular ejection (71). Long-term data supporting this indication remain sparse.

Investigational techniques may hold more promise. Some studies have suggested that biventricular pacing may improve hemodynamics, with a concomitant improvement in intermediate-term objective measures and subjective assessment. In the initial report of the Pacing Therapies for Congestive Heart Failure (PATH-CHF) study, biventricular and left ventricular pacing improved left ventricular inotropy and aortic pulse pressure. Maximal benefit was achieved with left ventricular pacing at the midlateral left ventricular pacing site. In the InSync study, there was increase in time in the 6-minute walk test, improvement in New York Heart Association (NYHA) classification, and patient quality of life with biventricular pacing. However, no definitive improvement in survival of these patients was documented in these early studies. Sudden cardiac death has been an important limiting factor in this regard. The combination of biventricular pacing with defibrillation capability is being considered in an effort to address this issue. Further investigation is under way to confirm these findings and define the role of biventricular pacing in this population.

His bundle pacing in patients with dilated cardiomyopathy and chronic atrial fibrillation has resulted in favorable hemodynamic effects, with reduction in left ventricular dimensions and improvement in ejection fraction (75). However, this procedure is technically difficult, with 20% of patients not able to achieve chronic pacing in an early report.

Pacing after Cardiac Transplantation

Transient sinus node dysfunction after cardiac transplantation is relatively common (76–78). Approximately 50% of patients demonstrate improvement in sinus node function within 6 to 12 months, but there are few predictors of outcome. Patients refractory to theophylline after more than 2 weeks beyond transplantation may be candidates for permanent DDDR pacing (Table 10-13). However, the use of bicaval anastomosis virtually eliminates this problem (79). Permanent pacing in this population is warranted only in patients with symptomatic, irreversible sinus node dysfunction, AV block, or both conditions.

Pacing after Atrioventricular Nodal Ablation

Patients with recurrent or permanent atrial fibrillation may undergo AV junctional ablation (80–82). DDDR or VVIR pacemaker systems, respectively, are inserted just before or after ablation in patients who develop complete heart block; these patients usually become device dependent. Programming of the correct rate response after ablation is important to prevent serious ventricular arrhythmias,

TABLE 10-13. PACING INDICATIONS AFTER CARDIAC TRANSPLANTATION

Class I
1. Symptomatic bradyarrhythmias or chronotropic incompetence not expected to resolve and other class I indications for permanent pacing

Class IIa
None

Class IIb
1. Symptomatic, bradyarrhythmias or chronotropic incompetence that, although transient, may persist for months and require intervention

Class III
1. Asymptomatic bradyarrhythmias after cardiac transplantation

Adapted from Gregoratos G, Cheitlin M, Conill A, et al. *Circulation* 1998;97:1325, with permission.

relieve symptoms, and improve quality of life (83). Improvement in the left ventricular ejection fraction in patients with depressed left ventricular function often improved quality of life after pacemaker insertion. Higher pacing rates may suppress polymorphic ventricular arrhythmias after AV junctional ablation.

Selection of the Appropriate Pacing System

Effective management of arrhythmias with pacing modalities depends on matching the appropriate device to the underlying electrophysiologic abnormalities (Fig. 10-11 and Table 10-14). Factors to be considered in selection of the appropriate mode for the patient's arrhythmia include the existence of intrinsic conduction system disease, ischemic heart disease, left ventricular dysfunction, the need for continuation of medications with bradycardic potential, anticipated activity level, operator expertise in implantation and programming, and cost. Pulse generator characteristics to be considered include single- versus dual-chamber devices, the presence of mode switching, unipolar versus bipolar configurations, presence and type of sensor for physiologic rate response, local availability of technical support, and cost.

Anticipating the progression of abnormalities in conduction and automaticity is an important consideration in selecting the appropriate pacing system. Selecting a pacemaker with more extensive capabilities than needed may obviate the need for subsequent reimplantation and allow for preemptive treatment of new ensuing arrhythmias.

Single-Chamber Pacing

The most widely used single-chamber pacing modes are AAI, AAIR, VVI, and VVIR. AAI (atrial-demand pacing) pacemakers are appropriate for sedentary patients with

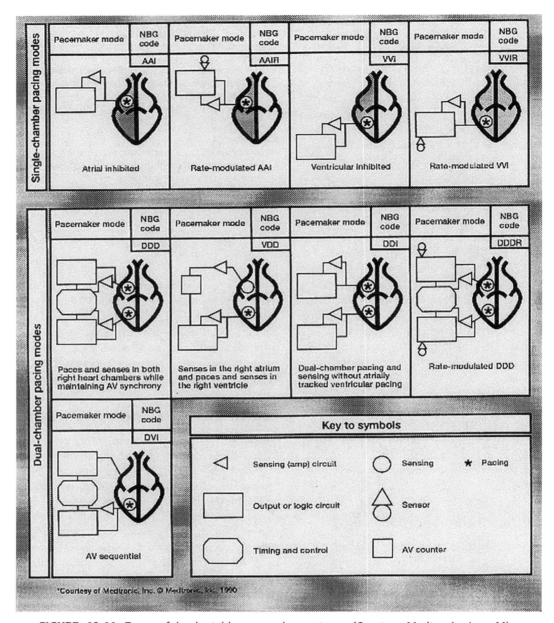

FIGURE 10-11. Types of implantable pacemaker systems. (Courtesy Medtronic, Inc., Minneapolis, MN.)

symptomatic sinus bradyarrhythmias who have intact AV conduction (Fig. 10-12).

The AAIR (rate-modulated AAI pacing) pacemakers are appropriate for patients, particularly those who are active, with chronotropic insufficiency. The VVI (ventricular-demand pacing) pacemakers are ideal in patients with persistent AV block and atrial arrhythmias, especially atrial fibrillation, if AV synchrony is not essential for symptomatic relief or hemodynamic stability (Fig. 10-13).

VVIR (rate-modulated VVI pacing) pacemakers are recommended in the subset of patients with the aforementioned electrophysiologic substrate who participate in daily physical activities. VVIR pacing is contraindicated in patients who have intact ventriculoatrial conduction because of the risk of pacemaker syndrome. Because of AV dyssynchrony, the symptoms of pacemaker syndrome can range from vague dizziness to overt syncope.

Dual-Chamber Pacing

Dual-chamber pacemakers provide the potential of sensing and pacing both chambers while maintaining AV synchrony (i.e., DDD pacing). Candidates for AAI pacing typically receive DDD pacemakers because of concerns about

TABLE 10-14. GUIDELINES FOR CHOICE OF PACEMAKER GENERATOR IN SELECTED INDICATIONS FOR PACING

Type of Pacemaker	Sinus Node Dysfunction	Atrioventricular Block	Neurally Mediated Syncope or Carotid Sinus Hypersensitivity
Single-chamber atrial	No suspected abnormality of atrioventricular (AV) conduction and not at increased risk for future AV block Maintenance of AV synchrony during pacing desired Rate response available if desired	Not appropriate	Not appropriate (unless AV block systematically excluded)
Single-chamber ventricular	Maintenance of AV synchrony during pacing not necessary Rate response available if desired	Chronic atrial fibrillation or other atrial tachyarrhythmia or maintenance of AV synchrony during pacing not necessary Rate response available if desired	Chronic atrial fibrillation or other atrial tachyarrhythmia Rate response available if desired
Dual-chamber	AV synchrony during pacing desired Suspected abnormality of AV conduction or increased risk for future AV block Rate response available if desired	AV synchrony during pacing desired Atrial pacing desired Rate response available if desired	Sinus mechanism present Rate response available if desired
Single-lead, atrial-sensing ventricular	Not appropriate	Normal sinus node function and no need for atrial pacing Desire to limit number of pacemaker leads	Not appropriate

Adapted from Gregoratos G, Cheitlin MD, Conill A, et al. *Circulation* 1998;97:1325, with permission.

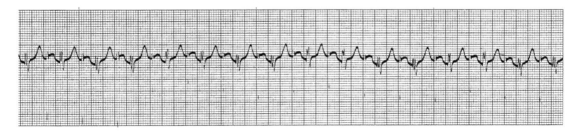

FIGURE 10-12. Types of implanted pacemaker systems. AAI: atrial-paced rhythm at 100 bpm. Atrioventricular conduction is intact, and each paced atrial event is followed by a native QRS.

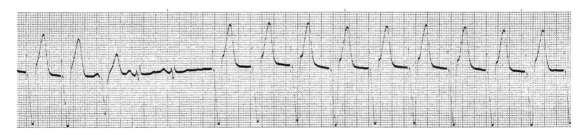

FIGURE 10-13. VVI: ventricular-paced rhythm at 90 bpm. Spontaneous ventricular events inhibit the ventricular output.

atrial lead stability or long-term AV conduction integrity. Dual-chamber pacemakers also obviate the risk of pacemaker syndrome in patients with intact ventriculoatrial conduction. However, pacemaker-mediated tachycardias due to ventriculoatrial conduction after ventricular premature beats or ventricular pacing can complicate this mode of pacing. These arrhythmias result from triggering of ventriculoatrial triggering after sensing retrograde atrial activation. They are addressed by appropriate blanking (i.e., inability to sense) after ventricular pacing.

The most widely used dual-chamber pacing modes are DDD, DDDR, DDI, and VDD. The DDD (P-synchronous pacing) pacemakers are indicated in patients who have persistent AV block with intact atrial function, particularly if retrograde ventriculoatrial conduction exists. Patients with sinus node dysfunction and borderline AV conduction should also be considered for DDD pacing (Fig. 10-14).

The DDDR (rate-responsive DDD pacing) pacemakers should be considered in physically active patients with the aforementioned electrophysiologic substrate who also have chronotropic insufficiency. Rate-modulated pacers employ sensors to determine the desired pacing rate. In newer pulse generators, sensor-driven algorithms allow the switch from DDDR to VVIR (i.e., *mode switching*) during supraventricular tachycardias, especially atrial fibrillation, to prevent inappropriate tracking of pathologic atrial electrical activity.

The DDI (dual-chamber–demand pacing) pacemakers provide AV sequential pacing and sensing of both chambers, but atrial sensing above the lower limit does not trigger ventricular pacing. Because tracking of atrial arrhythmias does not occur, this option may be useful in patients who alternate between sinus bradycardia and rapid atrial tachycardias. DDI pacing should not be employed in individuals with chronotropic competence and AV block, because any sinus rate above the lower rate limit results in loss of AV synchrony. To prevent the potential for AV dyssynchrony, these patients are typically managed in the DDD mode with the upper pacing limit restricted to a low rate.

The VDD (atrial-synchronous ventricular pacing) pacemakers have received heightened interest with the development of the "single-pass" lead. This one lead achieves atrial sensing and ventricular sensing and pacing. The distal end of the lead body is positioned in the right ventricle. The more proximal portion of the lead contains a pair of electrodes that lie within the right atrial cavity. The atrial signal sensed by this configuration may have a less consistent amplitude in comparison to dual-lead systems. The signal can vary considerably with posture. This mode of pacing is appropriate in patients with AV block and normal sinus node function but is relatively contraindicated in the presence of intact retrograde conduction (Fig. 10-15).

Most patients who have DDD pacemakers implanted for AV block have DDD devices that function in a VDD-like manner (i.e., atrial-synchronous ventricular pacing). Although VDD pacing offers no advantages to DDD pacing, interest in this pacemaker lies in the single-pass lead.

Rate-Adaptive Pacing

Rate-adaptive pacing permits physiologically appropriate electrical stimulation of the myocardium in response to the metabolic and circulatory demands of the body occurring during exercise or stress (84,85). In 1996, 83% of all generators implanted had rate-adaptive capabilities. In the elderly, who represent more than 85% of pacemaker recipients, rate-adaptive pacing offers benefits over fixed-rate ventricular pacing with respect to quality of life. In chronotropically incompetent patients, rate-adaptive pacing has improved exercise capacity and quality of life. The metabolic and circulatory burden is typically monitored by sensors (i.e., piezoelectric crystals) that detect motion, vibration, pressure, or acceleration. Newer sensors can measure minute ventilation or the QT interval. These sensors may provide a heart rate more responsive to the demands of the body. Although the common activity and accelerometer sensors respond more quickly at the onset of exercise, the respiration-based sensors respond slower but more smoothly.

Mode Switching

When atrial tachyarrhythmias occur in patients with conventional DDD or DDDR pacemakers, inappropriate atrial

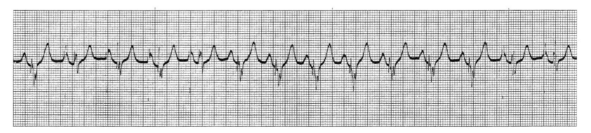

FIGURE 10-14. DDD: dual-chamber paced rhythm, atrial and ventricularly inhibited and atrially triggered. The lower rate limit is programmed to 85. The patient's spontaneous atrial rate is close to the lower rate limit. Atrially tracked ventricular pacing alternates with dual-chamber paced rhythm.

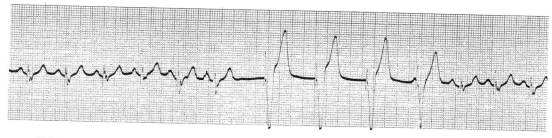

FIGURE 10-15. VDD: atrially tracked, ventricularly inhibited pacing. During sinus arrest, the escape is a ventricular-paced rhythm.

tracking may culminate in an undesirable acceleration of the ventricular pacing rate. Newer pulse generators incorporate sensor-driven algorithms to prevent tracking of the sustained atrial activity by "switching" the pacemaker mode from DDD or DDDR to VVI or VVIR (86). The algorithm reverts the pacemaker back to DDD or DDDR mode after termination of the atrial tachyarrhythmia.

Follow-up Evaluation and Assessment of Pacemaker Function

Patients with implantable cardiac pacemakers require organized and meticulous follow-up to ensure patient safety, optimal device performance, and detection of intervening clinical events that influence device function. Current generations of implantable pacemakers include significant functions that relate to arrhythmia monitoring, generator and lead system performance, and in the near term, even clinical data that are stored in device memory.

The need for organized follow-up should be discussed with patients before insertion of a permanent pacemaker system. It should be performed at outpatient clinics with appropriately trained personnel and instrumentation designed to ensure comprehensive device system follow-up. These facilities should have access to an inpatient pacemaker program for device replacement and troubleshooting. Pacemaker follow-up has several goals:

1. Monitoring device functions
2. Optimizing performance for maximal clinical effectiveness and system longevity
3. Minimizing complications
4. Anticipating replacement of system components
5. Ensuring timely intervention for clinical events
6. Patient education and support
7. Patient and device tracking

Pacemaker follow-up can be individualized but should include the elements needed for optimal results. Because pacemaker prescriptions are initiated at device system implantation, they should be recorded at implantation and reevaluated before hospital discharge. All prescriptions and system function should be reevaluated at 1 month after a new system implantation to ensure continuing appropriate function without intercurrent difficulties and after 3 months for finalization of the device parameters after lead system maturation. Subsequently, uncomplicated single-chamber systems are evaluated annually and dual-chamber systems at 6-month intervals. However, additional evaluations may be needed in the clinic as the clinical situation dictates. Transtelephonic follow-up is an important aid for these patients, particularly in unstable or pacemaker-dependent populations. This function is performed at monthly intervals in some programs.

The major elements of follow-up include pacemaker site inspection and evaluation of lead threshold and integrity using pacing threshold testing and impedance measurements. After implantation, the wound site should be checked within 1 week for proper healing and at each visit for evidence of infection or erosion. In general, lead thresholds rise immediately after implantation for 2 to 6 weeks and then decrease with lead maturation by 3 months. They usually settle at values somewhat greater than at implantation but may return to implantation levels. Programming should maintain a safety margin with output being at twice or thrice threshold levels. There is a diurnal variation in thresholds, and newer devices have features for automatic threshold measurements between clinical visits. Some newer devices can adjust output to minimal levels, achieving stable capture (i.e., *autocapture*) to maximize battery longevity. With careful attention to these parameters and features, device longevity can be significantly prolonged. Generator status was often evaluated by magnet pacing rates but is now more often judged using battery voltage and impedance measurements obtained at interrogation. Nevertheless, a magnet test remains part of the evaluation with a simultaneous rhythm strip, and a 12-lead ECG is obtained if needed. Device detection of intrinsic cardiac activity is measured using the sensed electrogram amplitudes in the atrium and ventricle, and the lowest amplitude detection parameter that consistently detects this electrogram is referred to as the *sensing threshold*. Absence of intrinsic activity, referred to as *pacemaker dependency*, should be documented for each patient.

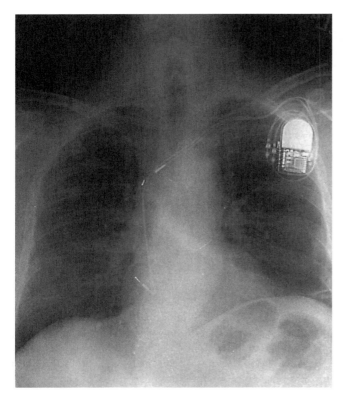

FIGURE 10-16. Posteroanterior chest radiograph demonstrates ventricular lead dislodgment into the right atrium.

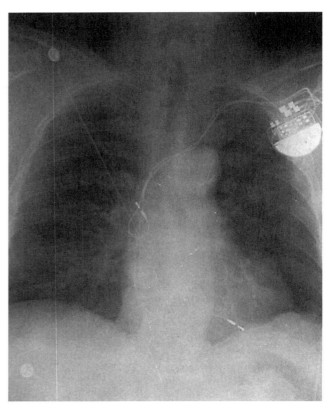

FIGURE 10-17. Posteroanterior chest radiograph demonstrates atrial lead dislodgment into the superior vena cava.

Posteroanterior and lateral chest radiographs should be obtained at implantation and considered annually. Lead position should be radiographically verified before hospital discharge. Radiography should be invariably performed if there are changes or abnormalities in system function that could involve lead system problems (Figs. 10-16 and 10-17).

Current pacemakers often include specialized functions that require interrogation and response. These include percentage pacing, spontaneous arrhythmias detected by such devices, and sensor functions. The behavior of individual rate-response sensors is beyond the scope of this discussion. Nevertheless, the common activity and accelerometer sensors respond quickly but abruptly at the onset of exercise, whereas respiration-based sensors respond slower but more smoothly. Exercise testing is necessary to ensure correct performance of these sensors at a full range of exercising heart rates. Some devices incorporate dual sensors, requiring specialized assessment and setup.

Pacemaker system surveillance is intensified if there are problems detected in the follow-up program related to its function or after a predetermined period based on manufacturers recommendations when generators approach end of life. The latter may require 3-monthly or even monthly follow-up to determine the exact timing of generator replacement.

Pacemaker Malfunction and Complications

Failure to Pace Appropriately

Pacing malfunctions can result from pulse generator stimulus output failure or inability of an appropriately timed stimulus to capture the myocardium (Fig. 10-18A). Differentiation is based on detection of pacing stimulus. In the latter situation, a pacing stimulus should be seen on the surface ECG or the telemetered intracardiac electrogram from the pacemaker. A full 12-lead ECG should be obtained before concluding there is no stimulus pulse, because bipolar stimuli can fail to be detected on an individual ECG lead.

Absence of the pacing stimulus output on an ECG recording can result from battery depletion, device malfunction due to system component failure (generator or lead), or inhibition of pacemaker output due to oversensing. Device diagnostics should indicate whether a pulse is being emitted by the generator, the battery is depleted (low voltage, high impedance) or there are sensed events. Alternatively, in the absence of a programmer and if the lead system is intact, placing the pulse generator in asynchronous mode by magnet application can show synchronous pacing stimuli, which may help differentiate the causes. If oversensing occurs, initiation of pacemaker output and capture

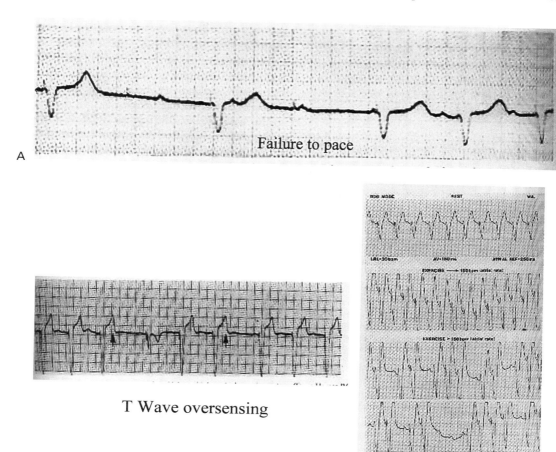

FIGURE 10-18. Complications of pacing systems. **A:** Failure to pace in response to the pacing stimulus. **B:** Oversensing of T wave and skeletal myopotentials during exercise with suppression of ventricular pacing output.

ensues in magnet mode. The absence of pacemaker output in magnet mode signifies battery depletion, lead fracture, or device component failure.

Failure to capture the myocardium can be caused by lead fracture or dislodgment, deterioration of lead insulation, increase in pacing threshold, battery depletion, or a loss of system integrity at the generator-lead interface (Figs. 10-16, 10-17, and 10-19). Device diagnostics often help elucidate whether pacing failure is related to lead or device malfunction. Impedance changes for one or more leads favor lead-related problems such as dislodgment, fracture or lead-generator connection disruption (i.e., increase in impedance), or insulation deterioration (i.e., decrease in impedance). Posteroanterior and lateral chest radiographs demonstrating the entire lead system from cardiac location to generator connection are needed to exclude these causes (Fig. 10-20).

Increasing the pacing stimulus output should initiate organized cardiac depolarizations if the tissue-electrode interface is involved because of an increase in stimulation threshold. Diaphragmatic stimulation by a ventricular lead should prompt concern regarding ventricular perforation, and echocardiographic studies are warranted to exclude pericardial effusion. In its most extreme form, cardiac tamponade can coexist with failure to capture. If the cause is still unknown despite all these studies, operative assessment of the leads, pulse generator, and their connections is warranted.

Failure to Sense Appropriately

Undersensing occurs when the pacemaker fails to appropriately recognize a spontaneous cardiac depolarization and emits an inappropriately timed stimulus output (Fig. 10-21). This can occur if the sensing circuit is disabled, such as by a magnet, or the sensing circuit input signal amplitude or wave shape is inadequate and does not pass through the sensing filter to trigger the threshold detector. Respiratory or other positional changes can affect the bipolar R-wave amplitude to cause undersensing. It is imperative to obtain adequate sensed signal amplitudes relative to generator circuit sensitivity thresholds to minimize these complications.

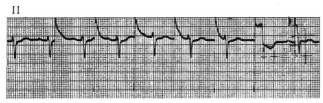

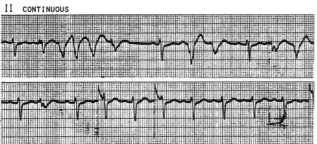

3 HOURS POST-IMPLANTATION PERMANENT PACEMAKER   A.S. 30 JULY, 1979

FIGURE 10-19. VVI pacing with lead dislodgment. This series of tracings demonstrates intermittent failure to sense and failure to capture, but when capture occurs, it results in a change in the expected morphology of the evoked potential, in this case showing an upright complex in lead II rather than the expected inverted complex if the lead were properly seated in the apex of the right ventricle. The unstable lead within the ventricle mechanically induces complex ventricular ectopy.

Lead repositioning may be needed. This problem can be corrected by increasing the sensitivity of the sensing circuit (i.e., lowering the sensing threshold).

Undersensing of cardiac events can result in inappropriately timed pacing, such as pacing on T waves, potentially triggering ventricular arrhythmias. In the immediate period after pacemaker insertion, undersensing can be caused by lead dislodgment or edema at the myocardium-lead interface. Undersensing may occur at a later stage because of fibrosis at the electrode-endomyocardial interface, lead fracture, or battery depletion. Improved lead designs with active fixation leads to prevent lead dislodgment and steroid-eluting electrodes, decreasing local tissue inflammation, and fibrotic repair have diminished the prevalence of these forms of sensing malfunction.

Oversensing occurs when the pacemaker senses unwanted physiologic or nonphysiologic signals (Fig. 10-18B). The sensing amplifier looks at the voltage difference across the electrodes (i.e., anode and cathode). The longer separation between the anode and cathode in unipolar systems creates a large sensing antenna. This results in excellent sensing of intracardiac signals with enhanced susceptibility to external signals, such as myopotentials from skeletal muscle (Fig. 10-18B). Oversensing is much less common in patients with bipolar pacing systems. These closely spaced electrodes make the sensing system relatively insensitive to far-field signals. Crosstalk, the inappropriate

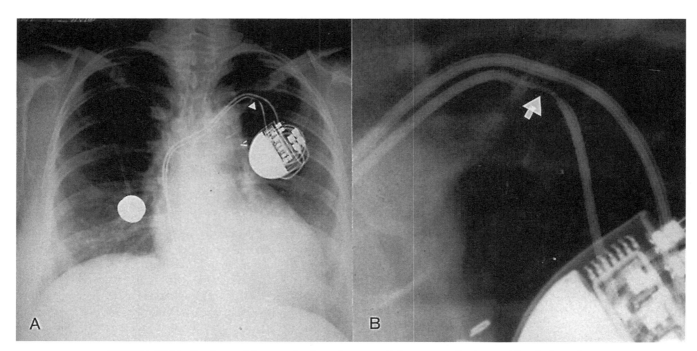

FIGURE 10-20. Fracture of the proximal conductor and damage to the internal insulation of a bipolar coaxial lead caused by rib-clavicle crush after implantation 6 months earlier by direct subclavian venipuncture. **A:** Full chest radiograph. **B:** Close-up view of the damaged area of the lead, showing the intact distal conductor with absence of the proximate conductor.

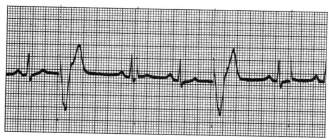

J.R. BUMC 683001 1-28-88

FIGURE 10-21. Undersensing with the pacemaker failing to sense native R waves occurring during the alert period. The stimuli that fail to capture do so because the myocardium is physiologically refractory at those times; hence, there is also functional noncapture. When the stimulus occurs at a time when the myocardium is capable of being depolarized, there is normal capture.

sensing of an atrial stimulus by the ventricular channel or vice versa, also occurs predominantly in unipolar systems (87) (Fig. 10-22).

Sensing of electrical events other than spontaneous cardiac depolarizations can inhibit normal pacemaker function. The diagnosis of oversensing is made by documenting electrocardiographically inappropriate inhibition of pacemaker output in the absence of a spontaneous cardiac event. These sensing errors occasionally may be resolved by protective mechanisms within the pulse generator if the event is recognized as being detected as distinct from a spontaneous cardiac depolarization. Oversensing commonly occurs as in some clinical scenarios, such as arm exercises causing myopotential interference or exposure to an electromagnetic field. System malfunction from a loose set screw, lead insulation break, lead conductor fracture, and current leaks may also result in oversensing. With bipolar leads, oversensing of near-field intracardiac signals (i.e., T

II

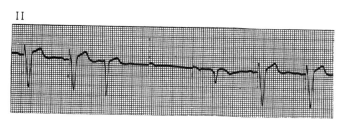

FIGURE 10-22. Crosstalk-mediated ventricular output inhibition in a dual-unipolar DDD pacing system. The first two and last two cycles show normal atrial synchronous ventricular pacing. After a ventricular ectopic beat, there is release of an atrial output pulse that captures the atrium but is not followed by a visible ventricular event, paced or sensed. The interval to the next atrial stimulus is slightly longer than the atrial escape interval, compatible with the ventricular channel having sensed an event right after the atrial output pulse was released. This second atrial stimulus is not followed by a visible ventricular event within the programmed atrioventricular delay. The patient is protected by a ventricular escape beat.

waves) can occur. This latter event can usually be managed by decreasing the sensitivity setting, such as by increasing the amplitude of the minimum sensed electrogram or prolonging the postventricular blanking period. P-wave oversensing is uncommon and may occur if the catheter location is near the right ventricular inflow tract. Repositioning the catheter is usually necessary.

Lead System Failure

Lead system failure manifests a potentially serious clinical dilemma, often requiring surgical intervention. Pacemaker lead fractures and lead insulation failures are relatively infrequent complications in the early history of system performance but can become more prevalent as a system ages. In contrast, lead dislodgment is most common in the immediate postoperative period. Impedance changes are useful in the diagnosis of lead-related complications because of lead conductor resistance or electrode-myocardial interface changes. A rise in impedance may reflect exit block or indicate complete or partial lead fracture, whereas a decline usually implies loss of insulation integrity in a lead fracture.

Lead dislodgment is a common lead system complication after implantation, occurring in 1% to 2% of atrial lead implants and in less than 1% of ventricular lead implants. Coronary sinus lead implants are particularly vulnerable, with more than 10% in some locations demonstrating these problems. It is best diagnosed by testing sensing and pacing in the newly implanted pacing system before hospital discharge and obtaining routine radiographs after system implantation (Figs. 10-16 and 10-17). Patients should be reevaluated at 1 and 3 months after system implantation for this purpose. Although minor dislodgment may be addressed by sensing and pacing reprogramming, significant dislodgments require reoperation and repositioning of the lead.

Lead conductor fracture occurs when there is a lack of electrical conductivity within the lead. A complete fracture manifests as complete absence of pacing stimuli as seen on the ECG. More commonly, an intermittent presentation is seen with failure of lead function periodically as the lead conductor intermittently fails to make electrical contact. There is intermittent presence of a pacing stimulus artifact on the ECG. An intermittent conductor fracture can show inappropriate sensing and erratic pacing. An overpenetrated chest radiograph may help to definitively confirm the presence of a fracture.

Lead insulation failure may occur because of implant technique issues or as a consequence of material failure, such as in polyurethane-insulated leads introduced in the 1970s. A disruption in the lead insulation of any magnitude may result in oversensing. A large break in the insulation may culminate in failure to capture because of current shunting and result in local stimulation into the tissue at the site of fracture. This can be seen as pectoral stimulation in patients with unipolar configurations (Fig. 10-19). Lead impedance is typically reduced and can correlate with the degree of insulation failure. Treatment entails lead replacement and, rarely, insulation repair.

Lead perforation is an important complication and should be monitored during system implantation and immediately after follow-up. It is identified by sensing and pacing difficulties despite apparent right heart positioning, pericardial or other extracardiac bleeding with a low cardiac output state, hypotension, or venous congestion with confirmatory evidence by echocardiographic or chest radiograph (Fig. 10-4). Repositioning of the lead is employed if feasible and deemed safe and usually results in resolution of the problem. Occasionally, draining of tamponade or closure of cardiac tear or injury by surgical intervention is needed. Open-chest surgery is sometimes needed to prevent serious morbidity or mortality. Prompt thoracic surgical consultation should be obtained in such patients.

Lead Removal

Extraction of previously implanted pacing leads is increasingly practiced. The primary indication for this procedure remains pacing system infection, as discussed subsequently (Table 10-15). An increasingly used indication is removal of leads demonstrating a failure mode, particularly with the potential for intracardiac injury. In one experience with the Accufix lead, a retention wire used for the preformed J fractured with extrusion, and intracardiac perforation occurred and warranted lead removal.

TABLE 10-15. INDICATIONS FOR PACEMAKER LEAD REMOVAL

Class I
Infection of lead (primary or secondary to pocket infection)
Malignant arrhythmias due to lead
Physical threat to patient
Absence of other venous access
Interference with device operation

Class II
Localized infection of generator
Chronic pain
Potential but not imminent threat
Interference with other therapy needed by patient
Nonfunctional leads in a young patient
Sterile lead section cut and isolated

Class III
Risk of removal outweighs lead retention risk
Single nonfunctional lead in older patient
Reusable and reliable lead
Relative Contraindications
Calcified leads
Patient is not a candidate for thoracotomy
Unavailable extraction equipment
Anomalous anatomy at insertion

Prophylactic removal is also practiced, but the risk-benefit ratio in noncompromised leads may not favor lead extraction. The risk of lead extraction procedures is estimated at 1% risk for major complications, including death. These procedures are best performed at experienced centers by physicians trained in such procedures.

Common Pacemaker Problems Related to System Performance on Follow-up

Several common pacing problems identified during follow-up are related to system performance.

Hysteresis

Hysteresis is a feature first introduced in single-chamber pacing systems and is being included in increasing numbers of dual-chamber pacing systems. It can be misinterpreted as a pacing system problem when pacing stimuli are absent. In a pacemaker programmed with hysteresis, the escape interval of the pacemaker is significantly longer than the rate at which it will pace, and the escape pacing rate is slower than the automatic basic pacing interval (88). The original goal of hysteresis was to allow the patient who only intermittently and infrequently required pacing support to remain in a normal native rhythm, even at low rates, when pacing was not required. When AV block developed such that pacing was required, sustained pacing at a very slow rate would be hemodynamically compromising. At these times, hysteresis would allow for the faster paced ventricular rate required (Fig. 10-23).

Frequent Mode Switching

Frequent mode switching is seen in newer dual-chamber pacemakers with this feature. The feature is designed to detect atrial arrhythmias and revert from the dual-chamber pacing mode to prevent inappropriate tracking of atrial signals in the DDD mode. This feature also may be activated if there is oversensing. Device interrogation of the event to see the atrial electrogram is essential to confirm the presence of an atrial arrhythmia and to evaluate for oversensing on the atrial channel. If atrial arrhythmias occur frequently,

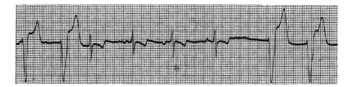

FIGURE 10-23. VVI pacing system programmed to a base rate of 70 bpm, with a hysteresis escape rate of 50 bpm. The native sinus rate preceding the pause is 68 bpm; the pacemaker escapes at a rate of 50 and then discharges at a rate of 70 ppm.

therapy is indicated based on the clinical scenario. Management of oversensing is performed using the guidelines indicated previously.

Proarrhythmic Syndromes

There are two forms of pacemaker-mediated proarrhythmia. The first can occur when undersensing and an inappropriate pacing stimulus trigger a supraventricular or ventricular tachycardia. After the tachycardia is initiated, the pacemaker becomes a bystander if inhibited by the arrhythmia or can continue to undersense and trigger during the arrhythmia (89).

In contrast, pacemaker-mediated tachycardias require active participation of the pacemaker to maintain the sustenance of the arrhythmia. Pacemaker-mediated tachycardias may occur in atrial fibrillation or flutter with some degree of AV block if the device senses the pathologic atrial activity and triggers a paced tachycardia near the maximum tracking rate (90) (Fig. 10-24). In effect, it functions as an accessory conduction pathway.

The classic form of pacemaker-mediated tachycardia, also referred to as *endless-loop tachycardia*, requires retrograde conduction from the ventricle to the atrium, with this atrial depolarization triggering the pacing output (91) (Fig. 10-25). Endless-loop tachycardia can only occur in patients who sustain ventriculoatrial conduction, have retrograde P waves that can be sensed by the atrial channel, or have an inciting trigger causing ventricular depolarization such as a ventricular ectopic beat.

Electrocardiographically, retrograde P waves are seen best in leads II, III, and aVF after the premature beat triggering the tachycardia and can help make the diagnosis (92). The resultant loss of AV synchrony may result in a constellation of symptoms referred to as pacemaker syndrome. Prolonging the blanking period after ventricular pacing or therapy to block ventriculoatrial conduction may be effective in resolving the problem.

Pacemaker Syndrome

Pacemaker syndrome is a clinical condition in patients treated by ventricular pacing characterized by symptoms of venous

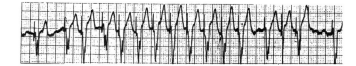

FIGURE 10-24. A form of pacemaker-mediated tachycardia in a patient with high-grade atrioventricular block, with a chronic VDD pacing system, who developed atrial fibrillation. The fibrillatory waves are being sensed on the atrial channel and interpreted as true P waves by the pacemaker, triggering ventricular outputs at rates up to the programmed maximum tracking rate.

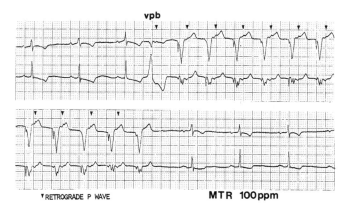

FIGURE 10-25. Classic induction of an endless-loop pacemaker-mediated tachycardia started by a ventricular premature beat (vpb) and running at the programmed maximum tracking rate (MTR). The downward arrowheads identify the retrograde P wave. The retrograde pathway fatigued, resulting in the spontaneous termination of this tachycardia and restoration of sinus rhythm. This was a dual unipolar pacing system. The diminutive pacing stimulus is an artifact of the high-frequency filters in the Holter recording system from which this rhythm was documented.

congestion and low forward cardiac output (93,94) (Fig. 10-26). These symptoms may include dyspnea, cough, chest discomfort, jugular venous distention with cannon a waves, nausea, fatigue with diminished exercise tolerance, dizziness, presyncope, and syncope. Diagnosis requires careful clinical evaluation being correlated with demonstration of ventricular pacing during the event. Ventricular pacing at rates comparable to sinus or atrial pacing produces significant (>30 mm Hg) decrease in blood pressure (Fig. 10-26). Invasive studies such as right heart catheterization and arterial pressure monitoring are occasionally necessary to confirm the diagnosis.

Pacemaker syndrome occurs more often in patients with impaired cardiac function because of diastolic or systolic abnormalities. It occurs in up to 30% of all patients implanted with ventricular-based pacing systems in prospective trials. It usually appears within 1 month and nearly always within 3 to 6 months of system implantation. Late appearance may be spurious or triggered by changes in ventricular function. Atrial or dual-chamber pacing is the treatment of choice in patients with pacemaker syndrome.

Pacemaker System Infection

Infection of the pacemaker system can be a serious and potentially fatal complication because of the risk of endocarditis and its sequelae. Local pocket infection most commonly occurs after implantation and is often caused by *Staphylococcus aureus*. Late infection is rarer, with *Staphylococcus epidermis* being the most likely culprit. The potential exists for development of subacute or acute bacterial endocarditis, suppurative myocarditis, and pancarditis. Patients with implanted pacemakers should receive prophylactic antibiotics when undergoing procedures with bacteremic

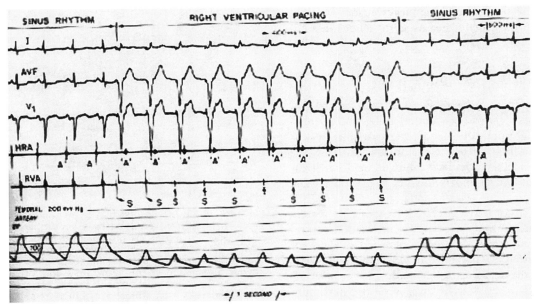

FIGURE 10-26. Pacemaker Syndrome Hemodynamic Impact. Pacemaker syndrome resulting from ventricular pacing in a patient with a noncompliant left ventricle.

potential, such as dental surgery, and if inadvertent invasion of the pocket region occurs with surgery in the same region as the pacing system.

Patients with pocket or system infection typically have subtle symptoms manifesting as a persistent febrile illness coupled with local signs of pocket swelling, erythema, or tenderness. The appearance of a collection in a pacemaker pocket is a source of immediate concern and should prompt consultation with a pacemaker surgeon. Symptoms of subacute bacterial endocarditis in a paced patient should prompt concern about a pacing system infection.

Erosion of the pacemaker pocket is a late surgical complication that can result in infection or occur because of infection. In the former situation, it occurs more often in excessively laterally located pockets or tightly sewn pockets with pressure at the generator's edges. As the unit erodes, it tends to get infected. If the unit is not infected, it is referred to as a *dry erosion.*

Initial treatment for infection includes broad-spectrum intravenous antibiotics, immediate removal of the pulse generator and lead system, and local pocket drainage with culture to direct long-term antibiotic therapy. After healing is complete, which may take 6 to 12 weeks, implantation of a new pacemaker system at a different site is performed. Temporary pacing may be necessary in dependent patients during the period that antibiotic therapy is needed.

Electromagnetic Interference

Electromagnetic interference usually results from high-frequency electrical signals (95–97). In the presence of elec-

tromagnetic interference, the sensing circuit has difficulty differentiating electrical noise from spontaneous cardiac depolarizations. When electromagnetic interference is sensed, it causes the pacemaker to function inappropriately, such as suppressing output or pacing in an asynchronous manner. This latter protective mechanism is employed in newer devices to avoid the potential for asystole. With improvements in circuit design, only strong electrical fields close to the pacemaker system can cause electromagnetic interference. Such exposure may occur in the medical environment with exposure to radiation therapy, magnetic resonance imaging, surgical procedures involving electrocautery, and direct current shock cardioversion.

Therapeutic radiation for a malignancy can cause unpredictable effects on implanted pacemakers (98,99). The radiation can punch holes in the silicon dioxide substrate that forms the basis of the integrated circuits that control the pacemaker.

The mechanism by which electrocautery, cardioversion, and defibrillation, all of which deliver a large amount of energy to the body, can damage the implanted pacing system is virtually identical (100–102). Occasionally, these techniques can damage the circuitry or reprogram the pacemaker. Manufacturers have incorporated a variety of circuits, most commonly employing Zener diodes, designed to protect the complex electronics of the pacemaker from a voltage surge of 12 V or greater.

When external cardioversion or defibrillation is performed, the paddles should be as far from the pulse generator as possible. In the pacemaker-dependent patient, programming the system to an asynchronous mode (VOO or

DOO) at the beginning of a surgical procedure has been recommended. Alternatively, a magnet placed over the pacemaker disables all sensing, producing a VOO or DOO mode.

Magnetic resonance imaging generates a very strong electromagnetic field, and although no pulse generator has been reported to be adversely programmed or damaged, pacing system inhibition and asynchronous behavior have been reported while the device is in the MRI field (103,104). Magnetic resonance imaging is contraindicated because of interference with the magnetic field by the device and should not be used for these patients.

Interaction between pacemakers and electronic surveillance systems using electromagnetic fields in the 10- to 300-Hz range has resulted in pacemaker inhibition, asystole in dependent patients, and crosstalk with resulting ECG patterns (105,106). In one report, interference with the pacemaker function of an implanted defibrillator has also been documented.

Interference introduced by cellular phones has been widely publicized but is largely restricted to some analog phone models with prolonged proximity to the pacemaker generator during active use (98,99). Typical use may involve placement in a shirt pocket and use of the device on the ipsilateral ear to the pacemaker. Newer digital phones do not have such interactions, and patients should be cautioned regarding the interaction of analog models with close exposure. Exposure of the implanted pacing system to any of these modalities or procedures should be avoided. Placement of a magnet over the generator can disable the sensing circuit and can be used for short-term protection.

REFERENCES

1. Furman S, Hayes DL, Holmes D Jr. *A practice of cardiac pacing,* 3rd ed. Armonk, NY: Futura Publishing, 1998.
2. Bernstein AD, Camm AJ, Fletcher RD, et al. The NASPE/BPEG generic pacemaker code for antibradyarrhythmic and adaptive-rate pacing and antitachyarrhythmia devices. *Pacing Clin Electrophysiol* 1987;10:794.
3. Bernstein AD, Camm AJ, Fisher JD, et al. The NASPE/BPEG defibrillator code. *Pacing Clin Electrophysiol* 1993;16:1776.
4. St Wirtz HD, et al. Reliability of different temporary myocardial pacing leads. *Thorac Cardiovasc Surg* 1989;37:163.
5. Haffajee CI. Temporary cardiac pacing: modes, evaluation of function, equipment and trouble shooting. *Cardiol Clin* 1985;6:515.
6. Gould BA, Marshall AJ. Noninvasive temporary pacemakers. *Pacing Clin Electrophysiol* 1988;11:1331.
7. Falk RH, Zoll PM, Zoll RH. Safety and efficacy of noninvasive cardiac pacing: a preliminary report. *N Engl J Med* 1983;309:1166.
8. Zoll PM, Zoll RH, Falk RH, et al. External noninvasive cardiac pacing: clinical trials. *Circulation* 1985;71:937.
9. Silver MD, Goldschlager N. Temporary transvenous cardiac pacing in the critical setting. *Chest* 1988;93:607.
10. Del Negro AA, Fletcher RD. Indications for and use of artificial cardiac pacemakers: part II. *Curr Probl Cardiol* 1978;3:1.
11. Col JJ, Weinberg SL, The incidence and mortality of intraventricular conduction defects in acute myocardial infarction. *Am J Cardiol* 1972;29:344–350.
11a. Goldberg R. Prognosis of acute myocardial infarction complicated by complete heart block: the Worcester Heart Attack Study. *Am J Cardiol* 1992;69:1135.
12. Hindman M. The clinical significance of bundle branch block complicating acute myocardial infarction. 1. Clinical characteristics, hospital mortality and one year follow-up. *Circulation* 1978;58:679.
13. Hindman MC, Wagner GS, Ja Ro M, et al. The clinical significance of bundle branch block complicating acute myocardial infarction. 2. Indication for temporary and permanent pacemaker insertion. *Circulation* 1978;58:689–699.
14. Lamas G. A simplified approach to predicting the occurrence of complete heart block during acute myocardial infarction. *Am J Cardiol* 1986;57:1213.
15. Gregoratos G, Cheitlin MD, Conill A, et al. ACC/AHA guidelines for implantation of cardiac pacemakers and antiarrhythmic devices: a report of the American College of Cardiology/American Heart Association Task Force on practice guidelines (Committee on Pacemaker Implantation). *J Am Coll Cardiol* 1998;31:1175–1209.
16. Dorostkar PC, Eldar M, Belhassen B, Scheinman MM. Long-term follow-up of patients with long-QT syndrome treated with beta-blockers and continuous pacing. *Circulation* 1999;100:2431.
17. Eldar M, Griffin JC, Van Hare G, et al. Combined use of beta adrenergic blocking agents and long-term cardiac pacing for patients with the long QT syndrome. *J Am Coll Cardiol* 1992;20:830–837.
18. Gerstenfeld EP, Hill MRS, French SN, et al. Evaluation of right atrial and biatrial temporary pacing for the prevention of atrial fibrillation after coronary artery bypass surgery. *J Am Coll Cardiol* 1999;33:1981.
19. Chung MK, Augostini RS, Asher CR, et al. Ineffectiveness and potential proarrhythmia of atrial pacing for atrial fibrillation prevention after coronary artery bypass grafting. *Ann Thorac Surg* 2000;69:1057.
20. Blommaert D, Gonzalez M, Mucumbitsi J, et al. Effective prevention of atrial fibrillation by continuous atrial overdrive pacing after coronary artery bypass surgery. *J Am Coll Cardiol* 2000;35:1411.
21. Greenberg MD, Katz NM, Iuliano S, et al. Atrial pacing for the prevention of atrial fibrillation after cardiovascular surgery. *J Am Coll Cardiol* 2000;35:1416.
22. Parsonnet V, Bernstein AD, Galasso AD. Cardiac pacing practices in the United States, 1985. *Am J Cardiol* 1988;62:71.
23. Albin G, Hayes DL, Holmes DR. Sinus node dysfunction in pediatric and young adult patients: treatment by implantation of a permanent pacemaker in 39 cases. Mayo Clin Proc 1985;60:667.
24. Skagen K, Hansen JF. The long term prognosis for patients with sinoatrial block treated with permanent pacemaker. *Acta Med Scand* 1975;199:13.
25. Connolly SJ, Kerr C, Gent M, et al. Effects of physiologic pacing versus ventricular pacing on the risk of stroke and death due to cardiovascular causes. Canadian Trial of Physiologic Pacing Investigators. *N Engl J Med* 2000;342:1385–1391.
26. Lamas G, Pashos CL, Normand SL, McNeil B. Permanent pacemaker selection and subsequent survival in elderly Medicare pacemaker recipients. *Circulation* 1995;91:1063–1069.
27. Lamas GA, Orav EJ, Stambler BS, et al, for the Pacemaker Selection in the Elderly Investigators. Quality of life and clinical outcomes in elderly patients treated with ventricular pacing as compared to dual-chamber pacing. *N Engl J Med* 1998;338:1097.

28. Andersen HR, Nielsen JC, Thomsen PEB, et al. Long-term follow-up of patients from a randomised trial of atrial versus ventricular pacing for sick-sinus syndrome. *Lancet* 1997;305:1210–1216.

29. Berger PB, Ruocco NA, Ryan TJ, et al. Incidence and prognostic implications of heart block complicating inferior myocardial infarction treated with thrombolytic therapy: results from TIMI II. *J Am Coll Cardiol* 1992;20:533–540.

30. Archbold RA, Sayer JW, Ray S, et al. Frequency and prognostic implications of conduction defects in acute myocardial infarction since the introduction of thrombolytic therapy. *Eur Heart J* 1998;19:893.

31. Harpaz D, Behar S, Gottlieb S, et al, for the SPRINT Study Group and the Israeli Thrombolytic Survey Group. Complete atrioventricular block complicating acute myocardial infarction in the thrombolytic era. *J Am Coll Cardiol* 1999;34:1721.

32. Newby KH, Pisano E, Krucoff MW, et al. Incidence and clinical relevance of the occurrence of bundle-branch block in patients treated with thrombolytic therapy. *Circulation* 1996;94:2424.

33. Rosen KM, Dhingra RC, Loeb HS, et al. Chronic heart block in adults: clinical and electrophysiological observations. *Arch Intern Med* 1973;131:663.

34. Michaelsson M, Jonzon A, Reisenfeld T. Isolated congenital complete atrioventricular block in adult life: a prospective study. *Circulation* 1995;92:442–449.

35. Pinsky WW, Gillette PC, Garson A Jr, McNamara DG. Diagnosis, management, and long-term results of patients with congenital complete atrioventricular block. *Pediatrics* 1982;69:728–733.

36. Mymin D, Mathewson FA, Tate RB, Manfreda J. The natural history of primary first-degree atrioventricular heart block. *N Engl J Med* 1986;315:1183–1187.

37. Morady F, Higgins J, Peters RW, et al. Electrophysiologic testing in bundle branch block and unexplained syncope. *Am J Cardiol* 1984;54:587–591.

38. Scheinman MM, Peters RW, Modin G, et al. Prognostic value of infranodal conduction time in patients with chronic bundle branch block. *Circulation* 1997;56:240–244.

39. Denes P, Dhingra RC, Wu D, et al. Sudden death in patients with chronic bifascicular block. *Arch Intern Med* 1977;137:1005–1010.

40. Dhingra RC, Denes P, Wu D, et al. The significance of second degree atrioventricular block and bundle branch block: observations regarding site and type of block. *Circulation* 1974;49:638–646.

41. Dhingra RC, Wyndham C, Bauernfiend R, et al. Significance of block distal to the His bundle induced by atrial pacing in patients with chronic bifascicular block, *Circulation* 1979;60:1455–1464.

42. Englund A, Bergfeldt L, Rehnqvist N, et al. Diagnostic value of programmed ventricular stimulation in patients with bifascicular block: a prospective study of patients with and without syncope. *J Am Coll Cardiol* 1995;26:1508–1515.

43. Ezri M, Lerman BB, Marchlinski FE, et al. Electrophysiologic evaluation of syncope in patients with bifascicular block. *Am Heart J* 1983;106:693–697.

44. McAnulty JH, Rahimtoola SH, Murphy E, et al. Natural history of "high risk" bundle branch block: final report of a prospective study. *N Engl J Med* 1982;307:137.

45. Strasberg B, Amat-Y-Leon F, Dhingra RC, et al. Natural history of chronic second-degree atrioventricular nodal block. *Circulation* 1981;63:1043–1049.

46. Olshansky B, Hahn EA, Hartz VL, et al, for the ESVEM Investigators. Clinical significance of syncope in the Electrocardiographic Study Versus Electrocardiographic Monitoring (ESVEM) trial. *Am Heart J* 1999;137:878.

47. Dhingra RC, Palileo E, Strasberg D, et al. Significance of the HV interval in 517 patients with chronic bifascicular block. *Circulation* 1981;64:1265.

48. Scheinman MM, Peters RW, Sauve MJ, et al. The value of the HQ interval in patients with bundle branch block and the role of prophylactic pacing. *Am J Cardiol* 1982;50:1316.

49. Sugrue DD, Gersh BJ, Holmes DR, et al. Symptomatic "isolated" carotid sinus hypersensitivity: natural history and results of treatment with anticholinergic drugs or pacemaker. *J Am Coll Cardiol* 1986;7:158–162.

50. Connolly SJ, Sheldon R, Roberts RS, Gent M, on behalf of the Vasovagal Pacemaker Study Investigators. The North American Vasovagal Pacemaker Study (VPS): a randomized trial of permanent cardiac pacing for the prevention of vasovagal syncope. *J Am Coll Cardiol* 1999;33:16–20.

51. Sutton R, Brignole M, Menozzi C, et al. Dual-chamber pacing in the treatment of neurally mediated tilt-positive cardioinhibitory syncope: pacemaker versus no therapy: a multicenter randomized study *Circulation* 2000;102:294.

52. Sra JS, Jazayeri MR, Avitall B, et al. Comparison of cardiac pacing with drug therapy in the treatment of neurocardiogenic (vasovagal) syncope with bradycardia or asystole. *N Engl J Med* 1993;328:1085–1090.

53. Peterssen ME, Chamberlain-Webber R, Fitzpatrick AP, et al. Permanent pacing for cardioinhibitory malignant vasovagal syndrome *Br Heart J* 1994;71:274–281.

54. Saksena S, Goldschlager N. *Electrical therapy for cardiac arrhythmias.* Philadelphia: WB Saunders, 1990.

55. Gillis AM, Wyse G, Connolly SJ, et al, for the Atrial Pacing Periablation for Paroxysmal Atrial Fibrillation (PA3) Study Investigators. Atrial pacing periablation for prevention of paroxysmal atrial fibrillation. *Circulation* 1999;99:2553.

56. Attuel P, Pellerin D, Mugica J, Coumel P. DDD pacing: an effective treatment modality for recurrent atrial arrhythmias. *Pacing Clin Electrophysiol* 1988;11:1647.

57. Garrigue S, Barold SS, Cazeau S, et al. Prevention of atrial arrhythmias during DDD pacing by atrial overdrive. *Pacing Clin Electrophysiol* 1998;21:1751.

58. Daubert C, Mabo P, Berder V, et al. Atrial tachyarrhythmias associated with high degree interatrial conduction block: prevention by permanent atrial resynchronization. *Eur J Clin Pacing Electrophysiol* 1994;4:435.

59. Prakask A, Delfaut P, Krol RB, Saksena S. Regional right and left atrial activation patterns during single- and dual-site atrial pacing in patients with atrial fibrillation. *Am J Cardiol* 1998;82:1197.

60. Saksena S, Prakash A, Hill M, et al. Prevention of recurrent atrial fibrillation with chronic dual-site right atrial pacing. *J Am Coll Cardiol* 1996;28:687.

61. Yu WC, Chen SA, Tai CT, et al. Effects of different atrial pacing modes on atrial electrophysiology: implicating the mechanism of biatrial pacing in the prevention of atrial fibrillation. *Circulation* 1997;96:2992.

62. Saksena S, Praksh A, Hill M, et al. Prevention of recurrent atrial fibrillation with chronic dual site right atrial pacing. *J Am Coll Cardiol* 1996;28:687–694.

63. Fananapazir L, Epstein ND, Curiel RV, et al. Long-term results of dual-chamber (DDD) pacing in obstructive hypertrophic cardiomyopathy: evidence for progressive symptomatic and hemodynamic improvement and reduction of left ventricular hypertrophy. *Circulation* 1994;90:2731–2742.

64. Gadler F, Linde C, Daubert C, et al. Significant improvement of quality of life following atrioventricular synchronous pacing

in patients with hypertrophic obstructive cardiomyopathy: data from 1 year of follow-up. PIC study group: Pacing In Cardiomyopathy. *Eur Heart J* 1999;20:1044.

65. Kappenberger L, Linde C, Daubert C, et al. Pacing in hypertrophic obstructive cardiomyopathy (PIC): a randomized crossover study. *Eur Heart J* 1997;18:1249–1256.

66. Maron BJ, Nishimura RA, McKenna WJ, et al, for the M-PATHY Study Investigators. Assessment of permanent dual-chamber pacing as a treatment for drug-refractory symptomatic patients with obstructive hypertrophic cardiomyopathy: a randomized, double-blind crossover study (M-PATHY). *Circulation* 1999;99:2927–2933.

67. Nishimura RA, Hayes DL, Ilstrup DM, et al. Effect of dual-chamber pacing on systolic and diastolic function in patients with hypertrophic cardiomyopathy: acute Doppler echocardiographic and catheterization hemodynamic study. *J Am Coll Cardiol* 1996;27:421–430.

68. Linde C, Gadler F, Edner M, et al. Results of atrioventricular synchronous pacing with optimized delay in patients with severe congestive heart failure *Am J Cardiol* 1995;75:919–923.

69. Brecker SJ, Xiao HB, Sparrow J, Gibson DG. Effects of dual-chamber pacing with short atrioventricular delay in dilated cardiomyopathy. *Lancet* 1992;340;1308–1312.

70. Nishimura RA, Hayes DL, Holmes DR, Tajik AJ. Mechanism of hemodynamic improvement by dual-chamber pacing for severe left ventricular dysfunction: an acute Doppler and catheterization study. *J Am Coll Cardiol* 1995;25:281–288.

71. Kerwin WF, Botvinick EH, O'Connell JW, et al. Ventricular contraction abnormalities in dilated cardiomyopathy: effect of biventricular pacing to correct interventricular dyssynchrony *J Am Coll Cardiol* 2000;35:1221.

72. Kass DA, Chen CH, Curry C, et al. Improved left ventricular mechanics from acute VDD pacing in patients with dilated cardiomyopathy and ventricular conduction delay. *Circulation* 1999;99:1567.

73. Gold MR, Feliciano Z, Gottlieb SS, et al. Dual chamber pacing with short atrioventricular delay in congestive heart failure: a randomized study *J Am Coll Cardiol* 1995;26:967–973.

74. Hochleitner M, Hortnagl H, Fridrich L, Gochnitzer F. Long-term efficacy of physiologic dual chamber pacing in the treatment of end stage idiopathic dilated cardiomyopathy. *Am J Cardiol* 1992;70:1320–1325.

75. Deshmukh P, Casavant DA, Romanyshyn M, Anderson K. Permanent, direct His-bundle pacing: a novel approach to cardiac pacing in patients with normal His-Purkinje activation. *Circulation* 2000;101:869–877.

76. Scott CD, Dark JH, McComb JM, et al. Sinus node function after cardiac transplantation. *J Am Coll Cardiol* 1994;24:1334–1341.

77. Jacquet L, Ziady G, Stein K, et al. Cardiac rhythm disturbances early after orthotopic heart transplantation: prevalence and clinical importance of the observed arrhythmias. *J Am Coll Cardiol* 1990;16:832.

78. Woodward DA, Conti JB, Mills RM, et al. Permanent atrial pacing in cardiac transplant patients. *Pacing Clin Electrophysiol* 1997;20:2398.

79. Aziz TM, Burgess MI, El-Gamel A, et al. Orthotopic cardiac transplantation technique: a survey of current practice [In process citation]. *Ann Thorac Surg* 1999;68:1242.

80. Gallagher JJ, Svenson R, Kasell SH, et al. Catheter technique for closed-chest ablation of the atrioventricular conduction system: a therapeutic alternative for the treatment of refractory supraventricular tachycardia. *N Engl J Med* 1982;306:194–200.

81. Williamson BD, Ching Man K, Daoud E, et al. Radiofrequency catheter modification of atrioventricular conduction to control the ventricular rate during atrial fibrillation. *N Engl J Med* 1994;331:910.

82. Curtis AB, Kutalek SP, Prior M, et al. Prevalence and characteristics of escape rhythms after radiofrequency ablation of the atrioventricular junction: results from the registry for AV junction ablation and pacing in atrial fibrillation. Ablate and Pace Trial Investigators. *Am Heart J* 2000;139:122.

83. Hamdan MH, Page RL, Sheehan CJ, et al. Increased sympathetic activity after atrioventricular junction ablation in patients with chronic atrial fibrillation. *J Am Coll Cardiol* 2000;36:151.

84. Higano ST, Hayes DL, Eisinger G. Sensor-driven rate smoothing in a DDDR pacemaker. *Pacing Clin Electrophysiol* 1989;12:922.

85. Hayes DL, Higano ST, Eisinger G. Electrocardiographic manifestations of a dual-chamber, rate-modulated (DDDR) pacemaker. *Pacing Clin Electrophysiol* 1989;12:555.

86. Kamalvand K, Tan K, Kotsakis A, et al. Is mode switching beneficial? A randomized study in patients with paroxysmal atrial tachyarrhythmias. *J Am Coll Cardiol* 1997;30:496.

87. Combs WJ, Reynolds DW, Sharma AD, Bennett TD. Cross-talk in bipolar pacemakers. *Pacing Clin Electrophysiol* 1989;12:1613.

88. Rosenqvist M, Vallin HO, Edhag KO. Rate hysteresis pacing: how valuable is it? A comparison of the stimulation rates of 70 and 50 bpm and rate hysteresis in patients with sinus node disease. *Pacing Clin Electrophysiol* 1984;7:332.

89. Luceri RM, Ramirez AV, Castellanos A, et al. Ventricular tachycardia produced by a normally functioning AV sequential demand (DVI) pacemaker with "committed" ventricular stimulation. *J Am Coll Cardiol* 1983;1:1177.

90. Greenspon AJ, Greenberg RM, Frankl WS. Tracking of atrial flutter during DDD pacing: another form of pacemaker-mediated tachycardia. *Pacing Clin Electrophysiol* 1984;7:955.

91. Frumin H, Furman S. Endless loop tachycardia started by an atrial premature complex in a patient with a dual chamber pacemaker. *J Am Coll Cardiol* 1985;5:707.

92. den Dulk K, Lindemans FW, Wellens HJ. Noninvasive evaluation of pacemaker circus movement tachycardias. *Am J Cardiol* 1984;53:537.

93. Ausubel K, Furman S. The pacemaker syndrome. *Ann Intern Med* 1985;103:420.

94. Heldman D, Mulvhill D, Nguyen H, et al. True incidence of pacemaker syndrome. *Pacing Clin Electrophysiol* 1990;13:1742.

95. Mathew P, Lewis C, Neglia J, et al. Interaction between electronic article surveillance systems and implantable defibrillators: insights from a fourth generation ICD. *Pacing Clin Electrophysiol* 1997;20:2857–2859.

96. Mugica J, Henry L, Podeur H. Study of interactions between permanent pacemakers and electronic antitheft surveillance systems. *Pacing Clin Electrophysiol* 2000;23:333.

97. Wilke A, Kruse T, Hesse H, et al. Interactions between pacemakers and security systems. *Pacing Clin Electrophysiol* 1998;21:1784.

98. Venselaar JL, Van Kerkoerle HL, Vet AJ. Radiation damage to pacemakers from radiotherapy. *Pacing Clin Electrophysiol* 1987;10:538.

99. Rodriguez F, Filimonov A, Henning A, et al. Radiation-induced effects in multiprogrammable pacemakers and implantable defibrillators. *Pacing Clin Electrophysiol* 1991;14:2143.

100. Levine PA, Balady GJ, Lazar HL, et al. Electrocautery and pacemakers: management of the paced patient subject to electrocautery. *Ann Thorac Surg* 1986;41:313.

101. Levine PA, Barold SS, Fletcher RD, Talbot P. Adverse acute and chronic effects of electrical defibrillation and cardioversion on implanted unipolar cardiac pacing systems. *J Am Coll Cardiol* 1983;1:1413.

102. Lamas GA, Antman EM, Gold JP, et al. Pacemaker backup-mode reversion and injury during cardiac surgery. *Ann Thorac Surg* 1986;41:155.

103. Hayes DL, Holmes DR, Gray JE. Effect of 1.5 Tesla nuclear magnetic resonance imaging scanner on implanted permanent pacemakers. *J Am Coll Cardiol* 1987;10:782.

104. Erlebacher JA, Cahill PT, Pannizzo F, Knowles RJ. Effect of magnetic resonance imaging on DDD pacemakers. *Am J Cardiol* 1986;57:437.

105. Irnrich W, Batz L, Muller R, et al. Electromagnetic interference of pacemakers by mobile phones. *Pacing Clin Electrophysiol* 1996;19:1431.

106. Hayes DL, Wang PJ, Reynolds D, et al. Interference with cardiac pacemakers by cellular telephones. *N Engl J Med* 1997;336:1473.

11

IMPLANTABLE CARDIOVERTER-DEFIBRILLATORS

N. A. MARK ESTES, III
DAVID CANNOM

In the three decades since Dr. Michel Morowski conceived of a miniature defibrillator, which would be implanted to detect and terminate ventricular tachycardia (VT) or ventricular fibrillation (VF), there has been a remarkable evolution of the technology and clinical utility of the implantable cardioverter-defibrillator (ICD) (1–5). Five years after the first human implant in 1980, the Food and Drug Administration (FDA) approved the ICD for widespread clinical use in February 1985. Since then, there have been multiple technological advances in the ICD, resulting in improved detections and therapy, enhanced stored diagnostic information, smaller size, and easier implantation (6–46). There also has been an evolution in lead technology, development of biphasic waveforms and the use of an active defibrillation electrode, resulting in reduction in the defibrillation energy requirements and device size.

During the last several years, multiple clinical reports and trials, which have incorporated the ICD as a therapy limb, have defined the risks and benefits of device therapy (46–73). This chapter provides an overview of the basic hardware, ICD function, diagnostic storage capabilities, indications, implantation techniques, complications, and follow-up of the ICD. In addition, the multiple clinical trials that have clarified the role of the ICD in the primary and secondary prevention of sudden cardiac death are reviewed (46–73).

The first-generation ICDs were capable of recognizing only VF and delivering committed high-energy shock therapy with only data about the total number of shocks stored and retrievable (2–5). Their use was reserved for individuals who had survived at least two episodes of cardiac arrest and had failed pharmacologic therapy (2). The first device implanted in a human in February 1980 sensed arrhythmias during a transcardiac (superior vena cava spring electrode to left ventricular apical epicardial patch) modified bipolar electrocardiographic signal. The initial device, known as the automatic implantable defibrillator, had no heart rate detection criteria and no cardioverting capability. It employed a relatively crude detection algorithm called the probability density function for arrhythmia sensing (3). The probability density function essentially assessed the amount of time the ventricular electrogram was at the isoelectric line. It was very sensitive and specific for VF but less sensitive for VT. Even with technical limitations in this early device, it became clear that it was effective in sensing and defibrillating VF. Subsequently, single-chamber VVI pacing capability was added to second-generation devices. With the addition of detection enhancements, antitachycardia pacing, low-energy cardioversion, and additional diagnostics including stored electrograms, so-called third-generation devices have provided a considerably wider range of programmability. Nonthoracotomy lead (NTL) systems, along with refinement of waveforms and use of "active can" devices, have resulted in lowering of the defibrillation thresholds (DFTs). Pectoral implantation of smaller devices has become routine, performed in the electrophysiology laboratory without the assistance of a cardiothoracic surgeon (3,16,22). More recently, dual-chamber, rate-responsive pacemakers with mode-switching capabilities have been incorporated into an ICD that is now capable of antitachycardia pacing, low-energy cardioversion, and high-energy defibrillation for ventricular arrhythmias. With the addition of cardioversion capability in the atrium for atrial fibrillation (74–81), atrial flutter, or other atrial arrhythmias, dual-chamber defibrillators currently offer bradycardia and tachycardia therapy for atrial and ventricular arrhythmias. The features of currently available generation devices are shown in Table 11-1.

N. A. Mark Estes, III: Department of Medicine, Tufts University School of Medicine, and the Department of Cardiac Arrhythmia Services, New England Medical Center Hospitals, Boston, Massachusetts 02111.

D. Cannom: Department of Cardiology, Hospital of the Good Samaritan, and the Department of Medicine, University of California at Los Angeles School of Medicine, Los Angeles, California 90017.

TABLE 11-1. AVAILABLE IMPLANTABLE CARDIOVERTER-DEFIBRILLATORS

Manufacturer	Model	Weight (g)	Volume (mL)	Maximum Energy	Brady Mode+	Detection Enhancements			
						Onset	Stability	Morph	AV
Biotronik									
	Micro Phylax	89	54	30 J	VVI	+	+	−	−
	Phylax AV*	109	69	30 J	DDD	+	+	−	+
ELA									
	Defender IV DR*	140	75	33 J	DDDR	+	+	−	+
Guidant									
	PRx III	179	97	34 J	VVI	+	+	−	−
	Mini	125	68	33 J	VVI	+	+	−	−
	Mini II	115	59	30 J	VVI	+	+	−	−
	Mini III	90	48	31 J	VVI	+	+	−	−
	Mini IV	78	39	31 J	VVI	+	+	−	−
	AV	150	79	33 J	DDD	+	+	−	+
	AV II	136	73	31 J	DDD	+	+	−	+
	AV II DR	136	73	31 J	DDDR	+	+	−	+
	AV III DR	108	58	31 J	DDDR	+	+	−	+
	VR	94	51	31 J	VVIR	+	+	−	−
Medtronic									
	Jewel	132	83	34 J	VVI	+	+	−	−
	Micro Jewel	116	72	34 J	VVI	+	+	−	−
	Micro Jewel II	97	54	30 J	VVI	+	+	+	−
	Gem	90	49	35 J	VVIR	+	+	+	−
	Gem DR	115	62	35 J	DDDR	+	+	−	+
	Gem II Dr	77	39	30 J	DDDR	+	+	−	+
	Jewel AF*	93	55	27 J	DDD	+	+	−	+
Ventritex									
	Cadet	129	73	750 V	VVI	+	+	−	−
	Contour	109	57	750 V	VVI	+	+	−	−
	Contour II	109	57	750 V	VVI	+	+	−	−
	Contour MD	109	57	750 V	VVI	+	+	+	−
	Angstrom II	90	44	750 V	VVI	+	+	−	−
	Angstrom MD	90	44	750 V	VVI	+	+	+	−
	Profile MD	70	34	800 V	VVI	+	+	+	−

*Investigational; +, bradycardia pacing mode.

BASIC HARDWARE: ELEMENTS OF AN ICD

In its most elemental form, the ICD consists of (a) a lead system for monitoring cardiac electrical signals and delivering electrical therapy and (b) a generator, which senses and interprets signals using logic circuitry and algorithms to make decisions regarding delivery of therapy (1–5). The generator is also a power source that finally delivers the desired therapy through the lead system. In contrast to output energies of pacemakers, which are on the order of 25 μJ per pulse, with associated current in the milliampere range, the ICD delivers shocks with energies on the order of approximately 30 J (1–5). To accomplish this, the device's battery must provide currents of 1 to 2 A for approximately 10 seconds to properly charge the high-voltage internal capacitors. The original ICD used mercury zinc batteries, although this battery technology had many limitations and could not reliably produce the high-energy current requirement (2). Lithium iodine batteries have been in use for more than two decades, but they are characterized by a large capacity but only a limited ability to provide a rapid charge (2). The optimal batteries for defibrillator application should have a low self-discharge rate and a predictable discharge characterization, should be safe and reliable for implantation, and should have the ability to deliver high-peak currents (2). Lithium vanadium pentoxide batteries, originally developed for NASA applications in the mid-1960s, were used for the first clinical implantable defibrillators (1–5). These batteries could sustain a current train of 2 A and had a capacity of 800 mA per hour. To guard against any leakage from components, manufacturers sealed the batteries inside a titanium case. Because the batteries provide only approximately 3.2 or 6.4 V when two are employed in a series, direct current to direct current voltage-converter circuits are used to generate the high voltage needed to charge the capacitors, which provide the high-energy shock. Since the late 1980s, lithium silver vanadium pentoxide, a further refinement in defibrillator battery technology, has become most commonly used (2). This technology provides better energy densities and lower internal resistance (2).

Capacitors represent the electronic components that store the electrical charge on the battery (2). In ICDs, a low-voltage battery is used to transport the necessary charge to the capacitors over a period of several seconds (1–5). The capacitors serve to accumulate and store the charge at a high voltage (up to 750 V). Therapy is then delivered by discharging the stored energy into the lead system for a relatively short time (approximately 10 ms) (1–5). The original capacitor used in devices were aluminum electrolytics and they were developed as an offshoot of photoflash units. These capacitors have been refined but still use aluminum electrolytic capacitors. They are two conductor plates separated by an insulator (1–5). Generally, they are constructed of two thinly rolled aluminum films separated by ammonium borate electrolyte. This results in the formation of aluminum oxide on the surface of the anode plate with the application of voltage (2). This oxide provides the thin dielectric layer, which separates the two conductive films to constitute a capacitor (2). The remaining electrode then functions as the cathode. Because deformation reduces the capacitor performance and results in a prolonged charge time, the dielectric layer must be periodically reformed by charging the capacitor. This occurs during the application of therapeutic shock or during periodic maintenance capacitor reformations (1–5).

Defibrillation Waveforms

Earlier ICDs incorporated a monophasic waveform for delivering defibrillating shocks. It has become clear that there are multiple advantages to biphasic waveforms, which are now routinely used in ICDs (7). Biphasic waveforms are associated with a lower DFT compared with that of the truncated monophasic shocks used in the older systems. The current generated by transvenous systems uses bipolar defibrillation between two coils, one located in the right ventricle and the other in a more proximal location (7,8). The two coils are generally placed on a single-pass transvenous lead (7,8). Biphasic waveforms, in addition to the bipolar defibrillation, have considerably lowered the defibrillation and energy requirements. More recently, ICDs have incorporated the titanium shell of the ICD can into the lead system. A shock is delivered between the shell (active or hot can) and the distal coil of the transvenously implanted lead with the coil located in the right ventricle (unipolar defibrillation).

ICD Evaluation

External implant support devices formerly played an important role in the assessment of DFTs, R waves, and thresholds at the time of implantation. They allowed for testing of R wave, threshold, and rate-sensing impedance, for sensing during ventricular arrhythmias, and for programming of specific waveforms for checking DFTs. However, implant support devices are rarely used at the time of ICD implantation. By contrast, device-based testing in which the ICD,

once placed in the pocket, is actually programmed with a sterile header is used in almost all implantations. This is possible because it is rare for the DFTs to be too high for initial device placement and because there is an algorithm available for self-testing of the device.

Communication with the ICD was initially performed by using a ring magnet (1–5). In the first-generation ICD, this controlled functions such as turning the device on and off. In addition, the charging cycle could be initiated and the charge time of the capacitors would be used as an indication of battery status. More recently, telemetry through the use of radiofrequency links has had the ability to control ICD functions. Currently, there is a wide range of programmability for detection, therapy, and diagnostics including high-fidelity reproductions of rate-sensing and shock electrograms from the defibrillating leads. These modifications permit a wide range of programmability, allowing physicians to tailor specific "tiered therapy" including antitachycardia pacing, low-energy cardioversion, and high-energy shocks and the retrieval of extensive diagnostic information from the ICD (23–29, 31,35).

Nonthoracotomy Lead Systems

The NTL systems have been associated with a marked reduction in implantation morbidity and mortality rates and a higher efficacy rate (44,59). Endocardial NTLs are implanted through the venous system using techniques similar to those used for the implantation of permanent pacemaker leads. These NTL systems sense the underlying myocardial activity in a bipolar fashion between a distal rate-sensing lead and a distal coil-integrated bipolar lead or between distal electrodes (dedicated bipolar). First-generation ICDs had no ventricular pacing for bradycardias, although second-generation ICDs had single-chamber ventricular pacing. However, if the patient had the clinical indication for pacing, a separately implanted pacemaker was used because ICD longevity could be significantly reduced by low-impedance pacing leads. More recently, single- and dual-chamber ICDs use high-impedance pacing electrode technology similar to that used in conventional pacing systems. This thereby allows permanent pacing through the ICD without the need for a separately implanted pacemaker. Developmental efforts are underway to optimize sensing by the atrial and ventricular leads, focusing on reduction in lead size using new materials and design, to improve handling characteristics, as controlled release of steroids and other substances to minimize pacing threshold rises can optimize sensing in the atrial and ventricular lead. In addition, new materials are being sought to improve long-term reliability (8,44,59). It is probable that pacing and shocking lead standards (IS-1 and DS-1) will be modified in the future to allow for reduction in connector/header size.

Detection Enhancements

Earlier ICDs were capable of delivering therapy based only on the patient's heart rate. Subsequently, a simple circuit with relatively modest computing requirements was developed to measure the probability density function (2). To minimize the delivery of inappropriate shocks for rhythms other than VT or VF, a number of detection enhancements have been added to the latest generation ICDs (23–29). With earlier devices, inappropriate shocks caused by sinus tachycardia, atrial fibrillation, or supraventricular arrhythmias occurred in approximately 30% to 40% of patients. To enhance the specificity of the ICD for detecting VT or VF, detection enhancements have been incorporated into algorithms in all current devices (23–29). These enhancements include onset, morphology, stability, and in dual-chamber devices, atrial lead discriminators. Typically with sinus tachycardia, the heart rate gradually accelerates (23–29), unlike with VT in which there is generally an abrupt increase in heart rate from the patient's baseline native rhythm (Fig. 11-1). Onset criteria were developed to discriminate sinus tachycardia from VT. To decrease inappropriate therapy for atrial fibrillation, stability algorithms have been developed to assess the degree of regularity or irregularity of the tachycardia. With these algorithms, consecutive R-R intervals are monitored and compared with an average of the preceding cycle length. These algorithms have the ability to discriminate VT from rapid atrial fibrillation (23–29). Morphology discrimination algorithms compare the morphology of the ventricular rate-sensing electrogram QRS complex with sinus rhythm when threshold heart rate is reached. During sinus rhythm, atrial fibrillation, and supraventricular arrhythmias, the conduction impulses pass through the atrioventricular node and the intracardiac electrogram morphology is similar to that in sinus rhythm when the rate exceeds the device rate cutoff (23–29). Occasionally, rate-related bundle branch blocks may change the morphology of the local electrograms during supraventricular arrhythmias, thereby decreasing the specificity of the algorithm.

In dual-chamber devices, the relationship of the atrial electrograms to the ventricular electrograms can be assessed (81–83) (Fig. 11-2A–D). A number of different sophisticated algorithms have been developed to assess whether the atrial rate is greater than the ventricular rate, thereby making it likely that the patient is having atrial fibrillation, atrial flutter, or atrial tachycardia. When the ventricular rate is greater than the atrial rate, it is extremely likely that the patient is having VT or VF (81–83). If there is 1 : 1 conduction through the atrioventricular node and the atrial electrogram precedes the ventricular electrogram with a PR shorter than the R-P interval, it is highly probable that this represents sinus tachycardia or supraventricular arrhythmias. The clinical use of these algorithms, which can be used alone or in conjunction with each other, is still being assessed. Onset and stability have been shown to increase the specificity of the ICD in classifying ventricular and atrial arrhythmias, but there is an associated decrease in sensitivity for VF and VT. It has been found that by refining the program of onset and stability, inappropriate treatment of atrial arrhythmias can be

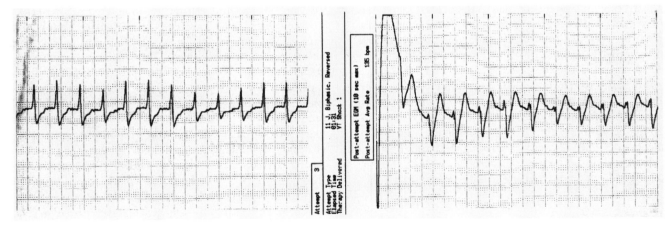

FIGURE 11-1. Shock therapy for sinus tachycardia. Stored shock electrograms from an implantable cardioverter-defibrillator are shown after the patient had received an asymptomatic shock. The patient had previously been documented to have therapy for sinus tachycardia with loop monitoring. Based on this, β-blocker therapy had been started and the rate cutoff for therapy had been increased from 130 to 145 beats per minute (bpm). A monitor zone had shown a gradual acceleration of the patient's rate to 148 bpm before the 11-J shock. The electrograms before shock therapy were identical to those in normal sinus rhythm from this patient. After an 11-J shock, the electrograms widen and shift axis, as is commonly observed transiently after shock delivery. The rhythm gradually slows. Based on this, the patient's β-blocker therapy was increased. However, because the patient had sustained monomorphic VT with a rate of 154 bpm, no change in the rate cutoff was made.

```
PG Configuration
Tachy Mode                          Monitor+Therapy
Tachy Zones                                        2
Last Programmed                     26-MAY-99 11:12
```

```
VT Zone

Initial Detection
 Rate                               170 to 210 bpm
  Interval                          353 to 286 ms
 Duration                                  2.5 sec
 Onset                                     OFF %
 And/Or                                    --
 Stability
  Inhibit if Unstable                      OFF ms
  Shock if Unstable                        OFF ms
 A Fib Rate Threshold                      OFF bpm
  A Fib Stability                          -- ms
 V Rate > A Rate                           --
 Sustained Rate Duration                   -- min:sec

Redetection
 Redetect Duration                         1.0 sec
 Post-shock Duration                       1.0 sec
 Post-shock Stability                      OFF ms
 Post-Shock A Fib Rate Threshold           OFF bpm
  Post-shock A Fib Stability               -- ms
 Post-shock V Rate > A Rate                --
 Post-shock Sustained Rate Duration        -- min:sec

ATP Therapy:                        ATP1        ATP2
 Scheme                          Ramp/Scan    Disabled
 Number of Bursts                    2          OFF




 Pulses per Burst
  Initial                            8         --
  Increment                          0         --
  Maximum                           --         --
 Coupling Interval                  81 %       -- --
  Decrement                          0 ms      -- ms
 Burst Cycle Length                 81 %       -- --
  Ramp Decrement                     6 ms      -- ms
  Scan Decrement                     6 ms      -- ms
 Minimum Interval                  200 ms      -- ms
 ATP Time-Out                     1:00 min:sec

Shock Therapy
 Shock 1                                     5 J
 Shock 2                                    31 J
 Max Shocks                                 31 J
```

```
VF Zone

Initial Detection
 Rate                               ≥ 210 bpm
  Interval                          ≤ 286 ms
 Duration                                1.0 sec

Redetection
 Redetect Duration                       1.0 sec
 Post-shock Duration                     1.0 sec

Shock Therapy
 Shock 1                                   31 J
 Shock 2                                   31 J
 Max Shocks                                31 J
```

A

FIGURE 11-2. A: Programmed parameters for dual-chamber tiered therapy in an implantable cardioverter-defibrillator (ICD). Programmed parameters for ventricular tachycardia (VT) and ventricular fibrillation (VF) detection and therapy are shown in a tiered-therapy ICD. The VT zone is configured to deliver therapy for rates of 170 to 210 beats per minute (bpm) with two bursts of antitachycardia pacing followed by low-energy cardioversion with 5 J followed by maximum shock therapy with 31 J. The VF zone is configured to deliver shock therapy for rates of more than 210 bpm with 31 J. **B:** Stored electrograms and event markers in a dual-chamber tiered-therapy ICD. Stored atrial **(top)** and ventricular **(middle)** rate-sensing electrograms and shock electrograms **(bottom)** from a dual-chamber tiered-therapy ICD. Event markers with arrows indicate atrial-sensed events *(AS)* with interval in milliseconds between events. Also, ventricular sensed *(VS)* and paced *(VP)* events and sensed ventricular electrograms in the VT zone *(VT)* for rates from 170 to 210 bpm are indicated. A premature ventricular contraction in normal sinus rhythm initiates VT with VA conduction. One burst of antitachycardia pacing results in termination of the VT with a posttherapy rate of 102 bpm and atrial sensing with ventricular pacing.

(continued on next page)

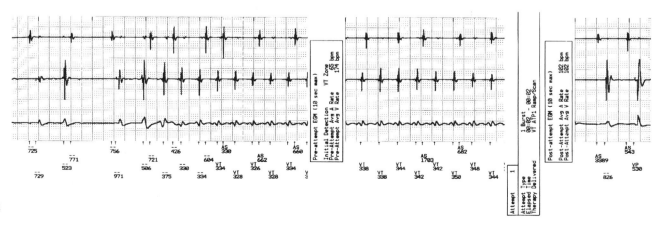

B

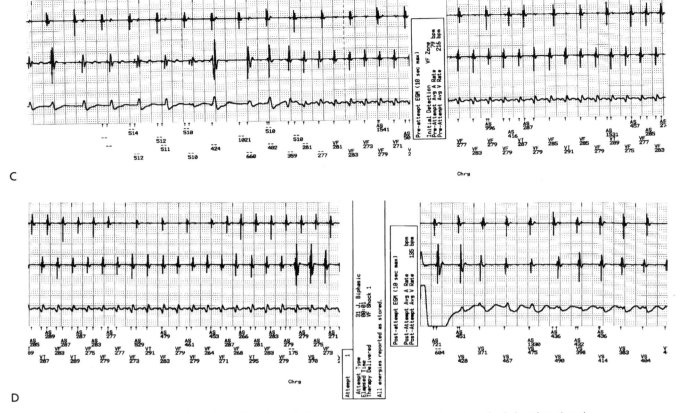

FIGURE 11-2. *(continued)* **C:** Stored electrograms and event markers in a dual-chamber tiered-therapy ICD. The stored electrograms and event markers are shown from the same ICD in Figure 11-2B and are displayed with an identical format. A premature ventricular contraction with a coupling interval of 424 ms initiates a rapid VT with a rate of 216 bpm and intermittent VA conduction. **D:** Maximum shock therapy, 31 J, results in restoration of normal sinus rhythm.

decreased by up to 95%. However, this is achieved at the expense of sensitivity for detection of VT with a resulting absolute decrease in sensitivity by as much as 10% (81–83). The inappropriate failure to detect VF or VT obviously can have life-threatening consequences. To that extent, clinicians are reluctant to use onset and stability criteria unless they have been proven safe in the individual patient (23–29, 81–83). Similarly, based on limited clinical data, morphology discrimination increases the specificity for detection of ventricular arrhythmias but at the cost of sensitivity. Further clinical research is needed to determine the optimal combination of programming detection enhancements.

Diagnostic Storage Capabilities

First-generation ICDs had only a simple counter that registered the number of therapy episodes (1–5). The diagnostic storage capabilities have grown exponentially since early devices. Electrophysiologists initially had to rely on the presence or absence of symptoms to assess the appropriateness of shocks. This classification scheme had many limitations, as 30% to 40% of all shocks were in fact for atrial fib-

rillation, sinus tachycardia, or supraventricular arrhythmic episodes (34–36,81–83). Today's devices provide extensive information regarding each episode including time, date, R-R intervals, shock-lead impedance, stored electrograms, and event markers (Tables 11-1 and 11-2). The use of R-R intervals alone was shown to confer a high degree of sensitivity and specificity for rhythm classification (23–29, 34–36,81–83). Atrial fibrillation is typically irregular with R-R intervals varying by more than 80 ms. Rapid ventricular rhythms (more than 200 beats per minute [bpm]) generally represent VT or VF (23–29,34–36,81–83). A gradual increase in the heart rate to the tachycardia zone commonly represents sinus tachycardia. By contrast, sudden onset of a regular tachycardia from the patient's baseline rhythm most likely represents supraventricular arrhythmias or monomorphic VT (23–29,34–36,81–83).

Information regarding the impedance for each shock lets the electrophysiologist assess the integrity of the high-voltage system. An increase in lead impedance of a high-voltage shock may indicate a lead fracture. A decrease in impedance generally represents an insulation break. Sensing and pacing abnormalities can be assessed from stored electrograms and

TABLE 11-2. STORED DIAGNOSTIC DATA

Implant data
  Device serial number and manufacturer
  Implant date
  Implanting physician
  Lead serial number and manufacturer
Shock counters
  Cumulative for device
  Since last cleared with dated cleared
  Number of detections in each zone
    Number of detections resulting in delivered therapy
    Number of detections resulting in aborted therapy
Episode data
  Rate, cycle length, date, and time of detected tachycardia
  Stability and onset of tachycardia
  Therapy delivered
  Energy delivered
  Shock impedance
  RR intervals
  Marker channels
  Electrograms
  Rate histograms
  Thresholds, R wave, P wave, lead impedances, percentage
    pacing

from real-time measures to identify sensing or pacing abnormalities (23–29,34–36,81–83). In this respect, the ability to distinguish signals that represent noise intrinsic to the system, such as environmental noise, has clinical utility in identifying factors that result in inappropriate therapy. The stored and real-time electrograms can be recorded from the shock or the rate-sensing lead.

The ability to store electrograms of the patient's rhythm before, during, and after an episode of tachycardia has been a major advance in classification of arrhythmias (Fig. 11-2A–D). When the morphology is different from the patient's native rhythm, it generally indicates a ventricular arrhythmia or aberrant conduction. Stored and real-time electrograms have clinical utility in assessing undersensing and oversensing, oversensing of T wave, environmental noise, and diaphragmatic signals that can result in device therapy or inhibition of pacing (23–29,34–36,81–83). In addition, analysis of stored electrograms have given valuable insights into the mechanism of onset of various supraventricular and ventricular arrhythmias (23–24,34–36,81–83). With the dual-chamber devices currently available, atrial and ventricular electrograms can be stored simultaneously, allowing assessment and refinement of detection algorithms, which rely on the atrioventricular relationship (81–83).

IMPROVEMENT IN TACHYCARDIA TERMINATION

Sustained monomorphic VT can usually be terminated by antitachycardia pacing or low-energy cardioversion with current-tiered therapy devices (3,33,44,46).

Antitachycardia Pacing

Multiple-pacing schemes have been evaluated to assess efficacy for termination (3,33,44,46). Refinement of antitachycardia pacing techniques has allowed for a greater success rate in termination of sustained tachycardias (3,33,44, 46). The strategies for antitachycardia pacing include single-capture methods such as scanning extrastimuli or multiple-capture techniques including multiple extrastimuli, burst, ramp (autodecremental), shifting bursts, scanning bursts, scanning ramps, and incremental-decremental pacing rates (3,33,44,46). The most useful algorithms employ simple burst pacing alone or in combination with adaptive or scanning algorithms (3,33,44,46). Adaptive modes introduce pacing as a percentage of the basic VT cycle length, typically in the range of 80% to 90% of the cycle length (3,33,44,46). This can be used with scanning that introduces each successive pacing train with increased prematurity until the tachycardia is terminated (3,33,44,46). Generally, antitachycardia pacing algorithms should be tested for efficacy with noninvasive programmed stimulation, although empiric antiarrhythmic pacing has been shown to have similar success rates to those of tested algorithms (3,33,44,46). Generally, tested or empirical pacing algorithms have success rates of approximately 90% in terminating sustained monomorphic VT with arrhythmia acceleration occurring in approximately 5% of tachycardias (3,33,44,46). No mode of pacing has proven clearly superior with regard to efficacy or risk of acceleration (3,33,44, 46).

The electrophysiologists have considerable flexibility in the number of stimuli, cycle length, coupling interval, and repetition sequences that can be programmed. Commonly, ramp pacing with 4 to 12 pulses are used with a rate-adaptive algorithm. The coupling interval is specified as the percentage of the cycle length of the tachycardia ranging from approximately 90% to 70% of the VT cycle length (3,33, 44,46). With a rate-adaptive algorithm, there is a decrement in the percentage of the tachycardia cycle length between trains. Some algorithms also allow for decrementing within each train. However, as one paces more rapidly, particularly at cycle lengths of less than 250 ms, a 1 : 1 relationship between the pacing stimulus and the ventricular capture may not occur, and acceleration of the tachycardia is more likely. It is generally recommended that the lower limit of such pacing trains be 70% of the VT cycle length. When acceleration does occur after antitachycardia pacing, cardioversion or defibrillation is used to reestablish sinus rhythm (3,33,44,46).

Tiered therapy or hierarchical antitachycardia therapy is incorporated into all current ICDs. Multiple zones of therapy are defined by the tachycardia rate, with the slower tachycardias, typically treated with antitachycardia pacing before low-energy cardioversion and finally high-energy shocks. A lower and upper rate for each zone is programmed. Many rapid tachycardias can be treated with more aggressive burst pacing techniques or low-energy cardioversion. Tachycardias that are rapid or accelerated by burst pacing are treated with high-energy cardioversion or defibrillation. A zone for "monitoring" has been incorporated into some devices, which allows for storage of events and a data log by the ICD without therapy delivery.

Low-Energy Cardioversion

In addition to antitachycardia pacing, low-energy cardioversion can be used to terminate episodes of hemodynamically tolerated sustained monomorphic VT (33,52). The success rate for low-energy cardioversion is approximately 90% and is similar to that seen with antitachycardia pacing. Most electrophysiologists consider low-energy cardioversion to be shocks in the range of 0.1 to 5 J. Low-energy cardioversion has been compared with antitachycardia pacing using decremental fixed-rate bursts (33,52). It has been determined that with slow tachycardias (those with a mean cycle length of less than 390 ms), cardioversion has an efficacy rate of approximately 85%, with acceleration occurring in 11% (33,52). Pacing is effective 80% of the time with a risk of acceleration of 6%. These investigators found a higher frequency of transient supraventricular arrhythmias after low-energy cardioversion (23%) (33,52). As the tachycardia accelerates with cycle lengths of less 270 ms, the efficacy of pacing decreases to 77% (33,52). When pacing failed, cardioversion increased efficacy by only 8%. These observations and others indicate that gains made by low-energy cardioversion are only modest once pacing has failed. It has also been found consistently that shocks with an energy of less than 0.5 J are tolerated by the nonsedated patient. However, as shock energy increases above this amount, there is considerable patient discomfort (33,52). Antitachycardia pacing has the advantage of using considerably less energy than low-energy cardioversion. Based on these considerations, most electrophysiologists prefer multiple attempts at antitachycardia pacing before using low-energy cardioversion.

INDICATIONS FOR IMPLANTATION OF AN ICD

The American College of Cardiology and the American Heart Association (ACC/AHA), working in collaboration with the North American Society of Pacing and Electrophysiology, have recently published guidelines for implantation of ICDs (48,50) (Table 11-3). These guidelines were based on many observational reports and randomized trials, which have assessed the use of the ICD in the prevention of sudden death and their impact on total mortality rate (48, 50). For patients with prior episodes of sustained VT or VF, or for individuals at extremely high risk for such arrhythmias, there has been a consistent trend toward reduction in

sudden cardiac death and improvement in total mortality rate with the ICD compared with those with pharmacologic therapy (48,50). The evolution of the NTL systems, improved waveforms, and smaller devices have allowed implantation by the electrophysiologist without a thoracotomy, resulting in lower implantation risks.

The ACC/AHA guidelines classify the data supporting their recommendations into three levels (50). Level A evidence is considered to be present if multiple randomized clinical trials involving many individuals are available. Level B evidence is present when data were derived from a limited number of clinical trials involving comparatively few patients or from well-designed data analysis of nonrandomized trials or observational data registry (50). Finally, evidence is classified as level C when expert opinion or expert consensus was the basis of the recommendation (50).

Outcomes after Implantation of the ICD for Secondary Prevention

It has been known for decades that patients with sustained VT or out-of-hospital cardiac arrest have an anticipated recurrence rate of 20% to 30% per year (5,65). However, through the 1980s and early 1990s, there was disagreement among electrophysiologists as to which therapy offered the best chance for patient survival. Various approaches were used including serial electrophysiologic-electropharmacologic treatment, empirical amiodarone, or ICD therapy (5, 65). It was clear from a retrospective analysis of sudden death survivors that patients who were sent home on antiarrhythmic therapy with suppression in the electrophysiologic laboratory had an unacceptably high subsequent mortality rate (5,65). Thus, because of disappointing outcomes with electrophysiologically guided or empirical antiarrhythmic therapy and ongoing concern about the cost of ICD therapy, various prospective randomized trials were designed in the late 1980s to assess the efficacy of the ICD and drug therapy.

These prospective randomized trials were terminated or completed within the last 2 years and indicate that ICD therapy is preferable to best-drug therapy in terms of overall survival and survival free of sudden death in the patient who has experienced out-of-hospital sudden death or sustained VT.

AVID Trial

The most widely heralded of these trials, the Antiarrhythmic Versus Implantable Defibrillator (AVID) trial, showed that ICD therapy reduced mortality rate compared with primarily amiodarone; the number of patients on the other drug in the trial, sotalol, was too small for analysis (42,47). The targeted patient group included those who were most seriously ill and (a) those with a cardiac arrest resulting from VF and not associated with an acute myocardial infarction, transient cause, or correctable cause; and (b)those with documented sustained VT with syncope or near syncope and an ejection

TABLE 11-3. INDICATIONS FOR ICD THERAPY

Class I (ICD is indicated by general consensus)
1. Cardiac arrest resulting from VF or VT not resulting from a transient or reversible cause
2. Spontaneous sustained VT
3. Syncope of undetermined origin with clinically relevant, hemodynamically significant sustained VT or VF induced at electrophysiologic study when drug therapy is ineffective, not tolerated, or not preferred
4. Nonsustained VT with coronary disease, prior MI, LV dysfunction, and inducible VF or sustained VT at electrophysiologic study that is not suppressible by a class I antiarrhythmic drug

Class IIa (weight of evidence/opinion is in favor of ICD implantation)
None

Class IIb (usefulness and efficacy is less well established by evidence and opinion)
1. Cardiac arrest presumed to be caused by VF when electrophysiologic testing is precluded by other medical conditions
2. Severe symptoms attributable to sustained ventricular tachyarrhythmias while awaiting cardiac transplantation
3. Familial VT with coronary artery disease, prior MI, and LV dysfunction, and inducible sustained VT or VF at electrophysiologic study
4. Nonsustained VT with coronary artery disease, prior MI, and LV dysfunction, and inducible sustained VT or VF at electrophysiologic study
5. Recurrent syncope of undetermined origin in the presence of ventricular dysfunction and inducible ventricular arrhythmias at electrophysiologic study when other causes of syncope have been excluded

Class III (evidence and general agreement that an ICD is not useful or effective and in some cases may be harmful)
1. Syncope of undetermined cause in a patient without inducible ventricular tachyarrhythmias
2. Incessant VT or VF
3. VF or VT resulting from arrhythmias amenable to surgical or catheter ablation: e.g., atrial arrhythmias associated with Wolff-Parkinson-White syndrome, right ventricular outflow tract VT, idiopathic left ventricular tachycardia, or fascicular VT
4. Ventricular tachyarrhythmias resulting from a transient or reversible disorder (e.g., acute MI, electrolyte imbalance, drugs, trauma)
5. Significant psychiatric illnesses that may be aggravated by device implantation or may preclude systematic follow-up
6. Terminal illnesses with projected life expectancy of <6 mo
7. Patients with coronary artery disease with LV dysfunction and prolonged QRS duration in the absence of spontaneous or inducible sustained or nonsustained VT who are undergoing coronary bypass surgery
8. NYHA class IV drug-refractory congestive heart failure in patients who are not candidates for cardiac transplantation

ICD, implantable cardioverterdefribrillator; VF, ventricular fibrillation; VT, ventricular tachycardia; MI, myocardial infarction; LV, left ventricular.
Source: Sabensa S, Chandran P, Shah Y, et al. Comparative efficacy of transvenous cardioversion and pacing in patients with sustained ventricular tachycardia; a prospective randomized crossover study. *Circulation* 1985;72:153-160, with permission.

fraction (EF) of less than 0.40 or systolic blood pressure of less than 80 mm Hg. Patients who had a cardiac arrest due to a correctable cause or syncope without a documented cardiac arrhythmia did not qualify for the trial, although based on subsequent findings perhaps should have been included. Patients who needed coronary revascularization but had a low EF (less than 0.40) could be entered in the trial after a bypass procedure was completed (42,47). The end point of the trial was total mortality, which was chosen to avoid ambiguities regarding cause of death. Secondary end points included analysis of cost and quality of life. The hypothesis tested was a null hypothesis that stated there would be no difference in overall mortality rates between patients who were treated with the ICD versus those receiving antiarrhythmic drug therapy. A sample size of 1,200 patients was estimated to be sufficient, assuming an event rate of 40% at 4 years in the control group with the ability to detect a 30% reduction in mortality rate (42,47).

The pilot phase of the trial was initiated in June 1993, and enrollment was prompt. By March 1997, there had been an enrollment of 1,000 more patients and the Data and Safety Monitoring Board ended the trial prematurely when

it saw a significant difference in primary outcome between the two groups (47). At that time, 1,016 patients had been randomized to the two treatment groups: one receiving an ICD and one receiving an antiarrhythmic drug, primarily amiodarone. In this trial, a very careful registry was kept. Of the 5,989 patients screened, 4,595 were entered in the registry (84). After lower risk restrictions (noneligible arrhythmias and medical exclusions) were removed, 2,225 patients were eligible for randomization (84). Various exclusions were encountered, including prior exposure to amiodarone, compliance exclusions, predetermined therapy, or patient resistance or refusal to be randomized, as well as patients presenting with nonqualifying ventricular arrhythmias. Initially, the investigators were concerned that the sickest patients were being withheld and given ICD therapy off protocol, but this did not appear to be the case. At a subsequent analysis of the registry data, the mortality rate of the patients who were excluded from the main trial was identical to that of those patients in the main trial (47,84). Thus, the patients who were in the main trial were (a) similar to the registry patients and (b) strikingly similar to patients who had previously been reported in the large retrospective ICD trials of the 1980s. These were patients who by and large had coronary disease with an ischemic cardiomyopathy and an EF in the 0.31 to 0.32 range. Of the patients randomized, 455 had VF, 561 had VT (216 with syncope), and 345 had VT with hemodynamic compromise and an EF of less than 0.40. During the index hospitalization, about 10% of the ICD group and about 12% of the drug group underwent coronary revascularization (47).

The randomization scheme was simple (42,47). Electrophysiologic testing for further risk stratification of the population was not required, but 572 of the 1,016 patients did undergo an electrophysiologic study. Of the patients studied, 384 (67%) had inducible VT. However, at 1 and 3 years, there was no difference in survival between those with and those without inducible arrhythmia (47).

The characteristics of the ICD group and the antiarrhythmic drug group were very similar (47). Most patients (81%) had underlying coronary disease and nearly one half of the patients had been in congestive failure. The left ventricular EF (LVEF) was 0.32 in the ICD group and 0.31 in the antiarrhythmic drug group. Only 7% of the ICD group and 12% of the drug group had New York Heart Association (NYHA) class III heart failure (47).

Of the patients assigned to the drug group, 356 began empirical amiodarone and were not considered eligible for sotalol therapy because of concerns about heart failure (47). A total of 74 patients were considered candidates for sotalol, but by the time of discharge, only 13 of the sotalol-treated group had adequate suppression of their arrhythmia and were receiving sotalol at the time of discharge. More patients were taking β blockers ($p < 0.001$) in the ICD limb compared with the amiodarone limb. Approximately 20% of patients had crossed over to or added the other therapy by 24 months. Adjustments for this imbalance in the Cox regression analysis slightly reduced the estimated beneficial effect of ICD on survival. The crossover rate was higher among those initially assigned to ICD use ($p < 0.001$) (47). These rates of crossover from the ICD group to drug therapy (25.7%) or from drug therapy to ICD (18.9%) at 2 years were relatively low and did not compromise the power of the study (47).

The AVID trial was stopped prematurely after a mean follow-up of 18.2 ± 12.2 months when 1,016 of the projected 1,200 patients were enrolled at the recommendation of the Data and Safety Monitoring Board. At the time the study was stopped, accrued death rates were $15.8\% \pm 3.2\%$ in the ICD group and $24\% \pm 3.7\%$ in the drug group (47). The survival benefit showed that patients treated with the ICD had a better survival throughout the course of the study than those in the antiarrhythmic drug group. Survival figures represented a decrease in death rate of $39\% \pm 20\%$ at 1 year, $27\% \pm 21\%$ at 2 years, and $31\% \pm 20\%$ at 3 years. The average length of additional life associated with ICD therapy was 2.7 months at 3 years. Subsequent subgroup analysis showed that the beneficial effect of the ICD was independent of congestive heart failure status, age, or β-blocker use (47,67,69).

Although patients with the ICD had better survival throughout the study, the effect was most prominent in patients with an EF of less than 0.35 (47,67,69). In patients with an EF of less than 0.35, the hazard ratio was less than 0.6, and in those with an EF of more than 0.35, the hazard ratio was approximately 0.9 (47,67,69). Thus, in the high EF population, any benefit of the ICD was not apparent statistically possibly because of the short follow-up. In patients with preserved left ventricular function, the survival benefit of the ICD may not be evident without longer follow-up (47,67,69). The improvement in survival was short lived and seen in the first 9 months of study with no additional survival advantage after 9 months (47,67,69). The AVID trial has very fundamental and important indications for clinical medicine (47,67,69). This trial defined the superiority of the ICD in the high-risk population with ventricular arrhythmias. It confirmed that the benefit of the ICD is short lived, although these figures appear more striking than in everyday clinical practice because of the design of the trial (47,67,69).

In subsequent analysis of the registry population, there were some interesting data (84). Various arrhythmia populations were not included in the trial because of concerns about their future risk. Three of these groups (patients with asymptomatic VT, patients with VT or VF resulting from a transient or correctable cause, and patients with unexplained syncope and subsequent inducible VT) had subsequent death rates of 13%, 13%, and 9%, respectively, which were very similar to the death rates of patients in the main trial (84). If the AVID trial were being redone, undoubtedly, these patients would be randomized as part of the main trial. These data certainly suggest that such patients should also be seriously considered for an ICD. This is particularly true of the patients with a transient correctable cause of cardiac arrest (84). Such patients have traditionally been treated with correction of electrolyte abnormalities, antiarrhythmic drug administration, or revascularization (84). This approach was certainly true of the patients in the AVID trial, where 42% were revascularized and 44% sent home on a β blocker (84). However, it is apparent that this is not adequate therapy and thought must be given to more completely treat these patients, perhaps with the use of an electrophysiologic study and ICD implantation directly.

CIDS Trial

The Canadian Implantable Defibrillator Study (CIDS) included 659 patients with documented VF, cardiac arrest with defibrillation, syncope, VT causing presyncope, or angina with an LVEF of less than 0.35 and monitored syncope with inducible VT (55,60,67,69,85). As in the AVID trial, this trial randomized patients to an ICD or amiodarone therapy; 328 patients were randomized to an ICD and 331 to amiodarone. At the conclusion of the trial, there was a modest reduction of mortality (20%) in the ICD group compared with that of the amiodarone group (8.3%

versus 10.2% per year; $p = 0.142$. Thus, the significance of ICD therapy was not as marked as it was in the AVID trial because the sample size was not adequate to show a difference (55,60,67,69,85). However, patients receiving an ICD had a nonsignificant 33% lower risk of sudden death (3% versus 4.5% per year); there were no differences between the groups with respect to other modes of death. In this trial, approximately 90% of patients with ICDs received concomitant β blocker, sotalol, or amiodarone therapy (55, 60,67,69,85).

To establish whether some subsets of patients might benefit from the ICD, the outcome of high-risk patients was analyzed (85a). A multivariate risk model identified age, LVEF, and NYHA class as independent predictors of risk and based on these parameters quartiles of risk were constructed. Patients in the highest risk quartile, those who had at least two risk factors (age of 70 or older, LVEF of less than or equal to 0.35, and NYHA class III or IV), had a significant reduction of death from the ICD compared with amiodarone (14.4% versus 30%); there was no benefit seen among patients in the other three quartiles.

CASH Trial

In the Cardiac Arrest Study Hamburg (CASH) trial, 346 patients were randomized to the ICD, amiodarone, and metoprolol or propafenone group; all patients were followed for at least 2 years (60,67,69,85). The propafenone limb was discontinued when an interim analysis showed an increased mortality rate with this drug. The final outcome of CASH was a reduction in mortality rate with ICD therapy of 37% compared with antiarrhythmic drugs (12.1% versus 19.6%; $p = 0.047$) with no difference in mortality rate between the amiodarone and metoprolol arms (60,67,69,85). The secondary end point of sudden death was also reduced by the ICD compared with drugs (2% versus 11%; $p < 0.001$). These results have been criticized because of the use of a one-sided t test. Furthermore, the trial was not powered to detect mortality rate differences between each of the pharmacologic treatment limbs. When each pharmacologic limb was compared separately to the ICD arm, no significant differences in all-cause mortality were noted (60,67,69,85).

Summary

Thus, CASH and CIDS supported the results of the AVID trial, although without the statistical power of the AVID result. When interpreted with the results of the CASH and AVID trials, it is likely that had there been more patients or longer follow-up, a total mortality benefit would have been found in the CIDS trial. However, CIDS and CASH (60, 67,69,85) confirmed the results of the AVID trial.

The ACC/AHA revised the guidelines for implantation of the ICD in 1998, largely because of the results of these three published trials (50). These recommendations are summarized in Table 11-2. They generally reflect the results

of the AVID trial, although already errors have slipped into these recommendations. For example, the recently presented Registry Data suggest that cardiac arrest resulting from a transient or reversible cause is associated with a risk as high as that for any other cause of a cardiac arrest and should be included as a class I indication (84).

Role of Prophylactic ICD in High-Risk Patients

A series of trials designed in the late 1980s and early 1990s analyzed the prophylactic role of the ICD in patients with depressed EF and various electrical markers who were at high risk but had not yet sustained an arrhythmic event.

MADIT Trial

The Multicenter Automatic Defibrillator Implantation Trial (MADIT) studied a very carefully selected group of post–myocardial infarction patients who were at high risk for future events (86). Previously published data from the 1980s suggested that the presence of nonsustained VT in a postinfarction patient carried a mortality risk of 14% at 12 months to 38% at 36 months. Thus, the MADIT study involved patients with coronary artery disease and a prior infarction who were 3 weeks removed from the myocardial infarction, had nonsustained VT on Holter (3 to 30 beats), had an EF of less than or equal to 0.35, and were inducible into sustained monomorphic VT or VF, which was not suppressed with procainamide (86). The MADIT study enrolled only 196 patients and randomized them to an ICD or conventional therapy. The mean EF of the conventional group was only 0.25 and that of the ICD group only 0.27. At a mean follow-up of 27 months, the trial was terminated prematurely when the ICD showed marked survival benefit over conventional therapy. During the course of the trial, there were 39 deaths in the conventional therapy arm and 15 deaths in the ICD arm (86). Thirteen of the deaths in the conventional arm resulted from a primary arrhythmia while only 3 deaths in the ICD arm were caused by a primary arrhythmia. Survival of all patients in the conventional group (all-cause mortality) was only 51% at 4 years, which is remarkably similar to that of a group of patients who already had an arrhythmic event (86). Also, the MADIT patients received frequent shocks from their ICDs, with 60% receiving device discharges at 2 years. Thus, it appears that properly selected high-risk patients can benefit as much from the ICD as patients who have already experienced a cardiac arrest.

The results of the MADIT trial were highly controversial at the time they were initially presented. A number of criticisms were noted. There was no registry of data, as in the AVID trial, so the total number of patients screened was not known (85,86). No data were kept on patients who were screened but were noninducible at electrophysiologic study or were inducible and suppressed with procainamide. A small substudy from three centers in the trial suggests that the 2-year mortality rate in this subset of patients was only about 8% (85,86). A high percentage of patients discontinued their amiodarone and there was a disproportionate use of β blockers (3 : 1 ratio) in the ICD arm (86). Finally, many clinicians were uncertain of what to do with the data in terms of screening many patients to identify the infrequent potential MADIT candidate (67,69,85,86). Such screening would involve doing Holter monitors on all post–myocardial infarction patients with an EF of less than 0.30.

To address the issue of primary prevention of sudden cardiac death, MADIT II is currently enrolling 1,200 patients with coronary artery disease and an LVEF of less than 0.30 to ICD versus conventional therapy without a specific antiarrhythmic drug (63). This study will randomize patients to ICD versus standard medical therapy by removing the criteria of inducibility of electrophysiologic study (63). Additionally, the Sudden Cardiac Death–Heart Failure Trial (SCD-HeFT) is a primary prevention trial in patients with ischemia and nonischemic cardiomyopathy, no history of cardiac arrest or sustained documented arrhythmia, an EF of less than 0.35, and NYHA functional class II/III heart failure (85). This trial will randomize patients to an ICD, amiodarone, or placebo with specific guidelines for maximizing other therapies known to improve survival such as β blockers, angiotensin-converting enzyme inhibitors, and cholesterol-lowering agents. In both trials, the primary end point is total mortality (63,67,69,85).

CABG Patch Trial

The Coronary Artery Bypass Graft Patch (CABG Patch) trial evaluated the efficacy of the ICD for reducing overall mortality in 900 patients undergoing surgical revascularization for severe coronary artery disease who had significant left ventricular dysfunction (EF of less than 0.36) and positive signal-average electrocardiogram results (87). Enrolled patients did not have a history of a sustained ventricular tachyarrhythmia or syncope. After an average follow-up of 32 months, there were 71 cardiac deaths in the defibrillator group and 72 cardiac deaths in the control group; there have been no reported differences in outcome in different subsets of patients.

Prophylactic therapy with the ICD did reduce arrhythmic-related death at 42 months by 45% (4% versus 6.9% in the control group) (88). However, because 71% of the deaths in this trial were not related to arrhythmia, this reduction did not have an impact on total mortality rate.

MUSTT Study

There was considerable anticipation of the results of another similar study, the Multicenter Unsustained Tachycardia Trial (MUSTT) (67,69,89). This trial assessed the efficacy of elec-

trophysiologic testing in a similar population, that is, patients with coronary disease, an EF of less than 0.40, and nonsustained VT on Holter monitor. An electrophysiologic study was done and patients who were inducible into sustained VT were randomized to electrophysiologically guided therapy or to no antiarrhythmic drug therapy (67,69,85,89). A series of antiarrhythmic drugs were tested in a logical but complicated fashion. If the patient did not respond to a medication, then the patient received an ICD. At the conclusion of the study, approximately 45% of the patients in the electrophysiologically guided arm were discharged on antiarrhythmic drug and 46% did not respond to antiarrhythmic drug and had an ICD implanted.

There were 353 patients discharged with no therapy and 351 who received electrophysiologically guided therapy, including an antiarrhythmic drug in 154 and an ICD in 161; the median follow-up was 39. The 2-year (12% versus 18%) and 5-year (25% versus 32%; $p = 0.04$) rates for the primary end point were lower for electrophysiologically guided therapy compared with those for no therapy. The secondary end point of total mortality was also lower at 5 years in the group receiving electrophysiologically guided therapy (42% versus 48%). The reduction in the primary and secondary end points in the electrophysiologically guided group was largely attributable to ICD therapy; at 5 years, the primary end point occurred in 9% of those receiving an ICD, compared with 37% of those receiving an antiarrhythmic drug, and the secondary end point occurred in 24% and 55%, respectively. There was no difference in outcome between patients receiving no therapy and those treated with an antiarrhythmic drug.

Because of the many patients involved in the MUSTT study (704 patients were inducible and randomized to electrophysiologically guided therapy or no antiarrhythmic therapy), there were enough ICD patients to compare the MUSTT results to the MADIT results (67,69,85,89). The MUSTT patients who received "a best drug" at electrophysiologic testing had a mortality rate virtually identical to that of the control population and very similar to that of the amiodarone arm of the MADIT trial (67,69,85,86,89). The patients in the MUSTT study who failed all drugs and went on to receive an ICD did extremely well and had a survival rate comparable to that of the ICD arm of the MADIT study (67,69,85,86,89). Thus, although an unintended consequence, the MUSTT study tended to confirm the MADIT study's results and opened the prospect of a new emphasis on prophylaxis ICD implantation in patients with coronary disease and an EF of less than 0.35 (MADIT study) or of 0.40 (MUSTT study). The MUSTT data again show the critical importance of prospective randomized trials to validate the concept that of all risk factors, EF is the most powerful (67,69,85). These trials again suggest that electrophysiologic testing is a powerful way to risk stratify, but it may be no more powerful than the presence of a low EF itself. The ACC/AHA 1998 guidelines already had included the MADIT data as a class I indication for ICD implantation (48,50). The MUSTT data further amplify this indication; however, it will again raise questions of how to screen for these patients, as in the post–thrombolytic era patients with such a low EF represent a small percentage of postinfarction patients.

One important conclusion from these trials is that the ICD is expensive therapy (12,47,56,72). Recent analysis of MADIT has focused on an economic analysis of health care services including hospitalizations, physician visits, medications, laboratory tests, and procedures during the trial. The analysis included cost for patients randomized to conventional therapy and to the ICD limb (12,47,56,72). The accumulated net costs for the 3.16 mean years of survival for the ICD group was $97,560, compared with the $75,980 for the 2.8 years of survival in the conventional limb. The authors concluded that the resulting cost-effectiveness ratio of $27,000 per life-year should compare favorably with other cardiac interventions and that the ICD is cost-effective in selected individuals at high risk for ventricular arrhythmias (12,47,56,72).

The cost data from the AVID trial demonstrated that patients in the antiarrhythmic or the ICD arm had a similar number of subsequent hospitalizations and physician encounters with the cost during 3 years in 1997 dollars $108,000 for the ICD arm and $76,000 for the antiarrhythmic drug arm (47). This difference in cost represents the cost of the ICD itself. However, there was no hidden benefit for the ICD in terms of reduced medical encounters over time (47). Although the final cost-effectiveness data have not been published, these data suggest that this will likely be in excess of $100,000 per life-years saved (47).

Role of ICD in Conditions Associated with Ventricular Tachyarrhythmias

A group of patients receiving a great deal of attention are those with familial or inherited conditions with a high risk for life-threatening ventricular arrhythmias, that is, those with ACC/AHA class IIb indication (50). Most electrophysiologists and cardiologists have seen an increasing number of such patients because of the wide dissemination of information by the media about the risk that many less widely known diagnoses carry. Such patients include those who have had a cardiac event (VF or syncope) associated with an uncommon diagnosis such as long QT syndrome, Brugada syndrome, or hypertrophic cardiomyopathy (70,73). Although the data are scant in these patient groups, most electrophysiologists now favor implantation of an ICD when the patient is symptomatic from serious ventricular arrhythmia or has experienced a sustained life-threatening arrhythmic event. More problematic are the asymptomatic patients or asymptomatic siblings of patients who have one of these conditions and have had a cardiac arrest. Prophylactic ICD implantation in these patient groups is being done more frequently, although without great scientific justification. However, the enormous emotional toll that such a death takes on a family is obvious and most electrophysiologists implant an ICD to avert another casualty in an afflicted family if the diagnosis can clearly be established by the usual techniques.

A recent retrospective multicenter study of the efficacy of the ICD in preventing sudden cardiac death in patients with hypertrophic cardiomyopathy was reported (70). Of 128 patients receiving the ICD, 32 had prior cardiac arrest or sustained VT (secondary prevention) and 85 had prophylactic implants because of risk factors such as family history of sudden cardiac death, syncope, or nonsustained VT (70). The rate of ICD discharge was 5% per year in the secondary prevention group and 11% per year in the primary prevention group. Based on these observations, the authors concluded that in selected high-risk patients with hypertrophic cardiomyopathy, ICDs are highly effective in terminating VT and VF and the use of the device is warranted (70).

The effectiveness and limitations of β-blocker therapy in patients with congenital long QT syndrome has recently been reported based on long-term follow-up data from 869 patients treated with β blockers, which included 113 patients with prior aborted cardiac arrest in whom β blocker was used for secondary prevention (73). Despite beta blockade, 14% would have another cardiac arrest (aborted or fatal) within 5 years on β blockers (73). Based on the high likelihood of experiencing recurrent aborted cardiac arrest or death despite β-blocker therapy, the authors recommend ICD therapy along with β blockers in these patients (73).

Summary

It is clear that the era of the ICD is with us largely because of the important scientific studies that have been summarized. The implantation rate of the ICD in the United States is currently 165 per million. This contrasts with 25 million in Canada and Western Europe and a much lower figure in the Far East. With the impact of the recently reported primary and secondary treatment studies, as well as the affirmation of the ACC/AHA guidelines, it is only a matter of time before general cardiologists and internists will view the ICD the same way that electrophysiologists do, that is, as first-line therapy for high-risk patients. Also, with the data being so clear and the national societies in complete agreement, it is likely that there will be little obstruction from governmental or private insurance payers when an ICD is indicated medically.

IMPLANTATION TECHNIQUES AND TESTING OF ICD FUNCTION

Currently, ICDs are placed in almost all instances with an NTL system, which uses a subclavian vein or cephalic vein access and pectoral implants (22,90–92). The placement of epicardial patches through a midline sternotomy, left lateral thoracotomy, subxiphoid, or subcostal approach has considerably greater morbidity or mortality than use of the NTL systems and accordingly they have been largely abandoned (22,90–92). When concomitant surgery is done through a midline sternotomy or lateral thoracotomy, the option of placement of epicardial patches and epicardial rate-sensing leads exists (22,90–92). However, most surgeons and electrophysiologist agree that placing a pectoral ICD with NTL at a separate procedure in individuals undergoing open-heart surgery is preferable to implantation at the time of thoracotomy. To incorporate the largest mass of the myocardium into the vector of defibrillation, it is generally agreed that placement of the NTL system in the left pectoral region with the lead inserted via the left subclavian vein is optimal (22,90–92). The lead is typically positioned at the right ventricular apex or in the apical portion of the right ventricular septum. Sensed R waves are determined during the patient's native rhythm using a pacemaker system analyzer. A minimum requirement for R-wave amplitude is 5 mV. It is essential that the ICD sense all of the ventricular depolarizations during the patient's native rhythm, VT, and VF to accurately determine the heart rate during these rhythms. With R waves of less than 5 mV, the potential for undersensing of the lower amplitude R waves of VF is a real concern (22,90–92). Occasionally, it is necessary to reposition the lead at a site other than the right ventricular apex or apical septum such as the midportion of the septum, inflow tract, or outflow tract to obtain an acceptable R wave. Once this is obtained, pacing threshold is assessed and should be less than 1.5 V at a 0.5-ms pulse width. The lead impedance should be repetitively measured to ensure that it is stable and in the range of 300 to 1,200 Ω and within specification of the individual lead manufacturer. The stability of lead impedance over multiple

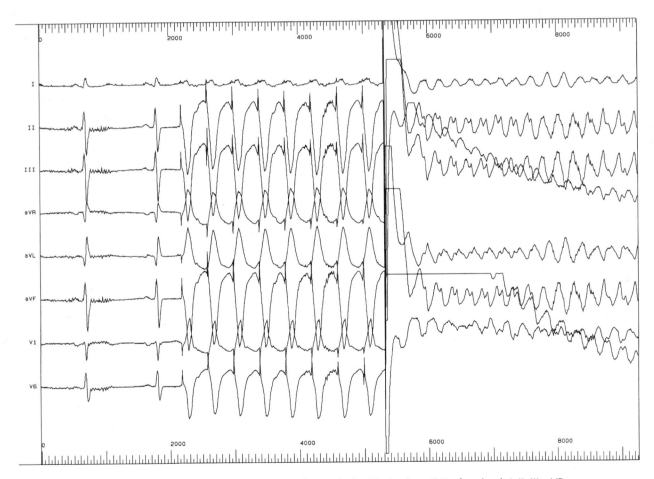

FIGURE 11-3. Induction of ventricular fibrillation (VF) with shock on T. Surface leads I, II, III, aVR, aVL, aVF, V₁, and V₆ are shown during induction of VF at the time of implantable cardioverter-defibrillator implantation. A drive of eight paced ventricular beats at a rate of 150 beats per minute at the right ventricular apex is followed by a 1-J shock with a coupling interval of 310 ms. This results in VF, which was subsequently terminated with a 15-J shock during defibrillation threshold testing.

measurements indicates a stable position at the endocardial surface as it interfaces with the lead. All measurements including R wave, impedance, and threshold should be rechecked after the lead is tied to the muscle or tunneled. All measurements are also repeated once the IS-1 connector is positioned into the header and the setscrew tightened into the ICD. Most commonly, a low-energy synchronized shock of approximately 1 J is delivered during the patient's native rhythm to assess the integrity of the high-voltage lead impedance before induction of any ventricular arrhythmias (22,90–92).

Determination of DFT is also a critical part of the initial testing; it requires the induction of VF. There are multiple different techniques for induction of VF noninvasively including programmed ventricular stimulation using extrastimuli, low-energy shocks critically timed in the vulnerable period of the T wave (Fig. 11-3) or high-frequency burst pacing (Figs. 11-4) and 11-5) (22,32,77, 90–92). Evaluation of the comparative defibrillation energy requirements using each of these techniques of induction has shown no significant difference. In individuals who have been taking amiodarone or sotalol, it may be difficult to induce VF and one would have to settle for testing of rapid VT or ventricular flutter for determination of DFTs (22,32, 90–92).

Two main strategies are used at the time of implantation to assess DFTs. One commonly used technique involves progressively stepping down the amount of energy to the point of failure of termination of VF (22,90–92). The DFT is defined as the minimum amount of energy that will terminate VF without failure at that energy level. An alternative technique, used by some electrophysiologists particularly in high-risk patients, involves only demonstrating an adequate safety margin between

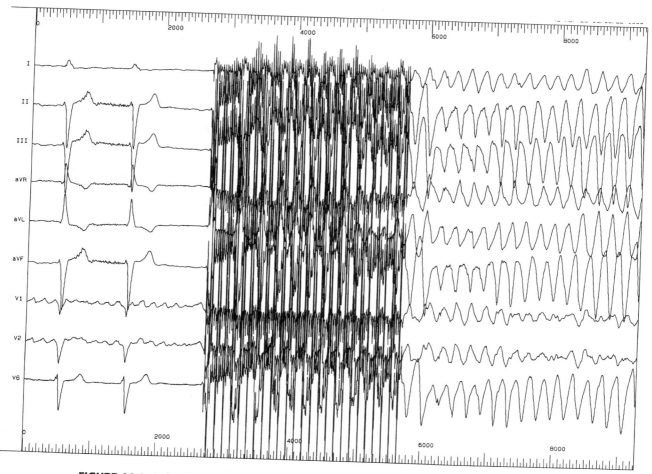

FIGURE 11-4. Induction of ventricular fibrillation (VF) with 50-Hz stimulation. Surface leads are shown with identical format as that in Figure 11-3. With delivery of approximately 3 seconds of 50-Hz stimulation, VF is induced, which was subsequently terminated with a 15-J shock during defibrillation threshold testing. Note intermittent failure to detect the ventricular electrogram during VF, as indicated by the absence of a sensing marker. This occasional undersensing occurs fairly commonly with VF but does not generally lead to delay in therapy.

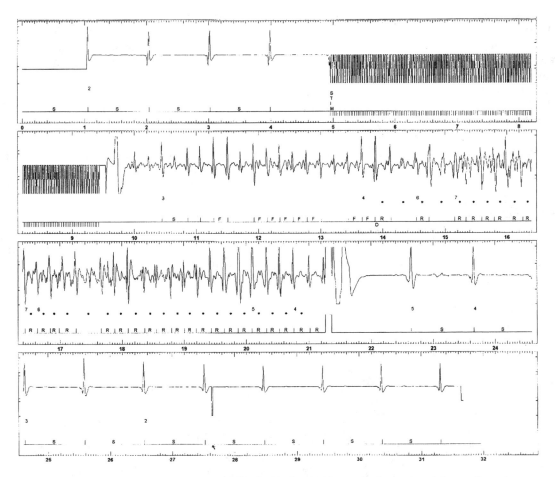

FIGURE 11-5. Induction of ventricular fibrillation by rapid ventricular pacing. Intracardiac rate-sensing ventricular electrograms are shown during normal sinus rhythm for the first four beats. Rapid ventricular pacing *(stim)* induces ventricular fibrillation. Despite intermittent undersensing of the fibrillation, as indicated by dropout of the "F" marker and reconfirmation, or the "R" marker, VF is sensed and terminated with a 37-J shock.

the shock energy tested at implantation and the maximum output of the device. Studies have demonstrated that the probability of successful termination of VF is more than 90% at twice the DFT and approximately 70% at the measured DFT. The advantage of the step-down approach is more precise determination of an actual DFT (22,90–92). In addition, this allows for assessment of the device's ability to redetect a ventricular arrhythmia immediately after a failed shock when there is commonly difficulty in sensing the ventricular electrograms. Clinically, acceptable DFTs for implantation are those that provide a safety margin of at least 10 J between the DFT and the maximum output of the device. DFTs average approximately 10 J with current NTL systems (22,90–92).

During intraoperative assessment of defibrillator function, the event marker channels can provide useful information for evaluating sensing with each induction of VT or VF. Not uncommonly, "dropout" or failure to detect elec-

trograms during fine VF, known as undersensing of VF, can result in nondetection or delayed detection (22,77,90–92). Many manufacturers recommend VF sensing testing by programming the device's sensitivity to the least sensitive setting at the time of implantation. Using this approach, the cardiologist is ensured that fine VF will be sensed at the more sensitive settings nominally used for the ICD. Because the amplitude of VF can decrease during a single episode or after a failed defibrillation attempt, many electrophysiologists prefer assessing sensing with long detection time and after at least one failed shock before high-energy rescue shock from the device (22,90–92).

Initially, defibrillation testing was performed at the time of epicardial lead system implantations or early NTL implantations using sterile high-voltage sensing cables attached to an external implant support device that mimics the function of the ICD (22,90–92). With development of NTL systems and modified waveforms, which are associated with lower DFTs, device-based testing is used. With this technique, the ICD is connected to the lead positioned at the right ventricular apex through the venous system and all testing is performed through the device using a programmer. Device-based testing offers multiple advantages including the ability to use marker channels and program sensitivities. Device-based testing significantly decreases the total implantation time, thereby reducing the risk of infection and other procedure morbidities (22,90–92).

ICD-PACEMAKER INTERACTIONS

Although single-chamber pacing has been available in ICDs for a decade, and dual-chamber pacing is currently available, it is occasionally necessary to implant an ICD in a patient with a preexisting permanent pacemaker. It is particularly important that the multiple types of potential interaction between the pacemaker and the ICD be assessed to minimize the risk of device-device interaction (40,93). The potential interaction between pacemakers and ICDs are summarized in Table 11-4. Based on these multiple potential interactions, most electrophysiologists feel it is far preferable to rely on current-generation ICDs for single- or dual-chamber pacing in individuals who need a pacemaker (40,92). Accordingly, the commonly used strategy has been to explant previously existing pacemakers in patients who need an ICD while relying on the ICD for its pacing functions to eliminate the potential for device-device interaction (40,92).

TABLE 11-4. POTENTIAL INTERACTIONS BETWEEN PACEMAKERS AND ICDS

Inhibition of ICD therapy
  Sensing of atrial or ventricular pacemaker stimuli during VT or VF by the ICD resulting in failure to detect the ventricular arrhythmia
Pacemaker malfunction from ICD shock
  Noise reversion mode
  Reprogramming of pacemaker
  Component damage
  Transient rise in pacing threshold
  Transient failure to capture
Inappropriate shock by ICD
  Sensing of atrial or ventricular pacemaker stimulus by the ICD resulting in detection criteria being met with delivery of therapy
  Inappropriate programming of maximal sensor rate of pacemaker into detection zone of ICD magnet testing resulting in detection of pacemaker stimuli

ICD, implantable cardioverterdefibrillator; VT, ventricular tachycardia; VF, ventricular fibrillation.

Complications

The use of thoracotomy lead systems, which required epicardial patches and rate-sensing leads and an abdominal implantation of the ICDs, was associated with a high surgical mortality rate of approximately 3% to 4%. This mortality rate occurred as a result of heart failure, acute myocardial infarction, respiratory failure, infection, and intractable ventricular arrhythmias. In individuals with poor left ventricular function or those undergoing concomitant surgery or those with prior amiodarone use, the morbidity or mortality rates were higher (93–96). Infection rates of 3% to 5% were noted consistently with abdominal implants with epicardial lead systems (93–96). In addition, pericarditis was common (10% to 15%) and atrial fibrillation was found in 20% to 25% of patients after patch implantation. Rarely, other potentially life-threatening complications such as myocardial infarction or stroke occurred (93,94). Because of the less-invasive nature and shorter duration of the procedure, the operative mortality rate of NTL systems is less than 1% (93,94). Morbidity occurs in approximately 1% to 2% of cases and is generally related to placement of the catheters in the intravascular space with the more common complications being pneumothorax, cardiac tamponade, or vascular complications including bleeding, thrombosis, or hematoma. The risk associated with ICD implantation increases with a thoracotomy approach, advanced age, concomitant cardiac surgery, comorbid illnesses, poor LVEF, and NYHA class III to IV heart failure (93,94).

Very few data exist regarding the long-term reliability of ICD lead; however, to date, with up to 6 years of follow-up in NTL lead systems, the rate of insulation breaks, dislodgment, and lead fractures appears to be acceptably low at less than 5%. Fortunately, the risk of infection has been dramatically reduced with implantation of pectoral devices. With abdominal implants and thoracotomy lead systems, infection rates are approximately 3% to 5% (93,94). This has been reduced to less than 1% with thoracotomy devices. Infection, which typically manifests in the first few weeks after implantation, mandates removal of the device and all leads, tissue débridement, and prolonged antibiotic therapy to cure the infection (93,94). The source of most infections is thought to be intraoperative contamination at the time of implantation. Accordingly, staphylococci are most commonly the source of infection from contamination with skin flora. Some infections from *Staphylococcus epidermidis* may manifest months after the procedure because of low virulence. NTL systems may be removed by extraction with or without the use of extraction sheaths in most cases (93,94). However, there is substantial risk with these extraction techniques of vascular complications and mortality. If the lead system cannot be removed by extraction techniques, a thoracotomy with surgical extraction may be warranted (94–96).

Among the potential long-term complications from ICD therapy are the psychologic distress that some patients may experience as a result of frequent ICD discharges (96). Adjustment disorders, major depression, panic reactions, and anxiety have been reported in some patients with ICDs. This psychopathology is responsive to reduction of ICD shocks, psychiatric counseling, and support from peers and family (96). In addition to the psychologic burdens, which these patients may encounter, the restrictions on activity, including driving, may have a negative impact on quality of life. Current guidelines are adhered to by cardiologists who recommend that these patients not drive for at least 6 months after implantation and each ICD discharge for a ventricular tachyarrhythmia (95,98).

Inappropriate therapy that is not delivered for VT or VF represents the most common adverse event associated with ICD use. Nonsustained VT, sinus tachycardia, supraventricular arrhythmias including atrial fibrillation and flutter, double sensing of ventricular activation, myopotentials, external magnetic fields, insulation defects, and lead fracture can cause inappropriate therapy (97).

Other complications that have been observed include the following:

1. An increase in the chronic DFT may occur with NTLs and is independent of waveform (monophasic or biphasic) (97a,97b). This problem may result from intense fibrosis and the cumulative acute damage produced by defibrillation discharges at the ICD electrode–myocardial interface (97c).
2. There are a number of shoulder-related problems with the pectoral approach to ICD implantation including decreased active shoulder motility, pain, reduced function, and insertion tendinitis. These complaints do not require additional intervention or surgical revision and often abate by 12 months after insertion (97d).
3. Twiddler's syndrome, in which twisting or rotating the device in its pocket results in lead dislodgment and device malfunction, can occur in patients with an ICD. It is most likely to develop when the device is implanted in the abdomen of an obese patient who is able to rotate it within the abdominal pocket (97e). Patients most often present with an increase in bradycardic pacing threshold or lead impedance; however, there is a possibility that the device will fail to sense and treat an arrhythmia. Careful suturing of the device to the fascia and matching pocket and device size is important to avoid this complication..
4. Because reliable function of the ICD depends on proper sensing of the electrical activity of the heart, a potential concern is electromagnetic interference from external sources, including cellular telephones, welding equipment, motor-generator systems, and surveillance systems. Functional evaluation of ICDs in the workplace has *not* demonstrated oversensing of an external electrical field (97f). However, because interference remains a concern, it is recommended that patients remain at least 2 feet from external electrical equipment, verify that the

equipment is properly grounded, and wear insulated gloves when using electrical devices.

ICD Follow-Up

The value of ventricular arrhythmias induction as part of routine follow-up in new-generation pectoral ICDs remains controversial (99–104). Based on several analyses, it is reasonable to conclude that with recent developments in ICD technology, it may not be necessary to perform routine predischarge or follow-up ICD evaluations in all patients with ICD implantations (94–104). Analysis of 153 patients with pectoral ICDs who had routine VF induced at predismissal, 3 months, and 1 year after implantation demonstrated important findings in 8.8%, 5.9%, and 3.8% of tested patients, respectively. VT induction at predischarge, 3 months, and 1 year after implantation resulted in programming changes in 37.4%, 28.1%, and 13.8% of tested patients, respectively (103).

Analysis of a larger database of predischarge ICD testing also demonstrated that routine testing rarely reveals dysfunctions (102). These investigators analyzed 1,007 ICD tests in 587 systems and 556 patients. The tests were performed routinely in 899, because of change in antiarrhythmic medication in 7% and because of suspected dysfunction of the ICD in 1%. During VF testing, four systems (0.4%) failed to defibrillate the patient. In three of these cases, abnormalities of the ICD had been ruled out before testing. In the 71 patients who had testing after the addition of antiarrhythmic drugs, the device failed to defibrillate two patients. Procedure-related complications occurred in 1.6% of cases. These authors recommended selective use of testing in individuals with suspected dysfunction or after the addition of class I or III antiarrhythmic drugs (102).

After implantation, a standard protocol for follow-up should be used in all patients. This should include assessment of wound integrity and staple or suture removal 7 to 10 days postimplantation (105). Subsequently, patients should be seen at 3-month intervals with inspection of the pacemaker site and palpation of the leads and ICD for any tenderness. Routinely, the sensing and pacing thresholds should be assessed with analysis of battery status, pacing lead impedance, and any episodes of therapy that the patient has received implantation (105). It is not necessary to deliver a shock to obtain a high-voltage impedance. If shock therapy has been delivered since the last follow-up, the information will be provided by the device about that shock. With some devices, the high-voltage lead impedance is automatically measured at regular intervals. All thresholds, R waves, and pacing and shock impedances should be compared with the values at the time of implantation.

A protocol for the evaluation of patients who receive their first shock should include evaluation within a few hours with a cardiac history, physical examination including blood pressure, a 12-lead electrocardiogram, and interrogation of the ICD. For patients who have received a previous shock, more elective evaluation of their clinical status and ICD is appropriate if they are feeling well. We typically advise patients to notify us immediately if they get a shock and plan on being seen within 24 hours of the therapy, unless they are feeling poorly, they have received multiple shocks, or this is their first shock. However, if the patient has any persistent symptoms of arrhythmia, shortness of breath, or chest pain after a shock, they are advised to be taken immediately to the nearest emergency ward (105). If they are feeling well, they can be more electively evaluated. At the time of evaluation, a detailed history focusing on any triggers of the arrhythmias such as emotional stress or physical exertion would be useful. All relevant information relative to the arrhythmia should be investigated and stored in the patient's permanent record. This would include all data log information such as R-R intervals, stored electrogram and high-voltage impedance, time of the episode, and the effective therapy. In those individuals who have a separate implanted pacemaker, full investigation and assessment of pacemaker function including atrial and ventricular thresholds should be performed after the patient has received an ICD shock to ensure continued normal function of the pacemaker (105).

Approximately 50% of patients experience spontaneous ICD shocks in the first 6 months after initial implantation. Subsequently, the rate of discharge is approximately 50% per year; this may be for a supraventricular or ventricular tachyarrhythmia. Many times, optimization of antiarrhythmic medications and programming of the ICDs reduce the frequency of shock therapy (105). The use of concomitant drugs, antitachycardia pacing, low-energy cardioversion, programming discrimination, and tachycardia detection criteria all influence the frequency of shock therapy (105, 106). In this regard, the tachycardia detection rate should be programmed at least 10 bpm above the maximum sinus or atrial fibrillation rate and at least 10 beats below the rate of the clinical VT. Occasionally, it is not possible to meet these criteria and cautious use of onset criteria, rate stability, and morphology may be helpful to discriminate VT and VF from sinus tachycardia, atrial tachycardia, or atrial fibrillation. Typically, devices are programmed to the noncommittal mode in which the device reconfirms the presence of the arrhythmia before delivering shock therapy (105). Most commonly, antitachycardia pacing and low-energy cardioversion is most successful when the VT rates are less than 220 bpm. More rapid arrhythmias or those that are hemodynamically poorly tolerated should be immediately treated with shock therapy.

Occasionally, a patient will receive inappropriate shocks for sinus tachycardia, atrial fibrillation, atrial tachycardia, supraventricular tachycardia, or long runs of nonsustained VT. Device malfunction or lead malfunction may also trigger shocks as a result of oversensing (97). All current devices have data logs and stored electrograms, which allow for the retrieval of information and determination of the appropri-

ateness of ICD discharges. When noise is detected as the cause of the shock, the electrophysiologist should carefully assess for diaphragmatic sensing by having the patient lean forward and strain while performing real-time telemetry of electrograms. With lead fractures and insulation breaks, positional maneuvers and manipulation of the generator and leads may intermittently reproduce the events, which can be captured on the real-time telemetry of electrograms with event markers (97). Maneuvers such as Valsalva, deep breathing, leaning forward and straining, coughing, or laughing may be necessary to reproduce diaphragmatic oversensing or lead problems. In the event of diaphragmatic oversensing, it is frequently possible to program the ICD to a less-sensitive mode to eliminate this problem. This should be done only if the device is shown to detect VF reliably.

However, if there is an insulation break or lead fracture, lead repair or replacement is mandatory (97). When patients receive repetitive shocks for VT or VF, atrial arrhythmias, or noise, it is frequently necessary to admit them to institute definitive therapy. In the event of frequent episodes of VT or VF and if antitachycardia pacing and low-energy cardioversion are not adequate to reduce the frequency of high-energy shock output, antiarrhythmic agents must be considered. Alternatively for sustained monomorphic VT, hybrid therapy with radiofrequency with ablation of the VT may be considered. One study of 21 patients with frequent ICD shocks caused by recurrent sustained VT despite antiarrhythmic drugs reported that ablation was effective in 76% of patients (105a). During a follow-up of 11 months, the frequency of ICD shocks per month decreased from 60 to 0.1 in this small study and was associated with an improvement in quality of life.

Occasionally, patients report the sensation of a discharge without an actual shock. Such "phantom shocks" are most commonly seen as the patient is about to go to sleep. In the devices of such individuals, the data log indicates the absence of any detected arrhythmia and any therapy. Such patients commonly respond well to reassurance and counseling (97).

ANTIARRHYTHMIC DRUG–ICD INTERACTIONS

Antiarrhythmic drug therapy for treatment of supraventricular or ventricular arrhythmias is needed in up to 50% of ICD patients. Most electrophysiologists attempt to use antitachycardia pacing to minimize the frequency of shock therapy for sustained monomorphic VT (40). However, in some patients, high frequency of ventricular arrhythmias requiring shock therapy mandate the use of concomitant antiarrhythmic agents. Drugs also can be used to treat ventricular arrhythmias for the purpose of enhancing the efficacy of antitachycardia pacing. Finally, drugs can be used to suppress atrial fibrillation, atrial flutter, atrial tachycardia, or supraventricular arrhythmias.

β-Blocker therapy is frequently used in patients with ICDs for their underlying cardiovascular condition. These β blockers also help prevent sinus tachycardia and slow rapid atrial fibrillation, which would cause an "overlap arrhythmia" with the patient's native rhythm accelerating into the VT or VF zone. There are very few prospective data on the prophylactic use of antiarrhythmic drugs to prevent device discharges in patients with ICDs. However, in one controlled study of prophylactic use of antiarrhythmic drug therapy after ICD implantation (19), there was no significant effect from the time to first clinical shock after implantation and shock-free interval in patients with antiarrhythmic agents. Another prospective randomized double-blinded placebo-controlled trial evaluated the role of the class III antiarrhythmia agent sotalol in patients with the ICD (71). In this trial, patients were stratified by LVEFs of less than or equal to 0.30 and more than or equal to 0.30 for three end points including the delivery of a first shock for any reason or death from any cause, the first appropriate shock for a ventricular arrhythmia or death from any cause, and the first inappropriate shock for a supraventricular arrhythmia or death from any cause (71). Compared with the placebo group, treatment with sotalol was associated with a lower risk of sudden death from any cause or the delivery of a first shock for any reason, death from any cause and delivery of first inappropriate shocks. Sotalol also decreased the mean frequency of shocks resulting from any cause (1.43 ± 3.53 shocks per year compared with 3.89 ± 10.65 in the placebo group; $p = 0.008$). The reduction in the risk of death or delivery of a shock for any reason did not differ significantly between patients with an EF of more than or less than 0.30 (71). Based on this trial, the investigators concluded that oral sotalol was effective and safe in reducing the risk of death or delivery of first ICD shock independent of left ventricular function (71).

Antiarrhythmic drugs can influence the rate of VT (Table 11-5). It is generally felt that slower VTs are easy to terminate with antitachycardia pacing. To that extent, some physicians will institute antiarrhythmic drugs in an effort to enhance the efficacy of antitachycardia pacing. With some drugs, there can be marked slowing of the VT rate to go below the ICD cutoff rate. To that extent, when an antiarrhythmic drug is instituted in the patient with an ICD, there should be thorough noninvasive testing to ensure appropriate detection and therapy.

Many antiarrhythmic drugs also alter the DFTs (Table 11-6). In some instances, the drugs may eliminate the safety margin and make shock therapy ineffective for VT or VF (40). Systematic evaluation of antiarrhythmic drugs has found that sodium channel active drugs are most likely to increase the energy requirements for successful defibrillation. It has been found in this respect that some drugs such as quinidine have a dose-related affect on DFTs. Metabolic factors such as acidosis can increase the affect of lidocaine on DFTs while respiratory alkalosis reverses lidocaine affect. Procainamide (NAPA) the metabolic product of procainamide, which has potassium channel-blocking effects, and sotalol, another potassium channel blocker, tend to decrease the DFTs. Amiodarone in most studies has caused elevation of DFTs. Verapamil and other calcium channel blockers have been noted to increase DFTs. It is well appreciated that antiarrhythmic drugs can also affect pacing thresholds, thus potentially alternating the efficacy of bradycardia and antitachycardia pacing. Finally, low sodium and potassium channel blockers can interfere with the sensing of VT and VF by slowing the tachycardia rate below the programmed detection rate. All antiarrhythmic drugs have the potential to decrease the impulse conduction velocity (dV/dT), prolong the QRS duration, and slow conduction. In some instances, these effects are sufficient to produce "double counting" of each QRS complex. The potential effects of antiarrhythmic drugs and DFTs are shown in Table 11-6.

TABLE 11-5. EFFECT OF ANTIARRHYTHMIC DRUGS ON VENTRICULAR TACHYCARDIA RATE

Weak
  β Blockers
  Tocainide
  Mexiletine
  Sotalol
Moderate
  Quinidine
  Procainamide
  Disopyramide
  Moricizine
Strong
  Ia & Ib combination
  Propafenone
  Encainide
  Flecainide
  Amiodarone

TABLE 11-6. ANTIARRHYTHMIC DRUG EFFECT ON DEFIBRILLATOR THRESHOLD

Decrease
  Sotalol
  N-acetylprocainamide
Variable
  Procainamide
  Bretylium
  Propafenone
Increase
  Lidocaine
  Phenytoin
  Flecainide
  Propranolol
  Mexiletine
  Verapamil
  Amiodarone
  Quinidine
  Disopyramide
  Moricizine

Patients with ICDs who have frequent episodes of VT despite pharmacologic therapy might be considered for catheter ablation as an adjunct to ICD therapy (105a,106, 107). In such patients, catheter mapping and ablation is a practical option only if the VT is monomorphic and hemodynamically tolerated for at least brief periods (106,107). The nature of the underlying structural heart disease and the size and configuration of the arrhythmia substrate determine the approach to mapping and ablation. Success rates vary from 90% with idiopathic right ventricular outflow tract VT to 40% to 60% with post–myocardial infarction VT (106, 107). Catheter ablation plays a useful role in controlling frequent episodes of VT or recurrent VT in selected patients with an ICD (106,107).

DUAL-CHAMBER DEVICES

Dual-chamber DDDR pacing has recently become available in ICD systems (Fig. 11-6). In addition to therapy for VT and VF, the dual-chamber device can provide dual-chamber, rate-responsive pacing (DDDR) for atrioventricular sequential pacing with mode-switching capacity (81,82). Up to 25% of patients with an ICD require concomitant single- or dual-chamber pacing. As noted previously, there are multiple potential interactions between ICD systems and separately implanted permanent pacemakers. Many electrophysiologists feel that dual-chamber pacing can offer potential benefit to individuals with sick sinus syndrome or atrioven-

tricular conduction disturbances who have VT or VF. In addition to the benefit of atrioventricular sequential pacing, dual-chamber pacing may play a role in prevention of atrial arrhythmias. Atrial tachyarrhythmias such as sinus tachycardia, atrial fibrillation, and supraventricular arrhythmias are relatively common problems in patients with ICDs and can cause inappropriate shocks. Dual-chamber devices incorporate algorithms that assess the relationship of the atrial activity in an effort to decrease the frequency of shocks for atrial arrhythmias (81,82). These discrimination algorithms can be selectively activated to use information regarding the relationship of the atrial and ventricular electrograms to discriminate between supraventricular arrhythmias and VT or VF. Using the sensed atrial and ventricular electrogram, the relationship of the atrial activity and the ventricular activity is analyzed by a complex algorithm in the ICD (Figs. 11-7 and 11-8). Studies of individuals with medically refractory heart failure and a dilated cardiomyopathy with prolonged PR intervals have shown a benefit from dual-chamber pacing with shorter atrioventricular delays (81,82). Accordingly, such individuals are now considered candidates for dual-chamber pacemakers as an indication for an ICD in a patient with dilated cardiomyopathy, first-degree atrioventricular block, and medically refractory heart failure (81,82).

Devices currently in clinical investigation will allow for shock therapy for VT, VF, atrial fibrillation, and other atrial arrhythmias. For patients with hypertrophic cardiomyopathy who are at risk or who have had sustained ventricular

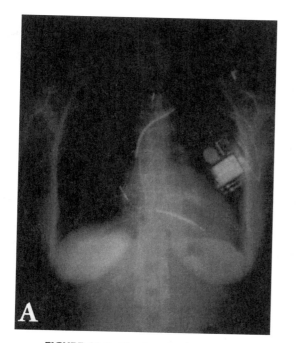
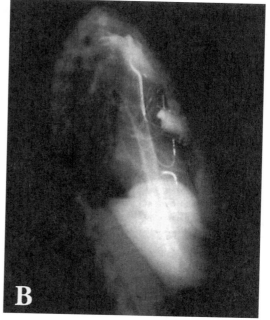

FIGURE 11-6. Chest x-ray of patient with a dual-chamber implantable cardioverter-defibrillator (ICD). Anteroposterior **(A)** and lateral **(B)** chest x-ray is shown from a patient with a dual-chamber ICD implanted in the left subpectoral area. The atrial lead is in the right atrial appendage and the ventricular lead at the right ventricular apex.

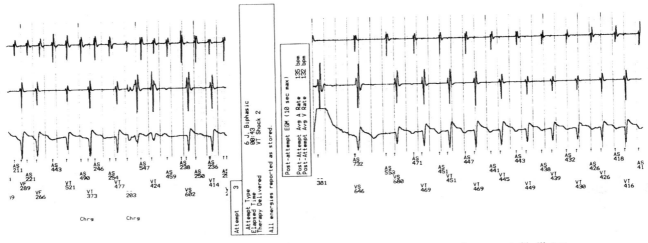

FIGURE 11-7. Stored electrograms from a dual-chamber implantable cardioverter-defibrillator. Intracardiac atrial rate-sensing lead electrograms **(top)**, ventricular rate-sensing electrograms **(middle)**, and ventricular shock electrograms **(bottom)** during rapid atrial fibrillation with a ventricular response of 139 beats per minute (bpm). In this individual, shock therapy had been programmed for rates of more than 130 bpm. A 6-J shock reestablishes normal sinus rhythm.

arrhythmias, there may be a symptomatic benefit by decreasing the outflow gradient with dual-chamber pacing with a short atrioventricular delay (81,82,108). Currently, multiple studies are evaluating the role of biventricular pacing for the treatment of heart failure, dual-sided atrial pacing for atrial fibrillation prevention, and algorithms for prevention of atrial and ventricular arrhythmias. It is likely that the results of these studies will have an impact on expanding indications of dual-chamber ICDs in the future. Improvements in rhythm discrimination, atrial therapies, integrated circuits, batteries, capacitors, and lead systems, as well as monitoring diagnostics and smaller size, are likely to be valued by the patient and the implanting physician and may result in a greater proportion of total ICDs being dual chamber as opposed to single chamber when implanted in the future (81,82,108,109).

ATRIAL CARDIOVERTER-DEFIBRILLATORS

Recently, an implantable atrial cardioverter-defibrillator has been developed and evaluated in a clinical trial. Like the

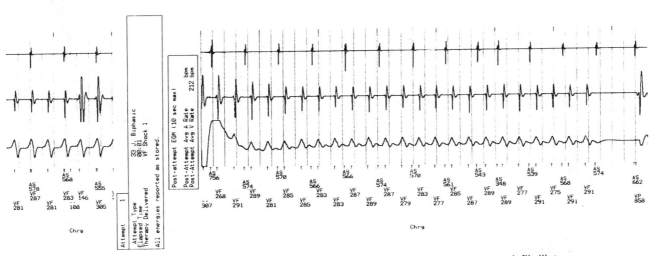

FIGURE 11-8. Stored electrograms from a dual-chamber implantable cardioverter-defibrillator. Stored intracardiac electrograms are shown from the atrial rate-sensing lead **(top)**, ventricular rate-sensing lead **(middle)**, and ventricular shock electrogram **(bottom)** during an episode of sustained monomorphic ventricular tachycardia (VT) with a heart rate of 212 beats per minute. Notice the dissociation of the atrial electrograms from the VT. A 33-J biphasic shock is delivered but fails to immediately terminate VT. The VT terminates approximately 6 seconds after shock therapy.

ICD, which is used for ventricular arrhythmias, the atrial cardioverter-defibrillator is a battery-powered device that is pectorally implanted (74–80). It is connected to an endocardial lead system that includes right atrial, coronary sinus, and right ventricular apical leads (74–80). With sensitive and specific algorithms, the device detects atrial fibrillation and delivers R-wave synchronous shocks to convert atrial fibrillation to sinus rhythm. The device also has the ability to pace the ventricle. The implantable atrial cardioverter-defibrillator can function in the automatic mode with detection and shock delivery with the onset of atrial fibrillation. Alternatively, it can be used in the patient or physician mode in which the detections and shock therapy are initiated electively with magnet applications over the device.

A multicenter prospective trial using the atrial cardioverter-defibrillator recently reported results of 51 patients with recurrent atrial fibrillation unresponsive to antiarrhythmic drugs (74–80). In this trial, patients were selected to be at low risk for ventricular arrhythmias; that is, it excluded patients with congestive heart failure, an LVEF of less than 0.40, myocardial infarction or CABG within 1 year, and documented nonsustained or sustained VT. The LVEF in this patient population was 0.58 ± 0.11. All patients were screened with atrial fibrillation testing before device implantation, and those with an atrial DFT of more than or equal to 240 V were excluded. Of 119 patients screened, 51 received the device. Reasons for not receiving a device included high atrial DFTs. In 43 patients in this study, all device testing and episodes of atrial fibrillation were terminated under physician observation. A total of 3,719 shocks were delivered including 3,049 during testing and 67 for spontaneous episodes of atrial fibrillation (74–80). Specificity of the detection algorithm was 100% and sensitivity was 92.3%. Forty-one patients had 231 episodes of atrial fibrillation; the device terminated 98% of the episodes. Early recurrence of atrial fibrillation occurred in 27% of episodes in 51% of patients. Overall, 48 of 51 patients received concomitant antiarrhythmic therapy for atrial fibrillation. Shock tolerability differed markedly among patients (74–80).

These preliminary results demonstrated that the atrial cardioverter-defibrillator can safely and effectively recognize and restore normal sinus rhythm in highly selected patients. Antiarrhythmic agents are still needed to suppress atrial fibrillation in most patients. Early recurrence of atrial fibrillation and shock tolerability remain issues that need further evaluation. The future role of the atrial cardioverter-defibrillator requires further investigation (74–80).

CONCLUSION AND FUTURE DEVELOPMENTS OF THE ICD

Although there has been remarkable progress in the technology and clinical uses of the ICD, it is probable that there will be continued significant progress. The several completed and ongoing trials on the use of the ICD for primary and secondary prevention of sudden cardiac death will provide guidelines for implantation of the ICD in the future. Ongoing clinical studies of the sensitivity and specificity and overall predictive accuracy of detection algorithms will likely result in selected employment of these discrimination algorithms in patients. Future devices will likely have expanded capacity for electrogram storage with the ability to simultaneously record from rate and defibrillation coils. Impedance measurements will be automated and threshold determinations for atrial and ventricular capture and sensing will likely be automated. In addition, there will likely be expansion of the capacity to perform transtelephonic monitoring for detection of lead problems and assessment of battery life. This will likely simplify patient follow-up dramatically. It is possible that there will be information included such as heart rate variability, ST-segment analysis, or electrical alternans to help predict and possibly prevent arrhythmia in pacing algorithms. As capacitor and battery technology continues to improve, the ICDs will likely get smaller. In addition, as DFTs trend downward because of improved waveforms and lead systems, there will be a tendency for ICDs to continue to have a reduction in size.

REFERENCES

1. Mirowski M, Reid PR, Mower M, et al. Termination of malignant ventricular arrhythmias with an implantable automatic defibrillator in human beings. *N Engl J Med* 1980;303:322–324.
2. Mower MM, Schumber B. Implantable cardioverter defibrillator and its basic principles. In: Podrid P, Kowey P, eds. *Cardiac arrhythmias: mechanisms, diagnosis, and management.* Philadelphia: Williams & Wilkins, 1995:689–699.
3. Cannom DS. Internal cardioverter-defibrillator: newer technology and newer devices: In: Podrid P, Kowey P, eds. *Cardiac arrhythmias: mechanism, diagnosis, and management.* Philadelphia: Williams & Wilkins, 1995:708–725.
4. Taylor E, Veltri EP. Clinical use of implantable cardioverter defibrillator: indications and outcomes. In: Podrid P, Kowey P, eds. *Cardiac arrhythmias: mechanism, diagnosis, and management.* Philadelphia: Williams & Wilkins, 1995:699–707.
5. Estes NAM III. Strategies for management of malignant ventricular arrhythmias: roles of pharmacotherapy, surgery, ablation, and the implantable cardioverter defibrillator. In: Estes NAM, Manolis A, Wang PJ, eds. *Implantable cardioverter defibrillators: a comprehensive textbook.* New York: Marcel Dekker Inc, 1994:229–257.
6. Winkle RA, Mead RH, Ruder MA, et al. Improved low energy defibrillation efficacy in man with the use of a biphasic truncated exponential waveform. *Am Heart J* 1989;117:122–127.
7. Bardy GH, Troutman C, Johnson G, et al. Electrode system influence on biphasic waveform defibrillation efficacy in humans. *Circulation* 1991;84:665–671.
8. Strickberger SA, Hummel JD, Horwood LE, et al. Effect of shock polarity on ventricular defibrillation threshold using a transvenous lead system. *J Am Coll Cardiol* 1994;24:1069–1072.
9. Leitch JW, Gillis AM, Wyse DG, et al. Reduction in defibrillator shocks with implantable device combining antitachycardia pacing and shock therapy. *J Am Coll Cardiol* 1991;18:145–151.
10. Winkle RA, Mead RH, Ruder MA, et al. Long-term outcome

with the automatic implantable cardioverter-defibrillator. *J Am Coll Cardiol* 1989;13:1353–1361.

11. Fogoros RN, Elson JJ, Bonnet CA, et al. Efficacy of the automatic implantable cardioverter-defibrillator in prolonging survival in patients with severe underlying cardiac disease. *J Am Coll Cardiol* 1990;16:381–386.

12. O'Donoghue S, Platia EV, Brooks-Robinson S, et al. Automatic implantable cardioverter-defibrillator: is early implantation cost-effective? *J Am Coll Cardiol* 1990;16:1258–1263.

13. Venditti FJ Jr, Martin DT, Vassolas G, et al. Rise in chronic defibrillation thresholds in nonthoracotomy implantable defibrillator. *Circulation* 1994;89:216–223.

14. Poole JE, Bardy GH, Dolack GL, et al. Serial defibrillation threshold measures in man: a prospective controlled study. *J Cardiovasc Electrophysiol* 1995;6:19–25.

15. Lehmann MH, Saksena S. Implantable cardioverter defibrillators in cardiovascular practice: report of the Policy Conference of the North American Society of Pacing and Electrophysiology. NASPE Policy Conference Committee. *Pace* 1991;14:969–979.

16. Naccarelli GV, Veltri EP. ICD implantation: intraoperative requirements. In: Naccarelli GV, Veltri EP, eds. *Implantable cardioverter-defibrillators*. Boston: Blackwell Science, 1993:53–65.

17. Naccarelli GV. Serial electrophysiologic guided drug testing versus ICD implantation in the survival of sudden cardiac death. In: Luceri R, ed. *Sudden cardiac death: strategies for the 1990s*. Miami: Peritus Publishing Co, 1992:57–72.

18. Luceri RM. Implantable defibrillators: physician's role after hospital discharge. In: Naccarelli GV, Veltri EP, eds. *Implantable cardioverter-defibrillators*. Boston: Blackwell Science, 1993:150–170.

19. Anderson JL, Karagounis LA, Roskelley M, et al. Effect of prophylactic antiarrhythmic therapy on time to implantable cardioverter-defibrillator discharge in patients with ventricular tachyarrhythmias. *Am J Cardiol* 1994;73:683–687.

20. Strickberger SA, Daoud EG, Davidson T, et al. Probability of successful defibrillation at multiples of the defibrillation energy requirement in patients with an implantable defibrillator. *Circulation* 1997;96:1217–1223.

21. Strickberger SA, Man KC, Souza J, et al. A prospective evaluation of two defibrillation safety margin techniques in patients with low defibrillation energy requirements. *J Cardiovasc Electrophysiol* 1998;9:41–46.

22. Grimm W, Timmann U, Menz V, et al. Simplified implantation of single-lead pectoral cardioverter defibrillators using device-based testing. *Am J Cardiol* 1998;81:503–506.

23. Neuzner J, Pitschner HF, Schlepper M. Programmable VT detection enhancements in implantable cardioverter defibrillator therapy. *Pace* 1995;18[Pt II]:539–546.

24. Swerdlow CD, Chen PS, Kass RM, et al. Discrimination of ventricular tachycardia from sinus tachycardia and atrial fibrillation in a tiered-therapy cardioverter-defibrillator. *J Am Coll Cardiol* 1994;23:1342–1355.

25. Reiter MJ, Mann DE. Sensing and tachyarrhythmias detection problems in implantable cardioverter defibrillators. *J Cardiovasc Electrophysiol* 1996;7(6):542–557.

26. Le Franc Pierre, Kus T, Vinet A, et al. Underdetection of ventricular tachycardia using a 40 ms stability criterion: effect of antiarrhythmic therapy. *Pace* 1997;20[Pt I]:2882–2892.

27. Barold HS, Newby KH, Tomassoni G, et al. Prospective evaluation of new and old criteria to discriminate between supraventricular and ventricular tachycardia in implantable defibrillators. *Pace* 1998;21:1347–1355.

28. Korte T, Jung W, Wolpert C, et al. A new classification algorithm for discrimination of ventricular from supraventricular tachycardia in a dual chamber implantable cardioverter defibrillator. *J Cardiovasc Electrophysiol* 1998;9(1):70–73.

29. Brugada J, Mont L, Figueiredo M, et al. Enhanced detection criteria in implantable defibrillators. *J Cardiovasc Electrophysiol* 1998;9(3):261–268.

30. Wieckhorst A, Buchwald A, Unterberg C. On the necessity of the invasive predischarge test after implantation of a cardioverter-defibrillator. *Am J Cardiol* 1998;81:933–935.

31. Stevenson SA, Jenkins JM, DiCarlo LA. Analysis of the intraventricular electrogram for differentiation of distinct monomorphic ventricular arrhythmias. *Pace* 1997;20:2730–2738.

32. Malkin RA, Johnson EE. The effect of inducing ventricular fibrillation with 50-Hz pacing versus T-wave stimulation on the ability to defibrillate. *Pace* 1998;21:1093–1097

33. Estes NAM III, Haugh CJ, Wang PJ, Manolis AS. Antitachycardia pacing and low-energy cardioversion: a clinical perspective. *Am Heart J* 1994;127:1038–1046.

34. Sarter BH, Callans DJ, Gottlieb CD, et al. Implantable defibrillator diagnostic storage capabilities: evolution, current status, and future utilization. *Pace* 1998;12:1287–1298.

35. Marchlinski FE, Callans DJ, Gottlieb CD, et al. Benefits and lessons learned from stored electrogram information in implantable defibrillators. *J Cardiovasc Electrophysiol* 1995;6(10): 832–851.

36. Jung J, Hohenberg G, Heisel A, et al. Discrimination of sinus rhythm, atrial flutter, and atrial fibrillation using bipolar endocardial signals. *J Cardiovasc Electrophysiol* 1998;9(7):689–695.

37. Markewitz A, Kaulbach H, Mattke S, et al. Influence of anodal electrode position on transvenous defibrillation efficacy in humans: a prospective randomised comparison. *Pace* 1997;20 [Pt 1]:2193–2199.

38. Gold MR, Foster AH, Shorofsky SR. Lead system optimization for transvenous defibrillation. *Am J Cardiol* 1997;80:1163–1167.

39. Natale A, Sra J, Axtell K, et al. Undetected ventricular fibrillation in transvenous implantable cardioverter-defibrillators. Prospective comparison of different lead system-device combinations. *Circulation* 1996;93:91–98.

40. Brode SE, Schwartzman D, Callans DJ, et al. ICD-antiarrhythmic drug and ICD-pacemaker interactions. *J Cardiovasc Electrophysiol* 1997;8:830–842.

41. van Rugge FP, Savalle LH, Schalij MJ. Subcutaneous single-incision implantation of cardioverter-defibrillators under local anesthesia by electrophysiologists in the electrophysiology laboratory. *Am J Cardiol* 1998;81:302–305.

42. AVID Investigators. Antiarrhythmics Versus Implantable Defibrillators (AVID): rationale, design, and methods. *Am J Cardiol* 1995;75:470–475.

43. Bigger JT Jr. Should defibrillators be implanted in high-risk patients without a previous sustained ventricular tachyarrhythmia? In: Naccarelli GV, Veltri EP, eds. *Implantable cardioverter-defibrillators*. Boston: Blackwell Science, 1993:284–317.

44. Morris MM, KenKnight BH, Warren JA, et al. A preview of implantable cardioverter defibrillator systems in the next millennium: an integrative cardiac rhythm management approach. *Am J Cardiol* 1999;83:48D–54D.

45. Trappe HJ, Achtelik M, Pfitzner P, et al. Single-chamber versus dual-chamber implantable cardioverter defibrillators: indications and clinical results. *Am J Cardiol* 1999;83:8D–16D.

46. Newman D, Dorian P, Hardy J. A randomized prospective comparison of ventricular antitachycardia pacing modalities. *Pace* 1992;15:506(abst).

47. The Antiarrhythmics Versus Implantable Defibrillators (AVID) Investigators. A comparison of antiarrhythmic-drug therapy with implantable defibrillators in patients resuscitated from near-fatal ventricular arrhythmias. *N Engl J Med* 1997;337:1576–1583.

48. Dreifus LS, Fisch C, Griffin JC, et al. Guidelines for implantation of cardiac pacemakers and antiarrhythmia devices. A report of the American College of Cardiology/American Heart Association Task Force on Assessment of Diagnostic and Therapeutic

Cardiovascular Procedures (Committee on Pacemaker Implantation). *J Am Coll Cardiol* 1991;18:1–13.

49. Link MS, Costeas XF, Griffith JL, et al. High incidence of appropriate implantable cardioverter-defibrillator therapy in patients with syncope of unknown etiology and inducible ventricular arrhythmias. *J Am Coll Cardiol* 1997;29:370–375.

50. Gregoratos G, Cheitlin MD, Conill A, et al. ACC/AHA guidelines for implantation of cardiac pacemakers and antiarrhythmic devices: a report of the American College of Cardiology/ American Heart Association Task Force on Practice Guidelines (Committee on Pacemaker Implantation). *J Am Coll Cardiol* 1998;31:1175–1209.

51. O'Donoghue S, Platia E. Device infection: prevention and treatment. In: Estes NAM, Manolis AS, Wang PJ, eds. *Implantable cardioverter defibrillator: a comprehensive textbook.* New York: Marcel Dekker Inc, 994:495–505.

52. Saksensa S, Chandran P, Shah Y, et al. Comparative efficacy of transvenous cardioversion and pacing in patients with sustained ventricular tachycardia: a prospective, randomized crossover study. *Circulation* 1985;72:153–160.

53. Bigger JT, Whang W, Rottman JN, et al. Mechanisms of death in the CABG Patch trial: a randomized trial of implantable cardiac defibrillator prophylaxis in patients at high risk of death after coronary artery bypass graft surgery. *Circulation* 1999;99: 1416–1421.

54. Bigger JT, for the Coronary Artery Bypass Graft (CABG) Patch Trial Investigators. Prophylactic use of implanted cardiac defibrillators in patients at risk for ventricular arrhythmias after coronary artery bypass graft surgery. *N Engl J Med* 1997;337: 1569–1575.

55. Connolly SJ, Gent M, Roberts RS, et al. Canadian Implantable Defibrillator Study (CIDS): study design and organization. *Am J Cardiol* 1993;72:103F–108F.

56. Mushlin AJ, Hall WJ, Zwanzinger J, et al. The cost effectiveness of automatic implantable cardioverter defibrillators. *Circulation* 1998;97:2179–2135.

57. Block M, Breithardt G. The implantable cardioverter defibrillator and primary prevention of sudden death: the Multicenter Automatic Defibrillator Implantation Trial and the Coronary Artery Bypass Graft (CABG) Patch Trial. *Am J Cardiol* 1999;83: 74D–78D.

58. Brugada P, Brugada R, Brugada J, et al. Use of prophylactic implantable cardioverter defibrillator for patients with normal hearts. *Am J Cardiol* 1999;83:98D–100D.

59. Cannom DS, Prystowsky EN. Management of ventricular arrhythmias: detection, drugs, and devices. *JAMA* 1999;281: 172–179.

60. Cappato R. Secondary prevention of sudden death: the Dutch study, the Antiarrhythmics Versus Implantable Defibrillators trial, the Cardiac Arrest Study Hamburg, and the Canadian Implantable Defibrillator Study. *Am J Cardiol* 1999; 83: 68D–73D.

61. Farre J. Navigation in the mega-trials waters; reflections on the Multicenter Automatic Defibrillator Implantation Trial and the Antiarrhythmics Versus Implantable Defibrillators study. *Am J Cardiol* 1999;83:5D–7D.

62. Maron BJ, Casey SA, Almquist AK. Aborted sudden cardiac death in hypertrophic cardiomyopathy. *J Cardiovasc Electrophysiol* 1999;10:263.

63. Moss AJ, Cannom DS, Daubert JP, et al. Multicenter Automatic Defibrillator Implantation Trial II (MADIT II): design and clinical protocol. *Ann Noninvasive Electrocardiol* 1994;4:83–91.

64. Nisam S. Can implantable defibrillators reduce non-arrhythmic mortality? *J Intervent Cardiac Electrophysiol* 1998;2:371–375.

65. Zipes DP, Wellens HJJ. Sudden cardiac death. *Circulation* 1998; 98:2334–2351.

66. Klein H, Auricchio A, Reek S, et al. New primary prevention trials of sudden cardiac death in patients with left ventricular dysfunction: SCD-HeFT and MADIT II. *Am J Cardiol* 1999; 83:91D–97D.

67. Zivin A, Bard GH. Implantable defibrillators and antiarrhythmic drugs in patients at risk for lethal arrhythmias. *Am J Cardiol* 1999;84:63R–68R.

68. Connolly S. Meta-analysis of antiarrhythmic drug trials. *Am J Cardiol* 1999;84:90R–93R.

69. Hohnloser SH. Implantable devices versus antiarrhythmic drug therapy in recurrent ventricular tachycardia and ventricular fibrillation. *Am J Cardiol* 1999;84:56R–62R.

70. Maron BJ, Shen WK, Link MS, et al. Efficacy of implantable cardioverter-defibrillators for the prevention of sudden death in patients with hypertrophic cardiomyopathy. *N Engl J Med* 2000;342:365–373.

71. Pacifico A, Hohnloser SH, William JH, et al, for the d,l-Sotalol Implantable Cardioverter-Defibrillator Study Group. Prevention of implantable-defibrillator shocks by treatment with sotalol. *N Engl J Med* 1999;340:1855–1862.

72. Mushlin AI, Zwanziger J, Gajary E, et al. Approach to cost-effectiveness assessment in the MADIT trial. Multicenter Automatic Defibrillator Implantation Trial. *Am J Cardiol* 1997;80:33F–41F.

73. Moss AJ, Zareba W, Hall J, et al. Effectiveness and limitations of β blocker therapy in congential long-QT syndrome. *Circulation* 2000;101:616–623.

74. Wellens HJJ, Lau CP, Berndt L, et al. Atrioverter: an implantable device for the treatment of atrial fibrillation. *Circulation* 1998;98(16):1651–1656.

75. Timmermans C, Rodriguez LM, Smeets JLRM, Wellens HJJ. Immediate re-initiation of atrial fibrillation following internal atrial defibrillation. *J Cardiovasc Electrophysiol* 1998;9:122–128.

76. Ammer R, Alt E, Ayers G, et al. Pain threshold for low energy intracardiac cardioversion of atrial fibrillation with low or no sedation. *Pacing Clin Electrophysiol* 1997;20:230–236.

77. Lok NS, Lau CP, Tse HF, Ayers GM. Clinical shock tolerability and effect of different right atrial electrode locations on efficacy of low energy human transvenous atrial defibrillation using an implantable lead system. *J Am Coll Cardiol* 1997;30:1324–1330.

78. Jung J, Heisel A, Fries R, Kollner V. Tolerability of internal low-energy shock strengths currently needed for endocardial atrial cardioversion. *Am J Cardiol* 1997;80:1489–1490.

79. Timmermans C, Ashish N, Rodriguez LM, et al. Use of sedation during cardioversion with implantable atrial defibrillator. *Circulation* 1999;100:1499–1501.

80. Timmermans C, Rodriguez LM, Ayers G, et al. Effects of butaphanol tartrate on shock-related discomfort during internal atrial defibrillation. *Circulation* 1999;99:1837–1842.

81. Kuhlkamp V, Dornberger V, Mewis C, et al. Clinical experience with the new detection algorithms for atrial fibrillation of a defibrillator with dual chamber sensing and pacing. *J Cardiovasc Electrophysiol* 1999;10:905–915.

82. Lavergne T, Daubert JC, Chanuin M, et al. Preliminary clinical experience with the first dual chamber pacemaker defibrillator. *Pacing Clin Electrophysiol* 1997;20:182–188.

83. Nair M, Saoudi N, Kroiss D, Letac B. Automatic arrhythmia detection using analysis of the atrioventricular association: application to a new generation of implantable defibrillators. *Circulation* 1997;95:967–973.

84. Anderson JL, Hallstrom AP, Epstein AE, et al, and the AVID Investigators. Design and results of the antiarrhythmic vs. implantable defibrillators (AVID) registry. *Circulation* 1999;99: 1692–1699.

85. Naccarelli GV, Wolbrette DL, Luck JC. Results of clinical trials: In: *Cardiac electrophysiology: from cell to bedside.* Zipes DP, Jalife J, eds. Philadelphia: WB Saunders, 2000:790–797.

85a. Sheldon R, Connolly S, Krahn A, et al, for the CIDS Investigators. Identification of patients most likely to benefit from implantable cardioverter-defibrillator therapy. The Canadian Implantable Defibrillator Study. *Circulation* 2000;101:1660.

86. Moss AJ, Hall WJ, Cannom DS, et al, for the Multicenter Automatic Defibrillator Implantation Trial Investigators. Improved survival with an implanted defibrillator in patients with coronary artery disease at high risk for ventricular arrhythmias. *N Engl J Med* 1996;335:1933–1940.

87. Bigger JT, for the Coronary Artery Bypass Graft (CABG) Patch Trial Investigators. Prophylactic use of implanted cardiac defibrillators in patients at high risk for ventricular arrhythmias after coronary artery bypass graft surgery. *N Engl J Med* 1997;337:1569.

88. Bigger JT, Whang W, Rottman JN, et al. Mechanisms of death in the CABG Patch trial: a randomized trial of implantable cardiac defibrillator prophylaxis in patients at high risk of death after coronary artery bypass graft surgery. *Circulation* 1999;99:1416.

89. Buxton AE, Fisher JO, Josephson ME, et al. Prevention of sudden death in patients with coronary artery disease: the Multicenter Unsustained Tachycardia Trial (MUSTT). *Prog Cardiovasc Dis* 1993;36:215–226.

90. Rastegar H, Bojar RM. Surgical techniques for the implantable cardioverter-defibrillator. In: Estes NAM, Manolis A, Wang PJ, eds. *Implantable cardioverter defibrillators: a comprehensive textbook.* New York: Marcel Dekker Inc, 1994:279–293.

91. Ellenbogen KA, Wood MA, Stambler BS. Intraoperative testing. In: Estes NAM, Manolis A, Wang PJ, eds. *Implantable cardioverter defibrillators: a comprehensive textbook.* New York: Marcel Dekker Inc, 1994:295–317.

92. Epstein AE, Shepard RB. Permanent pacemaker and implantable cardioverter-defibrillators: potential interactions. In: Estes NAM, Manolis A, Wang PJ, eds. *Implantable cardioverter defibrillators: a comprehensive textbook.* New York: Marcel Dekker Inc, 1994:479–494.

93. Haugh CJ, Wang PJ. Surgical complications of defibrillation implantation. In: Estes NAM, Manolis A, Wang PJ, eds. *Implantable cardioverter defibrillators: a comprehensive textbook.* New York: Marcel Dekker Inc, 1994:353–366.

94. Block M, Breithardt G. Implantable cardioverter-defibrillators: clinical aspects. In: Zipes DP, Jalife J, eds. *Cardiac electrophysiology: from cell to bedside.* Philadelphia: WB Saunders, 2000:958–970.

95. Epstein AE, Miles WM, Benditt DG, et al. Personal and public safety issues related to arrhythmias that may affect consciousness: implications for regulation and physician recommendations. A medical/scientific statement from the American Heart Association and the North American Society of Pacing and Electrophysiology. *Circulation* 1996;94:1147–1166.

96. Lampert R, Diwaker J, Burg M, et al. Destabilizing effects of mental stress on ventricular arrhythmias in patients with implantable cardioverter-defibrillators. *Circulation* 2000;101(2):158–164.

97. Lewis RJ, Veltri EP. Troubleshooting implanted devices. In: Estes NAM, Manolis A, Wang PJ, eds. *Implantable cardioverter defibrillators: a comprehensive textbook.* New York: Marcel Dekker Inc, 1994:445–478.

97a. Schwartzman, D, Nallamothu, N, Callans, DJ, et al. Postoperative lead-related complication in patients with nonthoracotomy defibrillation lead systems. *J Am Coll Cardiol* 1995;26:776.

97b. Martin DT, John R, Venditti FJ. Increase in defibrillation threshold in non-thoracotomy implanted defibrillators using a biphasic waveform. *Am J Cardiol* 1995;76:263.

97c. Epstein AE, Kay N, Plumb VJ, et al. Gross and microscopic pathologic changes associated with nonthoracotomy implantable defibrillator leads. *Circulation* 1998;98:1517.

97d. Korte T, Jung W, Schlippert U, et al. Prospective evaluation of shoulder-related problems in patients with pectoral cardioverter-defibrillator implantation. *Am Heart J* 1998;135:577.

97e. Boyle NG, Anselme F, Monahan KM, et al. Twiddler's syndrome variants in ICD patients. *Pacing Clin Electrophysiol* 1998;21:2685.

97f. Fetter JG, Benditt DG, Stanton MS. Electromagnetic interference from welding and motors on implantable cardioverter-defibrillators as tested in the electrically hostile work site. *J Am Coll Cardiol* 1996;28:423.

98. Larsen GC, Stupey MR, Walance CG, et al. Recurrent cardiac events in survivors of ventricular fibrillation or tachycardia: implications for driving restrictions. *JAMA* 1994;271:1335–1339.

99. Higgins SL, Rich DH, Haygood JR, et al. ICD restudy: results and potential benefit from routine predischarge and 2-month evaluation. *Pace* 1998;21:410–417.

100. Goldberger JJ, Horvath G, Inbar S, Kadish AH. Utility of predischarge and one-month transvenous implantable defibrillator tests. *Am J Cardiol* 1997;79:822–826.

101. Lewis RJ, Veltri EP. Predischarge testing of the ICD. In: Estes NAM, Manolis A, Wang PJ, eds. *Implantable cardioverter defibrillators: a comprehensive textbook.* New York: Marcel Dekker Inc, 1994:367–370.

102. Brunn J, Bocker M, Weber M, et al. Is there a need for routine testing of ICD defibrillation capacity? Results of more than 1000 studies. *Eur Heart J* 2000;21:162–169.

103. Glickson M, Luria D, Friedman PA, et al. Are routine arrhythmia inductions necessary in patients with pectoral implantable cardioverter defibrillators? *J Cardiovasc Electrophysiol* 2000;11:127–135.

104. Weiss DN, Zilo P, Luceri RM, et al. Predischarge arrhythmia induction testing of implantable defibrillators may be unnecessary in selected cases. *Am J Cardiol* 1997;80:1562–156.

105. Biblo LA, Carlson MA, Waldo AL. Follow up of patients with implantable cardioverter defibrillator devices. In: Estes NAM, Manolis A, Wang PJ, eds. *Implantable cardioverter defibrillators: a comprehensive textbook.* New York: Marcel Dekker Inc, 1994:425–436.

105a. Strickberger SA, Man KC, Daoud EG, et al. A prospective evaluation of catheter ablation of ventricular tachycardia as adjuvant therapy in patients with coronary artery disease and an implantable cardioverter-defibrillator. *Circulation* 1997;96:1525.

106. Stevenson WG, Friedman PL. Catheter ablation of ventricular tachycardia. In: Zipes DP, Jalife J, eds. *Cardiac electrophysiology: from cell to bedside.* Philadelphia: WB Saunders, 2000:1049–1056.

107. Kugler JD. Catheter ablation in pediatric patients. In: Zipes DP, Jalife J, eds. *Cardiac electrophysiology: from cell to bedside.* Philadelphia: WB Saunders, 2000:1056–1064.

108. Nair M, Saoudi N, Kroiss D, Letac B. Automatic arrhythmia identification using analysis of the atrioventricular association: application to a new generation of implantable defibrillators. *Circulation* 1997;95:967–973.

109. Hayes DL. Implantable pacemakers. In: Zipes DP, Jalife J, eds. *Cardiac electrophysiology: from cell to bedside.* Philadelphia: WB Saunders, 2000:974–982.

12

CATHETER AND SURGICAL ABLATION FOR CARDIAC ARRHYTHMIA

RONALD BERGER
MICHAEL D. LESH
HUGH CALKINS

For most cardiac arrhythmias, medical therapy with antiarrhythmic drugs is far from optimal. In addition to poor or sporadic efficacy, such drugs can be associated with bothersome and even fatal side effects, proarrhythmia, high cost, and inconvenience. In the past several decades, nonpharmacologic intervention, initially using a surgical approach and later employing closed-chest transvascular catheter ablation, has evolved to become the standard of care for an increasing number of arrhythmias. In this chapter, we discuss the concepts and results of ablation of cardiac arrhythmias.

By what general principle is it possible to ablate and cure a cardiac arrhythmia? If an arrhythmia is caused purely by an alteration in the functional properties of the myocardium or conduction system with no fixed relationship to cardiac anatomy, it would be difficult to ablate. Conversely, if a tachycardia involves an identifiable and specific region of cardiac anatomy, we can direct therapy to that region of the conducting tissue. Ablation can be thought of as an intervention that acts locally on cardiac tissue to abolish the anatomic substrate of a given cardiac arrhythmia, even if functional properties such as slow conduction or block are related to fixed anatomic structures. The goal of ablation is to cure cardiac arrhythmias by destroying areas of myocardial tissue or conduction system that are critical to the initiation or maintenance of a cardiac arrhythmia.

During the past 15 years, the varieties of cardiac arrhythmias that are amenable to an ablative approach have expanded greatly, which is a direct result of our advancing knowledge of the anatomic basis for the initiation or maintenance of such arrhythmias. We now recognize that tachycardias such as atrioventricular (AV) node reentry, atrial flutter, and atrial fibrillation have an anatomic substrate that can be altered by replacing conducting tissue with electrically inert tissue by means of surgical or catheter intervention.

In general, arrhythmias may be caused by any of several mechanisms, and the mode of ablative therapy depends on the mechanism. For example, some tachycardias involve a focal mechanism, for which a "point" ablative lesion suffices. Others involve macroreentry, and severing a relatively protected isthmus or conduction pathway with a linear lesion may be needed in these cases. Our understanding of the electrophysiology and anatomic substrates of arrhythmias has grown considerably in large part as a result of the detailed mapping required for successful ablation of these arrhythmias.

SURGICAL THERAPY

Overview

Arrhythmia surgery involves the use of a variety of surgical tools, including the scalpel, cryoablation (1–3), laser energy, radiofrequency energy, or other means of tissue destruction. Arrhythmia surgery usually requires a median sternotomy approach and general anesthesia and the need for cardiopulmonary bypass, with their associated risks and morbidity. However, the maze III procedure has been performed using minimally invasive surgery. The surgical treatment of cardiac arrhythmias has for the most part been replaced by catheter ablation. The most notable exception is atrial fibrillation, for which the surgical maze procedure remains a standard, although infrequently performed surgical procedure. Nevertheless, much was learned during the era of surgical arrhythmia therapy, and we briefly review the technique, results, and complications of arrhythmia surgery to place the current approach to catheter ablation in perspective.

R. Berger: Arrhythmia Service and Electrophysiology Laboratory, Johns Hopkins Hospital, Baltimore, Maryland 21287.

M. D. Lesh: Department of Medicine and Atrial Arrhythmia Center, University of California San Francisco, San Francisco, California 94143.

H. Calkins: Arrhythmia Service and Electrophysiology Laboratory, Johns Hopkins Hospital, Baltimore, Maryland 21287.

Surgical Treatment of Specific Arrhythmias

Atrial Flutter

Atrial flutter is a macroreentrant tachycardia confined to the right atrium. During the common form of atrial flutter, the reentrant wavefront travels superiorly up the interatrial septum and around the right atrium in a counterclockwise direction through a critical zone of slow conduction in the inferior right atrium among the tricuspid annulus, the inferior vena cava, and the os of the coronary sinus. The first treatment of atrial flutter with arrhythmia surgery was reported in 1986; atrial flutter was eliminated with cryosurgery in the region of the coronary sinus os (4). This important observation set the stage for catheter ablation of atrial flutter, first using direct current (DC) shock energy delivered in the low posteroseptal right atrium (5) and subsequently replaced by radiofrequency energy.

Atrial Fibrillation

The surgical maze procedure was developed by Cox and colleagues based on the multiple reentrant wavelet mechanism for atrial fibrillation, which proposes that atrial fibrillation is caused by the simultaneous presence of multiple, randomly wandering reentrant wavelets (6–15). The maze procedure creates lines of conduction block, resulting in areas too small to sustain reentry. This surgical procedure was developed with the goal of creating a generalized operative procedure that would interrupt all potential macroreentrant circuits and thereby cure atrial fibrillation. In developing this procedure, Cox and colleagues recognized that the complex nature of the multiple reentrant circuits responsible for atrial fibrillation would make a procedure that relied on detailed intraoperative mapping impractical. After extensive laboratory research, the maze procedure was first clinically applied in September 1987. Since then, several modifications in the surgical procedure have been made to maintain sinus node function and achieve restoration of atrial transport. The procedure, as performed today, is known as the maze III procedure and involves excision of the left and right atrial appendage, isolation of the pulmonary veins, and creation of several additional atrial incisions to interrupt intraatrial reentry but allow conduction of the sinus node impulse to the AV node along a specified route (6,8,) (Fig. 12-1).

As of October 1997, the maze procedure in one of its three forms has been carried out by Cox and colleagues in 190 patients (8). The average patient age was 54 ± 11 years. Paroxysmal atrial fibrillation was present in 58% and chronic atrial fibrillation in 42% of patients. The procedure was performed in conjunction with another cardiac procedure (i.e., mitral valve repair) in 34% of patients. During the first 3 months after surgery, approximately 50% of patients experienced recurrent atrial arrhythmias. As of the latest report,

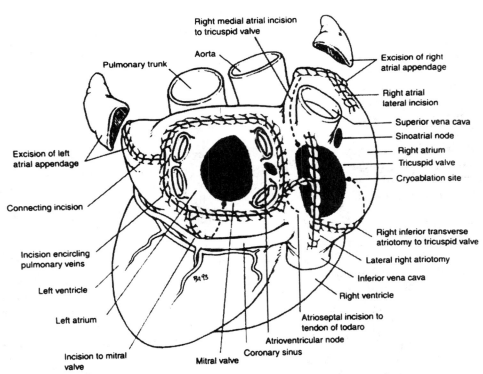

FIGURE 12-1. Schematic three-dimensional view of the heart, depicting the incisions of the maze 3 procedure. (Adapted from Cox JL, et al. Surgical therapy of cardiac arrhythmias. *Annu Rev Med* 1997;48:511–523, with permission.)

92% of patients followed longer than 3 months were in sinus rhythm without the need for concomitant antiarrhythmic therapy. Atrial fibrillation and flutter each recurred in 4% of patients and were subsequently controlled with antiarrhythmic therapy. Fifty-two patients (29%) also required a pacemaker before (*n* = 22) or after surgery because of underlying sick sinus syndrome identified preoperatively (*n* = 28) or as a complication of the procedure (*n* = 2). Based on a variety of types of evaluation, it is estimated that right atrial transport has been preserved in 98% of patients and left atrial transport in 92% of patients. Among the entire series of patients, a stroke (*N* = 1) or transient ischemic attack (*N* = 4) occurred in five patients. There were four perioperative deaths. Two of the deaths were caused by respiratory failure thought to be exacerbated by amiodarone therapy, one man died who also underwent a septal myotomy for treatment of hypertrophic cardiomyopathy, and one death resulted from delayed pericardial tamponade. Other reported complications included a low-output syndrome in 5 patients, myocardial infarction in 2, pancreatitis in 2, pneumonia in 10, bleeding in 11, and fluid retention in 29.

Several investigators have modified the maze procedure in an attempt to further improve the results of this operation. For example, Sueda and colleagues reported that surgical ablation of the left posterior atrium at the time of mitral valve surgery dramatically reduced the incidence of postoperative atrial fibrillation (16). Another technique, the radial approach, was developed to provide a more physiologic atrial activation-contraction sequence, thereby reducing the degree of left atrial dysfunction and optimizing the atrial contribution to left ventricular filling (17). In contrast to the maze procedure, in which the incisions desynchronize the activation sequence and often cut across the atrial coronary arteries, the incisions produced by the radial approach radiate from the sinus node toward the AV annular margins, paralleling the activation sequence and the atrial coronary arteries (18).

Most of these variants of the surgical maze procedure involve a subset of lesions, but all require isolation of the pulmonary vein region, and this may help us understand how the catheter-based interventions work. Given our knowledge of the role of pulmonary veins in initiation, it is tempting to speculate on whether the maze procedure and variants work to some extent by preventing initiating triggers rather than abolishing wavelets.

The remarkable success that has been achieved with the surgical maze procedure has provided an impetus to the development of catheter ablation systems specifically designed to facilitate a catheter-based maze procedure. Several of these systems are undergoing clinical evaluation (19).

Paroxysmal Supraventricular Tachycardia

Both common forms of paroxysmal supraventricular tachycardia (PSVT), atrioventricular nodal reentrant tachycardia (AVNRT) and atrioventricular reentrant tachycardia (AVRT)

which involves an accessory AV connection, have been treated with surgery.

The electrophysiologic substrate for AVNRT is provided by functional longitudinal dissociation of AV nodal conduction into two pathways; one usually has a rapid conduction velocity with a long effective refractory period, and the other has a slower conduction velocity and a longer effective refractory period. In 1979, a single case of unexpected surgical cure of AVNRT was reported in a patient with incessant symptoms after an unsuccessful attempt at surgical ablation of the AV node (20). This important observation suggested the possibility of developing a surgical procedure to ablate AVNRT while preserving AV conduction. A subsequent study demonstrated that a series of discrete cryolesions placed around the triangle of Koch were capable of altering the input pathways of the AV node, resulting in permanent prolongation of AV conduction in the experimental canine model (21). The first perinodal cryosurgery procedure was performed on a human in 1982 (22,23). Ross and colleagues subsequently reported on a surgical dissection technique in 1985 (24). Other modifications of these techniques have subsequently been reported (25–28).

The Wolff-Parkinson-White syndrome results from the presence of a small strip of working myocardium that bypasses the AV valve ring and serves as an electrical connection between the epicardial surface of the atrium and the ventricle. Sealy and colleagues reported the first successful surgical treatment of a patient with the Wolff-Parkinson-White syndrome in 1968 (29). Over the ensuing years, surgical ablation of accessory pathways to treat the Wolff-Parkinson-White syndrome and PSVT involving a concealed accessory pathway became a safe, effective, and commonly performed operation. Along with the development of improved surgical techniques came a better understanding of cardiac anatomy and of the anatomy and electrophysiologic characteristics of accessory pathways. This information paved the way for development of catheter ablation, which has largely eliminated the need for surgical ablation of accessory pathways. Today, only the rare patient who has failed multiple attempts at catheter ablation is considered an appropriate candidate for surgical ablation of an accessory pathway.

Two surgical approaches for interruption of accessory pathways have been developed. The endocardial approach was pioneered and perfected by Sealy, Gallagher, and Cox (30–32). This approach requires an atriotomy and is carried out under cardiopulmonary bypass and cold cardioplegic cardiac arrest. The alternative epicardial approach was developed and perfected by Guiraudon and colleagues (33–35). This technique combines epicardial exposure and cryoablation of the exposed AV junction. In contrast to the endocardial approach, it is performed on the normothermic beating heart and in most cases does not require the use of cardiopulmonary bypass.

The acute success rate for surgical ablation of accessory pathways approached 100%, with a complication rate of less than 5%. Despite the high efficacy and acceptable risk, this procedure has been replaced by catheter ablation because of the similar efficacy combined with lower cost and reduced patient morbidity (36–40).

Ventricular Tachyarrhythmias

Surgery for treatment of ventricular tachycardia (VT) was developed in the mid-1970s. The first surgical attempts were directed at VTs in patients without coronary artery disease (41–43). Shortly thereafter, attempts were made for surgical ablation of VT in the setting of a prior myocardial infarction. Initial studies revealed that a conventional aneurysmectomy was not effective in curing VT in a high proportion of patients (44). In the late 1970s, two surgical approaches were described: the encircling endocardial ventriculotomy (43–45) and the endocardial resection (46). Since then, these procedures have been modified by various investigators to improve the safety and efficacy of the operation.

The encircling endocardial ventriculotomy was developed by Guiradon and colleagues (43,45). This procedure was aimed at producing a fibrous barrier around the arrhythmogenic border zone, thereby confining the arrhythmogenic mechanism within the excluded area. Among the initial 29 patients who underwent this procedure, 4 died. One patient had an early recurrence, and three patients had late recurrences of VT. There were three late deaths. The procedure was later modified because it was determined that the extensive ventriculotomy was associated with development of left ventricular dysfunction (47,48). These modifications included the use of cryoablation directed at the border zone (49,50).

The treatment of ventricular tachycardia using a subendocardial resection was first described by Josephson (46). This operation involved preoperative or intraoperative mapping (or both) of a tachycardia site of origin and then a limited endocardial excision of the arrhythmogenic site. The excised tissue was approximately 5 cm². Approximately 70% of patients had no inducible VT at the time of predischarge electrophysiologic testing, and most of the remainder were rendered noninducible with the addition of antiarrhythmic drugs that had been ineffective preoperatively. Several modifications of this procedure have been described. This procedure is performed by opening the ventricle through the anterior or inferior scar or aneurysm. In 90% of cases, VT can be induced using standard programmed electrical stimulation. All tachycardias are mapped and surgically ablated, whether or not they have been observed clinically. After resection of the involved tissue, programmed electrical stimulation is repeated. The largest series includes 269 patients (51). Overall, VT was noninducible after surgery in approximately two thirds of patients. With antiarrhythmic drugs, more than 90% were noninducible. The perioperative mortality rate was 15%. Predictors of mortality included an ejection fraction of less than 0.20, emergency operation, and prior cardiac surgery. The 5-year actuarial survival was 60%.

Today, surgery for VT is rarely performed for several reasons. The development of advanced implantable devices that can detect and terminate most instances of VT and VF is perhaps the most important. The use of modern perimyocardial infarction care such as thrombolysis and acute coronary intervention seems to have reduced the incidence of sustained, hemodynamically tolerated VT, which typically requires a large infarct region or aneurysm.

CATHETER ABLATION

Overview

Since its initial description in 1982 (52), catheter ablation has evolved from a highly experimental technique to its present role as first-line therapy for many cardiac arrhythmias. During the 4-year period from 1989 through 1993, the number of patients undergoing catheter ablation procedures in the United States increased more than 30-fold from an estimated 450 procedures in 1989 to 15,000 procedures in 1993 (53). This evolution in the role of catheter ablation reflects in large part a change in the energy source used during catheter ablation procedures. Before 1989, catheter ablation was performed primarily with high-energy DC shocks. Typically, a multipolar electrode catheter was positioned in the heart and attached to a standard defibrillator. Under general anesthesia, 100 to 360 J of DC energy was delivered between the distal electrode and a patch placed on the patient's chest. This produced an explosive flash, heat, and increased pressure. Myocardial injury resulted from heat, barotrauma, and direct electrical injury. DC energy has been largely replaced with radiofrequency energy as the preferred energy source during catheter ablation procedures.

Principles of Catheter Ablation

Ablation procedures are performed in a specially equipped catheterization laboratory. Patients receive conscious sedation before and during the procedure. Two to five multipolar electrode catheters are inserted percutaneously under local anesthesia into a femoral, brachial, subclavian, or internal jugular vein and positioned in the heart under fluoroscopic guidance. Each electrode catheter has four or more electrodes. Typically, the most distal electrode pair is used for pacing and the delivery of critically timed extrastimuli, and the proximal electrodes are used to record electrograms from localized regions within the heart. During radiofrequency catheter ablation procedures, radiofrequency energy is delivered using an electrode catheter with a deflectable shaft and typically with a 4-mm distal electrode, although larger electrodes and those with irrigation or cooling are becoming available. Radiofrequency energy is usually delivered for 30 to 60 seconds between the distal electrode, and a patch is placed on the patient's back or chest (Fig. 12-2). Most catheter ablation systems in use today monitor the temperature of the ablation electrode and automatically adjust power output to achieve a targeted electrode temperature of between 60°C and 70°C. Knowledge of the electrode temperature at a particular ablation site is useful in determining whether an unsuccessful application of radiofrequency energy failed because of inaccurate mapping or inadequate heating. In the event of inadequate heating, additional applications of energy at the same site with improved catheter stability may result in success. Automatic adjustment of power output using closed-loop temperature control has been demonstrated to reduce the incidence of coagulum development, which may also facilitate catheter ablation by reducing the number of times the catheter has to be withdrawn from the body to have coagulum removed from the electrode tip (54).

Biophysics of Radiofrequency Catheter Ablation

Radiofrequency energy is a high-frequency, alternating electrical current. When used during catheter ablation procedures, it is delivered as a continuous, unmodulated, sinusoidal waveform with a frequency of approximately 500,000 cycles per second between the tip of an electrode

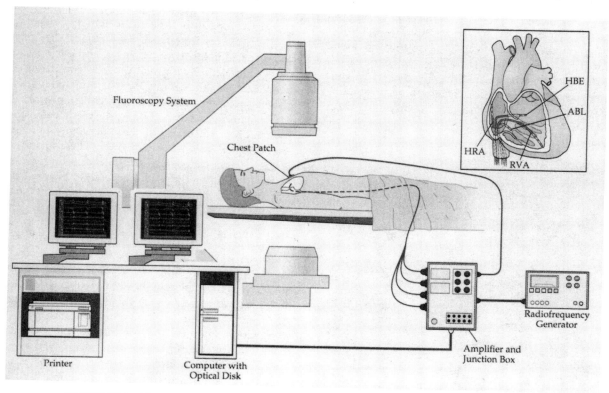

FIGURE 12-2. Schematic drawing of the equipment and usual approach to electrophysiology testing and catheter ablation. The patient is placed on a standard fluoroscopy table. Three to five electrode catheters are inserted percutaneously through the femoral vein and, in some cases, through the femoral artery, internal jugular vein, or subclavian vein. Each catheter contains four to eight electrodes. Each electrode is connected to a junction box, which is connected to the physiologic recorder that allows surface and intracardiac electrodes to be displayed on a monitor and recorded on a printer or optical disk; a stimulator, which is a device that allows electrical stimuli to be delivered to the heart at precise intervals; and the radiofrequency (RF) generator, which generates a sinusoidal wavefront with a frequency of about 500,000 Hz and a power output of as much as 50 W. The junction box allows the electrophysiologist to record, deliver stimuli, or deliver RF energy through any electrode. RF energy is typically delivered between the distal 4-mm tip of the ablation catheter and a large patch placed on the patient's back or chest. **Inset:** Typical position of the electrode catheters in the heart. During a standard diagnostic electrophysiology test, catheters are positioned in the high right atrium (HRA) near the sinus node, along the septal aspect of the tricuspid valve, and at the apex of the right ventricle. During catheter ablation procedures, an additional catheter is often positioned in the coronary sinus os to allow mapping of the left side of the heart. The placement of the ablation catheter depends on the type and precise location of the targeted ablation site. This figure shows the position that would be used to ablate a right-sided accessory pathway. ABL, ablation catheter; HBE, His bundle electrogram; RVA, right ventricular apex. (From Calkins H, et al. Catheter ablation of arrhythmias. In: Topol E, ed. *Scientific American Medicine*, Madison, NY: Scientific American Medicine, 1998, with permission.)

catheter and a ground plate positioned on the back or chest. Because the ground plate has a much larger surface area than the tip, current density is focused at the smaller electrode. Current flows into the tissue underlying the active electrode in alternating direction at high frequency. Resistive heating ensues as a result of ionic agitation in the tissue. The tissue underlying the ablation electrode, rather than the electrode itself, is the source of heat generation; this contrasts with a purely thermal source in which the probe itself is the source of heat and tissue destruction.

The heating of tissue during radiofrequency catheter ablation may be thought of as a two-step process: resistive heating followed by conductive heat transfer from the area of resistive heating to surrounding tissue. Because direct resistive heating falls precipitously with increasing distance from the ablation electrode, resistive heating is responsible for heating only a very narrow rim of tissue extending approximately 1 mm beyond the ablation electrode (55). Most of the lesion volume is determined by the relative contributions of conductive heat exchange into surrounding tissue and convective heat loss toward the relatively cooler moving blood (Fig. 12-3).

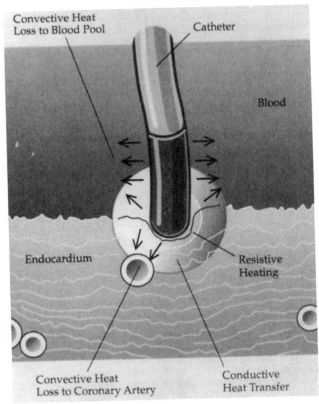

FIGURE 12-3. Schematic drawing of a radiofrequency ablation catheter positioned on the endocardium shows zones of resistive and conductive heating and convective heat loss from tissue into the blood pool and coronary arteries. (From Calkins H, et al. Catheter ablation of arrhythmias. In: Topol E, ed. *Scientific American Medicine*, Madison, NY: Scientific American Medicine, 1998, with permission.)

Thermal injury is the principal mechanism of tissue destruction during radiofrequency catheter ablation procedures. Elevation of tissue temperature results in desiccation and the denaturation of proteins and in coagulation of tissue and blood (56). Temperature-dependent depolarization of myocardial tissue and loss of excitability occurs at temperatures greater than 43°C. Reversible loss of excitability occurs at tissue temperatures between 43°C and 50°C. Irreversible tissue injury occurs at temperatures greater than 50°C (57). When the temperature at the electrode tissue interface exceeds 100°C, tissue immediately adjacent to the electrode desiccates, and plasma proteins denature to form a coagulum (58). The development of a coagulum results in a rapid increase in impedance that leads to a dramatic decrease in current density, thereby limiting further lesion growth. As a result of the need to achieve a tissue temperature of 50°C for irreversible tissue injury, the 100°C temperature ceiling for tissue heating, and the rapid decrease in tissue temperature with increasing distance from the ablation electrode, the lesions created during radiofrequency catheter ablation procedures are small (<5 mm) and have well-demarcated borders (Fig. 12-4). Methods for improved cooling of the electrode have been developed to allow delivery of higher radiofrequency power. These include the use of larger (8-mm) electrodes (59), which receive greater convective cooling by the blood, and saline-irrigated electrode tips, in which the electrode is actively cooled (60,61).

Hardware

Advances in catheter ablation have been facilitated by the development of equipment specifically designed for these procedures. The ablation part of the procedure is preceded by a diagnostic study, which entails the standard equipment of the electrophysiology laboratory: fluoroscopy, amplifiers with display monitor for intracardiac and surface electrograms, multipolar catheters for stimulation and electrogram acquisition, and a stimulator to provide pacing sequences to induce the target arrhythmia. The ablation itself requires additional catheters for the delivery of ablative energy, as well as a device that produces and regulates the ablative energy, and it may place additional requirements on the fluoroscopy and mapping systems.

Most of today's ablation catheters are specifically designed for the delivery of radiofrequency current, although ultrasonic (62–64), microwave (65–67), laser (68–71), and cryoablative (72) techniques have also been investigated. The catheter is manipulated to the appropriate site using a steering mechanism. In most catheters, this involves one or more pull wires that run the length of the catheter and control deflection of the catheter tip when tension is applied to these wires within the handle of the catheter. The operator moves the catheter tip within the heart using a combination of tip deflection and torque maneuvers. For radiofrequency ablation, the tip of the

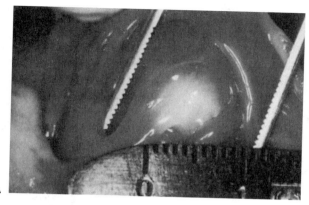
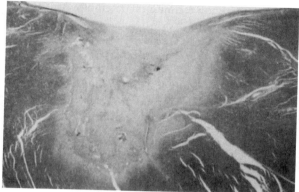

FIGURE 12-4. A: Photograph of a lesion created with radiofrequency energy 1 month earlier in a canine ventricle. The lesion is pale, is about 5 mm in diameter, and has smooth borders. (From Calkins H, et al. Catheter ablation of arrhythmias. In: Topol E, ed. *Scientific American Medicine*, Madison, NY: Scientific American Medicine, 1998, with permission.) **B:** Histologic section of the same lesion. The lesion has a distinct border surrounded by normal myocardium, is hemispherical, and shows extensive fibrosis. The lesion depth is 6 mm. (From Jumrussirikul P, Chen JT, Jenkins M, et al. Prospective comparison of temperature guided microwave and radiofrequency catheter ablation in the swine heart. *Pacing Clin Electrophysiol* 1998;21:1364–1374, with permission.)

catheter incorporates an electrode that is at least 4 mm long so that an adequate volume of myocardium can be heated with the delivery of ablative current.

The generator of radiofrequency ablative energy provides up to 50 W of unmodulated (constant amplitude) alternating current at a frequency of 350,000 to 500,000 Hz. The generator is connected to the ablation catheter, and the current is applied to achieve resistive heating within a rim of myocardium adjacent to the catheter tip electrode. Feedback control allows the generator to provide enough current to the tip electrode to heat the tissue adequately without getting so hot as to boil blood. Most ablation catheters have a thermistor or thermocouple in the tip electrode to monitor tip temperature, which serves as the feedback signal to the generator (54,73). Many ablation systems also monitor the electrical impedance between the catheter tip and reference electrodes and automatically discontinue energy delivery if the impedance rises above a preset ceiling, because it is indicative of coagulum formation around the tip electrode. Newer ablation systems provide for cooling of the tip electrode during energy delivery. This strategy allows for a higher current to be applied to the tip electrode without blood boiling around it. As a result, the adjacent myocardium in which resistive heating occurs gets hotter than it would have at lower levels of applied current, and a larger lesion can be produced. Tip cooling is achieved by infusion of saline through a lumen that runs the length of the catheter and within the tip (60,61).

As the range of ablatable arrhythmias has broadened, the ablation procedures have in some cases become more technically challenging. In such cases, particularly when targeting atrial tachycardias (ATs) or VTs, visualization of the catheter tip in relation to the cardiac anatomy is crucial. Because a single fluoroscopic view displays the catheter only

against the cardiac silhouette, biplane fluoroscopy is a useful, albeit expensive, addition to the electrophysiology laboratory. When the two fluoroscopic planes are placed orthogonal to each other, the position of the catheter in three-dimensional space can be inferred.

New technology has provided a means for nonfluoroscopic tracking of catheter tip position and orientation in three-dimensional space. The Biosense CARTO system comprises a set of three magnetic field–generating coils placed underneath the patient and catheters that include magnetic field sensors in the tip (74,75). The field-generating coils operate at different frequencies, and catheter tip position is determined by the sensed strength of the three separable fields, using much the same principle as in global positioning systems. The system displays the tip position on a rotatable stick figure image. Activation timing at each catheter location is also displayed as a color map.

Even with biplane fluoroscopy or the nonfluoroscopic mapping system described previously, the catheter tip cannot be visualized in relation to the actual endocardial surface or neighboring vascular structures. Although this may not be required in ablation procedures, it may facilitate catheter manipulation and avoid complications. Several investigators have employed intravascular ultrasound probes for this purpose (76–78) and used it in conjunction with fluoroscopy. Alternatively, magnetic resonance imaging may provide an entirely nonfluoroscopic means for visualizing anatomic structures and locating the ablation catheter tip in three-dimensional space (79).

Mapping

The process of determining the appropriate site or sites for delivery of ablative energy constitutes intracardiac mapping. Different mapping techniques are employed for different target arrhythmias.

Activation Mapping

Perhaps the most commonly used mapping technique is activation mapping. This method involves moving the steerable (or roving) catheter until the site of earliest activation is found. This technique is used, for example, in locating the site of an accessory pathway along the tricuspid or mitral annulus. If the pathway is manifest, the site of earliest ventricular activation can be sought during sinus rhythm or atrial pacing. It is important that the time measurement is referenced to a constant from beat to beat, such as the onset of the delta wave on a surface electrocardiogram (ECG) lead. It is not appropriate to measure the time from local atrial to local ventricular activation at a putative ablation site, because this time difference may be minimized at sites of relatively late atrial activation rather than early ventricular activation. Accessory pathways can also be mapped during ventricular pacing such that the site of earliest atrial activation is found. In this case, timing is typically referenced to the pacing artifact. However, it is often difficult to distinguish the atrial and ventricular deflections from each other at the optimal ablation site during retrograde activation, because continuous electrical activity is frequently observed at these sites (80). Anterograde (ventricular) and retrograde (atrial) activation mapping may not lead to identical anatomic sites, because many accessory pathways slant across the valve annulus (81). Mapping of manifest pathways is also facilitated by the finding of a Kent potential at the optimal ablation site (82,83).

Activation mapping is also used to identify ablation sites for automatic or triggered ATs or VTs. In this case, the appropriate atrial or ventricular chamber is determined by the P wave or QRS axis, respectively. A roving catheter is then manipulated within the chamber during tachycardia until the site of earliest activation is found. Timing is referenced to the P-wave or QRS onset in the surface ECG or to a reference catheter placed in the appropriate chamber (84–86). It is often difficult to keep track of the exact location of all sites tested and of the activation time at each of these sites. The Biosense CARTO system is designed specifically for this purpose (87). Activation mapping can also be facilitated by the use of catheters or insertable arrays with many electrodes. Halo catheters have up to 20 electrodes on a single catheter shaft and are frequently used to map activation along the right atrial septum or free wall. Deployable baskets of electrodes have been used to map ATs and VTs (88,89), as shown in Figure 12-5. Activation mapping can also be performed with a noncontact system made by Endocardial Solutions, Inc. The system comprises an inflatable balloon with 64 electrodes on the surface and software that computes and displays the endocardial activation sequence based on an inverse solution calculation (90).

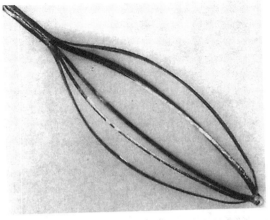

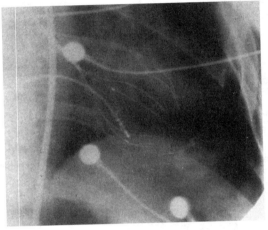

FIGURE 12-5. A: Basket-shaped mapping catheter. **B:** Left anterior oblique fluoroscopic image obtained after deployment of a 170-mL basket catheter. (From Schmitt C, Zrenner B, Schneider M, et al. Clinical experience with a novel multielectrode basket catheter in right atrial tachycardias. *Circulation* 1999;99:2414–2422, with permission.)

The electrograms used for activation mapping are usually bipolar. Bipolar electrograms are obtained by amplifying the voltage difference between the catheter tip electrode and a neighboring ring electrode 1 or 2 mm away. The signal is filtered to remove low-frequency (<30-Hz) activity associated with tissue repolarization and catheter movement. Activation is easily discerned as the time of first rapid deflection from the signal baseline. The greater the interelectrode spacing, the larger the electrogram amplitude is, although at the cost of diminished spatial resolution. Some workers prefer to map using unipolar electrograms. In this case, the signal from the tip electrode is measured against an indifferent electrode, typically placed on the body surface remote from the heart. The signal is low-pass filtered, and activation is taken as the point of maximum negative slope (91). Although activation is more difficult to discern in a unipolar electrogram, morphologic features in unipolar electrograms can be used to identify sites of origin of ectopic activity (92). Unipolar electrograms also allow determination of the quality of electrode-tissue contact (93).

Pace Mapping

Closely allied with activation mapping is the technique of pace mapping. Once the roving catheter is placed at a putative ablation site, the chamber is paced through the tip electrode. The activation sequence during pacing is then compared with that during beats of the tachycardia. In the case of ectopic VTs, such as those that arise in the right ventricular outflow tract, the comparison of paced and tachycardia beats is usually accomplished by examining the morphology of the QRS complex in all 12 standard surface ECG leads. When the paced complex matches the tachycardia in all 12 leads, ventricular activation is identical, and ablation is usually successful at that site (94). When using activation mapping for ectopic ATs, however, it is difficult to compare P-wave morphology of the paced and tachycardia beats because of the low amplitude of the P waves and interference from QRS complexes and T waves. In this case, the sequence of atrial activation is compared. Tracy and colleagues (95) showed that differences in the activation sequence between paced and tachycardia beats can be used to guide catheter movements to sites of progressively closer match and eventual ablation success.

Entrainment Mapping

Entrainment mapping is a technique that bears similarity to pace mapping but is used in reentrant ATs and VTs. During a reentrant tachycardia, pacing at a rate faster than the tachycardia from a bystander site (i.e., a site outside of the reentrant circuit) results in manifest entrainment (96). In this case, the activation sequence is altered because of

antidromic capture of some of the tissue within the paced chamber. However, if the pacing catheter is placed within the circuit or at a site connected to the circuit by a protected isthmus, the paced activation sequence matches that during tachycardia. This is called *concealed entrainment* (or entrainment with concealed fusion), and it results, for example, in a paced QRS morphology matching that during VT (Fig. 12-6). For concealed entrainment to occur, pacing must result in complete or nearly complete orthodromic capture of the paced chamber (97,98). Pacing into sinus rhythm (as opposed to the tachycardia) is generally not useful in mapping a reentrant tachycardia because substantial antidromic capture of the paced chamber is likely, resulting in alteration of the activation sequence compared with the tachycardia, even when pacing from sites within the circuit.

Other Methods

Distinguishing sites that are within the actual circuit from those connected by a protected alleyway requires additional mapping techniques. When entraining a tachycardia from within the circuit, the time from pacing artifact to onset of P wave (in atrial reentry) or QRS complex (in ventricular reentry) matches the time from spontaneous local activation of that site to P-wave or QRS onset during tachycardia. Entraining from sites in connected alleyways results in pace-to-P-wave or pace-to-QRS intervals that exceed the corresponding intervals from spontaneous activation to P-wave or QRS onset (98,99). Similarly, it is often helpful to measure the interval from the last pacing artifact until spontaneous local activation at the pacing site after cessation of a period of concealed entrainment. This measurement is called the *return cycle* or *postpacing interval*. It equals (or nearly equals) the tachycardia cycle length when pacing

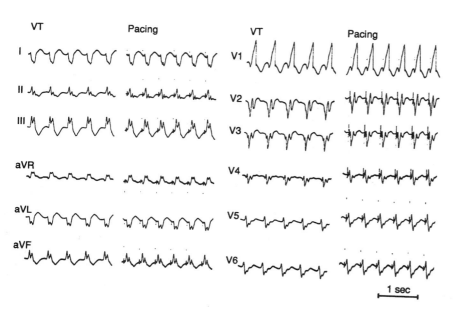

FIGURE 12-6. Pace mapping. The ventricular tachycardia (VT) induced in the electrophysiology laboratory had a right bundle branch block configuration and a cycle length of 480 ms. Pacing in the left ventricle at site 11 (anterior wall) at a cycle length of 400 ms resulted in QRS complexes similar or identical to the QRS complexes during VT in all leads except V_4 (pace map score, 11/12). After a 35-W application of radiofrequency energy at this site, the VT could no longer be induced by programmed ventricular stimulation. (From Morady F, Harvey M, Kalb-Fleisch ST, et al. *Circulation* 1993;87:363–372, with permission.)

from within the circuit, but it exceeds the tachycardia cycle length when pacing from a connected alleyway (98,99).

Some tachycardias call for a mapping strategy that is specific to the arrhythmia. For example, in AVNRT, sites for AV node modification are found using a combination of anatomic localization and electrogram characteristics. The catheter tip is placed on the septal aspect of the tricuspid annulus or just inside the coronary sinus ostium in search of sites where the local electrogram is more ventricular than atrial and the atrial component has fractionated activity or multiple deflections. Usually, at sites of successful AV node modification, junctional rhythms are observed during application of radiofrequency energy.

Ablation of typical atrial flutter is guided largely by anatomic positioning. The diagnosis of typical atrial flutter is made by activation or entrainment mapping such that involvement of the subeustachian isthmus in the right atrium is demonstrated (99,100). Ablative lesions are then placed along a line from the tricuspid annulus to the inferior vena cava until the arrhythmia terminates and bidirectional conduction block in the subeustachian isthmus is achieved (100–102).

Indications, Use, and Outcomes of Ablation

Atrial Tachycardia

The term *atrial tachycardia* refers to a group of arrhythmias confined to the atrium that have a rate less than 240 bpm and that are often difficult to control with standard antiarrhythmic medications. ATs, which have a focal site of origin or result from macroreentry involving a critical isthmus of atrial tissue, are amenable to cure with radiofrequency catheter ablation. From an ablation perspective, two major types of AT can be considered: focal (or ectopic) AT and scar-mediated (or incisional) AT.

Focal AT may manifest as a paroxysmal or a sustained arrhythmia. The mechanism of the tachycardia may be elu-

cidated by pharmacologic and pacing maneuvers, and it may be classified as automatic, triggered, or reentrant (103). The origin of these arrhythmias may be located in the right or left atrium, usually near the pulmonary vein orifices, right atrial appendage, or crista terminalis (104). In the automatic and triggered tachycardias, catheter ablation is performed by manipulating one or more steerable electrode catheters in the right or left atrium to identify the site of earliest atrial activation, usually at least 30 ms before onset of the P wave. The atrial activation sequence with pacing at that site should match the activation sequence during the clinical tachycardia. In the reentrant ATs, appropriate ablation sites are identified using the entrainment techniques described earlier. After the site is identified, 25 to 50 W of radiofrequency energy is delivered for 30 to 60 seconds.

Results of radiofrequency catheter ablation of focal ATs have been published in several series (103–109) and reviewed by Chen and colleagues (110). The success rate for ablation among a collective total of 252 patients reported in 16 relevant publications included in their review (110) was 93%. The collective recurrence rate was 7%. The Biosense CARTO system can facilitate mapping of sustained, focal ATs (85).

Incisional AT is mediated by macroreentry around the scar of a prior surgical atriotomy (Fig. 12-7). These tachycardias are frequently seen as late sequelae after surgical repair of congenital heart disease (111). Optimal ablation sites are those that occur within a protected isthmus of slow conduction that typically develops between one end of an atriotomy scar and a nearby anatomic barrier, such as the inferior vena cava, superior vena cava, or tricuspid annulus (112). The extent of the atriotomy scar may be mapped by identifying sites with distinct double potentials. The two deflections are widely separated near the middle of the scar and coalesce at the ends (113). Entrainment techniques are used to identify optimal ablation sites within the critical isthmus (114). The published clinical experience with catheter ablation is small. Among three series, ablation was

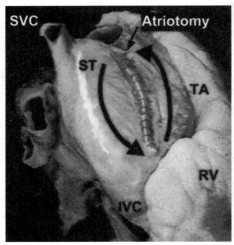 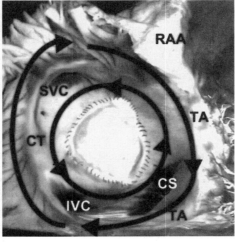

A,B

FIGURE 12-7. Mechanism of scar-mediated atrial flutter with atriotomy **(A)** or patch **(B)**. (See text for abbreviations.)

acutely successful in 33 (85%) of 39 patients (112–114), although recurrence of the ablated arrhythmia occurred in 6 of 13 patients in one series (112).

Inappropriate Sinus Tachycardia

Inappropriate sinus tachycardia (IST) is an ill-defined and uncommon clinical syndrome characterized by an increased resting heart rate and an exaggerated response to stress or exercise (115). The mechanism of this tachycardia is unknown, although it may involve a primary abnormality of the sinus node demonstrating enhanced automaticity or a primary autonomic disturbance with increased sympathetic activity and enhanced sinus node β-adrenergic sensitivity. The diagnosis of IST is one of exclusion. It most commonly occurs in young women.

It is important to distinguish IST from the postural orthostatic tachycardia syndrome (POTS). POTS is a type of dysautonomia that typically occurs in young women (116). It is defined as an increase of more than 28 bpm in the heart rate on standing, with associated symptoms of orthostatic intolerance such as lightheadedness and palpitations. Patients with POTS are treated primarily with increased salt intake, fludrocortisone, and midodrine (117). Catheter ablation does not have a role in the management of these patients.

The recognition that the sinus node region is a distributed complex exhibiting rate-dependent site differentiation allows for targeted ablation to eliminate the fastest sinus rates while maintaining some degree of sinus node function. This may require some fairly extensive ablation along up to 4 cm of the crista terminalis. The goal may be to modify sinus node function to prevent the fastest rates or to completely ablate the sinus node and implant a dual-chamber or atrial pacemaker. To overcome the limitations imposed by fluoroscopic imaging on the identification of endocardial landmarks and the spatial relationship of electrode catheters to such structures, some centers have explored the use of intracardiac echocardiography to identify endocardial structures such as the crista terminalis and particularly to guide mapping and ablation of sinus node tissue along the crista. The Biosense CARTO system may also be useful for identifying the sinus node region and the effect of ablation lesions on that area. Unfortunately, only about one half of affected patients receive symptomatic relief from sinus node ablation. Even after complete sinus node ablation and pacemaker implantation, some patients are symptomatic despite the absence of severe tachycardia (117). There are no specific guidelines to decide which patients with IST should undergo modification of the sinus node. However, this infrequently performed procedure should be reserved for the most highly symptomatic of patients (in whom POTS has been excluded) who have failed attempts at pharmacologic therapy and are willing to undergo a procedure with considerable risk of recurrence or

the need for a pacemaker and without assurance that their symptoms will be improved.

Atrial Flutter

Atrial flutter is an atrial arrhythmia characterized by a regular rate, a uniform morphology, and a rate greater than 240 bpm. Atrial flutter is usually accompanied by a fixed 2 : 1 ventricular response, and it is this rapid ventricular response that results in the most symptoms. Atrial flutter may be observed transiently after cardiac surgery or may persist for months to years. Many different forms of atrial flutter exist, which has led to multiple classification schemes. Atrial flutter can be classified as isthmus-dependent, non–isthmus-dependent, and atypical forms. In isthmus-dependent atrial flutter, the reentrant circuit involves the subeustachian isthmus in the inferior aspect of the right atrium between the tricuspid annulus and the eustachian valve (100). The complete circuit has been shown to also involve atrial septal tissue, the anterior roof of the right atrium, and the lateral wall of the atrium anterior to the crista terminalis (97,98,118) (Fig. 12-8). In isthmus-dependent flutter, activation proceeds along the atrial side of the tricuspid annulus in clockwise or counterclockwise direction (as viewed

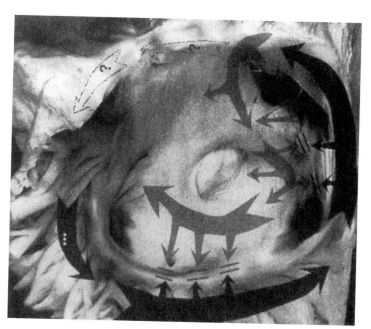

FIGURE 12-8. Diagram showing proposed circuit in type I atrial flutter with lines of block identified by double lines. Idealized depiction of the right atrial endocardium is viewed anterior to posterior through a reflected anterior wall. Arrows represent atrial activation sequence during atrial flutter. Areas within the reentrant circuit are marked by black arrows, whereas those not within the reentrant circuit are marked with gray arrows. The remainder of the circuit, which is not known, is marked by dotted arrows identified with a question mark. Lines of block are marked with double lines. (From Calkins H, et al. Catheter ablation of arrhythmias. In: Topol E, ed. *Scientific American Medicine*, Madison, NY: Scientific American Medicine, 1998, with permission.)

from the cardiac apex), and the subeustachian isthmus serves as a critical zone of slow conduction, enabling reentry to sustain. Counterclockwise isthmus-dependent flutter, also called common (type I) atrial flutter, is characterized by biphasic flutter waves in II, III, and aVF leads and an atrial rate of 250 to 320 bpm. Clockwise isthmus-dependent flutter (type II or uncommon flutter) is characterized by upright flutter waves in II, III, and aVF leads and an atrial rate of 250 to more than 320 bpm.

Non–isthmus-dependent flutter refers to any fixed reentrant atrial circuit that does not involve the sub-eustachian isthmus. The circuit often develops in the setting of scar tissue. This may represent microreentry within diseased tissue or macroreentry around a surgical scar. The latter differs from scar-mediated AT (described earlier) only in rate. Atypical atrial flutter involves an activation sequence that varies from one atrial beat to another. In this case, the reentrant pathway is not fixed, and the arrhythmia is mechanistically indistinguishable from coarse atrial fibrillation.

Isthmus-dependent and non–isthmus-dependent atrial flutters can be cured with catheter ablation. In isthmus-dependent flutter, the subeustachian isthmus represents an ablation target. Lesions are placed in one or more lines across the isthmus from the tricuspid annulus to eustachian valve [and usually continuing to the inferior vena cava until bidirectional conduction block in the isthmus is achieved (101)] (Fig. 12-9). In non–isthmus-dependent flutter, the slow conduction zone is identified with entrainment mapping and then becomes the ablation target. In contrast, atypical atrial flutter does not rely on an anatomically defined circuit and cannot be cured by ablation of a single target.

Catheter ablation of atrial flutter represents a rapidly developing area of interventional electrophysiology. The first successful ablation of atrial flutter, reported in 1986, was performed by employing cryosurgery in the region of the coronary sinus os (4). Subsequently, success rates of approximately 50% were obtained for catheter ablation of atrial flutter using DC shock energy delivered in the low posteroseptal right atrium (5). DC energy was later abandoned in favor of radiofrequency energy.

Catheter ablation of typical atrial flutter is performed using a deflectable ablation catheter positioned in the inferior right atrium, usually through the right femoral vein. In early series of these procedures, lesions were placed at putative exit sites of the slow conduction isthmus until atrial flutter terminated (119). Exit sites are consistently found just anterior or posterior to the coronary sinus ostium. Recurrence rates were relatively high with this approach, however. In subsequent work, the importance of achieving bidirectional conduction block in the subeustachian isthmus was established (120–121). Use of this strategy has led to an acute success rate of 100% and a recurrence rates of 7% in four published series (100,102,120,121). In these reports, clinical recurrence of atrial flutter was invariably

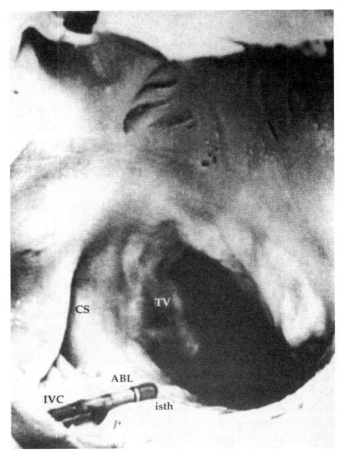

FIGURE 12-9. Position of the ablation catheter during ablation of atrial flutter is viewed from within the right atrium of a heart taken from a cadaver. Shown are the tricuspid annulus and the ostium of the coronary sinus (CS). The ablation catheter (ABL) is shown entering the right atrium from the inferior vena cava (IVC) and positioned along the isthmus (isth) of tissue that connects the tricuspid valve (TV) and the inferior vena cava. This isthmus represents a critical portion of the reentrant circuit during atrial flutter. Atrial flutter can be cured by delivering a series of radiofrequency lesions in a linear pattern along the isthmus to create a line of conduction block. (From Calkins H, et al. Catheter ablation of arrhythmias. In: Topol E, ed. *Scientific American Medicine*, Madison, NY: Scientific American Medicine, 1998, with permission.)

associated with loss of conduction block in the subeustachian isthmus. Using an end point of bidirectional isthmus block allows for application of radiofrequency lesions during normal sinus rhythm if preferred or if atrial flutter is paroxysmal and difficult to induce (120).

In some cases of typical atrial flutter, achieving bidirectional isthmus block can be challenging, which may be related to anatomic variations in some patients. For example, the subeustachian isthmus may constitute a deep valley between the tricuspid annulus and the eustachian valve and therefore may be difficult to fully navigate with standard ablation catheters. The floor of the isthmus may comprise relatively thick myocardial tissue that remains electrically intact with standard radiofrequency lesions. Jais and associates (122) showed that radiofrequency ablation using a cooled-tip catheter allows creation of conduction block in the subeustachian isthmus in cases resistant to standard ablation techniques. We prospectively compared cooled-tip and standard radiofrequency ablation for isthmus-dependent flutter and found that cooled-tip ablation allowed success with fewer lesions than with standard radiofrequency ablation and provided a useful alternative when ablation success could not be achieved with standard ablation catheters (123).

Some patients present with atrial fibrillation initially and then present with typical atrial flutter when treated with a class Ic or class III antiarrhythmic agent. These patients can be treated with catheter ablation to eliminate atrial flutter and usually remain arrhythmia free if maintained on the same antiarrhythmic drug therapy (124–126). Presumably, the antiarrhythmic drug slows conduction or prolongs refractoriness throughout the atria such that reentry can be maintained only when the subeustachian isthmus is included in the circuit. This hybrid treatment strategy may represent effective therapy for many patients with atrial fibrillation.

An unresolved issue in atrial flutter ablation is whether anticoagulation is required before or after the ablation procedure. Because thromboembolic events can be associated with cardioversion of atrial flutter (127,128), it seems appropriate to manage patients for ablation as if they are undergoing cardioversion. In our practice, we treat patients with coumadin for at least 4 weeks before ablation, discontinue the drug 3 days before the procedure, and restart it the night after. Anticoagulation is then continued for at least 1 month after the procedure.

Atrial Fibrillation

During the past 5 years, increasing attention has been focused on the development of catheter ablation techniques and ablation systems to cure atrial fibrillation. This endeavor has been fueled by several factors, including the clinical importance of atrial fibrillation because of its high prevalence in the general population, associated symptoms, stroke risk, and increased mortality, the limited efficacy, side effects, and risks associated with pharmacologic therapy, and demonstration of the feasibility of curing atrial fibrillation with catheter ablation techniques.

Swartz and colleagues are credited with being the first to demonstrate that chronic atrial fibrillation can be cured using catheter ablation techniques. In this landmark report, presented at the American Heart Association meeting in 1994, the investigators reported that creation of linear lesions in the right and left atrium results in a progressive increase in the organization of atrial activity until sinus rhythm is restored (129). The placement of the lesion lines was designed to emulate those placed surgically in the maze procedure developed by Cox (6). Almost simultaneous with Swartz's work,

Haissaguerre and colleagues began a series of investigations into the role of catheter ablation in the treatment of atrial fibrillation. An initial series of three patients who underwent successful ablation of atrial fibrillation was published in 1994 (130). Later that year, Haissaguerre and colleagues reported the successful ablation of paroxysmal atrial fibrillation in a patient with the creation of three linear lesions in the right atrium (two longitudinal and one transverse) using a specially designed 14-pole ablation catheter (131).

In a subsequent report on 45 patients with frequent drug-refractory episodes of atrial fibrillation, Haissaguerre and coworkers found that a purely right-sided ablation approach was successful in 33% of patients and that a higher success rate (60%) could be achieved with the addition of ablative lesions placed in the left atrium (132). The investigators found that linear lesions were often arrhythmogenic because of gaps in the ablative lines, yet many patients were ultimately cured with ablation of a single rapidly firing ectopic focus. These ectopic foci were found at the orifices of the left or right superior pulmonary veins or near the superior vena cava. The latter observation led the investigators to systematically attempt cure of paroxysmal atrial fibrillation by mapping and ablating individual foci of ectopic activity, first in a series of nine patients (133) and then in a series of 45 (134). In the larger series, long-term freedom from recurrent arrhythmia was achieved in 28 patients (62%). Ninety-four percent of the ectopic foci were mapped to the pulmonary veins, mostly the two superior pulmonary veins. Many of these foci were found well into the veins, outside of the cardiac silhouette, where myocardial bands are known to extend (135).

The feasibility of focal ablation for paroxysmal atrial fibrillation has also been confirmed by others (136). The investigators achieved an 88% long-term cure rate with ablation of foci in the pulmonary veins. The foci were generally found in the superior veins, most of which were well inside the veins (9 to 40 mm from the orifice). In a separate report, the same group described their experience in locating and ablating right atrial foci in eight patients with paroxysmal atrial fibrillation (137). These foci were found along the crista terminalis or near the coronary sinus ostium.

Despite the encouraging results in focal atrial fibrillation ablation reported, several obstacles remain. Mapping the ectopic foci requires the presence of frequent bursts of fibrillatory activity or at least of premature atrial beats. The site of earliest activity associated with these initiating beats must then be identified. Ideally, a site is found with local activity preceding the ectopic P wave by 40 to 160 ms (137). Provocative maneuvers, including isoproterenol and adenosine infusions and burst pacing, may be required to elicit atrial ectopy. However, it remains unclear whether provoked ectopy matches the type that occurs clinically. Because ectopic beats are fleeting, it is difficult to systematically map their origin. Some patients present in atrial fibrillation, requiring cardioversion so that a new onset of fibrillation can

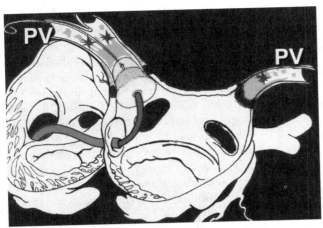

FIGURE 12-10. The balloon-tipped ablation catheter is designed for deployment at the ostium of the pulmonary vein. The safety and efficacy of creation of circumferential lesions on a purely anatomic basis is being investigated.

be mapped. These patients may require repeated cardioversions during the mapping and ablation procedure if each episode of fibrillation is sustained. It is also unknown what fraction of patients with paroxysmal atrial fibrillation has a focal source of the arrhythmia. Ablation systems are being developed using balloon-tipped ablation catheters that allow the rapid creation of circumferential lesions at the junction between the pulmonary veins and left atrium. If these systems are proven safe and effective, catheter ablation of focally initiated atrial fibrillation may become a routine procedure based only on anatomic considerations (Fig. 12-10).

Even more questions remain regarding ablation strategies for chronic atrial fibrillation. The initial experience reported by Swartz (129) was in patients with chronic atrial fibrillation. Given the success of the surgical maze procedure (8), the development of a practical catheter-based maze procedure appears to be a logical curative approach for chronic atrial fibrillation. However, this approach is limited by the lengthy procedure duration and fluoroscopy times; risk of complications, including thromboembolism; and proarrhythmia associated with incomplete lesion lines. Some of these difficulties may be alleviated by the development of specialized ablation systems designed to expedite application of continuous linear lesions (19,138).

Preexcitation Syndromes and Concealed Pathways

Accessory pathways are anomalous extranodal connections that connect the epicardial surface of the atrium and ventricle along the AV groove. Accessory pathways can be classified based on their location along the mitral or tricuspid annulus, type of conduction (decremental or nondecremental), and whether they are capable of antegrade conduction, retrograde conduction, or both. Accessory path-

ways that are capable only of retrograde conduction are concealed, whereas those capable of antegrade conduction demonstrate preexcitation on a standard ECG. The term Wolff-Parkinson-White syndrome is reserved for patients who have preexcitation and symptomatic tachyarrhythmias. Among patients with the Wolff-Parkinson-White syndrome, AVRT is the most common arrhythmia, occurring in 75% of patients. AVRT is further subclassified into orthodromic and antidromic AVRT. During orthodromic AVRT, the reentrant impulse uses the AV node and specialized conduction system for conduction from the atrium to the ventricle and uses the accessory pathway for conduction from the ventricle to the atrium. During antidromic AVRT, the reentrant impulse travels in the reverse direction, with conduction from the atrium to the ventricle occurring through the accessory pathway. Atrial fibrillation is a less common but potentially more serious arrhythmia in patients with the Wolff-Parkinson-White syndrome because it can result in a very rapid ventricular response and rarely result in ventricular fibrillation. The incidence of sudden cardiac death in patients with the Wolff-Parkinson-White syndrome has been estimated to be 0.15% per patient-year (139).

Catheter ablation of accessory pathways is performed in conjunction with a diagnostic electrophysiology test. The purpose of the electrophysiology test is to confirm the presence and location of an accessory pathway, determine its conduction characteristics, and define the role of the accessory pathway in the patient's clinical arrhythmia. Accurate localization of an accessory pathway is critical to the success of catheter ablation procedures. Among patients with preexcitation, preliminary localization of the accessory pathway can be determined based on the delta wave and QRS morphology (140). Mapping of concealed accessory pathways and more accurate localization of manifest accessory pathways require analysis of the retrograde atrial activation sequence or antegrade ventricular activation sequence. Right-sided and posteroseptal accessory pathways are typically localized and ablated using a steerable electrode catheter with a 4-mm distal electrode positioned along the tricuspid annulus or in the coronary sinus os from the inferior vena cava. The location of left-sided accessory pathways can be determined using a multipolar electrode catheter positioned in the coronary sinus, which runs parallel to the left AV groove, or with a steerable catheter positioned in the left atrium or ventricle. Once localized to a region of the heart, precise mapping and ablation is performed using a steerable, 4-mm, tipped electrode catheter positioned along the mitral annulus using the transeptal or retrograde aortic approach (Fig. 12-11). These two approaches for ablation of left-sided accessory pathways are associated with a similar rate of success and incidence of complications (37). The decision about which approach to employ is usually based on physician preference, although the transeptal approach may be preferable in the elderly and in young children. In

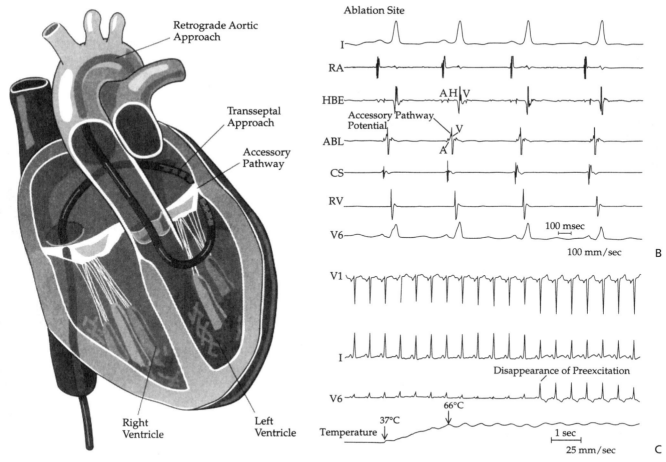

FIGURE 12-11. A: Two available approaches to ablate left-sided accessory pathways. The retrograde aortic approach involves inserting the ablation catheter into the femoral artery and traversing the aortic valve in the retrograde direction to enter the left ventricle. The ablation catheter is positioned against the ventricular aspect of the mitral valve at the site of the accessory pathway. The transseptal approach involves positioning a long transseptal sheath across the interatrial septum at the site of the foramen ovale. The ablation catheter is then passed through the sheath into the left atrium and positioned against the atrial aspect of the mitral valve at the site of the accessory pathway. **B:** The electrogram characteristics of a typical successful ablation site of an accessory pathway (ABL) are shown with the surface leads I and V$_6$ and intracardiac recordings obtained from the high right atrium (RA), the right ventricle apex (RV), an electrode catheter positioned to record a His bundle (HBE), and an electrode catheter positioned in the coronary sinus os (CS). The surface leads show a short PR interval and slurring of the upstroke of the QRS complex, which are characteristic of the preexcitation pattern observed in patients with the Wolff-Parkinson-White syndrome. The interval from the His bundle recording (H) to onset of the QRS complex is less than 50 ms, confirming the presence of preexcitation. At the successful ablation site, the ventricular electrogram (V) occurs very early relative to the onset of the QRS complex. There is a discrete deflection between the atrial (A) and the ventricular components of the electrogram recorded at the ablation site, which suggests an accessory pathway potential. **C:** Disappearance of preexcitation several seconds after onset of radiofrequency (RF) energy delivery to the site at which the electrogram in B was recorded. Shown are the surface leads V$_1$, I, and V$_6$ and the temperature recorded from the ablation catheter. The temperature recorded from the ablation electrode increases from 37°C to 66°C within 2 seconds of RF energy delivery. Preexcitation resolves several seconds thereafter. (From Calkins H, et al. Catheter ablation of arrhythmias. In: Topol E, ed. *Scientific American Medicine,* Madison, NY: Scientific American Medicine, 1998, with permission.)

rare instances, left-sided accessory pathways can only be ablated through the coronary sinus (141).

Appropriate sites for radiofrequency energy delivery during ablation of manifest accessory pathways are characterized by early ventricular activation, the presence of an accessory pathway potential, and stability of the local electrogram (80) (Fig. 12-11). Appropriate sites for energy delivery in patients with retrogradely conducting accessory pathways mapped during ventricular pacing or orthodromic AVRT are characterized by continuous electrical activity, the presence of accessory pathway potential, and electrogram stability. After an appropriate target site is identified, radiofrequency energy is delivered for 30 to 60 seconds with a target electrode temperature of 60°C to 70°C. At successful ablation sites, interruption of conduction through the accessory pathway usually occurs within 10 seconds and often within 2 seconds of the onset of radiofrequency energy delivery (Fig. 12-11).

The reported efficacy of catheter ablation of accessory pathways varies from 89% to 99%, with an overall success rate of approximately 93% to 95% (38,39,142–145). The success rate for catheter ablation of accessory pathways is highest for left free wall accessory pathways and lowest for posteroseptal and right free wall accessory pathways (145). After an initially successful procedure, recurrence of accessory pathway conduction occurs in approximately 7% of patients (145,146). Recurrence of conduction is more common after ablation of posteroseptal and right free wall pathways. Accessory pathways with recurrence of conduction can usually be successfully reablated. Complications associated with catheter ablation of accessory pathways may result from obtaining vascular access (e.g., hematomas, deep venous thrombosis, perforation of the aorta, arteriovenous fistula, pneumothorax), catheter manipulation (e.g., valvular damage, microemboli, perforation of the coronary sinus or myocardial wall, coronary dissection, thrombosis), or delivery of radiofrequency energy (e.g., AV block, myocardial perforation, coronary artery spasm or occlusion, transient ischemic attacks, cerebrovascular accidents). Complete heart block during ablation of an accessory pathway occurs in approximately 1% of patients and is observed most commonly after ablation of septal and posteroseptal accessory pathways. The overall incidence of complications varies between 1% and 4% (144). The incidence of procedure-related death is estimated to be less than 0.2% (145).

Atrioventricular Nodal Reentrant Tachycardia

AVNRT is a common arrhythmia that occurs in patients with two functionally distinct conduction pathways through the AV node, referred to as the fast and slow pathways. The slow pathway has a shorter refractory period than the fast pathway; both the fast and slow pathways are necessary to maintain AVNRT. The common form of AVNRT is typically initiated when an atrial premature beat blocks in the fast pathway, conducts down the slow pathway, and returns by the fast pathway to depolarize the atrium. During the uncommon form of AVNRT, the wavefront propagates in the opposite direction, conducting down the fast pathway and returning by the slow pathway. The fast pathway is located anteriorly along the septal portion of the tricuspid annulus, near the compact AV node, whereas the atrial insertion of the slow pathway is located more posteriorly along the tricuspid annulus, closer to the coronary sinus os.

AVNRT may be cured by ablation of the fast or the slow pathway. These alternative approaches are referred to as the anterior and the posterior approaches, respectively. The anterior approach targets the fast pathway. Catheter ablation is performed by locating an electrogram with a large His potential and then withdrawing the ablation catheter into the right atrium until the atrial signal is at least twice that of the ventricular signal (A to V ratio > 2) with a His potential no larger than 50 μV. Radiofrequency energy is then applied during sinus rhythm for 30 to 60 seconds while watching for prolongation in the PR interval. Energy delivery is immediately terminated if AV block occurs. Successful ablation of AVNRT using the anterior approach is characterized by lengthening of the PR interval and the inability to induce the tachycardia. Typically, there is elimination or marked attenuation of retrograde conduction during ventricular pacing. The AV block cycle length and the AV node effective refractory period are not usually altered during ablation of AVNRT using the anterior approach. Catheter ablation of AVNRT using the anterior approach is successful in approximately 90% of patients (147–149). Major limitations of the technique are the creation of inadvertent AV block in approximately 7% of patients and a 9% incidence of recurrence.

The posterior approach to ablation of AVNRT targets the slow pathway. The ablation catheter is directed into the right ventricle low, near the posterior septum, and is then withdrawn until an electrogram is recorded with a small atrial electrogram and a large ventricular electrogram (A to V ratio < 0.5). Specific ablation sites along the posterior portion of the tricuspid annulus can be selected based on the appearance of the local atrial electrogram or based strictly on anatomic factors. When using the electrogram-guided approach, fractionated atrial electrograms with a late "slow potential" are targeted (Fig. 12-12). When using the anatomic approach, the initial applications are delivered at the level of the coronary sinus os with subsequent applications of energy delivered to more superior sites. With either approach, junctional beats occurring during the application of radiofrequency energy are a marker for successful ablation. Successful ablation of AVNRT using the posterior approach is characterized by an increase in the AV block cycle length and in the AV node effective refractory period and elimination of inducible AVNRT. The posterior approach for ablation of AVNRT is effective in more than 95% to 97% of patients (145, 150–153). AV block is the most common complication,

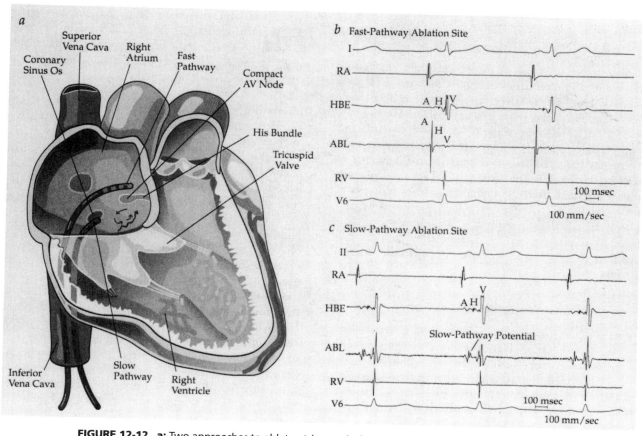

FIGURE 12-12. a: Two approaches to ablate atrioventricular nodal reentrant tachycardia (AVNRT). The anterior or fast-pathway approach involves positioning the catheter immediately proximal and anterior to the His bundle. The ablation catheter is positioned anterior to the coronary sinus os in the posterior or slow-pathway approach. A schematic drawing of the hypothesized reentrant circuit for AVNRT is also shown. **b:** The electrogram characteristics of a typical successful fast-pathway ablation site (ABL) are shown along with surface leads I and V₆ and intracardiac electrogram recordings obtained from the high right atrium (RA), the right ventricle apex (RV), and the electrode catheter positioned to record a His bundle (HBE). The His bundle recording shows a large ventricular electrogram (V) and a relatively large His bundle recording (H), whereas the fast-pathway ablation site has a large atrial electrogram (A), a small ventricular electrogram, and a diminutive His bundle recording. **c:** The electrogram characteristics of a successful slow-pathway ablation site are shown along with the surface leads I and V₆ and intracardiac recordings obtained from the high right atrium, the right ventricle apex, and the electrode catheter positioned to record a His bundle. At the ablation site, the ventricular electrogram is considerably larger than the atrial electrogram, and a distinct deflection consistent with a slow-pathway potential is seen immediately after the atrial electrogram. (From Calkins H, et al. Catheter ablation of arrhythmias. In: Topol E, ed. *Scientific American Medicine*, Madison, NY: Scientific American Medicine, 1998, with permission.)

occurring in 0.5% to 1% of patients. The incidence of recurrence after successful ablation of AVNRT using the posterior approach is approximately 3%. Because of the higher efficacy, the lower incidence of AV block and arrhythmia recurrence, and the greater likelihood of maintaining a normal PR interval during sinus rhythm, the posterior approach is the preferred approach to ablation of AVNRT.

Atrioventricular Junction

Theoretically, catheter ablation of the AV junction can eliminate any type of supraventricular arrhythmia that uses the AV node as part of the reentrant circuit and can slow the ventricular response to supraventricular arrhythmias confined to the atrium. In practice, complete catheter ablation of the AV junction is reserved for atrial fibrillation or atrial flutter that cannot be controlled with pharmacologic therapy and that results in a rapid ventricular response. The procedure is performed by positioning a steerable ablation catheter across the tricuspid annulus to record the largest His bundle electrogram associated with the largest atrial electrogram. A second electrode catheter is placed at the apex of the right ventricle for temporary pacing. After an appropriate target site is identified, radiofrequency energy is delivered for 30 to 60 seconds. If AV conduction remains unchanged, the catheter is repositioned, and a repeat attempt is made. If unsuccessful, a left-sided approach can be used (154). The ablation catheter is passed retrogradely across the aortic valve into the left ventricle and positioned immediately below the aortic valve to record a His bundle electrogram. Radiofrequency energy is then delivered in a standard fashion. The overall efficacy of catheter ablation of the AV junction using these two approaches 100% (145, 154–156). After ablation of the AV junction, a permanent rate-responsive pacemaker is inserted. Complication rates are generally less than 2%, with an estimated incidence of procedure-related death of 0.2% (145). Late sudden death has been reported after DC or radiofrequency ablation of the AV junction (145,157); this may be prevented by pacing the heart at a slightly faster rate. Because many of these patients have severe underlying heart disease, it is difficult to attribute these late sudden deaths directly to the ablation procedure.

Atrioventricular Nodal Modification

Another method for producing rate control in atrial fibrillation is to modify, not ablate, AV nodal conduction with radiofrequency energy. Most patients in whom this technique is performed do not require a permanent pacemaker (158,159). One study, for example, evaluated 19 patients with chronic or paroxysmal atrial fibrillation refractory to multiple medical trials (158). Short-term rate control was achieved in 14 by AV nodal modification without the production of pathologic AV block; 4 patients required a permanent pacemaker. During a mean 8-month follow-up, only 1 of the 14 patients had recurrence of symptomatic atrial fibrillation with a rapid rate that responded to a second modification procedure.

Although AV nodal modification may eliminate the need for a pacemaker, it is somewhat less successful than AV nodal ablation. One study compared these two techniques in 120 patients, 60 of whom underwent AV ablation and 60 of whom had modification (159). All patients undergoing AV nodal ablation had complete AV block produced; full or partial success with AV nodal modification was achieved in 57% of patients, and failure to produce adequate AV nodal modification induced complete AV block occurred in 15%. During a 26-month follow-up, recurrence of atrial fibrillation with a rapid rate was uncommon in both groups but occurred more frequently in those with AV nodal modification (12% versus 6% with AV nodal ablation). Although AV nodal modification achieves adequate slowing of the ventricular rate somewhat less often than AV nodal ablation, both approaches, when successful, are similarly effective for achieving long-term benefit.

Ventricular Tachycardias

The safety, efficacy, and clinical role of catheter ablation in the management of patients with ventricular arrhythmias critically depend on the specific type and mechanism of VT. Whereas catheter ablation is curative in patients with idiopathic VT or bundle branch reentry, catheter ablation of VT is considerably less effective in patients with coronary artery disease or cardiomyopathy.

Idiopathic Ventricular Tachycardia

Ventricular tachycardia occurring in patients without structural heart disease is commonly referred to as idiopathic VT. Idiopathic VT can be subclassified as repetitive monomorphic VT, paroxysmal sustained VT, and idiopathic left VT. Repetitive monomorphic VT is characterized by the presence of repetitive runs of nonsustained VT interspersed with sinus rhythm. These tachycardias typically have a left bundle branch block configuration with an inferiorly directed axis and arise from the outflow tract of the right ventricle (Fig. 12-13). Paroxysmal sustained VT is characterized by intermittent episodes of sustained VT. The VT morphology and site of origin are similar to that of repetitive monomorphic VT. Less commonly, idiopathic VT may arise from the left ventricle, usually along the posterior left ventricular septum one third of the distance from the apex to base. Idiopathic left VT typically has a right bundle branch configuration with a superior or rightward directed axis. Although the precise mechanism of these idiopathic VTs is unknown, they are often induced with exercise or a catecholamine infusion and are terminated with intravenous adenosine or verapamil, consistent with triggered activity.

Catheter ablation of idiopathic VT arising from the right ventricle is most commonly performed by positioning the ablation catheter into the right ventricle or right ventricular outflow tract using the inferior vena cava approach (Fig. 12-13). A retrograde aortic approach is most commonly used for ablation of idiopathic VT arising in the left ventricle. Selection of appropriate target sites can be guided by activation mapping or pace mapping. With activation mapping, the ablation catheter is manipulated to identify the earliest site of activation during VT, usually at least 25 ms before onset of the QRS complex. Pace mapping is performed by pacing at multiple ventricular sites during sinus rhythm to obtain an ECG morphology during pacing that is nearly identical to the ECG morphology of the clinical VT. Identification of a discrete potential preceding local ventricular activation, consistent with a Purkinje potential, may be useful in selecting ablation sites of idiopathic left VT. After an appropriate target site is identified, radiofrequency energy is delivered for 30 to 60 seconds (Fig. 12-13).

The reported efficacy of catheter ablation of idiopathic VT varies from 85% to 100%, with most series reporting success rates of 90% to 95% (160–162). Catheter ablation of idiopathic VT is more successful in patients with a single VT morphology arising in the right ventricular outflow tract compared with patients with multiple morphologies of

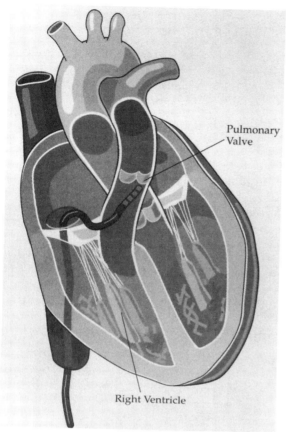

FIGURE 12-13. The ablation catheter is positioned to ablate idiopathic ventricular tachycardia arising from the outflow tract of the right ventricle. The most common site of origin of this type of ventricular tachycardia is on the septal aspect of the outflow tract immediately below the pulmonary valve. This type of ventricular tachycardia typically demonstrates a characteristic left bundle branch block pattern in lead V_1 with tall R waves observed in leads II, III, and aVF. Successful ablation sites are best identified for ablation of this type of idiopathic ventricular tachycardia by moving the catheter to various sites within the outflow tract and pacing from each site. Radiofrequency energy is delivered to the site, which results in a 12-lead morphology identical to that of the patient's clinical ventricular tachycardia. (From Calkins H, et al. Catheter ablation of arrhythmias. In: Topol E, ed. *Scientific American Medicine*, Madison, NY: Scientific American Medicine, 1998, with permission.)

VT or with VT arising from other sites (163). Although complications are rare, with most series reporting no complications, at least one patient death resulting from a torn outflow tract has been reported (161).

Bundle Branch Reentrant Tachycardia

Bundle branch reentry is an uncommon type of VT that is associated with conduction abnormalities of the His-Purkinje system and occurs most commonly in patients with a cardiomyopathy or severe left ventricular dysfunction. This type of VT results from reentry involving the bundle branches. Typically, the reentrant wavefront travels antegradely down the right bundle branch, traverses the septum, and returns

through the left bundle branch, resulting in a left bundle branch block morphology. Less commonly, the reentrant wavefront travels in the reverse direction, traveling first down the left bundle branch system and returning through the right bundle branch. Although selective ablation of the right or left bundle branch can cure this type of VT, the right bundle branch is more accessible and therefore is the preferred ablation target. Catheter ablation is performed by positioning the ablation catheter distal to the His bundle position to record a right bundle branch potential, where radiofrequency energy is delivered. Catheter ablation of bundle branch reentrant tachycardia is successfully accomplished in more than 95% of patients with most series reporting no arrhythmia recurrence and no complications (164,165).

Ventricular Tachycardia in Ischemic Heart Disease

VT in post–myocardial infarction patients results from a reentrant mechanism. Critical regions of slow myocardial conduction, created at infarct border zones, provide a substrate for reentry. These regions are characterized histologically by interspersed islands of viable myocardium and fibrosis. Although the feasibility of catheter ablation of VT in post–myocardial infarction patients has been demonstrated, success rates are considerably lower than in patients with idiopathic VT or bundle branch reentry. Less than 10% of patients in this group are candidates for catheter ablation because of the large size of the reentrant circuit; frequent presence of multiple types of VT in a given patient; hemodynamic instability during VT, preventing adequate VT localization; mid-myocardial or subepicardial locations of the arrhythmia circuit that may not be reached with the ablation catheter; and endocardial clot, preventing adequate delivery of radiofrequency energy.

Catheter ablation of VT in post–myocardial infarction patients is typically performed by positioning the ablation catheter into the left ventricle using a retrograde aortic approach, consistent with the high frequency with which this type of VT originates from the septum or free wall of the left ventricle. Rarely, the ablation catheter is positioned in the left ventricle using a transseptal approach. After the ablation catheter is within the left ventricle, mapping is performed to identify appropriate ablation sites. Three mapping strategies have been developed: pace mapping, entrainment mapping, and activation mapping. The technique of pace mapping has been previously described. Although the ability to map during sinus rhythm is advantageous, the accuracy of pace mapping is limited in patients with reentrant VT. Activation mapping attempts to identify an isolated mid-diastolic potential or to determine the site of earliest ventricular activation, usually more than 50 ms before onset of the QRS complex. Entrainment mapping is performed by ventricular pacing during VT. This technique is useful in identifying the zone of slow conduction critical to the reentrant circuit. An important limitation of activation and entrainment mapping is the need for the patient to remain in sustained VT during mapping. After an appropriate target site is identified, radiofrequency energy is delivered for 30 to 60 seconds. The U.S. food and Drug Administration approved a saline-irrigated catheter ablation system capable of creating larger lesions for use in the ablation of VT occurring in patients with structural heart disease (166).

The results of published series of catheter ablation of VT in patients with coronary artery disease must be interpreted with caution because the patient populations are small and highly selected, the definition of success varies among studies, and the duration of follow-up is short. The results of these studies report acute success rates of approximately 75% (167–169).

Only one prospective, multicenter clinical trial has been performed to evaluate the safety and efficacy of catheter ablation of VT occurring in patients with structural heart disease (166). The patient population included 146 patients who participated in the Cardiac Pathways Cooled RF Ablation clinical trial. The duration of follow-up was 243 ± 153 days. Catheter ablation was acutely successful, as defined prospectively by elimination of all mappable VTs, in 106 patients (75%). In 59 patients (41%), no VT of any type, mappable or unmappable, was inducible after ablation. Twelve patients (8%) experienced a major complication. After catheter ablation, 66 patients (46%) developed one or more episodes of a sustained ventricular arrhythmia. Clinical success, defined as a 75% reduction in VT frequency, was observed in 81% of patients.

Ventricular Tachycardia in Patients with Nonischemic Cardiomyopathy

In contrast to patients with VT in the setting of a prior myocardial infarction, in whom VT results most commonly from reentry, the electrophysiologic substrate in patients with dilated cardiomyopathies has not been well characterized. Although few data are available, catheter ablation is unlikely to play a curative role in this setting because of the progressive nature of most cardiomyopathies and the frequent absence of a fixed reentrant arrhythmia circuit or focal origin of VT that may be amenable to catheter ablation. Sustained VT can often not be reproducibly induced during electrophysiology testing, thereby eliminating a potential end point for catheter ablation (170).

The initial experience with radiofrequency catheter ablation in this setting has been disappointing. In one report, catheter ablation in eight patients with idiopathic dilated cardiomyopathy and incessant or recurrent and easily inducible VT was attempted (171). Catheter ablation of the targeted clinical VT was initially successful in each of four patients with incessant VT and in one of four patients with frequent recurrent VT, resulting in an overall immediate efficacy of 63%. However, 7 of 8 patients had inducible VT with a clinical or nonclinical morphology after the ablation procedure. Only two patients (25%) remained free of recurrent VT after discharge.

Catheter Ablation in Patients with an Implantable Cardioverter-Defibrillator

Catheter ablation is an alternative to antiarrhythmic drug therapy in patients with an implantable cardioverter-defibrillator (ICD) who experience frequent recurrences of VT. One study of 21 patients with frequent ICD shocks caused by recurrent sustained VT despite antiarrhythmic drugs reported that ablation was effective in 76% of patients (172). During a follow-up period of 11 months, the frequency of ICD shocks per month decreased from 60 to 0.1 in this small study and was associated with an improvement in quality of life.

AVNRT is uncommon in patients with an implantable ICD, but it can be a major problem when it occurs. Although ablation is an effective therapy, the endocardial lead of the ICD is located close to the site of ablation, making the procedure technically difficult. Successful ablation has been achieved using a long sheath to stabilize the ablation catheter without damage to the ICD or its leads (173).

Complications of Catheter Ablation

The potential risks and benefits of the procedure, as well as alternative treatment strategies, should be discussed in detail with the patient before proceeding. Patients must be aware that there is a small risk of emergency cardiac surgery, stroke, and death related to the procedure. Potential risks and approximate incidences include (174,175) those related to vascular access (2% to 4%), including bleeding, infection, hematoma, vascular injury, and thromboembolism, and to cardiac trauma, including myocardial perforation, infarction, and valvular damage (1% to 2%). The frequency of valvular complications is slightly higher with left-sided ablation using retrograde aortic technique (176).

The degree of myocardial injury is more accurately assessed by troponin I levels rather than creatine kinase-MB. Elevated troponin I levels, present in up to 68% of patients undergoing ablation, correlate with the number of radiofrequency lesions applied, the site of lesions (ventricular > atrial > annular lesions), and the approach to the left side (transaortic > transseptal) (177). However, the prognostic significance of asymptomatic elevations of troponin I remains unclear.

Other risks are thromboembolism, including stroke, systemic embolism, and pulmonary embolism (<1%); heart block requiring permanent pacemaker (1% to 2%); radiation exposure, including skin burn and risk of malignancy; and after ablation for atrial fibrillation, pulmonary hypertension due to pulmonary vein stenosis occurring near the junction with the left atrium (178).

New arrhythmias may occur because radiofrequency lesions themselves may serve as arrhythmogenic foci. Although a possibility, this problem has not been seen clinically. New atrial fibrillation has occurred in patients undergoing ablation for atrial flutter; it is possible, however, that this occurs primarily in patients predisposed to atrial fibrillation (179).

An inappropriate sinus tachycardia may occur in some patients after posteroseptal accessory pathway or AV nodal ablation, suggesting disruption of the parasympathetic or sympathetic inputs into the sinus and AV nodes (180–182). Death is a risk for approximately 0.1% to 0.3% of patients.

In a report of 1,050 patients who underwent catheter ablation using a temperature-controlled system, a major complication occurred in 3% and a minor complication in 8.2% (183). Predictors for a complication included structural heart disease and the presence of multiple targets for ablation.

CONCLUSIONS

Surgical ablation of cardiac arrhythmias played a critical role in the development of catheter ablation procedures. With the exception of the maze procedure for treatment of atrial fibrillation, arrhythmia surgery is no longer performed and is largely of historical interest. In contrast, the safety and efficacy of catheter ablation for treatment of most types of cardiac arrhythmias is well established. These arrhythmias or arrhythmia substrates include AVNRT, accessory pathways, focal AT, atrial flutter, idiopathic VT, and bundle branch reentry. Because of this, catheter ablation is considered an alternative to pharmacologic therapy in the treatment of these cardiac arrhythmias. The technique, safety, and efficacy of catheter ablation for treatment of atrial fibrillation and VT occurring in the setting of structural heart disease remains an area of active research. Although the potential for catheter ablation of these arrhythmias has been demonstrated, further research is needed to approach the remarkably high safety, efficacy, and clinical acceptance that have been seen with catheter ablation of other arrhythmias.

REFERENCES

1. Guiraudon GM, Klein GJ, Yee R. Surgery for cardiac tachyarrhythmias: ACE highlights. 1990;6:5–10.
2. Harrison L, Gallagher JJ, Kasell J, et al. Cryosurgical ablation of the AV node–His bundle: a new method for producing AV block. *Circulation* 1977;55:463.
3. Klein GJ, Harrison L, Ideker RF, et al. Reaction of the myocardium to cryosurgery: electrophysiology and arrhythmogenic potential. *Circulation* 1979;59:364–372.
4. Klein GJ, Guiraudon GM, Sharma AD, Milstein S. Demonstration of macroreentry and feasibility of operative therapy in the common type of atrial flutter. *Am J Cardiol* 1986;57:587–591.
5. Saoudi N, Atallah G, Kirkorian G, Touboul P. Catheter ablation of the atrial myocardium in human type I atrial flutter. *Circulation* 1990;81:762–771.
6. Cox JL, Canavan TE, Schuessler RB, et al. The surgical treatment of atrial fibrillation, 2: intraoperative electrophysiologic mapping and description of the electrophysiologic basis of atrial flutter and fibrillation. *J Thorac Cardiovasc Electrophysiol* 1991;101:406–426.
7. Cox JL, Boineau JP, Schuessier RB, et al. Successful surgical treatment of atrial fibrillation. *JAMA* 1991;266:1976–1980.
8. Sundt TM, Camillo CJ, Cox JL. The maze procedure for cure of atrial fibrillation. *Cardiol Clin* 1997;15:739–748.
9. Cox JL, Jaquiss RDB, Schuessler RB, Boineau JP. Modification of the maze procedure for atrial flutter and atrial fibrillation. *J Thorac Cardiovasc Surg* 1995;110:485–495.
10. Cox JL, Boineau JP, Schuessler RB, et al. Five-year experience with the maze procedure for atrial fibrillation. *Ann Thorac Surg* 1993;56:814–824.
11. Cox JL, Boineau JP, Schuessler RB, et al. From fisherman to fibrillation: an unbroken line of progress. *Ann Thorac Surg* 1994;58:1269–1273.
12. Moe GK, Rheinholdt WC, Abildskov J. A computer model of atrial fibrillation. *Arch Int Pharmacodyn Ther* 1962;140:183–188.
13. Moe GK, Rheinholdt WC, Abildskov J. A computer model of atrial fibrillation. *Am Heart J* 1964;67:200–220.
14. Konings KTS, Kirchof CJHJ, Smeets JRLM, et al. High density mapping of electrically induced atrial fibrillation in humans. *Circulation* 1994;89:1665–1680.
15. Scherf D. Studies on auricular tachycardia caused by aconitine administration. *Proc Soc Exp Biol Med* 1947;4:233–239.
16. Sueda T, Nagata H, Orihashi K, et al. Efficacy of a simple left atrial procedure for chronic atrial fibrillation in mitral valve operations. *Ann Thorac Surg* 1997;63:1070–1075.
17. Nitta T, Lee R, Watanabe H, et al. Radial approach: a new concept in surgical treatment for atrial fibrillation. II. Electrophysiologic effects and atrial contribution to ventricular filling. *Ann Thorac Surg* 1999;67:36–50.
18. Nitta T, Lee R, Schuessler RB, et al. Radial approach: a new concept in surgical treatment for atrial fibrillation. I. Concept, anatomic and physiologic bases and development of a procedure. *Ann Thorac Surg* 1999;67:27–35.
19. Calkins H, Hall J, Ellenbogen K, et al. A new system for catheter ablation of atrial fibrillation. *Am J Cardiol* 1999;83:227D–236D.
20. Pritchett ELC, Anderson RW, Benditt DG, et al. Reentry within the atrioventricular node: surgical cure with preservation of atrioventricular conduction. *Circulation* 1979;60:440–446.
21. Holman WL, Ikeshita M, Lease JG, et al. Elective prolongation of atrioventricular conduction by multiple cryolesions. *J Thorac Cardiovasc Surg* 1982;84:554–559.
22. Holman WL, Ikeshita M, Lease JG, et al. Cryosurgical modification of retrograde atrioventricular conduction: implications for the surgical treatment of atrioventricular nodal reentry tachycardia. *J Thorac Cardiovasc Surg* 1986;91:826–834.
23. Cox JL, Holman WL, Cain ME. Cryosurgical treatment of atrioventricular node reentrant tachycardia. *Circulation* 1987;76:1329–1336.
24. Ross DL, Johnson DC, Denniss AR, et al. Curative surgery for atrioventricular junctional (AAV nodal) reentrant tachycardia. *J Am Coll Cardiol* 1985;6:1383–1392.
25. Johnson DC, Nunn GR, Richards DA, et al. Surgical therapy for supraventricular tachycardia: a potential curable disorder. *J Thorac Cardiovasc Surg* 1987;93:913–918.
26. Gartman DM, Bardy GH, Williams AB, Ivey TD. Direct surgical treatment of atrioventricular node reentrant tachycardia. *J Thorac Cardiovasc Surg* 1989;98:63–72.
27. Fujimura O, Guiraudon GM, Yee R, et al. Operative therapy of atrioventricular node reentry and results of an anatomically guided procedure. *Am J Cardiol* 1989;64:1327–1332.
28. Guiraudon GM, Klein GJ, Sharma AD, et al. Skeletonization of the atrioventricular node for AV node reentrant tachycardia:

experience with 32 patients. *Ann Thorac Surg* 1990;49:565–573.

29. Sealy WC, Hattler BG, Blumenschein SD, et al. Surgical treatment of Wolff-Parkinson-White syndrome. *Ann Thorac Surg* 1969;8:1–11.

30. Sealy WC, Hattler BG, Blumennschein SD, et al. Surgical treatment of Wolff-Parkinson-White syndrome. *Ann Thorac Surg* 1969;8:1–11.

31. Sealy WC. Kent bundles in the anterior septal space. *Ann Thorac Surg* 1983;36:180–186.

32. Gallagher JJ, Sealy WC, Cox JL, et al. Results of surgery for pre-excitation in 200 cases. *Circulation* 1981;64[Suppl IV]:146A.

33. Guiraudon GM, Klein GJ, Gulamhusein S, et al. Surgical repair of Wolff-Parkinson-White syndrome: a new closed-heart technique. *Ann Thorac Surg* 1984;37:67–71.

34. Guiraudon GM, Klein GJ, Sharma AD, et al. Closed heart technique for Wolff-Parkinson-White syndrome: further experience and potential limitations. *Ann Thorac Surg* 1986;42:651–657.

35. Guiraudon GM, Klein GJ, Sharma AD, et al. Surgery for the Wolff-Parkinson-White syndrome: the epicardial approach. *Semin Thorac Cardiovasc Surg* 1989;1:21–33.

36. Calkins H, Langberg J, Sousa J, et al. Radiofrequency catheter ablation of accessory atrioventricular connections in 250 patients: abbreviated therapeutic approach to Wolff-Parkinson-White syndrome. *Circulation* 1992, 85:1337–1346.

37. Lesh MD, Van Hare G, Scheinman MM, Ports TA, Epstein LA. Comparison of the retrograde and transseptal methods for ablation of left free-wall accessory pathways. *J Am Coll Cardiol* 1993;22:542–549.

38. Jackman WM, Wang X, Friday KJ, et al. Catheter ablation of accessory atrioventricular pathways (Wolff-Parkinson-White syndrome) by radiofrequency current. *N Engl J Med* 1991;324:1605–1611.

39. Calkins H, Sousa J, El-Atassi R, et al. Diagnosis and cure of the Wolff-Parkinson-White syndrome or paroxysmal supraventricular tachycardias during a single electrophysiology test. *N Engl J Med* 1991;324:1612–1618.

40. De Buitleir M, Sousa J, Bolling SF, et al. Reduction in medical care cost associated with radiofrequency catheter ablation of accessory pathways. *Am J Cardiol* 1991;68:1656–1661.

41. Guiraudon G, Frank R, Fontaine G. Interet des cartographies dans le traitement chirurgical des tachycardies ventriculaires rebelles recidivantes. *Nouv Presse Med* 1974;3:321.

42. Fontaine G, Guiraudon G, Frank R, et al. La cartographie epicardique et le traitement chirurgical par simple entriculotomie de certaines tachycardies ventriculaires rebelles par reentree. *Arch Mal Coeur* 1975;68:113–124.

43. Guiraudon G, Fontaine G, Frank R, et al. Surgical treatment of ventricular tachycardia guided by ventricular mapping in 23 patients without coronary artery disease. *Ann Thorac Surg* 1981;32:439–450.

44. Couch OA. Cardiac aneurysm with ventricular tachycardia and subsequent excision of aneurysm. *Circulation* 1959;20:251–253.

45. Guiraudon G, Fontaine G, Frank R, et al. Encircling endocardial ventriculotomy: a new surgical treatment for life-threatening ventricular tachycardias resistant to medical treatment following myocardial infarction. *Ann Thorac Surg* 1978;26:438–444.

46. Josephson ME, Harken AH, Horowitz LN. Endocardial excision: a new surgical technique for the treatment of recurrent ventricular tachycardia. *Circulation* 1979;60:1430–1439.

47. Lawrie GM, Pacifico A, Kaushik R, et al. Factors predictive of results of direct ablative operations for drug-refractory ventricular tachycardia: analysis of 80 patients. *J Thorac Cardiovasc Surg* 1991;101:44–45.

48. Rokkas CK, Nitta T, Schuessler RB, et al. Human ventricular tachycardia: precise intraoperative localization with potential distribution mapping. *Ann Thorac Surg* 1994;57:1628–1635.

49. Miller JM, Gottlieb CD, Marchlinski FE, et al. Does ventricular tachycardia mapping influence the success of antiarrhythmic surgery? *J Am Coll Cardiol* 1988;11:112A.

50. Guiraudon GM, Thakur RK, Klein GJ, et al. Encircling endocardial cryoablation for ventricular tachycardia after myocardial infarction: experience with 33 patients. *Am Heart J* 1994;128:982–989.

51. Hargrove WC, Miller JM. Risk stratification and management of patients with recurrent ventricular tachycardia and other malignant ventricular arrhythmias. *Circulation* 1989;79:I-178–I-181.

52. Gallagher JJ, Svenson RH, Kasell JH, et al. Catheter technique for closed-chest ablation of the atrioventricular conduction system: a therapeutic alternative for the treatment of refractory supraventricular tachycardia. *N Engl J Med* 1982;306:194–200.

53. Scheinman, Melvin M. NASPE Survey on Catheter Ablation. From the Cardiac Electrophysiology Service, University of California, San Francisco, California. *Pacing Clin Electrophysiol* 1995;18:1474–1478.

54. Calkins H, Prystowsky E, Carlson M, et al, for the Atakr Multicenter Investigators Group. Temperature monitoring during radiofrequency catheter ablation procedures using closed loop control. *Circulation* 1994;90:1279–1286.

55. Haines DE, Watson DD, Verow AF. Electrode radius predicts lesion radius during radiofrequency energy heating: validation of a proposed thermodynamic model. *Circ Res* 1990;67:124–129.

56. Erez A, Shitzer A. Controlled destruction and temperature distributions in biological tissues subjected to monoactive electrocoagulation. *Trans ASME* 1980;102:42–49.

57. Nath S, Lynch C III, Whayne JG, Haines DE. Cellular electrophysiological effects of hyperthermia on isolated guinea pig papillary muscle: implications for catheter ablation. *Circulation* 1993;88[Pt I]:1826–1831.

58. Haines DE, Verow AF. Observations on electrode-tissue interface temperature and effect on electrical impedance during radiofrequency ablation of ventricular myocardium. *Circulation* 1990;82:1034–1038.

59. Otomo K, Yamanashi WS, Tondo C, et al. Why a large tip electrode makes a deeper radiofrequency lesion: effects of increase in electrode cooling and electrode-tissue interface area. *J Cardiovasc Electrophysiol* 1998;9:47–54.

60. Ruffy R, Imran MA, Santel DJ, Wharton JM. Radiofrequency delivery through a cooled catheter tip allows the creation of larger endomyocardial lesions in the ovine heart. *J Cardiovasc Electrophysiol* 1995;6:1089–1096.

61. Nakagawa H, Yamanashi WS, Pitha JV, et al. Comparison of *in vivo* tissue temperature profile and lesion geometry for radiofrequency ablation with a saline-irrigated electrode versus temperature control in a canine thigh muscle preparation. *Circulation* 1995;91:2264–2273.

62. Zimmer JE, Hynynen K, He DS, Marcus F. The feasibility of using ultrasound for cardiac ablation. *IEEE Trans Biomed Eng* 1995;42:891–897.

63. Nath S, Haines DE. Biophysics and pathology of catheter energy delivery systems. *Prog Cardiovasc Dis* 1995;37:185–204.

64. Lesh MD, Diederich C, Guerra PG, et al. An anatomic approach to prevention of atrial fibrillation: pulmonary vein isolation with through-the-balloon ultrasound ablation (TTB-USA). *Thorac Cardiovasc Surg* 1999;47[Suppl 3]:347–351.

65. Langberg JJ, Wonnell T, Chin MC, et al. Catheter ablation of the atrioventricular junction using a helical microwave antenna: a novel means of coupling energy to the endocardium. *Pacing Clin Electrophysiol* 1991;14:2105–2113.

66. Whayne JG, Nath S, Haines DE: Microwave catheter ablation of myocardium *in vitro*: assessment of the characteristics of tissue heating and injury. *Circulation* 1994;89:2390–2395.

67. Jumrussirikul P, Chen JT, Jenkins M, et al. Prospective comparison of temperature guided microwave and radiofrequency catheter ablation in the swine heart. *Pacing Clin Electrophysiol* 1998;21:1364–1374.

68. Vincent GM, Fox J, Benedick BA, et al. Laser catheter ablation of simulated ventricular tachycardia. *Lasers Surg Med* 1987;7: 421–425.

69. Haines DE. Thermal ablation of perfused porcine left ventricle *in vitro* with the neodymium- YAG laser hot tip catheter system. *Pacing Clin Electrophysiol* 1992;15:979–985.

70. Weber HP, Kaltenbrunner W, Heinze A, Steinbach K. Laser catheter coagulation of atrial myocardium for ablation of atrioventricular nodal reentrant tachycardia. *Eur Heart J* 1997;18: 487–495.

71. Keane D, Ruskin JN. Linear atrial ablation with a diode laser and fiberoptic catheter. *Circulation* 1999;100:e59–e60.

72. Dubuc M, Talajic M, Roy D, et al. Feasibility of cardiac cryoablation using a transvenous steerable electrode catheter. *J Interv Card Electrophysiol* 1998;2:285–292.

73. Dinerman J, Berger RD, Calkins H. Temperature monitoring during radiofrequency ablation. *J Cardiovasc Electrophysiol* 1996; 7:163–173.

74. Shpun S, Gepstein L, Hayam G, Ben-Haim SA. Guidance of radiofrequency endocardial ablation with real-time three-dimensional magnetic navigation system. *Circulation* 1997;96: 2016–2021.

75. Smeets JL, Ben-Haim SA, Rodriguez LM, et al. New method for nonfluoroscopic endocardial mapping in humans: accuracy assessment and first clinical results. *Circulation* 1998;97: 2426–2432.

76. Chu E, Fitzpatrick AP, Chin MC, et al. Radiofrequency catheter ablation guided by intracardiac echocardiography. *Circulation* 1994;89:1301–1305.

77. Kalman JM, Olgin JE, Karch MR, Lesh MD. Use of intracardiac echocardiography in interventional electrophysiology. *Pacing Clin Electrophysiol* 1997;20:2248–2262.

78. Daoud EG, Kalbfleisch SJ, Hummel JD. Intracardiac echocardiography to guide transseptal left heart catheterization for radiofrequency catheter ablation. *J Cardiovasc Electrophysiol* 1999;10:358–363.

79. Lardo AC, McVeigh ER, Atalar E, et al. Visualization and temporal characterization of radiofrequency ablation lesions using magnetic resonance imaging. 2001 (submitted).

80. Calkins H, Kim YN, Schmaltz S, et al. Electrogram criteria for identification of appropriate target sites for radiofrequency catheter ablation of accessory atrioventricular connections. *Circulation* 1992;85:565–573.

81. Jackman WM, Friday KJ, Fitzgerald DM, et al. Localization of left free-wall and posteroseptal accessory atrioventricular pathways by direct recording of accessory pathway activation. *Pacing Clin Electrophysiol* 1989;12:204–214.

82. Chen X, Borggrefe M, Shenasa M, et al. Characteristics of local electrogram predicting successful transcatheter radiofrequency ablation of left-sided accessory pathways. *J Am Coll Cardiol* 1992;20:656–665.

83. Berger RD, Nsah E, Calkins H. Signal-averaged intracardiac electrograms: a new method to detect Kent potentials. *J Cardiovasc Electrophysiol* 1997;8:155–160.

84. Davis J, Scheinman MM, Ruder MA, et al. Ablation of cardiac tissues by an electrode catheter technique for treatment of ectopic supraventricular tachycardia in adults. *Circulation* 1986; 74:1044–1053.

85. Poty H, Saoudi N, Haissaguerre M, et al. Radiofrequency

catheter ablation of atrial tachycardias. *Am Heart J* 1996;131: 481–489.

86. Coggins DL, Lee RJ, Sweeney J, et al. Radiofrequency catheter ablation as a cure for idiopathic tachycardia of both left and right ventricular origin. *J Am Coll Cardiol* 1994;23:1333–1341.

87. Kottkamp H, Hindricks G, Breithardt G, Borggrefe M. Three-dimensional electromagnetic catheter technology: electroanatomical mapping of the right atrium and ablation of ectopic atrial tachycardia. *J Cardiovasc Electrophysiol* 1997;8: 1332–1337.

88. Schmitt C, Zrenner B, Schneider M, et al. Clinical experience with a novel multielectrode basket catheter in right atrial tachycardias. *Circulation* 1999;99:2414–2422.

89. Schalij MJ, van Rugge FP, Siezenga M, van der Velde ET. Endocardial activation mapping of ventricular tachycardia in patients: first application of a 32-site bipolar mapping electrode catheter. *Circulation* 1998;98:2168–2179.

90. Schilling RJ, Peters NS, Davies DW. Mapping and ablation of ventricular tachycardia with the aid of a non-contact mapping system. *Heart* 1999;81:570–575.

91. Paul T, Moak JP, Morris C, Garson A. Epicardial mapping: how to measure local activation? *Pacing Clin Electrophysiol* 1990;13: 285–292.

92. Man KC, Daoud EG, Knight BP, et al. Accuracy of the unipolar electrogram for identification of the site of origin of ventricular activation. *J Cardiovasc Electrophysiol* 1997;8:974–979.

93. Fletcher R, Swartz J, Lee B, et al. Advances in catheter ablation of unipolar electrograms. *Pacing Clin Electrophysiol* 1989;12: 225–230.

94. Calkins H, Kalbfleisch SJ, el-Atassi R, et al. Relation between efficacy of radiofrequency catheter ablation and site of origin of idiopathic ventricular tachycardia. *Am J Cardiol* 1993;71: 827–833.

95. Tracy CM, Swartz JF, Fletcher RD, et al. Radiofrequency catheter ablation of ectopic atrial tachycardia using paced activation sequence mapping. *J Am Coll Cardiol* 1993;21:910–917.

96. Waldo AL, Henthorn RW, Plumb VJ, MacLean WA. Demonstration of the mechanism of transient entrainment and interruption of ventricular tachycardia with rapid atrial pacing. *J Am Coll Cardiol* 1984;3:422–430.

97. Waldo AL, Henthorn RW. Use of transient entrainment during ventricular tachycardia to localize a critical area in the reentry circuit for ablation. *Pacing Clin Electrophysiol* 1989;12:231–244.

98. Stevenson WG, Khan H, Sager P, et al. Identification of reentry circuit sites during catheter mapping and radiofrequency ablation of ventricular tachycardia late after myocardial infarction. *Circulation* 1993;88:1647–1670.

99. Olgin JE, Kalman JM, Fitzpatrick AP, Lesh MD. Role of right atrial endocardial structures as barriers to conduction during human type I atrial flutter: activation and entrainment mapping guided by intracardiac echocardiography. *Circulation* 1995;92: 1839–1848.

100. Nakagawa H, Lazzara R, Khastgir T, et al. Role of the tricuspid annulus and the eustachian valve/ridge on atrial flutter: relevance to catheter ablation of the septal isthmus and a new technique for rapid identification of ablation success. *Circulation* 1996;94:407–424.

101. Poty H, Saoudi N, Abdel Aziz A, et al. Radiofrequency catheter ablation of type 1 atrial flutter. Prediction of late success by electrophysiological criteria. *Circulation* 1995;92:1389–1392.

102. Tai CT, Chen SA, Chiang CE, et al. Electrophysiologic characteristics and radiofrequency catheter ablation in patients with clockwise atrial flutter. *J Cardiovasc Electrophysiol* 1997;8: 24–34.

103. Chen SA, Chiang CE, Yang CJ, et al. Sustained atrial tachycardia in adult patients. Electrophysiological characteristics, phar-

macological response, possible mechanisms, and effects of radiofrequency ablation. *Circulation* 1994;90:1262–1278.

104. Goldberger J, Kall J, Ehlert F, et al. Effectiveness of radiofrequency catheter ablation for treatment of atrial tachycardia. *Am J Cardiol* 1993;72:787–793.

105. Poty H, Saoudi N, Haissaguerre M, et al. Radiofrequency catheter ablation of atrial tachycardias. *Am Heart J* 1996;131:481–489.

106. Kay GN, Chong F, Epstein AE, et al. Radiofrequency ablation for treatment of primary atrial tachycardias. *J Am Coll Cardiol* 1993;21:901–909.

107. Lesh MD, Van Hare GF, Epstein LM, et al. Radiofrequency catheter ablation of atrial arrhythmias: results and mechanisms. *Circulation* 1994;89:1074–1089.

108. Sanders WE, Sorrentino RA, Greenfield RA, et al. Catheter ablation of sinoatrial node reentrant tachycardia. *J Am Coll Cardiol* 1994;23:926–934.

109. Chen S-A, Chiang C-E, Yang C-J, et al. Radiofrequency catheter ablation of sustained intra-atrial reentrant tachycardia in adult patients: identification of electrophysiology characteristics and endocardial mapping techniques. *Circulation* 1993;88:578–587.

110. Chen SA, Tai CT, Chiang CE, et al. Focal atrial tachycardia: reanalysis of the clinical and electrophysiologic characteristics and prediction of successful radiofrequency ablation. *J Cardiovasc Electrophysiol* 1998;9:355–365.

111. Lesh MD, Kalman JM, Saxon LA, Dorostkar PC. Electrophysiology of "incisional" reentrant atrial tachycardia complicating surgery for congenital heart disease. *Pacing Clin Electrophysiol* 1997;20:2107–2111.

112. Baker BM, Lindsay BD, Bromberg BI, et al. Catheter ablation of clinical intraatrial reentrant tachycardias resulting from previous atrial surgery: localizing and transecting the critical isthmus. *J Am Coll Cardiol* 1996;28:411–417.

113. Chinitz LA, Bernstein NE, O'Connor B, et al. Mapping reentry around atriotomy scars using double potentials. *Pacing Clin Electrophysiol* 1996;19:1978–1983.

114. Kalman JM, VanHare GF, Olgin JE, et al. Ablation of "incisional" reentrant atrial tachycardia complicating surgery for congenital heart disease: use of entrainment to define a critical isthmus of conduction. *Circulation* 1996;93:502–512.

115. Morillo CA, Klein GJ, Thakur RK, et al. Mechanism of "inappropriate" sinus tachycardia. Role of sympathovagal balance. *Circulation* 1994;90:873–877.

116. Low PA, Opfer-Gehrking TL, Textor SC, et al. Postural tachycardia syndrome (POTS). *Neurology* 1995;45[Suppl 5]:S19–S25.

117. Lee RJ, Kalman JM, Fitzpatrick AP, et al. Radiofrequency catheter modification of the sinus node for "inappropriate" sinus tachycardia. *Circulation* 1995;92:2919–2928.

118. Kalman JM, Olgin JE, Saxon LA, et al. Activation and entrainment mapping defines the tricuspid annulus as the anterior barrier in typical atrial flutter. *Circulation* 1996;94:398–406.

119. Feld GK, Fleck RP, Chen P-S, et al. Radiofrequency catheter ablation for the treatment of human type I atrial flutter: identification of a critical zone in the reentrant circuit by endocardial mapping techniques. *Circulation* 1992;86:1233–1240.

120. Poty H, Saoudi N, Nair M, et al. Radiofrequency catheter ablation of atrial flutter. Further insights into the various types of isthmus block: application to ablation during sinus rhythm. *Circulation* 1996;94:3204–3213.

121. Tai CT, Chen SA, Chiang CE, et al. Long-term outcome of radiofrequency catheter ablation for typical atrial flutter: risk prediction of recurrent arrhythmias. *J Cardiovasc Electrophysiol* 1998;9:115–121.

122. Jais P, Haissaguerre M, Shah DC, et al. Successful irrigated-tip catheter ablation of atrial flutter resistant to conventional radiofrequency ablation. *Circulation* 1998;98:835–838.

123. Atiga WL, Worley SJ, Hummel J, et al. Initial results of a prospective, randomized study of cooled RF versus standard RF ablation for typical atrial flutter. *Circulation* 1999;100:I-374A.

124. Huang DT, Monahan KM, Zimetbaum P, et al. Hybrid pharmacologic and ablative therapy: a novel and effective approach for the management of atrial fibrillation. *J Cardiovasc Electrophysiol* 1998;9:462–469.

125. Nabar A, Rodriguez LM, Timmermans C, et al. Effect of right atrial isthmus ablation on the occurrence of atrial fibrillation: observations in four patient groups having type I atrial flutter with or without associated atrial fibrillation. *Circulation* 1999;99:1441–1445.

126. Tai CT, Chiang CE, Lee SH, et al. Persistent atrial flutter in patients treated for atrial fibrillation with amiodarone and propafenone: electrophysiologic characteristics, radiofrequency catheter ablation, and risk prediction. *J Cardiovasc Electrophysiol* 1999;10:1180–1187.

127. Seidl K, Hauer B, Schwick NG, et al. Risk of thromboembolic events in patients with atrial flutter. *Am J Cardiol* 1998;82:580–583.

128. Lanzarotti CJ, Olshansky B. Thromboembolism in chronic atrial flutter: is the risk underestimated? *J Am Coll Cardiol* 1997;30:1506–1511.

129. Swartz JF, Pellersels G, Silvers J, et al. A catheter-based curative approach to atrial fibrillation in humans. *Circulation* 1994;90:I-335.

130. Haissaguerre M, Marcus FI, Fischer B, Clementy J. Radiofrequency catheter ablation in unusual mechanisms of atrial fibrillation: report of three cases. *J Cardiovasc Electrophysiol* 1994;5:743–751.

131. Haissaguerre M, Gencel L, Fischer B, et al. Successful catheter ablation of atrial fibrillation. *J Cardiovasc Electrophysiol* 1994;5:1045–1052.

132. Haissaguerre M, Jais P, Shah DC, et al. Right and left atrial radiofrequency catheter therapy of paroxysmal atrial fibrillation. *J Cardiovasc Electrophysiol* 1996;7:1132–1144.

133. Jais P, Haissaguerre M, Shah DC, et al. A focal source of atrial fibrillation treated by discrete radiofrequency ablation. *Circulation* 1997;95:572–576.

134. Haissaguerre M, Jais P, Shah DC, et al. Spontaneous initiation of atrial fibrillation by ectopic beats originating in the pulmonary veins. *N Engl J Med* 1998;339:659–666.

135. Nathan H, Eliakim M. The junction between the left atrium and the pulmonary veins: an anatomic study of human hearts. *Circulation* 1966;34:412–422.

136. Hsieh MH, Chen SA, Tai CT, et al. Double multielectrode mapping catheters facilitate radiofrequency catheter ablation of focal atrial fibrillation originating from pulmonary veins. *J Cardiovasc Electrophysiol* 1999;10:136–144.

137. Chen SA, Tai CT, Yu WC, et al. Right atrial focal atrial fibrillation: electrophysiologic characteristics and radiofrequency catheter ablation. *J Cardiovasc Electrophysiol* 1999;10:328–335.

138. Avitall B, Helms RW, Koblish JB, et al. The creation of linear contiguous lesions in the atria with an expandable loop catheter. *J Am Coll Cardiol* 1999;33:972–984.

139. Munger TM, Packer DL, Hammill SC, et al. A population study of the natural history of Wolff-Parkinson-White syndrome in Olmsted County, Minnesota, 1953–1989. *Circulation* 1993;87:866–873.

140. Fitzpatrick AP, Gonzales RP, Lesh MD, et al. New algorithm for the localization of accessory atrioventricular connections using a baseline electrocardiogram. *J Am Coll Cardiol* 1994;3:107–116.

141. Langberg JJ, Man C, Vorperian VR, et al. Recognition and

catheter ablation of subepicardial accessory pathways. *J Am Coll Cardiol* 1993;22:1100–1104.

142. Kuck KH, Schluter M, Geiger M, et al. Radiofrequency current catheter ablation of accessory atrioventricular pathways. *Lancet* 1991;337:1557–1561.

143. Kay GN, Epstein AE, Dailey SM, Plumb VJ. Role of radiofrequency ablation in the management of supraventricular arrhythmias: experience in 760 consecutive patients. *J Cardiovasc Electrophysiol* 1993;4:371–389.

144. Swartz JF, Tracy CM, Fletcher RD. Radiofrequency endocardial catheter ablation of accessory atrioventricular pathway atrial insertion sites. *Circulation* 1993;87:487–499.

145. Calkins H, Yong P, Miller JM, et al, for the Atakr Multicenter Investigators Group. Catheter ablation of accessory pathways, atrioventricular nodal reentrant tachycardia, and the atrioventricular junction: final results of a prospective, multicenter clinical trial. *Circulation* 1999;99:262–270.

146. Calkins H, Prystowsky E, Berger RD, et al, for the Atakr Multicenter Investigators Group. Recurrence of conduction following radiofrequency catheter ablation procedures: relationship to ablation target and electrode temperature. *J Cardiovasc Electrophysiol* 1996;7:704–712.

147. Jazayeri MR, Hempe SL, Sra JS, et al. Selective transcatheter ablation of the fast and slow pathways using radiofrequency energy in patients with atrioventricular nodal reentrant tachycardia. *Circulation* 1992;85:1318–1328.

148. Lee MA, Morady F, Kadish A, et al. Catheter modification of the atrioventricular junction with radiofrequency energy in patients with atrioventricular nodal reentry tachycardia. *Circulation* 1991;83:827–835.

149. Kottkamp H, Hindricks G, Willems S, et al. An anatomically and electrogram-guided stepwise approach for effective and safe catheter ablation of the fast pathway for elimination of atrioventricular node reentrant tachycardia. *J Am Coll Cardiol* 1995;25:974–983.

150. Haissaguerre M, Gaita F, Fischer B, et al. Elimination of atrioventricular nodal reentrant tachycardia using discrete slow potentials to guide application of radiofrequency energy. *Circulation* 1992,85:2162–2175.

151. Jackman WM, Beckman KJ, McClelland JH, et al. Treatment of supraventricular tachycardia due to atrioventricular nodal reentry by radiofrequency catheter ablation of slow-pathway conduction. *N Engl J Med* 1992;327:313–318.

152. Epstein LM, Lesh MD, Griffin JC, et al. A direct midseptal approach to slow atrioventricular nodal pathway ablation. *Pacing Clin Electrophysiol* 1995;18[Pt I]:57–64.

153. Kalbfleisch SJ, Strickberger SA, Williamson B, et al. Randomized comparison of anatomic and electrogram mapping approaches to ablation of the slow pathway of atrioventricular node reentrant tachycardia. *J Am Coll Cardiol* 1994;23:716–723.

154. Sousa J, El-Atassi R, Rosenheck S, et al. Radiofrequency catheter ablation of the atrioventricular junction from the left ventricle. *Circulation* 1991;84:567–571.

155. Morady F, Calkins H, Langberg JJ, et al. A prospective randomized comparison of direct current and radiofrequency ablation of the atrioventricular junction. *J Am Coll Cardiol* 1993;21:102–109.

156. Trohman RG, Simmons TW, Moore SL, et al. Catheter ablation of the atrioventricular junction using radiofrequency energy and a bilateral cardiac approach. *Am J Cardiol* 1992;70:1438–1443.

157. Evans GT Jr, Scheinman MM, Scheinman MM, et al. The percutaneous cardiac mapping and ablation registry: final summary of results. *Pacing Clin Electrophysiol* 1988;11:1621–1626.

158. Williamson BD, Ching Man K, Daoud E, et al. Radiofrequency catheter modification of atrioventricular conduction to control the ventricular rate during atrial fibrillation. *N Engl J Med* 1994;331:910.

159. Proclemer A, Della Bella P, Tondo C, et al. Radiofrequency ablation of atrioventricular junction and pacemaker implantation versus modulation of atrioventricular conduction in drug refractory atrial fibrillation. *Am J Cardiol* 1999;83:1437–1442.

160. Klein LS, Shih H-T, Hackett FK, et al. Radiofrequency catheter ablation of ventricular tachycardia in patients without structural heart disease. *Circulation* 1992;85:1666–1674.

161. Nakagawa H, Beckman KJ, McClelland JH, et al. Radiofrequency catheter ablation of idiopathic left ventricular tachycardia guided by a Purkinje potential. *Circulation* 1993;88:2607–2617.

162. Coggins DL, Lee RJ, Sweeney J, et al. Radiofrequency catheter ablation as a cure for idiopathic tachycardia of both left and right ventricular origin. *J Am Coll Cardiol* 1994;23:1333–1341.

163. Calkins H, Kalbfleisch SJ, El-Atassi R, et al. Relation between efficacy of radiofrequency catheter ablation and site of origin of idiopathic ventricular tachycardia. *Am J Cardiol* 1993;71:827–833.

164. Blanck Z, Dhala A, Deshpande S, et al. Bundle branch reentrant ventricular tachycardia: cumulative experience in 48 patients. *J Cardiovasc Electrophysiol* 1993;4:253–262.

165. Mehdirad AA, Keim S, Rist K, Tchou P. Long-term clinical outcome of right bundle branch radiofrequency catheter ablation for treatment of bundle branch reentrant ventricular tachycardia. *Pacing Clin Electrophysiol* 1995;18:2135–2143.

166. Calkins H, Epstein A, Ellenbogen KA, et al. Catheter ablation of VT using cooled RF energy: final results of a prospective multicenter clinical trial. *Circulation* 1999;100:I-374A.

167. Morady F, Harvey M, Kalbfleisch SJ, et al. Radiofrequency catheter ablation of ventricular tachycardia in patients with coronary artery disease. *Circulation* 1993;87:363–372.

168. Kim YH, Sosa-Suarez G, Trouton TG, et al. Treatment of ventricular tachycardia by transcatheter radiofrequency ablation in patients with ischemic heart disease. *Circulation* 1994;89:1094–1102.

169. Stevenson WG, Khan H, Sager P, et al. Identification of reentry circuit sites during catheter mapping and radiofrequency ablation of ventricular tachycardia late after myocardial infarction. *Circulation* 1993;88[Pt I]:1647–1670.

170. Das SK, Morady F, DiCarlo L Jr, et al. Prognostic usefulness of programmed ventricular stimulation in idiopathic dilated cardiomyopathy without symptomatic ventricular arrhythmias. *Am J Cardiol* 1986;58:998–1000.

171. Kottkamp H, Hindricks G, Chen X, et al. Radiofequency catheter ablation of sustained ventricular tachycardia in idiopathic dilated cardiomyopathy. *Circulation* 1995;92:1159–1168.

172. Strickberger SA, Man KC, Daoud EG, et al. A prospective evaluation of catheter ablation of ventricular tachycardia as adjuvant therapy in patients with coronary artery disease and an implantable cardioverter-defibrillator. *Circulation* 1997;96:1525–1531.

173. Kilborn, MJ, McGuire MA. Radiofrequency catheter ablation of atrioventricular junctional ("AV nodal") reentrant tachycardia in patients with implantable cardioverter defibrillators. *Pacing Clin Electrophysiol* 1998;21:2681–2684.

174. Kay GN, Epstein AE, Dailey SM. Role of radiofrequency ablation in the management of supraventricular arrhythmias: experience in 760 consecutive patients. *J Cardiovasc Electrophysiol* 1993;4:371–389.

175. Chen S-A, Chiang CE, Tai CT, et al. Complications of diagnostic electrophysiologic studies and radiofrequency catheter ablation in patients wit tachyarrhythmias: an eight-year survey of 3,966 consecutive procedures in tertiary referral center. *Am J Cardiol* 1996;77:41–46.

176. Olsson A, Darpo B, Bergfeldt L, et al. Frequency and long term follow-up of valvular insufficiency caused by retrograde aortic radiofrequency catheter ablation procedures. *Heart* 1999;81:292–296.

177. Manolis AS, Vassilikos V, Maounis T, et al. Detection of myocardial injury during radiofrequency catheter ablation by measuring serum cardiac troponin I levels: procedural correlates [In process citation]. *J Am Coll Cardiol* 1999;34:1099–1105.

178. Robbins IM, Colvin EV, Doyle TP, et al. Pulmonary vein stenosis after catheter ablation of atrial fibrillation. *Circulation* 1998;98:1769–1775.

179. Paydak H, Kall JG, Burke MC, et al. Atrial fibrillation after radiofrequency ablation of type I atrial flutter: time to onset, determinants, and clinical course. *Circulation* 1998;98:315–322.

180. Kocovic DZ, Harada T, Shea JB, et al. Alterations of heart rate and heart rate variability after radiofrequency catheter ablation of supraventricular tachycardia: delineation of parasympathetic pathways in the human heart. *Circulation* 1993;88:1671–1681.

181. Psychari SN, Theodorakis GN, Koutelou M, et al. Cardiac denervation after radiofrequency ablation of supraventricular tachycardias. *Am J Cardiol* 1998;81:725–731.

182. Hamdan MH, Page RL, Wasmund SL, et al. Selective parasympathetic denervation following posteroseptal ablation for atrioventricular nodal reentrant tachycardia or accessory pathways. *Am J Cardiol* 2000;85:875–878.

183. Calkins H, Yong P, Miller JM, et al. Catheter ablation of accessory pathways, atrioventricular nodal reentrant tachycardia, and the atrioventricular junction: final results of a prospective, multicenter clinical trial. *Circulation* 1999;99:262–270.

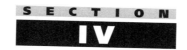

SECTION IV

SPECIFIC ARRHYTHMIAS

13

SINOATRIAL/ATRIAL TACHYARRHYTHMIAS

JEFFREY J. GOLDBERGER
ALAN H. KADISH

There are various tachyarrhythmias that arise from the atrium. These include sinoatrial reentry, inappropriate sinus tachycardia, atrial tachycardia (AT), atrial flutter, and atrial fibrillation. This chapter focuses on the first three of these arrhythmias (atrial flutter is discussed in Chapter 16, and atrial fibrillation is discussed in Chapter 15).

MULTIFOCAL ATRIAL TACHYCARDIA

Definition

Multifocal AT (MAT), also known as *chaotic AT,* is a disorder in atrial rhythm that is frequently caused by acute pulmonary or cardiac disease processes. Multiple foci within the atria are responsible for activation of the atria and lead to the appearance of multiple P-wave morphologies on the surface electrocardiogram (ECG) (Fig. 13-1). Thus, MAT is characterized by an atrial rate of more than 120 beats per minute (bpm) associated with at least three different P-wave morphologies.

Incidence/Prevalence

MAT has been noted in 0.05% to 0.38% of ECGs interpreted in hospitals (1–6). It is most commonly noted in an elderly population with a mean age in the upper sixties and seventies (1–8). The incidence of MAT in an outpatient setting has not been adequately studied, probably because of its association with acute illnesses. However, it is likely much less common in an outpatient setting. Common illnesses found in patients with MAT include chronic obstructive pulmonary disease (with or without an acute exacerbation), pneumonia, nonpulmonary infections, congestive heart failure, postoperative state, diabetes mellitus,

J. J. Goldberger: Department of Cardiology, Northwestern University Medical School, Chicago, Illinois 60611.
A. H. Kadish: Northwestern Memorial Hospital, Wesley Pavilion Cardiology, Chicago, Illinois 60611.

coronary artery disease, lung carcinoma, and pulmonary embolus (1–7,9,10). Chronic obstructive pulmonary disease and congestive heart failure account for the associated diseases in most patients. In patients admitted for acute respiratory decompensation of their underlying chronic obstructive pulmonary disease, the incidence of MAT has been reported between 6% and 17% (11,12).

Although MAT has a particularly strong association with advanced pulmonary disease, it has been noted in other settings, such as acute myocardial infarction (13), electrolyte imbalance—particularly hypokalemia and hypomagnesemia (14)—and mitral stenosis (15).

In the pediatric age-group, MAT is extremely uncommon. There are only sporadic reported cases in the literature (16–21). Most of these patients had no cardiac or pulmonary disease. However, congenital heart disease has been noted in some of these patients. Most cases resolved spontaneously. Nevertheless, the mortality rate in this group was fairly high at approximately 20%.

Etiology

Many factors contribute to the precipitation of MAT. The most common clinical precipitant is hypoxia resulting from an acute pulmonary or cardiac problem. Other conditions associated with increased sympathetic tone, such as acute myocardial infarction, sepsis, and the postoperative state, are also common precipitants of MAT. Electrolyte abnormalities, particularly hypokalemia and hypomagnesemia

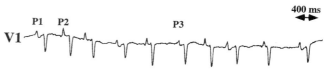

FIGURE 13-1. Electrocardiographic recording from lead V_1 of multifocal atrial tachycardia. Note the multiple P-wave morphologies (P_1 through P_3). In addition, there are multiple PR intervals as well as irregular R-R intervals.

(14), may play a role in precipitating MAT. Frequently in the setting of an acute exacerbation of chronic obstructive pulmonary disease, there may be a combination of these precipitants including hypoxia, elevated catecholamine levels, acidosis, and electrolyte abnormalities. Theophylline toxicity has also been suggested to precipitate MAT. In a study (8) of 16 patients with MAT treated with theophylline, MAT resolved when theophylline was discontinued. On rechallenge with increasing doses of intravenous aminophylline, there was a correlation between the theophylline level and the percentage of atrial ectopic beats until MAT was noted in all patients. This report provides the best evidence of the relation between theophylline and MAT.

Early reports suggested digoxin also played an etiologic role. However, many studies have now demonstrated that digoxin is not a likely precipitant of MAT. Finally, atrial distension has been suggested as an etiologic factor, but no confirmatory evidence is available.

ECG Characteristics

The diagnosis of MAT is made on the ECG when an AT (with a rate of more than 120 bpm) is noted with at least three different P-wave morphologies and with different P-P, PR, and R-R intervals (Fig. 13-1). There must be an isoelectric interval between P waves. When the atrial rate is slower (less than 100 bpm) and associated with three different P-wave morphologies, a diagnosis of wandering atrial pacemaker is appropriate (Fig. 13-2). Because of the varying intervals in MAT, the ventricular response may be irregularly irregular and the arrhythmia may be confused with

coarse atrial fibrillation. This distinction becomes more difficult because of the strong association of atrial fibrillation with MAT. Atrial fibrillation or flutter may be noted before or after MAT in approximately half the cases (1,2,4). It may be important to examine multiple ECG leads to confirm the diagnosis. Some degree of atrioventricular (AV) block is commonly noted during MAT. Typical ventricular rates during MAT range from 100 to 170 bpm.

Electrophysiologic Mechanisms

In MAT, multiple P-wave morphologies are noted, which is likely the result of the origination of impulses from multiple sites within the atria. No definitive data exist to delineate the mechanism of MAT. Abnormal automaticity at multiple atrial sites has been proposed as the mechanism (22). Alternatively, there is support for the role of triggered activity (23). Conditions such as hypoxia, hypercapnia, hypokalemia, hypomagnesemia, and increased sympathetic tone may lead to elevation of intracellular calcium. Elevation of intracellular calcium may lead to afterdepolarizations and triggered activity. In an *in vitro* study on the effects of theophylline on human atrial tissue (24), it was noted that theophylline caused delayed afterdepolarizations and triggered activity. This was blocked by pretreatment with diltiazem. Theophylline has also been shown to lead to elevated circulating catecholamine levels (25), which may precipitate triggered activity and abnormal automaticity. The clinical response of some patients with MAT to verapamil, as well as the findings of hypoxia, increased sympathetic tone, and the other metabolic abnormalities frequently noted in patients with MAT, suggest that intracellular calcium accumulation and triggered activity may be responsible for the genesis of this arrhythmia. However, verapamil can be used to successfully treat other arrhythmia mechanisms. Although it has been proposed that there may be multiple reentrant circuits leading to this arrhythmia, there is no verification of this mechanism. Anecdotal experience in patients with MAT suggests that it cannot be terminated or initiated with programmed stimulation, making reentry an unlikely mechanism.

Symptoms and Presentation/Physical Examination

Subjects with MAT predominantly have complaints related to their underlying disorder such as shortness of breath related to an exacerbation of chronic obstructive pulmonary disease or congestive heart failure. Patients may also have complaints related to the arrhythmia such as palpitations, light-headedness, and chest pain. It is critical to evaluate patients with MAT for evidence of clinical or hemodynamic compromise, such as myocardial ischemia, which would mandate more aggressive therapy specifically directed at controlling the arrhythmia. Given the advanced age and

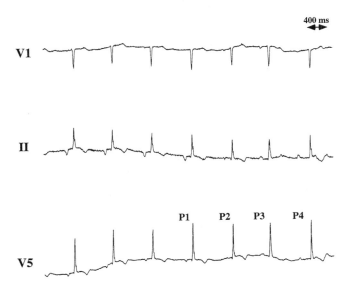

FIGURE 13-2. Simultaneous electrocardiographic recordings from leads V₁, II, and V₅. The tracing demonstrates a wandering atrial pacemaker. Four P-wave morphologies can be identified (P₁ through P₄). Because the rate is approximately 80 beats per minute, the diagnosis is "wandering atrial pacemaker" rather than "multifocal atrial tachycardia."

significant incidence of cardiac disease in these patients, they may not tolerate the rapid rates associated with MAT.

Physical examination findings are notable for an irregular and perhaps irregularly irregular pulse, often leading to the incorrect diagnosis of atrial fibrillation. The presence of *a* waves on the jugular venous pulsations may aid in the differentiation of MAT from atrial fibrillation. The predominant findings on physical examination are usually related to the underlying precipitating illness.

Prognostic/Clinical Significance

The finding of MAT is significant, as many studies have shown that these patients have a very high in-hospital mortality rate ranging from 29% to 56% (1–7,10,26). Death is not directly caused by the arrhythmia, but the severity of the underlying disease.

Methods for Evaluation

Typically, patients with MAT require no further evaluation beyond an ECG. There are no indications for performing electrophysiologic studies in patients with MAT. Typically, this arrhythmia cannot be induced or terminated in the electrophysiology laboratory. Lewis lead recordings or esophageal lead recordings may be helpful to distinguish MAT from atrial fibrillation. Electrophysiologic recordings during MAT would be expected to show an AT with varying pathways of atrial activation. In the single reported study (22) of the electrophysiologic evaluation of patients with chaotic AT, major findings included impaired intraatrial conduction and varying atrionodal conduction times. Eighty milligrams of lidocaine was administered intravenously in seven patients and resulted in short periods of sinus rhythm in six patients. The authors suggested that lidocaine was depressing multiple hyperexcitable atrial foci, leaving the sinus mechanism as the predominant rhythm.

Therapy

Treatment of this disorder should first be aimed at correcting the underlying physiologic derangements, which should include improvement in oxygenation and correction of electrolyte abnormalities. Occasionally, patients will require adjunctive therapy to control the tachycardia. Various treatment strategies have been attempted. Cardioversion is ineffective for MAT (13). Digoxin and type I antiarrhythmic agents have generally been ineffective for treatment of MAT.

β Blockers (26–30) and verapamil (26,27,31,32) have been described to be effective for treatment of MAT by either restoring sinus rhythm or slowing the rate. However, in a direct comparison of verapamil, metoprolol, and placebo, Arsura and colleagues (27) found that 20% of patients responded to placebo, 44% responded to verapamil,

and 89% responded to metoprolol. Five patients who did not respond to verapamil responded to metoprolol. Kastor (26) combined the results of several studies using verapamil and/or metoprolol for treatment of MAT. Verapamil was effective in 18 of 42 patients (43%), and metoprolol was effective in 30 of 38 patients (79%). Thus, metoprolol does appear to be more efficacious in patients with MAT. However, extreme caution must be exercised with the use of β blockers in patients with obstructive pulmonary disease, as many of these patients cannot tolerate β blockers. Esmolol, an ultrashort-acting β blocker, has been used effectively to control MAT (28); given its short half-life and the potential deleterious respiratory effects of β blockers in patients with MAT, a trial of esmolol may be warranted before treatment with other β blockers with longer half-lives. The effectiveness of β blockers is likely related to their antiadrenergic effects. Verapamil may be effective by lowering intracellular calcium or other unknown effects. Concomitant treatment with calcium may lead to less hypotension (32).

Flecainide has also been reported to be effective for MAT (33,34). Amiodarone has been reported to be effective for treatment of MAT in a limited number of cases (19,35). However, it seems unlikely that the typical patient with MAT would require amiodarone therapy. Magnesium therapy has also been shown to be effective in treating MAT, even in patients with normal serum magnesium levels (36–39). Although there is rarely a need to do so, catheter ablation may be used to treat this arrhythmia. AV nodal ablation and pacemaker implantation have been helpful in a few patients (40).

For those patients with pulmonary problems being treated with agents such as aminophylline or theophylline, which may be responsible for precipitating or exacerbating MAT, these agents should be discontinued and alternative therapy should be considered.

ATRIAL TACHYCARDIA
Definition

AT refers to one of several types of tachycardias that originate in the right or left atrium. Generally, these tachycardias have a rate between 150 and 250 bpm, although slower and faster rates of ATs have been observed. When the rate is less than 100 bpm and the P-wave morphology is not consistent with sinus rhythm, an ectopic atrial rhythm should be diagnosed. ATs may be brief and self-terminating, paroxysmal and sustained, or incessant. Historically, the term *paroxysmal AT* (PAT) had been used to describe all types of paroxysmal supraventricular tachycardia (41–43) including AV junctional reentrant tachycardia and orthodromic AV reentrant tachycardia using an accessory pathway. Now, this term should be applied only to patients whose tachycardia originates in the atrium. Multiple mechanisms and disease states can lead to AT. Because of the relative infrequency of

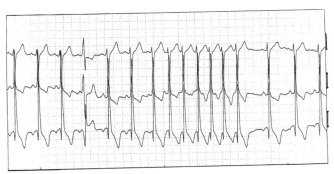

FIGURE 13-3. Holter monitor recording demonstrating a brief nonsustained run of atrial tachycardia lasting seven beats.

these arrhythmias, the multiple possibilities for classifying them, and the multitude of reports with few patients, there is substantial diversity in the literature regarding their clinical characteristics and treatment.

To discuss these tachycardias, we divide them into four syndromes: (a) short bursts of self-limited AT (Fig. 13-3); (b) paroxysmal sustained AT (Fig. 13-4); (c) incessant or near-incessant AT (Fig. 13-4); and (d) PAT with AV block, as can be seen in digitalis toxicity (Fig. 13-5). With the availability of assays for serum digoxin levels and an appreciation of drug interactions with digoxin, the incidence of digitalis toxicity has markedly decreased (44), making PAT with AV block less likely to be caused by digitalis toxicity.

Recently, it has been reported that short-lived episodes of tachycardias can arise from the pulmonary veins, superior vena cava, or ligament of Marshall. These tachycardias may be a precursor to the onset of atrial fibrillation. These tachycardias are discussed in Chapter 15.

Incidence/Prevalence

Short Bursts

Short bursts of AT occur occasionally on Holter monitoring in healthy subjects. In young adult subjects, nonsustained AT lasting 6 to 12 beats has been noted in 2% to 6% of cases (45–49). In a subset of 142 age-stratified patients with no cardiopulmonary disease from the Framingham study, "supraventricular tachycardia"—likely representing short bursts of AT (although not specifically stated)—was noted in 15% of subjects. In the healthy, active elderly population, short bursts of AT have been noted in 1% to 13% of subjects (50,51) with most episodes lasting less than five beats.

In patients with mitral valve prolapse, the incidence of AT has been reported to be between 3% and 29% (52–54), with a mean prevalence of approximately 20%. Winkle and colleagues (53) noted that the mean duration of these episodes was 5.6 ± 2.6 beats with a range of 3 to 11 beats. Though the incidence of AT appears higher in patients with mitral valve prolapse, in a direct comparison with patients

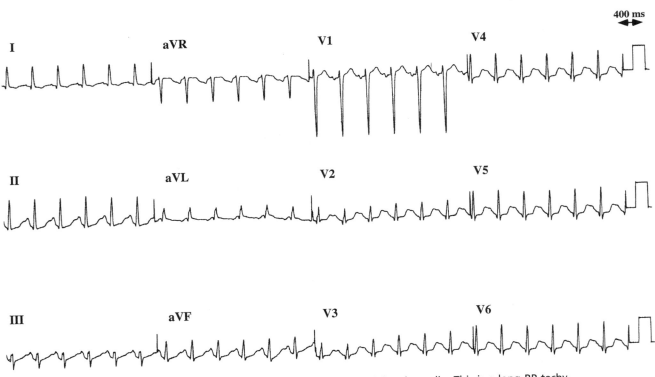

FIGURE 13-4. A 12-lead electrocardiogram (ECG) of atrial tachycardia. This is a long RP tachycardia. Examination of the 12-lead ECG reveals no information regarding the mechanism of the atrial tachycardia.

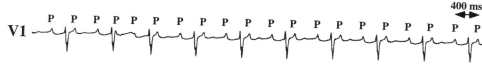

FIGURE 13-5. Electrocardiographic recording from V₁ of atrial tachycardia with 2 : 1 atrioventricular block. Although classically associated with digitalis toxicity, paroxysmal atrial tachycardia with block may be noted in patients with other types of sustained atrial tachycardias.

without mitral valve prolapse, Savage and colleagues (54) found no significant increase resulting from the high prevalence of AT in their control group. In several large series of unselected patients undergoing Holter monitoring (55–57), 5% to 12% were noted to have short bursts of AT with a mean duration of less than 6 seconds (55) or 10 beats (57). The rate of these tachycardias is generally slower than that for other types of supraventricular tachycardia, with a mean reported rate of approximately 115 bpm (55,57).

AT has been noted in the setting of acute myocardial infarction, present in 4% to 19% of patients (58–64). In some cases, the tachycardia may persist for prolonged periods, requiring specific therapy for treatment of hemodynamic deterioration (63). Although an increased mortality rate has been reported in patients with AT versus those without, this is related to the severity of the underlying infarction. Short bursts of AT lasting up to 8 seconds have been noted in 40% of patients with mitral stenosis (15). In hospitalized patients with chronic obstructive pulmonary disease, AT may be noted in 20% of patients (11). In general, this variety of AT represents a benign arrhythmia.

Paroxysmal Sustained Atrial Tachycardia

Paroxysmal sustained ATs account for approximately 10% to 15% of all cases of paroxysmal supraventricular tachycardia referred for electrophysiologic evaluation (65–68). Patients with AT are more likely to have organic heart disease than patients with other types of paroxysmal supraventricular tachycardia (67). The incidence of concomitant heart disease has been reported to vary from 30% to 100% (69–71) and includes coronary artery disease, valvular disease, congenital heart disease, and other cardiomyopathies. This type of AT has been reported in all age-groups, ranging from infants to the elderly (66,71,72). Multiple ATs (multiple foci) may be present in a significant percentage of patients.

Incessant Atrial Tachycardia

Incessant AT is a much rarer entity than PAT. This tachycardia is present more than half of the day (68). The exact prevalence of this disorder is difficult to gauge because of its low incidence. Southall and colleagues (73) noted one newborn with continuous supraventricular tachycardia out of

3,383 healthy newborns. Most reports have been in the pediatric age-group (74–80), although this arrhythmia has been documented in adults (81–86). In a series of ECGs in 3,554 asymptomatic male applicants for a pilot license, 12 (0.43%) were noted to have ectopic AT (defined as having a rate of more than 90 bpm) with heart rates ranging from 91 to 113 bpm (87). In the same report (87), 17 out of 3,700 (0.46%) symptomatic arrhythmia patients in the hospital showed ectopic AT with heart rates from 92 to 145 bpm. The incessant nature of these tachycardias may lead to tachycardia-related cardiomyopathies, which may improve dramatically when the tachycardia is controlled (74,75,79, 80,82,85,86,88–92).

Paroxysmal Atrial Tachycardia with Block

PAT with block has been noted in 0.25% to 0.40% of ECGs (93–96) recorded in large centers during several years. PAT with block may be associated with digitalis toxicity. The differentiation of this disorder from other varieties of atrial or sinus tachycardia may be difficult. Because of the presence of AV block, the nonconducted P wave may be obscured by the QRS complex or the T wave. Carotid sinus pressure or intravenous administration of adenosine may be used to increase the degree of AV block, allowing better visualization of the P waves. Similarly, esophageal lead recordings may be used to document the presence of AT with block. For the rare patients with digitalis-induced PAT with block at atrial rates of more than 250 bpm, differentiation from atrial flutter is essential. Patients with AT will have isoelectric intervals between P waves, rather than a continuously undulating baseline, producing the "sawtoothed" pattern of atrial flutter. In addition, discontinuation of digoxin or potassium repletion will slow the tachycardia and then cause digitalis-induced AT to terminate. Administration of digitalis will increase the atrial rate of digitalis-induced PAT (97).

In patients with PAT, discontinuation of digitalis does not always result in control of the arrhythmia. Although digitalis toxicity may have been responsible for 50% to 80% of cases of AT with block in the past (93–99), recent studies show a much lower incidence (44,100,101). Although digitalis toxicity should be suspected in a patient with PAT with block who is receiving digitalis, it is important to recognize that the AT may be a primary rhythm disorder requiring therapy. In the absence of digitalis toxicity, this tachycardia should be approached and treated in the same fashion as a paroxysmal sustained AT. As in patients with MAT, there is a high in-hospital mortality rate associated with PAT with block likely because of the severity of the underlying heart disease. The reported mortality rate has ranged from 20% to 60% (93–96,98,99,102–104). However, the mortality rates associated with this arrhythmia are likely significantly lower when the presence of digitalis toxicity is recognized (94,96), allowing for institution of appropriate therapy.

Etiology

Short Bursts

Short bursts of AT may occur in the setting of various precipitating factors. Myocardial ischemia or infarction, alcohol ingestion, hypoxia, theophylline toxicity, and electrolyte abnormalities (e.g., hypokalemia) may predispose to the short bursts of AT (11,12,64,105–107). However, in most cases, the arrhythmia is not associated with any clear precipitating factor.

Sustained Reentrant Atrial Tachycardia

Sustained reentrant ATs may be found in patients with previous atrial surgery such as those who have undergone procedures for correction of congenital heart disease (108–111). Multiple tachycardias may be present in these patients. Intraatrial reentry may also be noted in the setting of other structural heart diseases. In the report by Haines and DiMarco (72), only 2 of 19 patients with intraatrial reentrant tachycardia had no known cardiac disease. Other studies have found a lower incidence of heart disease (70,112), yet significantly more than patients with other types of reentrant paroxysmal supraventricular tachycardias (67). The cause of intraatrial reentrant tachycardia in the absence of structural heart disease is unknown.

Automatic Ectopic Atrial Tachycardia

The cause of automatic ectopic ATs is unclear. Pathologic findings of atrial tissue obtained from patients who have undergone surgery have revealed no structural abnormalities, but patchy fibrosis, cellular infiltration, abnormal myocytes, and fatty infiltration are present (113–115). The tachycardia may be incessant or may only be noted in the setting of catecholamine release or administration (82,83, 85,112,116). Frequently, there is an associated cardiomyopathy, but at presentation, it may be difficult to discern whether this is primary or secondary to the tachycardia. When the tachycardia is controlled, many patients will have marked improvements in ventricular function within several months, suggesting that the myopathy was secondary to the tachycardia. If ventricular function does not improve, it is likely that the myopathy is primary. Despite restoration of left ventricular function to normal, evidence of myocardial fibrosis has been noted 1 year after successful ablation (117). The high incidence of structural heart disease in patients with AT compared with other types of paroxysmal supraventricular tachycardia suggests that structural or functional abnormalities of the atria might predispose to AT.

Paroxysmal Atrial Tachycardia with Block

PAT with block is occasionally a result of digitalis toxicity. These patients usually have structural heart disease, providing the rationale for digitalis therapy. Hypokalemia and hypoxia may accentuate the toxic effects of digitalis. Pulmonary disease is also frequently noted in these patients (93,98,104).

ECG Characteristics

The ECG manifestations of AT are variable. The P wave in AT may be located preceding the QRS complex (Fig. 13-4, long RP tachycardia), during the QRS complex, or after the QRS complex (Fig. 13-6). Thus, the PR interval may be variable depending on the AV nodal conduction characteristics. As the ventricles are not a critical component of the tachycardia in AT, variable degrees of AV block may be noted as well. AV block may be useful in establishing the diagnosis, as AV block noted during tachycardia rules out the possibility of AV reentrant tachycardia and makes the diagnosis of AV junctional reentrant tachycardia less likely. The P-wave morphology on the surface ECG may not be a reliable indicator of the site of origin of the tachycardia (118,119), although recently various surface ECG techniques have been reported that may aid in the localization of these tachycardias (120,121). The ECG diagnosis of AT may be difficult to make, particularly if the P wave is hidden in the QRS complex; in which case, the diagnosis of AV junctional reentrant tachycardia must be strongly considered. Establishing the diagnosis may also be difficult if the P wave occurs in the ST segment; in which case, the diagnosis of AV reentrant tachycardia must be strongly considered. However, even in long RP tachycardias, other diagnoses such as atypical AV junctional reentrant tachycardia (fast/slow variety) or AV reentrant tachycardia using a slowly conducting accessory pathway need to be considered. The permanent form of junctional reciprocating tachycardia may appear identical to an incessant AT on the ECG. In patients with automatic ectopic AT, the tachycardia rate may vary throughout the day, because of alterations in autonomic tone. In PAT with block, AV block may be exhibited in a 2 : 1 or Wenckebach-like fashion (Fig. 13-7). If there is AV block, the ventricular rates are rarely more than 120 bpm.

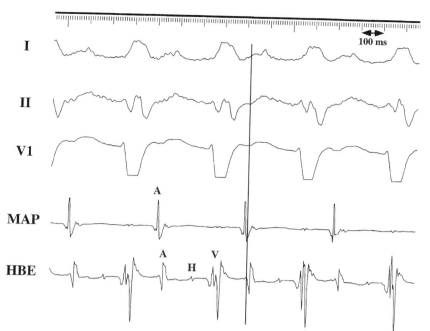

FIGURE 13-6. Simultaneous surface electrocardiographic recordings from leads I, II, and V₁, as well as intracardiac recordings from a mapping catheter *(MAP)* located in the inferolateral right atrium and the His bundle electrogram *(HBE)*. The atrial electrogram on the mapping catheter preceded the onset of the surface P wave by approximately 20 ms. Earliest atrial activation during automatic atrial tachycardia was at this site. Application of radiofrequency energy to this site resulted in successful ablation of the tachycardia.

Electrophysiologic Mechanisms

AT may be caused by any of the three potential mechanisms for tachyarrhythmias: reentry, abnormal automaticity, and triggered automaticity.

Short Bursts

The mechanism for short bursts of AT has not been studied. Based on their short duration and the presence of

"warm-up," it seems likely that abnormal automaticity is the mechanism. Nevertheless, triggered automaticity and reentry must be considered, particularly in patients with structural heart disease and acute medical problems.

Paroxysmal Sustained Atrial Tachycardia

Paroxysmal sustained ATs may also be caused by multiple mechanisms (68). Reentry within the atrium can occur

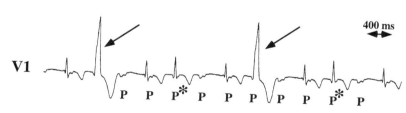

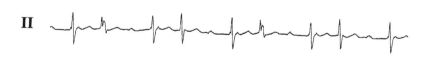

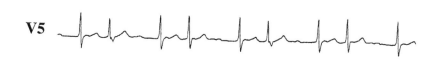

FIGURE 13-7. Simultaneous electrocardiographic recordings from leads V₁, II, and V₅ demonstrating an atrial tachycardia with type I, second-degree atrioventricular block (Wenckebach). The P waves are labeled. The blocked P waves are marked with an asterisk. The wide complex beats *(arrows)* may reflect aberrant conduction or premature ventricular depolarization.

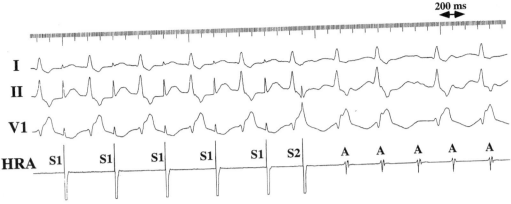

FIGURE 13-8. Simultaneous surface electrocardiographic recordings from leads I, II, and V₁, as well as intracardiac recordings from the high right atrium *(HRA)*. After an eight-beat drive train *(S1)* at a cycle length of 400 ms, an extrastimulus *(S2)* is introduced at a coupling interval of 290 ms and results in induction of atrial tachycardia at a cycle length of 290 ms *(A)*. Note the presence of atrioventricular block.

around anatomic and functional obstacles (122). Several investigators have described patients, many with structural heart disease, who had intraatrial reentrant tachycardias (67,69–72,112,123). Reentrant tachycardias are usually easily initiated and terminated with programmed stimulation (Fig. 13-8). These tachycardias are typically paroxysmal (69,72). In contrast, reports of automatic ATs state that they are repetitive or paroxysmal in 40% to 50% of cases. Automatic ATs are more often paroxysmal in adults compared with children (83,124). Catheter recordings from "automatic foci" in humans have shown the presence of a diastolic slope preceding the P wave (125). Microelectrode recordings from excised tissue from a patient with AT have also suggested an automatic mechanism for the tachycardia (114,115).

There are several reports that propose triggered activity as a potential mechanism for AT (68,126,127). Wellens and Brugada (68) reported a direct relationship between the prematurity of the tachycardia-initiating premature depolarization and the interval from the premature depolarization to the first beat of AT in 10 of 71 (14%) patients with AT. Because of this behavior characteristic for triggered activity and a clinical response in all these patients to treatment with verapamil, it was speculated that triggered activity accounted for the arrhythmia. Chen and colleagues (112) identified 9 of 36 (25%) patients with presumed triggered activity as the mechanism for AT based on the presence of afterdepolarizations on monophasic action potential recordings. Other electrophysiologic characteristics consistent with triggered activity were also noted. In one report (127), a patient with PAT underwent surgical excision of the right atrial appendage. Microelectrode studies on the excised tissue demonstrated afterdepolarizations and inducible triggered activity. Afterdepolarizations and triggered activity have also been reported from other microelectrode studies of diseased human atrium in patients

without a history of AT (128,129). Although these studies suggest that the atrium is capable of demonstrating triggered activity, they do not conclusively establish the mechanism of clinically occurring AT.

Incessant Atrial Tachycardia

Incessant AT is most likely caused by an automatic mechanism, although intraatrial reentry cannot be ruled out as a potential mechanism (123,130). In a report of 19 cases of intraatrial reentrant tachycardia (72), none of the patients were described as having incessant tachycardia. However, it has been reported that in up to half the patients with incessant ATs, the mechanism may be reentrant (130). Nevertheless, most reports link an automatic mechanism to this type of tachycardia. Automatic ATs are frequently incessant, particularly in children in whom most cases may be incessant tachycardias (71,74,75,78).

Paroxysmal Atrial Tachycardia with Block

The mechanism for PAT with block caused by digitalis intoxication has not been well characterized *in vivo.* Although early *in vitro* studies suggested that digitalis may increase automaticity by increasing diastolic depolarization (131,132), more recent evaluation of the data (133) suggests that this probably represented triggered automaticity (which requires an initiating beat and therefore does not represent true automaticity). More recent *in vitro* studies have also shown that digitalis induces delayed afterdepolarizations and triggered activity (134–136). Thus, it has been suspected that triggered automaticity is the mechanism for the *in vivo* arrhythmias. However, abnormal automaticity cannot be ruled out as a potential mechanism. PAT with block may not be related to digitalis toxicity and thus may be caused by any of the previously mentioned mechanisms for AT.

Effect of Pharmacologic Agents

Several investigators have systematically evaluated the effects of various pharmacologic agents on AT (72,112, 137–140). The most studied agent is adenosine. Adenosine effects include inhibition of adenyl cyclase and activation of the adenosine-sensitive potassium currents, thereby shortening action potential duration, hyperpolarizing atrial myocardium, and decreasing the amount of cyclic adenosine monophosphate. Adenosine may terminate AT or transiently suppress it. Most cases of automatic AT can be transiently suppressed with adenosine administration (112,137, 138,140). Most investigators have found that reentrant ATs are generally not affected by adenosine (72,138) unless there is a zone of decremental slow conduction within the atrium participating in the reentrant circuit (139). However, some intraatrial reentrant tachycardias may terminate with adenosine, such as those that originate near the AV nodal transitional area (141). Interestingly, Chen and colleagues (112) reported that adenosine terminated 24 out of 27 (89%) reentrant ATs, an effect that has not been demonstrated in other studies. Although it is difficult to differentiate AT caused by triggered activity from reentrant AT, in those settings when triggered activity was felt to be the mechanism, adenosine has generally terminated the tachycardia (112,138). Because of the multiple effects of adenosine, it is difficult to relate specific effects to specific tachycardia mechanisms.

Verapamil and β blockers may also have effects on various ATs. Chen and colleagues (112) reported that verapamil was effective in terminating most reentrant and triggered ATs while propanolol terminated all automatic and triggered ATs and half the reentrant ATs. Vagal maneuvers resulted in termination mostly of the triggered ATs.

Symptoms and Presentation/Physical Examination

Patients with short bursts of AT are mostly asymptomatic (55,57). However, they may develop palpitations. Patients with sustained ATs may have symptoms of palpitations, chest pain, near syncope, syncope, fatigue, shortness of breath, or exercise intolerance. In addition, patients with incessant tachycardia may develop congestive heart failure as a result of tachycardia-related myopathy. Patients with PAT with block resulting from digitalis toxicity may have other signs of digitalis toxicity. Because of the AV block, the ventricular response is rarely more than 120 bpm. Thus, symptoms related to the tachycardia may be minimal.

Physical examination may be useful in identifying potential underlying structural heart disease. It may also be important in detecting patients who have developed tachycardia-related myopathies. Otherwise, the physical examination results may be unremarkable. Findings during tachycardia will include a rapid rate if there is a 1 : 1 AV conduction. If there is AV block, multiple *a* waves may be noted in the jugular venous pulsations. Other findings during tachycardia depend on the patient's clinical presentation.

Prognostic/Clinical Significance

The significance of PATs is related to the symptoms they generate. Incessant ATs may cause tachycardia-related cardiomyopathy that may completely reverse with abolition of the tachycardia (74,75,79,80,82,85,86,88–92). A substantial portion of ectopic ATs (both incessant and paroxysmal) may resolve during a period of years. This has been well demonstrated in the pediatric population with approximately one third resolving during a period of several years (74,75,79,80). Resolution of AT with time has also been shown to occur in adults (87,142). Klersy and colleagues (142) followed 41 patients with ectopic AT and noted a spontaneous remission rate of 34% during a 5-year follow-up.

Methods for Evaluation

Electrophysiologic studies are not indicated or useful in patients with short bursts of AT or in patients with PAT resulting from digitalis toxicity. However, in patients with other types of paroxysmal or incessant ATs, electrophysiologic studies are frequently indicated to evaluate the mechanism of tachycardia and to aid in therapy. Although there may be some overlap regarding the findings during electrophysiologic studies for each of the tachycardia mechanisms, a presumptive mechanism can often be elucidated based on the tachycardia characteristics.

Atrial Tachycardia Caused by Abnormal Automaticity

AT caused by abnormal automaticity may be difficult to induce during electrophysiologic studies. It is most often noted spontaneously or after infusion of isoproterenol. Criteria that have been used for the electrophysiologic diagnosis of automatic ectopic ATs include the following (67,124, 143):

1. Spontaneous initiation without a relation to critical rates or coupling intervals.
2. The initial beat of spontaneous tachycardia is identical to subsequent beats.
3. Inability to initiate or terminate the tachycardia with atrial or ventricular programmed stimulation.
4. Demonstration of a "warm-up" phase at the initiation of tachycardia.
5. The ability to reset the tachycardia with early atrial premature depolarizations.
6. Suppression of the tachycardia by rapid atrial pacing.

Atrial Tachycardias Caused by Reentry

Reentrant ATs are frequently induced with atrial pacing. To differentiate these tachycardias from atrial flutter, an arbitrary cycle length cutoff of 250 ms has been used (72). It is important to differentiate these induced tachycardias from AV node reentry and AV reentry using an accessory AV bypass tract, as these tachyarrhythmias occur more commonly than AT. Helpful observations include the following:

1. Spontaneous or induced AV block does not affect the tachycardia. AV block may be induced by carotid sinus massage or adenosine infusion. This finding rules out AV reentry.
2. Bundle branch block aberration does not affect the tachycardia rate or the ventriculoatrial conduction intervals. If this finding is present, it suggests the presence of an AV reentrant tachycardia.
3. Mapping during AT may reveal the site of origin of the tachycardia. If the site of origin is away from the AV ring and the AV nodal region, this can rule out the possibilities of AV reentry or AV junctional reentry. However, ATs that arise from the low septal right atrium may be difficult to distinguish from AV node reentry (Fig. 13-9).
4. Application of premature ventricular depolarizations during tachycardia should not preexcite the atrium when the His bundle is refractory. This finding suggests the presence of an accessory pathway.
5. If the tachycardia is terminated by an applied premature ventricular depolarization, there should be retrograde conduction of the premature ventricular depolarization to the atrium. If the premature ventricular depolarization reliably fails to conduct to the atrium and terminates the tachycardia, AT can be ruled out (Fig. 13-10).
6. Spontaneous termination of the tachycardia in a patient who has not demonstrated AV block during tachycardia should be associated with intact AV conduction of the final tachycardia beat. If the tachycardia terminates spontaneously with a nonpremature atrial depolarization, the diagnosis of AT is unlikely .
7. Tachycardia initiation is not dependent on critical A-H interval prolongation. Of note, early atrial premature depolarizations may be required to initiate intraatrial reentry and may, therefore, be associated with prolonged A-H intervals. Thus, the presence of long A-H intervals during tachycardia induction does not rule out an AT.

The response of the tachycardia to atrial and ventricular pacing has also been reported to be helpful in identifying AT (144,145). Kadish and Morady (144) reported that a variable VA time on the first postpacing beat after atrial or ventricular pacing at increasing rates identified the tachycardia to be AT (versus AV nodal or orthodromic AV reentry). Knight and colleagues (145) reported that the appearance of two consecutive atrial depolarizations (without an intervening ventricular depolarization) after cessation of ventricular pacing was highly sensitive and specific for the identification of AT (versus AV nodal or orthodromic reentry).

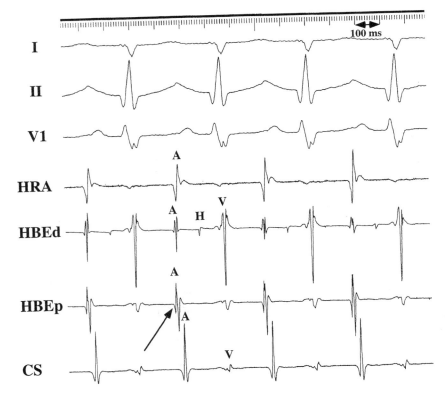

FIGURE 13-9. Simultaneous surface electrocardiographic recordings from leads I, II, and V₁, as well as intracardiac recordings from the high right atrium *(HRA)*, distal and proximal His bundle electrograms *(HBEd* and *HBEp*, respectively), and coronary sinus *(CS)* during atrial tachycardia. Earliest atrial activation was recorded in the proximal His bundle electrogram *(arrow)* suggesting the diagnosis of atypical atrioventricular nodal reentrant tachycardia. However, electrophysiologic maneuvers demonstrated that this was an atrial tachycardia that originated from the low septal right atrium.

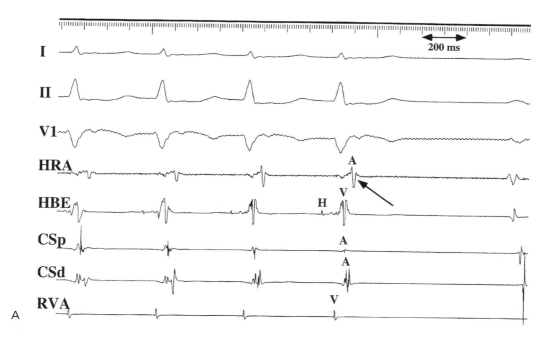

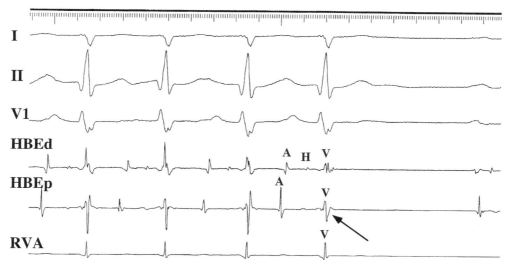

FIGURE 13-10. Simultaneous surface electrocardiographic recordings from leads I, II, and V₂, as well as the indicated intracardiac recordings (high right atrium *[HRA]*, His bundle electrograms including distal and proximal *[HBE, HBEd, HBEp]*, proximal and distal coronary sinus *[CSp, CSd]*, and right ventricular apex *[RVA]*). **A:** Atrioventricular (AV) nodal reentrant tachycardia. Note that the tachycardia spontaneously terminates with the last depolarization (*arrow*). It would be very unlikely for atrial tachycardia that did not previously demonstrate AV block to spontaneously terminate and develop AV block at the same time. Thus, tachycardias that terminate spontaneously with a final atrial depolarization do not likely represent atrial tachycardia. They are more likely to represent AV nodal or AV reentrant tachycardias that terminate as a result of spontaneous block in the AV node, which is the anterograde limb of those tachycardias. **B:** Spontaneous termination of an atrial tachycardia. In this case, the tachycardia spontaneously terminates with a ventricular depolarization (*arrow*). Spontaneous termination of atrial tachycardia will usually appear this way. However, other types of supraventricular tachycardia, such as AV nodal reentrant tachycardia or orthodromic AV reentrant tachycardia using an accessory pathway may also terminate spontaneously with a ventricular depolarization (representing block in the retrograde limb of those tachycardias).

Atrial Tachycardias Caused by Triggered Automaticity

Tachycardias caused by triggered automaticity may be induced with atrial pacing. There are no strict criteria to establish triggered activity as the tachycardia mechanism. There may be significant overlap in the electrophysiologic findings of ATs caused by triggered activity and those caused by reentry. As noted previously, the response to adenosine may not distinguish these mechanisms. However, a direct relationship between the paced cycle length or prematurity of the atrial premature depolarization that initiates tachycardia and the interval from the last paced beat to the first beat of the tachycardia suggests triggered activity. The utility of monophasic action potential recordings requires further exploration.

Atrial Mapping

Mapping of the atria during AT has been performed in patients undergoing surgical or catheter ablation for treatment of this arrhythmia. In a compilation of reported studies (71) that mapped AT (not caused by sinus node reentry, inappropriate sinus tachycardia, or atrial surgery), the atrial foci were right sided in 255 of 311 cases (82%). Right-sided ATs were mapped to the right atrial appendage (n = 32), high right atrial free wall (n = 52), mid or low free wall (n = 87), interatrial septum (n = 36), or coronary sinus ostium (n = 40). Left-sided ATs were mapped to the left atrial appendage (n = 7), the region of the pulmonary veins (n = 41), or the left atrial free wall (n = 6). There is no obvious explanation for the predominance of right-sided atrial foci.

Attempts have been made to further classify ATs based on location. The crista terminalis appears to be a frequent site of origin for these tachycardias (146). Other sites of special interest that have been described in the literature include the AV annulus (147) and the apex of the Koch triangle (148).

Therapy

Short bursts of AT only require therapy if the patient has intolerable symptoms. Reassurance of the benign nature of this rhythm and correction of potential precipitating factors may alleviate the symptoms.

Pharmacologic Therapy

If medications are required, first-line therapy should be a β blocker if there are no contraindications. Digoxin is not likely to be effective; however, it may be useful in slowing the ventricular response during AT. The efficacy of calcium channel blockers is not known. However, subgroups of patients, such as those whose AT is caused by triggered activity may respond to calcium channel blockers. The use of class Ia, Ic, or III antiarrhythmic agents must be balanced with the potential risks of proarrhythmia associated with these agents. They may significantly reduce the number of episodes of AT (149).

Both paroxysmal and incessant ATs are reported to be difficult to treat medically (76,79,81,150). Various agents including digoxin, β blockers, calcium channel blockers, class Ia antiarrhythmic agents, class Ic antiarrhythmic agents, class III antiarrhythmic agents including amiodarone, and combinations have all been used with varying success rates (34,74,75,79–81,151,152). As there are no controlled trials of medical therapy for AT, it is difficult to assess the relative efficacy of these agents. In general, the automatic tachycardias are more difficult to control with medications than the reentrant or triggered (34,68,81) tachycardias. Digitalis compounds are frequently used and may help control the ventricular response during tachycardia. β Blockers have been reported to control paroxysmal and incessant tachycardias (153,154), but the overall success rates are low (155). Class Ia agents have limited efficacy in patients with AT (155). Kunze and colleagues (81) reported successful therapy of chronic ectopic AT using encainide and flecainide in five patients who had failed after receiving four other antiarrhythmic drugs including amiodarone and verapamil. Other investigators (155–157) have also shown the type Ic agents to be somewhat effective in treating these tachycardias, with efficacy rates of approximately 50%. Amiodarone has been reported to be efficacious in reentrant and automatic ATs (74,75,155,158). Reports of a few patients have found moricizine and a combination of amiodarone and flecainide to be efficacious in patients with incessant AT (88,151). Direct current cardioversion may be considered in the patient with AT associated with hemodynamic compromise.

Surgical or Catheter Ablation

Other treatment options include catheter and surgical ablation. Although there have been many reports on the use of surgical therapy for automatic AT, most individual reports have generally included few patients. Hendry and colleagues (159) compiled 26 series of surgical treatment for automatic AT, which included a total of 76 patients. The cumulative success rate was 87%. More recent reports (150, 160,161) document success rates of more than 90%. The surgical approach has in general been individualized but includes open-heart and closed-heart procedures. Ablation has been performed by resection, isolation, cryogenic techniques, or laser techniques.

There have been multiple small reports of radiofrequency catheter ablation treatment for AT (82–86,92,108, 109,111,112,123,130,162), with the largest series including only 45 cases (116). Chen and colleagues (71) summarized the results of catheter ablation from multiple reports and noted a success rate of 92.9% (234 of 252 patients) with a recurrence rate of 7.3% (14 of 192 patients). The presence of cardiac disease, younger age, and multiple foci predicted recurrence. New mapping techniques, such as noncontact mapping and electroanatomic mapping (163, 164) may facilitate the three-dimensional mapping that is necessary for catheter ablation of this arrhythmia.

Digoxin Toxicity

AT caused by digitalis intoxication is treated by discontinuing digitalis therapy. Correction of electrolyte and other metabolic abnormalities should be undertaken. Administration of oral or intravenous potassium is a mainstay of therapy likely because of the loss of potassium induced by the concomitant diuretic therapy that most patients receive. A potpourri of other antiarrhythmic agents including procainamide and β blockers (96,165) has been successfully used as well. β Blockers may be particularly useful because digoxin toxic arrhythmias may be the result of an enhancement of sympathetic neural activity mediated by the central nervous system, resulting in enhanced automaticity or increased afterpotentials and triggered automaticity. There is a case report describing the successful use of direct current cardioversion to treat this arrhythmia (166).

Presently, if there is an urgent need to stop the tachycardia, intravenous administration of digoxin-specific antibodies should be strongly considered. Digoxin-specific antibody Fab fragments, purified from sheep IgG, rapidly bind to circulating. These antibody fragments are given intravenously during 30 minutes (unless cardiac arrest has occurred; in which case, the solution is given as a bolus) and in molar equivalency with estimated ingested digoxin (167).

SINOATRIAL TACHYCARDIAS

Definition

This category or subset of atrial tachyarrhythmias is generally defined by the presence of tachycardia with a P wave during tachycardia that is similar to that noted during normal sinus rhythm. These tachycardias may be reentrant and paroxysmal or incessant. Sinoatrial nodal reentrant tachycardia is defined by its mechanism (reentry involving the sinoatrial node) and generally has sudden onset and termination. Inappropriate sinus tachycardia is poorly defined. In general, the syndrome of inappropriate sinus tachycardia is defined as a sinus rate that is inappropriate for the associated physiologic condition, be it rest or mild exertion. Because these arrhythmias are uncommon causes of sustained supraventricular tachycardias, there are very few large clinical studies addressing these arrhythmias.

Prevalence

Although microelectrode studies of rabbit hearts (168,169) have demonstrated evidence of reentry within the sinus node,

all the reports of humans are presumptive, as this arrhythmia may be difficult to distinguish from other intraatrial reentrant tachycardias originating in the region of the sinus node. Nevertheless, several investigators (170–173) have described this finding in humans in a few patients (5 to 20) undergoing electrophysiologic testing. Among patients referred for electrophysiologic testing for paroxysmal supraventricular tachycardia (174), sustained sinoatrial nodal reentrant tachycardia has been reported in up to 17% of patients. Sanders and colleagues (175) identified 11 of 343 (3%) patients referred for radiofrequency ablation of paroxysmal supraventricular tachycardia who had inducible sustained sinoatrial nodal reentrant tachycardia. Most of these patients had other associated arrhythmias. However, an arrhythmia consistent with sustained sinoatrial nodal reentrant tachycardia was recorded in all but two of these patients. In our laboratory, sustained sinoatrial nodal reentrant tachycardia accounts for less than 1% of cases referred for catheter ablation of paroxysmal supraventricular tachycardia. As the rate of sinoatrial nodal reentrant tachycardias may be slower (average, 130 bpm; range, 90 to 240 bpm) than the rates of other paroxysmal supraventricular tachycardias, these arrhythmias may cause fewer symptoms and therefore may be underreported. In addition, there may be a tendency for these arrhythmias to be self-terminating and relatively brief. Thus, it is difficult to gauge their true prevalence.

Inappropriate sinus tachycardia is reported to be an uncommon disorder. The frequency of this arrhythmia will depend on the criteria used for its definition. It is clear that some patients may have accelerated sinus rates at rest associated with symptoms, but the rates may not be in a classic tachycardia range (i.e., 90 to 100 bpm). Many patients with palpitations undergo event monitoring; this shows sinus rhythm at rates of 90 to 100 bpm during symptoms at rest, which may represent an inappropriately elevated rate for these patients. In addition, patients only come to medical attention and classification if they have symptoms. It is also clear that there are patients with inappropriate sinus tachycardia who have no symptoms secondary to the accelerated rates. Because of underawareness of this syndrome and lack of established criteria, this syndrome may be underdiagnosed, particularly in patients with palpitations. Inappropriate sinus tachycardia has been predominantly reported in woman. There is also a suggestion that it occurs more frequently or more likely it is reported more frequently in health care workers.

Inappropriate sinus tachycardia has been described after catheter ablation for supraventricular tachycardias remote from the sinus node. We first described this in association with fast pathway AV nodal modification (176). Since then, several reports have documented this problem with an incidence of 6% to 10% (177–179). In most cases, the inappropriate sinus tachycardia subsides with time (177), usually within days, suggesting that it is a transient abnormality that develops as a result of the ablation procedure. Although it has been reported to occur after ablation at other sites, it most commonly occurs after ablations near the interatrial septum, anteriorly and posteriorly (162,177–179). It is the result of alterations in sympathetic and parasympathetic inputs into the sinus node. In patients with persistent inappropriate sinus tachycardia, it remains unclear whether these cases represent *de novo* inappropriate sinus tachycardia resulting from ablation or whether the problem coexisted with the other supraventricular tachycardia but went undetected.

Etiology

In patients with sinoatrial nodal reentry, it is not clear whether there are particular properties of the sinoatrial nodal tissues that predispose to this arrhythmia in some subgroups of patients. Concomitant heart disease is frequently noted but the relationship of heart disease or conduction system disease to the tachycardia is not firmly established.

Inappropriate sinus tachycardia is likely a disease of diverse origins. In theory, inappropriate sinus tachycardia may result from an intrinsic abnormality in sinus node function, extrinsic factors such as increased sympathetic tone or decreased parasympathetic tone, or a combination. Some patients with this disorder have been characterized by an elevation in intrinsic heart rate (180,181). The efferent cardiovagal reflex in response to the cold face test has been reported to be depressed (181). β-Adrenergic hypersensitivity to isoproterenol has also been found (181). A reduction in heart rate variability has been reported (182). Despite the array of abnormal autonomic findings, it is not possible to distinguish whether the abnormality is intrinsic or extrinsic to the sinus node. If there were an intrinsic abnormality in the sinus node, autonomic reflex responses may be abnormal. We evaluated the diurnal heart rate variation in patients with inappropriate sinus tachycardia (183). In patients with symptomatic inappropriate sinus tachycardia and average daily heart rate of 80 bpm, an exaggerated morning heart rate peak was evident, compared with those with inappropriate sinus tachycardia and average daily heart rate of more than 80 bpm. This would be consistent with either enhanced morning sympathetic tone or responsiveness in the former group. Based on the response of the heart rate and activation sequence to catheter ablation, Man and colleagues (184) described two distinct responses: progressive slowing of the heart rate with a cranial-caudal shift in activation sequence versus abrupt reduction in sinus rate without a change in sequence. These reports suggest that there are multiple mechanisms responsible for this syndrome.

The cause of inappropriate sinus tachycardia after catheter ablation is unclear. Heart rate variability has been reported to be decreased (162,179), unchanged (162,178), or increased (185) with radiofrequency ablation at septal sites either compared with preablation values or with values of patients who underwent ablation at nonseptal sites. Because there may be parasympathetic fibers that course through the area of the low interatrial septum before innervating the sinus node, it is an attractive hypothesis to consider that radiofrequency catheter ablation in this area damages these fibers with a resultant decrease in parasympathetic effect at the sinus node. However, there are insufficient data to support this hypothesis. Because the inappropriate sinus tachycardia in this setting resolves spontaneously in most cases, it must result from a transient abnormality induced by the ablation procedure.

ECG Characteristics

The ECG manifestations of sinoatrial nodal reentrant tachycardia and inappropriate sinus tachycardia are identical in that P-wave morphology is similar to that noted during sinus rhythm. In general, the rates of these tachycardias tend to be less than the rates noted in patients with paroxysmal supraventricular tachycardia. The rates are usually less than 150 bpm, but with sinoatrial nodal reentry, rates have been reported to be as high as 240 bpm. In some cases, relative "tachycardia" may be noted with rates as low as 90 bpm. The difference between rhythms at 90 bpm and normal sinus rhythm is identified by paroxysmal onset of the "tachycardia" in a patient who otherwise has sinus bradycardia. If a patient has underlying sinus rhythm at 50 to 60 bpm and sudden onset of a dysrhythmia at a rate of 90 bpm with a P-wave morphology identical to that noted during sinus rhythm, this could be classified as sinoatrial nodal reentrant tachycardia. In patients with inappropriate sinus tachycardia, the rates during symptoms may depend on whether the patient is at rest or involved in an activity. It is possible to observe symptoms with heart rates as low as 90 bpm if the patient is at rest. It may not be possible to completely differentiate either of these arrhythmias from perisinoatrial nodal arrhythmias such as intraatrial reentry or automatic ATs that originate near the sinus node. The differentiation of these arrhythmias is difficult by ECG and by intracardiac electrophysiologic recordings.

Electrophysiologic Mechanisms

Sinoatrial nodal reentrant beats were first identified in rabbit sinoatrial nodal preparations (168). The mechanism for sinoatrial nodal reentry is by definition reentry. Microelectrode studies have suggested that slowed conduction within the sinoatrial node is the critical finding allowing for reentry (169). The exact mechanism of this tachycardia in humans is unclear. Specifically, it is unknown whether the arrhythmia is confined completely to the sinoatrial node, involves sinoatrial nodal tissue and perisinoatrial nodal atrial tissue, or includes only atrial tissue in or near the sinoatrial node. Sinoatrial nodal reentrant tachycardias can be initiated and terminated with programmed atrial stimulation. They can be terminated by adenosine (138,186). In contrast, inappropriate sinus tachycardia, which is caused

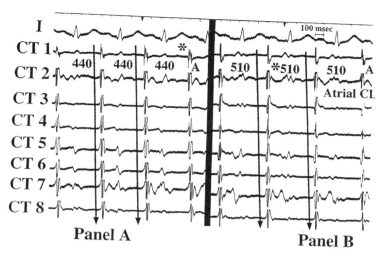

FIGURE 13-11. Electrophysiologic effects of adenosine in a patient with inappropriate sinus tachycardia. Simultaneous lead I with intracardiac electrograms from cranial *(CT1)* to caudal *(CT8)* sites along the crista terminalis. The atrial cycle lengths for 30 seconds before **(A)** and 10 seconds after **(B)** adenosine 6 mg was given are shown. Adenosine causes an increase in the atrial cycle length with a slight shift in the cranial to caudal crista activation. (*, earliest endocardial activation before and after adenosine.) (From Glatter KA, et al. Electrophysiologic effects of adenosine in patients with supraventricular tachycardia. *Circulation* 1999;99:1034, with permission.)

by increased sinus node automaticity, will slow with adenosine but not terminate (137). Adenosine administration may cause a slight cranial-caudal shift in activation sequence along the crista terminalis (Fig. 13-11). Inappropriate sinus tachycardia cannot be induced with programmed stimulation; isoproterenol is frequently used to initiate this abnormality in the electrophysiology laboratory. Man and colleagues (183) identified two types of responses to catheter ablation in patients with inappropriate sinus tachycardia. In one group of patients (n = 13), catheter ablation resulted in a cranial-caudal migration of earliest endocardial activation time from the high lateral right atrium as catheter ablation proceeded. In another group of patients (n = 9) with a successful outcome, there was a sudden reduction in sinus rate unaccompanied by migration of the site of earliest activation. This suggests that multiple electrophysiologic mechanisms may be in operation in patients with inappropriate sinus tachycardia.

Symptoms and Presentation/Physical Examination

Patients with sinoatrial nodal reentrant tachycardia or inappropriate sinus tachycardia may report palpitations, chest pain, shortness of breath, fatigue, light-headedness, or near syncope. Patients with inappropriate sinus tachycardia have been reported to have a higher level of somatization than patients with other types of paroxysmal supraventricular tachycardia (187). This excessive level of somatization may explain the excessive sensitivity of these patients to even a mild elevation of their heart rates. Physical examination results are often unremarkable in these patients, as they mostly have no structural heart disease.

Prognostic/Clinical Significance

These arrhythmias mostly have no significant adverse prognosis. They often present a significant nuisance to patients,

as they are associated with significant discomfort. The level of dysfunction associated with inappropriate sinus tachycardia may be quite advanced, as a few of these patients may actually be completely incapacitated by the rhythm problem (188).

Methods for Evaluation

The evaluation and treatment for sinoatrial nodal reentrant tachycardia is virtually identical to that for patients with other intraatrial reentrant tachycardias. For patients with inappropriate sinus tachycardia, it is critical to rule out secondary causes of sinus tachycardia. This should include evaluation for anemia and hyperthyroidism, and careful history and physical examination. Evaluation for structural heart disease should be undertaken as well.

Therapy

Reassurance of the benign nature of these rhythm problems is critical. Vagal maneuvers may be helpful in patients with sinoatrial nodal reentry. For patients who require additional therapy, β blockers and calcium channel blockers are the commonly used pharmacologic agents. In the very few patients in whom the effects of pharmacologic agents have been reported (171,174), intravenous verapamil, ouabain, and amiodarone have prevented induction of tachycardia, whereas intravenous propranolol has not. In long-term follow-up, these agents, as well as other type Ia, Ib, Ic, and III antiarrhythmic drugs, have been reported to be unsuccessful in the few patients who were referred for catheter ablation (175). There are no substantial data to assess the efficacy of these agents for treatment of these arrhythmias. Thus, it is important to weigh the risk-benefit ratio of using these agents for treatment of these arrhythmias.

Various nonpharmacologic approaches have been tried. Although various procedures have been used in the past, including surgical isolation of the sinoatrial node (188),

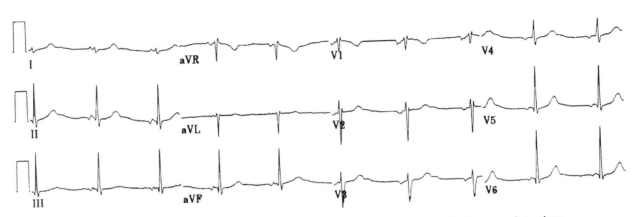

FIGURE 13-12. Electrocardiograms (ECGs) obtained from a patient with inappropriate sinus tachycardia before **(A)** and after **(B)** sinus node modification. In the preablation ECG, normal sinus rhythm is noted at a rate of 85 beats per minute (bpm). After ablation, there is an ectopic atrial rhythm at a heart rate of 55 bpm. Note the change in P-wave morphology.

occlusion of the sinoatrial nodal artery (189), and cryosurgical ablation in the region of the sinus node (190), currently the most widely used nonpharmacologic treatment is catheter ablation. Catheter ablation is typically performed by activation mapping and/or use of anatomic landmarks. Intracardiac echocardiography has been successfully used to identify the region of the sinus node on the superior portion of the crista terminalis to facilitate ablation procedures involving the sinus node (191,192). Newer three-dimensional mapping techniques (193) may also be useful to identify the site of impulse initiation in these patients. In general, the success rate for catheter ablation for treatment of sinoatrial nodal reentrant tachycardia exceeds 90% (83,175). For patients with inappropriate sinus tachycardia, the acute success rate has been reported to be 76% to 100% (184,192). However, long-term results are disappointing, with reported recurrence rates from 17% to 77% (184,192,194). This likely reflects the difficulty in titrating the degree of damage required in the region of the sinus node to control tachycar-

dia and prevent excessive bradycardia. Figure 13-12 shows ECGs from a patient who underwent successful sinus node modification. After ablation, there is an ectopic atrial rhythm at a rate of 55 bpm. A small percentage of patients will require atrial pacing after ablation because of excessive damage to the sinus node. If a direct ablation approach is ineffective, AV nodal ablation and pacemaker therapy can be considered in patients who have refractory symptomatology.

REFERENCES

1. Shine K, Kastor J, Yurchak P. Multifocal atrial tachycardia. Clinical and electrocardiographic features in 32 patients. *N Engl J Med* 1968;279(7):344–349.
2. Phillips J, Spano J, Burch G. Chaotic atrial mechanism. *Am Heart J* 1969;78(2):171–179.
3. Kones R, Phillips J, Hersh J. Mechanism and management of chaotic atrial mechanism. *Cardiology* 1974;59(2):92–101.
4. Lipson M, Naimi S. Multifocal atrial tachycardia (chaotic atrial

tachycardia): clinical associations and significance. *Circulation* 1970;42(3):397–407.

5. Habibzadeh M. Multifocal atrial tachycardia: a 66 month follow-up of 50 patients. *Heart Lung* 1980;9(2):328–335.

6. Scher D, Arsura E. Multifocal atrial tachycardia: mechanisms, clinical correlates, and treatment. *Am Heart J* 1989;118(3): 574–580.

7. Wang K, Goldfarb B, Gobel F, Richman H. Multifocal atrial tachycardia. *Arch Intern Med* 1977;137(2):161–164.

8. Levine J, Michael J, Guarnieri T. Multifocal atrial tachycardia: a toxic effect of theophylline. *Lancet* 1985;1:12–14.

9. Chung E. Appraisal of multifocal atrial tachycardia. *Br Heart J* 1971;33(4):500–504.

10. McCord J, Borzak S. Multifocal atrial tachycardia. *Chest* 1998; 113(1):203–209.

11. Holford F, Mithoefer J. Cardiac arrhythmias in hospitalized patients with chronic obstructive pulmonary disease. *Am Rev Respir Dis* 1973;108:879–885.

12. Hudson L, Kurt T, Petty T, Genton E. Arrhythmias associated with acute respiratory failure in patients with chronic airway obstruction. *Chest* 1973;63(5):661–665.

13. White R. Prehospital recognition of multifocal atrial tachycardia: association with acute myocardial infarction. *Ann Emerg Med* 1992;21(6):753–756.

14. Strickberger S, Miller C, Levine J. Multifocal atrial tachycardia from electrolyte imbalance. *Am Heart J* 1988;115(3):680–682.

15. Ramsdale D, Arumugam N, Singh S, et al. Holter monitoring in patients with mitral stenosis and sinus rhythm. *Eur Heart J* 1987;8(2):164–170.

16. Farooki Z, Green E. Multifocal atrial tachycardia in two neonates. *Br Heart J* 1977;39(8):872–874.

17. Bisset G, Seigel S, Gaum W, Kaplan S. Chaotic atrial tachycardia in childhood. *Am Heart J* 1981;101(3):268–272.

18. Liberthson R, Colan S. Multifocal or chaotic atrial rhythm. *Pediatr Cardiol* 1982;2:179–184.

19. Zeevi B, Berant M, Sclarovsky S, Blieden L. Treatment of multifocal atrial tachycardia with amiodarone in a child with congenital heart disease. *Am J Cardiol* 1986;57(4):344–345.

20. Southall D, Johnson A, Shinebourne E, et al. Frequency and outcome of disorders of cardiac rhythm and conduction in a population of newborn infants. *Pediatrics* 1981;68(1):58–66.

21. Yeager S, Hougen T, Levy A. Sudden death in infants with chaotic atrial rhythm. *Am J Dis Child* 1984;138:689–692.

22. Gavrilescu S, Luca C. Chaotic atrial rhythm. *Eur J Cardiol* 1974;2(2):153–159.

23. Marchlinski F, Miller J. Atrial arrhythmias exacerbated by theophylline. *Chest* 1985;88(6):931–934.

24. Lin C, Chuang I, Cheng K, Chiang B. Arrhythmogenic effects of theophylline in human atrial tissue. *Int J Cardiol* 1987;17: 289–297.

25. Kearney T, Manoguerra A, Curtis G, Ziegler M. Theophylline toxicity and the beta-adrenergic system. *Ann Intern Med* 1985; 102:766–769.

26. Kastor J. Multifocal atrial tachycardia. *N Engl J Med* 1990;322 (24):1713–1717.

27. Arsura E, Lefkin A, Scher D, et al. A randomized, double-blind, placebo-controlled study of verapamil and metoprolol in treatment of multifocal atrial tachycardia. *Am J Med* 1988;85(4): 519–524.

28. Hill G, Owens S. Esmolol in the treatment of multifocal atrial tachycardia. *Chest* 1992;101:1726–1728.

29. Arsura E, Solar M, Lefkin A, et al. Metoprolol in the treatment of multifocal atrial tachycardia. *Crit Care Med* 1987;15(6): 591–597.

30. Hazard P, Burnett C. Treatment of multifocal atrial tachycardia with metoprolol. *Crit Care Med* 1987;15(1):20–25.

31. Levine J, Michael J, Guarnieri T. Treatment of multifocal atrial tachycardia with verapamil. *N Engl J Med* 1985;312(1):21–25.

32. Salerno D, Anderson B, Sharkey P, Iber C. Intravenous verapamil for treatment of multifocal atrial tachycardia with and without calcium pretreatment. *Ann Intern Med* 1987;107(5): 623–628.

33. Barranco F, Sanchez M, Rodriguez J, Guerrero M. Efficacy of flecainide in patients with supraventricular arrhythmias and respiratory insufficiency. *Intensive Care Med* 1994;20:42–44.

34. Creamer J, Nathan A, Camm A. Successful treatment of atrial tachycardias with flecainide acetate. *Br Heart J* 1985;53: 164–166.

35. Kouvaras G, Cokkinos D, Halal G, et al. The effective treatment of multifocal atrial tachycardia with amiodarone. *Jpn Heart J* 1989;30(3):301–312.

36. Cohen L, Kitzes R, Shnaider H. Multifocal atrial tachycardia responsive to parenteral magnesium. *Magnesium Res* 1988;1(3-4): 239–242.

37. Iseri L, Allen B, Brodsky M. Magnesium therapy of cardiac arrhythmias in critical care medicine. *Magnesium* 1989;8(5-6): 299–306.

38. Iseri L, Fairshter R, Hardemann J, Brodsky M. Magnesium and potassium therapy in multifocal atrial tachycardia. *Am Heart J* 1985;110(4):789–794.

39. McCord J, Borzak S, Davis T, Gheorghiade M. Usefulness of intravenous magnesium for multifocal atrial tachycardia in patients with chronic obstructive pulmonary disease. *Am J Cardiol* 1998;81(1):91–93.

40. Tucker K, Law J, Rodriques M. Treatment of refractory recurrent multifocal atrial tachycardia with atrioventricular junction ablation and permanent pacing. *J Invasive Cardiol* 1995;7(7): 207–212.

41. Benson D, Dunnigan A, Benditt D. Follow-up evaluation of infant paroxysmal atrial tachycardia: transesophageal study. *Circulation* 1987;75(3):542–549.

42. Pritchett E, McCarthy E, Lee K. Clinical behavior of paroxysmal atrial tachycardia. *Am J Cardiol* 1988;62(6):3D–9D.

43. Waldo A, Plumb V, Arciniegas J, et al. Transient entrainment and interruption of the atrioventricular bypass pathway type of paroxysmal atrial tachycardia. *Circulation* 1983;67(1):73–83.

44. Kelly R, Smith T. Recognition and management of digitalis toxicity. *Am J Cardiol* 1992;69(18):108G–118G.

45. Sobotka P, Mayer J, Bauernfeind R, et al. Arrhythmias documented by 24-hour continuous ambulatory electrocardiographic monitoring in young women without apparent heart disease. *Am Heart J* 1981;101(6):753–759.

46. Romhilt D, Chaffin C, Choi S, Irby E. Arrhythmias on ambulatory electrocardiographic monitoring in women without apparent heart disease. *Am J Cardiol* 1984;54:582–586.

47. Raftery E, Cashman P. Long-term recording of the electrocardiogram in a normal population. *Postgrad Med* 1976;52(7): 32–37.

48. Brodsky M, Wu D, Denes P, et al. Arrhythmias documented by 24 hour continuous electrocardiographic monitoring in 50 male medical students without apparent heart disease. *Am J Cardiol* 1977;39(3):390–395.

49. Talan D, Bauernfeind R, Ashley W, et al. Twenty-four hour continuous ECG recordings in long-distance runners. *Chest* 1982;82(1):19–24.

50. Fleg J, Kennedy H. Cardiac arrhythmias in a healthy elderly population. *Chest* 1982;81(3):302.

51. Camm A, Evans K, Ward D, Martin A. The rhythm of the heart in active elderly subjects. *Am Heart J* 1980;99(5):598–603.

52. DeMaria A, Amsterdam E, Vismara L, et al. Arrhythmias in the mitral valve prolapse syndrome. *Ann Intern Med* 1976;84: 656–660.

53. Winkle R, Lopes M, Fitzgerald J, et al. Arrhythmias in patients with mitral valve prolapse. *Circulation* 1975;52(1):73–81.

54. Savage D, Levy D, Garrison R, et al. Mitral valve prolapse in the general population. *Am Heart J* 1983;106:582–586.

55. Shani J, Lichstein E, Jonas S, et al. Clinical significance of slow paroxysmal atrial tachycardia. *Am Heart J* 1983;106(3):478–483.

56. Tanabe T, Furuya H, Kanemoto N, et al. Holter system electrocardiographic studies on 617 cases. *Tokai J Exp Clin Med* 1980;5(1):73–82.

57. Stemple D, Fitzgerald J, Winkle R. Benign slow paroxysmal atrial tachycardia. *Ann Intern Med* 1977;87:44–48.

58. Meltzer L, Kitchell J. The incidence of arrhythmias associated with acute myocardial infarction. *Prog Cardiovasc Dis* 1966;9(1):50–63.

59. Lown B, Vassaux C, Hood W, et al. Unresolved problems in coronary care. *Am J Cardiol* 1967;20:494–508.

60. Julian D, Valentine P, Miller G. Disturbances of rate, rhythm and conduction in acute myocardial infarction. *Am J Med* 1964;37:915–927.

61. Kurland G, Pressman D. The incidence of arrhythmias in acute myocardial infarction studies with a constant monitoring system. *Circulation* 1965;31:834–841.

62. Cristal N, Szwarcberg J, Gueron M. Supraventricular arrhythmias in acute myocardial infarction. *Ann Intern Med* 1975;82:35–39.

63. Jewitt D, Raferty E, Balcon R, Oram S. Incidence and management of supraventricular arrhythmias after acute myocardial infarction. *Lancet* 1967;2:734–738.

64. Liberthson R, Salisbury K, Hutter A, DeSanctis R. Atrial tachyarrhythmias in acute myocardial infarction. *Am J Med* 1976;60:956–960.

65. Josephson M, Wellens H. Differential diagnosis of supraventricular tachycardia. *Cardiol Clin* 1990;8(3):411–442.

66. Ko J, Deal B, Strasburger J, Benson D. Supraventricular tachycardia mechanisms and their age distribution in pediatric patients. *Am J Cardiol* 1992;69(12):1028–1032.

67. Wu D, Denes P, Dhingra R, et al. Clinical, electrocardiographic and electrophysiologic observation in patients with paroxysmal supraventricular tachycardia. *Am J Cardiol* 1978;41:1045–1051.

68. Wellens H, Brugada P. Mechanisms of supraventricular tachycardia. *Am J Cardiol* 1988;62(6):10D–15D.

69. Wu D, Amat-Y-Leon F, Denes P, et al. Demonstration of sustained sinus and atrial re-entry as a mechanism of paroxysmal supraventricular tachycardia. *Circulation* 1975;51:234–243.

70. Coumel P, Flammang D, Attuel P, Leclercq J. Sustained intraatrial reentrant tachycardia: electrophysiologic study of 20 cases. *Clin Cardiol* 1979;2:167–178.

71. Chen S, Tai C, Chiang C, et al. Focal atrial tachycardia: reanalysis of the clinical and electrophysiologic characteristics and prediction of successful radiofrequency ablation. *J Cardiovasc Electrophysiol* 1998;9(4):355–365.

72. Haines D, DiMarco J. Sustained intraatrial reentrant tachycardia: clinical, electrocardiographic and electrophysiologic characteristics and long-term follow-up. *J Am Coll Cardiol* 1990;15(6):1345–1354.

73. Southall D, Richards J, Mitchell P, et al. Study of cardiac rhythm in healthy newborn infants. *Br Med J* 1980;43(1):14–20.

74. Mehta A, Sanchez G, Sacks E, et al. Ectopic automatic atrial tachycardia in children: clinical characteristics, management and follow-up. *J Am Coll Cardiol* 1988;11(2):379–385.

75. vonBernuth G, Engelhardt W, Kramer H, et al. Atrial automatic tachycardia in infancy and childhood. *Eur Heart J* 1992;13:1410–1415.

76. Garson A, Gillette P. Electrophysiologic studies of supraventric-

ular tachycardia in children. Clinical electrophysiologic correlations. *Am Heart J* 1981;102:233–250.

77. Gillette P. The mechanisms of supraventricular tachycardia in children. *Circulation* 1976;54:133–139.

78. Gillette P, Garson A. Electrophysiologic and pharmacologic characteristics of automatic ectopic atrial tachycardia. *Circulation* 1977;56(4):571–575.

79. Koike K, Hesslein P, Finlay C, et al. Atrial automatic tachycardia in children. *Am J Cardiol* 1988;61:1127–1130.

80. Naheed Z, Strasburger J, Benson D, Deal B. Natural history and management strategies of automatic atrial tachycardia in children. *Am J Cardiol* 1995;75:405–407.

81. Kunze K, Kuck K, Schluter M, Bleifeld W. Effect of encainide and flecainide on chronic ectopic atrial tachycardia. *J Am Coll Cardiol* 1986;7(5):1121–1126.

82. Goldberger J, Kall J, Ehlert F, et al. Effectiveness of radiofrequency catheter ablation for treatment of atrial tachycardia. *Am J Cardiol* 1993;72:787–793.

83. Kay G, Chong F, Epstein A, et al. Radiofrequency ablation for treatment of primary atrial tachycardias. *J Am Coll Cardiol* 1993;21(4):901–909.

84. Tracy C, Swartz J, Fletcher R, et al. Radiofrequency catheter ablation of ectopic atrial tachycardia using paced activation sequence mapping. *J Am Coll Cardiol* 1993;21(4):910–917.

85. Lesh M, Hare GV, Epsterin L, et al. Radiofrequency catheter ablation of atrial arrhythmias: Results and mechanisms. *Circulation* 1994;89(3):1074–1089.

86. Feld G. Catheter ablation for the treatment of atrial tachycardia. *Prog Cardiovasc Dis* 1995;37(4):205–224.

87. Poutiainen A, Koistinen M, Airaksinen K, et al. Prevalence and natural course of ectopic atrial tachycardia. *Eur Heart J* 1999;20(9):694–700.

88. Evans V, Garson A, Smith R, et al. Ethmozine (moricizine HCI): a promising drug for 'automatic' atrial ectopic tachycardia. *Am J Cardiol* 1987;60(11):83F–86F.

89. Chen S, Yang C, Chiang C, et al. Reversibility of left ventricular dysfunction after successful catheter ablation of supraventricular reentrant tachycardia. *Am Heart J* 1992;124(6):1512–1516.

90. Rabbani L, Wang P, Couper G, Friedman P. Time course of improvement in ventricular function after ablation of incessant automatic atrial tachycardia. *Am Heart J* 1991;121:816–819.

91. Chiladakis J, Vassilikos V, Maounis T, et al. Successful radiofrequency catheter ablation of automatic atrial tachycardia with regression of the cardiomyopathy picture. *Pacing Clin Electrophysiol* 1997;20[Suppl 4, Pt II]:953–959.

92. Walsh E, Saul J, Hulse J, et al. Transcatheter ablation of ectopic atrial tachycardia in young patients using radiofrequency current. *Circulation* 1992;86:1138–1146.

93. Burton C. Paroxysmal atrial tachycardia with atrioventricular block. *Can Med Assoc J* 1962;87:114–120.

94. Lown B, Marcus F, Levine H. Digitalis and atrial tachycardia with block. *N Engl J Med* 1959;260(7):301–309.

95. Freiermuth L, Jick S. Paroxysmal atrial tachycardia with atrioventricular block. *Am J Cardiol* 1958;1:584–591.

96. El-Sherif N. Supraventricular tachycardia with AV block. *Br Heart J* 1970;32:46–56.

97. Lown B, Wyatt N, Levine H. Paroxysmal atrial tachycardia with block. *Circulation* 1960;21:129–143.

98. Goldberg L, Bristow J, Parker B, Ritzmann L. Paroxysmal atrial tachycardia with atrioventricular block. *Circulation* 1960;21:499–504.

99. Lown B, Levine S. Current concepts in digitalis therapy. *N Engl J Med* 1954;250(19):819–832.

100. Storstein O, Hansteen V, Hatle L, et al. Studies on digitalis.

XIII. A prospective study of 649 patients on maintenance treatment with digitoxin. *Am Heart J* 1977;93(4):434–443.

101. Goren C, Denes P. The role of Holter monitoring in detecting digitalis-provoked arrhythmias. *Chest* 1981;79(5):555–558.

102. Harris E, Julian D, Oliver M. Atrial tachycardia with atrioventricular block due to digitalis poisoning. *Br Med J* 1960;2:1409–1413.

103. Oram S, Resnekov L, Davies P. Digitalis as a cause of paroxysmal atrial tachycardia with atrioventricular block. *Br Med J* 1960;2:1402–1409.

104. Agarwal B, Agrawal B. Digitalis induced paroxysmal atrial tachycardia with AV block. *Br Heart J* 1972;34:330–335.

105. Ettinger P, Wu C, DeLaCruz C, et al. Arrhythmias and the 'holiday heart': alcohol-associated cardiac rhythm disorders. *Am Heart J* 1978;95:555–562.

106. Buckingham T, Kennedy H, Goenjian A, et al. Cardiac arrhythmias in a population admitted to an acute alcoholic detoxification center. *Am Heart J* 1985;110(5):961–965.

107. Corazza L, Pastor B. Cardiac arrhythmias in chronic cor pulmonale. *N Engl J Med* 1958;259:862–868.

108. Triedman J, Saul J, Weindling S, Walsh E. Radiofrequency ablation of intra-atrial reentrant tachycardia after surgical palliation of congenital heart disease. *Circulation* 1995;91:707–714.

109. Kalman J, VanHare G, Olgin J, et al. Ablation of 'incisional' reentrant atrial tachycardia complicating surgery for congenital heart disease. Use of entrainment to define a critical isthmus of conduction. *Circulation* 1996;93(3):502–512.

110. Lesh M, Kalman J, Saxon L, Dorostkar P. Electrophysiology of 'incisional' reentrant atrial tachycardia complicating surgery for congenital heart disease. *Pacing Clin Electrophysiol* 1997;20 [Suppl 8, Pt II]:2107–2111.

111. Dorostkar P, Cheng J, Scheinman M. Electroanatomical mapping and ablation of the substrate supporting intraatrial reentrant tachycardia after palliation of complex congenital heart disease. *Pacing Clin Electrophysiol* 1998;21(9):1810–1819.

112. Chen S, Chiang C, Yang C, et al. Sustained atrial tachycardia in adult patients. Electrophysiological characteristics, pharmacological response, possible mechanisms, and effects of radiofrequency ablation. *Circulation* 1994;90(3):1262–1278.

113. McGuire M, Johnson D, Nunn G, et al. Surgical therapy for atrial tachycardia in adults. *J Am Coll Cardiol* 1989;14(7):1777–1782.

114. Josephson M, Spear J, Harken A, et al. Surgical excision of automatic atrial tachycardia: anatomic and electrophysiologic correlates. *Prog Cardiol* 1982;104:1076–1085.

115. deBakker J, Hauer R, Bakker P, et al. Abnormal automaticity as mechanism of atrial tachycardia in the human heart. Electrophysiologic and histologic correlation: a case report. *J Cardiovasc Electrophysiol* 1994;5:335–344.

116. Pappone C, Stabile G, deSimone A, et al. Role of catheter-induced mechanical trauma in localization of target sites of radiofrequency ablation in automatic atrial tachycardia. *J Am Coll Cardiol* 1996;27(5):1090–1097.

117. Tomita M, Ikeguchi S, Kagawa K, et al. Serial histopathologic myocardial findings in a patient with ectopic atrial tachycardia-induced cardiomyopathy. *J Cardiol* 1997;29(1):37–42.

118. MacLean W, Karp R, Kouchoukos N, et al. P waves during ectopic atrial rhythms in man: a study utilizing atrial pacing with fixed electrodes. *Circulation* 1975;52(3):426–434.

119. Tang C, Scheinman M, VanHare G, et al. Use of P wave configuration during atrial tachycardia to predict site of origin. *J Am Coll Cardiol* 1995;26(5):1315–1324.

120. SippensGroenewegen A, Roithinger F, Peeters H, et al. Body surface mapping of atrial arrhythmias. *J Electrocardiol* 1998;31 [Suppl]:85–91.

121. Tada H, Nogami A, Naito S, et al. Simple electrocardiographic criteria for identifying the site of origin of focal right atrial tachycardia. *Pacing Clin Electrophysiol* 1998;21[Suppl 11, Pt II]:2431–2439.

122. Allessie M, Bonke F, Schopman F. Circus movement in rabbit atrial muscle as a mechanism of tachycardia. *Circ Res* 1973;33:54–62.

123. Chen S, Chiang C, Yang C, et al. Radiofrequency catheter ablation of sustained intra-atrial reentrant tachycardia in adult patients: identification of electrophysiological characteristics and endocardial mapping techniques. *Circulation* 1993;88:578–587.

124. Goldreyer B, Gallagher J, Damato A. The electrophysiologic demonstration of atrial ectopic tachycardia in man. *Am Heart J* 1973;85:205–215.

125. Hariman R, Krongrad J, Boxer R, et al. A method for recording electrical activity of the sinoatrial node and automatic atrial foci during cardiac catheterization in humans. *Am J Cardiol* 1980;45:775–781.

126. Hluchy J, Milovsky V, Uhliarikova H. Triggered activity as the proposed mechanism of left atrial tachycardia induced by premature ventricular beats. *Int J Cardiol* 1992;34(3):342–345.

127. Wyndham C, Arnsdorf M, Levitsky S, et al. Successful surgical excision of focal paroxysmal atrial tachycardia. *Circulation* 1980;62(6):1365–1372.

128. Rabine L, Hordof A, Danilo P, et al. Mechanisms for impulse initiation in isolated human atrial fibers. *Circ Res* 1980;47:267–277.

129. Singer D, Baumgarten C, Eick RT. Cellular electrophysiology of ventricular and other dysrhythmias: studies on diseased and ischemic heart. *Prog Cardiovasc Dis* 1981;24(2):97–156.

130. Poty H, Saoudi N, Haissaguerre M, et al. Radiofrequency catheter ablation of atrial tachycardias. *Am Heart J* 1996;131(3):481–489.

131. Hogan P, Wittenberg S, Klocke F. Relationship of stimulation frequency to automaticity in the canine Purkinje fiber during ouabain administration. *Circ Res* 1973;32:377–384.

132. Vassalle M, Karis J, Hoffman B. Toxic effect of ouabain on Purkinje fibers and ventricular muscle fibers. *Am J Physiol* 1962;203(3):433–439.

133. Rosen M. Cellular electrophysiology of digitalis toxicity. *J Am Coll Cardiol* 1985;5(5):22A–34A.

134. Ferrier G. Digitalis arrhythmias: role of oscillatory afterpotentials. *Prog Cardiovasc Dis* 1977;19:459–474.

135. Rosen M, Fisch C, Hoffman B, et al. Can accelerated atrioventricular junctional escape rhythms be explained by delayed afterdepolarizations? *Am J Cardiol* 1980;45:1272–1284.

136. Kojima M, Sperelakis N. Effects of calcium channel blockers on ouabain-induced oscillatory afterpotentials in organ-cultured young embryonic chick hearts. *Eur J Pharmacol* 1986;122:65–73.

137. Glatter K, Cheng J, Dorostkar P, et al. Electrophysiologic effects of adenosine in patients with supraventricular tachycardia. *Circulation* 1999;99(8):1034–1040.

138. Engelstein E, Lippman N, Stein K, Lerman B. Mechanism-specific effects of adenosine on atrial tachycardia. *Circulation* 1994;89(6):2645–1654.

139. Markowitz S, Stein K, Mittal S, et al. Differential effects of adenosine on focal and macroreentrant atrial tachycardia. *J Cardiovasc Electrophysiol* 1999;10(4):489–502.

140. Kall J, Kopp D, Olshansky B, et al. Adenosine-sensitive atrial tachycardia. *Pacing Clin Electrophysiol* 1995;18(2):300–306.

141. Iesaka Y, Takahashi A, Goya M, et al. Adenosine-sensitive atrial reentrant tachycardia originating from the atrioventricular nodal transitional area. *J Cardiovasc Electrophysiol* 1997;8(8):854–864.

142. Klersy C, Chimienti M, Marangoni E, et al. Factors that predict

spontaneous remission of ectopic atrial tachycardia. *Eur Heart J* 1992;14(12):1654–1656.

143. Scheinman M, Basu D, Hollenberg M. Electrophysiologic studies in patients with persistent atrial tachycardia. *Circulation* 1974;50:266–273.

144. Kadish A, Morady F. The response of paroxysmal supraventricular tachycardia to overdrive atrial and ventricular pacing: can it help determine the tachycardia mechanism? *J Cardiovasc Electrophysiol* 1993;4(3):239–252.

145. Knight B, Zivin A, Souza J, et al. A technique for the rapid diagnosis of atrial tachycardia in the electrophysiology laboratory. *J Am Coll Cardiol* 1999;33(3):775–781.

146. Kalman J, Olgin J, Karch M, et al. 'Cristal tachycardias': origin of right atrial tachycardias from the crista terminalis identified by intracardiac echocardiography. *J Am Coll Cardiol* 1998;31: 451–459.

147. Nogami A, Suguta M, Tomita T, et al. Novel form of atrial tachycardia originating at the atrioventricular annulus. *Pacing Clin Electrophysiol* 1998;21(12):2691–2694.

148. Lai L, Lin J, Chen T, et al. Clinical, electrophysiological characteristics, and radiofrequency catheter ablation of atrial tachycardia near the apex of Koch's triangle. *Pacing Clin Electrophysiol* 1998;21(2):367–374.

149. Carrasco H, Vicuna A, Molina C, et al. Effect of low oral doses of disopyramide and amiodarone on ventricular and atrial arrhythmias of chagasic patients with advanced myocardial damage. *Int J Cardiol* 1985;9(4):425–438.

150. Prager N, Cox J, Lindsay B, et al. Long-term effectiveness of surgical treatment of ectopic atrial tachycardia. *J Am Coll Cardiol* 1993;22(1):85–92.

151. Dhala A, Case C, Gillette P. Evolving treatment strategies for managing atrial ectopic tachycardia in children. *Am J Cardiol* 1994;74(3):283–286.

152. Beaufort-Krol G, Bink-Boelkens M. Sotalol for atrial tachycardias after surgery for congenital heart disease. *Pacing Clin Electrophysiol* 1997;20[Suppl 8, Pt II]:2125–2129.

153. Stock J. Beta adrenergic blocking drugs in the clinical management of cardiac arrhythmias. *Am J Cardiol* 1966;18:444–449.

154. Harrison D, Griffin J, Fiene T. Effects of beta-adrenergic blockade with propranolol in patients with atrial arrhythmias. *N Engl J Med* 1965;273:410–415.

155. Coumel P, Leclercq J, Assayag P. European experience with the antiarrhythmic efficacy of propafenone for supraventricular and ventricular arrhythmias. *Am J Cardiol* 1984;54(9):60D–66D.

156. Brugada P, Abdollah H, Wellens H, Paulussen G. Suppression of incessant supraventricular tachycardia by intravenous and oral encainide. *J Am Coll Cardiol* 1984;4(6):1255–1260.

157. Pool P, Quart B. Treatment of ectopic atrial arrhythmias and premature atrial complexes in adults with encainide. *Am J Cardiol* 1988;62(19):60L–62L.

158. Kopelman H, Horowitz L. Efficacy and toxicity of amiodarone for the treatment of supraventricular tachyarrhythmias. *Prog Cardiovasc Dis* 1989;31(5):355–366.

159. Hendry P, Packer D, Anstadt M, et al. Surgical treatment of automatic atrial tachycardias. *Ann Thorac Surg* 1990;49: 253–260.

160. Bredikis J, Lekas R, Benetis R, et al. Diagnosis and surgical treatment of ectopic atrial tachycardia. *Eur J Cardiothorac Surg* 1991;5(4):199–204.

161. Graffigna A, Vigano M, Pagani F, Salerno G. Surgical treatment for ectopic atrial tachycardia. *Ann Thorac Surg* 1992;54: 338–343.

162. Pappone C, Stabile G, Oreto G, et al. Inappropriate sinus tachycardia after radiofrequency ablation of para-Hisian accessory pathways. *J Cardiovasc Electrophysiology* 1997;8(12):1357–1365.

163. Natale A, Breeding L, Tomassoni G, et al. Ablation of right and left ectopic atrial tachycardias using a three-dimensional nonfluoroscopic mapping system. *Am J Cardiol* 1998;82(8): 989–992.

164. Schmitt C, Zrenner B, Schneider M, et al. Clinical experience with a Novel multielectrode basket catheter in right atrial tachycardias. *Circulation* 1999;99(18):2414–2422.

165. Irons G, Ginn W, Orgain E. Use of a beta adrenergic receptor blocking agent (propranolol) in the treatment of cardiac arrhythmias. *Am J Med* 1967;43:161–170.

166. Corwin N, Klein M, Friedberg C. Countershock conversion of digitalis-associated paroxysmal atrial tachycardia with block. *Am Heart J* 1963;66:804–808.

167. Antman EM, Wenger TL, Butler VP, et al. Treatment of 150 cases of life-threatening digitalis intoxication with digoxin-specific Fab antibody fragments. Final report of a multicenter study. *Circulation* 1990;81:1744.

168. Allessie M, Bonke F. Direct demonstration of sinus node reentry in the rabbit heart. *Circ Res* 1979;44(4):557–568.

169. Han J, Malozzi A, Moe G. Sino-atrial reciprocation in the isolated rabbit heart. *Circ Res* 1968;12:355–362.

170. Weisfogel G, Batsford W, Paulay K, et al. Sinus node re-entrant tachycardia in man. *Am Heart J* 1975;90(3):295–304.

171. Curry P, Evans T, Krikler D. Paroxysmal reciprocating sinus tachycardia. *Eur J Cardiol* 1977;6(3):199–228.

172. Narula O. Sinus node reentry: a mechanism for supraventricular tachycardia. *Circulation* 1974;50:1114–1128.

173. Pahlajani D, Miller R, Serratto M. Sinus node re-entry and sinus node tachycardia. *Am Heart J* 1975;90(3):305–311.

174. Gomes J, Hariman R, Kang P, Chowdry I. Sustained symptomatic sinus node reentrant tachycardia: Incidence, clinical significance, electrophysiologic observations and the effects of antiarrhythmic agents. *J Am Coll Cardiol* 1985;5:45–57.

175. Sanders W, Sorrentino R, Greenfield R, et al. Catheter ablation of sinoatrial node reentrant tachycardia. *J Am Coll Cardiol* 1994;23(4):926–934.

176. Ehlert F, Goldberger J, Brooks R, et al. Persistent inappropriate sinus tachycardia after radiofrequency current catheter modification of the atrioventricular node. *Am J Cardiol* 1992;69: 1092–1095.

177. Skeberis V, Simonis F, Tsakonas K, et al. Inappropriate sinus tachycardia following radiofrequency ablation of AV nodal tachycardia: Incidence and clinical significance. *Pacing Clin Electrophysiol* 1994;17:924–927.

178. Madrid A, Mestre J, Moro C, et al. Heart rate variability and inappropriate sinus tachycardia after catheter ablation of supraventricular tachycardia. *Eur Heart J* 1995;16:1637–1640.

179. Kocovic D, Harada T, Shea J, et al. Alterations of heart rate and heart rate variability after radiofrequency catheter ablation of supraventricular tachycardia: delineation of parasympathetic pathways in the human heart. *Circulation* 1993;88[Suppl 4, Pt I]:1671–1681.

180. Bauernfeind R, Amat-Y-Leon F, Dhingra R, et al. Chronic nonparoxysmal sinus tachycardia in otherwise healthy persons. *Ann Intern Med* 1979;91:702–710.

181. Morillo C, Klein G, Thakur R, et al. Mechanism of 'inappropriate' sinus tachycardia: role of sympathovagal balance. *Circulation* 1994;90(2):873–877.

182. Castellanos A, Moleiro F, Chakko S, et al. Heart rate variability in inappropriate sinus tachycardia. *Am J Cardiol* 1998;82(4): 531–534.

183. Freher M, Kadish A, Passman R, et al. Heterogenous circadian heart rate patterns in inappropriate sinus tachycardia. 2000(abst) *(in press)*.

184. Man K, Knight B, Tse H, et al. Radiofrequency catheter ablation of inappropriate sinus tachycardia guided by activation mapping. *J Am Coll Cardiol* 2000;35(2):451–457.

185. Frey B, Heinz G, Kreiner G, et al. Increased heart rate variability after radiofrequency ablation. *Am J Cardiol* 1993;71: 1460–1461.
186. Griffith M, Garratt C, Ward D, Camm A. The effects of adenosine on sinus node reentrant tachycardia. *Clin Cardiol* 1989;12: 409–411.
187. Zivin A, Glick R, Knight B, et al. Psychiatric profile of patients with inappropriate sinus tachycardia. *Pacing Clin Electrophysiol* 1998;21[Suppl 4, Pt II]:923(abst).
188. Yee R, Guiraudon G, Gardner M, et al. Refractory paroxysmal sinus tachycardia: management by subtotal right atrial exclusion. *J Am Coll Cardiol* 1984;3(2):400–404.
189. dePaola A, Horowitz L, Vattimo A, et al. Sinus node artery occlusion for treatment of chronic nonparoxysmal sinus tachycardia. *Am J Cardiol* 1992;70:128–130.
190. Kerr C, Klein G, Guiraudon G, Webb J. Surgical therapy for sinoatrial reentrant tachycardia. *Pacing Clin Electrophysiol* 1988; 11(6):776–783.
191. Kalman J, Lee R, Fisher W, et al. Radiofrequency catheter modification of sinus pacemaker function guided by intracardiac echocardiography. *Circulation* 1995;92:3070–3081.
192. Lee R, Kalman J, Fitzpatrick A, et al. Radiofrequency catheter modification of the sinus node for "inappropriate" sinus tachycardia. *Circulation* 1995;92(10):2919–2928.
193. Leonelli F, Richey M, Beheiry S, et al. Tridimensional mapping: guided modification of the sinus node. *J Cardiovasc Electrophysiol* 1998;9(11):1214–1217.
194. Shinbane J, Lesh M, Scheinman M, et al. Long-term follow-up after radiofrequency sinus node modification for inappropriate sinus tachycardia. *J Am Coll Cardiol* 1997;29(2)[Suppl A]:199A.

14

ATRIOVENTRICULAR NODAL REENTRY

RICHARD I. FOGEL
ERIC N. PRYSTOWSKY

Paroxysmal supraventricular tachycardia (PSVT) is a relatively common condition that has been recognized as a distinct clinical entity for more than 80 years (1). Typically, it has a sudden onset and offset, and it is characterized electrocardiographically by regular R-R intervals with 1 : 1 atrioventricular (AV) conduction. Fifty years ago, Barker and Wilson (2) hypothesized that the AV node participated in the mechanism of the tachycardia and concluded that the mostly likely mechanism for this arrhythmia was reentry, based on the P-wave morphology, the response to vagal stimulation and digitalis, the alternation in the atrial cycle length, and the relative stability of the tachycardia rate. In the past 20 years, data from intracardiac electrophysiologic studies have elucidated the mechanisms responsible for PSVT.

This chapter reviews pertinent AV nodal anatomy and physiology, as well as the mechanism and treatment of one form of PSVT, atrioventricular node reentrant tachycardia (AVNRT).

ATRIOVENTRICULAR NODAL ANATOMY

The dissection of the AV node was described by Retzer (3), although Tawara (4) usually is given credit for a more thorough anatomic evaluation. In mammalian hearts from multiple species, Tawara (4) identified the AV node as a spindle-shaped, compact network of cells, called *knoten*, located anteriorly at the base of the intraatrial septum. More precisely, the AV node is located in a region called the triangle of Koch (5) (Fig. 14-1). The apex of this triangle is the membranous septum, the inferior border is the attachment of the septal tricuspid leaflet, and the superior border is the tendon of Todaro, a fibrous band running from the central fibrous body to the ostium of the coronary sinus.

Several pertinent histologic observations have been made. The actual AV node is somewhat larger than the

compact node described by Tawara (4), and it extends more posteriorly and superiorly, with no abrupt transition from atrial tissue. Anderson (6) described three basic types of cells within the AV node: transitional cells and the upper and lower nodal cells. Transitional cells form the superior, anterior, and posterior approaches to the AV node. Upper nodal cells are closely packed cells that correspond to the

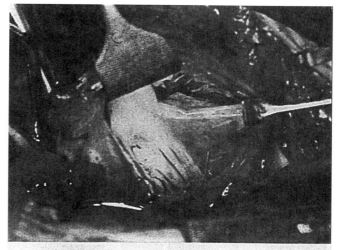

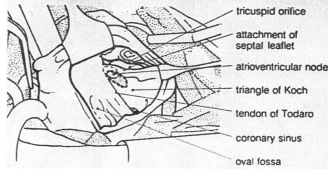

tricuspid orifice

attachment of
septal leaflet

atrioventricular node

triangle of Koch

tendon of Todaro

coronary sinus

oval fossa

FIGURE 14-1. Triangle of Koch. This view of the triangle of Koch is taken in the surgical orientation. It illustrates the margins of the triangle, including the attachment of the septal tricuspid leaflet and the tendon of Todaro. (From Wilcox BR, Anderson RH. *Surgical anatomy of the heart.* New York: Raven Press, 1985: 28, with permission.)

R. I. Fogel and E. N. Prystowsky: The Care Group, Northside Cardiology, Indianapolis, Indiana 46260.

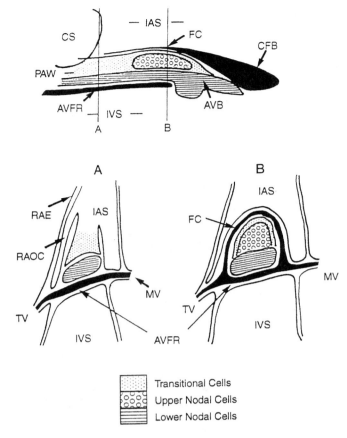

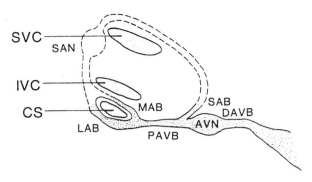

FIGURE 14-3. Schematic model of atrioventricular nodal inputs as proposed by Racker. The model proposes that the lateral atrionodal bundle (LAB), medial atrionodal bundle (MAB), and superior atrionodal bundle (SAB) are continuations of three internodal tracts running from the sinoatrial node to the atrioventricular node. AVN, atrioventricular node; CS, coronary sinus ostium; DAVB, distal atrionodal bundle; IVC, inferior vena cava; PAVB, proximal atrioventricular bundle; SAN, sinus node; SVC, superior vena cava. (From Racker DK. Atrioventricular node and input pathways: a correlated gross anatomical and histological study of the canine atrioventricular junctional region. *Anat Rec* 1989;224:353, with permission.)

Transitional Cells
Upper Nodal Cells
Lower Nodal Cells

FIGURE 14-2. Histologic representation of the rabbit atrioventricular (AV) node. These figures show the cellular anatomy of the rabbit AV node taken in long axis and coronal views. The septum *(top)* is viewed from the right side with the anterior portion to the right. A and B represent coronal sections as indicated. AVB, atrioventricular bundle; AVFR, atrioventricular fibrous ring; CFB, central fibrous body; CS, coronary sinus; FC, fibrous collar; IAS, interatrial septum; IVS, interventricular septum; MV, mitral valve; PAW, posterior atrial wall; RAE, right atrial endocardium; RAOC, right atrial overlay cells; TV, tricuspid valve. (From Anderson RH: Histologic and histochemical evidence concerning the presence of morphologically distinct cellular zones within the rabbit AV node. *Anat Rec* 1972;173:7–24, with permission.)

compact node of Tawara. Lower nodal cells form a tract running the length of the AV node and in direct continuity with the penetrating AV bundle of His (Fig. 14-2). One salient observation made was the scarcity of intracellular connections in the AV node (7). Classic intercalated disks were not present, although "junctional specializations between interdigitating protrusions of contiguous nodal cells" did occur (8). One hypothesis is that the lack of nexus may be partly responsible for AV nodal delay. Using a novel section plane parallel to the long axis of the AV node, Racker (9) identified three discrete inputs to the AV node region (Fig. 14-3). A proximal AV bundle is formed by a lateral and medial AV bundle, which runs laterally and medially to the coronary sinus ostium. A superior AV bun-

dle joins with the proximal AV bundle anteriorly but does not bypass the central compact AV node. Racker suggested that these three bundles are continuations of three internodal atrial tracts. However, this concept has not been universally accepted.

ATRIOVENTRICULAR NODAL PHYSIOLOGY

Electrical conduction slows dramatically within the AV node (10). Using microelectrodes, Hoffman and Cranefield (11) and Paes de Carvalho (12) studied the electrical activity of single fibers within the AV node and identified three cell types within the AV node based on activation times and transmembrane action potential characteristics. The N cells were centrally located and were in the zone where maximal conduction slowing occurred. The AN cells were proximally located and were transitional between the rapidly conducting atrial cells and the N zone. Similarly, NH cells were transitional between the N zone and the His bundle. Cells in the N zone were characterized by a lower resting potential, diastolic depolarization, markedly slower phase 0 upstroke, and longer repolarization (which often exceeded the action potential duration) than corresponding atrial cells (11,13). Initial studies suggested that the AN, N, and NH cells were topographically well localized, with discrete areas corresponding to the proximal, middle (compact) and distal AV node, respectively. However, subsequent work by Billette (14) showed that these cells were more generally dispersed in the AV nodal region.

Most AV nodal delay occurs within the N zone (15). This is the zone where block of premature atrial complexes occurs. However, the mechanism responsible for slowed AV nodal conduction and block remains controversial, and at least two theories have been advanced. In the first, AV nodal conduction is thought to be decremental (11). During propagation of the action potential, there is a progressive loss of action potential amplitude and upstroke velocity. Propagation fails under certain conditions, such as a closely coupled premature atrial complex. An alternative hypothesis proposed by Meijler and Janse (16) is that AV nodal activation occurs by electrotonic transmission over an inexcitable gap and that the distal AV node functions as an electronically mediated pacemaker. Evidence to support this hypothesis is derived from the observation that the PR interval shows remarkable consistency across many species and sizes of mammals. We favor the concept that the AV node conducts impulses from the atrium to the ventricle.

As physiologists continued to study the AV node, the complexity of conduction became apparent. Langendorf (17) described the phenomenon of concealed conduction in humans. With concealed conduction, a nonpropagated atrial or ventricular complex can alter subsequent conduction through the AV node. An example is the PR prolongation that occurs after interpolated ventricular premature beats. Hoffman and Cranefield (18) studied this phenomenon in the AV node by recording the electrical activity from many AV nodal cells during differing patterns of premature stimulation. They observed that a premature atrial beat within the AV node may conduct to the middle nodal cells and subsequently become extinguished by decremental conduction. However, these middle nodal cells also remain refractory, and subsequent beats encounter relatively refractory tissue as they are propagated.

To understand better patterns of AV nodal activation, several investigators performed studies in which they simultaneously recorded the electrical activity from many cells within the AV node. Janse (19), using rabbits, and Spach and colleagues (20), using dogs and rabbits, showed that there were two physiologically distinct inputs to the AV node, posteriorly by the crista terminalis and anteriorly through the intraatrial septum. The investigators (19,20) showed that there were different efficiencies of propagation over each of these input pathways, with one pathway usually predominating over the other. Van Capelle and coworkers (21) demonstrated that anterograde conduction and retrograde AV nodal conduction were not mirror images of each other. The shape of the action potential depended on the direction of propagation. The posterior input to the AV node was more prominent in a rabbit model (21). Mazgalev and associates (22), in an isolated, perfused rabbit heart model, concluded that the stimulation site (i.e., intraatrial septum versus crista terminalis) and the timing of AV nodal input determined conduction through the AV node. Zipes and colleagues (23) surgically isolated the anterior and posterior input from one another and showed that there was electrical summation of the anterior and posterior AV nodal

inputs and that the action potential upstroke was voltage dependent. Successful ablation of AV node reentry was performed from the left posterior atrial septum (24). Taken together, these studies suggest a complex pattern of AV nodal activation that is determined by the timing, direction, and amplitude of the electrical impulse as it enters the AV node.

STUDIES OF ATRIOVENTRICULAR NODE REENTRY

Basic Studies

In the late 1950s and earlier 1960s, several groups of investigators studied the response of the AV node to premature atrial stimulation. In a classic publication Moe and colleagues (25) graphed the ventricular response (V_1 through V_2) as a function of progressively decreased premature atrial complexes (A_1-A_2) in a dog heart. Three patterns of V_1-V_2 response were observed. The first pattern was a progressive decrease in V_1-V_2 as A_1-A_2 shortened, until a minimal V_1-V_2 plateau was reached. The second was a progressive decrease in V_1-V_2, followed by a subsequent gradual increase in V_1-V_2. In the third, there was a progressive decrease in V_1-V_2, but at a certain critical A_1-A_2, an abrupt increase in V_1-V_2 occurred. After this abrupt increase was seen, they also observed the occurrence of atrial echo beats. To explain these findings, the investigators hypothesized the existence of a dual AV transmission system. They postulated that there were two conduction pathways, fast and slow, through the AV node with different conduction velocities and refractory periods. Late premature atrial stimuli conducted preferentially over the fast pathway. As the A_1-A_2 was progressively shortened, A_2 was blocked in the fast pathway and then was conducted over the slow pathway. For this to occur, the fast pathway had to have a longer refractory period than the slow pathway. The AV node was longitudinally dissociated into two separate pathways. If there was sufficient conduction delay in the slow pathway, the fast pathway could recover excitability and allow retrograde conduction and an atrial echo. The investigators also speculated that, if this process could be sustained, it would provide a mechanism for reciprocal rhythm and nodal paroxysmal tachycardia as described by Barker and Wilson (2) (Fig. 14-4).

Watanabe and Dreifus (26) subsequently used multiple microelectrodes to study the physiology of the rabbit AV node in response to premature stimuli. They also observed that the AV node could be dissociated into two conduction pathways. Under appropriate conditions, one pathway had slowed but successful conduction, whereas the other pathway demonstrated decremental conduction and block. When the delay in the slow pathway was sufficient, the alternative pathway had time to repolarize, and echo beats occurred.

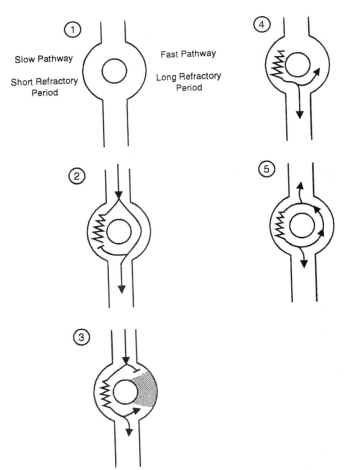

FIGURE 14-4. Hypothetical model of a dual atrioventricular (AV) nodal transmission system proposed by Mendez and Moe. In this model, two AV nodal pathways are represented, one with fast conduction and a relatively long refractory period and a second with slower conduction but shorter refractory period (1). A sinus impulse conducts over both pathways but reaches the bundle of His first by means of conduction over the fast pathway (2). A premature atrial depolarization finds the fast pathway still refractory and conducts over the slower AV nodal pathway (3). If the fast pathway has enough time to recover excitability, the impulse may reenter the fast pathway retrogradely and establish sustained reentry (4 and 5).

Mendez and Moe (27) systematically studied the dual AV conduction system and the atrial echo phenomenon in an *in vitro* rabbit heart preparation. They found that the upper part of the AV node could be functionally and spatially dissociated into two pathways. It was not uncommon for an atrial echo to occur without prior conduction to the ventricle. They concluded that the turn-around point and distal junction of the two pathways were located in the lower portion of the AV node. The investigators also believed that the atrium was a necessary component of the reentrant circuit.

In contrast, Mignone and Wallace (28), using a canine model, concluded that the atria were not needed in the reentrant circuit. They observed ventricular echo beats in response to premature ventricular stimulation. However, by introducing premature atrial complexes at the time of expected conduction of the ventricular beat, they observed that it was possible to render the atrium refractory without abolishing the ventricular echo. They did not, however, exclude the possibility that a thin rim of atrial tissue was necessary for reentry to occur.

Clinical Studies

Reciprocating rhythm, which is a sustained alternation of atrial and then ventricular activation, was described in humans by White (29) in 1915. Further clinical observations were provided by Barker and Wilson (2), who hypothesized that reciprocating rhythm was caused by sustained reentry in the AV node. Armed with the demonstration of a dual AV nodal conduction system in rabbits and dogs, investigators searched for the clinical counterpart in man. Schuilenberg and Durrer (30) described a patient who demonstrated spontaneous echo beats after premature atrial complexes. To study this phenomenon, the investigators introduced progressively closer coupled premature atrial stimuli during atrial pacing to elicit atrial echo beats. They elicited atrial echoes and observed that a marked delay in AV conduction with the atrial premature beat was a requisite for the occurrence of an echo.

Ventricular echo beats were also commonly described in the clinical literature. The ECG pattern was a ventricular premature beat with a retrograde P wave followed closely by another QRS complex with a narrow configuration suggesting a supraventricular origin. Schuilenberg and Durrer (31) studied three patients with premature ventricular stimulation to assess this phenomenon. They induced a ventricular echo, but only after the ventricular premature beat was conducted retrogradely with sufficient ventriculoatrial (VA) delay. The investigators postulated that dual AV node pathways were the explanation for the echo beats. One limitation of both studies, however, was the failure to record a His bundle potential and localize the area of critical delay in AV conduction that seemed to be a prerequisite for the echo phenomenon.

Rosen and coworkers (32) presented further evidence in support of a dual AV nodal conduction system in humans. The investigators described a patient who spontaneously manifested two separate, distinct PR intervals. Using His bundle recordings, they showed that there were two different atrial-His (A-H) intervals and a constant His-ventricular (H-V) interval. Because the A-H interval was considered a measure of AV nodal conduction, they concluded that their patient had two distinct AV nodal pathways. The investigators constructed an AV nodal function curve by plotting the H_1-H_2 interval on the ordinate as a function of the A_1-A_2 interval on the abscissa. Consistent with observations from animal studies, they observed that a critical A_1-A_2 interval produced a sudden increase or "jump" in the

H_1-H_2 curve, as well as in the A-H interval of the premature atrial beat. In this patient, no echo beats or supraventricular tachycardia were induced.

Bigger and Goldreyer (33) used programmed electrical stimulation to study the mechanism of PSVT in humans. In six patients without ventricular preexcitation, they analyzed the mechanisms by which PSVT was initiated and sustained. Supraventricular tachycardia spontaneously occurred after critically timed atrial premature complexes. Programmed atrial stimulation also initiated PSVT. In all cases, there was marked AV conduction delay preceding initiation of SVT, which the investigators thought was more essential than the prematurity of the initiating premature beat. All of their patients had intact VA conduction. However, in these studies, no His bundle recording was obtained, and the mechanism responsible for retrograde conduction was not clearly defined. Bigger and Goldreyer (33) concluded that reentry used the AV conduction system. However, they did not conclusively demonstrate the role of the AV node in the reentrant circuit.

Evidence of AV node reentry and dual AV nodal pathways in humans was provided by Denes and colleagues (34). Two patients with a history of PSVT and a normal PR interval at rest were studied using programmed atrial stimulation and His bundle recordings. Both patients showed evidence of a fast and slow AV nodal pathway, each with its own functional and effective refractory period. At relatively long A_1-A_2 intervals, conduction occurred over the fast pathway. At a critically short A_1-A_2 interval, there was an abrupt discontinuity and jump in the H_1-H_2 response. This was interpreted as the effective refractory period (ERP) of the fast AV nodal conducting system. Failure of conduction in the fast pathway was associated with conduction over the slow pathway and, if enough conduction delay occurred, subsequent atrial echo beats conducted retrogradely over the fast pathway. Sustained supraventricular tachycardia also occurred.

In a subsequent paper, Wu and associates (35) defined the determinants of fast and slow pathway conduction in patients with dual AV node pathways. One new observation was the variable refractoriness of the two pathways at different heart rates. For example, the ERP of the fast pathway could be shorter than the ERP of the slow pathway at one rate, but this could be reversed at a different rate. In our experience, the ERP of the fast pathway often is longer than the slow pathway at faster atrial paced rates.

Dual AV nodal pathways were thought to be a common finding and were demonstrated in many patients undergoing an electrophysiologic study for reasons other than SVT. Of 397 patients studied by Denes and coworkers (36), 41 had dual AV nodal pathways. Twenty-seven patients had dual pathways demonstrated at a cycle length close to the sinus cycle rate, and 14 others had dual AV nodal physiology demonstrated only at faster atrial paced cycle lengths. Seventeen of these 41 patients had a history of documented

PSVT, and atrial echo beats were demonstrated in 15. However, in the other 24 patients, no echo beats or PSVT occurred. The investigators concluded that dual AV nodal physiology, defined by a jump and discontinuity in the A_1-A_2/H_1-H_2 curve, was a relatively common electrophysiologic finding. Our bias is that most people without AV node reentry have the anatomic substrate for dual AV node conduction. Slow pathway conduction is not demonstrated at electrophysiology study because the fast-pathway anterograde ERP is always greater than the slow pathway ERP. However, in these same individuals, it is common to demonstrate retrograde dual AV node physiology with closely coupled premature ventricular complexes.

Denes and colleagues (37) investigated the electrophysiologic requisites for atrial echo beats and the induction of sustained AV node reentry. Of 38 patients with dual AV nodal physiology, only 21 had atrial echo beats induced. Of these 21 patients, 7 had only one atrial echo, and 14 had sustained reentry. Initiation of an atrial echo depended on the properties of retrograde conduction. Atrial echo beats were not induced in the 17 patients with poor or absent retrograde conduction. The capacity to have sustained reentry was determined by slow-pathway anterograde conduction. In patients with only one echo response, the impulse was extinguished anterogradely in the slow pathway. Sustained AVNRT was induced only when anterograde slow-pathway conduction was relatively good.

After these investigations, Wu and coworkers (38) reported three patients with an unusual form of AV node reentry with fast anterograde and slow retrograde conduction. Whereas the anterograde AV nodal function curves were continuous, premature ventricular stimulation revealed discontinuous VA conduction curves. The investigators hypothesized that the ERP of the retrograde fast pathway exceeded the ERP of the retrograde slow pathway. A critically timed premature ventricular complex blocked in the retrograde fast pathway, conducted over the slow pathway, and initiated AV node reentry (i.e., fast/slow AVNRT). This produced tachycardia with a long RP interval.

Sung and colleagues (39) later described five patients with this unusual variety of AV node reentry. In all patients, tachycardia was initiated with a premature ventricular complex that blocked in the retrograde fast pathway and conducted over the retrograde slow pathway.

CLINICAL ASPECTS AND DIAGNOSIS OF ATRIOVENTRICULAR NODE REENTRANT TACHYCARDIA

In patients with PSVT without ventricular preexcitation in sinus rhythm, AV nodal reentry is the most common mechanism of tachycardia, accounting for 60% or more of unknown tachycardias (40–43). Clinically, AVNRT can affect persons of virtually any age. Cases of children younger than 10 years old and of octogenarians have been described, but the onset of arrhythmia most often occurs beyond the fourth decade. In one study, the average age at presentation was 55 years, with a range of 24 to 81 years (43). This was statistically older than other patients with PSVT due to reentry over a concealed bypass tract. In general, there is a minor female predilection. Multiple investigators have also reported that there is no significant association with other structural heart disease.

Palpitations are the primary symptom during AV node reentry (44). The rate of the tachycardia is usually 150 to 200 bpm, although rates of up to 250 bpm can occur. Rapid ventricular rates may be associated with complaints of dyspnea, weakness, angina, lightheadedness, or even frank syncope. Some symptoms, such as neck pain, are related to the simultaneous contraction of the atria and ventricles against closed mitral and tricuspid valves. Episodes may last from seconds to hours, and many patients with sustained reentry require treatment to terminate the arrhythmia. Patients often relate various methods they have discovered that can terminate their arrhythmias. These include the Valsalva maneuver, carotid sinus massage, deep breathing quietly while lying down, and coughing. In essence, most successful maneuvers rely on enhanced vagal tone.

The physical examination is remarkable for the finding of a rapid, regular heart rate. Because of the simultaneous contraction of the atrium and ventricle, cannon A waves may be seen in the jugular venous waveform.

Electrocardiographic And Electrophysiologic Considerations

The resting electrocardiogram (ECG) is usually normal in patients with AVNRT. On rare occasions, a patient may spontaneously show two distinct PR intervals suggestive of dual AV pathways. One report describes the use of adenosine given intravenously during normal sinus rhythm to demonstrate two distinct PR intervals and suggests that this test may be used as a noninvasive marker of dual AV nodal physiology in patients with PSVT (45). In the usual (slow anterograde/fast retrograde conduction) form of AVNRT, ECG documentation of the initiation of AVNRT usually shows a premature atrial beat that conducts with marked delay to the ventricle, followed by the generation of a regular narrow QRS complex tachycardia (Fig. 14-5). Because atrial and ventricular activation are nearly simultaneous, distinct P waves are not usually visible. However, close inspection of lead V_1 often reveals a pseudo-r′ pattern because of deformation of the terminal portion of the QRS complex by the retrograde P wave (Figs. 14-5 and 14-6). It is rare for the usual form of AVNRT to be initiated by a spontaneous premature ventricular complex. If PSVT is induced by a single premature ventricular contraction, the physician should suspect AV reentry or an atypical variant

of AV nodal reentry. In the variant form, there is fast anterograde/slow retrograde AV nodal reentry, and inverted P waves occur close to the next QRS complex so that the RP : PR ratio is greater than 1. It is a type of "long RP tachycardia." In the intermediate form of AVNRT, also called slow/slow AVNRT, inverted P waves are clearly discernible after the QRS complex, and the RP : PR interval depends on the relative conduction time over both pathways.

AV node reentry most often occurs with a narrow QRS morphology similar to the QRS morphology recorded during normal sinus rhythm. Occasionally, functional right or left bundle branch block aberrancy may be present. In some cases, AV node reentry may occur in patients with ventricular preexcitation. Rarely, the accessory pathway is an innocent bystander (not used in the tachycardia circuit), and the tachycardia has a preexcited appearance similar to the QRS morphology seen in sinus rhythm. Differentiation of antidromic reciprocating tachycardia from AVNRT with a bystander accessory pathway requires electrophysiologic testing.

Other ECG changes may be seen during or after termination of AVNRT. Significant ST segment depression during tachycardia has been observed in 25% to 50% of patients with AVNRT, although it is more commonly seen in those with an atrioventricular reentrant tachycardia (AVRT) associated with an accessory pathway (45a,45b). With AVNRT, there is no correlation between the rate of the tachycardia and the presence or extent of ST segment changes. Although the presence of ST segment depression suggests myocardial ischemia, most patients do not have underlying coronary artery disease; in these patients, ST segment changes represent repolarization changes or retrograde atrial activation. However, one study found that 33% of patients with AVNRT older than 45 years of age did have coronary artery disease, even though symptoms were absent (45b).

Negative T waves newly acquired after the termination of AVNRT commonly are seen in the anterior or inferior leads and were present in about 40% of patients in one study (45c). They may be seen immediately on AVNRT termination or may develop within the first 6 hours, and they can persist for a variable duration (mean, 34 hours). The occurrence of negative T waves is not predicted by clinical parameters, tachycardia rate or duration, or the presence and extent of ST segment depression during the tachycardia. They are not the result of coronary artery disease but are repolarization abnormalities, probably because of ionic current alterations resulting from the rapid rate.

The purported electrophysiologic circuit of AV nodal reentry includes two conducting pathways in the AV node, one with fast conducting characteristics but a long refractory period and the second with slower conduction and a shorter refractory period (Fig. 14-4). However, there has been considerable debate about whether the reentrant cir-

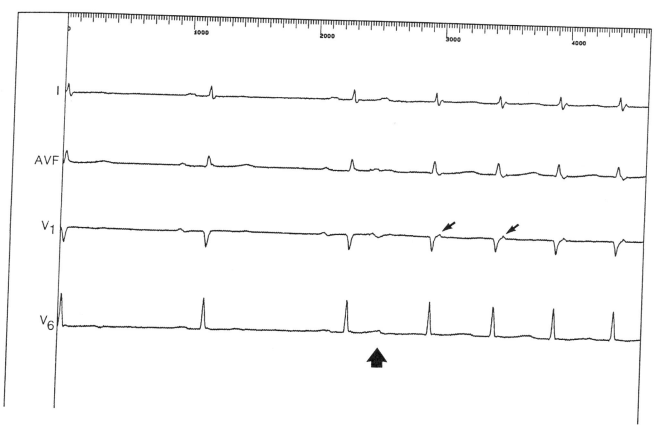

FIGURE 14-5. Initiation of atrioventricular nodal reentrant tachycardia (AVNRT) by a premature atrial beat. A premature atrial beat *(large arrow)* occurs that presumably blocks in the fast pathway and conducts with marked delay over the slow pathway to the ventricle. This initiates AVNRT. Also seen is the pseudo-r' in lead V_1 *(small arrows)*, representing retrograde depolarization of the atrium.

AVN Reentry

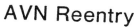

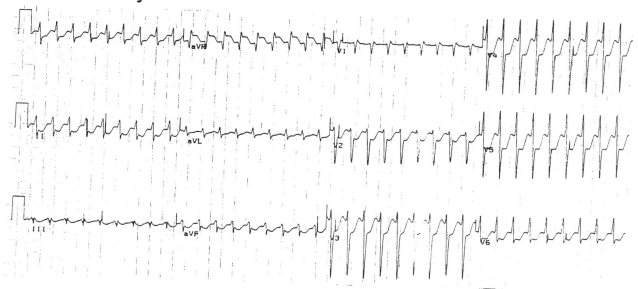

FIGURE 14-6. The 12-lead electrocardiogram of atrioventricular nodal reentrant tachycardia in a patient is typical. Notice the pseudo-r' in lead V_1, representing retrograde atrial activation. Distinct P waves in the ST segment are not present.

cuit is confined to the AV node or also includes atrial tissue, probably surrounding transitional cells. A common upper pathway is not consistent with the results of catheter ablation cure in the posterior atrial septum. It is unclear whether dual AV nodal pathways are ubiquitous but unrecognized in most patients or are a distinct pathologic entity. We think that most individuals have two distinct inputs to the AV node with the capability of conduction over a slow pathway.

Demonstration of dual AV nodal physiology using premature atrial stimuli in patients with PSVT is suggestive, but not diagnostic, of AV nodal reentry as the mechanism of tachycardia. Dual AV nodal physiology may occur in patients with AV reentry, and the slow pathway may be used for anterograde conduction during AVRT (46). Programmed atrial stimulation involves the introduction of a series of atrial extrastimuli at progressively earlier intervals starting late in diastole during sinus rhythm or atrial pacing. The hallmark of dual AV nodal physiology is a jump or discontinuity in the AV nodal function curve (A_1-A_2/H_1-H_2) or the AV nodal conduction curve (A_1-A_2/A_2-H_2) by at least 50 ms in response to a 10 ms decrement in the A_1-A_2 coupling interval (Figs. 14-7 and 14-8). The 50-ms increase is rather arbitrary and may differ depending on the paced rate used. A continuous AV nodal function curve does not exclude AVNRT and can occur in up to 30% of patients

subsequently proven to have AVNRT (47). For example, if a premature atrial complex blocks in the fast pathway and conducts over the slow pathway, but conduction time over the slow pathway is only slightly longer than that of the fast pathway, AVNRT could be initiated without a discontinuous curve. Changes in the atrial paced cycle length may cause unpredictable changes in the ERP of the fast and slow pathways. Although the AV node ERP generally increases in response to a shorter paced cycle length, the degree of increase in the ERP of the fast and slow pathway may differ at various heart rates. Dual AV nodal physiology and discontinuous AV nodal function curves may be present at one cycle length and absent at another. Dual AV node physiology often is easier to demonstrate at shorter paced cycle lengths, such as 400 ms, or with two premature atrial contractions.

Rarely, a 2 for 1 response may be seen in patients with dual AV nodal physiology in response to a premature atrial impulse (Fig. 14-9). In this instance, the fast and slow pathways are dissociated such that an impulse conducts simultaneously over the fast and slow pathways. For this phenomenon to occur, the impulse that conducts over the fast pathway must not penetrate retrogradely into the slow pathway and generally indicates poor retrograde, slow-pathway conduction (48).

In some patients with PSVT, dual AV nodal physiology is demonstrated, but neither echo beats nor tachycardia is initiated. Assuming AVNRT is the mechanism of the tachycardia, the conduction time over the slow pathway is too fast to allow recovery of the retrograde fast pathway, or retrograde conduction over the fast pathway is poor. Generation of greater AV nodal delay can often be accomplished with more closely coupled atrial extrastimuli or the use of two closely coupled atrial extrastimuli (Fig. 14-10). Facilitation of retrograde AV nodal conduction can usually be accomplished with pharmacologic measures. Isoproterenol and atropine can enhance anterograde and retrograde AV nodal conduction and enable the induction of sustained tachycardia.

Differential Diagnosis

Certain features are useful to diagnose the usual slow/fast form of AV node reentry. Atrial activation occurs simultaneously with or immediately after ventricular activation. The earliest VA interval is therefore usually less than 60 ms, and the V to high right atrial (V-HRA) interval is typically less than 90 ms (Fig. 14-11). P waves are not clearly visible but may occur at the end of the QRS complex, leading to the pseudo-r' in V_1 (Figs. 14-5 and 14-6). Retrograde atrial activation is concentric with the earliest atrial activation recorded in the interatrial septum. A critical A-H interval is necessary to initiate the tachycardia, and because the reentrant loop is small and at least partly

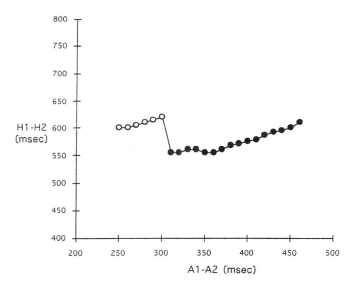

FIGURE 14-7. Atrioventricular (AV) nodal function curve in a patient with dual AV nodal pathways. As A_1-A_2 is progressively decremented, there is a plateau in the H_1-H_2 response *(solid circles)*. This is the functional refractory period of the fast pathway. At an A_1-A_2 of 300 ms, the effective refractory period (ERP) of the fast pathway is reached, and there is a jump of 70 ms to the slow pathway *(open circles)*. Concomitant with this jump is the development of atrioventricular nodal reentrant tachycardia. A_1-A_2 can be progressively decremented until the ERP of the slow pathway is attained at 250 ms.

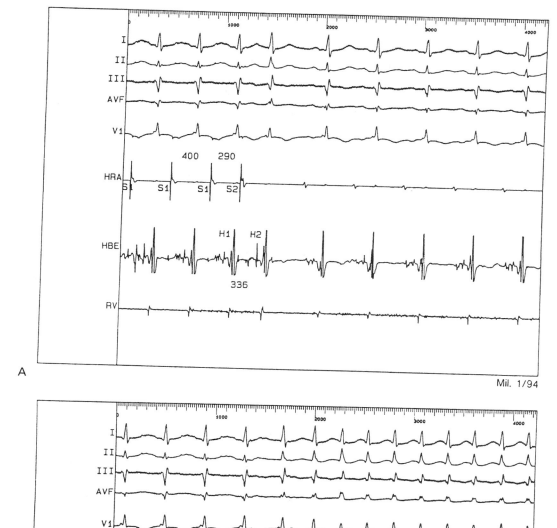

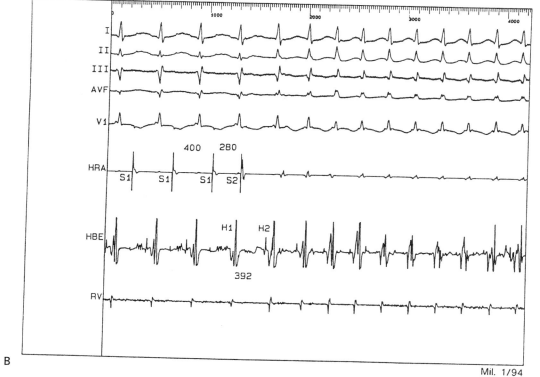

FIGURE 14-8. Electrophysiologic demonstration of dual atrioventricular (AV) nodal physiology and the initiation of atrioventricular nodal reentrant tachycardia (AVNRT). **A:** A premature atrial beat introduced with an A_1-A_2 coupling interval of 290 ms conducts with a H_1-H_2 response of 336 ms. **B:** At an A_1-A_2 coupling interval of 280 ms, there is a sudden jump in the H_1-H_2 response to 392 ms that is associated with the initiation of AVNRT.

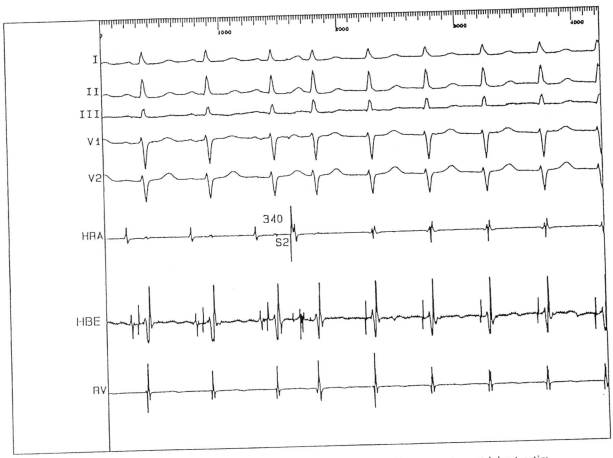

FIGURE 14-9. Induction of atrioventricular (AV) nodal reentry with a premature atrial extrastimulus results in two ventricular responses. An atrial extrastimulus delivered with a coupling interval of 340 ms results in conduction over the fast AV nodal pathway and simultaneous conduction over the slow AV nodal pathway. The impulse then retrogradely reenters the fast pathway to initiate atrioventricular nodal reentrant tachycardia. This pattern has been called the 2 for 1 phenomenon.

intranodal, only very early premature atrial or ventricular extrastimuli can penetrate the tachycardia circuit to reset it or terminate tachycardia. AVNRT often is a diagnosis of exclusion.

AVNRT of the unusual variety (fast anterograde/slow retrograde) also has a concentric retrograde atrial activation sequence; however, the RP interval is longer than the PR interval. The differential diagnosis of this long RP tachycardia also includes atrial tachycardia and various forms of AV reentry using a slowly conducting accessory pathway for retrograde conduction. Differentiation among these mechanisms of tachycardia may be difficult and is beyond the scope of this chapter. Several other features are characteristic of the unusual form of AVNRT: retrograde dual AV nodal function curves; reproducible initiation with premature ventricular beats, more commonly than with atrial premature beats; and initiation dependent on a critical H-A interval during retrograde, slow-pathway conduction.

AVNRT must be differentiated from other forms of narrow-complex supraventricular tachycardia with 1 : 1 AV conduction, including sinus node reentry, atrial tachycardia, and AV reentry over an accessory pathway (40–42). Certain clinical features can be helpful; however, the analysis of the surface electrocardiogram and invasive electrophysiologic studies can almost always distinguish among these mechanisms.

Sinus node reentrant tachycardia has a high-low atrial activation sequence, and the P-wave morphology is identical or very similar to the sinus P wave. Atrial tachycardias may be caused by abnormal automaticity, triggered automaticity, or reentry. Because they may occur from many locations within either atrium, the P-wave morphology is

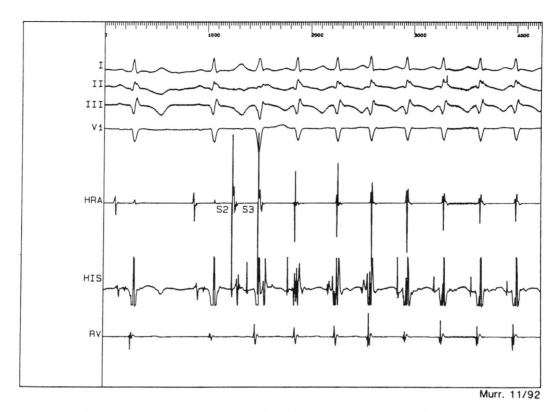

Murr. 11/92

FIGURE 14-10. Use of two atrial extrastimuli to initiate atrioventricular nodal reentrant tachy-cardia (AVNRT). Two atrial extrastimuli were introduced during normal sinus rhythm. Notice the marked prolongation of the A-H interval after S_3, associated with the initiation of AVNRT.

variable, and the sequence of atrial activation depends on the site of tachycardia origin. Consequently, a high-low or eccentric (i.e., not in the septum) atrial activation sequence distinguishes this tachycardia from AV nodal reentry. A rare exception is retrograde earliest atrial activation in the left atrial free wall in AVNRT (49). Continuation of the tachycardia in the presence of AV nodal block is typical for atrial tachycardia but rare for AVNRT. Drugs such as adenosine or verapamil often cause AV node block without termination of atrial tachycardia or just before termination (Fig. 14-12). Unfortunately, rare cases of AVNRT can persist with AV block, presumably because the circuit is proximal to the site of block. Regardless, the physician should always consider atrial tachycardia as the diagnosis of choice in this situation but perform other maneuvers to prove it. Introduction of closely coupled premature ventricular stimuli during tachycardia, which terminate the tachycardia without conduction to the atrium, effectively excludes atrial tachycardia (Fig. 14-13). The observation of His-to-His changes preceding and predicting changes from atrial electrogram to atrial electrogram during subtle cycle length variation during the tachycardia implies that the tachycardia is AV nodal dependent and excludes atrial tachycardia from the differ-

ential diagnosis (Fig. 14-14). These subtle changes in tachycardia cycle length are often seen immediately after tachycardia initiation or immediately before termination, especially if termination is caused by the administration of adenosine.

In orthodromic AV reentry, the AV node is part of the anterograde limb of the tachycardia circuit and the accessory pathway forms the retrograde limb. The P waves are usually seen after the QRS deflection in the early ST segment. The earliest VA interval during tachycardia is typically greater than 70 ms, and the V-HRA is more than 95 ms. Very short VA intervals are incompatible with AVRT. Atrial activation may be eccentric when the pathway is located on the right or left free wall, and this finding excludes AVNRT as the mechanism of an unknown tachycardia. In patients with septal accessory pathways and longer VA conduction times, the differentiation of AV node from AV reentry is considerably more difficult. Preexcitation of the atria during tachycardia with ventricular extrastimuli introduced when the His bundle is refractory confirms the presence of an accessory pathway but does not prove AVRT. AVRT is diagnosed when infra-AV nodal structures are demonstrated to be part of the tachycardia

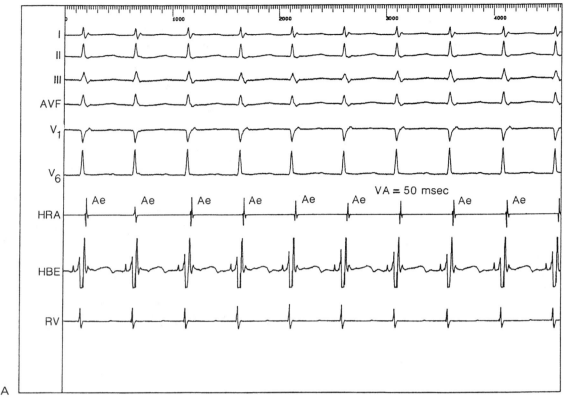

VA = 50 msec

A

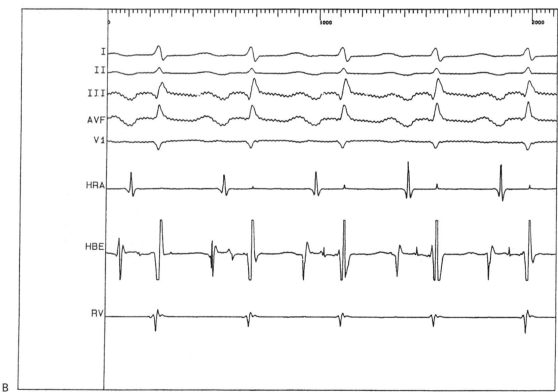

B

FIGURE 14-11. Electrophysiologic recordings during the usual and unusual varieties of atrioventricular nodal reentrant tachycardia (AVNRT). **A:** The usual variety of AVNRT is demonstrated with a V to high right atrial echo (Ae) interval of 50 ms. Notice the pseudo-r' in lead V₁ corresponding to retrograde atrial activation (Ae). **B:** An unusual variety of AVNRT is demonstrated. Notice the low-to-high atrial activation sequence, the long RP interval, and the inverted P waves in leads II, III, and aVF.

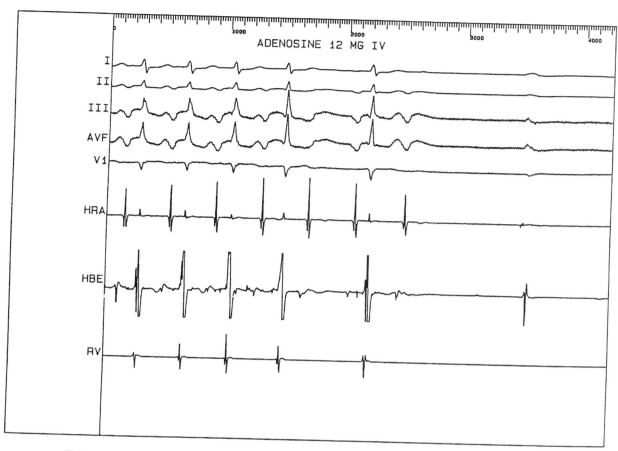

FIGURE 14-12. Use of adenosine in a patient with atrial tachycardia. Adenosine (12 mg) was given during tachycardia. There was a block of condition through the atrioventricular (AV) node with continuation of atrial activity, proving the mechanism of atrial tachycardia. Notice, however, the subsequent termination of tachycardia. In our experience, atrial tachycardias often terminate after adenosine administration. Termination of tachycardia with adenosine is not a specific marker for AV nodal–dependent arrhythmias, unless AV block precedes tachycardia termination.

circuit. Examples are increases in the VA interval during tachycardia with bundle branch block; an increase in the H-V interval associated with an increase in the H-A interval; and termination of the tachycardia with a premature ventricular complex that occurs with a His electrogram that is visible and unperturbed and that does not conduct to the atria.

MANAGEMENT

Autonomic Influences

For many years, it has been known that AV nodal conduction is under regulation by the autonomic nervous system. In 1913, Cohn and Lewis (50) demonstrated that vagal stimulation by carotid sinus massage could produce AV block. In 1944, Barker and Wilson (2) used the observation that vagal stimulation could terminate supraventricular tachycardia to conclude that the AV node was part of the

reentrant circuit. In interpreting data regarding the autonomic influences on AV nodal conduction, it is important to realize that AV conduction is rate dependent (51). An increase in heart rate during atrial pacing produces a progressive slowing of AV nodal conduction with an increase in the A-H interval. In contrast, when the sinus rate increases because of atropine (vagolytic) or isoproterenol (sympathomimetic), AV conduction is enhanced (52). Wenckebach AV node block is characteristic with incremental atrial pacing but rarely occurs with exercise because of vagal withdrawal and increased sympathetic tone. In general, the parasympathetic and sympathetic influences on AV node conduction at rest tend to be balanced (53,54). However, patients with intrinsic abnormalities of AV nodal conduction appear to be more sensitive to parasympathetic tone, the significance of which is not clear (55).

Because of the known influence of autonomic tone on AV nodal conduction, as well as the observation that vagal

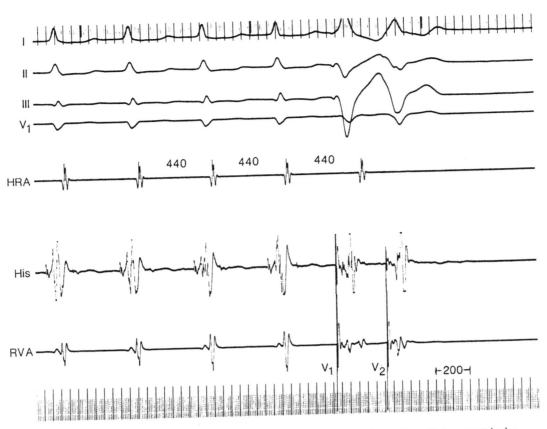

FIGURE 14-13. Termination of atrioventricular nodal reentrant tachycardia with two ventricular extrastimuli. The termination of tachycardia with ventricular extrastimuli that do not depolarize the atria effectively excludes atrial tachycardia as a mechanism. In this instance, the first ventricular premature extrastimulus (V_1) does not reset the tachycardia because the A-to-A cycle length is unperturbed. The second ventricular premature extrastimulus (V_2) results in tachycardia termination without depolarization of the atria. Because termination of tachycardia occurs with block in subatrial structures, atrial tachycardia is not the mechanism. The very short ventriculoatrial interval excludes atrioventricular (AV) reentry. AV node reentry is the diagnosis.

stimulation can terminate AV nodal–dependent tachycardias, maneuvers that increase vagal tone, such as a Valsalva maneuver or carotid sinus massage, have been used to terminate AVNRT. In the slow/fast form, the tachycardia typically terminates in the anterograde direction, often with a slight prolongation of the A-H interval immediately before tachycardia termination. In the fast/slow variety of AVNRT, the tachycardia typically terminates with block in the retrograde slow pathway. The effect of vagal maneuvers is most pronounced on the slow pathway.

Drugs that alter the autonomic nervous system have been studied in patients with AVNRT. Wellens and associates (56) investigated the effect of digoxin in 15 patients with AV nodal dependent tachycardia; 13 had AVNRT, and 2 had AVRT. They found that digitalis, an agent known to enhance parasympathetic tone, increased AV nodal conduction time and the ERP and functional refractory period (FRP) of the anterograde fast and slow pathways. In seven patients, no tachycardia could be initiated after digitalis, and in five others, the atrial extrastimuli zone of initiation

was decreased. The investigators also reported that chronic therapy with digitalis resulted in similar electrophysiologic results. However, in some patients, the ability to initiate AVNRT after digitalis seemed to be enhanced with the observation of a larger echo zone during premature atrial stimulation (56). This finding has been explained by the following hypothesis. Digitalis, through a vagal mechanism, induces slowing of AV conduction. In some patients, however, the degree of conduction slowing is minimal, but the ERP of the fast pathway increases to a greater extent than the ERP of the slow pathway. In this situation, the echo zone increases. Premature beats more easily block in the fast pathway allowing initiation of AVNRT. Mazgalev and colleagues (57) showed in a rabbit AV nodal preparation that postganglionic vagal stimulation could occasionally perturb intranodal conduction and allow AV node reentry to occur. However, vagal stimulation more frequently prevented or terminated AVNRT.

Vagolytic agents can improve anterograde and retrograde AV nodal function. Wu and coworkers (58) studied 14

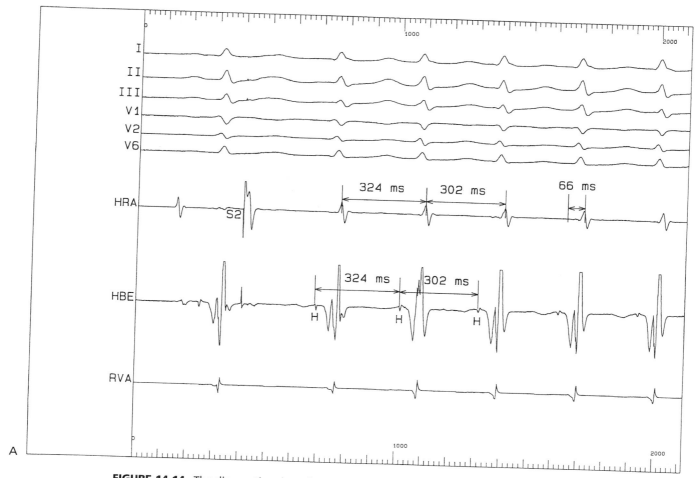

FIGURE 14-14. The diagnostic value of cycle length changes in the diagnosis of atrioventricular nodal reentrant tachycardia (AVNRT). **A:** A premature atrial extrastimulus, S_2, delivered during sinus rhythm conducts over the slow AV nodal pathway and initiates AVNRT. The cycle length varies from 324 to 302 ms between the first and second beats. Notice that the changes in the His-to-His intervals precede and predict the subsequent changes in atrial cycle length. This finding suggests that the AV node is a component of the tachycardia circuit and excludes atrial tachycardia from the differential diagnosis. The His-to-A interval is constant, indicating that the changes in cycle length result from changes in the A-H intervals. Changes in cycle length are associated with a constant H-A interval, inconsistent with an atrial tachycardia, and the ventriculoatrial interval is too short for atrioventricular reentrant tachycardia.

(continues on next page)

patients with a clinical history of PSVT and dual AV nodal pathways. Five patients had AVNRT induced in the baseline state. However, in seven patients, AVNRT was not induced because of poor retrograde, fast-pathway conduction. Atropine facilitated retrograde AV node conduction, and AVNRT was induced in all seven patients. These findings were corroborated by other investigators (59). Isoproterenol can also improve anterograde and retrograde AV nodal function. In one series, eight patients had AVNRT induced after the addition of isoproterenol, which improved retrograde, fast-pathway conduction (60).

Logic suggests that, if catecholamines can facilitate induction of AVNRT, sympathetic blockade may terminate or prevent its reinduction. In one study, propranolol acutely terminated AVNRT by creating block and slowed conduction in the anterograde slow pathway (61). Propranolol increased the ERP and FRP of the slow and fast pathways. In a manner similar to digitalis, propranolol can paradoxically increase the tachycardia induction echo zone by minimally slowing anterograde AV node conduction and increasing the refractory period of the fast pathway more than that of the slow pathway.

Pharmacologic Therapy

Digoxin and β-adrenergic blocking agents can be used clinically in the termination and prevention of AVNRT. These agents predominantly act through the autonomic nervous

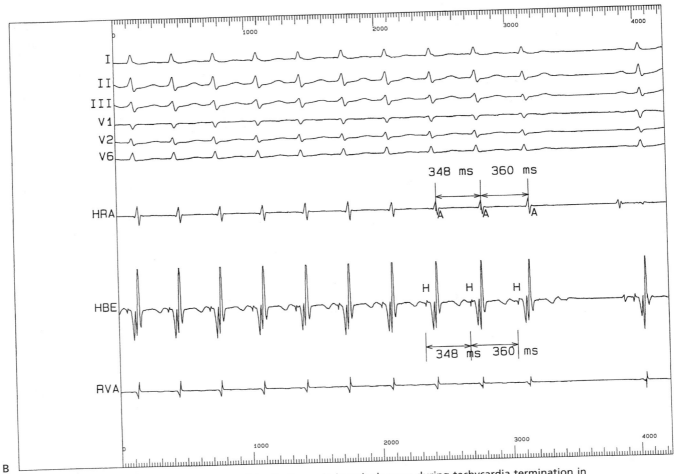

FIGURE 14-14. (continued) B: Similar cycle length changes during tachycardia termination in which His-to-His interval changes again precede and predict subsequent A-to-A changes.

system on the slow anterograde pathway. Other agents may act directly on this pathway. Verapamil is a calcium channel blocking agent that can terminate and prevent the induction of AVNRT (62–64). Verapamil slows conduction and prolongs refractoriness in the fast and slow pathways. The termination of AVNRT is usually caused by anterograde block but also occurs because of block in the retrograde fast pathway.

Adenosine, a purinergic blocker, is an agent that acutely and transiently causes AV nodal blockade (65,66). The effect is usually short lived because endogenous enzymes rapidly metabolize adenosine. Adenosine also exhibits a dose-related effect on AV nodal conduction. At lower doses, a gradual prolongation in the A-H interval is observed. At higher doses complete AV nodal block may be achieved. One group proposed the use of intravenous adenosine as a bedside test to identify patients with dual AV nodal physiology (45). Multiple studies have shown that adenosine is nearly 100% effective for terminating AV nodal–dependent arrhythmias. Usually, prolongation of the A-H interval occurs immediately before tachycardia termination. Because of its dramatic effect on AV nodal conduction, adenosine has been proposed as a diagnostic tool to differentiate AV nodal–depen-

dent from AV nodal–independent tachycardias. The development of AV block with perpetuation of the tachycardia indicates that the AV node is not a requisite part of the tachycardia circuit. However, adenosine can also terminate some types of atrial tachycardia (Fig. 14-12).

Many other agents have been employed in the therapy of AVNRT. In general, most sodium channel blocking agents can prevent AV nodal reentry. These include the Ia agents quinidine (67), procainamide (68), and disopyramide (69, 70); the Ic agents, including flecainide (71), encainide (72), propafenone (73,74), and Ethmozine (75); and the class III agents. Most commonly, these agents depress retrograde, fast-pathway conduction. Based on these observations, it has been speculated that the anterograde slow pathway is composed of slow channel tissue, and the retrograde pathway contains a mixture of fast and slow channel tissue (76).

Nonpharmacologic Therapy: Historical Perspectives

For many years, a significant controversy has existed concerning the anatomic boundaries of the reentrant circuit in

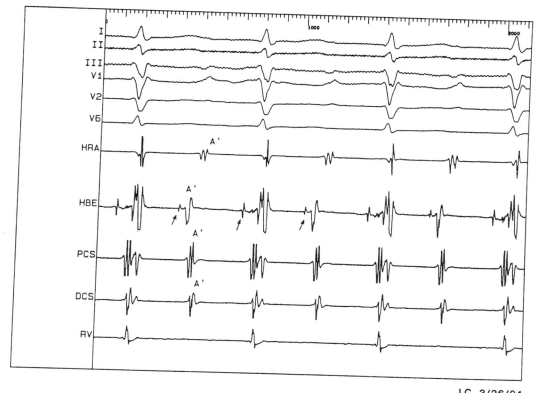

J.C. 3/26/91

FIGURE 14-15. Atrioventricular nodal reentrant tachycardia (AVNRT) with 2 : 1 block below the bundle of His. AVNRT occurs at a cycle length of 310 ms. The His bundle depolarization *(arrow)* precedes each atrial depolarization, and every other complex is conducted to the ventricle. This finding provides evidence that the ventricles are not a requisite part of the AVNRT circuit.

AVNRT (44). The observation of AVNRT with 2 :1 block below the bundle of His is well described (Fig. 14-15), and has been used as evidence to confirm that the ventricle is not part of the AVNRT circuit. Whether a very proximal part of the His bundle is used in the circuit cannot be excluded, but we do not think it is. However, the role of the atrium remains more contentious. In rare cases, the tachycardia may be initiated in the absence of an atrial echo and may persist in the presence of AV dissociation. These observations do not exclude the possibility that a small rim of atrial tissue near the AV node participates in the reentrant tachycardia, with intraatrial block preventing atrial activation.

Several observations favor the atrium being part of the reentrant circuit. In a microelectrode study in the rabbit, the reentrant circuit was mapped to the perinodal region and used the coronary sinus as a mechanical obstacle around which the AVNRT occurred (77). An early observation by Pritchett and colleagues (78) provided further data. In a patient with AV node reentry, they attempted surgically to ablate AV node conduction. However, anterograde conduction persisted postoperatively, with AV conduction being slower and markedly impaired in the anterograde and retrograde directions. This approach resulted in cure of the arrhythmia. The investigators con-

cluded that conduction in the fast and slow pathways was anatomically distinct and that it was possible to abolish AVNRT with operations on specific components of the AV conduction system.

This hypothesis was studied in a canine model by Holman and colleagues (79). They used strategically placed cryolesions in the peri-AV nodal region of the right atrium to modify AV nodal conduction. AV nodal conduction was slowed anterogradely and retrogradely without the development of AV block. Additional studies (80,81) showed that this cryosurgical procedure was capable of selectively ablating only one of the pathways of AV conduction, leaving some degree of conduction intact and disrupting the anatomic substrate necessary for AV node reentry. Ross and coworkers (82) reported the cure of AVNRT with this technique in humans. In 10 patients with AVNRT, cure was obtained with cryosurgical ablation of perinodal tissue. Five of seven patients also had dual AV nodal physiology abolished. Cox and associates (83) also described eight patients with classic AV node reentry and dual AV node curves preoperatively. Postoperatively, the patients had no AVNRT, and none had dual AV node function curves. It became clear that modification of the perinodal atrial tissue could result in cure of AVNRT.

Despite the intuitive appeal of "curing" AV node reentrant tachycardia by surgical modification of the AV node and its atrial input, this procedure did not receive widespread acceptance. However, catheter ablation to cure AVNRT has permanently changed the therapeutic approach to this arrhythmia. It has also offered compelling data implicating the atrium as part of the tachycardia circuit.

In 1981, Sung and coworkers (84) demonstrated that the fast and slow AV nodal pathways had different retrograde exit points into the right atrium. It was hypothesized that delivery of direct current energy at the site of earliest retrograde atrial activation could abolish preferentially the atrial insertion of the retrograde fast pathway. During tachycardia, this region was consistently localized to an area in the atrial septum, just anterior to the AV node. Haissaguerre and colleagues (85) reported results of direct current catheter ablation in this region in 21 patients with AVNRT. Treatment resulted in the preferential ablation or impairment of retrograde AV nodal conduction in all patients. Anterograde conduction was modified in 19 patients, and complete heart block occurred in 2 patients. Sixteen patients remained free of arrhythmia over a mean follow-up of 14 months. Epstein and associates (86) reported similar results using this technique in nine patients with drug-refractory AVNRT. Six of the nine patients had complete cure over a mean follow-up period of 12.3 months. No patient required permanent pacing, although one patient developed complete AV block, which persisted for several months. Three patients had complete retrograde block in the fast pathway, but three other patients had attenuation of only slow-pathway conduction, suggesting that it might be possible to modify selectively the slow pathway.

A prominent limitation to the use of direct current modification of the AV node was the uncontrolled delivery of an abrupt shock to the perinodal atrial region. Consequently, other energy sources for catheter ablation were investigated. Lee and coworkers (87) described the use of catheter-delivered radiofrequency energy for the controlled modification of the anterior fast pathway in humans (Fig. 14-16). They reported 39 patients who underwent this therapy. The ablation catheter was positioned anteriorly with a large atrial electrogram and very small His electrogram (<100 μV) recorded. The end points of energy delivery were first-degree AV block or the impairment of VA conduction. The investigators reported cure of the tachycardia in 32 of 39 patients and the development of complete AV block in 3 patients. In successfully treated patients, the mean A-H interval increased from 74 to 146 ms, and retrograde VA conduction was eliminated in all but one patient. In 17

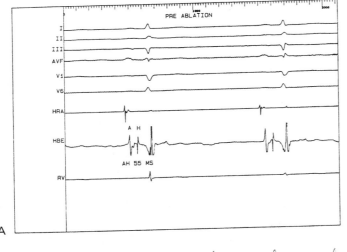

A

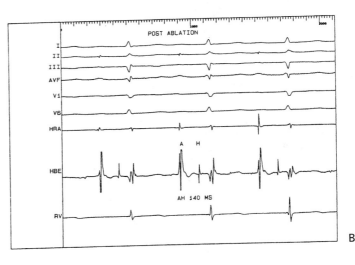

B

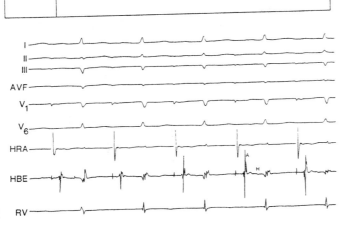

C

FIGURE 14-16. Atrioventricular nodal fast pathway modification. Before ablation, the A-H interval is 55 ms **(A)**. After delivery of radiofrequency energy for 30 seconds during atrial pacing at an appropriate anterior site with a large atrial and small His electrogram **(B)**, the A-H interval is prolonged to 140 ms **(C)**, representing ablation of the fast AV nodal pathway.

patients with dual AV nodal physiology before the procedure, 14 had continuous AV nodal function curves after the procedure. The investigators concluded that the delivery of radiofrequency energy could modify the AV node and successfully ablate the fast AV nodal pathway. However, the relatively high incidence of complete heart block in this region led other investigators to develop radiofrequency techniques for the ablation of the slow pathway.

The observations of Sung and associates (84) suggested that atrial tissue located posteriorly near the os of the coronary sinus may be part of the AVNRT circuit. Jackman and colleagues (88) performed detailed mapping of this posterior space and in variable posterior locations were able to identify a unique potential, which they called *Ap*. This potential was shown to be distinctly different from local atrial activation, and they thought it represented the activation of the atrial insertion of the slow pathway (Fig. 14-17). We do not think that this potential is activation of the slow pathway *per se*, but it may represent depolarization of atrial tissue overlying or adjacent to the slow pathway. It may result from anisotropic conduction in this region. Delivery of radiofrequency energy to this region in 80 patients with AVNRT and dual AV nodal pathways resulted in abolition or modification of the slow pathway in 78 patients. In one patient, the fast pathway was ablated, and in one patient, complete heart block resulted. Similar results with high success rates (> 95%) and a low incidence of complications (<1%) have been reported by several other groups (89–91a). In one histologic study of a patient who underwent cardiac transplant shortly after slow pathway modification, the lesion extended from the septal portion of the tricuspid annulus to the posterior border of the AV node but did not include the compact AV node (92). It appears that the slow pathway is composed of posterior approaches to the AV node but is distinct from the compact AV node. A caveat must be inserted in that the anatomic arrangements of the fast and slow pathways are not identical in different patients. Intraoperative ice mapping of the AV nodal region (93) and detailed mapping of the recorded area of the Ap potential (88) have identified variable posterior locations where destructive lesions can abolish or modify anterograde conduction over the slow pathway. These studies demonstrated that the slow pathway is, at least in part, anatomically separated from the fast pathway and that modification of perinodal atrial tissue can selectively affect changes in one or the other pathway. Figure 14-18 is an accepted concept of the anatomic circuit of AVNRT.

Radiofrequency Ablation

After the diagnosis of AVNRT is confirmed, we initially position the ablation catheter at the tricuspid annulus near the coronary sinus ostium, where we think the atrial inputs to the slow pathway are located. Optimal sites for radiofrequency ablation have a fractionated atrial electrogram with

an A to V ratio of 1 : 2 to 1 : 6. At stable target sites, radiofrequency energy is applied during normal sinus rhythm. We prefer to use ablation catheters with temperature feedback and to deliver radiofrequency energy in a ramped fashion; the power control mode is started at 15 to 20 W, and energy increases until 45°C to 50°C is obtained. Despite the ablation catheter being positioned posteriorly, we and others (88) have observed several instances in which even relatively low-energy application leads to transient AV block, presumably because the compact AV node is posteriorly displaced. In general, if radiofrequency energy is discontinued immediately on development of AV block, AV conduction returns to normal without any permanent AV nodal damage. During radiofrequency ablation, we monitor the temperature at the tip of the ablation catheter and the occurrence of enhanced junctional automaticity with 1 : 1 retrograde atrial conduction. If junctional complexes do not occur and the ablation temperature has reached 50°C, we discontinue the energy application and move the ablation catheter to a more anterior location. As the ablation catheter is moved anteriorly, the physician needs to be more cautious with energy application, and we usually start at a lower power.

The mechanism responsible for junctional complexes is not completely understood, but it appears to involve heating the junctional tissue and increasing the phase 4 automaticity of junctional cells. Junctional complexes appear to be a necessary but not sufficient condition for ablation success (94). Rarely, success is achieved without junctional complexes (95). Junctional rhythm should be accompanied by intact fast-pathway, retrograde conduction. Failure of a junctional beat to conduct to the atrium often portends the development of AV block and requires immediate discontinuation of energy application. A technical dilemma ensues when a patient has relatively poor retrograde, fast-pathway conduction (often as the result of sedation). Immediately before energy application, we assess VA conduction with incremental ventricular pacing. Poor retrograde conduction shifts our approach to one of two strategies. A low dose of isoproterenol can be infused. Unfortunately, this can result in hyperdynamic myocardial contraction and catheter instability. Alternatively, we apply radiofrequency energy as before, but as soon as junctional complexes occur, we pace the high right atrium at a rate faster than the junctional rate. We continue radiofrequency application during atrial pacing with close attention to AV conduction. If there is any prolongation of the PR interval or any development of a nonconducted atrial beat, the delivery of radiofrequency energy is immediately discontinued.

After the delivery of what appears to be a successful radiofrequency energy application, we retest the patient without and with isoproterenol to determine if AVNRT is inducible. We wait 30 to 60 minutes and retest to be certain that the ablation effects are not transient. In the early

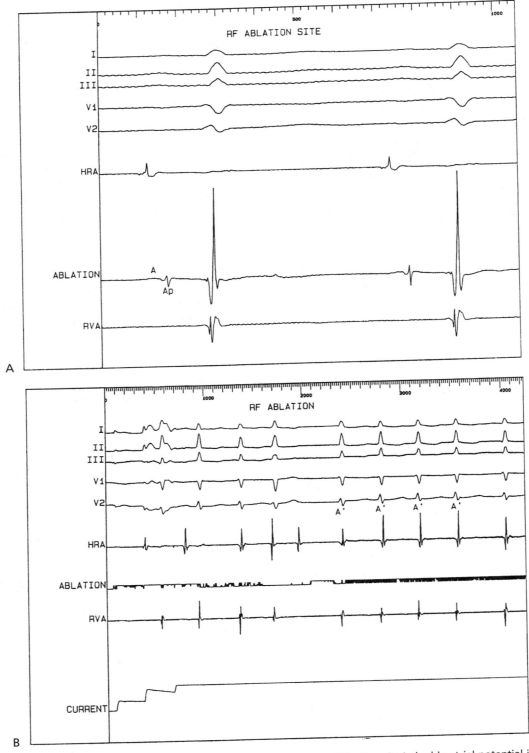

FIGURE 14-17. Atrioventricular (AV) nodal slow pathway modification. **A:** A double atrial potential is recorded on the distal bipolar electrode pair of the ablation catheter. The first low-amplitude potential (A) is thought to represent local atrial activation. The second, sharper potential (Ap) may represent activation of the posterior atrial inputs to the AV node. It is possible that the two atrial depolarizations occur because of anisotropic conduction. The first smaller deflection may represent transverse conduction, and the latter, more rapid deflection may represent longitudinal conduction. **B:** Delivery of radiofrequency energy at this site results in loss or markedly poor conduction over the slow pathway. A marker for success during ablation in this area is the occurrence of junctional beats associated with intact retrograde conduction to the atrium (A'). Junctional beats without retrograde conduction may indicate damage to the fast pathway, and continued energy delivery may result in complete heart block.

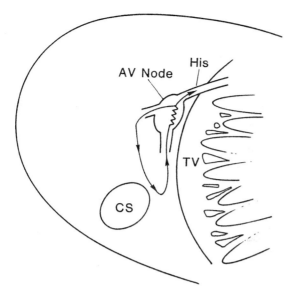

FIGURE 14-18. In this simplified model of the atrioventricular nodal reentrant tachycardia (AVNRT) reentrant circuit, the AV node has anterior and posterior atrial inputs. Based on the available data, we think that in most cases the anatomic substrate of AVNRT includes a small rim of posterior atrial tissue. As we learn more about AVNRT, this model will undoubtedly become more complex. (From Prystowsky EN, Klein GK. *Cardiac arrhythmias: an integrated approach for the clinician.* New York: McGraw-Hill, 1994:326, with permission.)

years of radiofrequency AV nodal modification, many investigators attempted to eliminate all evidence of slow-pathway conduction. However, later data from our group and others suggest that noninducibility and the presence of up to one AV nodal echo are associated with a very high cure rate with a low incidence of complications (96–99).

Approach to Therapy

AVNRT is the most common mechanism of PSVT. The AV node, rather than acting as a simple passive electrical conduit between the atrium and ventricle, has unique anatomic and electrophysiologic properties that allow it to be a critical part of the reentrant circuit. Pharmacologic and non-pharmacologic therapy are directed to selected components of the tachycardia circuit.

We recommend electrophysiologic testing to diagnose the mechanism of PSVT in patients with frequent or symptomatic episodes of tachycardia. Acute therapy for an episode of AVNRT should begin with methods to increase vagal tone such as carotid sinus massage or the Valsalva maneuver. The patient should be in a resting, supine position to enhance parasympathetic tone. If PSVT persists, intravenous adenosine or verapamil is given, which almost always restores sinus rhythm.

Chronic treatment can be palliative with drugs or curative with endocardial catheter ablation. We prefer to cure

patients and therefore recommend ablation as first-line therapy for almost all adult patients who have significant symptoms with AVNRT. Alternatively, the physician can prescribe drugs to try to prevent AVNRT. β-Adrenergic blockers, as well as verapamil and diltiazem, are often quite effective, usually more so than digitalis. Quinidine, disopyramide, flecainide, propafenone, and sotalol may also be given.

REFERENCES

1. Lewis T. Paroxysmal tachycardia. *Heart* 1909;1:43.
2. Barker PS, Wilson FN, Johnston FD. The mechanism of auricular paroxysmal tachycardia. *Am Heart J* 1943;4:435–445.
3. Retzer R. Quoted by Tawara : Ueber die musculose Verindung zwischen Vorhof und Ventrikel des Saugetierherzens. *Arch Anat Physiol Anat Abt* 1904;1:.
4. Tawara S. *Das Reizleitungssystem des Saugetierherzens: eine anatomisch-histologische Studie uber das Atrioventrikularbundel und die Purkinjeschen Faden.* Jena: G Fischer, 1906.
5. Koch W. Weitere Mitteilungen ueber den Sinusknoten des Herzens. *Verh Dtsch Ges Pathol* 1909;13:85–92.
6. Anderson RH. Histologic and histochemical evidence concerning the presence of morphologically distinct cellular zones with the rabbit atrioventricular node. *Anat Rec* 1972;173:7–24.
7. Sherf L, James TN, Woods WT. Function of the atrioventricular node considered on the basis of observed histology and fine structure. *J Am Coll Cardiol* 1985;5:770–780.
8. Thaemert JC. Fine structure of the atrioventricular node as viewed in serial sections. *Am J Anat* 1972;136:43–66.
9. Racker DK. Atrioventricular node and input pathways: a correlated gross anatomical and histological study of the canine atrioventricular junctional region. *Anat Rec* 1989;224:336–354.
10. De Mello WC. Passive electrical properties of the atrio-ventricular node. *Pflugers Arch* 1977;371:135–139.
11. Hoffman BF, Cranefield PF. The atrioventricular node. In: Hoffman BF, Cranefield PF, eds. *Electrophysiology of the heart.* New York: McGraw-Hill, 1960:132–174.
12. Paes de Carvalho A. Cellular electrophysiology of the atrial specialized tissues. In: Paes de Carvalho A, ed. *Symposium on the specialized tissues of the heart.* New York: Elsevier, 1961:115–129.
13. Hoffman BF, Paes de Carvalho A, Mello WC, Cranefield PF. Electrical activity of single fibers of the AV node. *Circ Res* 1958;7:11–18.
14. Billette J. Atrioventricular nodal activation during periodic premature stimulation of the atrium. *Am J Physiol* 1987;252:H163–H177.
15. Hoffman BF, Moore EN, Stuckey JH, Cranefield PF. Functional properties of the atrioventricular conduction system. *Circ Res* 1963;13:308–328.
16. Meijler FL, Janse MJ. Morphology and electrophysiology of the mammalian atrioventricular node. *Physiol Rev* 1988;68:608–647.
17. Langendorf R. Concealed AV conduction: the effect of blocked impulses on the formation and conduction of subsequent impulses. *Am Heart J* 1948;35:542–552.
18. Hoffman BF, Cranefield PF, Stuckey JH. Concealed conduction. *Circ Res* 1961;9:194–203.
19. Janse MJ. Influence of the direction of the atrial wave front on AV nodal transmission in isolated hearts of rabbits. *Circ Res* 1969;25:439–449.
20. Spach MS, Lieberman M, Scott JG, et al. Excitation sequences

of the atrial septum and the AV node in isolated hearts of the dog and rabbit. *Circ Res* 1971;29:156–172.

21. van Capelle FJL, Janse MJ, Varghese PJ, et al. Spread of excitation in the atrioventricular node of isolated rabbits hearts studied by multiple microelectrode recording. *Circ Res* 1972;31:602–616.

22. Mazgalev T, Dreifus LS, Iinuma H, Michelson EL. Effects of the site and timing of atrioventricular nodal input on atrioventricular conduction in the isolated perfused rabbit heart. *Circulation* 1984;70:748–759.

23. Zipes DP, Mendez C, Moe GK. Evidence for summation and voltage dependency in rabbit atrioventricular nodal fibers. *Circ Res* 1973;32:170–177.

24. Jais P, Haussaguerre M, Shah DC, et al. Successful radiofrequency ablation of a slow atrioventricular nodal pathway on the left posterior atrial septum. *Pacing Clin Electrophysiol* 1999;22:525–527.

25. Moe G, Preston JB, Burlington H. Physiologic evidence for a dual AV transmission system. *Circ Res* 1956;4:357–375.

26. Watanabe Y, Dreifus LS. Inhomogeneous conduction in the AV node. *Am Heart J* 1965;70:506–514.

27. Mendez C, Moe GK. Demonstration of a dual A-V nodal conduction system in the isolated rabbit heart. *Circ Res* 1966;19:378–393.

28. Mignone RJ, Wallace AG. Ventricular echoes—evidence for dissociation of conduction and reentry within the AV node. *Circ Res* 1966;19:636–648.

29. White P. A study of A-V rhythm following auricular flutter. *Arch Intern Med* 1915;16:516–535.

30. Schuilenburg RM, Durrer D. Atrial echo beats in the human heart elicited by induced atrial premature beats. *Circulation* 1968;37:680–693.

31. Schuilenburg RM, Durrer D. Ventricular echo beats in the human heart elicited by induced ventricular premature beats. *Circulation* 1969;40:337–347.

32. Rosen KM, Mehta A, Miller RA. Demonstration of dual atrioventricular nodal pathways in man. *Am J Cardiol* 1974;33:291–294.

33. Bigger JT, Goldreyer BN. The mechanism of supraventricular tachycardia. *Circulation* 1970;42:673–688.

34. Denes P, Wu D, Dhingra RC, et al. Demonstration of dual A-V nodal pathways in patients with paroxysmal supraventricular tachycardia. *Circulation* 1973;48:549–555.

35. Wu D, Denes P, Dhingra RC, et al. Determinants of fast and slow pathway conduction in patients with dual atrioventricular nodal pathways. *Circ Res* 1975;36:782–789.

36. Denes P, Wu D, Dhingra RC, et al. Dual atrioventricular nodal pathways—a common electrophysiological response. *Br Heart J* 1975;37:1069–1076.

37. Denes P, Wu D, Amat-y-Leon F, et al. The determinants of atrioventricular nodal reentrance with premature atrial stimulation in patients with dual A-V nodal pathways. *Circulation* 1977;56:253–259.

38. Wu D, Denes P, Amat-y-Leon F, et al. An unusual variety of atrioventricular nodal reentry due to retrograde dual atrioventricular pathways. *Circulation* 1977;56:50–59.

39. Sung RJ, Styperck JL, Myerburg RJ, Castellanos A. Initiation of two distinct forms of atrioventricular nodal reentrant tachycardia during programmed ventricular stimulation in man. *Am J Cardiol* 1978;42:404–415.

40. Akhtar M. Atrioventricular nodal reentrant tachycardia. *Med Clin North Am* 1984;68:819–830.

41. Josephson ME, Kastor JA. Supraventricular tachycardia: mechanisms and management. *Ann Intern Med* 1977;87:346–358.

42. Josephson ME. Supraventricular tachycardias. In: Josephson ME, ed. *Clinical cardiac electrophysiology*. Philadelphia: Lea and Febiger, 1993:269.

43. Wu D, Denes P, Amat-y-Leon F, et al. Clinical, electrocardiographic and electrophysiologic observations in patients with paroxysmal supraventricular tachycardia. *Am J Cardiol* 1978;41:1045–1051.

44. Josephson ME, Kastor JA. Paroxysmal supraventricular tachycardia: Is the atrium a necessary link? *Circulation* 1976;54:430.

45. Tebbenjohanns J, Niehaus M, Korte T, Drexler H. Noninvasive diagnosis in patients with undocumented tachycardias: value of adenosine test to predict AV nodal reentrant tachycardia. *J Cardiovasc Electrophysiol* 1999;10:916–923.

45a. Riva SI, Della Bella P, Fassini G, et al. Value of analysis of ST segment changes during tachycardia in determining type of narrow QRS complex tachycardia. *J Am Coll Cardiol* 1996;27:1480–1485.

45b. Gulec S, Ertab F, Karaoouz R, et al. Value of ST-segment depression during paroxysmal supraventricular tachycardia in the diagnosis of coronary artery disease. *Am J Cardiol* 1999;83:458.

45c. Paparella N, Ouyang F, Fuca G, et al. Significance of newly acquired negative T waves after interruption of paroxysmal reentrant supraventricular tachycardia with narrow QRS complex. *Am J Cardiol* 2000;85:261.

46. Pritchett ELC, Prystowsky EN, Benditt DG, Gallagher JJ. Dual atrioventricular nodal pathways in patients with the Wolff-Parkinson-White syndrome. *Br Heart J* 1980;43:7–13.

47. Sheahan RG, Klein GJ, Yee R. Atrioventricular node reentry with "smooth" AV node function curves: a different arrhythmia substrate? *Circulation* 1996;93:969–972.

48. Kertesz NJ, Fogel RI, Evans JJ, Prystowsky EN. Mechanisms of induction of atrioventricular node reentry by simultaneous conduction over fast and slow pathways. *Circulation* 1998;98:I-73.

49. Hwang C, Martin DJ, Goodman JS, et al. Atypical atrioventricular node reciprocating tachycardia masquerading as tachycardia using a left-sided accessory pathway. *J Am Coll Cardiol* 1997;30:218–225.

50. Cohn AE, Lewis T. The predominant influence of the left vagus nerve upon conduction between the auricles and ventricles in the dog. *J Exp Med* 1913;:239–247.

51. Prystowsky EN, Page RL. Electrophysiology and autonomic influences of the human atrioventricular node. In: *Electrophysiology of the sinoatrial and atrioventricular nodes*. Alan R Liss, 1988:259–277.

52. Lister JW, Stein E, Kosowsky BD, et al. Atrioventricular conduction in man—effect of rate, exercise, isoproterenol and atropine on the PR interval. *Am J Cardiol* 1965;16:516–523.

53. Levy MN, Zieske H. Autonomic control of cardiac pacemaker activity and atrioventricular transmission. *J Appl Physiol* 1969;27:465–470.

54. Prystowsky EN, Jackman WM, Rinkenberger RL, et al. Effect of autonomic blockade on ventricular refractoriness and atrioventricular nodal conduction in humans. *Circ Res* 1981;49:511–518.

55. Rahilly GT, Zipes DP, Naccarelli GV, et al. Autonomic blockade in patients with normal and abnormal atrioventricular nodal function. *Am J Cardiol* 1982;49[IV]:898.

56. Wellens HJJ, Durer DR, Liem KL, Lie KI. Effect of digitalis in patients with paroxysmal atrioventricular nodal tachycardia. *Circulation* 1975;52:779–788.

57. Mazgalev T, Dreifus LS, Michelson EL, Pelleg A. Effect of postganglionic vagal stimulation on the organization of atrioventricular nodal conduction in isolated rabbit heart tissue. *Circulation* 1986;74:869–880.

58. Wu D, Denes P, Baurnfeind R, et al. The effects of atropine on

induction and maintenance of atrioventricular nodal reentrant tachycardia. *Circulation* 1979;59:779–788.

59. Akhtar M, Damato AN, Batsford WP, et al. Induction of atrioventricular nodal reentrant tachycardia after atropine. *Am J Cardiol* 1975;36:286–291.

60. Brownstein SL, Hopson RC, Martins JB, et al. Usefulness of isoproterenol in facilitating atrioventricular nodal reentry tachycardia during electrophysiologic testing. *Am J Cardiol* 1988;61:1037–1041.

61. Wu D, Denes P, Dhingra RC, et al. The effects of propranolol on induction of A-V nodal reentrant paroxysmal tachycardia. *Circulation* 1974;50:665–677.

62. Sung RJ, Elser B, McAllister RG. Intravenous verapamil for termination of reentrant supraventricular tachycardia. *Ann Intern Med* 1980;93:682–689.

63. Rinkinberger RL, Prystowsky EN, Heger JJ, et al. Effect of IV and chronic oral verapamil administration in patients with a variety of supraventricular tachyarrhythmias. *Circulation* 1980;62:996–1010.

64. Reddy CP, McAllister RG. Effect of verapamil on retrograde conduction in atrioventricular nodal reentrant tachycardia. *Am J Cardiol* 1984;54:535–543.

65. Belardinelli L, Bellomi FL, Rubio R, Berne RM. Atrioventricular conduction disturbances during hypoxia. *Circ Res* 1980;47:684–691.

66. DiMarco JP, Sellers TD, Berne RM, et al. Adenosine: electrophysiologic effects and therapeutic use for terminating paroxysmal supraventricular tachycardia. *Circulation* 1983;68:1254–1263.

67. Wu D, Hung J, Kuo C, et al. Effects of quinidine on atrioventricular nodal reentrant paroxysmal tachycardia. *Circulation* 1981;64:823–831.

68. Shenasa M, Gilbert CJ, Schmidt DH, Akhtar M. Procainamide and retrograde atrioventricular nodal conduction in man. *Circulation* 1982;65:355–362.

69. Sethi KK, Jaishanka S, Khalilullah M, Gupta MP. Selective blockade of retrograde fast pathway by intravenous disopyramide in paroxysmal supraventricular tachycardia mediated by dual atrioventricular nodal pathways. *Br Heart J* 1983;49:532–543.

70. Brugada P, Wellens HJJ. Effects of intravenous and oral disopyramide on paroxysmal atrioventricular nodal tachycardia. *Am J Cardiol* 1984;53:88–92.

71. Bexton RS, Hellestems KJ, Nathan AW, et al. A comparison of the antiarrhythmic effects on AV junctional re-entrant tachycardia of oral and intravenous flecainide acetate. *Eur Heart J* 1983;4:92–102.

72. Niazi I, Naccarelli G, Dougherty A, et al. Treatment of atrioventricular node reentrant tachycardia with encainide: reversal of drug effect with isoproterenol. *J Am Coll Cardiol* 1989;13:904–910.

73. Garcia-Civera R, Sanjuan R, Morll S, et al. Effects of propafenone on induction and maintenance of atrioventricular nodal reentrant tachycardia. *Pacing Clin Electrophysiol* 1984;7:649–655.

74. Shen EN, Keung E, Huycke E, et al. Intravenous propafenone for termination of reentrant supraventricular tachycardia. *Ann Intern Med* 1986;105:655–661.

75. Chazov EI, Rosehshtraukh LV, Shugushev KK. Ethmozin: effects of intravenous drug administration on atrioventricular nodal reentrant tachycardia. *Am Heart J* 1984;108:483–489.

76. Sethi KK, Jaishanka S, Gupta MP. Salutary effects of intravenous ajmaline in patients with paroxysmal supraventricular tachycardia mediated by dual atrioventricular pathways: blockage of the retrograde fast pathway. *Circulation* 1984;70:876–883.

77. Mazgalev T, Dreifus LS, Bianchi J, Michelson EL. The mechanism of AV junctional reentry: role of the atrionodal junction. *Anat Rec* 1981;201:179–188.

78. Pritchett ELC, Anderson RW, Benditt DG, et al. Reentry within the atrioventricular node: surgical cure with preservation of atrioventricular conduction. *Circulation* 1979;60:440–446.

79. Holman WL, Ikeshita M, Lease JG, et al. Elective prolongation of atrioventricular conduction by multiple discrete cryolesions. *J Thorac Cardiovasc Surg* 1982;84:554–559.

80. Holman WL, Ikeshita M, Lease JG, et al. Alteration of antegrade atrioventricular conduction by cryoablation of peri-atrioventricular nodal tissue. *J Thorac Cardiovasc Surg* 1984;88:67–75.

81. Holman WL, Ikeshita M, Lease JG, et al. Cryosurgical modification of retrograde atrioventricular conduction. *J Thorac Cardiovasc Surg* 1986;91:826–834.

82. Ross DL, Johnson DC, Denniss AR, et al. Curative surgery for atrioventricular junctional ("AV nodal") reentrant tachycardia. *J Am Coll Cardiol* 1985;6:1383–1392.

83. Cox JL, Holman WL, Cain ME. Cryosurgical treatment of atrioventricular node reentrant tachycardia. *Circulation* 1987;76:1329–1336.

84. Sung RJ, Waxman HL, Saksena S, Juma Z. Sequence of retrograde atrial activation in patients with dual atrioventricular nodal pathways. *Circulation* 1981;64:1059–1067.

85. Haissaguerre M, Warin JF, Lemetayer P, et al. Closed-chest ablation of retrograde conduction in patients with atrioventricular nodal reentrant tachycardia. *N Engl J Med* 1989;320:426–433.

86. Epstein LM, Scheinman MM, Langberg JL, et al. Percutaneous catheter modification of the atrioventricular node. *Circulation* 1989;80:757–768.

87. Lee MA, Morady F, Kadish A, et al. Catheter modification of the atrioventricular junction with radiofrequency energy for control of atrioventricular nodal reentry tachycardia. *Circulation* 1991;83:827–835.

88. Jackman WM, Beckman KJ, McClelland JH, et al. Treatment of supraventricular tachycardia due to atrioventricular nodal reentry by radiofrequency catheter ablation of slow pathway conduction. *N Engl J Med* 1992;327:313–318.

89. Kay GN, Epstein AE, Dailey SM, Plumb VJ. Selective radiofrequency ablation of the slow pathway for the treatment of atrioventricular nodal reentrant tachycardia. *Circulation* 1992;85:1675–1688.

90. Wu D, Yeh S, Wang C, et al. A simple technique for selective radiofrequency ablation of the slow pathway in atrioventricular node reentrant tachycardia. *J Am Coll Cardiol* 1993;21:1612–1621.

91. Jazayeri MR, Hempe SL, Sra JS, et al. Selective transcatheter ablation of the fast and slow pathways using radiofrequency energy in patients with atrioventricular nodal reentrant tachycardia. *Circulation* 1992;85:1318–1328.

91a. Calkins H, Yong P, Miller JM, et al. Catheter ablation of accessory pathways, atrioventricular nodal reentrant tachycardia, and the atrioventricular junction: final results of a prospective, multicenter clinical trial. *Circulation* 1999;99:262.

92. Gamache C, Bharati S, Lev M, Lindsay B. Elimination of the slow pathway in atrioventricular nodal reentry by ablation of the posterior atrial approaches to the atrioventricular node: a histopathologic study. *Pacing Clin Electrophysiol* 1993;16:868(abst).

93. Keim S, Werner P, Jazayeri M, et al. Localization of the fast and slow pathways in atrioventricular nodal reentrant tachycardia by intraoperative ice mapping. *Circulation* 1992;86:919–925.

94. Thakur RK, Klein GJ, Yee R, et al. Junctional tachycardia: a useful marker during radiofrequency ablation for atrioventricu-

lar nodal reentrant tachycardia. *J Am Coll Cardiol* 1993;22: 1706.

95. Hseih MH, Chen SA, Tai CT, et al. Absence of junctional rhythm during successful slow-pathway ablation in patients with atrioventricular nodal reentrant tachycardia. *Circulation* 1998;98:2296–2300.

96. Manolis AS, Wang PJ, Estes NA III, et al. Radiofrequency ablation of slow pathway in patients with atrioventricular nodal reentrant tachycardia: do arrhythmia recurrences correlate with persistent slow pathway conduction or site of successful ablation? *Circulation* 1994;90:2815–2819.

97. Lindsay BD, Chung MK, Gamache C, et al. Therapeutic end points for the treatment of atrioventricular node reentrant tachycardia by catheter guided radiofrequency current. *J Am Coll Cardiol* 1993;22:733–740.

98. Chamberlain-Webber R, Hill JN, et al. Characteristics of successful posterior septal sites to cure atrioventricular node reentry using a thermistor controlled catheter system. *J Am Coll Cardiol* 1995;128A.

99. Prystowsky EN. Atrioventricular node reentry: physiology and radiofrequency Ablation. *Pacing Clin Electrophysiol* 1997;20 [Suppl II]:552–571.

15

ATRIAL FIBRILLATION

ARSHAD JAHANGIR
THOMAS M. MUNGER
DOUGLAS L. PACKER
HARRY J. G. M. CRIJNS

DEFINITION OF ATRIAL FIBRILLATION

The World Health Organization–ISFC task force's electrocardiographic (ECG) definition of atrial fibrillation (AF) is "an irregular, disorganized, electrical activity of the atria" (1). P waves are absent and the baseline consists of irregular waveforms, which continuously change in shape, duration, amplitude, and direction. Because the atrial rate is irregular, the ventricular response also is irregular. However, a regular ventricular rhythm does not exclude AF as a regular (sub)nodal focus or an artificial pacemaker rhythm may be present.

Classification of AF

AF may be classified according to its temporal presentation, mode of induction, attack rate, cause, and response to therapy. In the literature, there is no consensus concerning the classification of AF. Classification is essential to precisely delineate severity and variety of symptoms and their clinical consequences, as well as to enhance the evaluation of treatment strategies. The standard temporal classification includes a paroxysmal and a chronic form. However, the term *chronic* does not cover the temporal pattern comprehensively. After an initial attack of the arrhythmia, it will usually recur (2,3). This means that even paroxysmal AF is a chronic condition. Also, it is difficult to differentiate paroxysmal from chronic on first presentation. Usually, the type becomes clear only after follow-up.

A clinically useful classification is the so-called *3-P classification* proposed by Sopher and Camm (4).

1. AF that terminates spontaneously, with restoration of sinus rhythm, is defined as *paroxysmal*.

A. Jahangir, D. L. Packer, T. M. Munger: Department of Cardiology, Mayo Foundation, Rochester, Minnesota 55902.

H. J. G. Crijns: Department of Cardiology, University Hospital Groningen, 9700 RB Groningen, The Netherlands.

2. AF that can be successfully cardioverted, with the restoration of sinus rhythm, is indicated as *persistent*.
3. AF that is completely refractory to reversion or is allowed to continue it is classified as *permanent*. AF is therefore the underlying rhythm of choice for the patient.

The prevalence of intermittent or paroxysmal AF varies from 22% to 65% based on the population studied (5,6). About one fourth of the patients who have paroxysmal episodes progress to more persistent forms (6). The presence of valvular heart disease, left atrial or ventricular enlargement, ventricular hypertrophy, or systolic dysfunction increases the risk of progression to permanent AF (7).

The 3-P classification is based on the temporal pattern of the arrhythmia and the response to treatment and may be used regardless of the cause or symptoms. Most clinicians intuitively follow this classification because it matches with clinical practice. One must consider that with time, the arrhythmia may change from paroxysmal to persistent or permanent AF.

The duration of AF determines not only spontaneous conversion to sinus rhythm but also pharmacologic conversion (8) and the need for periconversion anticoagulation; 48 hours is important because beyond that point, oral anticoagulation is indicated if cardioversion is contemplated.

Paroxysmal AF may remain paroxysmal for a prolonged time, but it usually terminates within 24 to 48 hours (8,9). If left untreated, almost all cases of paroxysmal AF terminate spontaneously within 7 days; it is extremely rare that AF would still terminate spontaneously beyond 7 days (10). In a population admitted to the hospital, Danias and colleagues (9) found that almost 70% of those with AF for less than 72 hours converted spontaneously, with the highest conversion rate in patients with an arrhythmia duration of less than 24 hours. The arrhythmia duration was the only independent determinant of spontaneous conversion, whereas atrial size and ventricular function were not.

Therefore, with paroxysmal AF, the arrhythmia trigger is more important than the perpetuating substrate; that is, the atria are unable to harbor sufficient reentrant circuits to sustain AF. On the other hand, many patients with paroxysmal AF revert to persistent AF. Godtfredsen (11) found that 30% of patients with paroxysmal AF develop a chronic or persistent pattern within a few years. This suggests that AF is a progressive disease, which may be dictated by the underlying disease. However, more recently it has become clear that arrhythmia-related electrical, structural, and molecular remodeling also play a role (12–14).

EPIDIMIOLOGY OF AF

Age- and Gender-Specific Prevalence of AF

AF is the most common sustained cardiac arrhythmia encountered in clinical practice, affecting more than 2 million people in the United States (15–17). The incidence of AF strongly depends on age, with approximate doubling of incidence with each decade of life and a sharper rise in incidence in the very elderly (15–22) (Table 15-1 and Fig. 15-1A, B). AF is present in 0.4% of the general population, 2% to 3% of people older than 40 years, and 8% to 9% of those older than 80 years (15,22). The median age of individuals with AF is approximately 75 years, with two thirds occurring in individuals between 65 and 85 years of age, a group representing 11% of the U.S. population (21). The frequency of AF, for unclear reasons, appears to be increasing, independent of age and other risk factors (23). It is expected that with the aging of the population and improved survival of patients with myocardial infarction and heart failure, the number of patients with AF will continue to increase.

The incidence of AF at all ages is greater in men than women (17,18,20,23) (Table 15-1). However, because there are many more women than men older than 75 years in the general population, the absolute number of women in the elderly age group with AF is greater than the number of men (24). Approximately 60% of people with AF older than 75 years are women (21).

ETIOLOGY AND PREDISPOSING FACTORS

There are many etiologic factors that may be responsible for the occurrence of AF, explaining its frequency in the population. These include disease processes that cause changes of the atrial myocardium including distention, inflammation, hypertrophy, ischemia, fibrosis, or infiltration. There are normal age-related changes of the myocardium, perhaps accounting for the increased incidence of AF in the elderly. In most cases, AF occurs as a consequence of underlying cardiovascular disease, and in only a few cases is there no clinical or subclinical evidence of structural heart disease (19). The most powerful predictors of development of AF include dilated cardiomyopathy and the presence of heart failure, valvular heart disease (rheumatic, myxomatous, or congenital), hypertension, myocardial infarction, and advanced age (20,25). The presence of left atrial enlargement, ventricular hypertrophy, or systolic dysfunction (on echocardiogram) is also associated with an increased risk of AF (26,27). Other cardiac abnormalities associated with an increased risk of AF include myocardial infarction, hypertrophic cardiomyopathy (28), sick sinus syndrome, and the Wolff-Parkinson-White (WPW) syndrome (29). AF is commonly observed after cardiac surgery, with an incidence after coronary artery bypass surgery of 15% in patients

TABLE 15-1. INCIDENCE OF ATRIAL FIBRILLATION RELATED TO AGE AND SEX

Age (y)	Framingham (15,20) (N = 5,070) All	Western Australia (18) (N = 1,770) Men	Women	All	Rochester, MN (17) (N = 2,122) Men	Women	All	Cardiovascular Health Study (19) (N = 5,201) Men	Women	All
35–39	—	—	—	—	0	0	0	—	—	—
40–44	0.1	—	—	—	0	0	0	—	—	—
45–49	0.1	—	—	—	0.5	0.5	0.5	—	—	—
50–54	0.5	—	—	—	0.5	0.5	0.5	—	—	—
55–59	0.5	—	—	—	1.0	1.5	1.2	—	—	—
60–64	1.8	1.1	2.3	1.7	1.0	1.5	1.2	—	—	—
65–69	1.8	3.3	2.7	3.0	6.0	3.0	4.6	5.9	2.8	4.0
70–74	4.8	8.6	5.5	7.0	6.0	3.0	4.6	5.8	5.9	5.8
75–79	4.8	15.0	8.4	11.6	16.1	12.2	13.7	5.8	5.9	5.8
≥80	8.8	15.0	8.4	11.6	16.1	12.2	13.7	8.0	6.7	7.3

Note: Age-groups in the Framingham Study, in years, were 40–49, 50–59, 60–69, 70–79, and 80 or older. Age-groups in the Western Australia survey, in years, were 60–64, 65–69, 70–74, and 75 or older. Age-groups in the Rochester survey, in years, were 35–44, 45–54, 55–64, 65–74, and 75 or older. Age-groups in the Cardiovascular Health Study, in years, were 65–69, 70–79, and 80 or older.

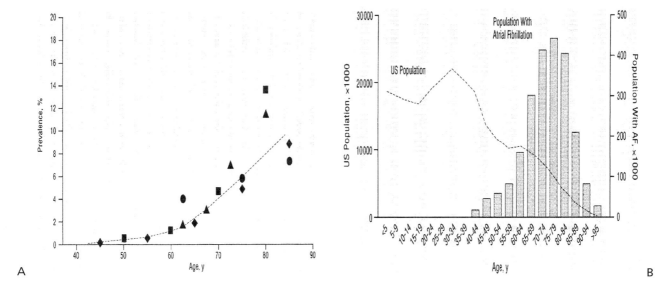

FIGURE 15-1. A: The values are plotted at the midpoint of the age range—i.e., the prevalence of atrial fibrillation from ages 60 to 69 years is plotted at 65 years. Prevalence for "over age 75 years" is plotted at 80 years. Prevalence for "over age 80 years" is plotted at 85 years. Also shown are the estimated prevalence values (*dotted line*) used to calculate absolute numbers of people with atrial fibrillation. Values are shown for the (*diamonds*) Framingham Study; the (*circles*) Cardiovascular Health Study; the (*squares*) Mayo Clinic Study, Rochester, Minnesota; and for (*triangles*) Busselton, Western Australia. **B:** Bars indicate numbers of people (×10³) with atrial fibrillation per 5-year age group (*right axis*). Dotted line indicates U.S. population (×10³) per 5-year age group (*left axis* 1991 census data). (From Feinberg WM, Blackshear JL, Laupacis A, et al. Prevalence, age distribution, and gender of patients with atrial fibrillation. Analysis and implications. *Arch Intern Med* 1995;155[5]:469–473, with permission.)

younger than 65 years to up to 30% in those older than 65 years (30). After valve replacement, the incidence of AF rises to 50% to 60% (30). In the Framingham Heart Study of 5,000 men and women followed biennially for 24 years or until death, rheumatic heart disease was the most powerful predictor of AF, followed by heart failure, hypertensive heart disease (hypertension with left ventricular hypertrophy on the ECG or cardiomegaly), and coronary heart disease (Table 15-2).

Although rheumatic mitral valve disease is the strongest precursor of AF, its present-day rarity in developed countries makes it accountable for only a very small proportion of the total cases. Indeed, overt cardiovascular disease in the Framingham Heart Study accounted for only 25% of cases of AF. The remaining patients presumably developed the arrhythmia as a result of hypertension without cardiomegaly or ECG evidence of hypertrophy or of other occult or noncardiac causes.

TABLE 15-2. RISK OF DEVELOPMENT OF ATRIAL FIBRILLATION (AF) BY CARDIOVASCULAR (CV) DISEASE STATUS IN 2,326 MEN AND 2,866 WOMEN AFTER 24 YEARS OF FOLLOW-UP IN THE FRAMINGHAM STUDY[a]

Predisposing Cardiovascular Disease	Chronic AF		Transient AF	
	Men	Women	Men	Women
Coronary heart disease	2.2[b]	0.5[c]	2.1[b]	4.5[b]
Hypertensive CV disease	4.7[b]	4.0[b]	4.4[b]	4.6[b]
Cardiac failure	8.5[b]	13.7[b]	8.2[b]	20.4[b]
Rheumatic heart disease	9.9[b]	27.5[b]	7.6[b]	24.3[b]
Any cardiovascular disease	3.2[b]	4.8[b]	4.4[b]	5.4[b]

[a]Two-year age-adjusted risk ratio. All patients with coronary heart disease, defined as prior infarction and angina, are included regardless of coexistence of other risk factors such as hypertension. Hypertensive cardiovascular disease is defined as hypertension with either evidence of left ventricular hypertrophy by cardiomegaly on x-ray or cardiac failure.
[b]$p < 0.05$.
[c]Not significant.

Several noncardiac disorders also increase the risk of AF, including hyperthyroidism (31), diabetes mellitus (20), and alcohol ingestion in some studies (19,20,32), and with increased vagal or sympathetic tone in susceptible individuals. Severe infection, pulmonary pathology, and massive pulmonary embolism may also contribute to AF occurrence (33). Potential contributors to the occurrence of AF are summarized in Table 15-3.

Lone AF

AF in the absence of recognizable structural heart disease or precipitating illnesses is referred to as *idiopathic AF* or *lone AF*. The reported prevalence of lone AF varies from 1.6% to 31%, depending on the definitions used in various studies and the intensity of investigation to identify underlying

TABLE 15-3. CARDIOVASCULAR AND NONCARDIOVASCULAR PRECIPITANTS OF ATRIAL FIBRILLATION

Atrial pressure elevation
  Mitral or tricuspid valve disease
  Myocardial disease (primary or secondary, leading to systolic or diastolic dysfunction)
  Semilunar valvular abnormalities (causing ventricular hypertrophy)
  Systemic or pulmonary hypertension (pulmonary embolism)
  Intracardiac tumors or thrombi
Atrial ischemia
  Coronary artery disease
Inflammatory or infiltrative atrial disease
  Pericarditis
  Amyloidosis
  Myocarditis
  Age-induced atrial fibrotic changes
Intoxicants
  Alcohol
  Carbon monoxide
  Poison gas
Increased sympathetic activity
  Hyperthyroidism
  Pheochromocytoma
  Anxiety
  Alcohol
  Exertion-induced
  Drugs
Increased parasympathetic activity
Primary or metastatic disease in or adjacent to the atrial wall
Postoperative
  Cardiac and pulmonary surgery
  Pericarditis
  Cardiac trauma
  Hypoxia
  Pneumonia
Congenital heart disease
  Particularly atrial septal defect
Neurogenic
  Subarachnoid hemorrhage
  Nonhemorrhagic, major stroke
Idiopathic

cardiovascular disease (33–36); approximately 30% to 40% of paroxysmal and 20% of persistent or chronic patients do not have a demonstrable underlying disease (3,37). In the Framingham Heart Study, in which hypertensive patients were not excluded and the mean age of the population was 70 years, the prevalence of lone AF was reported as 11%, with stroke risk four times that of baseline (34). However, in population-based studies, with exclusion of patients older than 60 years, the prevalence of lone AF is much lower (2.7%) with a more benign outcome without any excessive increase in stroke risk (35).

Acute Myocardial Infarction

AF is rarely a manifestation of an acute ischemic event and is not precipitated by angina or an acute myocardial infarction unless heart failure or pericarditis is also present. A common misperception is that patients who present to the emergency department with asymptomatic AF might have ischemia or myocardial infarction that is silent. This is not usually the case, and unless there are symptoms or ECG evidence of ischemia, these patients need not be admitted for suspected myocardial infarction.

However, AF complicates acute myocardial infarction in about 10% of cases; the incidence is higher when congestive heart failure (CHF) is present (20% versus 9% without CHF) (38). AF results in longer hospitalization and a more complicated hospital course than those for patients in sinus rhythm (25,39). Older age, higher peak creatine kinase levels, increased heart rate, presence of heart failure, and worse Killip class, more severe coronary artery disease, poorer reperfusion, and a lower ejection fraction are all associated with the development of AF after myocardial infarction (25,39,40). A history of hypertension, cerebrovascular disease, diabetes mellitus, and female gender are also predictive of AF in this setting (25).

The risk of in-hospital death, stroke, reinfarction, cardiogenic shock, heart failure, ventricular arrhythmia, and conduction disturbances, including asystole, is higher in patients who develop AF compared with those in sinus rhythm (25). This might be a reflection of a higher risk population with more ischemia caused by severe underlying coronary artery disease, lesser reperfusion or poor ventricular function combined with hemodynamic compromise from more severe ischemia, and the loss of atrial contraction. In one multivariant analysis, AF was not found to be an independent risk factor for death, but it was associated with older age, CHF, or cardiogenic shock, which are themselves factors for increased mortality rates.

Although development of AF has been associated with poor short-term outcome and increased mortality rates, the impact of AF on long-term mortality rates after acute myocardial infarction is controversial (41,42). An analysis of patients enrolled in the Global Utilization Streptokinase and Tissue Plasminogen Activator for Occluded coronary Arteries (GUSTO) I trial demonstrated that in-hospital, 30-day, and 1-year mortality rates were higher in those who developed AF after myocardial infarction than in those in sinus rhythm or with chronic AF (25). This was also observed in the TR Andolapril Cardiac Evaluation study in which AF, particularly when sustained, was associated with an increased 5-year mortality rate (relative risk, 1.3); this association persisted after adjusting for prognostic characteristics such as use of thrombolytic therapy, age, history of diabetes or hypertension, prior myocardial infarction, or CHF (38).

Rheumatic Valvular Heart Disease

The association between AF and rheumatic heart disease, particularly mitral stenosis or mitral regurgitation, is well established; AF is estimated to occur in about 40% of patients with mitral stenosis and 75% of those with mitral regurgitation (43). There is, however, no association between AF and mitral valve area, pulmonary artery wedge pressure, and total pulmonary vascular resistance, but there is an association with age and duration of mitral stenosis (44). In such patients, clinical factors associated with AF are increased left atrial size, P-wave abnormality on the ECG, PR-interval prolongation, and atrial premature beats. The occurrence of AF in patients with mitral valve disease often results in severe symptoms and a rapid clinical deterioration, often prompting surgical intervention.

AF is less commonly seen with aortic valve disease, unless CHF is present, and its occurrence suggests coexisting mitral valve disease (43). Isolated right-sided valvular lesions are much less frequently associated with AF, although the prevalence of AF related to right-sided lesions is unknown. Other nonrheumatic valvular causes of AF include congenital valve disease, mitral valve prolapse, and chordal or papillary muscle rupture. Endocarditis may provoke AF, particularly when it causes mitral regurgitation. However, endocarditis occurring in patients with AF is unusual.

Cardiomyopathy

There is a significant incidence of AF in patients with a dilated, congestive cardiomyopathy regardless of the cause; it is estimated to occur in 15% to 30% of patients during the course of their disease (20,45,46). In the Framingham Heart Study, heart failure was the most powerful independent predictor of AF, with a relative risk of approximately sixfold (20). Left ventricular dysfunction, even in the absence of symptoms, is predictive of AF (27). However, in most cases, AF is the result of heart failure and associated mitral or tricuspid regurgitation. The occurrence of AF in such patients often results in exacerbation of left ventricular dysfunction and CHF, because of the loss of atrial contraction and the rapid heart rate.

Other causes of cardiomyopathy are also associated with AF. These include Chagas disease, hemochromatosis, and

tumor or amyloid infiltration, particularly when these conditions involve the atrial myocardium (47). Senile amyloidosis of the left atrium has been implicated as a factor related to the increased incidence of AF in the elderly (48).

Hypertrophic Cardiomyopathy

Among patients with hypertrophic cardiomyopathy in which the left ventricle is significantly hypertrophic, stiffened, and noncompliant, similar to the situation with left ventricular hypertrophy caused by hypertension, AF may occur in up to 30% of cases; although episodes of AF are often brief and asymptomatic, this arrhythmia can result in substantial deterioration of functional status because of the loss of atrial contribution to ventricular filling, precipitating heart failure (28,49). In some patients, mitral regurgitation may also be present, another factor responsible for AF. The risk of thromboembolism with AF is also increased in this population. Although it has been suggested that AF in patients with a hypertrophic cardiomyopathy is of prognostic importance, this is controversial (28,50).

Sick Sinus Syndrome

Sinus node dysfunction, commonly termed *sick sinus syndrome,* involves a disorder of sinus node automaticity or sinoatrial conduction (51). It actually represents a spectrum of abnormalities; one form known as a *tachycardia-bradycardia syndrome* presents with a tachycardia (most commonly AF) that terminates abruptly and is followed by a long offset pause before the resumption of sinus rhythm (52). It is because of this offset pause and the resulting bradycardia that syncope may occur. Another form is a sinus bradycardia resulting in an escape tachyarrhythmia, often AF, known as a *bradytachycardia syndrome.*

Often a sick sinus syndrome is a part of general conduction system disease that also involves the AV node; when AV nodal involvement is also present, AF is associated with a slow ventricular response, even in the absence of AV nodal blocking drugs (53). It has been suggested that chronic AF is part of the natural history of a sick sinus syndrome, representing an end-stage rhythm, and that many patients, particularly the elderly, who are felt to have lone AF actually have a sick sinus syndrome as the underlying cause (53,54).

Many causes of sinus node dysfunction are identical to those of AF, making it difficult to distinguish between these two conditions.

Wolff-Parkinson-White Syndrome

It has been reported that 10% to more than 35% of patients with a preexcitation syndrome, particularly WPW, develop AF (55,56). Several factors predispose to WPW development, including closely coupled atrial premature and spontaneous ventricular premature beats, which may be conducted retrogradely by way of the accessory pathway, activating the atria (55). Impulses conducted by way of the accessory pathway can collide with those originating from the sinus node, setting up the potential for multiple wavefronts and hence AF (55). There is evidence that patients with WPW have intraatrial conduction abnormalities. The presence of antegrade conduction over the accessory pathway that has a short refractory period facilitates the occurrence of AF; after interruption of the accessory pathway, the incidence of AF is decreased (29,57). In patients with WPW, an atrioventricular (AV) reentrant tachycardia induced in the electrophysiology laboratory has been observed to degenerate into AF in approximately 15% of cases, and it is often precipitated by a premature beat occurring during the tachycardia (57,58). Excitation contraction feedback has also been suggested as a possible mechanism (59). When a reentrant tachycardia occurs, there is an increase in atrial pressure and volume. This stretch shortens the atrial refractory period and increases intraatrial conduction time, appropriate preconditions for establishing multiple reentrant circuits and AF.

In some patients with WPW syndrome, rapid conduction over the accessory pathway during AF may result in extreme ventricular rates and degeneration into ventricular fibrillation may occur in some patients, causing sudden death (60,61).

AF after Cardiac Surgery

AF is a common complication after cardiac surgery and is associated with an increased morbidity rate and prolonged hospital stay, because of hemodynamic compromise, increased risk of heart failure, thromboembolic events, and anticoagulant-related hemorrhagic complications (62). AF occurs in 15% to 33% of patients after coronary artery bypass surgery and in 38% to 64% after cardiac valvular surgery (30,63). The precise cause of postoperative AF is not known, but excessive catecholamine levels, along with pericardial inflammatory reaction, alterations in neurohormonal, and other metabolic factors, play a major role. Advanced age, presence of mitral stenosis, and left atrial enlargement independently predict the risk of AF in the postoperative setting (64).

The greater susceptibility to AF after valvular surgery reflects increased prevalence of structural and hemodynamic abnormalities such as atrial enlargement and fibrosis from aging and the long-standing valve disease. Usually postoperative AF is self-limited and more than 95% of patients who develop *de novo* AF after cardiac surgery are in normal sinus rhythm within 2 months after surgery (65).

Alcohol

Alcohol has long been suspected as a cause of AF in those with and without heart disease (66–68). It has been observed that most hospital admissions or emergency department visits for atrial arrhythmias occurred during weekends or holidays when alcohol intake was more marked. This was termed the *holiday heart syndrome* (32).

Alcohol can cause AF by several mechanisms including its acute effects on atrial refractoriness and conduction, as well as from the cumulative depressive effects of chronic alcohol consumption on myocardial function (69,70).

Alcohol may alter sympathetic and parasympathetic inputs into the heart, important factors in arrhythmogenesis. Although these may result from a direct effect of alcohol, autonomic changes, particularly activation of the sympathetic nervous system, generally accompany alcohol withdrawal.

Thyroid Abnormalities

Thyroid dysfunction, specifically hyperthyroidism, is frequently associated with AF (71); almost 3% of patients presenting to the emergency department with AF have hyperthyroidism as the cause, although the overall incidence of hyperthyroidism in patients with AF varies from 10% to 30%, and it is more common in the elderly (72). Hyperthyroidism in the elderly is often not obvious but is masked (apathetic hyperthyroidism). It has been suggested that many elderly patients with AF have occult or masked hyperthyroidism (73). It has also been observed that AF associated with hyperthyroidism is more common in patients older than 40 years (74).

The identification of hyperthyroidism as a precipitating factor of AF is important because there is evidence that with antithyroid therapy, 60% of patients may have spontaneous reversion of AF and maintenance of sinus rhythm (75). The conversion rate appears to be greater when hypothyroidism or a euthyroid state is produced more rapidly.

The mechanism for AF in hyperthyroidism is multifactorial, including the following:

1. A direct effect of thyroxin on the myocardium, resulting in a shortening of the action potential duration and the refractory period and an increase in automaticity.
2. An associated hypercatecholamine state that can directly cause arrhythmia or may do so indirectly by the development of hypertension and an increase in left atrial pressure and dimension.
3. Thyroxin causes an increase in β receptors and in adenyl cyclase activity, sensitizing the heart to the effect of circulating catecholamines (76).

Primary Electrical Abnormality

Primary electrical abnormality of the atrium with familial transmission of AF at a young age has also been recognized. Recently, abnormal genetic chromosomal loci have been identified at chromosome 10q (22–24) regions in three families with familial AF with autosomal dominant mode of inheritance (76a). However, the exact genetic abnormality in these patients remains undetermined.

PROGNOSTIC IMPLICATIONS OF AF

AF is a heterogeneous disorder with variable causes, clinical profiles, natural history, and outcomes. In patients with underlying cardiovascular disease, AF is associated with an approximate doubling of the all-cause mortality rate (77). Most of the excess mortality rate associated with AF is secondary to thromboembolic complications (15), deleterious effects on ventricular function (78), and proarrhythmia resulting from the use of antiarrhythmic medications (79). In the Framingham Heart Study, AF was a predictor of increased mortality rate, even after adjusting for several other risk factors of death including age, hypertension, smoking, diabetes, stroke or transient ischemic attacks (TIAs), myocardial infarction, heart failure, valvular heart disease, and ventricular hypertrophy (36). AF increased the likelihood of dying in all age groups, but the impact of AF on the risk of mortality was more prominent in women than men and the presence of AF diminished the female advantage in survival; the adjusted odds ratio for death with AF was 1.5 for men and 1.9 for women (36).

The mortality rate is low for patients without heart disease who have lone AF, which is most often paroxysmal (77). Unlike the Framingham data about permanent AF that was in general associated with heart disease, lone AF appears to have a benign prognosis (77). In the Framingham Heart Study, the annual mortality rate for patients without heart disease who had lone AF was 3.8% compared with 2.8% for patients without AF (15). However, after a mean follow-up of 8.5 years, cerebrovascular embolic events occurred in 2.8% of these patients, an incidence that was four to five times higher than that of the group without AF. Data from insurance companies suggest that mortality rate is fivefold higher in patients with lone AF that is chronic while mortality rate is not affected by the presence of paroxysmal AF. Lastly, the prognosis of lone AF is likely influenced by patient age, chronicity of the AF, and conversion from paroxysmal to chronic arrhythmia (80).

AF and the Development or Worsening of Heart Failure

One functional consequence of the fast and irregular atrial rhythm is that the atria are not contracting and hence the atrial contribution to ventricular filling (atrial kick) is lacking. Ventricular function becomes diminished because of rhythm irregularity and a shortened diastole (81,82). Cellular damage may contribute further to heart failure. This results from ventricular ischemia, calcium overload, and neurohumoral activation, particularly the induction of catecholamines and activation of the renin-angiotensin system (83,84).

AF could have adverse hemodynamic consequences in those with underlying left ventricular dysfunction and in those with normal left ventricular function because of the rapidity and the irregularity of the ventricular response (81,82,85). Reversible tachycardia-induced cardiomyopathy can occur in patients with AF and uncontrolled rapid ventricular response (86,87); ventricular function in these patients may improve with control of ventricular rate or reversion to sinus rhythm (88–90).

The extent to which AF causes heart failure in patients with previously normal ventricular function remains unclear. It is also not entirely clear whether the worse outcome observed in patients with AF in the presence of heart failure is merely a marker for more severe underlying disease or it actually influences overall prognosis and survival (91). Conflicting data have been reported from recent heart failure trials. In a study combining data from Vasodilator–Heart Failure Trial I and II, there was no adverse effect of AF on overall survival or incidence of sudden death in patients with mild to moderate heart failure treated with vasodilators (45). On the other hand, in a retrospective analysis of the Studies of Left Ventricular Dysfunction Prevention and Treatment Trials, AF in patients with asymptomatic and symptomatic left ventricular systolic dysfunction was associated with worsening of heart failure and an increased risk of all-cause mortality (78). This increase in overall mortality rate was largely a result of progressive heart failure and not arrhythmic death .

AF and Risk of Stroke

The risk of stroke in permanent AF varies greatly depending on age and coexisting disease (16,92). Because the prevalence of AF is much greater in the elderly, nonvalvular AF is the most powerful precursor of stroke in this population. As reported by the Framingham Heart Study, the risk of stroke in patients with nonrheumatic chronic AF is fivefold higher compared with that in patients in sinus rhythm, corresponding to a 4% to 5% annual incidence of stroke among those with AF (93).

The source of most emboli is the left atrium and its appendage. Most atrial thrombi are small and are often located within the trabeculated left atrial appendage, which in the fibrillating heart, is an important location for stagnation of blood, a predisposing factor for thrombus formation (94,95).

Compared with age-matched controls without AF, the risk of stroke is increased 17-fold in patients with permanent AF associated with rheumatic valvular disease and fivefold in those with nonrheumatic AF (93). The proportion of stroke resulting from AF increases steadily with age, rising from 6.5% for ages 50 to 59 years to approximately 31% for ages 80 to 89 years (16,93). The risk of stroke in patients with nonvalvular AF increases not only with advancing age, but also with the presence of hypertension, diabetes mellitus, female gender older than 75 years, previous TIAs or stroke, CHF, or presence of left ventricular dysfunction. Left atrial enlargement, mitral annular calcification, and increased left ventricular mass have been associated with a higher risk of stroke in some studies (27, 92,96,97). At least half of the strokes secondary to AF result in severe neurologic deficits or death (16,98). The risk of stroke in patients with AF younger than 65 years and none of the above risk factors is low (1% per year) and is similar to that of the general population (22,92).

The information regarding the risk of stroke has been derived mainly from patients with chronic or permanent AF; however, recent data suggest that the risk of thromboembolism is similar in patients with paroxysmal AF (22).

MORPHOLOGIC CHANGES IN THE ATRIUM PREDISPOSING TO AF

Despite varied causes, dilation of the atrium and increased fibrosis appear to be the common morphologic changes that result in the inhomogeneity of depolarization, conduction, and refractoriness of the atrial myocardium (99–102). During the normal aging process, various histologic changes occur within the atrium that also result in electrical inhomogeneity, including progressive proliferation of smooth muscle cells, increased deposition of elastic fibers and collagen with focal fibrosis, and deposition of amyloid within the atrial myocardium and the sinoatrial node (103). These changes and the reduced compliance of ventricles result in dilation of the atrium (100). Such changes predispose the atrium to inhomogeneous and slowed conduction, which increase nonuniform anisotropy and could result in AF (104).

In long-standing AF, further histologic changes are observed with fatty infiltration, loss of myofibrils, accumulation of glycogen, increase in mitochondrial size, and fragmentation of sarcoplasmic reticulum with myocyte hypertrophy and fibrosis (105,106). In a model of pacing-induced chronic AF, changes in protein expression similar to a dedifferentiation process, including reexpression of smooth muscle actin, decrease in cardiotoxin, and increase in titin have also been described (107). Structural changes in the atrium, some of which are reversible, not only increase predisposition to recurrent arrhythmias but also provide the substrate for prolonged atrial contractile dysfunction observed after cardioversion and restoration of sinus rhythm (105,108). The number of right atrial epicardial neurons in patients with long-standing AF is also decreased and could predispose to initiation or maintenance of AF by the autonomic nervous system (109,110).

Whether observed histologic changes in patients with long-standing AF represent underlying disease process and aging or are secondary to AF itself is not clear. The observation that restoration of sinus rhythm results in decrease in atrial volume independent of hemodynamic improvement does suggest that AF might contribute to the atrial myopathic changes including atrial enlargement (108,111).

ELECTROCARDIOGRAPHIC MANIFESTATIONS OF AF

The ECG diagnosis of AF is based on the presence of rapid, irregular, low-amplitude atrial activity with continuous variation in cycle length, morphology, and activation pattern of the fibrillatory waves. Because of the variable penetrance and conduction of the atrial impulses to the ventricles through the AV node, there is marked variability in ventricular cycle length. The ECG during AF could vary markedly among different patients and in the same patient at different times. Recent mapping studies have demonstrated variability of the actual local atrial activation responsible for these ECG manifestations. Three patterns of AF based on the atrial activation and temporal irregularity at any given site, representing a continuum of increasing complexities, have been described (112,113). Type I AF, which is most compatible with "coarse AF" seen on the surface ECG, exhibits the most homogenous activation pattern with a single broad wavefront, the least cycle length variation, the longest median fibrillatory cycle length, and only a few areas of slow conduction or conduction block. In contrast, type III AF, with the most complex activation pattern, exhibits multiple (three or more) simultaneously conducting fibrillatory wavelets within the mapping area with multiple areas of conduction block and slow conduction. The median fibrillatory interval (a measure of tissue refractoriness) is very short, with the greatest degree of beat-to-beat variation in cycle length. Type II AF is intermediate between type I and III with a single wave with longer or multiple lines of conduction block and/or slowing or with two wavelets simultaneously conducting across the mapping area. All three types of activation patterns could be present during a single episode of AF (112).

ELECTROPHYSIOLOGY OF AF

Three different electrophysiologic mechanisms for AF have been proposed (114) (Fig. 15-2):

1. Multiple reentrant wavefront simultaneously activating atria (115,116).
2. A single reentry circuit with variable rate and conduction within the atria or pulmonary veins (112,117;118).
3. Rapidly firing incoordinated ectopic foci within the atria or pulmonary veins (119–121).

It is now generally accepted that sustained AF commonly results from a critical number of simultaneously circulating reentrant wavelets that are dependent on the refractoriness

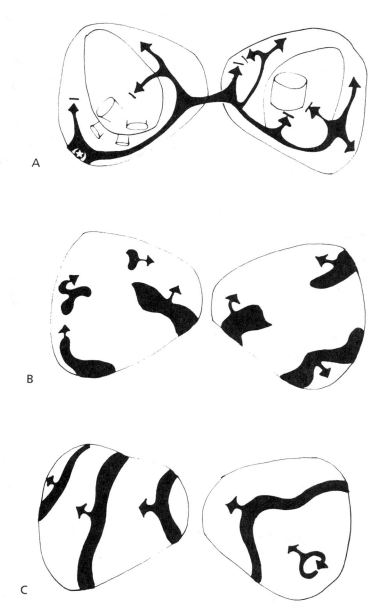

FIGURE 15-2. Schematic representation of different mechanisms that can result in atrial fibrillation. **A:** Rapid focal atrial tachycardia with fibrillatory conduction. **B:** Multiple wavelet reentry. **C:** Single microreentrant circuit. (From Janse MJ. Future prospects of antearrhythmic treatment based on experimental studies. *Eur Heart J* 1995;16[Suppl G]:2–6, with permission.)

and critical mass of the atrial tissue. The reentrant excitation could be a result of random reentry, in which a propagating wavelet reexcites an area that was previously excited by another wavelet, or leading circle reentry, in which the tissue is reexcited by the same wavefront that activated it before. Abnormal, rapidly discharging foci, particularly within the pulmonary veins, have been recently demonstrated to be the initiating mechanism in some patients (121).

Concept of Wavelength and AF

For reentry to occur, the reentrant impulse traveling around an area of block must be delayed enough to allow areas proximal to the block to recover from refractoriness. The wavelength of a circuit is defined as the minimum path length that can support reentry and is equal to the conduction velocity of the reentrant impulse around the circuit times the functional refractory period of the circuit (114, 122) (Fig. 15-3). The number of simultaneous reentrant circuits that can be accommodated in a given atrium thus depends on the wavelength, with a decrease in wavelength resulting in more circuits. A decrease in the wavelength below a critical level, either by slowing of conduction (depressed conduction or increased anisotropy) or by decrease in refractoriness, increases the propensity for reentry to be sustained. On the other hand, prolongation of wavelength by either accelerating conduction velocity or prolonging refractoriness favors termination of reentry and prevents its recurrence by decreases in the number of wavelets that can continue in the atrium at a time (123). The efficacy of various drugs in treating AF has been shown to correlate in the past with the changes in refractoriness and more importantly in wavelength that they produce at rapid rates (123,124) (Fig. 15-4). Similarly, by reducing the amount of excitable atrial tissue, either surgically or by catheter-based ablation procedures, one can decrease the number of reentrant fibrillatory wavelets to below the critical number needed to sustain AF, thus preventing its recurrence (118,125).

The Multiple-Wavelet Hypothesis

In 1962, Moe (126) proposed the multiple-wavelet hypothesis of AF, and later Moe and colleagues (116) in a com-

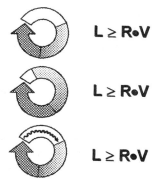

$$L \geq R \bullet V$$

$$L \geq R \bullet V$$

$$L \geq R \bullet V$$

FIGURE 15-3. Relation between refractory period, conduction velocity, and wavelength. The wavelength *(L)* for reentry is defined as the distance traveled by the depolarization wave during the refractory period and is equal to conduction velocity *(V)* times refractory period *(R)*. The number of simultaneous reentrant circuits that can be accommodated in a given atrium thus depends on the wavelength, with a decrease in wavelength resulting in a larger number of circuits.

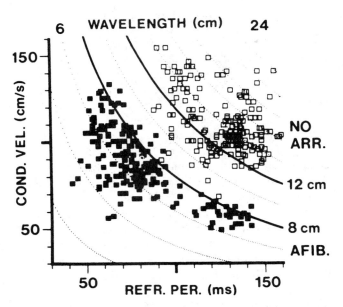

FIGURE 15-4. Relationship between induction of atrial arrhythmias, refractory period, conduction velocity, and wavelength of the initiating premature beat. Conduction velocity and refractory period were changed with drugs (acetylcholine, lidocaine, ouabain, propafenone, quinidine, sotalol) and atrial arrhythmia induction was attempted with programmed electrical stimulation. The predictive power of conduction velocity alone or refractory period duration alone for induction of arrhythmia was poor, as atrial arrhythmias could be induced over a wide range of refractory periods and conduction velocities. However, the wavelength correlated very well with inducibility of atrial arrhythmia, with clear separation of the inducible (*filled symbols*) and noninducible (*open symbols*) population. The critical wavelength where atrial arrhythmia was frequently induced was less than 8 cm, less frequently between 8 and 12 cm, and never more than 12 cm. (From Rensma PL, Allessie MA, Lammers WJ, et al. Length of excitation wave and susceptibility to reentrant atrial arrhythmias in normal conscious dogs. *Circ Res* 1988;62: 395–410, with permission.)

puter model with inhomogeneous refractoriness simulated fibrillation with irregular and tortuous impulse propagation, which was self-sustained and once initiated independent of the initiating event. The fibrillation in this model was reentrant with fractionation of wavefronts into multiple daughter wavelets around areas of conduction block, resulting in numerous microreentrant circuits. The persistence of fibrillation was dependent on the number of wavelets, which in turn depended on the tissue mass, refractoriness, and conduction velocity. Moe proposed that factors that increase the number of wavelets perpetuate arrhythmia, whereas those decreasing the number favor termination (127). Schyessler and colleagues confirmed this hypothesis in an acetylcholine-induced AF model and *in vivo* demonstrated multiple independently propagating wavelets causing AF (117). Each wavelet existed for a short period before extinction resulting from fusion or collision with other wavelets on reaching the border of the atria or refractory tissue with functional conduction block. New

wavelets were formed by division of a wave at a localized area of conduction block or by an offspring of waves traveling to the other atrium (115). At least in the dog atria, a critical number of four to six wavelets was required to maintain fibrillation (115). These results have been subsequently confirmed in humans using intraoperative mapping (118). Optical mapping and modeling studies have provided further insight into the complexity of the atrial architecture and the spatiotemporal discordance between endocardial and epicardial activation sequence and its contribution to excitation propagation and destabilization of reentrant wavefronts (128,129).

Electrical Remodeling of the Atrium

Paroxysmal AF becomes resistant to pharmacologic therapy as the duration of a paroxysm increases, often degenerating into a persistent form (130,131). In animal models of pacing-induced AF, the facilitative role of rapid atrial rate in the initiation and maintenance of sustained AF has been demonstrated; that is, "AF begets AF" (105,132). Artificial maintenance of AF results in prolongation of the individual paroxysms of AF and later development of sustained AF (132,133) (Fig. 15-5). The mechanisms underlying this increased susceptibility to AF is not fully understood but appears to be related to a progressive decrease in atrial refractoriness, increased heterogeneity in refractoriness within different regions of the atrium (134), and loss of the normal physiologic rate-dependent adaptation of refractoriness (132,135,136). Slowing of the conduction velocity also occurs within the atrium, but at a slower time course than changes in refractoriness (137). These changes in the electrophysiologic properties, termed *electrical remodeling* of the atrium (134,137), increase the vulnerability of the atrium to functional reentry. They are not only the cause but also the consequence of persistent rapid atrial rhythm, thus creating a condition in which AF perpetuates AF (132). The shortening of the refractory period, which occurs within minutes of rapid atrial pacing (138), and slowed conduction, which occurs after several days, promote AF by decreasing the wavelength, allowing continuation of multiple wavelets and stabilization of reentry (137). Similar electrophysiologic changes have been demonstrated in humans after induction of AF by programmed stimulation (138) and in patients with chronic AF (139–141). These electrophysiologic changes are reversible during the early stage with progressive normalization of refractoriness after restoration of sinus rhythm (132). These observations are the basis of the concept that prompt termination of an episode of AF—for example, by an atrial defibrillator—may prevent progressive remodeling of the atrium, slow the natural progression of the disease, and decrease the number of episodes of AF (142). Moreover, because these electrophysiologic changes persist for sometime after cardioversion, electrophysiologic conditions remain favorable for reinduc-

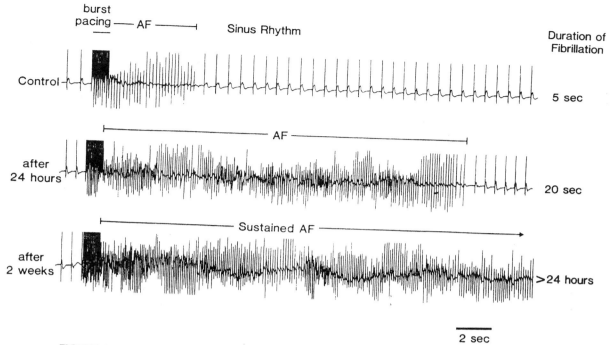

FIGURE 15-5. Prolongation of the duration of episodes of electrically induced atrial fibrillation (AF) after maintaining AF for 24 hours and 2 weeks. The three tracings show a single atrial electrogram recorded from the same goat during induction of AF by a 1-second burst of stimuli (50 Hz, four times the threshold). The goat **(top tracing)** has been in sinus rhythm all the time and AF self-terminated within 5 seconds. After the goat had been connected to the fibrillation pacemaker for 24 hours **(middle tracing)**, there was a clear prolongation of the duration of AF to 20 seconds. The **(bottom tracing)** was recorded after 2 weeks of electrically maintained atrial fibrillation. After induction of AF, this episode became sustained and did not terminate. (From Wijffels MCEF, Kirchhof CJHJ, Dorland R, Allessie MA. Atrial fibrillation begets atrial fibrillation: a study in awake, chronically instrumented goats. *Circulation* 1995;92:1954–1962, with permission.)

tion of AF immediately after cardioversion and may require more intense initial drug therapy to prevent reversion to AF (132,138,143).

Cellular Electrophysiology and Ionic Basis of Electrical Remodeling During AF

Substantial heterogeneity in action potential morphology and duration is present within different regions of the atrium (114), which is further increased during AF. At least three different types of action potential waveforms have been distinguished in atrial tissue (114). Cardiomyocytes with a distinct plateau or square action potential morphology, those without plateau or triangular action potential, and intermediate types have been demonstrated with variation in the amplitude and distribution of ionic currents (114,144) (Fig. 15-6). The decrease in refractoriness and the loss of rate adaptation of refractoriness in the atrium that occur with AF correlate with the reduction in action potential duration and its rate adaptation (145).

Although the mechanism of ionic changes and electrical remodeling is not fully understood, Ca^{2+} loading appears

to, at least partially, mediate some of the changes (146). Rapid atrial rates result in impairment of intracellular Ca^{2+} handling and a decrease in the rate of intracellular Ca^{2+} release, which has been suggested to contribute to decreased atrial contractility observed after restoration of sinus rhythm (147). Shortening of refractoriness with AF and increased propensity for reinduction of AF after conversion to sinus rhythm at least acutely could be blocked with verapamil and accentuated with hypercalcemia (146). Similarly, atrial contractile dysfunction after short-term AF can be reduced by verapamil and increased by the calcium agonist Bay K 8644 (148). Additional factors also play a role, because despite attenuation of pacing-induced changes in atrial refractoriness by verapamil, AF induction at least in the goat model is only minimally affected (149).

The role of atrial ischemia promoting AF is not clear and conflicting evidence exists as to whether atrial myocytes are ischemic during AF (148,150). Similarly, neurohumoral changes, including autonomic tone or concentration of atrial natriuretic factor, atrial stretch, or ischemia do not appear to play a significant role in the mediation of pacing-induced electrical remodeling (150).

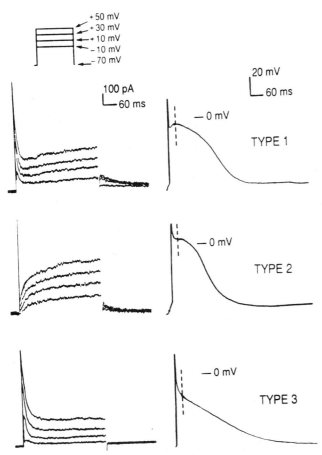

FIGURE 15-6. Variations among isolated human atrial myocytes in ionic currents **(left)** and action potential morphology **(right)**. Type 1 cells consistently have both I_k and I_{to} currents, type 2 cells only I_k currents, and type 3 cells only I_{to} currents. Ionic currents shown at the left were recorded from the same cells as the corresponding action potentials at the right. The consistent patterns suggest that variations in K^+ currents contribute importantly to action potential heterogeneity. (From Wang J, Bourne GW, Wang Z, et al. Comparative mechanisms of antiarrhythmic drug action in experimental atrial fibrillation. Importance of use-dependent effects on refractoriness. *Circulation* 1993;88:1030–1044, with permission.)

Focal AF

Although AF is commonly caused by microreentry, single or multiple rapidly discharging foci in the atrium or the pulmonary veins may activate the atrium irregularly and give the appearance of AF on the surface ECG (151). The rapid atrial rhythm could also generate conditions in the atrium that lead to microreentry and sustained AF. In experimental studies, local application of aconitine resulted in rapid atrial tachycardia, arising from a single focus at the site of application of the drug (119). Because of the rapidity of the focal discharge, uniform excitation of the remaining atrium is lost and rate-dependent conduction block develops, giving rise to "fibrillatory conduction" and irreg-

ularity in atrial activation. The presence of one or more sites of impulse generation from foci of enhanced automaticity during AF reduces the probability of simultaneous extinction of the wandering wavelets because of reinitiation of arrhythmia from the automatic focus (115). Thus, both mechanisms—a rapidly discharging ectopic focus (or foci) and multiple reentry—can coexist and cooperate in maintaining arrhythmia (115). These focal generators clinically become very important, as eliminating abnormal foci with catheter ablation provides the possibility of a cure in some patients with AF (121).

ROLE OF THE AUTONOMIC NERVOUS SYSTEM IN AF

The autonomic nervous system strongly affects initiation and persistence of AF and associated arrhythmia complaints. Several modalities of autonomic influence exist: vagal, adrenergic, and mixed.

Increases in parasympathetic or sympathetic nervous system activity can precipitate AF in certain patients, with vagal influences predominantly affecting patients with healthy hearts and adrenergic stimulation favoring microreentry or enhanced automaticity or triggered activity in patients with structural heart disease who have depressed vagal activity (152).

Parasympathetic Nervous System

The role of activation of the parasympathetic nervous system and acetylcholine in the initiation and perpetuation of AF has been recognized for a long time and has been used in experimental animal models to sustain AF (117, 153–155). Vagal stimulation may set the stage for reentry by shortening the wavelength through reduction of the atrial refractory period. Vagal effects on the refractory period are nonuniform, leading to dispersion of refractoriness.

Neurally released acetylcholine through activation of G-protein–gated potassium channels results in shortening of action potential duration and a decrease in refractoriness of the atrial myocardium (156,157). Because the distribution of vagal fibers within the atrium is inhomogeneous, the increase in vagal activity results in substantial dispersion of refractoriness in the atrium, which increases susceptibility to reentry and development of AF (158).

Vagal AF

Vagal AF usually starts in the night and stops during morning activities. It may also occur after stress, meals, or alcohol ingestion. Attacks may be terminated by exercise. The male-female ratio is 4 : 1 and the age at onset is 40 to 50 years. The syndrome of vagal fibrillation may be difficult to recognize because mixed forms that have adrenergic components exist. The absence of heart disease is considered typical for vagal fibrillation. It has been felt that in this situation, paroxysmal AF does not progress to chronic AF. Digoxin and β blockers, because of their vagotonic effects, may aggravate the syndrome. Class Ia agents may be particularly beneficial because of their vagolytic effects.

Holter monitoring studies have shown that the onset of the arrhythmia is preceded by mild bradycardia (a rate of less than 60 beats per minute [bpm]). Along with slowing of the sinus rate, premature atrial beats occur in increasing numbers. Initially, the attacks may be nonsustained with intermittent sinus rhythm for a few beats. The ventricular response usually is relatively low (100 to 120 bpm). Transition from fibrillation to flutter and flutter to fibrillation is not uncommon.

Sympathetic Nervous System

Increases in sympathetic nervous system activity (physical activity, emotional stress, or with hyperthyroidism or pheochromocytoma) can also result in AF in certain patients, although this is less common than parasympathetic influence (152). The exact mechanism by which the adrenergic system precipitates AF is not well understood. β-Adrenergic stimulation, by its direct effect on the myocardium and indirectly by the increase in heart rate or influence on cholinergic activity, results in reduction in the action potential duration, favoring development of AF (158). Sympathetic stimulation also enhances abnormal automaticity or triggered activity and, by the precipitation of focal atrial premature beats or atrial tachycardia, predisposes to or degenerates into AF (159). The interaction between the two autonomic systems, at the prejunctional and postjunctional level of the neuroeffector system, influences the electrophysiology of the atrium and may also play a facilitatory role in the initiation or maintenance of atrial arrhythmias (159).

Sympathetic AF

Adrenergic AF usually occurs in the daytime, particularly in the morning, during exercise, or periods of emotional stress. At rest, the arrhythmia tends to disappear. Most attacks terminate a few minutes after one has stopped exercising.

Adrenergic AF is usually preceded by an increase in the sinus rate. This increase is accompanied by atrial premature beats, often couplets and short salvos. Alternatively, a longer episode of regular tachycardia may precede the onset of AF. Flutter does not occur. The tachycardia may remain organized or convert to fibrillation. However, AF may be initiated by a single premature beat. The ventricular response usually is rapid, causing severe symptoms. β Blockers are the drugs of choice and patients usually are resistant to class Ia and Ic drugs. The response to amiodarone may vary.

THE HEMODYNAMICS OF AF

Although it has long been supposed that the loss of the "atrial kick" is the most important mechanism for altered cardiac function in AF, the hemodynamics of this arrhythmia are significantly more complicated, and multiple factors are responsible for changes in cardiac performance (Table 15-4). When considered together, these factors may result in a 15% to 25% decrease in stroke volume and cardiac output (160–163), a problem that may be significantly amplified by the presence of underlying heart disease; the emergence of AF may be causally related to the presence of underlying left ventricular dysfunction but in turn contributes to even greater functional myocardial impairment and accompanying symptoms.

The impact of AF on both exercise and resting cardiac output has also been examined in a number of studies conducted in catheterization laboratories (164). Conversion to sinus rhythm produced a 2% to 38% improvement in resting cardiac output and a 7% to 30% increase during exercise (165–170). The nature of the underlying disease of patients in some of these studies was highly variable and the observations made shortly after cardioversion. Because full restoration of atrial contraction may require several weeks, the magnitude of improvement may be even greater than previously thought.

Although there may be substantial interplay between contributors to hemodynamic impairment with AF, they are best understood when considered separately. First, the loss of atrial systole, as demonstrated in various studies, results in a decrease in cardiac output or transvalvular blood flow (171–175). The loss of this active process results in inadequate ventricular filling, particularly in the setting of rapid heart rates. This effect may be less critical in the absence of other underlying heart disease than when significant mitral valve disease or ventricular hypertrophy is present, associated with preexisting impediments to ventricular filling, in which the loss of atrial function can lead to marked hemodynamic deterioration (176).

Reductions in hemodynamic performance may also be related to a decreased interval of passive diastolic filling (177–179). With rapid ventricular rates, the diastolic interval

TABLE 15-4. CAUSES OF HEMODYNAMIC IMPAIRMENT IN ATRIAL FIBRILLATION

Loss of active atrial filling
Atrial stunning after cardioversion
Reduced passive filling time
Irregularity of cardiac cycles
Altered intrinsic myocardial contractility
Decreased restitution of ventricular contractility
Changes in sympathetic tone
Altered neurohumeral factors
Accompanying rate-related conduction abnormalities
Tachycardia-induced cardiomyopathy

of cardiac filling and coronary blood flow is foreshortened, contributing to an increase in wall stress and perhaps relative myocardial ischemia. It has been suggested that the reduction in ejection fraction that occurs with shorter R-R intervals in AF is not entirely compensated for by the increments in cardiac ejection accompanying longer R-R intervals (169,180).

Beyond the effect of a rapid ventricular response rate, the irregularity of cardiac activation also contributes to further impairment of ventricular function (167,180,181). This can be understood in terms of the dependency of stroke volume on the preceding R-R interval and its reverse dependency on the penultimate or pre-preceding R-R interval (167,178,182). Changes in ventricular ejection and cardiac output may be a result of beat-by-beat changes in preload. Acting by the Frank-Starling mechanism (183–185), longer preceding R-R intervals should be accompanied by larger end-diastolic volumes and augmented contraction. R-R-interval–dependent restitution of ventricular contractility or the interval-force relationship may also be operative when AF occurs (186–190) and may act in combination (182,191) with preload-dependent factors.

Post-extrasystolic potentiation and mechanical restitution also produce variations in left ventricular systolic performance over a broad range of AF intervals (183). However, this effect is likely to be dependent on the pre-preceding R-R interval. It is possible that the outflow from systolic activation may be greater in the setting of a short pre-preceding R-R interval in much the same way that an augmentation of contraction occurs with the beat after a premature complex (post-extrasystolic potentiation) (189). Other investigators have also provided evidence for an impact of mechanical restitution on beat-to-beat variation in hemodynamics in patients with chronic AF (191). These changes are manifested in the left ventricular dp/dt$_{max}$ and left ventricular ejection velocity integral (which is proportional to stroke volume) measured at the ascending aorta.

Other contributors to hemodynamic impairment may be operative. Abrupt changes in ventricular cycle length may have a direct effect on intrinsic myocardial contractility (179,180). With more rapid ventricular response rates, mitral regurgitation can occur. Although this process has been well described in the presence of other chronic supraventricular tachycardias, it appears to be less of an issue in the setting of AF, particularly if there is no underlying mitral valve disease (191). Neurohumoral and vasomotor factors may also be contributory (192–194). Increases in atrial natriuretic peptide may have an indirect effect on cardiac afterload. Increased sympathetic tone at the time of rapid ventricular response rates may similarly alter output through an afterload-incrementing mechanism. The emergence of bundle branch block during AF with rapid ventricular response rates could also modestly alter ventricular function at the most rapid rates.

Finally, in some patients with rapid ventricular response rates during a more prolonged time, tachycardia-induced

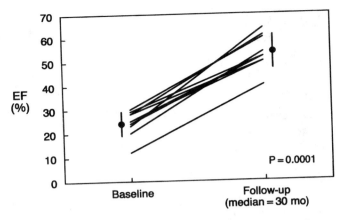

FIGURE 15-7. Improvement in tachycardia-induced cardiomyopathy after rate-controlled therapy for atrial fibrillation. At baseline, the injection fraction averaged 0.24 but rose to 0.52 at a median follow-up at 30 months.

cardiomyopathy may develop (86,87,195,196). In this situation, rapid heart rates likely result in effective subendocardial ischemia or depletion of high-energy phosphate substrates (197,198). This entity is manifest as a decrease in ejection fraction and a drop in stroke volume, related to increments in the end-diastolic and systolic volumes. Furthermore, its regression after restoration of sinus rhythm or slowing of heart rate is also well documented (86,199–202) (Fig. 15-7). Recent studies have demonstrated that this cardiomyopathic process reverses to a near-total extent during 1 month after control of tachycardia, although some patients continue to show slight ventricular dilation (200, 201,203). This improvement is also manifested by improvement in peak Vo$_2$ occurring during the same time frame. These changes require a longer time than the recovery of active atrial filling occurring within 1 to 2 weeks of restoration of sinus rhythm, indicating that simple improvement in atrial function is not the exclusive explanation for improvement in ventricular function (204).

Each of these factors may contribute to a patient's cardiac symptoms. In the absence of underlying heart disease, the many factors contribute little to hemodynamic deterioration. On the other hand, the additional impairment created by AF in patients with depressed ventricular function resulting from underlying disease, whether in the form of ischemic, dilated, or hypertrophic cardiomyopathy or valvular heart disease, may be sufficient to result in acute hemodynamic deterioration, heart failure, or hypotension.

APPROACH TO THE PATIENT WITH NEW-ONSET AF

In the patient with a first episode of AF, it is important to search for a cause, such as coronary artery disease, progression of heart failure, or extracardiac problems such as hyperthyroidism or periodic alcohol abuse.

Patients presenting with a new attack of paroxysmal AF (that lasting for less than or equal to 24 hours) in whom known heart disease, particularly valve disease, is present usually undergo pharmacologic or electrical conversion to sinus rhythm on the same day. Alternatively, one may adopt a wait-and-see approach because placebo-controlled studies show that most patients with new-onset AF convert to sinus rhythm spontaneously, without intervention, within 24 hours (8). Such a strategy is particularly applicable if the ventricular rate is well controlled and the patient has only minimal complaints. A β blocker or calcium antagonist may be given to reduce the ventricular rate, if indicated.

If the time of onset is not known or is longer than 24 hours, a wait-and-see approach is highly appropriate; rate control, depending on complaints, and anticoagulation should be instituted. It is important to search for underlying causes and institute appropriate therapy. Cardioversion should be performed after at least 3 weeks of adequate anticoagulation.

Pharmacologic therapy for patients with AF is directed at (a) controlling an inappropriately rapid ventricular response rate with drugs targeting the AV node, (b) preventing thromboembolic events with anticoagulants, and (c) restoring and maintaining sinus rhythm with membrane active antiarrhythmic drugs. Many patients require intervention in each area while others need nothing more than careful observation.

Heart rates in AF vary according to level of activity and time of day (205–207). Some patients who show appropriately controlled ventricular response rates at rest may develop excessively rapid rates with exertion (208–211). Others show substantial diurnal variability of heart rates with peak rates occurring in the early afternoon, whereas the slowest ventricular response rates typically occur during sleep (205,206). Some patients with rapid conduction through the AV node may be totally asymptomatic, although most note palpitations, exercise limitations, and fatigue. In some cases, dyspnea, dizziness, and chest pain may occur.

THERAPY TO CONTROL VENTRICULAR RATE

Rate control of AF depends on altering the conduction properties of the AV node with a pharmacologic agent, such as digoxin, a calcium channel blocker, or a β blocker, or with nonpharmacologic therapy, such as AV nodal ablation.

Digoxin

For the past century, the most common treatment has been the use of digoxin, which exerts its effects by an indirect action mediated by the vagus nerve (208,212). However, it has been observed that digoxin is relatively ineffective in individuals with the most rapid heart rates and for rate control during activity; although the resting ECG may show adequate rate control, uncontrolled rapid heart rates are seen with exertion and at times of sympathetic stimulation (207–210,212–214). In one study of 72 patients, Rawles and colleagues (207) found that digoxin did not alter the heart rates at the onset of a paroxysm of AF or during the paroxysm. This limited effect of digoxin may be a particular problem in younger, more active individuals or women in whom faster heart rates have been documented during AF (215). Additionally, the peak of digitalis effect does not occur for 6 to 9 hours after its intravenous or oral administration, limiting its usefulness for acute rate control (216,217). Digoxin may also aggravate the occurrence of AF; as a result of its vagotonic effect, it typically increases atrial excitability, depresses intraatrial conduction, and reduces atrial refractoriness, all of which create conditions conducive for maintenance of this arrhythmia.

Digoxin does appear to regularize the ventricular response, which makes a paroxysmal episode less symptomatic. One study by Hnatkova and colleagues (216) examined the distribution of R-R intervals in 45 patients receiving digoxin or placebo; there was a significant reduction in the variability of R-R–interval segments with active treatment.

β Blockers and Calcium Channel Blockers

There is extensive experience with the use of various β blockers (218–221), verapamil (219,220–224), and diltiazem (223–225) for controlling heart rate. β Blockers and calcium channel blockers substantially decrease rapid heart rates at rest and during activity and reduce symptoms; however, their impact on exercise tolerance is less consistent (Fig. 15-8). Patients receiving calcium channel blockers may have an improvement in exercise tolerance (222,223, 225–227); in contrast, β blockers produce a decrease in exercise tolerance in many patients (220,228).

Combination Therapy

In many patients, a single pharmacologic agent is ineffective for controlling the ventricular rate in AF; in these cases, patients may respond to combination therapy (225–231). Various studies have shown that oral β blockers when given in with digoxin have a highly beneficial effect on rapid heart rates. Similar studies have examined the utility of calcium channel blockers when used in with digoxin. Although an interaction between digoxin and verapamil may occur, this does not contraindicate their combined use but does mandate careful follow-up of patients so treated. Farshi and colleagues (222) have recently shown the greatest control of heart rates during exercise occurs with the combination of

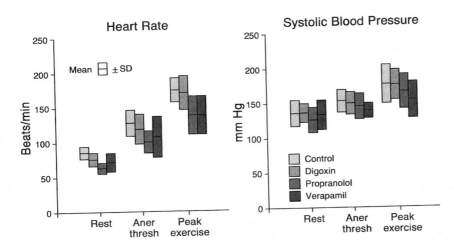

FIGURE 15-8. Heart rate and blood pressure response to exercise in atrial fibrillation patients. The **(left)** heart rate at rest, upon reaching the anaerobic threshold, and at peak exercise in patients treated with digoxin, propranolol, or verapamil. The calcium channel and β-blocker–treated patients showed better rate control during exercise than that seen with digoxin. The **(right)** systolic blood pressure at the same exercise points. Again calcium channel and β blockers showed a greater impact on blood pressure than digoxin. (From Matsuda M, Matsuda Y, Yamagiohi T, et al. Effects of digoxin, propranolol, and verapamil on exercise in patients with chronic isolated atrial fibrillation. *Cardiovasc Res* 1991;25: 453–457, with permission.)

digoxin and atenolol (Fig. 15-9). The combination of digoxin and diltiazem was also more effective than either drug alone. Similarly, Steinberg and colleagues (232) have documented a significant improvement in ventricular response rate at rest and during treadmill exercise testing with the addition of diltiazem to digoxin.

The outcome of digoxin–β-blocker combination therapy may be dependent on the specific β blocker used. Several studies have demonstrated that the combination of digoxin and a β blocker with intrinsic sympathomimetic activity has a beneficial effect on peak ventricular response rate while minimizing the effect of these agents at times of slowest heart rates (229,230). Reiffel (229) examined the effect of digoxin and pindolol (2.5 to 10 mg twice a day) on patients with heart rates of more than 160 bpm with activity and rates lower than 60 bpm during the night. In these patients, digitalis treatment alone resulted in further natural heart rate slowing to less than 40 bpm; in contrast, the addition of pindolol improved the minimum heart rate during AF to more than 45 bpm in most patients while control of maximum AF to rates of less than 140 bpm was achieved in all patients.

Therapy for Acute Control of Heart Rate

β Blockers or Calcium Channel Blockers

When rapid control of the heart rate is required acutely, intravenous administration of a β blocker (including esmolol, propranolol, or metoprolol) or a calcium channel blocker (primarily verapamil or diltiazem) is appropriate (Fig. 15-10) (233–242). As shown in Table 15-5, these agents are typically given as a small bolus, followed by a more prolonged maintenance infusion when required. Patients with marked hemodynamic compromise related to excessive ventricular response rate may require more urgent electrical cardioversion.

Intravenous Clonidine

Investigations have also suggested that intravenous clonidine, acting through a central nervous system mechanism, can effectively reduce rapid ventricular response rates. Roth and colleagues (243) demonstrated that 0.075 to 0.150 mg of intravenous clonidine decreased uncontrolled heart rates by 30 to 40 bpm. Although not typically used, this

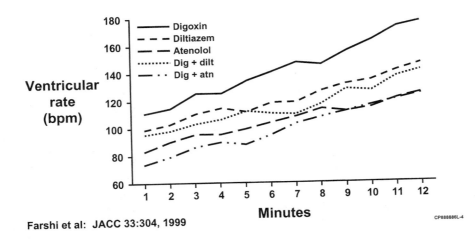

FIGURE 15-9. Impact of drug therapy on exercise ventricular rate in atrial fibrillation. Shown are the ventricular response rates at 1 to 12 minutes of exercise on digoxin, diltiazem, atenolol, or with the combination of digoxin and diltiazem, as well as digoxin and atenolol. Digoxin provided the least control of atrial fibrillation heart rate during exercise while therapy with atenolol plus digoxin was most effective. (From Farshi R, Kistner D, Sarma JS, et al. Ventricular rate control in chronic atrial fibrillation during daily activity and programmed exercise: a crossover open-label study of five drug regimens. *J Am Coll Cardiol* 1999;33[2]:304–310, with permission.)

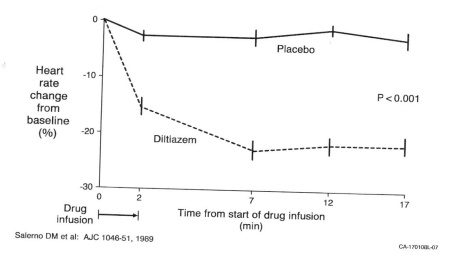

Salerno DM et al: AJC 1046-51, 1989

CA-170108L-07

FIGURE 15-10. Effect of intravenous dilti-azem on heart rate in atrial fibrillation. The ventricular response rate during atrial fibril-lation, displayed as heart rate changed from baseline, in individuals receiving placebo ver-sus diltiazem. A marked decrease in heart rate with intravenous diltiazem was seen at 2 minutes, with the further reduction at 7 min-utes ($p < 0.001$). (From Salerno DM, Dias VC, Kleiger RE, et al. Efficacy and safety of intra-venous diltiazem for treatment of atrial fib-rillation and atrial flutter. *Am J Cardiol* 1989; 63:1046–1251, with permission.)

approach may be useful when other more conventional agents fail to produce the desired effect.

Rate Control in WPW Syndrome

Important exceptions to the use of digoxin, β blockers, and calcium channel blockers for rate control are patients with WPW syndrome and those with anterograde conduction through an accessory pathway during AF. Although 10% to 40% of patients with an accessory pathway may develop AF, a smaller fraction of patients have accessory pathways with the propensity for rapid AV conduction during this arrhythmia. The administration of intravenous agents that block the AV node may actually result in an acceleration in the ventricular response rate, leading to a deterioration of AF to ventricular fibrillation. Such an occurrence has been reported in one third of individuals receiving digitalis (244) and has also been seen with the administration of intra-venous verapamil or adenosine (245–250).

Rate acceleration may be a result of a direct facilitatory effect on accessory pathway conduction and an indirect action from an increase in central sympathetic tone; in some cases, this is related to a drop in blood pressure

accompanying verapamil or β-blocker administration. Another factor responsible for the increase in ventricular rate is the withdrawal of beneficial concealed conduction into the accessory pathway from antegrade conduction of impulses through the AV node-His-Purkinje system; these impulses enter the accessory pathway retrogradely, colliding with impulses conducted in an antegrade along the acces-sory pathway (Fig. 15-11).

In the setting of WPW syndrome, intravenous pro-cainamide has been the most effective medication for block-ing AV nodal and accessory pathway conduction and for facilitating the conversion to sinus rhythm. The intravenous form of flecainide or propafenone is also used in Europe and Canada. Some data suggest that ibutilide may also have a beneficial effect on conduction through the accessory path-way and result in the restoration of sinus rhythm (251,252).

Role of Antiarrhythmic Drugs for Rate Control

Some class 1a membrane-active drugs such as pro-cainamide, quinidine, or disopyramide have direct and indirect effects on the AV conduction system and are not

TABLE 15-5. SLOWING VENTRICULAR RESPONSE RATES DURING ATRIAL FIBRILLATION

	Acutely (IV)	Chronically
Digoxin	1.0–1.5 mg	0.125–0.5 mg/d
Esmolol	0.5 mg/kg/1 min	
	0.05–0.3 mg/kg/min	
Verapamil	5–20 mg (incr)	120–360 mg SR/d
	0.005 mg/kg/min	
Diltiazem	0.25–0.35 mg/kg	120–240 mg SR/d
	5–15 mg/hr	

INCR, incremental; SR, sustained release.

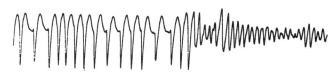

FIGURE 15-11. Effect of adenosine administered during preex-cited atrial fibrillation in a patient with a left free wall accessory pathway. Atrial fibrillation with a rapid ventricular response rate is seen at the beginning of the strip but deteriorates into ven-tricular fibrillation after the administration of 12 mg of adeno-sine. (From Exner DV, Muzyka T, Gillisam. Proarrhythmia in patients with the Wolff-Parkinson-White syndrome after stan-dard doses of IV adenosine. *Ann Intern Med* 1995;122:351–352, with permission.)

useful for the control of ventricular response rates in AF. The electrical activity during AF may also organize during therapy with class I agents and may lead to the emergence of atrial flutter in 5% to 15% of patients. With sufficient slowing of the atrial flutter rate, 1 : 1 conduction through the AV node occurs in up to 5% of patients (253,254).

In contrast, the class III antiarrhythmic agents sotalol and amiodarone may have a significant negative dromotropic effect on AV conduction. In part, this beneficial effect is a result of intrinsic β-blocking properties of these agents while amiodarone also has an appreciable calcium channel-blocking effect, particularly when given intravenously. In one comparison, Juul-Möller and colleagues (255) demonstrated a decrease in heart rate in patients treated with sotalol, whereas quinidine, even when given with digoxin, resulted in a 20- to 30-bpm increase in heart rate. Although not very effective in restoring sinus rhythm, intravenous amiodarone may be highly effective in slowing ventricular response rates in AF (256).

Recommendations for Rate Control

The most appropriate oral agent to use to control rapid heart rates in a specific patient will on the origin of AF, the underlying disease, and noncardiac factors such as presence of renal or hepatic disease. An algorithm for drug selection is given in Figure 15-12. For example, patients with thyrotoxicosis and a rapid ventricular response rate are more likely to respond to beta blockade. Similarly, those patients with a previous myocardial infarction or ongoing ischemia may benefit most from β blockers. In addition to a beneficial effect on the ventricular response rate, β blockers also decrease postinfarction mortality rates. If there is a contraindication to beta blockade, verapamil may be useful; diltiazem may increase mortality risk in these patients and should not be used (257,258).

In patients with a hypertrophic cardiomyopathy, β blockers and verapamil are useful in those with AF and have a beneficial effect on obstruction. In this situation, digoxin may be detrimental. In contrast, digoxin has been the main-

stay of therapy for AF accompanied by a fast ventricular response rate in the setting of a dilated cardiomyopathy. Other agents, particularly β blockers, may also be administered, albeit with greater difficulty; β blockers have also reduced mortality rates of patients with dilated cardiomyopathy, independent of AF (259–262).

In patients with no heart disease, β blockers or calcium channel blockers are typically well tolerated and highly beneficial. Verapamil may also blunt or prevent the profibrillatory electrical remodeling seen with AF.

Nonpharmacologic Therapy for Rate Control

Some patients continue to be symptomatic from persistently rapid heart rates despite the use of an AV nodal blocking agent; in these patients, nonpharmacologic therapy, primarily AV nodal ablation with radiofrequency energy, can be considered (263–265). A number of studies have shown success rates of more than 98% for the interruption of the AV conduction system and complete control of the patient's rate, an improvement in underlying ventricular function (266), and an improvement in symptoms (reduction in palpitations, dyspnea on exertion, and fatigue and improvement in exercise tolerance and duration) (267, 268) (Fig. 15-13). In addition to an improvement in quality of life, there is also a decrease in health care system utilization and cost, physician visits per year, hospitalizations per year, and antiarrhythmic drug use (269).

Although the risks of AV nodal ablation are low, patients receiving AV nodal ablation are effectively pacemaker-dependent. An increased risk of sudden death for a brief period of time after ablation has also been observed (270–272). The mechanism for sudden death may be related to the procedure itself and the resulting bradycardia, although some studies have suggested that it is more likely to be related to the underlying disease. It is possible that some patients with depressed ventricular function and prolonged repolarization develop a triggered ventricular rhythm related to the transition of rapid AF rates to signif-

Patient	Normal	Post MI/ ischemia	Hypertrophy/ hypertrophic myopathy	Dilated cardiomyopathy
1st choice	Verapamil Diltiazem	β-blockers	β-blockers Verapamil	Digoxin
2nd choice	β-blockers	Digoxin Verapamil	Diltiazem	β-blockers
Gray zone	Digoxin	Diltiazem	Digoxin	Verapamil Diltiazem

FIGURE 15-12. Drug approach for rate control in atrial fibrillation. Shown are candidate first and second choices for patients with healthy hearts, postinfarction or ischemic cardiomyopathies, hypertrophic cardiomyopathies, or dilated cardiomyopathies in failure. These choices are based on efficacy, safety, and tolerance.

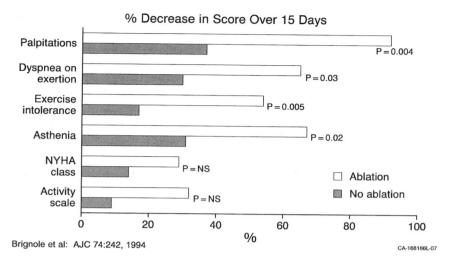

Brignole et al: AJC 74:242, 1994

FIGURE 15-13. Comparison of quality of life scores in atrial fibrillation patients treated with and without ablation. Shown are the percentage decreases in symptoms for more than 15 days. Atrioventricular nodal ablation granted symptomatic relief of palpitations, dyspnea on exertion, exercise intolerance, and general asthenia. (From Brignole, et al. Influence of atrioventricular radiofrequency ablation in patients with chronic atrial fibrillation and on quality of life and cardiac performance. *Am J Cardiol* 1994;74:242, with permission.)

icantly slower heart rates after ablation. In such a setting, the accompanying prolongation of repolarization may lead to a torsade-like rhythm abnormality. Although such a mechanism is yet to be proven clinically, the sudden death rate has been diminished by programming the pacemaker to a rate of 80 to 90 bpm during the first 2 to 4 weeks after ablation. It is hypothesized that this increment in heart rate results in more rapid repolarization, thus reducing the potential for bradycardia-mediated arrhythmias.

Several investigators have demonstrated that the AV node can be modified without completely eliminating AV conduction, thereby eliminating the need for permanent pacing (273,274). However, such procedures are time-consuming and have not received widespread physician acceptance; in addition, some patients have restoration of AV nodal conduction resulting in a recurrence of symptoms due to the rapid rate. Patients with significant underlying heart disease should be paced regardless of the outcome of this procedure to decrease the risk of bradycardia-dependent ventricular arrhythmias.

THERAPEUTIC OPTIONS FOR ARRHYTHMIA TERMINATION

After initial termination, AF often recurs within 1 year, even if prophylactic antiarrhythmic drugs are used. Several studies have shown that after initial presentation and successful termination of paroxysmal AF, nearly all patients had a recurrence for which further treatment was necessary after 4 years (2,3).

External Cardioversion

Direct current electrical cardioversion was introduced for chronic AF in 1962 by Lown and colleagues (275). It restores sinus rhythm in 70% to 90% of patients, particu-

larly in those with arrhythmia of short duration in whom the left atrium is small (276,277). Electrical cardioversion for chronic AF is unlikely to succeed in patients with AF for more than 3 years or those with a left atrial size of more than 60 mm on a long-axis echocardiographic view. To avoid the use of excessive energy levels (which may be counterproductive), the initial dose should be 100 J of stored energy; if the initial shock is not successful, a stepwise increase until the highest energy setting is usually followed. However, one study of 64 patients with AF for more than 48 hours suggested that the initial energy of 360 J was more effective than 100 or 200 J for reverting the arrhythmia (95% versus 14% and 39%, respectively), required the use of fewer shocks and less total cumulative energy, and was safe (278). It has been shown that biphasic defibrillation is more effective than monophasic shocks and lower energies are required. Biphasic defibrillation is particularly useful if transthoracic impedance is high (279).

Cardioversion (electrical or pharmacologic) of AF that has been present for more than 2 days requires oral anticoagulation, maintaining the international normalized ratio (INR) at 2 to 3 for at least 3 weeks before the intervention and for at least 4 weeks after the shock, because there is a period of atrial stunning after cardioversion (280,281). There is ample evidence that electrical cardioversion of AF with a known duration of less than 48 hours in patients with paroxysmal AdependF who do not have risk factors for embolism (heart failure, valvular heart disease, previous thromboembolism) is not associated with a significant thromboembolism risk.

For patients with AF of unknown duration, acute conversion after transesophageal echocardiographic exclusion of left atrial thrombi or spontaneous echo contrast has been advocated as an effective and safe approach (282). Patients are begun on heparin before cardioversion and continue oral anticoagulation for 3 weeks after the conversion. The Assessment of Cardioversion Using Transesophageal

Echocardiography acute trial compared a transesophageal-guided strategy with a conventional strategy in 1,222 patients with AF lasting more than 2 days who were undergoing electrical cardioversion, The primary end point events were ischemic stroke, TIA, and systemic embolization at an 8-week follow-up (283). There was no difference between the two strategies in the incidence of ischemic stroke (0.65% versus 0.33%), TIA (0.16% versus 0.17%), or all embolic events (0.81% versus 0.5%), suggesting that the transesophageal strategy is an alternative to a conventional approach.

Pretreatment with Antiarrhythmic Drugs

Drugs may be used to enhance the effectiveness of conversion and prevent immediate recurrences; at the very moment of electrical restoration of sinus rhythm, an adequate plasma level is present, suppressing acute relapses. Bianconi and colleagues (284) compared placebo with in-hospital loading with propafenone for 48 hours. Acute conversion was seen in 82% and 84% of patients, respectively. However, placebo was associated with more immediate recurrences 11% versus 0% on propafenone; at discharge, significantly more patients were in sinus rhythm on propafenone (53% versus 74%).

Oral and colleagues (285) compared treatment with placebo or intravenous ibutilide administered immediately before electrical cardioversion in 100 patients with persistent AF. Ibutilide pretreatment resulted in a 100% conversion rate compared with 72% in the placebo group; in addition, all patients initially resistant to electrical cardioversion responded after ibutilide treatment. Amiodarone may also be helpful in patients resistant to electrical cardioversion; 1 month of pretreatment with 600 mg of amiodarone daily in combination with electrical cardioversion produced sinus rhythm in 63% of patients (286).

Pretreatment with the calcium channel blocker verapamil may also improve outcome of cardioversion (287,288). In a nonrandomized retrospective study of 61 patients with persistent AF, multivariate analysis revealed that the use of intracellular calcium-lowering drugs during AF to control the ventricular rate was the only significant variable related to maintenance of sinus rhythm after cardioversion (287).

Internal Electrical Cardioversion

The use of internal electrical cardioversion involves the delivery of a high-energy transcatheter shock between the internal catheter electrode, which is used as a cathode and positioned remotely from the His bundle, and an anodal back plate. One prospective study, which compared external cardioversion (300 to 360 J stored energy) with internal cardioversion (200 to 300 J) showed that internal cardioversion was more effective for reverting AF (91% versus 67%), although long-term maintenance of sinus rhythm and complications did not differ between the two groups (289). Transcatheter cardioversion has gained popularity partly because it helps to circumvent general anesthesia. However, in view of the option of biphasic defibrillation (as well as other alternatives such as sequential bidirectional defibrillation), efficacy should not be an issue in the choice of mode of cardioversion.

Pharmacologic Therapy

Today pharmacologic conversion is primarily used to revert paroxysmal AF. Many trials have shown that class I and III antiarrhythmic drugs shorten the time to conversion and increase the number of patients who revert acutely (within, e.g., 30 minutes to 1 hour) or subacute (within a few hours to days). For reversion of AF, digoxin, β blockers, and calcium channel blockers are usually ineffective, while effective agents include the class I agents procainamide, flecainide, and propafenone and the class III agents ibutilide, dofetilide, and amiodarone. Sotalol is less effective (290) but has been used because it reduces the ventricular rate. Amiodarone is particularly recommended in patients with significant left ventricular dysfunction because it lacks significant negative inotropic effects (291).

Several studies have found that therapy with some drugs, such as ibutilide (290,292) and dofetilide (293), can result in the restoration of sinus rhythm in patients with persistent AF. Although with dofetilide or sotalol, for example, 3 days of in-hospital drug therapy may be required (294). Other studies have used amiodarone or propafenone to convert chronic fibrillation on an out-of-hospital basis, after in-hospital initiation (295,296). However, the use of out-of-hospital conversion involves safety issues, particularly for patients with underlying cardiac disease and those with drug-specific arrhythmogenic characteristics.

When evaluating the potential of a drug to revert AF to sinus rhythm, one must consider the conversion rate and time from start of treatment to achievement of sinus rhythm; the type of drug regimen, such as single bolus infusion or prolonged oral treatment, is also important. Paroxysmal fibrillation will convert earlier after start of treatment than persistent AF. Paroxysmal AF usually reverts after 1 to 2 hours, although some studies have found that reversion occurs after a few hours, up to 1 or 2 days; for example, amiodarone may produce sinus rhythm in more than 80% of paroxysmal patients within 24 hours, although the early conversion rate of within 1 hour is low. For other drugs, the cumulative dose may be important. The efficacy of flecainide may be enhanced if the initial bolus infusion is followed by an oral regime for 48 hours with a maximum dose of 700 mg (297).

In persistent AF, early conversion using electrical countershock is not always warranted and a trial of drug conversion may be preferred. Because persistent AF usually is resistant to drugs, a prolonged course of oral drug scheme is usually necessary (298).

TABLE 15-6. PROARRHYTHMIA DURING TREATMENT OF CHRONIC ATRIAL FIBRILLATION OR FLUTTER

Ventricular proarrhythmia
  Torsade de pointes
  Sustained monomorphic ventricular tachycardia
  Sustained polymorphic ventricular tachycardia without
    long QT
Atrial proarrhythmia
  Provocation of recurrence?
  Conversion of atrial fibrillation to flutter
Abnormalities of conduction or impulse formation
  Acceleration of ventricular rate
  Enhancement of atrioventricular nodal conduction
  Preferential accessory pathway conduction
  Atrioventricular block
  Abnormal sinus mechanisms after conversion to sinus rhythm

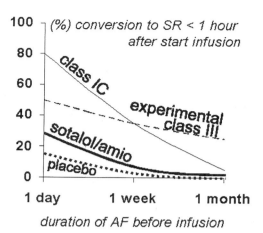

FIGURE 15-14. Considering time to conversion within 1 hour, the literature suggests a crossover concerning effectiveness of class Ic and class III drugs in relation to the preinfusion duration of atrial fibrillation. Sotalol performs relatively poorly no matter what the arrhythmia duration, although in a wait-and-see approach, this drug may be of some use above simple beta blockade. Because of its complicated pharmacokinetics, amiodarone has a too slow onset of action to produce early conversion. Hypothetical curves, however, are based on data as presented in the literature. Placebo curve derived from placebo-controlled conversion studies. Note that short-lasting atrial fibrillation (e.g., that lasting as long as 1 week) usually represents paroxysmal fibrillation.

The obvious disadvantages of a protracted course of drug therapy is that it is not often applicable to patients with severe complaints directly related to the AF and that it is time-consuming, particularly if ECG monitoring is required. Furthermore, membrane-active drugs may produce atrial or ventricular proarrhythmia (299–302) or as described in Table 15-6 negative dromotropic effects and acute heart failure, both of which necessitate in-hospital monitoring, particularly during treatment initiation. Class III drugs may unexpectedly produce bradycardia (sotalol, amiodarone) and sotalol and dofetilide may produce torsade de pointes. It is recommended, therefore, that dofetilide be started in the hospital and continued out-of-hospital only if significant QT prolongation is not present. With short-term infusion of intravenous drugs, these issues are less compelling because any case of proarrhythmia is immediately diagnosed and treated.

Arrhythmia duration is an important determinant of successful pharmacologic conversion (303–305). Class Ic drugs are extremely effective in the conversion of short-lasting paroxysmal AF. In patients with an arrhythmia duration of less than 24 hours, the conversion rate may be as high as 90% at 1 hour after intravenous flecainide or propafenone. By contrast, these drugs are rather ineffective in stopping persistent AF. Compared with class Ic agents, class III drugs are less effective for acute conversion of short-lasting AF (306) (Fig. 15-14). If AF is of short duration, class Ic drugs are more effective than class III agents. However, in AF that has lasted a few weeks or months, class III drugs seem more effective.

Quinidine

Quinidine has long been used to convert AF to sinus rhythm and to maintain the sinus rhythm. Approximately 10% to 15% of patients will convert to sinus rhythm with normal maintenance doses of quinidine, a response that is probably similar for oral procainamide and disopyramide. Each of these drugs has significant vagolytic effects; as a result, the patient must be carefully monitored because the ventricular response to AF may increase. Many patients require concurrent therapy with a β blocker, calcium channel blocker, or digoxin to slow AV nodal conduction. An important exception is in patients with organic disease of the AV node (which is common in sick sinus syndrome); drugs that further slow AV conduction should be used with caution in this setting.

The success rate is greater with higher drug doses. As an example, the use of increasing and frequent doses of quinidine was shown in 1950 to convert more than 80% of patients with AF (307). However, significant drug toxicity was also seen, including ventricular tachycardia at high plasma quinidine levels. A less aggressive but still high-dose regimen reduces toxicity, but the conversion rate falls to 60% (308).

The proarrhythmic potential of quinidine remains a concern in this setting. One study used QT-interval dispersion, as determined by measurements in multiple leads, as an index of susceptibility to developing ventricular arrhythmias (309). This parameter increased significantly during quinidine therapy but not sotalol therapy despite a comparable prolongation in the maximal QT interval. Quinidine converted 22 of 25 patients to sinus rhythm, compared with 17 of 25 patients on sotalol therapy. There were, however, three cases of torsade de pointes and one case of monomorphic ventricular tachycardia in the quinidine group; these arrhythmias did not occur in the sotalol group.

Procainamide

Intravenous procainamide has a similar success rate to that of quinidine, converting 20% to 60% of cases to sinus rhythm, particularly if the AF is of recent onset (310,311). Thus, procainamide is most useful in the hospitalized patient with acute AF.

Ibutilide

Ibutilide, only available for intravenous administration, is effective for terminating AF and atrial flutter. In controlled studies, the acute AF reversion rate was higher with ibutilide than with placebo (28% to 31% versus 0% to 2%); arrhythmia conversion occurred within a mean of 27 to 33 minutes after the start of the infusion (292,311,312). Conversion rates were higher in patients with shorter arrhythmia duration or a normal left atrial size. In comparative studies, ibutilide has been more effective for AF reversion than procainamide (51% versus 21%) (312) or intravenous sotalol (44% versus 11%) (313). Although the reversion rate with ibutilide is higher than that of placebo, it is still relatively low. As previously mentioned, the drug is more effective when given as pretreatment before cardioversion.

However, one potential side effect is torsade de pointes and the incidence is similar to sotalol. Of 180 patients who received 1.0 mg of ibutilide, followed by a second bolus of 0.5 or 1.0 mg after 10 minutes, the incidence of torsade de pointes was 8.3% (292).

Dofetilide

Dofetilide is of limited use for reversion of AF. In one study of 91 patients with AF or atrial flutter, the reversion rate was much lower for AF (14.5% versus 54%) (314). A second study of 96 patients found reversion in 24% of those with AF (versus 4% for placebo) compared with 64% (versus 0% for placebo) in those with flutter (315). Another trial, European and Australian Multicenter Evaluative Research on Atrial Fibrillation Dofetilide (EMERALD), found that the reversion rate with dofetilide was dose-related; pharmacologic reversion with dosages of 125, 250, and 500 µg twice daily occurred in 6%, 11%, and 29%, respectively, compared with a reversion rate of 5% with sotalol (315a). As with other class III agents, dofetilide can cause torsade de pointes, and in one study, the incidence was 3% (315). Given the high rate of adverse events, dofetilide is limited to patients who during in-hospital initiation do not exhibit (signs considered to be associated with) proarrhythmia. In addition, on the basis of renal function and drug response of the QT interval, preset dose reductions must be carried out.

Flecainide

Flecainide, a class Ic agent, is effective for reversion and prevention of AF. Intravenous flecainide (150 mg) acutely reverts recent-onset AF in up to 65% of patients and is more effective than procainamide, sotalol, propafenone, and amiodarone (316–318). However, the intravenous preparation is not available in the United States.

There are limited data that a single large oral dose of flecainide (300 mg) is effective for AF reversion. As an example, one study that randomized 79 patients to intravenous or large oral dose of flecainide found that the rate of reversion to sinus rhythm was the same at 2 hours (64% versus 68% for oral drug) and 8 hours after treatment (72% versus 75%); however, the mean time to reversion was shorter with intravenous drug (52 versus 110 minutes) (319).

Propafenone

Intravenous propafenone is used in Europe and elsewhere for the acute termination of AF; it is not available in the United States. In one study of 136 patients, the overall conversion rate was equal with propafenone or placebo (29% versus 17%) (320). The conversion rate was higher in patients with AF lasting less than or equal to 2 weeks (55% versus 43%) and in those with a left atrial diameter of less than 40 mm (38% versus 23%), but these differences were not statistically significant.

Other studies have demonstrated that oral propafenone is also an effective drug for reversion of AF to sinus rhythm. One study, for example, evaluated 283 patients with recent-onset (less than 72 hours) AF and clinical signs of heart failure (321). The patients were randomized to a single loading oral dose of propafenone (450 or 600 mg), digoxin (1 mg), or placebo, and 24-hour Holter monitoring was performed. Propafenone was more effective than digoxin or placebo in converting patients to sinus rhythm at 4 hours (57% versus 25% for digoxin or placebo). Digoxin and propafenone were also useful in reducing the ventricular response.

Similar findings were noted in a second study of 240 patients with recent-onset AF (less than or equal to 7 days) who were randomized to a single loading dose of propafenone or placebo (322). Approximately 80% of patients treated with propafenone reverted to sinus rhythm at 8 hours, compared with 56% of control patients (p = 0.02). The response to propafenone was the same in patients with and without structural heart disease. The administration of propafenone before electrical cardioversion does not alter the energy requirements for or the success rate of cardioversion (323).

Amiodarone

Intravenous amiodarone has been found to be effective for reversion of AF, converting 60% to 70% of patients to sinus rhythm in some trials (324). One study randomized 208 patients to placebo or intravenous amiodarone for 24 hours followed by oral drug for 4 weeks (325). At the end of the first 24 hours, reversion to sinus rhythm was more frequent with amiodarone (61% versus 40% for placebo). By the end of 1 month, more patients receiving amiodarone were in sinus rhythm (81% versus 40%). The only significant predictors of conversion were left atrial size and duration of AF.

However, amiodarone is relatively expensive and other studies have not confirmed its efficacy. One study, for example, randomized 100 patients with recent-onset AF to intravenous amiodarone or saline; there was no difference in rate of reversion to sinus rhythm at 24 hours (68% versus 60%) (326).

Oral amiodarone alone has also been evaluated. One study of 72 patients with recent-onset AF (less than 48 hours) found that a single oral dose of amiodarone (30 mg/kg) was more effective than placebo for restoring sinus rhythm after 8 and 24 hours (50% versus 20% and 87% versus 35%) (327). In contrast, in a study of 129 patients with AF or atrial flutter that was refractory to conventional antiarrhythmic drugs, only 18% of patients converted to sinus rhythm when treated with oral amiodarone at a dosage of 600 mg per day for 4 weeks, although there was a significant reduction in ventricular rate (328).

In summary, amiodarone is probably not as effective as class Ia or Ic agents for reverting AF, although it may be more effective for preventing recurrence. Pretreatment with oral amiodarone for 1 month before electrical cardioversion improves the reversion rate (88% versus 56% to 65% without pretreatment). Amiodarone has not yet been approved by the Food and Drug Administration for treatment of AF.

Sotalol

Intravenous sotalol may be effective for reversion of AF; however, it is not available in the United States. Preliminary reports have noted successful cardioversion in 29 of 40 patients (73%) with refractory AF resulting from various types of organic heart disease (329). The lower proarrhythmic potential with this drug makes it even more attractive.

However, intravenous sotalol appears to be less effective than intravenous flecainide or ibutilide for reversion of AF (313,330). One study, for example, compared intravenous flecainide with intravenous sotalol in 106 patients with AF for less than or equal to 6 months. The conversion rate within 2 hours of drug infusion was significantly higher with flecainide (52% versus 23%) (330). A metaanalysis found that oral sotalol was significantly less effective than quinidine for conversion of recent-onset (less than 48 hours) AF and was comparable to placebo for reversion of AF of more than 48 hours' duration (331).

Digoxin

Intravenous or oral digoxin has long been considered the drug of choice for rate control of AF as well as for pharma-

cologic reversion to sinus rhythm. Several small studies, however, have reported that the rate of conversion with digoxin is comparable to that of placebo, although conversion is earlier with digoxin and heart rate is slower (332, 333). Digoxin may restore sinus rhythm when AF is caused by CHF. In this setting, reversion is the result of improved hemodynamics and a reduction in left atrial pressure.

Calcium Channel Blockers

Although verapamil itself lacks specific antiarrhythmic properties considered essential for conversion, it has been suggested that it may support reversion to sinus rhythm in patients on quinidine (334) or class III agents (295,335). Innes and colleagues (334) pretreated patients with paroxysmal AF with verapamil or digoxin followed by quinidine; the conversion rates (within 6 hours) were 84% and 45%, respectively and average time to conversion was 185 and 368 minutes, respectively. Similarly, Tieleman and colleagues (295) found that verapamil enhanced conversion to sinus rhythm during 1 month of amiodarone therapy (600 mg daily) in 129 patients with persistent AF (median duration of 53 months; all patients had failed more than one previous cardioversion and more than one other antiarrhythmic drug). Conversion was achieved in 23 patients. These studies were nonrandomized and further research is needed before a definite role for calcium antagonists in the conversion of AF can be established.

Recommendations for Pharmacologic Therapy

Class Ic drugs are most appropriate for out-of-hospital conversion of intermittent paroxysmal AF because of their high efficacy. Self-administered oral drug conversion should, however, be applied only if the patient is clinically stable and if the specific drug appeared effective and safe after a few in-hospital trials. Conditions under which these class Ic drugs should be avoided include heart failure, presence of an impaired cardiac function or coronary artery disease with acute or chronic ischemia, and known sick sinus syndrome or AV conduction disturbances.

Implantable Atrial Defibrillator

An atrial defibrillator (atrioverter) is a device used to restore sinus rhythm by internal countershock (336). Shocks are delivered between two intracardiac leads. Shortening the attacks of atrial fibrillation by such a device may exert an antiarrhythmic effect by limiting remodeling. Patients with recurrent, but not too frequent, AF are thought to be candidates if conventional pharmacologic therapy fails. However, immediate relapses occur rather frequently and may limit the efficacy of this device. The degree of discomfort related to the shock usually is acceptable if not more than a few shocks are needed per episode (337).

THERAPY FOR ARRHYTHMIA PREVENTION

Some patients may not require antiarrhythmic therapy, particularly when AF is precipitated by transient noncardiac factors in susceptible subjects. These include infection, thyrotoxicosis, hypoxia, and alcohol, as well as several acute cardiac conditions, such as acute myocardial infarction, pericarditis, and exacerbation of heart failure. Very often therapy of the underlying cause or elimination of the provoking factor will prevent arrhythmia recurrence. Among patients with paroxysmal AF unassociated with a definable precipitating cause, many experience a relapse if left untreated. Even in patients receiving prophylactic therapy, the risk of recurrence is high; therefore, breakthrough arrhythmia does not equal treatment failure; rather the goal of treatment is to reduced arrhythmia frequency and improve quality of life (Fig. 15-15).

Patients with persistent AF usually undergo electrical cardioversion to restore sinus rhythm. Those with infrequent recurrences may be considered candidates for serial electrical treatment, which is often preferred over chronic antiarrhythmic drug therapy. However, if recurrences are frequent, chronic suppressive drug treatment may be necessary (Fig. 15-16). In this situation, appropriate therapy is either pharmacologic, using class Ia, Ic, or III antiarrhythmic agents, or nonpharmacologic, using a surgical or catheter ablation or an implantable device (pacemaker or implantable atrial defibrillator).

Pharmacologic Therapy

Each of the class Ia, Ic, or III antiarrhythmic drugs is effective for maintenance therapy to prevent recurrent AF.

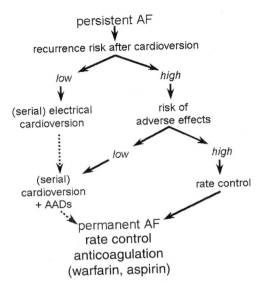

FIGURE 15-16. Flow chart for a rhythm versus rate control strategy in persistent atrial fibrillation (AF). Adverse effects include proarrhythmia, heart failure, and conduction problems. Serial electrical cardioversion represents a "season ticket" for cardioversion for those with infrequent recurrences of persistent AF. Dotted lines represent (*middle left*) transition from serial electrical cardioversion to serial electrical cardioversion with the addition of serial antiarrhythmic drug treatment if the former fails and (*lower left*) transition from serial treatment to permanent atrial fibrillation after failure of the former. Rate control (acceptance of permanent AF) is chosen as first option if the recurrence risk after cardioversion as well as the risk of adverse effects is considered too high.

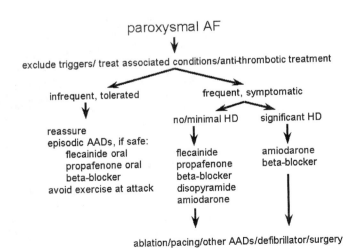

FIGURE 15-15. Flow chart showing treatment options for rhythm control in patients with paroxysmal atrial fibrillation. Depending on the arrhythmia burden, severity of arrhythmia complaints, and the perceived proarrhythmia risk, rate control should be considered an alternative for rhythm control using antiarrhythmic drugs. Attention should be given to vagal versus adrenergic mode of initiation, because this may affect choice of drug. HD, heart disease.

Digoxin

Digoxin is often continued on a long-term basis as prophylaxis against recurrent episodes of AF or in some cases for slowing the heart rate during a recurrent episode. However, digoxin is generally not effective for preventing recurrences of AF, a possible exception being AF secondary to heart failure. Digoxin is ineffective for controlling the heart rate during a paroxysmal episode. This is likely because at the onset of AF, there is activation of the sympathetic nervous system, a result of an initial reduction in cardiac output and blood pressure during AF, which counteracts the vagotonic effect of digoxin. Based on extended ambulatory monitoring, Rawles and colleagues (338) observed no difference in the number of episodes among 72 patients with frequent paroxysms of AF who were receiving digoxin therapy, compared with a similar group of patients not receiving the drug. The heart rate at the onset of the AF was similar (140 versus 130 bpm). The length of a paroxysm was longer in the digoxin group. These data are not unexpected because digoxin has no major direct action on the electrophysiologic properties of the atrial myocardium but exerts an indirect effect mediated by an increase in parasympathetic tone that may be profibrillatory in some patients.

Quinidine

A metaanalysis of six controlled trials showed that quinidine was superior to no treatment, with 50% of patients remaining in sinus rhythm compared with 25% of those on placebo, although the total mortality rate was significantly higher in the quinidine group, 2.9% versus 0.8% (339). Data from a registry also demonstrated a relatively high incidence of sudden death with quinidine, presumably resulting from torsade de pointes (340). Of 570 patients younger than 65 years, 6 patients died suddenly shortly after restoration of sinus rhythm.

Up to 30% of patients who were prescribed quinidine had intolerable side effects, most commonly diarrhea. These findings make it questionable whether there is still a role for quinidine as a first-line agent in the prophylaxis of AF.

Disopyramide

Disopyramide is an effective agent for preventing AF, although there are only a few studies reporting its use. Comparative trials are limited, but it appears to be as effective as quinidine. The usual dose is 100 to 200 mg orally three or four times a day. There is a long-acting preparation available that is administered at a dose of 100 to 300 mg orally twice daily. However, an important limitation to the use of disopyramide is its negative inotropic activity and the potential to worsen CHF, particularly in patients with a reduced left ventricular ejection fraction and a history of CHF resulting from systolic dysfunction. Unfortunately, a substantial number of patients with AF have CHF resulting from a dilated or congestive cardiomyopathy. Although in these patients, the maintenance of sinus rhythm is particularly important for better left ventricular function and hemodynamics stability, the potential risk of this drug far outweighs its benefit.

Procainamide

Oral procainamide is less effective than quinidine for preventing recurrent episodes of AF. Another limitation to its usefulness for chronic suppressive therapy is the high frequency of side effects, many of which occur during long-term therapy. Particularly important are a lupus-like syndrome and agranulocytosis.

Flecainide

Flecainide is effective for prevention of AF, although it is restricted for use in patients with a structurally normal heart. The usual dose is 50 to 200 mg orally twice daily. At one year, this agent prevents recurrent AF in 60% of patients and it prolongs the time to the first recurrence, from a mean of 3 days on placebo to 14.5 days on flecainide (341,342). Rasmussen and colleagues (343) administered a fairly large dose of flecainide (300 mg twice daily) and found a very high rate for maintenance of sinus rhythm

(81%) at 6 months, which may have been because of the high dose used. Response to this agent is not related to left atrial size, duration of AF, or the presence of underlying heart disease. This is in contrast to what has been observed with quinidine and other class Ia agents. Although the incidence of nuisance side effects is low, flecainide may worsen heart failure, even in the absence of a prior history of heart failure or when left ventricular function is not significantly impaired. Like other drugs, flecainide can aggravate arrhythmia, provoking a new ventricular arrhythmia or worsening atrial arrhythmia. Although the incidence of this complication is low in patients without structural heart disease who have AF, it is nevertheless an important concern.

Propafenone

Propafenone is effective for preventing recurrent episodes, although it is slightly less effective than flecainide. One study compared flecainide and propafenone in 200 patients, and at the end of 1 year, the therapeutic success rate was 79% with flecainide versus 63% with propafenone (344). In a double-blind placebo-controlled trial of 102 patients with chronic AF who were successfully converted to sinus rhythm, 67% of those receiving propafenone remained in normal sinus rhythm 6 months after cardioversion versus 35% taking placebo (345). The usual dose is 150 to 300 mg three times a day, although the drug can be administered twice daily. This drug is negatively inotropic and can precipitate CHF, particularly in patients with a history of CHF. Like all antiarrhythmic drugs, propafenone can aggravate arrhythmia, but the incidence of this complication in patients with AF is low (2.3%).

Sotalol

Only a few trials have evaluated sotalol, and they have showed that this drug is as effective as class Ia drugs. One study randomized 253 patients with AF or atrial flutter to placebo or three doses of sotalol (80, 120, or 160 mg twice daily); the recurrence rate at 1 year was 72%, 70%, 60%, and 55%, respectively, and the median times to recurrence were 27, 106, 119, and 175 days, respectively (346). As noted with other drugs, predictors of AF recurrence were the presence of coronary disease, duration of AF of more than 2 months before reversion, left atrial size of more than 60 mm, and older age. The mode of cardioversion had no impact on the recurrence rate.

A number of studies have compared the efficacy of sotalol with that of other antiarrhythmic drugs for preventing recurrent AF. When compared with quinidine, sotalol appears to be as effective in preventing recurrent AF; however, recurrences are associated with a slower ventricular rate with sotalol, presumably because of its β-blocking activity (347). One review of studies in which quinidine or sotalol were used for AF found that at 6 months, normal sinus rhythm was maintained in 50%, 53%, and 32% of patients receiving sotalol, quinidine, or no antiarrhythmic drug therapy (348). However, with long-term therapy, there was a trend for both agents to increase mortality rates (2.2%, 3%, and 1% for sotalol, quinidine, or no therapy); careful ECG monitoring during the first 4 to 7 days of therapy is recommended.

Sotalol has also been compared with propafenone in patients with recurrent AF after therapy with a class Ia antiarrhythmic drug (349). Both drugs were equally effective, with 30% to 37% remaining in sinus rhythm at 1 year. Another trial of patients with recurrent AF refractory to conventional therapy showed that staged care with propafenone and, if AF recurred, sotalol (or in some cases, both drugs) resulted in the maintenance of normal sinus rhythm at 6 months in 55% of patients; the incidence of side effects necessitating discontinuation of therapy was less than 10% with this regimen.

Sotalol appears to be less effective than amiodarone for maintaining normal sinus rhythm. In one randomized study of 70 patients cardioverted from AF, 71% of patients on low-dose amiodarone, compared with 40% of those receiving sotalol, were still in normal sinus rhythm at 12 months (350).

Amiodarone

The most effective agent for long-term prevention of paroxysmal AF is amiodarone and there is increasing evidence that low-dose amiodarone may become the drug of choice in the prevention of AF. However, it is not approved in the United States for supraventricular arrhythmia. Although this drug infrequently results in spontaneous reversion of chronic sustained AF to sinus rhythm, it will prevent recurrence after chronic AF is reverted electrically or a paroxysmal episode reverts spontaneously. The drug prevents recurrent AF at 1 year in more than 70% of patients while an additional 15% will have partial efficacy (i.e., paroxysmal AF occurs less frequently, is of briefer duration, or occurs at a slower rate). The Canadian Trial of AF randomized 403 patients who had at least one episode of AF within 6 months of entry to low-dose amiodarone, sotalol, or propafenone; after a mean follow-up of 16 months, the AF recurrence rate was lower with amiodarone (35% versus 63% for sotalol and propafenone) and the median time to recurrence was longer (more than 468 versus 98 days) (351). There was no difference among the three therapies in mortality or the incidence of side effects resulting in drug discontinuation (18% versus 11% for sotalol or propafenone).

The usual loading dosage is 600 mg daily for 3 to 4 weeks, followed by 400 mg for 2 to 4 weeks and a maintenance dose of 200 mg daily. Not infrequently, a dose administered every other day or every third day is effective. It has been reported that left atrial size, duration of AF, and the presence or absence of underlying heart disease are not related to the efficacy of this drug.

An important concern is the frequency of side effects. Although most are mild, often dose-related, and do not necessitate drug discontinuation, the potential for hepatic, thyroid, and pulmonary toxicity is a concern. The potential toxicity of this agent has limited its use for therapy of AF, an arrhythmia considered to be relatively benign. Generally low-dose amiodarone is effective for AF prevention; hence, serious side effects are infrequent because they may be related to the use of higher doses administered during a prolonged time. The occurrence of side effects does not appear to be related to the presence or severity of underlying heart disease. Interestingly, the incidence of arrhythmia aggravation is low despite that there is significant QT prolongation with this agent. Because AF often responds to low doses of amiodarone, the small risk of side effects, particularly serious ones, must be compared with the benefit of this agent, particularly in patients for whom the maintenance of sinus rhythm is important—for example, those with cardiomyopathy, poor left ventricular function, and CHF, or those with valvular heart disease.

Dofetilide

Dofetilide, a new pure class III agent, is effective for the prevention of AF or atrial flutter. The postcardioversion European and Australian Multicenter Evaluative Research on Atrial Fibrillation Dofetilide and Symptomatic Atrial Fibrillation Investigation and Randomized Evaluation of Dofetilide studies have found that at 6 to 12 months, 500 μg of dofetilide twice daily was more effective than 80 mg of sotalol twice daily or placebo; 60% to 70% remained in sinus rhythm on dofetilide, approximately 50% to 60% on sotalol, and 20% to 25% on placebo (352,353).

One concern with dofetilide is torsade de pointes or sudden death. However, a pooled analysis of 1,346 patients receiving dofetilide and 677 treated with placebo in randomized clinical trials of the treatment of supraventricular arrhythmias found that dofetilide was not associated with an increase in mortality (adjusted hazard ratio, 1.1) (354).

Dofetilide has been shown to reduce the incidence of heart failure in patients with AF and heart failure. Torp-Pedersen and colleagues (355) performed a randomized comparison of dofetilide and placebo in 1,518 patients with symptomatic CHF (Danish Investigations of Arrhythmia and Mortality–Congestive Heart Failure); dofetilide was associated with a lower incidence of AF than placebo after an average 18 months of follow-up (1.9% versus 6.6%). Additionally, dofetilide treatment was associated with a significantly reduced admission rate for heart failure.

Rate Control and Anticoagulation Versus Rhythm Control

Most often the treatment goal in highly symptomatic patients with recent-onset paroxysmal or persistent AF, even when episodes have been recurrent despite therapy, is pharmacologic or electrical conversion to sinus rhythm. However, it is not certain whether a strategy aimed at restoring sinus rhythm with antearrhythmic drugs is preferred to AF as the rhythm of choice using rate control and anticoagulation.

The strengths and weaknesses of repeated pharmacologic or electrical cardioversion versus maintenance of sinus rhythm with chronic antearrhythmia therapy are well known. The downside to cardioversion is the extremely frequent relapses of fibrillation, demanding further conversions, and institution of potentially harmful antiarrhythmic drugs. Even with serial electrical cardioversions and antiarrhythmic drug administration, only about 30% of patients with persistent fibrillation will maintain sinus rhythm for a substantial period. Additionally, many of these patients remain candidates for antithrombotic treatment because it is not certain whether asymptomatic episodes of AF are occurring despite the perception that persistent sinus rhythm is present. It has been observed that on ambulatory monitoring, asymptomatic episodes are far more common than symptomatic ones. Therefore, therapy to maintain sinus rhythm does not always eliminate the need for anticoagulation with its associated risk of bleeding. One observational study demonstrated that such an aggressive strategy to maintain sinus rhythm did not prevent the occurrence of heart failure (356).

There are a number of benefits to the maintenance of sinus rhythm, particularly an improvement in left ventricular function and prevention of a tachycardia-induced cardiomyopathy, a result of a slowing of heart rate and an increased ventricular filling time, restoration of atrial contraction, and regularization of the rhythm.

Conversely, accepting AF as the underlying rhythm results in the continued potential for heart failure, because rate control is often suboptimal, particularly with exercise, despite the use of AV nodal blocking drugs. Moreover, there is a continued risk, albeit small, of an embolism despite adequate anticoagulation.

There are several studies investigating whether rhythm control is superior to rate control with anticoagulation in regard to morbidity, mortality, and quality of life. Figures 15-15 and 15-16 provide schemes for rhythm and rate control in patients with paroxysmal and persistent AF.

1. The German Pharmacological Intervention in Atrial Fibrillation study randomized patients with persistent symptomatic AF of less than 1 year, to rate control with diltiazem or amiodarone or cardioversion (357). Preliminary results showed that the number of patients in sinus rhythm was significantly higher in the cardioversion group; however, although exercise duration was significantly better in those maintaining sinus rhythm, quality of life did not differ.
2. The Atrial Fibrillation Follow-up Investigation of Rhythm Management study group is comparing the strategies of rate control and anticoagulation with pre-

vention of AF in patients with a history of persistent or paroxysmal AF; all patients receive anticoagulation and are then randomized to rate control and continued anticoagulation or restoration and maintenance of sinus rhythm using antiarrhythmic drugs (358). The primary end point is mortality and secondary end points are thromboembolic complications, quality of life, and cost of therapy for both strategies.
3. The Netherlands Multicenter Rate Control Versus Electrical Cardioversion study was designed to address the issue of rate versus rhythm control in patients with persistent AF who have had recurrent AF despite one or two previous cardioversions; the primary end point is morbidity (359).

Surgical Therapy

The maze procedure, in which an electrical labyrinth is created in the atria, is an effective approach to the prevention of AF; the incisions are made so that the area between the scars is too small to sustain AF. One of the potential complications of the maze procedure is extensive damage to the atrial myocardium with resultant atrial dysfunction that may limit the hemodynamic benefit. A modification of the maze procedure has been developed in an attempt to ameliorate sinus nodal dysfunction and the occasionally observed poor left atrial function; because most atrial tissue is still electrically connected, a coordinated atrial contraction is usually preserved and atrial transport function is preserved (359a). Modification of the operation, the radial approach, has further reduced the amount of atrial damage (360). In contrast to the maze procedure, in which the incisions desynchronize the activation sequence and often cut across the atrial coronary arteries, the incisions produced by the radial approach radiate from the sinus node toward the AV annular margins, paralleling the activation sequence and the atrial coronary arteries.

In a 5-year experience in one center with 65 patients who had chronic AF, the procedure cured AF, restored AV synchrony, and preserved atrial transport function in 98% of patients, with only 9% requiring antiarrhythmic medications (361). Postoperative atrial pacemakers were implanted in 40% of cases, mostly for preoperative sick sinus syndrome but occasionally for iatrogenic sinus node injury. Encouraging results have also been obtained in a study from Japan (362). Another study of 48 patients found that at 6 and 12 months after surgery, there was a significant improvement in health-related quality of life.

The maze procedure may be an effective therapeutic approach in patients with drug refractory paroxysmal lone AF that occurs in the absence of any structural heart disease. In a study of 41 patients who underwent a maze procedure, for example, 85% of patients were arrhythmia free at the time of discharge (363). After a mean follow-up of 31 months,

95% of patients were free of paroxysmal AF, although 20% required an antiarrhythmic drug. There were no deaths or strokes and no changes on echocardiography; however, two patients developed a sick sinus syndrome and one patient had a nodal escape rhythm. All patients noted an improvement in quality of life and an increase in exercise capacity.

Catheter Ablation

The surgical experience has paved the way for radiofrequency catheter ablation of AF. Preliminary results of an initial experience using radiofrequency catheter ablation in an attempt to cure AF in more than 20 patients have been reported (364). Anatomically conforming introducers were used to guide the radiofrequency catheter along predesignated courses that would roughly reproduce the surgical "maze" procedure. A transseptal approach was used for left atrial ablation. The results were encouraging, but the procedure is very long and the radiation exposure is substantial.

The use of intracardiac echocardiography may permit more accurate targeting of lesions (365). Another possible approach is a nonfluoroscopic catheter-based electroanatomic mapping system, CARTO (Cordis-Biosense); this system has a magnetic field emitter and sensor and can create a replica of the anatomy of the cardiac chamber in which the tachycardia focus is located, permitting the deployment of anatomy-based linear transmural incisions (366).

In some patients, AF may be triggered by atrial ectopic beats, and identification and ablation of a single point of origin of these ectopic beats may be effective therapy; these foci are most often located near the pulmonary veins, which have been found to be nonspecifically dilated in these patients (367). In one study, 94% of the foci were within 2 to 4 cm of the pulmonary veins. After ablation of these foci, 62% of patients were free of AF and most of the recurrent AF was associated with recurrent ectopic beats. A second study of 90 patients found that most (69%) had multiple pulmonary vein foci, and the clinical success correlates with the number of arrhythmogenic foci (368). Success rates were 93%, 73%, and 55% in patients with one, two, and three or more foci, respectively.

In some patients, class Ic drugs or amiodarone may convert AF to atrial flutter. Classic flutter ablation may lead to complete suppression of the arrhythmia in most of these patients while drug treatment is continued; this has been termed *hybrid therapy* (368a).

Pacemakers

The role of pacing in preventing or terminating fibrillation in patients suffering from paroxysmal AF still is experimental. In patients requiring pacemakers for bradycardia, atrial pacing may be associated with a lower frequency of AF by producing a more homogeneous substrate (369–371). Pacing may also suppress premature atrial depolarizations, which serve as triggers for AF in some patients. Usually a hybrid approach is needed, combining pacing with drugs and ablation.

The Canadian Trial of Physiologic Pacing, which randomized 2,568 patients to a ventricular (VVI) or physiologic (AAI or DDD) pacemaker, found that the annual rate of AF was lower with physiologic pacing (5.3% versus 6.6%), for a relative risk reduction of 18%; the effect on the rate of AF was not apparent until 2 years after implantation (371). Another prospective trial of 225 patients with sick sinus syndrome compared atrial and ventricular pacing (372). After a 3-year follow-up, atrial pacing decreased the frequency of AF and the likelihood of thromboembolism (5% versus 17%), perhaps by maintaining AV synchrony, which prevents the development of right atrial electrical and left atrial mechanical remodeling and the potential for AF. Atrial pacing continued to confer a significantly lower risk for AF and thromboembolism than ventricular pacing at 8 years of follow-up (369).

In contrast, rate-adaptive atrial pacing does not prevent AF in the absence of symptomatic bradycardia. One study of 97 patients with drug-refractory paroxysmal AF found that the time to first episode of AF was shorter with atrial pacing (1.9 versus 4.2 days for no pacing) and the AF burden was greater (1 versus 0.32 hours per day) (373).

THROMBOEMBOLISM AND ROLE OF ANTICOAGULATION

Thromboembolism is the most important complication of AF (374); 85% of all systemic thromboemboli are secondary to AF while two thirds occur in the cerebrovascular circulation (375). Nonrheumatic AF accounts for approximately one third of all strokes per year in patients older than 65 years, and 50% of all strokes in patients older than 75 years; it is also the most common cause for deadly stroke in elderly women. In addition to causing clinical stroke with major deficit, AF is also associated with a higher frequency of silent cerebral infarctions detected by computed brain tomography.

In surviving elderly patients, stroke frequently leaves irreversible disability and dependency. In patients with AF who have not had a stroke, intraatrial thrombus can be observed on transesophageal echocardiography in 6% to 25%, underscoring the critical need for antithrombotic therapy with AF patients who are at risk of untoward events (376).

Risk Factors for Thromboembolic Events in Chronic AF

The risk of thromboembolic events is related to the patient group studied. In the absence of heart disease, the risk of stroke is low. The risk is also low in younger patients. In AF patients younger than 60 years, Kopecky and colleagues (35) demonstrated a very low risk of embolic complications (0.5%

per year), even in the absence of anticoagulant prophylaxis. In the Framingham Heart Study, the risk of events was closer to 1% to 2% per year. The difference between studies is related to the inclusion of patients with hypertension and diabetes in the analysis of lone AF in the latter study.

The prevalence of stroke associated with AF also increases strikingly with age. One study evaluated 27,202 men and women, aged 50 to 89, with a hospital diagnosis of AF and without a prior diagnosis of stroke (377). The stroke rate (percentage per patient per year) was 1.3% for those aged 50 to 59, 2.2% for those aged 60 to 69, 4.2% for those aged 70 to 79, and 5.1% for those aged 80 to 89. In the Framingham Heart Study, the stroke rate in individuals between the ages of 60 and 69 without AF was 9 per 1,000 patients while it was 42.5 per 1,000 in individuals with AF (378). In contrast, in patients older than 80 years, the stroke rate was 28.7 per 1,000 patients without AF but increased to 142.9 per 1,000 patients with AF.

There is an association between the risk of a thromboembolic event in AF and the presence of certain cardiovascular and endocrine diseases; these diseases include rheumatic mitral valvular disease, hypertension, dilated and hypertrophic cardiomyopathy, and hyperthyroidism (378). In the Framingham Heart Study, which followed participants for 34 years, the 2-year, age-adjusted incidence of stroke was 19 per 1,000 patients if hypertension was present, compared with only 5 per 1,000 patients without hypertension (relative risk, 3.4) (379). In those with coronary artery disease, the incidence was 25 per 1,000 with AF and 11 per 1,000 patients without AF (relative risk, 2.4). The 2-year, age-adjusted incidence of stroke was 4.3-fold higher in patients with heart failure. There is also a relationship between incidence of stroke and left atrial size in both men and women. In Framingham patients with a left atrium of 24 to 39 mm, the incidence of stroke during 6 years was 1.7%; the incidence was approximately 6% in those with a left atrial size of 44 to 74 mm.

Various other risk factors for thromboembolic events have been derived from recent clinical trials. These include age, hypertension, diabetes, prior cerebrovascular event (TIA or stroke), left atrial enlargement, poor left ventricular function, and female gender. In the absence of any risk factors, the annual incidence of a stroke is 2.5%; when one risk factor is present the incidence is 7.5% while the presence of two or more risk factors increases the annual incidence to 17.6%. Patients who have had an embolic stroke or event are at particularly high risk for recurrence; the recurrence rate ranges from 25% to 42%, with one half occurring within 2 weeks and another one quarter occurring within 4 months.

Echocardiographic parameters that identify high-risk individuals include spontaneous echo contrast, left atrial thrombus, left atrial dimension (width and length), aortic plaques, enlarged left atrial appendage surface areas, and diminished left atrial appendage Doppler velocities (380).

The risk of thromboembolic events in patients with paroxysmal AF has been less well established. Large randomized trials have failed to demonstrate that paroxysmal AF is an independent risk factor for thromboembolic events; however, the number of patients with paroxysmal AF in these studies was very small. Other small studies similarly failed to demonstrate excess risk in these individuals (379,381,382) while several other studies came to opposite conclusions (383,384). Hart and colleagues (385) compared the stroke rates of 460 patients with intermittent AF treated with aspirin or with aspirin and low-dose warfarin in the Stroke Prevention in Atrial Fibrillation trials (SPAF I through III) and 1,552 patients with sustained versus paroxysmal AF; patients with intermittent AF tended to be younger, were more often women, had shorter durations of AF, less frequent history of heart failure, and less moderate to severe left ventricular dysfunction. The ischemic stroke rate was 3.2 % per year among those with intermittent AF compared with 3.3% per year for those with sustained AF. With multivariate analysis, the strongest factors associated with stroke in patients with intermittent AF included age, hypertension, and prior stroke or TIA; the annual incidence of stroke among the 25% of the high-risk patients with intermittent AF was 7.8 per year. Therefore, there was no difference in observed stroke rates between those with intermittent versus sustained AF in this analysis, although those with intermittent AF were more frequently classified as lower risk than were those with the sustained arrhythmia. Thus, the data support that there is a significant risk in older patients with intermittent AF. Furthermore, it suggests that the risk factors used in the assessment of patients with chronic AF may apply equally well to patients with the paroxysmal form of arrhythmia. This presence of underlying disease and frequent asymptomatic recurrences of AF suggest that anticoagulation is important in these patients, although data that treatment alters outcome in these individuals are not available.

Therapy for Prevention of Stroke in Chronic AF

During the past 10 years, six randomized prospective trials have documented the beneficial effect of warfarin for reducing thromboembolic events in patients with nonrheumatic AF (386–394). These six studies (European Atrial Fibrillation Trial [EAFT], Canadian Atrial Fibrillation Anticoagulation [CAFA], SPINAF, SPAF I, AFASAK I, and BAATAF) enrolled 4,672 patients and demonstrated a 70% reduction of stroke with the use of warfarin (Table 15-1). This reduction was statistically significant in each of the studies except the CAFA study, which was terminated early because of the significant benefit of warfarin seen in other studies. It is important to note that the EAFT study enrolled only high-risk patients who had a prior cerebrovascular event.

In these studies, the event rate was less than 1% with and without warfarin therapy in patients younger than 65 years. With one or more risk factors, the event rate was nearly 5% in the control patients, but 2% in the warfarin-treated individuals. In subjects between the ages of 65 and 75 years, the event rate was 4% in the control group, but less than 1% in those on active therapy; if one or more risk factors were present in these individuals, the event rate was 6% in the control group and approximately 2% in treated individuals. Among patients older than 75 years, the risk of a thromboembolic event was 6% in the control group and 2% in warfarin-treated patients; if one or more risk factors were present, the event rate increased to nearly 8% but was less than 1% in warfarin-treated patients (397).

The occurrence of thromboembolic events in treated patients is also inversely related to the intensity of anticoagulation. Hylek and colleagues (395) demonstrated that stroke risk was very low in patients with an INR maintained between 2 and 4 while event rates rose steeply with INRs of less than 1.8.

Role of aspirin

Several studies directly compared the efficacy of warfarin with that of aspirin for preventing thromboembolic events (387,388,391). Two of these, the AFASAK I and EAFT trials, showed that the reduction in event rates was 40% greater with warfarin compared with aspirin. In the SPAF II trial (387), warfarin decreased stroke occurrence by approximately 30% more than aspirin in older and younger patients. The combination of aspirin and low-dose warfarin was compared with adjusted-dose warfarin in the SPAF II trial; full-dose warfarin adjusted to an INR of 2.0 to 3.0 was superior to low-dose warfarin (INR, 1.2 to 1.5) and aspirin given together (387). In addition to excess risk of thromboembolic events seen in this latter group, additional bleeding events were reported.

Bleeding Risk

The major complication of anticoagulation with warfarin is the potential for bleeding. However, the bleeding risk accompanying warfarin therapy in five large clinical trials was very low (393); of 1,236 control patients, 2 experienced an intracranial bleed while among 10 of 1,225 patients treated with warfarin, 6 developed a major intracerebral hemorrhage. A minor bleed occurred in 18 individuals in the control group and in 24 of warfarin-treated patients. The ISCOAT trial also examined the impact of warfarin anticoagulation in 2,745 patients in individuals less than 60 years of age (397a); 30 had a minor bleeding event while 5 developed a major bleed. In individuals 75 years or older, 46 (10%) had a minor bleeding complication while a major event was seen in only 10. A recent study showed that the most significant risk factor for an intracranial hemorrhage was the intensity of anticoagulation and was markedly enhanced when the INR was more than or equal to 4 (395,397b). Below a prothrombin time ratio of 2, the odds ratio for bleeding was close to 1.

Older patients may be at higher risk for hemorrhagic complications from long-term anticoagulant therapy, although this risk appears to be modest. In SPAF II (387), the annualized rate of intracranial hemorrhage in patients 75 years or older was only 1.8%, compared with 0.8% for aspirin. A subsequent analysis has suggested this bleeding rate can also be explained by the greater intensity of anticoagulation (INR target, 2.0 to 4.5) (397).

Use of Anticoagulation in AF

Despite the cost effectiveness and efficacy of anticoagulation in chronic AF, appropriate use of anticoagulation is low. From 1992, the National Ambulatory Medical Care Survey documented that only 34% of patients with AF were receiving anticoagulants from 1992 to 1993 (398). More recently, the Connecticut Peer Review Organization conducted a review of 635 Medicare patients age 65 or older who were hospitalized in 1994 with AF; about half had a principle diagnosis of stroke. Among those discharged after stroke, only 53% were prescribed warfarin while 68% received aspirin (399). This study demonstrates inadequate compliance with anticoagulation guidelines, even in patients with a significant risk for subsequent stroke. In another study, the rate of anticoagulation with warfarin was approximately 65% of patients in the 65 to 74 age group, although in those patients older than 75 years, only 45% were treated (400). It is obvious that there is hesitance to prescribe anticoagulants for elderly patients, although this remains a group in which maximal benefit occurs (401). Close follow-up of anticoagulation and maintaining the INR between 2 and 3 are the most effective means of decreasing the risk of hemorrhagic complications in this group of patients. The supplemental use of home monitoring kits may enhance this safety. Patient education also remains critical to reduce bleeding risk.

Use of Low-Molecular-Weight Heparin for Thromboembolic Prophylaxis

Low-molecular-weight heparin has the advantages that administration through the subcutaneous route is easier for outpatients and that there is less need for patient monitoring. The drug's efficacy has been demonstrated in patients who have deep venous thrombosis and in those who have acute coronary syndromes. Nonetheless, its efficacy for preventing embolization of intrachamber clots in patients with chronic fibrillation has not been comprehensively evaluated. A single study from 1993 examined the impact of low-molecular-weight heparin on the incidence of embolism in 75 AF patients; a daily subcutaneous injection (dose) of the study medication was given during 6 months (402). The incidence of embolic events was 8.6% with drug treatment, compared with 20% in the control group. In this small study, the benefit of low-molecular-weight heparin was similar to that seen with aspirin. However, the short-term use of this agent before cardioversion has not been studied and there are no studies comparing its efficacy to that of warfarin.

Treatment Recommendations in Chronic AF

Because the risk of thromboembolic events is low in patients younger than 65 years who have no risk factors for stroke, long-term anticoagulation with warfarin is not recommended; for these patients, aspirin may be considered but is not necessary. In patients with one or more risk factors for thromboembolic events, warfarin therapy is recommended. Warfarin therapy is recommended for all patients (with or without risk factors) older than 65 years. Careful monitoring of anticoagulation intensity is required to avoid bleeding risk in these patients; the recommended INR is 2 to 3.

Antithrombotic Therapy before Cardioversion

The well-established occurrence of embolic stroke as a complication of electrical or pharmacologic cardioversion of AF in the absence of anticoagulant therapy is also reduced by prior warfarin therapy. For example, a prospective cohort study from 30 years ago documented a 5.3% incidence of embolic events in patients not receiving warfarin, compared with 0.8% for those receiving anticoagulation (403). Other studies from the 1960s (404,405) have documented similar results, although no randomized trials comparing event rates with or without therapy have been conducted. All patients with heart disease, particularly mitral valve disease, require AF before conversion and anticoagulation before conversion is mandated in patients with nonrheumatic AF of more than 48 hours' duration, although only limited data supporting this time cutoff are available. In one study, Weigner and colleagues (406) examined the risk for thromboembolism associated with active restoration of sinus rhythm in patients with AF of less than 48 hours' duration. Of 357 patients, 107 patients converted spontaneously without event while 250 underwent pharmacologic or electrical conversion; central or peripheral thromboembolic events occurred in three individuals (1%). Although this rate is low, it is not negligible and suggests that in patients with risk factors for thromboembolic events, a 24-hour cutoff may be more reasonable.

The requisite duration of anticoagulant therapy before cardioversion has not been thoroughly studied, although the general recommendation is that at least 3 weeks of therapeutic anticoagulation is required to minimize stroke risk in patients with AF present for longer than 24 to 48 hours. This is based on the assumption that it takes approximately 3 weeks for thrombus to organize and adhere to the atrial wall once it has developed; anticoagulation prevents further thrombus formation. The therapeutic INR sought for patients who are to undergo chemical or electrical cardioversion is the same as that for chronic anticoagulation— an INR of 2 to 3. It is also known that there is a period of atrial stunning after reversion, and contractility does not return for 1 to 4 weeks after cardioversion (407,408). For this reason, it has been recommended that anticoagulation be continued for at least 1 month after cardioversion (409).

Most recurrences of AF occur the first 3 months after cardioversion. Recent data have also documented that at least 75% to 80% of AF episodes may be asymptomatic. In the worldwide Metrix atrial defibrillator experience, the occurrence of asymptomatic AF was assessed in 51 patients; only 19% of episodes were sufficiently symptomatic to prompt treatment while 81% were relatively asymptomatic and no therapy was instituted. Of those seeking treatment, the AF duration was nearly 40 hours but only 10 hours in those cases in which therapy was not required. These data suggest that the duration of postcardioversion anticoagulation be increased in patients at risk for thromboembolic events.

No prospective trials have examined the relative risk of a thromboembolic event with pharmacologic or direct current cardioversion. Retrospectively, Goldman suggested a comparable risk of embolization (1.5%) in patients converted from AF into sinus rhythm using quinidine rather than direct current cardioversion (410).

Role of Transesophageal Echocardiography

Transesophageal echocardiography (TEE) is used as an alternate means of identifying appropriate candidates for acute cardioversion without the use of a 3-week period of anticoagulation. In patients with AF for more than 48 hours, TEE documented left atrial appendage thrombus in 15% and a low blood velocity by Doppler in approximately 40% (282,411). Stoddard and colleagues (412) found that of 24 patients with recent embolic events, approximately 20% had left atrial thrombus. The true predictive power of TEE for detecting thrombus is difficult to assess. Observations at the time of surgery for mitral valve replacement have shown that the sensitivity of TEE for identifying intraatrial clot was 92% and the specificity was 98% (413). However, intracardiac clot may be underdetected because of their small size or the complexity of left atrial architecture (414).

The strongest support for a TEE-guided approach was provided by Manning and colleagues (411) in a 4.5-year prospective study. A total of 230 patients underwent TEE and intraatrial thrombus was identified in 15%, primarily located in the left atrial appendage; 95% of atrial thrombi visualized by TEE were not visualized by accompanying transthoracic echocardiography. Factors associated with left atrial thrombus included recent cerebrovascular event, decreased ejection fraction, spontaneous left atrial contrast (smoke), and rheumatic heart disease. Successful cardioversion to sinus rhythm was performed during heparin therapy in 186 of the 196 patients without thrombus and this was followed by at least 3 weeks of warfarin therapy; there were no thromboembolic events. All of the 34 patients with TEE-documented clots were placed on warfarin and there were no events after cardioversion.

Negative TEE findings, however, do not guarantee embolization-free cardioversion of AF or atrial flutter (413,415,416). In one multicenter retrospective study, 17 patients with AF but no demonstrable thrombus by TEE sustained a thromboembolic event after converting to normal sinus rhythm. This could have been because of the formation of clot in the chamber after conversion, as none of these patients was therapeutically anticoagulated at the time of the embolic event. Furthermore, in some cases, TEE was performed with monoplane probes. An alternative reason might have been that a thrombus in the left atrium went unrecognized, which could be related to the complicated architecture of the left atrial appendage.

The Assessment of Cardioversion Using Transesophageal Echocardiography trial compared a TEE-guided strategy with a conventional strategy in 1,222 patients with AF for more than 2 days who were undergoing electrical cardioversion (283). Patients assigned to the TEE-guided strategy were anticoagulated with heparin immediately before TEE and cardioversion; anticoagulation was continued for 4 weeks after cardioversion. If the initial TEE demonstrated thrombus, cardioversion was postponed and patients underwent routine anticoagulation for 3 weeks, at which time a second TEE was performed. Patients randomized to conventional strategy received 3 weeks of anticoagulation before cardioversion, followed by 4 weeks of anticoagulation after cardioversion. The primary end point events were ischemic stroke, TIA, and systemic embolization at an 8-week follow-up. There was no difference between the TEE and conventional groups in the incidence of ischemic stroke (0.65% versus 0.33%), TIA (0.16% versus 0.17%), or all embolic events (0.81% versus 0.5%) (417). Additionally, there was no difference in the incidence of major bleeding (0.8% versus 1.5%), all-cause mortality (2.4% versus 1%), or cardiac deaths (1.3% versus 0.66%). These data suggest that the TEE strategy is an alternative to a conventional approach; however, the study was underpowered to detect any differences as 2,900 patients were required.

Recommendations for Anticoagulation before Cardioversion

A reasonable approach to managing anticoagulation around the time of cardioversion is as follows:

1. For patients with no valvular heart disease who have AF known to be of less than 24 to 36 hours, no anticoagulation is needed.
2. For patients with nonvalvular AF of more than 24 to 36 hours or of unknown duration and those at high risk (valvular disease or high-risk features), 3 weeks of full-dose anticoagulation to an INR of 2 to 3 is strongly recommended before chemical or electrical cardioversion. A minimum of 1 month of therapeutic anticoagulation after cardioversion is required. An acceptable alternative to this approach is to screen patients by TEE for intra-atrial thrombus. If no clot is seen, the patient may be cardioverted while heparinized but still must receive at least 4 weeks of therapeutic anticoagulation after conversion.

The length of time needed to appropriately treat a patients with left atrial thrombus identified by TEE is unclear. Among patients with nonvalvular AF, the efficacy of prolonged anticoagulation before cardioversion appears to be largely related to resolution of left atrial thrombi. Resolution of thrombi occurs in more than 85% of these patients after 4 weeks of warfarin therapy (417); the time of resolution is more prolonged in patients with rheumatic mitral valve disease or chronic AF. These observations suggest that the benefit of anticoagulation is to cause thrombus resolution and to prevent new thrombus formation, rather than promote organization of the thrombus.

REFERENCES

1. Robles de Medina EO, Bernard R, Coumel P, et al. WHO-ISFC Task Force. Definition of terms related to cardiac rhythm. *Am Heart J* 1978;95:796–806.
2. Suttorp MJ, Kingma JH, Koomen EM, et al. Recurrence of paroxysmal atrial fibrillation or flutter after successful cardioversion in patients with normal left ventricular function. *Am J Cardiol* 1993;71:710–713.
3. Van Gelder IC, Crijns HJGM, Tieleman RG, et al. Value and limitation of electrical cardioversion in patients with chronic atrial fibrillation—importance of arrhythmia risk factors and oral anticoagulation. *Arch Intern Med* 1996;156:2585–2592.
4. Sopher SM, Camm AJ. Atrial fibrillation—maintenance of sinus rhythm versus rate control. *Am J Cardiol* 1996;77:24A–38A.
5. Levy S, Maarek M, Coumel P, et al. Characterization of different subsets of atrial fibrillation in general practice in France: the ALFA study. The College of French Cardiologists. *Circulation* 1999;99:3028–3035.
6. Takahashi N, Seki A, Imataka K, Fujii J. Clinical features of paroxysmal atrial fibrillation. An observation of 94 patients. *Jpn Heart J* 1981;22:143–149.
7. Godtfresen J. Atrial fibrillation: course and prognosis. A follow-up study of 1212 cases. In: Kulbertus HE, Olsson SB, Schlepper M, eds. *Atrial fibrillation*. Mölndal, Sweden: AB Hässle, 1982:134–145.
8. Fresco C, Proclemer A, for the PAFIT 2 Investigators. Management of recent onset atrial fibrillation. *Eur Heart J* 1996;17 [Suppl C]:41–47.
9. Danias PG, Caulfield TA, Weigner MJ, et al. Likelihood of spontaneous conversion of atrial fibrillation to sinus rhythm. *J Am Coll Cardiol* 1998;31:588–592.
10. Levy S, Breithardt G, Campbell RW, et al. Atrial fibrillation: current knowledge and recommendations for management. Working Group on Arrhythmias of the European Society of Cardiology. *Eur Heart J* 1998;19:1294–1320.

11. Godtfredsen J. *Atrial fibrillation. Etiology, course and prognosis. A follow-up study 1212 cases.* Copenhagen: Thesis University of Copenhagen, 1975.

12. Wijffels MCEF, Kirchhof CJHJ, Dorland R, Allessie MA. Atrial fibrillation begets atrial fibrillation: a study in awake, chronically instrumented goats. *Circulation* 1995;92:1954–1962.

13. Ausma J, Wijffels M, Thone F, et al. Structural changes of atrial myocardium due to sustained atrial fibrillation in the goat. *Circulation* 1997;96:3157–3163.

14. Brundel BJJM, Van Gelder IC, Henning RH, et al. Ion channel remodeling is related to intraoperative atrial flutter in patients with paroxysmal and persistent atrial fibrillation. *Circulation.* 2001;103:690–698.

15. Kannel WB, Abbott RD, Savage DD, McNamara PM. Epidemiologic features of chronic atrial fibrillation. The Framingham Study. *N Engl J Med* 1982;306:1018–1022.

16. Wolf PA, Abbott RD, Kannel WB. Atrial fibrillation as an independent risk factor for stroke: the Framingham Study. *Stroke* 1991;22:983–988.

17. Philips SJ, Whisnant J, O'Fallon WM, Frye RL. Prevalence of cardiovascular disease and diabetes in residents of Rochester, Minnesota. *Mayo Clin Proc* 1990;65:344–359.

18. Lake RR, Cullen KJ, deKlerk NH, et al. Atrial fibrillation in an elderly population. *Aust N Z J Med* 1989;19:321–326.

19. Furberg CD, Psaty BM, Manolio TA, et al. Prevalence of atrial fibrillation in elderly subjects: the Cardiovascular Health Study. *Am J Cardiol* 1994;74:238–241.

20. Benjamin EJ, Levy D, Vaziri SM, et al. Independent risk factors for atrial fibrillation in a population-based cohort. The Framingham Heart Study. *JAMA* 1994;271:840–844.

21. Feinberg WM, Blackshear JL, Laupacis A, et al. Prevalence, age distribution, and gender of patients with atrial fibrillation. Analysis and implications. *Arch Intern Med* 1995;155(5):469–473.

22. Atrial Fibrillation Investigators. Risk factors for stroke and efficacy of anti-thrombotic therapy in atrial fibrillation: analysis of pooled data from five randomized trials. *Arch Intern Med* 1994; 154:1449–1457.

23. Kannel WB, Wolf PA, Benjamin EJ, Levy D. Prevalence, incidence, prognosis, and predisposing conditions for atrial fibrillation: population-based estimates. *Am J Cardiol* 1998;82:2N–9N.

24. U.S. Bureau of the Census. *Statistical abstract of the United States: 1993,* 113th ed. Washington: U.S. Bureau of the Census, 1993:16.

25. Crenshaw BS, Ward SR, Granger CB, et al, for the GUSTO I Trial Investigators. Atrial fibrillation in the setting of acute myocardial infarction: the GUSTO I experience. *J Am Coll Cardiol* 1997;30:406–413.

26. Psaty BM, Manolio TA, Kuller LH, et al. Incidence of and risk factors for atrial fibrillation in older adults. *Circulation* 1997; 96:2455–2461.

27. Vaziri SM, Larson MG, Benjamin EJ, Levy D. Echocardiographic predictors of nonrheumatic atrial fibrillation. The Framingham Heart Study. *Circulation* 1994;89:724–730.

28. Robinson K, Frenneaux MP, Stockins B, et al. Atrial fibrillation in hypertrophic cardiomyopathy: a longitudinal study. *J Am Coll Cardiol* 1990;15:1279–1285.

29. Chen PS, Pressley JC, Tang AS, et al. New observations on atrial fibrillation before and after surgical treatment in patients with the Wolff-Parkinson-White syndrome. *J Am Coll Cardiol* 1992; 19:974–981.

30. Creswell LL, Schuessler RB, Rosenbloom M, Cox JL. Hazards of postoperative atrial arrhythmias. *Ann Thorac Surg* 1993;56: 539–549.

31. Sawin CT, Geller A, Wolf PA, et al. Low serum thyrotropin concentrations as a risk factor for atrial fibrillation in older persons. *N Engl J Med* 1994;331:1249–1252.

32. Ettinger PO. Holiday heart arrhythmias. *Int J Cardiol* 1984;5: 540–542.

33. Davidson E, Weinberger I, Rotenberg Z, et al. Causes and time of onset of atrial fibrillation. *Arch Intern Med* 1989;149:457–459.

34. Brand FN, Abott RD, Kannel WB, Wolf PA. Characteristics and prognosis of lone atrial fibrillation: 30-year follow-up in the Framingham Study. *JAMA* 1985;254:3449–3453.

35. Kopecky SL, Gersh BJ, McGoon MD, et al. The natural history of lone atrial fibrillation: a population–based study over three decades. *N Engl J Med* 1987;317:669–674.

36. Benjamin EJ, Wolf PA, D'Agostino RB, et al. Impact of atrial fibrillation on the risk of death: the Framingham Heart Study. *Circulation* 1998;98:946–952.

37. Murgatroyd FD, Gibson SM, Baiyan X, et al. Double-blind placebo-controlled trial of digoxin in symptomatic paroxysmal atrial fibrillation. *Circulation* 1999;99:2765–2770.

38. Pedersen OD, Bagger H, Kober L, Torp-Pedersen C. The occurrence and prognostic significance of atrial fibrillation/ flutter following acute myocardial infarction. TRACE Study Group. TR Andolapril Cardiac Evaluation. *Eur Heart J* 1999; 20:748–754.

39. Behar S, Zahavi Z, Goldbourt U, Reicher-Reiss H, and the SPRINT Study Group. Long-term prognosis of patients with paroxysmal atrial fibrillation complicating acute myocardial infarction. *Eur Heart J* 1992;13:45–50.

40. Goldberg RJ, Seeley D, Becker RC, et al. Impact of atrial fibrillation on the in-hospital and long-term survival of patients with acute myocardial infarction: a community-wide perspective. *Am Heart J* 1990, 119:996–1001.

41. Kobayashi Y, Katoh T, Takano T, Hayakawa H. Paroxysmal atrial fibrillation and flutter associated with acute myocardial infarction: hemodynamic evaluation in relation to the development of arrhythmias and prognosis. *Jpn Circ J* 1992; 56:1–11.

42. Liberthson RR, Salisbury KW, Hutter AM Jr, DeSanctis RW. Atrial tachyarrhythmias in acute myocardial infarction. *Am J Med* 1976;60:956–960.

43. Diker E, Aydogdu S, Ozdemir M, et al. Prevalence and predictors of atrial fibrillation in rheumatic heart disease. *Am J Cardiol* 1996;77:96.

44. Moreyra AE, Wilson AC, Deac R, et al. Factors associated with atrial fibrillation in patients with mitral stenosis: a cardiac catheterization study. *Am Heart J* 1998;135:138.

45. Carson PE, Johnson GR, Dunkman WB, et al, for the V-HeFT VA Cooperative Studies Group. The influence of atrial fibrillation on prognosis in mild to moderate heart failure. The V-HeFT Studies. *Circulation* 1993;87[Suppl VI]:102–110.

46. Stevenson WG, Stevenson LW, Middlekauff HR, et al. Improving survival for patients with atrial fibrillation and advanced heart failure. *J Am Coll Cardiol* 1996:28(6):1458–63.

47. Falk RH. Cardiac amyloidosis. *Prog Cardiol* 1989;2:143–156.

48. Hodkinson HM, Pomerance A. The clinical pathology of heart failure and atrial fibrillation in old age. *Postgrad Med* 1979;55: 251.

49. Cecchi F, Olivotto I, Montereggi A, et al. Hypertrophic cardiomyopathy in Tuscany: clinical course and outcome in an unselected regional population. *J Am Coll Cardiol* 1995;26:1529.

50. McKenna WJ, England D, Doi Y, et al. Arrhythmia in hypertrophic cardiomyopathy. 1. Influence on prognosis. *Br Heart J* 1981;46:168.

51. Bashur TT. Classification of sinus node dysfunction. *Am Heart J* 1985;110:1251–1258.

52. Kaplan BM, Langendorf R, Lev M, et al. Tachycardia-bradycardia syndrome (so called "sick sinus syndrome"). *Am J Cardiol* 1973;26:497–502.

53. Vallin H, Edhag V. Associated conduction disturbances in

patients with symptomatic sinus node disease. *Acta Med Scand* 1981;210:263–270.

54. Sutton R, Kenny RA. The natural history of sick sinus syndrome. *Pace* 1986;9:1110–1114.

55. Campbell RWF, Smith RA, Gallagher JJ, et al. Atrial fibrillation in the pre-excitation syndrome. *Am J Cardiol* 1977;40:514–520.

56. Bauernfiend RA, Wyndham CR, Swiryn SD, et al. Paroxysmal atrial fibrillation in the Wolff-Parkinson-White Syndrome. *Am J Cardiol* 1981;47:562–569.

57. Fuijimura O, Klein GJ, Yee R, et al. Mode of onset of atrial fibrillation in the Wolff-Parkinson-White syndrome: how important is the accessory pathway? *J Am Coll Cardiol* 1990;15: 1082–1086.

58. Morady F, Sledge C, Shen E, et al. Electrophysiologic testing in the management of patients with the Wolff-Parkinson-White syndrome and atrial fibrillation. *Am J Cardiol* 1973;51: 1623–1628.

59. Klein LS, Miles WM, Zipes DP. Effect of atrioventricular interval during pacing or reciprocating tachycardia in atrial size, pressure and refractory period: contraction excitation feedback in human atrium. *Circulation* 1990;82:60–68.

60. Gallastegui JL, Bauman JL, Hariman RJ. The predictive value of electrophysiologic studies in untreated patients with Wolff-Parkinson-White syndrome. *J Am Coll Cardiol* 1990;15: 640–647.

61. Klein GJ, Bashore TM, Sellers TD, et al. Ventricular fibrillation in the Wolff-Parkinson-White syndrome. *N Engl J Med* 1979; 301:1080–1085.

62. Ommen SR, Odell JA, Stanton MS. Atrial arrhythmias after cardio-thoracic surgery. *N Engl J Med* 1997;336:1429–1434.

63. Aranki SF, Shaw DP, Adams DH, et al. Predictors of atrial fibrillation after coronary artery surgery: current trends and impact on hospital resources. *Circulation* 1996;94:390–397.

64. Asher CR, Miller DP, Grimm RA, et al. Analysis of risk factors for development of atrial fibrillation early after cardiac valvular surgery. *Am J Cardiol* 1998;82:892–895.

65. Kowey PR. Atrial arrhythmias after cardiac surgery: Sisyphus revisited? *J Am Coll Cardiol* 1999;34:348–350.

66. Cohen EJ, Klatsky AL, Armstrong MA. Alcohol use and supraventricular arrhythmia. *Am J Cardiol* 1988;62:971–973.

67. Lowenstein AJ, Gaboer PA, Cramer J, et al. The role of alcohol in new onset atrial fibrillation. *Arch Intern Med* 1983;143: 1882–1885.

68. Koskinen P, Kupari M, Leonine H, et al. Alcohol and new onset atrial fibrillation: a case control study of a current series. *Br Heart J* 1987;57:468–473.

69. Gould L, Reddy LV, Becker W, et al. Electrophysiologic properties of alcohol in man. *J Electrocardiol* 1978;11:219–226.

70. Gimeno AL, Bimeno MD, Webb JL. Effects of alcohol on cellular membrane potential and contractility of isolated atrium. *Am J Physiol* 1962;203:194–196.

71. Forfar JC, Toft AD. Thyrotoxic atrial fibrillation: an under diagnosed condition. *Br Med J* 1982;285:909–910.

72. Cobbler JL, Williams MC, Greenland P. Thyrotoxicosis in institutionalized elderly patients with atrial fibrillation. *Arch Intern Med* 1984;144:1758–1770.

73. Thomas FS, Mozzferri EL, Skillman TK. Apathetic thyrotoxicosis: a distinct clinical and laboratory abnormality. *Ann Intern Med* 1970;72:679–685.

74. Iwasaki T, Naka H, Namatsu K, et al. Echocardiographic studies on the relationship between atrial fibrillation and atrial enlargement in patients with hyperthyroidism of Graves disease. *Cardiology* 1989;76:10–17.

75. Fortar JC, Feck CM, Miller HC, et al. Atrial fibrillation and isolated suppression of the pituitary thyroid axis to specific antithyroid therapy. *Int J Cardiol* 1981;1:43–48.

76. Williams LT, Lefkowitz RJ, Witanabe AM, et al. Thyroid hormone regulation of beta adrenergic receptor number. *J Biol Chem* 1977;252:2787.

76a. Brugada R, Tapscott T, Czernuszewicz GZ, et al. Identification of a genetic locus for familial atrial fibrillation. *N Engl J Med* 1997;336(13):905–911.

77. Kannel WB, Abbott RD, Savage DD. Coronary heart disease and atrial fibrillation: the Framingham Study. *Am Heart J* 1985; 106:386–396.

78. Dries DL, Exner DV, Gersh BJ, et al. Atrial fibrillation is associated with an increased risk for mortality and heart failure progression in patients with asymptomatic and symptomatic left ventricular systolic dysfunction: a retrospective analysis of the SOLVD trials. *J Am Coll Cardiol* 1998;32:3:695–703.

79. Flaker GC, Blackshear JL, McBride R, et al. Antiarrhythmic drug therapy and cardiac mortality in atrial fibrillation. *J Am Coll Cardiol* 1992;20:527–532.

80. Peterson P, Godtfredsen J. Embolic complications in paroxysmal atrial fibrillation. *Stroke* 1986;17:622–626.

81. Brookes CIO, White PA, Staples M, et al. Myocardial contractility is not constant during spontaneous atrial fibrillation. *Circulation* 1998;98:1762.

82. Daoud EG, Weiss R, Bahu M, et al. Effect of an irregular ventricular rhythm on cardiac output. *Am J Cardiol* 1996;78:1433.

83. Sun H, Gaspo R, Leblanc N, et al. Cellular mechanisms of atrial contractile dysfunction caused by sustained atrial tachycardia. *Circulation* 1998;98:719.

84. Yonemochi H, Yasunaga S, Teshima Y, et al. Rapid electrical stimulation of contraction reduces the density of beta-adrenergic receptors and responsiveness of cultured neonatal rat cardiomyocytes. Possible involvement of microtubule disassembly secondary to mechanical stress. *Circulation* 2000;101:2625.

85. Clark DM, Plumb VJ, Epstein AE, Kay GN. Hemodynamic effects of irregular sequence of ventricular cycle lengths during atrial fibrillation. *J Am Coll Cardiol* 1997;30:1039–1045.

86. Grogan M, Smith HC, Gersh BJ, Wood DL. Left ventricular dysfunction due to atrial fibrillation in patients initially believed to have idiopathic dilated cardiomyopathy. *Am J Cardiol* 1992; 69:1570–1573.

87. Packer DL, Bardy GH, Worley SJ, et al. Tachycardia-induced cardiomyopathy: a reversible form of left ventricular dysfunction. *Am J Cardiol* 1986;57:563–570.

88. Rodriguez LM, Smeets JL, Xie B, et al. Improvement in left ventricular function by ablation of atrioventricular nodal conduction in selected patients with lone atrial fibrillation. *Am J Cardiol* 1993;72:1137–1141.

89. Kieny JR, Sacrez A, Facello A, et al. Increase in radionuclide left ventricular ejection fraction after cardioversion of chronic atrial fibrillation in idiopathic dilated cardiomyopathy. *Eur Heart J* 1992;13:1290.

90. Twidale N, Sutton P, Kreiner G, et al. Improvement in left ventricular systolic function after successful radiofrequency His bundle ablation for drug refractory, chronic atrial fibrillation and recurrent atrial flutter. *Am J Cardiol* 1992;69:489.

91. Middlekauff HR, Stevenson WG, Stevenson LW. Prognostic significance of atrial fibrillation in advanced heart failure: a study of 390 patients. *Circulation* 1991;84:40–48.

92. Ezekowitz MD, Levine JA. Preventing stroke in patients with atrial fibrillation. *JAMA* 1999;281:1830–1835.

93. Wolf PA, Abbot RD, Kannel WB. Atrial fibrillation: a major contributor to stroke in the elderly. *Arch Intern Med* 1987;147: 1561–1564.

94. Jones EF, Calafiore P, McNeil JJ, et al. Atrial fibrillation with left atrial spontaneous contrast detected by transesophageal echocardiography is a potent risk factor for stroke. *Am J Cardiol* 1996;78:425.

95. Heppell RM, Berkin KE, McLenachan JM, Davies JA. Haemostatic and haemodynamic abnormalities associated with left atrial thrombosis in non-rheumatic atrial fibrillation. *Heart* 1997;77:407

96. The Stroke Prevention in Atrial Fibrillation Investigators Committee on Echocardiography. Transesophageal echocardiographic correlates of thromboembolism in high-risk patients with nonvalvular atrial fibrillation. *Ann Intern Med* 1998;128:639.

97. Atrial Fibrillation Investigators. Echocardiographic predictors of stroke in patients with atrial fibrillation. *Arch Intern Med* 1998;158:1316.

98. Wolf PA, Mitchell JB, Baker CS, et al. Impact of atrial fibrillation on mortality, stroke, and medical costs. *Arch Intern Med* 1998;158:229–234.

99. Davies MJ, Pomerance A. Pathology of atrial fibrillation in man. *Br Heart J* 1972;34:520–525.

100. Sanfilippo AJ, Abascal VM, Sheehan M, et al. Atrial enlargement as a consequence of atrial fibrillation. A prospective echocardiographic study. *Circulation* 1990;82:792–797.

101. Boutjdir M, Le Heuzey JY, Lavergne T, et al. Inhomogeneity of cellular refractoriness in human atrium: factor of arrhythmia? *Pace* 1986;9:1095–1100.

102. Ravelli F, Allessie M. Effects of atrial dilatation on refractory period and vulnerability to atrial fibrillation in the isolated Langendorff-perfused rabbit heart. *Circulation* 1997;96:1686–1695.

103. Lie JT, Hammond PI. Pathology of the senescent heart: anatomic observation on 237 autopsy studies of patients 90 to 105 years old. *Mayo Clin Proc* 1988;63:552–564.

104. Spach MS, Dolber PC. Relating extracellular potentials and their derivatives to anisotropic propagation at a microscopic level in human cardiac muscle. Evidence for electrical uncoupling of side-to-side fiber connections with increasing age. *Circ Res* 1986;58:356–371.

105. Ausma J, Wijffels M, Thone F, et al. Structural changes of atrial myocardium due to sustained atrial fibrillation in the goat. *Circulation* 1997;96:3157–3163.

106. Morillo CA, Klein GJ, Jones DL, Guiraudon CM. Chronic rapid atrial pacing. Structural, functional, and electrophysiological characteristics of a new model of sustained atrial fibrillation. *Circulation* 1995;91:1588–1595.

107. Ausma J, Wijffels M, van Eys G, et al. Dedifferentiation of atrial cardiomyocytes as a result of chronic atrial fibrillation. *Am J Pathol* 1997;151:985–997.

108. Manning WJ, Silverman DI. Atrial anatomy and function postcardioversion: insights from transthoracic and transesophageal echocardiography. *Prog Cardiovasc Dis* 1996;39:33–46.

109. Rossi L. Cardioneuropathy and extracardiac neural disease. *J Am Coll Cardiol* 1985;5:66B–70B.

110. Olgin JE, Sih HJ, Hanish S, et al. Heterogeneous atrial denervation creates substrate for sustained atrial fibrillation. *Circulation* 1998;98:2608–2614.

111. Goette A, Honeycutt C, Langberg JJ. Electrical remodeling in atrial fibrillation. Time course and mechanisms. *Circulation* 1996;94:2968–2974.

112. Konings KT, Kirchhof CJ, Smeets JR, et al. High-density mapping of electrically induced atrial fibrillation in humans. *Circulation* 1994;89:1665–1680.

113. Kumagai K, Khrestian, Waldo AL. Simultaneous multisite mapping studies during induced atrial fibrillation in the sterile pericarditis model. Insights into the mechanism of its maintenance. *Circulation* 1997;95:511.

114. Janse MJ, Allessie MA. Experimental observations on atrial fibrillation. In: Falk RH, Podrid PJ, eds. *Atrial fibrillation: mechanisms and management,* 2nd ed. Philadelphia: Lippincott–Raven Publishers, 1997:53–73.

115. Allessie MA, Lammers WJEP, Bonke FIM. Experimental evaluation of Moe's multiple wavelet hypothesis of atrial fibrillation. In: Zipes DP, Jalife J, eds. *Cardiac electrophysiology and arrhythmias.* Orlando, FL: Grune & Stratton, 1985:265–275.

116. Moe GK, Rheinboldt WC, Abildskov JA. A computer model of atrial fibrillation. *Am Heart J* 1964;67:200–220.

117. Schuessler RB, Grayson TM, Bromberg BI, et al. Cholinergically mediated tachyarrhythmias induced by a single extrastimulus in the isolated canine right atrium. *Circ Res* 1992;71: 1254–1267.

118. Cox JL, Canavan TE, Schuessler RB, et al. The surgical treatment of atrial fibrillation. II. Intraoperative electrophysiologic mapping and description of the electrophysiologic basis of atrial flutter and atrial fibrillation. *J Thorac Cardiovasc Surg* 1991;101: 406–426.

119. Scherf D. Studies on auricular tachycardia caused by aconitine administration. *Proc Soc Exp Biol Med* 1947;64:233–239.

120. Garrey WE. The nature of fibrillary contraction of the heart. Its relation to tissue mass and form. *Am J Physiol* 1914;33: 397–414.

121. Haissaguerre M, Jais P, Shah DC, et al. Spontaneous initiation of atrial fibrillation by ectopic beats originating in the pulmonary veins. *N Engl J Med* 1998;339:659–666.

122. Allessie MA, Bonke FI, Schopman FJ. Circus movement in rabbit atrial muscle as a mechanism of tachycardia. III. The "leading circle" concept: a new model of circus movement in cardiac tissue without the involvement of an anatomical obstacle. *Circ Res* 1977;41:9–18.

123. Rensma PL, Allessie MA, Lammers WJ, et al. Length of excitation wave and susceptibility to reentrant atrial arrhythmias in normal conscious dogs. *Circ Res* 1988;62:395–410.

124. Wang J, Bourne GW, Wang Z, et al. Comparative mechanisms of antiarrhythmic drug action in experimental atrial fibrillation. Importance of use-dependent effects on refractoriness. *Circulation* 1993;88:1030–1044.

125. Haissaguerre M, Jais P, Shah DC, et al. Right and left atrial radiofrequency catheter therapy of paroxysmal atrial fibrillation. *J Cardiovasc Electrophysiol* 1996;7:1132–1144.

126. Moe GK. On the multiple wavelet hypothesis of atrial fibrillation. *Arch Intern Pharmacodyn Ther* 1962;140:183–188.

127. Patel P, Jones D, Dupont E. Remodelling of atrial connexin 43 expression in human atrial fibrillation. *Eur Heart J* 1998;19: 465.

128. Gray RA, Pertsov AM, Jalife J. Incomplete reentry and epicardial breakthrough patterns during atrial fibrillation in the sheep heart. *Circulation* 1996;94:2649–2661.

129. Jalife J, Gray RA. Importance of the complex three-dimensional anatomic structure in propagation during atrial fibrillation. Saoudi N, Schels W, El-Sherif N, eds. *Atrial flutter and fibrillation: from basic to clinical application.* Armonk, NY: Futura Publishing, 1998:17–33.

130. Takahashi N, Seki A, Imataka K, Fujii J. Clinical features of paroxysmal atrial fibrillation. An observation of 94 patients. *Jpn Heart J* 1981;22:143–149.

131. Kopecky SL, Gersh BJ, McGoon MD, et al. The natural history of lone atrial fibrillation. A population-based study over three decades. *N Engl J Med* 1987;317:669–674.

132. Wijffels MC, Kirchhof CJ, Dorland R, Allessie MA. Atrial fibrillation begets atrial fibrillation. A study in awake chronically instrumented goats. *Circulation* 1995;92:1954–1968.

133. Ramdat Misier AR, Opthof T, van Hemel NM, et al. Increased dispersion of "refractoriness" in patients with idiopathic paroxysmal atrial fibrillation. *J Am Coll Cardiol* 1992;19:1531–1535.

134. Fareh S, Villemaire C, Nattel S. Importance of refractoriness heterogeneity in the enhanced vulnerability to atrial fibrillation induction caused by tachycardia-induced atrial electrical remodeling. *Circulation* 1998;98:2202–2209.

135. Wang J, Liu L, Feng J, Nattel S. Regional and functional factors determining induction and maintenance of atrial fibrillation in dogs. *Am J Physiol* 1996;271:H148–H158.

136. Fareh S, Bénardeau A, Thibault B, Nattel S. The T-type Ca²⁺ channel blocker mibefradil prevents the development of a substrate for atrial fibrillation by tachycardia-induced atrial remodeling in dogs. *Circulation* 1999;100:2191–2197.

137. Gaspo R, Bosch RF, Talajic M, Nattel S. Functional mechanisms underlying tachycardia-induced sustained atrial fibrillation in a chronic dog model. *Circulation* 1997;96:4027–4035.

138. Daoud EG, Bogun F, Goyal R, et al. Effect of atrial fibrillation on atrial refractoriness in humans. *Circulation* 1996;94:1600–1606.

139. Franz MR, Karasik PL, Li C, et al. Electrical remodeling of the human atrium: similar effects in patients with chronic atrial fibrillation and atrial flutter. *J Am Coll Cardiol* 1997;30:1785–1792.

140. Bosch RF, Zeng X, Grammer JB, et al. Ionic mechanisms of electrical remodeling in human atrial fibrillation. *Cardiovasc Res* 1999;44:121–131.

141. Attuel P, Childers R, Cauchemez B, et al. Failure in the rate adaption of the atrial refractory period: its relationship to vulnerability. *Int J Cardiol* 1958;2:179–197.

142. Wellens HJ, Lau CP, Luderitz B, et al. Atrioverter: an implantable device for the treatment of atrial fibrillation. *Circulation* 1998;98:1651–1656.

143. Tieleman RG, Van Gelder IC, Crijns HJ, et al. Early recurrences of atrial fibrillation after electrical cardioversion: a result of fibrillation-induced electrical remodeling of the atria? *J Am Coll Cardiol* 1998;31:167–173.

144. Feng J, Yue L, Wang Z, Nattel S. Ionic mechanisms of regional action potential heterogeneity in the canine right atrium. *Circ Res* 1998;83:541–551.

145. Yue L, Feng J, Gaspo R, et al. Ionic remodeling underlying action potential changes in a canine model of atrial fibrillation. *Circ Res* 1997;81:512–525.

146. Daoud EG, Knight BP, Weiss R, et al. Effect of verapamil and procainamide on atrial fibrillation-induced electrical remodeling in humans. *Circulation* 1997;96:1542–1550.

147. Sun H, Gaspo R, Leblanc N, Nattel S. Cellular mechanisms of atrial contractile dysfunction caused by sustained atrial tachycardia. *Circulation* 1998;98:719–727.

148. Leistad E, Aksnes G, Verburg E, Christensen G. Atrial contractile dysfunction after short-term atrial fibrillation is reduced by verapamil but increased by Bay K 8644. *Circulation* 1996;93:1747–1754.

149. Tieleman RG, De Langen C, Van Gelder IC, et al. Verapamil reduces tachycardia-induced electrical remodeling of the atria. *Circulation* 1997;95:1945–1953.

150. Wijffels MC, Kirchhof CJ, Dorland R, et al. Electrical remodeling due to atrial fibrillation in chronically instrumented conscious goats: roles of neurohumoral changes, ischemia, atrial stretch, and high rate of electrical activation. *Circulation* 1997;96:3710–3720.

151. Chen SA, Hsieh MH, Tai CT, et al. Initiation of atrial fibrillation by ectopic beats originating from the pulmonary veins: electrophysiological characteristics, pharmacological responses, and effects of radiofrequency ablation. *Circulation* 1999;100:1879.

152. Coumel P. The role of the autonomic nervous system in atrial flutter and fibrillation: clinical findings. In: Saoudi N, Schels W, El-Sherif N, eds. *Atrial flutter and fibrillation: from basic to clinical applications.* Armonk, NY: Futura Publishing, 1998:89–103.

153. Liu L, Nattel S. Differing sympathetic and vagal effects on atrial fibrillation in dogs: role of refractoriness heterogeneity. *Am J Physiol* 1997;273:H805.

154. Coumel P. Autonomic influences in atrial tachyarrhythmias. *J Cardiovasc Electrophysiol* 1996;7:999.

155. Geddes LA, Hinds M, Babbs CF, et al. Maintenance of atrial fibrillation in anesthetized and unanesthetized sheep using cholinergic drive. *Pacing Clin Electrophysiol* 1996;19:165.

156. Yamada M, Jahangir A, Hosoya Y, et al. GK* and brain G beta gamma activate muscarinic K⁺ channel through the same mechanism. *J Biol Chem* 1993;268:24551–24554.

157. Yamada M, Inanobe A, Kurachi Y. G protein regulation of potassium ion channels. *Pharmacol Rev* 1998;50:723–760.

158. Allessie R, Nusynowitz M, Abildskov J, Moe G. Non-uniform distribution of vagal effects on atrial refractory period. *Am J Physiol* 1958;194:406–410.

159. Levy MN. Autonomic nervous system in atrial flutter and fibrillation. In: Saoudi N, Schels W, El-Sherif N, eds. *Atrial flutter and fibrillation: from basic to clinical applications.* Armonk, NY: Futura Publishing, 1998:69–87.

160. Manning WJ, Leeman DE, Gotch PJ, Come PC. Pulsed Doppler evaluation of atrial mechanical function after electrical cardioversion of atrial fibrillation. *J Am Coll Cardiol* 1989;13:617–623.

161. Samet P, Bernstein W, Levine S. Significance of the atrial contribution to ventricular filling. *Am J Cardiol* 1965;15:195–202.

162. Rowlands DJ, Logan WF, Howitt G. Atrial function after cardioversion. *Am Heart J* 1967;74:149–160.

163. Shapiro W, Klein G. Alterations in cardiac function immediately following electoral conversion of atrial fibrillation to normal sinus rhythm. *Circulation* 1968;38:1074–1084.

164. Atwood JE. Exercise hemodynamics of atrial fibrillation. In: Falk RH, Podrid PJ, eds. *Atrial fibrillation: mechanisms and management.* New York: Raven Press, 1992:145–163.

165. Graettinger JS, Carleton RA, Muenster JJ. Circulatory consequences of changes in cardiac rhythm produced in patients by transthoracic direct-current shock. *J Clin Invest* 1964;43:2290–2302.

166. Killip T, Baer RA. Hemodynamic effects after reversion from atrial fibrillation to sinus rhythm by precordial shock. *J Clin Invest* 1966;45:658–671.

167. Lipkin DP, Frenneaux M, Steward R, et al. Delayed improvement in exercise capacity after cardioversion of atrial fibrillation to sinus rhythm. *Br Heart J* 1988;59:572–577.

168. Sacrez A, Kieny JR, Bouhouw JB, et al. Effect of cardioversion of atrial fibrillation on left ventricular function in dilated cardiomyopathy: a multicenter study [in French]. *Arch Mal Coeur* 1990;83:15–21.

169. Skinner NS, Mitchell JH, Wallace AG, Sarnoff SJ. Hemodynamic consequences of atrial fibrillation at constant ventricular rates. *Am J Med* 1964;36:342–350.

170. Alam A, Thorstrand C. Left ventricular function in patients with atrial fibrillation before and after cardioversion. *Am J Cardiol* 1992;69:694–696.

171. Braunwald E. Symposium on cardiac arrhythmias: introduction with comments on the hemodynamic significance of atrial systole. *Am J Med* 1964;37:665–669.

172. Morris JJ Jr, Entman M, North WC, et al. The changes in cardiac output with reversion of atrial fibrillation to sinus rhythm. *Circulation* 1965;31:670–678.

173. Resnekov L. Haemodynamic studies before and after electrical conversion of atrial fibrillation and flutter to sinus rhythm. *Br Heart J* 1967;29:700–708.

174. Khaja F, Parker JO. Hemodynamic effects of cardioversion in chronic atrial fibrillation. *Arch Intern Med* 1972;129:433–440.

175. Atwood JE, Myers J, Sullivan M, et al. The effect of cardioversion on maximal exercise capacity in patients with chronic atrial fibrillation. *Am Heart J* 1989;118:913–918.

176. Carleton RA, Graettinger JS. The hemodynamic role of the

atria with and without mitral stenosis. *Am J Med* 1967;42: 532–538.

177. Naito M, David M, Michelson EL, et al. The hemodynamic consequences of cardiac arrhythmias: evaluation of the relative roles of abnormal atrioventricular sequencing, irregularity of ventricular rhythm and atrial fibrillation in a canine model. *Am Heart J* 1983;106:284–291.

178. Herbert WJ. Cardiac output and the varying R-R interval of atrial fibrillation. *J Electrocardiol* 1973;6:131–135.

179. Kerr AJ, Simmonds MB, Stewart RAH. Influence of heart rate on stroke volume variability in atrial fibrillation in patients with normal and impaired left ventricular function. *Am J Cardiol* 1998;82:1496–1500.

180. Daoud EG, Weiss R, Bahu M, et al. Effect of an irregular ventricular rhythm on cardiac output. *Am J Cardiol* 1996;78: 1433–1436.

181. Clark DM, Plumb VJ, Epstein AE, Kay GN: Hemodynamic effects of an irregular sequence of ventricular cycle lengths during atrial fibrillation. *J Am Coll Cardiol* 1997;30:1039–1045.

182. Belenkie I. Beat-to-beat variability of echocardiographic measurements of left ventricular end diastolic diameter and performance. *J Clin Ultrasound* 1979;7:263–268.

183. Gosselink ATM, Blanksma PK, Crijns HJGM, et al. Left ventricular beat-to-beat performance in atrial fibrillation: contribution of Frank-Starling mechanism after short rather than long RR intervals. *J Am Coll Cardiol* 1995;26:1516–1521.

184. Buchbinder WC, Sugerman. Arterial blood pressure in case of auricular fibrillation, measured directly. *Arch Intern Med* 1940: 625–642.

185. Linderer T, Chatterjee K, Parmley WW, et al. Influence of atrial systole on the Frank-Starling relation and the end-diastolic pressure-diameter relation of the left ventricle. *Circulation* 1983;67: 1045–1053.

186. Meijler FL, Strackee J, van Capelle FJL, Du Perron JC. Computer analysis of the RR interval-contractility relationship during radon stimulation of the isolated heart. *Circ Res* 1968;22: 695–702.

187. Edmands RE, Greenspan K, Fisch C. The role of inotropic variation in ventricular function during atrial fibrillation. *J Clin Invest* 1970;49:738–746.

188. Gibson DG, Broder G, Sowton E. Effect of varying pulse interval in atrial fibrillation on left ventricular function in man. *Br Heart J* 1971;33:388–393.

189. Hardman SMC, Noble MIM, Seed WA. Postextrasystolic potentiation and its contribution to the beat-to-beat variation of the pulse during atrial fibrillation. *Circulation* 1992;86: 1223–1232.

190. Karliner JS, Gault JH, Bovchard RJ, Holzer J. Factors influencing the ejection fraction and the mean rate of circumferential fibre shortening during atrial fibrillation. *Cardiovasc Res* 1974; 8:18–25.

191. Hardman SM, Noble MI, Biggs T, Seed WA. Evidence for an influence of mechanical restitution on beat-to-beat variations in haemodynamics during chronic atrial fibrillation in patients. *Cardiovasc Res* 1998;38(1):82–90.

192. Erlebacher JA, Danner RL, Stelzer PE. Hypotension with ventricular pacing: an atria vasodepressor reflex in human beings. *J Am Coll Cardiol* 1984;4:550–555.

193. Noll B, Goke B, Simon B, Maisch B. Cardiac natriuretic peptide hormones during artificial cardiac pacemaker stimulation and left heart catheterization. *Clin Invest* 1992;70:1057–1060.

194. Ellenbogen KA, Thames MD, Mohanty PK. New insights into pacemaker syndrome gained from hemodynamic, humoral, and vascular responses during ventriculo-atrial pacing. *Am J Cardiol* 1990;65:53–59.

195. Brill IC. Auricular fibrillation with congestive heart failure and no other evidence of organic heart disease. *Am Heart J* 1937;13: 175.

196. Phillips E, Levine SA. Auricular fibrillation without other evidence of heart disease: a cause of reversible heart failure. *Am J Med* 1949;303:478–489.

197. Spinale FG, Holzgrefe HH, Murkherjee R, et al. LV and myocyte structure and function after early recovery from tachycardia induced cardiomyopathy. *Am J Physiol* 1995;268:H836.

198. Spinale FG, Clayton C, Tanaka R, et al. Myocardial Na$^+$,K$^{(+)}$-ATPase in tachycardia induced cardiomyopathy. *J Mol Cell Cardiol* 1992;24:277.

199. Heinz G, Siostrzonek P, Kreiner G, Gossinger H. Improvement in left ventricular systolic function after successful radiofrequency. His bundle ablation for drug refractory, chronic atrial fibrillation and recurrent atrial flutter. *Am J Cardiol* 1992;69: 489–492.

200. Lemery R, Brugada P, Cheriex E, Wellens HJJ. Reversibility of tachycardia-induced left ventricular dysfunction after closed-chest catheter ablation of the atrioventricular junction for intractable atrial fibrillation. *Am J Cardiol* 1987;60: 1406–1408.

201. Peters KG, Kienzle MG. Severe cardiomyopathy due to chronic rapidly conducted atrial fibrillation: complete recovery after restoration of sinus rhythm. *Am J Med* 1988;85:242–244.

202. McLaran CJ, Gersh BJ, Sugrue DD, et al. Tachycardia induced myocardial dysfunction. A reversible problem? *Br Heart J* 1985; 53:323–327.

203. Cruz FES, Cheriex EC, Smeets JLRM, et al. Reversibility of tachycardia-induced cardiomyopathy after cure of incessant supraventricular tachycardia. *J Am Coll Cardiol* 1990;16: 739–744.

204. Van Gelder IC, Crijns HJGM, Blanksma PK, et al. Time course of hemodynamic changes and improvement of exercise tolerance after cardioversion of chronic atrial fibrillation unassociated with cardiac valve disease. *Am J Cardiol* 1993;72:560–566.

205. Raeder EA. Circadian fluctuations in ventricular response to atrial fibrillation. *Am J Cardiol* 1990;66(12):1013–1016.

206. Sopher SM, Hnatova K, Waktare JE, et al. Circadian variation in atrial fibrillation in patients with frequent paroxysms. *Pace* 1998;21:2445–2449.

207. Rawles JM, Metcalfe MJ, Jennings K. Time of occurrence, duration, and ventricular rate of paroxysmal atrial fibrillation: the effect of digoxin. *Br Heart J* 1990;63:225–227.

208. Redfors A. Digoxin dosage and ventricular rate at rest and exercise in patients with atrial fibrillation. *Acta Med Scand* 1971; 190:321–333.

209. Bootsma BK, Hoelen AJ, Strackee J, Meijler FL. Analysis of the R-R intervals in patients with atrial fibrillation at rest and during exercise. *Circulation* 1970;41:783–794.

210. Botker HE, Toft P, Klitgaard NA, Simonsen EE. Influence of physical exercise on serum digoxin concentration and heart rate in patients with atrial fibrillation. *Br Heart J* 1991;65(5): 337–341.

211. Beasley R, Smith DA, McHaffie DJ. Exercise heart rates at different serum digoxin concentrations in patients with atrial fibrillation. *Br Med J (Clin Res Ed)* 1985;290(6461):9–11.

212. Goodman DJ, Rossen RM, Cannom DS, et al. Effect of digoxin on atrioventricular conduction: studies in patients with and without cardiac autonomic innervation. *Circulation* 1975;51: 251–256.

213. Falk RH, Leavitt JI. Digoxin for atrial fibrillation: a drug whose time has gone? *Ann Intern Med* 1991;114:573–575.

214. Goldman S, Brobst P, Selzer A, Cohn K. Inefficacy of therapeutic serum levels of digoxin in controlling the ventricular rate in atrial fibrillation. *Am J Cardiol* 1975;35:651–655.

215. Hnatkova K, Waktare JE, Murgatroyd FD, et al. Age and gen-

der influences on rate and duration of paroxysmal atrial fibrillation. *Pace* 1998;21(11, Pt 2):2455–2458.

216. Hnatkova K, Murgatroyd FD, Poloniecki J, et al. Mid- and long-term similarity of ventricular response to paroxysmal atrial fibrillation: digoxin versus placebo. *Pace* 1998;21(9): 1735–1740.

217. Falk RH, Knowlton AA, Bernard SA, et al. Digoxin for converting recent-onset atrial fibrillation to sinus rhythm. A randomized double-blinded trial. *Ann Intern Med* 1987;106: 503–506.

218. Stafford RS, Robson DC, Misra B, et al. Rate control and sinus rhythm maintenance in atrial fibrillation: natural trends in medication use. *Arch Intern Med* 1998;158(19):2144–2148.

219. Lundstrom T, Moor E, Ryden L. Differential effects of xamoterol and verapamil on ventricular rate regulation in patients with chronic atrial fibrillation. *Am Heart J* 1992;124(4): 917–923.

220. Lewis RV, McMurray J, McDevitt DG. Effects of atenolol, verapamil, and xamoterol on heart rate and exercise tolerance in digitalized patients with chronic atrial fibrillation. *J Cardiac Pharmacol* 1989;13(1):1–6.

221. DiBianco R, Morganroth J, Freitag JA, et al. Effects of nadolol on the spontaneous and exercise-provoked heart rate of patients with chronic atrial fibrillation receiving stable dosages of digoxin. *Am Heart J* 1984;108:1121–1127.

222. Farshi R, Kistner D, Sarma JS, et al. Ventricular rate control in chronic atrial fibrillation during daily activity and programmed exercise: a crossover open-label study of five drug regimens. *J Am Coll Cardiol* 1999;33(2):304–310.

223. Lewis RV, Irvine N, McDevitt DG. Relationships between heart rate, exercise tolerance and cardiac output in atrial fibrillation: the effects of treatment with digoxin, verapamil, and diltiazem. *Eur Heart J* 1988;9(7):777–781.

224. Botto GL, Bonini W, Broffoni T. Modulation of ventricular rate in permanent atrial fibrillation: randomized, crossover study of the effects of slow-release formulations of gallopamil, diltiazem, or verapamil. *Clin Cardiol* 1998;21(11):837–840.

225. Roth A, Harrison E, Mitani G, et al. Efficacy of medium and high-dose diltiazem alone and in combination with digoxin for control of heart rate at rest and during exercise in patients with chronic atrial fibrillation. *Circulation* 1986;73:316–324.

226. Piepho RW, Culbertson VL, Rhodes RS. Drug interactions with the calcium-entry blockers. *Circulation* 1987;75[Supp 5]: V181–V194.

227. David D, Segni ED, Klein HO, Kaplinsky E. Inefficacy of digitalis in the control of heart rate in patients with chronic atrial fibrillation: beneficial effect of an added beta adrenergic blocking agent. *Am J Cardiol* 1979;44:1378–1382.

228. Matsuda M, Matsuda Y, Yamagiohi T, et al. Effects of digoxin, propranolol, and verapamil on exercise in patients with chronic isolated atrial fibrillation. *Cardiovasc Res* 1991;25:453–457.

229. Reiffel JA. Improved rate control in atrial fibrillation. *Am Heart J* 1992;123[Suppl 4, Pt 1]:1094–1098.

230. James MA, Channer KS, Papouchado M, Rees JR. Improved control of atrial fibrillation with combined pindolol and digoxin therapy. *Eur Heart J* 1989;10:83–90.

231. Hsieh MH, Chen SA, Wen ZC, et al. Effects of antiarrhythmogenic drugs on variability of ventricular rate and exercise performance in chronic atrial fibrillation complicated with ventricular arrhythmias. *Int J Cardiol* 1998;64(1):37–45.

232. Steinberg JS, Katz RJ, Bren GB, et al. Efficacy of oral diltiazem to control ventricular response in chronic atrial fibrillation at rest and during exercise. *J Am Coll Cardiol* 1987;9(2):405–411.

233. Lundstrom T, Ryden L: Ventricular rate control and exercise performance in chronic atrial fibrillation: effects of diltiazem and verapamil. *J Am Coll Cardiol* 1990, 16:86–90.

234. Lang R, Klein H, Segni E, et al. Verapamil improves exercise capacity in chronic atrial fibrillation: double-blind crossover study. *Am Heart J* 1983;105:820–824.

235. Atwood JE, Sullivan M, Forbes S, et al. Effects of beta-adrenergic blockade on exercise performance in patients with chronic atrial fibrillation. *J Am Coll Cardiol* 1987;10:314–320.

236. Anderson S, Blanski L, Byrd RC, et al. Comparison of the efficacy and safety of esmolol, a short-acting beta-blocker, with placebo in the treatment of supraventricular tachyarrhythmias: the Esmolol vs Placebo Multicenter Study Group. *Am Heart J* 1986;111:42–48.

237. Rinkenberger RL, Prystowsky EN, Heger JJ, et al. Effects of intravenous and chronic oral verapamil administration in patients with supraventricular tachyarrhythmias. *Circulation* 1980;62:996–1010.

238. Waxman HL, Myerburg RJ, Appel R, Sung RJ. Verapamil for control of ventricular rate in paroxysmal supraventricular tachycardia and atrial fibrillation or flutter: a double-blind randomized cross-over study. *Ann Intern Med* 1981;94:1–6.

239. Reiter MJ, Shand DG, Aanonsen LM, et al. Pharmacokinetics of verapamil: experience with a sustained intravenous infusion regimen. *Am J Cardiol* 1982;50:716–721.

240. Ellenbogen KA, Dias VC, Plumb VJ, et al. A placebo-controlled trial of continuous intravenous diltiazem infusion for 24-hour heart rate control during atrial fibrillation and atrial flutter: a multicenter study. *J Am Coll Cardiol* 1991;18:891–897.

241. Salerno DM, Dias VC, Kleiger RE, et al. Efficacy and safety of intravenous diltiazem for treatment of atrial fibrillation and atrial flutter. *Am J Cardiol* 1989;63:1246–1251.

242. Heywood JT, Graham B, Marais GE, Jutzy KR. Effects of intravenous diltiazem on rapid atrial fibrillation accompanied by congestive heart failure. *Am J Cardiol* 1991;67:1150–1152.

243. Roth A, Kaluski E, Felner S, et al. Clonidine for patients with rapid atrial fibrillation. *Ann Intern Med* 1992;116:388–390.

244. Sellers TD, Bashore TM, Gallagher JJ. Digitalis in the preexcitation syndrome. Analysis during atrial fibrillation. *Circulation* 1977;56:260–267.

245. Rinkenberger RL, Prystowsky EN, Heger JJ, et al. Effects of intravenous and chronic oral verapamil administration in patients with supraventricular tachyarrhythmias. *Circulation* 1980;62:996–1010.

246. McGovern B, Garan H, Ruskin JN. Precipitation of cardiac arrest by verapamil in patients with Wolff-Parkinson-White syndrome. *Ann Intern Med* 1986;104:791.

247. Gulamhusein S, Ko P, Klein GJ. Ventricular fibrillation following verapamil in the Wolff-Parkinson-White syndrome. *Brief Commun* 1983;106:145.

248. Jacob AS, Nielsen DH, Gianelly RE. Fatal ventricular fibrillation following verapamil in Wolff-Parkinson-White syndrome with atrial fibrillation. *Ann Emerg Med* 1985;14:159.

249. Rowland TW. Augmented ventricular rate following verapamil treatment for atrial fibrillation with Wolff-Parkinson-White syndrome. *Pediatrics* 1983;72:245.

250. Exner DV, Muzyka T, Gillis AM. Proarrhythmia in patients with the Wolff-Parkinson-White syndrome after standard doses of intravenous adenosine. *Ann Intern Med* 1995;122:351–352.

251. Glatter KA, Dorostkar P, Cheng J, Scheinman MM. Use of Ibutilide to terminate atrial fibrillation in patients with accessory pathways. *Circulation* 1998;I-103:525.

252. Varriale P, Sedighi A, Mirzaietehrane M. Ibutilide for termination of atrial fibrillation in the Wolff-Parkinson-White syndrome. *Pacing Clin Electrophysiol* 1999;22:1267.

253. Murdock CJ, Kyles AE, Yeung-Lai-Wah JA, et al. Atrial flutter in patients treated for atrial fibrillation with propafenone. *Am J Cardiol* 1990;66(7):755–757.

254. Feld GK, Chen PS, Nicod P, et al. Possible atrial proarrhythmic

effects of class 1c antiarrhythmic drugs. *Am J Cardiol* 1990;66 (3):378–383.

255. Juul-Möller, Edvardsson N, Rehnqvist-Ahlberg N. Sotalol versus quinidine for the maintenance of sinus rhythm after direct current conversion of atrial fibrillation. *Circulation* 1990;82: 1932–1939.

256. Donovan KD, Powers BM, Hockings BE, et al. Intravenous flecainide versus amiodarone for recent onset atrial fibrillation. *Am J Cardiol* 1995;75:693

257. Messerli FH. "Cardioprotection"—not all calcium antagonists are created equal: second round. *Am J Cardiol* 1997;79(6): 788–789.

258. The Multicenter Diltiazem Postinfarctoon Trial Research Group. The effect of diltiazem on mortality and reinfarction after myocardial infarction. *N Engl J Med* 1988;319:385–392.

259. Packer M, Bristow MR, Cohn JN, et al. The effect of carvedilol on morbidity and mortality in patients with chronic heart failure. U.S. Carvedilol Heart Failure Study Group. *N Engl J Med* 1996;334(21):1349–1355.

260. CIBIS II Investigators: The cardiac insufficiency bisoprolol study II (CIBIS II): a randomized trial. *Lancet* 1999;353:9–13.

261. MERIT Investigators. Effect of metoprolol CR/XL in chronic heart failure: Metoprolol CR/XL Randomized Intervention Trial in Congestive Heart Failure (MERIT-CHF). *Lancet* 1999; 12:353:1988–1989.

262. Sharpe N. Benefit of beta-blockers for heart failure: proven in 1999. *Lancet* 1999;353(9169):1988–1989.

263. Scheinman MM, Morady F, Hess DS, Gonzalez R. Catheter-induced ablation of the atrioventricular junction to control refractory supraventricular arrhythmias. *JAMA* 1982;248: 851–855.

264. Gallagher JJ, Svenson RH, Kasell JH, et al. Catheter technique for closed-chest ablation of the atrioventricular conduction system: a therapeutic alternative for the treatment of refractory supraventricular tachycardia. *N Engl J Med* 1982;306:194–200.

265. Langberg JJ, Chin MC, Rosenqvist M, et al. Catheter ablation of the atrioventricular junction with radiofrequency energy. *Circulation* 1989;80:1527–1535.

266. Rodrigues LM, Smeets JL, Xie B, et al. Improvement in left ventricular function by ablation of atrioventricular nodal conduction in selected patients with lone atrial fibrillation. *Am J Cardiol* 1993;72(15):1137–1141.

267. Brignoli M, Gianfranchi L, Menozzi C, et al. Influence of atrioventricular junction radiofrequency ablation in patients with chronic atrial fibrillation and flutter on quality of life and cardiac performance. *AJR Am J Roentgenol* 1994;74(3):242–246.

268. Kay GN, Bubien RS, Epstein AE, Plumb VJ. Effect of catheter ablation of the atrioventricular junction on quality of life and exercise tolerance in paroxysmal atrial fibrillation. *Am J Cardiol* 1988;62[Pt 1]:741–744.

269. Fitzpatrick AP, Kourouyan HD, Siu A, et al. Quality of life and outcomes after radiofrequency His-bundle catheter ablation and permanent pacemaker implantation: impact of treatment in paroxysmal and established atrial fibrillation. *Am Heart J* 1996; 131(3):499–507.

270. DeLima G, Talajic M, Dubuc M, et al. Malignant ventricular arrhythmias after atrioventricular nodal ablation. A long-term follow-up study. *Circulation* 1996;94:I682.

271. Olgin JE, Scheinman MM. Comparison of high energy direct current and radiofrequency catheter ablation of atrioventricular junction. *J Am Coll Cardiol* 1993;21(3):557–564.

272. Geelen P, Brugada J, Andries E, Brugada P. Ventricular fibrillation and sudden death after radiofrequency catheter ablation of the atrioventricular junction. *Pace* 1997;20:343–348.

273. Williamson BD, Man KC, Daoud E, et al. Radiofrequency catheter modification of atrioventricular conduction to control

the ventricular rate during atrial fibrillation. *N Engl J Med* 1994;334:910–917.

274. Feld GK, Fleck RP, Fujimura O, et al. Control of rapid ventricular response by radiofrequency catheter modification of the atrioventricular node in patients with medically refractory atrial fibrillation. *Circulation* 1994;90:2299–2307.

275. Lown B, Amarasingham R, Neuman J. New method for terminating cardiac arrhythmias. *JAMA* 1962;182:548–555.

276. Lown B. Electrical cardioversion of cardiac arrhythmias. *Br Heart J* 1967;29:469–487.

277. Van Gelder IC, Crijns HJ, Van Gilst WH, et al. Prediction of uneventful cardioversion and maintenance of sinus rhythm from direct-current electrical cardioversion of chronic atrial fibrillation and flutter. *Am J Cardiol* 1991;68(July 1):41–46.

278. Joglar JA, Hamdan MH, Ramaswamy K, et al. Initial energy for elective external cardioversion of persistent atrial fibrillation. *Am J Cardiol* 2000;86:348.

279. Mittal S, Ayati S, Stein KM, et al. Transthoracic cardioversion of atrial fibrillation: a comparison of rectilinear biphasic versus damped sine wave monophasic shocks. *Circulation* 2000;101: 1282–1287.

280. Grimm RA, Stewart WJ, Maloney JD, et al. Impact of electrical cardioversion for atrial fibrillation on left atrial appendage function and spontaneous echo contrast: characterization by simultaneous transesophageal echocardiography. *J Am Coll Cardiol* 1993;22:1359–1366.

281. Fatkin D, Kelly RP, Feneley MP. Relations between left atrial appendage blood flow velocity, spontaneous echocardiographic contrast and thromboembolic risk *in vivo*. *J Am Coll Cardiol* 1994;23:961–969.

282. Manning WJ, Silverman DI, Keighly CS, et al. Transesophageal echocardiographically facilitated early cardioversion from atrial fibrillation using short-term anticoagulation: final results of a prospective 4.5 year study. *J Am Coll Cardiol* 1995; 25:1354–1361.

283. Klein AL, Grimm RA, Black IW, et al. Cardioversion guided by transesophageal echocardiography: the ACUTE pilot study. A randomized, controlled trial. Assessment of Cardioversion Using Transesophageal Echocardiography. *Ann Intern Med* 1997;126: 200–209.

284. Bianconi L, Mennuni M, Lukic V, et al. Effects of oral propafenone administration before electrical cardioversion of chronic atrial fibrillation: a placebo-controlled study. *J Am Coll Cardiol* 1996;28:700.

285. Oral H, Souza JJ, Michaud GF, et al. Facilitating transthoracic cardioversion of atrial fibrillation with ibutilide pretreatment. *N Engl J Med* 1999;340:1849–1854.

286. Van Noord T, Van Gelder IC, Schoonderwoerd BA, Crijns HJGM. Immediate reinitiation of atrial fibrillation after electrical cardioversion predicts subsequent pharmacological and electrical conversion to sinus rhythm on amiodarone. *Am J Cardiol* 2000;86:1384–1385.

287. Tieleman RG, van Gelder IC, Crijns HJGM, et al. Early recurrences of atrial fibrillation after electrical cardioversion: a result of fibrillation-induced electrical remodeling of the trial? *J Am Coll Cardiol* 1998;31:167–173.

288. De Simone A, Stabile G, Vitale DF, et al. Pretreatment with verapamil in patients with persistent or chronic atrial fibrillation who underwent electrical cardioversion. *J Am Coll Cardiol* 1999;34:810–881.

289. Levy S, Lauribe P, Dolla E, et al. A randomized comparison of external and internal cardioversion of chronic atrial fibrillation. *Circulation* 1992;86:1415.

290. Vos MA, Golitsyn SR, Stangl K, et al, for the Ibutilide/Sotalol Comparator Study Group. Superiority of ibutilide (a new class III agent) over dl-sotalol in the converting atrial flutter and fib-

rillation. A multicenter trial with 300 patients. *Heart* 1998;79:568–575.

291. Hou ZY, Chang MS, Chen CY, et al. Acute treatment of recent-onset atrial fibrillation and flutter with a tailored dosing regimen of intravenous amiodarone. A randomized, digoxin-controlled study. *Eur Heart J* 1995;16:521–528.

292. Stambler BS, Wood MA, Ellenbogen KA, et al, and the Ibutilide Repeat Dose Study Investigators. Efficacy and safety of repeated intravenous doses of ibutilide for rapid conversion of atrial flutter or fibrillation. *Circulation* 1996;94:1613–1621.

293. McClellan KJ, Markham A. Dofetilide: a review of its use in atrial fibrillation and atrial flutter. *Drugs* 1999;58:1043–1059.

294. Hohnloser SH, Van Loo A, Baedeker F. Efficacy and proarrhythmic hazards of pharmacologic cardioversion of atrial fibrillation: prospective comparison of sotalol versus quinidine. *J Am Coll Cardiol* 1995;26:852–858.

295. Tieleman RG, Gosselink ATM, Crijns HJGM, et al. Efficacy, safety and determinants of conversion of atrial fibrillation and flutter with oral amiodarone. *Am J Cardiol* 1997;79:53–57.

296. Bianconi L, Mennuni M, Lukic V, et al. Effect of oral propafenone administration before electrical cardioversion of chronic atrial fibrillation: placebo controlled study. *J Am Coll Cardiol* 1996;28:700–706.

297. Goy JJ, Grbic M, Hurni M, et al. Conversion of supraventricular arrhythmias to sinus rhythm using flecainide. *Eur Heart J* 1985;6:518–524.

298. Kochiadakis GE, Igoumenidis NE, Parthenakis FI, et al. Amiodarone versus propafenone for conversion of chronic atrial fibrillation: results of a randomized, controlled study. *J Am Coll Cardiol* 1999;33:966–971.

299. Levine JH, Morganroth J, Kadish AH. Mechanism and risk factors for proarrhythmia with type Ia compared with Ic antiarrhythmic drug therapy. *Circulation* 1989;80:1063–1069.

300. Flaker GC, Blackshear JL, McBride R, et al, for the Stroke Prevention in Atrial Fibrillation Investigators. Antiarrhythmic drug therapy and cardiac mortality in atrial fibrillation. *J Am Coll Cardiol* 1992;20:527–532.

301. London F, Howell M. Atrial flutter: 1 to 1 conduction during treatment with quinidine and digitalis. *Am Heart J* 1954;48:152–155.

302. Crijns HJGM, Van Gelder IC, Lie KI. Supraventricular tachycardia mimicking ventricular tachycardia during flecainide treatment. *Am J Cardiol* 1988;62:1303–1306.

303. Parkinson J, Campbell M. The quinidine treatment of auricular fibrillation. *Q J Med* 1929;22:281–303.

304. Fenster PE, Comess KA, Marsh R, et al. Conversion of atrial fibrillation to sinus rhythm by acute intravenous procainamide infusion. *Am Heart J* 1983;106:501–504.

305. Fresco C, Proclemer A, for the PAFIT 2 Investigators. Management of recent onset atrial fibrillation. *Eur Heart J* 1996;17 [Suppl C]:41–47.

306. Reisinger J, Gatterer E, Heinze G, et al. Prospective comparison of flecainide versus sotalol for immediate cardioversion of atrial fibrillation. *Am J Cardiol* 1998;81:1450–1454.

307. Sokolow M, Edgar AL. Blood quinidine concentrations as a guide in the treatment of cardiac arrhythmias. *Circulation* 1950;1:576.

308. Borgeat A, Goy JJ, Maendly R, et al. Flecainide versus quinidine for conversion of atrial fibrillation to sinus rhythm. *Am J Cardiol* 1986;58:496.

309. Hohnloser SH, Baedeker F, van de Loo A. Quinidine or sotalol-induced changes in QT-dispersion during pharmacologic conversion therapy of atrial fibrillation: link to proarrhythmia as assessed in a prospective randomized trial. *J Am Coll Cardiol* 1995;25:66A(abst).

310. Fenster PE, Comess KA, Marsh R, et al. Conversion of atrial

fibrillation to sinus rhythm by acute intravenous procainamide infusion. *Am Heart J* 1983;106:501.

311. Abi-Mansour P, Carberry PA, McCowan RJ, et al, and the Study Investigators. Conversion efficacy and safety of repeated doses of ibutilide in patients with atrial flutter and atrial fibrillation. *Am Heart J* 1998;136:632.

312. Volgman AS, Carberry PA, Stambler B, et al. Conversion efficacy and safety of intravenous ibutilide compared with intravenous procainamide in patients with atrial flutter or fibrillation. *J Am Coll Cardiol* 1998;31:1414.

313. Vos MA, Golitsyn SR, Stangl K, et al, for the Ibutilide/Sotalol Comparator Study Group. Superiority of ibutilide (a new class III agent) over dl-sotalol in converting atrial flutter and atrial fibrillation. *Heart* 1998;79:568.

314. Falk RH, Pollak A, Singh SN, et al, for the Intravenous Dofetilide Investigators. Intravenous dofetilide, a class III antiarrhythmic agent, for the termination of sustained atrial fibrillation or flutter. *J Am Coll Cardiol* 1997;29:385.

315. Norgaard BL, Wachtell K, Christiansen PD, et al, and the Danish Dofetilide in Atrial Fibrillation and Flutter Study Group. Efficacy and safety of intravenously administered dofetilide in acute termination of atrial fibrillation and flutter; a multicenter, randomized, double-blind, placebo-controlled trial. *Am Heart J* 1999;137:1062.

315a. Greenbaum R, Campbell TF, Channg KS, et al., for the EMERALD investigators. Conversion of AF and maintenance of sinus rhythm by dofetilide (abst). *Eur Heart J* 1998;19(abst suppl):661.

316. Reisinger J, Gatterer E, Heinze G, et al. Prospective comparison of flecainide versus sotalol for immediate conversion of atrial fibrillation. *Am J Cardiol* 1998;81:1450.

317. Madrid AH, Moro C, Marin-Huerta E, et al. Comparison of flecainide and procainamide in cardioversion of atrial fibrillation. *Eur Heart J* 1993;14:1127.

318. Donovan KD, Power BM, Hockings BE, et al. Intravenous flecainide versus amiodarone for recent-onset atrial fibrillation. *Am J Cardiol* 1995;75:693.

319. Alp NJ, Bell JA, Shahi M. Randomised double blind trial of oral versus intravenous flecainide for the cardioversion of acute atrial fibrillation. *Heart* 2000;84:37.

320. Stroobandt R, Stiels B, Hoebrechts R, for the Propafenone Atrial Fibrillation Trial Investigators. Propafenone for conversion and prophylaxis of atrial fibrillation. *Am J Cardiol* 1997;79:418.

321. Botto GL, Bonini W, Broffoni T, et al. Conversion of recent onset atrial fibrillation with single loading oral dose of propafenone: is in-hospital admission absolutely necessary? *Pacing Clin Electrophysiol* 1996;19:1939.

322. Boriani G, Biffi M, Capucci A, et al. Oral propafenone to convert recent-onset atrial fibrillation in patients with and without underlying heart disease. A randomized, controlled trial. *Ann Intern Med* 1997;126:621.

323. Bianconi L, Mennuni M, Lukic V, et al. Effects of oral propafenone administration before electrical cardioversion of chronic atrial fibrillation: a placebo-controlled study. *J Am Coll Cardiol* 1996;28:700.

324. Vietti-Ramus G, Veglio F, Marchisio U, et al. Efficacy and safety of short term intravenous amiodarone in supraventricular tachyarrhythmias. *Int J Cardiol* 1992;35:77.

325. Vardas PE, Kochiadakis GE, Igoumenidis NE, et al. Amiodarone as a first-choice drug for restoring sinus rhythm in patients with atrial fibrillation: a randomized, controlled study. *Chest* 2000;117:1538.

326. Galve E, Rius T, Ballester R, et al. Intravenous amiodarone in the treatment of recent-onset atrial fibrillation. Results of a randomized, controlled trial. *J Am Coll Cardiol* 1996;27:1079.

327. Peuhkurinen K, Niemela M, Ylitalo A, et al. Effectiveness of

amiodarone as a single oral dose for recent-onset atrial fibrillation. *Am J Cardiol* 2000;85:462.

328. Tieleman RG, Gosselink ATM, Crijns HJGM, et al. Efficacy, safety, and determinants of conversion of atrial fibrillation and flutter with oral amiodarone. *Am J Cardiol* 1997;79:53.

329. Krol RB, Varanasi S, Mathew P, Saksena S. Safety and efficacy of sotalol in drug refractory atrial fibrillation/flutter. *J Am Coll Cardiol* 1995; 25:66A(abst).

330. Reisinger J, Gatterer E, Heinze G, et al. Prospective comparison of flecainide versus sotalol for immediate conversion of atrial fibrillation. *Am J Cardiol* 1998;81:1450.

331. Ferreira E, Sunderji R, Gin K. Is oral sotalol effective in converting atrial fibrillation to sinus rhythm? *Pharmacotherapy* 1997;17:1233.

332. Jordaens L, Trouerbach J, Calle P, et al. Conversion of atrial fibrillation to sinus rhythm and rate control by digoxin in comparison to placebo. *Eur Heart J* 1997;18:643.

333. The Digitalis in Acute Atrial Fibrillation (DAAF) Trial Group. Intravenous digoxin in acute atrial fibrillation. Results of a randomized, placebo-controlled multicentre trial in 239 patients. *Eur Heart J* 1997;18:649.

334. Innes GD, Vertesi L, Dillon EC, Metcalfe C. Effectiveness of verapamil-quinidine versus digoxin-quinidine in the emergency department treatment of paroxysmal atrial fibrillation. *Ann Emerg Med* 1997;29:126–134.

335. Houltz B, Darpo B, Swedberg K, et al. Effects of the I_{kr}-blocker almokalant and predictors of conversion of chronic atrial tachyarrhythmias to sinus rhythm. A prospective study. *Cardiovasc Drugs Ther* 1999;13:329–338.

336. Wellens HJ, Lau CP, Luderitz B, et al. Atrioverter: an implantable device for the treatment of atrial fibrillation. *Circulation* 1998;98:1651–1656.

337. Timmermans C, Nabar A, Rodriguez LM, et al. Use of sedation during cardioversion with the implantable atrial defibrillator. *Circulation* 1999;100:1499–1501.

338. Rawles JM, Metcalfe MJ, Jennings K. Time of occurrence, duration and ventricular rate of paroxysmal atrial fibrillation: the effect of digoxin. *Br Heart J* 1990;63:225–227.

339. Coplen SE, Antman EM, Berlin JA, et al. Efficacy and safety of quinidine therapy for maintenance of sinus rhythm. A meta-analysis of randomized control trials. *Circulation* 1990;82:1106–1116.

340. Carlsson J, Tebbe U, Rox J, et al. Cardioversion of atrial fibrillation in the elderly. *Am J Cardiol* 1996;78:1380–1384.

341. Van Gelder IC, Crijns HJ, Van Gilst WH, et al. Efficacy and safety of flecainide acetate in the maintenance of sinus rhythm after electrical cardioversion of chronic atrial fibrillation or atrial flutter. *Am J Cardiol* 1989;64:1317–1321.

342. Touboul P, Aliot E, Brembilla-Perrot B. Flecainide in the prevention of atrial fibrillation after cardioversion: comparison with quinidine. *Circulation* 1991;84:II127.

343. Rasmussen K, Andersen A, Abrahamsen AM, et al. Flecainide versus disopyramide in maintaining sinus rhythm following conversion of chronic atrial fibrillation. *Eur Heart J* 1988;9 [Suppl 1]:52(abst).

344. Antman EM, Beamer AD, Cantillon C, et al. Therapy of refractory symptomatic atrial fibrillation and flutter: a staged care approach with new antiarrhythmic drugs. *J Am Coll Cardiol* 1990;15:698.

345. Stroobandt R, Stiels B, Hoebrechts R. Propafenone Atrial Fibrillation Trial Investigators. *Am J Cardiol* 1997;79:418.

346. Benditt DG, Williams JH, Jin J, et al. Maintenance of sinus rhythm with oral d,l-sotalol therapy in patients with symptomatic atrial fibrillation and/or atrial flutter. d,l-Sotalol Atrial Fibrillation/Flutter Study Group. *Am J Cardiol* 1999; 84:270.

347. Juul-Möller S, Edvardsson N, Rehnqvist-Ahlberg N. Sotalol versus quinidine for the maintenance of sinus rhythm after direct current conversion of atrial fibrillation. *Circulation* 1990; 82:1932–1939.

348. Southworth MR, Zarembski D, Viana M, Bauman J. Comparison of sotalol versus quinidine for maintenance of normal sinus rhythm in patients with chronic atrial fibrillation. *Am J Cardiol* 1999;83:1629.

349. Reimold SC, Cantillon CO, Friedman PL, Antman EM. Propafenone versus sotalol for suppression of recurrent symptomatic atrial fibrillation. *Am J Cardiol* 1993;71:558.

350. Kochiadakis GE, Igoumenidis, Marketou ME, et al. Low-dose amiodarone versus sotalol for suppression of recurrent symptomatic atrial fibrillation. *Am J Cardiol* 1998;81:995.

351. Roy D, Talajic M, Dorian P, et al. Amiodarone to prevent recurrence of atrial fibrillation. Canadian Trial of Atrial Fibrillation Investigators. *N Engl J Med* 2000;342:913.

352. Dalrymple HW, Campbell TJ, Channer KS, et al. Maintenance of sinus rhythm by dofetilide improves quality of life. The EMERALD (European and Australian Multicenter Evaluative Research on Atrial Fibrillation Dofetilide) Study. *Circulation* 1998;98:I13.

353. Singh SN, Berk M, Yellen L, et al. Efficacy and safety of oral dofetilide in maintaining sinus rhythm: 12 months follow-up results of SAFIRE-D. *Circulation* 1999;100:I501.

354. Pritchett EL, Wilkinson WE. Effect of dofetilide on survival in patients with supraventricular arrhythmias. *Am Heart J* 1999; 138:994.

355. Torp-Pedersen C, Moller M, Bloch-Thomsen PE, et al. Dofetilide in patients with congestive heart failure and left ventricular dysfunction. Danish Investigations of Arrhythmia and Mortality on Dofetilide Study Group. *N Engl J Med* 1999;341:857.

356. Tuinenburg AE, Van Gelder IC, Van Den Berg MB, et al. Lack of prevention of heart failure by serial electrical cardioversion therapy in patients with persistent atrial fibrillation. *Heart* 1999;82:486–493.

357. Hohnloser SH, Kuck KH, Lilienthal J. Rhythm or rate control in atrial fibrillation—Phamacological Intervention in Atrial Fibrillation (PIAF): a randomised trial. *Lancet* 2000;356(9244):1789–1794.

358. The AFFIRM Investigators. Atrial fibrillation following investigation of rhythm management—the AFFIRM Study design. *Am J Cardiol* 1997;79:1198.

359. Abhilakh Missier KA, Van Gelder IC, Crijns HJGM, Kingma JH, Kamp O, Bosker HA, Tijssen JGP. Rate control versus electrical cardioversion for persistent atrial fibrillation: the RACE study design. *Eur Heart J* 1999;20:1184 (abst).

359a. Cox JL, Ad N. New surgical and catheter-based modifications of the maze procedure. *Semin Thorac Cardiovasc Surg* 2000;12:68–73.

360. Nitta T, Lee R, Schuessler RB, et al. Radial approach: a new concept in surgical treatment for atrial fibrillation I. Concept, anatomic and physiologic bases and development of a procedure. *Ann Thorac Surg* 1999;67(1):27–35.

361. Cox JL, Boineau JP, Schuessler RB, et al. Five year experience with the maze procedure for atrial fibrillation. *Ann Thorac Surg* 1993;56:814.

362. Kosakai Y, Kawaguchi AT, Isobe F, et al. Modified maze procedure for patients with atrial fibrillation undergoing simultaneous open heart surgery. *Circulation* 1995;92:II359.

363. Jessurun ER, van Hemel NM, Defauw JA, et al. Results of maze surgery for lone paroxysmal atrial fibrillation. *Circulation* 2000; 101:1559.

364. Swartz JF, Pellersels G, Silvers J, et al. A catheter-based curative approach to atrial fibrillation in humans. *Circulation* 1994;90:I(abst).

365. Olgin JE, Kalman JM, Chin M, et al. Electrophysiologic effects of long, linear atrial lesions placed under intracardiac ultrasound guidance. *Circulation* 1997;96:2715.

366. Pappone C, Oreto G, Lamberti F, et al. Catheter ablation of paroxysmal atrial fibrillation using a 3D mapping system. *Circulation* 1999;100:1203.

367. Lin WS, Prakash VS, Tai CT, et al. Pulmonary vein morphology in patients with paroxysmal atrial fibrillation initiated by ectopic beats originating from the pulmonary veins: implications for catheter ablation. *Circulation* 2000;101:1274.

368. Haissaguerre M, Jais P, Shah DC, et al. Electrophysiological end point for catheter ablation of atrial fibrillation initiated from multiple pulmonary venous foci. *Circulation* 2000;101:1409.

368a. Schumacher B, Jung W, Lewalter T, et al. Radiofrequency ablation of atrial flutter due to administration of class IC antiarrhythmic drugs for atrial fibrillation. *Am J Cardiol* 1999;83(5):710–713.

369. Andersen HR, Nielsen JC, Thomsen PEB, et al. Long-term follow-up of patients from a randomised trial of atrial versus ventricular pacing for sick sinus syndrome. *Lancet* 1997;350:1210.

370. Mattioli AV, Vivoli S, Mattioli G. Influence of pacing modalities on the incidence of atrial fibrillation in patients without prior atrial fibrillation: a prospective study. *Eur Heart J* 1998;19:282.

371. Connolly SJ, Kerr CR, Gent M, et al. Effects of physiologic pacing versus ventricular pacing on the risk of stroke and death due to cardiovascular causes. Canadian Trial of Physiologic Pacing Investigators. *N Engl J Med* 2000;342:1385.

372. Andersen HR, Thuesen L, Bagger JP, et al. Prospective randomized trial of atrial versus ventricular pacing in sick sinus syndrome. *Lancet* 1994;344:1523.

373. Gillis AM, Wyse G, Connolly SJ, et al, for the Atrial Pacing Periablation for Paroxysmal Atrial Fibrillation (PA3) Study Investigators. Atrial pacing periablation for prevention of paroxysmal atrial fibrillation. *Circulation* 1999;99:2553.

374. Abbott WM, Maloney RD, McCafe CC, et al. Arterial embolism: a 44-year perspective. *Am J Surg* 1982;243:460–464.

375. Hinton RC, Kistler JP, Fallon JT, et al. Influence of etiology of atrial fibrillation on incidence of systemic embolism. *Am J Cardiol* 1977;40:509–513.

376. Grimm RA, Stewart WJ, Black IW, et al. Should all patients undergo transesophageal echocardiography before electrical cardioversion of atrial fibrillation? *J Am Coll Cardiol* 1994;23:533–541.

377. Frost L, Engholm G, Johnsen S, et al. Incident stroke after discharge from hospital with a diagnosis of atrial fibrillation. *Am J Med* 2000;108:36.

378. Wolf PA, Dawber TR, Thomas HE, Kannel WB. Epidemiologic assessment of chronic atrial fibrillation and risk of stroke: the Framingham Study. *Neurology* 1978;28:973–77.

379. Kannell WB, Abbott RD, Savage DD, McNamara P. Coronary heart disease and atrial fibrillation: the Framingham Study. *Am Heart J* 1983;106:389–396.

380. The Stroke Prevention in Atrial Fibrillation investigator's committee on echocardiography. Transesophageal echocardiographic correlates of thromboembolism in high-risk patients with nonvalvular atrial fibrillation. *Ann Intern Med* 1998;128:639–647.

381. Treseder AS, Sastey BSD, Thomas TPL, et al. Atrial fibrillation and stroke in elderly hospitalized patients. *Age Aging* 1986;15:89–92.

382. Phillips SJ, Whisnant JP, O'Fallon WM, Frye RL. Prevalence of cardiovascular disease and diabetes mellitus in residents of Rochester, Minnesota. *Mayo Clin Proc* 1990;75:344–357.

383. Nakajima K, Incinose M. Ischemic stroke in elderly patients with paroxysmal atrial fibrillation. *Jpn J Geriatr* 1996;33:273–277.

384. Roy D, Marchand E, Ganne P, et al. Usefulness of anticoagulant therapy in the prevention of embolic complications of atrial fibrillation. *Am Heart J* 1986;112:1039–1043.

385. Hart RG, Pearce LA, Rothbart RM, et al. Stroke with intermittent atrial fibrillation: incidence and predictors during aspirin therapy. *J Am Coll Cardiol* 2000;35(1):183–187.

386. Stroke Prevention in Atrial Fibrillation Investigators. Stroke Prevention in Atrial Fibrillation Study: final results. *Circulation* 1991;84:527–539.

387. Stroke Prevention in Atrial Fibrillation Investigators. Warfarin versus aspirin for prevention of thromboembolism in atrial fibrillation: stroke prevention in atrial fibrillation II study. *Lancet* 1994;343:687–691.

388. EAFT Study Group. European Atrial Fibrillation Trial: Secondary prevention of vascular events in patients with non-rheumatic atrial fibrillation and a recent transient ischemic attack or minor ischemic stroke. *Lancet* 1993;342:1255–1262.

389. Connolly SJ, Laupacis A, Gent M, et al, for the CAFA Study Co-Investigators. Canadian Atrial Fibrillation Anticoagulation (CAFA) Study. *J Am Coll Cardiol* 1991;18:349–355.

390. Ezekowitz MD, Bridgers SL, James KE, et al. For the Veterans Affairs Stroke Prevention in Non-rheumatic Atrial Fibrillation Investigators. Warfarin in the prevention of stroke associated with non-rheumatic atrial fibrillation. *N Engl J Med* 1992;327:1406–1412.

391. Peterson P, Boysen G, Godtfredsen J, et al. Placebo controlled, randomized trial of Warfarin and aspirin for prevention of thromboembolic complications in chronic atrial fibrillation: the Copenhagen AFASAK Study. *Lancet* 1989;1:175–178.

392. Boston Area Anticoagulation Trial for Atrial Fibrillation Investigators. The effect of low-dose warfarin on the risk of stroke in patients with non-rheumatic atrial fibrillation. *N Engl J Med* 1990;323:1505–1511.

393. Atrial Fibrillation Investigators Risk Factors for Stroke and Efficacy of Antithrombotic Therapy in Atrial Fibrillation: Analysis of pooled data from five randomized control trials. *Arch Intern Med* 1994;155:1449–1457.

394. Stroke Prevention in Atrial Fibrillation Investigators. Adjusted dose warfarin versus low intensity, fixed dose warfarin plus aspiring for high risk patients with atrial fibrillation: Stroke Prevention in Atrial Fibrillation III randomized clinical trial. *Lancet* 1996;348:633–638.

395. Hylek EM, Singer DE. Risk factors for intracranial hemorrhage in outpatients taking warfarin. *Ann Intern Med* 1994;120:897–902.

396. Stroke Prevention in Atrial Fibrillation Investigators. Bleeding during antithrombotic therapy in patients with atrial fibrillation. *Arch Intern Med* 1996;156:409–416.

397. Risk factors for stroke and efficacy of antithrombotic therapy in atrial fibrillation. Analysis of pooled data from five randomized controlled trials. *Arch Intern Med* 1994;154(13):1449–1457.

397a. Palareti G, Manotti C, DAngelo A, et al. Thrombotic events during oral anticoagulant treatment: results of the inception-cohort, prospective, collaborative ISCOAT study: ISCOAT study group (Italian Study on Complications of Oral Anticoagulant Therapy). *Thromb Haemost* 1997;78(6):1438–1443.

397b. Hylek EM, Skates SJ, Sheehan MA, et al. An analysis of the lowest effective intensity of prophylactic anticoagulation for patients with non-rheumatic atrial fibrillation. *N Engl J Med* 1996;335:540–546.

398. Stafford RS, Singer DE. National patterns of warfarin use in atrial fibrillation. *Arch Intern Med* 1996;156:2537–2541.

399. Brass LM, Krumholz HM, Scinto JD, et al. Warfarin use fol-

lowing ischemic stroke among Medicare patients with atrial fibrillation. *Arch Intern Med* 1998;158:2093–2100.

400. Gordian ME, Muston HJ. Antithrombotic therapy for stroke prevention among Medicare beneficiaries hospitalized in Alaska with atrial fibrillation. *Alaska Med* 1998;40:79–84.

401. Gurwitz JH, Avorn J, Roth-Begnan D, et al. Aging and anticoagulant response to warfarin therapy. *Ann Intern Med* 1992;116: 901–904.

402. Harenberg J, Weuster B, Pfitzer M, et al. Prophylaxis of embolic events in patients with atrial fibrillation using low molecular weight heparin. *Semin Thromb Hemost* 1993;19[Suppl 1]: 116–121.

403. Bjerkelund C, Orning O. The efficacy of anticoagulant therapy in preventing embolism related to DC electrical cardioversion of atrial fibrillation. *Am J Cardiol* 1969;23:208–216.

404. Resnekov L, McDonald L. Complications of 220 patients with cardiac dysrhythmias treated by phase DC shock and indications for electroversion. *Br Heart J* 1967;29:926–936.

405. Navab A, Ladue JS. Post conversion systemic arterial embolization. *Am J Cardiol* 1965;16:52–53.

406. Weigner WJ, Caulfield TA, Danias PG, et al. Risk for clinical thromboembolism associated with conversion to sinus rhythm in patients with atrial fibrillation lasting less than 48 hours. *Ann Intern Med* 1997;126:615–620.

407. Ikram H, Nixon PG, Arcan TE. Left atrial function after electrical conversion to sinus rhythm. *Br Heart J* 1968;30:80–83.

408. Padraig GO, Puleo PR, Bolli R, et al. Return of atrial mechanical function following electrocardioversion of atrial dysrhythmias. *Am Heart J* 1990;120:353–359.

409. Prystowsky EN, Benson W, Fuster V, et al. Management of patients with atrial fibrillation: a statement for healthcare professionals from the Subcommittee on Electrocardiography and Electrophysiology, American Heart Association. *Circulation* 1996;93:1262–1277.

410. Goldman MJ. The management of chronic atrial fibrillation: indications and methods of conversion to sinus rhythm. *Prog Cardiovasc Dis* 1959;2:465–579.

411. Manning WJ, Silverman DI, Keijhly CS, et al. Transesophageal echocardiography facilitated early cardioversion from atrial fibrillation using short-term anticoagulation: final results of prospective 4.5-year study. *J Am Coll Cardiol* 1995;25: 1354–1361.

412. Stoddard MF, Dawkins PR, Prince CR, Ammash NM. Left atrial appendage thrombus is not uncommon in patients with acute atrial fibrillation and a recent embolic event: a TEE study. *J Am Coll Cardiol* 1995;25:452–459.

413. Black I, Fatkin D, Sagar K, et al. Exclusion of atrial thrombus by transesophageal echocardiography does not preclude embolism after cardioversion of atrial fibrillation; a multi-center trial. *Circulation* 1994;89:2509–2513.

414. Blackshear JL, Zabalgoitia M, Pennock G, et al. Warfarin safety and efficacy in patients with thoracic aortic plaque and atrial fibrillation. SPAF-TEE investigators. Stroke Prevention in Atrial Fibrillation–Transesophageal Echocardiography. *Am J Cardiol* 1999;83:453–455.

415. Moreyra E, Finkelhor RS, Cebul RD. Limitations of transesophageal echocardiography and the risk assessment of patients before anticoagulant cardioversion from atrial fibrillation and flutter: an analysis of tool trials. *Am Heart J* 1995; 129:71–75.

416. Lanzarotti CJ, Olshansky B. Thromboembolism and chronic atrial flutter: is the risk underestimated? *J Am Coll Cardiol* 1997; 30:1506–1511.

417. Collins LJ, Silverman DI, Douglas PS, Manning WJ. Cardioversion of nonrheumatic atrial fibrillation: reduced thromboembolic complications with 4 weeks of pre-cardioversion anticoagulation are related to atrial thrombus resolution. *Circulation* 1995;92:160.

16

ATRIAL FLUTTER

ALBERT L. WALDO

Atrial flutter has been recognized for about eight decades (1). Despite this duration, remarkably little was known about its mechanism until relatively recently, and techniques for its diagnosis and management had changed little over the years. The mechanism was thought to be a single focus firing rapidly or some form of reentry (2). The diagnosis rested largely with the 12-lead electrocardiogram (ECG). The treatment centered on the use of a digitalis preparation to slow atrioventricular (AV) nodal conduction and control the ventricular response rate and on the use of quinidine or procainamide to convert the rhythm to sinus rhythm or to prevent recurrence of the rhythm after sinus rhythm was restored. The past two decades have brought considerable change. Studies have provided insights into the mechanism of atrial flutter (2), some old techniques to diagnose atrial flutter have been significantly refined, and some new ones have evolved (3).

Beginning with the advent of direct current (DC) cardioversion in the 1960s (4,5), significant improvements in therapy of atrial flutter have been developed, including the addition of β blockers and calcium channel blockers as an adjunct to or in lieu of digitalis therapy in an effort to control ventricular response rate to atrial flutter (6–8), new antiarrhythmic agents that can be used to revert and prevent atrial flutter (9–12), pacing techniques to interrupt or suppress atrial flutter (3), catheter ablation techniques to cure atrial flutter (13–15) or to control the ventricular response rate (16), surgical ablative therapy (17–19), and even an implantable atrial DC cardioverter (20).

Since the first description of atrial flutter by Jolly and Ritchie in 1911 (1), little had changed in its characterization except for a distinction between so-called typical and atypical flutter (21). Atypical atrial flutter was described as having positive P waves in ECG leads II, III, and aVF, whereas typical atrial flutter had the classic negative saw-toothed flutter waves in ECG leads II, III, and aVF. The

atrial rate during atypical atrial flutter was sometimes slower than typical atrial flutter. Both rhythms are caused by the same reentrant mechanism.

Subsequently, the studies of Wells and colleagues (22) demonstrated two types of atrial flutter: type I (usual) and type II (very rapid) (Fig. 16-1). Type I atrial flutter can always be entrained and interrupted by rapid atrial pacing, but this is not the case with type II atrial flutter (3,22,23). The two types of atrial flutter can also be differentiated on the basis of atrial rates. In the absence of drug therapy, type I atrial flutter is characterized by a range of atrial rates of 240 to 340 bpm, and type II atrial flutter is characterized by a range of 340 to 433 bpm (3,22), although there probably is overlap in the upper range of rates of type I with the lower range rates of type II. There is almost certainly some flexibility in the upper range of atrial rates of type II and the lower range atrial rates in type I.

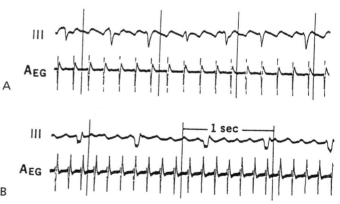

FIGURE 16-1. Simultaneous recording of electrocardiographic lead III and a bipolar atrial electrogram (AEG) during type I atrial flutter with an atrial rate of 296 bpm **(A)** and type II atrial flutter and a rate of 420 bpm **(B)**. In each example, notice the constant beat-to-beat cycle length, polarity, morphology, and amplitude of recorded atrial electrogram signal characteristic of atrial flutter. (Adapted from Wells JL Jr, MacLean WAH, James TN, Waldo AL. Characterization of atrial flutter: studies in man after open heart surgery using fixed atrial electrodes. *Circulation* 1979;60:665–673, with permission.)

A. L. Waldo: Department of Cardiology, School of Medicine, Case Western Reserve University and University Hospitals of Cleveland, Cleveland, Ohio 44106.

Little is known about the natural history and treatment of type II atrial flutter, although it is beginning to be understood. It appears to be a localized atrial rhythm, probably reentrant, which is so rapid that it generates fibrillatory conduction to significant portions of the atria (i.e., it produces atrial fibrillation) (24,25). But because not enough is known about this rhythm clinically, the remainder of this chapter deals almost entirely with type I atrial flutter.

Much new information about the mechanisms of atrial flutter has brought about a growing and even confusing atrial flutter nomenclature. A European Society of Cardiology/North American Society of Pacing and Electrophysiology Working Group (26) has offered a new atrial flutter classification based on mechanism. Usual atrial flutter, in which the reentrant impulses travel up the atrial septum and down the right atrial free wall, is called (as it was previously called) *typical atrial flutter*, and atrial flutter that uses the same circuit but in the opposite direction is called *reverse typical atrial flutter* (Fig. 16-2). These rhythms have previously also been called counterclockwise and clockwise atrial flutter, respectively, because when viewed in the right anterior oblique projection fluoroscopically, the reentrant impulses appear to travel in those directions. They have also been called common and uncommon or rare atrial flutter, respectively. Atrial flutter in which the reentrant circuit is confined to the left atrium is called *left atrial flutter*. Reentry around an incisional line of block in the rate range of atrial flutter is called *incisional atrial reentry*. All other forms of reentrant atrial tachycardia in the rate range of atrial flutter that were not previously described are called *atypical atrial flutter*. This new nomenclature does not include the terms type I and type II atrial flutter, although all types of reentrant atrial flutter that can be entrained and interrupted by atrial pacing would be classified as type I.

INCIDENCE AND CLINICAL SETTING

Atrial flutter is primarily paroxysmal, lasting for variable periods of time, usually seconds to hours but occasionally 1 day or longer. Persistent atrial flutter (i.e., atrial flutter as a stable, chronic rhythm) is unusual, because atrial flutter usually reverts to sinus rhythm or atrial fibrillation spontaneously or as a result of therapy. However, atrial flutter has been reported to be present for more than 20 years (27).

The incidence of atrial flutter is uncertain. Several series of hospital-reviewed ECGs (27) have reported an incidence of 1 of 238 patients up to a rate of 1 of every 81 patients. Atrial flutter is said to be more common in male than in female patients, with a reported ratio of 4.7 : 1 (27). Although it is more common when the atria are abnormal, it can occur in patients with ostensibly normal atria. A unique setting in which atrial flutter occurs commonly is during the first week after open-heart surgery. In these patients, there is about a 30% incidence of supraventricular tachyarrhythmias, of which about one third are atrial flutter (3). Atrial flutter is also associated with chronic obstructive pulmonary disease, mitral or tricuspid valve disease, thyrotoxicosis, and after repair of certain congenital cardiac lesions that include large incisions or suture lines in the right atrium (e.g., Mustard procedure, Fontan procedure) (28–32). It is also associated with any condition resulting in enlargement of the atria for any reason, especially the right atrium (27,30,32). Atrial flutter is commonly associated with atrial fibrillation (27–30,32). The two rhythms often occur in the same patient, and the rhythm may shift between flutter and fibrillation. In its paroxysmal form, atrial flutter is associated with antecedent premature atrial beats.

CLINICAL SIGNIFICANCE

Atrial flutter is largely a nuisance arrhythmia. Its clinical significance lies largely in its association with a rapid ventricular response rate that is difficult to control, its frequent association with atrial fibrillation, and its association with the potential for clot formation in the atria.

The rapid ventricular response rate is important because it is principally responsible for the symptoms associated with atrial flutter. If the duration of the rapid ventricular response rate is prolonged, it may be associated with ventricular dilatation and congestive heart failure. It is one of the causes of a dilated cardiomyopathy, known as a *tachycardia-mediated cardiomyopathy*. Like atrial fibrillation, atrial flutter is associated with the potential for clot formation in the atria (33–36). This condition is associated with an incidence of systemic emboli, including stroke, that is

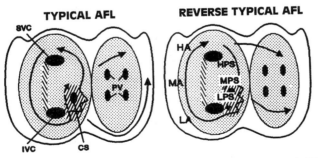

FIGURE 16-2. A: Atrial activation in typical atrial flutter (AFL). **B:** Activation in reverse typical AFL. The atria are represented schematically in a left anterior oblique view, from the tricuspid *(left)* and mitral rings. The endocardium is shaded, and the openings of the superior (SVC) and inferior vena cava (IVC), coronary sinus (CS), and pulmonary veins (PV) are shown. The direction of activation is shown by the arrows. Dashed areas mark the approximate location of zones of slow conduction and block. Lettering in **B** marks the low (LPS), middle (MPS), and high (HPS) posteroseptal wall. (Adapted from Cosío FG, Arribas F, Lopez-Gil M. Radiofrequency ablation of atrial flutter. *J Cardiovasc Electrophysiol* 1996;7:60–70, with permission.)

similar to that of atrial fibrillation. When associated with an underlying bundle branch block or aberrant ventricular conduction, atrial flutter must be differentiated from ventricular tachycardia, and in the presence of the Wolff-Parkinson-White syndrome or a very short PR interval (≤0.115 second) in the absence of a delta wave (i.e., Lown-Ganong-Levine syndrome), it may be associated with 1 : 1 AV conduction and a rapid ventricular response with or without associated QRS aberrancy.

MECHANISMS OF ATRIAL FLUTTER

There are a large number of studies, principally in experimental models but also in humans, indicating that most atrial flutter results from reentry in the right atrium. On the basis of studies in experimental animals and on vector analysis of human ECGs, Lewis and colleagues (37) concluded that atrial flutter was the result of circus movement in the atria. Many years later, Rosenblueth and Garcia-Ramos (38) created a lesion between the venae cavae that occasionally extended into a portion of the free wall of the right atrium and then induced intraatrial reentrant atrial flutter, which they thought was occurring around the obstacle created by the atrial lesion. In the presence of a more extensive Y lesion in the right atrium, atrial flutter can be explained by circus movement around the tricuspid valve annulus (39,40). The latter may have a clinical counterpart in the atrial flutter that is often seen after repair of complex congenital heart disease that requires several large incisions in the right atrium (28–31). Other canine right atrial lesion models have been developed (41–43) in which the reentrant wavefront travels around a lesion, amply demonstrating that this form of reentrant excitation around an atrial lesion can cause atrial flutter.

Almost from its recognition as a clinical entity, a single focus firing rapidly has been thought to be a possible mechanism of atrial flutter, even by Lewis, who later changed his mind (44). Experimental evidence to support this idea came from the studies of Scherf and colleagues (45–47), later confirmed by Kimura and coworkers (48), in which atrial flutter was shown to occur in the canine atria after the application of aconitine. Whether there is a clinical counterpart to this model is uncertain, although focal atrial tachycardias are now recognized (49).

Models that have not required application of substances or creation of primary atrial lesions are of special interest because they may be considered more likely to be the experimental counterparts of spontaneous atrial flutter in patients. The acetylcholine model studies of Allessie and associates in the canine heart (50,51) showed that atrial flutter due to intraatrial reentry could occur superiorly or inferiorly in either atrium and could occur in the absence of an anatomic obstacle. However, the atrial flutter cycle length was very short (<100 ms), suggesting that this might

be a model for type II atrial flutter. In studies of several other models of atrial flutter in the canine heart (52–63), the reentrant circuit was confined to the right atrium. The canine model of mitral regurgitation described by Cox and associates (64) showed several reentrant circuits, including one resulting from reentry confined to the right atrium in which the reentrant circuit had no anatomic obstacle. A limitation of most of these experimental studies is that minimal or no mapping of the intraatrial septum was performed. However, Boyden's studies, which included mapping of the atrial septum, demonstrated that the septum sometimes was involved in the reentrant circuit (54,65). The initial sequential site mapping studies of the sterile pericarditis model also suggested that the atrial septum sometimes might be involved (56). However, the studies in the sterile pericarditis model by Uno and colleagues (66), who recorded systematically from the atrial septum, showed that the reentrant atrial flutter circuit involved the atrial septum as part of a single-loop reentrant circuit or as part of a figure-of-eight reentry circuit (Figs. 16-3 and 16-4). Whether there is a clinical counterpart of this functional figure-of-eight reentrant circuit is uncertain (although we think likely). Shah and associates (67) demonstrated figure-of-eight reentry in patients in the presence of a lesion (i.e., line of block) in the right atrial free wall.

Mapping studies of atrial flutter in humans have been performed since the 1950s. Prinzmetal and coworkers (68), using photographic techniques during exposure of the heart during thoracic surgery, and Wellens and coworkers (69), using sequential site epicardial mapping techniques during cardiac surgery, suggested that atrial flutter was caused by a single site firing rapidly. That a single focus firing rapidly in patients could generate the classic clinical ECG of atrial flutter was shown by Rosen and colleagues (70). Nevertheless, these conclusions have not been supported by numerous other mapping studies in patients, primarily using electrode catheter techniques during electrophysiologic studies. As summarized by Rytand (71), catheter mapping studies in the 1950s and 1960s initially supported the notion that atrial flutter is an intraatrial reentrant rhythm in which an activation wavefront travels in a caudocranial direction in the left atrium and in a craniocaudal direction in the right atrium. However, mapping studies by Puech and colleagues (21,72) suggested that the entire duration of the atrial flutter cycle length could be explained by activation of the right atrium alone and that atrial flutter could be explained by circus movement in the right atrium.

The demonstration of transient entrainment and interruption of atrial flutter in humans (3,23,73–75) provided strong evidence that atrial flutter is an intraatrial reentrant rhythm with an excitable gap. Results of mapping studies, often in concert with atrial pacing, have been consistent with the conclusion that the usual atrial flutter reentrant circuit is confined to the right atrium. The studies of Cosío and coworkers (76–78), Olshansky and associates (79,80),

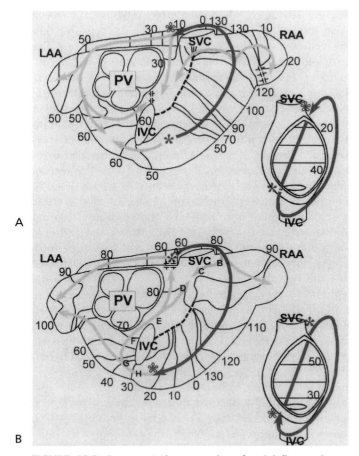

FIGURE 16-3. Representative examples of atrial flutter due to one reentrant circuit in the canine sterile pericarditis model. **A:** Isochronous map (atrial epicardium, left; atrial septum, right) from dog with induced, sustained atrial flutter demonstrating a single reentrant circuit in which reentrant circuit travels down the atrial septum and up the right atrial free wall. In this and subsequent activation maps, arrows indicate the direction of activation of the various wavefronts, gray arrows indicate daughter wavefronts generated by the reentrant circuit, isochrones are at 10-ms intervals, the thick dashed line indicates line of functional block, the dark asterisk indicates epicardial breakthrough of septal activation, and the white asterisk indicates site of reentry from epicardium to atrial septum. Numbers equal activation times in milliseconds. IVC, inferior vena cava; LAA, left atrial appendage; PV, pulmonary veins; RAA, right atrial appendage; SVC, superior vena cava. The T bar indicates block. **B:** Isochronous map from a different dog with induced, sustained atrial flutter demonstrating a single reentrant circuit in which reentrant circuit travels up atrial septum and down right atrial free wall. (Adapted from Uno K, Kumagai K, Khrestian C, Waldo AL. New insights regarding the atrial flutter reentrant circuit. Studies in the canine sterile pericarditis model. *Circulation* 1999;100:1354–1360, with permission.)

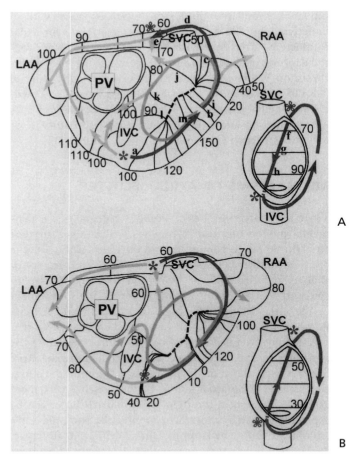

FIGURE 16-4. Representative examples of atrial flutter due to figure-of-eight reentry in the canine sterile pericarditis model. **A:** Isochronous map (atrial epicardium, left; atrial septum, right) from an episode of induced, sustained atrial flutter in a dog. It demonstrates figure-of-eight reentry in which the right atrial free wall reentrant circuit circulates in a counterclockwise direction and a reentrant circuit involving the atrial septum travels down the interatrial septum and up the right atrial free wall. All lines and arrows are as described in Figure 16-3. **B:** Isochronous map from an episode of sustained atrial flutter in another dog that demonstrated figure-of-eight reentry in which the right atrial free wall reentrant circuit circulated clockwise and a reentrant circuit involving the atrial septum traveled up the interatrial septum to Bachmann's bundle and then down the right atrial free wall. (Adapted from Uno K, Kumagai K, Khrestian C, Waldo AL. New insights regarding the atrial flutter reentrant circuit. Studies in the canine sterile pericarditis model. *Circulation* 1999;100:1354–1360, with permission.)

and Klein and colleagues (17) indicated that the reentrant circuit of typical atrial flutter in humans involves reentrant excitation in the right atrium, with the impulse traveling in a caudocranial direction in the interatrial septum and a craniocaudal direction in the right atrial free wall (Fig. 16-2), much as suggested by Puech and coworkers (21,72). Reverse typical atrial flutter was shown to be caused by

activation of the same reentrant circuit, although in the opposite direction from that just described (81). The studies of Cosío and coworkers (76–78,81) and Olshansky and colleagues (79,80) provided evidence that an area of slow conduction is present in the posteroinferior aspect of the reentrant circuit and that a critical area of block is present in the region between the vena cavae. Based on data from catheter mapping studies that included entrainment mapping, the area of slow conduction in the reentrant circuit is thought to be localized principally in an isthmus bounded by the inferior vena cava, the coronary sinus ostium, eustachian ridge, and the tricuspid annulus (13–15,78,82–84). The areas of block that permit the reentrant wavefront to circulate without short circuiting itself have been largely defined and include the orifice of the inferior vena cava (i.e., fixed block), the region of the crista terminalis (i.e., intercaval block, probably functional), and probably the orifice of the superior vena cava (i.e., fixed block) (77,78,85,86) (Fig. 16-2). The role of the eustachian ridge and the tricuspid ring as boundaries or regions of block for the reentrant circuit has also been demonstrated (13–15,78,82–86) (Fig. 16-2).

In sum, the reentrant circuit in 90% of clinical presentations of atrial flutter is as just described. Other locations for an atrial flutter reentrant circuit in patients may occur in the right atrial free wall, most often as a consequence of reentry around a surgical incision made during surgical repair of a congenital defect; around the pulmonary veins in the left atrium, with reentry likely around all or some of the veins; and around the tricuspid valve annulus, much as described in the animal model. Still other atypical atrial flutter reentrant circuits have been described, including one in the inferior atrial septum (87), one in the inferior left atrium (88), and one involving functional block in the right atrial free wall (89). Future studies using the more sophisticated contemporary mapping techniques now available should provide better data, so that an improved understanding of these reentrant circuits in patients can be expected.

ASSOCIATED SYMPTOMS AND HEMODYNAMIC EFFECTS

The symptoms associated with atrial flutter depend considerably on the presence or absence of underlying heart disease and on the ventricular response rate during atrial flutter. A rapid ventricular rate commonly is associated with palpitations, lightheadedness, dizziness, shortness of breath, weakness, faintness, and sometimes with overt syncope. If the ventricular rate is very fast, anginal pain may develop, particularly in the presence of underlying ischemic heart disease, but even in the absence of underlying ischemic heart disease, pain may occur if the rate is fast enough and the duration long enough (90). In patients with underlying heart disease, the presence of a rapid ventricular rate may induce signs and symptoms of congestive heart failure. Even in patients without underlying heart disease, if the rapid ventricular rate persists for prolonged periods, signs and symptoms of congestive heart failure may occur as a result of a tachycardia-mediated cardiomyopathy.

Hemodynamic effects depend on underlying disease, the ventricular rate, the duration of the rhythm, concurrent medications, and whether the patient is at rest or is exerting himself or herself. However, the hemodynamic effects of the arrhythmia are largely related to ventricular rate (90). At rapid ventricular rates, there is usually a decline in cardiac output. Blood pressure may also be substantially reduced. The abrupt onset of increased rates is known to affect blood pressure, typically with an initial decline and subsequent rise. The response of the blood pressure depends in large measure on peripheral adaptation. The initial decline in blood pressure with the rapid rate associated with the onset of the tachycardia may be associated with presyncope or with syncope in some cases. There may also be a significant reduction in coronary blood flow and a rate-related increment in myocardial oxygen consumption despite maintenance of baseline cardiac output. Because coronary artery blood flow occurs during diastole that is shortened during a tachycardia, the reduction in coronary artery flow is inversely proportional to ventricular rate and decreases progressively to a maximum of 60% of baseline. During atrial flutter, if the ventricular rate is rapid, this reduction in coronary flow is induced by changes in systolic and diastolic function. First, the diastolic interval is significantly shortened, thereby reducing the time for coronary flow, which occurs during diastole. Second, the mean aortic pressure declines, so that coronary artery perfusion pressure is reduced. Third, if there is associated ischemia or diastolic dysfunction, left ventricular end-diastolic pressure rises as the rapid ventricular rate continues. The decrease in coronary artery flow occurs in the face of an increase in myocardial oxygen consumption resulting from the enhanced rate of contraction. This combination of factors explains the frequent association of symptomatic ischemia with supraventricular tachycardias, including atrial flutter (90).

DIAGNOSIS
Physical Examination

During atrial flutter, there is commonly a regular ventricular response to the rapid atrial rate, typically 2 : 1 or 4 : 1 and infrequently 1 : 1. During a paroxysm of atrial flutter, it is common for the peripheral pulse and the rate ausculted from the precordium to be regular and often rapid. However, atrial flutter also can be associated with an irregular ventricular response rate. Results of the physical examination may mimic those for atrial fibrillation in that there may be an irregular ventricular rate ausculted at the precordium associated with an irregular peripheral pulse rate with dropped beats (i.e., the apical ventricular rate is greater than the peripheral ventricular rate). Examination of the neck may reveal jugular venous pulsations that demonstrate prominent "a" or flutter waves occurring at the same rate as atrial activation.

Other signs during the physical examination primarily are related to the presence or absence of congestive heart failure. The latter runs the gamut from frank pulmonary edema to respiratory rales and right-sided heart failure. Hypotension may exist, particularly if the ventricular rate is rapid.

Electrocardiographic Manifestations and Diagnostic Features

Atrial flutter usually can be diagnosed from the ECG. Classically, the examiner looks for so-called flutter waves, principally in ECG leads II, III, and aVF and in V_1. Flutter waves appear as atrial complexes of constant morphology, polarity, and cycle length in a rate range from 240 to 340 bpm (22). The atrial rate may be slower if the rhythm is present in the face of therapy with antiarrhythmic drugs such as quinidine, procainamide, disopyramide, flecainide, propafenone, moricizine, or amiodarone; however, these agents do not alter the morphology of the flutter waves. Classically, in the inferior leads (II, III, and aVF), the appearance of a picket fence because the leads are primarily negative (Fig. 16-5). If the ventricular response to atrial flutter is equal to that of the atrial flutter rate (i.e., there is 1 : 1 AV conduction), it may be difficult to identify flutter waves in the ECG leads because they may be temporally superimposed on other ECG deflections such as the QRS complex or the T wave.

Although the physician may suspect atrial flutter, in the presence of a narrow QRS complex with 2 : 1 AV conduc-

tion, it must be differentiated from sinus tachycardia, AV nodal reentrant tachycardia, AV reentrant tachycardia involving an accessory AV connection, an atrial tachycardia with 1 : 1 AV conduction, an accelerated AV junctional tachycardia, and sinus node reentrant tachycardia. In such cases, vagal maneuvers or other transient interventions are recommended to provide transient increased AV block while recording the ECG, thereby revealing the underlying flutter waves. In the presence of a wide QRS complex, it must be differentiated from all of the previous rhythms in the presence of an underlying bundle branch block or aberrant ventricular conduction and from ventricular tachycardia or antegrade conduction over an accessory AV connection.

The ventricular response rate to atrial flutter commonly is 2 : 1 or 4 : 1, but it may be irregular, and rarely, it may even be 1 : 1. The latter may be seen in patients with Wolff-Parkinson-White syndrome when the accessory AV connection is capable of conducting impulses at rapid rates from the atria to the ventricles. The 1 : 1 AV conduction pattern may also be present in patients who have a very short PR interval during sinus rhythm because of enhanced AV nodal conduction or the Lown-Ganong-Levine syndrome. AV conduction may become 1 : 1 during exertion or in the presence of therapy with catecholamines or sympathomimetic amines administered as therapy for another underlying clin-

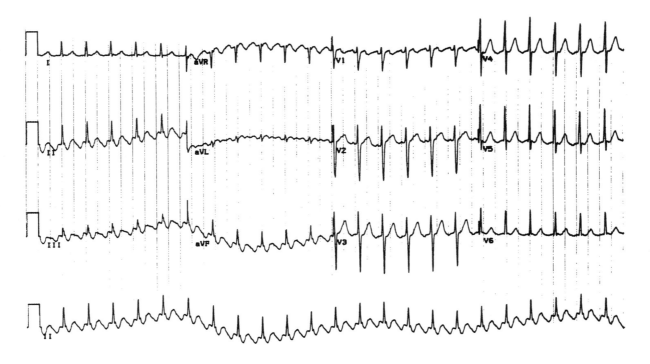

FIGURE 16-5. A 12-lead electrocardiogram of a typical case of type I atrial flutter. The atrial rate is 300 bpm, and the ventricular rate is 150 bpm; 2 : 1 atrioventricular block is present. Notice how the atrial activity is best seen in leads II, III, and aVF and is barely perceptible in lead I. (From Waldo AL, Kastor JA. Atrial flutter. In: Kastor JA, ed. *Arrhythmias*. Philadelphia: WB Saunders, 1994:105–115, with permission.)

ical problem. In the presence of therapy with a class Ia or particularly a class Ic antiarrhythmic agent, the atrial flutter rate may slow be enough to allow 1 : 1 AV conduction.

The atrial flutter rate and ventricular response rate may be affected by the presence of drug therapy. In the presence of an antiarrhythmic agent that slows the atrial flutter rate, especially Ic agents or moricizine, the atrial flutter rate may be 200 ± 20 bpm. With a slower than usual atrial flutter rate, the ventricular response rate paradoxically increases, such as from 150 bpm with 2 : 1 AV block to 200 bpm with 1 : 1 AV nodal conduction. With drugs that slow conduction through the AV node (e.g., digitalis, β-blocking agent, calcium channel blocker), the ventricular response rate to atrial flutter may be remarkably slow. Any of the latter drugs, if present in too high a plasma concentration, may cause complete heart block, such that no atrial flutter beats are conducted to the ventricle.

The QRS complex during atrial flutter is most commonly identical to the QRS complex during sinus rhythm because atrial flutter is a supraventricular rhythm. However, atrial flutter beats may be conducted aberrantly to the ventricles, thereby manifesting a functional bundle branch block morphology, most commonly a right bundle branch. Even when conducted normally, the QRS complex may be distorted by temporal superimposition of flutter waves in the QRS complex (Fig. 16-6). The QRS complex may "grow" a new R wave, S wave, Q wave, or a taller R or S wave.

The ECG in sinus rhythm rarely provides any clues to the propensity to develop atrial flutter except for the presence of premature atrial beats. Occasionally, the examiner may see a P mitrale or P pulmonale, providing evidence of left or right atrial enlargement, respectively. If the patient

presented with 1 : 1 AV conduction of atrial flutter, the examiner should look for a short PR interval with a delta wave during previous or subsequent sinus rhythm because of the presence of Wolff-Parkinson-White syndrome or a short PR interval (≤0.115 second) without a delta wave, formerly called the Lown-Ganong-Levine syndrome. Some patients with atrial flutter may demonstrate sinus bradycardia or other manifestations of sick sinus syndrome when the ECG is recorded during sinus rhythm. Sinus node dysfunction and bradycardia can predispose to tachycardia (i.e., tachycardia-bradycardia syndrome). Diagnosing the presence of sick sinus syndrome is important because when the atrial flutter terminates abruptly in the presence of underlying sinus node dysfunction, there may be an associated prolonged period of asystole before the sinus node or any escape pacemaker fires. When that happens, it may result in syncope, with all its potential adverse consequences.

Diagnosis of Suspected Atrial Flutter

When atrial flutter is suspected, it is recommended that the diagnosis be clearly established before initiating therapy, unless the tachycardia is clinically life threatening, such as when associated with pulmonary edema or with 1 : 1 AV conduction, perhaps because of Wolff-Parkinson-White syndrome. The presence of saw-toothed flutter waves in the ECG, particularly ECG leads II, III and aVF, remains the standard for the diagnosis of typical atrial flutter (Figs. 16-5 and 16-6). If the diagnosis is not clear from a standard ECG and circumstances permit, any of a number of vagal maneuvers (e.g., carotid sinus pressure, Valsalva maneuver, invoking the diving reflex) that prolong AV conduction and slow the ventricular response rate transiently may be used while recording the ECG (preferably at least lead II or V₁). This should permit atrial flutter complexes to be readily appreciated in the ECG. If the diagnosis remains unclear after a vagal maneuver and if permitted by the clinical situation, any of the following diagnostic maneuvers may be used. First, an electrogram may be recorded directly from the atria by placement of an esophageal electrode, by transvenous placement of a catheter electrode, or by use of a temporary atrial epicardial wire electrode placed at the time of open-heart surgery, which is the preferred choice for these patients. Second, a pharmacologic agent such as adenosine, esmolol, verapamil, diltiazem, or edrophonium may be administered intravenously to prolong AV conduction transiently, thereby revealing the atrial complexes in the ECG. The advantage of the first option is that it permits the definitive diagnosis to be made and provides an opportunity to treat the atrial flutter with rapid atrial pacing. The advantage of the second option is that it does not require any invasive procedure. Esmolol, verapamil, or diltiazem can be administered continuously, and virtually always safely, to slow the ventricular response rate, giving the clinician additional time to determine the next course of ther-

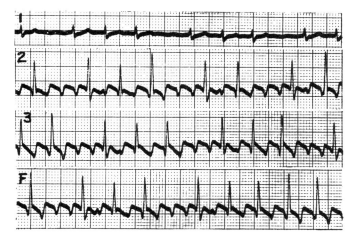

FIGURE 16-6. Atrial flutter with atrioventricular block varying between 2 : 1 and 4 : 1. Notice the lack of evidence of atrial activity in lead I and the superimposition of atrial flutter complexes on the QRS complexes, such that q waves and s waves appear and disappear. (Adapted from Marriott HJL. Atrial arrhythmias. In: Marriott HJL. *Practical electrocardiography*, 3rd ed. Baltimore: Williams & Wilkins, 1962:119, with permission.)

apy. However, in the presence of a wide QRS complex tachycardia that may represent a ventricular tachycardia or a supraventricular tachycardia with aberrant ventricular conduction because of a rate-related or underlying bundle branch block or intraventricular conduction defect or the presence of AV conduction over an accessory AV connection, drug intervention to establish the diagnosis of atrial flutter is fraught with difficulties and dangers and usually is contraindicated.

CLINICAL ELECTROPHYSIOLOGY

For patients with paroxysms of tachycardia in whom atrial flutter is suspected but has not been documented with an ECG, 24-hour ambulatory (Holter) monitoring is recommended for initial evaluation. However, for some patients, the episodes of tachycardia are sufficiently infrequent that the documentation requires use of an event recorder such as a transtelephonic monitor. Until recently, cardiac electrophysiologic studies during cardiac catheterization were not used routinely to characterize atrial flutter. They have become more important because of the advent of safe and effective catheter ablation procedures to cure atrial flutter. However, no standards for use of programmed stimulation for the initiation of atrial flutter have evolved. The most reliable method is to pace the atria very rapidly to initiate atrial fibrillation, which then usually evolves to atrial flutter (91). Initiation of atrial flutter by introducing premature atrial beats after a train of eight paced beats is much less reliable, and despite a known history of atrial flutter, using these techniques still may not induce atrial flutter.

Mapping studies of atrial flutter are generally performed to identify the location of the reentrant circuit, particularly to identify a vulnerable portion of the reentrant circuit that can be ablated to provide a cure of atrial flutter. This location is thought to be an isthmus between the tricuspid valve orifice and the orifice of the inferior vena cava or the coronary sinus (13–15,78,82–86) in typical and reverse typical atrial flutter. However, with the recognition of incisional reentrant atrial flutter, left atrial flutter, and truly atypical forms of atrial flutter, mapping studies are an important part of the electrophysiologic workup of clinically important atrial flutter.

MANAGEMENT OF ATRIAL FLUTTER

Acute Treatment of Atrial Flutter

When the diagnosis of atrial flutter is established, three options are available to restore sinus rhythm: administer antiarrhythmic drug therapy, initiate DC cardioversion, or initiate rapid atrial pacing to interrupt atrial flutter. In large measure, the treatment depends on the clinical status of the patient. In the past, the preferred option to interrupt atrial flutter was DC cardioversion or rapid atrial pacing. The introduction of ibutilide has provided another viable option; use of this antiarrhythmic drug is associated with a 60% likelihood of converting atrial flutter to sinus rhythm (92,93). Because ibutilide prolongs ventricular repolarization, and consequently the Q-T interval, there is a small incidence of torsade de pointes associated with its use (93,94). However, such episodes are usually self-limited and of brief duration because of the short half-life of this drug. Nevertheless, the physician should be prepared to administer intravenous magnesium and even perform DC cardioversion to treat a prolonged episode of torsade de pointes or ventricular fibrillation if either occurs when using ibutilide.

Intravenous procainamide is sometimes useful in converting atrial flutter to normal sinus rhythm (95), and several studies suggest that a single large oral dose of flecainide (300 mg) or propafenone (600 mg) may successfully cardiovert atrial flutter to sinus rhythm, although most of the data are from patients with atrial fibrillation (96,97). Drug therapy may be given before initiating DC cardioversion or rapid atrial pacing to slow the ventricular response rate (i.e., with a β blocker or a calcium channel blocker or digoxin); to enhance the efficacy of rapid atrial pacing in restoring sinus rhythm (i.e., use of procainamide, disopyramide, or ibutilide [98–100]); or to enhance the likelihood that sinus rhythm will be sustained after effective DC cardioversion (i.e., use of a class Ia or a class Ic or class III antiarrhythmic agent).

For many years, standard initial treatment was aggressive administration of a digitalis preparation, usually intravenously, until atrial flutter converted to atrial fibrillation with a controlled ventricular response rate or converted to sinus rhythm. This treatment mode is no longer the treatment of choice, except perhaps in the presence of severe left ventricular dysfunction (3). When rapid control of the ventricular response rate during atrial flutter is desirable, it can usually and readily be accomplished by using an intravenous calcium channel blocking agent (e.g., verapamil, diltiazem) or an intravenous β-blocking agent (e.g., esmolol).

Selection of acute therapy for atrial flutter with DC cardioversion, atrial pacing, or intravenous ibutilide depends on the clinical presentation of the patient and on the clinical availability and ease of applying these techniques. Because DC cardioversion requires administration of an anesthetic agent, it may be undesirable in the patient who presents with atrial flutter after having recently eaten or the patient who has severe chronic obstructive lung disease. Such patients are best treated with ibutilide or rapid atrial pacing to interrupt atrial flutter or with agents to slow the ventricular response rate. For the patient who develops atrial flutter after open-heart surgery, use of the temporary atrial epicardial wire electrodes to perform rapid atrial pacing to restore sinus rhythm generally is the treatment of choice, although intravenous ibutilide has been quite effective in this circumstance (3,94).

Techniques of Rapid Atrial Pacing to Interrupt Atrial Flutter

Several atrial pacing techniques are available and effective (3). During typical atrial flutter, pacing is best performed from the high right atrium, because the appearance of positive atrial complexes (i.e., flutter waves) in ECG lead II is the hallmark of interruption of atrial flutter (3,23). When using the ramp atrial pacing technique, bipolar atrial pacing is initiated at a rate about 10 bpm faster than the spontaneous atrial rate, and the ECG lead II is recorded continuously. After demonstrating atrial capture, the atrial pacing rate is gradually increased until the atrial complexes in ECG lead II become positive (Fig. 16-7). Atrial pacing then may be abruptly terminated, or the pacing rate may be rapidly slowed to a desirable atrial pacing rate. The latter permits control of the atrial rhythm and may be invaluable in the presence of underlying sick sinus syndrome.

Another satisfactory method is the constant-rate pacing technique. Because the most successful rate for interruption of type I atrial flutter is approximately 120% to 130% of the spontaneous atrial rate (3,23), when this technique is used, rapid atrial pacing is best initiated at a rate within this percentage range of the spontaneous atrial flutter rate and continued for 15 to 30 seconds or until the atrial complexes in ECG lead II become positive. Pacing then is abruptly terminated or rapidly slowed to a desirable atrial pacing rate. If pacing at the initially selected rate does not interrupt atrial flutter, the atrial pacing rate should be increased by 5- to 10-bpm increments until atrial flutter is successfully interrupted. A more conservative approach would be to initiate pacing at a rate 10 bpm faster than the spontaneous atrial rate, and if atrial flutter has not been interrupted after termination of pacing, the atrial pacing rate is then increased by 5- to 10-bpm increments until atrial flutter is successfully interrupted (Fig. 16-8 and 16-9).

Regardless of the pacing technique used, when the atria are paced at rates faster than the spontaneous rate, the atrial flutter may not be interrupted despite achieving atrial capture during pacing. This should not be considered evidence that rapid atrial pacing will be unsuccessful. Rather, it means that the pacing rates selected have transiently entrained the atrial flutter (3,23,73–75) and indicates that pacing at a more rapid rate is required to interrupt the atrial flutter. Occasionally, atrial pacing rates higher than 400 bpm may be required to interrupt atrial flutter. When using the constant-rate pacing technique, a critical duration of pacing (average, 11 seconds) at the critical pacing rate is required (3,23,74,75). Whether using epicardial or endocardial pacing techniques, the stimu-

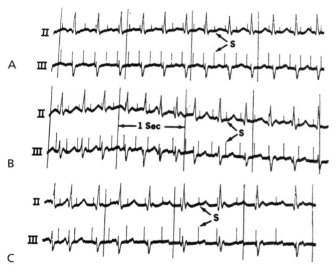

FIGURE 16-7. Electrocardiogram leads II and III recorded from a patient during rapid high right atrial pacing to treat atrial flutter (intrinsic atrial flutter rate of 294 bpm). Previously, pacing had been initiated at a rate of 309 bpm and increased to a rate of 355 bpm but had failed to interrupt the atrial flutter. During the previous ramp pacing, the atrial complexes became biphasic only in leads II and III. Then pacing was reinitiated (**A**) at a rate of 350 bpm and increased to a rate of 382 bpm. The atrial complexes became completely positive in leads II and III when the pacing rate reached about 370 bpm. When the pacing rate was slowed from 382 bpm to a rate below the rate of the spontaneous atrial flutter, atrial capture was maintained (**B** and **C**). Atrial capture was maintained as the pacing rate was decreased ultimately to a rate of 110 bpm (not shown). Time lines are at 1-second intervals. S, stimulus artifact. (From Waldo AL, MacLean WAH, Karp RB, et al. Entrainment and interruption of atrial flutter with atrial pacing: studies in man following open heart surgery. *Circulation* 1977;56:737–745, with permission.)

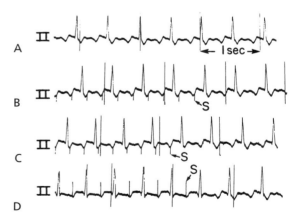

FIGURE 16-8. Electrocardiographic lead II was recorded from a patient with classic (type I) atrial flutter (atrial cycle length of 264 ms) (**A**) and at the end of 30 seconds of rapid atrial pacing from a high right atrial site at a cycle length of 254 ms (**B**), at a cycle length of 242 ms (**C**), and at a cycle length of 232 ms (**D**). The atrial flutter was transiently entrained at each pacing rate. When comparing the morphology of the atrial complexes during atrial pacing at each cycle length, especially comparing the atrial complexes during atrial pacing in **D** with those in **A** and **B**, notice that progressive fusion has occurred. S, stimulus artifact. Time lines are at 1-second intervals. (Modified from Waldo AL, MacLean WAH, Karp RB, et al. Entrainment and interruption of atrial flutter with atrial pacing: studies in man following open heart surgery. *Circulation* 1977;56:737–745, with permission.)

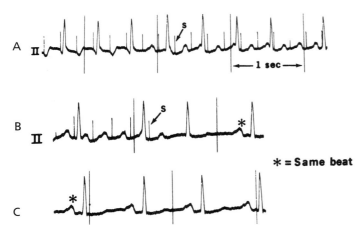

FIGURE 16-9. A: Electrocardiographic lead II was recorded in the same patient as in Figure 16-8 during high right atrial pacing from the same site at a cycle length of 224 ms. With the seventh atrial beat in this tracing and after 22 seconds of atrial pacing at a constant rate, the atrial complexes suddenly became positive. **B:** Electrocardiographic lead II was recorded at the termination of atrial pacing in the same patient. With abrupt termination of pacing, sinus rhythm occurs. **C:** The first beat *(asterisk)* is identical to the last beat in *B (asterisk).* S, stimulus artifact. Time lines are at 1-second intervals. (Adapted from Waldo AL, MacLean WAH, Karp RB, et al. Entrainment and interruption of atrial flutter with atrial pacing: studies in man following open heart surgery. *Circulation* 1977;56:737–745, with permission.)

lus strength required for atrial capture at the rapid rates necessary to interrupt atrial flutter are usually high (3,101), and a loss of capture or a failure to capture the atria may occur unless a sufficient stimulus strength is applied. It is recommended that pacing be initiated with a stimulus strength of at least 10 mA. However, it is not unusual to require up to 20 mA, and occasionally, an even stronger stimulus strength may be required (3).

When esophageal pacing is used to interrupt atrial flutter, the previous suggestions apply but with two important exceptions. First, to capture the atria, the stimulus must be at least 9 to 10 ms long and the stimulus strength up to 30 mA (102). Use of a pacemaker without these characteristics decreases the likelihood of successful capture of the atria. Second, because pacing through the esophagus tends to be somewhat painful (usually causing a stinging sensation), pacing should be as brief as possible, and a pacing rate likely to interrupt atrial flutter should be selected at the outset to minimize the number of pacing attempts required to interrupt atrial flutter. Before initiating rapid pacing of any sort, it is recommended that pacing be initiated at a relatively slow rate to demonstrate that no ventricular capture is inadvertently produced.

Pacing Precipitation of Inadvertent and Deliberate Atrial Fibrillation

Despite appropriate care taken in performing any of the pacing techniques, rapid atrial pacing provokes atrial fibril-

lation in some patients. Most often, atrial fibrillation so precipitated is transient, lasting seconds to minutes, before spontaneously converting to sinus rhythm. For the few patients in whom atrial fibrillation persists, it is usually a more desirable rhythm because atrial fibrillation is almost always associated with a slower ventricular response rate than atrial flutter. The ventricular response rate to atrial fibrillation can almost always be more easily controlled with standard agents. For patients in whom atrial flutter recurs despite its successful interruption by rapid atrial pacing, continuous rapid atrial pacing to precipitate and sustain atrial fibrillation may be indicated on a temporary basis in selected patients, most commonly in patients after open-heart surgery (Fig. 16-10), until pharmacologic control of atrial flutter is achieved (3,103).

When atrial pacing is performed after initiation of therapy with a class Ia antiarrhythmic agent (e.g., procainamide, disopyramide) or ibutilide, there is a very high incidence of successful conversion of atrial flutter to sinus

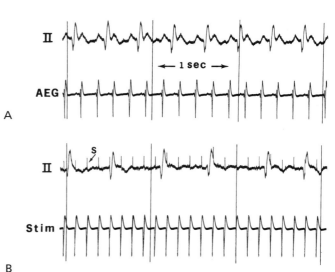

FIGURE 16-10. A: Electrocardiographic lead II was recorded simultaneously with a bipolar atrial electrogram (AEG) during type I atrial flutter at a rate of 320 bpm with 2 : 1 atrioventricular (AV) conduction, producing a ventricular rate of 160 bpm. In this patient after open-heart surgery, the atrial flutter was interrupted successfully on several occasions with rapid atrial pacing, but it recurred each time. **B:** Continuous rapid atrial pacing at 450 bpm was initiated. Pacing at this rate precipitated and sustained atrial fibrillation and was associated with a slowing of the ventricular rate to about 120 bpm. Digoxin was then administered to further slow the ventricular rate. Continuous rapid atrial pacing to sustain atrial fibrillation for control of ventricular rate was required for 26 hours in this patient (longer than usual) while antiarrhythmic drug therapy (digoxin and quinidine) was administered. After rapid atrial pacing was terminated, atrial fibrillation spontaneously converted to sinus rhythm within several minutes (not shown). S, stimulus artifact. Time lines are at 1-second intervals. (Adapted from Waldo AL, MacLean WAH, Karp RB, et al. Continuous rapid atrial pacing to control recurrent or sustained supraventricular tachycardias following open heart surgery. *Circulation* 1976;54:245–250, with permission.)

rhythm without any period of atrial fibrillation (98–100). When using rapid atrial pacing, use of one of these agents is recommended.

Direct Current Cardioversion to Convert Atrial Flutter to Sinus Rhythm

DC cardioversion of atrial flutter to sinus rhythm has a very high likelihood of success. It may also require as little as 25 J of energy, although a strength of at least 50 J is generally recommended because it is more often successful. Because a strength of 100 J is virtually always successful and never harmful, it should be considered as the initial shock strength. The high degree of success avoids the need for delivery of a second shock in case the first was unsuccessful because its strength was too low.

Intravenous Ibutilide to Convert Atrial Flutter to Sinus Rhythm

One milligram of ibutilide is given *slowly* (over 5 to 10 minutes) while monitoring the ECG carefully. If the rhythm does not convert to sinus rhythm, a second 1-mg intravenous infusion is administered over 5 to 10 minutes. If torsade de pointes develops, it generally is of no clinical consequence because it usually consists of very short runs. However, the physician must be prepared to perform prompt DC cardioversion if a sustained episode develops, and uncommonly, intravenous magnesium must be administered to prevent recurrent torsade de pointes. Because the distribution half-life of ibutilide is so short (90 minutes), any adverse effects usually are quite short lived and almost always occur within the first hour of administration (93).

Chronic Treatment of Atrial Flutter

Catheter Ablation Therapy

Two types of catheter ablation have been used for the treatment of chronic or recurrent atrial flutter. One type is radiofrequency ablation to cure atrial flutter. Advances in mapping and ablation techniques have improved the efficacy of this technique to about 95%, with little subsequent recurrence for patients with typical or reverse typical atrial flutter (13–15,84,104–107), making it the treatment of choice in most patients. Treatment of atrial flutter with ablation may result in an improvement in left ventricular function by reversing a tachycardia-mediated cardiomyopathy (108). The technique first involves mapping the atria during atrial flutter to identify the location of the reentrant circuit and a critical isthmus in the atrial flutter reentrant circuit. When the latter area is identified, radiofrequency energy is delivered through the catheter electrode to create a bidirectional line of block across it. For typical or reverse typical atrial flutter, ablation of a critical isthmus between the inferior vena cava–eustachian ridge–coronary sinus

ostium and tricuspid valve (Fig. 16-2) has proven most efficacious, but this isthmus may be difficult to ablate completely (84,104–107). The latter was the principal reason for the ablation failures and recurrences of typical or reverse typical atrial flutter. Fortunately, combined entrainment pacing and mapping techniques permit the reliable demonstration that this isthmus is a part of the reentrant circuit, and testing can demonstrate the presence of complete bidirectional conduction block in this isthmus (106,107). When the latter is demonstrated, successful ablation of atrial flutter has been accomplished.

Similar to what has been observed after reversion of chronic atrial fibrillation, atrial stunning and spontaneous echo contrast on transesophageal echocardiography may be seen after radiofrequency ablation of chronic atrial flutter; these abnormalities are not present in patients with paroxysmal atrial flutter, suggesting that atrial stunning is related to the duration of the arrhythmia and not the mode of reversion (109). These changes resolved after 3 weeks of sinus rhythm.

Successful ablation of the atrial flutter reentrant circuit does not prevent recurrence or the new appearance of atrial fibrillation, which occurs in up to 36% of patients (110, 111). The risk appears to increase dramatically in patients with a history of atrial fibrillation and reduced left ventricular ejection fraction; in one report, 74% of such patients developed atrial fibrillation (112). These data suggest that atrial fibrillation may be a trigger for rather than a consequence of atrial flutter in some patients.

When incisional reentrant atrial flutter is identified by electrophysiologic mapping techniques, a vulnerable isthmus usually can be identified and successfully ablated using radiofrequency catheter ablation techniques (113–115). Even though incisional atrial reentry is suspected, studies (107) have shown that most atrial flutter that occurs chronically after congenital heart surgery uses the atrial flutter isthmus, making the latter the preferred ablation target. There is insufficient information available to discuss the likely efficacy of successful radiofrequency ablation techniques to cure left atrial flutter or atypical atrial flutter, although contemporary electrophysiologic mapping techniques are capable of identifying the location of their reentrant circuits, making effective ablation therapy a good possibility.

For patients with atrial flutter in the presence of an accessory AV connection (Wolff-Parkinson-White syndrome), especially with a history of 1 : 1 conduction of atrial flutter impulses to the ventricles through the accessory AV connection, catheter ablation of the accessory AV connection is the treatment of choice. There is a high likelihood that, with successful ablation of the accessory AV connection, the atrial flutter no longer recurs (116).

A second technique, not often used primarily to treat atrial flutter, is His bundle ablation to create a high degree of AV block, usually a third-degree AV block. This technique eliminates the rapid ventricular response rates to atrial flutter (16). However, it does not prevent the atrial flutter, and it requires placement of a pacemaker system. For patients in whom catheter ablation of atrial flutter is unsuccessful and in whom antiarrhythmic drug therapy is ineffective or is not tolerated or in whom atrial flutter with a clinically unacceptable rapid ventricular response rate recurs despite antiarrhythmic drug therapy, producing third-degree AV block or a high degree of AV block provides a successful form of therapy. Selection of a pacemaker in such circumstances should be tailored to the needs of the patient and may include a single-chamber, rate-responsive, ventricular pacemaker or a dual-chamber pacemaker with mode switching capability.

Drug Therapy

It may be difficult to suppress atrial flutter completely with any antiarrhythmic drug therapy. Based on available long-term data, there appears to be a limited ability to maintain sinus rhythm without occasional to frequent recurrence of atrial flutter, even when multiple agents are used (117). When considering antiarrhythmic drug efficacy, an important measure should be the frequency of recurrence of atrial flutter rather than a single recurrent episode. For instance, recurrence only one time per year probably should be considered quite reasonable therapy.

For a long time, standard treatment consisted of administration of a class Ia antiarrhythmic agent (e.g., quinidine, procainamide, disopyramide) in an effort to prevent recurrence. However, studies indicate that the type Ic antiarrhythmic agents (e.g., flecainide, propafenone) are as effective and perhaps more effective than class Ia agents (9,10). They are better tolerated and have less organ toxicity. Principally because of their serious adverse effects in The Cardiac Arrhythmia Suppression Trial I (CAST I) (118), it is widely acknowledged that type Ic agents should not be used in the presence of underlying ischemic heart disease. This notion has also been extrapolated to the presence of underlying structural heart disease. However, because of their efficacy, class Ic agents should be considered early on for long-term suppression of atrial flutter in the absence of structural heart disease. Moricizine, a drug with Ia, Ib, and Ic properties, also may be effective in the treatment of atrial flutter, and based on the long-term data from CAST II (119), in which mortality with moricizine and placebo were no different, perhaps it can be considered in patients with atrial flutter and coronary artery disease.

Class III antiarrhythmic agents (e.g., amiodarone, sotalol, dofetilide) may be quite effective (12,120,121). When using sotalol or dofetilide, care must be taken to prevent QT interval prolongation much beyond 500 ms to avoid precipitation of torsade de pointes, and these drugs probably should not be given if the baseline corrected QT is more than 460 ms for men and more than 440 ms for women. Amiodarone appears to be quite effective (12), but its potential toxicity is a well-recognized concern, making widespread long-term use of this drug to treat atrial flutter problematic (122). The use of amiodarone as the drug of first choice probably should be limited to patients with congestive heart failure due to markedly depressed left ventricular function (e.g., ejection fraction <0.30).

A "drug-induced" form of atrial flutter (123,124) can occur in patients treated for atrial fibrillation with a class Ic agent, although it may also occur occasionally in patients treated with amiodarone or a class Ia agent (125). In these cases, when the atrial flutter is mapped electrophysiologically, its reentrant circuit is that of typical or reverse typical atrial flutter and is therefore vulnerable to effective ablative therapy. In patients treated with a Ic agent, maintenance of this drug therapy plus successful ablation of the atrial flutter isthmus results in an approximately 70% success rate in prevention of recurrent atrial fibrillation and atrial flutter (123,124). This therapy should be considered for patients who present with drug-induced atrial flutter.

Anticoagulant Therapy

Although one study found neither atrial clot formation nor stroke associated with atrial flutter in a relatively small cohort of patients after open-heart surgery (126), other studies indicate that the incidence of stroke associated with atrial flutter approaches that of atrial fibrillation (33–36). The fact that atrial flutter and atrial fibrillation often coexist in patients simply adds clinical weight to this consideration. In two studies that used transesophageal echocardiography in patients with atrial flutter, a high incidence of spontaneous echo contrast and atrial thrombi was documented, as were striking abnormalities in the left atrial appendage (127,128). In patients with atrial flutter, daily warfarin therapy to achieve an international normalized ratio (INR) of 2 to 3 is recommended using the same criteria as for atrial fibrillation.

Implanted Antitachycardia Pacemaker

For selected patients, consideration should be given to implantation of a permanent antitachycardia pacemaker to treat recurrent atrial flutter. Although the published series of patients with these devices has been small, they nevertheless have shown to be effective in interrupting recurrent atrial flutter with return to sinus rhythm (129,130). In properly selected patients, the ability to interrupt atrial flutter promptly whenever it recurs should provide safe and effective treatment. Because precipitation of atrial fibrillation is always a potential problem when using any form of pacing to treat atrial flutter, if any pacing-induced episodes of atrial fibrillation are clinically unacceptable, placement of a permanent antitachycardia pacemaker to treat atrial flutter should be avoided. To decrease or eliminate an incidence of inadvertent precipitation of atrial fibrillation, chronic use of an antiarrhythmic drug may be desirable (98,99). Chronic antiarrhythmic drug therapy may be required to decrease the incidence of recurrent atrial flutter.

Surgical Therapy

Much as for catheter ablation of a critical portion of the atrial flutter reentrant circuit, acceptable surgical therapy awaits more definitive understanding of the mechanism of atrial flutter and the location of the critical portions of its reentry circuit. However, Klein and coworkers (17) and Guiraudon and associates (131) described operated patients in whom intraoperative mapping demonstrated an area of slow conduction or a gap in activation during atrial flutter. This area was between the coronary sinus orifice and the tricuspid annulus. Cryoablation of the region successfully prevented recurrent atrial flutter in two. However, the third patient had subsequent symptomatic atrial fibrillation. Similarities between the surgical data and the catheter ablation data are apparent. However, the efficacy of radiofrequency ablation using catheter techniques almost certainly obviates the need for surgical ablation.

For patients with Wolff-Parkinson-White syndrome, when catheter ablation of the accessory AV connections is not successful but is still desirable, surgical ablation should be considered as a therapeutic option; this includes patients with 1 : 1 AV conduction of atrial flutter (116).

CONCLUSIONS

Atrial flutter is caused by some form of reentrant excitation, usually in the right atrium. It is usually easily diagnosed. Acute treatment consists of obtaining rapid control of the ventricular response rate and restoring sinus rhythm, although precipitation of atrial fibrillation occasionally may be useful. Radiofrequency catheter ablation therapy provides an excellent chance for cure, although atrial fibrillation may subsequently occur after an ostensibly successful ablative procedure. Alternatively, antiarrhythmic drug therapy to suppress recurrent atrial flutter episodes may be useful, recognizing that occasional recurrences are common despite therapy. Radiofrequency ablation of the His bundle with placement of an appropriate pacemaker system may be useful in selected patients. Anticoagulation with warfarin in patients with chronic or recurrent atrial flutter is recommended using the same criteria as for atrial fibrillation.

ACKNOWLEDGMENTS

This work was supported in part by grant RO1 HL38408 from the National Institutes of Health and the National Heart, Lung, and Blood Institute in Bethesda, Maryland, and by a grant from the Wuliger Foundation in Cleveland, Ohio.

REFERENCES

1. Jolly WA, Ritchie WJ. Auricular flutter and fibrillation. *Heart* 1911;2:177–221.
2. Waldo AL. Mechanisms of atrial fibrillation, atrial flutter, and ectopic atrial tachycardia—a brief review. *Circulation* 1987;75 [Suppl III]:37–40.
3. Waldo AL, MacLean WAH. *Diagnosis and treatment of arrhythmias following open heart surgery—emphasis on the use of epicardial wire electrodes.* New York: Futura Publishing, 1980.
4. Morris JJ, Kong Y, North WC, McIntosh HD. Experience with "cardioversion" of atrial fibrillation and flutter. *Am J Cardiol* 1964;14:94–100.
5. Castellanos A, Lemberg L, Gosselin A, Fonseca UJ. Evaluation of countershock treatment of atrial flutter. *Arch Intern Med* 1965;115:426–433.
6. Zipes DP. Management of cardiac arrhythmia: pharmacological, electrical and surgical techniques. In: Braunwald E, ed. *Heart disease: a textbook of cardiovascular medicine,* 3rd ed. Philadelphia: WB Saunders, 1988:621–657.
7. The Esmolol Research Group. Intravenous esmolol for the treatment of supraventricular tachyarrhythmia: results of a multi center, baseline-controlled safety and efficacy study of 160 patients. *Am Heart J* 1986;112:498–505.
8. Plumb VJ, Karp RB, Kouchoukos NT, et al. Verapamil therapy of atrial fibrillation and atrial flutter following open heart surgery. *J Thorac Cardiovasc Surg* 1982;83:590–596.
9. Anderson JL, Gilbert EM, Alpert BL, et al, for the Flecainide Supraventricular Tachycardia Study Group. Prevention of symptomatic recurrences of paroxysmal atrial fibrillation in patients initially tolerating antiarrhythmic therapy: a multicenter, double-blind, crossover study of flecainide and placebo using transtelephonic monitoring. *Circulation* 1989;80:1557–1570.
10. Pritchett ELC, McCarthy EA, Wilkinson WE. Propafenone treatment of symptomatic paroxysmal supraventricular arrhythmias: a randomized, placebo-controlled, crossover trial in patients tolerating oral therapy. *Ann Intern Med* 1991;114:539–544.
11. Reimold SC, Cantillon CO, Friedman PL, Antman EM. Propafenone versus sotalol for suppression of recurrent symptomatic atrial fibrillation. *Am J Cardiol* 1993;71:558–563.
12. Gosselink ATM, Crijns HJGM, Van Gelder K, et al. Low dose amiodarone for maintenance of sinus rhythm after cardioversion of atrial fibrillation or flutter. *JAMA* 1992;267:3289–3293.
13. Saoudi N, Atallah G, Kirkorian G, Touboul P. Catheter ablation of the atrial myocardium in human type I atrial flutter. *Circulation* 1990;81:762–771.
14. Cosío FG, Lopez-Gil M, Giocolea A, et al. Radiofrequency ablation of the inferior vena cava-tricuspid valve isthmus in common atrial flutter. *Am J Cardiol* 1993;71:705–709.
15. Feld GK, Fleck P, Cheng P-S, et al. Radiofrequency catheter ablation for the treatment of human type I atrial flutter: identification of a critical zone in the reentrant circuit by endocardial mapping techniques. *Circulation* 1992;86:1233–1240.
16. Scheinman MM. Catheter techniques for ablation of supraventricular tachycardia. *N Engl J Med* 1989;320:460–461.
17. Klein GJ, Guiraudon GM, Sharma AD, Milstein S. Demonstration of macroreentry and feasibility of operative therapy in the common type of atrial flutter. *Am J Cardiol* 1986;57:587–591.
18. Leitch JW, Klein GH, Yee R, Guiraudon GM. Sinus node-atrio-ventricular node isolation: long term results with the corridor operation for atrial fibrillation. *J Am Coll Cardiol* 19891;17:970–975.
19. Cox JG. The surgical treatment of atrial fibrillation. *J Thorac Cardiovasc Surg* 1991;101:584–592.
20. Wellens HJJ, Lau C-P, Luderitz B, et al, for the METRIX Investigators. Atrioverter: an implantable device for the treatment of atrial fibrillation *Circulation* 1998;98:1651–1656.
21. Puech P, Latour H, Grolleau R. Le flutter et ses limites. *Arch Mal Coeur* 1970;63:116–144.

22. Wells JL Jr, MacLean WAH, James TN, Waldo AL. Characterization of atrial flutter: studies in man after open heart surgery using fixed atrial electrodes. *Circulation* 1979;60:665–673.

23. Waldo AL, MacLean WAH, Karp RB, et al. Entrainment and interruption of atrial flutter with atrial pacing: studies in man following open-heart surgery. *Circulation* 1977;56:737–745.

24. Waldo AL, Cooper Waldo AL, Cooper TB. Spontaneous onset of type I atrial flutter in patients. *J Am Coll Cardiol.* 1996;28: 707–712.

25. Matsuo K, Tomita Y, Khrestian CM, Waldo AL. A new mechanism of sustained atrial fibrillation: studies in the sterile pericarditis model. *Circulation* 1998;98:I-209(abstr).

26. Saoudi N, Cosío F, Chen SA, et al. A new classification of atrial tachycardias based on electrophysiologic mechanisms. *Eur J Cardiol (in press).*

27. Bellet S. *Clinical disorders of the heart beat.* Philadelphia: Lea & Febiger, 1963:144–145.

28. Flinn CJ, Wolff GS, Dick M II, et al. Cardiac rhythm after the Mustard operation for complete transposition of the great arteries. *N Engl J Med* 1984;310:1625–1638.

29. Bink-Boelkens MThE, Velvia H, van der Heide JJH, et al. Dysrhythmias after atrial surgery in children. *Am Heart J* 1983;106: 125–130.

30. Waldo AL. Clinical evaluation in therapy of patients with atrial fibrillation or flutter. In: Scheinman MM, ed. *Cardiology clinics: supraventricular tachycardia.* 1990;8:479–490.

31. Garson A Jr, Bink-Boelkens M, Hesslein PS, et al. Atrial flutter in the young: a collaborative study of 380 cases. *J Am Coll Cardiol* 1985;6:871–878.

32. Camm AJ. The recognition and management of tachyarrhythmias. In: Julian DG, Camm AJ, Fox KM, et al, eds. *Diseases of the heart.* London: Bailliere Tindall, 1989:509–583.

33. Wood KA, Eisenberg SJ, Kalman JM, et al. Risk of thromboembolism in chronic atrial flutter. *Am J Cardiol* 1997;79: 1043–1047.

34. Yuan Z, Biblo L, Bowlin S, Rimm A. Atrial flutter, a risk for stroke. *J Am Coll Cardiol* 1997;29[Suppl A]:471A(abstr).

35. Weiss R, Marcovitz P, Knight BP, et al. Acute changes in spontaneous echo contrast and atrial function after cardioversion of persistent atrial flutter. *Am J Cardiol* 1998;82:1052–1055.

36. Seidl K, Haver B, Schwick NG, et al. Risk of thromboembolic events in patients with atrial flutter. *Am J Cardiol* 1998;82: 580–584.

37. Lewis T. *The mechanism and graphic registration of the heart beat,* 3rd ed. London: Shaw & Sons, 1925:295–306.

38. Rosenblueth A, Garcia-Ramos J. Studies on flutter and fibrillation. II. The influence of artificial obstacles on experimental auricular flutter. *Am Heart J* 1947;33:677–684.

39. Frame LH, Page RL, Hoffman BF. Atrial reentry around an anatomic barrier with a partially refractory excitable gap: a canine model of atrial flutter. *Circ Res* 1986;58:495–511.

40. Frame LH, Page RL, Boyden PA, et al. Circus movement in the canine atrium around the tricuspid ring during experimental atrial flutter and during reentry *in vivo. Circulation* 1987;76: 1155–1175.

41. Yamashita T, Inoue H, Nozaki A, Sugimoto T. Role of anatomic architecture in sustained atrial reentry and double potentials. *Am Heart J* 1992;124:938–946.

42. Feld GK, Shahandeh-Rad F. Mechanism of double potentials recorded during sustained atrial flutter in the canine right atrial crush-injury model. *Circulation* 1992;86:628–641.

43. Shimizu A, Igarashi M, Rudy Y, Waldo AL. Insights into atrial flutter from experimental models. *Pacing Clin Electrophysiol* 1991;14:627(abst).

44. Lewis T. *Clinical disorders of the heart beat,* 4th ed. New York: Paul B Hoeber, 1918:73–83.

45. Scherf D. Studies on auricular tachycardia caused by aconitine administration. *Proc Exp Biol Med* 1947;64:233–239.

46. Scherf D, Terranova R. Mechanism of auricular flutter and fibrillation. *Am J Physiol* 1949;159:137–142.

47. Scherf D, Romano FJ, Terranova R. Experimental studies on auricular flutter and auricular fibrillation. *Am Heart J* 1958; 36:241–251.

48. Kimura E, Kato K, Murao S, et al. Experimental studies on the mechanism of auricular flutter. *Tohoku J Exp Med* 1954;60: 197–207.

49. Callans DJ, Schwartzman D, Gottlieb CD, Marchlinski FE. Insights into the electrophysiology of atrial arrhythmias gained by the catheter ablation experience. Part II. Learning while burning. *J Cardiovasc Electrophysiol* 1995;6:229–243.

50. Allessie M, Lammers W, Smeets J, et al. Total mapping of atrial excitation during acetylcholine-induced atrial flutter and fibrillation in the isolated canine heart. In: Kulbertus HE, Olsson SB, Schlepper M, eds. *Atrial fibrillation.* Molndal, Sweden: AB Hassell, 1982:44–59.

51. Allessie MA, Lammers WJEP, Bonke FIM, Hollen J. Intraatrial reentry as a mechanism for atrial flutter induced by acetylcholine in rapid pacing in the dog. *Circulation* 1984;70:123–135.

52. Boineau JP, Schuessler RB, Mooney CR, et al. Natural and evoked atrial flutter due to circus movement in dogs. *Am J Cardiol* 1980;45:1167–1181.

53. Boyden PA, Hoffman BF. The effects on atrial electrophysiology and structure of surgically induced right atrial enlargement in dogs. *Circ Res* 1981;49:1319–1331.

54. Boyden PA. Activation sequence during atrial flutter in dogs with surgically induced right atrial enlargement. I. Observations during sustained rhythms. *Circ Res* 1988;62:596–608.

55. Pagé P, Plumb VJ, Okumura K, Waldo AL. A new model of atrial flutter. *J Am Coll Cardiol* 1986;8:872–879.

56. Okumura K, Plumb VJ, Pagé PL, Waldo AL. Atrial activation sequence during atrial flutter in the canine pericarditis model and its effects on the polarity of the flutter wave in the electrocardiogram. *J Am Coll Cardiol* 1991;17:509–518.

57. Shimizu A, Nozaki A, Rudy Y, Waldo AL. Onset of induced atrial flutter in the canine pericarditis model. *J Am Coll Cardiol* 1991;17:1223–1234.

58. Shimizu A, Nozaki A, Rudy Y, Waldo AL. Multiplexing studies of effects of rapid atrial pacing on the area of slow conduction during atrial flutter in canine pericarditis model. *Circulation* 1991;83:983–994.

59. Ortiz J, Igarashi M, Gonzalez HX, et al. Mechanism of spontaneous termination of atrial flutter in the canine sterile pericarditis model. *Circulation* 1993;88:1866–1877.

60. Shimizu A, Nozaki A, Rudy Y, Waldo AL. Characterization of double potentials in a functionally determined reentrant circuit: multiplexing studies during interruption of atrial flutter in the canine pericarditis model. *J Am Coll Cardiol,* 1993;22:2022–2032.

61. Ortiz J, Niwano S, Abe H, et al. Mapping the conversion of atrial flutter to atrial fibrillation and atrial fibrillation to atrial flutter—insights into mechanism. *Circ Res* 2001 *(in press).*

62. Pagé PL, Hassanahzadeh H, Cardinal R. Transitions among atrial fibrillation, atrial flutter and sinus rhythm during procainamide infusion and vagal stimulation in dogs with sterile pericarditis. *Can J Physiol Pharmacol* 1991;69:15–24.

63. Schoels W, Restivo M, Caref EB, et al. Circus movement atrial flutter in the canine sterile pericarditis model. *Circulation* 1991; 83:1716–1730.

64. Cox JL, Canaven TE, Schuessler RB, et al. The surgical treatment of atrial fibrillation. II. Intraoperative electrophysiologic mapping and description of the electrophysiologic basis of atrial flutter and atrial fibrillation. *J Thorac Cardiovasc Surg* 1991;101: 406–426.

65. Boyden PA. Studies in animal models of atrial flutter: tricuspid regurgitation model. In: Waldo AL, Touboul P, eds. *Atrial flutter: advances in mechanisms and management.* Armonk, NY: Futura Publishing, 1966:137–157.

66. Uno K, Kumagai K, Khrestian C, Waldo AL. New insights regarding the atrial flutter reentrant circuit. Studies in the canine sterile pericarditis model. *Circulation* 1999;100:1354–1360.

67. Shah D, Jais P, Takahasi A, et al. Dual-loop intra-atrial reentry in humans. *Circulation* 2000;101:631–639.

68. Prinzmetal M, Corday E, Oblath RW, et al. Auricular flutter. *Am J Med* 1951;11:410–430.

69. Wellens HJJ, Janse MJ, van Dam RTH, Durrer D. Epicardial excitation of the atria in a patient with atrial flutter. *Br Heart J* 1971;33:233–237.

70. Rosen K, Lau SH, Damato AN. Simulation of atrial flutter by rapid coronary sinus pacing. *Am Heart J* 1969;78:635–642.

71. Rytand DA. The circus movement (entrapped circuit wave) hypothesis of atrial flutter. *Arch Intern Med* 1966;65:125–159.

72. Puech P. *L'Activite electrique auriculaire normale et pathologique.* Paris: Masson, 1956:214–240.

73. Inoue H, Matsuo H, Takayanagi K, Murao S. Clinical and experimental studies of the effects of extrastimulation and rapid pacing on atrial flutter: evidence of macroreentry with an excitable gap. *Am J Cardiol* 1981;48:623–631.

74. Waldo AL. Cardiac pacing: role in diagnosis and treatment of disorders of cardiac rhythm and conduction. In: Rosen MR, Hoffman BF, eds. *Cardiac therapy.* Boston: Martinus Nijhoff, 1983:299–336.

75. Waldo AL, Plumb VJ, Henthorn RW. Observations on the mechanism of atrial flutter. In: Surawicz B, Reddy CP, Prystowsky EN, eds. *Tachycardias.* The Hague: Martinus Nijhoff, 1984:213–229.

76. Cosío FG, Arribas F, Palacios J, et al. Fragmented electrograms and continuous electrical activity in atrial flutter. *Am J Cardiol* 1986;57:1309–1314.

77. Cosío FG, Arribas F, Barbero JM, et al. Validation of double-spike electrograms as markers of conduction delay or block in atrial flutter. *Am J Cardiol* 1988;61:775–780.

78. Cosío FG. Endocardial mapping of atrial flutter. *In*: Touboul P, Waldo AL, eds. *Atrial arrhythmias.* St. Louis: Mosby–Year Book, 1990:229–240.

79. Olshansky B, Okumura K, Henthorn RW, Waldo AL. Characterization of double potentials in human atrial flutter: studies during transient entrainment. *J Am Coll Cardiol* 1990;15: 833–841.

80. Olshansky B, Okumura K, Hess PG, Waldo AL. Demonstration of an area of slow conduction in human atrial flutter. *J Am Coll Cardiol* 1990;16:1639–1648.

81. Cosío FG, Goicolea A, Lopez-Gil M, et al. Atrial endocardial mapping in the rare form of atrial flutter. *Am J Cardiol* 1990; 66:715–720.

82. Kalman JM, Olgin JE, Saxon LA, et al. Activation and entrainment mapping defines the tricuspid annulus as the anterior boundary in atrial flutter. *Circulation* 1996;94:398–406.

83. Nakagawa H, Lazzara R, Khastgir T, et al. Role of the tricuspid annulus and the Eustachian valve/ridge on atrial flutter: relevance to catheter ablation of the septal isthmus and a new technique for rapid identification of ablation success. *Circulation* 1996;94:407–424.

84. Cosío FG, Arribas F, Lopez-Gil M, Palacios J. Atrial flutter mapping and ablation: I. Studying atrial flutter mechanisms by mapping and entrainment. *Pacing Clin Electrophysiol* 1996;19: 841–853.

85. Olgin JE, Kalman JM, Fitzpatrick AP, Lesh MD. Role of right atrial endocardial structures as barriers to conduction during human type I atrial flutter: activation and entrainment mapping

86. Shah DC, Jais P, Haissaguerre M, et al. Three dimensional mapping of the common atrial flutter circuit in the right atrium. *Circulation* 1997;96:3904–3912.

87. Cheng J, Cabeen WR Jr, Scheinman MM. Right atrial flutter due to lower loop reentry: mechanism and anatomic substrates. *Circulation* 1999;99:1700–1705.

88. Olgin JE, Jayachandran JV, Engesstein E, et al. Atrial macroreentry involving the myocardium of the coronary sinus: a unique mechanism for atypical flutter. *J Cardiovasc Electrophysiol* 1998; 9:1094–1099.

89. Kall JG, Rubenstein DS, Kopp DE, et al. Atypical atrial flutter originating in the right atrial free wall. *Circulation.* 2000 Jan 25;101(3):270–279.

90. Switzer DF, Waldo AL, Henthorn RW. Hemodynamic effects of tachycardia: a supraventricular tachycardia. In: Saksena S, Goldschlager N, eds. *Electrical therapy for cardiac arrhythmias.* Philadelphia: WB Saunders, 1990:467–477.

91. Watson MM, Josephson ME. Atrial flutter. I. Electrophysiologic substrates and modes of initiation and termination. *Am J Cardiol* 1980;45:732–741.

92. Ellenbogen KA, Clemo HF, Stambler BS, et al. Efficacy of ibutilide for termination of atrial fibrillation and flutter. *Am J Cardiol* 1996;78[Suppl 8A]:42–45.

93. Stambler BS, Wood MA, Ellenbogen KA, et al. Efficacy and safety of repeated intravenous doses of ibutilide for rapid conversion of atrial flutter or fibrillation. *Circulation* 1996;94: 1613–1621.

94. Kowey PR, Vanderlugt JI, Luderer JR. Safety and risk/benefit analysis of ibutilide for acute conversion of atrial fibrillation/flutter. *Am J Cardiol* 1996;78[Suppl 8A]:42–45.

95. Fenster PE, Comess KA, Marsh R, et al. Conversion of atrial fibrillation to sinus rhythm by acute intravenous procainamide infusion. *Am Heart J* 1983;106:501–504.

96. Capucci A, Boriani G, Botto GL, et al. Conversion of recent-onset atrial fibrillation by a single oral loading dose of propafenone. *Am J Cardiol* 1994;74:503–505.

97. Capucci A, Lenzi T, Boriani G, et al. Effectiveness of loading oral flecainide for converting recent-onset atrial fibrillation to sinus rhythm in patients without organic heart disease or with only systemic hypertension. *Am J Cardiol* 1992;70:69–72.

98. Olshansky B, Okumura K, Hess PG, et al. Use of procainamide with rapid atrial pacing for successful conversion of atrial flutter to sinus rhythm. *J Am Coll Cardiol* 1988;11:359–364.

99. Camm J, Ward D, Spurrell R. Response of atrial flutter to overdrive atrial pacing and intravenous disopyramide phosphate singly and in combination. *Br Heart J* 1980;44:240–247.

100. Stambler BS, Wood MA, Ellenbogen KA. Comparative efficacy of intravenous ibutilide versus procainamide for enhancing termination of atrial flutter by atrial overdrive pacing. *Am J Cardiol* 1996;77:960–966.

101. Plumb VJ, Karp RB, James TN, Waldo AL. Atrial excitability and conduction during rapid atrial pacing. *Circulation* 1981;63: 1140–1149.

102. Benson DW, Sanford M, Dunnigan A, Benditt DG. Transesophageal atrial pacing threshold: role of interelectrode spacing, pulse width and catheter insertion depth. *Am J Cardiol* 1984;53:63–67.

103. Waldo AL, MacLean WAH, Karp RB, et al. Continuous rapid atrial pacing to control recurrent or sustained supraventricular tachycardias following open-heart surgery. *Circulation* 1976;54: 245–250.

104. Poty H, Saoudi N, Abdel Aziz A. Radiofrequency ablation of type 1 atrial flutter: prediction of late success by electrophysiological criteria. *Circulation* 1995;92:1389–1392.

105. Cosío FG, Arribas F, Lopez-Gil M, Gonzalez D. Atrial flutter mapping and ablation. II. Radiofrequency ablation of atrial flutter circuits. *Pacing Clin Electrophysiol* 1996;19:965–975.

106. Cauchemez B, Haissaguerre M, Fischer B, et al. Electrophysiological effects of catheter ablation of inferior vena cava–tricuspid annulus isthmus in common atrial flutter. *Circulation* 1996;93:284–294.

107. Poty H, Saoudi N, Nair M, et al. Radiofrequency catheter ablation of atrial flutter: further insights in to the various types of isthmus block: application to ablation during sinus rhythm. *Circulation* 1996;94:3204–3213.

108. Luchsinger JA, Steinberg JS. Resolution of cardiomyopathy after ablation of atrial flutter. *J Am Coll Cardiol* 1998;32:205–210.

109. Sparks PB, Jayaprakash S, Vohra JK, et al. Left atrial "stunning" following radiofrequency catheter ablation of chronic atrial flutter. *J Am Coll Cardiol* 1998;32:468–475.

110. Anselme F, Saudi N, Poty H, et al. Radiofrequency catheter ablation of common atrial flutter: significance of palpitations and quality-of-life evaluation in patients with proven isthmus block. *Circulation* 1999;99:534–540.

111. Paydak H, Kall JG, Burke MC, et al. Atrial fibrillation after radiofrequency ablation of type I atrial flutter: time to onset, determinants, and clinical course. *Circulation* 1998;98:315.

112. Paydak H, Kall JG, Burke MC, et al. Atrial fibrillation after radiofrequency ablation of type I atrial flutter: time to onset, determinants, and clinical course. *Circulation* 1998;98:315.

113. Triedman JK, Saul JP, Weindling SN, Walsh EP. Radiofrequency ablation of intra-atrial reentrant tachycardia after surgical palliation of congenital heart disease. *Circulation* 1995;91:707–714.

114. Van Hare GF, Lesh MD, Ross BA, et al. Mapping and radiofrequency ablation of intraatrial reentrant tachycardia after the Senning or Mustard procedure for transposition of the great arteries. *Am J Cardiol* 1996;77:985–991.

115. Chan DP, Van Hare GF, Carlson MD, et al. Importance of the typical atrial flutter isthmus in post-operative intra-atrial reentrant. *Circulation* 2001 (in press).

116. Waldo AL, Akhtar M, Benditt DG, et al. Appropriate electrophysiologic study and treatment of patients with the Wolff-Parkinson-White syndrome. *J Am Coll Cardiol* 1988;11:1124–1129.

117. The NHLBI Working Group on Atrial Fibrillation (Antman E, DiMarco J, Domanski MJ, et al). Atrial fibrillation: current understandings and research imperative. *J Am Coll Cardiol* 1993;22:1830–1834.

118. The Cardiac Arrhythmia Suppression Trial (CAST) Investigators. Effect of encainide and flecainide on mortality in a randomized trial of arrhythmia suppression after myocardial infarction. *N Engl J Med* 1989;321:406–412.

119. The Cardiac Arrhythmia Suppression Trial-II (CAST) Investigators. Effect of the antiarrhythmic agent moricizine on survival after myocardial infarction. *N Engl J Med* 1992;327:227–233.

120. Benditt DG, Williams JH, Jin J, et al. Maintenance of sinus rhythm with oral d,l -sotalol therapy in patients with symptomatic atrial fibrillation and/or atrial flutter. *Am J Cardiol* 1999;84:270–277.

121. Singh SN, Berk MR, Yellen LG, et al. Efficacy and safety of oral dofetilide in maintaining normal sinus rhythm in patients with atrial fibrillation: a multicenter study. *Circulation* 1997;96:I-38(abstr).

122. Podrid PJ. Amiodarone: reevaluation of an old drug. *Ann Intern Med* 1995;122:689–700.

123. Huang DT, Monohan KM, Zimetbaum P, et al. Hybrid pharmacologic and ablative therapy: a novel and effective approach for the management of atrial fibrillation. *J Cardiovasc Electrophysiol* 1998;9:462–467.

124. Nabar A, Rodriguez LM, Timmermans C, et al. Radiofrequency ablation of class IC atrial flutter in patients with resistant atrial fibrillation. *Am J Cardiol* 1999;83:785–787.

125. Reithmann C, Hoffmann E, Spitzlberger G, et al. Catheter ablation of atrial flutter due to amiodarone therapy for paroxysmal atrial fibrillation. *Eur Heart J* 2000;21:565.

126. Arnold AZ, Mick MJ, Mazurck RP, et al. Role of prophylactic anticoagulation for direct current cardioversion in patients with atrial fibrillation or atrial flutter. *J Am Coll Cardiol* 1992;19:851–855.

127. Grimm RA, Stewart WJ, Arheart KL, et al. Left atrial appendage "stunning" after electrical cardioversion of atrial flutter: an attenuated response compared with atrial fibrillation as the mechanism for lower susceptibility to thromboembolic events. *J Am Coll Cardiol* 1997;29:582–589.

128. Irani WN, Grayburn PA, Afridi I. Prevalence of thrombus, spontaneous echo contrast, and atrial stunning in patients undergoing cardioversion of atrial flutter: a prospective study using transesophageal echocardiography. *J Am Coll Cardiol* 1997;29:582–589.

129. Barold SS, Wyndham CRC, Kappenberger LL, et al. Implanted atrial pacemakers for paroxysmal atrial flutter: long term efficacy. *Ann Intern Med* 1987;107:144–149.

130. Goicolea A, Cosío FG, Lopez-Gil M, Kallmeyer C. Conversion of recurrent atrial flutter with implanted pacemakers programmable to high rate AOO mode. *Eur J Card Pacing Electrophysiol* 1992;2;19–21.

131. Guiraudon GM, Klein GJ, Sharma AD, Yee R. Surgical alternatives for supraventricular tachycardias. *Am J Cardiol* 1989;64:92J–96J.

17

TACHYCARDIAS IN WOLFF-PARKINSON-WHITE SYNDROME

ROGER A. MARINCHAK
SETH J. RIALS

In 1930, Louis Wolff, Sir John Parkinson, and Paul Dudley White published a seminal article describing 11 patients who suffered attacks of tachycardia associated with a sinus rhythm electrocardiographic (ECG) pattern of "bundle branch block with short PR interval" (1). Earlier isolated case reports of patients with paroxysmal tachycardias who also possessed this unique and peculiar ECG finding had been published since 1915 (2–4). However, it was not until 1943 through 1944, when Wood and colleagues (5) and Ohnell (6) independently correlated the ECG features of preexcitation with anatomic evidence for the existence of anomalous bundles of conducting tissue that bypassed all or part of the atrioventricular (AV) conduction system.

In the latter half of the 20th century, our understanding of the anatomic and pathophysiologic features of the preexcitation syndromes grew impressively, as did the treatment options for these entities. This progress in no small measure resulted from the advent of intracardiac recording and stimulating techniques in concert with surgical and catheter-based ablation therapies. Advances in antiarrhythmic drug development have been of benefit, but proliferation of catheter ablation therapy in particular has provided the opportunity to offer a cure with relatively low morbidity and mortality risks for patients suffering tachycardias caused by anomalous AV conduction pathways. This chapter reviews the pathogenesis of accessory pathways and the anatomic, pathophysiologic, diagnostic, and therapeutic features that are common and unique to each associated tachyarrhythmia.

PATHOGENESIS OF ACCESSORY PATHWAYS AND PREEXCITATION

The Wolff-Parkinson-White (WPW) syndrome can be viewed as a congenital heart disease characterized by the presence of one or more rests of excitable cardiac tissue providing electrical continuity between atria and ventricles while bypassing all or part of the normal AV conduction system (7–9). The classic accessory pathway is the AV bypass tract, or Kent bundle, that directly connects atrial and ventricular myocardium, bypassing the AV node-His-Purkinje system. Variant accessory pathways include those that connect the atrium to the distal or compact AV node (i.e., James fiber), the atrium to the His bundle (i.e., Brechenmacher fiber), and the AV node or His bundle to the distal Purkinje fibers or ventricular myocardium (i.e., Mahaim fiber) (10,11).

The hallmark of AV accessory pathway function during sinus rhythm is preexcitation: depolarization of all or part of the ventricles earlier than expected if conduction has occurred only over the normal AV conduction system. The classic ECG pattern of preexcitation in sinus rhythm is characterized by an abnormally short PR interval and a prolonged QRS complex duration. The intraventricular conduction delay begins with the onset of the QRS complex, in contrast to intraventricular conduction defects such as left or right bundle branch block, in which the delay occurs throughout or during the terminal portion of the QRS complex. The resultant slurred upstroke or downstroke comprising the initial part of the preexcited QRS complex is known as the *delta wave* (12,13) (Fig. 17-1).

AV bypass tracts usually exhibit rapid, nondecremental conduction, a property that is shared with normal His-Purkinje tissue and atrial or ventricular myocardium. Conduction velocity in the bypass tract remains constant as long as impulses propagate into it at a time interval greater than its refractory period (14). In contrast, the AV node conducts decrementally so that conduction time is inversely

R. A. Marinchak: Department of Clinical Cardiac Electrophysiology, Thomas Jefferson University School of Medicine, Wynnewood, Pennsylvania 19096.

S. J. Rials: Heart Care, Inc., Columbus, Ohio 43214.

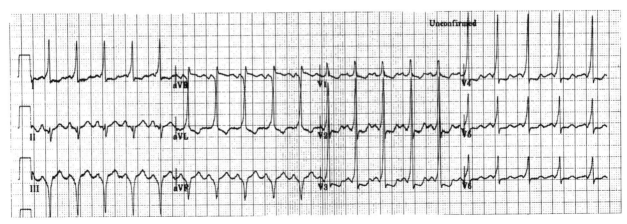

FIGURE 17-1. A 12-lead electrocardiogram recorded during sinus rhythm from a patient with a left posterior accessory pathway. The PR interval is short at 0.10 seconds, and a delta wave is present, comprising the initial 40 ms of the QRS complex and prolonging its duration to 0.12 seconds. The polarity of the delta wave is positive in leads I, aVL, and V_1 through V_6 and negative in leads II, III, aVF, and aVR, as predicted for a left posterior accessory pathway by the ECG classification of accessory pathway location depicted in Figure 17-5.

proportional to the cycle length of impulse input propagating through the node (15). AV bypass tracts may uncommonly display decremental antegrade or retrograde conduction; this was reported in 8% of patients in one large series (16). Because AV accessory pathways bypass the AV node and usually exhibit nondecremental antegrade conduction, ventricular activation begins earlier than expected if depolarization has only resulted from normal AV conduction. The time to ventricular activation onset also remains constant, regardless of the input stimulus cycle length, as long as the latter is less than the bypass tract's refractory period. Preexcited ventricular conduction spreads from the AV bypass tract's ventricular insertion point by direct muscle fiber–to–muscle fiber conduction; this process is inherently slower than when ventricular depolarization results from rapid His-Purkinje system conduction (17). Consequently, as more myocardium is depolarized through the accessory pathway, the more prominent is the delta wave, which represents the early preexcitation, and the more prolonged is the QRS duration because of more direct muscle fiber conduction (Fig. 17-2A).

A shorter than expected preexcited PR interval need not be abnormally short in an absolute sense (14). The degree to which the PR interval is shorter than normal and the extent to which ventricular preexcitation occurs depend on several factors, including the relationship between antegrade conduction times and refractory periods of the AV bypass tract and the normal AV conduction system (especially the AV node, which is importantly and variably influenced by the autonomic nervous system); the atrial insertion point of the AV bypass tract with respect to the normal AV conduction system; the site of atrial impulse origin; interatrial conduction time; and atrial refractoriness (14). Because of these factors, preexcitation may be less apparent

during sinus tachycardia when sympathetic tone is high and vagal tone is low, resulting in a short AV node conduction time. An AV bypass tract that crosses the AV groove in the left lateral region may also result in inapparent preexcitation and minimal PR interval shortening during sinus rhythm. This results from the greater interatrial distance required for impulse propagation from the sinus node to the left atrial insertion of the bypass tract compared with the closer, centrally located atrial input into the AV node (Fig. 17-3).

Intermittent preexcitation should be distinguished from day-to-day variability in preexcitation or inapparent preexcitation resulting from the factors described previously (14). True intermittent preexcitation is characterized by abrupt loss of the delta wave, normalization of the QRS duration, and an increase in the PR interval during a continuous ECG recording, often despite only minor variations in the resting sinus rhythm heart rate. This finding is usually a reliable sign that the AV bypass tract has a relatively long refractory period and is unlikely to mediate a rapid, preexcited ventricular response during atrial fibrillation (18). The same inference can be made about "preexcitation alternans" or the "concertina" form of preexcitation (Fig. 17-4). In the former situation, the delta wave manifests in an abrupt on-off fashion on a beat-to-beat basis, while in the latter, a cyclic pattern occurs that consists of preexcitation becoming progressively more prominent over a number of QRS complex cycles; this is followed by a gradual diminution in the degree of preexcitation as QRS cycles continue, all at a fairly constant rate (18–20).

Although they usually conduct bidirectionally, AV bypass tracts may be capable of propagating impulses in only one direction (14,16,21–24). Antegrade-only conducting bypass tracts are uncommon, often cross the right AV groove, and frequently possess decremental conduction

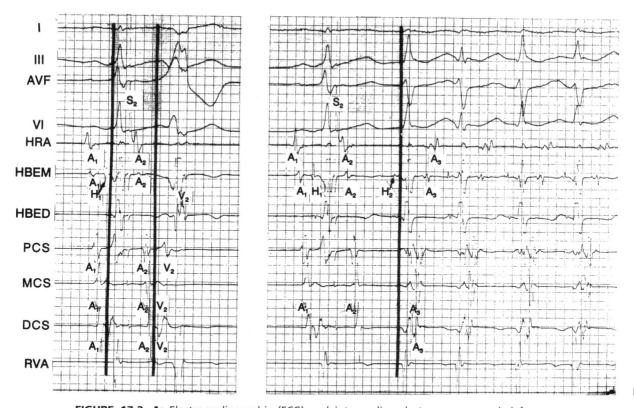

FIGURE 17-2. A: Electrocardiographic (ECG) and intracardiac electrograms recorded from a patient with a left posterolateral accessory pathway. ECG leads I, III, aVF, and V₁ are shown with electrograms recorded from the high right atrium (HRA); middle (HBEM) and distal (HBED) His bundle regions; proximal (PCS), middle (MCS), and distal (DCS) coronary sinus; and the right ventricular apex (RVA). During sinus rhythm, the atrial impulse (A₁) is conducted to the ventricles largely through the atrioventricular (AV) node-His-Purkinje system. Preexcitation is minimal, although the H-V interval is abnormally short (duration of 25 ms measured from the His potential to the onset of ventricular activation marked by the long vertical line before the first QRS complex). A premature stimulus (S₂), delivered in the HRA, yields an atrial premature impulse (A₂) that is conducted largely through the accessory pathway to produce a maximally preexcited QRS complex. Local ventricular activation (V₂) is recorded first on the MCS electrogram, consistent with the accessory pathway's left posterolateral ventricular insertion point. Decremental AV node conduction causes the AV node conduction time (A₂-H₂) to increase after the premature A₂, but the His potential is obscured by the simultaneously inscribed, larger, and preexcited V₂. Notice that the interval from S₂ to the earliest V₂ *(second long vertical line)* is identical to the sinus rhythm PR interval of 170 ms and in accord with the nondecremental conduction properties of the accessory pathway. **B:** A premature S₂ delivered in the HRA, 10 ms earlier than the S₂ shown in **(A)**, causes the resultant A₂ to block in the accessory pathway and defines the accessory pathway's antegrade effective refractory period (280 ms, measured as the A₁-A₂ interval recorded from the MCS, the site closest to the accessory pathway's atrial insertion point). A₂ still conducts decrementally through the AV node (A₂-H₂ 290 ms versus A₁-H₁ 100 ms) and initiates orthodromic atrioventricular reentrant tachycardia (OAVRT). Notice during OAVRT that the earliest retrograde atrial activation (A₃) is recorded from the DCS, suggesting that the accessory pathway courses in an oblique direction across the AV sulcus and results in an atrial insertion of the accessory pathway that is more lateral than the ventricular insertion. During OAVRT, the QRS complexes are not preexcited and have an H-V interval of 40 ms (measured from His potential to onset of ventricular activation, marked by the long vertical line before the first tachycardia QRS complex) compared with an H-V interval of 25 ms during sinus rhythm. The second QRS complex during tachycardia is conducted with slight aberration through the His-Purkinje system and is followed by a normal, nonpreexcited third QRS complex, probably as a result of the longer A-H (and therefore H-H) interval before the third tachycardia QRS complex. ECG leads and electrogram abbreviations are same as in **A**.

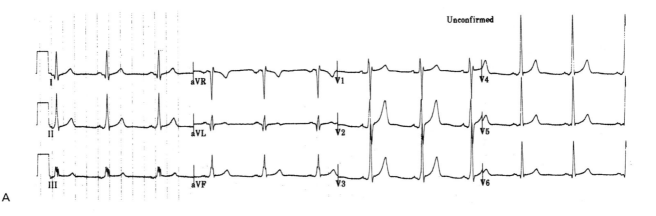

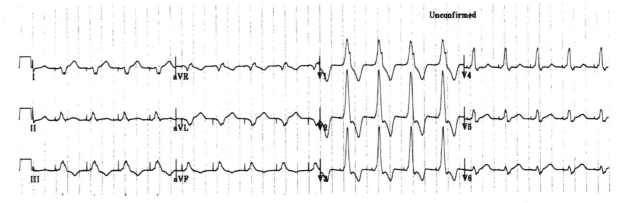

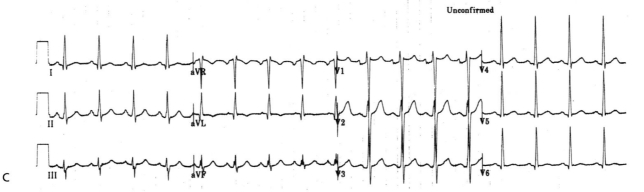

FIGURE 17-3. A: A 12-lead electrocardiogram (ECG) recorded during sinus rhythm from a patient with a left lateral accessory pathway. Preexcitation is barely discernible as delta waves that appear as slightly slurred, positive QRS onsets in leads II, III, aVF, V₃, V₄, and V₅. The q wave in aVL is somewhat prominent, and the R-wave transition in the precordial leads is shifted rightward (Rs in lead V₂) as additional subtle indicators of preexcitation. Note that the PR interval (0.13 second) and QRS duration (0.10 second) are not, respectively, abnormally short and prolonged in the absolute sense. **B:** A 12-lead ECG recorded from the same patient as in **A** during pacing from the coronary sinus at a rate of 110 bpm. The proximity of the pacing site to the accessory pathway's atrial insertion point and decremental atrioventricular (AV) node conduction during atrial pacing favor near-maximal preexcitation. The paced P wave partially overlaps the QRS onset and is negative in lead I and positive in aVR (as would be expected when pacing from a left atrial site). **C:** A 12-lead ECG recorded during sinus rhythm from the same patient after a successful radiofrequency energy catheter ablation procedure. Comparison with **A** permits appreciation of the subtle differences between the original, slightly preexcited ECG and the now normal-appearing ECG. The PR interval is increased to 0.16 second, and the QRS duration is decreased to 0.08 second in the absence of preexcitation.

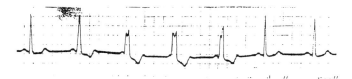

FIGURE 17-4. A single-lead rhythm strip demonstrates the concertina form of preexcitation. A mild degree of sinus arrhythmia is present, with the rate varying from 58 to 63 bpm (corresponding to a cycle length varying from 1040 to 960 ms). A cyclic increase and decrease in the degree of preexcitation manifests as variable PR interval shortening and QRS duration prolongation. (From Bellet S. *Clinical disorders of the heart beat,* 2nd ed. Philadelphia: Lea & Febiger, 1963:446, with permission.)

properties (14,16,23,25,26). Bypass tracts that conduct only in the retrograde direction have a reported incidence as high as 16% (21). Because they do not preexcite the ventricles, the surface ECG during sinus rhythm appears normal, resulting in these pathways being labeled "concealed." Most concealed AV bypass tracts conduct nondecrementally, serve as a conduit for retrograde ventriculoatrial (VA) conduction, and cause arrhythmias (21,27). Reasons for why AV bypass tracts may conduct unidirectionally include long refractory periods and conduction times, concealed conduction through the AV node-His-Purkinje system, degenerative fibrosis, and *impedance mismatch* (22,24). The latter term was coined to describe the situation in which a narrow strip of accessory pathway tissue generates an insufficient voltage wavefront at its insertion point to depolarize the large mass of ventricular or atrial tissue (22,24,28).

ANATOMIC CONSIDERATIONS

The gross anatomy of AV bypass tracts can be considered in two planes that run transversely at the level of and parallel to the AV groove and that run longitudinally, perpendicular to the AV groove (29). In the transverse plane, bypass tracts can cross the AV groove anywhere except between the left and right fibrous trigones because atrial myocardium is not in direct juxtaposition with ventricular myocardium in this region. The remainder of the transverse plane can then be divided into quadrants consisting of the left free wall, posteroseptal space, right free wall, and anteroseptal space (29,30). The distribution of accessory pathways within these regions is not homogeneous; 46% to 60% of bypass tracts are found within the left free wall space, 25% within the posteroseptal and midseptal spaces, 13% to 21% within the right free wall space, and 2% within the anteroseptal space (21,31,32). The left and right free wall spaces can be further subdivided into anterior, anterolateral, lateral, posterolateral, and posterior regions. Distinctive, fully preexcited QRS patterns have been validated during surgical and endocardial catheter mapping and ablation of accessory pathways within each of these subdivisions (33–38) (Fig.

17-5). Detailed knowledge of accessory pathway location is of vital importance to the interventional electrophysiologist performing catheter ablation procedures (39).

Accessory pathway anatomy in the longitudinal plane can be most easily understood by studying a longitudinal section of the left free wall region (Fig. 17-6). AV bypass tracts usu-

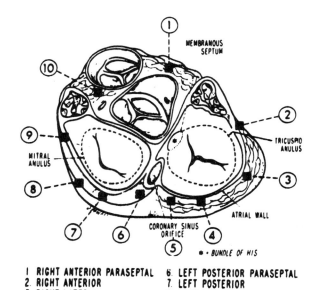

DELTA WAVE POLARITY

	I	II	III	AVR	AVL	AVF	V1	V2	V3	V4	V5	V6
①	+	+	+(±)	-	±(+)	+	±	±	+(±)	+	+	+
②	+	+	-(±)	-	+(±)	±(-)	±	+(±)	+(±)	+	+	+
③	+	±(-)	-	-	+	-(±)	±	±	±	+	+	+
④	+	-	-	-	+	-	±(+)	±	+	+	+	+
⑤	+	-	-	-(+)	+	-	±	+	+	+	+	+
⑥	+	-	-	-	+	-	+	+	+	+	+	+
⑦	+	-	-	±(+)	+	-	+	+	+	+	+	-(±)
⑧	-(±)	±	±	±(+)	-(±)	±	+	+	+	+	-(±)	-(±)
⑨	-(±)	+	+	-	-(±)	+	+	+	+	+	+	+
⑩	+	+	+(±)	-	±	+	±(+)	+	+	+	+	+

± = Initial 40 msec delta wave isoelectric
+ = Initial 40 msec delta wave positive
- = Initial 40 msec delta wave negative

1. RIGHT ANTERIOR PARASEPTAL
2. RIGHT ANTERIOR
3. RIGHT LATERAL
4. RIGHT POSTERIOR
5. RIGHT PARASEPTAL
6. LEFT POSTERIOR PARASEPTAL
7. LEFT POSTERIOR
8. LEFT LATERAL
9. LEFT ANTERIOR
10. LEFT ANTERIOR PARASEPTAL

FIGURE 17-5. Electrocardiographic (ECG) classification of accessory pathway locations in the Wolff-Parkinson-White syndrome. The delta wave polarities caused by preexcitation resulting from accessory pathways located at the designated sites in the atrioventricular sulcus are indicated for the 12 standard ECG leads. These data were derived by analyzing the initial 40 ms of the QRS complex and are valid for single accessory pathways without superimposed QRS abnormalities resulting from hypertrophy, infarction, intraventricular conduction delay, and other factors. (From Gallagher JJ, Pritchett ELC, Sealy WC, et al. The preexcitation syndromes. *Prog Cardiovasc Dis* 1978;20:298, with permission.)

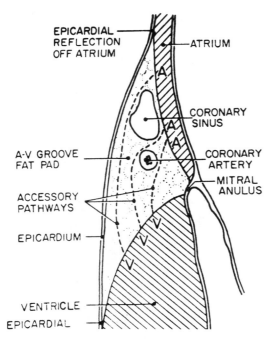

FIGURE 17-6. A diagrammatic, longitudinal cross section of the left heart's free wall at the level of the atrioventricular (AV) sulcus. Accessory pathways can course through the AV groove fat pad at variable depths in relation to the mitral annulus and the epicardium overlying the AV sulcus. (From Cox JL. The surgical management of cardiac arrhythmias. In: Sabiston DS Jr, Spencer FC, eds. *Gibbon's surgery of the chest.* Philadelphia: WB Saunders, 1990:1872, with permission.)

ally exist between the annulus fibrosus and the epicardial reflection off the atrial and ventricular walls, confined within the AV groove subepicardial fat of the right and left free walls, the anteroseptal space, and the posteroseptal space. Accessory pathways insert directly into the atrial and basal ventricular myocardium, although they may course through the AV sulcus at a depth that ranges most commonly from subendocardial to subepicardial in location (29). The existence of vascular structures, including the circumflex coronary artery and coronary sinus in the left free wall space, the coronary sinus, middle cardiac vein, and posterior descending artery in the posteroseptal space, and the right coronary artery in the anteroseptal and right free wall spaces, should also be identified. AV bypass tracts may run in an oblique course rather than absolutely perpendicular to the transverse plane of the AV groove (40) (Fig. 17-2).

Bypass tracts may also exist as "broad bands" of tissue rather than discrete, hairlike structures (29). Reports have described accessory pathways connecting atrial and ventricular myocardium at some distance from the AV sulcus (41,42). In these instances, the pathways appeared to be bridging the atrial appendages to subjacent ventricular myocardium. The anatomic association of posteroseptal accessory pathways with anomalies of the coronary sinus anatomy, particularly diverticula, has been described (43).

Most patients with AV bypass tracts do not have a coexisting structural cardiac abnormality beyond that which may result from age-related, acquired cardiac disease (14). When a congenital heart disease is associated with an accessory pathway, the latter is more likely to have a right-sided than left-sided location (44,45). Ebstein's anomaly is the congenital lesion most strongly associated with WPW syndrome. Up to 10% of afflicted patients may have one or more accessory pathways; most are located in the right free wall and right posteroseptal spaces (44–47). An association between mitral valve prolapse and left-sided bypass tracts has been reported, but it may reflect the random coexistence of these two relatively common conditions (14,33).

EPIDEMIOLOGY OF PREEXCITATION

The prevalence of manifest AV bypass tracts detectable on the ECG is reported to be 0.15% to 0.25% in the general population (48–50). However, among first-degree relatives of patients with WPW syndrome, the prevalence is increased to 0.55%; a family history of preexcitation is also associated with an increased probability of affected family members having multiple accessory pathways (51). Multiple accessory pathways have been found in as many as 13% of patients with the WPW syndrome, who comprise large referral populations (52,53). The population prevalence of WPW syndrome may be decreasing as more affected individuals undergo curative catheter ablation (54). The incidence of preexcitation appears to be substantially lower than the prevalence. The only population study examining this parameter in a diverse population of residents of Olmsted County, Minnesota, from 1953 through 1989, reported an annual incidence of newly diagnosed cases of WPW syndrome of only 0.004% (32). The incidence among male patients was twice that among female patients and highest in the first year of life, with a secondary peak in young adulthood. Preexcitation occurring within the general population or a patient cohort may be intermittent and even disappear permanently over time (32,49). In the Olmsted County population, 22% of individuals who ultimately had an ECG recorded demonstrating preexcitation had an initially negative tracing. In 40% of this subgroup, late and persistent loss of preexcitation occurred on subsequent ECGs. Ultimate symptom status in initially asymptomatic individuals did not correlate with baseline intermittent preexcitation but was importantly affected by age at the time preexcitation was discovered; one third of asymptomatic individuals younger than 40 years of age when preexcitation was identified eventually had symptoms, compared with no one 40 years of age and older (32). Intermittent and persistent loss of preexcitation may indicate that the accessory pathway possesses a relatively longer baseline refractory period and possibly may be more susceptible to age-related degenerative changes and variation in autonomic tone (18,32).

PATHOPHYSIOLOGY OF TACHYCARDIAS ASSOCIATED WITH ATRIOVENTRICULAR ACCESSORY PATHWAYS

Tachycardias associated with accessory pathways can be classified as those in which the bypass tract is necessary for initiation and maintenance of the tachycardia and those in which the bypass tract acts as a "bystander," providing a route of conduction from the anatomic site of tachycardia origin to other regions of the heart (55).

Tachycardias Requiring an Atrioventricular Bypass Tract for Arrhythmia Initiation and Maintenance: Atrioventricular Reentrant Tachycardia

Atrioventricular reentrant tachycardia (AVRT) is a macroreentrant tachycardia with an anatomically defined circuit that consists of two distinct pathways, the normal AV conduction system and an AV bypass tract, linked by common proximal (i.e., atria) and distal (ventricles) tissues. If sufficient differences in conduction time and refractoriness exist between the normal conduction system and the bypass tract, a properly timed premature impulse of atrial, junctional, or ventricular origin can initiate reentry. Orthodromic AVRT (OAVRT) can be initiated by atrial or ventricular premature depolarizations (APDs or VPDs). APDs initiating tachycardia block antegradely in the bypass tract and conduct relatively slowly into the ventricles over the AV node-His-Purkinje system; the AV node is invariably the site of antegrade conduction delay.

The impulse then retrogradely penetrates into the AV bypass tract, reentering the atria at the atrial insertion of the pathway to complete the first reentrant loop (14) (Fig. 17-7). VPDs initiate tachycardia by blocking in the AV node-His-Purkinje system while conducting retrogradely over the bypass tract into the atria; the impulse then conducts antegradely back to the ventricles through

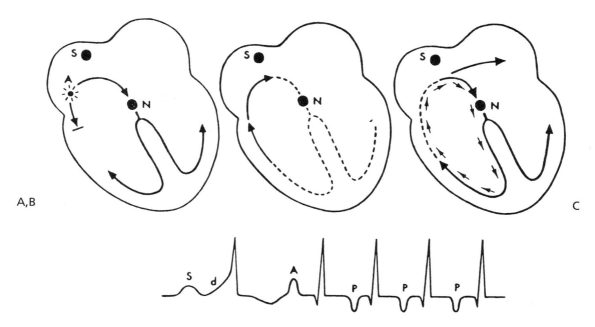

FIGURE 17-7. Schematic of initiation and maintenance of orthoventricular reentrant tachycardia (OAVRT). A diagrammatic electrocardiogram recording shows the first P wave of sinus node (S) origin yielding a preexcited QRS complex with a delta wave (d) and short PR interval. **A:** An ectopic atrial premature depolarization (A) blocks antegradely in the bypass tract but still conducts through the atrioventricular (AV) node (N) and His-Purkinje system to the ventricles. This causes the second QRS complex to appear nonpreexcited as it follows the premature A with a longer PR interval. **B:** The premature impulse continues to conduct retrogradely through the bypass tract because the latter has had time to recover excitability during the preceding period of antegrade impulse conduction through the AV node and His-Purkinje system. **C:** The retrogradely conducted impulse has activated the atria from the bypass tract's atrial insertion point and generated the first retrograde P wave (P) of OAVRT. Reentrant penetration of the impulse into the AV node and His-Purkinje system then occurs, with maintenance of OAVRT determined by the conduction velocities and refractory periods of all tissues comprising the reentrant circuit and the circuit length. The RP interval during OAVRT reflects the relatively long distance that the reentrant impulse must propagate from ventricles to atria. (From Chung EK. Wolff-Parkinson-White syndrome: current views. *Am J Med* 1977;62:261, with permission.)

the normal AV conduction system to complete the reentrant circuit (14,56). The QRS complex during OAVRT is not preexcited because ventricular activation is occurring only through the AV node and His-Purkinje system. However, the QRS duration may be prolonged during OAVRT when there is chronic or rate-related bundle branch block.

During antidromic AVRT (AAVRT), the ventricles are activated antegradely through the AV bypass tract, followed by retrograde conduction over the AV node-His-Purkinje system; the QRS complex during AAVRT is therefore fully preexcited (Fig. 17-8). Initiation of AAVRT by APDs requires that they occur at a coupling interval that is longer than the antegrade refractory period of the bypass tract but shorter than the refractory period of the AV node-His-Purkinje system; the converse would be true if a VPD were to induce the tachycardia (14). Susceptibility to AAVRT also appears to depend on the existence of at least a 4-cm transverse separation between the bypass tract and the normal AV conduction system. Consequently, most AAVRTs use a left-sided bypass tract as the antegrade route for conduction (14,39,55).

Tachycardias Not Requiring an Atrioventricular Bypass Tract for Initiation and Maintenance of the Arrhythmia: Atrial Fibrillation or Flutter, Atrioventricular Node Reentrant Tachycardia, and Ventricular Tachycardia

Atrial tachycardias, junctional tachycardias (including AVNRT), and ventricular tachycardias can all coexist with a bypass tract; the bypass tract can serve as a bystander route for ventricular or atrial activation during these tachycardias. AVNRT and ventricular tachycardia have disparate prevalences among patients with the WPW syndrome. Dual AV node pathway conduction physiology has been reported in up to 12% of patients with WPW syndrome, although spontaneous sustained AVNRT is less common (57–59). Coexisting ventricular tachycardia is uncommon because patients with WPW syndrome tend to present with arrhythmia symptoms at a younger age and less commonly have structural heart disease (14,44,45).

During atrial fibrillation and atrial flutter, the accessory pathway functions as a route for conducting atrial impulses

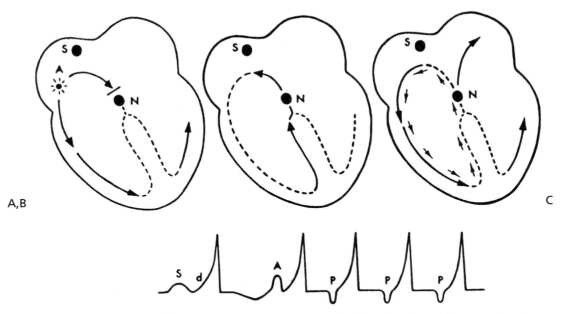

FIGURE 17-8. Schematic of initiation and maintenance of antidromic atrioventricular reentrant tachycardia (AAVRT). The layout and abbreviations are identical to those depicted in Figure 17-7. **A:** The premature atrial depolarization (A) blocks antegradely in the AV node but still conducts through the bypass tract to the ventricles. The second QRS complex after the premature A is therefore fully preexcited with a short PR interval. **B:** The premature impulse continues to conduct retrogradely through the His-Purkinje system and the AV node because these tissues have recovered excitability. **C:** The retrograde-conducted impulse has activated the atria, starting from the centrally located AV node's atrial insertion point. Reentrant penetration of the impulse into the bypass tract then occurs with maintenance of AAVRT determined by the same factors described for orthodromic atrioventricular reentrant tachycardia in Figure 17-7. (From Chung EK. Wolff-Parkinson-White syndrome: current views. *Am J Med* 1977;62:261, with permission.)

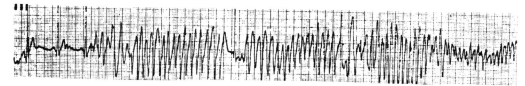

FIGURE 17-9. Electrocardiographic lead III monitor recording of preexcited atrial fibrillation (AF) degenerating into ventricular fibrillation (VF) in a patient with a left free wall accessory pathway. Preexcitation is not readily apparent during sinus rhythm. After the third sinus rhythm-generated QRS complex, an atrial premature depolarization (ectopic P wave distorting the T wave after the third QRS complex) initiates AF that is conducted with an extremely rapid ventricular response; nearly all of the QRS complexes are preexcited, and the R-R intervals are as short as 120 ms. On the right-hand side of the recording, the rhythm degenerates into VF. (From Dreifus LS, Wellens HJ, Watanabe Y, et al. Sinus bradycardia and atrial fibrillation associated with the Wolff-Parkinson-White syndrome. *Am J Cardiol* 1976;38:151, with permission.)

into the ventricles. If the pathway has a short antegrade refractory period, a rapid ventricular rate response can occur with degeneration of the rhythm to ventricular fibrillation (60,61) (Fig. 17-9). In particular, a shortest preexcited R-R interval of less than 250 ms during spontaneous or induced atrial fibrillation has been retrospectively correlated with an increased risk of cardiac arrest and sudden death. This risk also appears to be increased in patients who have more than one accessory pathway (61). The ventricular rate during preexcited atrial fibrillation is also determined by the degree to which the AV node-His-Purkinje system "competes" with the bypass tract for ventricular activation. Concealed retrograde conduction into the bypass tract plays an important protective role in modulating the ventricular rate response during preexcited atrial fibrillation (62–64).

The 40% frequency with which paroxysmal atrial fibrillation afflicts patients with the WPW syndrome is striking because of the low prevalence of coexisting structural heart disease (14,44,45,65,66). The AV bypass tract may be related to the genesis of atrial fibrillation because most patients undergoing bypass tract ablation are cured of AVRT and atrial fibrillation (67). One study demonstrated that the presence during electrophysiologic testing of multiple accessory pathways or arborizing atrial insertions of a single pathway was associated with a 69% prevalence of clinical episodes of atrial fibrillation, compared with a 23% prevalence when only a single pathway and atrial insertion were detected (68). Vulnerability to atrial fibrillation may ultimately require a functioning bypass tract and susceptibility to AVRT in most instances, but only in those patients with coexisting idiopathic atrial electrical abnormalities (55). Despite the fear of catastrophic hemodynamic instability engendered by preexcited atrial fibrillation, it is nonetheless reassuring that the annual incidence of sudden death of patients with WPW syndrome is quite low, ranging from 0.15% to 0.39% in several large series (32,69–71). Cardiac arrest as the first symptomatic manifestation of WPW syndrome is distinctly unusual (32).

ELECTROCARDIOGRAPHIC AND ELECTROPHYSIOLOGIC MANIFESTATIONS OF ATRIOVENTRICULAR ACCESSORY PATHWAYS AND ASSOCIATED TACHYCARDIAS

The tachyarrhythmias associated with AV accessory pathways display a diverse spectrum of morphologic characteristics and functional patterns.

Atrioventricular Bypass Tract Function During Sinus Rhythm, Atrial Pacing or Extrastimulation, and Ventricular Pacing or Extrastimulation

During preexcited sinus rhythm, the His-ventricular (H-V) interval is abnormally short and the QRS duration prolonged. The PR and AV intervals also are shortened to an extent that is equal to the degree of H-V interval abbreviation. With increasing preexcitation, the H-V interval progressively shortens (usually achieving negative values), whereas the QRS duration lengthens, and the PR interval remains constant. During complete preexcitation, the His bundle potential is often overlapped and masked by the larger amplitude of the local ventricular electrogram (Fig. 17-2A).

Analysis of the preexcited QRS complex pattern and corresponding electrograms recorded from the AV sulcus is invaluable for localizing the ventricular insertion of the AV accessory pathway (14,39). However, this technique can result in erroneous conclusions when multiple bypass tracts, preexisting intraventricular conduction delay, hypertrophy, drugs, electrolyte imbalance, and myocardial infarction or fibrosis are present (14) (Fig. 17-5). Pacing from the right and left atria while documenting the site of stimulation that yields the shortest stimulus–to–delta wave interval is also useful (33,72) (Fig. 17-10). Body surface isopotential mapping has been described as a useful technique for noninvasive localization of the ventricular insertion of bypass tracts (73–76). Invasive but nonfluoroscopically guided endocar-

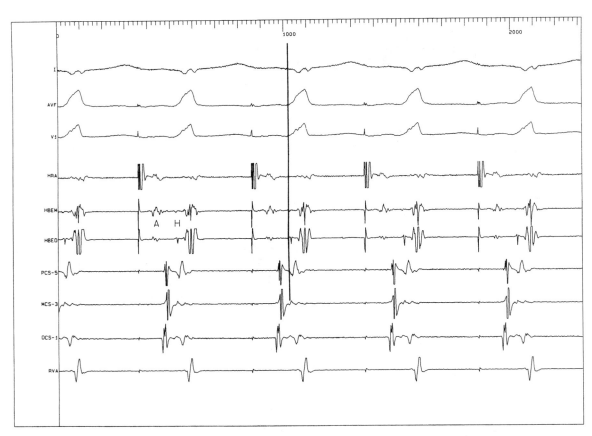

FIGURE 17-10. Electrocardiographic (ECG) and intracardiac electrogram recordings obtained from a patient with a left lateral accessory pathway during right atrial pacing at a cycle length of 500 ms. ECG leads I, aVF, and V$_1$ are shown with electrograms labeled as in Figure 17-2. A His bundle potential (H) is recorded after the onset *(long vertical line)* of the preexcited QRS complex, yielding an H-V interval of −10 ms. The earliest ventricular electrogram is recorded at the middle coronary sinus (MCS) site, consistent with a left lateral accessory pathway location.

dial mapping of accessory pathway location and contiguous mapping or ablation catheter positioning have been performed within an artificially generated electromagnetic field (77). Optimum positioning of a mapping catheter with closely spaced bipoles along the annuli of the mitral and tricuspid valves or within the coronary sinus tributaries in the posteroseptal region usually permits recording of an accessory pathway potential (40) (Fig. 17-11).

Analysis of VA conduction and the retrograde atrial activation sequence aids in identifying the atrial insertion point of an accessory pathway. This should ideally be performed during OAVRT, because the accessory pathway serves as the sole route for retrograde conduction into the atria (Fig. 17-2B). Ventricular pacing and extrastimulation can also be used to assess retrograde VA conduction, provided that retrograde conduction through the AV node is not present during these maneuvers (14).

Retrograde VA conduction over the AV node-His-Purkinje system is decremental and results in a normal sequence of retrograde atrial activation; the atrial electrogram recorded by the His bundle catheter is inscribed first, fol-

lowed by centrifugal spread of atrial activation from that point (78,79). In contrast, most AV bypass tracts conduct retrogradely in a nondecremental manner; the VA conduction time over a classic AV bypass tract remains constant at all ventricular pacing rates and extrastimulus coupling intervals, allowing conduction to occur. Left- and right-sided bypass tracts also can activate the atria in an eccentric fashion (14,39). The atrial insertion of an AV bypass tract should be sought by analyzing atrial electrograms recorded directly from a catheter placed on the tricuspid annulus and indirectly from the mitral annulus through the coronary sinus during OAVRT and ventricular pacing or extrastimulation (39).

Atrial and ventricular pacing should be performed at increasing rates until loss of 1 : 1 antegrade or retrograde conduction occurs within the normal AV conduction system and the bypass tract (Fig. 17-12). In addition to inducing AVRT, these maneuvers permit identification of the "weak" and "strong" limbs of conduction maintaining AVRT, as well as determination of the AV bypass tract's ability to mediate a rapid ventricular response during

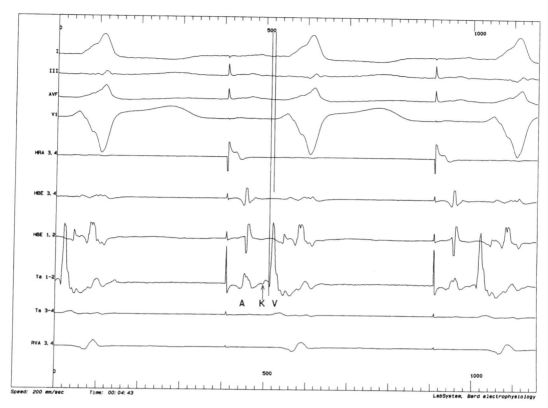

FIGURE 17-11. Surface electrocardiographic (ECG) and intracardiac electrograms recorded at 200 mm/sec during atrial pacing at a cycle length of 500 ms. Surface ECG leads I, II, aVF, and V_1 are displayed along with intracardiac electrograms recorded from the high right atrium (HRA 3, 4), His bundle region proximally (HBE 3, 4) and distally (HBE 1, 2), tricuspid annulus by means of the distal (Ta 1, 2) and proximal (Ta 3, 4) bipoles of a deflectable-tip ablation catheter, and the right ventricular apex (RVA 3, 4). The local intracardiac electrogram recorded from the tricuspid annulus (Ta 1-2) at the site of successful radiofrequency current application to ablate a right lateral accessory pathway is displayed. Ta 1-2 displays atrial (A) and ventricular (V) electrograms with an A to V ratio of less than 1.0, suggesting that the recording bipoles are located on the ventricular side of the tricuspid annulus. Between A and V is a low-amplitude potential (K) that represents accessory pathway depolarization. The local V potential is recorded 16 ms before the onset of the surface ECG delta wave activity.

atrial fibrillation and atrial flutter (14,80). Atrial pacing should be performed as close as possible to the putative atrial insertion of the AV bypass tract (14). Ventricular pacing is generally performed at the right ventricular apex; however, intraventricular conduction time should be taken into consideration when analyzing the response to this maneuver (81).

Antegrade and retrograde accessory pathway refractory periods should be measured as close as possible to the bypass tract using the extrastimulus technique in the atria and ventricles (14) (Fig. 17-2). The extrastimulus should be systematically delivered in 10- to 20-ms decrements until refractoriness occurs at the extrastimulation site. Bypass tracts that maintain 1 : 1 retrograde conduction at ventricular paced cycle lengths less than 300 ms and with retrograde refractory periods less than 300 ms tend to mediate very rapid OAVRT. Similarly, the minimum atrial-paced cycle length maintaining 1 : 1 preexcited ventricular con-

duction and the antegrade refractory period of the bypass tract are strongly correlated with the shortest preexcited R-R interval and mean R-R interval during atrial fibrillation (14,61,82). However, the best reflection of an accessory pathway's ability to mediate a malignant, rapid ventricular rate during atrial fibrillation is to measure the mean ventricular rate and shortest preexcited R-R interval of atrial fibrillation induced in the laboratory.

The detection of multiple bypass tracts can be a challenging task. The presence of more than one preexcited QRS pattern during sinus rhythm, incremental atrial pacing, or atrial fibrillation is helpful. Additional diagnostic clues include changing retrograde P wave, atrial electrogram, and atrial activation patterns during OAVRT; discordance of more than 1 to 2 cm between atrial and ventricular bypass insertion points mapped during OAVRT and AAVRT; a spontaneous change between OAVRT and AAVRT or between two AAVRTs having different preex-

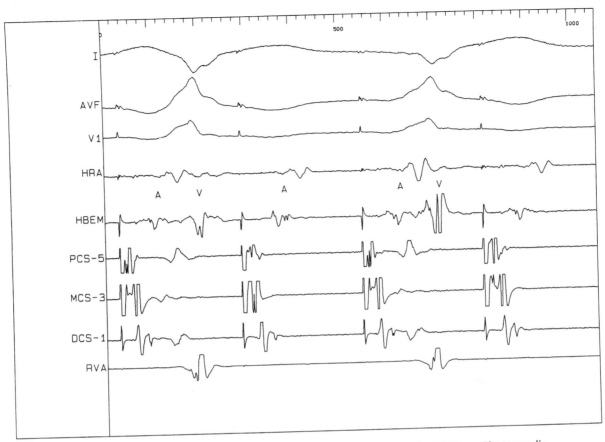

FIGURE 17-12. Atrial pacing from the coronary sinus at a cycle length of 260 ms. Electrocardiographic leads I, aVF, and V₁ are shown with electrograms labeled as in Figure 17-2. A 2 : 1 atrioventricular block is present in the accessory pathway.

cited QRS patterns; and an abrupt change in preexcited QRS configuration during atrial extrastimulation, incremental pacing, or after antiarrhythmic drug administration (14,35,37,39,52,53).

Administration of isoproterenol during the electrophysiologic study can help induce arrhythmia and unmask potentially dangerous catecholamine facilitation of accessory pathway function (83,84). Antiarrhythmic drugs and exercise testing have been used as noninvasive screening tests to assess an accessory pathway's propensity to mediate a rapid ventricular response during atrial fibrillation (85–87). An intravenous dose of procainamide that causes complete loss of preexcitation has good positive predictive value in identifying a bypass tract with a relatively long (>270 to 300 ms) antegrade refractory period and a low likelihood of mediating a rapid, preexcited ventricular response during atrial fibrillation (14,85). However, failure of antiarrhythmic drug infusion to eliminate preexcitation does not predict that the pathway has a short (<250 ms) refractory period (86–88). Adenosine transiently depresses AV node conduction while usually having no effect on accessory pathways that conduct nondecrementally. Administration of adenosine during the electrophysiologic study or ECG monitoring is therefore useful in transiently unmasking preexcitation. Adenosine may cause enhanced susceptibility to atrial fibrillation and OAVRT or promote incessant behavior of OAVRT (89,90). Exercise uncommonly causes abrupt loss of preexcitation as the sinus rhythm rate increases (Fig. 17-13). More often, preexcitation becomes inapparent because increasing sympathetic tone and decreasing vagal tone enhance AV node conduction. However, when true loss of preexcitation occurs abruptly during exercise testing, it is a fairly reassuring but imperfect sign that the bypass tract is unlikely to conduct atrial fibrillation with a rapid ventricular response.

Electrophysiologic Testing in Asymptomatic Individuals

The indication for performing diagnostic electrophysiologic testing on truly asymptomatic individuals who are found by chance to have preexcitation on their ECG remains a controversial issue. Two studies that addressed

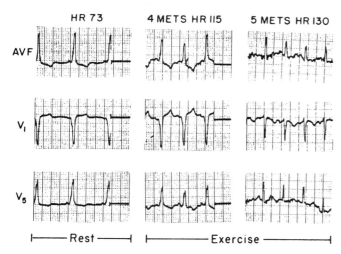

FIGURE 17-13. Electrocardiographic recordings of leads aVF, V_1, and V_5 during an exercise test conducted with a patient with an antegradely conducting right anterior accessory pathway. Preexcitation is apparent at rest and during the initial stages of exercise. As the sinus rhythm rate reaches 130 bpm, abrupt loss of preexcitation develops with relative lengthening of the PR interval, shortening of the QRS duration, and normalization of the QRS pattern. METS, metabolic equivalents. (From Strasberg B, Ashley WW, Wyndham CR, et al. Treadmill exercise testing in the Wolff-Parkinson-White syndrome. *Am J Cardiol* 1980;45:745, with permission.)

this issue demonstrated that a sizable minority of asymptomatic individuals with preexcitation were found at electrophysiologic testing to have bypass tracts with potential for conducting rapidly if atrial fibrillation were to develop in the future. However, over a considerable follow-up period, only a small number of individuals actually developed unmonitored symptoms or documented tachyarrhythmias. Reassuringly, there were no individuals during follow-up who suffered sudden death or were resuscitated from cardiac arrest (69,91). These data, in concert with the low prevalence of WPW syndrome and the even lower incidence of associated cardiac arrest, support the notion that the positive predictive value of diagnostic electrophysiologic testing for selecting asymptomatic individuals with preexcitation at risk for future, hemodynamically destabilizing arrhythmia is too low to justify a policy of wholesale implementation. Exceptions to this recommendation may include asymptomatic individuals engaged in occupations or activities that put other individuals in potential jeopardy, such as pilots, heavy equipment operators, and mass ground transit chauffeurs, or when large financial investments are an issue, such as professional athletes (54). An argument could also be advanced for studying asymptomatic individuals with preexcitation if they are a first-degree relative of a patient with WPW syndrome, particularly if the patient suffered a cardiac arrest related to WPW syndrome or has been identified as having multiple AV bypass tracts.

Orthodromic Atrioventricular Reentrant Tachycardia

OAVRT comprises 95% of the reentrant tachycardias associated with the WPW syndrome (14,55). Because OAVRT incorporates the entire heart within its macroreentrant circuit, tachycardia initiation, termination, and reset are easily invoked by spontaneous APDs, VPDs, or rapid atrial and ventricular pacing. Intracardiac recordings during electrophysiologic testing show that the APD inducing OAVRT is conducted with an increased atrial-His (A-H) interval compared with the A-H intervals during the preceding atrial drive train or sinus rhythm. The tachycardia QRS complexes after the APD are nonpreexcited, with a normal H-V interval and QRS duration or, not uncommonly, an initially prolonged H-V interval and QRS duration resulting from functional aberrant conduction. After the first nonpreexcited QRS complex, retrograde atrial activation occurs in a pattern consistent with the bypass tract's site of atrial insertion. Initiation of OAVRT in the presence of a concealed accessory pathway follows the same rules except that preexcitation is not present during the preceding atrial drive train or sinus rhythm (21) (Fig. 17-14).

When a VPD initiates OAVRT, the AV node-His-Purkinje system must have a longer retrograde refractory period than the AV bypass tract. The tachycardia-inducing VPD conducts retrogradely and activates the atria in a pattern consistent with the atrial insertion point of the accessory pathway. A nonpreexcited QRS complex then follows as a result of antegrade AV node-His-Purkinje system conduction (Fig. 17-15).

OAVRT tends to be a rapid tachycardia, with rates ranging from 150 to more than 250 bpm. A beat-to-beat oscillation in QRS amplitude (i.e., QRS alternans) may be present in up to 38% of cases (92,93). The mechanism for QRS alternans is not clear but may in part result from oscillations in the relative refractory period of the His-Purkinje system (52,94). ST segment depression may also occur during OAVRT, even in young individuals who are unlikely to have coronary artery disease. Such ST segment abnormalities appear to result from autonomic nervous system influences, coexisting intraventricular conduction delays, a longer VA interval, or a retrograde P of longer duration that overlaps with the ST segment (95). The location of the ST segment changes may vary with the location of the accessory pathway. ST segment depression in V_3 to V_6 is almost invariably seen with a left lateral pathway, ST segment depression and a negative T wave in the inferior leads is associated with a posteroseptal or posterior accessory pathway, and a negative or notched T wave in V_2 or V_3 with a positive retrograde P wave in at least two inferior leads suggests an anteroseptal tract (95,96). However, ST segment depression occurring during OAVRT episodes in older patients or associated with symptoms of ischemia mandates considering the possibility of coexisting coronary disease.

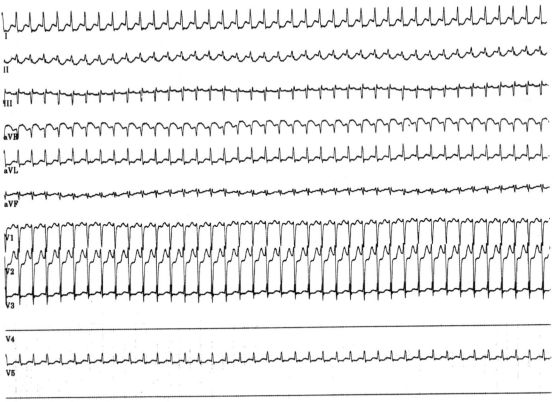

A   V6

Unconfirmed

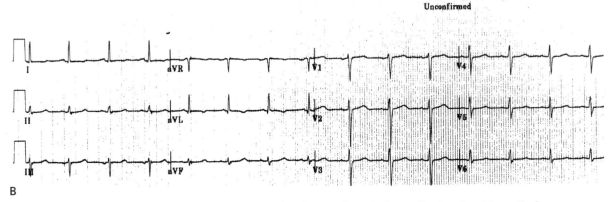

B

FIGURE 17-14. A: Electrocardiographic (ECG) recording during orthodromic atrioventicular reentrant tachycardia (OAVRT) obtained from a patient with a concealed right free wall accessory pathway (leads V₄ and V₆ are not recorded). The tachycardia cycle length is 250 ms. Retrogradely conducted P waves during tachycardia having an RP interval less than half of the tachycardia's R-R interval are most readily seen in lead V₁; the early portion of the ST-T segment in this lead is negative, giving the T wave a biphasic appearance. This results from the superimposition of the tachycardia's retrograde P wave on the ST-T segment. Compare the appearance of the ST-T segment in lead V₁ with that recorded during sinus rhythm as shown in **B**. **B:** ECG recording obtained during sinus rhythm from the same patient as in **A**. Because the accessory pathway conducts only retrogradely, preexcitation is absent.

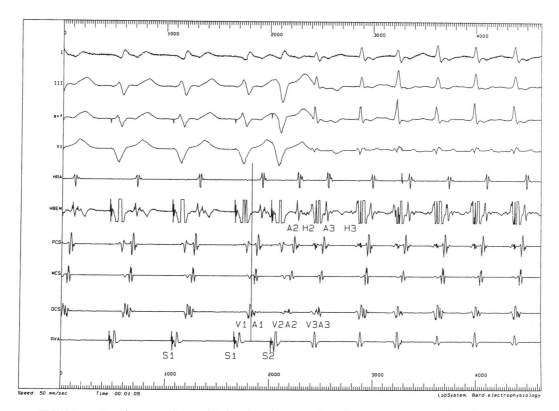

FIGURE 17-15. Electrocardiographic (ECG) and intracardiac electrograms recorded at 50 mm/sec during induction of orthodromic atrioventricular reentrant tachycardia (OAVRT) using ventricular extrastimulation. The labeling of the surface ECG leads and intracardiac electrogram is identical to that in Figure 17-2. The first three QRS complexes are paced (S_1) from the right ventricular apex (RVA) at a cycle length of 600 ms. Retrograde ventriculoatrial (VA) conduction results in eccentric atrial activation, with the earliest atrial electrogram (A_1) recorded from the distal coronary sinus (DCS), consistent with retrograde conduction occurring over a left lateral accessory pathway. A premature stimulus (S_2) is delivered from the RVA at an S_1S_2 interval of 350 ms and is conducted to the atria with the same retrograde atrial activation sequence for A_2 as was true for A_1. A_2 is followed by a His potential (H_2) and ventricular electrogram (V_3) with a corresponding, nonpre-excited QRS complex that exhibits right bundle branch block aberrant conduction. V_3 is followed by sustained OAVRT that has a cycle length of 375 ms. The retrograde atrial activation sequence, VA interval duration, and atrial electrogram pattern during OAVRT are identical to those during ventricular pacing. Notice that A_2-H_2 is considerably shorter (80 ms) than A_3-H_3 (230 ms) and all subsequent A-H intervals during OAVRT; the short A_2-H_2 interval probably results from retrograde His-Purkinje conduction block occurring after the S_2 and V_2, thereby permitting V_2 to conduct retrogradely solely through the accessory pathway and encounter the atrioventricular node in a state of fully recovered excitability.

The relationship and timing of atrial and ventricular activation are important diagnostic features of OAVRT. Because the atria and ventricles are part of a macroreentrant circuit and have a 1 : 1 relationship with each other, observing AV dissociation or intermittent AV block during a tachycardia excludes an AV reentrant mechanism. The ECG recorded during tachycardia shows P waves inscribed within the ST-T wave segment with an RP interval that is usually less than one half of the tachycardia R-R interval (Fig. 17-14A). The RP interval remains constant, regardless of the tachycardia cycle length (39).

Spontaneous or induced functional bundle branch block occurring during OAVRT can yield a diagnostically useful phenomenon. If bundle branch block exists ipsilateral to a free wall bypass tract, the reentrant impulse is forced to traverse a greater distance from the ventricular insertion of the antegrade-conducting Purkinje fibers to the ventricular insertion of the bypass tract. As a result, the global VA interval during the tachycardia must increase, usually by at least 35 ms (96) (Fig. 17-16). The tachycardia cycle length may also increase, although little or no change may occur because of an offsetting decrease in the A-H interval (21,39). In contrast, bundle branch block occurring contralateral to a free wall AV bypass tract exerts no effect on the VA interval and the tachycardia cycle length.

A VPD delivered late in the diastolic interval of OAVRT, when the His bundle has been rendered refractory from antegrade tachycardia activation, can advance atrial activa-

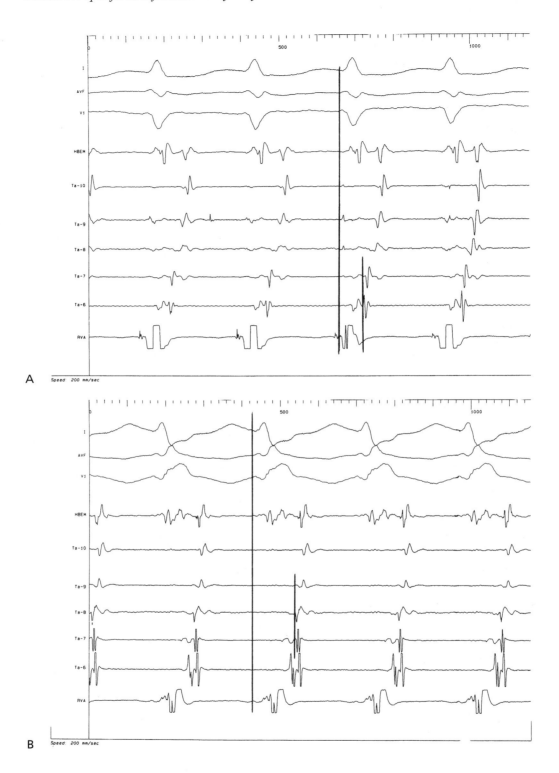

tion while preserving the retrograde atrial activation pattern existing during tachycardia. If the same VPD also resets the tachycardia, a bypass tract must exist and be necessary for tachycardia maintenance; retrograde conduction of such a VPD could occur only over an accessory pathway because the His bundle is still refractory (97) (Fig. 17-17).

Termination of OAVRT results when block occurs within the AV node-His-Purkinje system or the accessory pathway (98,99). An APD usually terminates the tachycardia by blocking antegradely (in the orthodromic direction) within the AV node while colliding retrogradely (in the antidromic direction) with the previous tachycardia depolarization wavefront, usually within the atria or bypass tract. Tachycardia termination caused by a VPD usually occurs when the extrastimulus blocks orthodromically within the bypass tract and collides antidromically with the previous tachycardia depolarization wavefront in the AV node-His-Purkinje system (87).

Spontaneous tachycardia termination occurring after a retrograde P wave on the surface ECG and an atrial electrogram not followed by a His potential on the intracardiac recording indicates that conduction block occurred within the AV node. Tachycardia termination occurring after a QRS complex and ventricular electrogram not followed by a retrograde P wave and atrial electrogram implies that block occurred within the bypass tract (98,99). In most instances, spontaneous block occurs within the AV node. Cycle length alternans may be seen immediately before the occurrence of AV node block and tachycardia termination, during which long-short oscillations occur in the tachycardia cycle length and A-H interval while the H-V and VA intervals remain constant. Spontaneous block occurring within the AV bypass tract is uncommonly observed during very rapid OAVRT. However, accessory pathways exhibiting slow, decremental retrograde conduction may be the site of block and tachycardia termination after the same autonomic and pharmacologic perturbations that affect the AV node (100–102).

Permanent Junctional Reciprocating Tachycardia

Permanent junctional reciprocating tachycardia (PJRT) occurs at rates between 120 and 200 bpm with a usually normal QRS duration; distinguishing features are its tendency to exhibit incessant behavior and the QRS/P wave relationship (55,103). The arrhythmia is an OAVRT mediated by a concealed AV bypass tract with slow and decremental conduction properties (103–105). The bypass tract is usually located within the posteroseptal region, although other portions of the AV sulcus may also harbor this unique pathway (104–107). Slow, retrograde conduction over the pathway causes the RP interval during PJRT to be long, usually greater than one half of the tachycardia's R-R interval. P waves resulting from retrograde conduction are easily seen on the ECG (Fig. 17-18).

Because the accessory pathway is anatomically separate from the AV node-His-Purkinje system, a ventricular extrastimulus delivered late in diastole during tachycardia when the His bundle is refractory can easily reset the next atrial activation and tachycardia cycle (39,55). This response cannot occur during uncommon fast/slow AVNRT or atrial tachycardia and is useful for differentiating between these three forms of long RP supraventricular tachycardia (101). Because the accessory pathway conducts decrementally during PJRT, the atrial electrogram and tachycardia cycle length reset response to the VPD may be one of delayed activation, rather than advancement (39).

The reason for the incessant nature of PJRT is not clear. Its onset and rate are quite sensitive to changes in autonomic tone and sinus rhythm rate. Spontaneous PJRT initiation and induction during electrophysiologic testing often occur after only trivial increases in the rate of sinus rhythm or atrial overdrive pacing (55). Tachycardia termination occurring spontaneously or after vagomimetic maneuvers frequently results from block in the accessory pathway; the ECG and intracardiac recordings show the last tachycardia event as a QRS com-

FIGURE 17-16. A: Electrocardiographic (ECG) and intracardiac electrogram recordings obtained during the same orthodromic atrioventricular reentrant tachycardia (OAVRT) displayed in Figure 17-14A from a patient with a concealed right free wall accessory pathway. ECG leads I, aVF, and V₁ are displayed along with electrograms recorded from the middle His bundle region (HBEM), the right ventricular apex (RVA), and five sites circumferentially around the tricuspid annulus (Ta). A His bundle potential is not well seen on the HBEM electrogram because of catheter displacement away from the septum during tachycardia. The shortest ventriculoatrial (VA) interval recorded from the earliest ventricular activation (long vertical line) to the earliest atrial activation (short vertical line) is 125 ms at site Ta 6, which corresponds anatomically to the right anterior tricuspid annulus. The tachycardia cycle length is 250 ms. **B:** The same OAVRT as in **A** with spontaneously occurring right bundle branch block aberrant conduction. The His bundle potential is not seen. Because of the accessory pathway's right free wall location, the reentrant impulse must propagate over a greater intraventricular distance from the left bundle branch's terminal Purkinje fibers to the right ventricular insertion of the accessory pathway. The VA interval during tachycardia has therefore increased to 220 ms. Displacement of the tricuspid annulus mapping catheter has caused the recording electrodes labeled Ta 8 to be positioned over the right anterior tricuspid annulus. The tachycardia cycle length (270 ms) has increased by only 20 ms because the increased VA interval has resulted in a shorter atrioventricular node conduction time and corresponding A-H interval.

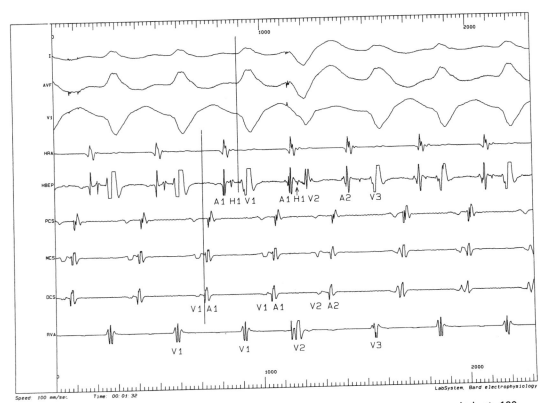

FIGURE 17-17. Electrocardiographic (ECG) and intracardiac electrograms recorded at 100 mm/sec during orthodromic atrioventicular reentrant tachycardia (OAVRT) that is conducted antegradely with left bundle branch block aberrant conduction with a tachycardia cycle length of 320 ms. The labeling of the surface ECG leads and intracardiac electrograms is identical to that in Figure 17-2. The earliest retrograde atrial electrogram (A_1) is recorded from the distal coronary sinus (DCS), consistent with a left lateral accessory pathway serving as the retrograde limb of conduction during OAVRT. A ventricular extrastimulus is delivered from the right ventricular apex (RVA) after the third V_1, with a resultant V_1-V_2 coupling interval of 250 ms. Despite the fact that the His bundle (H_1) was depolarized by antegrade conduction during OAVRT through the atrioventricular (AV) node 10 ms after the extrastimulus *(arrow)*, V_2 conducts retrogradely to the atria with the same atrial activation sequence, atrial electrogram pattern, and nearly the same ventriculoatrial (VA) interval duration as during OAVRT. The A_1-A_2 interval (275 ms) is less than the OAVRT cycle length, and the V_1-V_3 interval (630 ms) is less than twice the tachycardia cycle length. The ventricular extrastimulus advanced the atrial activation sequence and reset the tachycardia. Taken together, these findings prove that an AV bypass tract is conducting retrogradely during the tachycardia and is an obligatory participant in tachycardia maintenance.

plex and ventricular electrogram without a subsequent P wave and atrial electrogram (Fig. 17-18). Chronic suppression of PJRT is usually not possible with drugs, and ablation of the accessory pathway is often necessary to achieve arrhythmia control (55,105,106). Among tachycardias afflicting infants and children, PJRT figures prominently. The incessant behavior of PJRT may also result in dilated cardiomyopathy and congestive heart failure that are potentially reversible if the accessory pathway can be ablated (55,108).

Antidromic Atrioventricular Reentrant Tachycardia

AAVRT is the least common arrhythmia associated with WPW syndrome, occurring in only 5% to 10% of these patients (55,109–112). The tachycardia is characterized by a wide QRS complex that is fully preexcited and with usually regular R-R intervals, occurring at rates up to 250 bpm (111,112). AAVRT can result in diagnostic and therapeutic uncertainty because the differential diagnosis includes all other wide QRS tachycardias, such as ventricular tachycardia, any supraventricular tachycardia conducted aberrantly, and tachycardias of atrial and junctional origin with bystander accessory pathway activation of the ventricles (55) (Fig. 17-19). During intervening sinus rhythm, preexcitation may be relatively inapparent because AAVRTs frequently use left-sided bypass tracts as the antegrade route for conduction (14). Demonstrating an identical, preexcited QRS pattern during AAVRT and atrial pacing near the atrial insertion of the accessory pathway is diagnostically helpful if additional antegrade-conducting accessory pathways are not present (37,55). However, the prevalence of

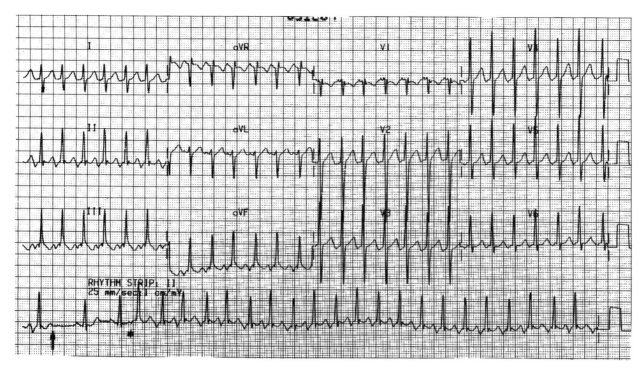

FIGURE 17-18. A 12-lead electrocardiogram (ECG) and lead II rhythm strip recording obtained from a patient with the permanent form of junctional reciprocating tachycardia (PJRT). The patient had been experiencing incessant palpitations for months during periods of emotional and physical stress before undergoing this ECG recording. The arrhythmia appears as a regular tachycardia at a rate of 165 bpm (cycle length of 360 ms) with a normal QRS duration. The tachycardia's P waves that result from retrograde conduction over the accessory pathway are readily seen as inverted deflections occurring after the T wave in leads II, III, and aVF and positive P waves in leads aVR, aVL, and V_1. The long R-P interval is consistent with the long conduction time that is characteristic of the accessory pathway that mediates this arrhythmia. The tachycardia's tendency to terminate spontaneously and recur incessantly is demonstrated in the lead II rhythm strip. Arrhythmia termination occurs after the first QRS complex because spontaneous block develops in the accessory pathway; the arrow marks where the next retrogradely conducted P wave would have been inscribed if block and tachycardia termination had not occurred. After two sinus depolarizations, a spontaneous atrial premature depolarization (*asterisk*) reinitiates PJRT.

multiple accessory pathways in patients who experience AAVRT may range from 33% to 60% (14,33,45,109).

If only one antegrade-conducting AV bypass tract exists, the AV node-His-Purkinje system must be the route for retrograde atrial activation during AAVRT. During tachycardia, the earliest retrograde atrial activation is inscribed at the His bundle recording site, and the sequence of retrograde atrial activation is normal. A 1 : 1 VA conduction relationship exists, because there is obligatory participation of the atria and ventricles in the reentrant circuit. Atrial and ventricular extrastimuli advance, respectively, the next set of ventricular and atrial electrograms as well as the entire tachycardia cycle while preserving the tachycardia's electrogram activation sequence. The width of the preexcited QRS complex and the amplitude of the ST-T wave segment usually obscure the retrograde P wave inscribed on the surface ECG.

The H-V interval is negative, with a retrograde His potential inscribed immediately preceding the local ventricular electrogram or occurring simultaneously with and obscured by the larger-amplitude ventricular electrogram

(14,112) (Fig. 17-20). As with OAVRT, tachycardia termination can occur after properly timed atrial and ventricular extrastimuli. Spontaneous termination can also follow block occurring within the accessory pathway or the AV node-His-Purkinje system (14,109,110).

Atrial Fibrillation and Atrial Flutter

Atrial fibrillation may be the index arrhythmia in up to 20% of patients with WPW syndrome and is usually paroxysmal in nature (14,44,45,65,66). Patients with bypass tracts causing overt preexcitation seem to be more prone to atrial fibrillation than patients whose bypass tracts are concealed (14). The accessory pathway's ability to mediate a rapid and hemodynamically unstable preexcited ventricular response is what determines the clinical mode of presentation with atrial fibrillation in the WPW syndrome (55). Ventricular fibrillation resulting from preexcited atrial fibrillation is rare as the first symptomatic arrhythmia occurring in an individual not previously known to have WPW

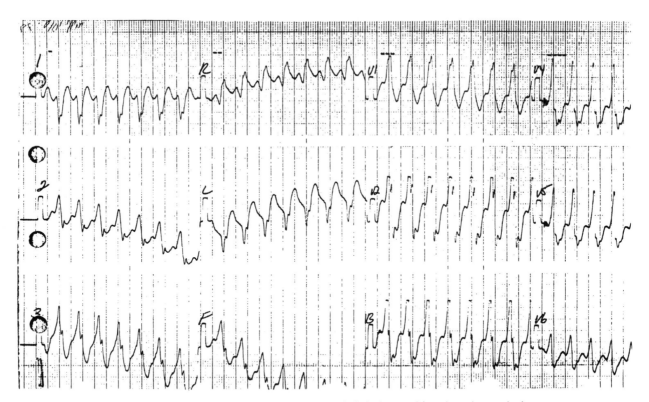

FIGURE 17-19. A 12-lead electrocardiogram recorded during antidromic atrioventricular reentrant tachycardia from a patient with a single left lateral accessory pathway. The tachycardia cannot be distinguished from ventricular tachycardia without concomitant intracardiac electrogram recordings and analysis of the response to programmed stimulation and pacing.

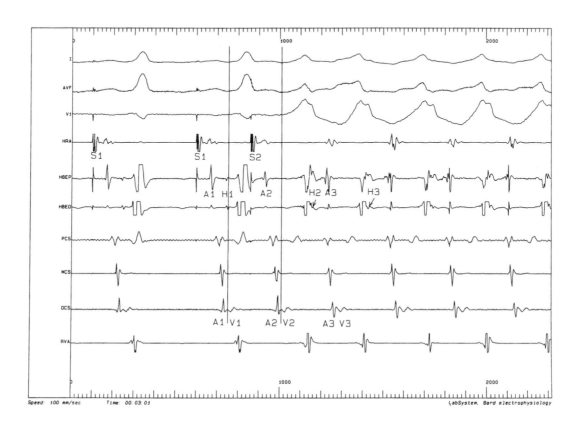

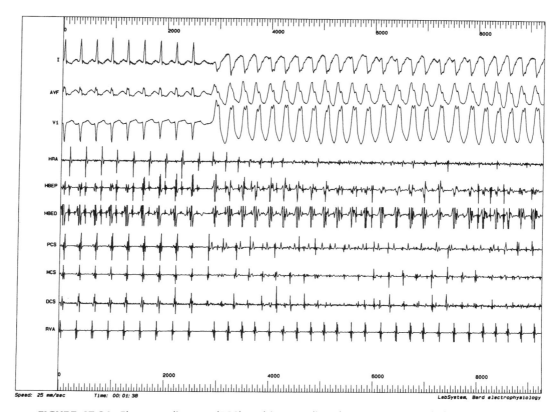

FIGURE 17-21. Electrocardiogram (ECG) and intracardiac electrograms recorded at 25 mm/sec during spontaneous degeneration of orthodromic atrioventricular reentrant tachycardia (OAVRT) into preexcited atrial fibrillation (AF). The labeling of the surface ECG leads and intracardiac electrograms is similar to that in Figure 17-2. In the left-hand portion of the figure, OAVRT is present at a cycle length of 310 ms. This is followed by the abrupt onset of a rapid atrial tachycardia that quickly degenerates into a preexcited AF that has a mean ventricular rate of 220 bpm. The initially relatively discrete and organized atrial electrograms at the onset of atrial tachycardia rapidly change to low-amplitude, fractionated, and continuous electrical activity that is most readily apparent in the high right atrium (HRA) recording site. During AF, all of the QRS complexes are preexcited, and the shortest R-R interval is 240 ms. The rapid ventricular response created by the left lateral accessory pathway's short antegrade refractory period creates a pseudo-regularized appearance to the R-R intervals at a recording speed of 25 mm/sec.

syndrome. Most patients with WPW syndrome who have atrial fibrillation have had preexisting episodes of AVRT. Paroxysmal and chronic atrial flutter are less common than paroxysmal atrial fibrillation in WPW syndrome (55).

The ECG during preexcited atrial fibrillation exhibits an irregular ventricular response; however, a sustained, rapid ventricular rate greater than 180 to 200 bpm often creates pseudo-regularized R-R intervals when the ECG is recorded at 25 mm/sec (Fig. 17-21). The atrial electrograms recorded during preexcited atrial fibrillation are not different in appearance from those recorded in the absence of preexcitation. Not uncommonly, atrial fibrillation in WPW syndrome may secondarily occur by degenerating from a rapid OAVRT (Figs. 17-21 and 17-22). The ventricular rate dur-

FIGURE 17-20. Electrocardiogram (ECG) and intracardiac electrograms recorded at 100 mm/sec during induction of antidromic atrioventricular (AV) reentrant tachycardia (AAVRT). The labeling of the surface ECG and intracardiac electrograms is similar to that in Figure 17-2. An extrastimulus (S2) is delivered in the high right atrium (HRA) at a coupling interval of 260 ms after an initial atrial drive train at a cycle length of 500 ms. During atrial drive, the QRS complexes are conducted with partial preexcitation, and an H-V interval (H1 to first vertical line) of 10 ms. The earliest V1 is recorded from the distal coronary sinus (DCS), consistent with antegrade conduction through a left lateral accessory pathway. After S2, the resultant A2 blocks antegradely in the AV node and conducts solely through the accessory pathway to the ventricle, yielding a fully preexcited QRS complex. Retrograde conduction occurs through the His-Purkinje system (H2, *arrow*) and the AV node (H2-A3) to initiate the first AAVRT cycle; the retrograde atrial activation sequence is inscribed first at the His bundle electrogram (HBE) recording sites. The subsequent retrograde His bundle potentials (H3) are visible as deflections that follow the local ventricular electrogram at the distal HBE recording site. The tachycardia cycle length is 290 ms.

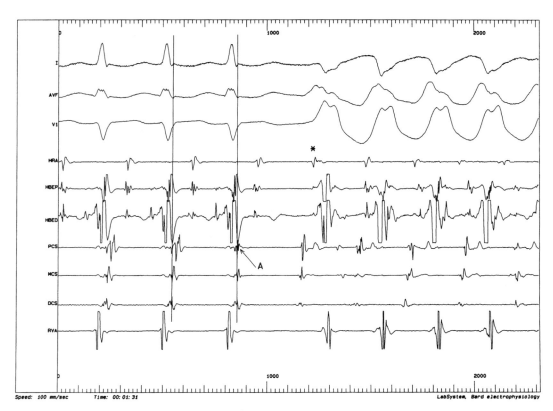

FIGURE 17-22. A detailed view of how the orthodromic atrioventicular reentrant tachycardia (OAVRT) spontaneously degenerates into atrial fibrillation (AF), recorded at 100 mm/sec. The labeling of the surface electrocardiographic leads and intracardiac electrograms is unchanged from that shown in Figure 17-21. The second QRS complex followed by a vertical line shows that the retrograde atrial activation sequence during OAVRT starts at the distal coronary sinus (DCS), consistent with the accessory pathway's left lateral atrial insertion. After the third QRS complex, retrograde atrial activation over the accessory pathway activates all atrial sites except for the proximal coronary sinus (PCS) and, possibly, the middle coronary sinus (MCS). The PCS and MCS display atrial electrograms that have different patterns from the preceding ones during OAVRT; the atrial activity (A) at the PCS also occurs prematurely at 290 ms; notice the location of the relation of the PCS electrogram (A) to the second vertical reference line versus the preceding atrial depolarization reference line relationship. This spontaneous local atrial premature depolarization (APD) blocks in the atrioventricular (AV) node and renders the node refractory to conducting the atrial depolarization resulting from OAVRT that still captures other atrial recording sites such as the high right atrium (HRA), proximal (HBEP) and distal (HBED) His bundle regions, and the DCS. After this spontaneous APD, a rapid atrial tachycardia *(asterisk)* develops that has a cycle length of 220 ms and conducts in a 1:1 fashion to the ventricles through the accessory pathway. The atrial electrograms during the tachycardia occur earliest in the DCS and vary considerably in appearance with intervening low-amplitude, fractionated activity as a prelude to rapid degeneration into AF.

ing preexcited atrial fibrillation can vary considerably; the important rate-modulating effects of autonomic tone and the interplay between refractoriness and conduction in the AV node-His-Purkinje system versus those variables within the bypass tract have already been discussed.

Repetitive retrograde concealed conduction into the bypass tract during preexcited atrial fibrillation may also result in a slower ventricular rate response than would be predicted, based on the accessory pathway's antegrade refractory period and shortest atrial pacing cycle length maintaining 1:1 preexcited conduction (14). These factors also influence the

degree to which QRS complexes are totally preexcited or variably exist as fusion of normal and preexcited QRS complexes (Fig. 17-23). Detecting the presence of more than one preexcited QRS pattern during atrial fibrillation also aids in identifying multiple bypass tracts (35). The total absence of preexcited QRS complexes during atrial fibrillation, despite the presence of (often intermittent) preexcitation during sinus rhythm is also a reassuring sign that the antegrade refractory period of the bypass tract is long and the pathway unlikely to mediate a rapid ventricular response during spontaneous atrial fibrillation (14).

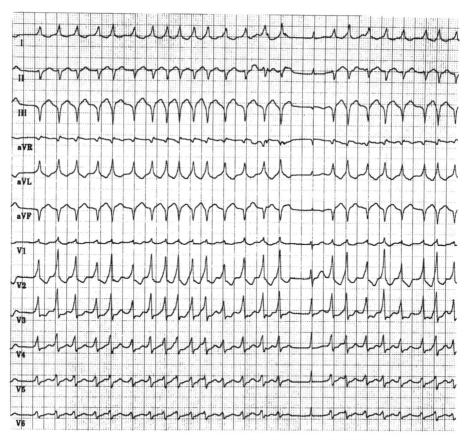

FIGURE 17-23. A 12-lead electrocardiogram recorded during atrial fibrillation from a patient with a left lateral accessory pathway. All preexcited QRS complexes have the same appearance. The shortest preexcited R-R interval is 220 ms, and the mean ventricular rate is 180 bpm. An isolated QRS complex is conducted without preexcitation.

THERAPY FOR ARRHYTHMIAS ASSOCIATED WITH WOLFF-PARKINSON-WHITE SYNDROME

Treatment options for patients with WPW syndrome include pharmacologic agents, antitachycardia devices, catheter and surgical ablation, and combinations of these therapies. The past decade has been marked by a dramatic shift in the relative degree to which these therapies are employed for primary and secondary tachyarrhythmia prevention and management.

Pharmacologic Therapy

The rational choice of an antiarrhythmic drug depends on making a correct arrhythmia diagnosis and defining the electrophysiologic properties of the arrhythmia's trigger for initiation and substrate for maintenance. For WPW syndrome, in addition to choosing drugs that decrease the frequency of ectopy initiating tachycardia, the physician would ideally wish to select an antiarrhythmic drug that has the most potent depressant action on the "weakest link" of an AVRT circuit. Performing atrial and ventricular pacing at incremental rates faster than that of the AVRT and noting the paced cycle lengths causing block in the antegrade and retrograde limbs of conduction can define a "safety factor" for conduction over these routes. The conduction pathway having the greater difference between the tachycardia cycle length and the paced cycle length causing block in that pathway can be considered the strong limb of conduction. Conversely, the weak limb of the AVRT circuit is the pathway with the longer refractory period or more tenuous conduction properties (80).

Orthodromic Atrioventricular Reentrant Tachycardia: Acute Drug Therapy

The AV node is usually the weak link of this arrhythmia. Relatively specific therapies that lengthen AV node refractoriness and depress conduction are therefore desirable to cause the reentrant wave to block in the node and terminate the tachycardia. Transient depression of AV node function engendered by carotid sinus massage and a Valsalva maneuver may also be sufficient to cause AV node block and tachycardia termination (113).

Intravenous administration of verapamil is an effective means of causing acute termination of OAVRT, provided that the patient is not profoundly hypotensive or suffering from congestive heart failure associated with severely depressed ventricular systolic function (114,115). Intravenous adenosine is equally effective in acutely terminating OAVRT (89,116,117). Its ultrashort duration of action is preferable for the patient whose hemodynamic state is more tenuous before resorting to emergent DC cardioversion. However, adenosine's proclivity to cause atrial ectopy that could reinitiate OAVRT after acute termination of tachycardia and transiently increase vulnerability to atrial fibrillation is disadvantageous compared with verapamil (89,90,118).

Agents of second choice include β-blocking drugs available for intravenous administration: propranolol, metoprolol, and esmolol (80,119,120). Intravenous digoxin's prolonged time to onset of action and peak effect, coupled with low potency, make it a less attractive treatment alternative (121).

Intravenous procainamide is an important alternate second-choice drug. Unlike the other agents listed, procainamide depresses conduction in all cardiac tissues and prolongs refractoriness in the atria, ventricles, bypass tract, and the His-Purkinje system while having no effect or causing slight shortening of the AV node refractory period (122,123). Procainamide is the drug of choice if the OAVRT presents as a hemodynamically tolerated, wide QRS complex tachycardia due to functional or preexisting bundle branch block and the arrhythmia diagnosis is in doubt. Intravenous procainamide is the safest, if not most efficacious, drug to administer for acute treatment of an unknown wide QRS tachycardia (124).

Orthodromic Atrioventricular Reentrant Tachycardia: Chronic Drug Therapy

An antiarrhythmic drug's efficacy for preventing OAVRT is predicated on its ability to alter the electrophysiologic properties of the reentrant circuit to render reentry incapable of sustaining itself. Antiectopic activity is also desirable to decrease the number of tachycardia-triggering APDs and VPDs. Chronic drug therapy usually requires continuous dosing at regular intervals. However, some patients with infrequent episodes of OAVRT that are not overly symptomatic or hemodynamically destabilizing may be served equally well by an intermittent, short-term oral-drug regimen that is taken when needed to effect termination of tachycardia episodes (125). Patients requiring chronic drug treatment are potentially committed to indefinite antiarrhythmic drug prophylaxis. The optimum drug must have a high efficacy rate and a low risk for causing adverse effects,

especially serious cardiac and noncardiac organ toxicity. Cardiac organ toxicity tends to be less of concern when treating patients without structural heart disease, especially those who are young. However, this risk increases as the patient ages. The class Ic antiarrhythmic drugs possess the most favorable efficacy and tolerance records (126–131). Flecainide and propafenone are approved antiarrhythmic drugs available for chronically suppressing and delaying time to recurrence of OAVRT in patients who have no structural heart disease.

Second-line drugs for suppression of OAVRT include agents with AV node-specific activity such as β blockers, calcium channel blockers, and digoxin. These agents may be inadequate as monotherapy because of their inability to directly slow conduction and increase retrograde refractoriness in the accessory pathway. They also do not reduce the frequency of arrhythmia-triggering atrial and ventricular ectopy and do not prolong antegrade refractoriness in the bypass tract (114,115,119,120).

However, a β blocker may be a useful adjunct to a class Ic antiarrhythmic drug by preventing attenuation of drug effect caused by endogenous catecholamine release during tachycardia episodes (132). The class Ia antiarrhythmic drugs are alternative choices to Ic agents because of their generally less potent ability to lengthen refractoriness and slow conduction in the accessory pathway (123,133,134). These drugs tend to minimally prolong refractoriness in the AV node and possess a higher likelihood of causing serious organ toxicity and intolerable noncardiac adverse effects, limiting long-term drug tolerance.

Amiodarone has multiple electrophysiologic effects that make it effective for suppressing OAVRT (135–138). These include antiadrenergic activity, prolongation of repolarization and voltage-dependent refractoriness, and blockade of the fast and slow inward currents. These effects slow conduction and lengthen refractoriness in all cardiac tissue involved in the macroreentrant circuit of AVRT. However, clinical studies do not clearly show that amiodarone is superior in antiarrhythmic efficacy to class Ic drugs used alone or in combination with a β-blocking drug. The drug's well-known ability to cause serious organ-toxic side effects can be minimized by using low-maintenance doses of 200 to 300 mg/day or less (139,140). However, intolerable noncardiac adverse effects that limit quality of life, at the very least, eventually occur in 30% to 93% of patients and require drug withdrawal in many individuals (135,140). Amiodarone therapy is best reserved for preventing OAVRT in otherwise drug-refractory, elderly patients with comorbidities who refuse or are judged to be poor-risk candidates to undergo ablation therapy.

Sotalol has also been shown to have clinical efficacy in preventing OAVRT (141,142). An incidence of torsade de pointes as high as 4% is the main serious adverse effect. This risk is greatest among patients with advanced structural heart disease who have decreased ventricular function and congestive heart failure.

Antidromic Atrioventricular Reentrant Tachycardia: Acute and Chronic Drug Therapy

Retrograde AV node conduction may be the weak link during AAVRT. However, intravenously administered AV node–blocking drugs such as β blockers, calcium channel blockers, adenosine, and digoxin should be avoided to effect acute termination of tachycardia. Unless the arrhythmia is known to be AAVRT with certainty before treatment is initiated, the patient should be considered to have an undiagnosed wide QRS tachycardia. AAVRT can also degenerate into atrial fibrillation after drug administration, especially if adenosine is administered (89). A bypass tract capable of supporting AAVRT may have a short antegrade refractory period, and the resultant ventricular response during preexcited atrial fibrillation may be hemodynamically even more destabilizing. The intravenous drug of choice for acute treatment to terminate AAVRT is therefore procainamide. Even if it does not cause outright tachycardia termination, intravenous procainamide can at least slow the tachycardia rate and improve or probably not worsen the patient's hemodynamic state (124). When considering drug therapy for chronic suppression, it is emphasized that the accessory pathway mediating antegrade conduction during AAVRT is also capable of serving as the limb for antegrade preexcited conduction during atrial fibrillation. Drugs of utility must therefore depress conduction and prolong refractoriness in the accessory pathway. The class Ic drugs are again the agents of choice in the absence of contraindications; class Ia drugs and amiodarone would be less desirable second choices for reasons previously mentioned.

Atrial Fibrillation: Acute Drug Therapy

The goals of acute drug therapy for preexcited atrial fibrillation are prompt control of the ventricular response and stabilization of the patient's hemodynamic state. Treatment of preexcited atrial fibrillation requires a parenteral drug with rapid onset of action that lengthens antegrade refractoriness and slows conduction in the accessory pathway and the AV node-His-Purkinje system. Flecainide and propafenone are highly efficacious when used for these purposes, but the parenteral formulations of these drugs are not approved for use in the United States (143–145). Intravenously administered procainamide is therefore the drug of choice. However, preliminary experience with ibutilide, a class III antiarrhythmic agent available only for intravenous use, has suggested that it is an effective therapy for terminating atrial fibrillation and atrial flutter in patients with a preexcitation syndrome (146). It also has the advantage of being devoid of a negative hemodynamic effect. AV node–specific antiarrhythmic drugs that are normally used to control the ventricular rate during nonpreexcited atrial fibrillation are contraindicated. When used alone, intravenous β-blocking drugs do not increase bypass tract refractoriness. β-Blocker–mediated inhibition of AV node conduction may also enhance the preexcited ventricular rate response by decreasing the degree of concealed retrograde conduction into the bypass tract. A bypass tract with a short antegrade refractory period that was initially competing with the AV node could then become the dominant route for antegrade conduction.

Intravenous digoxin is contraindicated because of its unpredictable effect on bypass tract refractoriness (147). Digoxin's vagomimetic action lengthens AV node refractoriness and reduces concealed retrograde conduction into the bypass tract. A slow time to onset of action and peak effect also make digoxin an unacceptable drug to use when rapid ventricular rate control is required. Intravenous verapamil is the most unsafe AV node blocker to administer during preexcited atrial fibrillation (148–150). Intravenous verapamil lengthens AV node refractoriness, decreases concealed conduction into the accessory pathway, and has no direct depressant effect on the pathway. Myocardial contractility and systemic vascular resistance are also reduced; these latter effects may cause a reflex increase in already elevated sympathetic tone that further shortens accessory pathway refractoriness. Precipitation of cardiac arrest by degeneration of preexcited atrial fibrillation to ventricular fibrillation has been reported after intravenous verapamil administration. Intravenous adenosine causes a similar effect, albeit of much shorter duration.

Atrial Fibrillation: Chronic Drug Therapy

The drug selected for suppressing paroxysmal atrial fibrillation in WPW syndrome should possess antiectopic activity to suppress APDs and VPDs, which can directly induce atrial fibrillation and AVRT that may degenerate into atrial fibrillation. The drug must also provide adequate background protection against a rapid ventricular response by lengthening refractoriness in the accessory pathway and the AV node-His-Purkinje system if atrial fibrillation intermittently breaks through. Class Ic drugs appear to possess the best electrophysiologic profile for achieving these goals if no cardiac contraindications exist (151,152). Class Ia drugs are less potent and have greater noncardiac adverse and organ toxicity risks. The class III agents sotalol and dofetilide are also effective for maintaining sinus rhythm, and they appear to be as effective as class Ic agents (153–155). Amiodarone is useful when class Ic or Ia drugs are ineffective or not tolerated and when ablation therapies are inappropriate or have failed (156,157).

Antitachycardia Devices

Antitachycardia device therapy includes the use of external direct current (DC) cardioverters, temporary pacemakers, and permanently implanted antitachycardia pacemakers that can be manually or automatically activated to terminate arrhythmia. External DC cardioversion may be emergently required when a patient presents with hemodynamically destabilizing tachycardia or when initially prescribed therapy is ineffective or causes abrupt worsening of the patient's condition. AVRTs lend themselves well to pacemaker termination because the entire heart is involved in the reentrant circuit. Temporary pacemaker stimulation of the right atrium or ventricle or transesophageal pacing are alternatives to DC cardioversion if an AVRT episode persists after initial attempts to terminate it with an intravenous antiarrhythmic drug (158) (Fig. 17-24); this approach assumes that the patient is in a hemodynamic state that allows time to insert a transvenous pacing catheter or can tolerate swallowing a transesophageal pacing electrode. The risk of inducing preexcited atrial fibrillation with a rapid ventricular response during attempts to pace-terminate AVRT is particularly likely when delivering multiple atrial extrastimuli at close coupling intervals or when rapidly pacing the atrium at rates in excess of 250 bpm (159,160). This risk may be reduced by first administering intravenous procainamide to slow the tachycardia rate and lengthen bypass tract refractoriness (161,162). Atrial flutter conducted with preexcitation can also be pace-terminated after the ventricles have been drug-protected from 1 : 1 AV conduction and the atrial flutter rate decreased (158,162). Conventional rapid pacing stimulation is not effective for termination of atrial fibrillation.

Chronic preventive treatment of AVRT with permanently implanted pacemakers has become rare since catheter ablation therapy has evolved (163). Such therapy is also contraindicated for patients with WPW syndrome who have manifest preexcitation caused by accessory pathways with a short antegrade refractory period because of the risk of inadvertently precipitating atrial fibrillation during automatic or manually activated pacing attempts to terminate AVRT. Antitachycardia pacemakers do not prevent AVRT and frequently have relatively poor long-term efficacy, especially if tachycardia episodes occur frequently, are very symptomatic, or tend to reoccur quickly after being transiently pace-terminated.

Ablation Therapy

Ablation therapy plays a dominant role in the treatment of patients with WPW syndrome. Before the advent of radiofrequency energy–mediated catheter ablation, surgical ablation of AV bypass tracts was the standard technique that provided a true cure for patients suffering from drug-refractory WPW syndrome. The success rate for WPW surgery had been nearly 100%, with an operative mortality rate of less than 1% (29,30). However, the proliferation of catheter-based ablation therapy caused surgical ablation procedures for WPW syndrome to dwindle to a low level such that surgical expertise may no longer be capable of yielding the cited outcome results. This is of particular concern when confronted with a severely symptomatic, drug-refractory WPW syndrome patient who has failed several attempts at catheter-based ablation therapy, despite performance by operators at centers with track records of high procedural volume and efficacy.

Radiofrequency catheter–mediated ablation is the procedure of choice for curing most patients with WPW syndrome who experience highly symptomatic or frequent arrhythmia episodes, particularly when they are poorly responsive to antiarrhythmic drug therapy (Fig. 17-25). The procedure can be accomplished with success rates of 95%, recurrence rates of 6%, and major complications rates of less than 2% (164–166). A new nonfluoroscopic catheter-based electroanatomic mapping system, CARTO, has a magnetic field emitter and sensor and can create a replica of the anatomy of the cardiac chamber in which the tachycardia focus is located, permitting more precise localization of the arrhythmia focus and the accessory pathway (167). However, the presence of structural heart disease (especially with decreased left ventricular function) and multiple accessory pathways, which may be present in up to 13% of patients, predicts an increased risk of mortality and serious morbidity (166,168). Ablation of multiple pathways requires more procedure time and greater radiation exposure (168). A compelling argument has been made for the cost-effectiveness of catheter ablation therapy compared with the cost of prolonged and unsuccessful attempts at treatment with multiple antiarrhythmic drugs (169). This is especially true for those with a history of a cardiac arrest or symptomatic atrial fibrillation (170).

Patients with WPW syndrome who experience only infrequent and minimally symptomatic episodes of OAVRT, particularly if terminated by properly and self-performed vagomimetic maneuvers, should be encouraged to

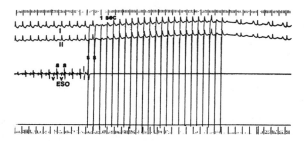

FIGURE 17-24. Transesophageal pacing of the left atrium in an infant to terminate a rapid (cycle length of 220 ms) orthodromic atrioventricular reentrant tachycardia (OAVRT). Two surface electrocardiographic leads are displayed along with a recording obtained from the esophagus (ESO) by means of the pacing electrode at 25 mm/sec. On the ESO recording, the atrial electrogram (a) is of greater amplitude than the ventricular electrogram (v) because of the proximity of the left atrium to the esophagus. The v-to-a electrogram relationship is consistent with the RP interval timing of an OAVRT. A rapid train of pacing pulses is delivered at a cycle length of 180 ms that captures the atria and produces variable atrioventricular block as shown on the surface electrocardiogram. The tachycardia is terminated by the pacing train, evidenced by the resumption of sinus rhythm after pacing ceases. (From Jenkins JM, Dick M, Collins S, et al. Use of the pill electrode for transesophageal atrial pacing. *Pacing Clin Electrophysiol* 1985;8:523, with permission.)

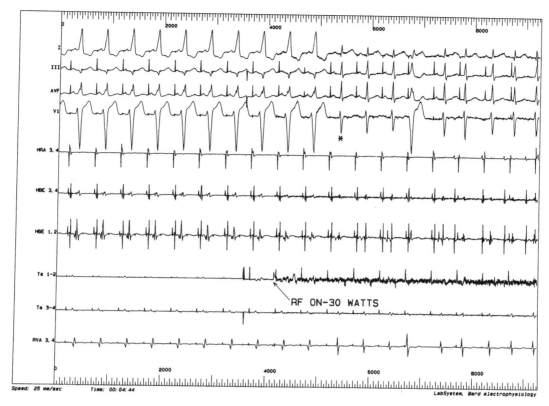

FIGURE 17-25. Surface electrocardiogram (ECG) and intracardiac electrograms recorded at 25 mm/sec during radiofrequency (RF) energy catheter-mediated ablation of a right lateral accessory pathway. Labeling of the surface ECG leads and intracardiac electrograms is identical to that in Figure 17-11. Pacing from the high right atrium (HRA) at a cycle length of 500 ms is performed to maximize preexcited arterioventricular conduction to facilitate localization of the accessory pathway where it crosses the tricuspid annulus. RF current is applied at a power setting of 30 W by means of the distal tip electrode of the ablation catheter, and within 1.2 seconds of onset of RF current delivery, preexcitation disappears *(asterisk)* as the accessory pathway is ablated. RF current was applied for a total duration of 45 seconds.

consider "cocktail" treatment—large, single-dose pharmacologic therapy, taken when needed, to assist in terminating acute episodes of tachycardia. However, such patients with manifest preexcitation may still warrant electrophysiologic testing to ensure that their accessory pathway lacks antegrade conduction properties capable of mediating a dangerously rapid ventricular rate response in case preexcited atrial fibrillation develops in the future. In such cases and for patients with moderately symptomatic WPW syndrome declining first-round chronic antiarrhythmic drug therapy, radiofrequency energy–catheter ablation may be appropriate at the same electrophysiologic testing session if the procedural risk is deemed low enough and discussed in advance with the patient.

REFERENCES

1. Wolff L, Parkinson J, White PD. Bundle-branch block with short P-R interval in healthy young people prone to paroxysmal tachycardia. *Am Heart J* 1930;5:685–704.
2. Wilson FN. A case in which the vagus influenced the form of the ventricular complex of the electrocardiogram. *Arch Intern Med* 1915;16:1008–1027.
3. Wedd AM. Paroxysmal tachycardia with reference to Normotopic tachycardia and the role of the intrinsic cardiac nerves. *Arch Intern Med* 1921;27:571–590.
4. Hamburger WW. Bundle branch block: four cases of intraventricular block showing some interesting and unusual clinical features. *Med Clin North Am* 1929;13:343–362.
5. Wood FC, Wolferth CC, Geckeler GD. Histological demonstration of accessory muscular connections between auricle and ventricle in a case of short P-R interval and prolonged QRS complex. *Am Heart J* 1943;25:454–462.
6. Ohnell RF. Preexcitation, a cardiac abnormality. *Acta Med Scand* 1944;152[Suppl]:1–167.
7. Anderson RH, Becker AE. *The development of the heart: cardiac anatomy.* London: Gower Medical Publishing, 1980:1–10.
8. Anderson RH, Becker AE. Anatomy of the conduction tissues and accessory atrioventricular connections. In: Zipes DP, Jalife J, eds. *Cardiac electrophysiology.* Philadelphia: WB Saunders, 1990:240–248.
9. Anderson RH, Becker AE, Wenink ACG, Janse MJ. The development of the cardiac specialized tissue. In: Wellens HJJ, Lie KI, Janse MJ, eds. *The conduction system of the heart: structure,*

function, and clinical implications. Philadelphia: Lea & Febiger, 1976:3–28.

10. Waller BF. Clinicopathological correlations of the human cardiac conduction system. In: Zipes DP, Jalife J, eds. *Cardiac electrophysiology*. Philadelphia: WB Saunders, 1990:249–269.

11. Anderson RH, Becker AE, Brechenmacher C, Davies MJ, Rossi L. Ventricular pre-excitation: a proposed nomenclature for its substrates. *Eur J Cardiol* 1975;3:27–36.

12. Ferrer MI. Preexcitation. *Am J Med* 1977;62:715–730.

13. Chung EK. Wolff-Parkinson-White syndrome: current views. *Am J Med* 1977;62:252–266.

14. Josephson ME. Preexcitation syndromes. In: *Clinical cardiac electrophysiology*. Philadelphia: Lea & Febiger, 1993:311–416.

15. Prystowsky EN, Page RL. Electrophysiology and autonomic influences of the human atrioventricular node. In: Mazgalev T, Dreifus L, Michelson EL, eds. *Electrophysiology of the sinoatrial and atrioventricular nodes*. New York: Alan R Liss, 1988: 259–277.

16. Murdock CJ, Leitch JW, Teo WS, et al. Characteristics of accessory pathways exhibiting decremental conduction. *Am J Cardiol* 1991;67:506–510.

17. Bayes de Luna A. Cardiac electrophysiology. In: *Textbook of clinical electrocardiography*. Dordrecht, The Netherlands: Martinus Nijhoff, 1987:1–29.

18. Klein GJ, Gulamhusein SS. Intermittent preexcitation in the Wolff-Parkinson-White syndrome. *Am J Cardiol* 1983;52: 292–296.

19. German LD, Gallagher JJ. Functional properties of accessory atrioventricular pathways in Wolff-Parkinson-White syndrome: clinical implications. *Am J Med* 1984;76:1079–1086.

20. Nalos PC, Deng Z, Gang ES, et al. Intermittent preexcitation: clinical recognition and management. *Pract Cardiol* 1985;11: 49–67.

21. Ross DL, Uther JB. Diagnosis of concealed accessory pathways in supraventricular tachycardia. *Pacing Clin Electrophysiol* 1984; 7:1069–1085.

22. Klein GJ, Hackel DB, Gallagher JJ. Anatomic substrate of impaired antegrade conduction over an accessory atrio-ventricular pathway in the Wolff-Parkinson-White syndrome. *Circulation* 1980;61:1249–1256.

23. Gallagher JJ, Sealy WC, Kasell J. Intraoperative mapping studies in the Wolff-Parkinson-White syndrome. *Pacing Clin Electrophysiol* 1979;2:523–537.

24. Winters SL, Gomes JA. Intracardiac electrode catheter recordings of atrioventricular bypass tracts in Wolff-Parkinson-White syndrome: techniques, electrophysiologic characteristics and demonstration of concealed and decremental propagation. *J Am Coll Cardiol* 1986;7:1392–1403.

25. Tchou P, Lehmann MH, Jazayeri M, Akhtar M. Atriofascicular connection or a nodoventricular Mahaim fiber? Electrophysiologic elucidation of the pathway and associated reentrant circuit. *Circulation* 1988;77:837–848.

26. Gilette PC, Garson A Jr, Cooley DA, McNamara DG. Prolonged and decremental antegrade conduction properties in right anterior accessory connections: wide QRS antidromic tachycardia of left bundle branch block pattern without Wolff-Parkinson-White configuration in sinus rhythm. *Am Heart J* 1982;103:66–74.

27. Gilette PC. Concealed anomalous cardiac conduction pathways: a frequent cause of supraventricular tachycardia. *Am J Cardiol* 1977;40:848–852.

28. de la Fuente D, Sasyniuk B, Moe GK. Conduction through a narrow isthmus in isolated canine atrial tissue: a model of the W-P-W syndrome. *Circulation* 1971;44:803–809.

29. Ferguson TB, Cox JL. Surgical treatment for the Wolff-Parkinson-White syndrome: the endocardial approach. In: Zipes DP,

Jalife J, eds. *Cardiac electrophysiology*. Philadelphia: WB Saunders, 1990:897–907.

30. Cox JL, Gallagher JJ, Cain ME. Experience with 118 consecutive patients undergoing surgery for Wolff-Parkinson-White syndrome. *J Thorac Cardiovasc Surg* 1985;90:490–501.

31. Cain ME, Cox JL. Surgical treatment of supraventricular arrhythmias. In: Platia E, ed. *Management of cardiac arrhythmias: the nonpharmacologic approach*. Philadelphia: JB Lippincott, 1987:304–339.

32. Munger TM, Packer DL, Hammill SC, et al. A population study of the natural history of Wolff-Parkinson-White syndrome in Olmsted County, Minnesota, 1953–1989. *Circulation* 1993;87:866–873.

33. Gallagher JJ, Pritchett ELC, Sealy WC, et al. The preexcitation syndromes. *Prog Cardiovasc Dis* 1978;20:285–327.

34. Reddy GV, Schamroth L. The localization of bypass tracts in the Wolff-Parkinson-White syndrome from the surface electrocardiogram. *Am Heart J* 1987;113:984–993.

35. Fananapazir L, German LD, Gallagher JJ, et al. Importance of preexcited QRS morphology during induced atrial fibrillation to the diagnosis and localization of multiple accessory pathways. *Circulation* 1990;81:578–585.

36. Lindsay BD, Crossen KJ, Cain ME. Concordance of distinguishing electrocardiographic features during sinus rhythm with the location of accessory pathways in the Wolff-Parkinson-White syndrome. *Am J Cardiol* 1987;59:1093–1102.

37. Milstein S, Sharma AD, Guiraudon GM, Klein GJ. An algorithm for the electrocardiographic localization of accessory pathways in the Wolff-Parkinson-White syndrome. *Pacing Clin Electrophysiol* 1987;10:555–563.

38. Arruda MS, McClelland JH, Wang X, et al. Development and validation of an ECG algorithm for identifying accessory pathway ablation site in Wolff-Parkinson-White syndrome. *J Cardiovasc Electrophysiol* 1998;9:2–12.

39. Cain ME, Luke RA, Lindsay BD. Diagnosis and localization of accessory pathways. *Pacing Clin Electrophysiol* 1992;15:801–824.

40. Jackman WM, Friday KJ, Fitzgerald DM, et al. Localization of left free-wall and posteroseptal accessory atrioventricular pathways by direct recording of accessory pathway activation. *Pacing Clin Electrophysiol* 1989;12:204–214.

41. Lam C, Schweikert R, Kanagaratnam L, et al. Radiofrequency ablation of a right atrial appendage-ventricular accessory pathway by transcutaneous epicardial instrumentation. *J Cardiovasc Electrophysiol* 2000;11(10)1170–1173.

42. Kuck KH, Schluter M, Siebels J, et al. Right-sided epicardial accessory pathways-rare but there. *Circulation* 1994;90:I-127.

43. Lesh MD, Van HG, Kao AK, et al. Radiofrequency catheter ablation for Wolff-Parkinson-White syndrome associated with a coronary sinus diverticulum. *Pacing Clin Electrophysiol* 1991;14: 1479–1484.

44. Deal BJ, Keane JF, Gillette PC, Garson A Jr. Wolff-Parkinson-White syndrome and supraventricular tachycardia during infancy: Management and follow-up. *J Am Coll Cardiol* 1985;5:130–135.

45. Scheibler GL, Adams P, Anderson RC. The Wolff-Parkinson-White syndrome in infants and children: a review and a report of 28 cases. *Pediatrics* 1959;24:585–603.

46. Lev M, Gibson S, Miller RA. Ebstein's disease with Wolff-Parkinson-White syndrome. *Am Heart J* 1955;49:724–741.

47. Cappato R, Hebe J, Weib C, et al. Radiofrequency current ablation of accessory pathways in Ebstein's anomaly. *J Am Coll Cardiol* 1993;21:172A.

48. Chung K-Y, Walsh TJ, Massie E. Wolff-Parkinson-White syndrome. *Am Heart J* 1965;69:116–133.

49. Krahn AD, Manfreda J, Tate RB, et al. The natural history of electrocardiographic preexcitation in men: the Manitoba follow-up study. *Ann Intern Med* 1992;116:456–460.

50. Sorbo MD, Buja GF, Miorelli M, et al. Prevalence of Wolff-Parkinson-White syndrome in a population of 116,452 young males. *G Ital Cardiol* 1995;25:681–687.

51. Vidaillet HJ Jr, Pressley JC, Henke E, et al. Familial occurrence of accessory atrioventricular pathways (preexcitation syndrome). *N Engl J Med* 1987;317:65–69.

52. Gallagher JJ, Sealy WC, Kasell J, Wallace AG. Multiple accessory pathways in patients with the preexcitation syndrome. *Circulation* 1976;54:571–591.

53. Colavita PG, Packer DL, Pressley JC, et al. Frequency, diagnosis, and clinical characteristics of patients with multiple accessory atrioventricular pathways. *Am J Cardiol* 1987;59:601–606.

54. Miller JM. Wolff-Parkinson-White syndrome, its variants, and concealed bypass tracts. *Card Electrophysiol Rev* 1997;1:86–89.

55. Yee R, Klein GJ, Sharma AD, et al. Tachycardia associated with accessory atrioventricular pathways. In: Zipes DP, Jalife J, eds. *Cardiac electrophysiology.* Philadelphia: WB Saunders, 1990: 463–472.

56. Akhtar M, Lehmann MH, Denker ST, et al. Electrophysiologic mechanisms of orthodromic tachycardia initiation during ventricular pacing in the Wolff-Parkinson-White syndrome. *J Am Coll Cardiol* 1987;9:89–100.

57. Sung RJ, Styperek JL. Electrophysiologic identification of dual atrioventricular nodal pathway conduction in patients with reciprocating tachycardia using anomalous bypass tracts. *Circulation* 1979;60:1464–1476.

58. Yee R, Klein GJ. Atrioventricular nodal reentry in the Wolff-Parkinson-White syndrome. *J Electrocardiol* 1985;18:295–298.

59. Reyes W, Milstein S, Dunnigan A, et al. Indications for modification of coexisting dual atrioventricular node pathways in patients undergoing surgical ablation of accessory atrioventricular connections. *J Am Coll Cardiol* 1991;17:1561–1567.

60. Dreifus LS, Haiat R, Watanabe Y, et al. Ventricular fibrillation: a possible mechanism of sudden death in patients with Wolff-Parkinson-White syndrome. *Circulation* 1971;43:520–527.

61. Klein GJ, Bashore TM, Sellers TD, et al. Ventricular fibrillation in the Wolff-Parkinson-White syndrome. *N Engl J Med* 1979; 301:1080–1085.

62. Klein GJ, Yee R, Sharma AD. Concealed conduction in accessory atrioventricular pathways: An important determinant of the expression of arrhythmias in patients with Wolff-Parkinson-White syndrome. *Circulation* 1984;70:402–411.

63. Prystowsky EN, Pritchett ELC, Gallagher JJ. Concealed conduction preventing anterograde preexcitation in Wolff-Parkinson-White syndrome. *Am J Cardiol* 1984;53:960–961.

64. Chen P-S, Prystowsky EN. Role of concealed and supernormal conductions during atrial fibrillation in the preexcitation syndrome. *Am J Cardiol* 1991;68:1329–1334.

65. Campbell RWF, Smith R, Gallagher JJ, et al. Atrial fibrillation in the preexcitation syndrome. *Am J Cardiol* 1977;40:514–520.

66. Wellens HJ, Durrer D. Wolff-Parkinson-White syndrome and atrial fibrillation. *Am J Cardiol* 1974;34:777–782.

67. Sharma AD, Klein GJ, Guiraudon GM, Milstein S. Atrial fibrillation in patients with Wolff-Parkinson-White syndrome: incidence after surgical ablation of the accessory pathway. *Circulation* 1985;72:161–169.

68. Iesaka Y, Yamane T, Takahashi A, et al. Retrograde multiple and multifiber accessory pathway conduction in the Wolff-Parkinson-White syndrome: potential precipitating factor of atrial fibrillation. *J Cardiovasc Electrophysiol* 1998;9:141–151.

69. Leitch JW, Klein GJ, Yee R, Murdock C. Prognostic value of electrophysiology testing in asymptomatic patients with Wolff-Parkinson-White pattern. *Circulation* 1990;82:1718–1723.

70. Smith RF. The Wolff-Parkinson-White syndrome as an aviation risk. *Circulation* 1990;82:1718–1723.

71. Gilette PC, Garson A Jr, Kugler JD. Wolff-Parkinson-White syndrome in children: electrophysiologic and pharmacologic characteristics. *Circulation* 1979;60:1487–1495.

72. Denes P, Wyndham CR, Amat-y-Leon F, et al. Atrial pacing at multiple sites in the Wolff-Parkinson-White syndrome. *Br Heart J* 1977;39:506–514.

73. Benson WD, Sterba R, Gallagher JJ, et al. Localization of the site of ventricular pre-excitation with body surface maps in patients with Wolff-Parkinson-White syndrome. *Circulation* 1982;65: 1259–1268.

74. Kamakura S, Shimomura K, Ohe T, et al. The role of initial minimum potentials on body surface maps in predicting the site of accessory pathways in patients with Wolff-Parkinson-White syndrome. *Circulation* 1986;74:89–96.

75. Liebman J, Zeno JA, Olshansky B, et al. Electrocardiographic body surface potential mapping in the Wolff-Parkinson-White syndrome: noninvasive determination of the ventricular insertion sites of accessory atrioventricular connections. *Circulation* 1991;83:886–901.

76. Dubuc M, Nadeau R, Tremblay G, et al. Pace mapping using body surface potential maps to guide catheter ablation of accessory pathways in patients with Wolff-Parkinson-White syndrome. *Circulation* 1993;87:135–143.

77. Worley SJ. Use of a real-time three-dimensional magnetic navigation system for radiofrequency ablation of accessory pathways. *Pacing Clin Electrophysiol* 1998;21:1636–1645.

78. Josephson ME, Scharf DL, Kastor JA, Kitchen JG III. Atrial endocardial activation in man. Electrode catheter technique for endocardial mapping. *Am J Cardiol* 1977;39:972–981.

79. Amat-y-Leon F, Dhingra R, Wu D, et al. Catheter mapping of retrograde atrial activation. Observations during ventricular pacing and A-V nodal reentrant paroxysmal tachycardia. *Br Heart J* 1976;38:355–362.

80. Jackman WM, Friday KJ, Fitzgerald DM, et al. Use of intracardiac recordings to determine the site of drug action in paroxysmal supraventricular tachycardia. *Am J Cardiol* 1988;62:8L–19L.

81. Benditt DG, Benson DW Jr, Dunnigan A, et al. Role of extrastimulus site and tachycardia cycle length in inducibility of atrial preexcitation by premature ventricular stimulation during reciprocating tachycardia. *Am J Cardiol* 1987;60:811–819.

82. Wellens HJJ, Durrer D. Relation between refractory period of the accessory pathway and ventricular frequency during atrial fibrillation in patients with the Wolff-Parkinson-White syndrome. *Am J Cardiol* 1974;33:178.

83. Wellens HJJ, Brugada P, Roy D, et al. Effect of isoproterenol on the antegrade refractory period of the accessory pathway in patients with the Wolff-Parkinson-White syndrome. *Am J Cardiol* 1982;50:180–184.

84. Helmy I, Scheinman MM, Herre JM, et al. Electrophysiologic effects of isoproterenol in patients with atrioventricular reentrant tachycardia treated with isoproterenol. *J Am Coll Cardiol* 1990;16:1649–1655.

85. Wellens HJJ, Braat S, Brugada P, et al. Use of procainamide in patients with the Wolff-Parkinson-White syndrome to disclose a short refractory period of the accessory pathway. *Am J Cardiol* 1982;50;1087–1089.

86. Wellens HJJ, Bar FW, Dassen WRM, et al. Effect of drugs in the Wolff-Parkinson-White syndrome: importance of initial length of effective refractory period of the accessory pathway. *Am J Cardiol* 1980;46:665–669.

87. Critelli G, Gallagher JJ, Perticone F, et al. Evaluation of noninvasive tests for identifying patients with preexcitation syndrome at risk of rapid ventricular response. *Am Heart J* 1984;108:905–909.

88. Fananapazir L, Packer DL, German LD, et al. Procainamide infusion test: inability to identify patients with Wolff-Parkinson-White syndrome who are at potential risk for sudden death. *Circulation* 1988;77:1291–1296.

89. Belardinelli L, Berne RM. The cardiac effects of adenosine. *Prog Cardiovasc Dis* 1989;32:73–97.

90. Dougherty AH, Gilman JK, Wiggins S, et al. Provocation of atrioventricular reentry tachycardia: a paradoxical effect of adenosine. *Pacing Clin Electrophysiol* 1993;16:8–12.

91. Brembilla-Perrot B, Ghawi P. Electrophysiological characteristics of asymptomatic Wolff-Parkinson-White syndrome. *Eur Heart J* 1993;14:511–515.

92. Green M, Heddle B, Dassen W, et al. Value of QRS alternation in determining the site of origin of narrow QRS supraventricular tachycardia. *Circulation* 1983;68:368–373.

93. Kay GN, Pressley JC, Packer DL, et al. Value of the 12-lead electrocardiogram in discriminating atrioventricular nodal reciprocating tachycardia from circus movement atrioventricular tachycardia utilizing a retrograde accessory pathway. *Am J Cardiol* 1987;59:296–300.

94. Tchou PJ, Lehmann MJ, Dongas J, et al. Effect of sudden rate acceleration on the human His-Purkinje system: adaptation of refractoriness in a damped oscillatory pattern. *Circulation* 1986; 73:920–929.

95. Nelson SD, Kou WH, Annesley T, et al. Significance of ST segment depression during paroxysmal supraventricular tachycardia. *J Am Coll Cardiol* 1988;12:383–387.

96. Riva SI, Della Bella P, Fassini G, et al. Value of analysis of ST segment changes during tachycardia in determining type of narrow QRS complex tachycardia. *J Am Coll Cardiol* 1996;27:1480.

97. Scheinman MM, Wang YS, Van Har GF, et al. Electrocardiographic and electrophysiologic characteristics of anterior, midseptal, and right anterior free wall accessory pathways. *J Am Coll Cardiol* 1992; 20:1220–1229.

98. Pritchett ELC, Tonkin AM, Dugan FA, et al. Ventriculo-atrial conduction time during reciprocating tachycardia with intermittent bundle branch block in Wolff-Parkinson-White syndrome. *Br Heart J* 1976;38:1058–1064.

99. Benditt DG, Benson DW Jr, Dunnigan A, et al. Role of extrastimulus site and tachycardia cycle length in inducibility of atrial preexcitation by premature ventricular stimulation during reciprocating tachycardia. *Am J Cardiol* 1987;60:811–819.

100. Ross DL, Farre J, Bar FWHM, et al. Spontaneous termination of circus movement tachycardia using an atrioventricular pathway: incidence, site of block and mechanism. *Circulation* 1981; 63:1129–1139.

101. Brugada P, Bar FWHM, Vanagt EJ, Wellens HJJ. Observations on mechanism of circus movement tachycardia in the Wolff-Parkinson-White syndrome: role of different tachycardia circuits and sites of block in maintenance of tachycardia. *Pacing Clin Electrophysiol* 1981;4:507–516.

102. Farre J, Ross D, Wiener I, et al. Reciprocal tachycardias using accessory pathways with long conduction times. *Am J Cardiol* 1979;44:1099–1109.

103. Brugada P, Farre J, Green M, et al. Observations in patients with supraventricular tachycardia having a P-R interval shorter than the R-P interval: differentiation between atrial tachycardia and reciprocating atrioventricular tachycardia using an accessory pathway with long conduction times. *Am Heart J* 1984; 107:556–570.

104. Rosenthal M, Oseran DS, Gant E, et al. Verapamil-induced retrograde conduction block in a concealed atrioventricular bypass tract. *Am J Cardiol* 1985;55:1222–1223.

105. Brugada P, Vanagt EJ, Bar FW, Wellens HJJ. Incessant reciprocating atrioventricular tachycardia: factors playing a role in the mechanism of the arrhythmia. *Pacing Clin Electrophysiol* 1980;3:670–677.

106. Critelli G, Gallagher JJ, Monda V, et al. Anatomic and electrophysiologic substrate in the permanent form of junctional reciprocating tachycardia. *Circulation* 1984;69:269–277.

107. Guarnieri T, Sealy WC, Kasell JH, et al. The non-pharmacologic management of the permanent form of junctional reciprocating tachycardia. *Circulation* 1984;69:269–277.

108. Ticho BS, Saul JP, Hulse JE, et al. Variable location of accessory pathways associated with the permanent form of junctional reciprocating tachycardia and confirmation with radiofrequency ablation. *Am J Cardiol* 1992;70:1559–1564.

109. Okumura K, Henthorn R, Epstein AE, et al. "Incessant" atrioventricular (AV) reciprocating tachycardia utilizing left lateral AV bypass pathway with a long retrograde conduction time. *Pacing Clin Electrophysiol* 1986;9:332–342.

110. Packer DL, Bardy GH, Worley SJ, et al. Tachycardia induced cardiomyopathy: a reversible form of left ventricular dysfunction. *Am J Cardiol* 1986;57:563–570.

111. Bardy GH, Packer DL, German LD, Gallagher JJ. Preexcited reciprocating tachycardia in patients with Wolff-Parkinson-White syndrome: incidence and mechanisms. *Circulation* 1984; 70:377–391.

112. Kuck K-H, Brugada P, Wellens HJJ. Observations on the antidromic type of circus movement tachycardia in the Wolff-Parkinson-White syndrome. *J Am Coll Cardiol* 1983;2: 1003–1010.

113. Mehta D, Wafa S, Ward DE, Camm AJ. Relative efficacy of various physical manoeuvres in the termination of junctional tachycardia. *Lancet* 1988;1(8596):1181–1185.

114. Rinkenberger RL, Prystowsky EN, Heger JJ, et al. Effects of intravenous and chronic oral verapamil administration in patients with supraventricular tachyarrhythmias. *Circulation* 1980;62:996–1010.

115. Sung RJ, Elser B, McAllister RG Jr. Intravenous verapamil for termination of reentrant supraventricular tachycardias: intracardiac studies correlated with plasma verapamil concentrations. *Ann Intern Med* 1980;93:682–689.

116. DiMarco JP, Sellers TD, Lerman BB, et al. Diagnostic and therapeutic use of adenosine in patients with supraventricular tachyarrhythmias. *J Am Coll Cardiol* 1985;6:417–425.

117. Dimarco JP, Sellers TD, Berne RM, et al. Adenosine: electrophysiologic effects and therapeutic use for terminating paroxysmal supraventricular tachycardia. *Circulation* 1983;68:1254–1263.

118. Dimarco JP, Miles W, Akhtar M, et al. Adenosine for paroxysmal supraventricular tachycardia: dose ranging and comparison with verapamil. *Ann Intern Med* 1990;113:104–110.

119. Kowey PR, Friehling TD, Marinchak RA. Electrophysiology of beta blockers in supraventricular arrhythmias. *Am J Cardiol* 1987;60:32D–38D.

120. Anderson S, Blanski L, Byrd RC, et al. Comparison of the efficacy and safety of esmolol, a short acting beta blocker with placebo in the treatment of supraventricular arrhythmias. *Am Heart J* 1986;111:42–48.

121. Smith TW. Digitalis: mechanisms of action and clinical use. *N Engl J Med* 1988;318:358–365.

122. Josephson ME, Caracta AR, Ricciutti MA, et al. Electrophysiological properties of procainamide in man. *Am J Cardiol* 1974;33:596–603.

123. Mandel WJ, Laks MM, Obayashi K, et al. The Wolff-Parkinson-White syndrome: pharmacologic effects of procainamide. *Am Heart J* 1975;90:744–754.

124. Wellens HJ. The wide QRS tachycardia. *Ann Intern Med* 1986;104(6):879.

125. Margolis B, DeSilva RA, Lown B. Episodic drug treatment in the management of paroxysmal arrhythmias. *Am J Cardiol* 1980;45:621–626.

126. Kim SS, Lal R, Ruffy R. Treatment of paroxysmal reentrant supraventricular tachycardia with flecainide acetate. *Am J Cardiol* 1986;58:80–85.

127. Ward DE, Jones S, Shinebourne EA. Use of flecainide acetate

for refractory junctional tachycardias in children with Wolff-Parkinson-White syndrome. *Am J Cardiol* 1986;57:787–790.

128. Prystowsky EN, Klein GJ, Rinkenberger RL, et al. Clinical efficacy and electrophysiologic effects of encainide in patients with the Wolff-Parkinson-White syndrome. *Circulation* 1984;69: 278–287.

129. Kunze K-P, Kuck K-H, Schluter M, et al. Electrophysiologic and clinical effects of intravenous and oral encainide in accessory atrioventricular pathway. *Am J Cardiol* 1984;54:323–329.

130. Ludmer PL, McGowan NE, Antman EM, Friedman PL. Efficacy of propafenone in Wolff-Parkinson-White syndrome: electrophysiologic findings and long-term followup. *J Am Coll Cardiol* 1987;9:1357–1363.

131. Musto B, D'Onofio A, Cavallaro C, Musto A. Electro-physiological effects and clinical efficacy of propafenone in children with recurrent paroxysmal supraventricular tachycardia. *Circulation* 1988;78:863–869.

132. Manolis AS, Estes NAM III. Reversal of electro-physiologic effects of flecainide on the accessory pathway by isoproterenol in the Wolff-Parkinson-White syndrome. *Am J Cardiol* 1989; 64:194–198.

133. Kerr CR, Prystowsky EN, Smith WM, et al. Electrophysiological effects of disopyramide phosphate in patients with Wolff-Parkinson-White syndrome. *Circulation* 1982;65:869–878.

134. Wellens HJJ, Durrer D. Effects of procainamide, quinidine, and ajmaline in the Wolff-Parkinson-White syndrome. *Circulation* 1974;50:114–120.

135. Mason JW. Amiodarone. *N Engl J Med* 1987;316:455–466.

136. Rosenbaum MD, Chiale PA, Ryba D, Elizari MV. Control of tachyarrhythmias associated with Wolff-Parkinson-White syndrome by amiodarone hydrochloride. *Am J Cardiol* 1974;34: 215–223.

137. Wellens HJJ, Lie KI, Bar FW, et al. Effect of amiodarone in the Wolff-Parkinson-White syndrome. *Am J Cardiol* 1976;38: 189–194.

138. Feld GK, Nademanee K, Weiss J, et al. Electrophysiologic basis for the suppression by amiodarone of orthodromic supraventricular tachycardia complicating pre-excitation syndromes. *J Am Coll Cardiol* 1984;3:1298–1307.

139. Kowey PR, Friehling TD, Marinchak RA, et al. Safety and efficacy of amiodarone: the low dose perspective. *Chest* 1988;93:54–59.

140. Hamer AWF, Arkles LB, Johns JA. Beneficial effects of low dose amiodarone in patients with congestive heart failure: a placebo-controlled trial. *J Am Coll Cardiol* 1989;14:1768–1774.

141. Mitchell LB, Wyse G, Duff HJ. Electropharmacology of sotalol in patients with Wolff-Parkinson-White syndrome. *Circulation* 1987;76:810–818.

142. Kunze KP, Schluter M, Kuck KH. Sotalol in patients with Wolff-Parkinson-White syndrome. *Circulation* 1987;75:1050–1057.

143. Bianconi L, Boccadamo R, Pappalardo A, et al. Effectiveness of intravenous propafenone for conversion of atrial fibrillation and flutter of recent onset. *Am J Cardiol* 1989;64:335–338.

144. Suttorp MJ, Kingma JH, Jessurun ER, et al. The value of class IC antiarrhythmic drugs for acute conversion of paroxysmal atrial fibrillation or flutter to sinus rhythm. *J Am Coll Cardiol* 1990;16:1722–1727.

145. Suttorp MJ, Kingma JH, Lie-A-Huen L, Mast EG. Intravenous flecainide versus verapamil for acute conversion of paroxysmal atrial fibrillation or flutter to sinus rhythm. *Am J Cardiol* 1989; 63:693–696.

146. Varriale P, Sedighi A, Mirzaietehrane M. Ibutilide for termination of atrial fibrillation in the Wolff-Parkinson-White syndrome. *Pacing Clin Electrophysiol* 1999; 22:1267.

147. Sellers TD Jr, Bashore TM, Gallagher JJ. Digitalis in preexcitation syndrome: analysis during atrial fibrillation. *Circulation* 1977;56:260–267.

148. Garratt C, Antoniou A, Ward D, Camm AJ. Misuse of verapamil in pre-excited atrial fibrillation. *Lancet* 1989;1(8634): 367–369.

149. Gulamhusein S, Ko P, Carruthers SG, Klein GJ. Acceleration of the ventricular response during atrial fibrillation in the Wolff-Parkinson-White syndrome after verapamil. *Circulation* 1982; 348–354.

150. McGovern B, Garan H, Ruskin JN. Precipitation of cardiac arrest by verapamil in patients with Wolff-Parkinson-White syndrome. *Ann Intern Med* 1986;104:791–794.

151. Chouty F, Coumel P. Oral flecainide for prophylaxis of paroxysmal atrial fibrillation. *Am J Cardiol* 1988;62:35D–37D.

152. Antman EM, Beamer AD, Cantillon C, et al. Long-term oral propafenone therapy for suppression of refractory symptomatic atrial fibrillation and atrial flutter. *J Am Coll Cardiol* 1988;12: 1005–1011 [published erratum appears in *J Am Coll Cardiol* 1989;13:26].

153. Southworth MR, Zarembski D, Viana M, Bauman J. Comparison of sotalol versus quinidine for maintenance of normal sinus rhythm in patients with chronic atrial fibrillation. *Am J Cardiol* 1999; 83:1629–1632.

154. Singh S, Berk M, Yellen L, et al. Efficacy and safety of oral dofetilide in maintaining normal sinus rhythm in patients with atrial fibrillation/flutter: a multicentre study. *Eur Heart J* 1998; 19[Suppl]:363(abst).

155. Greenbaum R, Campbell TJ, Channer KS, et al, for the EMERALD Investigators. Conversion of AF and maintenance of sinus rhythm by dofetilide. *Eur Heart J* 1998; 19[Suppl]:661(abst).

156. Kappenberger LJ, Fromer MA, Steinbrunn W, Shenasa M. Efficacy of amiodarone in the Wolff-Parkinson-White syndrome with rapid ventricular response via the accessory pathway during atrial fibrillation. *Am J Cardiol* 1984;54:330–335.

157. Feld GK, Nademanee K, Stevenson W, et al. Clinical and electrophysiologic effects of amiodarone in patients with atrial fibrillation complicating the Wolff-Parkinson-White syndrome. *Am Heart J* 1988;115:102–107.

158. Crawford W, Plumb VJ, Epstein AE, Kay GN. Prospective evaluation of transesophageal pacing for the interruption of atrial flutter. *Am J Med* 1989;86:663–667.

159. Lau CP, Cornu E, Camm AJ. Fatal and nonfatal cardiac arrest in patients with an implanted antitachycardia device for the treatment of supraventricular tachycardia. *Am J Cardiol* 1988; 61:919–921.

160. DeBelder MA, Malik M, Ward DE, Camm AJ. Pacing modalities for tachycardia termination. *Pacing Clin Electrophysiol* 1990; 13:231–248.

161. Naccarelli GV, Zipes DP, Rahilly GT, et al. Influence of tachycardia cycle length and antiarrhythmic drugs on pacing termination and acceleration of ventricular tachycardia. *Am Heart J* 1983;105:1–5.

162. Olshansky B, Okumura K, Hess PR, et al. Use of procainamide with rapid atrial pacing for successful conversion of atrial flutter to sinus rhythm. *J Am Coll Cardiol* 1988;11:359–364.

163. Fisher JD, Kim SG, Mercando AD. Electrical devices for the treatment of arrhythmias. *Am J Cardiol* 1988;61:45A–57A.

164. Scheinman MM. Catheter ablation for cardiac arrhythmias, personnel, and facilities. *Pacing Clin Electrophysiol* 1992;15: 715–721.

165. Kay GN, Epstein AE, Dailey SM, Plumb VJ. Role of radiofrequency ablation in the management of supraventricular arrhythmias: experience in 760 consecutive patients. *J Cardiovasc Electrophysiol* 1993;4:371–398.

166. Calkins H, Yong P, Miller JM, et al. Catheter ablation of accessory pathways, atrioventricular nodal reentrant tachycardia, and the atrioventricular junction. *Circulation* 1999;99: 262–270.

167. Worley SJ. Use of a real-time three dimensional magnetic navigational system for radiofrequency ablation of accessory pathways. *Pacing Clin Electrophysiol* 1998;21:1636.

168. Calkins H, Langberg J, Sousa J. Radiofrequency catheter ablation of accessory atrioventricular connection in 250 patients: abbreviated therapeutic approach to Wolff-Parkinson-White syndrome. *Circulation* 1992; 85:1337–1346.

169. de Buitleir M, Sousa J, Bolling SF, et al. Reduction in medical care cost associated with radiofrequency catheter ablation of accessory pathways. *Am J Cardiol* 1991;68:1656–166.

170. Hogenhuis W, Stevens SK, Wang P, et al. Cost-effectiveness of radiofrequency ablation compared with other strategies in Wolff-Parkinson-White syndrome. *Circulation* 1993;88[Pt 2]:II-437–446.

18

VENTRICULAR PREMATURE DEPOLARIZATIONS AND NONSUSTAINED VENTRICULAR TACHYCARDIA

ALFRED E. BUXTON
JAMES DUC

Ventricular premature depolarizations (VPDs) occur commonly. Nonsustained ventricular tachycardia (NSVT) occurs less often. Both entities are seen in a broad spectrum of patients, ranging from subjects with no heart disease to those with severe cardiac dysfunction. The management of patients with VPDs or NSVT poses unique challenges to the clinician. Unlike most arrhythmias that a physician encounters, VPDs and NSVT are frequently not associated with symptoms. However, in some settings, these arrhythmias are associated with increased risk for sudden death. Before the physician initiates therapy or pursues further evaluation, it is necessary to examine the therapeutic goals. Is the aim to make the patient feel better by controlling symptoms, or is the goal to prolong life because of a perceived mortality risk associated with the arrhythmia? It is not always easy to determine whether an arrhythmia is responsible for symptoms, and prolonged ambulatory electrocardiographic (ECG) monitoring may be required to document an association. Even if an association between one of these arrhythmias and symptoms is documented, the decision to initiate antiarrhythmic therapy must be tempered by the realization that pharmacologic antiarrhythmic therapy may relieve symptoms but can increase mortality in the presence of certain types of cardiac disease. When dealing with one of these arrhythmias, it is axiomatic that the physician treat the patient, not the electrocardiogram.

ELECTROCARDIOGRAPHIC CHARACTERISTICS

VPDs and NSVT may be discovered during physical examination or by ECG monitoring of ambulatory patients or during in-hospital telemetry. VPDs are recognized by their ECG appearance. The ECG characteristics of a VPD include a QRS duration of at least 120 ms, bizarre morphology, and a T wave in the opposite direction from the main QRS vector. However, a VPD originating from the contralateral ventricle in a patient with a preexisting bundle branch block may result in a QRS complex narrower than that of the sinus and a pseudo-normalized T wave in a patient with a prior myocardial infarction. Their origin in the ventricular myocardium below the specialized conduction system accounts for the abnormal morphology. The increase in width of the QRS complex is explained in part by ventricular electrical activation spreading from myofibril to myofibril, a process that is inherently slower than activation spread using the His-Purkinje system. Depending on the presence and type of structural cardiac disease and on the site of origin of the VPD within the ventricle, the spread of activation may involve the His-Purkinje system to a variable extent, and this spread using the specialized conduction system can modulate the QRS width.

VPDs may be followed by pauses, and the pause may or may not be fully compensatory. If the VPD conducts retrogradely to the atrium and resets the sinus node, the pause will not be fully compensatory. If the VPD does not conduct retrogradely, and the AV node is refractory at the time of the next sinus impulse, a fully compensatory pause results (i.e., the R-R interval surrounding the VPD is twice the sinus R-R interval). An interpolated VPD is one that does not affect the underlying ventricular rate because its

A.E. Buxton and J. Duc: Division of Cardiology, Brown University School of Medicine, Providence, Rhode Island 02912.

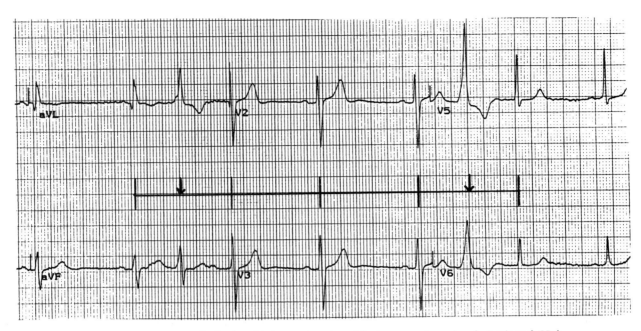

FIGURE 18-1. Sinus arrhythmia with interpolated ventricular premature depolarizations (VPDs). The underlying sinus rate is unaffected by the presence of the VPD. The P-R interval after the VPDs is prolonged, an indication of concealed conduction, most likely into the atrioventricular node.

timing is such that the function of the sinus node and AV conduction system are not disturbed (Fig. 18-1). Multifocal premature ventricular contractions may originate from various sites or may originate from one site if there are differing exit points into the ventricular myocardium or changes in the pattern or direction of myocardial activation. VPDs may have coupling intervals fixed to the preceding beat,

which is usually thought to indicate a reentrant mechanism. Other VPDs have variable coupling to the preceding sinus complex. This finding suggests parasystole, an independently discharging, autonomous focus. Parasystole may be caused by an automatic or triggered mechanism, may be modulated by other coincident cardiac rhythms, or may be irregular because of exit block (Fig. 18-2). Exit block may

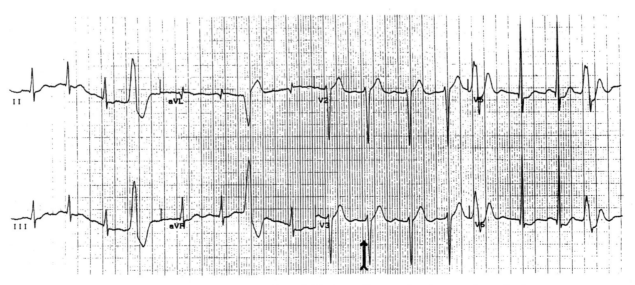

FIGURE 18-2. Ventricular parasystole. The exit block manifests as the absence of an ectopic complex determined by the prior interectopic intervals *(arrow)*.

result from variable conduction in the tissue causing the ectopic rhythm itself or from refractoriness of ventricular myocardium surrounding the parasystolic focus, and therefore no evidence of ventricular activation manifests electrocardiographically. The focus may appear to be independent and not influenced by external impulses, exhibiting apparent entrance block. In other cases, the behavior of the ectopic rhythm may be modulated by other impulses.

VPDs that begin at or near the apex of the T wave are said to exhibit the R on T phenomenon (Fig. 18-3). Although Wolff and Lown originally described the phenomenon as carrying a grave prognosis because of the association with ventricular fibrillation, much of their work was based on their experience in the basic laboratory where dogs were rendered ischemic by coronary artery occlusion or in patients with an acute myocardial infarction who were in the cardiac care unit (1). Since that original description, several studies have shown that late-coupled VPDs are at least as likely to initiate repetitive ventricular arrhythmia in humans (2–5). However, these studies did not involve patients with acute ischemia, and they evaluated the association between early or late VPDs and ventricular tachycardia, not ventricular fibrillation. The R on T VPD may have importance and is associated with a risk of ventricular fibrillation in a patient with ongoing ischemia.

Several specific VPD patterns have been described. *Ventricular bigeminy* refers to a persistent alternation of normal and premature beats (Fig. 18-4). Because the coupling intervals between normal and ectopic beats are constant, it is assumed that the mechanism is reentry. When bigeminy occurs in patients with compromised ventricular function, especially in patients with an intrinsically slow sinus rate, the alternating loss of an effective contraction can cause hemodynamic embarrassment. This is one of the few situations in which VPDs may compromise cardiac output. Trigeminal and quadrigemal patterns have also been described but rarely cause severe symptoms and have no known independent prognostic importance.

The pause after a VPD or retrograde concealment into one of the bundle branches resulting from a VPD may

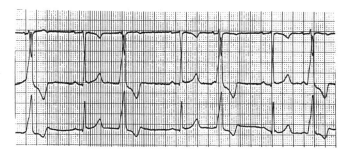

FIGURE 18-4. Ventricular bigeminy.

allow normal conduction of the subsequent supraventricular beat (Fig. 18-5). This normalization may permit the diagnosis of otherwise covert conditions. VPDs with a qR pattern may unmask an infarction otherwise not obvious in supraventricular complexes (Fig.18- 6).

NSVT is most commonly defined as a run of three or more consecutive ventricular complexes at a rate greater than 100 bpm that terminates spontaneously within 30 seconds. Although this definition sets arbitrary limits, it is useful by providing a framework within which to communicate. Episodes of NSVT typically are brief, lasting 3 to 10 beats (6–12). Ventricular rates usually range from 100 to 200 bpm.

The frequency with which episodes of NSVT occur seems to be influenced by the type of underlying heart disease. Most patients with coronary artery disease and prior myocardial infarction have infrequent episodes of NSVT, usually one or two daily (10,12–14). This also appears to be true of patients with hypertrophic cardiomyopathy (8,15). In contrast, in patients with nonischemic dilated cardiomyopathy, NSVT tends to occur with a higher frequency, typically two or more episodes detected over 24 hours (8,16,17). Patients with NSVT tend to have a higher fre-

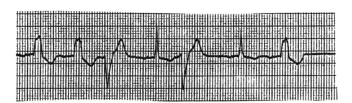

FIGURE 18-5. Example of a ventricular premature depolarization (VPD) causing normalization of the following QRS complex. The patient has an underlying left bundle branch block (LBBB). A VPD (third beat) is followed by a compensatory pause and a QRS complex that has a narrow (normalized) QRS complex. Another VPD is followed by a normal QRS complex and then a QRS with a LBBB. This patient has a rate-related LBBB, and when the rate is slower, ventricular conduction is normal.

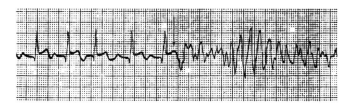

FIGURE 18-3. R on T ventricular premature depolarization initiating ventricular fibrillation.

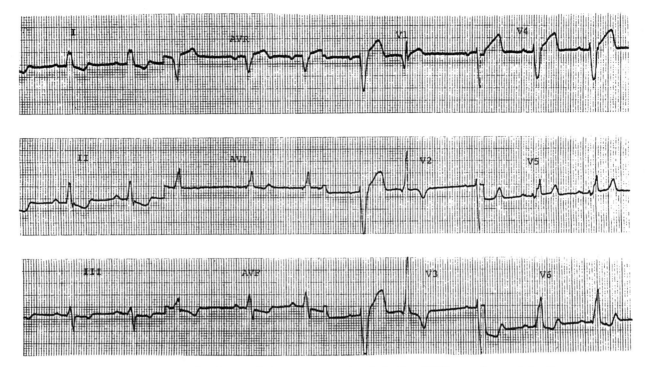

FIGURE 18-6. Example of a ventricular premature depolarization (VPD) revealing an infarction pattern. The underlying rhythm is sinus with a complete left bundle branch block (LBBB). In leads V₁ through V₃, a VPD having a QR pattern suggests a previous anterior myocardial infarction not otherwise evident because of the LBBB.

quency of isolated VPDs when compared with patients without NSVT (10,13,18).

As is the case with sustained ventricular tachycardia, most episodes of NSVT are initiated with late-coupled VPDs (4,6,9–11,18,19) (Fig. 18-7). In general, there appears to be no association between the ambient sinus rate and the initiation of NSVT (6,8,10,11).

The ECG morphology of NSVT may be uniform and constant or can be polymorphic, varying constantly during individual episodes. There does not appear to be any relationship between the morphologic characteristics and the

type of underlying heart disease, with two exceptions. First, when episodes of NSVT arise during acute myocardial ischemia, they often appear polymorphic. Episodes of ventricular tachycardia associated with the long QT syndrome are also typically polymorphic (Fig. 18-8). Second, a unique subtype of NSVT, which usually appears in persons without obvious structural heart disease, has a left bundle branch block pattern with an inferior frontal plane axis (20–22) (Fig. 18-9). Patients with this arrhythmia exhibit a range of arrhythmias, including isolated ventricular premature complexes, nonsustained tachycardia episodes, and rarely, sustained ventricular tachycardia, all having this same morphology. In some patients, this arrhythmia occurs as periods of incessant NSVT, characteristic of the syndrome of repetitive monomorphic ventricular tachycardia. Consistent with this ECG appearance is the demonstration by endocardial catheter mapping that this tachycardia originates in the right ventricular outflow tract (21).

CLINICAL MANIFESTATIONS

The most common symptoms resulting from VPDs and NSVT are palpitations. These seem to result from the hypercontractility of the postectopic beat or a feeling that

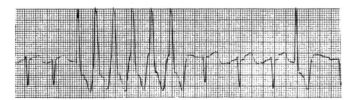

FIGURE 18-7. Typical episode of nonsustained ventricular tachycardia in a patient with chronic coronary artery disease. The tachycardia appears to have a uniform morphology in this single monitor lead. The initial complex of the arrhythmia is a late-coupled ventricular premature beat.

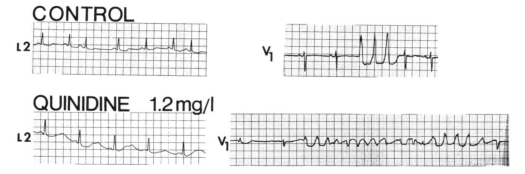

FIGURE 18-8. Polymorphic ventricular tachycardia resulting from quinidine-induced long QT syndrome. The top tracings were recorded in the baseline state in the absence of antiarrhythmic drugs. The patient had asymptomatic, brief runs of nonsustained ventricular tachycardia that appeared monomorphic in lead V_1. After initiation of quinidine therapy, the patient developed longer runs of polymorphic ventricular tachycardia. Electrocardiographic recordings from leads 2 (L_2) and V_1 are shown in the baseline state and after initiation of quinidine. Notice the marked prolongation of the QT interval in the presence of quinidine.

the heart has stopped because of the postectopic pause. VPDs and NSVT can also cause a pounding sensation in the neck, lightheadedness, or near syncope. NSVT may cause syncope if the rate and duration are prolonged sufficiently to cause a marked decrease in cerebral blood flow. There is great variability in when the symptoms are most prominent, although a quiet environment, such as at night before sleep, may make patients more aware of their ectopy. VPDs and NSVT arising from the right ventricle are provoked by exercise in some patients (21). The palpitations that the patient feels may provoke anxiety that many times causes a vicious cycle of palpitations, anxiety, catecholamine

surges, and more ectopy. Affected patients may report dizziness that is not related to any fall in cerebral perfusion pressure or blood flow.

VPDs may facilitate the diagnosis of certain cardiac conditions. For example, patients who have hypertrophic obstructive cardiomyopathy have an increased outflow tract gradient during the more forceful contraction that follows the compensatory pause. Dubbed the Brockenbrough sign, it can be responsible for an increase in the intensity of the heart murmur characteristic of this entity, as well as for an increase in the gradient as measured in the echocardiography or catheterization laboratory (23) (Fig. 18-10). VPDs

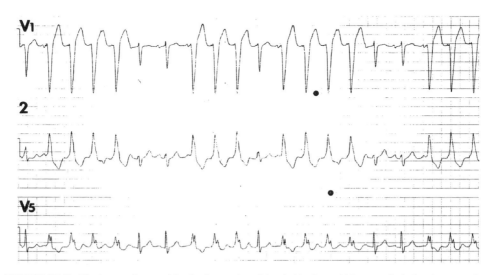

FIGURE 18-9. Electrocardiographic rhythm strip of leads V_1, 2, and V_5 recorded simultaneously. The morphology is typical of tachycardia originating in the right ventricular outflow tract in a patient without structural heart disease: left bundle branch pattern with an inferiorly directed frontal plane QRS axis. The pattern is typical of repetitive monomorphic ventricular tachycardia. Notice that the sinus QRS complexes have a normal pattern.

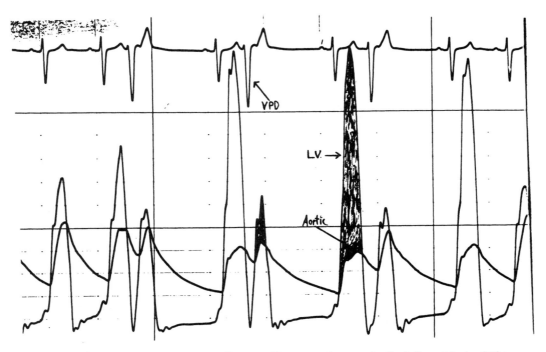

FIGURE 18-10. The Brockenbrough effect manifests as an increase in the left ventricular (LV) to aortic gradient on the beat after a ventricular premature depolarization.

may precipitate pulsus alternans, a marker of severe left ventricular dysfunction.

PREVALENCE

The prevalence of VPDs and NSVT is directly related to the detection methods and to the patient population studied. On a resting 12-lead ECG, less than 5% of patients with no known heart disease have been found to have VPDs (24,25). When the ECG is sampled for longer periods, such as using 24-hour continuous ambulatory monitoring, VPDs are found in 50% of apparently healthy individuals (26,27), suggesting that VPD frequency is a function of sampling time. The prevalence of NSVT depends on the presence, type, and severity of underlying heart disease (Table 18-1). NSVT is recorded during 24-hour monitoring in 0% to 3% of healthy, asymptomatic subjects, without a significant difference between men and women (27–36).

Aging appears to increase the prevalence of VPDs and NSVT, independent of the presence of heart disease (24,27,37). In one analysis, 11% of apparently healthy elderly subjects demonstrated NSVT during 24-hour monitoring (37). The prevalence of VPDs and NSVT in patients with coronary artery disease depends on the stage of the disease in which monitoring is performed. The prevalence of ectopy and NSVT is greatest within 48 hours of acute infarction, when up to 90% of patients have ectopy and 45% exhibit NSVT (38,39). After the first 48 hours, during the first month after myocardial infarction, the prevalence of NSVT dropped to 7% from 16% in the prethrombolytic era (9–12,15,40) (Table 18-2). In the presence of thrombolytic therapy, 6.8% of patients had NSVT on 24-hour monitoring 2 weeks after infarction (41). The incidence then remained fairly constant over the first year after infarction (11).

TABLE 18-1. PREVALENCE OF NONSUSTAINED VENTRICULAR TACHYCARDIA IN ASYMPTOMATIC SUBJECTS

Study	Type of Subjects	Frequency (%)
Hinkle et al. (28)	Middle-aged men	3.2
Califf et al. (36)	No coronary disease on angiography	0
Romhilt et al. (34)	Healthy women	1
Pilcher et al. (33)	Healthy runners	1
Kantelip et al. (29)	All elderly (age >80 years)	2

TABLE 18-2. PREVALENCE OF NONSUSTAINED VENTRICULAR TACHYCARDIA IN THE LATE HOSPITAL PHASE OF MYOCARDIAL INFARCTION

Study	VT Frequency (%)	Time of Recording from Onset of MI (days)
Vismara et al. (87)	8	11
Anderson et al. (9)	7	14
Kleiger et al. (93)	12	28
Bigger et al. (10)	12	10–20
Maggioni et al. (41)	6.8	17

MI, myocardial infarction; VT, ventricular tachycardia.

The prevalence and type of ectopy are related to the degree of left ventricular dysfunction in ambulatory patients. As the left ventricular ejection fraction progressively decreases, the prevalence of ventricular ectopy and NSVT increases (36). Among ambulatory patients with coronary disease, 5% have NSVT on 24 hours of monitoring, but the incidence increases to about 15% of patients with ejection fractions of less than 0.40 (37). Conversely, about 75% of patients with NSVT have ejection fractions of less than 0.40 (37).

NSVT and ventricular ectopy occur infrequently in patients with hypertensive left ventricular hypertrophy (2% to 12%) and rheumatic heart disease (7%) when these processes are not complicated by congestive heart failure (8,42,43). NSVT occurs much more often (17% to 28%) in patients with idiopathic hypertrophic cardiomyopathy (8,14,44–48) (Table 18-3). The presence of NSVT in patients with idiopathic hypertrophic cardiomyopathy is not related to pulmonary capillary wedge pressure or the degree of obstruction but may be related to septal thickness (46,49–51).

TABLE 18-3. PREVALENCE OF NONSUSTAINED VENTRICULAR TACHYCARDIA IN PATIENTS WITH CARDIOMYOPATHY

Study	Type of Subjects	Frequency (%)
Savage et al. (46)	HCM	19
Mulrow et al. (44)	HCM	22
Huang et al. (19)	DCM	60
Suyama et al. (8)	DCM	46
Neri et al. (16)	DCM	43
Olshausen et al. (52)	DCM	42
Singh et al. (54)	DCM	80
Doval et al. (53)	DCM	33.5

DCM, dilated cardiomyopathy; HCM, hypertrophic cardiomyopathy.

The highest prevalence of ventricular ectopy and NSVT is seen in patients with nonischemic dilated cardiomyopathy. In this case, almost all patients have ventricular ectopy, and about one half have NSVT (8,16,17,19,52) (Table 18-3). Some of these studies correlated an increased prevalence with more advanced disease. A difficulty in interpreting the true prevalence of ectopy and NSVT in patients with idiopathic dilated cardiomyopathy is that many of these studies included patients with heart failure, without accurately distinguishing between coronary and noncoronary disease as the cause. Trials of patients with congestive heart failure documented NSVT in 30% to 80% of patients (53–55). Several factors have been implicated as contributing to the occurrence of ventricular arrhythmias in patients with ventricular dysfunction and heart failure, including the presence of localized fibrosis, abnormal wall stress, heightened sympathetic tone, and electrolyte abnormalities.

Ventricular arrhythmias in patients with valvular heart disease and well-preserved left ventricular function are uncommon. The most common valvular lesion associated with VPDs is mitral valve prolapse, and frequent or complex ventricular ectopy has been reported in 43% to 56% of adults based on ambulatory monitoring (56). The occurrence of NSVT in this setting correlates best with the presence of mitral regurgitation (57). Postulated mechanisms for ventricular ectopy include abnormal tension on the papillary muscles, mechanical irritation of the endocardium by thickened chordae tendineae, alterations in autonomic tone or circulating catecholamines, and abnormalities of repolarization.

In congenital heart disease, ventricular ectopy can result from the primary defect or as a result of surgical repair. VPDs occur commonly in patients with poor right ventricular hemodynamics (58,59). The one congenital defect consistently associated with frequent ventricular ectopy is repaired tetralogy of Fallot.

There is diurnal variability of VPD frequency; they are more common in the morning than during the night. For this reason, at least 24 hours of ambulatory monitoring are necessary to document and quantitate VPDs. There are wide hourly and daily fluctuations in the absolute number of VPDs and occurrence of NSVT on ambulatory ECG recording (60–65). As a result of this enormous random variability, a single 24-hour monitoring session may fail to detect NSVT in patients having the arrhythmia at other times. This limits the utility of 24-hour monitoring periods for risk stratification, and it makes assessment of the effects of an intervention, such as pharmacologic antiarrhythmic therapy, on suppression of spontaneous ventricular arrhythmias subject to error, unless prolonged periods of monitoring in the baseline state are performed (Table 18-4). Random variability in the frequency of all forms of ventricular ectopy (e.g., isolated VPDs, couplets and runs of NSVT) is common (61).

TABLE 18-4. VARIABILITY OF ARRHYTHMIA: MINIMAL REDUCTION NECESSARY TO DEFINE DRUG EFFICACY

Study	N	Interval between Monitoring	Minimal Reduction (%)		
			VPDs	Couplets	NSVT
Michelson and Morganroth (61)	20	1 d		75	65
Pratt et al. (64)	110	1 d	78	83	77
Pratt et al. (65)	26	17 mo	50	65	83
Toivonen (62)	20	4 d–9 mo	65–100	78–100	
Anastttasiou-Nana et al. (63)	47	1 d	55	75[a]	
		1 wk	85	95[a]	
		2 wk	86	92[a]	
		3 wk	93	95[a]	
		4 wk	96	94[a]	
		>1 y	96	98[a]	
		No. of control monitoring days			
Morganroth et al. (60)	15	1 d	83		
		3 d	73		
		7 d	49		

NSVT, nonsustained ventricular tachycardia; VPDs, ventricular premature depolarizations.
[a]Repetitive forms.

MECHANISMS

The mechanisms responsible for the genesis of VPDs and NSVT probably are similar to the mechanisms that cause sustained tachyarrhythmias, but there is little direct evidence supporting the various mechanisms in humans. Much of our information regarding mechanisms of these arrhythmias has been derived indirectly from observations of spontaneous arrhythmia patterns. Animal studies have shown that VPDs may arise because of abnormalities in impulse generation, conduction, or both (66). Abnormal automaticity refers to spontaneous depolarization occurring when the resting cell membranes are partially depolarized. Such conditions arise in the presence of electrolyte abnormalities or acute ischemia and may be enhanced by endogenous or exogenous catecholamines. These conditions favor a lowering of the diastolic transmembrane voltage, resulting in premature depolarization. The principal site of VPD development caused by abnormal automaticity is the Purkinje fiber layer.

Triggered activity seems to be responsible for VPD and NSVT development in two principal clinical settings. Early afterdepolarizations arising in Purkinje cells or ventricular myocardium are responsible for the initiation of most episodes of polymorphic ventricular tachycardia (i.e., torsade de pointes) associated with congenital and acquired long QT syndrome (67). If repetitive firing allows these afterdepolarizations to reach threshold potential, VPDs and NSVT can be generated that under the proper conditions may perpetuate, sometimes in a reentrant pattern (68). The second setting in which triggered activity appears to be responsible for VPDs and NSVT is the syndrome of right ventricular outflow tract arrhythmias (69). Most of these tachycardias are suppressed by adenosine. This information, combined with the response of the arrhythmia to other pharmacologic agents and to pacing, suggests that the mechanism is triggered activity mediated by increased intracellular levels of cyclic AMP (yielding increased levels of intracellular calcium ions) (70).

Other settings in which experimental data suggest focal, nonreentrant mechanisms underlying NSVT are nonischemic and ischemic dilated cardiomyopathies. NSVT in a rabbit model of dilated cardiomyopathy appears to originate in the subendocardium (71). Likewise, similar mechanisms seem to be operative in a canine model of ischemic cardiomyopathy (72). The relation of these observations to clinical arrhythmias is not clear.

Reentrant VPDs occur in the setting of conduction delay and unidirectional block that are characteristically seen in patients with a healed myocardial infarction. A wavefront may perpetuate under the correct set of circumstances, such as the administration of drugs that prolong conduction. It seems likely that reentry also accounts for NSVT in the setting of chronic coronary artery disease. Subjects with NSVT and coronary artery disease have endocardial activation abnormalities that are a reflection of slow conduction, one of the prerequisites for reentry (73). These abnormalities are similar to those found in patients with spontaneous sustained ventricular tachycardia occurring after myocardial infarction. Even in this setting, the mechanisms responsible for NSVT identified in experimental models may differ from those responsible for inducible and spontaneous sustained ventricular tachycardia.

A combination of abnormalities of conduction and impulse generation can provoke parasystole. An automatic or triggered focus in one of the ventricles fires at a rate independent of the sinus mechanism. The focus is expressed when the sinus impulse does not penetrate this site of ventricular activity or its surrounding myocardium (i.e., entrance block); the myocardium can therefore be activated by the parasystolic impulse. However, the parasystolic focus may be modulated, entrained, or annihilated by the sinus mechanism, therefore not always displaying its classic features (74) (Fig. 18-2). The outcome of these interfering factors includes a variation in the parasystolic rate, its transient disappearance, or its abrupt termination.

PROGNOSTIC SIGNIFICANCE

The prognostic significance of VPDs and NSVT depends on the presence, type, and severity of underlying heart disease. However, it is not clear in most cases whether episodes of NSVT have a cause-and-effect relationship with the sustained ventricular tachycardias that are known to precipitate sudden death or whether they merely reflect an epiphenomenon indicating overall poor cardiac function.

Ventricular Premature Depolarizations and Nonsustained Ventricular Tachycardia in a Normal Population

The presence of ventricular ectopy and NSVT in apparently healthy individuals does not correlate with an increased risk for sudden death (36,75). This lack of association extends to the elderly as well (37). There does not appear to be any association with right ventricular outflow tract tachycardia and sudden death in otherwise healthy subjects (21,22,76,77).

Ventricular Premature Depolarizations and Nonsustained Ventricular Tachycardia in Patients with Nonischemic Dilated Cardiomyopathy

In general, patients with dilated cardiomyopathy are at considerable risk of sudden death and overall cardiac mortality, with 1-year mortality rates reported as high as 40% to 50% (19,78–81). The prognostic significance of VPDs and NSVT is variable, with little evidence that the occurrence of these arrhythmias is related specifically to an increased risk for sudden death, although they do correlate with increased overall cardiac mortality (16,17,19,32,53–55,78–81) (Table 18-5 and Fig. 18-11). This lack of association may result from the ubiquitous nature of NSVT in this population and the high overall mortality rates. However, one study of patients with congestive heart failure found an excess risk of sudden death among patients with NSVT (53) (Fig. 18-12).

TABLE 18-5. PROGNOSTIC SIGNIFICANCE OF NONSUSTAINED VENTRICULAR TACHYCARDIA IN PATIENTS WITH IDIOPATHIC DILATED CARDIOMYOPATHY

Study	Patients with NSVT: Cardiac Deaths That Were Sudden (%)	Patients without NSVT: Cardiac Deaths That Were Sudden (%)
Huang et al. (19)	50	100
Unverferth et al. (80)	100	100
Neri et al. (16)	9	43
Olshausen et al. (52)	33	80
Doval et al. (53)	47	28

NSVT, nonsustained ventricular tachycardia.

Ventricular Premature Depolarizations and Nonsustained Ventricular Tachycardia in Patients with Hypertrophic Cardiomyopathy

Patients with left ventricular hypertrophy (LVH) have more ventricular ectopy and are at increased risk of sudden cardiac death compared with individuals with hypertension and no hypertrophy. The Framingham Study demonstrated an eightfold increase in cardiovascular mortality in patients with LVH and a doubling of this risk with ECG evidence of repolarization abnormalities (82). This relationship exists independent of coexisting coronary artery disease (83). In patients with only echocardiographic evidence of LVH, the tendency to increased ventricular ectopy has not been as consistent (43,84).

Sudden death is a significant cause of mortality for patients with idiopathic hypertrophic cardiomyopathy, with a yearly incidence of 2% to 3% in selected referral populations (85). There is a 70% chance of discovering NSVT in patients who have experienced syncope or survived cardiac arrest, compared with a 20% prevalence in those without such a history (14,85). For patients with hypertrophic cardiomyopathy and NSVT, the yearly sudden death mortality rate is reported to be 8% to 10%, compared with 1% for patients without NSVT (14,85). Unfortunately, most reports of patients with hypertrophic cardiomyopathy have originated from two specialized centers and are based on highly selected referral populations. It may be difficult to extrapolate these data to individual patients. A closer approximation of the risks in more general populations may be derived from a study in Italy, which reported over an average follow-up period of 4.8 years, a sudden death incidence of 1.4% yearly for patients with NSVT versus 0.6% for patients without ventricular tachycardia (86).

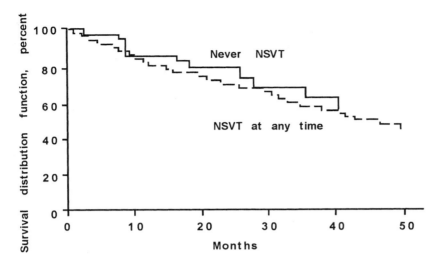

FIGURE 18-11. Percent survival with and without NSVT (nonsustained ventricular tachycardia) and heart failure. (From Singh SN, Fisher SG, Carson PE, et al, for the Department of Veterans Affairs CHF-STAT Investigators. Prevalence and significance of nonsustained ventricular tachycardia in patients with premature ventricular contractions and heart failure treated with vasodilator therapy. *J Am Coll Cardiol* 1998;32:942–947, with permission.)

Ventricular Premature Depolarizations and Nonsustained Ventricular Tachycardia in Patients with Coronary Artery Disease

The prognostic significance of NSVT with underlying coronary artery disease depends on the time the arrhythmia is discovered in the course of the disease. The occurrence of NSVT during the first 24 to 48 hours of acute myocardial infarction was not thought previously to carry an increased risk for cardiac mortality or sudden death in hospital or over the long term (39,87,88). However, one analysis demonstrated that the occurrence of NSVT may have adverse prognostic significance when it occurs 13 or more hours after the onset of infarction (89).

The occurrence of NSVT in the first month after myocardial infarction more than doubles the risk of subsequent sudden death when compared with patients without NSVT. In the prethrombolytic era, frequent VPDs and NSVT were shown repeatedly to be independent risk factors for overall cardiac death and sudden death (9,10,

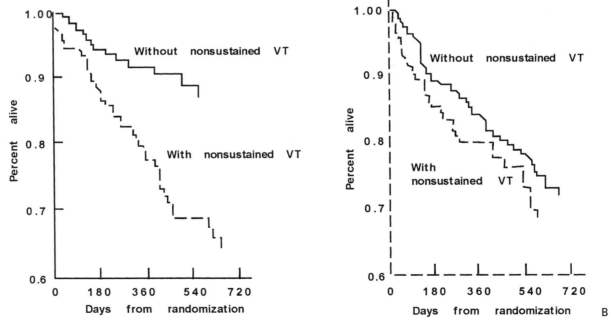

FIGURE 18-12. A: Nonsustained ventricular tachycardia (VT) and sudden death. **B:** Nonsustained VT and progressive heart failure death. (From Doval HC, Nul DR, Grancelli HO, et al, for the GESICA-GEMA Investigators. Nonsustained ventricular tachycardia in severe heart failure. Independent marker of increased mortality due to sudden death. *Circulation* 1996;94:3198–3203, with permission.)

15,40,90,91). Three-year cumulative mortality rates were 33% versus 15% for patients with and without NSVT, respectively (15). NSVT detected 3 months to 1 year after myocardial infarction is also associated with a significantly higher mortality rate (91,92).

Although the overall incidence of cardiac mortality and sudden death is higher among patients with NSVT, the proportion of sudden death compared with overall cardiac mortality is not increased in patients with frequent ectopy or NSVT (9,10,93) (Table 18-6). This observation raises the question of the specificity of NSVT as a marker for subsequent arrhythmic events rather than a marker for overall poor cardiac function. Because of this, the discovery of NSVT in an individual patient cannot be taken as evidence that the patient is at risk specifically for sudden death, as opposed to nonsudden cardiac death, such as caused by progressive congestive heart failure or recurrent myocardial infarction. More specific data, such as those derived from electrophysiologic testing, are required to make this determination.

Data from trials performed in the thrombolytic era are consistent with the data from the multicenter studies performed before the use of thrombolytic therapy in the prethrombolytic era. The GISSI-2 trial reported a 6.8% prevalence of NSVT in a population of subjects who had received thrombolytic therapy (41). In univariate analysis, NSVT was associated with a significantly increased risk of sudden death and overall cardiac mortality during an average follow-up of 6 months after infarction. However, in a multivariate analysis, although frequent and complex ventricular ectopy remained a significant risk factor, NSVT failed to carry prognostic significance. The study investigators suggest two possible explanations for these findings. First, thrombolytic therapy may somehow modify the myocardial substrate. Second, the extreme variability and low frequency of the occurrence of NSVT during 24-hour Holter monitoring may decrease its utility as a marker.

Role of Programmed Electrical Stimulation in Patients with Nonsustained Ventricular Tachycardia

Patients with Nonischemic Dilated Cardiomyopathy

In patients with nonischemic dilated cardiomyopathy, results of programmed electrical stimulation have been discouraging (94–97). Sustained ventricular tachycardia is seldom induced in asymptomatic patients with dilated cardiomyopathy, and there is no correlation between inducibility of sustained ventricular tachycardia and subsequent arrhythmic events or total cardiac mortality. Sudden death occurs more frequently among patients without inducible ventricular tachycardia than those with inducible arrhythmias. There appears to be no role for programmed electrical stimulation as a prognostic tool in this group of patients.

Patients with Hypertrophic Cardiomyopathy

In high-risk patients with hypertrophic cardiomyopathy, inducible ventricular tachycardia indicates a poorer prognosis over a 28-month follow-up period (98). In the subset of patients with NSVT on Holter monitoring, those who did not have induction of sustained ventricular tachycardia had a 3% mortality rate compared with 20% for inducible patients. However, this was a highly selected population of patients, with the majority having survived episodes of cardiac arrest, syncope, or having a strong family history for sudden death. It is not clear whether inducible ventricular tachycardia has independent prognostic utility for asymptomatic patients with a negative family history for sudden death. However, two groups of investigators have found a correlation between history of cardiac arrest and the development of fractionated electrograms in response to ventricular stimulation in this setting (99,100).

Patients with Coronary Artery Disease

Results from many studies suggest that programmed electrical stimulation may have a useful role in risk stratification of patients with coronary artery disease and NSVT whose left ventricular ejection fraction is 0.40 or less. Several small studies documented that patients with normal and depressed ejection fractions who did not have inducible sustained ventricular tachycardia developed arrhythmic events (i.e., sudden death and spontaneous sustained ventricular tachycardia) at rates approximating 10% over 1- to 2-year follow-up periods (101–104). The Multicenter Unsustained Tachycardia Trial (MUSTT) evaluated the utility of programmed stimulation in 2,202 patients with coronary artery disease, left ventricular ejection fraction of 0.40 or less and asymptomatic spontaneous NSVT. This trial demonstrated that in patients without inducible sustained

TABLE 18-6. PROGNOSTIC SIGNIFICANCE OF NONSUSTAINED VENTRICULAR TACHYCARDIA IN PATIENTS WITH RECENT MYOCARDIAL INFARCTION

Study	Patients with NSVT: Cardiac Deaths That Were Sudden (%)	Patients without NSVT: Cardiac Deaths That Were Sudden (%)
Anderson et al. (9)	73	64
Kleiger et al. (93)	33	64
Bigger et al. (10)	58	75
Bigger et al. (15)	70	58
Maggioni et al. (41)	39	32

NSVT, nonsustained ventricular tachycardia.

ventricular tachycardia arrhythmic death or cardiac arrest rates occurred in 12% and 24% over 2- and 5-year follow-up periods, respectively. The rate of arrhythmic events in patients without inducible sustained ventricular tachycardia was significantly lower than that occurring in patients with inducible tachycardia.

Patients with inducible ventricular tachycardia are at significantly increased risk for sudden death. Earlier studies were limited in their ability to demonstrate the positive predictive value of inducible sustained ventricular tachycardia, because of small size, and lack of treatment control (101–104). However, the MUSTT randomized 704 patients having inducible sustained ventricular tachycardia to one of two therapy arms (105). One group received appropriate cardiac therapy without any specific antiarrhythmic treatment. This group experienced arrhythmic death or cardiac arrest rates of 18% and 32% over 2- and 5-year follow-up periods, respectively. The risk of arrhythmic events in this group was significantly greater than that occurring in the patients without inducible sustained ventricular tachycardia.

In summary, the results of programmed electrical stimulation in the coronary artery disease population are encouraging. Programmed electrical stimulation appears capable of stratifying the risk for future sudden death among patients with a depressed ejection fraction and NSVT (106). Patients with inducible sustained ventricular tachycardia are at significant risk for sudden death and merit treatment with implanted defibrillators. Pharmacologic antiarrhythmic therapy does not appear to be capable of reducing the risk of sudden death in this population.

Prognostic Significance of the Signal-Averaged Electrocardiogram in Patients with Nonsustained Ventricular Tachycardia

The signal-averaged electrocardiogram is a noninvasive test that identifies low-amplitude, high-frequency signals originating in myocardial regions that have slow conduction, resulting in delayed activation. These signals have been correlated with the presence of inducible sustained ventricular tachycardia. Although a variety of techniques have been used, including analysis of signals in the time and frequency domain, most data in this patient population have been derived using time-domain signal-processing techniques. The signal-averaged ECG variables that have been examined are the filtered QRS duration, the presence of late potentials (i.e., signals in the terminal 40 ms of the filtered QRS complex having a mean amplitude of less than 20 to 25 µV), and the duration of the low-amplitude signal in the terminal 40 ms of the filtered QRS complex.

Studies of heterogeneous patient populations with NSVT, complex ventricular ectopy, or both conditions correlate abnormal signal-averaged electrocardiograms with inducibility of sustained ventricular tachycardia with 92% to 100% sensitivity and 75% to 88% specificity (107,108). The negative predictive accuracy in predicting inducibility has been found to be as high as 91% (109,110). However, to obtain meaningful data, the investigation must take into account historical information such as the presence, type, and extent of underlying heart disease. It is essential to study patients with similar types of underlying heart disease.

Patients with Idiopathic Dilated Cardiomyopathy

In patients with NSVT and idiopathic dilated cardiomyopathy, the presence of late potentials correlates with induction of sustained ventricular tachycardia by programmed electrical stimulation with a sensitivity and specificity of 66% and 86%, respectively (109,111). No study has examined the potential correlation between the signal-averaged electrocardiogram and sudden death in patients with NSVT and nonischemic dilated cardiomyopathy, although two reports have examined this question in patients with advanced congestive heart failure due to nonischemic dilated cardiomyopathy (112,113). One study found a fair correlation between abnormalities of the conventional time-domain signal-averaged electrocardiogram and subsequent sudden death (112). However, the other found a poor correlation between signal-averaged ECG abnormalities and sudden death. The prognostic utility of the signal-averaged electrocardiogram in this population remains unclear.

Survivors of Myocardial Infarction with Nonsustained Ventricular Tachycardia

Several earlier studies suggested that the signal-averaged electrocardiogram may identify patients with prior myocardial infarction likely to have ventricular tachycardia inducible by programmed stimulation (108–110,114,115). In contrast, analysis of signal-averaged electrocardiograms of patients enrolled in the MUSTT showed a poor correlation with the presence of inducible sustained ventricular tachycardia (116). However, preliminary analysis correlating abnormalities of the signal-averaged electrocardiogram with survival in the same trial suggest that this test may prove to be useful for risk stratification in this population (117,118).

TREATMENT

The two indications for treating VPDs or NSVT are relief of associated symptoms and reduction in the risk of sudden cardiac death.

Symptom Relief

The first step in deciding whether to initiate therapy for a patient with VPDs or NSVT is to determine whether significant symptoms attributable to the arrhythmia are present. If symptoms can be clearly correlated with either arrhythmia, regardless of the presence or type of underlying heart disease, treatment may be appropriate to make the patient feel better, although not to improve survival. In general, no antiarrhythmic agents can be considered to be specific for the treatment of symptomatic ventricular ectopy or NSVT. Groups I and III antiarrhythmic drugs, β-adrenergic blocking agents and calcium channel blockers, have been used with various degrees of success. Because the symptoms produced by these arrhythmias are usually mild, our first choice is to explain the nature of the arrhythmia to the patient, then explain the potential side effects and toxicities associated with antiarrhythmic drugs, and try to treat with reassurance. Only if one of these arrhythmias clearly compromises the quality of a patient's life do we initiate specific therapy. Our first choice of therapy for these arrhythmias is almost always a β-adrenergic antagonist or a calcium channel blocking agent. In light of progressively accumulating data demonstrating risks of type I antiarrhythmic agents in patients with a variety of structural heart disease, our usual choice of treatment for these relatively uncommon patients with symptomatic ectopy or NSVT is amiodarone.

Repetitive monomorphic ventricular tachycardia originating in the right ventricular outflow tract may respond to β blockade in up to 50% of patients tested. Verapamil, propafenone, and amiodarone have also been used with variable success (20–22). Many patients with this syndrome have frequent episodes of spontaneous tachycardia so that the efficacy of therapy can be judged with the systematic use of repeated ambulatory monitoring or electrophysiologic testing. As a rule, if a symptomatic patient with this type of arrhythmia does not respond to β-adrenergic or calcium channel blocking agents, we recommend electrophysiologic study with radiofrequency catheter ablation (119). In this setting, catheter ablation has a very low risk and should be successful in more than 80% of cases.

Reduction in Sudden Cardiac Death

The second potential indication for treatment is to reduce the risk of sudden death that has been associated with the presence of NSVT in certain patients with structural heart disease. In this case, it is important to understand what is being treated. In general, for prevention of sudden death, the physician does not treat ventricular ectopy or NSVT, because these arrhythmias are not lethal. Rather, the physician treats a presumed substrate for sustained tachyarrhythmias with which the VPDs or NSVT are associated. Prevention of sudden death has met with various degrees of success, depending on the type of therapy used and underlying heart disease.

Congestive Heart Failure

The prophylactic use of antiarrhythmic agents in patients with congestive heart failure has been discouraging, having no clear benefit in a number of small older studies (120). The Veterans Administration Heart Failure Trial (CHF-STAT) studied the effects of empiric therapy with amiodarone in patients with 10 asymptomatic VPDs per hour (121). The cause of heart failure was coronary artery disease in 71% of patients in this trial. The effect of amiodarone on survival in this study was neutral, even among patients with documented NSVT. One noteworthy aspect of these results was the fact that amiodarone did effectively suppress ventricular ectopy. Although amiodarone had no beneficial effect on survival of the patients with coronary artery disease, there was a trend for improved survival of patients with nonischemic cardiomyopathy (Fig. 18-13). These results contrast with those of the GESICA trial of amiodarone in patients with conges-

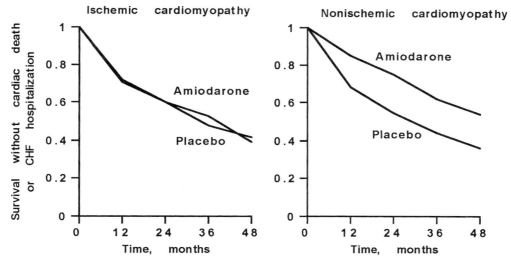

FIGURE 18-13. Outcome of patients in CHF-STAT according to cardiomyopathy type (From Singh SN, Fletcher RD, Fisher SG, et al, for the Survival Trial of Antiarrhythmic Therapy in Congestive Heart Failure (CHF-STAT). Amiodarone in patients with congestive heart failure and asymptomatic ventricular arrhythmia. *N Engl J Med* 1995;333:77–82, with permission.)

tive heart failure; this trial found a survival benefit associated with amiodarone therapy (122) (Fig. 18-14). However, the GESICA trial differed from the CHF-STAT study in that patients were not required to have arrhythmias to gain entry. Congestive heart failure was attributed to coronary artery disease in only 39% of participants in this trial; it is possible that this accounts for the difference in outcome between the two studies.

Nevertheless, meta-analysis of 13 randomized amiodarone trials involving 6,553 patients found that amiodarone reduced total mortality from congestive heart failure by 13% and arrhythmic or sudden death by 29% (122a) (Fig. 18-15). The effectiveness of amiodarone was not influenced by left ventricular ejection fraction, New York Heart Association (NYHA) class, or the presence of asymptomatic arrhythmias on Holter monitoring. The most common serious side effect of amiodarone was hypothyroidism (net absolute difference of 5.9%), and the excess risk of pulmonary toxicity from amiodarone was 1%.

A second meta-analysis of 15 randomized trials involving 5,864 patients reported similar results. The overall reductions in total, cardiac, and sudden death mortality were 19%, 23%, and 30%, respectively, and for patients with congestive heart failure, the reductions were 22%, 25%, and 23%, respectively (122b). There was a trend toward a greater risk reduction in the trials requiring evidence of ventricular ectopy than in the remaining trials (25% versus 10%).

Hypertrophic Cardiomyopathy

The benefit of antiarrhythmics in the setting of hypertrophic cardiomyopathy is also unclear. McKenna and colleagues reported a possible benefit of amiodarone over conventional antiarrhythmics in patients with hypertrophic cardiomyopathy and ventricular tachycardia (48). However, this study design was retrospective with historical controls, and another report failed to confirm these findings (123).

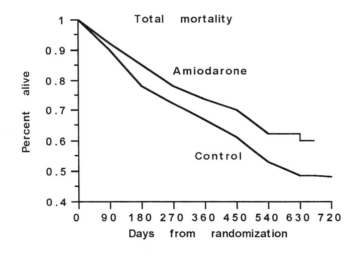

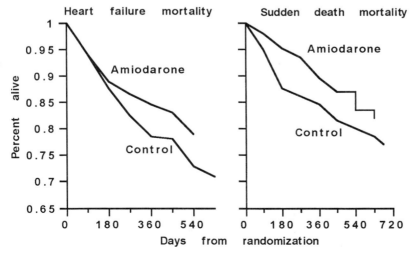

FIGURE 18-14. Outcomes in patients with congestive heart failure treated and not treated with low-dose amiodarone. (From Doval HC, Nul DR, Grancelli HO, et al. Randomized trial of low-dose amiodarone in severe congestive heart failure. *Lancet* 1994;344:493–498, with permission.)

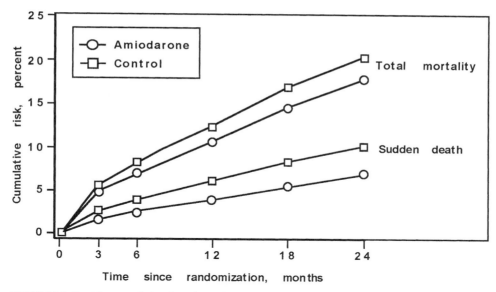

FIGURE 18-15. Meta-analysis of studies of amiodarone. (From Amiodarone Trials Meta-analysis Investigators. Effect of prophylactic amiodarone on mortality after acute myocardial infarction and in congestive heart failure: meta-analysis of individual data from 6500 patients in randomized trials. *Lancet* 1997;350:14127–1423, with permission.)

Coronary Artery Disease and Myocardial Infarction

Pharmacologic therapy guided by Holter monitoring has been used in an attempt to reduce the risk of sudden death in the setting of VPDs or NSVT and a recent myocardial infarction. The largest and best designed trial is the Cardiac Arrhythmia Suppression Trial (CAST), which evaluated the effect of encainide, flecainide, and moricizine in patients within 2 years of acute myocardial infarction who had an average of six or more VPDs per hour detected on Holter monitors (124,125). Runs of NSVT, lasting up to 15 beats, were seen in 20% of patients randomized to therapy. To be

randomized to active therapy or placebo, patients had to demonstrate suppression of ventricular ectopy and NSVT using rigid criteria. Patients who were in the active treatment group, receiving encainide or flecainide, had a 4.5% sudden death rate over 10 months, compared with 1.2% for placebo controls (Fig. 18-16). The overall mortality was increased in similar proportions in the active treatment group. In subgroup analysis, the presence of NSVT was associated with a higher total mortality or sudden death rate in the active treatment group when compared with patients without NSVT, but the difference did not reach statistical significance. However, patients in the active treatment group who had more than one run per day of NSVT on the baseline

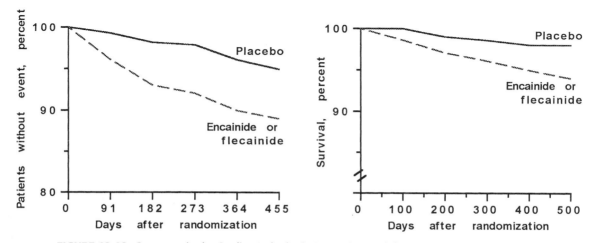

FIGURE 18-16. Outcomes in the Cardiac Arrhythmia Supression Trial. (From CAST Investigators. Preliminary report: effect of encainide and flecainide on mortality in a randomized trial of arrhythmia suppression after myocardial infarction. *N Engl J Med* 1989;321:406–412, with permission.)

Holter recording had a significantly higher rate of sudden death compared with patients with a single run or none. No such difference was observed in the placebo group. Although these results are compelling, only one half of the randomized patients had a left ventricular ejection fraction less than 0.40, and a minority of patients had NSVT. The results cannot necessarily be extrapolated to the highest-risk group of myocardial infarction survivors. As a result of the increased mortality with encainide and flecainide, CAST was stopped prematurely. However, the study was redesigned, using only moricizine (CAST II). This study was also stopped prematurely when moricizine also failed to show any survival advantage over placebo therapy (125).

The efficacy of empiric amiodarone in the post–myocardial infarction population has been evaluated in two large randomized trials (126,127). Although the trials were very different in their protocols and they differed somewhat in entry criteria, they arrived at virtually identical results. The European Myocardial Infarction Amiodarone Trial (EMIAT)

enrolled patients with recent infarction who had left ventricular ejection fractions of 0.40 or less without screening for ventricular ectopy. The Canadian Myocardial Infarction Amiodarone Trial (CAMIAT) enrolled patients with recent infarction who had 10 or fewer VPDs per hour or NSVT without regard for left ventricular ejection fraction. In each case, amiodarone had a neutral effect on total mortality but did reduce the risk of sudden death (Figs. 18-17 and 18-18). Empiric therapy with amiodarone cannot be relied on to improve survival in high-risk patients with recent myocardial infarction. However, because there was no adverse effect on survival, as has been observed during earlier trials with type I antiarrhythmic agents, amiodarone can be regarded as relatively safe to suppress symptomatic arrhythmias, such as atrial fibrillation, in this population.

Two meta-analyses of randomized trials of amiodarone found similar results for patients after acute myocardial infarction (122a,122b). In one analysis of eight trials and more than 5,000 patients, the reduction in total mortality

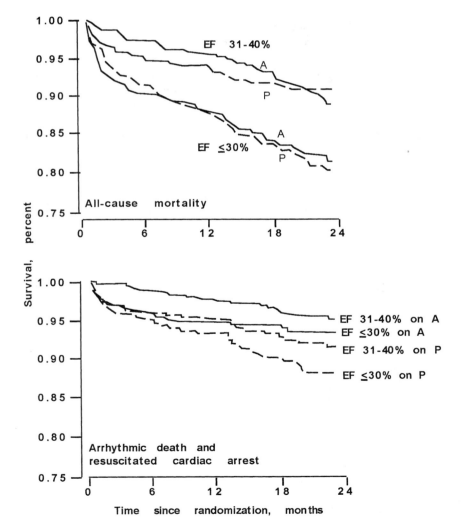

FIGURE 18-17. Outcomes in EMIAT. A, amiodarone; EF, ejection fraction; P, placebo. (From Julian DG, Camm AJ, Franglin G, et al. Randomized trial of effect of amiodarone on mortality in patients with left-ventricular dysfunction after recent myocardial infarction: EMIAT. *Lancet* 1997;349:667–674, with permission.)

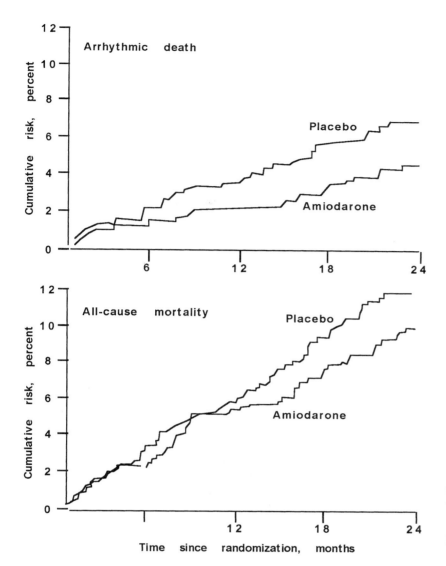

FIGURE 18-18. Outcome in CAMIAT. (From Cairns JA, Connolly SJ, Roberts R, et al. Randomized trial of outcome after myocardial infarction in patients with frequent or repetitive ventricular premature depolarizations: CAMIAT. *Lancet* 1997;349:675–682, with permission.)

and arrhythmic or sudden death with amiodarone was 8% and 35%, respectively (122a) (Fig. 18-15). The effectiveness of amiodarone was not influenced by left ventricular ejection fraction, NYHA class, or detection of asymptomatic arrhythmias by Holter monitoring. The most common serious side effect of amiodarone was hypothyroidism, and the excess risk of pulmonary toxicity from amiodarone was 1%. The second analysis of 15 randomized trials involving 5,864 patients reported that reductions for the amiodarone groups in total, cardiac, and sudden death mortality after myocardial infarction were 21%, 21%, and 38%, respectively (122b). There was a trend toward a greater risk reduction in those trials requiring evidence of ventricular ectopy than in the remaining studies.

Results from several nonrandomized, uncontrolled studies suggested that the response to antiarrhythmic therapy guided by programmed stimulation in patients with NSVT and coronary artery disease might be of significant value in improving survival (101–104). MUSTT randomized 704 patients having inducible sustained ventricular tachycardia to no therapy or electrophysiologically guided antiarrhythmic drug therapy (105). After a 5-year follow-up, the control group that received no antiarrhythmic treatment experienced a 32% arrhythmic death or arrest rate. In the active treatment group, the arrhythmic event rate was 25%; the relative risk of arrhythmic events was reduced by 27% (absolute risk reduction, 7%) compared with the group that received no antiarrhythmic therapy. A second major finding of this study was that pharmacologic antiarrhythmic therapy guided by the electrophysiologic test conferred no survival benefit because the improvement in survival associated with electrophysiologically guided therapy was entirely the result of treatment with implanted defibrillators (Fig. 18-19).

These results are consistent with those of a second study, the Multicenter Automatic Defibrillator Implantation Trial (MADIT), which examined the relative survival benefits of

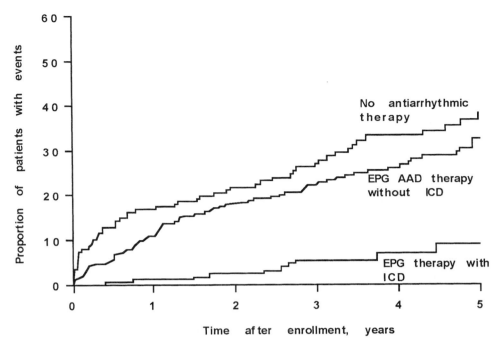

FIGURE 18-19. Arrhythmic events in MUSTT. EPG, electrophysiologically guided; AAD, antiarrhythmia drug. ICD, implantable cardioverter-defibrillator. (From Buxton AE, Lee KL, Fisher JD, Josephson ME, et al, for the Multicenter Unsustained Tachycardia Trial Investigators. A randomized study of the prevention of sudden death in patients with coronary artery disease. *N Engl J Med* 1999;341:1882–1890, with permission.)

implanted defibrillators compared with "conventional" pharmacologic antiarrhythmic therapy in a patient population similar to that studied in the MUSTT trial. (106). This trial involved 196 patients with previous myocardial infarction, an ejection fraction of less than 0.35, spontaneous NSVT, and inducible sustained ventricular tachycardia that could not be suppressed by intravenous procainamide. Patients were randomized to therapy with an implantable

defibrillator or pharmacologic antiarrhythmic therapy, primarily empiric amiodarone. The primary end point in this trial was total mortality, rather than sudden death. After a 27-month follow-up, patients randomized to defibrillator therapy in this trial experienced a 54% reduction in total mortality compared with patients randomized to pharmacologic therapy (15.8% versus 38.6%) (Fig. 18-20). The 2-year total mortality rate of 32% for patients randomized to

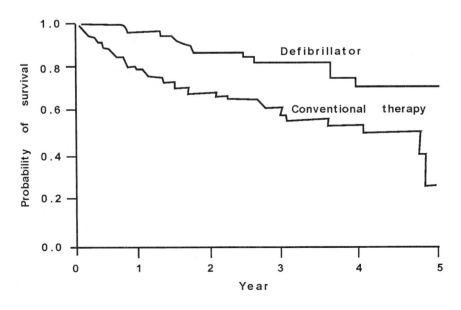

FIGURE 18-20. Total mortality in MADIT. (From Moss AJ, Hall WJ, Cannom DS, et al. Improved survival with an implanted defibrillator in patients with coronary disease at high risk for ventricular arrhythmia. *N Engl J Med* 1996;335:19–33, with permission.)

the conventional (pharmacologic) therapy arm was similar to that of patients in the MUSTT study randomized to no antiarrhythmic therapy (28%). The mortality rate for the control group in MADIT was also similar to that observed for MUSTT patients randomized to electrophysiologically guided antiarrhythmic therapy who were not treated with a defibrillator (33%).

Based on these results, it seems reasonable at this time to perform electrophysiologic testing in patients with previous myocardial infarction and left ventricular ejection fractions less than 0.40 who have NSVT. If sustained ventricular tachycardia is induced, an implantable cardioverter-defibrillator should be recommended rather than pharmacologic antiarrhythmic therapy.

CONCLUSIONS

Management of the patient with VPDs or NSVT depends on the presence or absence of symptoms due to the arrhythmia and on the presence and type of structural heart disease. If debilitating symptoms are present and reassurance alone does not succeed, pharmacologic antiarrhythmic therapy may be initiated. Medications such as β blockers and calcium channel blockers are reasonable first-line agents because of their low side-effect profiles. If these agents fail to relieve symptoms, the physician should consider radiofrequency catheter ablation. Efficacy may be determined by resolution of symptoms and confirmed by follow-up Holter monitors, event monitors, or repeated exercise testing.

The asymptomatic patient represents a more troublesome category for management. Subjects without underlying heart disease in whom VPDs or NSVT is discovered fortuitously do not require treatment. Likewise, we do not recommend antiarrhythmic therapy for patients with idiopathic dilated cardiomyopathy, because there is no evidence that asymptomatic patients with NSVT in this setting are at higher risk for sudden death, and no treatment modality has shown evidence for a reduction in the significant risk of sudden death.

In patients with hypertrophic cardiomyopathy, NSVT may have value for predicting sudden death, but the positive predictive value of NSVT for predicting sudden death is low, and no treatment has been shown to benefit asymptomatic patients. We therefore do not advocate further study or antiarrhythmic therapy for such patients.

In asymptomatic patients with coronary artery disease and significant left ventricular dysfunction, the presence of frequent or complex VPDs or NSVT indicates a significantly increased risk for sudden death. The first step in managing this group of patients is to evaluate for the presence of reversible ischemia; if present, ischemia should be treated appropriately using revascularization or pharmacologic therapy. If NSVT persists after optimal treatment of

ischemia, the next step is to evaluate left ventricular function. If the ejection fraction is greater than 0.40, no further evaluation or therapy is indicated. If the patient has an ejection fraction less than or equal to 0.40, electrophysiologic testing should be used to stratify the risk and to guide therapy. If sustained ventricular tachycardia is inducible, an implantable cardioverter-defibrillator is indicated. β-adrenergic blocking agents and angiotensin-converting enzyme (ACE) inhibitors have improved survival modestly, reducing the rates of sudden and nonsudden death in this high-risk group of patients. They should be used whenever possible.

REFERENCES

1. Wolff GA, Veith F, Lown B. A vulnerable period for ventricular tachycardia following myocardial infarction. *Cardiovasc Res* 1968;2:111–121.
2. De Soyza N, Bissett JK, Kane JJ, et al. Ectopic ventricular prematurity and its relationship to ventricular tachycardia in acute myocardial infarction in man. *Circulation* 1974;50:529–533.
3. Roberts R, Ambos HD, Loh CW, Sobel BE. Initiation of repetitive ventricular depolarizations by relatively late premature complexes in patients with acute myocardial infarction. *Am J Cardiol* 1978;41:678–683.
4. Berger MD, Waxman HL, Buxton AE, et al. Spontaneous compared with induced onset of sustained ventricular tachycardia. *Circulation* 1988;78:885–892.
5. Kempf FC, Josephson ME. Cardiac arrest recorded on ambulatory electrocardiograms. *Am J Cardiol* 1984;53:1577–1582.
6. Winkle RA, Derrington DC, Schroeder JS. Characteristics of ventricular tachycardia in ambulatory patients. *Am J Cardiol* 1977;39:487–492.
7. Buxton AE, Waxman HL, Marchlinski FE, Josephson ME. Electrophysiologic studies in NSVT: relation to underlying heart disease. *Am J Cardiol* 1983;52:985–991.
8. Suyama A, Anan T, Araki H, et al. Prevalence of ventricular tachycardia in patients with different underlying heart disease: a study by Holter ECG monitoring. *Am Heart J* 1986;112:44–51.
9. Anderson KP, DeCamilla J, Moss AJ. Clinical significance of ventricular tachycardia (3 beats or longer) detected during ambulatory monitoring after myocardial infarction. *Circulation* 1978;57:890–897.
10. Bigger JT, Weld FM, Rolnitzky LM. Prevalence, characteristics and significance of ventricular tachycardia (three or more complexes) detected with ambulatory electrocardiographic recording in the late hospital phase of acute myocardial infarction. *Am J Cardiol* 1981;48:815–823.
11. Moeller M, Nielsen BL, Fabricius J. Paroxysmal ventricular tachycardia during repeated 24-hour ambulatory electrocardiographic monitoring of post-myocardial infarction patients. *Br Heart J* 1980;43:447–453.
12. Denes P, Gillis AM, Pawitan Y, et al, for the CAST Investigators. Prevalence, characteristics and significance of ventricular premature complexes and ventricular tachycardia detected by 24-hour continuous electrocardiographic recording in the Cardiac Arrhythmia Suppression Trial. *Am J Cardiol* 1991;68:887–896.
13. Pratt CM, Hallstrom A, Theroux P, et al, for the CAPS Investigators. Avoiding interpretive pitfalls when assessing arrhythmia suppression after myocardial infarction: insights from the long-term observations of the placebo-treated patients in the Cardiac Arrhythmia Pilot Study. *J Am Coll Cardiol* 1991;17:1–8.
14. Maron BJ, Savage DD, Wolfson JK, Epstein SE. Prognostic sig-

nificance of 24 hour ambulatory electrocardiographic monitoring in patients with hypertrophic cardiomyopathy: a prospective Study. *Am J Cardiol* 1981;48:252–257.

15. Bigger JT, Fleiss JL, Rolnitzky LM, for the Multicenter Post-Infarction Research Group. Prevalence, characteristics and significance of ventricular tachycardia detected by 24-hour continuous electrocardiographic recordings in the late hospital phase of acute myocardial infarction. *Am J Cardiol* 1986;58:1151–1160.

16. Neri R, Mestroni L, Salvi A, Camerini F. Arrhythmias in dilated cardiomyopathy. *Postgrad Med J* 1986;62:593–597.

17. Meinertz T, Hofmann T, Kasper W, et al. Significance of ventricular arrhythmias in idiopathic dilated cardiomyopathy. *Am J Cardiol* 1984;53:902–907.

18. Thanavaro S, Kleiger RE, Miller JP, et al. Coupling interval and types of ventricular ectopy associated with ventricular runs. *Am Heart J* 1983;106:484–491.

19. Huang SK, Messer JV, Denes P. Significance of ventricular tachycardia in idiopathic dilated cardiomyopathy: observations in 35 patients. *Am J Cardiol* 1983;51:507–512.

20. Ritchie AH, Kerr CR, Qi A, et al. NSVT arising from the right ventricular outflow tract. *Am J Cardiol* 1989;64:594–598.

21. Buxton AE, Waxman HL, Marchlinski FE, et al. Right Ventricular tachycardia: clinical and electrophysiologic characteristics. *Circulation* 1983;68:917–927.

22. Buxton AE, Marchlinski FE, Doherty JU, et al. Repetitive, monomorphic ventricular tachycardia: clinical and electrophysiologic characteristics in patients with and patients without organic heart disease. *Am J Cardiol* 1984;54:997–1002.

23. Grossman W. Profiles in dilated (congestive) and hypertrophic cardiomyopathies. In: Grossman W, Baim DS, eds. *Cardiac catheterization, angiography, and intervention.* Philadelphia: Lea & Febiger, 1991:618–632.

24. Hiss RG, Lamb LE. Electrocardiographic findings in 122,043 individuals. *Circulation* 1962;25:947–961.

25. Chiang BN, Perlman LV, Ostrander LD, Epstein FH. Relationship of premature systoles to coronary heart disease and sudden death in the Tecumseh Epidemiologic Study. *Ann Intern Med* 1969;70:1159–1166.

26. Sobotka PA, Mayer JH, Bauernfeind RA, et al. Arrhythmias documented by 24-hour continuous ambulatory electrocardiographic monitoring in young women without apparent heart disease. *Am Heart J* 1981;101:753–759.

27. Brodsky M, Wu D, Denes P, et al. Arrhythmias documented by 24 hour continuous electrocardiographic monitoring in 50 male medical students without apparent heart disease. *Am J Cardiol* 1977;39:390–395.

28. Hinkle LE, Carver ST, Stevens M. The frequency of asymptomatic disturbances of cardiac rhythm and conduction in middle-aged men. *Am J Cardiol* 1969;24:629–650.

29. Kantelip JP, Sage E, Duchene-Marullaz P. Findings on ambulatory electrocardiographic monitoring in subjects older than 80 years. *Am J Cardiol* 1986;57:398–401.

30. Kennedy HL, Underhill SJ. Frequent or complex ventricular ectopy in apparently healthy subjects. *Am J Cardiol* 1976;38:141–148.

31. Kostis JB, McCrone K, Moreyra AE, et al. Premature ventricular complexes in the absence of identifiable heart disease. *Circulation* 1981;6:1351–1356.

32. Pantano JA, Oriel RJ. Prevalence and nature of cardiac arrhythmias in apparently normal well-trained runners. *Am Heart J* 1982;104:762–768.

33. Pilcher GF, Cook AJ, Johnston BL, Fletcher GF. Twenty-four-hour continuous electrocardiography during exercise and free activity in 80 apparently healthy runners. *Am J Cardiol* 1983;52:859–861.

34. Romhilt DW, Chaffin C, Choi SC, Irby EC. Arrhythmias on ambulatory electrocardiographic monitoring in women without apparent heart disease. *Am J Cardiol* 1984;54:582–586.

35. Takada H, Mikawa T, Murayama M, et al. Range of ventricular ectopic complexes in healthy subjects studied with repeated ambulatory electrocardiographic recordings. *Am J Cardiol* 1989;63:184–186.

36. Califf RM, McKinnis RA, Burks J, et al. Prognostic implications of ventricular arrhythmias during 24 hour ambulatory monitoring in patients undergoing cardiac catheterization for coronary artery disease. *Am J Cardiol* 1982;50:23–31.

37. Wajngarten M, Grupi C, Bellotti GM, et al. Frequency and significance of cardiac rhythm disturbances in healthy elderly individuals. *J Electrocardiol* 1990;23:171–176.

38. Campbell R, Murray A, Julian DG. Ventricular arrhythmias in the first 12 hours of acute myocardial infarction. *Br Heart J* 1981;46:351–357.

39. De Soyza N, Bennett FA, Murphy ML, et al. The relationship of paroxysmal ventricular tachycardia complicating the acute phase and ventricular arrhythmia during the late hospital phase of myocardial infarction to long-term survival. *Am J Med* 1978;64:377–381.

40. Bigger JT, Fleiss JL, Kleiger R, et al, for the Multicenter Post-Infarction Research Group. The relationships among ventricular arrhythmias, left ventricular dysfunction, and mortality in the 2 years after myocardial infarction. *Circulation* 1984;69:250–258.

41. Maggioni AP, Zuanetti G, Franzosi MG, et al, on behalf of GISSI-2 Investigators. Prevalence and prognostic significance of ventricular arrhythmias after acute myocardial infarction in the fibrinolytic era: GISSI-2 results. *Circulation* 1993;87:312–322.

42. Pringle SD, Dunn FG, Macfarlane PW, et al. Significance of ventricular arrhythmias in systemic hypertension with left ventricular hypertrophy. *Am J Cardiol* 1992;69:913–917.

43. Levy D, Anderson KM, Savage DD. Risk of ventricular arrhythmias in left ventricular hypertrophy: the Framingham Heart Study. *Am J Cardiol* 1987;60:560–565.

44. Mulrow JP, Healy MJ, McKenna WJ. Variability of ventricular arrhythmias in hypertrophic cardiomyopathy and implications for treatment. *Am J Cardiol* 1986;58:615–618.

45. Newman H, Sugrue D, Oakley C, et al. Relation of left ventricular function and prognosis in hypertrophic cardiomyopathy: an angiographic study. *J Am Coll Cardiol* 1985;5:1064–1074.

46. Savage DD, Seides SF, Maron BJ, et al. Prevalence of arrhythmias during 24-hour electrocardiographic monitoring and exercise testing in patients with obstructive and nonobstructive cardiomyopathy. *Circulation* 1979;59:866–875.

47. McKenna WJ, England D, Doi YL, et al. Arrhythmia in hypertrophic cardiomyopathy I: influence on prognosis. *Br Heart J* 1981;46:168–172.

48. McKenna WJ, Oakley C, Krikler DM, Goodwin JF. Improved survival with amiodarone in patients with hypertrophic cardiomyopathy and ventricular tachycardia. *Br Heart J* 1985;53:412–416.

49. Maron BJ, Roberts WC, Epstein SE. Sudden death in hypertrophic cardiomyopathy: a profile of 78 patients. *Circulation* 1982;65:1388–1394.

50. Maron BJ, Fananapazir L. Sudden cardiac death in hypertrophic cardiomyopathy. *Circulation* 1992;85[Suppl I]:I-57–I-63.

51. McKenna WJ, Chetty S, Oakley CM, Goodwin JF. Arrhythmia in hypertrophic cardiomyopathy: exercise and 48 hour ambulatory electrocardiographic assessment with and without beta adrenergic blocking therapy. *Am J Cardiol* 1980;45:1–5.

52. Olshausen KV, Stienen U, Math D, et al. Long-term prognostic significance of ventricular arrhythmias in idiopathic dilated cardiomyopathy. *Am J Cardiol* 1988;61:146–151.

53. Doval HC, Nul DR, Grancelli HO, et al, for the GESICA-GEMA Investigators. Nonsustained ventricular tachycardia in severe heart failure. Independent marker of increased mortality due to sudden death. *Circulation* 1996;94:3198–3203.

54. Singh SN, Fisher SG, Carson PE, et al, for the Department of Veterans Affairs CHF-STAT Investigators. Prevalence and significance of nonsustained ventricular tachycardia in patients with premature ventricular contractions and heart failure treated with vasodilator therapy. *J Am Coll Cardiol* 1998;32: 942–947.

55. Teerlink JR, Jalaluddin M, Anderson S, et al, on behalf of the PROMISE Investigators. Ambulatory ventricular arrhythmias in patients with heart failure do not specifically predict an increased risk of sudden death. *Circulation* 2000;101:40–46.

56. Kligfield P, Levy D, Devereux RB, Savage DD. Arrhythmias and sudden death in mitral valve prolapse. *Am Heart J* 1987; 113:1298–1307.

57. Kligfield P, Hochreiter C, Niles N, et al. Relation of sudden death in pure mitral regurgitation, with and without mitral valve prolapse, to repetitive ventricular arrhythmias and right and left ventricular ejection fractions. *Am J Cardiol* 1987;60:397–399.

58. Garson A, Porter CJ, Gillette PC, McNamara DG. Induction of ventricular tachycardia during electrophysiologic study after repair of tetralogy of Fallot. *J Am Coll Cardiol* 1983;1: 1493–1502.

59. Garson A, Nihill MR, McNamara DG, Cooley DA. Status of the adult and adolescent after repair of tetralogy of Fallot. *Circulation* 1979;59:1232–1240.

60. Morganroth J, Michelson EL, Horowitz LN, et al. Limitations of routine long term electrocardiographic monitoring to assess ventricular ectopic frequency. *Circulation* 1978;58:408–414.

61. Michelson EL, Morganroth J. Spontaneous variability of complex ventricular arrhythmias detected by long-term electrocardiographic recording. *Circulation* 1980;61:690–695.

62. Toivonin L. Spontaneous variability in the frequency of ventricular premature complexes over prolonged intervals and implications for antiarrhythmic treatment. *Am J Cardiol* 1987; 60:608–612.

63. Anastasiou-Nana MI, Minlove RL, Nanas JN, Anderson JL. Changes in spontaneous variability of ventricular ectopic activity as a function of time in patients with chronic arrhythmias. *Circulation* 1988;78:286–295.

64. Pratt CM, Slymen DJ, Wierman AM, et al. Analysis of the spontaneous variability of ventricular arrhythmias: consecutive ambulatory electrocardiographic recordings of ventricular tachycardia. *Am J Cardiol* 1985;56:67–72.

65. Pratt CM, Delclos G, Wierman AM, et al. The changing baseline of complex ventricular arrhythmias: a new consideration in assessing long-term antiarrhythmic drug therapy. *N Engl J Med* 1985;313:1444–1449.

66. Peters NC, Cabo C, Wit AL. Arrhythmogenic mechanisms: automaticity, triggered activity, and reentry. In: Zipes DP, Jalife J, eds. *Cardiac electrophysiology: from cell to bedside*. Philadelphia: WB Saunders, 2000:345–356.

67. Roden DM, Lazzara R, Rosen M, et al, for the SADS Foundation Task Force on LQTS. Multiple mechanisms in the long QT syndrome: current knowledge, gaps, and future directions. *Circulation* 1996;94:1996–2012.

68. El-Sherif N, Turitto G. The long QT syndrome and torsade de pointes. *Pacing Clin Electrophysiol* 1999;22:91–110.

69. Buxton AE, Waxman HL, Marchlinski FE, et al. Right ventricular tachycardia: clinical and electrophysiologic characteristics. *Circulation* 1983;68:917–927.

70. Lerman BB, Stein K, Engelstein ED, et al. Mechanism of repetitive monomorphic ventricular tachycardia. *Circulation* 1995; 92:421–429.

71. Pogwizd SM. Nonreentrant mechanisms underlying spontaneous ventricular arrhythmias in a model of nonischemic heart failure in rabbits. *Circulation* 1995;92:1034.

72. Pogwizd SM. Focal mechanisms underlying ventricular tachycardia during prolonged ischemic cardiomyopathy. *Circulation* 1994;90:1441.

73. Buxton AE, Kleiman RB, Kindwall KE, Josephson ME. Endocardial mapping during sinus rhythm in patients with coronary artery disease and nonsustained ventricular tachycardia. *Am J Cardiol* 1993;71:695–698.

74. Castellanos A, Moleiro F, Saoudi NC, Myerburg RJ. Parasystole. In: Zipes DP, Jalife J, eds. *Cardiac electrophysiology: from cell to bedside*. Philadelphia: WB Saunders, 2000:690–690.

75. Kennedy HL, Whitlock JA, Sprague MK, et al. Long-term follow-up of asymptomatic healthy subjects with frequent and complex ventricular ectopy. *N Engl J Med* 1985;312:193–197.

77. Ritchie AH, Kerr CR, Qi A, Yeung-Lai-Wah JA. Nonsustained ventricular tachycardia arising from the right ventricular outflow tract. *Am J Cardiol* 1989;64:594–598.

78. Gradman A, Deedwania P, Cody R, et al, for The Captopril-Digoxin Study Group. Predictors of total mortality and sudden death in mild to moderate heart failure. *J Am Coll Cardiol* 1989;14:564–570.

79. Holmes J, Kubo SH, Cody RJ, Kligfield P. Arrhythmias in ischemic and nonischemic dilated cardiomyopathy: prediction of mortality by ambulatory electrocardiography. *Am J Cardiol* 1985;55:146–151.

80. Unverferth DV, Magorien RD, Moeschberger ML, et al. Factors influencing the one-year mortality of dilated cardiomyopathy. *Am J Cardiol* 1984;54:147–152.

81. Wilson JR, Schwartz JS, St. John Sutton M, et al. Prognosis in severe heart failure: Relation to hemodynamic measurements and ventricular ectopic activity. *J Am Coll Cardiol* 1983;2:403–410.

82. Kannel WB. Prevalence and natural history of electrocardiographic left ventricular hypertrophy. *Am J Med* 1983;74:4–11.

83. Cooper RS, Simmons BE, Castaner A, et al. Left ventricular hypertrophy is associated with worse survival independent of ventricular function and number of coronary arteries severely narrowed. *Am J Cardiol* 1990;65:441–445.

84. Lavie CJ, Nunez BD, Garavaglia GE, Messerli FH. Hypertensive concentric left ventricular hypertrophy: when is ventricular ectopic activity increased? *S Med J* 1988;81:696–700.

85. Maron BJ, Fananapazir L. Sudden cardiac death in hypertrophic cardiomyopathy. *Circulation* 1992;85[Suppl I]:I-57–I-63.

86. Spirito P, Rapezzi C, Autore C, et al. Prognosis of asymptomatic patients with hypertrophic cardiomyopathy and nonsustained ventricular tachycardia. *Circulation* 1994;90:2743.

87. Vismara LA, Amsterdam EA, Mason DT. Relation of ventricular arrhythmias in the late hospital phase of acute myocardial infarction to sudden death after hospital discharge. *Am J Med* 1975;59:6–12.

88. Eldar M, Sievner Z, Goldbourt U, et al, for the SPRINT Study Group. Primary ventricular tachycardia in acute myocardial infarction: clinical characteristics and mortality. *Ann Intern Med* 1992;117:31–36.

89. Cheema AN, Sheu K, Parker M, et al. Nonsustained ventricular tachycardia in the setting of acute myocardial infarction: tachycardia characteristics and their prognostic significance. *Circulation* 1998;98:2030–2036.

90. Gomes JA, Winters SL, Stewart D, et al. A new noninvasive index to predict sustained ventricular tachycardia and sudden death in the first year after myocardial infarction: based on signal-averaged electrocardiogram, radionuclide ejection fraction and Holter monitoring. *J Am Coll Cardiol* 1987;10:349–357.

91. Tominaga S, Blackburn H, for The Coronary Drug Project Research Group. Prognostic importance of premature beats fol-

lowing myocardial infarction: experience in the Coronary Drug Project. *JAMA* 1973;223:1116–1124.

92. Hallstrom AP, Bigger JT, Roden D, et al. Prognostic significance of ventricular premature depolarizations measured 1 year after myocardial infarction in patients with early postinfarction asymptomatic ventricular arrhythmia. *J Am Coll Cardiol* 1992; 20:259–264.

93. Kleiger RE, Miller JP, Thanavaro S, et al. Relationship between clinical features of acute myocardial infarction and ventricular runs 2 weeks to 1 year after infarction. *Circulation* 1981;63: 64–70.

94. Meinertz T, Treese N, Kasper W, et al. Determinants of prognosis in idiopathic dilated cardiomyopathy as determined by programmed electrical stimulation. *Am J Cardiol* 1985;56: 337–341.

95. Poll DS, Marchlinski FE, Buxton AE, et al. Usefulness of programmed stimulation in idiopathic dilated cardiomyopathy. *Am J Cardiol* 1986;58:992–997.

96. Stamato NJ, O'Connell JB, Murdock DK, et al. The response of patients with complex ventricular arrhythmias secondary to dilated cardiomyopathy to programmed electrical stimulation. *Am Heart J.* 1986;112:505–508.

97. Das SK, Morady F, DiCarlo L, et al. Prognostic usefulness of programmed ventricular stimulation in idiopathic dilated cardiomyopathy without symptomatic ventricular arrhythmias. *Am J Cardiol* 1986;58:998–1000.

98. Fananapazir L, Chang AC, Epstein SE, McAreavey D. Prognostic determinants in hypertrophic cardiomyopathy: prospective evaluation of a therapeutic strategy based on clinical, Holter, hemodynamic, and electrophysiologic findings. *Circulation* 1992;86:730–740.

99. Saumarez RC, Slade AKB, Grace AA, et al. The significance of paced electrogram fractionation in hypertrophic cardiomyopathy: a prospective study. *Circulation* 1995;91:2762–2768.

100. Watson RM, Schwartz JL, Maron BJ, et al. Inducible polymorphic ventricular tachycardia and ventricular fibrillation in a subgroup of patients with hypertrophic cardiomyopathy at high risk for sudden death. *J Am Coll Cardiol* 1987;10:761–764.

101. Buxton AE, Marchlinski FE, Flores BT, et al. Nonsustained ventricular tachycardia in patients with coronary artery disease: role of electrophysiologic study. *Circulation* 1987;75:1178–1185.

102. Klein RC, Machell C. Use of electrophysiologic testing in patients with nonsustained ventricular tachycardia: prognostic and therapeutic implications. *J Am Coll Cardiol* 1989;14: 155–161.

103. Wilber DJ, Olshansky B, Moran JF, Scanlon PJ. Electrophysiologic testing and nonsustained ventricular tachycardia: use and limitations in patients with coronary artery disease and impaired ventricular function. *Circulation* 1990;82:350–358.

104. Kowey PR, Waxman HL, Greenspon A, et al, for the Philadelphia Arrhythmia Group. Value of electrophysiologic testing in patients with previous myocardial infarction and nonsustained ventricular tachycardia. *Am J Cardiol* 1990;65:594–598.

105. Buxton AE, Lee KL, Fisher JD, Josephson ME, et al, for the Multicenter Unsustained Tachycardia Trial Investigators. A randomized study of the prevention of sudden death in patients with coronary artery disease. *N Engl J Med* 1999;341:1882–1890.

106. Moss AJ, Hall WJ, Cannom DS, et al. Improved survival with an implanted defibrillator in patients with coronary disease at high risk for ventricular arrhythmia. *N Engl J Med* 1996;335: 19–33.

107. Nalos PC, Gang ES, Mandel WJ, et al. The signal-averaged electrocardiogram as a screening test for inducibility of sustained ventricular tachycardia in high risk patients: a prospective study. *J Am Coll Cardiol* 1987;9:539–548.

108. Winters SL, Stewart D, Targonski A, Gomes JA. Role of signal averaging of the surface QRS complex in selecting patients with nonsustained ventricular tachycardia and high grade ventricular arrhythmias for programmed ventricular stimulation. *J Am Coll Cardiol* 1988;12:1481–1487.

109. Turitto G, Fontaine JM, Ursell SN, et al. Value of the signal-averaged electrocardiogram as a predictor of the results of programmed stimulation in nonsustained ventricular tachycardia. *Am J Cardiol* 1988;61:1272–1278.

110. Turitto G, Fontaine JM, Ursell SN, et al. Risk stratification and management of patients with organic heart disease and nonsustained ventricular tachycardia: role of programmed stimulation, left ventricular ejection fraction, and the signal-averaged electrocardiogram. *Am J Med* 1990;88:35–41.

111. Poll DS, Marchlinski FE, Falcone RA, et al. Abnormal signal-averaged electrocardiograms in patients with nonischemic congestive cardiomyopathy: relationship to sustained ventricular tachyarrhythmias. *Circulation* 1985;72:1308–1313.

112. Keeling PJ, Kulakowski P, Yi G, Slade AKB, et al. Usefulness of signal-averaged electrocardiogram in idiopathic dilated cardiomyopathy for identifying patients with ventricular arrhythmias. *Am J Cardiol* 1993;72:78–84.

113. Mancini DM, Wong KL, Simson MB. Prognostic value of an abnormal signal-averaged electrocardiogram in patients with nonischemic congestive cardiomyopathy. *Circulation* 1993;87: 1083–1092.

114. Gomes JA, Winters SL, Stewart D, et al. A new noninvasive index to predict sustained ventricular tachycardia and sudden death in the first year after myocardial infarction: based on signal-averaged electrocardiogram, radionuclide ejection fraction and Holter monitoring. *J Am Coll Cardiol* 1987;10: 349–357.

115. Buxton AE, Simson MB, Falcone RA, et al. Results of signal-averaged electrocardiography and electrophysiologic study in patients with nonsustained ventricular tachycardia after healing of acute myocardial infarction. *Am J Cardiol* 1987;60:80–85.

116. Cain ME, Gomes JA, Hafley GE, et al, for the MUSTT Investigators. Performance of the signal-averaged ECG in identifying patients inducible into sustained ventricular tachycardia. *Circulation* 1996;94[Suppl I]:I–451 (Abs).

117. Cain ME, Gomes JA, Hafley GE, et al. Performance of the signal-averaged ECG and electrophysiologic testing in identifying patients vulnerable to arrhythmic or cardiac death. *Circulation* 1999;100:1–244 (Abs).

118. Gomes JA, Cain MF, Buxton AE, et al. The signal averaged ECG is a powerful predictor of Outcome in The Multicenter Unsustained Tachycardia Trial. *Circulation* 1999;100:1–244.

119. Klein LS, Shih HTS, Hackett FK, et al. Radiofrequency catheter ablation of ventricular tachycardia in patients without structural heart disease. *Circulation* 1992;85:1666–1674.

120. Chakko CS, Gheorghiade M. Ventricular arrhythmias in severe heart failure: incidence, significance, and effectiveness of antiarrhythmic therapy. *Am Heart J* 1985;109;497–504.

121. Singh SN, Fletcher RD, Fisher SG, et al, for the Survival Trial of Antiarrhythmic Therapy in Congestive Heart Failure (CHF-STAT). Amiodarone in patients with congestive heart failure and asymptomatic ventricular arrhythmia. *N Engl J Med* 1995; 333:77–82.

122. Doval HC, Nul DR, Grancelli HO, et al. Randomized trial of low-dose amiodarone in severe congestive heart failure. *Lancet* 1994;344:493–498.

122a. Amiodarone Trials Meta-analysis Investigators. Effect of prophylactic amiodarone on mortality after acute myocardial infarction and in congestive heart failure: meta-analysis of individual data from 6500 patients in randomized trials. *Lancet* 1997;350:1417–1423.

122b. Sim, I, McDonald, KM, Lavori, PW, et al. Quantitative

overview of randomized trials of amiodarone to prevent sudden cardiac death. *Circulation* 1997;96:2823–2829.

123. Fananapazir L, Leon MB, Bonow RO, et al. Sudden death during empiric amiodarone therapy in symptomatic hypertrophic cardiomyopathy. *Am J Cardiol* 1991;67:169–174.

124. CAST Investigators. Preliminary report: effect of encainide and flecainide on mortality in a randomized trial of arrhythmia suppression after myocardial infarction. *N Engl J Med* 1989;321:406–412.

125. CAST II Investigators. Effect of the antiarrhythmic agent moricizine on survival after myocardial infarction. *N Engl J Med* 1992;327:227–233.

127. Julian DG, Camm AJ, Franglin G, et al. Randomized trial of effect of amiodarone on mortality in patients with left-ventricular dysfunction after recent myocardial infarction: EMIAT. *Lancet* 1997;349:667–674.

128. Cairns JA, Connolly SJ, Roberts R, et al. Randomized trial of outcome after myocardial infarction in patients with frequent or repetitive ventricular premature depolarizations: CAMIAT. *Lancet* 1997;349:675–682.

SUSTAINED MONOMORPHIC VENTRICULAR TACHYCARDIA

DAVID MARTIN
J. MARCUS WHARTON

DEFINITION

Sustained *monomorphic* ventricular tachycardia (VT) is defined as an arrhythmia with a rate of more than 100 beats per minute (bpm) that originates solely in the ventricles. The QRS complexes during monomorphic VT have a single, uniform morphology, different from that generated by supraventricular activation. The QRS morphology may change from one episode to the next or even abruptly during a single episode (pleomorphism) (1). However, beat-to-beat change in QRS morphology is referred to as *polymorphic VT*. Although polymorphic VT may be clinically associated with monomorphic VT, a number of other specific causes of polymorphic VT must be considered, particularly ischemia or a prolonged QT interval, as discussed in Chapter 20.

Monomorphic VT is frequently classified by its duration. Sustained VT has arbitrarily been defined as that lasting more than 30 seconds or as that being associated with hypotension and lasting less than 30 seconds because of the need for cardioversion; VT is considered nonsustained when it terminates spontaneously in less than 30 seconds. Nonsustained VT is frequently a predictor of a high risk for sustained VT or ventricular fibrillation and is discussed in detail in Chapter 18. If a monomorphic ventricular arrhythmia has a rate of less than 100 bpm (some authors have used 120 bpm) (2,3), the arrhythmia is called *accelerated idioventricular rhythm*. Monomorphic VT at a fast rate (more than 270 bpm) is usually called *ventricular flutter*, because at this rate, the QRS morphology may appear sinusoidal; that is, the QRS complexes and T waves are indistinguishable.

PREVALENCE

Sustained monomorphic VT occurs as a consequence of any disorder affecting the ventricles. Given the very high prevalence of ischemic heart disease in industrial countries, VT is seen most commonly in patients with prior myocardial infarction. The prevalence of monomorphic VT in the general population has not been well characterized. Sudden cardiac death, most of which results from VT or ventricular fibrillation, accounts for at least 300,000 deaths per year in the United States (4), and hemodynamically tolerated VT occurs in an unknown additional number of patients. Because most large outcome studies combine the diagnoses of sustained monomorphic VT, polymorphic VT, and ventricular fibrillation into a single category of "serious or life-threatening ventricular arrhythmia," the ability to establish a true prevalence of monomorphic VT is limited. This grouping may be inappropriate because the pathophysiologic mechanisms and prognosis of these arrhythmias are not necessarily the same (4,5).

Acute Myocardial Infarction

Although the incidence and prevalence of sustained monomorphic VT may not be well characterized in the general population, it has been well studied in specific subgroups. The best studied subgroup includes patients with coronary artery disease, particularly patients with prior myocardial infarction and reduced left ventricular function (6–8). Sustained monomorphic VT occurs infrequently during the acute phase of myocardial infarction, with estimated prevalence of 0.3% to 2.8% (9–11); episodes of accelerated idioventricular rhythm are more frequent, particularly in patients receiving thrombolytic therapy and the incidence of this arrhythmia may be as high as 50%. Although ventricular fibrillation that occurs within the first 48 hours of myocardial infarction does not appear to provide important long-term prognostic information, VT during this period has been associated with an increased 1-year mortality rate (9–11). Thus, patients with acute myocardial infarction complicated by monomorphic VT may be at risk for recurrent VT during long-term follow-up and may deserve further evaluation before discharge, but this issue remains controversial.

D. Martin and J. M. Wharton: Department of Cardiology, Duke University Medical Center, Durham, North Carolina 27710.

Chronic Coronary Artery Disease

More commonly, patients with sustained monomorphic VT present without acute myocardial infarction, although they typically have a history of chronic coronary artery disease, often with a healed myocardial infarction, and may have a left ventricular aneurysm (7,12–14). Sustained VT and sudden cardiac death account for approximately one half of the mortality rate for patients with ischemic heart disease (4). Although the risk of VT is highest in the first year after myocardial infarction, ranging from 3% to 5% (11), patients may present with sustained monomorphic VT 15 to 20 years later in the absence of any intervening events (12). Patients with sustained monomorphic VT have lower ejection fractions than those of patients who present with nonsustained VT or sudden cardiac death (8). Because the extent of myocardial damage and the degree of left ventricular impairment are the most important prognostic indicators of VT development after myocardial infarction (15–17), the incidence of sustained monomorphic VT after myocardial infarction will likely decrease as gains are made in therapies that reduce infarct size and preserve myocardium (18,19).

Other Types of Heart Disease

In addition to ischemic heart disease, any other cardiac disease may predispose patients to the risk of sustained monomorphic VT. VT has been associated with dilated and hypertrophic cardiomyopathies (20,21), arrhythmogenic right ventricular dysplasia (22), infiltrative cardiomyopathies such as sarcoidosis (23), valvular heart disease, acute myocarditis (24), congenital heart disease usually after surgical repair (22), metabolic cardiac disease (25), and primary or metastatic cardiac tumors (26,27).

Normal Heart

Although sustained VT usually occurs in patients with structurally abnormal hearts, it may also occur in patients with "normal hearts," as assessed by traditional functional and imaging modalities (28). However, the presentation of a patient with VT should always initiate a detailed evaluation in search of structural and functional cardiac abnormalities. This "idiopathic" form represents approximately 10% of all patients referred for evaluation of VT (28a). The mean age of patients who have idiopathic VT is younger than that of patients with VT secondary to underlying heart disease.

PATHOGENESIS

Although VT may be caused by any mechanism, such as reentry, triggered activity, or abnormal automaticity, it is presumed that most VTs are generated by reentry, particularly when it occurs in the setting of ischemic heart disease (29–31).

Reentry

Scar formed by myocardial infarction or other processes provides the anatomic substrate for most reentrant VT (31,32). Areas of fibrosis interspersed between viable myocardium may provide the substrate for macroreentry and microreentry in several ways. First, the area of scar isolates corridors of abnormal conduction from the more uniform wavefront of activation in the remainder of the ventricles (Fig. 19-1) (32–35). These isolated bundles of conducting myocardium are often associated with slowed conduction, which may under appropriate modulatory influences result in such delay that the wavefront arrives at the distal terminus of the bundle to encounter fully repolarized myocardium, allowing formation of a reentrant circuit (Fig. 19-2) (32,33). These areas of slow conduction within muscle bundles surrounded by fibrosis may be caused by partially depolarized myocardium, particularly acutely after infarction. However, animal studies of healed infarction demonstrate normal resting potential of cells in these isolated bundles (34). Slow conduction appears to be a result of the relative paucity of gap junctions connecting cells within the bundle, resulting in delayed cell-cell activation (34–36). Regardless of the mechanism, delayed conduction is a critical component for reentry within the myocardium. In addition, infarction with dense fibrosis may isolate thin sheets of myocardium, which appears to accentuate the anisotropic properties of the ventricular myocardium. In canine models, premature stimulation may result in functional lines of block running parallel to fiber orientation within the sheet of myocardium with reentry established around these barriers, typically in a figure-of-eight pattern (Fig. 19-3) (37,38). Without premature stimulation of the region, no areas of constant block can be demonstrated. Thus, fibrosis provides a backdrop for reentry around anatomic, or fixed, regions of block and around functional, or nonfixed, regions of block. Clearly the two processes may be operative in the same patient with different tachycardias or even for genesis of the same tachycardia.

Fractionation and slowing of the wavefront of activation by interspersed fibrous tissue at the border of the infarct generates low-amplitude, prolonged, multicomponent electrograms that may extend beyond the end of the surface QRS (Fig. 19-1) (39–41). These complex fractionated potentials are frequently recorded at sites of VT during endocardial mapping during sinus rhythm but commonly occur at sites not involved in arrhythmogenesis (40,41). Late potentials detected by signal-average electrocardiography (SAECG) are generated by areas of delayed activation around the infarcted or fibrous zone and thus serve as a

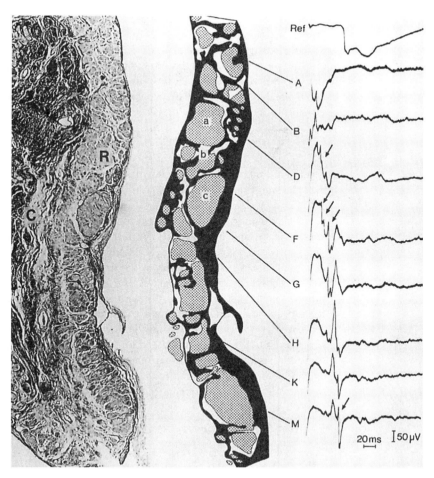

FIGURE 19-1. A strip of papillary muscle **(left)** near the site of origin of ventricular tachycardia resected from a patient undergoing surgical ablation. The section is cut perpendicular to the myocardial bundles *(R)* that survive in the area of fibrosis *(C)*. A schematic of the section **(middle)** with stippled areas representing viable muscle and black areas of fibrosis. Fractionated electrograms **(right)** recorded at various sites along the length of the section of tissue. The fractionated electrograms are caused by discontinuous, or nonsynchronous, conduction along the various bundles of myocardium at any particular site. Note the interconnections between myocardial bundles, creating the potential for multiple reentrant loops within this substrate. (From de Bakker JM, van Capelle FJ, Janse MJ, et al. Reentry as a cause of ventricular tachycardia in patients with chronic ischemic heart disease: electrophysiologic and anatomic correlation. *Circulation* 1988;77:589–606, with permission.)

noninvasive marker of substrate potentially capable of sustaining VT (40,41).

In the setting of a prior myocardial infarction, the substrate for reentrant VT typically occurs near the endocardium (31). However, the mid-myocardium or epicardium can be involved, and may be more commonly involved with nonischemic processes (42). Regions of fibrosis may separate bundles of myocardium in a complex of multiple interconnected tracts, generating the substrate for multiple interrelated reentrant circuits (32,33). Larger infarctions may generate spatially distinct sites of reentry at multiple locations along the circumference of the border zone (31). Thus, patients who have VT in the setting of prior infarction may have multiple spontaneously occurring VTs or multiple inducible VTs during electrophysiologic testing.

A specific form of VT, bundle branch reentrant VT, occurs with ischemic and nonischemic heart disease (43, 44). The heart disease is usually severe with cardiomegaly and a history of congestive heart failure. Patients with bundle branch block reentrant VT often have a baseline nonspecific conduction delay or left bundle branch block

(LBBB), and all have a prolonged His-ventricle (HV) time. The arrhythmia begins when one or more premature ventricular beats arise and conduct into the right bundle branch, where retrograde activation is blocked because of refractoriness from the preceding normally conducted antegrade beat, and into the left bundle branch, which has a shorter refractory period than that of the right bundle branch. As a result, the impulse conducts retrogradely up the left bundle branch to the bundle of His, leading to activation of the bundle of His and the recording of a His deflection during electrophysiologic study. The impulse then conducts retrogradely into the atrioventricular (AV) node, often to the atrium, and antegradely down the right bundle branch. If the right bundle branch has recovered its excitability, a reentrant circuit is established and a tachycardia may be established.

Triggered Activity

Mechanisms of arrhythmogenesis other than reentry are possible and may be more common with nonischemic heart disease or in the absence of heart disease (45–47). Cases

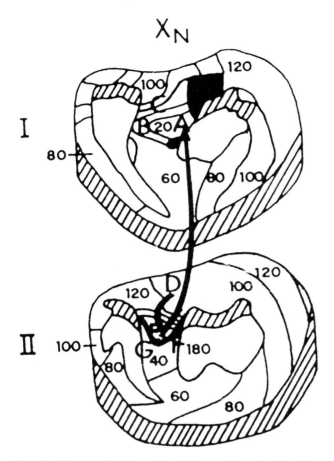

FIGURE 19-2. Detailed view of an intramural reentrant pathway during ventricular tachycardia (VT) obtained by three-dimensional mapping intraoperatively in a patient undergoing surgical ablation. Shown are the isochronal patterns reconstructed onto diagrams of two adjacent sections of the heart. Note the slow conduction (*crowded isochronal lines*) in the midseptum. The activation wavefront moves clockwise around an area of block (*between D and G*), which is represented by a thick line, and moves into a bounded corridor in the midseptum. Initiation of the subsequent VT beat occurs on the left ventricular endocardial side of the anterior septum (*long arrow*) of the more basal section of the heart. The pattern then repeats itself to sustain VT. (From Pogwizd SM, et al *Circulation* 1992;86:1872–1887, with permission.)

with VT having properties suggestive of triggered activity or abnormal automaticity have been reported (28). In particular, triggered activity has been convincingly demonstrated to be the mechanism of idiopathic right ventricular outflow tract (RVOT) tachycardias (47). However, in most clinically encountered cases of VT, the mechanism can only be inferred by results of electrophysiologic and pharmacologic testing.

Modulating Factors

The factors responsible for allowing the spontaneous occurrence of VT are poorly understood. There are a number of possible modulating factors: ischemia; changes in auto-nomic tone, particularly an increase in sympathetic neural inputs and circulating catecholamines; electrolyte disturbances, particularly hypokalemia; drugs; and loading conditions, with an increased stretch on the myocardial and elevated left ventricular wall tension, resulting in "electrical mechanical feedback," as may occur with left ventricular dilation in heart failure (4,48,49).

Ischemia

Although ischemic heart disease is the most common setting for monomorphic VT, ischemia infrequently precipitates episodes of VT (50,51). Small-vessel ischemia could possibly play a modulating role. Ischemia may increase the number of ventricular ectopic beats, which could induce VT in susceptible individuals. From a clinical standpoint, treatment of ischemia with revascularization infrequently eliminates the risk of recurrent monomorphic VT and should not be considered sole therapy for a patient presenting with VT (52,53). It has been presumed that premature ventricular contractions generated at one site were responsible for initiating VT that was maintained by a second site. Although this may occur, some studies have suggested that many episodes of VT occur by modulation of the substrate to allow spontaneous initiation from the site of maintenance (54).

Sympathetic Nervous System

Increased sympathetic tone has clearly been shown to enhance all potential mechanisms of VT; it can cause an increase in abnormal automaticity, enhance triggered activity, or alter the electrophysiologic properties of the myocardium and increase the predisposition for reentry (46,55). Sympathetic denervation of the border zone after myocardial infarction with resultant denervation supersensitivity may facilitate the effect of ambient catecholamines to provoke triggers for VT initiation and modulate reentrant circuits (55). One study suggests that regional increases in sympathetic nerves may also be related to scarring and the spontaneous occurrence of ventricular arrhythmias (56). Review of recordings before the onset of VT frequently demonstrate an increase in the heart rate, suggesting sympathetic facilitation (46,57). β-adrenergic blockade will attenuate all of the effects of sympathetic nervous system facilitation of VT. Nevertheless, β blockers do not prevent induction of VT during electrophysiologic testing (58); however, the frequency of clinically occurring episodes may be reduced (59) and the circadian increase in VT during the late morning is eliminated (60). In addition, some β blockers have been shown to decrease the risk of sudden cardiac death, total mortality rate, implantable cardioverter-defibrillator (ICD) shock frequency (61,62), and reinfarction in patients with ischemic disease and VT (63). However, a recent subanalysis of data from the Antiarrhythmics Versus Implantable Defibrillators (AVID) trial suggested that β

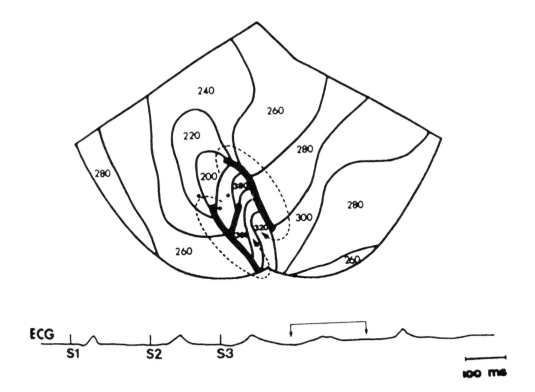

FIGURE 19-3. Figure-of-eight reentry during induced ventricular tachycardia (VT) in the canine infarct model. Shown is a planar diagram of the canine right and left ventricular epicardium as if sectioned along the posterior interventricular septum. The right ventricular epicardium is on the left side of the diagram and LV on the right, with anterior in the middle and posterior on either side. The diagram shows the isochronal map of activation during VT. Note that clockwise reentry (*dotted arrow*) occurs around a midanterior left ventricular line of functional block and counterclockwise reentry around the lower line of functional block. The two reentrant pathways define a figure-of-eight pattern. During sinus rhythm, the lines of block were not present. (From Mehra R, Zeiler RH, Gough WB, El-Sherif N. Reentrant ventricular arrhythmias in the late myocardial infarction period. 9. Electrophysiologic-anatomic correlation of reentrant circuits. *Circulation* 1983;67:11–24, with permission.)

blockers did not alter survival in patients receiving specific therapy with an ICD or amiodarone (64).

Sympathetic tone has also been shown to attenuate the effect of class I and III antiarrhythmic drugs, by reversing many of their depressant effects on impulse conduction and repolarization (65). Because beta blockade prevents this attenuation, its use may prevent partial reversal of antiarrhythmic drug effects during periods of stress and may improve long-term efficacy. Lastly, beta blockade appears to decrease the risk of proarrhythmia with class I and III antiarrhythmic drugs (66,67). All of this information suggests that beta blockade should be used whenever possible in patients with heart disease and VT.

CLINICAL PRESENTATION

Patients with sustained monomorphic VT present with a wide spectrum of signs and symptoms. The arrhythmia may rarely be detected as an incidental finding, particularly in

patients with a structurally normal heart, but usually patients with VT present with palpitations, with symptoms of reduced cardiac output and hypotension—including light-headedness, dizziness, altered mentation, visual disturbances, diaphoresis, or presyncope—or with hemodynamic collapse, syncope, and sudden death. Persistent VT may precipitate heart failure, particularly in patients with depressed left ventricular function, angina, or infarction. If blood pressure cannot be maintained during VT, cardiovascular collapse and cardiogenic shock will occur and the VT may degenerate into ventricular fibrillation. In patients with incessant, but relatively asymptomatic VT, as may occur in idiopathic VT syndromes, tachycardia-induced cardiomyopathy may occur and be reversed by pharmacologic or ablation suppression of the tachycardia (68,69). Patients on antiarrhythmic drugs such as amiodarone may develop very slow, but frequently near-incessant, VT with rates of less than 100 bpm, which is entirely asymptomatic.

The hemodynamic consequences associated with VT are related to a number of factors. Such factors include the ven-

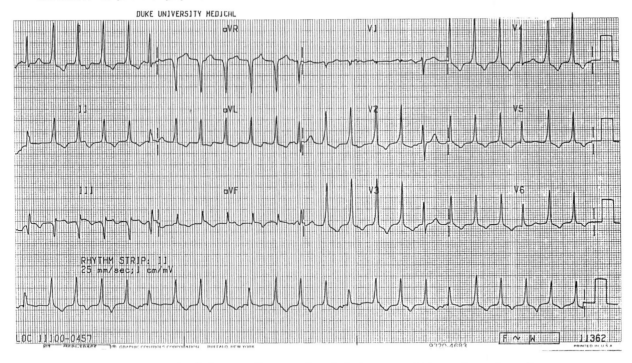

J.S. 2482995 53 yo F with palpitations

FIGURE 19-4. A 12-lead electrocardiogram of a relatively narrow QRS complex tachycardia, at first glance resembling a supraventricular tachycardia. However, on closer scrutiny, evidence of atrioventricular dissociation can be seen, with capture complexes occurring approximately every four to five QRS complexes (e.g., first, sixth, and tenth complexes) that are clearly preceded by a P wave. The QRS complexes of ventricular tachycardia have a slightly slurred upstroke, differentiating them from the capture complexes. Note the deep Q wave and ST elevation in the capture complex in lead III, from the patient's prior inferior myocardial infarction.

tricular rate, the presence and severity of structural or functional heart disease, the duration of VT, the presence and severity of peripheral vascular disease, the loss of AV synchrony, and the effect of the altered sequence of ventricular activation on systolic function (70,71). The interaction of these factors to generate hemodynamic instability is hard to predict. Clearly, the severity of underlying heart disease greatly affects the patient's tolerance of VT. Even relatively slow VT may result in hemodynamic collapse of patients with marked left ventricular systolic or diastolic dysfunction. Alteration of the sequence of ventricular activation during VT and the loss of AV synchrony can affect ventricular contractility, stroke volume, and cardiac output. In addition, the development of ischemia during the rapid ventricular rate may further alter left ventricular function.

CLINICAL EVALUATION

Patients presenting with sustained monomorphic VT and severe hemodynamic or clinical compromise need immediate electrical cardioversion. However, if the patient is clinically stable in the arrhythmia, a minimum amount of diag-

nostic information should be obtained before initiating therapy. The history, physical examination, and 12-lead ECG can all provide information that will help one confirm the diagnosis of VT versus supraventricular tachycardia with intraventricular conduction delay. As discussed later in this chapter, the 12-lead ECG during tachycardia to determine the QRS morphology may be helpful for establishing a diagnosis and a prolonged rhythm strip may facilitate identification of AV dissociation or fusion and capture beats. Furthermore, vagomimetic maneuvers or adenosine may be useful adjuncts in the diagnosis of wide-complex tachycardia by causing high-grade ventriculoatrial block and promoting identification of AV dissociation during ECG recording (72). Termination of the tachycardia with adenosine suggests a supraventricular mechanism, although adenosine-responsive VT (RVOT tachycardia) and coincidental termination of VT cannot be excluded (28). Acute pharmacologic termination of VT is discussed later in this chapter.

Physical Examination

The physical examination during VT generally adds little to the diagnosis other than the critical assessment of the rate of the arrhythmia and of the patient's tolerance to it (73,74). Specific findings during VT include evidence of AV dissociation, particularly the presence of cannon *a* waves that occur because of intermittent retrograde propulsion of blood during atrial contraction against a closed AV valve. This may occur sporadically in the setting of complete ventriculoatrial dissociation, after every beat if there is a 1 : 1 ventriculoatrial conduction, or in variable relationship if second or high-grade ventriculoatrial block is present. The carotid or peripheral pulses are often diminished in amplitude but may vary in intensity if intermittent periods of atrial and ventricular synchronization occur to augment cardiac output. Similarly, the intensity of the first heart sound may vary with the degree of AV association, although this can be difficult to appreciate when the rate is rapid. Garratt and colleagues (74) demonstrated that detection of AV dissociation in the jugular venous waveform had the highest sensitivity of these three physical findings for detection of VT, whereas detection of variability in the first heart sound had greatest specificity (74). Variability in the pulse pressure was not very sensitive or specific. Additionally, the first and second heart sounds may be variably split, and third and fourth heart sounds may be intermittently heard (73). Although these findings may be helpful in suggesting the diagnosis, the most useful tool is ECG monitoring.

Diagnostic Evaluation

After acute treatment of the VT, reversible causes of arrhythmia should be sought and a thorough diagnostic evaluation to exclude structural heart disease is warranted. Even young, otherwise healthy, patients need a thorough workup to exclude entities such as undiagnosed cardiomyopathy, anomalous origin of a coronary artery, hypertrophic cardiomyopathy, or arrhythmogenic right ventricular dysplasia. The diagnostic evaluation will generally include one or more of the following: echocardiography, exercise treadmill testing, ambulatory ECG monitoring, SAECG, coronary angiography, endomyocardial biopsy, or magnetic resonance imaging (MRI), depending partly on the clinical history and presentation. After the cardiac function and structure have been characterized, the tachycardia will often require further evaluation in an electrophysiologic study.

Electrocardiogram

Monomorphic VT typically generates a wide QRS complex tachycardia, usually with a QRS width of more than 0.12 seconds. However, the QRS may be relatively narrow (75), typically for tachycardias arising from the basal ventricular septum and may be incorrectly diagnosed and treated as a supraventricular tachycardia (Figs. 19-4 and 19-5). Akhtar and colleagues (7) demonstrated that a wide-complex tachycardia occurring in a patients with ischemic heart disease was almost always VT. However, in the setting of preexisting bundle branch block, if the QRS morphology is the same as that

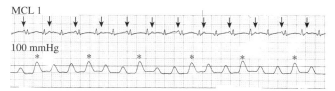

FIGURE 19-5. Single MCL₁ lead of an apparent narrow-complex tachycardia; however, other recording leads demonstrated a wide QRS complex (not shown). Careful scrutiny of the MCL₁ lead shown also demonstrates obvious atrioventricular (AV) dissociation (*arrows*). The radial artery pressure tracing is shown below the rhythm strip. Note that the systolic blood pressure for most complexes is less than 100 mm Hg. However, every third pressure recording is distinctly higher. Before each of these increases, AV synchrony is maintained with a P wave preceding the QRS complex (although there is no evidence of fusion or capture). This illustrates the significance of AV synchrony for maintaining hemodynamic stability during ventricular tachycardia.

during sinus rhythm, a supraventricular mechanism is likely (76). However, rare cases of bundle branch reentry with a QRS morphology identical to that in sinus rhythm have been reported (77). Although very uncommon, if the QRS complex is *narrower* during tachycardia than during sinus rhythm, VT is the probable diagnosis (78).

The ECG hallmark for the diagnosis of VT is demonstration of AV dissociation directly or indirectly by demonstrating fusion or capture complexes (Fig. 19-6). However, up to 40% of cases may have intact ventriculoatrial conduction during VT, preventing demonstration of ventriculoatrial dissociation (79). More often, the QRS-T-wave complexes obscure atrial activity and prevent identification of AV dissociation even when it is present. However, variability in the ST and T waves may be present, reflecting superimposed P waves and changes in ventricular repolarization, and subtle unrelated changes in the QRS morphology may occur, reflecting changes in the direction of ventricle depolarization. Esophageal lead recordings easily allow identification of atrial activity to confirm AV dissociation but are rarely used (80). The tachycardia rate is usually constant but may exhibit some variability. Marked variability in the tachycardia rate is unusual and suggests an alternative mechanism such as atrial fibrillation. Although there is often dissociation, in some cases of VT, there is retrograde AV nodal conduction. There may be a 1 : 1 retrograde conduction, a 2 : 1 retrograde conduction, or a second-degree retrograde block (79). The presence of an intermittent retrograde block, as with complete AV dissociation, is virtually diagnostic of VT.

The specific QRS morphology during wide-complex tachycardia may be helpful for distinguishing VT from supraventricular tachycardia with aberrancy (81–83). The mean frontal plane axis is generally not helpful unless it is in the far superior quadrant (−90° to −180°), which is highly specific but not sensitive for VT (7); a change in the axis, particularly a leftward shift, compared with that seen during sinus rhythm, is very suggestive of VT. Based on the QRS mor-

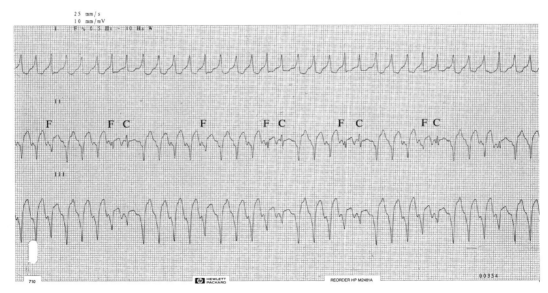

FIGURE 19-6. Leads I, II, and III during a wide-complex tachycardia in a 57-year-old man with a prior inferior myocardial infarction. Lead I demonstrates a relatively uniform QRS morphology. However, occasional pairs of narrower complexes are seen (*arrows*) with the faint suggestion of a P wave before the second complex in each pair. Review of leads II and III could almost suggest a polymorphic ventricular tachycardia, but the progressive narrowing of the QRS is associated with preceding P waves with progressive fusion (*F*) or supraventricular capture (*C*). Atrioventricular dissociation with fusion and capture beats are the hallmark of the diagnosis of ventricular tachycardia.

phology in lead V_1, VT may resemble an LBBB or a right bundle branch block (RBBB) morphology. VT having an LBBB morphology suggests an origin in the right ventricle, and an RBBB morphology from the left ventricle, but VT arising from or adjacent to either side of the septum may generate either pattern (1). Wellens and colleagues (80) demonstrated that the more the QRS morphology deviated from anticipated RBBB or LBBB patterns, the more likely the rhythm reflected VT. Thus, for an RBBB morphology tachycardia, the presence of a triphasic rSR′ in lead V_1 or qRs in lead V_6 suggested supraventricular tachycardia with a typical RBBB. However, monophasic R or RR′ complexes or biphasic QR or RS complexes were more often seen in VT (82). For an LBBB tachycardia, atypical characteristics such as the presence of a Q wave of any size in lead V_6 suggested VT, as did prolongation of the RS_{nadir} to more than 60 ms and/or notching of the S downstroke in lead V_1 or V_2 (81). For patients with LBBB morphology in the setting of healthy hearts, the LBBB criteria for VT diagnosis are less sensitive (83). With all of the morphologic criteria, there is considerable overlap of QRS morphologies that limits the utility of these criteria.

Building on the work of others (80,81), Brugada and colleagues described an algorithm for diagnosing VT that had a sensitivity of 99% and a specificity of 97% (82). According to this algorithm, if the ECG demonstrates any of the following four VT criteria, the diagnosis is VT:

1. Absence of an RS complex in all precordial leads.
2. RS_{nadir} interval of more than 100 ms in any precordial lead with an RS complex.
3. Presence of AV dissociation.
4. Morphology criteria for VT present in precordial leads V_1 or V_2 and V_6.

Only one of the above criteria needs to be satisfied to make the diagnosis of VT. If *not one* of these criteria is satisfied, the diagnosis is most likely supraventricular tachycardia with altered intraventricular activation. This algorithm cannot be applied to patients with Wolff-Parkinson-White syndrome, in which the anterograde conduction across the accessory pathway during tachycardia results in "ectopic" ventricular activation, which may fulfill these criteria. The algorithm also cannot be applied to patients taking antiarrhythmic drugs (particularly those in class Ic) because of the potential for drug-induced peripheral conduction abnormalities that may resemble VT. Furthermore, the first two criteria have less specificity in patients with preexisting intraventricular conduction defects (85). Given the number of exceptions and the need to establish the correct diagnosis, ECG criteria are only suggestive of VT and confirmation depends on other means, such as electrophysiologic testing.

The recognition of the bundle branch block pattern of monomorphic VT also has some clinical utility for suggesting possible specific VT syndromes (see discussion later in this chapter). Table 19-1 lists the various specific syndromes that need to be considered with VT having an RBBB or LBBB pattern. Clearly, the most common cause for either is ischemic heart disease. However, identification of specific types of VT may suggest clinical approaches that differ

TABLE 19-1. SPECIFIC SYNDROMES OF MONOMORPHIC VENTRICULAR TACHYCARDIA ASSOCIATED WITH LEFT AND RIGHT BUNDLE BRANCH BLOCK QRS MORPHOLOGIES

Left Bundle Branch Block	Right Bundle Branch Block
Ischemic heart disease	Ischemic heart disease
Nonischemic heart disease	Nonischemic heart disease
Arrhythmogenic right ventricular dysplasia	Idiopathic left posterior fascicular ventricular tachycardia
Bundle branch reentrant tachycardia	Bundle branch reentrant tachycardia
Idiopathic right ventricular outflow tract tachycardia	Fascicular reentrant tachycardia

from the treatment strategy for VT occurring in the setting of ischemic or nonischemic heart disease.

Signal-Average Electrocardiogram

The SAECG generally demonstrates evidence of late potentials in patients with sustained VT and ischemic heart disease (18,40,86). However, for patients with nonischemic heart disease, the findings may be more variable (87,88). The presence of bundle branch blocks, intraventricular conduction delays (89), and atrial fibrillation preclude reliable determination of late potentials, limiting application of this technique. The presence or absence of late potentials on the SAECG are only indirect data, suggestive, but not diagnostic, for the presence or absence of VT, respectively. Thus, the SAECG plays a limited role in the evaluation of patients with VT, although it may serve as a useful screening tool in the assessment of right ventricular dysplasia (22) or some patients with unexplained syncope (90).

Exercise Testing

Exercise stress testing probably has it greatest utility in assessing for the presence of ischemia in patients presenting with VT. However, some patients give a clear history of VT that is principally associated with exercise (Fig. 19-7) (91–93). These patients may have VT mechanisms that are facilitated by excess catecholamines. However, exercise is a complex physiologic event, and VT provocation may be secondary to other changes such as altered loading conditions, withdrawal of parasympathetic tone, ischemia, or some combination of these factors. Although the term *exercise-induced VT* is often used as if it represented a specific origin, this is not the case. Increased sympathetic tone and other changes that occur with exercise potentially may facilitate all mechanisms of VT; thus, the finding of exercise provocation of VT is not mechanism specific (94). However, types of VT that are often provoked with exercise include idiopathic RVOT tachycardia, which is usually catecholamine sensitive and exercise provoked (93); VT secondary to arrhythmogenic right ventricular dysplasia; idiopathic left posterior fascicular VT may

occur with exercise; and occasionally ischemic or nonischemic VT (22,91,92). Thus, exercise provocation of VT is also not specific for a categorical diagnosis of VT. Despite these limitations, patients with a history of symptoms associated with exercise should undergo exercise stress testing to see whether the arrhythmia is provoked. Careful 12-lead ECG recordings during provoked VT may suggest a specific cause of VT and guide further evaluation and therapy. Exercise provocation of VT may be reproducible enough to serve as a means of assessing pharmacologic end points (95).

Holter and Event Monitoring

Because sustained monomorphic VT generally occurs infrequently and sporadically, Holter monitoring has little utility in documenting the occurrence of this arrhythmia (50). For instance, in patients with syncope, Holter monitoring established the diagnosis of VT in less than 1% of cases (96). Holter recordings may suggest the risk of VT by the presence of frequent premature ventricular contractions and nonsustained VT; however, confirmation is needed by electrophysiologic testing or long-term event monitoring. In

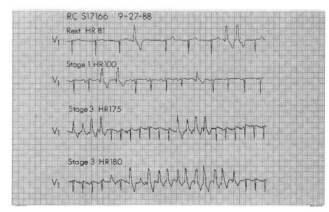

FIGURE 19-7. Lead V₁ rhythm strips from various stages of exercise in a young patient with exercise-induced palpitations. Note occasional premature ventricular contractions and couplets with a right bundle branch morphology at rest, with increasing nonsustained ventricular tachycardia with peak exertion.

Holter recordings demonstrating the spontaneous onset of monomorphic VT, ischemic ST segments are rarely seen before the event, suggesting that ischemia is rarely the cause of monomorphic VT initiation (50,51). In patients suspected of having VT but in whom the diagnosis has not been established by traditional monitoring and electrophysiologic testing, external or implantable loop monitoring may be an appropriate means of establishing the diagnosis in patients not suspected of risk of sudden death (97,98).

Electrophysiologic Studies

The electrophysiologic study on the other hand is the most effective means of establishing the diagnosis (Fig. 19-8). Patients with prior myocardial infarction and a history of sustained monomorphic VT who undergo electrophysiologic study almost always have inducible VT, although the reproducibility of VT is higher in those with slower monomorphic VT (rates of less than 250 bpm) than faster monomorphic VT or polymorphic VT (99,100). In some studies of patients with ischemic heart disease, up to 5% of patients with clinically occurring VT were not inducible (99,100). Thus, noninducibility does not exclude the diagnosis. The clinically occurring morphology of VT is frequently not the same as the morphology of the induced VT

during electrophysiologic testing. However, this is partly related to the limited number of induction attempts during routine diagnostic studies. When extensive reinitiation is performed, as during attempts at curative ablation, the clinically occurring VT is usually inducible, along with VTs that have not been seen to occur spontaneously. Thus, electrophysiologic testing remains the principle means of establishing a diagnosis of VT in the setting of ischemic heart disease. However, in patients with nonischemic cardiomyopathy and documented monomorphic VT, the rates of induction of VT are more variable, ranging from 25% to 70% (101–103). The relatively high false-negative rates must be kept in mind when interpreting electrophysiologic study results in these patients.

The role of the electrophysiologic study in evaluating patients with monomorphic VT is several-fold. First, it is used to establish the diagnosis of VT when the diagnosis is uncertain. Second, electrophysiologic study can be used to stratify patients with respect to arrhythmia risk. In the situation of patients who present with hemodynamically stable, sustained VT, electrophysiologic study can help determine the number and hemodynamic consequences of VT to determine whether medical options are a reasonable alternative or whether an ICD should be offered as primary therapy. In patients with prior myocardial infarction and

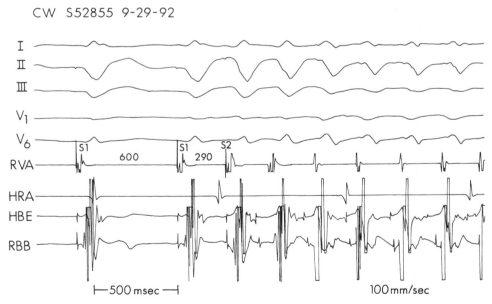

FIGURE 19-8. Surface electrocardiographic recordings from leads I, II, III, V₁, and V₆, as well as intracardiac electrographic recordings from the right ventricular apex *(RVA)*, high right atrium *(HRA)*, His bundle electrogram *(HBE)*, and right bundle branch *(RBB)* during the induction of bundle branch reentrant ventricular tachycardia (VT) during programmed ventricular extrastimulation using a single extrastimulus. The drive train (S1) is at 600 ms before delivery of the single extrastimulus (S2) with a coupling interval of 290 ms. Note that atrial activation in the HRA is dissociated from ventricular activation, confirming the diagnosis of VT. Also note the sharp deflection well before the ventricular deflections that are seen initially on the HBE and then on the RBB recording. This represents the His bundle with a right bundle potential, which is present before ventricular activation, confirming the diagnosis of bundle branch reentrant tachycardia.

left ventricular dysfunction with nonsustained VT, or in patients with heart disease and syncope, induction of sustained VT at electrophysiologic study suggests a high-risk group with an improved survival rate with an ICD (104,105). Third, electrophysiologic study can be used to establish the mechanism of the tachycardia, which may in some cases be useful in guiding appropriate therapy (e.g., for bundle branch reentrant tachycardia [BBRT] or idiopathic RVOT tachycardia). However, the utility of this application is limited in most cases.

The electrophysiologic study may also be used as a means of assessing the effectiveness of pharmacologic therapies. This last application for electrophysiologic study has recently fallen out of favor. Several clinical trials have suggested that serial electrophysiologic study to guide antiarrhythmic drug therapy is associated with relatively high rates of recurrent VT, even when optimal therapy is suggested by acute testing (106–110). The Electrophysiologic Study Versus Electrocardiographic Monitoring (ESVEM) trial prospectively compared electrophysiologically guided antiarrhythmic drug therapy with traditional Holter monitoring–guided therapy (107,108). Despite earlier retrospective data to the contrary, the ESVEM trial demonstrated no difference in recurrence rates of VT with either approach (Fig. 19-9). A randomized comparison of empirical β-blocker therapy with electrophysiologically guided medical therapy demonstrated no difference in the global strategies,

although patients rendered noninducible on medical therapy had the lowest recurrence rates of VT (106). Furthermore, electrophysiologic study–guided therapy identifies a potentially effective agent in only a few of the patients tested, and requires serial drug testing and repeated electrophysiologic studies, which result in prolonged hospitalizations and increased medical costs. Given the equivocal results of the electrophysiologic study–guided approach, it is rarely used but has been replaced by empirically given amiodarone or ICD implantation. However, in selected patients with a limited number of hemodynamically well-tolerated monomorphic VTs and relatively well-preserved left ventricular function, electrophysiologic study on therapy may be considered to assess the likelihood of VT recurrence (109).

The optimal protocol for inducing sustained monomorphic VT in the electrophysiologic laboratory has been a source of debate. A number of variables have been considered through the years in an attempt to maximize the tests' sensitivity without provoking nonclinical arrhythmias (111–118). These variables include the rate and length of the drive train, the number of extrastimuli and their current strength, the site of stimulation (including left ventricular stimulation), the role of burst pacing or infusion of isoproterenol, and the number of times stimulation should be repeated. A standard protocol would include drive trains of eight beats at 400 to 600 ms with up to three extrastimuli

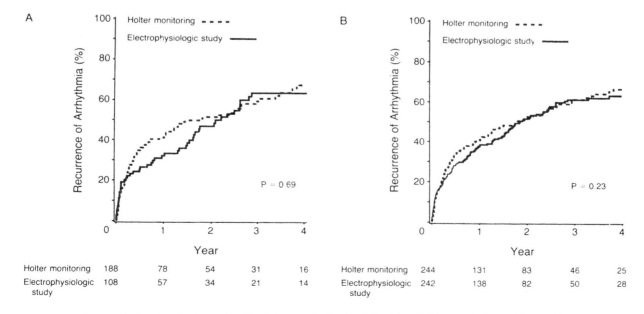

FIGURE 19-9. Percentage of patients in the Electrophysiologic Study Versus Electrocardiographic Monitoring trial with recurrent ventricular tachyarrhythmia when antiarrhythmic therapy was guided by Holter monitoring or electrophysiologic study. **A:** Only patients who achieved a therapeutic end point were compared. **B:** All patients were compared by intention-to-treat analysis. In either panel, there were no significant differences in recurrence rates between the two means of directing therapy. (From Mason JW, et al. *N Engl J Med* 1993;329:445–451, with permission.)

at currents of twice that of the diastolic threshold delivered at two right ventricular sites. An abbreviated protocol to just assess inducibility would include triple extrastimuli at a rapid drive train such as 350 ms (117). Clinical situations exist in which the electrophysiologic study may need to be tailored to the patient. For example, infusing high-dose isoproterenol may not be required in routine electrophysiologic studies, but it may be helpful when studying a competitive athlete suspected of having VT (115).

Determination of the Mechanism of VT

As mentioned previously, electrophysiologic testing can be used to determine the presumed mechanism of VT (Table 19-2). Each of the known mechanisms of VT has anticipated responses to specific pacing maneuvers and pharmacologic agents. In particular, VT caused by reentry or triggered activity should be inducible with premature extrastimuli or rapid pacing (118). Premature or burst ventricular stimulation will terminate reentrant or triggered VT. However, automatic VTs are neither provoked nor terminated by ventricular pacing maneuvers (119). However, many reentrant VTs also cannot be initiated by pacing techniques, possibly because of protective entrance block from the paced activation wavefront. Rapid burst pacing during an automatic VT may result in transient overdrive suppression, during which the VT would be transiently terminated and then demonstrate a gradual resumption and acceleration of its rate.

Reentrant VT demonstrates classic characteristics of entrainment and resetting (120–123). During resetting, a single premature stimulus enters a reentrant circuit to activate the excitable gap of the circuit to alter, or reset, the return cycle of the subsequent beat (122,123). The return cycle may remain unchanged with progressively premature extrastimuli, or it may increase (122,123). The latter implies that the wavefront encounters partially refractory tissue in at least part of the reentrant circuit. Entrainment requires overdrive pacing during VT. The criteria for entrainment include the following (120):

1. Fixed fusion complexes at a given paced cycle length.
2. Progressive degrees of fusion at faster paced cycle lengths.
3. Resumption of the tachycardia on cessation of pacing with a nonfused QRS complex, which is captured but not entrained.
4. Termination of the tachycardia on cessation of pacing at a critical rate.

Concealed entrainment refers to entrainment without evidence of surface or intracardiac fusion and occurs when pacing from sites within a protected isthmus of the tachycardia circuit (Fig. 19-10) (121). It may also occur at adjacent bystander sites that are not involved in the tachycardia circuit (121). Demonstrating concealed entrainment may be useful when attempting catheter ablation (see discussion later in this chapter).

Mapping Ventricular Tachycardia

Mapping VT begins with an analysis of the 12-lead ECG recordings during tachycardia (1,124). In general, an RBBB pattern indicates an origin in the left ventricle. Although in patients with healthy hearts, an LBBB pattern suggests an origin in the right ventricle, this is not the case in patients with healed myocardial infarction. In these patients, VT with an LBBB morphology more likely originates in the left ventricle with epicardial breakthrough in the septum (1). Determining the location of the tachycardia is aided by considering the frontal plane axis. For example, an inferior axis suggests a superior origin of the tachycardia, whereas a superior axis suggests the opposite. One may consider the precordial leads. A QS pattern during tachycardia in the lateral precordial leads, for instance, suggests that the ventricular wavefront is moving away from the apex of the heart, indicating the VT origin is near the apex.

TABLE 19-2. ELECTROPHYSIOLOGIC AND ELECTROPHARMACOLOGIC MEANS TO DETERMINE THE MECHANISM OF VENTRICULAR TACHYCARDIA

Characteristic	Reentry	Triggered Activity	Automaticity
Electrophysiologic			
Induction with PES/BP	Yes	Yes	No
Termination with PES/BP	Yes	Yes	No
Transient overdrive suppression	No	No	Yes
Resetting	Yes	Yes	No
Entrainment	Yes	No	No
DAD with MAP	No	Yes	No
Electropharmacologic			
β Blockers	No	Yes	Yes
Verapamil	No	Yes	No
Adenosine	No	Yes	No

DAD, delayed after depolarization; BP, burst pacing; PES, premature extrastimulus.

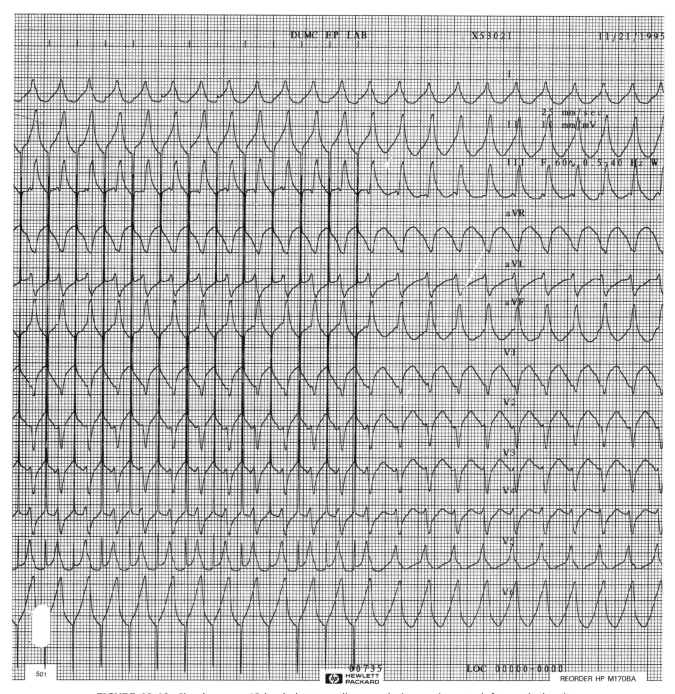

FIGURE 19-10. Simultaneous 12-lead electrocardiogram during pacing at a left ventricular site having a mid-diastolic potential during ventricular tachycardia (VT) with a left bundle branch block and normal axis morphology. Note the sharp artifacts during pacing, which disappear when pacing is terminated. During pacing, the evoked QRS pattern is the same as that during VT, but the rate has been accelerated to the pacing rate. Thus, pacing at the mid-diastolic potential is activating an excitable gap and advancing activation out of the bounded corridor of slow conduction to generate a QRS identical to that during VT without pacing. Acceleration of the VT cycle length to the paced cycle length without changing the QRS morphology is known as *concealed entrainment* and suggests a narrow bounded corridor amenable to ablation.

Pace mapping is an invasive technique for locating the origin of the tachycardia that involves placing a mapping catheter near the origin of the VT (Fig. 19-11) (125,126). Pacing at this site should generate QRS complexes resembling those during VT. The closer the QRS morphology during pace mapping to that during VT, the closer the catheter is to the origin of the tachycardia. Ideally, concordance should occur in 12 of 12 leads on the surface ECG, although this is frequently not achievable. Pace mapping is particularly useful in patients with poorly tolerated or non-sustained VT.

With activation mapping, the mapping catheter is advanced to the site with earliest endocardial activation preceding the QRS complex during tachycardia (Fig. 19-12) (1,121,127). Such early activation reflects the site from which electrical systole emanates. This assumption holds true whether the mechanism is focal (automatic, triggered) or reentrant. Prepotentials can precede the QRS by tens to hun-

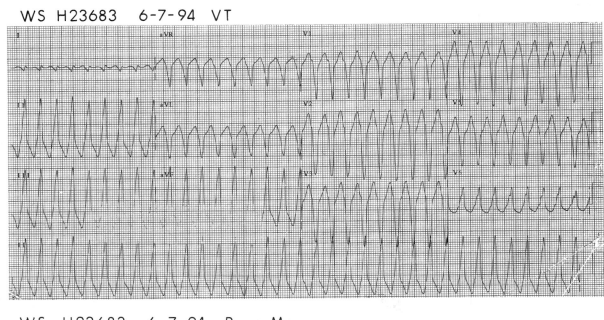

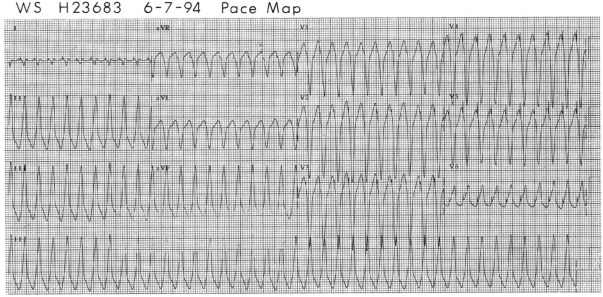

FIGURE 19-11. A: A 12-lead electrocardiogram of idiopathic right ventricular outflow tract tachycardia with a left bundle branch block and a right axis deviation pattern. **B:** Pace mapping at a similar rate as that of the ventricular tachycardia at the site of successful ablation reveals concordance of QRS morphology between paced and spontaneous ventricular tachycardia beats in all 12 leads.

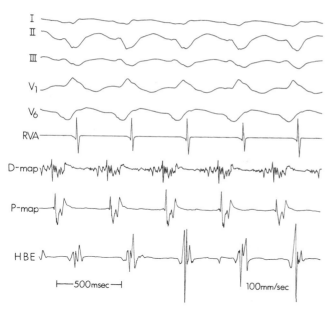

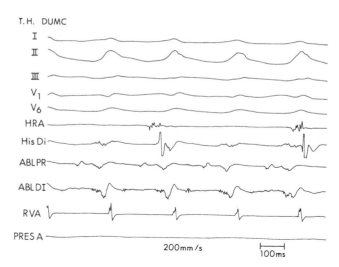

FIGURE 19-13. Discrete mid-diastolic potential occurring in early diastole in ventricular tachycardia on the distal ablation lead *(ABL DI)* and later on the proximal *(ABL PR)*. Pacing at this site resulted in concealed entrainment (Fig. 19-10).

FIGURE 19-12. Surface electrocardiographic and intracardiac electrographic recordings during ventricular tachycardia in a patient with a prior anterior myocardial infarction. Note the QRS morphology has a right bundle branch block and far superior axis with a QS in lead V₆ consistent with a left ventricular apical origin. On the distal mapping catheter *(D map)* at the site of successful ablation, there is a markedly fractionated electrogram that spans most of diastole into early systole. The proximal mapping catheter *(P map)* has a more normal appearing electrogram with an onset the same as that of the QRS complex. The distal mapping electrode thus is recording from the distal half of the diastolic zone of conduction and the proximal is probably closer to the exit site of the tachycardia into healthier periinfarct tissue.

dreds of milliseconds. Such prepotentials may merge into the major ventricular deflection, or there may be an intervening isoelectric segment, in which case, the potentials are called mid-diastolic potentials (Fig. 19-13) (127). Mid-diastolic potentials occur in reentrant VT and are thought to represent areas of slow and fractionated conduction in the distal zone of slow conduction (121,127,128). When combined with concealed entrainment, the presence of mid-diastolic potentials that cannot be dissociated from the tachycardia may be useful in identifying successful sites for ablation (121). Demonstrating concealed entrainment identifies a middle or proximal site within the zone of slow conduction and has been reported to increase the success rate of radiofrequency ablation by about threefold (121,127,128). For nonreentrant VT, ablation is performed at the site that shows earliest activation.

Demonstrating fractionated endocardial electrograms during sinus rhythm is another technique used to identify potential sites of VT origin. Sites of prior infarction frequently have complex patterns, including fractionation, split potentials, decreased amplitude, and prolonged duration, with electrogram components extending beyond the end of the surface QRS complex (39). Such areas are thought to serve as substrates for reentry and thus could identify regions

critical for the maintenance of VT. Although such areas could be targeted for ablation, this mapping technique is limited because similar electrograms often occur in regions not associated with the reentrant VT circuit. The other methods listed previously provide more direct approaches to mapping.

Nonfluoroscopic electroanatomic mapping is a new technique, which is based on the use of a special catheter with a locatable sensor tip, connected to a mapping and navigation system (129). An external magnetic field is created by an ultralow magnetic field emitter, usually located under the table where the patient lies. A miniature magnetic field sensor at the tip of the catheter can determine the location (x, y, z coordinates) and the orientation (roll, pitch, and yaw) of the catheter. The catheter generates an accurate and individualized three-dimensional reconstruction of the chamber size and local geometry, in addition to the usual local electrograms (130). The system can generate isochrones of electrical activity as color-coded static maps or animated dynamic maps of activation wavefront. These pictures can define the reentrant circuits during VT and the site of origin or breakthrough of ectopic activity with centrifugal, monoregional, or asymmetric spread of electrical activity (131,132). An additional advantage is local electrogram voltage mapping during sinus, paced, or any other rhythm that defines anatomically correct regions of no voltage (presumed scar), low voltage, and "normal" voltage.

THERAPY

Acute Therapy

The acute therapy for sustained monomorphic VT depends on the degree of hemodynamic tolerance. For clinically unstable patients, electrical cardioversion is indicated. If the patient is hemodynamically stable during VT, pharmacologic therapy is usually attempted before electrical cardioversion. Although lidocaine has in the past been considered the agent of choice for treatment of VT, recent studies have suggested only modest efficacy (133–137). Intravenous procainamide, sotalol, and amiodarone have much greater efficacy (134,137–141). The recently published guidelines from the American Heart Association and International Liaison Committee on Resuscitation recommend intravenous procainamide, sotalol, or amiodarone as frontline therapy for hemodynamically stable VT in lieu of lidocaine (141). Lidocaine can be considered in combination with procainamide or amiodarone if the latter are ineffective alone. Bretylium has been shown to have a similar efficacy to that of intravenous amiodarone for ventricular tachyarrhythmias, although it was associated with more hypotension (142). However, bretylium is no longer available for use. Intravenous amiodarone has been shown to have a dose-related decrease in arrhythmia recurrences (143). Intravenous dofetilide and ibutilide are effective treatments of VT, although their use is primarily for termination of atrial tachyarrhythmia (144,145).

For recurrent monomorphic VT that cannot be controlled with other oral or intravenous conventional agents, such as patients with ICDs receiving multiple shocks, several studies suggest that intravenous amiodarone is the drug of choice (140–143,146). Intravenous sotalol is also an effective alternative but is not available in the United States (134,138,147). Treatment of underlying ischemia and heart failure and decreasing sympathetic facilitation of VT are also critical components to acute therapies. Adjunctive use of β blockers is very effective for blocking sympathetic facilitation of VT in combination with antiarrhythmic agents. In the postoperative or intensive care unit setting, eliminating or decreasing the use of inotropic or adrenergic agents allows easier pharmacologic control of VT. In the acute setting, the judicious use of sedative-hypnotic agents to lower anxiety may facilitate management.

Chronic Therapy

Chronic therapy to prevent VT can involve the use of antiarrhythmic drugs, an ICD, or radiofrequency catheter ablation; in some patients, a combination of these approaches may be necessary.

Antiarrhythmic Drugs

A number of trials have evaluated the efficacy of antiarrhythmic therapy in the long-term management of patients with sustained monomorphic VT or other serious ventricular arrhythmia. A common theme of these studies is that for ethical reasons, no placebo-controlled group was used. This lack of a placebo control makes the results difficult to interpret because, as found in the Cardiac Arrhythmia Suppression Trial (148), antiarrhythmic therapy, despite demonstrating efficacy in suppressing arrhythmia, may increase the incidence of arrhythmic-related deaths, ischemic death, and overall mortality rate relative to placebo. Omitting this concern from analysis, class Ia, Ib, Ic, and III antiarrhythmic drugs all have antiarrhythmic efficacy. Combination therapy using different classes of antiarrhythmic drugs may also be effective (149) but is rarely used.

Of the antiarrhythmic agents, available data suggest that the class III drugs are superior to the class I drugs for treatment of monomorphic VT. In the ESVEM trial (107,108), sotalol was superior to all the other class I agents with which it was compared. Similarly, in the Cardiac Arrest in Seattle: Conventional versus Amiodarone Drug Evaluation (CASCADE) trial, amiodarone was superior to the class Ia agents with which it was compared (150). This suggests that sotalol or amiodarone is the preferred treatment for patients with monomorphic VT. Although there are no adequate trials comparing amiodarone with sotalol, several small trials have suggested similar efficacy (151–153). However, the negative inotropic properties of sotalol limit its usage as treatment of VT in patients with significant left ventricular dysfunction (154). The long-term efficacy of the newer class III drugs such as dofetilide has not been adequately evaluated.

Implantable Cardioverter-Defibrillator

Three large-scale prospective trials have suggested that ICD therapy improves survival rates compared with amiodarone in patients with hemodynamically unstable VT (154–157). The AVID trial has helped clarify the treatment of serious ventricular arrhythmias (154,155). This study compared the ICD with empirical amiodarone (a small proportion of patients received sotalol) in patients with (a) near-fatal ventricular fibrillation, (b) sustained VT with syncope, or (c) sustained VT with an ejection fraction of 0.40 or less and symptoms suggesting severe hemodynamic compromise. Overall, the survival rate was significantly higher with the ICD, with estimates of 89.3% as compared with 82.3% in the antiarrhythmic drug group at 1 year, and 75.4% versus 64.1% at 3 years (Fig. 19-14) (154). Based on these results, the ICD has become the treatment of choice in patients presenting with sustained monomorphic VT and hemodynamic compromise, with antiarrhythmic drug therapy used as an adjunct. Similar outcomes have been suggested in two other trials (Canadian Implantable Defibrillator Study and Cardiac Arrest Study Hamburg) of hemodynamically unstable ventricular arrhythmias (156,157).

However, none of these trials addresses therapy for patients with hemodynamically tolerated VT, and optimal therapy for this group remains to be defined. Studies have suggested that patients with slow or well-tolerated VT may have survival rates similar to those without inducible VT (109). However, controlled data are not available. Never-

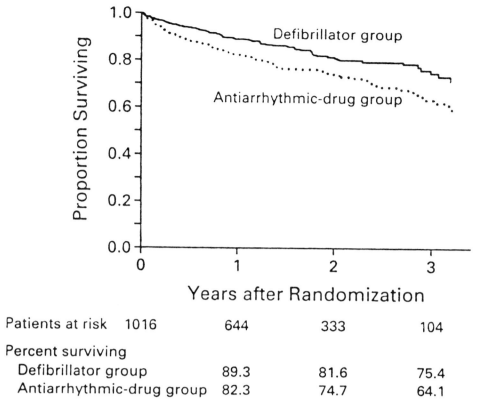

FIGURE 19-14. Survival in the Antiarrhythmics Versus Implantable Defibrillators (AVID) trial for patients with hemodynamically unstable ventricular tachyarrhythmias treated with an implantable cardioverter-defibrillator (ICD) versus antiarrhythmic drug therapy (essentially amiodarone). Note the improved survival in the patients treated with an ICD. (From AVID Investigators. A comparison of antiarrhythmic drug therapy with implantable defibrillators in patients resuscitated from near-fatal ventricular arrhythmias. The Antiarrhythmics Versus Implantable Defibrillators [AVID] Investigators. *N Engl J Med* 1997;337:1576–1583, with permission.)

theless, if the results of two clinical trials that evaluated prophylactic ICD in patients with prior myocardial infarction, depressed ejection fraction, nonsustained VT, and inducible sustained VT can be generalized to patients who present with sustained monomorphic VT, then survival benefit from ICD implantation could be anticipated (104,105).

Radiofrequency Catheter Ablation

For patients with recurrent VT despite antiarrhythmic and ICD therapy, and for patients with symptomatic idiopathic VT, radiofrequency catheter ablation is a therapeutic option (Fig. 19-15). This therapy is generally not an option in patients with hemodynamically unstable VT, as most ablation techniques require that patients be in sustained VT for prolonged periods to map the tachycardia, and recurrence rates are high (158–161). However, techniques are being developed for ablating hemodynamically unstable VT by mapping during sinus rhythm using pace mapping or searching for fractionated electrograms (162,163); a newer technique involves an electroanatomic mapping system (164).

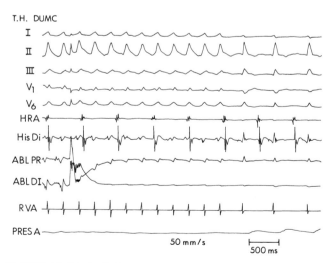

FIGURE 19-15. Radiofrequency ablation of ventricular tachycardia (VT). The distal ablation lead (*ABL DI*) is located at a site showing entrainment (Fig. 19-10) and mid-diastolic potentials. The VT is terminated within 2 seconds of turning on a radiofrequency current (note artifact on ablation leads). (PRES A is the right femoral artery pressure recording.)

Results of clinical studies suggest that radiofrequency ablation may be successful in ablating selected VT morphologies in patients with ischemic disease, with success rates varying from 50% to 90% depending on a number of factors (158–161). However, most still have inducible VT that may recur clinically, so implantation of an ICD is probably preferable as a backup (159). Success rates for ablation of VT in the setting of nonischemic cardiomyopathy are less impressive (161), unless the patient has bundle branch reentry (see later discussion). Despite the modest results for ablation of VT in the setting of heart disease, idiopathic VT has very high success rates for ablation, in excess of 90% (28). Surgical ablation is rarely used today, given its high morbidity and mortality rates.

SPECIFIC VENTRICULAR TACHYCARDIA SYNDROMES

Bundle Branch Reentrant Tachycardia

The reentrant circuit of some monomorphic VTs may predominantly involve the bundle branches (BBRT) or the left anterior or posterior fascicles (reentrant fascicular tachycardia).

Bundle Branch Reentrant Tachycardia

BBRT is by far the more common of the two, although the two may occur together (165). During BBRT, anterograde conduction typically proceeds down the right bundle branch, initially activating the right ventricle to generate an LBBB–left anterior descending QRS morphology tachycardia, retrogradely activating the left bundle branch to reenter the right bundle branch at the junction with the distal His bundle (Fig. 19-16) (166–168). The His bundle is not a critical part of the circuit but is retrogradely activated during tachycardia. However, because the anterograde conduction across the right bundle is relatively normal, the His deflection will proceed the inscription of the QRS complex with an interval equal to or slightly longer than the HV interval during sinus rhythm (Fig. 19-8). This could potentially suggest a supraventricular mechanism, if not for the fact that AV dissociation is almost always present. Less commonly, anterograde conduction proceeds down the left bundle branch, with retrograde activation up the right bundle branch, generating an RBBB morphology tachycardia (169,170).

BBRT occurs most commonly in patients with dilated cardiomyopathy; and in those patients with BBRT, dilated cardiomyopathy has been reported to be present in 45% to 95% of cases (171,172). BBRT, however, may occur in patients without dilated cardiomyopathy, and BBRT has been reported to be the mechanism of monomorphic VT in up to 41% of patients with nonischemic dilated cardiomyopathies (169,173). Bundle branch reentry usually results in a rapid VT, and syncope or even sudden cardiac death in

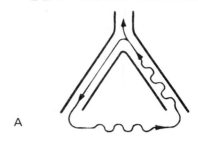

BBR-LBBB PATTERN

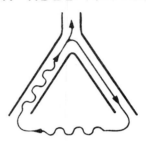

BBR-RBBB PATTERN

FIGURE 19-16. Diagram of the reentrant circuit during counterclockwise **(A)** and clockwise **(B)** reentry using the bundle branches. The more commonly encountered variant is counterclockwise reentry, which generates a left bundle branch block tachycardia. The clockwise pattern generates a right bundle branch block tachycardia and is seen much less frequently.

most patients (172). The ECG during supraventricular rhythm usually demonstrates a nonspecific or left ventricular intraventricular conduction delay, indicating disease within the bundle branches, which is necessary for imposing retrograde conduction delay of sufficient magnitude to allow anterograde reentry of the contralateral bundle branch.

Bundle branch reentry can only be diagnosed using intracardiac recordings. Conduction abnormalities in the His-Purkinje system, as reflected by HV interval prolongation, are invariably present and reflect the intraventricular conduction delays seen on the surface ECG (171). Premature stimulation of the ventricles is the usual method by which sustained BBRT is induced in the laboratory. Characteristic features of BBRT include the following (171):

1. His bundle potential before each QRS.
2. An HV interval equal to or greater than the HV interval during sinus rhythm.
3. Changes in the His-to-His interval precede changes in the ventricle-to-ventricle interval (this is an important criterion for separating BBRT from other VTs that incidentally retrogradely activate the bundle branches as "innocent bystanders").
4. A critical ventricle-to-His (VH) delay occurs at the initiation of tachycardia (representing both retrograde block in

one bundle branch and increasing retrograde conduction delay in the contralateral, unblocked bundle branch).

5. The tachycardia can be terminated by a critically timed pacing-induced extrastimulus in the His-Purkinje system.

Although BBRT should be suspected in any patient who has a dilated cardiomyopathy with syncope or sudden death, it should also be considered as the cause of any sustained monomorphic VT when the patient has conduction abnormalities during supraventricular rhythm or has an LBBB morphology tachycardia. Narasimhan and colleagues (169) reported that BBRT may occur as soon as a few days after aortic or mitral valve surgery, even in patients with normal left ventricular function. Identifying BBRT as the mechanism of VT is important because it may be easily cured by radiofrequency ablation of the right or left bundle branch (173,174). Unfortunately, patients with BBRT frequently have other inducible intramyocardial VTs, requiring additional treatment.

Reentrant Fascicular Tachycardia

Reentrant fascicular tachycardias involve reentry presumptively within interconnected branches of the left-sided fascicular network (165,175). Whether reentry occurs solely within the Purkinje network or within Purkinje fibers with interposed myocardium is not known. Reentrant fascicular tachycardias occur in similar situations as BBRT, although the patient may have a full RBBB or LBBB during supraventricular rhythm, and the two arrhythmias may occur in the same patient (165). The diagnosis is suggested by early activation of the His bundle during VT (VH of less than 50 ms), implying proximity of the His bundle to the critical limb of the reentrant circuit. The diagnosis is confirmed by demonstration of a Purkinje potential preceding ventricular activation during VT. Ablation at this site may eliminate the fascicular tachycardia (165). The localized ("intrafascicular") nature of this circuit distinguishes the tachycardia from interfascicular tachycardia in which the circuit involves anterograde conduction over one fascicle (e.g., left posterior) and retrograde conduction over another fascicle (e.g., left anterior) (165,175).

Arrhythmogenic Right Ventricular Dysplasia

Arrhythmogenic right ventricular dysplasia (ARVD) was first described in the late 1970s by Guy Fontaine and coworkers (176). In ARVD patients, the endocardium and epicardium are normally separated, but the right ventricular myocardium has been replaced by adipocytes (177,178). The pathologic picture of ARVD is in distinct contrast to Uhl's anomaly (parchment thin right ventricle), in which there is fusion of the endocardium and epicardium as a result of congenital absence of the right ventricular

myocardium (179). With ARVD, the fatty replacement of myocardium is patchy initially and may involve relatively small areas of myocardium. With time, the process may progress to involve most of the right ventricle and even the left ventricle. However, initially, ARVD involves the right ventricle only, with a particular predilection for the apex, outflow tract, and lateral base of the right ventricle (the so-called "triangle of dysplasia") (177). Little is known about the pathogenesis of ARVD or the factors responsible for its progression in some patients. Thiene and colleagues (178) have demonstrated evidence of an acute myocardium inflammation in some patients, suggesting a smoldering myocarditis of some origin followed by an abnormal healing process of fatty, rather than fibrous, tissue replacement. A family history of ARVD or sudden death occurs in about half of the patients, with genetic analysis suggesting an autosomal dominant pattern of inheritance and in some cases a definable genetic defect (179–184).

Because ARVD is a cause of ventricular arrhythmias and sudden death, the disorder should be considered in any patient who presents with syncope, particularly if the syncope occurred during exercise (177). ARVD is most common in young adult men but can be observed at any age and in both sexes. Some cases are familial and a genetic origin appears to account for some cases (180–184). Because of their preserved left ventricular function, many patients with ARVD and VT experience symptoms that last several minutes without complete loss of consciousness. However, sudden death may occur and this appears more common during sports or strenuous exertion. VT in patients with ARVD usually has an LBBB QRS configuration with a variable axis, depending on its site of origin in the right ventricle. These patients may have several monomorphic VTs with different LBBB morphologies. The presence of RBBB morphology VTs suggests progression of the disease or a process other than ARVD.

The diagnosis of ARVD may be difficult to confirm. The physical examination findings are usually normal. The 12-lead ECG results in sinus rhythm are often normal. T wave inversion in the anterior precordial leads and incomplete or complete RBBB are the most common patterns associated with ARVD (177,185), but the 12-lead ECG results are often normal. In the right precordial leads, the distinct but small amplitude potentials, called *epsilon waves,* may occur at, or shortly after, the termination of the QRS complex in less than one third of cases (Fig. 19-17) (176). Epsilon waves are secondary to delayed activation of myocardial fibers in the right ventricle. Patients with ARVD almost always have late potentials detected by SAECG, again reflecting delayed right ventricular activation in areas of fatty infiltration. However, nonspecific late potentials may be the most sensitive marker of ARVD (186,187) and provide an effective screening test for ARVD. If ARVD is suspected and the SAECG results are abnormal, then further studies are needed to confirm or exclude the diagnosis.

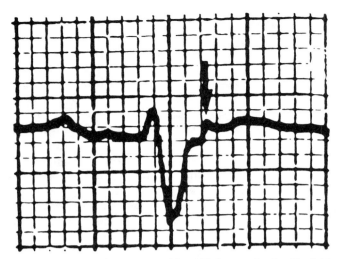

FIGURE 19-17. Enlargement of lead V₁ in a patient with right ventricular dysplasia. Note the deflection (*epsilon wave*) occurring after the end of the QRS complex. (From Reiter MI, et al. *Am J Cardiol* 1983;51:113–121, with permission.)

Imaging techniques such as echocardiography, radionuclide angiography, computed tomography, MRI, or ventricular angiography may be helpful in confirming the diagnosis by demonstrating right ventricular dilation, hypokinesia, or localized dyskinetic or aneurysmal segments (22,188–191). Left ventricular function is usually normal early in the disease presentation. The presence of left ventricular function should raise the possibility of other more diffuse cardiomyopathic processes. Although echocardiography is frequently considered an effective screening tool, its results are usually normal early in the presentation of the disease. Thus, right ventricular abnormalities suggest the diagnosis, but normal echocardiogram results do not exclude the diagnosis. Some experts have suggested that MRI is the most effective means of establishing the diagnosis, by demonstration of right ventricular wall motion abnormalities on cine–magnetic resonance angiography and the presence of a bright myocardial T2 signal suggesting intramyocardial fat on gated MRI (191). However, MRI studies require considerable expertise to interpret, and idiopathic RVOT tachycardia may be associated with right ventricular wall motion abnormalities and confused for ARVD, or vice versa (192). In our experience, multiplane right ventriculography is probably the optimal diagnostic test. However, the diagnosis is usually made by weighing the results of multiple tests.

One or more VTs with an LBBB morphology can usually be induced with programmed ventricular extrastimulation during electrophysiologic study, occasionally with isoproterenol to facilitate induction (193). Induction of VT with more than one morphology is inconsistent with idiopathic RVOT tachycardia. As with patients with healed myocardial infarction, delayed, doubled, and fragmented potentials may be recorded from the myopathic

areas. The ability to induce the VT, the presence of marked presystolic or mid-diastolic activity during tachycardia, and the demonstration of concealed entrainment from the latter areas suggest reentry as the mechanism of VT (176,194).

ARVD may be treated with antiarrhythmic drugs, an implantable defibrillator, catheter ablation, or surgery (177). Surgery involving a simple ventriculotomy or disarticulation of the right ventricle has been used (177,195), but the advent of the ICD has virtually eliminated the need for surgery. Because the disease tends to be progressive, antiarrhythmic drugs and catheter ablation are generally reserved as adjunctive therapy. The prognosis of patients with ARVD is unclear, as few studies have investigated the long-term evolution of the disease (196,197). Family members of ARVD patients should be screened for the disease. In a series of 20 cases at the Mayo Clinic, 30% of first-order relatives who were screened were affected (198).

Idiopathic Ventricular Tachycardia

VT occurring in the setting of an apparently healthy heart as determined by conventional imaging and functional studies is called *idiopathic VT.* Among all cases of diagnosed sustained VT, the proportion of patients without overt heart disease is approximately 10% to 15%. The mean age of patients with VT and apparently healthy hearts is about 35 years. Importantly, the heart in these syndromes is not normal, but the abnormalities are only electrophysiologic, possibly associated with structural changes that are not identifiable by present means. Idiopathic VTs are relatively uncommon and represent a heterogeneous group of disorders, the two most common of which are idiopathic RVOT tachycardia and idiopathic left posterior fascicular tachycardia.

Although the detection of sustained monomorphic VT in an otherwise healthy person is often alarming, the course of such patients is generally benign, assuming that heart disease has been adequately excluded.

Idiopathic Right Ventricular Outflow Tract Tachycardia

Idiopathic RVOT tachycardia may clinically present as paroxysmal sustained VT, repetitive nonsustained monomorphic VT, or frequent premature ventricular contractions with occasional nonsustained VT (Fig. 19-18) (28,93, 199). Patients may be asymptomatic or present with symptoms that range from palpitations to dizziness and syncope (200–202). In some cases, there is spontaneous remission of arrhythmia (203). Idiopathic RVOT tachycardia appears to have a benign course, although isolated cases of sudden death have been reported (201,204); these cases may have represented undiagnosed cases of right ventricular dysplasia. Because patients with right ventricular dysplasia may present like patients with idiopathic RVOT tachycardia, and

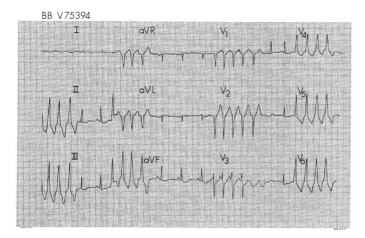

BB V75394

FIGURE 19-18. Repetitive runs of left bundle branch block nonsustained ventricular tachycardia initiated by infusion of isoproterenol. Note the relatively narrow left bundle branch morphology with a normal QRS transition in the mid-precordial leads. However, the frontal plane axis is rightward, and the QRS complexes in the inferior leads have a peculiar narrow and pointed appearance. These QRS morphology features and the repetitive nonsustained episodes with adrenergic stimulation are typical of catecholamine-sensitive, idiopathic right ventricular outflow tract tachycardia.

because these arrhythmias have significant differences in treatment and long-term prognosis, it is important that ARVD be excluded in patients suspected of having idiopathic RVOT tachycardia (28,187,190).

As its name implies, idiopathic RVOT tachycardia has a focal origin in the outflow tract of the right ventricle, usually along the septal aspects just below the pulmonary valve. This tachycardia has a characteristic QRS morphology with a relatively narrow LBBB and inferior and right axis deviation (Fig. 19-18) (202). The QRS width is usually narrower and the amplitude higher than that with VT in the setting of chronic myocardial infarction or other cardiomyopathies (204). The QRS complex morphology in the inferior leads shows a very characteristic pyramidal shape, characteristic of an origin immediately beneath the pulmonary valve. Occasional cases are shown to arise from the left ventricular outflow tract (LVOT), typically just beneath the aortic valve. Although still maintaining the inferiorly directed axis, the tachycardia may have an RBBB pattern in VT in lead V_1 or an LBBB pattern with an early transition at leads V_2 to V_3 to a dominant R complex (205).

Idiopathic RVOT tachycardia is catecholamine sensitive and thus is characteristically exercise- or stress-induced (28,93). The occurrence, frequency, and duration of premature ventricular contractions and nonsustained VT increase with increasing heart rate, further suggesting catecholamine dependence (46). The tachycardia is typically suppressed by calcium channel blockers, beta blockade, increased vagal tone, and adenosine. This clinical and pharmacologic profile suggests that the underlying mechanism of this arrhythmia

is a cyclic adenosine monophosphate–mediated triggered activity resulting from delayed afterdepolarizations (93).

Treatment of paroxysmal sustained RVOT tachycardia depends on patient symptoms. If symptoms are infrequent and mild, no treatment may be necessary. If symptoms include highly symptomatic palpitations, presyncope, or syncope, pharmacologic therapy or catheter ablation may be used. Given that triggered activity is the probable mechanism of the tachycardia, effective suppression may be obtained with verapamil or a β blocker in about 50% of patients (206–210). Calcium channel blockers and β blockers may be used synergistically. The low risk of proarrhythmia or serious side effects with these medications makes them appropriate front-line therapies in most patients. Other potentially effective therapies include class Ia agents (disopyramide, procainamide, quinidine), class Ic agents (flecainide, propafenone), and class III agents (sotalol, amiodarone) (202,206,208,209). Nonpharmacologic therapy includes radiofrequency catheter ablation, which has a success rate of more than 90% (211–213).

Idiopathic Left Posterior Fascicular Tachycardia

Idiopathic left posterior fascicular tachycardia is the most common form of idiopathic left VT. The tachycardia arises from a verapamil-sensitive, adenosine-insensitive reentrant mechanism involving the Purkinje network near the left posterior fascicle (214–216). Given its origin along the inferior midseptal left ventricle, the QRS morphology during tachycardia has an RBBB and left axis deviation pattern (Fig. 19-19) (214,215). Left anterior fascicular tachycardia may also occur and except for its location (right inferior axis on 12-lead ECG) is similar to the posterior fascicular type (217). The absence of adenosine sensitivity helps distinguish this VT from idiopathic LVOT tachycardia. Patients generally present between the ages of 15 and 40 years with palpitations, but they may present with presyncope or syncope (216,218,219). The QRS duration is shorter (less than 140 ms) than that seen in VT associated with structural heart disease (220). The tachycardia typically may occur at rest, but catecholamine dependence is not uncommon (221,222). The tachycardia can be incessant and may cause tachycardia-induced cardiomyopathy (68). As with other forms of VT in the setting of a healthy heart, the prognosis of patients with this arrhythmia is favorable (223).

Although the exact anatomic circuit has not been defined, the tachycardia appears to be generated at least in part within the left posterior (or anterior) fascicle. Fascicular dependence is suggested by induction of VT with atrial (in addition to ventricular) pacing (218), the early appearance of a retrogradely activated His bundle potential (VH of less than 40 ms) during VT, and at the site of successful ablation the demonstration of Purkinje potentials preceding by 20 to 30 msec the onset of the QRS during sinus rhythm and VT

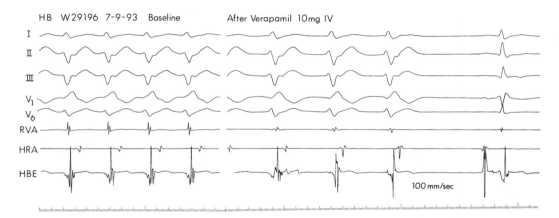

FIGURE 19-19. Right bundle branch block and left axis–deviated ventricular tachycardia (VT) occurring in a young patient with a healthy heart. **Left:** VT in the baseline state with a cycle length of 340 ms. **Right:** The VT after intravenous administration of 10 mg of verapamil, which slows the cycle length to 480 ms before termination. Note that the last complex on the far right side of the recording is a sinus beat. Also note the small His deflection buried in the initial portion of the ventricular electrogram on the His bundle electrogram *(HBE)* recording.

(221). Although its verapamil sensitivity was once thought to suggest triggered activity as the underlying cause (214), studies demonstrating classic entrainment confirm that the mechanism is reentrant (224,225). The verapamil-sensitive reentrant mechanism is not sensitive to adenosine or increased parasympathetic tone, a clinical characteristic useful to distinguish idiopathic left posterior (or anterior) fascicular VT from idiopathic RVOT or LVOT tachycardia (226,227).

Therapy for idiopathic left posterior fascicular tachycardia can be pharmacologic or nonpharmacologic. Although verapamil works well acutely, it is not universally effective as chronic therapy, particularly in highly symptomatic patients (223). Class I antiarrhythmics and β blockers are typically ineffective, although class III drugs are reported to be effective in about 50% of patients (204). As an alternative to chronic medical therapy, radiofrequency ablation may be offered and has a success rate of about 90% (221,222).

SUMMARY AND RECOMMENDATIONS

Although most patients with sustained monomorphic VT have a history of coronary artery disease and depressed left ventricular function, this arrhythmia represents a heterogenous group of disorders. It occurs in patients with other types of structural heart disease and in those with structurally normal hearts. The presentation of patients with sustained monomorphic VT is varied, as are the ECG features that suggest the diagnosis. Patients may require an electrophysiologic study to confirm the ventricular origin of a wide QRS complex tachycardia and to determine the mechanism of VT. Treatment must be individualized in accordance with the patient's symptoms during VT and the subsequent risk of death. Patients with structurally normal

hearts may often be treated with medications as initial therapy, although catheter ablation is a viable alternative in many patients. Patients with structural heart disease typically require implantation of an ICD as first-line therapy, with antiarrhythmics and catheter ablation used as adjunctive therapy.

Our ability to understand the causes, pathogenesis, and prognosis of ventricular arrhythmias at the personal and population levels is limited by the fact that many outcome studies in humans have grouped all ventricular tachyarrhythmias together. Future research should distinguish between the various types of ventricular arrhythmias. At a minimum, monomorphic VT, polymorphic VT, and ventricular fibrillation should be distinguished. When possible, and particularly important for monomorphic VT, the rate, duration, axis, and QRS morphology should also be recorded. Such specification will allow researchers to elucidate etiologic mechanisms more precisely and assess prognosis more accurately, thus ensuring continued improvement in our armamentarium for treating patients with ventricular tachyarrhythmias.

REFERENCES

1. Josephson ME, Horowitz LN, et al. Recurrent sustained ventricular tachycardia. 4. Pleomorphism. *Circulation* 1979;59:459–468.
2. Massumi RA, Ali N. Accelerated isorhythmic ventricular rhythms. *Am J Cardiol* 1970;26:170–185.
3. Denes P, Gillis AM, Pawitan Y, et al, and the CAST Investigators. Prevalence, characteristics and significance of ventricular premature complexes and ventricular tachycardia detected by 24-hour continuous electrocardiographic recording in the Cardiac Arrhythmia Suppression Trial. *Am J Cardiol* 1991;68:887–896.

4. Myerburg RJ, Kessler KM, Kimura S, et al. Life-threatening ventricular arrhythmias: The link between epidemiology and pathophysiology. In: Zipes DP, Jalife J, eds. *Cardiac electrophysiology: from cells to bedside.* Philadelphia: WB Saunders, 1995: 723–731.

5. Adhar GC, Larson LW, Bardy GH, Greene HL. Sustained ventricular arrhythmias: differences between survivors of cardiac arrest and patients with recurrent sustained ventricular tachycardia. *J Am Coll Cardiol* 1988;12:159–165.

6. Cohen M, Wiener I, Pichard A, et al. Determinants of ventricular tachycardia in patients with coronary artery disease and ventricular aneurysm. Clinical, hemodynamic, and angiographic factors. *Am J Cardiol* 1983;51:61–64.

7. Akhtar M, Shenasa M, Jazayeri M, et al. Wide QRS complex tachycardia. Reappraisal of a common clinical problem. *Ann Intern Med* 1988;109:905–912.

8. Eldar M, Sievner Z, Goldbourt U, et al, for the SPRINT Study Group. Primary ventricular tachycardia in acute myocardial infarction: clinical characteristics and mortality. *Ann Intern Med* 1992;117:31–36.

9. Newby KH, Thompson T, Stebbins A, et al, for the GUSTO Investigators. Sustained ventricular arrhythmias in patients receiving thrombolytic therapy: incidence and outcomes. *Circulation* 1998;98:2567–2573.

10. Mont L, Cinca J, Blanch P, et al. Predisposing factors and prognostic value of sustained monomorphic ventricular tachycardia in the early phase of acute myocardial infarction. *J Am Coll Cardiol* 1996;28:1670–1676.

11. Stevenson WG, Brugada P, Waldecker B, et al. Clinical, angiographic, and electrophysiologic findings in patients with aborted sudden death as compared with patients with sustained ventricular tachycardia after myocardial infarction. *Circulation* 1985;71:1146–1152.

12. Denniss AR, Ross DL, Richards DA, et al. Differences between patients with ventricular tachycardia and ventricular fibrillation as assessed by signal-averaged electrocardiogram, radionuclide ventriculography and cardiac mapping. *J Am Coll Cardiol* 1988;11:276–283.

13. Bolick DR, Hackel DB, Reimer KA, Ideker RE. Quantitative analysis of myocardial infarct structure in patients with ventricular tachycardia. *Circulation* 1986;74:1266–1279.

14. Mukharji J, Rude RE, Poole WK, et al. Risk factors for sudden death after acute myocardial infarction: two-year follow-up. *Am J Cardiol* 1984;54:31–36.

15. Marchlinski FE. Ventricular tachycardia associated with coronary artery disease. In: Zipes DP, Rowlands DJ, eds. *Progress in cardiology.* Philadelphia: Lea & Febiger, 1988:231–253.

16. Swerdlow CD, Winkle RA, Mason JW. Determinants of survival in patients with ventricular tachyarrhythmias. *N Engl J Med* 1983;308:1436–1442.

17. Lampert S, Lown B, Graboys TB, et al. Determinants of survival in patients with malignant ventricular arrhythmia associated with coronary artery disease. *Am J Cardiol* 1988;61:791–797.

18. Pedretti RF, Colombo E, Sarzi BS, Caru B. Effect of thrombolysis on heart rate variability and life-threatening ventricular arrhythmias in survivors of acute myocardial infarction. *J Am Coll Cardiol* 1994;23:19–26.

19. Hohnloser SH, Franck P, Klingenheben T, et al. Open infarct artery, late potentials, and other prognostic factors in patients after acute myocardial infarction in the thrombolytic era. A prospective trial. *Circulation* 1994;90:1747–1756.

20. Bansch D, Bocker D, Brunn J, et al. Cluster of ventricular tachycardias signify impaired survival in patients with idiopathic dilated cardiomyopathy and implantable cardioverter defibrillators. *J Am Coll Cardiol* 2000;36:566–573.

21. Elliott PM, Sharma S, Varnava A, et al. Survival after cardiac arrest or sustained ventricular tachycardia in patients with hypertrophic cardiomyopathy. *J Am Coll Cardiol* 1999;33: 1596–1601.

22. Nibley C, Wharton JM. Ventricular tachycardias with left bundle branch block morphology. *Pace* 1995;18:334–356.

23. Winters SL, Coheh M, Greenberg S, et al. Sustained ventricular tachycardia associated with sarcoidosis: assessment of the underlying cardiac anatomy and the prospective utility of programmed ventricular stimulation, drug therapy and an implantable antitachycardia device. *J Am Coll Cardiol* 1991;18:937–943.

24. Friedman RA, Kearney CL, Moak JP, et al. Persistence of ventricular arrhythmia after resolution of occult myocarditis in children and young adults. *J Am Coll Cardiol* 1994;24:780–783.

25. DeLonlay-Debeney P, Fournet JC, Bonnet D. Fatty acid betaoxidation deficiency masquerading as fulminant myocarditis. *Int J Cardiol* 1998;65:287–289.

26. Fukushima KK, Mitani T, Hashimoto K, et al. Ventricular tachycardia in a patient with cardiac lipoma. *J Cardiovasc Electrophysiol* 1999;10:1161.

27. Mager A, Strasberg B, Zlotikamien B, et al. Life-threatening ventricular tachycardia as the presenting symptom of metastatic cardiac disease. *Clin Cardiol* 1991;14:696–698.

28. Vergara I, Wharton JM. Ventricular tachycardia and fibrillation in normal hearts. *Curr Opinions Cardiol* 1998;13:9–19.

28a. Brooks R, Burgess JH. Idiopathic ventricular tachycardia: a review. *Medicine* 1988;67:271.

29. Pogwizd SM, Corr PB. Reentrant and nonreentrant mechanisms contribute to arrhythmogenesis during early myocardial ischemia: Results of three dimensional mapping. *Circ Res* 1987; 61:352–371.

30. Richardson AW, Callans DJ, Josephson ME. Electrophysiology of postinfarction ventricular tachycardia: a paradigm of stable reentry. *J Cardiovasc Electrophysiol* 1999;10:1288–1292.

31. Stevenson WG. Ventricular tachycardia after myocardial infarction: from arrhythmia surgery to catheter ablation. *J Cardiovasc Electrophysiol* 1995;6:942–950.

32. de Bakker JM, van Capelle FJ, Janse MJ, et al. Reentry as a cause of ventricular tachycardia in patients with chronic ischemic heart disease: electrophysiologic and anatomic correlation. *Circulation* 1988;77:589–606.

33. de Bakker JM, van Capelle FJ, Janse MJ, et al. Slow conduction in the infarcted human heart. `Zigzag` course of activation. *Circulation* 1993;88:915–926.

34. Gardner PI, Ursell PC, Fenoglio JJ Jr, Wit AL. Electrophysiologic and anatomic basis for fractionated electrograms recorded from healed myocardial infarcts. *Circulation* 1985;72:596–611.

35. Spear JF, Balke CW, Lesh MD, et al. Effect of cellular uncoupling by heptanal on conduction in infarcted myocardium. *Circ Res* 1990;66:202–217.

36. Peters NS, Coromilas J, Severs NJ, Wit AL. Disturbed connexin 43 gap junction distribution correlates with the location of reentrant circuits in the epicardial border zone of healing canine infarcts that cause ventricular tachycardia. *Circulation* 1997;95: 988–996.

37. Mehra R, Zeiler RH, Gough WB, El-Sherif N. Reentrant ventricular arrhythmias in the late myocardial infarction period. 9. Electrophysiologic-anatomic correlation of reentrant circuits. *Circulation* 1983;67:11–24.

38. Dillon SM, Allessie MA, Ursell PC, Wit AL. Influences of anisotropic tissue structure on reentrant circuits in epicardial border zones of subacute canine infarcts. *Circ Res* 1988;63:182–206.

39. Cassidy DM, Vassallo JA, Miller JM, et al. Endocardial catheter mapping in patients in sinus rhythm: relationship to underlying heart disease and ventricular arrhythmias. *Circulation* 1986;73: 645–652.

40. Vaitkus PT, Kindwall KE, Marchlinski FE, et al. Differences in

electrophysiological substrate in patients with coronary artery disease and cardiac arrest or ventricular tachycardia. Insights from endocardial mapping and signal-averaged electrocardiography. *Circulation* 1991;84:672–678.

41. Hood MA, Pogwizd SM, Peirick J, Cain ME. Contribution of myocardium responsible for ventricular tachycardia to abnormalities detected by analysis of signal-averaged ECGs. *Circulation* 1992;86:1888–1901.

42. Blanchard SM, Walcott GP, Wharton JM, Ideker RE. Why is catheter ablation less successful than surgery for treating ventricular tachycardia that results from coronary artery disease? *Pace* 1994;17[Pt I]:2315–2335.

43. Lloyd EA, Zipes DP, Heger JJ, Prystowsky EN. Sustained ventricular tachycardia due to bundle branch reentry. *Am Heart J* 1982;104:1095.

44. Caceres J, Jazayeri M, McKinnie J, et al. Sustained bundle branch reentry as a mechanism of clinical tachycardia. *Circulation* 1989;79:256.

45. Sung RJ, Shapiro WA, Shen EN, et al. Effects of verapamil on ventricular tachycardias possibly caused by reentry, automaticity, and triggered activity. *J Clin Invest* 1983;72:350–360.

46. Stein KM, Karagounis LA, Markowitz SM, et al. Heart rate changes preceding ventricular ectopy in patients with ventricular tachycardia caused by reentry, triggered activity, and automaticity. *Am Heart J* 1998;136:425–534.

47. Lerman BB, Stein K, Engelstein ED, et al. Mechanism of repetitive monomorphic ventricular tachycardia. *Circulation* 1995; 92:421.

48. Dean JW, Lab MJ. Arrhythmia in heart failure: role of mechanically induced changes in electrophysiology. *Lancet* 1989;1: 1309.

49. Reiter MJ, Landers M, Zetelaki Z, et al. Electrophysiologic effects of acute dilatation in the isolated rabbit heart. Cycle length–dependent effects on ventricular refractoriness and conduction velocity. *Circulation* 1997;96:4050.

50. De Luna AB, Coumel P, Leclercq J. Ambulatory sudden cardiac death: mechanisms of production of fatal arrhythmias on the basis of data from 157 cases. *Am Heart J* 1989;117:151–159.

51. Currie P, Saltissi S. Transient myocardial ischemia after acute myocardial infarction does not induce ventricular arrhythmias. *Br Heart J* 1993;69:303–307.

52. Kelly P, Ruskin JN, Vlahakes GJ, et al. Surgical coronary revascularization in survivors of prehospital cardiac arrest: its effect on inducible ventricular arrhythmias and long-term survival. *J Am Coll Cardiol* 1990;15:267–273.

53. Manolis AS, Rastegar H, Estes NA III. Effects of coronary artery bypass grafting on ventricular arrhythmias: results with electrophysiological testing and long-term follow-up. *Pace* 1993;16:984–991.

54. Bardy GH, Olson WH. Clinical characteristics of spontaneous onset sustained ventricular tachycardia and ventricular fibrillation in survivors of cardiac arrest. In: Zipes DP, Jalife J, eds. *Cardiac electrophysiology: from cells to bedside.* Philadelphia: WB Saunders, 1990:778–790.

55. Zipes DP. Sympathetic stimulation and arrhythmias. *N Engl J Med* 1991;325:656–657.

56. Coa JM, Fishbein MC, Han JB, et al. Relationship between regional cardiac hyperinnervation and ventricular arrhythmias. *Circulation* 2000;101:1960–1969.

57. Nemec J, Hammill SC, Shen WK. Increase in heart rate precedes episodes of ventricular tachycardia and ventricular fibrillation in patients with implantable cardioverter defibrillators: analysis of spontaneous ventricular tachycardia database. *Pace* 1999;22:1729–1738.

58. Leclercq JF, Leenhardt A, Lemarec H, et al. Predictive value of electrophysiologic studies during treatment of ventricular tachycardia with the beta-blocking agent nadolol. The Working Group on Arrhythmias of the French Society of Cardiology. *J Am Coll Cardiol* 1990;16:413–417.

59. Ogunyankin KO, Singh BN. Mortality reduction by antiadrenergic modulation of arrhythmogenic substrate: significance of combining beta blockers and amiodarone. *Am J Cardiol* 1999; 84(9A):76R–82R.

60. Behrens S, Ehlers C, Bruggemann T, et al. Modification of the circadian pattern of ventricular tachyarrhythmias by beta-blocker therapy. *Clin Cardiol* 1997;20:253–257.

61. Kuhlkamp V, Mewis C, Mermi J, et al. Suppression of sustained ventricular tachyarrhythmias: a comparison of d,l-sotalol with no antiarrhythmic drug treatment. *J Am Coll Cardiol* 1999;33:46.

62. Pacifico A, Hohnloser SH, Williams JH, et al, for the d,l-Sotalol Implantable Cardioverter-Defibrillator Study Group. Prevention of implantable-defibrillator shocks by pretreatment with sotalol. *N Engl J Med* 1999;340:1855

63. Szabo BM, Crijns HJ, Wiesfeld AC, et al. Predictors of mortality in patients with sustained ventricular tachycardia or ventricular fibrillation and depressed ventricular function: importance of beta-blockade. *Am Heart J* 1995;130:281–286.

64. Exner DV, Reiffel JA, Epstein AE, et al. Beta-blocker use and survival in patients with ventricular fibrillation or symptomatic ventricular tachycardia: the Antiarrhythmics Versus Implantable Defibrillator (AVID) trial. *J Am Coll Cardiol* 1999;34:325–333.

65. Sager PT. Modulation of antiarrhythmic drug effects by beta-adrenergic sympathetic stimulation. *Am J Cardiol* 1998;82(4A): 20I–30I.

66. Kennedy HL. Beta-blocker prevention of proarrhythmia and proischemia: clues from CAST, CAMIAT, and EMIAT. *Am J Cardiol* 1997;80:1208–1211.

67. Myerburg RJ, Kissler KM, Cox MM, et al. Reversal of proarrhythmic effects of flecainide acetate and encainide hydrochloride on propranolol. *Circulation* 1990;80:1571.

68. Singh B, Kaul U, Talwar KK, Wasir HS. Reversibility of "tachycardia induced cardiomyopathy" following the cure of idiopathic left ventricular tachycardia using radiofrequency energy. *Pace* 1996;19:1391–1392.

69. Vijgen J, Hill P, Biblo LE, Carlson MD. Tachycardia-induced cardiomyopathy secondary to right ventricular outflow tract ventricular tachycardia: improvement of left ventricular systolic function after radiofrequency catheter ablation of the arrhythmia. *J Cardiovasc Electrophysiol* 1997;8:445.

70. Hamer AW, Zaher CA, Rubin SA, et al. Hemodynamic benefits of synchronized 1 : 1 atrial pacing during sustained ventricular tachycardia with severely depressed left ventricular function in coronary artery disease. *Am J Cardiol* 1985;55:990–994.

71. Saksena S, Ciccone JM, Craelius W, et al. Studies on left ventricular function during sustained ventricular tachycardia. *J Am Coll Cardiol* 1984;4:501–508.

72. Rankin AC, Oldroyd KG, Chong E, et al. Value and limitation of adenosine in the diagnosis of narrow and broad complex tachycardias. *Br Heart J* 1989;62:195–203.

73. Mandel WJ. Sustained monomorphic ventricular tachycardia. In: Podrid PJ, Kowey PR, eds. *Cardiac arrhythmia: mechanisms, diagnosis, and management.* Baltimore: Williams & Wilkins, 1995: 919–935.

74. Garratt CJ, Griffith MJ, Young G, et al. Value of physical signs in the diagnosis of ventricular tachycardia. *Circulation* 1994; 90:3103–3107.

75. Hayes JJ, Stewart RB, Green HL, Bardy GH. Narrow QRS ventricular tachycardia. *Ann Intern Med* 1991;114:460–463.

76. Dongas J, Lehman MH, Mahmud R, et al. Value of preexisting bundle branch block in the electrocardiographic differentiation of supraventricular from ventricular origin of wide QRS tachycardia. *Am J Cardiol* 1985;55:717–721.

77. Oreto G, Smeets JLRM, Rodriguez L-M, et al. Wide complex tachycardia with atrioventricular dissociation and QRS morphology identical to that of sinus rhythm: a manifestation of bundle branch reentry. *Heart* 1996;76:541–547.

78. Ward DE, Camm AJ. *Clinical electrophysiology of the heart.* London: Edward Arnold, 1987.

79. Shaw M, Nieman JT, Haskell RJ, et al. Esophageal electrocardiography in acute cardiac care. Efficacy and diagnostic value of a new technique. *Am J Med* 1987;82:689–696.

80. Wellens HJJ, Bar RWHM, Lie KI. The value of the electrocardiogram in the differential diagnosis of a tachycardia with a widened QRS complex. *Am J Med* 1978;64:27–33.

81. Kindwell I, Brown J, Josephson ME. Electrocardiographic criteria for ventricular tachycardia in wide complex left bundle branch block morphology tachycardias. *Am J Cardiol* 1988;61: 1279–1283.

82. Brugada P, Brugada J, Mont L, et al. A new approach to the differential diagnosis of a regular tachycardia with a wide QRS complex. *Circulation* 1991;83:1649–1659.

83. Reddy CP, Khorasanchian A. Intraventricular reentry with narrow QRS complex. *Circulation* 1980;61:641–647.

84. Griffith MJ, De Belder MA, Linker NJ, et al. Difficulties in the use of electrocardiographic criteria for the differential diagnosis of left bundle branch block pattern tachycardia in patients with a structurally normal heart. *Eur Heart J* 1992;13:478–483.

85. Alberca T, Almendral J, Sanz P, et al. Evaluation of the specificity of morphological electrocardiographic criteria for the differential diagnosis of wide QRS complex tachycardia in patients with intraventricular conduction defects. *Circulation* 1997;96: 3527–3533.

86. Martinez-Rubio A, Shenasa M, Borgreffe M, et al. Electrophysiologic variables characterizing the induction of ventricular tachycardia versus ventricular fibrillation after myocardial infarction: relation between ventricular late potentials and coupling intervals for the induction of sustained ventricular tachyarrhythmias. *J Am Coll Cardiol* 1993;21:1624–1631.

87. Turitto G, Ahuja RK, Caref EB, el-Sherif N. Risk stratification for arrhythmic events in patients with nonischemic dilated cardiomyopathy and nonsustained ventricular tachycardia: role of programmed stimulation and the signal-averaged electrocardiogram. *J Am Coll Cardiol* 1994;24:1523–1528.

88. Brembilla-Perrot B, Terrier de la Chaise A, Jacquemin L, et al. The signal-averaged electrocardiogram is of limited value in patients with bundle branch block and dilated cardiomyopathy in predicting inducible ventricular tachycardia or death. *Am J Cardiol* 1997;79:154–159.

89. Ommen SR, Hammill SC, Bailey KR. Failure of signal-averaged electrocardiography with use of time-domain variables to predict inducible ventricular tachycardia in patients with conduction defects. *Mayo Clin Proc* 1995;70:132–136.

90. Steinberg JS, Prystowski E, Freedman RA, et al. Use of the signal-averaged electrocardiogram for predicting inducible ventricular tachycardia in patients with unexplained syncope: relation to clinical variables in a multivariate analysis. *J Am Coll Cardiol* 1994;23:99–106.

91. Rodriguez LM, Waleffe A, Brugada P, et al. Exercise-induced sustained symptomatic ventricular tachycardia: incidence, clinical, angiographic and electrophysiologic characteristics. *Eur Heart J* 1990;11:225–232.

92. O-Hara GE, Brugada P, Rodriguez LM, et al. Incidence, pathophysiology and prognosis of exercise-induced sustained ventricular tachycardia associated with healed myocardial infarction. *Am J Cardiol* 1992;70:875–878.

93. Lerman BB, Stein KM, Markowitz SM. Idiopathic right ventricular outflow tract tachycardia: a clinical approach. *Pace* 1996;19:2120–2137.

94. Sung RJ, Shen EN, Morady F, et al. Electrophysiologic mechanism of exercise-induced sustained ventricular tachycardia. *Am J Cardiol* 1983;51:525–530.

95. Woelfel A, Foster JR, Simpson RJ Jr, Gettes LS. Reproducibility and treatment of exercise-induced ventricular tachycardia. *Am J Cardiol* 1984;53:751–756.

96. Gradman AH, Batsford WP, Rieur EC, et al. Ambulatory electrocardiographic correlates of ventricular inducibility during programmed stimulation. *J Am Coll Cardiol* 1985;5:1087–1093.

97. Linzer M, Pritchett EL, Pontinen M, et al. Incremental diagnostic yield of loop electrocardiographic recorders in unexplained syncope. *Am J Cardiol* 1990;66:214–219.

98. Krahn AD, Klein GJ, Yee R, et al. Use of an extended monitoring strategy in patients with problematic syncope. Reveal Investigators. *Circulation* 1999;99:406–410.

99. Volgman AS, Zheutlin TA, Mattioni TA, et al. Reproducibility of programmed electrical stimulation responses in patients with ventricular tachycardia or fibrillation associated with coronary artery disease. *Am J Cardiol* 1992;70:758–763.

100. Bhandari AK, Hong R, Kulick D, et al. Day to day reproducibility of electrically inducible ventricular arrhythmias in survivors of acute myocardial infarction. *J Am Coll Cardiol* 1990;15:1075–1081.

101. Kron J, Hart M, Schual-Berke S, et al. Idiopathic dilated cardiomyopathy. Role of programmed electrical stimulation and Holter monitoring in predicting those at risk of sudden death. *Chest* 1988;93:85–90.

102. Brembilla-Perrot B, Donetti J, de la Chaise AT, et al. Diagnostic value of ventricular stimulation in patients with idiopathic dilated cardiomyopathy. *Am Heart J* 1991;121:1124–1131.

103. Chen X, Shenasa M, Borggrefe M, et al. Role of programmed ventricular stimulation in patients with idiopathic dilated cardiomyopathy and documented sustained ventricular tachyarrhythmias: inducibility and prognostic value in 102 patients. *Eur Heart J* 1994;15:76.

104. Moss AJ, Hall WJ, Cannom DS, et al. Improved survival with an implanted defibrillator in patients with coronary disease at high risk for ventricular arrhythmia. Multicenter Automatic Defibrillator Implantation Trial Investigators. *N Engl J Med* 1996;335:1933–1940.

105. Buxton AE, Lee KL, Fisher JD, et al. A randomized study of the prevention of sudden death in patients with coronary artery disease. Multicenter Unsustained Tachycardia Trial Investigators. *N Engl J Med* 1999;341:1882–1890.

106. Steinbeck G, Andresen D, Bach P, et al. A comparison of electrophysiologically guided antiarrhythmic drug therapy with beta-blocker therapy in patients with symptomatic, sustained ventricular tachyarrhythmias. *N Engl J Med* 1992;327:987–992.

107. ESVEM Investigators. The ESVEM trial. Electrophysiologic Study Versus Electrocardiographic Monitoring for selection of antiarrhythmic therapy of ventricular arrhythmias. *Circulation* 1989;79:1354–1360.

108. ESVEM Investigators. Determinants of predicted efficacy of antiarrhythmic drugs in the Electrophysiologic Study Versus Electrocardiographic Monitoring trial. *Circulation* 1993;87: 323–329.

109. Waller TJ, Kay HR, Spielman SR, et al. Reduction in sudden death and total mortality by antiarrhythmic therapy evaluated by electrophysiologic drug testing: criteria of efficacy in patients with sustained ventricular tachycardia. *J Am Coll Cardiol* 1987; 10:83–89.

110. Kim SG, Seiden SW, Felder SD, et al. Is programmed stimulation of value in predicting the long-term success of antiarrhythmic therapy for ventricular tachycardia? *N Engl J Med* 1986; 315:356–362.

111. Buxton AE, Waxman HL, Marchlinski FE, et al. Role of triple

extrastimuli during electrophysiologic study of patients with documented sustained ventricular tachyarrhythmias. *Circulation* 1984;69:532–540.

112. Morady F, DiCarlo L, Winston S, et al. A prospective comparison of triple extrastimuli and left ventricular stimulation in studies of ventricular tachycardia induction. *Circulation* 1984;70:52–57.

113. Brugada P, Abdollah H, Heddle B, Wellens HJ. Results of a ventricular stimulation protocol using a maximum of 4 premature stimuli in patients without documented or suspected ventricular arrhythmias. *Am J Cardiol* 1983;52:1214–1218.

114. Doherty JU, Kienzle MG, Buxton AE, et al. Discordant results of programmed ventricular stimulation at different right ventricular sites in patients with and without spontaneous sustained ventricular tachycardia: a prospective study of 56 patients. *Am J Cardiol* 1984;54:336–342.

115. Freedman RA, Swerdlow CD, Echt DS, et al. Facilitation of ventricular tachyarrhythmia induction by isoproterenol. *Am J Cardiol* 1984;54:765–770.

116. Morady F, Dicarlo LAJ, Liem LB, et al. Effects of high stimulation current on the induction of ventricular tachycardia. *Am J Cardiol* 1985;56:73–78.

117. Morady F, Kadish A, de Buitleir M, et al. Prospective comparison of a conventional and an accelerated protocol for programmed stimulation in patients with coronary artery disease. *Circulation* 1991;83:764–773.

118. Brugada P, Wellens HJ. The role of triggered activity in clinical ventricular arrhythmias. *Pace* 1984;7:260–271.

119. Delacretaz E, Stevenson WG, Ellison KE, et al. Mapping and radiofrequency catheter ablation of the three types of sustained monomorphic ventricular tachycardia in nonischemic heart disease. *J Cardiovasc Electrophysiol* 2000;11:11–17.

120. MacLean WA, Plumb VJ, Waldo AL. Transient entrainment and interruption of ventricular tachycardia. *Pacing Clin Electrophysiol* 1981;4:358–366.

121. Stevenson WG, Khan H, Sager P, et al. Identification of reentry circuit sites during catheter mapping and radiofrequency ablation of ventricular tachycardia late after myocardial infarction. *Circulation* 1993;88:1647–1670.

122. Almendral JM, Stamato NJ, Rosenthal ME, et al. Resetting response patterns during sustained ventricular tachycardia: relationship to the excitable gap. *Circulation* 1986;74:722–730.

123. Almendral JM, Rosenthal ME, Stamato NJ, et al. Analysis of the resetting phenomenon in sustained uniform ventricular tachycardia: incidence and relation to termination. *J Am Coll Cardiol* 1986;8:294–300.

124. Kuchar DL, Ruskin JN, Garan H. Electrocardiographic localization of the site of origin of ventricular tachycardia in patients with prior myocardial infarction. *J Am Coll Cardiol* 1989;13:893–903.

125. Goyal R, Harvey M, Daoud EG, et al. Effect of coupling interval and pacing cycle length on morphology of paced ventricular complexes. Implications for pace mapping. *Circulation* 1996;94:2843–2849.

126. Stevenson WG, Sager PT, Natterson PD, et al. Relation of pace mapping QRS configuration and conduction delay to ventricular tachycardia reentry circuits in human infarct scars. *J Am Coll Cardiol* 1995;26:481–488.

127. Fitzgerald DM, Friday KJ, Wah JA, et al. Electrogram patterns predicting successful catheter ablation of ventricular tachycardia. *Circulation* 1988;77:806–814.

128. Bogun F, Bahu M, Knight BP, et al. Comparison of effective and ineffective target sites that demonstrate concealed entrainment in patients with coronary artery disease undergoing radiofrequency ablation of ventricular tachycardia. *Circulation* 1997;95:183–190.

129. Gepstein L, Hayam G, Ben-Haim BA. A novel method for nonfluoroscopic catheter-based electroanatomical mapping of the heart. *Circulation* 1997;95:1611–1622.

130. Smeets JLRM, Ben-Haim SA, Rodrigues LM, et al. New method for nonfluoroscopic endocardial mapping in humans: accuracy assessment and first clinical results. *Circulation* 1998;97:2426.

131. Friedman PA, Packer DL, Hammill SC. Catheter ablation of mitral isthmus ventricular tachycardia using electroanatomically guided linear lesions. *J Cardiovasc Electrophysiol* 2000;11:466–471.

132. Nademanee K, Kosar EM. A nonfluoroscopic catheter-based mapping technique to ablate focal ventricular tachycardia. *Pacing Clin Electrophysiol* 1998;21:1442.

133. Griffith MJ, Linker NJ, Garratt CJ, et al. Relative efficacy and safety of intravenous drugs for termination of sustained ventricular tachycardia. *Lancet* 1990;336:670–673.

134. Ho DS, Zecchin R, Richards DA, et al. Double-blind trial of lignocaine versus sotalol for acute termination of spontaneous sustained ventricular tachycardia. *Lancet* 1994;344:18–23.

135. Nasir N Jr, Taylor A, Doyle TK, Pacifico A. Evaluation of intravenous lidocaine for the termination of sustained monomorphic ventricular tachycardia in patients with coronary artery disease with or without healed myocardial infarction. *Am J Cardiol* 1994;74:1183–1186.

136. Singh BN. Acute management of ventricular arrhythmias: role of antiarrhythmic agents. *Pharmacotherapy* 1997;17[Pt 2]:56S–64S.

137. Kowey PR, Marinchak RA, Rials SJ, Bharucha DB. Intravenous antiarrhythmic therapy in the acute control of in-hospital destabilizing ventricular tachycardia and fibrillation. *Am J Cardiol* 1999;84:46R–51R.

138. Gorgels AP, van dem Dool A, Hofs A, et al. Comparison of procainamide and lidocaine in terminating sustained monomorphic ventricular tachycardia. *Am J Cardiol* 1996;78:43–46.

139. Kudenchuk PJ, Cobb LA, Copass MK, et al. Amiodarone for resuscitation after out-of-hospital cardiac arrest due to ventricular fibrillation. *N Engl J Med* 1999;341:871–878.

140. Levine JH, Massumi A, Scheinman MM, et al. Intravenous amiodarone for recurrent sustained hypotensive ventricular tachyarrhythmias. Intravenous Amiodarone Multicenter Trial Group. *J Am Coll Cardiol* 1996;27:67–75.

141. Guidelines 2000 for Cardiopulmonary Resuscitation and Emergency Cardiovascular Care. International Consensus on Science. Part 6: Advanced Cardiovascular Life Support. *Circulation* 2000;102:I86.

142. Kowey PR, Levine JH, Herre JM, et al. Randomized, double-blind comparison of intravenous amiodarone and bretylium in the treatment of patients with recurrent, hemodynamically destabilizing ventricular tachycardia or fibrillation. The Intravenous Amiodarone Multicenter Investigators Group. *Circulation* 1995;92:3255–3263.

143. Credner SC, Klingenheben T, Mauss O, et al. Electrical storm in patients with transvenous implantable cardioverter-defibrillators: incidence, management and prognostic implications. *J Am Coll Cardiol* 1998;32:1909–1915.

144. Echt DS, Lee JT, Murray KT, et al. A randomized, double-blind, placebo-controlled, dose-ranging study of dofetilide in patients with inducible sustained ventricular tachycardia. *J Cardiovasc Electrophysiol* 1995;6:687–699.

145. Wood MA, Stambler BS, Ellenbogen KA, et al. Suppression of inducible ventricular tachycardia by ibutilide in patients with coronary artery disease. Ibutilide Investigators. *Am Heart J* 1998;135:1048–1054.

146. Kowey PR. An overview of antiarrhythmic drug management of electrical storm. *Can J Cardiol* 1996;12[Suppl B]:3B–8B.

147. Singh BN, Kehoe R, Woosley RL, et al. Multicenter trial of sotalol compared with procainamide in the suppression of inducible ventricular tachycardia: a double-blind, randomized parallel evaluation. Sotalol Multicenter Study Group. *Am Heart J* 1995;129:87–97.

148. CAST Investigators. Preliminary report: effect of encainide and flecainide on mortality in a randomized trial of arrhythmia suppression after myocardial infarction. The Cardiac Arrhythmia Suppression Trial (CAST) Investigators. *N Engl J Med* 1989; 321:406–412.

149. Greenspan AM, Spielman SR, Horowitz LN. Combination antiarrhythmic drug therapy for ventricular tachyarrhythmias. *Pace* 1986;9:565–576.

150. Greene HL, for the CASCADE Investigators. The CASCADE study: randomized antiarrhythmic drug therapy in survivors of cardiac arrest in Seattle. *Am J Cardiol* 1993;72:70F–74F.

151. Amiodarone Vs Sotalol Study Group. Multicentre randomized trial of sotalol vs amiodarone for chronic malignant ventricular tachyarrhythmias. *Eur Heart J* 1989;10:685–694.

152. Kavoor P, Eiper V, Byth K, et al. Comparison of sotalol with amiodarone for long-term treatment of spontaneous sustained ventricular tachyarrhythmias based on coronary artery disease. *Eur Heart J* 1999;20:364–374.

153. Man KC, Williamson BD, Niebauer M, et al. Electrophysiologic effects of sotalol and amiodarone in patients with sustained monomorphic ventricular tachycardia. *Am J Cardiol* 1994;74:1119–1123.

154. AVID Investigators. A comparison of antiarrhythmic-drug therapy with implantable defibrillators in patients resuscitated from near-fatal ventricular arrhythmias. The Antiarrhythmics Versus Implantable Defibrillators (AVID) Investigators. *N Engl J Med* 1997;337:1576–1583.

155. Domanski MJ, Sakseena S, Epstein AE, et al. Relative effectiveness of the implantable cardioverter-defibrillator and antiarrhythmic drugs in patients with varying degrees of left ventricular dysfunction who have survived malignant ventricular arrhythmias. AVID Investigators. Antiarrhythmics Versus Implantable Defibrillators. *J Am Coll Cardiol* 1999;34:1090–1095.

156. Connolly SJ, Gent M, Roberts RS, et al. Canadian Implantable Defibrillator Study (CIDS): a randomized trial of the implantable cardioverter defibrillator against amiodarone. *Circulation* 2000;101:1297.

157. Kuck KH, Cappato R, Siebels J, Ruppel R, for the CASH Investigators. Randomized comparison of antiarrhythmic drug therapy with implantable defibrillators in patients resuscitated from cardiac arrest. The Cardiac Arrest Study Hamburg (CASH). *Circulation* 2000;102:748.

158. Stevenson WG, Friedman PL, Kocovic D, et al. Radiofrequency catheter ablation of ventricular tachycardia after myocardial infarction. *Circulation* 1998;98:308–314.

159. Rothman SA, Hsia HH, Cossu SF, et al. Radiofrequency catheter ablation of postinfarction ventricular tachycardia: long-term success and the significance of inducible nonclinical arrhythmias. *Circulation* 1997;96:3499–3508.

160. Strickberger SA, Man KC, Daoud EG, et al. A prospective evaluation of catheter ablation of ventricular tachycardia as adjuvant therapy in patients with coronary artery disease and an implantable cardioverter-defibrillator. *Circulation* 1997;96: 1525–1531.

161. Kottkamp H, Hindricks G, Chen X, et al. Radiofrequency catheter ablation of sustained ventricular tachycardia in idiopathic dilated cardiomyopathy. *Circulation* 1995;92:1159–1168.

162. Ellison KE, Stevenson WG, Sweeney MMO, et al. Catheter ablation for hemodynamically unstable monomorphic ventricular tachycardia. *J Cardiovasc Electrophysiol* 2000;11:41–44.

163. Marchlinski FE, Callans DJ, Gottlieb CD, Zado E. Linear abla-

164. Smeets JLRM, Ben-Haim SA, Rodrigues LM, et al. New method for nonfluoroscopic endocardial mapping in humans: accuracy assessment and first clinical results. *Circulation* 1998;97:2426.

165. Simons GR, Sorrentino RA, Zimerman LI, et al. Bundle branch reentry tachycardia and possible sustained interfascicular reentry tachycardia with a shared unusual induction pattern. *J Cardiovasc Electrophysiol* 1996;7:44–50.

166. Reddy CP, Slack JD. Recurrent sustained ventricular tachycardia: report of a case with His-bundle branches reentry as the mechanism. *Eur J Cardiol* 1980;11:23–31.

167. Lloyd EA, Zipes DP, Heger JJ, Prystowsky EN. Sustained ventricular tachycardia due to bundle branch reentry. *Am Heart J* 1982;104:1095–1097.

168. Touboul P, Kirkorian G, Atallah G, Moleur P. Bundle branch reentry: a possible mechanism of ventricular tachycardia. *Circulation* 1983;67:674–680.

169. Narasimhan C, Jazayeri MR, Sra J, et al. Ventricular tachycardia in valvular heart disease: facilitation of sustained bundle-branch reentry by valve surgery. *Circulation* 1997;96:4307–4313.

170. Akhtar M, Gilbert C, Wolf FG, Schmidt DH. Reentry within the His-Purkinje system. Elucidation of reentrant circuit using right bundle branch and His bundle recordings. *Circulation* 1978;58:295–304.

171. Caceres J, Jazayeri M, McKinnie J, et al. Sustained bundle branch reentry as a mechanism of clinical tachycardia. *Circulation* 1989;79:256–270.

172. Blanck Z, Dhala A, Deshpande S, et al. Bundle branch reentrant ventricular tachycardia: cumulative experience in 48 patients. *J Cardiovasc Electrophysiol* 1993;4:253–262.

173. Tchou P, Jazayeri M, Denker S, et al. Transcatheter electrical ablation of right bundle branch. A method of treating macroreentrant ventricular tachycardia attributed to bundle branch reentry. *Circulation* 1988;78:246–257.

174. Touboul P, Kirkorian G, Atallah G, et al. Bundle branch reentrant tachycardia treated by electrical ablation of the right bundle branch. *J Am Coll Cardiol* 1986;7:1404–1409.

175. Crijns HJ, Smeets JL, Rodriguez LM, et al. Cure of interfascicular reentrant ventricular tachycardia by ablation of the anterior fascicle of the left bundle branch. *J Cardiovasc Electrophysiol* 1995;6:486–492.

176. Fontaine G, Guiraudon G, Frank R, et al. Stimulation studies and epicardial mapping in VT: study of mechanisms and selection for surgery. In: Kulbertus HE, ed. *Reentrant arrhythmias.* Lancaster: MTP Publishers, 1977:334–350.

177. Marcus FI, Fontaine GH, Guiraudon G, et al. Right ventricular dysplasia: a report of 24 adult cases. *Circulation* 1982;65: 384–398.

178. Thiene G, Nava A, Corrado D, et al. Right ventricular cardiomyopathy and sudden death in young people. *N Engl J Med* 1988;318:129–133.

179. Gerlis LM, Schmidt-Ott SC, Ho SY, Anderson RH. Dysplastic conditions of the right ventricular myocardium: Uhl's anomaly vs arrhythmogenic right ventricular dysplasia. *Br Heart J* 1993;69:142–150.

180. Ruder MA, Winston SA, Davis JC, et al. Arrhythmogenic right ventricular dysplasia in a family. *Am J Cardiol* 1985;56:799–800.

181. Rampazzo A, Nava A, Miorin M, et al. ARVD4, a new locus for arrhythmogenic right ventricular cardiomyopathy, maps to chromosome 2 long arm. *Genomics* 1997;45:259–263.

182. Rampazzo A, Nava A, Erne P, et al. A new locus for arrhythmogenic right ventricular cardiomyopathy (ARVD2) maps to chromosome 1q42-q43. *Hum Mol Genetics* 1995;4:2151–2154.

183. Rampazzo A, Nava A, Danieli GA, et al. The gene for arrhyth-

mogenic right ventricular cardiomyopathy maps to chromosome 14q23-q24. *Hum Mol Genetics* 1994;3:959–962.

184. Ahmad F, Li D, Karibe A, et al. Localization of a gene responsible for arrhythmogenic right ventricular dysplasia to chromosome 3p23. *Circulation* 1998;98:2791–2795.

185. Manyari DE, Klein GJ, Gulamhusein S, et al. Arrhythmogenic right ventricular dysplasia: a generalized cardiomyopathy? *Circulation* 1983;68:251–257.

186. Kinoshita O, Fontaine G, Rosas F, et al. Time- and frequency-domain analyses of the signal-averaged ECG in patients with arrhythmogenic right ventricular dysplasia. *Circulation* 1995; 91:715–721.

187. Turrini P, Angelini A, Thiene G, et al. Late potentials and ventricular arrhythmias in arrhythmogenic right ventricular cardiomyopathy. *Am J Cardiol* 1999;83:1214–1219.

188. Hamada S, Takamiya M, Ohe T, Ueda H. Arrhythmogenic right ventricular dysplasia: evaluation with electron-beam CT. *Radiology* 1993;187:723–727.

189. Blake LM, Scheinman MM, Higgins CB. MR features of arrhythmogenic right ventricular dysplasia. *AJR Am J Roentgenol* 1994;162:809–812.

190. Daliento L, Rizzoli G, Thiene G, et al. Diagnostic accuracy of right ventriculography in arrhythmogenic right ventricular cardiomyopathy. *Am J Cardiol* 1990;66:741–745.

191. Auffermann W, Wichter T, Breithardt G, et al. Arrhythmogenic right ventricular disease: MR imaging vs angiography. *AJR Am J Roentgenol* 1993;161:549–555.

192. McKenna WJ, Thiene G, Nava A, et al. Diagnosis of arrhythmogenic right ventricular dysplasia/cardiomyopathy. Task Force of the Working Group Myocardial and Pericardial Disease of the European Society of Cardiology and of the Scientific Council on Cardiomyopathies of the International Society and Federation of Cardiology. *Br Heart J* 1994;71:215–218.

193. Haissaguerre M, Le Metayer P, D'Ivernois C, et al. Distinctive response of arrhythmogenic right ventricular disease to high dose isoproterenol. *Pacing Clin Electrophysiol* 1990;13:2119–2126.

194. Di Biase M, Favale S, Massari V, et al. Programmed stimulation in patients with minor forms of right ventricular dysplasia. *Eur Heart J* 1989;10[Suppl D]:49–53.

195. Guiraudon GM, Klein GJ, Gulamhusein SS, et al. Total disconnection of the right ventricular free wall: surgical treatment of right ventricular tachycardia associated with right ventricular dysplasia. *Circulation* 1983;67:463–470.

196. Higuchi S, Caglar NM, Shimada R, et al. 16-year follow-up of arrhythmogenic right ventricular dysplasia. *Am Heart J* 1984; 108:1363–1365.

197. Lemery R, Brugada P, Janssen J, et al. Nonischemic sustained ventricular tachycardia: clinical outcome in 12 patients with arrhythmogenic right ventricular dysplasia. *J Am Coll Cardiol* 1989;14:96–105.

198. Kullo IJ, Edwards WD, Seward JB. Right ventricular dysplasia: the Mayo Clinic experience. *Mayo Clin Proc* 1995;70:541–548.

199. Lerman BB, Stein K, Engelstein ED, et al. Mechanism of repetitive monomorphic ventricular tachycardia. *Circulation* 1995; 92:421–429.

200. Buxton AE, Marchlinski FE, Doherty JU, et al. Repetitive, monomorphic ventricular tachycardia: clinical and electrophysiologic characteristics in patients with and patients without organic heart disease. *Am J Cardiol* 1984;54:997–1002.

201. Deal BJ, Miller SM, Scagliotti D, et al. Ventricular tachycardia in a young population without overt heart disease. *Circulation* 1986;73:1111–1118.

202. Proclemer A, Ciani R, Feruglio GA. Right ventricular tachycardia with left bundle branch block and inferior axis morphology: clinical and arrhythmological characteristics in 15 patients. *Pace* 1989;12:977–989.

203. Rahilly GT, Prystowsky EN, Zipes DP, et al. Clinical and electrophysiologic findings in patients with repetitive monomorphic ventricular tachycardia and otherwise normal electrocardiogram. *Am J Cardiol* 1982;50:459–468.

204. Mont L, Seixas T, Brugada P, et al. The electrocardiographic, clinical, and electrophysiologic spectrum of idiopathic monomorphic ventricular tachycardia. *Am Heart J* 1992;124:746–753.

205. Shimoike E, Ohnishi Y, Ueda N, et al. Radiofrequency catheter ablation of left ventricular outflow tract tachycardia from the coronary cusp: a new approach to the tachycardia focus. *J Cardiovasc Electrophysiol* 1999;10:1005–1009.

206. Buxton AE, Waxman HL, Marchlinski FE, et al. Right ventricular tachycardia: clinical and electrophysiologic characteristics. *Circulation* 1983;68:917–927.

207. Goy JJ, Tauxe F, Fromer M, et al. Ten-years follow-up of 20 patients with idiopathic ventricular tachycardia. *Pace* 1990; 13(9):1142–1147.

208. Mont L, Seixas T, Brugada P, et al. Clinical and electrophysiologic characteristics of exercise-related idiopathic ventricular tachycardia. *Am J Cardiol* 1991;68:897–900.

209. Gill JS, Mehta D, Ward DE, Camm AJ. Efficacy of flecainide, sotalol, and verapamil in the treatment of right ventricular tachycardia in patients without overt cardiac abnormality. *Br Heart J* 1992;68:392–397.

210. Gill JS, Ward DE, Camm AJ. Comparison of verapamil and diltiazem in the suppression of idiopathic ventricular tachycardia. *Pace* 1992;15:2122–2126.

211. Morady F, Kadish AH, DiCarlo L, et al. Long-term results of catheter ablation of idiopathic right ventricular tachycardia. *Circulation* 1990;82:2093–2099.

212. Stevenson WG, Nademanee K, Weiss JN, Wiener I. Treatment of catecholamine-sensitive right ventricular tachycardia by endocardial catheter ablation. *J Am Coll Cardiol* 1990;16: 752–755.

213. Rodriguez LM, Smeets JL, Timmermans C, Wellens HJ. Predictors for successful ablation of right- and left-sided idiopathic ventricular tachycardia. *Am J Cardiol* 1997;79:309–314.

214. Zipes DP, Foster PR, Troup PJ, Pedersen DH. Atrial induction of ventricular tachycardia: reentry versus triggered automaticity. *Am J Cardiol* 1979;44:1–8.

215. Belhassen B, Rotmensch HH, Laniado S. Response of recurrent sustained ventricular tachycardia to verapamil. *Br Heart J* 1981;46:679–682.

216. Ward DE, Nathan AW, Camm AJ. Fascicular tachycardia sensitive to calcium antagonists. *Eur Heart J* 1984;5:896–905.

217. Green LS, Lux RL, Ershler PR, et al. Resolution of pace mapping stimulus site separation using body surface potentials. *Circulation* 1994;90:462–468.

218. German LD, Packer DL, Bardy GH, Gallagher JJ. Ventricular tachycardia induced by atrial stimulation in patients without symptomatic cardiac disease. *Am J Cardiol* 1983;52:1202–1207.

219. Ohe T, Shimomura K, Aihara N, et al. Idiopathic sustained left ventricular tachycardia: clinical and electrophysiologic characteristics. *Circulation* 1988;77:560–568.

220. Andrade FR, Eslami M, Elias J, et al. Diagnostic clues from the surface ECG to identify idiopathic (fascicular) ventricular tachycardia: correlation with electrophysiologic findings. *J Cardiovasc Electrophysiol* 1996;7:2–8.

221. Nakagawa H, Beckman KJ, McClelland JH, et al. Radiofrequency catheter ablation of idiopathic left ventricular tachycardia guided by a Purkinje potential. *Circulation* 1993;88:2607–2617.

222. Kottkamp H, Chen X, Hindricks G, et al. Idiopathic left ventricular tachycardia: new insights into electrophysiological characteristics and radiofrequency catheter ablation. *Pace* 1995;18: 1285–1297.

223. Ohe T, Aihara N, Kamakura S, et al. Long-term outcome of

verapamil-sensitive sustained left ventricular tachycardia in patients without structural heart disease. *J Am Coll Cardiol* 1995;25:54–58.

224. Okumura K, Yamabe H, Tsuchiya T, et al. Characteristics of slow conduction zone demonstrated during entrainment of idiopathic ventricular tachycardia of left ventricular origin. *Am J Cardiol* 1996;77:379–383.

225. Okumura K, Matsuyama K, Miyagi H, et al. Entrainment of idiopathic ventricular tachycardia of left ventricular origin with evidence for reentry with an area of slow conduction and effect of verapamil. *Am J Cardiol* 1988;62:727–732.

226. Ng KS, Wen MS, Yeh SJ, et al. The effects of adenosine on idiopathic ventricular tachycardia. *Am J Cardiol* 1994;74:195–197.

227. Griffith MJ, Garratt CJ, Rowland E, et al. Effects of intravenous adenosine on verapamil-sensitive "idiopathic" ventricular tachycardia. *Am J Cardiol* 1994;73:759–764.

20

POLYMORPHOUS VENTRICULAR TACHYCARDIA, INCLUDING TORSADE DE POINTES

STEFAN H. HOHNLOSER

Polymorphous ventricular tachycardia (VT) is defined as a VT with unstable, continuously changing QRS complex morphology in any electrocardiographic (ECG) lead (1). In many instances, recording of more than one ECG lead is necessary to appreciate the fluctuations in beat-to-beat QRS morphology. The rate of polymorphous VT ranges from 100 bpm (2) up to 250 bpm (3). The definition of sustained polymorphous VT is similar to that of sustained monomorphic VT (i.e., VT lasting ≥30 seconds) (2). Many prolonged episodes of polymorphous VT are associated with hemodynamic compromise, and particularly those with a rate of 200 bpm or less often degenerate into ventricular fibrillation (4). However, most episodes of polymorphous VT terminate spontaneously. Although polymorphous VT is usually viewed as having a more ominous prognosis than monomorphic VT, spontaneous polymorphous VT and polymorphous VT induced in the electrophysiologic laboratory by programmed electrical stimulation may have different prognostic significance.

The electrophysiologic mechanisms underlying polymorphous VT have been the focus of intense research. There is more than one electrophysiologic mechanism for polymorphous VT, and an understanding of these mechanisms can help in selecting the most appropriate therapy for individual patients. Polymorphous VT can be classified by whether there is an associated prolonged QT or QTU segment in the ECG recording. With few exceptions, the electrophysiologic mechanisms of these two types of polymorphous VT are different. The association of a prolonged QT or QTU interval also avoids the unnecessary confusion regarding the use of the term polymorphous VT or torsade de pointes (TdP). TdP is a term used to describe a distinctive form of polymorphous VT associated with congenital or acquired QT prolongation with an ECG pattern of nonuniform, but still organized, electrical activity, with progressive changes in morphology, amplitude, and polarity of the QRS complexes whose peaks twist around the isoelectric baseline (5) (Fig. 20-1). The term TdP should be reserved to describe polymorphous VT in the setting of the congenital or acquired long QT syndrome. However, not all patients with the long QT syndrome have polymorphous VT with the classic TdP configuration, whereas some patients without a prolonged QT interval may present with TdP (6). This chapter reviews the electrophysiologic mechanisms, clinical presentation, and management of polymorphous VT.

ELECTROCARDIOGRAPHIC CHARACTERISTICS OF POLYMORPHOUS VENTRICULAR TACHYCARDIA

Whereas the ECG description of polymorphous VT is a VT with unstable, continuously changing QRS complex morphology in any ECG lead (1), the definition of TdP comprises several interesting ECG features, including QT prolongation, rate dependence of TdP, initiating sequences, and TU-wave abnormalities, including T-wave alternans (TWA).

Rate Dependence of Torsade de Pointes

TdP exhibits a typical rate dependence. In many instances, significant sinus bradycardia, bradyarrhythmias such as complete atrioventricular (AV) block (7,8), and even abrupt prolongation of the R-R interval (9) have been reported to trigger its onset. In contrast, faster heart rates such as those obtained by atrial or ventricular pacing or by the administration of isoproterenol, have been demonstrated to terminate TdP and to prevent its recurrence.

Initiating Sequences of Torsade de Pointes

In many instances of TdP in the setting of the acquired or congenital long QT syndrome, a peculiar initiating

S. H. Hohnloser: Department of Medicine, Division of Cardiology, J. W. Goethe University, 60590 Frankfurt, Germany.

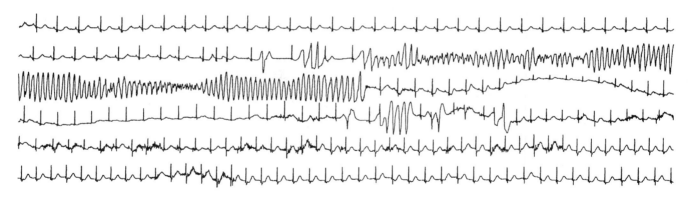

FIGURE 20-1. Polymorphous ventricular tachycardia of the torsade de pointes type documented during continuous electrocardiographic monitoring. The tracing was obtained in a patient treated with quinidine for conversion of atrial fibrillation. The arrhythmia occurred 6 hours after successful restoration of sinus rhythm.

sequence of the polymorphous VT has been observed. TdP is frequently preceded by a variable period of bigeminal rhythm due to one or two premature complexes coupled to the prolonged QT segment of the preceding basic beat. The typical pattern of this short-long-short sequence (Fig. 20-2) was first described by Kay and colleagues (10) and subsequently confirmed by other groups (4,9). In a study by Locati and coworkers (4), TdP tachycardias associated with the acquired long QT syndrome were documented with Holter monitoring of 12 patients. Detailed analysis of these Holter recordings revealed that typical short-long sequences preceded the onset of all arrhythmias. The investigators could show that specific characteristics of the observed long-short sequence were related to the severity of subsequent arrhythmias (i.e., salvos of ventricular extrasystoles versus episodes of TdP). In essence, the shorter the short interval and the longer the following pause, the more likely was the occurrence of more complex arrhythmias such as nonsustained episodes of TdP. These observations are generally in agreement with the characteristic profile of pause-dependent, early afterdepolarization-induced triggered activity.

T-Wave Alternans

Another typical feature of TdP initiation in the setting of the long QT syndrome is represented by marked alterations of the TU wave. It has long been recognized that tachycardia-dependent TWA occurs in patients with the congenital or acquired form of the long QT syndrome and may precede the onset of polymorphous VT (11,12). An example of such an episode of macroscopic TWA is shown in Figure 20-3. A total of 4,656 ECG recordings from 2,442 patients enrolled in the International Long QT Syndrome Registry were reviewed for the presence of TWA (13). TWA was identified in 30 patients of whom 25 had a corrected QT (QTc) interval longer than 500 ms. There was a strong association between QTc prolongation and TWA (odds ratio of 1.23 per 10-ms increase in QTc). Specifically, a patient with

a QTc interval of 600 ms would have a 22-fold greater likelihood of having TWA than a patient with a QTc interval of 450 ms (13). Patients with marked (biphasic) TWA had significantly longer QTc values than those with minor (monophasic) beat-to-beat changes in the configuration of

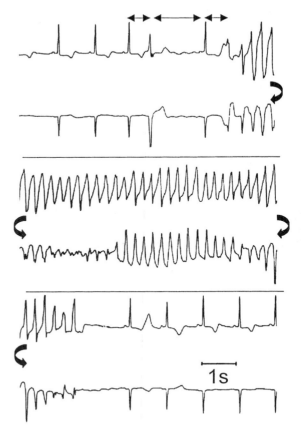

FIGURE 20-2. Continuous Holter monitoring (two channels shown) of a patient with sotalol-induced torsade de pointes. The arrows indicate the typical short-long-short initiating sequence of torsade de pointes. Notice the marked QTU alteration in the first sinus beat after cessation of torsade de pointes.

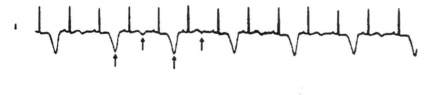

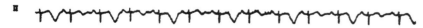

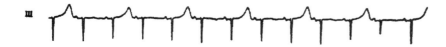

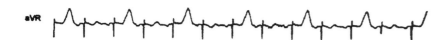

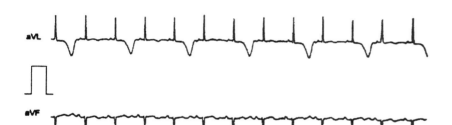

FIGURE 20-3. Macroscopic T-wave alternans in a patient with severe hypomagnesemia in the setting of dilative cardiomyopathy. Shortly after this electrocardiogram was recorded, the patient developed torsade de pointes that could be controlled by intravenous administration of magnesium sulfate.

the T wave. Although overt (i.e., macroscopic) TWA appears to be a relatively rare phenomenon in the clinical setting, it is a typical ECG finding associated with the congenital or acquired long QT syndrome complicated by TdP. Digital signal processing techniques have made it possible to detect subtle degrees (i.e., microvolt) of TWA not readily seen on the surface ECG recording (14). This indicates that the phenomenon may be more prevalent than previously recognized and may represent an important marker of vulnerability to ventricular tachyarrhythmias not specifically linked to prolonged repolarization (15,16).

ELECTROPHYSIOLOGIC MECHANISMS OF POLYMORPHOUS VENTRICULAR TACHYCARDIA ASSOCIATED WITH PROLONGED REPOLARIZATION

Significant advances have been made in elucidating the electrophysiologic mechanisms of TdP. Two hypotheses have been proposed to explain abnormally prolonged repolarization in the congenital long QT syndrome: a sympathetic imbalance or an intrinsic (or acquired) abnormality

of ionic currents underlying ventricular repolarization. The sympathetic imbalance theory proposes that reduced right cardiac sympathetic innervation (presumably congenital) results in reflex elevation of left cardiac sympathetic activity (17). The imbalance then results in marked dispersion of repolarization in different regions of the heart that could promote ventricular tachyarrhythmias, most likely based on a reentrant mechanism. However, the experimental evidence for sympathetic imbalance has been questioned (18). Moreover, clinical studies of sympathetic innervation patterns determined by *meta*-iodobenzylguanidine (MIBG) scintigraphy in patients with the long QT syndrome have reported conflicting results (19,20).

Ionic Mechanisms

Advances in elucidating the ionic basis of the various forms of the congenital long QT syndrome have shifted research activities toward the hypothesis that abnormalities in the ionic currents underlying cardiac repolarization are responsible for the ECG and electrophysiologic mechanisms underlying the congenital and the acquired long QT syndrome. The molecular findings for various forms of the congenital long QT syndrome are discussed elsewhere in this book, but it appears appropriate to review here the electrophysiologic findings that are responsible for the occurrence of polymorphous VT.

Two principal electrophysiologic mechanisms underlying polymorphous VT in the setting of prolonged cardiac repolarization have been proposed: dispersion of repolarization and early afterdepolarizations (EADs) (21). Indirect *in vivo* and *in vitro* evidence have suggested that EADs and dispersion of repolarization may be mechanisms for TdP in the congenital and acquired long QT syndromes. In a series of carefully conducted experimental studies, El Sherif and coworkers developed an *in vivo* canine model of the long QT syndrome and TdP using neurotoxin anthopleurin-A (AP-A) and a sea anemone toxin (ATXII) (22,23). These agents act by slowing sodium-channel inactivation, resulting in a sustained inward current during the plateau and prolongation of the action potential duration. This model is considered a surrogate of the LQT3 form of the congenital long QT syndrome, which is caused by a mutation in the gene *(SCN5A)* for the sodium channel subunit. Nevertheless, the basic electrophysiologic mechanisms of TdP in this model seem to apply, with some necessary modifications, to all forms of congenital and acquired long QT syndrome (24).

The model incorporates high-resolution, tridimensional mapping of activation and repolarization patterns in canines exposed to AP-A that develop QT prolongation and polymorphous VT. In a first series of experiments, El Sherif and coworkers could for the first time demonstrate the *in vivo* existence of spatial dispersion of repolarization in the ventricular wall and differences in regional recovery in response to cycle-length changes (25). These phenomena were markedly accentuated after AP-A administration. Analysis of tridimensional activation patterns revealed that single ectopic beats, couplets, and the initial beat of polymorphous VT consistently arose as focal activity from a subendocardial site. In contrast, subsequent beats were caused by successive subendocardial focal activity, reentrant excitation, or a combination of mechanisms. Reentrant excitation was caused by infringement of focal activity on the spatial dispersion of repolarization that resulted in conduction block and circulating wavefronts. Based on previous *in vitro* work of the same investigators, it appeared reasonable to assume that the focal activity represented the extracellular manifestation of a conducted EAD arising from a subendocardial Purkinje fiber. These observations were extended in a subsequent study from the same laboratory (26). More detailed mapping confirmed the initiating tachycardia beat to be caused by subendocardial activity; in contrast to the previous report, it was demonstrated that all fast polymorphous VTs were caused by successive reentrant excitation initiated by subendocardial focal activity (26). In no instance was a combination of focal and reentrant excitation observed.

The marked dispersion of repolarization across the left ventricular wall was caused by the differential response of mid-myocardial cell layers to the pharmacologic agent used to prolong action potential duration. This observation corresponds to findings reported previously by Antzelevitch and coworkers (27,28). In a series of *in vitro* experiments, investigators demonstrated differences in channel constituents, rate dependence, and pharmacologic sensitivity of mid-myocardial M cells compared with subepicardial and subendocardial cells (27,28). Using microelectrodes and patch-clamp techniques, the investigators showed that erythromycin produced a much more pronounced prolongation of the action potential duration in M cells than in endocardial or epicardial cells, resulting in the development of a large dispersion of repolarization across the ventricular wall (29). In this setting, a polymorphous VT closely resembling TdP was readily and reproducibly induced.

Studies have aimed at elucidating the electrophysiologic mechanisms underlying the typical ECG features of TdP (30). For this purpose, the AP-A model of the long QT syndrome was used to obtain tridimensional isochronal maps of ventricular activation constructed from 256 bipolar electrograms recorded from 64 plunge-needle electrodes; detailed maps of 26 episodes of nonsustained TdP could be analyzed. The tachycardia was always initiated by a subendocardial focal activity giving rise to subsequent reentrant excitation. In 22 of 26 episodes, the transition in the QRS axis coincided with the transient bifurcation of a predominantly single rotating scroll into two simultaneous scrolls involving the right and the left ventricle. The initiating mechanism for the bifurcation of the single wavefront was the development of functional conduction block between the anterior or posterior right ventricular free wall and the interventricular septum. These experiments provided direct evidence about the electrophysiologic mechanisms for the characteristic periodic transition of the QRS axis during TdP in the long QT syndrome.

The cause of the characteristic long-short initiating sequence of TdP has been evaluated in the same model (24). The bigeminal beats consistently arose from subendocardial focal activity from the same or different sites. TdP resulted from encroachment of the subendocardial focal activity on a substrate of dispersion of repolarization to induce reentrant arrhythmias. A slight lengthening of the preceding cycle produced an increased dispersion of repolarization at key sites because of a differential increase of local repolarization at M zones compared with epicardial zones (24). This created *de novo* arcs of block and slowed conduction, resulting in the initiation of reentry. The arrhythmogenic potential of QT or T alternans was also studied in the AP-A model, the surrogate model for LQT3 (31). In these experiments, it was shown that the arrhythmogenic potential of alternans was mainly caused by the greater degree of spatial dispersion of repolarization during alternans than during slower heart rates that were not associated with alternans. Marked alternans in local electrograms was observed without manifest alteration of the QT-T segment on the surface ECG.

Sympathetic Imbalance

The role of adrenergic stimulation in the genesis of TdP in the setting of the long QT syndrome was investigated by Shimizu and Antzelevitch using an arterially perfused wedge of canine left ventricle (32). The investigators used chromanol 293B, a specific I_{Ks} blocker, to simulate the chromosome 11–linked LQT1 form of the congenital long QT syndrome. Administration of this compound prolonged action potential duration in subepicardial, subendocardial, and M cells without an increase of transmural dispersion of repolarization. Isoproterenol administration, however, resulted in an abbreviation of action potential duration in epicardial and endocardial cells but not in M cells, resulting in a widening of the T wave on the ECG and in a marked increase in transmural dispersion of repolarization (32). Only under these experimental conditions were spontaneous and electrically induced TdP tachycardias observed. These results suggest that a deficiency of I_{Ks} alone may not be sufficient to induce TdP but that the addition of β-adrenergic stimulation predisposes the myocardium to the development of TdP by increasing transmural dispersion of repolarization. The most likely mechanism for this effort is a large augmentation of residual I_{Ks} in epicardial and endocardial cells but not in M cells, in which this current is intrinsically weak. Moreover, these data provide a mechanistic understanding of the cellular basis for the therapeutic actions of β-adrenergic antagonists in patients with the LQT1 form of the congenital long QT syndrome.

In summary, a wealth of *in vitro* and *in vivo* experimental data has increased the knowledge concerning the electrophysiologic mechanisms underlying polymorphous VT of the TdP type in the setting of prolonged ventricular repolarization. Appreciation of these data can help to tailor therapy to the needs of individual patients with congenital or acquired long QT syndromes.

CLINICAL CONDITIONS ASSOCIATED WITH TORSADE DE POINTES

Several clinical conditions are characterized by a prolongation of ventricular repolarization that may be associated with TdP. They can be divided into two categories: the congenital long QT syndrome, including the Jervell and Lange-Nielsen variant and the Romano-Ward variant, and the acquired long QT syndrome that is mainly iatrogenic, such as that caused by administration of drugs that can prolong the action potential duration.

Congenital Long QT Syndrome

The congenital long QT syndrome is characterized by marked prolongation of the QT interval together with morphologic abnormalities of the T wave and by the occurrence of syncopal episodes and sudden cardiac death (17). The

arrhythmia responsible for syncope is most often TdP, which may degenerate into ventricular fibrillation. In the idiopathic long QT syndrome, TdP can begin without changes in heart rate and without specific sequences such as the short-long-short sequence.

Genetic Factors

As demonstrated during the past 5 to 7 years, the long QT syndrome can be caused by mutations of several genes. The molecular background of this syndrome is discussed in detail in Chapter 4.1. Briefly, four genes have been identified and several mutations have been reported for each gene. A fifth gene locus at chromosome 4q 25-27 has been described in one family, but the gene itself has not been reported (Table 20-1). *KVLQT1 (KCNQ1)*, *minK (KCNE1)*, and *HERG (KCNH2)* encode for potassium channels (24). *SCN5A* encodes for the cardiac sodium channel. KVLQT1 and minK proteins coassemble to form I_{Ks}, the slowly activating delayed rectifier K channel. Most of these mutations are not confined to a single location but are found at various positions within each gene in different families. This genetic heterogeneity may contribute to the variability in the clinical presentation. Some families have long QT syndromes that are not linked to any of these gene loci. No abnormalities in the calcium ion channel, I_{to}, or I_p have been demonstrated in patients with the long QT syndrome (33). A significant number of sporadic cases, such as patients with syncope or a prolonged QT interval, do not have evidence of familial involvement.

Prevalence and Clinical Presentation of the Idiopathic Long QT Syndrome

An estimated 1 in 10,000 persons is a gene carrier for the long QT syndrome. In the United States, long QT syndrome is considered to be responsible for 3,000 to 4,000 sudden deaths of children and young adults each year (34). Syncope occurs in approximately two thirds of the gene carriers. However, asymptomatic and symptomatic persons may exist in families with the same genotype and muta-

TABLE 20-1. GENES ASSOCIATED WITH THE LONG QT SYNDROME

Disease	Gene (Alias)	Chromosome	Ion channel
LQT1	*KVLQT1*[a] (*KCNQ1*)	11p15.5	I_{Ks} subunit
LQT2	*KCNH2*	7q35-36	I_{Kr}
LQT3	*SCN5A*	3q21-24	Na
LQT4	*LQT4*	4q25-27	Unknown
LQT5	*KCNE1*	21q22.1-22.2	I_{Ks} subunit

[a]Homozygous carriers of novel mutations of *KVLQT1* have Jervell and Lange-Nielsen syndrome.
Adapted from El-Sherif N, Turitto G. The long QT syndrome and torsade de pointes. *Pacing Clin Electrophysiol* 1999;22:91–110, with permission.

tions. Symptoms begin most often during the preteen and teenage years, but onset may occur during the first days of life or, uncommonly, as late as 40 to 50 years of age (24).

The typical clinical presentation of idiopathic long QT syndrome is characterized by the occurrence of syncope or cardiac arrest, often precipitated by emotional, exertional, or auditory arousal stress in a young, otherwise healthy individual with a prolonged QT interval on the surface ECG recording (17). The syncopal episodes are frequently misinterpreted as a seizure disorder. In the absence of appropriate therapy, the syncopal episodes recur, and fatal cardiac arrest eventually may take place. When family screening is performed, prolonged QT intervals may be detected together with a family history of syncopal spells or unexplained sudden death.

Two variants of the syndrome have been identified: the Jervell and Lange-Nielsen surdocardiac syndrome with congenital deafness and the more frequent Romano-Ward syndrome, which has similar cardiac features but normal hearing. A significant number of cases are sporadic; these patients have syncope or a prolonged QT interval but no evidence of familial involvement.

The International LQTS Registry prospectively enrolled 3,343 individuals from 328 families in which one or more family members were identified as having long QT syndrome (35). This population was equally divided between affected (QTc >0.44 second) and unaffected (QTc ≤0.44 second) individuals. Table 20-2 contains the criteria for the diagnosis of the idiopathic long QT interval (36). In one

report, probands (i.e., the first family member identified as having long QT syndrome) were younger, were more likely to be female, and had a higher frequency of prior cardiac events such as syncope or aborted sudden death, congenital deafness, sinus bradycardia, a QTc interval of more than 0.50 second, and ventricular tachyarrhythmias when compared with affected family members. By age 12, 50% of the probands, 8% of the affected family members, and 2% of the unaffected family members experienced one or more cardiac events. The mortality rate was highest for young patients (57% by 20 years of age) who had a history of syncope and significant QT prolongation. During follow-up, the event rates among probands were 5% per year for syncope and 0.9% annually for cardiac death. Independent risk factors for subsequent cardiac events were the length of the QT interval, heart rate, and history of a cardiac event (35). In Table 20-2, the present diagnostic criteria for diagnosis of the idiopathic long QT interval are summarized (36).

Acquired Long QT Syndromes

TdP may be observed in various forms of the acquired forms of prolonged QT interval, which is more frequent than the idiopathic long QT syndrome. A variety of clinical conditions and drug-induced, acquired QT syndromes are subsequently discussed according to the cause of QT interval prolongation (Table 20-3). TdP in association with drug-induced prolongation of repolarization usually shows all classic ECG features discussed earlier, including QT pro-

TABLE 20-2. 1993 LONG QT SYNDROME DIAGNOSTIC CRITERIA

Criteria	Points
ECG findings	
A. QTc	
≥480 ms	3
460–470 ms	2
450 ms (males)	1
B. Torsade de pointes	2
C. T-wave alternans	1
D. Notched T wave in three leads	1
E. Low heart rate for age	0.5
Clinical history	
A. Syncope	
With stress	2
Without stress	1
B. Congenital deafness	0.5
Family history	
A. Family members with definite LQTS	1
B. Unexplained sudden cardiac death by age 30 among immediate family members	0.5
Scoring	
≤1 point	Low probability of LQTS
2–3 points	Intermediate probability of LQTS
≥4 points	High probability of LQTS

Adapted from Schwartz PJ, Moss AJ, Vincent GM, Crampton RS. Diagnostic criteria for the long QT syndrome. *Circulation* 1993;88:782–784. with permission.

TABLE 20-3. DRUGS AND PRECIPITATING CLINICAL CONDITIONS ASSOCIATED WITH THE AQUIRED LONG QT SYNDROME AND TORSADE DE POINTES

Drugs
  Antiarrhythmic drugs that prolong repolarization
    Class IA substances (quinidine, disopyramide,
      procainamide)
    Class III substances (d,l-sotalol, amiodarone,
      N-acetylprocainamide, bretylium, sematilide, ibutilide,
      dofetilide, azimilide, and others)
  Adenosine
  Prenylamine
  Bepridil
  Lidoflazine
  Terodiline
  Tricyclic and tetracyclic antidepressants (e.g. amitriptyline,
    imipramine, doxepin)
  Phenothiazines (thioridazine, chlorpromazine)
  Haloperidol
  Chloral hydrate
  Nonsedating antihistamines (terfenidine, astemizole,
    diphenyhydramine)
  Antibiotics (erythromycin, trimethoprim-sulfamethoxazole)
  Antifungals (ketoconazole, fluconazole)
  Chemotherapeutics (e.g., pentamidine)
  Serotonin antagonists (e.g., ketanserin)
  Papaverine
  Vasopressin
  Cisapride
Electrolyte abnormalities
  Hypokalemia
  Hypomagnesemia
Bradyarrhythmias
  Sinus node dysfunction
  Atrioventricular block
Altered nutritional states
  Anorexia nervosa
  Diets
Cerebrovascular diseases
  Intracranial and subarachnoidal hemorrhage
  Stroke
  Encephalitis
Hypothyroidism

longation, prominent U waves, TU-wave abnormalities, TWA, and slow heart rate.

Antiarrhythmic Drugs

TdP may develop with all antiarrhythmic drugs that block sodium or potassium channels and prolong repolarization.

Sodium Channel Blockers

Quinidine-associated TdP is probably the most widely recognized form of drug-related proarrhythmia. As early as 1964, Selzer and Wray described quinidine-associated TdP in eight patients; all of them were receiving quinidine for atrial fibrillation. The investigators called this condition *quinidine syncope* (37). The estimated prevalence of TdP in quinidine-treated patients is between 1.5% and 8% of treatment attempts (38). Roden and associates reported in 1986 that TdP during quinidine exposure occurred when plasma concentrations of the drug were low, when the drug was given for only a short period, and when additional predisposing conditions such as hypokalemia were present (9). In patients receiving quinidine for treatment of atrial fibrillation, TdP tends to occur most commonly shortly after restoration of sinus rhythm (9,39). In a meta-analysis of placebo-controlled trials of atrial fibrillation treatment, quinidine administration was shown to result in an increased mortality when compared with placebo, most likely because of its propensity to cause TdP (40). Other sodium channel blocking antiarrhythmic drugs that have been associated with the occurrence of TdP are disopyramide and procainamide, although precise data on the prevalence of polymorphous VT during treatment with these agents are lacking.

Potassium Channel Blockers

The focus of antiarrhythmic drug therapy has shifted from the widespread use of class I antiarrhythmic agents to an increasingly frequent administration of class III compounds, which block potassium channels and prolong repolarization. Because the clinical use of these agents is expected to increase even more during the coming years, it is mandatory that the risks of proarrhythmic events and TdP in particular are carefully explored. This information is available for compounds such as racemic d,l-sotalol, amiodarone and dofetilide; however, only limited data have been reported for newer drugs such as azimilide, ambasilide, and others.

d,l-Sotalol

Sotalol is a class III agent with dual properties: propensity to competitively block β receptors and the ability to prolong cardiac repolarization. It is a racemic mixture of the dextro and levo isomers, both of which have equal potency for prolonging the action potential duration (41). However, the l isomer retains nonselective competitive β-receptor activity, resulting in an additional significant class II action of the racemic compound with an important bradycardic effect. Sotalol has been found to prolong repolarization in all cardiac tissues in a dose-dependent fashion (41). Sotalol's effect on repolarization is predominantly caused by a block of the rapid component of the delayed rectifier potassium current (I_{Kr}) with no effect on the slow component (I_{Ks}).

In one of the first studies of its kind, Soyka and colleagues examined data on the proarrhythmic potential of sotalol from 12 controlled clinical studies involving 1,288 patients with ventricular arrhythmias (42). The overall incidence of proarrhythmic reactions was 4.3% (56 patients), with almost one half of the cases demonstrating TdP (24 patients). From several clinical factors examined, baseline QTc and QTc after 1 week of therapy were longer in patients developing proarrhythmic events than those without. In an extension of this study, in 1,363 patients with a history of sustained VT or fibrillation, Hohnloser and coworkers found an overall incidence of proarrhythmia of 5.9% (43). TdP was the most commonly encountered proarrhythmic reaction (56 patients; incidence of 4.1%). When these serious proarrhythmic events were correlated with the daily doses taken by the patients, a clear dose dependence became evident. When doses up to 320 mg/day were used, the incidence of proarrhythmia was 1.8%. This incidence increased to 4.5% when dosages up to 480 mg/day were administered and up to 6.8% when drug doses exceeded 640 mg/day (43). The following clinical variables were found to correlate with the risk of TdP: dose, baseline arrhythmia (i.e., sustained VT versus others), history of congestive heart failure, cardiomegaly, New York Heart Association (NYHA) functional class, baseline prolongation of QTc, and elevated serum creatinine. In a stepwise logistic regression analysis, the parameters with the strongest correlation were gender ($p < 0.0001$), arrhythmia type ($p < 0.0001$), dose ($p < 0.001$), history of congestive heart failure ($p < 0.001$), and high serum creatinine level ($p < 0.05$). In all patient subgroups examined, the incidence of TdP was higher among female than male patients. Although the reason for such a female preponderance is not entirely clear, a gender relationship has been reported for other cardiovascular drugs. The fact that the baseline QT interval tends to be longer in women compared with men, as found by Merri and associates (44), may in part account for the observed higher incidence of TdP among women.

Amiodarone

In the mind of many clinicians, amiodarone is considered to be the most effective agent for the control of supraventricular and ventricular tachyarrhythmias. As reviewed in detail elsewhere (45), therapy with amiodarone was found to be associated with a remarkably low incidence of ventricular proarrhythmic events. An overall incidence of proarrhythmic effects of 2% as judged by the individual investigators was found when 17 studies, including a total of more than 2,800 patients, were examined. TdP was reported at a frequency of 0.7% of treatment attempts (45). Moreover, the analysis of eight published randomized controlled trials of amiodarone revealed no episodes of ventricular proarrhythmia in any of these trials.

The precise mechanism for this low incidence of amiodarone-associated proarrhythmia, particularly TdP, remains speculative but is almost certainly multifactorial. In addition to the increase in action potential duration by block of the delayed rectifier potassium current I_K, the drug blocks the fast sodium current and the slow inward calcium current mediated through the L-type calcium channel. Amiodarone also exhibits noncompetitive β-adrenergic antagonistic properties. In particular, the calcium channel–blocking effect may play a major role with respect to the low incidence of amiodarone-induced TdP. Because initiation of this arrhythmia

may be caused by calcium-dependent EADs, the reduced availability of calcium influx as a result of the amiodarone-induced block of the L-type calcium channels may explain the lack of development of TdP tachycardias despite a marked prolongation of repolarization associated with a significant bradycardic effect. However, that bepridil, a calcium channel blocker that also blocks Na$^+$ and K$^+$ channels, readily produces TdP especially in the presence of hypokalemia indicates that the role of L-type calcium channels in the genesis of TdP may not be the sole mechanism responsible for this form of proarrhythmia. Amiodarone can reduce or even abolish EADs induced by barium or electrically in isolated cardiac preparations. These effects have not been seen with other class III agents. Similarly, amiodarone differs from other class III agents in not exhibiting reverse use-dependency; there is no lengthening of the QT interval at slower heart rates, unlike the effect of agents that do exhibit reverse use-dependency in which the QT interval lengthens at slower heart rates. Amiodarone lengthens the action potential duration to a lesser extent in Purkinje fibers than in the ventricular muscle, an action that tends to decrease disparity of ventricular recovery, another decisive factor for the genesis of TdP.

Newer Class III Substances

A variety of newer class III drugs have been evaluated clinically. Ibutilide fumarate, a methane sulfonamide derivative with structural similarities to the antiarrhythmic compounds d,l-sotalol and dofetilide exerts potent class III effects by activating a slow Na$^+$ inward current during the plateau of the action potential and block of the rapid component of the delayed rectifier potassium current (46). This compound is available in the United States for cardioversion of atrial fibrillation and atrial flutter. In several well-designed, randomized comparative studies, its efficacy in cardioverting atrial flutter was found to be 50% to 70%, whereas atrial fibrillation was terminated in approximately 30% to 50% of cases (47–49). The major adverse effect associated with the use of this novel antiarrhythmic agent is its propensity to cause TdP. The incidence of this side effect averages 4.3%, with individual incidence rates reported from prospective studies as high as 7% (50). TdP occurs early after dosing, and death is rare. Known risk factors for this side effect should be carefully evaluated in each patient before ibutilide is administered.

Dofetilide, another new class III agent, is a highly selective I_{Kr} blocker that increases repolarization and refractoriness in the atria and in the ventricles. This new antiarrhythmic compound has been extensively studied in patients at high risk for sudden death (51,52) and in patients with atrial fibrillation (53–55). The summarized experience from the two atrial fibrillation trials demonstrates a 0.7% incidence of TdP, with most proarrhythmic reactions occurring during the first few days of drug exposure. However, all patients were exposed to dofetilide while being in hospital for the first 3 to 6 days, and the drug was stopped when QT prolongation occurred.

Although many of these new class III substances have not been evaluated in large patient samples, the available evidence indicates that the prevalence of TdP is similar with these new compounds compared with older drugs that prolong repolarization. For instance, the estimated incidence of TdP is 0.5% to 8% with quinidine, 0.5% to 6% with d,l-sotalol, and up to 6% with ibutilide (38).

Psychoactive Drugs

Drugs such as phenothiazines and tricyclic antidepressants can cause QT prolongation and TdP (56,57). In a report by Sharma and colleagues (58), intravenous application of haloperidol was associated with a significant risk of QT prolongation and development of TdP. The incidence of TdP was substantial if doses above 35 mg/day were used. The risk of TdP is greatly enhanced in patients who are concomitantly treated with diuretics that may cause hypokalemia. Patients with known structural heart disease who are treated with psychoactive drugs need to be monitored closely to identify ECG patterns suggestive of the acquired long QT syndrome.

Macrolide Antibiotics

Several antiinfective agents can cause QT prolongation leading to the development of TdP. Macrolide antibiotics are most frequently mentioned. Intravenous erythromycin has been shown several times to produce QT prolongation in individuals without structural heart disease and to exacerbate repolarization alterations in patients affected by the congenital QT syndrome (59–61). One experimental study demonstrated that erythromycin prolonged action potential duration to a greater extent in M cells than in endocardial or epicardial cells (29). This increase in dispersion of ventricular repolarization favored the occurrence of TdP, explaining the clinical observations.

Antihistamines

Several reports have shown that administration of antihistamines such as terfenadine may precipitate TdP, particularly when used in patients with baseline prolonged QT interval or at high dosages (62–66). Concomitant administration of some antibiotics or antifungal agents, such as ketoconazole, alters the metabolism of these agents, resulting in their accumulation in the plasma. Woosley and colleagues showed that terfenadine blocks I_{Kr}, similar to quinidine, prolonging action potential duration (65).

Other Drugs

Other drugs used for various indications have been associated with the acquired long QT syndrome. One of the most pertinent in this regard is cisapride, a gastrointestinal prokinetic agent (67). In an analysis of 348 cases reported, Zipes and coworkers identified 250 individuals who developed QT prolongation while on cisapride (68). In most cases, other important cofactors were identified; among these, inhibition of the cytochrome P450 3A4 was the most frequent (47% of cases), followed by electrolyte disturbances (32%) and coadministration of other QT prolonging drugs (23%). The investigators concluded that recognizable and often preventable cofactors were present in most cisapride-associated long QT syndromes. Conversely, the risk of drug-induced long QT syndrome diminishes greatly when the drug is used appropriately.

Risk Factors for Drug-Induced Acquired Long QT Syndrome and Torsade de Pointes

Various clinical conditions known to increase the risk for TdP are summarized in Table 20-4. One important factor is high drug concentrations, which is best exemplified by the experience with terfenadine (66) or cisapride (67) when they accumulate in plasma because of coadministration of a drug that inhibits their biotransformation to noncardioactive metabolites. Another example is the higher sotalol-associated TdP incidence found in patients with impaired renal function that allows sotalol accumulation in plasma (41). However, it is much more difficult to predict TdP in the absence of high plasma levels. Roden introduced an interesting concept to address this issue that he called *repolarization reserve* (38). He postulates that the normal heart has mechanisms to effect rapid and regularized repolarization that runs essentially no risk of setting up reentrant circuits or of generating EADs. The delayed rectifier currents I_{Kr} and I_{Ks} are major contributors to such stable repolarization. Risk factors such as those summarized in Table 20-4 reduce this repolarization reserve, enhancing the likelihood that the added stress (e.g., an I_{Kr}-blocking drug, a subtle genetic defect) is sufficient to precipitate TdP in individual

TABLE 20-4. RISK FACTORS FOR DRUG-INDUCED TORSADE DE POINTES

Female gender
Hypokalemia, hypomagnesemia
Bradycardia
Recent conversion from atrial fibrillation
History of congestive heart failure, depressed left ventricular ejection fraction
Myocardial hypertrophy
Diuretic use
High drug dose or concentrations (except quinidine)
Rapid intravenous drug infusion
Drug-free electrocardiogram
  QT prolongation
  T-wave abnormalities
  Bradycardia
Electrocardiogram during drug administration
  Marked QT prolongation
  T-wave morphology changes
Congenital long QT syndrome

patients. Another clinically relevant example is the period immediately after conversion of atrial fibrillation; it can be hypothesized that one possible mechanism is that neuro-hormonal activation, known to stimulate I_{Ks}, is withdrawn after successful cardioversion, reducing repolarization reserve. The concept of reduced repolarization reserve appears to be a unifying hypothesis that helps to explain several established clinical risk factors for the genesis of TdP.

Genetic Considerations in Acquired Long QT Syndrome

It has long been postulated that drug-induced acquired QT syndrome might represent a genetically determined "forme fruste" of the long QT syndrome (33). A relatively large number of individuals who carry silent mutations on long QT syndrome genes can be identified (33). These individuals, whose long QT syndrome mutations by themselves produce an alteration in repolarizing currents that is insufficient to prolong the QT interval at rest, may be particularly sensitive to any drug that affects potassium currents. This idea agrees with the concept of reduced repolarization reserve (38). As pointed out by Priori and colleagues (33), the combination of even a modest degree of I_{Kr} blockade induced by a variety of drugs and the silent mutations could produce a major prolongation in action potential duration and QT interval that may ultimately result in TdP. A few patients with drug-induced QT syndrome and underlying mutations on long QT syndrome genes have been identified. The rarity of this phenomenon precludes genetic testing in all patients with the acquired long QT syndrome, except when there are other indications to do so.

Role of Bradyarrhythmias in Torsade de Pointes

Bradycardia caused by sinus node dysfunction or high-degree AV block may also be associated with TdP. In susceptible individuals, arrhythmias are precipitated at heart rates that are well tolerated by most patients. An interesting study on this subject was published by Kurita and associates (7). The investigators studied six patients with bradycardia-associated TdP and compared the findings with those observed in eight patients with bradycardia without TdP. Patients in both groups presented with comparable rates during escape rhythm, but the TdP patients had significantly longer QT intervals. After pacemaker implantation for therapy of AV block, the pacemaker frequency was varied between 50 and 100 bpm; patients presenting with bradycardia-associated TdP continued to manifest prolonged QT intervals at slow pacing rates compared with the control group. The investigators concluded that patients with complete AV block who develop TdP have a bradycardia-dependent repolarization abnormality that may account for the electrical vulnerability of the heart.

Bradycardia-associated TdP and sudden cardiac death have also been reported in patients who had AV node catheter ablation for drug-refractory atrial fibrillation (69,70). In a report by Geelen and colleagues of 100 consecutive patients in whom postablation pacing was not set at a stimulation rate of more than 90 bpm, 6 of 100 patients had recurrent TdP, ventricular fibrillation, or both conditions after the ablation procedure. The arrhythmias occurred most commonly during episodes of slow ventricular escape rhythms or during slow ventricular pacing. With appropriate pacing at a rate of 90 bpm in the subsequent 135 patients undergoing AV node ablation at the same institution, no instance of sudden death or TdP was observed (69). These findings strongly suggest a bradycardia-dependent mechanism for these polymorphous VTs.

Cerebrovascular Diseases

A variety of cerebrovascular disorders, including subarachnoidal hemorrhage, cerebral strokes, encephalitis, and intracranial trauma, occasionally have been associated with QT interval prolongation and TdP. For instance, in a larger series of patients with subarachnoidal hemorrhage, a 3.8% incidence of TdP was observed (71). As a general rule, in most patients with QT prolongation associated with cerebrovascular disorders, the prolongation of repolarization is usually a transient phenomenon that tends to normalize within days or weeks.

Polymorphous Ventricular Tachycardia in the Absence of Prolonged Cardiac Repolarization

Polymorphous VT without concomitant QT prolongation is observed in patients with or without structural heart disease. This may be more common than TdP due to prolonged cardiac repolarization. The arrhythmia may be asymptomatic and discovered on ambulatory ECG monitoring, but prolonged episodes can degenerate into ventricular fibrillation. Unfortunately, much less information, such as the underlying electrophysiologic mechanisms of the arrhythmia, is available for these patients.

Torsade de Pointes in the Setting of a Short QT Interval

Leenhardt and coworkers described 14 patients without structural heart disease who presented with syncope related to a typical ECG pattern of TdP (72). However, in none of these patients was there evidence of a prolonged QT interval, and the polymorphous VT manifested with the unusual finding of an extremely short coupling interval of the first beat. TdP subsequently degenerated into ventricular fibrillation in 10 cases. The arrhythmia was reproduced by programmed electrical stimulation in only 2 of 14 patients.

During the follow-up period of 7 years, four patients died suddenly. The investigators reported inefficacy of all antiarrhythmic drugs, including β blockers and amiodarone. Implantation of an automatic defibrillator was advocated as the therapy of choice. This report emphasized the need to clinically recognize these peculiar ECG patterns, because these patients had a poor prognosis if left untreated.

Polymorphous Ventricular Tachycardia in Ischemic Heart Disease

Despite the high prevalence of ischemic heart disease, there are only occasional case reports of patients with acute coronary syndromes complicated by polymorphous VT (Fig. 20-4). During a 2.9-year period, Wolfe and colleagues observed 11 patients who developed polymorphous VT 1 to 13 days after suffering acute myocardial infarction (73). In contrast to drug-associated TdP, none of the 11 patients had sinus bradycardia immediately before the onset of polymorphous VT, and only 3 showed a sinus pause. The QT and the rate-corrected QTc interval were normal or only minimally prolonged. However, 9 of 11 patients had symptoms or ECG signs of recurrent myocardial ischemia. Although commonly used antiarrhythmic drugs, such as lidocaine or β-blocking drugs, were ineffective in suppressing recurrent VT episodes, some patients responded to intravenous amiodarone. Acute coronary revascularization proved to be effective in otherwise unresponsive patients.

Polymorphous VT may also occur in patients with acute myocardial ischemia caused by coronary artery spasm and Prinzmetal angina. For instance, Myerburg and associates reported their findings for five patients with aborted sudden death in the absence of significant coronary artery disease (74). In these patients, silent ischemic events caused by induced or spontaneous focal coronary artery spasm (or both) were associated with the initiation of serious ventricular tachyarrhythmias. The characteristic arrhythmia observed during ischemia or on reperfusion was polymorphous VT that, in some patients, degenerated into ventricular fibrillation or flutter. Therapy with calcium channel antagonists aimed at the prevention of recurrent coronary artery spasm and tested in the catheter laboratory was successful in preventing the episodes of spasm and arrhythmias in all patients. Nishizaki and colleagues studied 14 patients with vasospastic angina by means of programmed electrical stimulation (75). At baseline, 6 of 14 patients had polymorphous VT induced, and in 1 additional patient, ventricular fibrillation was provoked. After administration of isosorbide dinitrate, polymorphous VT was only induced in the patient with ventricular fibrillation, whereas the VT in all other patients was rendered noninducible. These studies provide evidence that vasospastic angina may be associated with increased electrical instability that most commonly manifests as polymorphous VT.

Polymorphous Ventricular Tachycardia Induced during Electrophysiologic Testing

Polymorphous VT is a frequently observed as a response to programmed electrical stimulation (Fig. 20-5). In patients without spontaneous sustained arrhythmias or structural heart disease, polymorphous VT is the most frequently induced arrhythmia, and the incidence of induction increases with the number of extrastimuli used (76). In this patient cohort, induction of polymorphous VT is considered a nonspecific response to aggressive stimulation protocols (76). However, in patients with documented spontaneous episodes of polymorphous VT, the arrhythmia was found to be reproducible on electrophysiologic testing when patients were excluded who presented with TdP in the setting of the congenital or acquired long QT syndrome (77).

In patients with underlying structural heart disease, the prognostic significance of induced polymorphous VT remains uncertain. In survivors of cardiac arrest, polymorphous VT may represent a meaningful end point of programmed stimulation. In patients with structural heart disease, in whom the clinical problem probably is not polymorphous VT, the induction of this arrhythmia elicited by multiple extrastimuli at close coupling intervals is considered a nonspecific response (78–80). Several reports have suggested that polymorphous VT induced at electrophysiologic testing can be converted to monomorphic VT by administration of procainamide (2,77). This finding argues in favor of a reentrant mechanism underlying the induced polymorphous VT. Moreover, in some selected patients, this conversion to monomorphic VT may allow detailed mapping of the arrhythmia resulting in ablative therapy (2).

THERAPY FOR POLYMORPHOUS VENTRICULAR TACHYCARDIA

Torsade de Pointes with Prolonged Ventricular Repolarization

Therapeutic concepts for termination and prevention of recurrence of TdP can be derived from the electrophysiologic mechanisms underlying its initiation. The initiating beat of TdP always arises as focal activity from a subendocardial site and is most likely caused by an EAD. These EADs result from an excess of inward over outward currents during the plateau and phase 3 of the action potential, resulting in a delay or interruption of repolarization. Any intervention able to reduce plateau inward currents (e.g., I_{CaL}) or increase outward current (e.g., I_K) is likely to prevent EADs, preventing the initiation of TdP. EADs are more likely to arise at low heart rates or after prolonged pauses, when action potential duration is maximal.

Based on these considerations, the following therapeutic concepts are recommended to terminate TdP and to prevent early recurrences. In the case of the acquired QT syndrome complicated by TdP, the first and most important therapeutic step is discontinuation of all medications potentially causing prolongation of ventricular repolarization.

Acceleration of Heart Rate

The best practical option to enhance outward currents is to increase heart rate. For this purpose, infusion of isoproterenol has been proposed to maintain heart rates of 100 to 120 bpm (81). However, isoproterenol infusion by itself carries some risk, particularly in patients with coronary artery disease. It is generally contraindicated in patients with hypertension, angina pectoris, or myocardial infarction. Moreover, it may favor the genesis of ventricular tachyarrhythmias. Alternative therapies to increase heart rate must be considered. Administration of atropine has yielded variable therapeutic effects, and it is often difficult to maintain the target heart rate over the period necessary for washout of the offending agent (82). The treatment of choice during the acute phase is temporary pacing. Atrial or ventricular pacing at rates of 100 to 120 bpm has interrupted bradycardia-associated TdP and prevented early recurrences during washout of the offending substance (82). Atrial pacing may offer advantages in patients with hemodynamic compromise, whereas ventricular pacing is preferred in most patients because of the more stable electrode position (82). The only disadvantages of pacing are the requirement of skilled personnel and difficulty of inserting the electrode without fluoroscopy in the emergency room where patients with TdP are initially seen. However, isoproterenol infusion can be used until fluoroscopy is available. Whether a permanent pacemaker should be implanted must be decided on an individual basis.

Magnesium Sulfate

A therapeutic means to reduce inward currents and shorten the action potential is represented by the administration of magnesium sulfate at intravenous dosages of 2 to 3 g (82,83). This has been effective in suppressing drug-induced TdP even in patients with normal serum magnesium levels. The bolus injection can be repeated if needed after 10 to 15 minutes. If TdP is abolished, constant magnesium sulfate infusion at a dose of 2 to 10 mg/min is initiated to allow the time necessary for washout of the offending drug. The calcium-blocking properties of magnesium may inhibit the triggered activity resulting in the genesis of EADs.

Long-Term Therapy

Long-term therapy for patients with acquired long QT syndrome and TdP primarily involves avoiding exposure to the precipitating agents and medications. Specific treatment using drugs or devices is not warranted unless the patient has a history of additional arrhythmias. In patients with congenital long QT syndrome, the primary therapeutic goal is to prevent recurrent syncope and sudden cardiac death. It is beyond the scope of this chapter to discuss all potential therapeutic avenues for the various forms of congenital QT syndrome, particularly because they continue to evolve. In brief, three treatment modalities are successfully used in this condition: administration of β blockers, left cervicothoracic sympathetic ganglionectomy, and device therapy using pacemakers, defibrillators, or both. However, therapy must be individualized to each patient. Some excellent review articles detail the therapeutic options for the various patient subsets with this syndrome (17).

Polymorphous Ventricular Tachycardia in the Absence of Prolonged Repolarization

Therapy for patients with documented polymorphous VT in the absence of the congenital or acquired long QT syndrome is guided by the clinical presentation and the presence of underlying structural heart disease. For instance, in patients with vasospastic angina and polymorphous VT, adequate therapy aimed at prevention of recurrent vasospasm is an important therapeutic step. In survivors of cardiac arrest due to polymorphous VT, the therapy of choice is implantation of a cardioverter-defibrillator (84,85). In patients presenting with aborted sudden death due to polymorphous VT or ventricular fibrillation in the absence of structural heart disease, vasospastic angina, or other obvious precipitating causes, therapy with the implantable cardioverter-defibrillator is likewise considered to be the primary treatment option.

CONCLUSIONS

Polymorphous VT is associated with an increased risk of sudden death. The arrhythmia is characterized by various electrophysiologic mechanisms and clinical presentations. The initial step in the management of these patients is to identify the presence or absence of a prolonged QTU segment. The term TdP is reserved for polymorphous VT in the presence of prolonged ventricular repolarization. The long QT syndrome can be congenital or acquired. In the former, various mutations (mostly missense mutations) resulting in specific defects in ionic currents responsible for the repolarization process have been identified. The acquired form can be caused by nearly every drug that prolongs repolarization.

Patients with congenital long QT syndrome can be managed by a strategy that includes β blockers, left cervicotho-

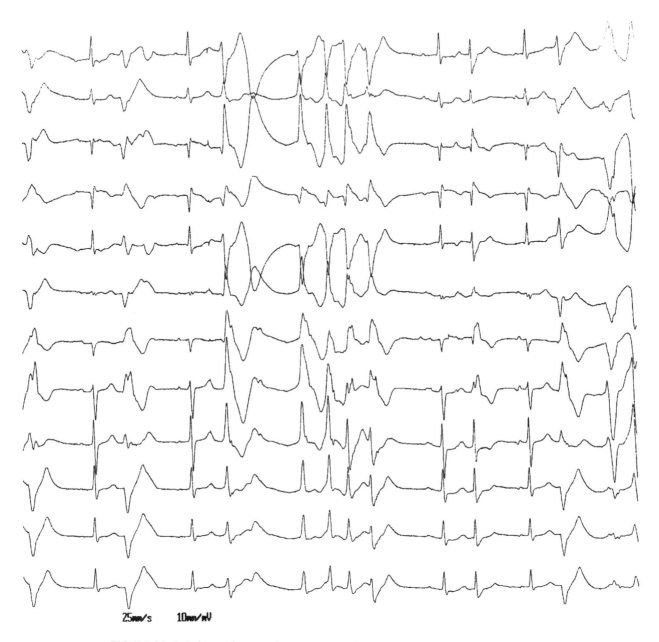

25mm/s   10mm/mV

FIGURE 20-4. Polymorphous VT in a patient with triple vessel coronary artery disease.

racic sympathectomy, and permanent cardiac pacing or an implantable cardioverter-defibrillator. The acquired long QT syndrome is managed by withdrawal of the offending agent, increasing the heart rate by isoproterenol infusion or pacing, and administration of intravenous magnesium sulfate along with the correction of predisposing conditions such as hypokalemia.

The prevalence, precise electrophysiologic mechanisms, and optimal treatment strategies for polymorphous VT in the absence of prolonged ventricular repolarization are ill defined. In many patients, however, long-term therapy consists of implantation of a cardioverter-defibrillator because the recurrence rate of these arrhythmias seems to be significant.

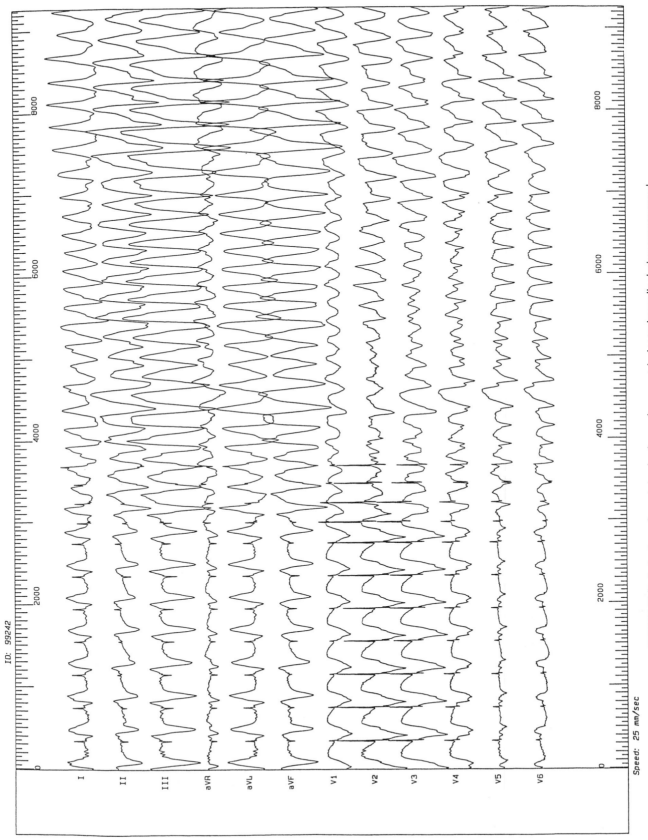

FIGURE 20-5. Induction of a sustained polymorphous ventricular tachycardia during programmed ventricular stimulation in a patient with aborted sudden death due to ventricular fibrillation in the setting of dilative cardiomyopathy. Shown are the 12 surface electrocardiographic leads.

REFERENCES

1. Waldo AL, Akhtar M, Brugada P, et al. The minimally appropriate electrophysiologic study for the initial assessment of patients with documented sustained monomorphic ventricular tachycardia. *J Am Coll Cardiol* 1985;6:1174–1177.
2. Buxton AE, Josephson ME, Marchlinski FE, Miller JM. Polymorphic ventricular tachycardia induced by programmed stimulation: response to procainamide. *J Am Coll Cardiol* 1993;21:90–98.
3. Nguyen PT, Scheinman MM, Seger J. Polymorphous ventricular tachycardia: clinical characterization, therapy, and the QT interval. *Circulation* 1986;74:340–349.
4. Locati EH, Maison-Blanche P, Dejode P, et al. Spontaneous sequences of onset of torsade de pointes in patients with acquired prolonged repolarization: quantitative analysis of Holter recordings. *J Am Coll Cardiol* 1995;25:1564–1575.
5. Dessertenne F. La tachycardie ventriculaire a deux foyers opposes variable. *Arch Mal Coeur* 1966;59:263–272.
6. Roden DM, Lazzara R, Rosen M, et al. Multiple mechanisms in the long QT syndrome: current knowledge, gaps, and future directions. *Circulation* 1996;94:1996–2012.
7. Kurita T, Ohe T, Marui N, et al. Bradycardia induced abnormal QT prolongation in patients with complete atrioventricular block with torsade de pointes. *Am J Cardiol* 1992;9:628–633.
8. Shimizu W, Tanaka KM, Suenaga K, Wakamoto A. Bradycardia-dependent early after-depolarizations in a patient with QTU prolongation and torsade de pointes in association with marked bradycardia and hypokalemia. *Pacing Clin Electrophysiol* 1991;14:1105–1111.
9. Roden DM, Woosley RL, Primm RK. Incidence and clinical features of the quinidine-associated long QT syndrome: implications for patient care. *Am Heart J* 1986;111:1088–1093.
10. Kay GN, Plumb VJ, Arciniegas JG, et al. Torsade de pointes: the long-short initiating sequence and other clinical features. *Am J Cardiol* 1983;2:806–817.
11. Schwartz PJ. Idiopathic long QT syndrome: progress and questions. *Am Heart J* 1985;109:399–411.
12. Habbab MA, El-Sherif N. TU alternans, long QTU, and torsade de pointes: clinical and experimental observations. *Pacing Clin Electrophysiol* 1992;15:916–931.
13. Zareba W, Moss AJ, Le Cessie S, Hall WJ. T wave alternans in idiopathic long QT syndrome. *J Am Coll Cardiol* 1994;23:1541–1546.
14. Rosenbaum D, Albrecht P, Cohen RJ. Predicting sudden cardiac death from T wave alternans of the surface electrocardiogram: promise and pitfalls. *J Cardiovasc Electrophysiol* 1996;7:1095–1111.
15. Rosenbaum DS, Jackson LE, Smith GM, et al. Electrical alternans and vulnerability to ventricular arrhythmias. *N Engl J Med* 1994;330:235–241.
16. Hohnloser SH, Klingenheben T, Li Y-G, et al. T wave alternans as a predictor of recurrent ventricular tachyarrhythmias in ICD recipients: prospective comparison with conventional risk markers. *J Cardiovasc Electrophysiol* 1998;9:1258–1268.
17. Schwartz PJ, Locati EH, Napolitano C, Priori SG. The long QT syndrome. In: Zipes DP, Jalife J, eds. *Cardiac electrophysiology: from cell to bedside.* Philadelphia: WB Saunders, 1995:788–811.
18. Zipes DP. The long QT syndrome: a Rosetta stone for sympathetic related ventricular tachyarrhythmias. *Circulation* 1991;84:1414–1419.
19. Gohl K, Feistel H, Weikl A, et al. Congenital myocardial sympathetic dysinnervation: a structured defect of idiopathic long QT syndrome. *Pacing Clin Electrophysiol* 1991;14:754(abst).
20. Zipes DP. Influence of myocardial ischemia and infarction on automatic innervation of the heart. *Circulation* 1990;82:1095–1105.

21. Surawicz B. Electrophysiologic substrate of torsade de pointes: dispersion of repolarization or early afterdepolarization? *J Am Coll Cardiol* 1989;14:172–184.
22. El-Sherif N, Zeiler RH, Craelius W, et al. QTU prolongation and polymorphic ventricular tachyarrhythmias due to bradycardia-dependent early afterdepolarizations. *Circ Res* 1988;63:286–305.
23. Boutjdir M, El-Sharif N. Pharmacological evaluation of early afterdepolarizations induced by sea anemone toxin (ATXII) in dog heart. *Cardiovasc Res* 1991;25:815–819.
24. El-Sherif N, Turitto G. The long QT syndrome and torsade de pointes. *Pacing Clin Electrophysiol* 1999;22:91–110.
25. El-Sherif N, Caref EB, Yin H, Restivo M. The electrophysiological mechanism of ventricular arrhythmias in the long QT syndrome. *Circ Res* 1996;79:474–492.
26. El-Sherif N, Chinushi M, Caref EB, et al. Electrophysiological mechanism of the characteristic ECG morphology of torsade de pointes tachyarrhythmias in the long QT syndrome. Detailed analysis of ventricular tridimensional activation patterns. *Circulation* 1997;96:4392–4399.
27. Antzelevitch C, Sicouri S. Clinical relevance of cardiac arrhythmias generated by afterdepolarization: role of M cells in the generation of U waves, triggered activity and torsade de pointes. *J Am Coll Cardiol* 1994;23:259–277.
28. Antzelevitch C, Shimizu W, Yan GX, et al. The M cell: its contribution to the ECG and to normal and abnormal electrical function of the heart. *J Cardiovasc Electrophysiol* 1999;10:1124–1152.
29. Antzelevitch C, Sun ZQ, Zhang ZQ, Yan GX. Cellular and ionic mechanisms underlying erythromycin-induced long QT intervals and torsade de pointes. *J Am Coll Cardiol* 1996;28:1836–1848.
30. El-Sherif N, Chinushi M, Restivo M, et al. Electrophysiologic basis of the arrhythmogenicity of short-long cardiac sequences that precede ventricular tachyarrhythmias in the long QT syndrome. *Pacing Clin Electrophysiol* 1998;21:852(abst).
31. Chinushi M, Restivo M, Caref EB, El-Sherif N. Electrophysiological basis of arrhythmogenicity of QT/T alternans in the long QT syndrome: tridimensional analysis of the kinetics of cardiac repolarization. *Circ Res* 1998;83:614–628.
32. Shimizu W, Antzelevitch C. Cellular basis for the ECG features of the LQT1 form of the long QT syndrome: effects of β-adrenergic agonists and antagonists and sodium channel blockers on transmural dispersion of repolarization and torsade de pointes. *Circulation* 1998;98:2314–2322.
33. Priori SG, Barhanin J, Hauer RNW, et al. Genetic and molecular basis of cardiac arrhythmias. *Eur Heart J* 1999;20:174–195.
34. Vincent GM. The molecular basis of the long QT syndrome: genes causing fainting and sudden death. *Annu Rev Med* 1998;49:263–274.
35. Moss AJ, Schwartz PJ, Crampton RS, et al. The long QT syndrome: prospective longitudinal study of 328 families. *Circulation* 1991;84:1136–1144.
36. Schwartz PJ, Moss AJ, Vincent GM, Crampton RS. Diagnostic criteria for the long QT syndrome. *Circulation* 1993;88:782–784.
37. Selzer A, Wray HW. Quinidine syncope. *Circulation* 1964;30:17–23.
38. Roden DM. Taking the "idio" out of "idiosyncratic": predicting torsade de pointes. *Pacing Clin Electrophysiol* 1998;21:1029–1034.
39. Hohnloser SH, van de Loo A, Baedeker F. Efficacy and proarrhythmic hazards of pharmacologic cardioversion of atrial fibrillation: prospective comparison of sotalol versus quinidine. *J Am Coll Cardiol* 1995;26:852–858.
40. Coplen SE, Antman EM, Berlin JA, et al. Efficacy and safety of quinidine therapy for maintenance of sinus rhythm after cardioversion: a meta-analysis of randomized control trials. *Circulation* 1990;82:1106–1116.

41. Hohnloser SH, Woosley RL. Sotalol. *N Engl J Med* 1994;331: 31–38.

42. Soyka LF, Wirz C, Spangenburg RB. Clinical safety profile of sotalol in patients with arrhythmias. *Am J Cardiol* 1990;65: 74A.

43. Hohnloser SH, Arendts W, Quart B. Incidence, type, and dose-dependence of proarrhythmic events during sotalol therapy in patients treated for sustained VT/VF. *Pacing Clin Electrophysiol* 1992;15:551.

44. Merri M, Benhorin J, Alberti M, et al. Electrocardiographic quantitation of ventricular repolarization. *Circulation* 1989;80: 1301–1308.

45. Hohnloser SH, Klingenheben T, Singh BN. Amiodarone-associated proarrhythmic effects: a review with special reference to torsade de pointes tachycardia. *Ann Intern Med* 1994;121: 529–535.

46. Naccarelli GV, Lee KS, Gibson JK, Vanderlugt J. Electrophysiology and pharmacology of ibutilide. *Am J Cardiol* 1996;78[Suppl 8A]:12–16.

47. Stambler BS, Wood MA, Ellenbogen KA, et al. Efficacy and safety of intravenous doses of ibutilide for rapid conversion of atrial flutter or fibrillation. *Circulation* 1996;94:1613–1621.

48. Volgman AS, Carberry PA, Stambler B, et al. Conversion efficacy and safety of intravenous ibutilide compared with intravenous procainamide in patients with atrial flutter or fibrillation. *J Am Coll Cardiol.* 1998;31:1414–1419.

49. Stambler BS, Wood MA, Ellenbogen KA. Antiarrhythmic actions of intravenous ibutilide compared with procainamide during human atrial flutter and fibrillation. *Circulation* 1997;96: 4298–1306.

50. Kowey PR, Vanderlugt JT, Luderer JR. Safety and risk/benefit analysis of ibutilide for acute conversion of atrial fibrillation/flutter. *Am J Cardiol* 1996;78[Suppl 8A]:46–52.

51. Torp-Pedersen C, Moller M, Bloch-Thomsen, et al. Dofetilide in patients with congestive heart failure and left ventricular dysfunction. *N Engl J Med* 1999;341:857–865.

52. Kober L, for the DIAMOND Study Group. A clinical trial of dofetilide in patients with acute myocardial infarction and left ventricular dysfunction—the DIAMOND MI study. *Eur Heart J* 1998;19[Suppl]:90.

53. Pedersen OD, for the DIAMOND Study Group. Dofetilide in the treatment of atrial fibrillation in patients with impaired left ventricular function. *Eur Heart J* 1998; 19[Suppl]:363.

54. Singh SN, Berk MR, Yellen LG, et al. Efficacy and safety of oral dofetilide in maintaining normal sinus rhythm in patients with atrial fibrillation/flutter: a multicenter study. *Circulation* 1997;96[Suppl I]:I-383.

55. Greenbaum RA, Campbell TJ, Channer KS, et al. Conversion of atrial fibrillation and maintenance of sinus rhythm by dofetilide. The EMERALD study. *Circulation* 1998;98[Suppl I]:I-633.

56. Moore TM, Book MH. Sudden death in phenothiazine therapy: a clinico-pathologic study of 12 cases. *Psychiatr Q* 1970;44: 384–402.

57. Metzger E, Friedman R. Prolongation of the corrected QT and torsade de pointes cardiac arrhythmias associated with intravenous haloperidol in the medically ill. *J Clin Psychopharmacol* 1993;13:128–132.

58. Sharma ND, Rosman HS, Padhi ID, Tisdale JE. Torsades de pointes associated with intravenous haloperidol in critically ill patients. *Am J Cardiol* 1998;81:238–240.

59. McComb JM, Campbell NPS, Cleland J. Recurrent ventricular tachycardia associated with QT prolongation after mitral valve replacement and its association with intravenous administration of erythromycin. *Am J Cardiol* 1984;54:922–923.

60. Freedman RA, Andersen KP, Green LS, Mason JW. Effect of ery-

thromycin on ventricular arrhythmias and ventricular repolarization in idiopathic long QT syndrome. *Am J Cardiol* 1987;59:168–169.

61. Nattel S, Ranger S, Talajic M, et al. Erythromycin-induced long QT syndrome: concordance with quinidine and underlying cellular electrophysiologic mechanisms. *Am J Med* 1990;89: 235–238.

62. Sakemi H, Van Natta B. Torsade de pointes induced by astemizole in a patient with prolongation of the QT interval. *Am Heart J* 1993;125:1436–1438.

63. Zimmermann M, Duruz H, Guinand O, et al. Torsade de pointes after treatment with terfenadine and ketoconazole. *Eur Heart J* 1992;13:1002–1003.

64. Pohjola-Sintonen S, Viitasalo M, Toivonen L, Neuvonen P. Torsades de pointes after terfenadine-itraconazole interaction. *Br Med J* 1993;306:186–188.

65. Woosley RL, Chen Y, Freiman JP, Gillis RA. Mechanism of the cardiotoxic actions of terfenadine. *JAMA* 1993;269:1532–1536.

66. Monahan BP, Ferguson CL, Killeavy ES, et al. Torsades de pointes occurring in association with terfenadine use. *JAMA* 1990;264:2788–2790.

67. Wysowski DK, Bacsanyi J. Cisapride and fatal arrhythmia. *N Engl J Med* 1996;335:290–291.

68. Zipes DP, Barbey JT, Lazzara R. Review of spontaneous adverse event reports of serious ventricular arrhythmias, QT prolongation, syncope, and sudden death in patients treated with cisapride. *Circulation* 1999;100(Suppl I)I–308.

69. Geelen P, Brugada J, Andries E, Brugada P. Ventricular fibrillation and sudden death after radiofrequency catheter ablation of the atrioventricular junction. *Pacing Clin Electrophysiol* 1997; 20:343–348.

70. Darpö B, Walfridsson H, Aunes M, et al. Incidence of sudden death after radiofrequency ablation of the atrioventricular junction for atrial fibrillation. *Am J Cardiol* 1997;80:1174–1177.

71. DiPasquale G, Pinelli GA, Andreoli A, et al. Torsade de pointes and ventricular flutter-fibrillation following spontaneous cerebral subarachnoid hemorrhage. *Int J Cardiol* 1988;18:163–172.

72. Leenhardt A, Glaser E, Burguera M, et al. Short-coupled variant of torsade de pointes: a new electrocardiography entity in the spectrum of idiopathic ventricular tachyarrhythmias? *Circulation* 1994;89:206–215.

73. Wolfe CL, Nibley C, Bhandari A, et al. Polymorphous ventricular tachycardia associated with acute myocardial infarction. *Circulation* 1991;84:1543–1551.

74. Myerburg RJ, Kessler KM, Mallon SM, et al. Life-threatening ventricular arrhythmias in patients with silent myocardial ischemia due to coronary artery spasm. *N Engl J Med* 1992;326: 1451–1455.

75. Nishizali M, Arita M, Sakurada H, et al. Induction of polymorphic ventricular tachycardia by programmed ventricular stimulation in vasospastic angina pectoris. *Am J Cardiol* 1996;77:355–360.

76. Wellens HJJ, Brugada P, Stevenson WG. Programmed electrical stimulation: its role in the management of ventricular arrhythmias in coronary heart disease. *Prog Cardiovasc Dis* 1986;29: 165–180.

77. Horowitz LN, Greenspan AM, Spielman SR, et al. Torsade de pointes: electrophysiologic studies in patients without transient pharmacologic or metabolic abnormalities. *Circulation* 1981; 309:1120–1128.

78. Brugada P, Green M, Abdollah H, Wellens HJJ. Significance of ventricular arrhythmias initiated by programmed ventricular stimulation: the importance of the type of ventricular arrhythmia induced and the number of premature stimuli required. *Circulation* 1984;69:87–92.

79. Buxton AE, Waxman HL, Marchlinski FE, et al. Role of triple extrastimuli during electrophysiologic study of patients with

documented sustained ventricular tachyarrhythmias. *Circulation* 1984;69:532–540.

80. DiCarlo LA, Morady F, Schwartz AB, et al. Clinical significance of ventricular fibrillation-flutter induced by ventricular programmed stimulation. *Am Heart J* 1985;109:959–963.

81. Keren A, Tzivoni D, Gavish D, et al. Etiology, warning signs, and therapy of torsades de pointes: a study of 10 patients. *Circulation* 1981;64:1167–1174.

82. Keren A, Tzivoni D. Torsades de pointes: prevention and therapy. *Cardiovasc Drugs Ther* 1991;5:509–514.

83. Tzivoni D, Banai S, Schuger C, et al. Treatment of torsade de pointes with magnesium sulfate. *Circulation* 1988;77:392–397.

84. The Antiarrhythmics Versus Implantable Defibrillators (AVID) Investigators. A comparison of antiarrhythmic-drug therapy with implantable defibrillators in patients resuscitated from near-fatal ventricular arrhythmias. *N Engl J Med* 1997;337:1576–1583.

85. Siebels J, Cappato R, Rüppel R, et al, and the CASH Investigators. Preliminary results of the cardiac arrest study Hamburg (CASH). *Am J Cardiol* 1993;72:109F–113F.

21

SUDDEN CARDIAC DEATH

PHILIP J. PODRID
PETER R. KOWEY

Sudden cardiac death (SCD), usually the result of a ventricular tachyarrhythmia, ventricular tachycardia (VT), or ventricular fibrillation (VF), accounts for 50% of the mortality due to coronary artery disease (CAD). Because CAD accounts for about 35% of total mortality, SCD is the cause of death of 15% of patients each year, accounting for 350,000 to 400,000 deaths annually (1–4).

DEFINITION AND INCIDENCE OF SUDDEN DEATH

Various criteria are used to define SCD in the medical literature. However, the one developed by the World Health Organization has been widely accepted: sudden collapse occurring within 1 hour of symptoms (5). However, as the name implies, SCD is instantaneous, and most individuals become unconscious within seconds to minutes as a result of insufficient cerebral blood flow. There are usually no premonitory symptoms. Symptoms, if present, are nonspecific and include chest discomfort, palpitations, shortness of breath, and weakness.

SCD is a rare event, even among older adults. It has been estimated that about 30 SCDs per million persons occur each week in industrialized countries (5). The incidence increases with age and is two to three times higher among men than women (Fig. 21-1). The annual incidence among men without prior clinically recognized heart disease who are between 70 and 79 years old is 34 cases per 10,000; the annual incidence among the same group of women is 13 cases per 10,000. The incidence of SCD is increased sixfold to 10-fold in the presence of clinically recognized heart disease; it is increased twofold to fourfold in the presence of risk factors for CAD.

Epidemiologic studies have shown that a substantial proportion of these deaths occur out of the hospital; a high proportion of SCDs occurs as a first expression of previously silent underlying disease or in patients whose first clinical manifestation has been unrecognized (e.g., silent infarction). Identification of risk factors specific for SCD is an issue of major public health concern because an accurate prediction of potential SCD victims within the general population would permit more efficient preventive interventions (6).

ARRHYTHMIC MECHANISM OF SUDDEN CARDIAC DEATH

The exact mechanism of collapse in an individual patient is often impossible to establish because patients who die suddenly are seldom under close observation. As a result, the mechanism can only be inferred, based on information obtained after the process has been initiated. However, there have been many cases in which the initiating event has been witnessed or recorded (7,8). Spontaneous nonsustained arrhythmias are often present for a variable period before the development of a sustained ventricular tachyarrhythmia, which includes the following:

1. A sustained monomorphic VT can accelerate to a rapid rate and then degenerate into VF (Fig. 21-2). However, the relationship between monomorphic VT and sudden death has been debated, with some studies finding this arrhythmia in only a minority of patients with SCD (9,10). Ambulatory monitoring and electrophysiologic studies have suggested that some cases of VF begin with a brief, but variable, period of an organized VF.
2. A sustained polymorphic VT can degenerate into VF. This is most often the result of underlying ischemia, although it may be because of acquired or congenital QT prolongation.
3. VF can develop as a primary event.
4. A bradyarrhythmia or asystole is an important but less common cause of SCD (7,11).

P. J. Podrid: Department of Medicine, Boston University Medical School, Boston, Massachusetts 02118.
P. R. Kowey: Department of Medicine, Jefferson Medical College, Philadelphia, Pennsylvania 19107.

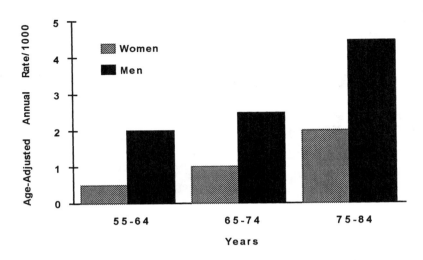

FIGURE 21-1. Incidence of sudden death by age and gender. During a 38-year follow-up of subjects in the Framingham Heart Study, the annual incidence of sudden death increases with age for men and women. However, at each age, the incidence of sudden death is higher for men than women. (Adapted from Kannell WB, Wilson PWF, D'Agostino RB, et al. Sudden coronary death in women. *Am Heart J* 1998;136:205, with permission.)

VF is the rhythm most frequently recorded at the inception of a cardiac arrest (Fig. 21-2). It appears to be the result of multiple localized areas of microreentry resulting in the absence of any organized electrical activity (12). One animal study found that the most likely mechanism is rotating spiral waves (13). This almost always occurs because of underlying myocardial disease, which is often diffuse, resulting in heterogeneity of depolarization and dispersion of repolarization; usually a triggering event is necessary to precipitate the arrhythmia in a vulnerable heart (14). This disparity of electrophysiologic properties is a precondition for reentry. The diversity in conduction and recovery parameters results in fragmentation of the impulse as it travels through the myocardium, and this produces multiple areas of localized

reentry or multiple wavelets of myocardial activation (12). Because there is no organized electrical activity or myocardial depolarization, there is no uniform ventricular contraction—hence, failure of the heart to generate a cardiac output. With the development of global ischemia, the rate of VF decreases because of changes in the electrophysiologic properties of the myocardium resulting from acidosis and hyperkalemia (13).

On the electrocardiogram (ECG), there is an absence of QRS complexes, but there are high-frequency undulations or fibrillatory waves that are regular in amplitude and periodicity, occurring at a rate of greater than 320 bpm. At the very onset of VF, the fibrillatory waves may be coarse, having a tall amplitude and appearing to be regular. The QRS complexes are indistinguishable from T waves, and they appear to be sinusoidal. This may represent a brief period of unorganized ventricular flutter with rates of more than 240 bpm. However, the fibrillatory waves rapidly become finer and more regular in amplitude, duration, and cycle length. Over several minutes, they may become so fine that there does not appear to be any electrical activity.

A bradyarrhythmia or asystole is an important, but less common cause for sudden death and is observed in about 10% of cases of sudden death documented by ambulatory monitoring (7). A bradyarrhythmia is more often associated with nonischemic cardiomyopathy and congestive heart failure (11). In some cases, a profound bradyarrhythmia results in a polymorphous ventricular tachyarrhythmia resembling torsade de pointes. When the patient collapses in an unmonitored setting and the exact onset of the etiologic arrhythmia is uncertain and probably remote, asystole is often the first rhythm observed (15). However, this may be the result of VF that has been present for several minutes, culminating in loss of all electrical activity as a result of hypoxia, acidosis, and death of myocardial tissue. This is of particular importance, because in such cases the chance of successful resuscitation and establishment of sinus rhythm is small, and very few

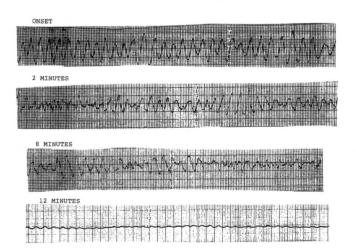

FIGURE 21-2. Ambulatory monitor recording during an episode of ventricular fibrillation (VF). At the onset, the QRS complexes are regular, are widened, and have a tall amplitude, suggesting an organized ventricular tachycardia. Over a brief period, the rhythm becomes more disorganized and is coarse VF, culminating in fine VF and asystole.

of these patients (<10%) survive to hospital discharge. In contrast, patients who were found in a sustained ventricular tachyarrhythmia, especially VT, have a better outcome.

CAUSES OF SUDDEN CARDIAC DEATH

Many cardiac and noncardiac causes for a sustained ventricular tachyarrhythmia can result in SCD (Table 21-1). However, most patients who experience SCD have an underlying cardiac abnormality, particularly chronic coronary heart disease (3). The incidence of sudden death is related to the clinical manifestations of preexisting CAD; the rate is highest for those with a prior myocardial infarction (MI) and intermediate for those who have angina without a prior MI.

Regardless of gender, symptoms of an acute ischemic episode are generally absent, and the collapse typically occurs instantaneously and without any warning (3). Approximately 75% to 80% of patients have no ECG changes or enzyme abnormalities after resuscitation that suggest an acute MI as a precipitating factor. When such changes are present, it is often impossible to establish whether an acute MI caused VF or the VF resulted in myocardial damage because of the absence of coronary artery blood flow. VF usually should be considered a primary process or an electrical accident rather than a consequence of a coronary event.

TABLE 21-1. CAUSES OF SUDDEN CARDIAC DEATH

Cardiac—ischemic
  Coronary artery disease with myocardial infarction or angina
  Coronary artery embolism
  Nonatherogenic coronary artery disease
  Coronary artery spasm
Cardiac—nonischemic
  Coronary artery disease without myocardial infarction or angina
  Cardiomyopathy (obstructive, nonobstructive, nonischemic)
  Valvular heart disease
  Congenital heart disease
  Prolonged QT syndrome
  Preexcitation syndrome
  Complete heart block
  Arrhythmogenic right ventricular dysplasia
  Myocarditis
  Acute pericardial tamponade
  Acute myocardial rupture
Noncardiac
  Sudden infant death syndrome
  Drowning
  Pickwickian syndrome
  Pulmonary embolism
  Drug-induced
  Airway obstruction
  No structural heart disease (primary electrical disease)

Myocardial Ischemia and Infarction

Acute myocardial ischemia or infarction can be a precipitating event for VF. Acute MI is associated with an approximate 15% risk of VF within the first 24 to 48 hours, with the incidence falling to only 3% over the next several days (16). When an MI provokes VF, symptoms of the MI are present for minutes to hours before SCD occurs; more than 80% of VF episodes occur within the first 6 hours (17). Some patients have unstable coronary lesions or coronary spasm that may be responsible for acute ischemic events, short of infarction, and that could cause electrical instability (18,19). One autopsy study of men and women with CAD who died suddenly found that approximately one half had an acute coronary thrombus and one half had severe narrowing of the coronary artery by an atherosclerotic plaque without acute thrombosis (i.e., stable plaque) (20,21). Among those with acute thrombosis, the cause was rupture of a vulnerable plaque (i.e., thin fibrous cap overlying a lipid-rich core) or erosion of a fibrous plaque rich in smooth-muscle cells and proteoglycans. In another autopsy study of patients with CAD who had SCD, acute plaque rupture or hemorrhage into the plaque, without evidence of MI, was seen more in patients who died during exertion than in those who died while at rest (72% versus 23%) (22).

Heart Failure

The presence of heart failure, regardless of cause, increases overall mortality and the incidence of SCD in men and women. In a 38-year follow-up of patients in the Framingham Heart Study, the incidence of SCD among those with heart failure, compared with those without heart failure, was increased fivefold in either sex, although the absolute risk in women was only one-third that of men (23). The SCD potential in men and women with heart failure was as great as that in patients with overt CAD (13.7 and 3.8 versus 12.9 and 2.4 per 1,000 patients, respectively).

Myocardial Abnormalities

Hypertension with left ventricular hypertrophy, often associated with diastolic dysfunction, appears to increase the risk of SCD independently of underlying ischemia. In one study, for example, patients with hypertension and left ventricular hypertrophy who died suddenly had less extensive CAD and were less likely to have thrombi in the coronary vessels than normotensives who had SCD (24). These findings suggest that the hypertrophied myocardium is more susceptible than normal myocardium to the effects of ischemia (24).

Hereditary and acquired diseases of the myocardium are associated with an increased risk of SCD. Hereditary abnormalities of the myocardium include hypertrophic cardiomyopathy, dilated cardiomyopathy, and arrhythmogenic right ventricular dysplasia (ARVD). Acquired structural heart disease associated with abnormalities of the myocardium, such as aortic stenosis, also may be involved in the pathogenesis of SCD.

Absence of Structural Heart Disease: Primary Electrical Disease

Rarely, SCD occurs in patients younger than 40 years of age who have no evidence of structural heart disease (25,26). However, in approximately 90% of these cases, autopsy reveals evidence of previously unrecognized heart disease, including myocarditis, hypertrophic cardiomyopathy, ARVD, sarcoidosis, or asymptomatic CAD (27,28). The remaining 10% of patients have idiopathic VF, also called *primary electrical disease*. Despite the absence of structural heart disease, these patients are at a significant risk for a recurrent episode, reported at 37% during a 43-month period in one study (29).

Brugada Syndrome

Some patients with idiopathic VF have Brugada syndrome, which is associated with a peculiar ECG pattern consisting of a right bundle branch block and ST segment elevation in V_1 to V_3 (30). Affected men outnumber affected women, and most affected individuals are Asian (31). All clinical manifestations of this syndrome are related to life-threatening ventricular arrhythmias, and SCD may be the first and only clinical event, as occurs in 47% of patients. Arrhythmic events generally occur between ages 22 and 65 and are more common at night than in the day and during sleep than while awake (30–33). In general, the QT interval is normal; positive late potentials on a signal-averaged ECG are a common finding, and programmed electrical stimulation reproducibly induces VT or VF in almost all patients.

Brugada syndrome may represent a functional abnormality of the electrical activity of the heart (i.e., primary electrical disease) or an early subclinical manifestation of ARVD (32). Like ARVD, Brugada syndrome is consistent with autosomal dominant inheritance with variable expression; however, it is not related to the same genetic abnormalities that have been associated with ARVD. Mutations in the cardiac sodium channel gene, *SCN5A*, have been found in three families with Brugada syndrome; this is the same gene responsible for long QT syndrome type 3, but the mutation is found at sites other than those known to contribute the long QT syndrome (34).

There are no specific pharmacologic treatments for preventing SCD in the Brugada syndrome. The implantable cardioverter-defibrillator (ICD) appears to be the only effective therapy.

Commotio Cordis

SCD has been described in young athletes who have been struck in the precordium with a projectile object such as a baseball, hockey puck, or fist (35). This phenomenon, called commotio cordis, most commonly affects young adults without preexisting heart disease, and there is usually no structural damage to the chest wall, thoracic cavity, or heart. When documented, the most common arrhythmia is VF, although complete heart block and an idioventricular rhythm have also been described. One study described an animal model in which low-energy blows to the chest wall delivered during repolarization, just before the peak of the T wave, produced VF, whereas blows delivered during depolarization, during the QRS complex, produced transient complete heart block followed by ST segment elevation (36). The frequency of VF was related to the hardness of the projectile.

Familial Form

A family history of MI or primary cardiac arrest is associated with an increased risk for primary cardiac arrest (37). For example, one study found that the rate of MI and SCD among relative of patients with a primary cardiac arrest was 50% higher than in first-degree relatives of the control subjects (risk ratio = 1.46). In a multivariate logistic model, family history of MI or SCD was associated with primary cardiac arrest even after adjustment for other common risk factors.

Conduction System Abnormalities

Hereditary and acquired abnormalities of cardiac conduction, including ventricular conduction delays and prolongation of the QT interval, are associated with an increased risk of SCD. However, many of these electrophysiologic abnormalities occur most commonly in adults with CAD, and because most cases of SCD occur in the setting of structural heart disease, isolated abnormalities of cardiac conduction probably account for only a small proportion (<5%) of SCD among adults in the community (38). Several drugs, primarily the antiarrhythmic agents, slow and prolong cardiac conduction and can alter the risk of SCD even in the absence of underlying heart disease.

Congenital Long QT Syndrome

Affected individuals with a congenital long QT syndrome have an increased risk of SCD. Multiple mutations have been identified in a number of genes related to myocardial potassium channels (LQT1 [*KCNQ1*], LQT2 [*KCNH2*], and LQT5 [*KCNQ5*]) and sodium channels (LQT3 [*SCN5A*] and LQT4 [*LQT4*]) (39). The mutations result in abnormalities of depolarization or repolarization of myocardial cells, and they are associated with ECG abnormalities, syncope, and SCD.

The mutations in different genes may influence the response to specific therapies in families with a long QT syndrome (40). However, screening for gene mutations in patients with known long QT syndrome is not recommended because more than 40 genetic mutations have been identified, and different mutations have been found in the same family. Nevertheless, the molecular biology of the familial long QT syndrome provides important insights into the pathogenesis of the life-threatening ventricular arrhythmia that results in SCD. Whether environmental factors, such as exercise, diet, and drugs, interact with molecular variants in these and other genes to contribute to the risk of SCD remains unknown.

CLINICAL RISK FACTORS FOR SUDDEN CARDIAC DEATH

Various clinical characteristics and other factors are associated with an increased risk of SCD among persons without prior clinically recognized heart disease (41–45). Most risk factors for CAD are also risk factors for SCD (Fig. 21-3). The role of factors that influence the cardiac vulnerability to

potential triggers of SCD is becoming clearer. The available evidence suggests that the occurrence of SCD among adults is likely to result from interaction between underlying structural heart disease and the resulting electrophysiologic abnormalities and triggers for life-threatening arrhythmia.

The major established risk factors for CAD, including hypercholesterolemia, hypertension, cigarette smoking, physical inactivity, obesity, diabetes mellitus, and family history of MI, also are risk factors for SCD. Data from several studies have found that SCD is significantly and positively associated with obesity, cigarette smoking, high pulse rate, and strenuous physical activity. Additional factors include chronic heart disease, left ventricular hypertrophy as determined by ECG, enlarged heart as assessed by chest radiography, heart failure, and heavy alcohol consumption (46).

Pooled data indicate that SCD is the initial and terminal manifestation of CAD in more than one half of all SCD victims. The incidence of SCD was four times greater among those who had known CAD at baseline than those who did not. However, the proportion of coronary deaths

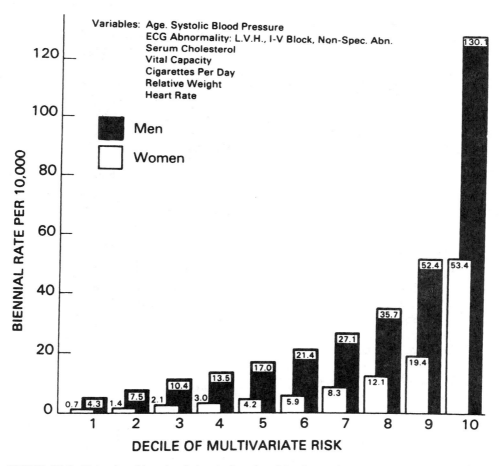

FIGURE 21-3. Risk of sudden death by decile of multivariate risk: a 26-year follow-up in the Framingham Study. I-V, intraventricular; LVH, left ventricular hypertrophy; Non-Spec. Abn., nonspecific abnormality. (From Kannel WB, Schatzkin A. Sudden death: lessons from subsets in population studies. *J Am Coll Cardiol* 1985;5:141B–149B, with permission.)

that were sudden was not significantly different among those who had recognized CAD at baseline examination from those who had not.

Sex is a factor in the incidence of SCD. The Framingham Study found that the incidence of SCD was significantly lower among women than men, but 64% of all SCD in women occurred without prior clinically apparent CAD, indicating that SCD was often the first and last manifestation of CAD in women (23). Among clinical characteristics, left ventricular hypertrophy was found as the strongest predictor of SCD in this group of women. Another U.S. study found that cigarette smoking was the strongest risk factor in the incidence of SCD among women; all of those 45 years old or younger who died suddenly were heavy smokers (21).

Most epidemiologic studies indicated that blacks have a higher incidence of SCD than whites (47–50). The reasons for this difference are not fully explained. It has been suggested that different levels of health care delivery provided for blacks and whites may be a strong contributor to the difference (51). Further epidemiologic studies are needed to provide better insights into risk factors and incidence of SCD among men and women of different races and ethnic origins.

Despite a large number of epidemiologic studies that have shown a strong relationship of major risk factors (blood pressure, serum cholesterol, cigarette smoking, body weight, physical activity) to the incidence of CAD in general, and SCD in particular, there is as yet not a single or a set of risk factors identified as being specific for SCD. Until risk factors specific for SCD are found, prediction of SCD in the general population remains a matter of predicting SCD on the basis of standard risk factors, with continued difficulty in identifying the specific individuals at risk. This creates a problem regarding the limited efficiency of preventive interventions and the ability of such interventions to impact on the large numbers of SCD candidates hidden within the general population.

TRIGGERS FOR SUDDEN DEATH

A number of transient risk factors, acting in concert with underlying myocardial electrical instability, can provoke VF. These include electrolyte disturbances, pH changes, antiarrhythmic drugs, ischemia, autonomic nervous system activation, an increase in circulating catecholamines, and psychosocial stress factors (Fig. 21-4). Other factors such as heavy alcohol and caffeine consumption and specific pharmacologic therapies may also trigger SCD (46,52,53); however, few studies have examined the transient risk associated with these possible triggers.

Electrolyte Disturbances

Any reversible metabolic abnormalities, but especially hypokalemia and hypomagnesemia, may predispose to ven-

tricular tachyarrhythmias (54,55). However, by themselves these abnormalities are often insufficient to be solely responsible for sudden death. The only setting in which hypokalemia definitely plays a role is during an acute MI (56). It is potentially hazardous to ascribe a cardiac arrest to an electrolyte or metabolic derangement alone, unless there is compelling evidence of an association. Mistaken attribution of a major arrhythmia to an innocent laboratory abnormality places the patient at a high risk of recurrence.

It should also be appreciated that hypokalemia immediately after resuscitation may be a result of the cardiac arrest rather than a cause (4). Catecholamines (particularly epinephrine) stimulate the β_2-adrenergic receptors, which drive potassium into the cells, thereby lowering the plasma potassium concentration.

Heart Failure and Myocardial Ischemia

Most patients who experience SCD have left ventricular dysfunction and a history of heart failure (57). Active overt or silent ischemia occasionally is the provoking factor for SCD (58). In one study, 84 patients resuscitated from SCD underwent immediate coronary angiography (59). Significant CAD was found in 60 patients; 40 (48%) had an acute occlusion. Occlusion existed in 87% of those who had ST segment elevation on ECG and chest pain before the cardiac arrest, compared with 39% without these features. However, for most patients who survive an episode of SCD, an ischemic event cannot be regarded as the critical factor, even though the patient may have significant underlying CAD (60).

Drugs

Antiarrhythmic Drugs

Antiarrhythmic drugs can themselves contribute to the likelihood of an event (61,62). This is particularly true in the patient with a recent MI, as was observed with flecainide and encainide in the Cardiac Arrhythmia Suppression Trial (CAST) (63), or the patient with heart failure (64). Of particular concern is the patient who has had a cardiac arrest while receiving an antiarrhythmic drug. It is very difficult to be certain in many of these cases if the arrest was provoked by the drug or occurred despite its use. This dilemma is especially difficult in making decisions about chronic therapy for such patients.

Other Drugs

The use of an illicit drug such as cocaine can directly cause arrhythmia or produce coronary artery vasospasm and ischemia (65,66). Drugs that prolonged QT interval may be associated with the risk of torsade des pointes and SCD. It has been postulated that drug-induced long QT syndrome might represent a genetically mediated "forme fruste" of the syndrome; support for this theory comes

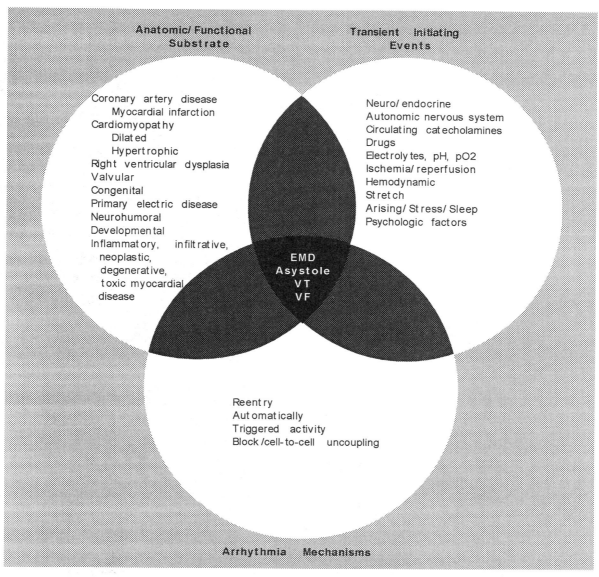

FIGURE 21-4. Interaction of factors for sudden death. The Venn diagram shows the interaction of anatomic or functional substrate abnormalities and transient risk factors that modulate the arrhythmogenic mechanisms capable of causing sudden cardiac death.

from an observation that there is a relatively large number of individuals who carry silent mutations on long QT syndrome genes (i.e., gene carriers with a low penetrance) (67–69). In such individuals, the long QT syndrome mutations may produce an alteration in repolarizing currents that is insufficient to prolong the QT interval at rest but that becomes prolonged by any drug that affects potassium currents.

Exercise

The risk of SCD is transiently increased during strenuous exercise compared with other situations (70). The magni-

tude of the transient increase in risk during acute exercise is lower among men who are regular exercisers than among men for whom exercise is unusual. The transient increase in risk during exercise is outweighed by a reduction in the risk of SCD at other times. There is an overall reduction in the risk of SCD among strenuous exercisers compared with sedentary men.

Psychosocial Stress

Clinical observations have long suggested a possible relation between acutely stressful situations and the risk of SCD. Major disasters, such as earthquakes and war, result in a rapid, transient increase in the rate of SCD in populations (71,72). Emotional stress may lower the threshold for arrhythmia directly and secondary to the provocation of transient myocardial ischemia. A circadian variation has been found for SCD that parallels that of MI, with a peak in the morning (73,74). It has been suggested that a primary arrhythmic event is more likely to occur in the morning because increased adrenergic activity at this time may increase electrical instability or induce myocardial ischemia without infarction. Sympathetic nervous system stimulation increases cardiac vulnerability in the normal and ischemic heart (75,76).

OUTCOME OF RESUSCITATION

There is an association between the arrhythmic mechanism for SCD and the outcome of resuscitation. When the initial rhythm is asystole or electrical-mechanical dissociation (i.e., pulseless electrical activity), the likelihood of successful resuscitation is low, and when it is performed out of hospital, very few of these patients (<10%) survive to hospitalization (77) (Table 21-2). Several studies have found that virtually none of these patients survives to be discharged from the hospital (78). The poor outcome probably reflects the prolonged duration of the cardiac arrest, usually more than 4 minutes, and the presence of severe and irreversible myocardial damage. The myocardial damage and extinction of electrical activity result from severe tissue hypoxemia, metabolic acidosis, and hyperkalemia that develop rapidly. Ultimately, there is irreversible damage of other organs.

The outcome is much better when the initial rhythm is a sustained ventricular tachyarrhythmia. Approximately 25% of patients with VF survive to be discharged (79). In comparison, the survival rate for those with hemodynamically unstable VT is 65% to 70% (80). The prognosis may be better for patients found in monomorphic VT because of the potential of some systemic perfusion during this more organized arrhythmia. Patients with VT tend to have a lower incidence of a remote MI and a higher ejection fraction compared with those with VF (81).

The outcome of patients with bradycardia due to a very slow idioventricular rhythm or asystole is poor, and in many studies, none of these patients survives to hospital discharge. This probably reflects the prolonged duration of the cardiac arrest, which is usually more than 4 minutes, and the presence of severe and irreversible myocardial damage. The myocardial damage and extinction of electrical activity result from severe tissue hypoxemia, metabolic acidosis, and hyperkalemia that develop rapidly. Ultimately, there is also irreversible damage of other organs.

Patients who have SCD caused by electrical-mechanical dissociation (i.e., pulseless electrical activity) also have a poor outcome. In one study of 150 such patients, 35 patients (23%) were resuscitated and survived to hospital admission (82). However, 19 of these patients died in hospital, and only 16 (11%) were discharged.

Outcome of Noncardiac Sudden Death

Although the most frequent mechanism for SCD is a ventricular tachyarrhythmia resulting from underlying heart

TABLE 21-2. CARDIOPULMONARY RESUSCITATION

Study	Group	N	Successful CPR (%)	Discharged (%)
Liberthson et al. (91)	Outpatient	301	99 (33)	42 (14)
Thompson et al. (85)	Outpatient	316	199 (63)	88 (28)
Fusgen et al. (210)	Outpatient	335	335 (100)	23 (7)
Bachman et al. (211)	Outpatient (witnessed)	283	37 (13)	14 (5)
Taffet et al. (92)	Inpatient and outpatient	399	160 (40)	24 (6)
Bedell et al. (93)	Inpatient	294	129 (44)	41 (14)
Bayer et al. (212)	Inpatient and outpatient (elderly)	95	37 (39)	16 (17)
Murphy et al. (94)	Inpatient and outpatient (elderly)	503	110 (22)	19 (4)
Myerburg et al. (89)	Outpatient	352	200 (57)	67 (19)
Ritter et al. (95)	Outpatient	2,142	407 (19)	171 (8)
Greene et al. (96)	Outpatient	447	268 (60)	89 (20)
Roberts et al. (97)	Inpatient	310	115 (37)	30 (10)
Tortolani et al. (98)	Inpatient	470	153 (33)	69 (15)
Marwick et al. (99)	Inpatient	710	198 (28)	92 (13)
Rosenberg et al. (213)	Inpatient	349	188 (54)	81 (23)
Burns et al. (100)	Inpatient	122	56 (46)	9 (7)
Total		7,428	2,691 (36)	875 (12)

disease, one study reported that noncardiac causes accounted for 34% of cases (83). Trauma, nontraumatic bleeding, intoxication, near drowning, and pulmonary embolism were the most common noncardiac causes of SCD in this study, and 40% of patients were successfully resuscitated and hospitalized. However, only 11% were discharged from the hospital, and only 6% were neurologically intact or had mild disability.

Factors Related to the Outcome of Resuscitation

SCD is a catastrophic event, and VF in the human heart does not terminate spontaneously; survival therefore depends on prompt cardiopulmonary resuscitation (CPR). The only effective way to reestablish organized electrical activity and myocardial contraction is prompt electrical defibrillation.

It has been estimated that ischemic changes begin with the onset of the ventricular arrhythmia resulting from the absence of tissue perfusion. Organ damage becomes irreversible after approximately 4 minutes of VF and cessation of cardiac output (84). As a result, the longer the duration of the cardiac arrest, the lower is the likelihood of resuscitation or survival, even if initial resuscitation is successful. The Seattle Heart Watch program reported the percentage of patients discharged alive was significantly higher among those with CPR initiated at the scene by a bystander trained in CPR compared with CPR initiated by emergency medical personnel (43% versus 22%, *p* < 0.001) (85). The most important reason for the improvement in survival was that earlier CPR and prompt defibrillation were associated with less damage to the central nervous system (Fig. 21-5). More patients with bystander-initiated CPR were conscious at the time of hospital admission (50% versus 9%), and more regained consciousness by the end of hospitalization (81% versus 52%) (85).

These observations were confirmed by a second and larger study that analyzed data from 1,872 patients with a witnessed cardiac arrest due to VF (86). Overall, 31% of patients survived to hospital discharge. Lower age, bystander-initiated CPR, and shorter intervals between collapse and CPR with defibrillation were significantly associated with survival. Another study found that performing CPR for at least 90 seconds before defibrillation improved survival, especially in patients for whom the initial response interval was longer than 4 minutes (27% versus 17% without prior CPR) (87).

Optimizing the emergency medical system within a community and reducing the response interval to within 8 minutes can improve the survival to hospital discharge. This was observed in one study of 6,331 patients who had an out-of-hospital cardiac arrest; the overall survival to hospital discharge improved by 33% after the response time was

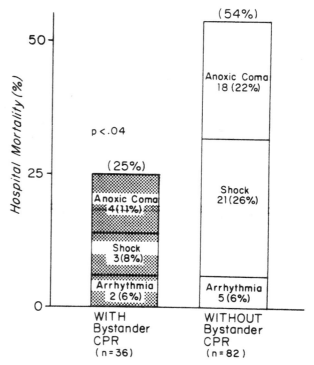

FIGURE 21-5. Hospital mortality among 118 patients initially resuscitated from out-of-hospital sudden cardiac death. Mortality was significantly lower among patients receiving bystander cardiopulmonary resuscitation (CPR) compared with those not receiving CPR from a bystander, primarily because of a lower incidence of death from shock and anoxic coma. (From Thompson RG, Hallstrom AP, Cobb LA. Bystander-initiated cardiopulmonary resuscitation in the management of ventricular fibrillation. *Ann Intern Med* 1979;90:737–740, with permission.)

shortened (5.2% versus 3.9%), representing an additional 21 lives saved (88).

Causes of In-Hospital Mortality

The cause of death in hospital is most often noncardiac, usually resulting from anoxic encephalopathy or respiratory complications from long-term respirator dependence (89). Only about 10% of patients die of recurrent arrhythmia, whereas approximately 30% die of a low cardiac output or cardiogenic shock. Recurrence of severe arrhythmia in the hospital is associated with a poor outcome (90).

Risk Factors for Mortality

Despite the efforts of emergency personnel, resuscitation is successful in only one third of patients, and only about 10% of all patients are ultimately discharged from the hospital (91–95). In addition to later onset of CPR, several factors are associated with a poor outcome with CPR, as shown in (Table 21-3) (96–102).

TABLE 21-3. CARDIOPULMONARY RESUSCITATION OUTCOMES

Risk Factors for Poor Outcome of CPR
- Later onset of CPR
- Absence of any vital signs
- Sepsis
- Cerebrovascular accident with severe neurologic deficit
- Cancer or Alzheimer's disease
- History of more than two chronic diseases
- History of cardiac disease
- An initial rhythm of asystole or electromechanical dissociation
- CPR lasting more 5 minutes

Poor Prognostic Features of Survivors of CPR
- Persistent coma after CPR
- Hypotension, pneumonia, or renal failure after CPR
- Need for intubation or pressors
- Class 3 or 4 congestive heart failure
- Older age

EVALUATION AND MANAGEMENT OF THE CARDIAC SUDDEN DEATH VICTIM

Management of the SCD victim involves acute resuscitation, immediate evaluation, and prompt therapy for the patients surviving to the hospital, In-hospital management is needed to prevent a recurrent episode (Table 21-4).

TABLE 21-4. MANAGEMENT OF THE SUDDEN DEATH SURVIVOR

Diagnostic Evaluation
1. Establish the nature and extent of heart disease.
2. Evaluate left ventricular function.
3. Establish the presence of metabolic abnormalities and prior drug use.
4. Evaluate for underlying ischemia.
5. Establish presence and extent of neurologic or psychologic abnormalities.
6. Establish type, frequency, and reproducibility of ventricular and supraventricular arrhythmia in a drug-free state with ambulatory monitoring, exercise testing, and electrophysiologic testing.

Therapeutic Management
1. Discontinue drugs, especially antiarrhythmic drugs (if possible).
2. Correct metabolic and electrolyte abnormalities.
3. Evaluate for precipitating factors.
4. Optimize left ventricular function.
5. Control symptoms of active ischemia.
6. Apply interventions for neurologic and psychologic states.
7. Use primary therapy of implantable cardioverter-defibrillator (ICD); consider amiodarone as primary therapy for selected patients (based on nature of arrhythmia and left ventricular function).
8. Consider adjunctive therapy (e.g., ablation, antiarrhythmic drugs) for patients with spontaneous arrhythmia that causes symptoms or interferes with ICD function.

Cardiac Resuscitation

The occurrence of VF and SCD is a catastrophic event during which there is no active cardiac contraction and no cardiac output. VF in the human heart does not spontaneously terminate, and survival therefore depends on prompt CPR and reestablishment of organized electrical activity and a stable sinus or supraventricular rhythm. The only effective approach to terminating VF is defibrillation using transthoracic energy in a nonsynchronized fashion (103). Although defibrillation is lifesaving, direct current shock to the heart delivered transthoracically or epicardially can generate free radicals, which may be in part responsible for defibrillation injury (104). The generation of free radicals is related to the peak energy of an individual shock, not the cumulative energy delivered. The amount of energy required usually is between 200 and 400 J delivered with a monophasic waveform or 120 to 200 J delivered with a biphasic waveform (105). The initial success of defibrillation depends directly on the duration of the arrhythmia (106). When VF has been present for seconds to a few minutes and the fibrillatory waves are coarse, the success rate is high. However, as VF continues for a longer period, the fibrillatory waves become finer as the result of a depletion of myocardial epinephrine stores, and the ability to terminate arrhythmia is decreased (107). When VF continues for more than 4 minutes, there is irreversible damage of the central nervous system and other organs, which affects survival even if there is initially successful defibrillation (108). Guidelines for CPR have been established by the American Heart Association and are revised periodically. They call for prompt evaluation of state of consciousness followed by an assessment of airway, efforts of mechanical ventilation, direct cardiac compression, and electrical defibrillation.

Active Compression-Decompression

Meaningful survival after cardiac arrest depends on providing minimal levels of blood flow to vital organs (109). In particular, coronary perfusion pressure appears to correlate most closely with the success of resuscitation (110). Optimally performed standard manual CPR is barely able to achieve the minimal coronary perfusion pressure required to sustain life. On the basis of an anecdotal case report of successful resuscitation using a toilet plunger, Cohen and others developed a hand-held suction cup as an adjunct to standard manual CPR (111). Use of this device in active compression-decompression (ACD) CPR involves a compression phase, as in conventional CPR, but the passive relaxation phase is replaced by active decompression where the chest wall is lifted upward by the suction cup. Active decompression can rapidly decrease intrathoracic pressure and may thereby increase venous return to the heart (112).

ACD CPR has been shown to improve pulmonary ventilation, cardiopulmonary flow, and vital organ perfusion in animal models and human subjects after cardiac arrest (113, 114). However, several randomized trials have failed to demonstrate a statistically significant improvement in hospital discharge rate, the most important clinical outcome.

Adjunctive Drug Therapy

There has been an increasing interest in determining the relative value of adjuvant drug therapy during cardiac resuscitation. Although several interventions have been recommended in the guidelines prepared by the American Heart Association, most of these do not have sufficient evidence to support their routine use.

The administration of bicarbonate in patients who have lactic acidemia and large anion gaps seems logical, but the efficacy of sodium bicarbonate administration has been a source of controversy (115,116). Only one prospective, randomized, double-blinded trial of 502 adults with asystole or VF refractory to an initial defibrillation attempt has examined the use of buffering agents in the treatment of out-of-hospital cardiac arrest (117). When patients treated with saline or a mixture of sodium bicarbonate, tromethamine, and phosphate were compared, no significant differences were observed in the rates of survival to intensive care unit admission (36% versus 36%) or survival to hospital discharge (14% versus 10%).

Likewise, patients who had inadequate blood pressures after restoration of an organized rhythm frequently required the use of pressor agents such as epinephrine, norepinephrine, or dopamine. Use of high-dose pressor agents, especially high-dose epinephrine, as a routine, appears to be associated with an adverse outcome and is not recommended as a routine therapy for cardiac arrest (118–120). The routine use of drugs such as magnesium has not con-

ferred a benefit, although magnesium is indicated for drug-induced torsade des pointes (121).

A particular point of controversy has been the use of antiarrhythmic drugs for patients who have recalcitrant VF or in whom the arrhythmia occurs soon after restoration of sinus rhythm. Lidocaine, bretylium, and procainamide have been listed in the most recent version of the Advanced Cardiac Life Support guidelines published by the American Heart Association. Within the published literature, there is little evidence to support their use. Controlled trials with limited numbers of patients have shown lidocaine and bretylium to be ineffective for this indication. Procainamide, although useful for the termination of sustained monomorphic VT, has not been studied specifically in patients with cardiac arrest or VF in any systematic fashion. Intravenous amiodarone has been better studied for this indication, and results indicate that it may have value in improving the chances of survival to the hospital admission, although not necessarily for improving total mortality. In a prospective trial, 504 patients with cardiac arrest due to VF or pulseless VT who were not resuscitated after at least three defibrillation shocks were randomized to intravenous amiodarone (300 mg) or placebo (122). Although the mean time to resuscitation and number of shocks delivered were the same, the rate of survival to hospitalization was greater for the amiodarone group (44% versus 34%, *p* = 0.03), especially for patients who had a transient return of pulse during defibrillation and then received amiodarone (64% versus 41%) (Fig. 21-6). However, the incidence of hypotension (59% versus 48%) and bradycardia requiring therapy (41% versus 25%) was greater with amiodarone therapy compared with placebo. More than 50% of patients who survived to discharge had no neurologic

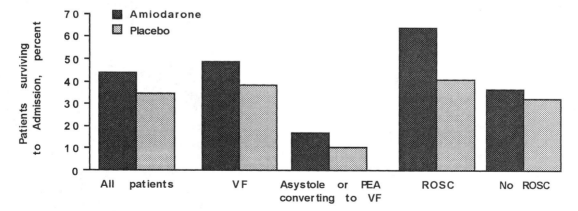

FIGURE 21-6. Among 504 patients with an out-of-hospital cardiac arrest who did not respond to at least three defibrillation shocks and were randomized to amiodarone or placebo, the survival to hospitalization was greater for those receiving amiodarone (44% versus 34% for placebo, *p* = 0.03). Survival was greater with amiodarone for those with ventricular fibrillation (VF) (49% versus 39%) or pulseless electrical activity (PEA) (17% versus 12%), especially in those with return of spontaneous circulation (ROSC) before administration of the study drug (65% versus 41%); there was no significant benefit in those with no ROSC (38% versus 33%). (Adapted from Kudenchuk PJ, Cobb LA, Copass MK, et al. Amiodarone for resuscitation after out-of-hospital cardiac arrest due to ventricular fibrillation. *N Engl J Med* 1999;341:871, with permission.)

impairment. This study was not properly powered to assess total mortality or other outcomes. Studies are in progress to determine the relative value of amiodarone versus other antiarrhythmic drugs as first-line therapy for patients who have failed initial attempts of resuscitation.

Patient Evaluation

The evaluation of the patient who has had a cardiac arrest begins immediately after resuscitation. The physician needs to identify any obvious provoking factors that might have led to the event and to correct them so as to prevent an immediate recurrence. As soon as historical information can be obtained, the patient and family should be questioned about previous diagnoses of heart disease; the use of any medication, especially cardioactive drugs such as antiarrhythmics, diuretics, and digoxin; and antecedent symptoms, especially evidence of ischemia. Unfortunately, cardiac arrest is often not witnessed, or if there are observers, they are often unaware of any symptoms that may have preceded the event. The patient resuscitated from VF often has retrograde amnesia and is unable to remember anything that occurred before the cardiac arrest. Retrograde amnesia may extend from several minutes to many hours or days before the collapse. A coherent history of chest pain or palpitations that heralded the event may not be ascertainable.

Metabolic Abnormalities

Any reversible metabolic abnormalities should be identified and corrected, particularly hypokalemia or hypomagnesemia, because such electrolyte imbalances can predispose to ventricular tachyarrhythmias (123,124). However, hypokalemia may be present immediately after resuscitation as a result of the cardiac arrest rather than its cause (125). This condition is caused by a transit decrease in serum potassium as a result of an increase in catecholamine levels and stimulation of the β_2 receptors, an increase in insulin secretion, and acidosis-mediated hydrogen potassium exchange. It is especially hazardous to ascribe a cardiac arrest to an electrolyte or metabolic derangement alone unless there is particularly compelling evidence of an association. Mistaken attribution of the major arrhythmia to an innocent laboratory abnormality places the untreated patient at a high risk for recurrence.

Prior Drug Use

The use of cardioactive drugs in victims of cardiac arrest is a particular problem. Drugs that could affect ventricular electrical properties should be discontinued, if possible, before a full assessment of the patient's susceptibility to a recurrent event. Of particular concern are patients who have had cardiac arrest while receiving an antiarrhythmic drug. It is difficult to be certain in many of these cases if the arrest was provoked by the drug or occurred despite its use

(126,127). This dilemma is especially important for making decisions about chronic drug therapy for such patients.

Left Ventricular Function

Many patients who experience cardiac arrest have left ventricular dysfunction and a history of heart failure (128). Before any baseline evaluation, overt congestive heart failure needs to be treated and left ventricular function optimized. This process includes therapy with digoxin, diuretics, angiotensin-converting enzyme (ACE) inhibitors, and β blockers as generally indicated.

Because global left ventricular dysfunction due to myocardial stunning may occur as a result of the cardiac arrest and successful CPR, baseline evaluation of left ventricular function should be performed at least 48 hours after resuscitation (129). It has been reported that the severity of myocardial dysfunction after resuscitation in animals is related in part to the energy used for defibrillation (130).

Myocardial Ischemia

Active ischemia must be aggressively treated with aspirin, β blockers, nitrates, and calcium channel blockers or, if necessary, with revascularization using percutaneous interventions or bypass surgery. Infrequently, active overt or silent ischemia is the provoking factor for the sudden death episode, and revascularization is the only therapy necessary (131). This may be particularly applicable to the patient who has CAD with normal left ventricular function and a documented ischemic episode before the cardiac arrest. However, for most patients who survive an episode, an ischemic event cannot be regarded as the causative factor, even though the patient may have significant underlying CAD. For such patients, revascularization is an adjunctive, not primary, therapy. A full arrhythmia evaluation is still necessary (132).

Underlying Heart Disease

After the patient has been stabilized, it is particularly important to establish the nature and extent of underlying heart disease and left ventricular function by physical examination, imaging techniques, and cardiac catheterization if indicated. Although coronary heart disease is the most frequent type of disease associated with VF, patients with many other cardiac disease states can develop this arrhythmia (Table 21-1). Determining the nature of the underlying heart disease is important for several reasons (Fig. 21-7). It may expose a significant abnormality that contributed to the acute event and that requires therapy, such aortic stenosis, a severe proximal coronary artery lesion, acute myocarditis, or hypertrophic cardiomyopathy. The nature of the cardiac abnormality and severity of left ventricular dysfunction may be helpful in deciding whether there is any value to performing invasive electrophysiologic testing for

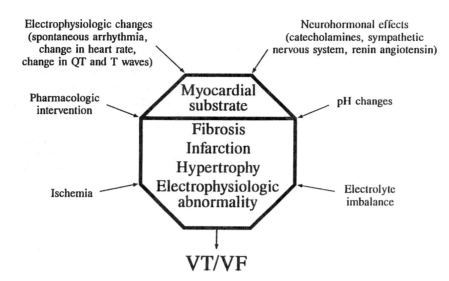

FIGURE 21-7. In the schematic of sudden death, there is an interaction between the damaged and abnormal myocardium and several other factors that may be responsible for the precipitation of ventricular tachycardia (VT) or ventricular fibrillation (VF).

the purposes of selecting an antiarrhythmic drug rather than implanting an ICD. For example, electrophysiologic testing is less useful in patients with nonischemic cardiomyopathy than in those who have had a prior MI. Similarly, antiarrhythmic drugs are less effective and more likely to cause significant cardiac toxicity in patients with heart failure and significant left ventricular dysfunction. Coronary revascularization in patients after cardiac arrest is a useful procedure that may, in concert with a direct arrhythmia approach, have an important effect on prolonging life.

Neurologic Examination

Patients who have been resuscitated from SCD should undergo a complete neurologic examination, which is important to establish the nature and extent of impairment resulting from the arrest. It is also important to exclude conditions that could mimic an arrhythmic event such as a seizure disorder.

Equally important is an assessment of a patient's psychologic state, which often becomes a concern to the patient and the family, particularly after hospital discharge. Patients who have been resuscitated from SCD frequently have emotional problems and anxieties that prevent them from resuming a normal and active life and that can interfere with family interactions. Such potential problems should be identified and discussed with the patient and the family before discharge. Support groups that include individuals who have received an implantable device have become increasingly popular and useful in making proper long-term adjustments (133).

Arrhythmia Evaluation

After an underlying condition has been diagnosed and treated appropriately, an arrhythmia evaluation follows; there has been substantial evolution in the approach in recent years. Previously, an extensive evaluation was undertaken,

including ambulatory monitoring, signal-averaged electrocardiography, exercise testing, and invasive electrophysiologic study, but it is now believed, based on the results of clinical trials, that SCD victims are best served by treatment with an ICD (134–136). Arrhythmia evaluation and testing using noninvasive or invasive techniques are reserved for cases in which there is some uncertainty about the cause or the mechanism of SCD, and for those cases in which a number of reasons exist for preferring an antiarrhythmic drug therapy over an implantable device. This group can include patients with relatively well-preserved left ventricular function whose cardiac arrest was initiated by monomorphic VT, patients who for technical reasons cannot have a device implantation, and the very elderly patient with a terminal disease for whom device therapy is not expected to provide adequate benefit to justify risk and expense of device implantation.

Noninvasive techniques, including ambulatory recording of the ECG and exercise testing, have largely been abandoned because they do not add substantially to the decision to implant a device versus prescribe an antiarrhythmic drug. Knowledge of conduction system disease is of considerably less importance with the advent of implantable devices, which can also provide single- or dual-chamber pacemaker support. Current devices have the ability to record and store electrograms during spontaneous arrhythmias that cause device activation and inappropriate or appropriate shock delivery. Aside from an ischemia assessment, only rare patients require preimplantation exercise testing for arrhythmia assessment. Postimplantation testing may be important to determine the device response to rapid rates, especially if there is an anticipation that the patient will resume a high level of activity soon after device implantation.

Other noninvasive methods, such as determining the signal-averaged ECG, heart rate variability, baroreceptor sensitivity, and T-wave alternans, all have some value for predicting the patient at risk for a cardiac arrest, but they have little value in the management of the SCD victim (Fig. 21-7).

LONG-TERM THERAPY OF THE SUDDEN DEATH SURVIVOR

Pharmacologic Therapy

Electrophysiologic testing is employed for the determination of the inducibility and characteristics of a ventricular tachyarrhythmia before initiation of antiarrhythmic drug therapy. With compelling evidence from randomized trials completed over the past few years, there is increasing emphasis on the use of implantable devices over antiarrhythmic drugs for the treatment of patients who have cardiac arrest caused by VF (134–136). The most notable exception to this approach are patients who have monomorphic VT documented to degenerate into VF, especially in the setting of relatively well-preserved left ventricular function (137,138). For these individuals, an argument can be made for the use of antiarrhythmic drug therapy guided by the results of programmed stimulation. For the very elderly and sickly individuals who are not candidates for implantable devices, empiric administration of oral amiodarone appears to be the treatment of choice. Data from several nonrandomized trials suggested amiodarone may be the most effective drug for this indication with the least chance of causing significant toxicity in an elderly population with concurrent diseases. Whether the empiric use of amiodarone improves survivorship in this highly selected patient population has never been studied specifically. However, the results of the Cardiac Arrest in Seattle: Conventional versus Amiodarone Drug Evaluation (CASCADE) study, a randomized trial comparing the effects of conventional antiarrhythmic drug therapy with empiric amiodarone, suggest that this option may be preferred to empiric use of other membrane active drugs (139) (Fig. 21-8).

Although there are no data to support the use of conventional antiarrhythmic drugs as primary therapy for the cardiac arrest victim, pharmacologic therapy is frequently employed for patients who already have a device implantation (140–143). Adjunctive antiarrhythmic drug therapy may be employed for several reasons:

1. The drug may be expected to decrease the frequency of supraventricular arrhythmia, particularly atrial fibrillation that causes symptoms or is of a sufficient rate to cause device activation and firing (Fig. 21-9). With the advent of devices that can also perform atrial defibrillation, antiarrhythmic drugs, which lower the atrial defibrillation threshold, may be particularly valuable.
2. Antiarrhythmic drugs may reduce the level of ventricular arrhythmia to reduce symptoms caused by nonsustained forms or to reduce the frequency of VT that triggers ICD shocks (Fig. 21-9).
3. Antiarrhythmic drugs may slow the rate of VT to permit efficient pace termination, avoiding the need for unpleasant cardioversion or defibrillation shocks.
4. Some antiarrhythmic drugs, particularly class III agents, can reduce the ventricular defibrillation threshold, which may benefit patients who have a narrow margin between the energy required and deliverable for termination of ventricular tachyarrhythmias (144).

Despite the preeminence of device therapy for patients with cardiac arrest caused by VF, there may be an expanding role of antiarrhythmic drugs in the treatment of arrhythmias that already have occurred in patients with device implantation and perhaps as prophylactic therapy. The growing evidence in the literature indicates that concomitant antiarrhythmic drug therapy may help prevent arrhythmias that may cause loss of consciousness or psychologic harm (143).

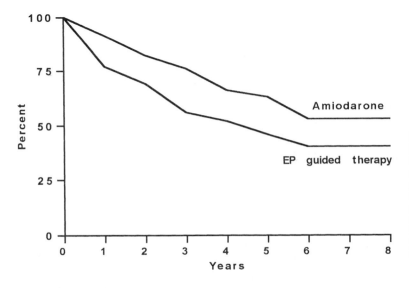

FIGURE 21-8. The Cardiac Arrest in Seattle: Conventional versus Amiodarone Drug Evaluation (CASCADE) trial. Compared with 115 survivors of sudden cardiac death receiving conventional antiarrhythmic agents selected by electrophysiologic testing, 113 patients treated with amiodarone had a significantly greater survival free of a cardiac event, including cardiac mortality, resuscitated cardiac arrest, or implanted defibrillator shock. (Adapted from the CASCADE Investigators. Randomized antiarrhythmic drug therapy in survivors of cardiac arrest [the CASCADE study]. *Am J Cardiol* 1993;72:280, with permission).

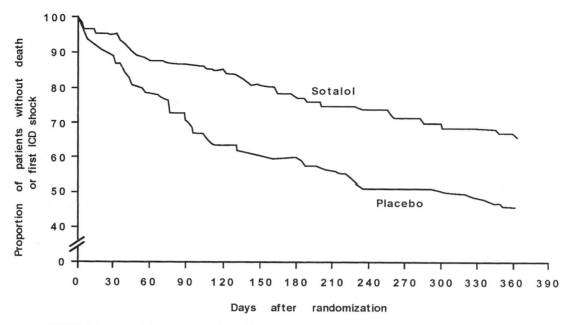

FIGURE 21-9. Sotalol with an implantable cardioverter-defibrillator (ICD). Among 302 patients with an ICD, sotalol reduced the risk of death or the delivery of a first shock for any reason by 48% compared with placebo (*p*< 0.001). (Data from Pacifico A, Hohnloser SH, Williams JH, et al, for the d,l-Sotalol Implantable Cardioverter-Defibrillator Study Group. Prevention of implantable-defibrillator shocks by pretreatment with sotalol. *N Engl J Med* 1999;340:1855.)

Nonpharmacologic Therapy

Comprehensive therapy of a patient with cardiac arrest must include correction of the heart disease underlying the genesis of the arrhythmia. Therapy includes revascularization for patients with CAD, surgical techniques for the correction of valvular heart disease, and pacemaker implantation if necessary for patients with malignant bradyarrhythmias that may have triggered a tachyarrhythmic event.

Although other modalities are available, the ICD has become the keystone of primary therapy for patients after cardiac arrest. Several other modalities have been used in the past and, if nothing else, have historical interest. Each of these is reviewed briefly.

Arrhythmic Surgery

The first report of the surgical approach for therapy of ventricular arrhythmia was in 1959 by Couch, who resected a ventricular aneurysm in a patient with VT (145). During the 1970s, there were many reports about the use of coronary artery bypass grafting alone, with aneurysmectomy as a primary therapy for SCD (146). Unfortunately, the success rate of this approach was low. In the 1970s, there were reports of the utility of endocardial resection techniques for abolition of sustained VT that could be initiated in the electrophysiology laboratory and replicated in the operating room (147). Various techniques of resection were employed, including endo-

cardial mapping with resection of a circumscribed zone of endocardium versus encircling endocardial ventriculotomy, which isolated an aneurysm or area of infarcted myocardium electrically from the rest of the myocardium by a surgical incision made around the entire border of the scar. Unfortunately, surgical mortality for this procedure was significant, as was the chance of recurrence; these operations have largely been abandoned (148). The incidence of discrete aneurysm formation after acute MI appears to have been severely reduced with the advent of thrombolytic therapy and other methods of prompt coronary revascularization.

Catheter Ablation

Catheter ablation techniques have been employed with increasing frequency for the management of certain forms of ventricular tachyarrhythmia (149,150). Rarely do these idiopathic forms of VT lead to cardiac arrest. The applicability of catheter techniques for patients who have had cardiac arrest is limited, because successful ablation presumes a well-tolerated ventricular tachyarrhythmia that can be easily mapped and ablated in a catheterization laboratory; this is not the case for patients who have had unstable VT or for those with VF (Fig. 21-10). Nevertheless, the development of multisite mapping systems that may permit rapid localization at the site of activation of highly unstable VT may make this methodology more applicable (151,152). A principal limita-

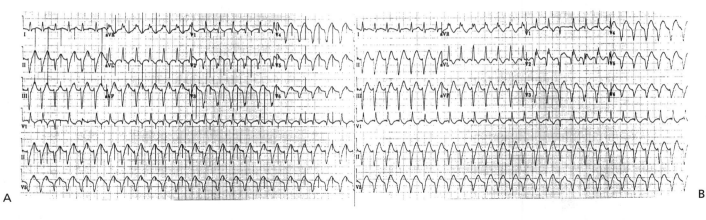

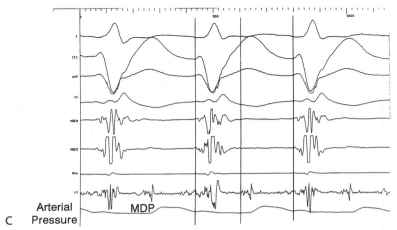

FIGURE 21-10. A: Example of ventricular mapping. Twelve-lead electrocardiogram of patient's clinical ventricular tachycardia (VT) induced in the electrophysiology laboratory. Notice the fusion beat (third beat in lead V$_1$). **B:** Pace map from the apical inferoseptal border of an anteroapical aneurysm. Notice the nearly identical morphology compared with the clinical arrhythmia. A stimulus to QRS latency of 180 ms is also apparent, suggesting that the mapping catheter was a recording from an area of slow conduction responsible for the VT. **C:** Surface and intracardiac electrograms during VT. Notice the low-amplitude, continuous, fractionated electrogram recorded from the left ventricular bipolar mapping catheter, with more discrete, broad electrograms in the body of the QRS. There is also a mid-diastolic potential (MDP) 185 ms before QRS onset. This is the same site at which pacing was carried out in **B.**

tion of this technique, especially in patients who have had a cardiac arrest, is that the disease process usually leading to cardiac arrest, which is most often an ischemic or nonischemic cardiomyopathy, is a progressive multisite disease that is likely to recur in another form or another location. This problem may be obviated by the ability to produce larger lesions. Currently, the use of catheter ablation techniques in patients with a history of cardiac arrest is limited to those who have already have an implanted device and continue to have episodes of VT that trigger frequent device activation and that can be adequately localized, mapped, and ablated (153). More widespread application of so-called hybrid therapy or adjuvant ablation therapy is not possible until the procedure is rendered safer with the use of better mapping techniques and catheter designs to deliver longer and larger linear lesions in strategic areas of the ventricle.

Implantable Defibrillator

The implantable defibrillator is a well-established and highly effective therapy for patients who have experienced SCD and is discussed in Chapter 11. Although the device does not prevent the arrhythmia, it reverses it automatically and promptly when it occurs. The device is indicated as a primary treatment modality for those who have experienced SCD because of sustained VT or VF. Failure of antecedent antiarrhythmic drug therapy is not a prerequisite for implantation of a defibrillator, and patients no longer need to be subjected to electrophysiologic testing to determine the inducibility of ventricular arrhythmia before a decision is made to implant the device. These developments are based on data from randomized clinical trials that have clearly shown the benefit of implantable defibrillators in cardiac arrest victims, especially those with low ejection fractions and in the absence of diseases that would otherwise limit longevity (134–138).

Several technologic advances since the first-generation devices have greatly facilitated the applicability of defibrillators to a progressively larger number of potential recipients. There is no longer a need for a thoracotomy for device implantation, because devices can be implanted transvenously and placed in an infraclavicular pocket, similar to the technique used for pacemaker implantation. This advance was facilitated by the development of transvenous leads, which could be placed in the endocardium with the ability to deliver adequate energy for defibrillation, and by the availability of progressively smaller devices that could be placed in a pectoral pocket (154–156). The ability to deliver adequate energy through a single lead was likewise facilitated by the development of biphasic waveforms, rather than the monophasic waveforms that were used with the original devices (105). The devices also make possible the storage of electrogram information, which allows adequate diagnosis of arrhythmias for which defibrillation shock therapy or pacing therapy is delivered (157).

Current-generation implantable defibrillators have the ability to deliver bradycardia pacing (158,159). This is a particularly important development in the SCD population, because malignant bradyarrhythmias may be the cause of cardiac arrest in a substantial number of patients. Bradycardia may occur as a primary event and may trigger a ventricular tachyarrhythmia; it may also occur after delivery of a high-energy shock, delaying patient recovery and perhaps leading to neurologic impairment. Pacing can be carried out in the ventricle or atrium with modern defibrillators. The preservation of atrioventricular synchrony has obvious hemodynamic advantage for patients with structural heart disease. The availability of atrial leads permits more precise detection algorithms to prevent the delivery of inappropriate shocks to patients with supraventricular arrhythmias that may overlap with VT detect zones, causing inappropriate device discharge (157). Modern devices can deliver *tiered therapy*. Patients who have a well-tolerated VT may undergo multiple attempts at ventricular burst pacing for arrhythmia determination before the delivery of uncomfortable cardioversion or defibrillation shocks (Fig. 21-11).

Despite technologic advances, devices still have several problems that will not likely be completely solved in the immediate future. These include complications from the lead system, such as infection, extrusion, erosion, lead or insulation fracture or failure, all of which can interfere with effective device function and may be associated with dire consequences (160–164). The generator itself may undergo random component failure or other complications, which interfere with detection or delivery of effec-

tive therapy or in rare cases lead to delivery of inappropriate therapy such as ultrarapid pacing or frequent device discharges. Defibrillation thresholds in the atrium and the ventricle are highly vulnerable to changes from drug use or metabolic derangements (165–167). Patients who have defibrillators have a change in lifestyle, such as the inability to drive or return to work (168,169), and may experience severe psychologic reactions to device discharge; many require extensive counseling (170–173). All of these potential difficulties with device therapy mandate comprehensive and expert testing of the device at the time of its implantation and on an ongoing basis, including comprehensive interrogation of the device and the lead system during office evaluation on a quarterly basis in addition to reevaluation of the defibrillation thresholds and the device's ability to terminate VF after arrhythmia initiation, perhaps annually. The ability of the device to induce ventricular tachyarrhythmias on demand makes such testing technically feasible and relatively well accepted by patients.

During the past several years, several completed randomized clinical trials have proven that the implantable defibrillator does have an overall mortality benefit in patients who have experienced a malignant tachyarrhythmia, including cardiac arrest (134–136) (Figs. 21-12 and 21-13). The magnitude of the benefit— a 20% to 30% reduction in the mortality rate—appears consistent across trials. It is not yet clear if we can define populations who may derive maximum benefit. We do know that the benefits of the device may be lost at the extremes of left ventricular function (137,138). For example, patients with CAD who experience a cardiac arrest have good left ventricular function (left ventricular ejection fraction >0.35) and are completely revascularized have a very low event rate, at which it is difficult to prove significant added benefit of an implantable device over therapy with an antiarrhythmic drug such as amiodarone (Fig. 21-14). In contrast, patients with very low ejection fractions (<20%) have a high mortality rate as a result of nonarrhythmic cardiac causes, especially heart failure, that offsets the benefit of the device, which would only be expected to reduce the incidence of sudden death in these patients. Completed clinical trials do not provide clear information about how adjuvant drug therapy may influence outcome, because a large number of patients in these trials crossed over from drug to device therapy. The completed trials were of relatively short duration and therefore do not answer the question about the long-term benefit of device therapy, especially given the potential for mechanical problems that may occur after several years of device use. Because several of the trials, such as the Antiarrhythmics Versus Implantable Defibrillator (AVID) study, were interrupted prematurely, there are no reliable cost-effectiveness data available to assess the benefit to society of implanting devices compared with the use of antiarrhythmic drugs in patients who have had a cardiac arrest.

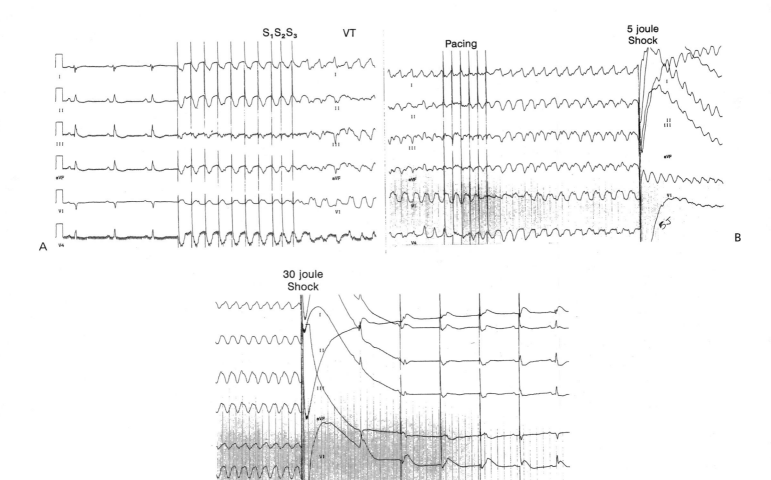

FIGURE 21-11. Tiered device therapy. **A:** Induction of a right bundle branch ventricular tachycardia (VT) with a train of eight paced beats (cycle length, 400 ms) with two premature extrastimuli (S_2-S_3) delivered noninvasively be means of a tiered implanted device. **B:** The VT is automatically sensed by the device, previously programmed to deliver a burst of ventricular pacing for an arrhythmia of this rate (zone 1). Because pacing does not terminate the arrhythmia, the device goes on to deliver zone 2 therapy, a 5-J synchronized shock that causes an accelerated and more disorganized arrhythmia. **C:** Although VT reorganizes spontaneously, the device recharged its capacitors to deliver zone 3 therapy, in this case a 30-J shock that converts VT to sinus rhythm. The device had also been programmed to temporarily deliver pacing therapy at a demand rate of approximately 50 bpm until the sinus mechanism recovered (last beat of tracing).

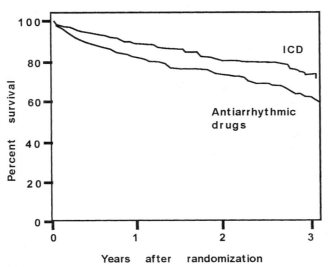

FIGURE 21-12. The Antiarrhythmics Versus Implantable Defibrillator trial randomized 1,016 patients with a history of ventricular fibrillation, ventricular tachycardia, or syncope thought to be caused by arrhythmia to an implantable cardioverter-defibrillator (ICD) or to antiarrhythmic therapy (sotalol or amiodarone). After a 3-year follow-up, survival was significantly better in the ICD group ($p < 0.02$), but the improvement in mean survival was only 2.6 months. (Adapted from The Antiarrhythmics Versus Implantable Defibrillator [AVID] Investigators. A comparison of antiarrhythmic-drug therapy with implantable defibrillators in patients resuscitated from near-fatal ventricular arrhythmias. *N Engl J Med* 1997;337:1576, with permission.)

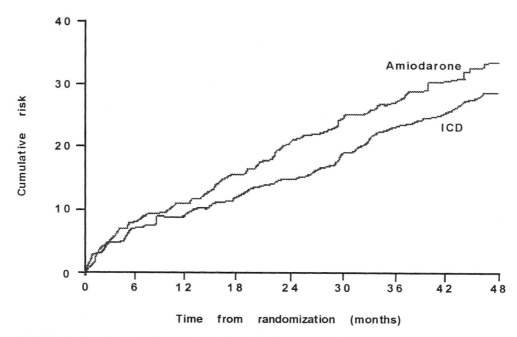

FIGURE 21-13. The Canadian Implantable Defibrillator Study (CIDS) randomized 659 patients with sustained ventricular tachyarrhythmia or syncope judged to be caused by an arrhythmia to an implantable cardioverter-defibrillator (ICD) or to amiodarone. After a 5-year follow-up, there was an insignificant reduction in total mortality with the ICD (8.3% versus 10.2% per year with amiodarone, *p* = 0.142). (Data from Connolly SJ, Gent M, Roberts RS, et al, for the CIDS Investigators. Canadian Implantable Defibrillator Study [CIDS]: a randomized trial of the implantable cardioverter defibrillator against amiodarone. *Circulation* 2000;101;1297, with permission.)

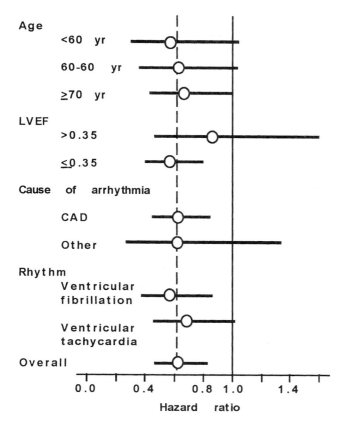

FIGURE 21-14. Antiarrhythmics Versus Implantable Defibrillator (AVID) subset analysis. Subset analysis of 1,013 survivors of sudden death or hemodynamically significant ventricular tachycardia entered into the AVID trial shows that the hazard ratios for death from any cause with the implantable cardioverter-defibrillator compared with amiodarone are not significantly different for any of the prespecified subgroups. (Adapted from The Antiarrhythmics Versus Implantable Defibrillator [AVID] Investigators. A comparison of antiarrhythmic-drug therapy with implantable defibrillators in patients resuscitated from near-fatal ventricular arrhythmias. *N Engl J Med* 1997;337:1576, with permission.)

Given the reduction in mortality and improvement in quality of life that have been ascribed to device therapy in these trials, it is unlikely that these issues will be important enough to interfere with recommendation that implantable devices are the mainstay of therapy for patients who have had resuscitated out-of-hospital arrest. However, longer-term trials of device therapy are important to understand nonmortality end points such as the need for hospitalization, psychologic well-being, and use, especially in patients who receive device therapy versus those who receive device and drug therapy in randomized trials.

PRIMARY PREVENTION OF SUDDEN CARDIAC DEATH IN THE GENERAL POPULATION

Administration of prompt and effective CPR, as well as other emergency medical interventions in the community, have substantially improved the prognosis of out-of-hospital cardiac arrest victims. Long-term survival of these patients, however, is still very poor. Although 30% to 50% of individuals with out-of-hospital SCD are admitted to a hospital alive, only one half of them survive to discharge (1,101,102).

These observations provide the rationale for attempts at primary prevention. This effort consists of accurate identification of potential victims and effective preventive interventions. Because many of the traditional risk factors associated with the development of CAD are also associated with SCD, clinical and public health efforts that promote the effective treatment of hypercholesterolemia and hypertension, a heart-healthy diet, regular exercise, smoking cessation, and moderation of alcohol consumption are likely to reduce the incidence of SCD (174). However, screening of asymptomatic patients with 12-lead electrocardiography, exercise stress testing, Holter monitoring, or echocardiography to identify those at high risk for SCD is not recommended, in part because of the limited sensitivity of the tests and the low incidence of SCD in the community (Fig. 21-15).

Efforts to identify persons in the general population who are at high risk for SCD can be justified only if the applied

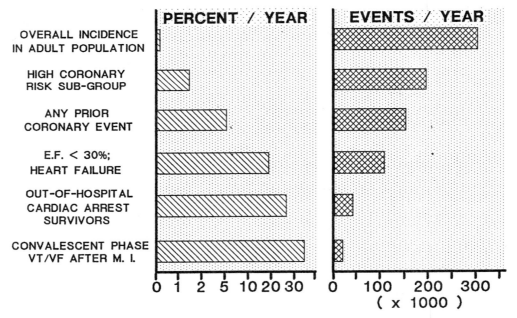

FIGURE 21-15. The relationship between annual incidence and total number of sudden cardiac deaths (SCDs) among population subgroups. Approximation of incidence figures (percentage per year) and the total number of events per year is shown for the overall adult population in the United States and for increasingly higher-risk subgroups. The overall adult population has an estimated sudden death incidence of 0.1% to 0.2% per year. Within subgroups identified by increasingly powerful risk factors, the incidence increases progressively but is accompanied by a progressive decrease in the total number of events. There is an inverse relationship between incidence and total number of events because of the progressively smaller denominator pool in the highest-risk subgroup categories. Successful interventions among larger population subgroups will require specific markers to identify higher-risk clusters within the lower-risk subgroups. The horizontal axis for the incidence figures is nonlinear and should be interpreted accordingly. E.F., ejection fraction; M.I., myocardial infarction; VT/VF, ventricular tachycardia/ventricular fibrillation. (From Myerburg RJ, Kessler KM, Castellanos A. Sudden cardiac death: structure, function, and time-dependence of risk. *Circulation* 1992;85[Suppl 1–2]:1–10, with permission.)

measures prevent fatal outcomes. A major criticism in the past was the lack of valid evidence that intervention trials aimed at controlling standard risk factors reduced the incidence of coronary heart disease, including SCD, and lowered total mortality rates.

Several published trials suggest that intervention to reduce risk factors can reduce the incidence of SCD and coronary mortality. As an example, a multifactorial, controlled, randomized trial from the Belgian component of the World Health Organization evaluated the effect of efforts aimed at reducing serum cholesterol by dietary changes, increasing physical activity, and controlling smoking, hypertension, and weight (in those who were overweight) on risk factors and mortality (175). Compared with the control group, the intervention group had significant reductions in the incidence of coronary heart disease and coronary mortality. The difference in mortality was most pronounced in the first 6 years of the study.

A basic problem in the application of these studies to sudden death is that most interventions do not directly affect the transient pathophysiologic event that initiates potentially fatal arrhythmias. Instead, they attempt to alter and prevent underlying disease. Current epidemiologic efforts to decrease the incidence of lethal arrhythmias are limited by the inability to clearly identify the transient factors responsible for the initiation of sudden death.

Lipid Lowering

Reduction of high blood cholesterol with a 3-hydroxy-3-methylglutaryl coenzyme A (HMG CoA) reductase inhibitor reduces CAD mortality (176). However, lipid-lowering trials have not reported the effects of treatment on SCD. Nevertheless, given the proportion of CAD mortality that results from SCD, particularly among middle-aged persons, it is likely that the primary prevention of CAD through the reduction of high levels of low-density lipoprotein (LDL) cholesterol also will reduce the risk of SCD.

The dietary intake of long-chain n-3 polyunsaturated fatty acids (i.e., eicosapentaenoic acid and docosahexaenoic acid) from fish is associated a reduction in LDL-cholesterol and a reduced risk of SCD, possibly by reducing vulnerability to life-threatening cardiac arrhythmia (177). The consumption of one to two fish meals per week, the equivalent of 3 ounces of salmon or 6 ounces of albacore tuna per week, is associated with a 50% reduction in the risk of SCD after taking into account potential confounding factors (177). However, there is little evidence that the intake of more than one to two servings of fish per week is better than the intake of modest amounts of fish. Similarly, the benefit and risk of pharmacologic doses of n-3 fatty acids found in fish-oil supplements (approximately 10 to 20 times the nutritional dose from fish) on the risk of SCD remains unclear.

Antihypertensive Therapy

Treatment of hypertension with low-dose thiazide diuretics reduces the incidence of SCD, particularly when potential toxic effects of drug therapy are minimized. Unexpected findings from the Multiple Risk Factor Intervention Trial and the results of early meta-analyses raised concerns about a potential adverse effect of high-dose thiazide diuretic therapy on the risk of SCD. However, the results of an observational study and a meta-analysis of clinical trials that used low-dose thiazide diuretic therapy suggest that the treatment of hypertension with currently recommended doses of thiazide diuretics (12.5 mg and 25 mg hydrochlorthiazide), with appropriate attention to potential adverse metabolic effects, particularly hypokalemia, is likely to reduce the risk of CAD mortality and SCD (178,179).

There is no evidence that other antihypertensive agents, including β-adrenergic blockers, dihydropyridine or nondihydropyridine calcium channel blockers, ACE inhibitors, or α-adrenergic blockers are superior or even equivalent to low-dose thiazide diuretic therapy in reducing CAD mortality or SCD in hypertensive patients with left ventricular hypertrophy. However, β blockers and the ACE inhibitors do reduce overall and sudden death mortality in patients with recent MI and those with congestive heart failure (180–184). Spironolactone reduces overall mortality by 36% and SCD mortality by 29% in patients with heart failure (185). The improvement in mortality rates was seen in all patient subsets, including those with an ischemic or nonischemic cause for congestive heart failure.

Lifestyle Modification

Several lifestyle modifications can reduce the incidence of CAD and hence SCD. Clinical trials of smoking cessation have not focused on major disease outcomes, in part because intervention and follow-up of large populations for long periods are needed to assess an effect. Nevertheless, based on the observations that the risk of SCD is particularly high among current smokers and declines rapidly after stopping smoking, smoking cessation should be viewed as an important component of efforts to reduce the risk of SCD.

There are no data from long-term exercise intervention trials among apparently healthy persons that focus on major disease end points. Nevertheless, regular exercise should be encouraged for the primary prevention of CAD and SCD, because the cardiac benefits of regular exercise outweigh the transient increase in risk during strenuous exercise (186).

Patients should be advised to pay appropriate attention to potential symptoms of CAD, even if they have engaged in regular exercise without limitations for an extended period. Patients with known heart disease should be encouraged to engage in regular exercise in a supervised setting, such as a cardiac rehabilitation program.

It also is reasonable to recommend moderation of alcohol intake (e.g., no more than one to two drinks per day, avoidance of binge drinking). As an example, a report from the Physicians Health Study evaluated 21,537 men who provided information on their alcohol intake and were also free of cardiovascular disease (187). Compared with men who rarely or never drank, those who had two to four drinks per week or five to six drinks per week had a significantly reduced risk for sudden death (relative risks of 0.40 and 0.21, respectively); the risk approached unity at two drinks per day. Heavy alcohol consumption (six or more drinks per day) or binge drinking increases the risk for sudden death (188).

Modest dietary intake of long-chain n-3 polyunsaturated fatty acids from fish may reduce vulnerability to life-threatening ventricular arrhythmia in the setting of potential triggers. However, additional clinical trial data are needed to confirm the potential protective effect of modest intake of long-chain n-3 polyunsaturated fatty acids on the risk of SCD.

Epidemiologic studies suggest a positive association between average dietary intake of saturated fat in the population and the population rates of SCD. However, it is not known if reduction of dietary intake of saturated fatty acids reduces the vulnerability to VF. Nevertheless, given available experimental evidence in animals and other benefits of reducing saturated fat intake, the reduction of saturated fatty acids also seems prudent.

Few studies have specifically assessed the risk of SCD related to caffeine consumption. However, moderation of caffeine intake (i.e., consumption of fewer than five cups of coffee per day) seems appropriate (189).

Family History of Sudden Death

A family history of MI and SCD is associated with a 1.5-fold increased risk of SCD, but the increase in risk is not explained by traditional risk factors that tend to aggregate in families such as hypercholesterolemia, hypertension, diabetes mellitus, and obesity (190). The magnitude of the increased risk associated with a family history is modest compared with the twofold to fivefold increased risk associated with other modifiable risk factors such as physical inactivity and current cigarette smoking. Few studies have examined potential gene-environment interactions related to the risk of SCD. Nevertheless, it is likely that interactions of genetic factors (i.e., mutations in specific genes) and environmental factors influence this risk.

PRIMARY PREVENTION OF SUDDEN DEATH IN PATIENTS WITH HEART DISEASE

Much attention is given to the management of the patient resuscitated from SCD; however, a superior but more difficult strategy is to first identify those patients with heart disease who are at risk for sudden death but in whom such an event has not yet occurred and then attempt to prevent the potentially fatal initial arrhythmia (191). Several primary prevention trials have evaluated the role of therapeutic interventions in the prevention of sudden death among high-risk patients (192). Different populations have been examined, including patients with a history of MI, congestive heart failure, cardiomyopathy, ventricular ectopy, or a combination of these disorders.

Antiarrhythmic Agents after Myocardial Infarction

Prophylactic therapy with β blockers is an effective therapy for preventing overall and sudden death mortality in post–MI patients (184,193). However, several antiarrhythmic drug trials in postinfarction patients have reported an increase in mortality in patients treated with drugs such as encainide, flecainide, or d-sotalol (184,194,195). One exception may be amiodarone, which has been evaluated in two large trials, the European Myocardial Infarction Amiodarone Trial (EMIAT), which evaluated survivors of MI who had a left ventricular ejection fraction of 0.40 or less (Fig. 21-16), and the Canadian Myocardial Infarction Amiodarone Trial (CAMIAT), which evaluated survivors of MI who had frequent or repetitive ventricular premature depolarizations (196,197) (Fig. 21-17). In both reports, the administration of amiodarone was associated with a reduction in sudden death mortality, but there was no significant change in overall and cardiac mortality rates. However, subset analysis of patients in EMIAT showed that amiodarone reduced total mortality rates for patients with an ejection fraction of less than 0.30, with arrhythmia identified on initial Holter monitoring, or with concurrent β-blocker therapy (198). It also reduced mortality rates for patients with absent heart rate variability (199). In contrast, there was a trend toward an increase in total mortality in patients without these features.

Two meta-analyses of trials of postinfarction patients showed that, compared with usual care, amiodarone reduced the total mortality rate by 13% to 19% and sudden death mortality rate by 29% to 30% (200,201) (Fig. 21-18).

Amiodarone in Congestive Heart Failure

In general class I and III antiarrhythmic agents are ineffective and potentially hazardous in patients with heart failure. Several studies have shown that β blockers are effective in these patients and they improve survival rates and reduce the incidence of SCD (180,181).

The role of amiodarone in patients with cardiomyopathy, congestive heart failure, and frequent ventricular arrhythmias is uncertain. Two large trials, Congestive Heart Failure–Survival Trial of Antiarrhythmic Therapy (CHF-STAT) and Grupo de Estudio de la Sobrevida en la Insuficencia Cardiaca en Argentina (GESICA) trial, appeared to produce conflicting results (202,203) (Figs. 21-19 and Fig. 21-20). However, both trials suggested that amiodarone might reduce mortality in patients with nonischemic cardiomyopathy.

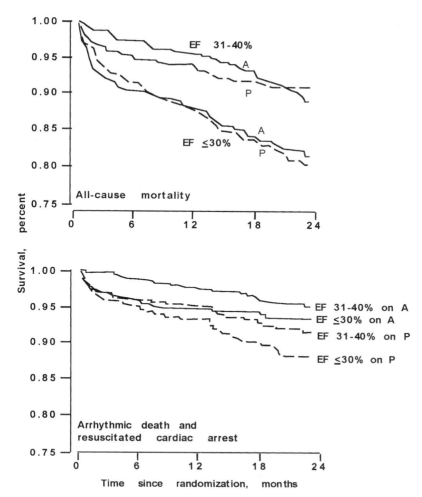

FIGURE 21-16. The effect of amiodarone in 1,486 postmyocardial patients who were randomized to amiodarone (A) or placebo (P) in the European Myocardial Infarction Amiodarone Trial (EMIAT). When analyzed by baseline ejection fraction (EF), amiodarone had no effect on all-cause mortality *(top)*, but reduced the incidence of arrhythmic death or resuscitated cardiac arrest *(bottom)*. The benefit was greatest for patients with an ejection fraction of less than 0.30 *(dashed lines)*. (Adapted from Julian DG, Camm AJ, Frangin G, et al. Randomised trial of effect of amiodarone on mortality in patients with left-ventricular dysfunction after recent myocardial infarction: EMIAT. *Lancet* 1997;349:667, with permission.)

Two meta-analyses of trials of postinfarction patients have shown that, compared with usual care, amiodarone reduced total mortality by 13% to 22% and sudden death mortality by 23% to 29% (200,201) (Fig. 21-18).

Use of Implantable Cardioverter-Defibrillators in High-Risk Patients

An alternative therapy to antiarrhythmic agents in the patient at risk for SCD is the ICD. Three trials have evaluated the prophylactic use this modality.

Multicenter Automatic Defibrillator Trial

The Multicenter Automatic Defibrillator Trial (MADIT) enrolled 196 patients with a prior MI, nonsustained ventricular tachycardia (NSVT), left ventricular dysfunction (ejection fraction <0.35), a positive signal-averaged ECG, and inducible sustained monomorphic VT that was unresponsive to intravenous procainamide. These patients were randomized to pharmacologic therapy or an ICD (204).

The major findings at 27-month follow-up were significant reductions in the incidence of overall mortality, cardiac mortality, and arrhythmic deaths in the patients treated with an ICD (Fig. 21-21). The average survival for the ICD group over a 4-year period was 3.7 years, compared with 2.8 years for the conventionally treated patients; the incremental cost effectiveness ratio was $27,000 per life-year saved (205).

Several important limitations to this study, in addition to its small size, limit its applicability. First, by enrolling only patients in whom inducible sustained VT was not suppressed or slowed by the administration of procainamide, the study selected patients who were less likely to respond to antiarrhythmic drugs. Second, two factors other than true benefit may have contributed to the better outcome in the ICD group. Twenty-three percent of patients receiving conventional therapy were not taking any antiarrhythmic drugs at the last follow-up, and more patients given the ICD were taking a β blocker at 1 month (8% versus 26%) and at the last follow-up visit (5% versus 27%). It is possible that β blockade itself confers a survival benefit. Third,

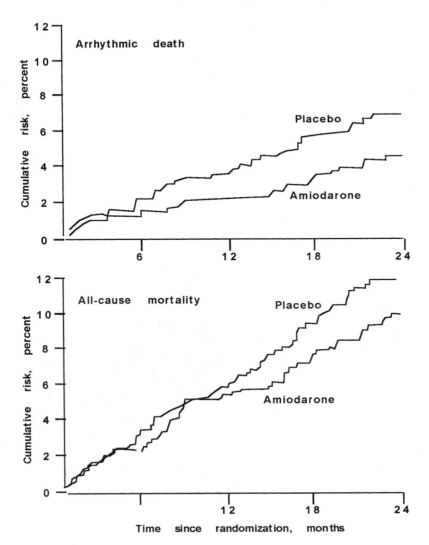

FIGURE 21-17. Effect of amiodarone versus placebo in 1202 postmyocardial infarction patients with ventricular ectopy in the Canadian Myocardial Infarction Amiodarone Trial (CAMIAT). By an intention to treat analysis, amiodarone produced a significant reduction in arrhythmic death (*top*, $p = 0.016$) but no change in all-cause mortality *(bottom)*. (Adapted from Cairns JA, Connolly SJ, Roberts R, et al. Randomised trial of outcome after myocardial infarction in patients with frequent or repetitive ventricular premature depolarisations: CAMIAT. *Lancet* 1997;349: 675, with permission.)

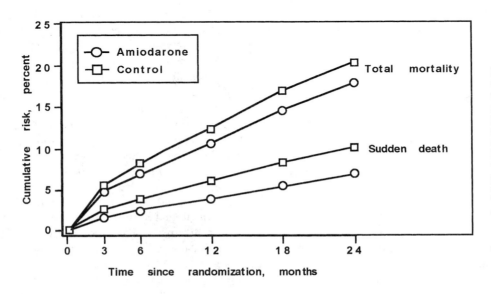

FIGURE 21-18. A meta-analysis of randomized trials involving 6,553 patients with congestive heart failure or a recent myocardial infarction shows that, compared with placebo or usual care, amiodarone reduced total mortality by 13% ($p = 0.03$) and sudden death mortality by 29% ($p = 0.0003$). There was no difference in treatment effect between postinfarction or congestive heart failure trials. (Adapted from Amiodarone Trials Meta-analysis Investigators. Effect of prophylactic amiodarone on mortality after acute myocardial infarction and in congestive heart failure: meta-analysis of individual data from 6500 patients in randomized trials. *Lancet* 1997;350: 1417, with permission.)

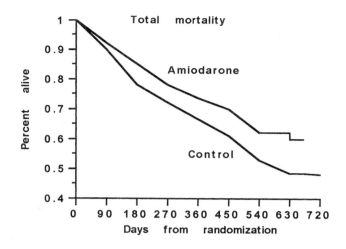

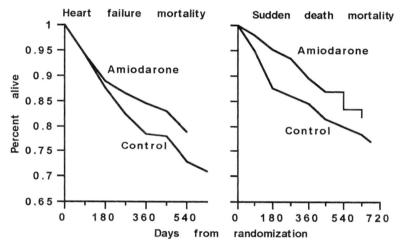

FIGURE 21-19. Kaplan-Meier curves for total mortality *(top)*, death from progressive heart failure *(left)*, or sudden death *(right)* in the GESICA trial. Patients with congestive heart failure and episodes of nonsustained ventricular tachycardia (NSVT) on ambulatory monitoring were randomized to therapy with amiodarone or placebo. All outcomes were improved in the amiodarone group. (Adapted from Doval HC, Nul DR, Grancelli HO, et al. Randomised trial of low dose amiodarone in severe congestive heart failure. *Lancet* 1994;344:493, with permission.)

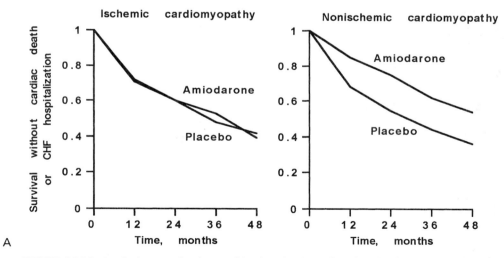

FIGURE 21-20. Survival curves for the combined end points of cardiac death and hospitalization due to heart failure in patients in the Congestive Heart Failure–Survival Trial of Antiarrhythmic Therapy (CHF-STAT) trial with congestive heart failure and more than 10 ventricular premature beats per hour. The data are presented separately for those with an ischemic **(A)** or nonischemic **(B)** cause for the cardiomyopathy. There was a 46% reduction in events in the nonischemic group but no difference in patients with an ischemic cause. (Adapted from Massie BM, Fisher SG, Radford M, et al. Effect of amiodarone on clinical status and left ventricular functon in patients with congestive heart failure. CHF-STAT Investigators. *Circulation* 1996;93(12):2128–2134, with permission.)

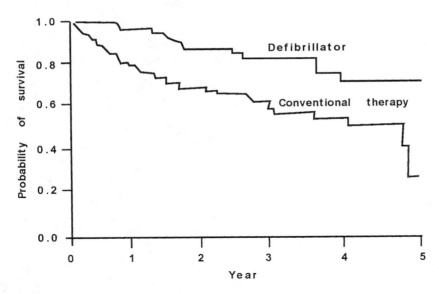

FIGURE 21-21. Kaplan-Meier cumulative survival curves for the Multicenter Automatic Defibrillator Trial (MADIT) show that selected high-risk patients (i.e., prior infarction, left ventricular ejection fraction < 0.35, nonsustained ventricular tachyarrhythmia not suppressible with procainamide) have a better survival rate with an implantable defibrillator than with conventional therapy with antiarrhythmic drugs (p = 0.009). (Adapted from Moss AJ, Hall WJ, Cannom DS, et al, for the Multicenter Automatic Defibrillator Implantation Trial Investigators. Improved survival with an implanted defibrillator in patients with coronary disease at high risk for ventricular arrhythmia. *N Engl J Med* 1996; 335;1933, with permission.)

by comparing the ICD to antiarrhythmic drugs that may increase mortality through their proarrhythmic effect, it was not demonstrated that the ICD was better than no therapy. However, the mortality rate in the "conventional therapy" group was 32% at 2 years, a value that is in accord with previously reported results for high-risk patients. Amiodarone did not appear to confer an increased mortality in this trial, and the results probably reflected a survival benefit of the ICD.

Based on the results of MADIT, the U.S. Food and Drug Administration approved the prophylactic use of the automatic defibrillator in patients who meet the entry criteria for MADIT. However, it remains unclear how many patients with a recent MI would be candidates for a prophylactic ICD based on MADIT criteria; data from the CAST suggest that between 0.3% and 1.1% of patients are at high enough risk to benefit from a prophylactic ICD (206).

Coronary Artery Bypass Graft Patch Trial

The Coronary Artery Bypass Graft (CABG) Patch trial evaluated the efficacy of the ICD for reducing overall mortality in 900 patients undergoing surgical revascularization for severe CAD who had significant left ventricular dysfunction (ejection fraction <0.36) and a positive signal-averaged ECG (207). Enrolled patients did not have a history of a sustained ventricular tachyarrhythmia or syncope. After an average follow-up of 32 months, there were 71 cardiac deaths in the defibrillator group and 72 cardiac deaths in the control group (Fig. 21-22). There have been no reported differences in outcome for different subsets of patients.

Prophylactic therapy with the ICD did reduce arrhythmic death at 42 months by 45% (4% versus 6.9% in the control group) (208). However, because 71% of the deaths

in this trial were nonarrhythmic, this reduction did not impact total mortality.

Multicenter Unsustained Tachycardia Trial

The Multicenter Unsustained Tachycardia Trial (MUSTT) involved 704 patients with coronary disease, asymptomatic NSVT, a left ventricular ejection fraction of 0.40, and inducible sustained VT (209). Patients were randomized to no therapy or electrophysiologically guided antiarrhythmic

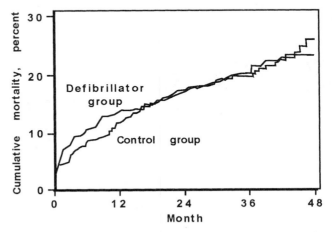

FIGURE 21-22. The Coronary Artery Bypass Graft (CABG) Patch trial randomized 900 patients with a low ejection fraction and a positive signal-averaged electrocardiogram to an implantable cardioverter-defibrillator or to no defibrillator after CABG surgery. There was no difference in mortality at a mean follow-up of 32 months. (Adapted from Bigger JT, for the Coronary Artery Bypass Graft [CABG] Patch Trial Investigators. Prophylactic use of implanted cardiac defibrillators in patients at high risk for ventricular arrhythmias after coronary artery bypass graft surgery. *N Engl J Med* 1997;337:1569, with permission.)

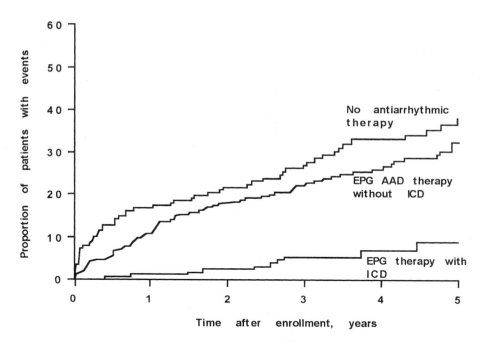

FIGURE 21-23. The Multicenter Unsustained Tachycardia Trial (MUSTT) enrolled 704 patients with coronary artery disease, nonsustained ventricular tachycardia (VT), and a left ventricular ejection fraction of less than 0.40 who had sustained VT induced during electrophysiologic (EP) study. Kaplan-Meier estimates show that the incidence of cardiac arrest or death from arrhythmia is significantly lower for those receiving an implantable cardioverter-defibrillator (ICD) compared with those receiving no therapy or those with EP-guided (EPG) antiarrhythmic drug (AAD) therapy (9% versus 32% and 25%, respectively; *p* < 0.001 for both ICD versus EP guided AAD without ICD and for ICD versus no antiarrhythmic therapy). (Data from Buxton AE, Lee KL, Fisher JD, et al, for the Multicenter Unsustained Tachycardia Trial Investigators. A randomized study of the prevention of sudden death in patients with coronary artery disease. *N Engl J Med* 1999;341:1882, with permission.)

therapy that included an antiarrhythmic agent (i.e., class Ia with or without mexiletine, propafenone, sotalol, or amiodarone) or an ICD if at least one antiarrhythmic agent was ineffective. The primary end point was arrhythmic death or resuscitated cardiac arrest.

There were 353 patients discharged with no therapy and 351 who received electrophysiologically guided therapy, including an antiarrhythmic drug in 154 and an ICD in 161; the median follow-up was 39 months. The 2-year (12% versus 18%) and 5-year (25% versus 32%, *p* = 0.04) event rates for the primary end point (arrhythmic death or resuscitated cardiac arrest) were lower for electrophysiologically guided therapy compared with no therapy. The secondary end point of total mortality was also lower at 5 years in the group receiving electrophysiologically guided therapy (42% versus 48%).

The reduction in the primary and secondary end points in the electrophysiologically guided group was largely attributable to ICD therapy; at 5 years, the primary end point occurred for 9% of those receiving an ICD, compared with 37% of those receiving an antiarrhythmic drug, and the secondary end point occurred for 24% and 55%, respectively. There was no difference in outcome between patients receiving no therapy and those treated with an antiarrhythmic drug (Fig. 21-23).

REFERENCES

1. Lown B, Wolf M. Approaches to sudden death from coronary heart disease. *Circulation* 1971;44:130–142.
2. Goldstein S. The necessity of a uniform definition of sudden cardiac death: witnessed death within one hour of the onset of acute symptoms. *Am Heart J* 1982;103:156–159.
3. Epstein SE, Quyyumi AA, Bonow RO. Sudden cardiac death without warning: possible mechanisms and implications for screening asymptomatic populations. *N Engl J Med* 1989;321:320–324.
4. Kannel WB, Schatzkin A. Sudden death: lessons for subsets in population studies. *J Am Coll Cardiol* 1985;5[Suppl 6]:141B–149B.
5. WHO Scientific Group Report. Sudden cardiac death. *World Health Organ Tech Rep Ser* 1985:726.
6. Myerburg RJ, Kessler KM, Kimura S, Castellanos A. Sudden cardiac death: future approaches based on identification and control of transient risk factors. *J Cardiovasc Electrophysiol* 1992;3:626–640.
7. Bayes de Luna A, Coumel P, Leclercq JF. Ambulatory sudden cardiac death: mechanisms of production of fatal arrhythmia on the basis of data from 157 cases. *Am Heart J* 1989;117:151–159.
8. Dubner SJ, Pinski S, Palma S, et al. Ambulatory electrocardiographic findings in out-of-hospital cardiac arrest secondary to coronary artery disease. *Am J Cardiol* 1989;64:801–806.
9. Kempf FC, Josephson ME. Cardiac arrest recorded on ambulatory electrocardiograms. *Am J Cardiol* 1984;53:1577–1582.
10. Weaver WD, Hill D, Fahrenbruch CE, et al. Use of the automatic external defibrillator in the management of out-of-hospital cardiac arrest. *N Engl J Med* 1988;319:661–666.
11. Luu M, Stevenson WG, Stevenson LW, et al. Diverse mechanisms of unexpected cardiac arrest in advanced heart failure. *Circulation* 1989;80:1675–1680.
12. Kuo CS, Munakata K, Reddy P, Surawicz B. Characteristics and possible mechanism of ventricular arrhythmia dependent on the dispersion of action potential durations. *Circulation* 1983;67:1356.
13. Mandapati R, Asano Y, Baxter WT, et al. Quantification of effects of global ischemia on dynamics of ventricular fibrillation in isolated rabbit heart. *Circulation* 1998;98:1688.
14. Kuo CS, Amlie JP, Munakata K, et al. Dispersions of monophasic action potential durations and activation times during atrial pacing, ventricular pacing and ventricular premature stimulation in canine ventricles. *Cardiovasc Res* 1983;17:152.
15. Cummins RO, Ornato JP, Thies WH, Pepe PE. Improving sur-

vival from sudden cardiac arrest: the "chain of survival" concept. *Circulation* 1991;83:1832.

16. Tofler GH, Stone PH, Muller JE, et al. Prognosis after cardiac arrest due to ventricular tachycardia or VF associated with acute myocardial infarction (the MILIS Study). *Am J Cardiol* 1987; 60:755–761.

17. Goldberg RJ, Gore JM, Haffajee CI, et al. Outcome after cardiac arrest during acute myocardial infarction. *Am J Cardiol* 1987;59:251–255.

18. Stevenson WG, Wiener I, Yeatman L, et al. Complicated atherosclerotic lesions: a potential cause of ischemic ventricular arrhythmias in cardiac arrest survivors who do not have inducible ventricular tachycardia. *Am Heart J* 1988;116:1–6.

19. Spaulding CM, Joly LM, Rosenberg A, et al. Immediate coronary angiography in survivors of out-of-hospital cardiac arrest. *N Engl J Med* 1997;336:1629.

20. Burke AP, Farb A, Malcom GT, et al. Coronary risk factors and plaque morphology in men with coronary disease who die suddenly. *N Engl J Med* 1997;336:1276.

21. Burke AP, Farb A, Malcom GT, et al. Effect of risk factors on the mechanism of acute thrombosis and sudden coronary death in women. *Circulation* 1998;97:2110.

22. Burke AP, Farb A, Malcom GT, et al. Plaque rupture and sudden death related to exertion in men with coronary artery disease. *JAMA* 1999;281:921.

23. Kannel WB, Wilson PWF, D'Agostino RB, et al. Sudden coronary death in women. *Am Heart J* 1998;136:205.

24. Burke AP, Fard A, Liang YH, et al. Effect of hypertension and cardiac hypertrophy on coronary artery morphology in sudden cardiac death. *Circulation* 1996;94:3138.

25. Viskin S, Belhassen B. Idiopathic ventricular fibrillation. *Am Heart J* 1990;120:661.

26. Drory Y, Turetz Y, Hiss Y, et al. Sudden unexpected death in persons less than 40 years of age. *Am J Cardiol* 1991;68:1388.

27. Topaz O, Edwards JE. Pathologic features of sudden death in children, adolescents and young adults. *Chest* 1985;87:476.

28. Neuspiel DR, Kuller LH. Sudden unexpected cardiac death in childhood and adolescence. *JAMA* 1985;254:1321.

29. Wever RF, Hauer RNW, Oomen A, et al. Unfavorable outcome in patients with primary electrical disease who survived an episode of ventricular fibrillation. *Circulation* 1993;88:1021.

30. Brugada P, Brugada J. Right bundle branch block, persistent ST segment elevation and sudden cardiac death: a distinct clinical and electrocardiographic syndrome. *J Am Coll Cardiol* 1992;20:1391.

31. Alings M, Wilde A. "Brugada" syndrome: clinical data and suggested pathophysiologic mechanism. *Circulation* 1999;99:666.

32. Gussak I, Antzelevitch C, Bjerregaard P, et al. The Brugada syndrome: clinical, electrophysiologic and genetic aspects. *J Am Coll Cardiol* 1999;33:5.

33. Matsuo K, Kurita M, Inagaki M, et al. The circadian pattern to the development of ventricular fibrillation in patients with Brugada syndrome. *Eur Heart J* 1999;20:465.

34. Chen Q, Kirsch GE, Zhang D, et al. Genetic basis and molecular mechanisms for idiopathic ventricular fibrillation. *Nature* 1998;392:293.

35. Maron BJ, Poliac LC, Kaplan JA, et al. Blunt impact to the chest leading to sudden death from cardiac arrest during sports activities. *N Engl J Med* 1995;333:337.

36. Link MS, Wang PJ, Pandian NG, et al. An experimental model of sudden death due to low-energy chest-wall impact (commotio cordis). *N Engl J Med* 1998;338:1805.

37. Friedlander Y, Siscovick DS, Weinmann S, et al. Family history as a risk factor for primary cardiac arrest. *Circulation* 1998;97:155.

38. Siscovick DS, Raghunathan TE, Psaty BM, et al. Clinically

silent electrocardiographic abnormalities and the risk of primary cardiac arrest among hypertensive patients. *Circulation* 1996;94:1329.

39. Grace AA, Chien KR. Congenital long QT syndromes: toward molecular dissection of arrhythmia substrates. *Circulation* 1995; 92:2786.

40. Compton SJ, Lux RL, Ramsey MR, et al. Genetically defined therapy of inherited long QT-syndrome: correction of abnormal repolarization by potassium. *Circulation* 1996;94:1018.

41. Siscovick DS, Weiss NS, Hallstrom AP, et al. Physical activity and primary cardiac arrest. *JAMA* 1982;248:3113.

42. Friedlander Y, Siscovick DS, Weinmann S, et al. Family history as a risk factor for primary cardiac arrest. *Circulation* 1998;97:155.

43. Siscovick DS, Weiss NS, Fletcher RH, Lasky T. The incidence of primary cardiac arrest during vigorous exercise. *N Engl J Med* 1984;311:874.

44. Jouven X, Desnos M, Guerot C, Ducimetiere P. Predicting sudden death in the population: the Paris Prospective Study I. *Circulation* 1999;99:1978.

45. Kannel WB, Thomas HE Jr. Sudden coronary death: the Framingham Study. *Ann N Y Acad Sci* 1982;382:3.

46. Wannamethee G, Shaper AG. Alcohol and sudden cardiac death. *Br Heart J* 1992;68:443.

47. Gillum RF. Coronary artery disease in black populations: mortality and morbidity. *Am Heart J* 1982;104:839–845.

48. Williams RA. Sudden cardiac death in blacks, including black athletes. *Cardiovasc Clin* 1991;21:297–320.

49. Hagstrom RM, Federspiel CF, Ho YC. Incidence of myocardial infarction and sudden cardiac death from coronary heart disease in Nashville, Tennessee. *Circulation* 1971;44:884–889.

50. Keil JE, Loadholt CB, Winrich MC, et al. Incidence of coronary heart disease in blacks in Charleston, South Carolina. *Am Heart J* 1984;108:79–81.

51. Kuller L, Cooper M, Perper J, et al. Myocardial infarction and sudden death in an urban community. *Bull NY Acad Med* 1973; 49:532–556.

52. Weinmann S, Siscovick DS, Raghunathan TE, et al. Caffeine intake in relation to the risk of primary cardiac arrest. *Epidemiology* 1997;8:505.

53. Roden DM. Taking the "idio" out of "idiosyncratic": predicting torsades de pointes. *Pacing Clin Electrophysiol* 1998;21:1029.

54. Siscovick DS, Raghunathan TE, Psaty BM, et al. Diuretic therapy for hypertension and risk of primary cardiac arrest. *N Engl J Med* 1994;330:1852.

55. Hoes AW, Grobbee DE, Lubsen J, et al. Diuretics, beta blockers and the risk for sudden cardiac death in hypertensive patients. *Ann Intern Med* 1995;123:481.

56. Gettes LS. Electrolyte abnormalities underlying lethal and ventricular arrhythmias. *Circulation* 1992;85[Suppl I]:I-70.

57. Stevenson WG, Middlekauff HR, Stevenson LW, et al. Significance of aborted cardiac arrest and sustained ventricular tachycardia in patients referred for treatment therapy of advanced heart failure. *Am Heart J* 1992;124:123.

58. Kelly P, Ruskin JN, Vlahakes GJ, et al. Surgical coronary revascularization in survivors of prehospital cardiac arrest: its effect on inducible ventricular arrhythmias and long-term survival. *J Am Coll Cardiol* 1990;15:267.

59. Spaulding CM, Joly LM, Rosenberg A, et al. Immediate coronary angiography in survivors of out-of-hospital cardiac arrest. *N Engl J Med* 1997;336:1629.

60. Natale A, Sra J, Axtell K, et al. Ventricular fibrillation and polymorphic ventricular tachycardia with critical coronary artery stenosis: does bypass surgery suffice? *J Cardiovasc Electrophysiol* 1994;5:988.

61. Velebit V, Podrid PJ, Lown B, et al. Aggravation and provoca-

tion of ventricular arrhythmia by antiarrhythmic drugs. *Circulation* 1982;65:886.

62. Ruskin JN, McGovern B, Garan H, et al. Antiarrhythmic drugs: a possible cause of out-of-hospital cardiac arrest. *N Engl J Med* 1983;309:1302.

63. Echt DS, Liebson PR, Mitchell LB, et al. Mortality and morbidity in patients receiving encainide, flecainide, or placebo: the Cardiac Arrhythmia Suppression Trial. *N Engl J Med* 1991;324:781.

64. Baker GC, Blackshear JL, McBride R, et al. Antiarrhythmic therapy and cardiac mortality in atrial fibrillation: the Stroke Prevention in Atrial Fibrillation Investigators. *J Am Coll Cardiol* 1992;20:527

65. Kloner RA, Hale S, Alker K, et al. Effects of acute and chronic cocaine use on the heart. *Circulation* 1992;85:407.

66. Bauman JL, Grawe JJ, Winecoff AP, et al. Cocaine-related sudden cardiac death: a hypothesis correlating basic science and clinical observations. *J Clin Pharmacol* 1994;34:902.

67. Priori SG, Napolitano C, Schwartz PJ. Low penetrance in the long-QT syndrome: clinical impact. *Circulation* 1999;99:529.

68. Vincent GM, Timothy KM, Leppert M, et al. The spectrum of symptoms and QT intervals in carriers of the gene for long QT syndrome. *N Engl J Med* 1992;327:846.

69. Donger C, Denjoy I, Berhet M, et al. KVLQT1 C-terminal missense mutation causes a forme fruste long-QT syndrome. *Circulation* 1997;96:2778.

70. Siscovick DS, Weiss NS, Fletcher RH, Lasky T. The incidence of primary cardiac arrest during vigorous exercise. *N Engl J Med* 1984;311:874.

71. Trichopoulos D, Katsouyanni K, Zavitsanos X, et al. Psychological stress and fatal heart attack: the Athens (1981) earthquake; natural experiment. *Lancet* 1983;1:441.

72. Kark JD, Goldman S, Epstein L. Iraqi missile attacks on Israel: the association of mortality with a life-threatening stressor. *JAMA* 1995;273:1208.

73. Tofler GH, Gebara OCE, Mittleman MA, et al. Morning peak in ventricular tachyarrhythmias detected by time of implantable cardioverter/defibrillator therapy. *Circulation* 1995;92:1203.

74. Muller JE, Ludmer PL, Willich SN, et al. Circadian variation in the frequency of sudden cardiac death. *Circulation* 1987;75:131.

75. Verrier RL, Thompson PL, Lown B. Ventricular vulnerability during sympathetic stimulation: role of heart rate and blood pressure. *Cardiovasc Res* 1974;8:602.

76. Lown B, Verrier RL, Corbalan R. Psychologic stress and threshold for repetitive ventricular response. *Science* 1973;182:834.

77. Weaver WD, Cobb LA, Hallstrom AP, et al. Factors influencing survival after out-of-hospital cardiac arrest. *J Am Coll Cardiol* 1986;7:752.

78. Gray WA, Capone RJ, Most AS. Unsuccessful emergency resuscitation: are continued efforts in the emergency department justified? *N Engl J Med* 1991;325:1393.

79. de Vreede-Swagemakers JJM, Gorgels APM, Dubois-Arbouz WI, et al. Circumstances and causes of out-of-hospital cardiac arrest in sudden death survivors. *Heart* 1998;79:356.

80. Goldstein S, Landis JR, Leighton R, et al. Characteristics of the resuscitated out-of-hospital cardiac arrest victim with coronary heart disease. *Circulation* 1981;64:977.

81. Adhar GC, Larson LW, Bardy GH, et al. Sustained ventricular arrhythmias: difference between survivors of cardiac arrest and patients with recurrent ventricular tachycardia. *J Am Coll Cardiol* 1988;12:159.

82. Levine RL, Wayne MA, Miller CC. End-tidal carbon dioxide and outcome of out-of-hospital cardiac arrest. *N Engl J Med* 1997;337:301.

83. Kuisma M, Alaspaa A. Out-of-hospital cardiac arrest of non-cardiac origin: epidemiology and outcome. *Eur Heart J* 1997;18:1122.

84. Olson DW, LaRochelle J, Fark D, et al. EMT-defibrillation: the Wisconsin experience. *Ann Emerg Med* 1989;18:806.

85. Thompson RG, Hallstrom AP, Cobb LA. Bystander-initiated cardiopulmonary resuscitation in the management of ventricular fibrillation. *Ann Intern Med* 1979;90:737.

86. Valenzuela TD, Roe DJ, Cretin S, et al. Estimating effectiveness of cardiac arrest interventions: a logistic regression survival model. *Circulation* 1997;96:3308.

87. Stiell IG, Wells GA, Field BJ, et al, for the OPALS Study Group. Improved out-of-hospital cardiac arrest survival through the inexpensive optimization of an existing defibrillation program: OPALS study phase II. *JAMA* 1999;281:1175.

88. Cobb LA, Fahrenbruch CE, Walsh TR, et al. Influence of cardiopulmonary resuscitation prior to defibrillation in patients with out-of-hospital ventricular fibrillation. *JAMA* 1999;281:1182.

89. Myerburg RJ, Conde CA, Sung RJ, et al. Clinical, electrophysiologic, and hemodynamic profile of patients resuscitated from prehospital cardiac arrest. *Am J Med* 1980;68:568.

90. Myerburg RJ, Kessler KM, Zaman L, et al. Survivors of prehospital cardiac arrest. *JAMA* 1982;247:1485.

91. Liberthson RR, Nagel EL, Hirschman JC, Nussenfeld SR. Prehospital ventricular fibrillation. *N Engl J Med* 1974;291:317.

92. Taffet GE, Teasdale TA, Luchi RJ. In-hospital cardiopulmonary resuscitation. *JAMA* 1988;260:2069.

93. Bedell SE, Delbanco TL, Cook EF, et al. Survival after cardiopulmonary resuscitation in the hospital. *N Engl J Med* 1983;309:569.

94. Murphy DJ, Murray AM, Robinson BE, et al. Outcomes of cardiopulmonary resuscitation in the elderly. *Ann Intern Med* 1989;111:199.

95. Ritter G, Wolfe RA, Goldstein S, et al. The effect of bystander CPR on survival in out-of-hospital cardiac arrest victims. *Am Heart J* 1985;110:932.

96. Greene HL. Sudden arrhythmic cardiac death-mechanism, resuscitation and classification: the Seattle perspective. *Am J Cardiol* 1990;65:43.

97. Roberts D, Landolfo G, Light HB, et al. Early predictors of mortality for hospitalized patients suffering cardiopulmonary arrest. *Chest* 1990;97:413.

98. Tortolani AJ, Resucci DA, Rosati RJ, et al. In-hospital cardiopulmonary: patient arrest and resuscitation factors associated with survival. *Resuscitation* 1990;20:115.

99. Marwick TH, Case CC, Siskind V, et al. Prediction of survival from resuscitation: a prognostic index derived from multivariate logistic model analysis. *Resuscitation* 1991;22:122.

100. Burns R, Graney MJ, Nichols LO. Prediction of in-hospital cardiopulmonary arrest outcome. *Arch Intern Med* 1989;149:1318.

101. Thompson RJ, McCullough PA, Kahn JK, et al. Prediction of death and neurologic outcome in the emergency department in out-of-hospital cardiac arrest survivors. *Am J Cardiol* 1998;81:17.

102. Weaver WD, Cobb LA, Hallstrom AP, et al. Factors influencing survival after out-of-hospital cardiac arrest. *J Am Coll Cardiol* 1986;7:752.

103. Chen PS, Wolf PD, Ideker RE. Mechanism of cardiac defibrillation: a different point of view. *Circulation* 1991;84:913.

104. Caterine MR, Spencer KT, Pagan-Carlo LA, et al. Direct current shocks to the heart generate free radicals: an electron paramagnetic resonance study. *J Am Coll Cardiol* 1996;28:1598.

105. Walcott GP, Melnick SB, Chapman FW, et al. Relative efficacy of monophasic and biphasic waveforms for transthoracic defibrillation after short and long durations of ventricular fibrillation. *Circulation* 1998;98:2210.

106. Winkle RA, Mead RH, Ruder MA, et al. Effect of duration of ventricular fibrillation on defibrillation efficacy in humans. *Circulation* 1990;81:1477.

107. Niemann JT, Cairns CB, Sharma J, et al. Treatment of prolonged ventricular fibrillation: immediate countershock versus high-dose epinephrine and CPR preceding countershock. *Circulation* 1992;85:281.

108. Baum RS, Alvarez H, Cobb LA. Survival after resuscitation from out-of-hospital ventricular fibrillation. *Circulation* 1974; 50:1231.

109. Safar P. Cerebral resuscitation after cardiac arrest: a review. *Circulation* 1986;74[Suppl IV]:IV-138.

110. Paradis NA, Martin G, Rivers E, et al. Coronary perfusion pressure and the return of spontaneous circulation in human cardiopulmonary resuscitation. *JAMA* 1990;263:1106.

111. Cohen TJ, Tucker KJ, Redberg RF, et al. Active compression-decompression resuscitation: a novel method of cardiopulmonary resuscitation. *Am Heart J* 1992;124:1145.

112. Chang MW, Coffeen P, Lurie KG, et al. Active compression-decompression CPR improves vital organ perfusion in a dog model of ventricular fibrillation. *Chest* 1994;106:1250.

113. Shultz JJ, Coffeen P, Sweeney M, et al. Evaluation of standard and active compression-decompression CPR in an acute human model of ventricular fibrillation. *Circulation* 1994;89:684.

114. Cohen TJ, Tucker KJ, Lurie KG, et al. Active compression-decompression resuscitation: a new method of cardiopulmonary resuscitation. *JAMA* 1992;267:2916.

115. Weisfeldt ML, Guerci AD. Sodium bicarbonate in CPR. *JAMA* 1991;266:2129.

116. Levy MM. An evidenced-based evaluation of the use of sodium bicarbonate during cardiopulmonary resuscitation. *Crit Care Clin* 1998;14:457.

117. Dybvik T, Strand T, Steen PA. Buffer therapy during out-of-hospital cardiopulmonary resuscitation. *Resuscitation* 1995;29: 89.

118. Stiell IG, Hebert MD, Weitzman BN, et al. High dose epinephrine in adult cardiac arrest. *N Engl J Med* 1992;327:1045.

119. Brown CG, Martin DR, Pepe PE, et al. A comparison of standard-dose and high dose epinephrine in cardiac arrest outside the hospital: the multicenter high-dose epinephrine study group. *N Engl J Med* 1992;327:1051.

120. Callaham M, Madsen CD, Barton CW, et al. A randomized clinical trial of high-dose epinephrine and norepinephrine vs standard-dose epinephrine in prehospital cardiac arrest. *JAMA* 1992;268:2667.

121. Banai S, Tzivoni D. Drug therapy for torsades de pointes. *J Cardiovasc Electrophysiol* 1993;4:206.

122. Kudenchuk PJ, Cobb LA, Copass MK, et al. Amiodarone for resuscitation after out-of-hospital cardiac arrest due to ventricular fibrillation. *N Engl J Med* 1999;341:871.

123. Siscovick DS, Raghunathan TE, Psaty BM, et al. Diuretic therapy for hypertension and risk of primary cardiac arrest. *N Engl J Med* 1994;330:1852.

124. Hoes AW, Grobbee DE, Lubsen J, et al. Diuretics, beta blockers and the risk for sudden cardiac death in hypertensive patients. *Ann Intern Med* 1995;123:481.

125. Salerno DM, Asinger RW, Elsperger J, et al. Frequency of hypokalemia after successfully resuscitated out-of-hospital cardiac arrest compared with that in transmural acute myocardial infarction. *Am J Cardiol* 1987;59:84.

126. Velebit V, Podrid PJ, Lown B, et al. Aggravation and provocation of ventricular arrhythmia by antiarrhythmic drugs. *Circulation* 1982;65:886.

127. Ruskin JN, McGovern B, Garan H, et al. Antiarrhythmic drugs: a possible cause of out-of-hospital cardiac arrest. *N Engl J Med* 1983;309:1302.

128. Stevenson WG, Middlekauff HR, Stevenson LW, et al. Significance of aborted cardiac arrest and sustained ventricular tachycardia in patients referred for treatment therapy of advanced heart failure. *Am Heart J* 1992;124:123.

129. Kern KB, Hilwig RW, Rhee KH, et al. Myocardial dysfunction following resuscitation from cardiac arrest: an example of global myocardial stunning. *J Am Coll Cardiol* 1996;28:232.

130. Xie J, Weil MH, Sun S, et al. High-energy defibrillation increases the severity of postresuscitation myocardial dysfunction. *Circulation* 1997;96:683.

131. Kelly P, Ruskin JN, Vlahakes GJ, et al. Surgical coronary revascularization in survivors of prehospital cardiac arrest: its effect on inducible ventricular arrhythmias and long-term survival. *J Am Coll Cardiol* 1990;15:267.

132. Natale A, Sra J, Axtell K, et al. Ventricular fibrillation and polymorphic ventricular tachycardia with critical coronary artery stenosis: does bypass surgery suffice? *J Cardiovasc Electrophysiol* 1994;5:988.

133. Keren R, Aarons D, Veltri EP. Anxiety and depression in patients with life-threatening ventricular arrhythmias: impact of the implantable cardioverter-defibrillator. *Pacing Clin Electrophysiol* 1991;14:181.

134. Siebels J, Cappato R, Ruppel R, et al. Preliminary results of the Cardiac Arrest Survival in Hamburg (CASH) study. CASH Investigators. *Am J Cardiol* 1993;72:109F.

135. Connolly SJ, Gent M, Roberts RS, et al, for the CIDS Investigators. Canadian Implantable Defibrillator Study (CIDS): a randomized trial of the implantable cardioverter defibrillator against amiodarone. *Circulation* 2000;101:1297.

136. The Antiarrhythmics Versus Implantable Defibrillator (AVID) Investigators. A comparison of antiarrhythmic-drug therapy with implantable defibrillators in patients resuscitated from near-fatal ventricular arrhythmias. *N Engl J Med* 1997;337: 1576.

137. Sheldon R, Connolly S, Krahn A, et al. Identification of patients most likely to benefit from implantable cardioverter-defibrillator therapy: the Canadian Implantable Defibrillator Study. *Circulation* 2000;101:1660.

138. Domanski MJ, Saksena S, Epstein AE, et al. Relative effectiveness of the implantable cardioverter-defibrillator and antiarrhythmic drugs in patients with varying degrees of left ventricular dysfunction who have survived malignant ventricular arrhythmias. *J Am Coll Cardiol* 1999;34:1090.

139. The CASCADE Investigators. Randomized antiarrhythmic drug therapy in survivors of cardiac arrest (the CASCADE Study). *Am J Cardiol* 1993;72:280.

140. Knilans TK, Prystowsky EN. Antiarrhythmic drug therapy in the management of cardiac arrest survivors. *Circulation* 1992; 85:I118.

141. Manz M, Jung W, Luderitz B. Interaction between drugs and devices: experimental and clinical studies. *Am Heart J* 1994; 127:978.

142. Kuhlkamp V, Mewis C, Mermi J, et al. Suppression of sustained ventricular tachyarrhythmias: a comparison of d,l-sotalol with no antiarrhythmic drug treatment. *J Am Coll Cardiol* 1999; 33:46.

143. Pacifico A, Hohnloser SH, Williams JH, et al, for the d,l-Sotalol Implantable Cardioverter-Defibrillator Study Group. Prevention of implantable-defibrillator shocks by pretreatment with sotalol. *N Engl J Med* 1999;340:1855.

144. Jung W, Manz W, Luderitz B. Effects of antiarrhythmic drugs on defibrillation thresholds in patients with the implantable cardioverter-defibrillator. *Pacing Clin Electrophysiol* 1992;15: 645.

145. Couch AWE. Cardiac aneurysm with ventricular tachycardia and subsequent excision of aneurysm. *Circulation* 1959;20:251.

146. Cox JL. Patient selection criteria and results of surgery for refractory ischemic ventricular tachycardia. *Circulation* 1989;79 [Suppl I]:I-163.
147. Josephson ME, Harken AH, Horowitz LN. Endocardial excision: a new surgical technique of the treatment of recurrent ventricular tachycardia. *Circulation* 1979;60:1430.
148. Ungerleider RM, Holman WL, Calcagno D, et al. Encircling endocardial ventriculotomy (EEV) for refractory ischemic ventricular tachycardia. III. Effects on regional left ventricular function. *J Thorac Cardiovasc Surg* 1982;83:857.
149. Klein LS, Shih HT, Hackett FK, et al. Radiofrequency catheter ablation of ventricular tachycardia in patients without structural heart disease. *Circulation* 1992;85:1666.
150. Morady F, Harvey M, Kalbfleish SJ, et al. Radiofrequency catheter ablation of ventricular tachycardia in patients with coronary artery disease. *Circulation* 1993;87:363.
151. Schalij MJ, van Rugge FP, Siezenga M, et al. Endocardial activation mapping of ventricular tachycardia in patients: first application of a 32-site bipolar mapping electrode catheter. *Circulation* 1998;98:2168.
152. Nademanee K, Kosar EM. A nonfluoroscopic catheter-based mapping technique to ablate focal ventricular tachycardia. *Pacing Clin Electrophysiol* 1998;21:1442.
153. Strickberger SA, Man KC, Daoud EG, et al. A prospective evaluation of catheter ablation of ventricular tachycardia as adjuvant therapy in patients with coronary artery disease and an implantable cardioverter-defibrillator. *Circulation* 1997;96:1525.
154. Pacifico A, Johnson JW, Stanton MS, et al, for the Jewel 7219D Investigators. Comparison of results in two implantable defibrillators. *Am J Cardiol* 1998;82:875.
155. Anvari A, Stix G, Grabenwoger M, et al. Comparison of three cardioverter defibrillator implantation techniques: initial results with transvenous pectoral implantation. *Pacing Clin Electrophysiol* 1996;19:1061.
156. Fenelon G, Huvelle E, Brugada P, for the European Ventak Mini Investigator Group. Initial clinical experience with a new small sized third-generation implantable cardioverter defibrillator: results of a multicenter study. *Pacing Clin Electrophysiol* 1997;20:2967.
157. Swerdlow CD, Schsls W, Dijkman, B, et al, for the Worldwide Jewel AF Investigators. Detection of atrial fibrillation and flutter by dual-chamber implantable cardioverter-defibrillator. *Circulation* 2000;101:878.
158. Geelen P, Lorga A, Chauvin M, et al. The value of DDD pacing in patients with an implantable cardioverter defibrillator. *Pacing Clin Electrophysiol* 1997;20:177.
159. Higgins SL, Pak JP, Barone J, et al. The first year experience with the dual chamber ICD. *Pacing Clin Electrophysiol* 2000;23:18.
160. Jafar MZ, Schloss EJ, Mehdirad AA, et al. Long-term survival and complications in patients with malignant ventricular tachyarrhythmias: treatment with a nonthoracotomy implantable cardioverter defibrillator with or without a subcutaneous patch. *Pacing Clin Electrophysiol* 1997;20:1305.
161. Smith PN, Vidaillet HJ, Hayes JJ, et al, for the Endotak Lead Clinical Investigators. Infection with nonthoracotomy implantable cardioverter defibrillators: can these be prevented? *Pacing Clin Electrophysiol* 1998;21:42.
162. Samuels LE, Samuels FL, Kaufman MS, et al. Management of infected implantable cardiac defibrillators. *Ann Thorac Surg* 1997;64:1702.
163. Brady PA, Friedman PA, Trusty JM, et al. High failure rate for an epicardial implantable cardioverter-defibrillator lead: implications for long-term follow-up of patients with an implantable cardioverter-defibrillator. *J Am Coll Cardiol* 1998;31:616.
164. Mehta D, Nayak HM, Singson M, et al. Late complications in patients with pectoral defibrillator implants with transvenous defibrillator lead systems: high incidence of insulation breakdown. *Pacing Clin Electrophysiol* 1998;21:1893.
165. Schwartzman D, Nallamothu N, Callans DJ, et al. Postoperative lead-related complication in patients with nonthoracotomy defibrillation lead systems. *J Am Coll Cardiol* 1995;26:776.
166. Martin DT, John R, Venditti FJ. Increase in defibrillation threshold in non-thoracotomy implanted defibrillators using a biphasic waveform. *Am J Cardiol* 1995;76:263.
167. Zhou L, Chen BP, Kluger J, et al. Effects of amiodarone and its active metabolite desethylamidarone on the ventricular defibrillation threshold. *J Am Coll Cardiol* 1998;31:1672.
168. Luderitz B, Jung W, Deister A, et al. Patient acceptance of the implantable cardioverter-defibrillator in ventricular tachyarrhythmias. *Pacing Clin Electrophysiol* 1993;16:1815.
169. Kalbfleisch KR, Lehmann MH, Steinman RT, et al. Reemployment following implantation of the automatic cardioverter-defibrillator. *Am J Cardiol* 1989;64:199.
170. Burgess ES, Quigley JF, Moran G, et al. Predictors of psychosocial adjustment in patients with implantable cardioverter defibrillators. *Pacing Clin Electrophysiol* 1997;20:1790.
171. Namerow PB, Firth BR, Heywood GM, et al, for the CABG Patch Trial Investigators and Coordinators. Quality-of-life six months after CABG surgery in patients randomized to ICD versus no ICD therapy: findings from the CABG Patch trial. *Pacing Clin Electrophysiol* 1999;22:1305.
172. Bourke JP, Turkington D, Thomas G, et al. Florid psychopathology in patients receiving shocks from implanted cardioverter-defibrillators. *Heart* 1997;78:581.
173. Kohn CS, Petrucci RJ, Baessler C, et al. The effect of psychological intervention on patients' long-term adjustment to the ICD: a prospective study. *Pacing Clin Electrophysiol* 2000;23:450.
174. DiMarco JP, Haines DE. Sudden cardiac death. *Curr Probl Cardiol* 1990;15:183.
175. De Backer G, Kornitzer M, Dramiax M, et al. The Belgian Heart Disease Prevention Project: 10-year mortality follow-up. *Eur Heart J* 1988;9:238.
176. Shepherd J, Cobbe SM, Ford I, et al. Prevention of coronary heart disease with pravastatin in men with hypercholesterolemia. West of Scotland Coronary Prevention Study Group. *N Engl J Med* 1995;333:1301.
177. Siscovick DS, Raghunathan TE, King I, et al. Dietary intake and cell membrane levels of long-chain n-3 polyunsaturated fatty acids and the risk of primary cardiac arrest. *JAMA* 1995;274:1363.
178. Siscovick DS, Raghunathan TE, Psaty BM, et al. Diuretic therapy for hypertension and the risk of primary cardiac arrest. *N Engl J Med* 1994;330:1852.
179. Psaty BM, Smith NL, Siscovick DS, et al. Health outcomes associated with antihypertensive therapies used as first-line agents: a systematic review and meta-analysis. *JAMA* 1997;277:739.
180. MERIT-HF Study Group. Effect of metoprolol CR/XL in chronic heart failure: Metoprolol CR/XL Randomised Intervention Trial in Congestive Heart Failure (MERIT-HF). *Lancet* 1999;353:2001.
181. Packer M, Bristow MR, Cohn JN, et al, for the US Carvedilol Heart Failure Study Group. The effect of carvedilol on morbidity and mortality in patients with chronic heart failure. *N Engl J Med* 1996;334:1349.
182. Cleland JGF, Erhardt L, Murray G, et al, on behalf of the AIRE Study Investigators. Effect of ramipril on morbidity and mode of death among survivors of acute myocardial infarction with clinical evidence of heart failure: a report from the AIRE Study Investigators. *Eur Heart J* 1997;18:41.

183. Kober L, Torp-Pedersen C, Carlsen JE, et al. A clinical trial of the angiotensin-converting-enzyme inhibitor trandolapril in patients with left ventricular dysfunction after myocardial infarction. *N Engl J Med* 1995;333:1670.

184. Teo KK, Yusuf S, Furberg CD. Effects of prophylactic antiarrhythmic drug therapy in acute myocardial infarction: An overview of results from randomized controlled trials. *JAMA* 1993;270:1589.

185. Pitt B, Zannad F, Remme WJ, et al, for the Randomized Aldactone Evaluation Study Investigators. The effect of spironolactone on morbidity and mortality in patients with severe heart failure. *N Engl J Med* 1999;341:709.

186. Shephard RJ, Balady GJ. Exercise as cardiovascular therapy. *Circulation* 1999;99:963.

187. Albert CM, Manson JE, Cook NR, et al. Moderate alcohol consumption and the risk of sudden cardiac death among US male physicians. *Circulation* 1999;100:944.

188. Wannamethee G, Shaper AG. Alcohol and sudden cardiac death. *Br Heart J* 1992;68:443.

189. Weinmann S, Siscovick DS, Raghunathan TE, et al. Caffeine intake in relation to the risk of primary cardiac arrest. *Epidemiology* 1997;8:505.

190. Friedlander Y, Siscovick DS, Weinmann S, et al. Family history as a risk factor for primary cardiac arrest. *Circulation* 1998;97:155.

191. Kowey PR, Marinchak RA, Rials SJ. Sudden death prevention after myocardial infarction: What are the choices? *J Cardiovasc Electrophysiol* 1991;2[Suppl]:S192.

192. Hamalainen H, Luurila OJ, Kallio V, et al. Long-term reduction in sudden deaths after a multifactorial intervention programme in patients with myocardial infarction: 10-year results of a controlled investigation. *Eur Heart J* 1989;10:55.

193. Gottlieb SS, McCarter RJ, Vogel RA. Effect of beta-blockade on mortality among high-risk and low-risk patients after myocardial infarction. *N Engl J Med* 1998;339:489.

194. Echt DS, Liebson PR, Mitchell LB, et al. Mortality and morbidity in patients receiving encainide, flecainide or placebo. The Cardiac Arrhythmia Suppression Trial. *N Engl J Med* 1991;324:781.

195. Waldo AL, Camm AJ, deTruyter H, et al, for the SWORD Investigators. Effect of d-sotalol on mortality in patients with left ventricular dysfunction after recent and remote myocardial infarction. *Lancet* 1996;348:7.

196. Julian DG, Camm AJ, Frangin G, et al. Randomised trial of effect of amiodarone on mortality in patients with left-ventricular dysfunction after recent myocardial infarction: EMIAT. *Lancet* 1997;349:667.

197. Cairns JA, Connolly SJ, Roberts R, et al. Randomised trial of outcome after myocardial infarction in patients with frequent or repetitive ventricular premature depolarisations: CAMIAT. *Lancet* 1997;349:675.

198. Janse MJ, Malik M, Camm AJ, et al, on behalf of the EMIAT Investigators. Identification of post acute myocardial infarction patients with potential benefit from prophylactic treatment with amiodarone: a substudy of EMIAT (the European Myocardial Infarct Amiodarone Trial). *Eur Heart J* 1998;19:85.

199. Malik M, Camm AJ, Janse MJ, et al. Depressed heart rate variability identifies postinfarction patients who might benefit from prophylactic treatment with amiodarone: a substudy of EMIAT (The European Myocardial Infarct Amiodarone Trial) [In process citation]. *J Am Coll Cardiol* 2000;35:1263.

200. Amiodarone Trials Meta-analysis Investigators. Effect of prophylactic amiodarone on mortality after acute myocardial infarction and in congestive heart failure: meta-analysis of individual data from 6500 patients in randomized trials. *Lancet* 1997;350:1417.

201. Sim I, McDonald KM, Lavori PW, et al. Quantitative overview of randomized trials of amiodarone to prevent sudden cardiac death. *Circulation* 1997;96:2823.

202. Singh SN, Fletcher RD, Fisher SG, et al. Amiodarone in patients with congestive heart failure and asymptomatic ventricular arrhythmia. *N Engl J Med* 1995;333:77.

203. Doval HC, Nul DR, Grancelli HO, et al. Randomised trial of low dose amiodarone in severe congestive heart failure. *Lancet* 1994;344:493.

204. Moss AJ, Hall WJ, Cannom DS, et al. Improved survival with an implanted defibrillator in patients with coronary disease at high risk for ventricular arrhythmia. *N Engl J Med* 1996;335:1933.

205. Muschlin AI, Hall J, Zwanziger J, et al, for the MADIT Investigators. The cost-effectiveness of automatic cardiac defibrillators: results from MADIT. *Circulation* 1998;97:2129.

206. Every NR, Hlatky MA, McDonald KM, et al. Estimating the proportion of post-myocardial infarction patients who may benefit from prophylactic implantable defibrillator placement from analysis of the CAST registry. *Am J Cardiol* 1998;82:683.

207. Bigger JT, for the Coronary Artery Bypass Graft (CABG) Patch Trial Investigators. Prophylactic use of implanted cardiac defibrillators in patients at high risk for ventricular arrhythmias after coronary artery bypass graft surgery. *N Engl J Med* 1997;337:1569.

208. Bigger JT, Whang W, Rottman JN, et al. Mechanisms of death in the CABG Patch trial: a randomized trial of implantable cardiac defibrillator prophylaxis in patients at high risk of death after coronary artery bypass graft surgery. *Circulation* 1999;99:1416.

209. Buxton AE, Lee KL, Fisher JD, et al, for the Multicenter Unsustained Tachycardia Trial Investigators. A randomized study of the prevention of sudden death in patients with coronary artery disease. *N Engl J Med* 1999;341:1882.

210. Fusgen I, Summa JD. How much sense is there in an attempt to resuscitate an aged person. *Gerontology* 1978;24:37–45.

211. Bachman JW, MacDonald GS, O'Brien PC. A study of out-of-hospital cardiac arrest in northeastern Minnesota. *JAMA* 1986;256:477–783.

212. Bayer AJ, Ang HC, Pathy MSJ. Cardiac arrests in a geriatric unit. *Age and aging* 1985;14:271–276.

213. Rosenberg M, Wang C, Hoffman-Wilde S, Hickham D. Results of cardiopulmonary resuscitation failure to predict survival in two community hospitals. *Arch Intern Med* 1993;153:1370–1375.

22

SINUS NODE FUNCTION AND DYSFUNCTION

JAMES A. REIFFEL

SINUS RHYTHM

Normal Sinus Rhythm

Sinus rhythm is the dominant rhythm in the normal heart. Normal sinus rhythm (NSR) is defined by a physiologically normal atrial rate (60 to 100 bpm while awake and sedentary) and a P-wave vector on the electrocardiogram indicating a high lateral right atrial origin (upright in leads I, II, III, AVL, and AVF). Sinus rhythm usually results from impulse initiation by spontaneously depolarizing P cells within the sinoatrial node (SAN) (1,2) and conduction of the impulse through the node and out to the atrium. Under certain circumstances, as has been shown during electrical mapping intraoperatively under general anesthesia (3), impulse initiation may shift to areas around but outside of the histologically defined, spindle-shaped SAN (2). Although all P cell regions within the SAN have properties of automaticity, usually one group is dominant (i.e., has the most rapid firing rate at any instant and serves as the cardiac pacemaker), while the other P cell regions remain latent as they are reset by or interfered with by impulses generated by the dominant focus. Whether the dominant focus is a single cell or nest of cells with the most rapid rate of depolarization or whether it really is several groups of cells electrotonically linked remains uncertain (4–8).

In infants and children, sinus rates are age related. Sinus rates in children are higher than in adults and decline through childhood. However, the age-related decline in resting rate does not continue through adulthood (9). Although intrinsic SAN function does decrease during the adult years, it is balanced by a progressive decrease in parasympathetic influence (10) and α_1 receptor sensitivity (11).

In NSR, impulse initiation in the dominant pacemaker region is followed by impulse conduction through the node and the perinodal region out to the atrium (1,2). The sinus node possesses automatic and conductive properties. Under physiologic conditions, automaticity and conduction are enhanced by sympathetic input, are depressed by parasympathetic input (12–15), and are subject to a continually shifting balance between the autonomic limbs. Normal SAN function is also modulated by several additional factors, including adrenal catecholamines, thyroxin, temperature, pH, and electrolyte status. When parasympathetic (vagal) influence is blocked pharmacologically with atropine or by transplantation (i.e., denervation) (16), sinus rate increases, sometimes by more than 50%. However, it does not exceed 120 bpm in normal subjects. With total pharmacologic autonomic denervation using atropine and propranolol, the intrinsic sinus rate in normal subjects is usually higher than before such blockade, is generally less than 100 bpm, and can be predicted by this formula: intrinsic heart rate (IHR) = 118.1 − (0.57 × age) (17). At rest, parasympathetic influence usually predominates, whereas with physiologic stress, such as exercise, vagal withdrawal and adrenergic stimulation combine to increase sinus rates.

Sinus Arrhythmia

During NSR, the cyclical changes in sinus rate that are synchronized to breathing and autonomically mediated are called *sinus arrhythmia* (Fig. 22-1). Respiratory phasic changes in cardiac parasympathetic nerve traffic result in alterations in P cell automaticity, conduction velocity within and around the SAN, and shifts in the region of the dominant pacemaker (18). These factors, which have been confirmed by directly recorded sinus node electrograms in humans (19), result in the cyclical changes in sinus rate as determined by atrial cycle lengths (i.e., P-wave to P-wave intervals). Sinus arrhythmia is most pronounced in the young and decreases as parasympathetic influence on the SAN decreases with age (10). Exercise (i.e., vagal withdrawal), parasympathetic blockade (i.e., atropine), or denervation (i.e., transplantation) can abolish sinus arrhythmia. When marked, sinus arrhythmia can be difficult to distinguish from sinus pauses or atrial ectopy and can be

J. A. Reiffel: Department of Medicine, Division of Cardiology, Columbia University, New York, New York 10032.

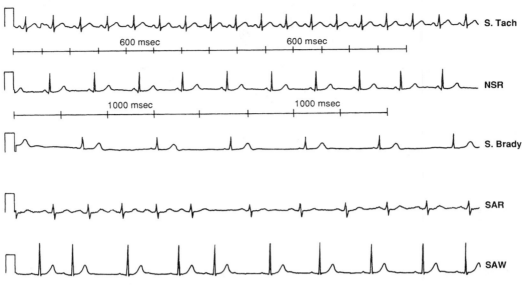

FIGURE 22-1. Electrocardiographic rhythm strips. Rhythm strips *(top to bottom)* demonstrate sinus tachycardia (S. Tach) (P-P intervals < 600 ms), normal sinus rhythm (NSR) (P-P intervals between 600 and 1,000 ms), and sinus bradycardia (S. Brady) (P-P intervals > 100 ms). Sinus arrhythmia (SAR) and sinoatrial Wenckebach (SAW) are also demonstrated.

sensed as palpitations by some patients. Treatment consists of reassurance.

The range of variation in sinus cycle length (SCL) (normalized by dividing by the average SCL and the maximal change in SCL between any two consecutive cycles) is greater in patients with sinus node dysfunction than in normal subjects (20). This variation probably is related to periods of bradycardia or pathologic pauses in such patients. Conversely, a decrease in the cycle-to-cycle variation (i.e., *heart rate variability*) during moderate or prolonged periods of monitoring can also reflect pathophysiology. For example, decreased heart rate variability, which probably reflects decreased absolute or relative parasympathetic nerve traffic and increased sympathetic influence, has been associated with an adverse prognosis after myocardial infarction (21,22).

Vagal activity is also a dominant factor in the circadian variation in sinus rate that occurs with the daily sleep-wake cycle. Enhanced vagal activity in normal subjects during sleep can result in sinus rates less than 40 bpm, pauses longer than 1.5 seconds, and sinoatrial (SA) and atrioventricular (AV) nodal Wenckebach patterns. Commonly, circadian variation is attenuated in the presence of sinus node disease (23).

Sinus Tachycardia

Electrocardiographically defined sinus rates greater than 100 bpm are called *sinus tachycardia* (Fig. 22-1). Sinus tachycardia may be physiologic, pathologic, or pharmacologic. Vagal withdrawal, enhanced catecholamines, thyro-

toxicosis, fever, and pharmacologic stimulants can all enhance sinus node automaticity and thereby increase the sinus rate. During exercise, the sinus rate should increase progressively in normal individuals proportionately to the isotonic load until an age-related maximum is achieved. This upper rate, which is approximately 220 bpm minus the age in years, is an effect mediated by vagal withdrawal, adrenergic stimulation, and possibly by mechanical effects of decreased atrial stretch and altered sinus node artery pulse pressure (4,24). The rate limit of approximately 200 bpm in young adults is probably not incidental. Rather, it likely relates to SAN refractory, excitability, and conductive properties. In normal subjects, the duration of sinus node depolarization, as determined by sinus node electrography, is 100 to 150 ms (25). However, because time dependence exists in the SAN (26), recovery of excitability outlasts the voltage excursion of sinus node action potentials by more than 100 ms, and because intranodal conduction velocity is exceedingly slow, normally less than 0.05 m/sec (7,27–29), an intercycle time frame of less than 300 ms (heart rate >200 bpm) would be difficult to achieve.

The blunting of maximal sinus rate with age is normal; however, a greater degree of blunting of maximal achievable sinus rate with disease is not and is called *chronotropic incompetence* (30,31). Chronotropic incompetence may result in symptoms of exertional fatigue or dyspnea. Many drugs and disease can alter the sinus rate directly or through autonomic interaction. Conditioning by isotonic (aerobic) exercise reduces the resting heart rate through augmented peripheral muscle efficiency and therefore improves the adequacy of a lower resting cardiac output, as well as by enhancing vagal tone and reducing sympathetic neural inputs. Physical conditioning typically results in slow sinus rates at rest (<60 bpm). Rates of 50 to 60 bpm while awake or less than 40 bpm during sleep are expected in normal subjects. Conditioning does not reduce the maximal achievable sinus rate with exercise; rather, it prolongs the amount of aerobic exercise time before obtaining the maximal rate and reduces the cardiac output and sinus rate required for any submaximal level of activity.

Sinus tachycardia may be pathologic in several circumstances. Pathologic sinus tachycardia is recognized when sinus tachycardia is inappropriate for the level of activity. Most commonly, pathologic sinus tachycardia is mediated by increased levels of sympathetic nerve traffic or circulating catecholamines, thyrotoxicosis, or the ingestion of agents with sympathomimetic or direct stimulating effects. These compounds include caffeine or cocaine. Each of these factors reflects enhanced automaticity. Typically, there are other signs of catecholamine, thyroxin, or stimulant excess, such as tremor, sweating, increased cardiac output, esthesia, and chest discomfort. The so-called hyperkinetic heart syndrome probably reflects such pathophysiology. Removal of the offending agent or β-blocker administration usually ameliorates the symptom. Sinus tachycardia, which is usually transient and probably caused by altered parasympathetic input (32), has been reported after radiofrequency ablation in the AV nodal region (33). Occasionally, persistent sinus tachycardia is pathologic and idiopathic (34). I have seen two cases of persistent inappropriate sinus tachycardia that followed a combination of chemotherapy and thoracic radiotherapy: one for Hodgkin's disease and one for breast carcinoma. Although the mechanism is uncertain, inflammatory changes or destruction of vagal fibers may be postulated. Perhaps paradoxically, pathologic sinus tachycardia can also result from disordered SA conduction. As in the AV node, regions of impaired conduction can serve as a substrate for reentry, and reentry in the SAN region can manifest as paroxysmal sinus tachycardia.

Sinus Bradycardia

Sinus bradycardia is a sinus rhythm rate of less than 60 bpm (Fig. 22-1). Sinus bradycardia, like sinus tachycardia, may be physiologic, pathologic, or pharmacologic. Sinus bradycardia is a physiologic response to conditioning and a normal response to periods of increased parasympathetic tone. Enhanced parasympathetic tone itself may be physiologic, as during sleep (35,36), or may be pathologic. The latter may be triggered by gastrointestinal, genitourinary, pharyngeal, or other disorders involving tissues that are richly innervated by the vagus, or it may represent an enhanced sensitivity to or disproportionate increase in or response to vagal traffic triggered by normal reflexes, such as baroreceptor stimulation. Vagally induced sinus bradycardia may be

responsive to atropine, but it needs to be treated only if symptomatic. Atropine doses of less than 0.5 mg may cause a paradoxical increase in vagally induced bradycardia. These effects are mediated by central nervous system actions and should be avoided. Physiologic sinus bradycardia should be distinguished from pathologic bradycardia because of differences in treatment and prognosis. Findings that may indicate physiologic sinus bradycardia are correlations of the bradycardia with physiologic increases in vagal tone, such as sleep, micturition, nausea and vomiting, or sinus bradycardia in a well-conditioned individual, such as one who participates regularly in aerobic exercise. Physiologic sinus bradycardia should be reversible with atropine because the efferent mechanism involves vagotonia. Sinus bradycardia under other circumstances, particularly in the setting of coexisting pathologic disorders involving the myocardium, coronary flow, or components of the conduction system distal to the sinus node, suggest a pathologic rather than a physiologic mechanism, as does sinus bradycardia in the setting of cardioactive drugs or central nervous system disorders. Pathologic and symptomatic sinus bradycardias are part of the constellation of sinus node disorders collectively known as sick sinus syndrome (SSS).

Mechanistically, sinus bradycardia usually results from a decrease in the automatic firing rate of sinus node P cells. When physiologic, it usually reflects acetylcholine's actions of decreasing the rate of diastolic depolarization or hyperpolarizing the membrane, causing a shift away from threshold (12,13). Sinus node exit block may also cause sinus bradycardia if the degree of conduction block is stable; although this may be acetylcholine induced, it more commonly represents pathophysiology in my experience. Pathologically and pharmacologically induced sinus bradycardia are discussed later as part of SSS.

SINUS NODE REENTRY

In many ways, the SAN is functionally similar to the AV node (see Chapter 23). Resting potentials less negative than those of Purkinje tissue or working myocardial cells, "slow channel"-dependent action potentials, and a structurally complex node all promote slow rates of intranodal and perinodal conduction. Similarly, both nodes demonstrate decremental conduction (i.e., decreasing conduction velocity in association with premature stimuli of increasing prematurity during relative refractoriness), inequalities in bidirectional conduction, and occasionally "dual-pathway" properties (27,37–40). As in the AV node (41), the presence of decremental conduction with premature stimulation (some regions may slow, some may block) and the existence of more than one "functional" pathway for conduction within the SAN region (4,27) provide the potential conditions to support reentry: slow conduction and unidirectional block.

Sinus node reentry has been demonstrated and mapped in atrial preparations (27,42–45), and reentry in the sinus node region has been confirmed in humans (37,46–53). In clinical practice, paroxysmal supraventricular tachycardia (PSVT) due to sinus node reentry is uncommon (Fig. 22-2). In the experience of Wellens, only 10% of patients who undergo clinical electrophysiologic study for tachycardias have sinus node reentry (53). Others, however, have reported slightly higher frequencies (46,54,55), but in my experience, it is much less common. With the increase in AV nodal reentrant PSVT and atrioventricular reentrant tachycardia being referred for ablative therapy, sinus node reentrant tachycardias appear to represent less than 5% of PSVT seen in the laboratory. Current techniques do not allow us to tell *in vivo* how much of the reentrant pathway is within the node versus in the perinodal tissue. In general, the cycle length of PSVT due to sinus node reentry is generally longer (i.e., the rate is slower) than with other PSVTs. Rates of 110 to 150 bpm, often with some cycle-to-cycle variation, are most common. Symptoms such as palpitations or dizziness are less frequent and severe than with other, more rapid PSVTs. At least when studied in the clinical electrophysiology laboratory, sinus node reentry typically is self-terminating in one to six beats and is sustained only infrequently.

Sinus node reentry can be presumed when several electrocardiographic (ECG) and intracardiac atrial electrogram criteria are fulfilled (56). First, the sinus node return cycle length after an atrial premature depolarization (APD) is shorter than what would occur with an interpolated APD. Second, when visible (i.e., not buried in the preceding QRST complex), the echo beat P-wave vector in multiple ECG leads and its atrial activation sequence are the same as in sinus rhythm, and the RP′ : P′R ratio is greater than 1. Third, for single echoes, the postecho sinus return cycle should exceed the basic SCL. Fourth, neither atrial-His (A-H) prolongation nor AV conduction are prerequisites to inducing or supporting the reentrant beats. When sustained, sinus node reentrant tachycardia usually responds to the same drugs that suppress AV nodal reentry (e.g., digitalis, β blockers, verapamil, diltiazem, class I or III antiarrhythmics) and usually can be terminated by "vagal maneuvers" and antitachycardia pacing algorithms. Radiofrequency ablation may be attempted as a cure. My colleagues and I have employed it, guided by careful sinus node identification, although injury to the sinus node is a risk, thereby justifying it only in resistant cases (Fig. 22-3).

SINUS NODE DYSFUNCTION: SICK SINUS SYNDROME

Sinus node dysfunction (SND) (57–61) exists when nonphysiologic alterations in sinus rhythm are present. SND encompasses disordered SAN automaticity and SA conduction. The recognition of SND, or *sick sinus syndrome*, a term popularized by Ferrer (62), is by ECG evidence. The patient may or may not have symptoms. The recognition of SND is important in terms of the mechanism and treatment of symptoms, the initiation of cardioactive pharmaceuticals, and the prognosis.

Recognition

Electrocardiographically, SND is recognized by the appearance of any or all of the following: inappropriate sinus bradycardia, sinus pauses (representing impaired automaticity or SA exit block), or alternating periods of sinus bradyarrhythmias and nonsinus tachyarrhythmias (49,62,63). This finding may present as a bradycardia followed by an escape tachyarrhythmia (i.e., the bradycardia-tachycardia syndrome [Fig. 22-4]) or as a tachyarrhythmia that after termination is followed by a long offset pause (i.e., the tachycardia-bradycardia syndrome [Fig. 22-5]).Most commonly, the tachyarrhythmia is paroxysmal atrial fibrillation or flutter. Because dysfunction of other segments of the cardiac conduction system, particularly the AV junction, frequently coexist with SND, several additional ECG findings should suggest the possibility of concomitant SND (64–69), including atrial fibrillation or flutter with a slow ventricular rate in the absence of drugs, other AV nodal conduction disorders, APDs with prolonged post-APD pauses, and atrial fibrillation in the absence of any demonstrable associated cardiac disorder or known extracardiac cause (i.e., lone atrial fibrillation). Lone atrial fibrillation can represent a default or escape rhythm in the setting of persistent sinus nodal arrest or exit block. The latter is important to recognize because

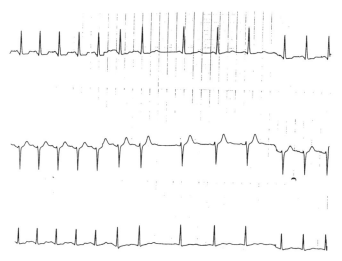

FIGURE 22-2. Example of sinus node reentry. Notice the abrupt onset and offset of the arrhythmia, the same PR interval, and the P waves, which are identical in sinus rhythm and during the tachycardia.

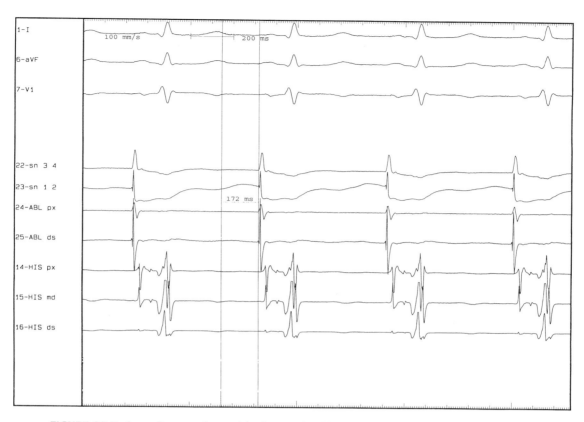

FIGURE 22-3. Recordings used to guide sinus node ablation. The patient is a 32-year-old with symptomatic inappropriate sinus tachycardia that is unresponsive to tolerated medical therapy. Sinus node ablation provided a cure. The level of the dominant portion of the sinus node was identified by the sinus node potential on a sinus node electrogram and early atrial activation on a mapping catheter. The ablation catheter was then used to create a line of block across the sinus node region at this level, guided by sites of the earliest atrial signals, and then a vertical more posterior line across the exit region and access route for Bachmann's bundle. Shown from top to bottom are electrocardiographic leads I, aVF, V₁; proximal (SN 3,4) and distal (SN 1,2) electrograms off a sinus node (SN) mapping catheter; proximal (PX) and distal (DS) electrograms on the ablation (AB) catheters, and three His bundle electrograms (proximal, middle, distal).

direct current or pharmacologically mediated cardioversion may result in asystole or marked bradyarrhythmias rather than NSR under these circumstances. Automaticity of AV junctional ventricular pacemakers is often depressed in SSS, and escape rhythms are slower than expected. Sinus "bradycardia" may be relative rather than absolute, presenting as NSR with chronotropic incompetence.

During sinus rhythm, pathologic sinus pauses may result from SA arrest or exit block. Sinus arrest, a disorder of automaticity, is recognized as pauses that are out of proportion to sinus arrhythmia and that are not multiples of the basic underlying cycle length (Figs. 22-6 and 22-7). This pattern contrasts with that of sinus node exit block, a disorder of conduction, which exists when an impulse generated within

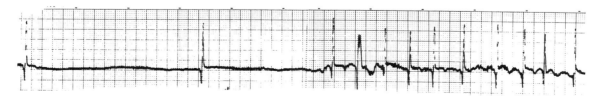

FIGURE 22-4. Example of a bradycardia-tachycardia syndrome. As a result of sinus node dysfunction, the patient has a slow junctional rhythm at a rate of approximately 20 bpm, resulting in atrial fibrillation.

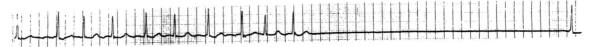

FIGURE 22-5. Example of a tachycardia-bradycardia syndrome. The initial rhythm is atrial fibrillation, which terminates abruptly. This is followed by a 6.3-second pause and a junctional beat.

the SAN fails to conduct out to the atrium or does so slowly (Figs. 22-6 and 22-7). First-degree sinus node exit block can be identified by intracardiac electrophysiologic studies but cannot be recognized on the routine electrocardiogram, on which sinus node depolarization is not visible. Although sinus node depolarization may be visible on appropriately obtained signal-averaged electrocardiograms, my colleagues and I have found that any degree of sinus arrhythmia precludes accurate measurements. First-degree sinus node exit block, a prolongation of SA conduction time, is analogous to the prolonged PR interval seen when AV nodal conduction is slow. Analogous to AV nodal conduction is type I and type II second-degree sinus node exit block. Type I sinus node exit block is recognized by Wenckebach periodically of P-P intervals (i.e., a progressive shortening of consecutive P-P intervals until one abruptly lengthens), similar to the R-R interval periodicity in AV Wenckebach (Fig. 22-1). Type II second-degree sinus node exit block is recognized by an abrupt P-P interval lengthening to a value that is a multiple of (e.g., twice, three times, four times) the basic SCL. Third-degree SAN exit block and cessation of automaticity, both of which are rare, can cause atrial standstill in the absence of an escape rhythm (70).

Prevalence

Because sinus bradyarrhythmias are often asymptomatic and may be physiologic rather than dysfunctional, it is impossible to determine the frequency of SND within any population. In screening studies such as cardiovascular detection programs, the incidence has been less than 0.2% (71–73). However, the absence of routine, prolonged ambulatory monitoring in most such programs should

underestimate the true incidence. In contrast, if the examiner does not distinguish between pathologic and physiologic sinus bradyarrhythmias, the incidence is substantial. For example, in a University of Illinois study of 50 normal young men and women (35), 24% of men and 8% of women had rates less than 50 bpm with sleep. (The average, maximum, and minimum waking and sleeping heart rates were also higher in women than in men.) Other studies reveal that sinus pauses in excess of 2 seconds can occur in apparently normal subjects (35,36,72–76) and in up to 37% of trained athletes. Pauses in excess of 3 seconds (77–80), however, are rare in normal subjects, frequently correlate with symptoms, and should provoke clinical assessment.

Significance

The recognition of SND is important in several respects. First and foremost is its relationship to symptoms (60,67,79–83). If sinus rates are sufficiently slow or pauses are sufficiently long as to impair cerebral or peripheral blood flow, symptoms will ensue. The extent of bradycardia or length of pause that results in symptoms, however, varies among individuals because stroke volume, peripheral resistance, and local vascular patency also contribute to the extent of regional blood flow at any heart rate. Chronotropic incompetence often leads to exertional fatigue or dyspnea. Symptoms associated with undue resting bradycardia most commonly are fatigue, dizziness, or minor personality changes. Symptoms most commonly associated with undue pauses are dizziness, syncope, or manifestations of escape rhythms. All of these symptoms are nonspecific; many processes can produce identical symptoms, and no symptom

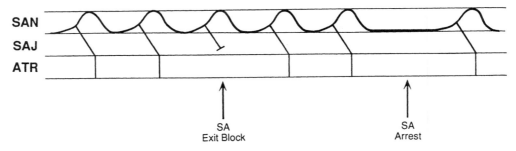

FIGURE 22-6. The schematic differentiates sinoatrial exit block from sinoatrial arrest. The sinus node action potential is shown in the sinoatrial node (SAN) ladder on the ladder diagram. ATR, atrium; SAJ, sinoatrial junction.

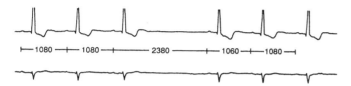

FIGURE 22-7. An electrocardiogram rhythm strip illustrates a sinus pause. The interval measurements are used to determine whether it is caused by sinoatrial (SA) exit block or SA arrest.

is therefore specific for SND. Accordingly, the treatment of symptomatic SND requires documentation of the association between the dysrhythmia and the symptom or the reasonable exclusion of alternate explanations for the symptom. Rarely, marked sinus bradycardia causes dyspnea or worsened angina that reflects the associated increase in ventricular filling and diastolic pressure.

The recognition of SND is also important for concomitant therapy. An asymptomatic bradycardia may become symptomatic if worsened by the administration of an agent that depresses the sinus node (84–123) (Table 22-1). Many of these agents, such as digitalis, the β blockers, verapamil, diltiazem, and the class I and III antiarrhythmics are used in the treatment of paroxysmal supraventricular tachyarrhythmias. In patients with the bradycardia-tachycardia syndrome, however, reduction of or control of the tachycardia may occur at the expense of worsening of the bradycardia. Digitalis is the less apt to worsen sinus bradycardia than β or calcium channel blockers in SND patients in our experience (93). Pindolol is tolerated in most patients (124) because of its intrinsic sympathomimetic actions and is probably the drug of choice for ventricular rate control in SND patients

TABLE 22-1. CARDIOACTIVE DRUGS THAT MAY INDUCE OR WORSEN SINUS NODE DYSFUNCTION

β Blockers
Calcium channel blockers (e.g., verapamil, diltiazem)
Sympatholytic antihypertensives (e.g., α-methyldopa, clonidine, guanabenz, reserpine)
Cimetidine
Lithium
Phenothiazines (rarely)
Antihistamines
Antidepressants
Antiarrhythmic agents
  May cause sinus node dysfunction (SND) in normal subjects: amiodarone
  Frequently worsens *mild* SND: flecainide, propafenone, sotalol
  Infrequently worsens *mild* SND: digitalis, quinidine, procainamide, disopyramide,[a] moricizine
  Rarely worsens *mild* SND: lidocaine, phenytoin, mexiletine, tocainide
Opioid blockers

[a]The anticholinergic properties of disopyramide may reduce the risk of SND.

who have periods of atrial fibrillation. Frequently, pacemaker implantation is pursued to support antiarrhythmic therapy in patients with asymptomatic SND.

SND is also important to recognize because of the potential for embolism. The bradycardia-tachycardia syndrome has had sufficiently high incidence of systemic emboli reported (125–136) that anticoagulation should be used. Similarly, right atrial thrombi have been documented when underlying atrial disorders coexist with SND (129).

Some data suggest that SND may have an adverse prognosis as regards mortality (130–136). However, when SND is idiopathic and unassociated with apparent underlying structural heart disease or more distal conduction system dysfunction, the mortality rate may not be increased (134), although symptoms may develop or worsen with time. If atrial fibrillation becomes persistent as a default rhythm in SSS (137,138), the prognosis of atrial fibrillation itself comes in to play.

Etiology and Pathophysiology

Because SSS is not a disease itself but rather a set of pathophysiologic dysrhythmias, it can have several diverse etiologic instigators (1,2,12,58,60,61,63,82,84,103,139–161). Disordered SAN automaticity or conduction can result from hypothermia, severe electrolyte disturbance, ischemia, or pharmacologic depression. SND may also be caused by myxedema or, rarely, Graves disease; infiltrative disorders such as amyloidosis, tumor, or hemochromatosis; myocarditis or pericarditis; or intracranial hypertension. It has been associated with obstructive jaundice, Duchenne or myotonic dystrophy, Friedreich's ataxia, mitral valve prolapse, hypertrophic cardiomyopathy, pheochromocytoma, and autoantibodies to the SAN (162). SND may also result from a secondary (e.g., lupus erythematosus, scleroderma) or primary (e.g., fatty or fibrotic replacement) degenerative process, trauma, familial inheritance, or prior cardiac surgery, such as the Mustard procedure (157,158). SND may result from coronary artery disease. Sinus bradycardia and pauses, often transient, may occur in the acute phase of myocardial infarction (163–166), particularly inferior or lateral. Whether this is because of impairment of flow in the sinus node artery (usually a branch of the right or circumflex coronary artery), because of the release of acetylcholine from infarcted cells, or because of the initiation of neural reflexes is rarely clear. High-grade stenosis of the sinus node artery is uncommon (149–152).

SND may result from states of increased parasympathetic influence. Often, the inciting cause is apparent, such as a hypersensitive carotid sinus syndrome, gastrointestinal distress, or a genitourinary disorder. The link among these causes is a condition involving tissue with rich vagal innervation. It may also be one component of micturition or cough syncope. Autonomically mediated SND may occur *de novo*, or an autonomic component may be a factor additive to the effect of disease or drug. The determination of an autonomic cause or component can be ascertained by observing the results of carotid massage or the induction of enhanced vagal as by means of facial ice water immersion, hypertension induced by phenylephrine infusion, tilt-table testing, or the phases of the Valsalva maneuver. Similarly, it may be assessed by studying the effects of parasympathetic blockade or total autonomic blockade with atropine or atropine plus propranolol, respectively, as discussed earlier. If SND persists after autonomic denervation, as determined by an abnormal intrinsic heart rate or abnormal electrophysiologic tests after such blockade, the presence of an underlying intrinsic (nonautonomic) component is confirmed. Practically, however, determination of the role of vagally induced dysfunction is important only when the underlying disorder (e.g., hypertensive carotid sinus that could be surgically denervated) can be identified. Because vagal blockade with an oral belladonna compound is rarely tolerated chronically, therapy of SND is independent of mechanism in most cases. Through the years, my colleagues and I have had occasional patients in whom symptoms have been prevented by selective use of prophylactic pharmacotherapy, such as an oral belladonna derivative before exercise in a patient with vagally mediated, symptomatic, chronotropic incompetence or with an agent that may initiate reflex sympathetic activation, such as hydralazine. However, vagally induced vasodepression, in contrast to bradycardia, does not usually respond to atropine-like agents.

Careful attention to the search for etiologic disorders or a vagal component should be given during each history obtained or physical examination performed in patients with known or suspected SND.

Diagnostic Evaluation

Therapy for SND usually is required only for symptom relief or to support concomitant drug therapy (60). However, the relationship between the dysrhythmia and the symptoms should be established as clearly as possible, because many of the common symptoms are nonspecific and need not indicate SND and because periods of sinus bradycardia or pauses are common in normal individuals, particularly during sleep or with other periods of high vagal tone. Because symptoms are typically brief or intermittent, they are rarely present during routine electrocardiograms. More often, prolonged ambulatory ECG recordings or transtelephonic event recordings are needed to capture a symptomatic episode (61,167–174). Documentation of symptoms simultaneously with a bradydysrhythmia is a strong enough piece of evidence to declare a relationship between the two and to pursue therapy. In the case of suspected chronotropic incompetence, an exercise electrocardiogram may similarly be diagnostic (175–180). In patients with hypersensitive carotid sinus syndrome, appropriate symptoms (e.g., symptoms associated with shaving, head turning, buttoning a collar, tying a tie) coupled with a

hypersensitive response on physical examination can establish a diagnosis. The hypersensitive response on physical examination is represented by a pause in excess of 3 seconds in response to moderate unilateral massage of 5 seconds.

Noninvasive techniques are often inadequate because of the transient nature of symptoms. In an early study using Holter recordings for patients with known SSS, the sensitivity was only 60% to 75% (168). Similarly, in a study of 44 symptomatic patients, Stern and colleagues achieved a diagnosis in only 48% despite an average duration of almost 6 days of continuous recordings (170). Chronotropic incompetence may vary (perhaps with autonomic tone); exercise test reproducibility is limited (181,182), and a normal response may not exclude SND.

When ambulatory ECG surveillance with Holter, memory loop, or patient-applied event recorders fails to capture a symptomatic episode or fails to reveal a bradycardia severe enough in itself to warrant therapy (i.e., rate <30 bpm or pauses >3 seconds), electrophysiologic techniques are used (12,56,183–193).

Electrophysiologic studies are designed to be diagnostic, demonstrating the severity of SND and, if possible, provoking the clinical symptoms. Electrophysiologic studies can also be used to provide prognostic information. When performed serially, electrophysiologic studies can provide information about the efficacy, safety, or intolerance of proposed medications for concurrent disorders. For example, serial electrophysiologic studies (i.e., before and after drug administration) can be used to tell whether a drug may worsen a bradycardia or a posttachycardic pause if it fails to prevent the paroxysmal tachycardia itself. Acute drug studies using intravenous or oral agents are highly predictive of long-term effects in patients with SND. Sinus node pauses after overdrive pacing in the electrophysiologic laboratory closely approximate pauses after spontaneous tachyarrhythmias (194) before and after drug administration.

The target of electrophysiologic evaluation of the SAN is an assessment of automaticity, conduction, occasionally refractoriness, and possible associated tachyarrhythmias and conduction defects. A detailed review of sinus node electrophysiologic testing is beyond the scope of this chapter, but an overview is presented. Several in-depth reviews are listed among the references (56,183–186).

No technique purely assesses automaticity. However, the heart rate response after atropine and the behavior of sinus rhythm after overdrive atrial pacing come the closest. In normal individuals, incremental dosing of atropine produces progressively more rapid sinus rates until all vagal influence is abolished. In our experience, at this point, the sinus rate plateaus at about 110 to 120 bpm. In patients with intrinsic SND, this peak rate is lower. A sinus rate that does not exceed 90 bpm after atropine is indicative of intrinsic SND (195,196). However, those with autonomically mediated extrinsic SND appear normal by this test. If the baseline bradycardia results from SA exit block (e.g., 2 : 1) and the

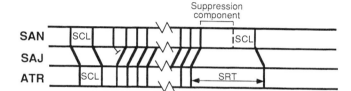

FIGURE 22-8. A schematic of the events in the sinoatrial node (SAN), sinoatrial (SA) junction (SAJ), and atrium during normal sinus rhythm *(left of break indicators)* and during atrial overdrive pacing culminating in measurement of the sinus node recovery time. ATR, atrium; SCL, sinus cycle length; SRT, sinus recovery time (on the atrial catheter).

atropine reverses the conduction defect, the sinus rate also improves, although not simply from enhanced automaticity.

Overdrive pacing is probably the most commonly used single test to screen for SND in the electrophysiology laboratory. It is based on observations made in the tortoise heart more than a century ago (197), which revealed that cardiac

pacemakers can be suppressed by overdrive stimulation and take a finite and reproducible time to recover their normal automatic firing rate after such overdrive suppression. In clinical practice, this technique uses trains of atrial pacing (usually 30 to 60 seconds) at several cycle lengths shorter than the spontaneous SCL to suppress the sinus node. After termination of pacing, the interval until the recovery of the first sinus beat is measured (Figs. 22-8 and 22-9). Occasionally, the interval to the complete return of the prepacing sinus rate is also assessed (198). In our laboratory, cycle lengths such as 400, 500, 600, 700, 800, 900, and 1,000 ms are used. This technique assumes that the paced impulses conduct into the sinus node and continuously reset and suppress the pacemaker focus. After termination of pacing, the speed of recovery of a sinus impulse is taken as an index of sinus node function—reflecting in large part automaticity. In theory, the more disordered are the automatic properties of the SAN, the more severely it is suppressed by overdrive, the slower it recovers, and the longer

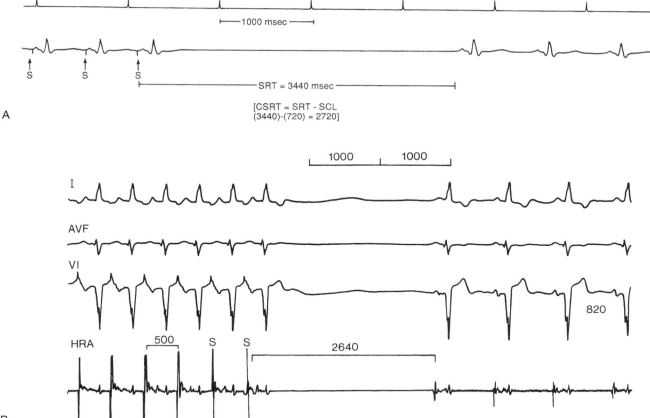

FIGURE 22-9. A: A lead II rhythm strip shows the sinus recovery time (SRT) after the last three paced beats of 30 seconds of overdrive pacing. Calculation of the corrected sinus node recovery time (CSRT) is demonstrated. S, stimulus. **B:** The sinus node recovery time (2,640 ms) is shown after the last six beats of a 30-second pacing run (cycle length = 500 ms; s, stimulus). The spontaneous sinus cycle length was 820 ms. The 100-ms time markers are at the top, above electrocardiographic leads I, aVF, and V₁, and the high right atrial electrogram (HRA). The CSRT for this pacing run would be 2640 − 820 = 1820 ms, which is very abnormal.

is the postpacing pause. However, the impulse, once formed, must conduct out of the node, and prolonged postpacing pauses have also been documented to occasionally reflect postpacing exit delay or exit block for one or more impulses (199,200).

To facilitate interpatient comparisons, because the absolute value of the postpacing pause is not the same in patients with different native sinus rates, the longest pause is usually normalized or "corrected," most often by subtracting the prepacing SCL. A corrected sinus node recovery time ($SNRT_C$) obtained in this way is less than 525 ms in normal subjects (201). (The absolute value taken in normal subjects varies a little among laboratories.) In truth, however, overdrive pacing is more complex than just an assessment of suppression of automaticity. Rapid atrial pacing reflexively initiates vagal activation, which depresses AV nodal and SA nodal conduction. The increase in A-H intervals and eventual development of AV node Wenckebach patterns with incremental atrial pacing is a commonly recognized manifestation of the former. Atriosinus entrance block can also occur with incremental atrial pacing, in which case all atrial-paced impulses may not penetrate the sinus node (193). The same would be true if perinodal or intranodal conduction were impaired by disease. It is for this reason that multiple pacing rates must be used to determine the maximal obtainable sinus recovery time, and it is for this reason that, in the setting of disease or substantial vagotonia, the maximally recorded sinus recovery time may appear normal despite dysfunction. If impaired conduction sufficiently limits sinus nodal penetration by the paced impulses, the node is not suppressed, and recovery intervals are not prolonged. Such "falsely shortened" sinus node recovery times reduce the sensitivity of sinus recovery time assessment to the range of 55% to 75% (185). Fortunately, in most such circumstances, the longest recovery time is observed at a fairly long paced cycle length rather than at a rapid pacing rate, especially if the reproducibility of postpacing pauses is assessed at each paced cycle length tested and the average of those obtained at each cycle length is considered (193,202). Other evidence of SND obtained from postpacing observations are secondary pauses: cycles after the first with cycle lengths longer than that of the first. These secondary pauses are not seen in normal subjects, but their utility in symptom assessment is uncertain (183,198, 200,203).

When the postpacing pause is long enough to induce the patient's clinical symptoms, the diagnosis and mechanism of symptoms are clearly established, and therapy goals will be clear. When the postpacing pauses are sufficiently long to establish SND, but the link to symptom remains undocumented, interpretation must be handled like the interpretation of notable but asymptomatic sinus bradycardia on ambulatory monitoring. Therapy is usually pursued when alternative explanations for the symptoms have been excluded. Although $SNRT_C$ values greater than 525 ms are abnormal, there is no single value that, if exceeded, always correlates with symptoms.

Because determination of the $SNRT_C$ is not in itself highly sensitive for SND, although a prolonged $SNRT_C$ has high specificity, additional electrophysiologic tests have been developed. These focus on SAN properties other than automaticity. Most frequently, they involve assessment of SA conduction. One clue to disordered SA conduction is when the longest sinus node recovery times occur at the slowest pacing rates. However, SA conduction can also be assessed without the stress of overdrive pacing and its inherent increase in vagal tone. The earliest methods to determine the time it takes an impulse to conduct from the dominant pacemaker region of the sinus node out to the atrium, the SA conduction time (SACT), were all indirect. They used observations made during atrial premature stimulation or during short trains of slow atrial pacing to calculate the SACT (204–209). These two stimulation approaches assume that, after a beat that retrogradely captures the SAN in the absence of overdrive suppression, the return sinus cycle as measured on the atrial electrogram encompasses the conduction time from the atrial paced beat into the SAN, the SCL after reset of the pacemaker focus by the atrial beat, and the conduction time of the next sinus beat out of the node (Fig. 22-10).

If the SCL of this recovery beat within the node is the same as the average SCL, the atrial cycle equals the SCL plus the SACT into and out of the node. One half of the difference between the post-APD atrial cycle length and the average SCL approximates the average unidirectional SACT. Referenced texts provide additional and specific details regarding these techniques (183–185). Using such approaches, the average SACT is generally less than 120 to 130 ms and has been found to be abnormal in some patients with normal $SNRT_C$ values (183,184,210). SACT values longer than 130 ms represent first-degree SA exit block. In this regard, the SACT calculation has been of

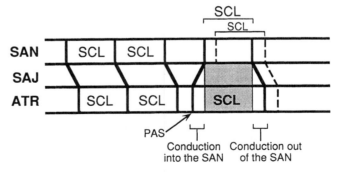

FIGURE 22-10. The sinoatrial conduction time (SACT) is calculated from the return cycle after a stimulated atrial beat that penetrates and resets the sinoatrial node pacemaker region. The dotted lines indicate where the sinus impulse would have occurred had the premature beat not been placed. ATR, atrium; PAS, premature atrial stimulus; SAJ, sinoatrial junction; SAN, sinoatrial node; SCL, sinus cycle length.

diagnostic and prognostic value. Occasionally, patterns of 2 : 1 or more advanced SA block are precipitated by atrial premature stimuli or slow atrial pacing and can replicate spontaneous long pauses or symptoms. In such cases, SACT testing helps to identify the need for therapy; hence its interpretation and utility parallels that of the $SNRT_C$.

We and others have developed a direct technique to determine SACT. Sinus node electrograms can be recorded using appropriate catheter placement and filters (39,211–214). By directly visualizing the depolarization of the sinus node as well as atrial activation on such sinus node electrograms, the SACT can be directly measured (Fig. 22-3).

Recognition of abnormal SA conduction can be useful as a direct determinant of SND or as a factor in falsely short sinus node recovery times, but it helps in the attempt to improve the sensitivity of $SNRT_C$ testing. When SA entrance block has limited overdrive suppression and hence has falsely shortened the sinus node recovery time, repetition of the overdrive pacing runs after the administration of atropine (to prevent or alleviate vagally induced depression of SA conduction) may reveal the inherent defect in automaticity and produce long and diagnostic pauses (215). This should be performed when $SNRT_C$ values are normal, but the longest ones occur at a long paced cycle length or when the SACT is prolonged.

For diagnostic purposes, when the previous constellation of electrophysiologic tests is used to confirm SND in the absence of clear noninvasive documentation, the sensitivity is variable. Individual reports for $SNRT_C$ or SACT have ranged from 18% to 75%, (184,192,203,216–218), with an increase generally reported when the tests are used in combination. The specificity probably approximates 90%. In patients with syncope of uncertain origin, the combination of electrophysiologic tests is more likely to document SND than is a 24-hour Holter monitor recording (184).

For prognostic purposes, abnormal electrophysiologic test results are also useful. Gann and colleagues (219,220) reported a significant incidence (60%) of symptom development during follow-up among patients with asymptomatic sinus bradycardia who had prolonged $SNRT_C$ values. Similar findings using multiple sinus node electrophysiologic test results have been reported by our group (183,210). Conversely, patients with asymptomatic sinus bradycardia but a normal $SNRT_C$ had a less than 30% incidence of subsequent symptom development in Gann's series. In patients who are already symptomatic, pacemaker implantation is associated with resolution of symptoms in more than 90% of those with prolonged $SNRT_C$ values (183,210).

In addition to determining the SACT and examining observations made during overdrive atrial pacing, assessment of the duration of sinus node refractory periods has been suggested as having clinical utility (184,221–223). Its role remains uncertain and underexamined, however, and it is not widely used. My colleagues and I later showed that the duration of the sinus node depolarization on sinus node electro-

grams (Fig. 22-11) is prolonged in patients with modest or severe SND and has direct clinical utility (186). The duration of the sinus node depolarization is prolonged when the P cells' action potentials are prolonged, automaticity is impaired, or intrasinus or perisinus impulse conduction is slow. As such, it correlates closely with the findings of an abnormal $SNRT_C$ or SACT. It is probably not a more sensitive identifier of SND than is an abnormal $SNRT_C$ or SACT, but it may be quicker to determine in some patients and is not subject to the "pseudonormalization" seen with the $SNRT_C$ when entrance block exists.

One additional test for SND has been proposed (224). In 1992, Resh and associates reported the use of intravenous adenosine (150 μg/kg) to expose SND. An increase in SCL of longer than 675 ms after adenosine had similar sensitivity (69%) and specificity (100%) to that of a prolonged $SNRT_C$. However, the number of patients studied was small (12 controls and 11 with SSS). In 1999, Burnett and coworkers (225) published similar results (sensitivity of 80%, specificity of 97%) for another small series (10 patients and 67 controls) using a $SNRT_C$ of 550 ms as abnormal. Because of limited experience, the optimal role of this intervention remains uncertain. As with the $SNRT_C$ itself, a modestly high false-negative rate (36%) may limit its utility.

Therapy

Therapy for SND usually is based on symptoms. In general, a bradycardia or a pause of sinus origin that is asymptomatic requires no therapy. Exceptions to this rule occur when the physician must add an agent for the treatment of

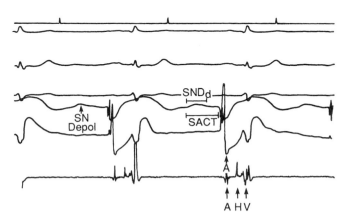

FIGURE 22-11. A human sinus node electrogram (SNE). From top to bottom are shown 1,000-ms time marker; electrocardiographic leads I, aVF, and V_1; the human sinus node electrogram; a high right atrial electrogram 1 cm proximal to the SNE; and the His bundle electrogram, where atrial (a), His bundle (H), and ventricular (V) depolarizations are indicated. On the SNE, the sinus node depolarization (SN Depol) denotes the measurement of the sinoatrial conduction time (SACT), and the duration of the sinus node depolarization (SND_d) is depicted.

a concomitant disorder, such as a tachyarrhythmia or hypertension, and that agent has a likelihood of worsening the SND significantly (Table 22-1). Prophylactic treatment of the SND is then justifiable. When the degree of the bradycardia or the length of the pause is so severe that any further worsening is likely to produce symptoms or place the patient at risk for an escape rhythm that is potentially serious or life threatening, another exception exists. Acceptable indications for pacemaker implantation in this respect, for example, are rates in the thirties or pauses in excess of 3 seconds.

Specific corrective therapy is possible only when a reversible cause has been established. For example, sinus bradycardia due to myxedema resolves with the treatment of the hypothyroidism. Similarly, the hypersensitive carotid sinus syndrome may resolve with carotid sinus denervation. However, in most circumstances, therapy must be aimed at symptom prevention, independent of the cause. When the pathophysiologic mechanism is parasympathetic excess, belladonna alkaloids, such as atropine and its congeners, may be tried prophylactically or therapeutically (226). However, most patients with SND are older and have intrinsic SAN dysfunction or do not tolerate the anticholinergic side effects, such as constipation, sicca, visual blurring, prostatism, lethargy, or confusion. Such patients may also have a discrete contraindication to these agents, such as glaucoma, sluggish bowel, angina, prostate hypertrophy, or obstructive pulmonary disease. Anticholinergics are generally used as emergency intravenous therapy in younger patients or for prophylactic or short-term treatment. Occasionally, agents that produce sympathetic activation in response to drug-induced vasodilation (e.g., hydralazine) or β blockers with intrinsic sympathomimetic activity (124) may help reduce or prevent sinus bradycardia. There have been no reported studies linking the efficacy of such agents to the mechanism of the bradycardia. However, it is likely that patients with intrinsic SND are less responsive. For most patients with SSS, pacemaker implantation is the therapy of choice (53, 134,153,164,227–235). Underlying disease pathophysiology, ventricular compliance characteristics, the status of associated conduction defects and arrhythmias, and the status of ventriculoatrial (VA) conduction are important considerations in selecting pacemaker nodes and sites (231–234).

Pacemaker therapy for SSS is directed at symptoms (81,137,138,153,230), not at longevity (132,133,236–239). The progression of effectively treated SSS is determined by the associated heart disease, such as left ventricular dysfunction, myocardial ischemia, or valvular disorder, and longevity is usually not prolonged for patients with SSS by pacemaker insertion. Quality of life, however, may be notably enhanced when pacemaker insertion is directed at symptom relief, and the symptoms have been adequately correlated with SND as the mechanism.

In the presence of associated AV conduction defects (which are common and usually AV nodal in origin), pacing must be ventricular or dual chamber. In its absence, atrial pacing may suffice, particularly when AV nodal conduction is found to be normal at detailed electrophysiologic testing. When the disorder being treated manifests as occasional pauses, an AAI or VVI pacer to prevent such pauses may be all that is initially needed. Some patients, however, develop persistent bradycardia with time and begin to pace most or all of the time. This possibility and the status of VA conduction should be considered before pacer implantation in terms of potential pacing modes and lead sites that should be available. In the presence of frequent or persistent sinus bradycardia, whether initial or later in the course, attention to the hemodynamics of pacing is required, and dual-chamber devices often are necessary. In the presence of chronotropic incompetence (which should be looked for before pacer implantation), a rate-responsive unit such as VVIR or DDDR is optimal and is needed for full symptom relief. AAIR devices are occasionally useful but are less predictably effective if AV conduction becomes impaired over time. In the presence of atrial tachycardias such as paroxysmal atrial fibrillation, DDDR with mode switching, DDI(R), or VVI(R) features may be necessary. The specific modes depend on the type of tachycardia, status of AV and VA conduction, and status of chronotropic competence. Because atrial fibrillation is a common, long-term sequela of SND, this possibility should be considered before pacemaker implantation. In the bradycardia-tachycardia patients, atrial pacing at a rate in the middle to upper normal range (e.g., 80 to 85 bpm) with an AAI or dual-chamber device (perhaps enhanced by septal or dual-site atrial pacing) often reduces and occasionally eliminates the paroxysmal fibrillating periods (185,229,232,233). Because so many issues must be considered before implanting a pacemaker for SND, the decision about type and features of the device to be implanted should be reviewed with or by a physician knowledgeable about current pacemaker methodology (234).

REFERENCES

1. Bouman LN, Jongsma HJ. Structure and function of the sino-atrial node: a review. *Eur Heart J* 1986;7:94–104.
2. James TN. The sinus node. *Am J Cardiol* 1977;40:965–986.
3. Boineau HP, Canavan TE, Schuessler RB, et al. Demonstration of a widely distributed atrial pacemaker complex in the heart. *Circulation* 1988;77:1221–1237.
4. Sano T, Sawanobori T, Adinya H. Mechanism of rhythm determination among pacemaker cells of the mammalian sinus node. *Am J Physiol* 1978;235:H379–H384.
5. Jalife J. Mutual entrainment and electrical coupling mechanisms for synchronous firing of rabbit sinoatrial pacemaker. *J Physiol* 1984;356:221–243.
6. Michael DC, Matyas EP, Jalife J. Mechanisms of sinoatrial pacemaker synchronization: a new hypothesis. *Circ Res* 1987;61:704–714.
7. Bonke FIM, Kirchhoff CJHJ, Allessie MA, et al. Impulse propagation from the S-A node to the ventricles. *Experientia* 1987;43:1044–1049.

8. Michael DC, Matyas EP, Jalife J. Experimental and mathematical observations on pacemaker interactions as a mechanism of synchronization in the sinoatrial node. In: Zipes DP, Jalife J, eds. *Cardiac electrophysiology: from cell to bedside.* Philadelphia: WB Saunders, 1990:182–192.

9. Padeletti L, Micheluci A, Franchi F, Fradella GA. Sinoatrial function in old age. *Acta Cardiol (Brux)* 1982;37:11–21.

10. de Marneffe M, Jacobs P, Haardt R, Englert M. Variations of normal sinus node function in relation to age: role of autonomic influence. *Eur Heart J* 1986;7:662–672.

11. Saitoh H, Nomura A, Osaka M, et al. Effects of α_1-adrenergic stimulation on human sinus node automaticity. *J Am Coll Cardiol* 1993;21:860–897.

12. Strauss HC, Prystowsky EN, Scheinman MM. Sino-atrial and atrial electrogenesis. *Prog Cardiovasc Dis* 1977;19:385–404.

13. Prystowsky EN, Grant AO, Wallace AG, et al. An analysis of the effects of acetylcholine on conduction and refractoriness in the rabbit sinus node. *Circ Res* 1979;44:112–140.

14. Bouman LN, Mackaay AJC, Bleeker WK, et al. Pacemaker shifts in the sinus node: effects of vagal stimulation, temperature and reduction of extracellular calcium. In: Bonke FIM, ed. *The sinus node: function and clinical relevance.* The Hague: Martinus Nijhoff, 1978:245–247.

15. Lu HH, Lange G, McBrooks C. Factors controlling pacemaker action in cells of the sinoatrial node. *Circ Res* 1965;17:460–471.

16. Bexton RS, Nathan AW, Hellestrand KJ, et al. Sinoatrial function after cardiac transplantation. *J Am Coll Cardiol* 1984;3:712–723.

17. Jose AD, Collison D. The normal range, and determinants, of the intrinsic heart rate in man. *Cardiovasc Res* 1970;4:160–167.

18. Harriman RJ, Hoffman BF. Effects of ouabain and vagal stimulation on sinus nodal function in conscious dogs. *Circ Res* 1982;51:760–768.

19. Reiffel JA, Bigger JT Jr. The relationship between sinoatrial conduction time and sinus cycle length revisited. *J Electrophysiol* 1987;1:290–299.

20. Bergfeldt BL, Edhag KO, Solders G, Vallin HO. Analyses of sinus cycle variation: a new method for evaluation of suspected sinus node dysfunction. *Am Heart J* 1987;114:321–327.

21. Malik M, Camm AJ. Heart rate variability. *Clin Cardiol* 1990;13:570–576.

22. Kleiger RE, Miller JP, Bigger JT, Moss AJ. Decreased heart rate variability and its association with increased mortality after acute myocardial infarction. *Am J Cardiol* 1987;59:256–262.

23. Alboni JA, Uberti ED, Codeca L, et al. Circadian variations of sinus rate in subjects with sinus node dysfunction. *Chronobiologia* 1982;9:173–183.

24. Ushiyama J, McBrooks C. Interaction of oscillators: effect of sinusoidal stretching of the sinoatrial node on nodal rhythm. *J Electrocardiol* 1977;10:39–44.

25. Reiffel JA, Zimmerman G. The duration of the sinus node depolarization on transvenous sinus node electrograms can identify sinus node dysfunction and can suggest its severity. *Pacing Clin Electrophysiol* 1989;12:1746–1756.

26. Reiffel JA, Cook JA, Meissner MD. Evidence suggesting time dependent recovery of excitability in the in vivo human sinus node. *Am J Cardiol* 1991;68:798–800.

27. Kirchoff CJHJ, Bonke FIM, Allessie MA. Sinus node reentry: fact or fiction. In: Brugada P, Wellens HJJ, eds. *Cardiac arrhythmias: where to go from here?* Mount Kisco, NY: Futura Publishing, 1987:53–65.

28. Paes de Cervallo A. Cellular electrophysiology of the atrial specialized tissues. In: Paes de Carvallo A, deMellow C, Hoffman BF, eds. *The specialized tissues of the heart.* Amsterdam: Elsevier, 1962.

29. Sano T, Yamogishi S. Spread of excitation from the sinus node. *Circ Res* 1965;16:423–430.

30. Vallin HO, Edhag KO. Heart rate responses in patients with sinus node disease compared to controls: physiological implications and diagnostic possibilities. *Clin Cardiol* 1980;3:391–398.

31. Abbott JA, Hirschfeld DS, Kunkel FW, et al. Graded exercise testing in patients with sinus node dysfunction. *Am J Med* 1977;62:330–338.

32. Kocovic D, Shea J, Friedman PL, et al. Evidence for parasympathetic denervation of the sinus node after radiofrequency modification of the A-V node in patients with A-V nodal reentry. *J Am Coll Cardiol* 1993;21[Suppl A]:50A.

33. Skeberis V, Simonis F, Andries E, et al. Inappropriate sinus tachycardia after radiofrequency ablation of AV nodal tachycardia, incidence and clinical significance. *J Am Coll Cardiol* 1993;21[Suppl A]:358A.

34. Bauernfeind RA, Amat-y-Leon F, Dhingra RC, et al. Chronic nonparoxysmal sinus tachycardia in otherwise healthy persons. *Ann Intern Med* 1979;91:702–710.

35. Brodsky M, Wu D, Denes P, et al. Arrhythmias documented by 24 hour continuous electrocardiographic monitoring in 50 male medical students without apparent heart disease. *Am J Cardiol* 1977;39:390–405.

36. Romano M, Clariia M, Onofrio E, et al. Heart rate, PR, and QT intervals in normal children: a 24 hour Holter monitoring study. *Clin Cardiol* 1988;11:839–842.

37. Reiffel JA, Bigger JT Jr, Ferrick K, et al. Sinus node echoes and concealed conduction: additional sinus node phenomena confirmed in man by direct sinus node electrography. *J Electrocardiol* 1985;18:259–266.

38. Reiffel JA. Further evidence for decremental conduction in the sinoatrial junction. *J Electrocardiol* 1984;17:104–105.

39. Reiffel JA, Bigger JT Jr. Current status of direct recordings of the sinus node electrogram in man. *Pacing Clin Electrophysiol* 1983;6:1143–1150.

40. Tzivoni D, Jordan J, Mandel WJ, et al. A second zone of compensation during atrial premature stimulation: evidence for decremental conduction in the sinoatrial junction. *J Electrocardiol* 1982;15:317–324.

41. Josephson ME, Seides SF. *Clinical cardiac electrophysiology: techniques and interpretation.* Philadelphia: Lea & Febiger, 1979:152.

42. Allessie MA, Bonke FIM. Direct demonstration of sinus node reentry in the rabbit heart. *Circ Res* 1979;44:557–568.

43. Allessie MA, Bonke FIM. Re-entry within the sinoatrial node as demonstrated by multiple micro-electrode recordings in the isolated rabbit heart. In: Bonke FIM, ed. *The sinus node: structure, function and clinical relevance.* The Hague: Martinus Nijhoff, 1978:409–421.

44. Childers R, Arnsdord M, DeLa Fuenta D, et al. Sinus nodal echoes: clinical case report and canine studies. *Am J Cardiol* 1973;90:1114–1128.

45. Strauss HC, Geer MR. Sinoatrial node reentry. In: Kulbertus HE, ed. *Reentrant arrhythmias: mechanisms and treatment.* Lancaster, UK: MTP Press, 1977:39–42.

46. Gomes JA, Hariman RJ, Kang PS, Chowdry IH. Sustained symptomatic sinus node reentrant tachycardia: incidence, clinical significance, electrophysiologic observations and the effects of antiarrhythmic agents. *J Am Coll Cardiol* 1985;5:45–57.

47. Breithardt G, Seipel L. Further evidence for the site of reentry in so-called sinus node reentrant tachycardia in man. *Eur J Cardiol* 1980;11:105–113.

48. Weisfogel GM, Batsford WP, Paulay KL, et al. Sinus node reentrant tachycardia in man. *Am Heart J* 1975;90:295–304.

49. Goldreyer BN. Sinus node dysfunction—a physiologic consideration of arrhythmias involving the sinus node. *Cardiovasc Clin* 1974;6:179–198.

50. Narula OS. Sinus node re-entry: a mechanism for supraventricular tachycardia. *Circulation* 1974;50:1114–1128.

51. Curry PVL, Krikler DM. Paroxysmal reciprocating sinus tachycardia. In: Kulbertus HE, ed. *Reentrant arrhythmias: mechanisms and treatments.* Lancaster, UK: MTP Press, 1977:39–62.

52. Romano S, Pisapia A, Pozzoni L, et al. Echo intrasinual: demonstration par enregistrement direct de pontentiel sinsual par voie endocavitaire. *Arch Mal Coeur* 1986;79:1337–1342.

53. Wellens HJJ. Role of sinus re-entry in the genesis of sustained cardiac arrhythmias. In: Bonke FIM, ed. *The sinus node: structure, function and clinical relevance.* The Hague: Martinus Nijhoff, 1978:422–427.

54. Dhingra RC, Wyndham C, Amat-y-Leon F, et al. Sinus nodal responses to atrial extrastimuli in patients without apparent sinus node disease. *Am J Cardiol* 1975;36:445–452.

55. Wellens HJJ. General conclusions. In: Bonke FIM, ed. *The sinus node: structure, function and clinical relevance.* The Hague: Martinus Nijhoff, 1978:428.

56. Reiffel JA. Clinical electrophysiology of the sinus node in man. *Prog Clin Biol Res* 1988;275:239–257.

57. Swiryn S, McDonough T, Hueter DC. Sinus node function and dysfunction. *Med Clin North Am* 1984;68:935–954.

58. Bashur TT. Classification of sinus node dysfunction. *Am Heart J* 1985;110:1251–1256.

59. Dhingra RC. Sinus node dysfunction. *Pacing Clin Electrophysiol* 1983;6:1062–1069.

60. Bigger JT Jr, Reiffel JA. Sick sinus syndrome. *Annu Rev Med* 1979;30:91–118.

61. Szatmary L, Barnay C, Medvedowsky JL, et al. Holter monitoring in the complex analysis of sinus node dysfunction. *Acta Cardiol (Brux)* 1982;37:427–440.

62. Ferrer MI. The sick sinus syndrome. *Circulation* 1973;47:635–641.

63. Jordan JA, Yamaguchi I, Mandel WJ. Studies on the mechanism of sinus node dysfunction in the sick sinus syndrome. *Circulation* 1978;57:217–223.

64. Rakovec P. Sinoatrial conduction time in patients with atrioventricular block. *Cardiology* 1981;68:161–166.

65. Vallin H, Edhag O. Associated conduction disturbances in patients with symptomatic sinus node disease. *Acta Med Scand* 1981;210:263–270.

66. Wyse DG, McAnulty JH, Rahimtoola SH, Murphy ES. Electrophysiologic abnormalities of the sinus node and atrium in patients with bundle branch block. *Circulation* 1979;60:413–420.

67. Rosenqvist M, Vallin H, Edhad O. Clinical and electrophysiologic course of sinus node disease: five-year follow up study. *Am Heart J* 1985;109:513–522.

68. van Mechelen R, Segers S, Hagemeijer F. Serial electrophysiologic studies after single chamber atrial pacemaker implantation in patients with symptomatic sinus node dysfunction. *Eur Heart J* 1984;5:628–636.

69. Hayes DL, Furman S. Stability of AV conduction in sick sinus syndrome patients with implanted atrial pacemakers. *Am Heart J* 1984;106:644–647.

70. Wu D, Yea SJ, Lin FC, et al. Sinus automaticity and sinoatrial conduction in severe symptomatic sick sinus syndrome. *J Am Coll Cardiol* 1992;19:335–364.

71. Kulbertus HE, de Leval-Rutten F, Demoulin JC. Sino-atrial disease: a report on 13 cases. *J Electrocardiol* 1973;5:303–312.

72. Bigger JT Jr, Reiffel JA, Coromilas J. Ambulatory electrocardiography. In: Platia E, ed. *Non-pharmacologic management of cardiac arrhythmias.* Philadelphia: JB Lippincott, 1986:36–61.

73. Sobotka PA, Mayer JH, Bauernfeind RA, et al. Arrhythmias documented by 24 hour continuous ambulatory electrocardiographic monitoring in young women without apparent heart disease. *Am Heart J* 1981;101:753–759.

74. Talan DA, Bauernfeind RA, Ashley WW, et al. Twenty-four continuous ECG recordings in long-distance runners. *Chest* 1982;82:19–24.

75. Viitasalo MT, Kala R, Eisale A. Ambulatory electrocardiographic recording in endurance athletes. *Br Heart J* 1982;47:213–220.

76. Hattori M, Toyama J, Ito A, et al. Comparative evaluation of depressed automaticity in sick sinus syndrome by Holter monitoring and overdrive suppression test. *Am Heart J* 1983;105:587–592.

77. Fleg JL, Kennedy HL. Cardiac arrhythmias in a healthy elderly population. *Chest* 1982;82:302–307.

78. Scott O, Williams GJ, Fiddler GI. Results of 24 hour ambulatory monitoring of electrocardiogram in 131 healthy boys ages 10 to 13 years. *Br Heart J* 1980;44:304–308.

79. Ector H, Rolies L, DeGeest H. Dynamic electrocardiography and ventricular pauses of 3 seconds and more: etiology and therapeutic implications. *Pacing Clin Electrophysiol* 1983;6:548–551.

80. Hilgard J, Ezri MD, Denes P. Significance of ventricular pauses of three seconds or more detected on twenty-four hour Holter records. *Am J Cardiol* 1985;55:1005–1008.

81. Simonsen E, Nielson JS, Nielsen BL. Sinus node dysfunction in 128 patients: a retrospective study with follow-up. *Acta Med Scand* 1980;208:343–348.

82. Ferrer MI. The etiology and natural history of sinus node disorders. *Arch Intern Med* 1982;142:371–372.

83. Kerr CR, Grant AO, Wenger TL, Strauss HC. Sinus node dysfunction. *Cardiol Clin* 1983;1:187–207.

84. Alpert MA, Flaker GC. Arrhythmias associated with sinus node dysfunction: pathogenesis, recognition, and management. *JAMA* 1983;250:2160–2166.

85. Leir CV, Johnson TM, Hashimoto H, Schaal SF. Effects of commonly used cardioactive drugs on atrial and sinoatrial conduction in man. *J Cardiovasc Pharmacol* 1980;2:553–566.

86. Vera Z, Awan NA, Mason DT. Assessment of oral quinidine effects on sinus node function in sick sinus syndrome patients. *Am Heart J* 1982;103:80–84.

87. Goldberg D, Reiffel JA, Davis JC, et al. Electrophysiologic effects of procainamide on sinus node function in patients with and without sinus node disease. *Am Heart J* 1982;103:75–79.

88. Tsuchioka Y, Yamaoka K, Hashimoto M, et al. Electrophysiological effects of diphenylhydantoin in patients with sinus node dysfunction. *Jpn Heart J* 1986;7:334–340.

89. Bolognesi R, Benedini G, Ferari R, Visioli O. Inhibitory effect of acute and chronic administration of digitalis on the sick sinus node. *Eur Heart J* 1986;7:334–340.

90. Gomes JA, Kang PS, El Sherif N. Effects of digitalis on the human sick sinus node after pharmacologic autonomic blockade. *Am J Cardiol* 1981;48:783–788.

91. Alboni P, Shantha N, Filippi I, et al. Clinical effects of digoxin on sinus node and atrioventricular node function after pharmacologic autonomic blockade. *Am Heart J* 1984;108:1255–1261.

92. Vera Z, Miller RR, McMillin D, Mason DT. Effects of digitalis on sinus nodal function in patients with sick sinus syndrome. *Am J Cardiol* 1978;41:318–323.

93. Reiffel JA, Bigger JT Jr, Cramer M. Effects of digoxin on sinus nodal function before and after vagal blockade in patients with sinus nodal dysfunction: a clue to the mechanisms of the action of digitalis on the sinus node. *Am J Cardiol* 1979;43:983–989.

94. Shugushev KK, Rosenshtraukh LV, Smetnev AS. Electrophysiologic effects of ethmozin on sinus node function in patients with and without sinus node dysfunction. *Clin Cardiol* 1986;9:443–448.

95. Rakovec P, Jakopin J, Rode P, et al. Electrophysiologic effects of ethmozin on sinus nodal function in patients with and without sinus node dysfunction. *Eur Heart J* 1984;5:243–246.

96. LaBarre A, Strauss HC, Scheinman MM, et al. Electrophysiologic effects of disopyramide phosphate on sinus node function in patients with sinus node dysfunction. *Circulation* 1979;59: 448–454.

97. Dhingra RC, Deedwania PC, Cummings JM, et al. Electrophysiologic effects of lidocaine on sinus node and atrium in patients with and without sinoatrial dysfunction. *Circulation* 1978;57:448–454.

98. Davis JC, Reiffel JA, Bigger JT Jr. Sinus node dysfunction caused by methyldopa and digoxin. *JAMA* 1981;245:1241–1243.

99. Rector WG, Jarzobski JA, Levin HS. Sinus node dysfunction associated with lithium therapy: report of a case and a review of the literature. *Nebr Med J* 1979;64:193.

100. Engle TR, Luck JC. Histamine 2 receptor antagonism by cimetidine and sinus-node function. *N Engl J Med* 1979; 391:L591–592.

101. Valette H, Barnay C, Lopez M, et al. Effects of intravenous diltiazem on sinus node function and atrioventricular conduction in patients. *J Cardiovasc Pharmacol* 1983;5:62–66.

102. Seipel L, Breithardt G. Electrophysiological actions of calcium antagonists in the heart. *Cardiology* 1982;69:105–116.

103. Strauss HC, Scheinman MM, LaBarre A, et al. Review of the significance of drugs in the sick sinus syndrome. In: Bonke FIM, ed. *The sinus node: structure, function and clinical relevance.* The Hague: Martinus Nijhoff, 1978:103–111.

104. Engel TR, Schaal SF. Digitalis in the sick sinus syndrome: the effect of digitalis on sinoatrial automaticity and atrioventricular conduction. *Circulation* 1973;43:1201–1207.

105. Margolis JR, Strauss HC, Miller HC, et al. Digitalis and the sick sinus syndrome: clinical and electrophysiologic documentation of a severe toxic effect on sinus node function. *Circulation* 1975;52:162–169.

106. Dhingra RC, Amat-y-Leon F, Wyndham C, et al. The electrophysiological effects of ouabain on sinus node and atrium in man. *J Clin Invest* 1975;56:555–562.

107. Ten Eick RE, Hoffman BF. Chronotropic effects of cardiac glycosides in cats, dogs, and rabbits. *Circ Res* 1969;24:365–378.

108. Smith TW, Haber E. Digitalis. *N Engl J Med* 1972;289:945–952.

109. Geer MR, Wagner GS, Waxman M, et al. Chronotropic effect of acetylstrophanthidin infusion in the canine sinus nodal artery. *Ann J Cardiol* 1977;39:684–689.

110. Kao A, Kreitt JM, Detloff BLS, et al. Bromocriptine treatment for digitalis-induced ventricular tachyarrhythmias: studies in a canine model. *J Am Coll Cardiol* 1984;4:1188–1194.

111. Strauss HC, Gilbert M, Svenson RH, et al. Electrophysiologic effects of propranolol on sinus node function in patients with sinus node dysfunction. *Circulation* 1976;54:454–459.

112. Narula OS, Vasquez M, Shantha N, et al. Effect of propranolol on normal and abnormal sinus node function. In: Bonke FIM, ed. *The sinus node: structure, function and clinical relevance.* The Hague: Martinus Nijhoff, 1978:113–128.

113. Mottee G, Bellanger P, Vogal M, et al. Asystole suivie de choc cardiogenique apres injection inraveinuse de verpamil. *Ann Cardiol Angeiol (Paris)* 1975;24:157–162.

114. Unger AH, Sklarhoff HJ. Fatalities following intravenous use of sodium diphenylhydantoin for cardiac arrhythmias. *JAMA* 1967;200:335–336.

115. Grayzel J, Angeles J. Sino-atrial block in man provoked by quinidine. *J Electrocardiol* 1972;5:289–294.

116. Josephson ME, Caracta AR, Lau SH, et al. Electrophysiologic properties of procainamide in man. *Am J Cardiol* 1974;33: 596–603.

117. Seipel L, Both A, Breithardt G, et al. Action of antiarrhythmic drugs on His bundle electrogram and sinus node function. *Acta Cardiol Suppl* 1967;48:251–267.

118. Hirschfeld DS, Ueda CT, Rowland M, et al. Clinical and electrophysiological effects of intravenous quinidine in man. *Br Heart J* 1977;39:309–316.

119. Vik-Mo H, Ohm OJ, Lund-Johansen P. Electrophysiological effects of flecainide acetate in patients with sinus nodal dysfunction. *Am J Cardiol* 1982;50:1090–1094.

120. Touboul P, Atallah G, Gressard A, et al. Effects of amiodarone on sinus node in man. *Br Heart J* 1979;42:573–578.

121. Wellens HJJ, Cats V, Duren DR. Symptomatic sinus node abnormalities following lithium carbonate therapy. *Am J Med* 1975;59:285–287.

122. Wilson JR, Kraus ES, Bailas MM, et al. Reversible sinus node abnormalities due to lithium carbonate therapy. *N Engl J Med* 1976;294:1223–1224.

123. Reding P, Devroede C, Barbier P. Bradycardia after cimetidine [Letter]. *Lancet* 1977;2:1227.

124. Strickberger SA, Fisher D, Lamas GA, et al. Comparison of effects of propranolol versus pindolol on sinus rate and pacing frequency in sick sinus syndrome. *Am J Cardiol* 1993;71:53–56.

125. Bathen J, Sparr S, Rokseth R. Embolism in sinoatrial disease. *Acta Med Scand* 1983;1:187–207.

126. Fairfax AJ, Lambert CD, Leatham A. Systemic embolism in chronic sinoatrial disorder. *N Engl J Med* 1986;295:190–192.

127. Rubenstein JJ, Schulman CL, Yurchak PM, et al. Clinical spectrum of the sick sinus syndrome. *Circulation* 1972;46:5–13.

128. Sutton R, Kenny RA. The natural history of sick sinus syndrome. *Pacing Clin Electrophysiol* 1986;9:1110–1114.

129. Lesiak M, Grajek S, Pyda M. Unusual location of mural thrombi in the right atrium caused by pathological changes in the sinoatrial node. *Kardiol Pol* 1990;33:49–53.

130. Fisher JD, Furman S, Escher DJW. Pacing in the sick sinus syndrome: profile and prognosis. In: Feruglio G, ed. *Cardiac pacing, electrophysiology and pacemaker technology.* Rome: Padova Piccin, 1982:519–520.

131. Simon AB, Janz N. Symptomatic bradyarrhythmias in the adult: natural history following ventricular pacemaker implantation. *Pacing Clin Electrophysiol* 1982;5:372–383.

132. Hauser RG, Jones J, Edwards LM, et al. Prognosis of patients paced for AV block or sinoatrial disease in the absence of ventricular tachycardia. *Pacing Clin Electrophysiol* 1983;6:123(abst).

133. Alt E, Volker R, Wirtzfeld A, et al. Survival and follow-up after pacemaker implantation: a comparison of patients with sick sinus syndrome, complete heart block and atrial fibrillation. *Pacing Clin Electrophysiol* 1985;8:849–855.

134. Skagen K, Hansen JR. The long-term prognosis for patients with sinoatrial block treated with permanent pacemaker. *Acta Med Scand* 1975;199:13–15.

135. Areosty JM, Cohen SI, Morkin E. Bradytachycardia syndrome: results in twenty-eight patients treated by combined pharmacologic therapy and pacemaker implantation. *Chest* 1974;66: 257–263.

136. Shaw DB, Holman RR, Gowers JI. Survival in sinoatrial disorder (sick-sinus syndrome). *Br Med J* 1980;280:139–141.

137. Alpert MA, Katti SK. Natural history of sinus node dysfunction after permanent pacemaker implantation. *South Med J* 1982;75: 1182–1188.

138. Ferrer MI. The natural history of the sick sinus syndrome. *J Chron Dis* 1972;25:313–315.

139. Thery C, Gosselin B, Lekieffre J, Warembourg H. Pathology of sinoatrial node: correlations with electrocardiographic findings in 111 patients. *Am Heart J* 1977;93:735–740.

140. Bashour TT, Kabbani SS, Brewster HP, et al. Sinus node dysfunction during coronary vasospastic angina. *Am Heart J* 1984; 108:1056–1059.

141. Szatmary L, Czako E, Solti F, Szabo Z. Autonomic sinus node dysfunction and its treatment. *Acta Cardiol (Brux)* 1984;39: 209–220.

142. Szatmary L, Torresani J. Autonomic sinus node dysfunction documented by Holter monitoring studies in 21 patients. *Acta Med Hung* 1983;40:25–31.

143. Nair CK, Sketch MH, Desai R, et al. High prevalence of symptomatic bradyarrhythmias due to atrioventricular node-fascicular and sinus node-atrial disease in patients with mitral annular calcification. *Am Heart J* 1982;103:226–229.

144. Talano JV, Euler D, Randall WC, et al. Sinus node dysfunction: an overview with emphasis on autonomic and pharmacologic consideration. *Am J Med* 1978;64:773–781.

145. Chiche P, Lellouch A, Denizeau JP. Autonomic influences and cardiac conduction in patients with sinus node disease. *Cardiology* 1976;611:98–112.

146. Chung EK. Sick sinus syndrome: current views. *Mod Concepts Cardiovasc Dis* 1980;61–66.

147. Davies MJ, Pomerance A. Quantitative study of aging changes in the human sinoatrial node and internodal tract. *Br Heart J* 1972;34:150–152.

148. Jordan J, Yamaguchi J, Mandel WJ. Characteristics of sinoatrial conduction in patients with coronary artery disease. *Circulation* 1988;55:569–574.

149. Engel TR, Meister SG, Feitosa GS, et al. Appraisal of sinus node artery disease. *Circulation* 1975;52:286–291.

150. Evans R, Shaw DB. Pathological studies in sinoatrial disorder (sick sinus syndrome). *Br Heart J* 1977;39:778–786.

151. Demoulin J-C, Kulbertus HE. Pathological correlates of atrial arrhythmias. In: Kilbertus HE, ed. *Reentrant arrhythmias: mechanisms and treatment.* Lancaster, UK: MTP Press, 1976:99–113.

152. Demoulin J-C, Kulbertus HE. Histopathological correlates of sinoatrial disease. *Br Heart J* 1978;40:1384–1389.

153. Kaplan BM, Langendorf R, Lev M, et al. Tachycardia-bradycardia syndrome (so-called "sick sinus syndrome"). *Am J Cardiol* 1973;26:497–508.

154. Rasmussen K. Chronic sinus node disease: natural course and indication for pacing. *Eur Heart J* 1982;1:455–459.

155. Tan ATH, Ee BK, Mah PK, et al. Diffuse conduction abnormalities in an adolescent with familial sinus node disease. *Pacing Clin Electrophysiol* 1981;4:645–649.

156. Surawicz B, Harriman RJ. Follow-up of the family with congenital absence of sinus rhythm. *Am J Cardiol* 1988;61:467–469.

157. Greenwood RD, Rosenthal A, Sloss LJ, et al. Sick sinus syndrome after surgery for congenital heart disease. *Circulation* 1975;52:208–213.

158. Gilette PC, Kugler JD, Garson AT Jr, et al. Mechanisms of cardiac arrhythmias after the Mustard operation for transposition of the great arteries. *Am J Cardiol* 1980;45:1225–1230.

159. Desai JM, Scheinman MM, Strauss HC, et al. Electrophysiologic effects of combined autonomic blockade in patients with sinus node disease. *Circulation* 1981;63:953–960.

160. Scheinman MM, Strauss HC, Evans GT, et al. Adverse effects of sympatholytic agents in patients with hypertension and sinus node dysfunction. *Am J Med* 1978;64:1013–1020.

161. Benditt DG, Benson DW Jr, Dunnigan A, et al. Drug therapy in sinus node dysfunction. In: Rapaport E, ed. *Cardiology update.* New York: Elsevier, 1984:79–101.

162. Maisch B, Lotze U, Schneider J, Kochsrek K. Antibodies to the human sinus node in sick sinus syndrome. *Pacing Clin Electrophysiol* 1986;9:1101–1109.

163. Adgey AAJ, Gedees JS, Mulholland HC, et al. Incidence, significance and management of early bradyarrhythmia, complicating acute myocardial infarction. *Lancet* 1968;2:1097–1101.

164. Rokseth R, Hatle L. Sinus arrest in acute myocardial infarction. *Br Heart J* 1971;33:639–642.

165. Parameswaran R, Ohe T, Goldberg H. Sinus node dysfunction in acute myocardial infarction. *Br Heart J* 1976;38:93–96.

166. Hatle L, Bathen J, Rokseth R. Sinoatrial disease in acute myocardial infarction: long-term prognosis. *Br Heart J* 1976;38:410–414.

167. Szatmary L, Jouve A, Pinot JJ, Torresani J. Comparative study of electrophysiological and Holter monitoring data in estimating sinoatrial function: significance of intrinsic heart rate in disclosing autonomic sinus node dysfunction. *Cardiology* 1983;70:184–193.

168. Reiffel JA, Bigger JT Jr, Cramer M, Reid DS. Ability of Holter electrocardiographic recording and atrial stimulation to detect sinus nodal dysfunction in symptomatic and asymptomatic patients with sinus bradycardia. *Am J Cardiol* 1977;40:189–194.

169. Crook BR, Cashman PM, Stott FD, Raftery EB. Tape monitoring of the electrocardiogram in ambulant patients with sinoatrial disease. *Br Heart J* 1973;35:1009–1013.

170. Stern S, Ben-Shachar G, Tzivoni D, et al. Detection of transient arrhythmias by continuous long-term recording of electrocardiograms of active subjects. *Isr J Med Sci* 1970;6:103–112.

171. Brodsky M, Wu D, Denes P, et al. Arrhythmias documented by 24 hour continuous electrocardiographic monitoring in 50 male medical students without apparent heart disease. *Am J Cardiol* 1977;39:390–396.

172. Johansson BW. Long-term ECG in ambulatory clinical practice. *Eur J Cardiol* 1977;5:39–48.

173. Ledieffre J, Libersa C, Caron J, et al. Electrocardiographic aspects of sinus node dysfunction: use of the Holter electrocardiographic recording. In: Levy S, Scheinman MM, eds. *Cardiac arrhythmias: from diagnosis to therapy.* Mount Kisco, NY: Futura Publishing, 1984:73–76.

174. Grodman RS, Capone RJ, Most AS. Arrhythmia surveillance by transtelephonic monitoring: comparison with Holter monitoring in symptomatic ambulatory patients. *Am Heart J* 1979;98:459–464.

175. Fowler NO, Fenton JC, Conway GF. Syncope and cerebral dysfunction caused by bradycardia without atrioventricular block. *Am Heart J* 1970;80:303–312.

176. Eraut D, Shaw DB. Sinus bradycardia. *Br Heart J* 1971;33:742–749.

177. Holden W, McAnulty JW, Rahimtoola SN. Characterization of heart rate response to exercise in the sick sinus syndrome. *Br Heart J* 1978;40:923–930.

178. Valin HO, Edhag KO. Heart rate responses in patients with sinus node disease compared to controls: physiological implications and diagnostic possibilities. *Clin Cardiol* 1980;3:391–398.

179. Johnston FA, Robinson JF, Fyfe T. Exercise testing in the diagnosis of sick sinus syndrome in the elderly: implications for treatment. *Pacing Clin Electrophysiol* 1987;10:831–838.

180. Abbott JA. Hirschfeld DS, Kunkel FW, et al. Graded exercise testing in patients with sinus node dysfunction. *Am J Med* 1977;62:330–338.

181. Buetikofer J, Fetter J, Milstein S, et al. Variability of sinoatrial rate-response during exercise: impact on assessment of chronotropic competence in sinus node dysfunction. *Pacing Clin Electrophysiol* 1988;11:531(abst).

182. Benditt DG, Buetikofer J, Fetter J, et al. Variability of sinoatrial rate-response during exercise testing in sinus node dysfunction. *Pacing Clin Electrophysiol* 1988;11:298(abst).

183. Reiffel JA. Electrophysiologic evaluation of sinus node function. *Cardiol Clin* 1986;4:401–416.

184. Reiffel JA, Ferrick K, Zimmerman J, Bigger JT Jr. Electrophysiologic studies of the sinus node and atria. *Cardiovasc Clin* 1985;16:37–59.

185. Benditt DG, Milstein S, Goldstein M, et al. Sinus node dysfunction: pathophysiology, clinical features, evaluation, and treatment. In: Zipes DP, Jalife J, eds. *Cardiac electrophysiology: from cell to bedside.* Philadelphia: WB Saunders, 1990:708–734.

186. Reiffel JA, Juehnert M. Electrophysiologic testing of sinus node

function: diagnostic and prognostic application (including updated information from sinus node electrograms). *Pacing Clin Electrophysiol* 1994;17:349–365.

187. Strauss HC, Grant AO, Scheinman MM, et al. The use of cardiac stimulation techniques to evaluate sinus node dysfunction. In: Little RC, ed. *Physiology of atrial pacemakers.* Mount Kisco, NY: Futura Publishing, 1980:339–365.

188. Tonkin AM, Heddle WF. Electrophysiological testing of sinus node function. *Pacing Clin Electrophysiol* 1984;5:637–648.

189. Mandel WJ, Hayakawa H, Allen HN, et al. Assessment of sinus node function in patients with sick sinus syndrome. *Circulation* 1972;46:761–769.

190. Jordan J, Yamaguchi I, Mandel WJ, et al. Comparative effects of overdrive on sinus and subsidiary pacemaker function. *Am Heart J* 1977;3:367–374.

191. Kulvertus HE, De Leval-Rutten F, Mary L, et al. Sinus node recovery time in the elderly. *Br Heart J* 1975;37:420–425.

192. Pop T, Fleischmann D. Measurement of sinus node recovery time after atrial pacing. In: Bonke FIM, ed. *The sinus node: structure, function and clinical relevance.* The Hague: Martinus Nijhoff, 1978:23–35.

193. Reiffel JA, Gang E, Bigger JR Jr, et al. Sinus node recovery time related to paced cycle length in normals and patients with sinoatrial dysfunction. *Am Heart J* 1982;104:746–752.

194. Gang E, Reiffel JA, Livelli FD Jr, Bigger JT Jr. Sinus node recovery time following the spontaneous termination of supraventricular tachycardia and following overdrive pacing: a comparison. *Am Heart J* 1983;105:210–215.

195. Dhingra RC, Amat-y-Leon F, Wyndham C, et al. Electrophysiologic effects of atropine on human sinus node and atrium. *Am J Cardiol* 1976;38:429–434.

196. Cappato R, Alboni P, Paparella N, et al. Bedside evaluation of sinus bradycardia: usefulness of atropine test in discriminating organic from autonomic involvement of sinus automaticity. *Am Heart J* 1987;114:1384–1288.

197. Gaskell WM. On the innervation of the heart with special reference to the tortoise. *J Physiol (Lond)* 1984;4:43–127.

198. Delius W, Wirtzfeld A. Significance of sinus node recovery time in sick sinus syndrome. In: Luderitz B, ed. *Cardiac pacing.* Berlin: Springer-Verlag, 1976:25–32.

199. Gang ES, Oseran DS, Mandel WJ, Peter T. Sinus node electrogram in patients with the hypersensitive carotid sinus syndrome. *J Am Coll Cardiol* 1985;5:1484–1490.

200. Schmidt G, Mashima S, Takayanagi K, Murao S. Studies on the mechanisms of secondary pause after high rate atrial pacing. *J Electrocardiol* 1984;17:79–84.

201. Narula OS, Samet P, Javier R. Significance of the sinus node recovery time. *Circulation* 1972;45:140–158.

202. Reiffel JA, Gang E, Livelli FD Jr, et al. Clinical and electrophysiologic characteristics of sinoatrial entrance block evaluated by direct sinus node electrography: prevalence, relation to antegrade sinoatrial conduction time, and relevance to sinus node disease. *Am Heart J* 1981;102:1011–1014.

203. Benditt DG, Strauss HC, Scheinman MM, et al. Analysis of secondary pauses following termination of rapid atrial pacing in man. *Circulation* 1976;54:436–441.

204. Narula OS, Shanttha N, Vasquez M, et al. A new method for measurement of sinoatrial conduction time. *Circulation* 1978; 58:706–714.

205. Strauss HC, Saroff AL, Bigger JR Jr, Giardina EG. Premature atrial stimulation as a key to the understanding of sinoatrial conduction in man. *Circulation* 1973;47:86–93.

206. Gomes JAC, Kang PS, El-Sherif N. The sinus node electrogram in patients with and without sick sinus syndrome: techniques and correlation between directly measured and indirectly estimated sino-atrial conduction time. *Circulation* 1982;66:864–867.

207. Gomed JAC, Winters SL. The origins of the sinus node pacemaker complex in man: demonstration of dominant and subsidiary foci. *J Am Coll Cardiol* 1987;9:45–52.

208. Kirkorian G, Touboul P, Atallah G, et al. Premature atrial stimulation during regular atrial pacing: a new approach to the study of the sinus node. *Am J Cardiol* 1984;54:109–114.

209. Grant AO, Kirkorian G, Benditt DG, et al. The estimation of sinoatrial conduction time in rabbit heart by the constant atrial pacing technique. *Circulation* 1979;60:597–604.

210. Reiffel JA, Ferrick K, Bigger JT Jr. Sinus node dysfunction: diagnostic and therapeutic pacing. *Intelligence Rep Card Pacing Electrophysiol* 1983;1:1–5.

211. Reiffel JA, Gang E, Glicklich J, et al. The human sinus node electrogram: a transvenous catheter technique and a comparison of directly measured and indirectly estimated sinoatrial conduction time in adults. *Circulation* 1980;62:1324–1334.

212. Gomes JAC, Hariman RI, Chowdry IA. New application of direct sinus node recordings in man: assessment of sinus node recovery time. *Circulation* 1984;70:663–671.

213. Hariman RJ, Krongrad E, Boxer RA, et al. Method for recording electrical activity of the sinoatrial node and automatic atrial foci during cardiac catheterization in human subjects. *Am J Cardiol* 1978;45:775–781.

214. Juillard A, Guillerm F, Chuong HV, et al. Sinus node electrogram recording in 59 patients. Comparison with simulation. *Br Heart J* 1983;50:75–84.

215. Reiffel JA, Bigger JT Jr, Giardina EGV. "Parodoxical" prolongation of sinus nodal recovery time after atropine in the sick sinus syndrome. *Am J Cardiol* 1975;36:98–104.

216. Gupta PK, Lichstein E, Chadd KD, et al. Appraisal of sinus nodal recovery time in patients with sick sinus syndrome. *Am J Cardiol* 1974;34:265–270.

217. Szatmary L, Medvedowsky J-L, Barnay C, et al. Electrophysiological classification of normal and pathological sinus node function. *Acta Med Acad Sci Hung* 1982;39:47–61.

218. Fujimora O, Yee R, Klein GJ, et al. The diagnostic sensitivity of electrophysiologic testing in patients with syncope caused by transient bradycardia. *N Engl J Med* 1989;321:1703–1707.

219. Gann D, Tolentino R, Samet P. Electrophysiologic evaluation of elderly patients with sinus bradycardia. *Arch Intern Med* 1979; 90:24–32.

220. Gann D, Samet P. Diagnostic and prognostic value of intracardiac electrophysiological studies: ten years of experience. *Bull Physiopathol Respir* 1979;15:839–860.

221. Kerr CR, Strauss HC. The measurement of sinus node refractoriness in man. *Circulation* 1984;68:1231–1237.

222. Kerr CR, Strauss HC, Aiama N. Effect of basic pacing cycle length on sinus node refractoriness in the rabbit. *Am J Cardiol* 1985;56:162–167.

223. Kerr CR. Effect of pacing cycle length and autonomic blockade on sinus node refractoriness. *Am J Cardiol* 1988;62:1192–1196.

224. Resh W, Feuer J, Wesley RC Jr. Intravenous asdenosine: a noninvasive diagnostic test for sick sinus syndrome. *Pacing Clin Electrophysiol* 1982;15:2068–2072.

225. Burnett D, Abi-Samra F, Vacek JL. Use of intravenous adenosine as a noninvasive diagnostic test for sick sinus syndrome. *Am Heart J* 1999;137:435–438.

226. Schweitzer P, Mark H. The effect of atropine on cardiac arrhythmias and conduction. Part 2. *Am Heart J* 1980;100: 255–261.

227. Albin G, Hayes DL, Holmes DR. Sinus node dysfunction in pediatric and young adult patients: treatment by implantation of a permanent pacemaker in 39 cases. *Mayo Clin Proc* 1985;60: 667–672.

228. Sasaki S, Takeuchi A, Ohzeki M, et al. Long-term follow up of paced patients with sick sinus syndrome. In: Steinback K,

Glogar D, Laszkovics A, et al, eds. *Cardiac pacing. Proceedings of the VIIth World Symposium on Cardiac Pacing.* Darmstadt: Steinkopff Verlag, 1983:85–90.

229. Conde CA, Leppo J, Lipski J, et al. Effectiveness of pacemaker treatment in the bradycardia-tachycardia syndrome. *Am J Cardiol* 1973;32:209–214.

230. Simon AG, Zloto AE. Symptomatic sinus node disease: natural history after permanent ventricular pacing. *Pacing Clin Electrophysiol* 1979;2:305–314.

231. Rosenqvist M, Brandt J, Schuller H. Atrial versus ventricular pacing in sinus node disease: a treatment comparison study. *Am Heart J* 1986;111:292–297.

232. Stone JM, Bhakta RD, Lutgen J. Dual chamber sequential pacing management of sinus node dysfunction: advantages over single-chamber pacing. *Am Heart J* 1982;104:1319–1327.

233. Mong HH. The bradyarrhythmias: current indications for permanent pacing (Part I). *Pacing Clin Electrophysiol* 1981;4: 432–442.

234. Reiffel JA. Clinical evaluation of the prospective pacemaker patient. In: Saksena S, Goldschlager N, eds. *Electrical therapy for cardiac arrhythmias: pacing, antitachycardia device, catheter ablation.* Philadelphia: WB Saunders, 1990:139–153.

235. Hartel G, Talvensaari T. Treatment of sinoatrial syndrome with permanent cardiac pacing in 90 patients. *Acta Med Scand* 1975; 198:341–347.

236. Moss AJ, Davis RJ. Brady-tachy syndrome. *Prog Cardiovasc Dis* 1974;16:439–454.

237. Wohl AJ, Laborrde J, Atkins JM, et al. Prognosis of patients permanently paced for sick sinus syndrome. *Arch Intern Med* 1976;136:406–408.

238. Scheinman MM, Strauss HC, Abbott JA. Electrophysiologic testing for patients with sinus node dysfunction. *J Electrocardiol* 1979;12:211–216.

239. Lichstein E, Aithal H, Jonas S, et al. Natural history of severe sinus bradycardia discovered by a 24 hour Holter monitoring. *Pacing Clin Electrophysiol* 1982;5:185–189.

23

ATRIOVENTRICULAR NODAL CONDUCTION ABNORMALITIES

MORTON F. ARNSDORF
RALPH VERDINO

ANATOMY OF THE ATRIOVENTRICULAR NODE

Sunao Tawara authored a remarkable study of the cardiac conduction system in 1906 (1). Even today this article is a standard reference for workers in this field, and Anderson and Ho (2) believe that much confusion and debate could have been avoided if investigators had followed the criteria of Tawara. The anatomy of the atrioventricular (AV) node has been reviewed recently, and there are differences of opinion concerning its structure and function (2–4). The atria are normally functionally isolated from the ventricles by the annuli fibrosi and conduction from the atria to the ventricles is through the AV node. During inscription of the P wave, the impulse enters the AV node, but the magnitude of the nodal signal is too small to produce a surface electrocardiographic (ECG) deflection and an isoelectric period follows the P wave.

The anatomy and cell types of the AV node are complex, and much debate still exists. The AV node is located beneath the endocardium of the right atrium and above the insertion of the septal leaflet of the tricuspid valve. It is located anterior to the ostium of the coronary sinus and near the "fast" perinodal fibers that are involved in AV nodal reentrant tachycardias.

The AV node consists of a number of cell types. Paes de Carvalho and De Almeida (5) separated the AV node into three functional zones: AN, N, and NH, representing cells considered *nodal* (N) cells, which presumably make up the major population in the compact AV node and transitional cells (AN) between the node and the atria and (NH) those between the node and the bundle of His. Anatomically, they considered the node as a three-layered structure arranged in parallel with the fibrous annulus. In this scheme, the slowest speed of propagation was thought to be in the N zone. Bil-

lette and Shrier (4) have further subdivided these zones into six cell groups based on their response to premature atrial activation: the AN, ANCO, ANL, N, NH, and H regions. AN cells have action potentials with a phase of rapid depolarization and rapid and slow repolarization. ANCO cells are lower in amplitude and are notched. ANL cells are similar to AN and N cells. N cells, compared with ANL cells, have a slower rate of rise, a smaller amplitude, and a less negative resting potential. H cells have action potentials that look like those of Purkinje fibers with a well-developed phase 0 through 4. The N and NH cells in the central node are responsible for about 50% of the delay.

Janse and colleagues (6) consider the AV node to consist of transitional, midnodal, and lower nodal cells, which are analogous to the cells types in the scheme by Paes de Carvalho and De Almeida. The major difference in schemes is that the N zone, according to Janse and colleagues, is thought to be confined to a small, central area that is surrounded at its anterior, superior, and posterior margins by the AN zone. Inferiorly, contact is made with NH and H cells.

Anderson and Ho (2) consider the AV junction to include the compact AV node and transitional cells that are located between the compact AV node and the atrium. In their view, transitional cells are situated between the atrial myocytes of the right side of the primary atrial septum. These transitional cells, in the view of Anderson and Ho (2), can extend anteriorly or inferiorly and posteriorly. The anterior run can be traced from the anterior and superior rim of the fossa ovalis toward the septal leaflet of the tricuspid valve, forming in part the atrial border of the Koch triangle. This area contains the so-called *fast pathways*. The inferior and posterior run consists of the transitional cells that are part of the "slow pathway." The distal portion of the AV node becomes the penetrating portion of the His bundle when it enters the central fibrous body. These authors underscore the likely importance of cell-cell orientation, the location of gap junctions, and the characteristics of ionic channels. These factors would create anisotropic conduction.

M. F. Arnsdorf and R. Verdino: Department of Cardiology, University of Chicago Hospital, Chicago, Illinois 60637.

INTRODUCTORY ELECTROPHYSIOLOGY

At this point, it is useful to make a few comments concerning the cellular electrophysiology of the AV node. As discussed already, there are a number of cell types, each of which has a somewhat different but characteristic action potential. For the clinician, however, it is useful to consider the AV node as a single entity with conduction determined largely by cells that depend on the slow inward calcium current (I_{Ca}) for phase 0 depolarization, which along with geometric considerations, results in a slow conduction velocity, realizing that the fast and slow pathways as well as the His bundle have different electrophysiologic properties.

More specifically, the kinetically fast sodium current (I_{Na}), which is responsible for the rapid depolarization phase of tissues of the atria, His-Purkinje system, and ventricles, is not evident. In the AV node, phase 0 depolarization is dominantly caused by the I_{Ca}, carried by a Ca^{2+} channel (l type). The repolarization of the action potential and reactivation of the calcium channel are complex. In the AV node, the I_{Ca} recovers slowly, and reactivation cannot occur until well into electrical diastole, limiting the rate at which action potentials can be reinitiated. In the AV node, this property would limit the maximal impulse rate and thereby protect the ventricles in case of atrial fibrillation or flutter.

The intracardiac ECG allows assessment of the function of the AV node, because the structure is bracketed by the recording of the low atrial, or A wave, and the deflection caused by activation of the bundle of His. Spontaneously or with pacing the heart at a fixed rate, the A-H time (and PR interval) will remain constant until the relative refractory period (RRP) is encroached upon, at which time the A-H time will increase,

indicating slower conduction in the AV node. If the heart rate is increased further, one of two events occur. Most commonly, A-H transmission will fail because the atrial impulse is now encroaching upon the effective refractory period (ERP) of the AV node, and the A wave will not be followed by an H spike. In some individuals, there will be a discontinuous jump to a new steady state in which the A-H interval is quite long. This is typical of dual AV nodal physiology in which there are two pathways with different conduction velocities and different refractory periods; the dual AV nodal physiology underlies reentrant AV nodal tachycardia.

The same type of observations are made if the atria are paced at a fixed cycle length and progressively premature atria are introduced. Panel A of Figure 23-1 shows that as the time between the last basic driven stimulus (A1) and the premature electrical atrial depolarization (A2), the response to each stimulus recorded in the His bundle (H1 and H2, respectively) decreases equally, resulting in a line of identity. With sufficient prematurity, a decrease in the A_1-A_2 interval results in a smaller decrease or even an increase in the H_1-H_2 interval, indicating that the AV node is now in its RRP. The A_1-A_2 interval that fails to conduct through the AV node defines the ERP. The same type of "J" configuration is seen in panel B, but at a critical A_1-A^2 interval, there is a sudden jump to another pathway characterized by a much longer A-H interval. The jump is from a pathway with faster conduction (F) to one with slower conduction (S), compatible with a dual-pathway physiology. Inspection of the curve also reveals that the F pathway has a longer refractory period than the S pathway. Echo beats and sustained AV nodal reentry can occur after the jump to the S pathway.

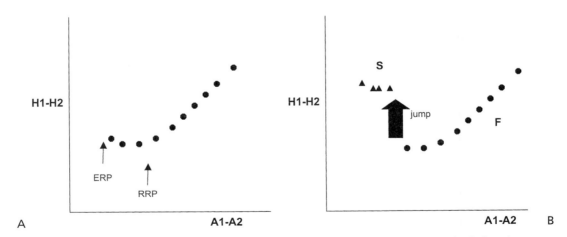

FIGURE 23-1. Diagrammatic representations of curves assessing the electrophysiologic function of the atrioventricular (AV) node. A1 is the last atrial depolarization in a string of basic electrically induced beats having the same cycle length. An electrical premature depolarization is triggered off the last A1, and this is called A2. On emerging from the AV node, a His potential *(H)* is noted; in this case, A1 gives rise to H1 and A2 to H2. The plot is of H_1-H_2 as a function of A_1-A_2. These two recording sites bracket the AV node. ERP, effective refractory period; RRP, relative refractory period; F, fast pathway; S, slow pathway. See text for discussion of **(A)** common AV nodal electrophysiology and **(B)** dual AV nodal physiology.

Figure 23-2 is an intracardiac recording of a "jump" from a "fast" pathway to a "slow" pathway. The top tracing is the high right atrial electrogram (HRA) and the lower tracing is the His bundle electrogram. The atria were paced at a cycle length of 360 ms, and the atrial electrogram is prominent in the HRA tracing. Note that the first three beats show an increasing A-H time of 91, 101, and 116 ms. This rate results in increasing encroachment on the RRP of the "fast" pathway and shows some characteristics of the Wenckebach phenomenon. The fourth and fifth beats show a sudden large jump to a much slower pathway with A-H times of 279 and 289 ms, respectively. The HV time remained constant.

Autonomic modulation of the AV node is also important with both vagal and adrenergic inputs (6). These inputs and the key location of cells that depend on I_{Ca} underlie the pharmacologic actions of digitalis that increases vagal tone, atropine that blocks vagal tone, β adrenoreceptor blockers, and calcium antagonists among other drugs.

Concealed Conduction

Concealed conduction is a common electrophysiologic event in which there is incomplete penetration of the AV junction with an unexpected effect on the next beat, or as stated by Pick and Langendorf, "The conduction was called concealed because in the surface ECG its presence was recognized only indirectly, by its aftereffects" (7). As discussed in the last section, the conduction velocity and the refractoriness of the AV node are very sensitive to the frequency and prematurity of beats with complicated relationships describing the input and output across the AV node. Mechanistically, the refractoriness caused by the incompletely conducted beat in the AV junction may affect (a) conduction on the subsequent beat by causing delay, block, repetitive concealment, rarely enhancement, and sometimes reentry, and (b) impulse formation in the subsequent beat by resetting a dominant pacemaker.

Examples of the effect on conduction include atrial flutter with a 2 : 1 AV conduction in which concealed conduction causes the block of alternate beats and the prolongation of the flutter-wave R interval of the conducted beats; the prolongation caused by a preceding atrial premature beat that partially penetrates the AV node; and a Mobitz type I (Wenckebach) second-degree block at the level of the AV node. Similarly, an infranodal beat arising in the His bundle, fascicles, or terminal Purkinje fibers may incompletely penetrate the AV junction by retrograde depolarization. An example of the effect on impulse formation of the subsequent beat includes a sinus beat penetrating the AV junction without causing ventricular depolarization but sufficiently to reset a junctional pacemaker or cause a pseudo-AV block on the ECG.

Atrioventricular Dissociation and Block

The most rapid pacemaker that reaches ventricular tissue is responsible for the heart beat. Usually, this is the pacemaker in the sinoatrial (SA) node, which is located in the high right atrium near the junction with the superior vena cava. The propagating wavefront activates the right atrium and then the left atrium, producing the P wave, and during the ECG, a silent period on the surface ECG (the PR segment) slowly

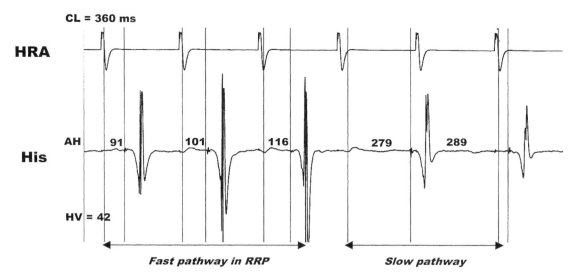

FIGURE 23-2. Intracardiac recording of a "jump" from a "fast" pathway to a "slow" pathway. Shown are **(top trace)** the high right atrial electrogram *(HRA)* and **(bottom trace)** the His bundle electrogram. The atria were paced at a cycle length of 360 ms. The A-H intervals are indicated by the numbers (in milliseconds). The first three beats show an increasing A-H time of 91, 101, and 116 ms, representing a rate-induced progressive increase in the refractoriness of the "fast" pathway. The fourth and fifth beats show a sudden jump to a much slower pathway with A-H times of 279 and 289 ms, respectively. The HV time was constant at 42 ms.

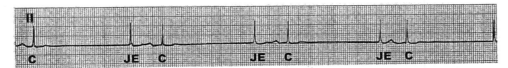

FIGURE 23-3. Marked sinus bradycardia with a variable PR interval that captures the ventricles *(C)* but is sufficiently slow so a junctional escape appears *(JE)*. The sinus and the junctional rates are depressed, at rates of approximately 30 and 38 beats per minute, respectively. Notice that the last P wave falls in the T wave of the JE and that it has a longer PR interval than elsewhere; the PR explained by concealed conduction into the atrioventricular (AV) node from the JE that renders the AV node relatively refractory and causes the PR interval to prolong.

traverses the AV node, conducts rapidly through the His bundle, the right and left fascicles of the bundles, and the terminal web of Purkinje fibers. The ventricles are then activated by impulses emerging from the terminal Purkinje fibers, resulting in the QRS complex. The advent of intracardiac ECG does allow for the recording of SA nodal, His bundle, bundle branch, and other potentials.

AV dissociation describes the "independence" between the atrial and ventricular beats, which may occur for a single beat or many beats (8). The AV conduction system consists of two parts: the AV node and the infranodal His bundle branch (or fascicular) of the His-Purkinje system.

The AV dissociation is complete if no supraventricular beat successfully traverses the AV conduction system and therefore fails to capture the ventricle at times in the cardiac cycle when a successful capture would be anticipated. AV dissociation is called *incomplete* when a supraventricular beat at times does traverse the AV conduction system, successfully capturing the ventricles.

AV dissociation can be caused by the slowing of the sinus rate below the rate of a lower pacemaker, usually junctional; acceleration of a lower pacemaker then competes with antegradely conducting beats (Fig. 23-7). The occurrence of AV block, which can be defined as a delay or interruption in the transmission of an impulse from the atria to the ventricles, is caused by an anatomic or functional impairment in the conduction system or by some combination of these two mechanisms.

AV dissociation is not synonymous with AV block (8,9). AV block is the most commonly encountered type of AV dissociation and is most related to the topic of bradyarrhythmias. These events can be seen with antegrade AV conduction, with retrograde ventriculoatrial (VA) conduction, or with both.

Terminology of AV Block

The conduction through the AV node can be delayed, intermittent, or absent. The commonly used terminology includes first-degree (slowed conduction and prolongation of the PR interval without missed beats) (Fig. 23-4), second-degree (missed beats, often in a regular pattern, e.g., 2 : 1, 3 : 2, or higher degrees of block) (Figs. 23-5 through 23-7), and third-degree or complete AV block (no relation-

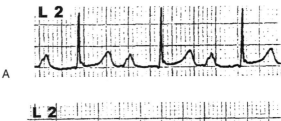

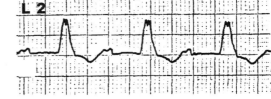

FIGURE 23-4. First-degree atrioventricular block in electrocardiographic lead II. **A:** PR duration of 0.306 seconds and a QRS duration of 0.08 seconds. **B:** PR duration of 0.40 seconds and a QRS duration of 0.15 seconds. (From Arnsdorf MF. First degree AV block. In: Rose B, Arnsdorf MF, Gersh B, et al, eds. *UpToDate in medicine*, vol 7.2 [Computerized database]. Wellesley, MA: UpToDate, Inc, 1999, with permission.)

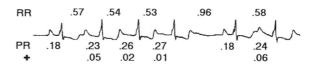

FIGURE 23-5. Classic Mobitz type I (Wenckebach) second-degree atrioventricular block. R-R, the interval between the QRS complexes; PR, the interval between the P wave and the QRS complex; and the increment (+) in the PR interval for each successive beat. See text for discussion. (From Arnsdorf MF. Second degree AV block, Mobitz type I [Wenckebach block]. In: Rose B, Arnesdorf MF, Gersh B, et al., eds. *UpToDate in medicine*, vol 7.2 [Computerized database]. Wellesley, MA: UpToDate, Inc, 1999, with permission.)

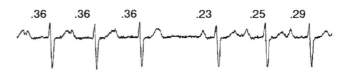

FIGURE 23-6. Long (17:16) atypical Mobitz type I (Wenckebach) second-degree atrioventricular block. For the reasons discussed in the text, it is important to scrutinize the PR intervals immediately before and after the dropped QRS complex. Otherwise, this tracing might be misdiagnosed as a Mobitz type II block. (From Arnsdorf MF. Second degree AV block, Mobitz type I [Wenckebach block]. In: Rose B, Arnsdorf MF, Gersh B, et al, eds. *UpToDate in medicine*, [Computerized database]. Wellesley, MA: UpToDate, Inc, 2001, with permission.)

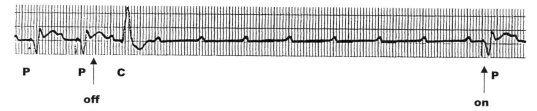

FIGURE 23-7. Mobitz type II second-degree atrioventricular block in which a series of P waves failed to conduct to the ventricles. P, beats paced by an artificial pacemaker that is turned off (*first arrow marked "off"*) and after the failure of conduction, "on" (*second arrow marked "on"*); C, a capture of the ventricle with a normal PR interval and a left bundle branch block pattern. (From Arnsdorf MF. Second degree AV Block, Mobitz type II. In: Rose B, Arnsdorf MF, Gersh B, et al, eds. *UpToDate in medicine,* [Computerized database]. Wellesley, MA: UpToDate, Inc, 1999, with permission.)

ship between the atrial and ventricular depolarizations) (Fig. 23-8).

Wenckebach (10) and Hay (11) independently used the jugular *a* and *c* waves to describe two types of second-degree AV block. Wenckebach (12) had previously described the phenomenon, which now bears his name, as a progressive increase in the a-c interval that preceded a nonconducted *a* wave. Wenckebach called the pauses recorded on the sphygmogram "Luciani periods," after the Italian physiologist who had described group beating with varying intervals between individual beats in the frog heart in 1872 (13,14).

Mobitz in 1924 divided second-degree heart block as determined by the ECG into two types (15). Mobitz type I second-degree AV block was characterized by a progressive PR interval prolongation preceded a nonconducted P wave; the phenomenon was described earlier by Wenckebach using pressure tracings (12) (Figs. 23-4 and 23-5).

Mobitz type II second-degree AV block was characterized by the PR interval remaining unchanged before one or more P waves that suddenly failed to conduct to the ventricles (Fig. 23-6). The Wenckebach type of second-degree AV block (Mobitz type I) is more common in the AV node while the Mobitz type II block is more common in the infranodal conduction system.

A 2 : 1 AV block can be considered a third type of second-degree heart block; it is a term applied when the mechanism (Mobitz type I or II) cannot be determined. High-

degree heart block is a term used to described a more advanced degree of AV block in which there is some conduction through the AV node for some beats while at other times, there is complete AV dissociation.

Third-degree, or complete, heart block is characterized by the failure of any atrial impulses reaching the ventricle (Figs. 23-8 and 23-9). Escape rhythms occur when a pacemaker other than the sinus node has sufficient time to depolarize, attain threshold, and produce a depolarization. In complete heart block, the escape rhythm that controls the ventricles can occur at any level below that of the conduction block, and the morphology of the QRS complex can help determine the location at which this is occurring—for example, a narrow complex originating in the AV junction or His bundle or wide complex from a ventricular focus.

All three degrees of heart block may be congenital or acquired. Lev (16) divided congenital heart block into two types: one occurring in a congenitally malformed heart and the other in an otherwise healthy heart. These are considered in more detail later in this chapter.

Bradyarrhythmias and Tachyarrhythmias

Bradyarrhythmias may arise when the impulse is blocked in the AV node and the lower escape pacemakers are slow, with symptoms depending on the hemodynamic consequences of the bradycardia. The AV block can be transient or per-

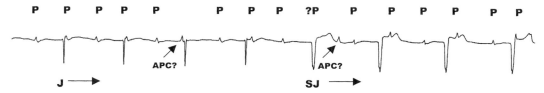

FIGURE 23-8. Complete heart block. The P waves are independent of the QRS complexes. The first four ventricular depolarizations (*J*) have a narrow QRS complex and arise from the His or junction above the bifurcation of the bundle branches. The rate of the junctional beats begins at about 50 beats per minute (bpm) and then slows below the rate of a lower, subjunctional pacemaker (*SJ*), which assumes control of the ventricles at a rate of about 43 bpm. Likely, the QRS is fusing with the P wave (*?P*). The first beat marked (*APC?*) resets the sinus node. The second is interpolated and does not affect the sinus rate.

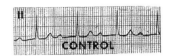

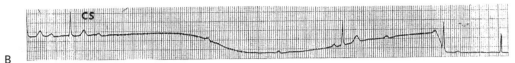

FIGURE 23-9. Intense vagal discharge as a cause of atrioventricular (AV) dissociation. **A:** Control with a prolonged PR interval. **B:** Carotid sinus massage results in a marked slowing of the sinus node, the failure of AV nodal transmission, and an inappropriately slow lower pacemaker. The asystolic period is 5.6 seconds. From Childers RC. Classification of cardiac dysrhythmias. *Med Clin North Am* 1976;60:3, with permission.)

manent. With first- and second-degree AV block, the setting is usually that of a slow sinus or atrial bradyarrhythmia in which conduction to the ventricles is impaired or intermittent and the lower escape pacemaker is sufficiently slow to produce a bradycardia.

When third-degree AV block is present, no beats are being transmitted from the atria to the ventricles. The ventricles are controlled by a junctional or subjunctional pacemaker. Frequently, the lower escape pacemaker is sluggish, resulting in a junctional or subjunctional bradycardia.

Tachyarrhythmias may arise when reentrant loops involve the AV node, such as AV nodal reentrant tachycardia and AV reentrant tachycardia (see Chapter 14)]. PR segment prolongation is often associated with these arrhythmias. AV nodal conduction abnormalities may also be associated. Bradycardia, tachycardias, and AV conduction disturbances may coexist in the so-called sick sinus syndrome.

Lown (17) first used the term *sick sinus syndrome* in 1967 to describe the sluggish return of SA nodal activity in some patients after direct-current (DC) electroversion. The term was later applied to a clinical syndrome characterized by chronic SA nodal dysfunction, a sluggish or absent SA nodal pacemaker after DC electroversion, frequently depressed escape pacemakers, and in more than 50% AV conduction disturbances (18,19). In more than half of cases, there is an alternating bradycardia and atrial tachyarrhythmias, with atrial fibrillation being the most common arrhythmia. In the absence of drugs that slow AV conduction, atrial fibrillation with a slow ventricular response reflects associated dysfunction of the AV node. Spontaneous reversion or DC cardioversion will typically produce a slow and often unstable sinus rhythm.

INCIDENCE AND PREVALENCE OF AV BLOCK

First-Degree AV Block

First-degree AV block is defined as PR-interval prolongation; the PR interval may be prolonged to more than 0.2

seconds in the absence of apparent heart disease (20–24) (Fig. 23-3). For example, first-degree AV block with PR intervals as long as 280 ms has been reported in 1.6% of healthy aviators (24). These individuals had a QRS complex within the normal duration range, and the prognosis was benign (24). Mathewson and colleagues (25) followed nearly 4,000 pilots for 27 years; 148 had first-degree AV block, and the morbidity and mortality rates in this group were the same as those for individuals with a normal PR interval (25). First-degree and second-degree (type I, Wenckebach) AV block is often present in healthy subjects, particularly during sleep (21,26–32), likely reflecting alterations in autonomic tone with enhancement of vagal tone.

Familial heart block is an autosomal dominant condition with incomplete penetrance in which AV nodal conduction disturbances progress through the years, and it is sometimes associated with fascicular or bundle branch block, eventually resulting in a high degree of AV block or even complete heart block with syncope and sudden death being not uncommon occurrences (33–35). The prognosis is not as benign if the delay is infranodal, with the possibility of it progressing to second-degree and eventually third-degree AV block.

Second-Degree AV Block

Mobitz Type I (Wenckebach)

Second-degree (type I, Wenckebach) AV block is often present in healthy subjects, particularly in athletes and during sleep (21,26–32) (Figs. 23-5 and 23-6). In healthy individuals, this largely reflects alterations in autonomic tone, with enhanced vagal effect. Most studies suggest a benign prognosis (22,27,32). However, one study of 16 infants with a second-degree type I AV block found that seven progressed to third-degree block (29).

The incidence of the location of block in second-degree Mobitz type I (Wenckebach) has been estimated as being the AV node in 72%, the bundle of His in 9%, and the bundle branches in 19% (36).

Mobitz Type II

The location of block in second-degree Mobitz type II block has been estimated to be in the bundle of His and bundle branches in about 20% and 80% of patients, respectively; it rarely occurs in the AV node (36) (Fig. 23-7). Type II block is permanent and frequently progresses to a higher degree of block or even complete heart block (37–41). Furthermore, at least two thirds of patients with this disorder have bifascicular or even trifascicular disease (42,43). The percentage of patients progressing to a higher degree of block requiring insertion of a pacemaker is uncertain, varying in part because of the presence or absence of other conduction disturbances. In one study, for example, 9 of 15 patients with Mobitz type II block had a preexisting bundle branch block, which was located distal to the bundle of His; of these patients, six had syncope within 6 months and received a pacemaker (39). The remaining three also received a pacemaker because of the development of congestive heart failure. There are only limited data on patients with type II block and a narrow QRS complex, but we have seen a number of cases that progressed to symptomatic heart block.

2 : 1 AV Block

A 2 : 1 AV block is quite common. The estimated incidence of the location of block in 2 : 1 AV block is 27% in the AV node, 23% in the bundle of His, and 50% in the bundle branches (36).

Third-Degree, or Complete, AV Block

Third-degree, or complete, AV block can be congenital or acquired (Figs. 23-8 through 23-10). Congenital complete heart block was first described in 1901 by Morquio, who also noted the familial occurrence and the association with Stokes-Adams attacks and death (44). The presence of fetal bradycardia (40 to 80 beats per minute [bpm]) as a manifestation of complete heart block was first noted in 1921 (45) and is currently the initial sign of this disorder in many cases. The incidence of congenital heart block is approximately 1 of 25,000 live births, but the incidence is higher in children with congenital heart disease (0.4% to 0.9%) (46).

The location of block in third-degree AV block in the general cardiologic population has been estimated based on the duration of the QRS complex and intracardiac recordings. In situations in which the QRS of the escape rhythm is narrow (less than 0.12 seconds), the interruption in conduction was found to be 48% in the AV

node and 52% in the bundle of His (36). About 6% of patients with a myocardial infarction develop third-degree AV block (see later discussion). In comparison, the block is in the fascicles or bundle of His in more than 80% of cases when the QRS is widened to more than 0.12 seconds (36).

ETIOLOGY OF AV BLOCK

A large number of processes can affect the AV conduction system. The most common are fibrosis and sclerosis (sclerodegenerative changes) of the conduction system and ischemic heart disease.

Fibrosis and Sclerosis

Fibrosis and sclerosis of the conduction system account for about one half of AV block cases and may be the result of several conditions that often cannot be distinguished clinically (47). Lenègre disease is a sclerodegenerative disease of the conduction system with some predilection in individuals older than 50 years for the right bundle branch and the left anterior fascicle (48). It is frequently associated with slow progression to complete heart block.

Lev disease is caused by fibrosis or calcification extending from any of the fibrous structures adjacent to the conduction system into the conduction system (16,49). Fibrosis of the top of the muscular septum is a common cause of right bundle branch block (RBBB) with left anterior fascicular block in the elderly patient. Calcification or fibrosis can also extend from the mitral or aortic valve rings into the conduction system. Involvement of the mitral ring or the central fibrous body, for example, may be the most common cause of complete heart block with a narrow QRS complex in the elderly patient. Aortic valve calcification, on the other hand, can invade the bundle of His, the right or left bundle branch, and the left anterior fascicle. Thus, the QRS complex may be prolonged.

Ischemic Heart Disease

The blood supply to the AV node is supplied by the AV nodal artery, which arises from the posterior descending branch of the right coronary artery in 85% to 90% of individuals and from the left circumflex artery in the remainder. Collateral circulation to the AV node arises from the left or the right coronary artery. The bundle of His has a dual blood supply from the AV nodal artery and the first septal branch of the anterior descending coronary artery.

About 40% of the cases of AV block have ischemic heart disease as the underlying cause (47). Conduction can be disturbed with chronic ischemic disease or during an acute myocardial infarction (50–54). About 20% of patients with

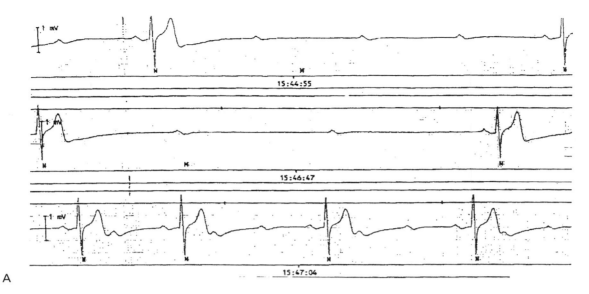

A

B

1 s

FIGURE 23-10. Intense vagal discharge as a cause of atrioventricular (AV) dissociation resulting from pain in a young man. **A:** Telemetry strip. **B:** Section of recordings on full disclosure. Note the profound AV dissociation with a return to a sinus tachycardia. Time bar equals 1 second. (From Fox W, Stein E. *Cardiac rhythm disturbances: a step-by-step approach.* Philadelphia: Lea & Febiger, 1983, with permission.)

an acute myocardial infarction develop AV block: 8% with first degree; 5% with second degree; and 6% with third degree (52–54).

AV block associated with inferior wall myocardial infarction—including first-degree, second-degree (Mobitz type I), and complete heart block—is located above the His bundle in 90% of patients (54a); this is why complete heart block often results in only a modest usually transient bradycardia with junctional or escape rhythm rates of more than 40 bpm. It is not uncommon, however, for the junctional pacemaker that controls the ventricles to accelerate to more than 60 bpm. The QRS complex is narrow in this setting and is associated with a low mortality rate.

AV block associated with anterior myocardial infarction—including first-degree, second-degree (Mobitz type II), or complete heart block—is more often located below the AV node. Chronic heart block with anterior myocardial infarction generally occurs abruptly in the first 24 hours. It can develop without warning or may be preceded by the development of an RBBB with a left anterior fascicular block or a left posterior fascicular block (bifascicular or trifascicular block) (55). The escape rhythm is wide and unstable and the event is associated with a high mortality rate from arrhythmias and pump failure.

Most serious conduction disturbances occur with anteroseptal myocardial infarction, and the degree of arrhythmic complications is directly related to the extent of infarction. It is usually symptomatic and has been associated with a mortality rate near 80%, partly because of a greater loss of functioning myocardium. The current mortality rate may be somewhat less as a result of improvements in the management of congestive heart failure and cardiogenic shock, but the risk remains substantial.

Conduction disturbance in inferior myocardial infarction can occur acutely or after hours or days. Sinus bradycardia, Mobitz type I (Wenckebach), and complete heart block are commonly seen, because the SA node, AV node, and His bundle are primarily supplied by the right coronary artery. Complete heart block with inferior myocardial infarction generally results from an intranodal lesion. It is associated with a narrow QRS complex and develops progressively from first- to second- to third-degree block. It often results in an asymptomatic bradycardia (40 to 60 bpm) and is usually transient, resolving within 5 to 7 days.

Intraventricular conduction disturbances, including bundle and fascicular blocks, also occur in 10% to 20% of cases of acute myocardial infarction (55–61). Left bundle branch block and RBBB with left anterior fascicle block are most common, each occurring in about one third of patients with an intraventricular conduction disturbance (57). RBBB with or without left posterior fascicular block and alternating bundle branch block are less frequently seen while isolated left anterior or posterior fascicle block is distinctly unusual.

Drugs

Several families of drugs can affect conduction and cause AV block. Drugs that affect the calcium-dependent cells in the AV node can slow conduction. The calcium channel antagonists diltiazem and verapamil slow conduction and increase the refractoriness of the AV node. The dihydropyridines have little or no effect. The difference is likely related to voltage-dependent conductances.

The autonomic nervous system may strongly influence AV nodal electrophysiology. Digoxin acts by increasing vagal tone. A sequence of ECGs during atrial fibrillation in the presence of digitalis excess are shown in Figure 23-11 and discussed later in this chapter.

β-Adrenoreceptor blockers cause a blockade or withdrawal of sympathetic tone with a relative increase in vagal tone. Amiodarone and propafenone can slow AV nodal conduction through several mechanisms including antagonism of calcium channels and β-adrenoreceptors. Adenosine, an antagonist of the α receptor, activates an outward repolarizing current and decreases an inward calcium current, which in turn hyperpolarizes a depolarized cell and shortens the duration of the action potential.

In comparison, antiarrhythmic drugs that modulate the sodium channel such as quinidine, procainamide, and disopyramide can produce block in the more distal His-Purkinje system. Some of these drugs, including the three mentioned, also have a potent atropine-like effect and may speed conduction through the AV node while hindering infranodal conduction, resulting in a decrease in the A-H interval and an increase in the HV interval with the PR interval remaining largely unchanged.

Increased Vagal Tone

Pain, carotid sinus massage, or hypersensitive carotid sinus syndrome can have a strong vagotonic effect that results in slowing of the sinus rate or the development of AV block. Vagal tone can be high during sleep and sufficient to produce a Wenckebach type of AV conduction disturbance in the healthy heart. ECGs showing intense vagal tone in patients during carotid massage and pain are shown in Figures 23-9 and 23-10 and are discussed in the related text in this chapter.

Valvular Disease

As already mentioned, calcification and fibrosis of the aortic or mitral valve rings can extend into the conduction system. AV block is not uncommonly associated with replacement of a calcified aortic or mitral valve, closure of a ventricular septal defect, or other surgical procedures (16, 62–65).

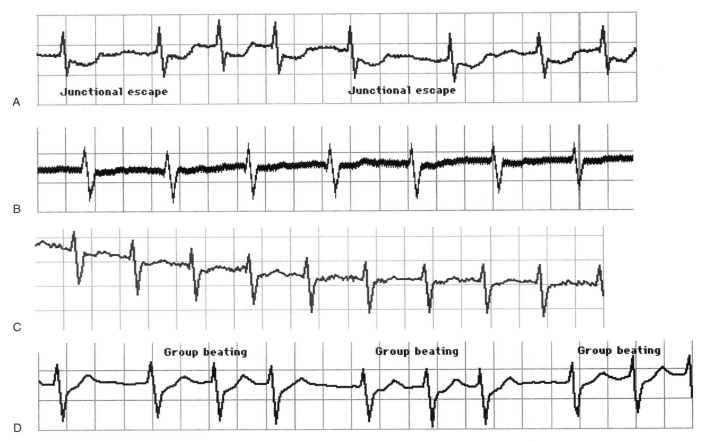

FIGURE 23-11. Atrial fibrillation and complete atrioventricular (AV) dissociation resulting from digitalis excess. **A:** Atrial fibrillation and junctional escapes. Note the irregularly irregular rhythm and the equal intervals of the junctional escape. **B:** Atrial fibrillation; complete AV block resulting from digitalis toxicity with the ventricles being controlled by an accelerated junctional pacemaker. **C:** Atrial fibrillation; AV block with the ventricles being controlled by an even faster junctional pacemaker. Note again the regular R-R intervals. **D:** Atrial fibrillation; complete AV block, the ventricles are controlled at an accelerated rate by a junctional pacemaker and the ventricular response shows group beating suggesting a Wenckebach-type conduction delay around or below the spontaneous pacemaker site. (From Arnsdorf MF. Electrocardiographic and electrophysiologic features of atrial fibrillation II. In: Rose B, Arnsdorf MF, Gersh B, et al, eds. UpToDate in medicine, vol 7.2 [Computerized database]. Wellesley, MA: UpToDate, Inc, 1999, with permission.)

Cardiomyopathies and Infiltrative Processes

Cardiomyopathies, including hypertrophic obstructive cardiomyopathy and infiltrative processes such as amyloidosis and sarcoidosis, can result in AV conduction disturbances (49,66). About 30% of individuals with hypertrophic cardiomyopathy also have His-Purkinje dysfunction (67).

Infiltrative malignancies, such as Hodgkin's disease, other lymphomas, and multiple myeloma, may also cause AV block. AV conduction disturbances may occur in the myotonic dystrophies (68).

AV block may result from tumors, hemochromatosis, and connective tissue disorders including lupus erythematosus, progressive systemic sclerosis, dermatomyositis, rheumatoid arthritis, and ankylosing spondylitis and hypothyroidism. Neurodegenerative diseases such as Duchenne progressive muscular dystrophy can also interfere with the conduction system.

Rarely, Paget disease may cause AV block, likely secondary to metastatic calcifications in the heart. Conduction abnormalities including complete and incomplete AV block and bundle branch block are more common in patients with severe Paget disease compared with healthy subjects (22% versus 4% and 20% versus 2.5%, respectively) (69).

Myocarditis

Myocarditis in a variety of inflammatory disorders may lead to AV block. These include rheumatic fever, Lyme disease, relapsing fever, diphtheria, viruses, systemic lupus erythematosus, toxoplasmosis, bacterial endocarditis, syphilis, numerous fungal diseases, and other causes. The list is long and has been well reviewed (70). The development of AV block with some causes of myocarditis may be a poor prognostic sign.

Infective Endocarditis

Infective endocarditis may cause an AV conduction disturbance. This is most common with a staphylococcal infection that involves the aortic valve and extends into the AV node (16).

Electrolyte Imbalance

Electrolyte change may affect AV conduction (71). The ratio of the intracellular to extracellular potassium concentration is about 35, so small changes in the extracellular concentration are greatly leveraged. An increasing $[K]o$ makes the resting potential less negative, inactivates the sodium channels, and alters repolarization. The result is a decrease in the conduction velocity in the atrial, His-Purkinje, and ventricular cells. There may be a transient acceleration in AV conduction at $[K]o$ of 5.5 to 6. Above this level, conduction begins to slow, an artificial pacemaker may no longer be able to capture the myocardium, fascicular block may appear, and asystole may result. Rarely, hyperkalemia may cause a conduction disturbance, presumably in the median fascicle of the left bundle, which mimics an anteroseptal myocardial infarction (72).

Infranodal Purkinje fibers have a paradoxical J-shaped relationship if the resting potential is plotted as a function of $[K]o$, so sodium channels may be inactivated at a high and a low $[K]o$. Significant AV block and intraventricular conduction disturbances may appear at a $[K]o$ of 2.7 or less.

Alterations in calcium levels are usually not associated with conduction disturbances. Extreme hypocalcemia may cause intermittent SA block, 2 : 1 AV block, and complete AV block. Severe hypercalcemia has been associated with sinus arrest and a Wenckebach AV nodal block.

Trauma

Trauma resulting from surgery or chest wall injury causes AV block. Intentional trauma may be used therapeutically, as in the use of AV nodal ablation to treat a patient with atrial fibrillation and a rapid ventricular response. Or it may be unintentional, such as heart block resulting from fast pathway ablation. An unusual case of myocardial bridging as a cause of paroxysmal AV block has been reported (73).

Congenital Heart Disease

Congenital complete heart block may be an isolated lesion or may be associated with other types of congenital heart disease, particularly congenitally corrected transposition of the great arteries. In the presence of congenital cardiac malformations. Lev and colleagues (74) has separated the congenital conditions into two categories. The first is the otherwise healthy heart and the second includes those situations that are associated with other types of congenital heart disease (75). When the heart is healthy, the cause of the conduction defect may be immune complexes that cross the placenta (i.e., anti-Ro/SSA and anti-La/SSB antibodies), fetal myocarditis, or idiopathic necrosis (76).

In the otherwise healthy heart, the type and location of the complete heart block depend on the histology of the junctional area (75). The most common types are (a) discontinuity between the atrial tissues and a hypoplastic nodal–bundle axis, (b) the AV node is normally formed but is discontinuous from the ventricular specialized tissues, and (c) the bundle branches are discontinuous from the branching bundle.

ECG MANIFESTATIONS
First-Degree AV Block

The PR interval includes activation of the atrium, AV node, His bundle, bundle branches and fascicles, and terminal Purkinje fibers. The normal range for the PR interval is between 120 and 200 ms (0.12 to 0.20 or even 0.21 seconds at slow rates) and tends to shorten with increases in heart rate resulting partly from rate-related and sympathetically mediated shortening of action potentials. As a rough approximation, the PR interval in most adults is approximately 210 ms at a rate of less than 70 bpm, 200 ms between 70 and 100 bpm, 180 to 190 ms between 100 and 130 bpm, and 170 ms at more than 130 bpm. Children younger than 14 years tend to have a PR interval of about 140 ms. Figure 23-4A shows a first-degree block with a normal QRS duration and Figure 23-4B displays first-degree AV block with a wide QRS complex. PR-interval prolongation most often occurs in the AV node, but the delay is likely to be infranodal in the presence of a wide QRS complex. This is discussed in more detail later in this chapter.

Second-Degree AV Block

In second-degree block, some atrial impulses fail to reach the ventricles. As already mentioned, Wenckebach in 1899 described a progressive delay between the atrial and the ventricular contraction and the eventual failure of an atrial beat to reach the ventricle (12). Twenty-five years later, Mobitz divided second-degree heart block, as determined by the ECG, into two types (15). Type I block was the phenomenon described by Wenckebach, which now was translated into ECG terms in which progressive PR-interval prolongation preceded a nonconducted P wave. Type II block was the phenomenon in which the PR interval remained unchanged before the P wave that suddenly failed to conduct to the ventricles.

Mobitz Type I (Wenckebach)

Classic Mobitz type I or Wenckebach block most commonly occurs in the AV node but may reflect a delay in the transmission of an impulse from the SA node to the atrium or in any part of the conduction system. It can be observed with antegrade AV conduction, retrograde VA conduction across the AV node, or as part of exit block with ectopic and parasystolic pacemakers. In the AV node, concealed conduction causes refractoriness in the AV junction that often is patterned.

The input must be fairly constant, and this input is usually the SA nodal pacemaker, which initiates atrial depolarization; however, the pacemaker providing the input may be an ectopic atrial focus. There needs to be an area of increasing conduction delay resulting in a nonconducted impulse (a "dropped beat"), and this occurs most commonly in the AV node. The P-P interval is constant but the PR interval is shortest in the first beat in the cycle and increases with each ensuing beat. The largest absolute increase in delay occurs in the first beat, a lesser increase in delay occurs in the second beat, and so forth. The impulse eventually conducts very slowly and block occurs, resulting in a dropped beat and in this case no QRS complex. If the pause between the last conducted beat and the first apparent beat of the next cycle is very long, the first beat may be a junctional escape, rather than a conducted beat; in this situation, the second beat of the new cycle will almost invariably have a PR interval shorter than that of the last conducted beat that preceded the dropped beat. Although the output (the P-P interval) will have a constant rate, in this case the QRS-QRS interval (more commonly called the R-R interval) usually decreases with each beat of the cycle; the shortening R-R interval results from the decreasing increment in delay of AV nodal conduction.

Figure 23-5 shows an ECG recording of a classic AV nodal Wenckebach block. The PR interval of beat one in a cycle increases by 0.05 seconds, thereby increasing the PR interval from 0.18 to 0.23 seconds. The PR interval of the next beat increases by 0.03 seconds, resulting in an increase in the PR interval from 0.23 to 0.26 seconds. As

a result, the R-R interval shortens and continues to do so as long as the increment of each successive beat is smaller than that of the beat that preceded it. Thus, the R-R interval that follows the blocked beat is longer than the R-R interval that precedes the dropped beat. Moreover, the cycle of the dropped beat is less than the summed cycles of any two previous cycles. This also results from the incremental conduction delay, as the P wave that is not conducted is closer to the preceding QRS than any other in the cycle. The classic Wenckebach pattern occurs usually with AV conduction ratios of 3 : 2, 4 : 3, or 5 : 4. This gives rise to a clustering of beats (group beating) with decreasing R-R intervals that tend to repeat. Not infrequently, mixed ratios occur.

AV conduction ratios of more than 7 : 6 usually show the atypical rather than the classic pattern. The progressive increment in PR interval becomes unpredictable and the PR interval remains prolonged but is constant. The most common explanation is that the sinus rate changes, which in turn influences the PR interval through hemodynamic and autonomic effects. The PR interval is still longest in the beat before the dropped beat and shortest in the first beat of the cycle, and then increases in the second beat. Figure 23-6 shows the dropped beat in a 17 : 16 AV Wenckebach. Note that the PR interval is quite constant at 0.36 seconds before the P wave that is not conducted. The next beat has a PR interval of 0.23 seconds, which may be conducted or may result from the similarity in escape times of the sinus node and the junction. The second and third beats after the pause are conducted with PR intervals of 0.25 and 0.29 seconds, respectively (Fig. 23-6).

The ECG cannot define with certainty the site of the Mobitz type I block, although the classic pattern favors the AV node as the site of delay. The diagnosis cannot be made from the ECG if there is 2 : 1 AV block, because type I (increasing PR interval) and type II (constant PR interval) cannot be distinguished if there is only one conducted beat in the cycle. In this setting, a long rhythm strip should be obtained or a previous ECG examined to try to find a 3 : 2 cycle. The administration of atropine also may induce 3 : 2 conduction.

The 2 : 1 AV response in atrial flutter, however, is almost invariably at the level of the AV node. Concealed conduction of the apparently blocked atrial impulses may prolong the time from the flutter wave to the QRS complex, at times causing alternation of the ventricular cycle length depending on the penetrance of the AV node.

If the ventricles are controlled by a pacemaker in the His bundle or below the His bundle, retrograde conduction may occur, which may partially or impartially penetrate the AV node. Retrograde VA Wenckebach is not an uncommon event, and if the RP interval gets sufficiently long, a ventricular echo beat may result.

Mobitz Type II

Type II block in which the PR interval remains unchanged before the P wave or several P waves that suddenly fail to conduct to the ventricles. The PR interval may be within the normal range or slightly prolonged.

Figure 23-7 is an interesting example of a Mobitz type II second-degree AV block in which a series of P waves failed to conduct to the ventricles. The first two beats are paced (P) by an artificial pacemaker, and the arrow indicates when the pacemaker was turned off. This is followed by a P wave that captures the ventricles producing a wide QRS complex (C), identical to that of the left bundle branch block pattern the patient had before the need for an artificial pacemaker. After the single conducted sinus beat, eight P waves that fail to reach the ventricles are observed. The artificial pacemaker is then turned on, resulting in a QRS complex.

Third-Degree AV Dissociation and Block

As mentioned earlier, AV dissociation describes the "independence" between the atrial and the ventricular beat, which may occur for one beat or continue for many beats (8). If no supraventricular beat traverses the AV conduction system at a time in the cardiac cycle when it would be expected to do so, this is complete AV dissociation. AV dissociation is called *incomplete* when a supraventricular beat at times does traverse the AV conduction system, successfully capturing the ventricles.

AV dissociation can be caused by the slowing of the sinus rate below the rate of a lower pacemaker and the acceleration of a lower pacemaker, usually junctional in the presence of an AV node that can carry impulses, which then competes with antegradely conducting beats in the presence of a conducting AV node; the occurrence of AV block can be defined as a delay or interruption in the transmission of an impulse from the atria to the ventricles because of an anatomic or functional impairment in the conduction system or some combination of the above (Fig. 23-3).

The slowing of the sinus rate below that of an AV junctional pacemaker that then activates the ventricles has been called *dissociation by default*. Figure 23-3 shows a very slow sinus rate that, however, captures the ventricles (C). The sinus node is very slow, allowing a pacemaker in the junction time to attain threshold, traverse the infranodal conduction system, and activate the ventricles producing a QRS complex; and this is termed a *junctional escape* rhythm.

Retrograde VA conduction may occur. *Interference dissociation* refers to the situation in which the atrial and junctional rates are nearly identical, so they will block each other from above and below by rendering the AV junction refractory to both impulses. For example, in the presence of similar rates, the P wave may not conduct because of the physiologic refractoriness in the AV node induced by the preceding firing of the subsidiary pacemaker. This results in the independent beating of the atria and ventricles that has an appearance suggestive of 1 : 1 conduction. The PR interval is shorter than expected for rate and manifests changes that reflect alterations in the sinus rate. The term *isorhythmic dissociation* is used to describe such a 1 : 1 relationship that persists for a period usually longer than that of the standard ECG recording.

Synchronization and accrochage refer to situations in which some influence holds two pacemakers in phase. Accrochage can be considered a short episode of synchronization. This is poorly understood but may be related to baroreceptor and mechanical factors that likely occur in isorhythmic dissociation. Another possibility is synchronization resulting from electrotonic interactions or a pacemaker firing in which one pacemaker resets the other, resulting in "pseudocoupling." Supernormal excitability may be another mechanism for synchronization. There may be a period during late phase 3 in which the activation threshold is lower than that at other times during the cardiac cycle. A normally subthreshold pacemaker (spontaneous or artificial) may become suprathreshold during this period of supernormal excitability. Because supernormal excitability occurs in a small window at the end of the T wave or at the beginning of isoelectric diastole, "pseudocoupling" would be present. Some good examples of these unusual events are found in the classic books of Pick and Langendorf (7) and of Fisch (78).

More commonly, however, the rates differ sufficiently that from time to time, atrial activation is not blocked in the AV conduction system, and this transmitted beat captures the ventricle; hence, the name *ventricular capture* or Dressler beat. Retrograde atrial capture by an impulse arising in the junction of ventricles may occur. Ventricular capture by a sinus beat appears as a short R-R interval in which the QRS complex is preceded by a normal P wave. Occasionally, fusion may occur between the sinus and the ventricular pacemakers, which results in fusion between the retrograde P and the sinus P wave. If ventricular or atrial capture occurs, this is called *incomplete AV dissociation*.

AV dissociation resulting from an acceleration of the AV junctional pacemaker above the sinus rate has been called *dissociation by usurpation* (75). Generally, the same rules apply as those for *dissociation by default* in that spontaneous pacemakers of similar rates will cause interference dissociation while pacemakers of differing rates allow ventricular or atrial captures. A long rhythm strip is useful for making these diagnoses. Common causes of an accelerated junctional rhythm are a myocardial infarction, usually inferior, and digitalis toxicity.

As discussed already, AV dissociation is not synonymous with AV block (8,9). Complete AV block refers to an anatomic conduction block. AV block is the most commonly encountered type of AV dissociation. The anatomic interruption may be in the AV node, the junction, in the bundle of His, and in the bundle branches and fascicles. The sinus pacemaker normally beats at a rate faster than the junctional or infranodal pacemakers. In the presence of complete heart block, the more rapid P waves are unrelated to the slower QRS complexes. The block may be above or below the bifurcation of the fascicular bundle branch systems. If above, the QRS complex will be normal in pattern unless there is a preexisting bundle or fascicular block; the rate of junctional escape rhythms is usually 45 to 60 bpm. These pacemakers high in the junction, such as the bundle of His, may respond to changes in autonomic balance. If below, the QRS has the pattern of an idioventricular rhythm being wide, often with abnormalities in the ST segment and T waves; the rate of the ventricular escape rhythm is usually 30 to 45 bpm.

Figure 23-8 shows the complete heart block as recorded in lead V$_1$. Note that the P waves are independent of the QRS complexes. The first four ventricular depolarizations (J) have a narrow QRS complex and the last four have a wider QRS complex; suggesting that the narrow beats arise from the His bundle or junction above the bifurcation of the bundle branches and that the wide beats are subjunctional (SJ).

The rate of the junctional beats begins at about 50 bpm and then slows below the rate of a lower, subjunctional pacemaker (SJ), which assumes control of the ventricles at a rate of about 43 bpm. Additionally, it is likely that the fifth QRS obscures the P wave that is in fusion with the QRS complex (?P). Two beats that are most likely atrial premature contractions are noted (APC?); the first resets the sinus node while the second is interpolated and does not affect the sinus node.

As mentioned previously, intense vagal tone may produce AV dissociation. Figure 23-9 shows a control tracing (A) and the recording during carotid sinus massage (CS). Note the marked negatively chronotropic effect on the sinus node, the complete AV dissociation, and the absence of an appropriately timed lower junctional or subjunctional escape pacemaker. The first QRS may be a very long junctional escape because the PR is likely to be too short to successfully conduct through the AV node.

Telemetry caught the intense vagal surge that pain caused in a young man (Fig. 23-10). Figure 23-10A shows some of the telemetry strips that document AV dissociation and block. No junctional pacemaker emerged spontaneously. Figure 23-10B is from the full-disclosure recording, which shows the slow rate followed by a sinus tachycardia.

A ventriculophasic sinus arrhythmia may be found in second- and third-degree AV block. This refers to a shortened P-P interval that surrounds a QRS complex as compared with a pair that does not contain a QRS complex. For reasons that are not clear, the prematurity of the P wave after the QRS complex has a positive chronotropic effect on the sinus node. Perhaps the ventricular activation and contraction affects the baroreceptor, the sinus node, and the atrial stretch reflexes.

Atrial fibrillation and digitalis excess are an issue that can trap the unwary. The ventricular response—the R-R interval—is characteristically irregularly irregular in atrial fibrillation. The R-R interval may be regular with AV dissociation or block, a setting in which a lower junctional, subjunctional, or ventricular pacemaker assumes control of the ventricles. A more complicated scenario can result if complete AV block exists and a type I block is present between the spontaneous pacemaker and the ventricles, resulting in group beating in the presence of atrial fibrillation (Fig. 23-11A–D).

ELECTROPHYSIOLOGIC MECHANISMS

First-Degree AV Block

A long PR interval associated with a narrow or wide P wave but a narrow QRS complex on ECG strongly implicates the AV node as being the site of the conduction delay. The A wave on the intracardiac ECG records activation of the low right atrium in the vicinity of the AV node, so it serves as a good marker for the beginning of AV nodal activation. The H wave is the His bundle deflection, so the HV interval represents a good measure of the infranodal conduction time. The A-H time is usually between 50 and 100 ms, and the HV time is between 35 and 55 ms.

A long PR interval associated with a wide QRS complex (20 ms) may be associated with delayed conduction in the AV node or bundle of His but most often involves the bundle branches (36,42). Two levels of conduction delay are present in about two thirds of patients studied (36,42,77, 78). For example, RBBB alone is associated with a normal PR interval. When the PR interval in prolonged, there is also a conduction delay in the AV node, His bundle, or left bundle branch. Similarly, when first-degree AV block occurs in a patient with bifascicular block (e.g., RBBB plus left anterior or posterior fascicular block), the prolongation of the PR interval is a result of a conduction delay in the remaining fascicle or the AV node. Some authors suggest that His bundle ECG studies be performed in these patients with several areas of conduction delay because of the common progression to complete heart block and syncope. A permanent pacemaker may be implanted if the HV interval is more than 75 to 100 ms (see later discussion) (8,77,79).

The PR interval may be prolonged because of an intraatrial conduction delay. The activation of the atrium by the sinus is indicated by the beginning of the P wave and depolarization of the low right atrial myocardium near the AV node is reflected by the intracardiac recording of the A wave. The P-A–interval prolongation resulting in a long PR interval is commonly seen in congenital heart disease.

Second-Degree AV Block

Mobitz Type I (Wenckebach)

The site of block is in the AV node in most cases (70% to 75%), with the remaining cases involving the His bundle, bundle branches, or fascicles (19). His bundle ECG can localize the site of the Mobitz type I block. If the block is occurring in the AV node, the A-H intervals will go through the same sequence described previously for the PR interval. If, however, the block is occurring in the His bundle, there will usually be two His potentials (H and H′) because of the slowing of conduction. In this setting, the H-H′ interval will prolong before the H′ interval and the subsequent QRS complex is dropped. Wenckebach in the bundles can be detected by demonstrating an increase in the interval between the His electrogram and the bundle potential. Thus, the A-H, H-H′, and HV—or H-bundle potentials—allow the site of even a 2 : 1 block to be established.

Figure 23-12 shows an intracardiac recording during Mobitz type I (Wenckebach) second-degree block. The A-H time increases progressively until a beat is dropped. The failure of the third A wave to produce an H spike indicates that the block is in the AV node. The fourth QRS complex is likely a junctional escape given the short A-H time. The cycle then resumed.

Mobitz Type II

Mobitz types I and II AV block differ importantly in the site of conduction delay. As mentioned, type I most often involves the AV node. The conduction failure in type II is always below the AV node, occurring in the bundle of His in about 20% of cases and in the bundle branches in the remainder (19). Patients with bundle branch involvement may also have shifts in the mean QRS axis and QRS widening depending on the location of the block.

Type II conduction defects have been studied with His bundle ECG. The nonconducted A wave is followed by a His spike, and not infrequently, a split His potential resulting from slowed intra-Hisian conduction on the conducted beat. Rarely, a proximal His block will not demonstrate a His potential with the nonconducted beat, falsely suggesting that the block is in the AV node. Figure 23-13 is an intracardiac recording that shows a block distal to the bundle of His. The surface ECG showed a 2 : 1 AV block with a widened QRS, so it was suspected that this was a Mobitz type II block. Both the A-H and HV intervals were constant on the conducted beats.

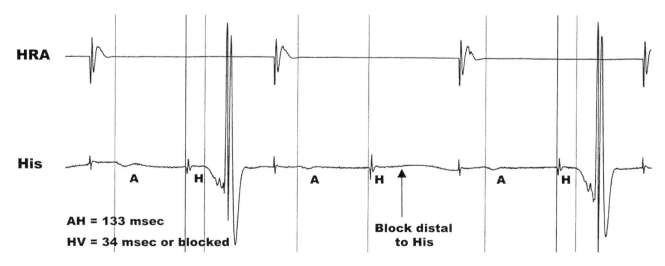

FIGURE 23-12. Intracardiac electrocardiograms of a Mobitz type I (Wenckebach) second-degree atrioventricular (AV) block at the level of the AV node. The two intracardiac recording sites were near the His bundle. Note the progressive increase in the A-H interval before the dropped beat. The block was in the AV node because no H spike was recorded. The spike after the arrow is the stimulus *(St)* spike, with the greatest increment being in the first beat. The HV interval remained constant. The fourth QRS is most likely a junctional escape, with an A-H time of 40 ms and an HV time of 60 ms.

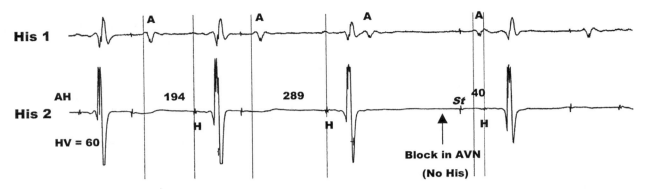

FIGURE 23-13. Intracardiac electrograms from the high right atrium *(HRA)* and bundle of His *(His)* of a Mobitz type II second-degree atrioventricular (AV) block distal to the bundle of His. The A-H time remains constant throughout. The dropped beat shows an "a" and H potential, but no V wave demonstrating that the conduction block is distal to the recording site in the bundle of His.

Third-Degree AV Dissociation and Block

AV dissociation caused by competing pacemakers will eventually show capture beats. Intracardiac ECGs are rarely needed to make this diagnosis.

Similarly, the lack of relationship between the supraventricular and the idionodal or idioventricular beats in complete AV block is almost always apparent from the surface ECG. If the block is at the level of the AV node, the atrial electrogram will not be followed by a His bundle potential. The escape activation, however, may be preceded by a His spike depending on the level of the block and the escape pacemaker. Figure 23-12 shows complete heart block at the level of the bundle of His. The A wave and initial H spike have a variable association while the ventricles are controlled by a spontaneous pacemaker in the bundle of His, as demonstrated by the coupled H and V waves throughout the recording.

SYMPTOMS AND PHYSICAL EXAMINATION

First-degree AV block in itself does not produce symptoms. It, however, may be an indicator of sick sinus syndrome, which is often associated with AV nodal disease and sluggish lower pacemakers, or the potential for atrial fibrillation. It may also be an indicator of significant infranodal disease if the PR prolongation is associated with a wide QRS complex or a combination of conduction defects such as a fascicular and a bundle branch block. These individuals are at a higher risk for a Mobitz type II AV block.

Uncomplicated Mobitz type I block does not produce symptoms. If, however, the sinus rate is slow and the ratio small (2 : 1 or 3 : 2 block), there may be a significant reduction in cardiac output and symptoms of hypoperfusion (including angina or syncope) or heart failure. Some patients sense the irregularity in their heartbeats.

Patients with Mobitz type II block may have symptoms related to a slow rate, like those with type I, and may feel irregularities in their heart rhythm. Of greater concern is that a Mobitz type II second-degree heart block may suddenly become complete heart block, resulting in syncope. Note the ECG in Figure 23-7 in which a beat with a normal PR interval is followed by complete heart block resulting from the lack of a lower pacemaker escaping to control the ventricles.

Complete heart block results in a lack of normal AV synchrony, which may diminish the cardiac output by as much as 25%. The rate of the spontaneous pacemaker is often quite slow. Cannon waves may be present when the atria intermittently contract against a closed tricuspid valve, and the pressure may differ depending on the amount of filling resulting from the position of the P and QRS waves in the cardiac cycle. The only mechanism for increasing cardiac output is often dilation and hypertrophy. Patients may develop symptoms associated with a slow rate and a decreased cardiac output such as congestive heart failure, angina pectoris, supraventricular arrhythmias, and sometimes, ventricular arrhythmias.

PROGNOSTIC IMPLICATIONS IN DIFFERENT DISEASE STATES

There is little information regarding the prognosis of patients with first-degree AV block at the level of the AV node, compared with that for a block at the bundle of His. Interestingly, patients with first-degree AV block at the bundle of His may be more likely to develop higher degrees of block. The presence of a wide QRS in the presence of a long PR interval increases the likelihood of infranodal delay.

Mobitz type I (Wenckebach) second-degree AV block can occur in healthy subjects with high vagal tone (as in young subjects or athletes during sleep). The prognosis is excellent in this setting, as studies of healthy subjects and athletes suggest that progressive block does not appear to occur. Mobitz type I block can also be seen with intrinsic AV nodal disease, after the administration of AV nodal blocking agents (digoxin, verapamil, diltiazem, β blockers), in patients with myocarditis, and in association with acute inferior myocardial infarction or ischemia. The right coronary artery supplies the inferior and posterior walls as well as the AV node (in about 90% of individuals) and the SA node (in about 50%). Thus, sinus bradycardia (resulting from involvement of the SA node and in some cases increased vagal tone) and Mobitz type I block (resulting from ischemia of the AV node) are not uncommon complications of an inferior myocardial infarction. These findings are associated with increased mortality rates, presumably because of a larger infarct size. The infarct does not typically extend to the AV node because of collaterals from the left coronary system. If, however, there is substantial left-sided coronary disease, right-sided coronary occlusion may lead to complete heart block.

Uncomplicated Mobitz type I block does not produce symptoms. If, however, the sinus rate is slow and the ratio small (2 : 1 or 3 : 2 block), there may be a significant reduction in cardiac output and symptoms of hypoperfusion (including angina or syncope) or heart failure.

Mobitz type II second-degree AV block may progress to a higher degree of block. The incidence of progression to a higher degree of block that requires the need for a pacemaker is uncertain (80,81). The presence or absence of other conduction disturbances may provide a clue to prognosis. In one study, for example, 9 of 15 patients with Mobitz type II block had preexisting bundle branch block with a block distal to the bundle of His (80). Six of nine had syncope within 6 months and received a pacemaker; the remaining three were also paced because of the development of congestive heart failure. There are only limited data about patients with type II block and a narrow QRS complex, but we have seen a number of cases that progressed to symptomatic heart block.

The prognostic significance of third-degree AV dissociation and block depends largely on the cause. It is beyond the scope of this chapter to discuss the myriad clinical situations that cause AV dissociation and heart block, but a few comments are in order. With many causes, such as those with electrolyte imbalance and drug excess, the dissociation or block is transient. The rate of the spontaneous pacemaker is important to determine whether syncope, heart failure, or other symptoms attributable to a slow rate occur. Infranodal AV block caused by coronary artery occlusion, on the other hand, has a poor prognosis because much myocardium is usually damaged. Congenital complete heart block may occur with other abnormalities or with an otherwise healthy heart. Patients usually remain asymptomatic until late childhood or adolescence, at which time they often require an electronic pacemaker.

INDICATION FOR AND EVALUATION WITH ELECTROPHYSIOLOGIC STUDIES

The electrophysiologic study is the definitive procedure to examine the conduction properties of the AV node. In the typical electrophysiologic study, multipolar electrode catheters are placed from the femoral veins into the heart under fluoroscopic guidance. Typically, a quadripolar catheter is placed in the high right atrium and another into the right ventricle, although the latter catheter may be omitted to conserve resources. The atrial catheter can be manipulated into the ventricle for the ventricular pacing part of the procedure. Another catheter (tripolar, quadripolar, or octapolar) is placed across the tricuspid valve to record an atrial depolarization spike, a His potential, and a ventricular depolarization spike.

The AV and HV intervals are measured during the patient's baseline rhythm. Often, this may prove diagnostic in determining the site of block in a patient with evidence of heart block. The normal value for the AV interval is 55 to 135 ms while a normal HV interval is 35 to 55 ms. In patients with prolonged PR intervals, the site of delay is usually in the AV node but can occasionally be infra-Hisian. A prolonged HV interval signifies distal conduction disease and a higher propensity to complete heart block. The intracardiac ECG in patients presenting with ECG evidence of type I second-degree heart block will often demonstrate gradual prolongation in the A-H interval until the dropped beat. The His bundle electrogram of the nonconducted P wave will show an atrial spike without a His or ventricular electrogram. Care must be taken to ensure that the His catheter is correctly positioned and not recording a right bundle potential or the latter part of a split His potential. In these cases, the lack of a spike after the atrial deflection may be mistakenly classified as *proximal heart block* when it is distal block, because conduction is intact through the AV node and actually blocks intra-His or infra-His.

After careful observations of the conduction properties in the baseline state, the clinician can obtain the physiology of the AV node using programmed stimulation of the atrium and the ventricle. The Wenckebach cycle of the AV node is obtained by progressively increasing the pacing rate of the atrium and observing progressive lengthening of the AV interval with subsequent block at the AV node (an atrial deflection followed by no His and ventricular deflections). The maximal 1 : 1 conduction for the AV node depends on the autonomic state of the patient, but a Wenckebach cycle of more than 505 ms (less than 118 bpm) is considered abnormal. The effective refractory of the AV node is determined by programmed stimulation of the atrium by gradually decreasing the coupling of a premature impulse until the impulse conducts to the atrium and not to the His bundle.

The most recent American College of Cardiology and the American Heart Association (ACC/AHA) guidelines for clinical intracardiac electrophysiologic and catheter ablation procedures were published in 1995 (82). These guidelines use a classification scheme with three classes (class I, general agreement that electrophysiologic study is useful and important for patient treatment; class II, conditions for which electrophysiologic study are frequently performed, but there is less certainty about the usefulness of the data obtained; class III, general agreement that electrophysiologic study results do not provide useful information and are not warranted for patients with these conditions).

The electrophysiologic study is indicated for patients who are symptomatic (usually who have experienced syncope or near syncope) in whom His-Purkinje block is suspected as a cause of symptoms but in whom the diagnosis has not been established by noninvasive monitoring. If a patient's symptoms are indeed correlated with ECG findings of AV block, the ACC/AHA Task Force classifies this as a class III indication. This indicates that the diagnostic study is not warranted, and a therapeutic intervention such as permanent pacemaker implantation should be performed. However, some physicians question this classification. Even in patients with documented AV nodal disease by ECG, ventricular tachyarrhythmias or occasionally supraventricular tachyarrhythmias may explain the cause of symptoms, particularly in the presence of a cardiomyopathy. Treatment with a pacemaker may fail to prevent further symptoms or sudden death, and implantation of a dual-chamber pacing defibrillator may be lifesaving. Therefore, the electrophysiologic study may indeed be indicated in this situation, not to document the presence of significant heart block but to determine the patient's risk for other arrhythmias. The ACC/AHA guidelines do consider this in the second class I indication. Patients with second- or third-degree heart block who are treated with pacemakers who remain symptomatic and in whom another arrhythmia is suspected as a cause of symptoms should receive electrophysiologic testing in hopes of finding a tachyarrhythmic cause of their symptoms.

A class II indication offered by the task force includes patients who are thought to have pseudo-AV block. Premature, concealed junctional depolarizations may make the ECG results suggestive of advanced heart block. If asymptomatic, these patients require no further intervention. The second class II intervention is rather broad and includes patients with second- and third-degree AV block in whom knowledge of the site of block or its mechanism or response to pharmacologic or other temporary intervention may help direct therapy or assess prognosis.

Finally, patients with transient AV block associated with sinus slowing (e.g., nocturnal) type I second-degree AV block) should not undergo electrophysiologic testing.

In summary, electrophysiologic studies should be performed for patients with symptoms thought to have signif-

icant heart block but without noninvasive documentation or for patients with noninvasive documentation of AV nodal disease with or without pacemakers in whom another arrhythmia is thought to be related to clinical scenario.

TREATMENT AND INDICATIONS FOR PACING

Because pharmacologic therapy that can specifically act to improve a chronic AV conduction defect largely does not exist, the main therapeutic modality employed for patients with AV nodal disease is the implantation of a permanent pacemaker. The ACC\AHA guidelines are a detailed consensus statement from various experts in the field of cardiac pacing and electrophysiology (83). As mentioned, the recommendations are divided into three classes according to the advice of the committee. Class II recommendations include conditions for which there is conflicting evidence and/or a divergence of opinion about the usefulness or efficacy of a procedure or treatment and are further divided into an *a* and a *b* level. The former (Class IIa) is designated for recommendations in which the weight of the evidence is in favor of the usefulness/efficacy whereas the data for the class IIb recommendations are less well established.

The latest document contains a new classification algorithm for the level of evidence of each recommendation. Recommendations are based on data derived (a) from multiple randomized clinical trials involving many individuals, (b) from a limited number of trials involving comparatively few patients or from well-designed data analyses of nonrandomized studies or observational data registries, and (c) from a consensus opinion of experts. Because few large-scale randomized trials have been performed for patients with AV nodal disease, most of the recommendations fall into the latter two categories, with a significant portion of the recommendations based on a consensus opinion of experts in the field. Also, randomized trials are lacking in the field of pacing, as alternative therapies largely do not exist.

First-Degree AV Block

The ACC/AHA guidelines for the implantation of cardiac pacemakers and antiarrhythmic devices do not recommend a pacemaker for most cases of first-degree AV block (83). It does, however, place the patient with a markedly prolonged HV interval (more than 100 ms) and pacing-induced infra-His block in class II, in which permanent pacemakers are frequently used, but there is divergence of opinion regarding the necessity for their insertion (84). The contrary view is that a pacemaker should be inserted if the first-degree AV block results from HV prolongation of more than 75 or 100 ms (8,85).

Second-Degree AV Block

Second-degree AV block regardless of the type or site of block with associated symptomatic bradycardia is a class I indication for pacing (84). For the asymptomatic patient, there are two recommendations that fall into class IIa. It is generally agreed that Mobitz type II second-degree heart block requires permanent pacing because it represents distal conduction disease rather than solely AV nodal disease and has a propensity to result in complete heart block. For Mobitz type I second-degree heart block (Wenckebach), symptoms are generally required for agreement for pacing. If, however, a patient with asymptomatic Mobitz type I second-degree AV block demonstrates block at the intra- or infra-Hisian level, as may be found incidentally at electrophysiologic study performed for other indications, the committee classifies this as a class IIa indication. Asymptomatic patients with Mobitz type I second-degree AV block with block at the supra-Hisian level, or those not known to be intra- or infra-Hisian should not receive pacemakers. Also, patients with AV block that is expected to resolve and unlikely to recur, as in those associated with drug toxicity or Lyme disease, should not receive permanent pacemakers. However, in some cases of Lyme disease, prolonged temporary pacing for symptomatic complete heart block may be required.

Third-Degree AV Block

Nonrandomized studies published as early as 30 years ago strongly suggest that the implantation of a permanent pacemaker improves survival in patients with third-degree heart block, particularly if syncope has occurred. Although many of the class I recommendations for patients with AV nodal disease are for symptomatic patients, they also include third-degree heart block with documented periods of asystole for 3.0 seconds or any escape rate at less than 40 bpm in awake, symptom-free patients. Third-degree AV block with average awake ventricular rates of 40 bpm or faster in asymptomatic patients is considered a class IIa indication for permanent pacing.

High-Degree Heart Block Associated with an Acute Myocardial Infarction

The indications for pacing in patients with acute myocardial infarction remain a concern for physicians involved in their care. With the advent of widespread use of thrombolytic therapy and acute angioplasty for patients presenting with acute myocardial infarction, the need for temporary and permanent pacing has markedly decreased (86). However, the long- and short-term mortality rates for these patients remain significantly high compared with those of patients not requiring pacing. This finding is related to the location and size of the infarction. Because the blood supply to the AV node is usually by way of the right coronary artery, patients with acute inferior myocardial infarctions are more likely to demonstrate AV nodal block than patients with anterior wall myocardial infarcts (87). Early AV block (within 24 hours of hospital admission) is less likely to respond to atropine and therefore is more likely to require temporary pacing than late AV block (more than 24 hours into the hospital course). It also portends higher morbidity and mortality rates (88). Endogenous adenosine may play a role in bradyarrhythmias associated with myocardial ischemia, particularly with inferior infarctions. Short-term treatment with theophylline has been successful in restoring 1 : 1 AV conduction in patients with inferior infarcts who are refractory to atropine or in whom atropine is thought to be contraindicated (89). Conduction through the AV node usually returns within several days postinfarction, and permanent pacing may not be required. For patients who remain in heart block, dual-chamber pacing is the preferred treatment.

Heart block associated with anterior infarction carries a high mortality rate because of the large amount of myocardium often involved. Despite advances in the treatment of acute anterior myocardial infarction from 1975 to 1988, complete heart block continued to have a higher in-hospital mortality rate (90). Even after multivariate regression analysis, patients with complete heart block and anterior infarctions had an in-hospital mortality rate that was more than twice that of patients without heart block. Heart block complicating anterior infarction is less likely to be transient, and permanent pacing is usually required when patients are otherwise ready for hospital discharge.

REFERENCES

1. Tawara S. *Das Reizleitungssystem des Säuegetierherzens.* Jena: Gustav Fischer, 1906.
2. Anderson RH, Ho SY. The architecture of the sinus node, the atrioventricular conduction axis and the internodal atrial myocardium. *J Cardiovasc Electrophysiol* 1998;9:1233–1248.
3. Racker DK. Atrial node and input pathways: a correlated gross anatomical and histological study of the canine atrioventricular junctional region. *Anat Rec* 1989;224:336–354.
4. Billette J, Shrier A. Atrioventricular nodal activation and functional properties. In: Zipes DP, Jalife J, eds. *Cardiac electrophysiology: from cell to bedside,* 2nd ed. Philadelphia: WB Saunders, 1995:216–228.
5. Paes de Carvalho A, De Almeida DF. Spread of activity through the atrioventricular node. *Circ Res* 1960;8:801–809.
6. Janse MF, van Capelle FJL, Anderson RH, et al. Electrophysiology and structure of the atrioventricular node of the isolated rabbit heart. In: Wellens HJJ, Lie KI, Janse MJ, eds. *The conduction system of the heart: structure, function and clinical implications.* Philadelphia: Lea & Febiger, 1976:296–315.
7. Pick A, Langendorf R. *Interpretation of complex arrhythmias.* Philadelphia: Lea & Febiger, 1979.
8. Bär FW, Den Dulk K, Wellens HJJ. Atrioventricular dissociation. In: MacFarlane PW, Lawrie TDV, eds. *Comprehensive elec-*

trocardiology: theory and practice in health and disease, 1st ed, vol 2. New York: Pergamon Press, 1989:933–959.

9. WHO/ISFC Task Force. Definition of terms related to cardiac rhythm. *Am Heart J* 1978;95:796–806.

10. Wenckebach KF. Beiträge zur Kenntnis der menschlichlichen Herztätigkeit. *Arch Anat Phys (Physiol Abth)* 1906:297–354.

11. Hay J. Bradycardia and cardiac arrhythmia produced by depression of certain functions of the heart. *Lancet* 1906;1:139.

12. Wenckebach KF. Zur Analyse der unregelmässigen Pulses. *Ztschr Klin Med* 1899;36:181–199.

13. Luciani L. Eine periodische Fuktion des isolierten Froschherzens. *Arb Physiol Anstalt* 1872;7:113.

14. Burch GE, DePasquale NP, Howell JD. *A history of electrocardiography.* San Francisco: Norman Publishing, 1990.

15. Mobitz W. Über die unvollständige Störung der Erregungsüberleitung zwischen Vorhof und Kammer des menschlichen Herzens. *Z Gesamte Exp Med* 1924;41:180–237.

16. Lev M. The pathology of complete atrioventricular block. *Prog Cardiovasc Dis* 1964;6:317–326.

17. Lown B. Electrical reversion of cardiac arrhythmias. Brit Heart J 1967;29:469.

18. Rosen KM, Loeb HS, Sinno MZ, et al. Cardiac conduction in patients with symptomatic sinus node disease. *Circulation* 1971; 43:836.

19. Narula OS. Atrioventricular conduction defects in patients with sinus bradycardia: analysis by His bundle recordings. *Circulation* 1971;44:1096.

20. Scherf D, Dix JH. The effects of posture on A-V conduction. *Am J Cardiol* 1962;43:494–506.

21. Johnson RL, Averill KH, Lamb LE. Electrocardiographic findings in 67,375 asymptomatic subjects: VII. Atrioventricular block. *Am J Cardiol* 1960;6:153–177.

22. Viitasalo MT, Kala R, Eisalo A. Ambulatory electrocardiographic recording in endurance athletes. *Br Heart J* 1982;47:213–220.

23. Graybiel A, McFarland RA, Gates DC, Webster FA. Analysis of the electrocardiogram obtained from 1000 young healthy aviators. *Am Heart J* 1944;27:524–549.

24. Packard JM, Graettinger JS, Graybiel A. Analysis of the electrocardiograms obtained from 1000 healthy aviators: ten year follow-up. *Circulation* 1954;10:384–400.

25. Mathewson FA, Rabkin SW, Hsu P. Atrioventricular heart block: 27 year follow-up experience. *Trans Assoc Life Insur Med Dir Am* 1976;60:110.

26. Grossman M. Second degree heart block with Wenckebach phenomenon: its occurrence over a period of several years in a young healthy adult. *Am Heart J* 1958;56:607–610.

27. Meyles I, Kaplinsky E, Yahini JH, et al. Wenckebach A-V block: a frequent feature following heavy physical training. *Am Heart J* 1975;90:426–430.

28 Brodsky M, Wu D, Denes P, et al. Arrhythmias documented by 24 hour continuous electrocardiographic monitoring in 50 male medical students without apparent heart disease. *Am J Cardiol* 1977;39:390.

29. Young D, Eisenberg R, Fish B, Fisher JD. Wenckebach atrioventricular block (Mobitz type I) in children and adolescents. *Am J Cardiol* 1977;40:393–399.

30. Otsuka K, Ichimaru Y, Yanaga T. Studies of arrhythmias by 24-hour polygraphic recordings: relation between atrioventricular block and sleep states. *Am Heart J* 1983;105:934–940.

31. Dickinson DF, Scott O. Ambulatory electrocardiographic monitoring in 100 healthy teenage boys. *Br Heart J* 1984;51:179–183.

32. Zeppili P, Fenici R, Sassara M, et al. Wenckebach second degree A-V block in top-ranking athletes: an old problem revisited. *Am Heart J* 1980;100:281–294.

33. Husson GS, Blackman MS, Rogers MC, et al. Familial congenital bundle branch system disease. *Am J Cardiol* 1973;32:365.

34. Waxman MB, Catching JD, Felderhof CH, et al. Familial atrioventricular heart block: an autosomal dominant trait. *Circulation* 1975;51:226.

35. Reid JM, Coleman EN, Doig W. Complete congenital heart block. Report of 35 cases. *Br Heart J* 1982;48:236–239.

36. Peuch P, Grolleau R, Guimond C. Incidence of different types of A-V block and their localization by His bundle recordings. In: Wellens HJJ, Lie KI, Janse MJ, eds. *The conduction system of the heart.* Leiden: Stenfert Kroese, 1976:467–484.

37. Donoso E, Adler LN, Friedberg CK. Unusual forms of second-degree atrioventricular block, including Mobitz type II block, associated with the Morgagni-Adams-Stokes syndrome. *Am Heart J* 1964;67:150–157.

38. Dhingra RC, Denes P, Wu D, et al. The significance of second degree atrioventricular block and bundle branch block: observations regarding site and type of block. *Circulation* 1974;49:638–646.

39. Strasberg B, Amat-Y-Leon F, Dhingra RC, et al. Natural history of chronic second degree atrioventricular nodal block. *Circulation* 1981;63:1043–1049.

40. Dhingra RC, Palileo E, Strasberg B, et al. Significance of the HV interval in 517 patients with chronic bifascicular block. *Circulation* 1981;63:1040.

41. Clarke M, Sutton R, Ward D, et al. Recommendations for pacemaker prescription for symptomatic bradycardia. *Br Heart J* 1991;66:185.

42. Peuch P. The value in intracardiac recordings. In: Krikler D, Godwin JF, eds. *Cardiac arrhythmias.* Philadelphia: WB Saunders, 1975:81.

43. Peuch P, Wainwright RJ. Clinical electrophysiology of atrioventricular block. *Cardiol Clin* 1983;1:209.

44. Morquio L. Sur une maladie infantile et familiale characterisée par des modifications permanentes du pouls, des attaques syncopales et epileptiforme et la mort subite. *Arch Méd d'Enfants* 1901; 4:467.

45. White P, Eustis R. Congenital heart block. *AJDC* 1921;22:299.

46. Michaelsson M, Engle AM. Congenital complete heart block: an international study of the natural history. *Cardiovasc Clin* 1972; 4:85–101.

47. Zoob M, Smith KS. The aetiology of complete heart-block. *Br Med J* 1963;2:1149–1153.

48. Lenegre J. Etiology and pathology of bilateral bundle branch block in relation to complete heart block. *Prog Cardiovasc Dis* 1964;6:409–444.

49. Lev M. Anatomic basis for atrioventricular block. *Am J Med* 1964;37:742–748.

50. Begg FR, Magovern GJ, Cushing WJ, et al. Selective cine coronary arteriography in patients with complete heart block. *J Thorac Cardiovasc Surg* 1969;57:9–16.

51. Simon AB, Zloto AE. Atrioventricular block: natural history after permanent ventricular pacing. *Am J Cardiol* 1978;41:500–507.

52. Penton GB, Miller H, Levine SA. Some clinical features of complete heart block. *Circulation* 1956;13:801–824.

53. Wright JC, Hejtmancik MR, Herrmann GR, Shields AH. A clinical study of complete heart block. *Am Heart J* 1956;52:369–378.

54. Rowe JC, White PD. Complete heart block: a follow-up study. *Ann Intern Med* 1958;49:260–270.

54a. Feigl D. Early and late atrioventricular block in acute inferior myocardial infarction. *J Am Coll Cardiol* 1984; 4:35–38.

55. Hindman MC, Wagner GS, Jaro M, et al. The clinical significance of bundle branch block complicating acute myocardial

infarction. 1. Clinical characteristics, hospital mortality and one-year followup. *Circulation* 1978;58:679–688.

56. Sugiura T, Iwasaka T, Hasegawa T, Matsutani M, et al. Factors associated with persistent and transient fascicular blocks in anterior wall acute myocardial infarction. *Am J Cardiol* 1989; 63:784–787.

57. Mullins CB, Atkins JM. Prognosis and management of ventricular conduction block in acute myocardial infarction. *Modif Conc Cardiovasc Dis* 1976;45:129.

58. Hindman MC, Wagner GS, Jaro M, et al. The clinical significance of bundle branch block complicating acute myocardial infarction. 2. Indications for temporary and permanent pacemaker insertion. *Circulation* 1978;58:689–699.

59. Hindman MC, Wagner GS, Jaro M, et al. The clinical significance of bundle branch block complicating acute myocardial infarction. I. Clinical characteristics, hospital mortality, and one-year follow-up. *Circulation* 1978;58:679–694.

60. Scheinman MM, Gonzalez RP. Fascicular block and acute myocardial infarction. *JAMA* 1980;244:2646.

61. Dubois C, Pierard LA, Smeets J-P, et al. Short- and long-term prognostic importance of complete bundle-branch block complicating acute myocardial infarction. *Clin Cardiol* 1988;11:292.

62. Sanoudos G, Reed GE. Late heart block in aortic valve replacement. *J Cardiovasc Surg* 1974;15:475–478.

63. Rosen KM, Mehta A, Rahimtoola SH, Miller RA. Sites of congenital and surgical heart block as defined by His bundle electrocardiography. *Circulation* 1971;44:833–841.

64. Furman S, Young D. Cardiac pacing in children and adolescents. *Am J Cardiol* 1977;39:350–358.

65. Hofschire PJ, Nicoloff DM, Moller JH. Postoperative complete heart block in 64 children treated with and without cardiac pacing. *Am J Cardiol* 1977;39:559–562.

66. Harris A, Davies M, Redwood D, et al. Aetiology of chronic heart block: a clinico-pathological correlation in 65 cases. *Br Heart J* 1969;31:206–218.

67. Fananapazir L, Tracy CM, Leon MB, et al. Electrophysiologic abnormalities in patients with hypertrophic cardiomyopathy. A consecutive analysis in 155 patients. *Circulation* 1989;80: 1259–1268.

68. Olofsson B-O, Forsberg H, Andersson S, et al. Electrocardiographic findings in myotonic dystrophy. *Br Heart J* 1988;59: 47–52.

69. Hultgren HN. Osteitis deformans (Paget's disease) and calcific disease of heart valves. *Am J Cardiol* 1998;81:1461–1464.

70. Wynne J, Braunwald EB. The cardiomyopathies and myocarditises: toxic, chemical and physical damage to the heart. In: Braunwald E, ed. *Heart disease: a textbook of cardiovascular medicine,* 4th ed. Philadelphia: WB Saunders, 1992:1394–1450.

71. Harumi K, Chen CY. Miscellaneous electrocardiographic topics. In: MacFarlane PW, Veitch Lawrie TD, eds. *Comprehensive electrocardiology,* vol 1. New York: Pergamon Press, 1989: 671–728.

72. Arnsdorf MF. Electrocardiographic pattern of anteroseptal myocardial infarction mimicked by a hyperkalemia-induced disturbance of impulse conduction. *Arch Intern Med* 1976;136: 1161–1163.

73. Den Dulk K, Brugada P, Braat S, et al. Myocardial bridging as a cause of paroxysmal atrioventricular block. *J Am Coll Cardiol* 1983;1:965–969.

74. Lev M, Silverman J, Fitzmaurice FM, et al. Lack of connection between the atria and the more peripheral conduction system in congenital atrioventricular block. *Am J Cardiol* 1971;27: 481–490.

75. Ross BA. Congenital complete atrioventricular block. *Pediatr Clin North Am* 1990;37:69.

76. Buyon JP, Hiebert R, Copel J, et al. Autoimmune-associated congenital heart block: demographics, mortality, morbidity and recurrence rates obtained from a National Neonatal Lupus Registry. *J Am Coll Cardiol* 1998;31:1658.

77. Dunn MI, Lipman BS. *Lipman-Massie clinical electrocardiography,* 8th ed. Chicago: Year Book, 1989.

78. Fisch C. *Electrocardiography of arrhythmias.* Philadelphia: Lea & Febiger, 1990.

79. Guimond C, Puech P. Intra-His bundle blocks (102 cases). *Eur J Cardiol* 1976;4:481–493.

80. Levites R, Haft J. Significance of first degree heart block (prolonged P-R interval) in bifascicular block. *Am J Cardiol* 1974;34: 259–264.

81. Strasberg B, Amat-Y-Leon F, Dhingra RC, et al. Natural history of chronic second-degree atrioventricular nodal block. *Circulation* 1981;63:1043–1049.

82. Zipes DP, DiMarco JP, Gillette PC, et al. Guidelines for clinical intracardiac electrophysiological and catheter ablation procedures: a report of the American College of Cardiology/American Heart Association Task Force on Practice Guidelines (Committee on Clinical Intracardiac Electrophysiologic and Catheter Ablation Procedures. *Circulation* 1995;49:673–691.

83. Gregoratos G, Chetlin MD, Conil A, et al. ACC/AHA guidelines for the implantation of cardiac pacemakers and antiarrhythmic devices. A report of the American College of Cardiology/American Heart Association Task Force on Practice Guidelines (Committee on Pacemaker Implantation). JACC 1998;31:1175–1209.

84. Dreifus LS, Fisch C, Griffin JC, Gillette PC, Mason JW, Parsonnet V. Guidelines for implantation of cardiac pacemakers and antiarrhythmia devices: A report of the American College of Cardiology/American Heart Association Task Force on Assessment of Diagnostic and Therapeutic Cardiovascular Procedures (Committee on Pacemaker Implantation). *J Am Coll Cardiol* 1991;18:1–13.

85. Scheinman MM, Peters RW, Modin G, et al. Prognostic value of infranodal conduction time in patients with chronic bundle branch block. *Circulation* 1977;56:240–244.

86. Berger PB, Ruocco NA Jr, Ryan TJ, et al. Incidence and prognostic implications of heart block complicating inferior myocardial infarction treated with thrombolytic therapy. *J Am Coll Cardiol* 1992;20:533–540.

87. Rotman M, Wagner GS, Wallace AG. Bradyarrhythmias in acute myocardial infarction. *Circulation* 1972;45:703.

88. Sclarlovsky S, Strasberg B, Hirshberg A, et al. Advanced early and late atrioventricular block in acute inferior wall myocardial infarction. *Am Heart J* 1984;108:19–24.

89. Bertolet BD, McMurtrie EB, Hill JA, Belardinelli L. Theophylline for the treatment of atrioventricular block after myocardial infarction. *Ann Intern Med* 1995;123:509–511.

90. Goldberg RJ, Zevallos JC, Yarzebski J, et al. Prognosis of acute myocardial infarction complicated by complete heart block (the Worcester Heart Attack Study). *Am J Cardiol* 1992;69: 1135–1141.

24

HIS-PURKINJE DISEASE

PABLO DENES

The His-Purkinje system is composed of specialized cardiac tissue that extends from the atrioventricular (AV) node to the terminal Purkinje fibers with their insertion into the ventricular myocardium. It is an "electronic highway" that transmits and distributes the depolarizing impulses to the ventricular working myocardium so that contraction can proceed in a synchronized and effective manner. Disruption of this network may result in dissociation between atrial and ventricular contraction or in an asynchronous sequence of ventricular depolarization and contraction, or it may become the site for the origin of abnormal impulses. It is well recognized that the His-Purkinje system has intrinsic automaticity, which is suppressed under normal circumstances by sinus node automaticity [1]. The His-Purkinje system may also be a site of abnormal automaticity and reentry, resulting in rapid ventricular rhythms [1].

ELECTROPHYSIOLOGIC PROPERTIES

The tissue of the His-Purkinje system generates a fast action potential, so the impulse conduction velocity through this tissue is rapid, approximately 1 to 3 m per second. It is notable that in 1928, Schmitt and Erlanger [2] suggested that the His-Purkinje ventricular junction might be a site of origin of reentrant ventricular extrasystoles. This model of reentry has been widely accepted and used to exemplify the circus movement reentry process. The hypothesis is partly based on the particular geometrical arrangement of the terminal Purkinje fibers and the ventricular muscle. An area of depressed conduction within the terminal Purkinje branch can become the site of unidirectional block, and slow conduction through this loop allows successful reentry, resulting in coupled ventricular extrasystoles. The His-Purkinje system and its specialized network-like architecture have served as a model

for a novel interpretation of cardiac arrhythmias based on the chaos theory [3,4].

Beyond the historical and the futuristic concepts of the involvement of the His-Purkinje system in the genesis of arrhythmias, there are other well-defined concepts that are unique to its electrophysiologic properties. One interesting observation in the organization of the His-Purkinje system is that the duration of the action potentials has been shown to prolong as one progresses more distally in the conduction system [5]. This progressive prolongation of the duration of action potentials is paralleled by a progressive prolongation of refractory periods. The longest refractory periods reside in the most distal sites of the ventricular conduction system [5]. This gradual prolongation of refractoriness has been termed the *gate phenomenon* [5]. Originally, it was thought that the gate, located at the distal Purkinje fibers, would limit the passage of premature impulses from the ventricular specialized conduction system to the ventricular myocardium or in the reverse direction [5]. Lazzara and colleagues [6] evaluated the gate hypothesis, using a preparation that included the entire ventricular conduction system. They confirmed the findings that the action potential durations increased progressively from the His bundle to the distal His-Purkinje fibers along the main right bundle branch and moderator band, the anterior border fibers of the left bundle branch and anterior false tendons, and the posterior fibers of the left bundle branch and posterior false tendons. The action potential duration near the termination of the false tendons was the longest in the system. The interior fibers of the left bundle branch had action potentials that were shorter in duration than those of the right bundle branch or the border fibers of the left bundle branch. They also found that fibers with short action potential duration provided the quickest pathway to the septal myocardium. They noted that when premature stimulation was applied to the His bundle, the block or delay was localized to the proximal 1 to 2 cm of the main bundle branches. The delay that was encountered at the proximal level frequently allowed recovery of the distal sites for conduction.

Another area of investigation that has yielded interesting information regarding special electrophysiologic properties

P. Denes: Department of Cardiology, Northwestern University Hospital, Chicago, Illinois 60637.

of the His-Purkinje system is the presence of supernormal excitability and conduction in this tissue. A supernormal period of excitability occurs during ventricular recovery and is manifest as a decrease in the intensity of the electrical current required to reexcite the myocardium. It is postulated that during the late phase of recovery, the threshold potential has recovered more completely than the membrane potential and a lesser degree of additional depolarization is needed to reach threshold. Spear and Moore (7) in 1974 reported on the supernormal period of excitability of and conduction in the His-Purkinje system of the dog. They noted that the period of supernormal excitability was voltage-dependent and terminated at full repolarization. The supernormal period of excitability is restricted to the bundle branches of the Purkinje system and is not found in the His bundle or ventricular myocardium. A direct correlation was also observed between the period of supernormal excitability and a period of increased conduction velocity.

ANATOMY OF THE HIS-PURKINJE CONDUCTION SYSTEM

In a comprehensive article, Titus (8) described the normal anatomy of the human cardiac conduction system. The His bundle is a direct continuation of the terminal portion of the AV node. A clear demarcation between the end of the node and the beginning of the bundle cannot be made. This region is defined as *the junction*. The His bundle proceeds through the fibrous AV ring (penetrating bundle) at the level of the central fibrous body of the heart. It proceeds around the posterior inferior portion of the membranous ventricular septum and straddles on the summit of the ventricular septum. Over the septum, it may be more to the left or to the right side of the septum. From this region, fibers of the left bundle branch begin to divide from the common bundle. This region is defined as the *branching portion* of the His bundle. The common AV bundle or His bundle is approximately 6 to 20 mm in length and 1.5 to 2 mm in diameter.

The left bundle at its origin is not a discrete branch of the common bundle but a series of fascicles given off over a relatively long extent. These muscular fascicles in the aggregate make up the left bundle branch. The left bundle branch demonstrates a marked variation in its origin and subsequent course (9). At its origin, the width may range from 5 to 15 mm from the beginning to the last fascicle to be given off. The predivisional left bundle divides into two or more branches, which cascade down the left ventricular septum in a fanlike configuration with multiple interconnections. The posterior (inferior) fascicle is short and wide, covering the posterior portion of the intraventricular septum. The anterior (superior) fascicle at its origin has a close anatomic relation to the proximal right bundle branch. The more distal ramifications and connection of these fibers and their distribution in the subendocardium of the anterior, posterior, and lateral free

left ventricular walls are difficult to identify in humans (8). An additional anatomically distinct fascicle, the septal fascicle, was described by Demoulin and Kulbertus (10). Although anatomically less clear, there is strong electrocardiographic (ECG) evidence for the trifascicular nature of the intraventricular conduction system in humans (11).

The right bundle branch is a more compact structure at its origin than the left bundle branch. It is the part of the common bundle that comes off most distant from the AV node. Its initial course over the right side of the septum is subendocardial and it is directed toward the anterior papillary muscle of the right ventricle, where it divides into fascicles that spread over the right ventricular myocardium. The right bundle branch is about 1 mm in diameter. In a limited number of human hearts, the right bundle separates from the common bundle before the origin of the left anterior fascicle is completed. In most other specimens, it is a direct continuation of the common bundle.

Blood Supply

The blood supply of the His bundle and proximal parts of the bundle branches originates from the right and left coronary systems (12). The arteries involved are the septal perforating branches of left anterior and posterior descending coronary arteries. The His bundle, the proximal right bundle branch, and the predivisional portion of the left bundle branch and its posterior fascicle receive dual blood supply from branches of the anterior and posterior descending coronary artery. The blood supply to the anterior fascicle of the left bundle branch is usually from the septal perforating branches of the left anterior descending coronary artery.

ETIOLOGY OF HIS-PURKINJE DISEASE

Alteration of the electrophysiologic properties of the His-Purkinje system may be chronic and irreversible as a result of structural changes caused by a disease process or may be an acute and reversible situation.

Structural

The strategic location of the His bundle and proximal bundle branches makes them vulnerable to disease processes that involve the central fibrous body, the mitral valve ring, the tricuspid valve ring, the aortic valve ring, and the ventricular septum. Calcific lesions involving these structures are frequently associated with fascicular block and bundle branch block (BBB) or even AV block. The cause of valvular involvement may be related to rheumatic heart disease or a degenerative, calcific, aging process of the left side of the cardiac skeleton. Hypertension is usually associated with fibrosis of the ventricular septum and accelerated degenerative changes of the annulus fibrosus and central fibrous body. Ischemic lesions resulting from disease of the left anterior descending or posterior descending arteries and their septal branches are important to the causes of intraventricular conduction disturbances. Other disease processes associated with myocardial scarring, such as dilated cardiomyopathy, are frequently associated with conduction disturbances. Pathologic processes such as inflammatory disease (lupus, scleroderma, ankylosing spondylitis), infectious agents (viral, bacterial, fungal), and infiltrative disease (amyloidosis, hemochromatosis, sarcoidosis) can affect the conduction system. Varying degrees of AV conduction block are the most common manifestation of Lyme carditis; bundle branch and fascicular blocks may also be seen (12a). The frequency of asymptomatic heart block, BBB, or fascicular block is unknown. The highest risk for progression to complete heart block, which may develop rapidly, occurs in patients with a PR interval of more than 0.3 seconds (12b). Electrophysiologic studies have usually found block occurring above the bundle of His, often within the AV node. However, block can occur at different levels within the conducting system. Sinoatrial node dysfunction (manifested as sinoatrial nodal block), abnormal nodal recovery time, intraatrial block, and fascicular block and BBB have been described (12b–12d). Some of the hereditary neuromuscular disorders may also be associated with pathologic His-Purkinje block (13). Neoplastic diseases of the heart (e.g., carcinoma, sarcoma, and leukemia) secondary to metastasis to the septum may cause block or conduction defects. In the presence of endocarditis with an abscess formation, the development of BBB and AV block have serious prognostic implications (14).

Primary conduction disease in the elderly has been defined as Lev disease, and in the young, it has been labeled Lenègre disease (15,16). Lev has called attention to the significance of the effect of the aging process and the hemodynamic stress on the cardiac skeleton. He described this pathologic process, which involves the aortic and mitral valve rings, the central fibrous body, and the summit of the ventricular septum, as "sclerosis of the left side of the cardiac skeleton." Lenègre in his investigation had emphasized the idiopathic nature of the conduction disease observed in pathologic specimens from younger patients.

The conduction system can also be involved in congenital heart disease such as the ostium primum type of atrial septal defect. There are also patients with otherwise healthy hearts but with congenital conduction disease. These usually involve the right bundle branch or the left anterior fascicle of the left bundle branch. Greenspahn and colleagues (17) examined the familial factors in the occurrence of bifascicular block. They evaluated 134 first- and second-degree relatives of 44 patients with chronic bifascicular block. These relatives were evaluated for the presence or absence of cardiac disease and conduction defects. A randomly chosen control population of employed volunteers was used for comparison. The study group had a significantly greater frequency of conduction defects than the control group. This study suggested that there was a familiar tendency to conduction disease among relatives of patients with chronic bifascicular block. Davies and colleagues (18) reviewed the origin of chronic AV block and found that 38% had an idiopathic cause (primary conduction disease), 21% had miscellaneous causes (myocarditis, inflammatory, infiltrative, congenital), 17% had associated coronary artery disease, 13% had dilated cardiomyopathy, and 11% had calcific AV block.

Acute Reversible Causes

The origin of His-Purkinje disease may also be related to acute and reversible causes. Antiarrhythmic drugs of class Ia, Ic, and III are known to affect the refractory period and conduction time of the His-Purkinje system. They can prolong the QRS duration and the HV interval. Hyperkalemia is known to slow conduction in the His-Purkinje system and the ventricular myocardium because of its hypopolarizing effect on the cell membrane. Hyperkalemia can induce an axis shift in the frontal QRS plane or produce bizarre nonspecific intraventricular conduction blocks or even transient advanced or complete heart block. Hypoxia and acidosis can exaggerate the effect of hyperkalemia. Mechanical trauma resulting from catheter manipulation in the right ventricular outflow tract can also produce transient depression of His-Purkinje conduction.

MECHANISM OF HIS-PURKINJE DISEASE

The basic mechanism of conduction block in the His-Purkinje system is under investigation. Several electrophysiologic changes have been invoked including prolongation of refractoriness of individual cells, the presence of postrepolarization refractoriness, decremental conduction of the tissue, and changes in excitability (19,20). Gonzales and colleagues (21), using an ischemically damaged canine His-Purkinje system model, examined the determinants of Mobitz type II AV block. They showed that the conduction block that appeared at a rapidly paced rate was associated with a decrease in the amplitude of the action potential and asynchronous cellular activation, resulting in dissociation of the electrical activity in the bundle. At slow rates of pacing, the action potential amplitude was 85 mV, and only a few cells (10%) showed dissociation of electrical activity within the bundle. At fast-paced rates during 1 : 1 conduction, the action potential amplitude decreased by 31% and the frequency of cellular dissociation increased to 57%. The frequency of dissociation closely correlated with the reduction of action potential amplitude; the lower the action potential amplitude, the greater the dissociation. The decreased action potential amplitude preceded the onset of a 2 : 1 block. Once a 2 : 1 block occurred, the amplitude of the action potential returned to normal levels and the frequency of dissociation returned to baseline. Interestingly, the site of block was not constant but showed a dynamic behavior with a spatial shifting in response to changes in paced rate or introduction of extrastimuli. The dissociated cells do not actively participate in the conduction process and resemble the "dead-end pathways" that normally exist in the AV node. The AV node also has low-amplitude action potentials, a low-level resting membrane potential, increased intercellular resistance, and a low safety factor for conduction. The study by Gonzalez and colleagues (21) showed that at fast rates in an ischemically damaged His-Purkinje system, the propagation of the depolarization wavefront is impaired. This finding was associated with low-amplitude action potentials and functional dissociation of cellular activation. The decreased action potential amplitude results in a reduced electronic input (source currents) to the distal segment and this may lead to block. The increased resistance, secondary to the ischemic process—intracellular and extracellular—may promote functional dissociation among the neighboring cells.

ECG MANIFESTATIONS AND DIAGNOSIS OF INTRAVENTRICULAR CONDUCTION DEFECTS

Rosenbaum and colleagues (11) popularized the concept of the trifascicular nature of the intraventricular conduction system. Many of the observations were based on ECG recordings. They proposed that the system consists of the right bundle branch and a left bundle that subdivides into anterior and posterior fascicles. Although more recently the existence of a fourth septal fascicle has been proposed, its origin and constancy have not been well defined.

The ECG presence of a BBB or fascicular block indicates a delay in ventricular activation. This delay may represent a complete block in the bundle branch or fascicle or a partial block with delayed conduction. It is the effect of the delay in depolarization that is observed on the surface ECG. Occasionally, this delay results from slow conduction within a localized portion of the myocardium, not necessarily including the bundle branch or fascicles. In this case, the block has been termed a *parietal block.*

Right BBB (RBBB) is characterized by a prolonged QRS duration of 0.12 seconds or more associated with abnormal terminal QRS forces directed anteriorly and to the right, indicating delayed activation of the right ventricle. These terminal forces will produce an R, rSR′, or qR wave in lead V_1; wide, slurred S waves in leads I, aVL, V_5, and V_6; and a wide terminal r wave in lead aVR.

Left BBB (LBBB) is characterized by a prolonged QRS duration of 0.12 seconds or more and delays in initial and mid QRS forces, which are directed posteriorly and to the left, indicating delayed left ventricular activation. This results in a broad, notched R wave without q waves in leads I, aVL, and V_6 and an rS pattern in lead V_1 (Fig. 24-1).

Left anterior fascicular block (LAFB) is characterized by a minimally prolonged QRS duration of 0.09 to 1.0 seconds and a leftward axis shift of −45 degrees or more. The initial QRS activation is directed inferiorly to the right, resulting in a qR in leads I and aVL and an rS pattern in leads II, III, and aVF (Fig. 24-2).

Left posterior fascicular block (LPFB) is characterized by a minimally prolonged QRS duration of 0.9 to 1.0 seconds with a rightward axis deviation of 90 degrees or more. The initial QRS forces are directed superiorly, resulting in a qR pattern in leads II, III, and aVF and an rS in leads I and aVL. Other causes of rightward axis deviation such as right ventricular hypertrophy must be excluded before making this diagnosis.

Nonspecific intraventricular conduction delay is characterized by a prolonged QRS duration in the absence of a specific bundle branch or fascicular block pattern. This type of widened QRS complex probably represents additional intramyocardial conduction delay and not an isolated lesion of the conduction system.

Combinations of RBBB and LAFB or RBBB and LPFB are defined as bifascicular blocks (Figs. 24-3 and 24-4).

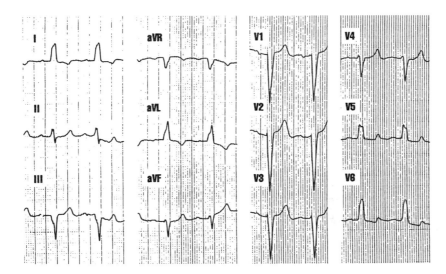

FIGURE 24-1. Complete left bundle branch block. A 12-lead electrocardiographic recording (paper speed 25 mm per second) showing a wide QRS complex with M-shaped morphology in leads I and aVL.

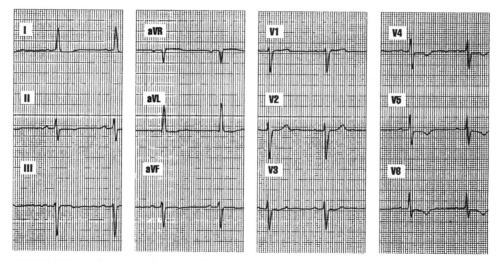

FIGURE 24-2. Left anterior fascicular block. Note that there is a left axis deviation (–45 degrees) in the frontal plane with a small q in lead aVL.

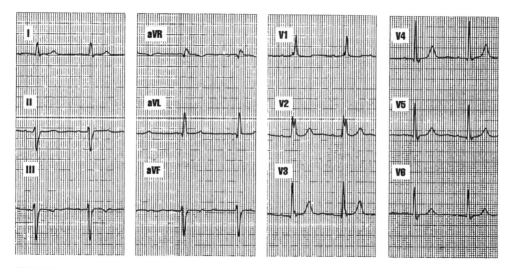

FIGURE 24-3. Bifascicular block. Right bundle branch block and left anterior fascicular block. Frontal plane QRS axis of –60 degrees.

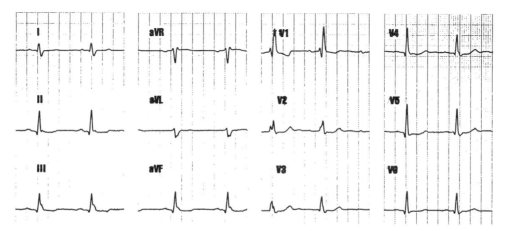

FIGURE 24-4. Bifascicular block. Right bundle branch block and left posterior fascicular block. Note wide QRS complexes with rSR′ in lead V$_1$ and small q waves in leads II, III, and aVF and frontal plane QRS axis of +100 degrees.

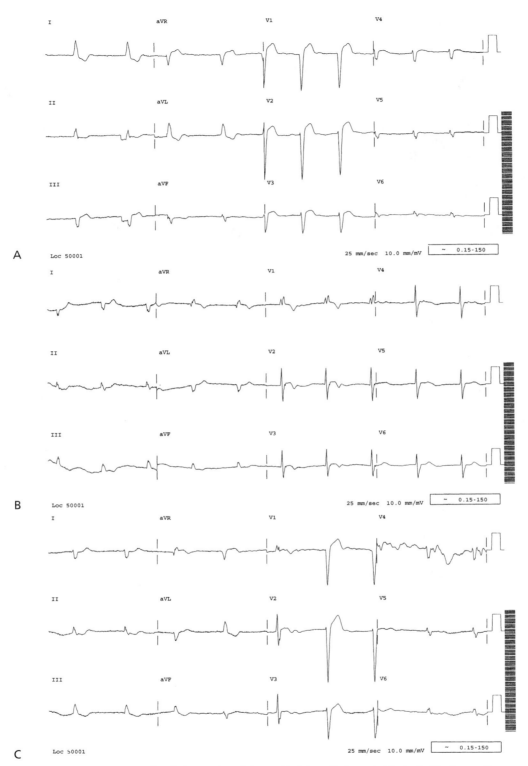

FIGURE 24-5. Example of alternating right and left bundle branch block. **A:** Electrocardiogram (ECG) showing atrial fibrillation with a slow ventricular response. The QRS complexes have a left bundle branch morphology. **B:** On the following day, a second ECG was recorded. The QRS complexes now show a right bundle branch morphology and the axis is rightward, diagnostic of a left posterior fascicular block. **C:** Two days later, another ECG was recorded. The underlying rhythm is still atrial fibrillation but QRS complexes are seen with a right and a left bundle branch morphology.

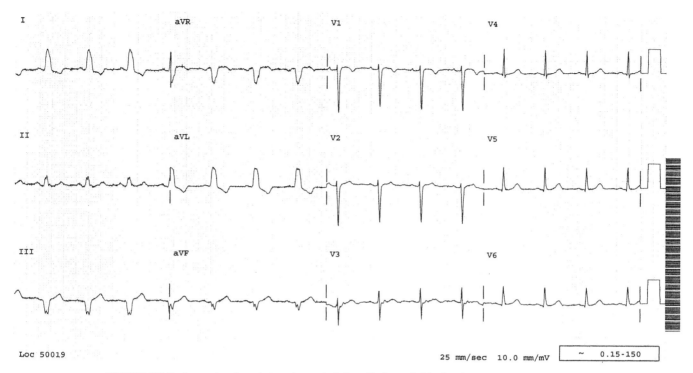

Loc 50019

25 mm/sec   10.0 mm/mV   ~ 0.15-150

FIGURE 24-6. Example of an intermittent left bundle branch block. The QRS complexes in the limb leads have a left bundle branch morphology while the complexes in the precordial leads show normal conduction. The PR and R-R intervals are identical throughout.

Most authors will classify complete LBBB as *bifascicular,* although some argue that lesions before the division of the left bundle (predivisional block) are not truly bifascicular.

Alternating BBB is an ECG pattern in which LBBB and RBBB conduction patterns are present on the same or different tracings of one patient (Fig. 24-5). Intermittent BBB is present when normal intraventricular conduction alternates with BBB or fascicular block patterns (Fig. 24-6).

First-degree AV block is defined as an abnormal prolongation of the PR interval (more than 0.20 seconds). Second-degree AV block has been classified on the basis of standard ECG findings into two types: Type I (Wenckebach phenomenon) is characterized by progressive prolongation of the PR interval before the blocked P wave (Fig. 24-7), and type II block (Mobitz) is characterized by a constant PR interval before the blocked beat (Fig. 24-8). AV block

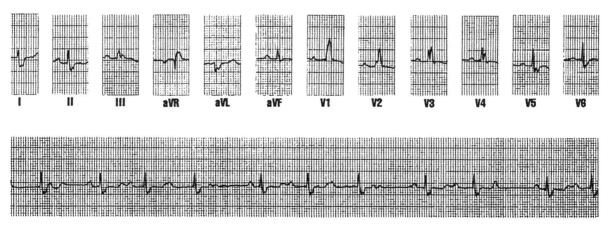

FIGURE 24-7. Type I (Wenckebach) second-degree atrioventricular block (4 : 3 and 3 : 2). Note that the QRS is wide and has right bundle branch block morphology. There are intermittently blocked P waves. There is lengthening of the PR interval before the blocked P wave. The site of block is uncertain; it may be in the atrioventricular node or in the His-Purkinje system.

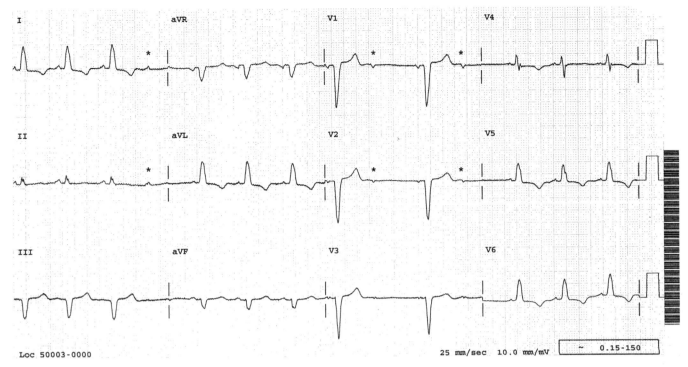

FIGURE 24-8. Example of Mobitz type II second-degree (atrioventricular) heart block. The rhythm is sinus, but there are several nonconducted P waves—that is, a P wave not followed by a QRS complex (*asterisks*). The PR and P-P intervals are constant (0.16) before and after the atrioventricular block.

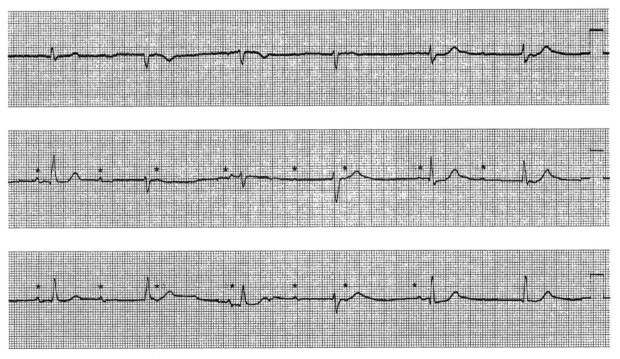

FIGURE 24-9. Example of complete, or third-degree, heart block. The atrial rate is 60 beats per minute and the ventricular rate is 38 beats per minute (*asterisks* indicate P waves).

with a 2 : 1 conduction ratio is not classified as type I or II because there is only one conducted P wave. AV blocks with two or more consecutive blocked P waves are classified as high-degree blocks and described as a ratio between P waves and QRS complexes (e.g., 3 : 1 and 4 : 1). Complete AV block is present when there is total dissociation between P waves and QRS complexes (Fig. 24-9).

CHRONIC INTRAVENTICULAR BLOCK

Prevalence of Chronic Intraventricular Blocks

In the general population, LAFB is the most common intraventricular conduction defect (prevalence, 4.5%). Isolated LPFB is a rare ECG finding. The prevalence of RBBB is from 1.15% to 3.19%, and for LBBB, the prevalence is 1% (22,23). The incidence of BBB increases with age. In a prospective study of 855 men followed for 30 years, the incidence of RBBB was 0.8% in subjects at age 50, 9.9% by age 75, and 11.3% by age 80; the incidence of an LBBB was 0.4% at age 50, 2.3% by age 75, and 5.7% by age 80. There was no significant association with the presence of ischemic heart disease, myocardial infarction, or cardiovascular deaths. It was suggested that BBB correlates strongly with age and is a marker of a slowly progressive degenerative disease that also affects the myocardium (23a). However, LBBB may be associated with significant and advanced heart disease.

Significance of Chronic Intraventricular Blocks

The clinical significance of a BBB found on the ECG depends on the population under investigation. The Framingham Study is perhaps the most representative of the population that is seen by clinicians (24,25). The 5,209 subjects who were free of cardiovascular disease at the time of initial entry were followed prospectively for 18 years (24,25). BBB developed in 125 patients during follow-up, yielding an overall incidence rate of 2.4% and an annual incidence rate of 0.13%.

Seventy patients developed RBBB, and the appearance of a BBB in these patients was not associated with any overt acute clinical event (24). Most of the patients who developed the conduction defect were hypertensive. Compared with a matched control group without an RBBB, the incidence of coronary artery disease was 2.5 times greater, the incidence of congestive heart failure was 4 times greater, and the cardiovascular mortality rate was 3 times higher than that of the group with no RBBB. Fifty patients developed an LBBB (25). In contrast to RBBB, 48% of the cases had a clinically diagnosable vascular event at the time of developing the LBBB. There was also a strong association between the presence of an LBBB and the occurrence of

hypertension, cardiomegaly, and coronary artery disease in these patients. The cumulative mortality rate was 50% within 10 years, which was 5 times more than that of the population at large without an LBBB.

In contrast to the above study, Rotman and Triebwasser (26) reported a group of 519 subjects with a BBB in the United States Air Force School of Aerospace Medicine; 394 subjects had an RBBB and 125 had an LBBB. Most subjects were young, asymptomatic, and without apparent cardiovascular disease. There were no sudden deaths and the overall mortality rate was 4% during a mean follow-up of 10 years. The incidence of progression to AV block in asymptomatic Air Force personnel with an RBBB was 0.25% versus 1% for those who had an LBBB.

Natural History of Conduction Abnormalities

Retrospective ECG studies examined the prognosis of patients with a chronic BBB. Lasser and colleagues (27) found a 1% prevalence of RBBB and LAFB in a retrospective study of hospital records. There was a 9% progression to complete heart block during an unspecified time. Scanlon and colleagues (28) included in their study patients with an RBBB associated with an LAFB or an LPFB. They found that 14% progressed to complete heart block. DePasquale and Bruno (29) reported a 6% incidence of progression to AV block (second or third degree) in 83 patients with an RBBB and LAFB.

The natural history and management of patients with chronic intraventricular conduction disease and the risk of advanced heart block during noncardiac surgery was studied by Pastore and colleagues (30). They reviewed the risk of progression to advanced AV block during anesthesia in 44 patients with an RBBB and LAFB. All patients had continuous ECG monitoring throughout anesthesia and operation, as well as during surgical recovery. They found only one episode of transient complete heart block in 52 operative procedures in these patients. Their conclusion was that temporary pacing is rarely required in patients with chronic bifascicular block who undergo noncardiac surgery and should not be routinely used.

Exercise Testing and Left Bundle Branch Block

Transient, exercise-induced LBBB occurs in approximately 0.5% of exercise stress tests. Although its significance has been uncertain, one study analyzed 70 episodes of this phenomenon, which occurred in the context of 17,277 exercise tests and found that exercise-induced LBBB was an independent predictor of death and major cardiac events (30a). The 4-year cumulative event rate was 19% and 10% for those with or without exercise-induced LBBB, respectively (relative risk, 2.78).

In patients with an LBBB, ECG during exercise stress testing is of limited value for the diagnosis of coronary heart disease because ECG changes cannot be evaluated. The results of exercise perfusion imaging with thallium or sestamibi have also been disappointing because specificity is low, primarily because of false-positive septal perfusion abnormalities.

In comparison, myocardial imaging with vasodilators such as adenosine or dipyridamole may improve the accuracy of perfusion imaging in patients with an LBBB, enhancing the ability to predict outcome (30b). Exercise echocardiography is extremely accurate for diagnosing coronary heart disease in the presence of an LBBB, particularly for detecting left anterior coronary artery and multivessel disease (30c).

INTRAVENTRICULAR BLOCKS RESULTING FROM ACUTE MYOCARDIAL INFARCTION

Conduction disturbances are well-recognized complications of acute myocardial infarction. They are induced by an autonomic imbalance or ischemia and necrosis of the conduction system. It is important to recognize which situations are transient and which are likely to progress to irreversible and symptomatic high-degree block. The use of reperfusion with thrombolytic therapy or angioplasty has reduced the incidence of BBB associated with a myocardial infarction, although its prognostic significance has not been affected.

Acute Conduction Blocks in the Prethrombolytic Era

Codini (31) reviewed reports published since 1970 on the overall incidence of intraventricular blocks during acute myocardial infarction, their progression to high-degree AV block, and the associated mortality rate. A total of 46,235 cases of acute myocardial infarction was reported. The overall incidence of intraventricular conduction block varied between 10% and 35% with an average of 19%. The mortality rate of patients with intraventricular conduction defects was twice that of patients without an intraventricular conduction block.

LAFB is the most common type of intraventricular conduction defect (7%) and LPFB is the rarest. Isolated fascicular blocks do not appear to worsen the course of acute myocardial infarction. LBBB is the second most common form of intraventricular conduction defect, with an average incidence of 4%. The progression to third-degree heart block is 9% and there is a high in-hospital mortality rate (41%) associated with this conduction defect. Isolated RBBB has a frequency of 2%. The progression to complete AV block is 19%. The associated mortality rate is 50%. In the presence of nonadjacent bifascicular blocks, such as

RBBB and LAFB, RBBB and LPFB, and alternating BBB, pathologic examination reveals extensive necrosis of the intraventricular septum. The progression to complete heart block in these patients is markedly increased (RBBB and LAFB, 36%; RBBB and LPFB, 39%; and alternating BBB, 40%). The mortality rate associated with bifascicular block is very high: 51% for RBBB and LAFB, 68% for RBBB and LPFB, and 70% for alternating BBB.

Transient intraventricular blocks during an acute myocardial infarction appear to have a more favorable clinical course and prognosis (32). Patients with delayed-onset or short-lasting BBB have a significantly lower mortality risk. The presence of an old versus a new intraventricular block also seems to influence outcome. The progression to third-degree AV block is twice as frequent in patients with new intraventricular blocks than in patients with old intraventricular blocks (22% versus 13%). The mortality rate for patients with a new intraventricular block is slightly higher than that for those with an existing block (43% versus 36%), although both carry a high in-hospital mortality rate.

Hindman and colleagues (33,34) identified three ECG variables that could define groups at low, intermediate, and high risk for progression to advanced or complete AV block. These variables were (a) first-degree AV block, (b) "new" BBB, and (c) bilateral BBB. The lowest risk group had a 10% to 13% incidence of progression and it was defined by having only one of the three variables present. The intermediate risk group had a progression rate of 19% to 20% and the group was defined as having any two of the variables present except for new bilateral BBB. The highest risk group had a progression rate of 31% to 38% and had either all three variables present or a new bilateral BBB.

The long-term prognosis of patients who have permanent or transient complete heart block in association with an intraventricular block during an acute myocardial infarction is ominous. Hindman and colleagues (34) retrospectively reviewed the outcome of patients who had episodes of high-degree AV block complicating an acute myocardial infarction associated with an intraventricular block. Twenty patients were discharged without permanent pacemakers. Seven of these patients subsequently developed high-degree AV block and 10 died suddenly. In the group of 29 patients who received permanent pacing, only 3 sudden deaths occurred.

The experience of other authors appears to be at variance with the results of the previously described study. Ginks and colleagues (35) reported on 25 hospital survivors of acute myocardial infarction and intraventricular block complicated by transient third-degree block. Two of 4 patients who received a permanent pacemaker died suddenly, and 3 of 21 patients discharged without a pacemaker also experienced sudden death. The issue of the use of permanent pacemakers was further complicated by the fact that not all of the sudden deaths in this population were necessarily caused by a recurrent heart block and asystole. In a retrospective study by Lie and colleagues (36), 14 of 30 patients after an acute myocardial infarction complicated by an RBBB or LBBB developed late in-hospital ventricular fibrillation. In a separate cohort followed prospectively by these authors, 17 of 47 patients with acute myocardial infarction and BBB developed ventricular fibrillation within 6 weeks while being monitored for arrhythmias.

Acute Conduction Blocks with Thrombolytic Therapy

The major thrombolytic trials have not reported detailed descriptions of the types and frequency of conduction disease associated with acute revascularization for acute myocardial infarction. The available data suggest that the incidence of complete heart block in patients with an acute myocardial infarction is lower with thrombolytic therapy (3.7% to 5%) and the incidence of complete heart block or second-degree AV block is from 7.3% to 9.5% (36a–36d). However, the poorer prognosis associated with complete heart block has not been altered by the current strategy of immediate revascularization (36a–36e).

There are limited data regarding the incidence and prognostic significance of BBB in patients with an acute myocardial infarction treated with thrombolytic agents; however, data suggest that the incidence and prognosis has not been altered by revascularization (36d). One study evaluated 681 patients from one institution entered into 2 thrombolytic trials (36f). The incidence of transient BBB was 18.% while persistent BBB occurred in 5.3% of patients. Fifty-four percent of BBBs resulted from occlusion of the left anterior descending artery. BBB was associated with lower ejection fractions, larger infarctions, and more diseased vessels. RBBB was most common, occurring in 13% of patients, followed by LBBB in 7% and alternating BBB. The mortality rate was higher in the presence of a persistent BBB and in those in whom the conduction abnormality was transient (19% and 6%, respectively) versus patients without BBBs (4%).

A different study of 1,238 patients found that the incidence and significance of an RBBB in patients receiving thrombolytic therapy are similar to those reported in the prethrombolytic era (36g).

Non–Q-wave Myocardial Infarction

Most studies reporting the incidence and prognostic significance of high-degree AV block after a myocardial infarction have not distinguished between Q-wave and non–Q-wave infarction. One study reported on 610 patients with a first non–Q-wave infarction and observed that second- or third-degree AV block developed in 45 patients (7%) (36h). Compared with patients without block, these patients had a higher rate of cardiac arrest, heart failure, elevation of cardiac enzymes, and in-hospital mortality, but there was no

difference in 1- or 5-year mortality rate. These findings suggest that high-degree AV block in patients with a non–Q-wave myocardial infarction is associated with a larger and more complicated infarctions, as is the case in patients with Q-wave myocardial infarction.

CLINICAL ELECTROPHYSIOLOGIC MANIFESTATIONS AND DIAGNOSIS

Recording of His Bundle Electrogram, Conduction Times, Refractory Period, and Aberrancy

The technique of His bundle recording in humans was described in 1969 by Scherlag and colleagues (37) (Fig. 24-10). Electrode catheters are introduced percutaneously, advanced to the right side of the heart, and positioned across the tricuspid valve. Appropriate amplification and frequency filtering (40 to 500 Hz) of the recorded signal allows recording of a His bundle potential (H potential). The His bundle electrogram needs to be differentiated from atrial and right bundle branch electrograms. The relative amplitude of the recorded atrial and ventricular electrograms is helpful in differentiating His potentials from right bundle potentials (38). An absent or small atrial electrogram suggests that the right bundle potential is being recorded. Prominent atrial and ventricular electrograms are consistent with an AV location of the catheter and a His bundle recording. Rapid atrial pacing is useful in delineating the atrial and His bundle potentials. Atrial pacing prolongs the A-H interval (AV nodal conduction) but will not affect the atrial potential. The verification of His bundle deflection can also be performed by direct pacing of the His bundle.

The PR interval can be divided into three subintervals with the recording of the His potential (Fig. 24-10). The P-A interval is a measure of intraatrial (high to low right atrium) conduction time. The A-H interval is a measure of the AV nodal conduction time; the HV interval, measured from the onset of His potential to the onset of ventricular activation, as determined from the earliest deflection of the surface QRS, is a measure of conduction time through the His bundle (distal to the recording site) and bundle branches. In patients with a BBB, the HV interval reflects conduction time in the functioning bundle branch.

Kupersmith and colleagues (39) directly measured the conduction intervals and the conduction velocity of the human cardiac conduction system during open-heart surgery. There was an increase in the HV interval with increasing age. The HV interval, recorded from the proximal His bundle, for infants varies from 13 to 27 ms, and for those 15 years of age and older, the normal interval is from 35 to 54 ms. With catheter techniques, an HV interval of 55 ms is the upper limit of normal (40). This suggests that

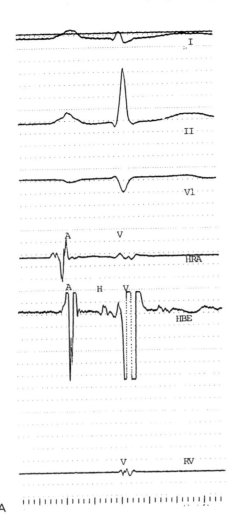

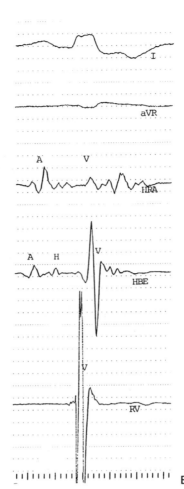

FIGURE 24-10. Example of His bundle recording. **A:** A typical recording from an electrophysiologic test including three surface electrocardiogram (ECG) leads (I, II, V1): a high right atrial (HRA) electrogram; His bundle electrogram (HBE), and a right ventricular electrogram (RV) recorded at the right ventricular apex. The A-H interval is 58 ms and the HV is 58 ms. **B:** A recording from a patient with a left bundle branch block who presented with syncope. Seen are two surface ECG leads (I, aVR) and tracings from HRA, HBE, and RV. Note an A-H interval of 90 ms and a prolonged HV interval of 110 ms. (A, atrial electrogram; H, His bundle electrogram; V, ventricular electrogram.)

most His bundle electrograms recorded by the catheter technique are from the proximal His bundle. The HV interval recorded from the distal His bundle varies from 18 to 35 ms. The right bundle to ventricle interval varies from 18 to 30 ms and the left bundle to ventricle interval from 20 to 39 ms. The conduction velocity in the His bundle was determined and averages 1.5 m per second (range, 1.3 to 1.7 m per second). The duration of the His potential varies from 10 to 20 ms.

Atrial pacing can be used to stress the conduction system and uncover abnormalities not apparent during sinus rhythm. Atrial pacing at rapid rates does not affect the His bundle potential or the HV interval under normal conditions (40). The development of block distal to the His bundle during rapid atrial pacing is a definite abnormal finding and indicates His-Purkinje disease (41) (Fig. 24-11).

The refractory period of the His-Purkinje system is rate-dependent, and as the rate increases, the refractory period of the His-Purkinje system and the ventricular muscle decreases (42). The cycle length dependency of the refractory period of the His-Purkinje system accounts for a num-

ber of ECG and electrophysiologic observations, such as aberrant conduction and the gap phenomenon (43,44). At long cycle lengths (slow rates), a premature atrial beat will be blocked or delayed in the region of the His-Purkinje system with the longest refractory period (6). Aberrant conduction of premature supraventricular impulses mostly exhibits an RBBB pattern (80% to 90%), although some may have an LBBB aberration or both patterns may be observed (45).

The Ashman phenomenon is an example of aberrancy resulting caused by the physiologic changes of the conduction system's refractory periods that are associated with the heart rate or R-R–interval cycle length. There may be aberrant conduction as the result of a long R-R interval followed by a short cycle. Because the refractory period of the bundles increases during the long R-R interval, the QRS complex, which ends the long pause, will be conducted normally; however, if the next QRS complex occurs after a short coupling interval, it may be conducted aberrantly because one of the bundles is still refractory as a result of a lengthening of the refractory period. This sequence occurs

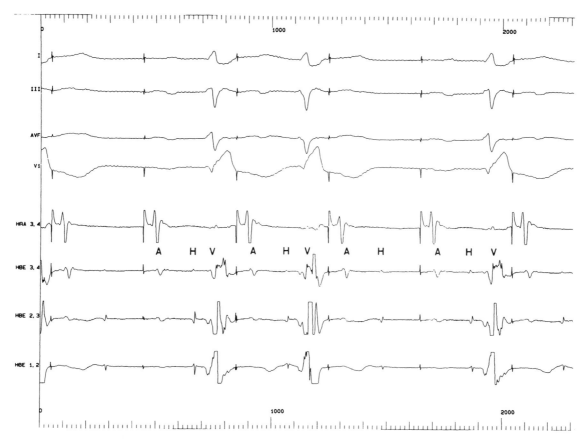

FIGURE 24-11. Infra-Hisian block during atrial pacing in a patient with a right bundle branch block and left anterior fascicular block. The first and fourth atrial paced beats are conducted to the His bundle but not to the ventricle (the His spike is seen, but there is no ventricular electrogram after it). Loss of distal conduction is sudden, not decremental. Atrioventricular nodal conduction times (A-H interval) are constant. (HBE, His bundle electrograms recorded from proximal [3,4] and distal [1,2] poles; HRA, high right atrial signals recorded from proximal poles [3,4].)

during atrial fibrillation when there are frequent episodes of long-short R-R cycle lengths; the aberrancy may be present for one beat and have a morphology that resembles a ventricular premature beat, or it may involve several sequential complexes, suggesting a ventricular tachycardia.

Occasionally, axis shifts are seen without the appearance of a BBB. Most of these axis shifts are leftward, indicating a delay in the left anterior fascicle. At other times, a combination of RBBB and leftward shift of axis is noted simultaneously, consistent with block or delay in the right bundle branch and left anterior fascicle of the left bundle (45). Even intra-Hisian block with a split His potential or a distal to His bundle block (bilateral BBB) can be seen with a premature atrial stimulation (45).

The presence of aberrancy, conduction delays, and blocks is dependent on multiple factors including the preceding cycle, conduction time of the AV node, refractoriness of the His-Purkinje system, and presence of catecholamines. A long preceding cycle, rapid AV nodal conduction, and long His-Purkinje refractoriness promote

aberrancy, whereas a short preceding cycle length, delayed AV nodal conduction, or block will prevent aberrancy of premature beats in the His-Purkinje system. The site of functional block during aberrancy has been localized to the proximal bundle branches (45). Catecholamines tend to restore or improve conduction in the His-Purkinje system.

Atrioventricular Blocks

Electrophysiological Criteria

First-Degree Atrioventricular Block

During first-degree AV block (PR interval of more than 0.20 seconds), the delay most commonly occurs in the AV node (46). However, occasionally in the presence of a narrow QRS, PR prolongation is related to a delay in the His bundle, with recording of split His potentials (HH′ interval) (Fig. 24-12). Prolongation of the HV interval in the presence of a wide QRS denotes disease in the His bundle or the bundle branches. Prolongation of the HV interval

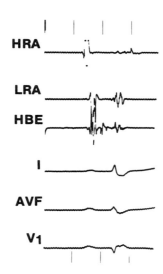

FIGURE 24-12. Fragmented His bundle potential in a patient with syncope, narrow QRS complex, and a normal PR interval. (HBE, His bundle electrogram; HRA, high right atrium; LRA, low right atrium.)

accounting by itself for first-degree AV block is quite rare. Most commonly, first-degree AV block represents a combination of prolongation of intraatrial, AV nodal, and His-Purkinje conduction times.

Second-Degree Atrioventricular Block

During second-degree AV block, the His bundle recording can delineate three sites of block: (a) a block proximal to the His potential (AV nodal), (b) a block within the His potential (intra-Hisian), in which the conducted beats demon-strate two His potentials, one proximal and another distal (the P wave is followed by the proximal His potential), and (c) a block distal to the His potential (trifascicular block), in which the blocked P wave is followed by a His potential (47) (Fig. 24-13). The clinical significance of second-degree AV block is related to the site of block rather than the ECG type of block (48,49). The presence of type I block with a narrow QRS is usually associated with an AV nodal block and rarely with an intra-Hisian block. In the presence of a wide QRS, a type I block usually occurs in the AV node but may occur in the His bundle or in the conducting bundle branch. In the latter case, progressive HH' or HV prolongation is present before the blocked P wave. Typically, type II AV block in the presence of a narrow QRS represents intra-Hisian block and in the presence of BBB reflects a distal to His bundle block (trifascicular block).

In summary, type I block usually represents AV nodal block (72%) and less commonly intra-Hisian block (8%) or infra-Hisian block (20%) (50,51). Type II AV block most commonly represents infra-Hisian block (71%) and less commonly intra-Hisian block (29%) (50,51). In the presence of a 2:1 and 3:1 block, the site of block is infra-Hisian in 51% of cases, intra-Hisian in 20%, and AV nodal in 29% (50,51).

It is the site of block and not necessarily the type of block that determines the prognosis. The prognosis of second-degree intra-Hisian block is controversial (52,53). In one series, heart failure and syncope occurred early during follow-up in patients who were not treated (52). However, another study failed to confirm these observations (53). Chronic second-degree block distal to the His bundle has a poor prognosis with most patients, becoming symptomatic with syncope (49).

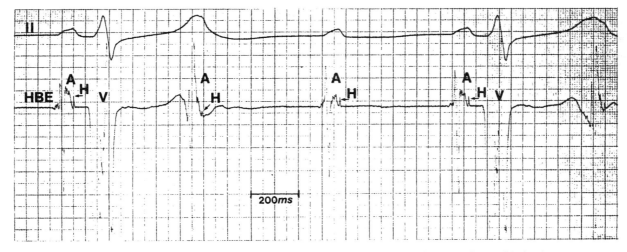

FIGURE 24-13. Advanced infra-Hisian atrioventricular block (3:1). Electrocardiographic lead II and the His bundle electrograms (HBEs) are shown. Atrial (A), His (H), and ventricular (V) electrograms are labeled. The paper speed is 100 mm per second. Note that the HV interval is prolonged (70 ms) on the conducted beats. The blocked beats show an atrial electrogram (A) followed by a His electrogram (H). The block is distal to H.

Complete Heart Block

In complete heart block, the use of His bundle recording allows the delineation of three sites of block: (a) proximal to His (AV node), (b) intra-Hisian (split His potential), and (c) distal to the His bundle (complete trifascicular block). The site of complete heart block cannot be accurately predicted from the surface ECG. In patients with AV nodal or intra-Hisian block, the escape rhythm may have narrow or wide QRS complexes. In patients with a block distal to the His bundle, the escape rhythm always has wide QRS complexes. The distribution of the site of block in complete heart block varies with different series (54,55). It is AV nodal in 14% to 35%, intra-Hisian in 14% to 18%, and distal to the His bundle in 49% to 72% of cases. Patients with complete heart block are frequently symptomatic with dizziness, syncope, or congestive heart failure. A distal site of block is frequently correlated with syncopal manifestation. The incidence of syncope is 29% in AV nodal block, 25% in intra-Hisian block, and 71% in a block distal to the His bundle (54).

Chronic Intraventricular Blocks

Significance of the HV Interval

In patients with chronic intraventricular blocks on the surface ECG, measurement of the HV interval is helpful because it has prognostic significance in these patients. In patients with bifascicular block, the HV interval reflects the function of the remaining fascicle, and the prolongation of the HV interval suggests the presence of trifascicular disease. In a review article of studies on bifascicular block, HV prolongation in patients with bifascicular block has been reported to occur with varying incidences: for RBBB, 7%; for LBBB, 50% to 80%; for RBBB and LAFB, 15% to 50%; and for RBBB and LPFB, 29% to 80% (25). There have been several major prospective studies that examined the natural history of chronic BBB and the role of electrophysiologic studies in predicting progression to advanced AV block or sudden death (56–58).

The study of Peters and Scheinman (56) included 313 patients (mean age of 66 years and a mean follow-up of 34 months) with chronic isolated BBB (right or left), RBBB and LAFB, RBBB and LPFB, and nonspecific intraventricular conduction defects. Group 1 had an HV interval of 30 to 54 ms (97 patients); group 2 had an HV interval of 55 to 69 ms (99 patients); and group 3 had an HV interval of 70 ms or more (117 patients). Eighty percent of patients had organic heart disease, most (75%) of which was coronary in origin. Transient neurologic symptoms were present in approximately 60% of all patients and syncope was present in 40%. The follow-up observations demonstrated progression to second- and third-degree AV block in 4% of group 1, 2% of group 2, and 12% of group 3 patients. Seventeen patients had an HV interval of more than 100 ms. Of these 17, 4 (24%) had progression to AV block. Repeated electrophysiologic studies were carried out in 20 patients who

developed AV block. The site of the block was distal to the His bundle in 12 (60%) patients, and in the remaining patients (40%), the site of the block was AV nodal. Approximately two thirds of patients with an HV interval of 70 ms or more (group 3) were paced prophylactically. The prophylactically paced group (62 patients) with a long HV interval (70 ms or more) was compared with the group who did not receive pacemaker therapy (37 patients); relief of syncope occurred in 88% of the paced group and 55% of the unpaced group ($p < 0.05$). Although pacing relieved symptoms of syncope in some patients with a chronic BBB and a long HV interval, there was no difference in the incidence of sudden death between the paced and the unpaced group (19% versus 16%, respectively). This lack of decrease in sudden death by pacing in patients with a chronic bifascicular block is most likely secondary to a mechanism of sudden death other than asystole in these patient groups.

The study of Dhingra and colleagues (57) included 517 patients (mean age of 62 years) with a mean follow-up of 26 months. The study included patients with a chronic bifascicular block (LBBB, RBBB and LAFB, RBBB and LPFB). Patients with HV intervals of less than 55 ms (319 patients) were compared with those with prolonged HV intervals of 55 ms or more (198 patients). In this study, 80% of all patients had organic heart disease, two thirds of which had either hypertension or arteriosclerotic heart disease. Syncope was present in approximately 15% of patients. Progression to second- or third-degree AV block occurred in 2% of patients with normal HV intervals and 6.5% of patients who demonstrated prolonged HV intervals. Cumulative 7-year incidence of spontaneous AV block was 10% in the group with normal HV intervals and 20% in the group with prolonged HV intervals ($p < 0.0005$). The site of AV block was considered to be distal in 33% of patients in the group with normal HV intervals and in 70% of patients in the group with prolonged HV intervals. The sudden death mortality rate was 15% in the group with normal HV intervals and 20% in the patients who had prolonged HV intervals.

This study also examined the incidence of AV block with the different types of intraventricular conduction defect. They found that in patients with RBBB and LAFB, the progression rate was 5%, in those with RBBB and LPFB, the rate of progression was 5%, and in those with LBBB, it was only 2% (59). These incidences of progression for a chronic AV conduction defect are significantly lower than incidences encountered in previously reported retrospective studies. In an earlier study, Dhingra and colleagues (60) reported that a markedly prolonged HV interval (80 ms or more) in patients with a bifascicular block was associated with a low incidence (6%) of progression to AV block. The cumulative incidence of sudden cardiac death was 10%, 13%, and 16% during the first, second, and third year of follow-up, respectively (61). In patients with an LBBB, the 3-year cumulative incidence of sudden death was 35%

while it was 11% for those with RBBB and LAFB, and 7% for those with RBBB and LPFB (61). Compared with the survivors, the following findings were significantly more frequent in the sudden cardiac death group: angina, previous myocardial infarction, presence of heart failure, cardiomegaly, presence of an LBBB on the ECG, presence of ventricular premature beats, and ventricular tachycardia (61). Ventricular fibrillation was the cause of death in four cases in which terminal ECG documentation was available. It was concluded that sudden cardiac death in patients with a bifascicular block is likely to be related to the occurrence of ventricular fibrillation and not heart block.

The third major prospective study of patients with a chronic BBB was reported by McAnulty and colleagues (58). They studied 351 patients (mean age of 63 years) with a mean follow-up of 42 months. The study included patients with a chronic bifascicular block. Organic heart disease was present in 74% of patients. Of these, 44% had coronary artery disease. Syncope was present in 31% of patients. Prolongation of the HV interval (more than 55 ms) was present in 54% of cases. The incidence of heart block was 4.9% in patients with prolonged HV intervals (more than 55 ms) and 1.9% for those with normal HV intervals. The 3-year cumulative incidence of sudden death was 18%. An evaluation of the circumstances of sudden death indicated that 73% of these were unrelated to bradyarrhythmias. Patients with an LBBB had a 36% total mortality rate and a 17% sudden death rate. Patients with an RBBB and left axis deviation had a 39% total mortality rate and a 16% sudden cardiac death rate. Patients with an RBBB and right axis deviation had a 28% total mortality rate and a 14% sudden cardiac death rate. Prolonged PR intervals (more than 0.20 seconds) in those patients with a BBB was associated with doubling of mortality and sudden death rates.

In summary, these prospective studies of patients with organic heart disease and BBBs demonstrate that there is a high prevalence of HV prolongation. However, despite the high prevalence of trifascicular disease, the overall rate is 2% to 4% per year. The progression to heart block is higher in those patients with HV prolongation. There is a high total mortality rate associated with intraventricular conduction defect, and half of the mortality rate is related to sudden death. The available evidence suggests that sudden death is more likely related to ventricular tachyarrhythmias and not the development of heart block.

To improve the accuracy of electrophysiologic studies in patients with a chronic BBB, investigators have used various means to stress the conduction system (41,62). The development of a block distal to the His bundle during incremental atrial pacing has been shown to predict the occurrence of spontaneous AV block (Fig. 24-11). Dhingra and colleagues (41) reported this finding in 4% (21) of 496 patients with a chronic bifascicular block. Of 15 patients who developed a distal block during intact AV nodal conduction, 8 developed spontaneous AV block and 2 died suddenly during a mean

follow-up of 3.4 years. Several pharmacologic agents have been used to stress the conduction system. Development of an AV block during intravenous administration of ajmaline has been shown to predict spontaneous occurrence of a distal block in patients with a chronic BBB (62).

The prognostic significance of the HV interval in primary conduction disease has also been evaluated. In their prospective study of 86 patients with a chronic bifascicular block without clinical evidence of organic heart disease (primary conduction disease), Dhingra and colleagues (63) reported that the incidence of HV prolongation (more than 55 ms) was 21% in patients with primary conduction disease and 41% in patients with organic heart disease ($p < 0.001$). Ninety percent of patients with primary conduction disease had an RBBB as opposed to 72% of patients with organic heart disease ($p < 0.01$). Progression to an AV block occurred in 3% of patients with primary conduction disease and 7% of patients with organic heart disease. The cumulative incidence of sudden death during a 3-year period was 6% in the patients with primary conduction disease and 17% in patients with organic heart disease ($p < 0.001$). It is concluded that patients with a bifascicular block in the presence of primary conduction disease have significantly lower incidences of electrophysiologic abnormalities, subsequent AV block, and sudden death than those of patients with organic heart disease.

Bundle Branch Block Resulting from Longitudinal Dissociation in the His Bundle

The appearance of a complete BBB pattern on the ECG has been assumed to be related to disease in the corresponding bundle branch. The concept that a BBB pattern on the ECG can result from disease within the His bundle had been postulated but not proven until the advent of His bundle recordings (64). It was observed that in patients with a complete LBBB pattern, pacing from the proximal His bundle reproduces the LBBB morphology, whereas pacing from the distal His bundle results in normalization of intraventricular conduction (64,65). It is suggested that the LBBB pattern in these cases is a result of an intra-Hisian lesion that involves the fibers destined to be part of the left bundle branch. Pacing distal to the lesion normalizes the intraventricular conduction. The pathologic mechanism for this may be a direct injury to the His bundle fibers destined to form part of the left bundle branch or a disruption of the transverse interconnections between strands of conducting fibers within the His bundle (66).

Intraventricular Block Resulting from Acute Myocardial Infarction

Significance of HV Interval

The use of His bundle recordings during acute myocardial infarction and the importance of the HV interval have been evaluated by Lie and colleagues (32). They showed that prolongation of the HV interval in the presence of BBB during an acute anteroseptal myocardial infarction is associated with a high risk of complete heart block and an increased mortality risk. However, prolongation of the HV interval in patients with acute myocardial infarction and a BBB is rarely used as an indication for temporary pacing, probably because the measurement of the HV interval already requires the same invasive procedure that is needed for placement of a temporary pacemaker.

Intermittent Bundle Branch Block

Unstable, or intermittent, BBB has been a subject of interest to electrocardiographers. Intermittent BBB may be heart rate–dependent, in which case, it is defined as rate-dependent BBB or unrelated to changes in heart rate. Most of the

electrophysiologic observations in humans have been made in rate-dependent BBB (67). Rate-dependent BBB is diagnosed when the BBB appears at a critical heart rate (Figs. 24-14 and 24-15). This should be differentiated from a functional BBB, in which the block is dependent on a preceding long cycle length (68). Functional BBB (aberrancy) may be a physiologic response, while rate-dependent BBB is most commonly seen in patients with heart disease. Rosenbaum and colleagues (69) described cases of intermittent rate-dependent BBB, in which a block was shown to occur at rapid and slow rates with an intermediate range of normal conduction. The tachycardia-dependent branch block was termed *phase 3 block* whereas the bradycardia-dependent BBB was defined as *phase 4 block* (Fig. 24-16). Clinical electrophysiologic observations in patients with tachycardia-dependent BBB have shown that the refractory period of the bundle branch is prolonged when compared

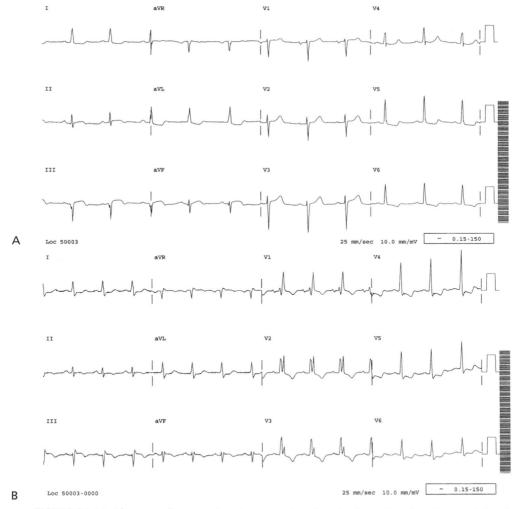

FIGURE 24-14. Electrocardiograms showing examples of a rate-dependent bundle branch block. **A:** In sinus rhythm at a rate of 66 beats per minute, the QRS complexes have a normal duration and there is no conduction abnormality. **B:** With sinus tachycardia at a rate of 105 beats per minute, there is a right bundle branch block.

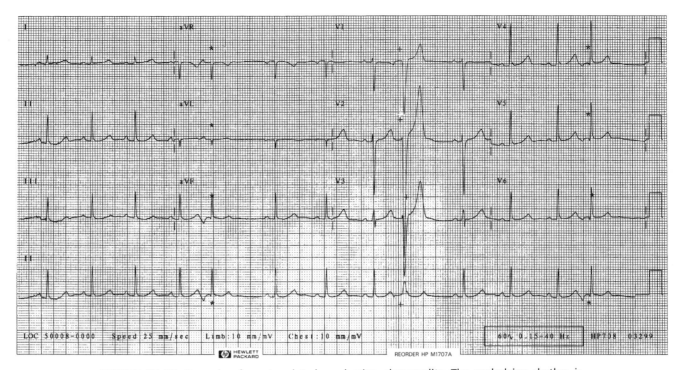

FIGURE 24-15. Example of a rate-related conduction abnormality. The underlying rhythm is sinus. There are atrial premature beats (APBs), which are normally conducted (*asterisks*), and in leads V$_1$ through V$_3$, there is an APB *(+)* with a shorter coupling interval, which is conducted aberrantly with a left bundle branch block morphology.

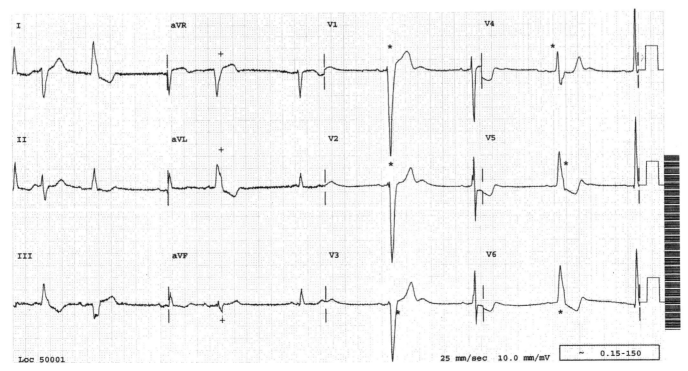

FIGURE 24-16. Example of a phase 4 or bradycardia-dependent bundle branch block. The patient is in sinus rhythm with QRS complexes that are normal. Seen in leads V$_1$ through V$_3$ and V$_4$ through V$_6$ are sinus QRS complexes after a long R-R interval that have a left bundle branch morphology (*asterisks*). There is also evidence of phase 3 or rate-related aberration—that is, the atrial premature complex in leads aVR, aVL, and aVF *(+)* also has a left bundle branch morphology.

with that of patients without conduction disease (67). The expected decrease in refractory period with shortening of cycle length, which is seen in the normal His-Purkinje system, is frequently not present (67). The critical heart rate (cycle length) for the onset of BBB and reversion to normal conduction during incremental and decremental atrial pacing differs by 50 to 190 ms (67).

The onset of a BBB in patients with a tachycardia-dependent block depends on the refractory period of the bundle branch and its response to the change in cycle length. It has been postulated that the retrograde concealment of the impulse in the blocked bundle branch accounts for this difference in paced cycle length between onset of BBB and resumption of normal conduction (68). Therefore, the hysteresis curves relating the onset and loss of rate-dependent BBB should parallel the transseptal conduction time. The 50- to 190-ms difference in the cycle length at the onset of BBB and resumption of normal conduction during rapid atrial pacing corresponds to the transseptal conduction time in humans (67).

The mechanism of a bradycardia-dependent BBB is more complex. The original explanation by Rosenbaum and colleagues (69) attributed the presence of a bradycardia-dependent BBB to hypopolarization and spontaneous diastolic depolarization of the Purkinje fibers distal to the area of block. Antzelevitch and colleagues (70) in very elegant experimental studies, using the sucrose gap preparation, demonstrated that there were two parameters that determined the success of propagation of an impulse across an area of impaired conduction. These parameters are the intensity of the current proximal to the area of block and the excitability of the tissue distal to the block. They demonstrated that a time-dependent decline of electrotonic input of the proximal to the distal segment plays an important role in the manifestation of a late diastolic block (70). The rate of recovery of excitability of the distal site is the other major determinant of a phase 4 block. When spontaneous diastolic repolarization occurs in the area distal to the block, impulse conduction is accelerated or facilitated (70). When the pacemaker is situated at a site proximal to the zone of depressed conduction, the distal segment demonstrates impaired conduction because of a decrease in the amplitude of the proximal response, resulting in a phase 4 block. Time-dependent changes of the amplitude of the proximal site may also occur independently of spontaneous diastolic depolarization. Catecholamines improve conduction related to a *phase 3 block,* probably related to the hyperpolarizing effect of catecholamines on the diseased His-Purkinje fibers (71), and may impair conduction related to a *phase 4 block.*

An additional interesting observation made originally by Rosenbaum and colleagues (69) in patients with an intermittent LBBB was the presence of deeply inverted T waves in the precordial leads during the period of normal conduction. They attributed this finding to extensive ischemia of the septum, accounting for the intermittent

BBB and the T-wave changes. Denes and colleagues (72) subsequently reported on similar findings in patients with an intermittent LBBB. However, they provided a different explanation. The coronary angiographic studies in their patients showed that many of them had healthy coronary arteries. They demonstrated that the severity and duration of T-wave changes directly correlated with the duration of the BBB conduction pattern before normalization. Denes and colleagues (72) suggested that the mechanism of T-wave changes seen in these cases is related to the abnormal ventricular activation (left bundle branch pattern) with persistent abnormal repolarization beyond the abnormality of ventricular activation. The mechanism by which the heart muscle would "remember" the activation abnormality associated with an LBBB pattern is not known. Similar observations have been reported in patients after right ventricular pacing (73).

Pseudoatrioventricular Block

A special type of AV block that on the ECG may present as an intermittent first-degree block or a second-degree type I or type II block is called the *pseudo-AV block* (74). His bundle recordings in these cases reveal the presence of concealed and manifest junctional premature beats. These premature His bundle depolarizations fail to propagate to the ventricle and remain concealed on the surface ECG. The presence of a pseudo-AV block frequently coexists with distal AV conduction disease, which accounts for the presence of concealed His extrasystoles and the block.

Bundle Branch Reentrant Sustained Ventricular Tachycardia

The diseased His-Purkinje system can also be the cause of tachyarrhythmias (ventricular tachycardia); this occurs most commonly in patients with a dilated cardiomyopathy. Schmitt and Erlanger (2) suggested that depressed conduction within the terminal portion of the Purkinje system could be a site for reentrant ventricular extrasystoles (microreentry). Another anatomic substrate for reentry in the ventricle involves the His bundle and bundle branches (macroreentry). This anatomic model for macroreentry in humans was demonstrated by Akhtar and colleagues (75) in 1974. The clinical importance of this reentry model was reported later. Tchou and colleagues (76,76a) described seven patients with bundle branch reentrant ventricular tachycardia. During sinus rhythm, these patients had an intraventricular conduction defect of the LBBB type with prolonged HV intervals. During ventricular tachycardia, a His potential preceded the QRS. In these cases, ablation of the right bundle branch prevented the occurrence of ventricular tachycardia. Further discussion of this entity can be found in Chapter 19.

HISTOLOGIC AND ELECTROPHYSIOLOGIC CORRELATION

The 12-lead ECG frequently underestimates the extent of the conduction disease. Demoulin and Kulbertus (10) found severe diffuse disease on the left side of the conduction system in hearts of patients whose ECG demonstrated an LAFB. Thus, the ECG pattern of an LAFB may be a marker for diffuse left-sided conduction disease. Takagi and Okada (77) examined hearts of hypertensive cases. They found a good correlation between an abnormal left axis (less than −30) and pathologic disease of the anterior radiation of the left bundle branch.

Bharati and Lev (78) reviewed the results of their own examinations of pathologic specimens from patients with conduction disease who had undergone prior electrophysiologic evaluation. The correlation between prolongation of the His potential, or split H potential, was evaluated in three cases. In one case, there was marked fibrosis in the penetrating and branching portion of the AV bundle. In the second case, a calcific lesion was impinging on the His bundle with fairly normal proximal and distal segments. The third patient had a cardiac stab wound with demonstration of a split His potential during electrophysiologic studies. There was disease in the distal portion of the His bundle, which was replaced with fibroelastic tissue. There were four cases of a complete heart block distal to the His bundle. They all showed marked pathologic involvement of both bundle branches. In a case of an LBBB and 2 : 1 block distal to the His bundle, there was marked fibrosis of the penetrating portion of the bundle and slight fibrosis of the branching portion. There were four cases of an LBBB with a prolonged HV interval. All of these showed pathologic changes at the beginning of the left bundle branch and significant changes in the right bundle branch. Three cases of an RBBB with left axis deviation and prolonged HV interval showed marked pathologic changes in both bundle branches. However, the left axis deviation did not necessarily correspond with a greater involvement of the anterior fibers compared with the posterior fascicular fibers. A case of alternating BBB with a normal HV interval showed moderate atherosclerosis and fibroelastosis in the penetrating and branching portion of the His bundle. There was also marked fibrosis at the bifurcation with the first portion of the left bundle, which was replaced by fibroelastic tissue. The right bundle showed marked fibrosis in the first and second portion.

Based on these observations, we can state that in chronic conduction disease, electrophysiologic abnormalities are paralleled by pathologically identifiable disease. In contrast, pathologically identifiable disease may not always correlate with electrophysiologic or ECG abnormalities. The amount of normal or diseased conduction fibers that are required to maintain AV conduction has not been defined. The ability to maintain conduction also depends on other physiologic factors (79).

INDICATION FOR ELECTROPHYSIOLOGIC TESTING

Recommendations for the use of electrophysiologic testing have been published by a task force formed jointly by the American College of Cardiology and the American Heart Association (ACC/AHA) (Tables 24-1 and 24-2) (80). They are categorized into three classes:

Class I refers to the general agreement that electrophysiologic study provides information that is very useful and important in the clinical management of the patient and should be done.

Class II refers to conditions for which electrophysiologic studies are frequently performed, but there is less certainty about the clinical usefulness of the information that is obtained. (Experts are divided in their opinion of whether electrophysiologic studies for these conditions should be done.)

Class III refers to conditions for which there is general agreement that electrophysiologic studies do not provide useful information and should not be done.

TABLE 24-1. ELECTROPHYSIOLOGIC STUDY IN ACQUIRED ATRIOVENTRICULAR BLOCK

Class I
  (a) Symptomatic patients (syncope or near syncope) in whom His-Purkinje block, which is not established with electrocardiographic recordings, is suspected as a cause of symptoms.
  (b) Patients with second- or third-degree atrioventricular block treated with a pacemaker who remain symptomatic and in whom ventricular tachyarrhythmia is suspected as a cause of symptoms.
Class II
  (a) Patients with second- or third-degree atrioventricular block in whom knowledge of the site or mechanism of block or both may help to direct therapy or assess prognosis.
  (b) Patients with suspected concealed junctional extrasystoles as a cause of second- or third-degree atrioventricular block (pseudoatrioventricular block).
Class III
  (a) Patients in whom the symptoms and presence of atrioventricular block are correlated with electrocardiography results.
  (b) Asymptomatic patients with transient atrioventricular block associated with sinus slowing or increased vagal tone (nocturnal type I second-degree atrioventricular block).

TABLE 24-2. ELECTROPHYSIOLOGIC STUDIES IN PATIENTS WITH CHRONIC INTRAVENTRICULAR CONDUCTION DELAY

Class I
  Symptomatic patients with bundle branch block in whom
  ventricular arrhythmias are suspected to cause the
  symptoms. The study is not designed to evaluate
  intraventricular conduction delay itself but the inducibility
  of sustained ventricular tachyarrhythmias.
Class II
  Symptomatic patients with bundle branch block in whom
  knowledge of the site, severity of conduction delay, or
  response to drugs may help to direct therapy or assess
  prognosis.
Class III
  (a) Asymptomatic patients with intraventricular conduction
      delay.
  (b) Symptomatic patients with intraventricular conduction
      delay whose symptoms can be casually related to
      electrocardiographically documented events.

TABLE 24-3. RECOMMENDATIONS FOR PLACEMENT OF TRANSCUTANEOUS PATCHES AND ACTIVE (DEMAND) TRANSCUTANEOUS PACING IN MYOCARDIAL INFARCTION

Class I
  1. Sinus bradycardia (rate <50 bpm) with symptoms of
     hypotension (systolic blood pressure <80 mm Hg)
     unresponsive to drug therapy[b].
  2. Mobitz type II second-degree atrioventricular (AV) block[b].
  3. Third-degree heart block[b].
  4. Bilateral bundle branch block (BBB) (alternating BBB, or
     RBBB and alternating left anterior fascicular block [LAFB],
     left posterior fascicular block [LPFB]) (irrespective of time
     of onset)[a].
  5. Newly acquired or age-indeterminate LBBB, BBB and LAFB,
     RBBB and LPFB[a].
  6. RBBB or LBBB and first-degree AV block[a].
Class IIa
  1. Stable bradycardia (systolic blood pressure >90 mm Hg, no
     hemodynamic compromise, or compromise responsive to
     initial drug therapy)[a].
  2. Newly acquired or age-indeterminate RBBB[a].
Class IIb.
  1. Newly acquired or age-indeterminate first-degree AV
     block[a].
Class III
  1. Uncomplicated acute myocardial infarction without
     evidence of conduction system disease.

[a]Apply patches and attach system; system is in active or standby
mode to allow immediate use on demand as required. In facilities
in which transvenous pacing or expertise are not available to place
an IV system, consideration should be given to transporting the
patient to one equipped and competent in placing transvenous
systems.
[b]Transcutaneous patches applied; system may be attached and
activated within a brief time if needed. Transcutaneous pacing may
be very helpful as an urgent expedient. Because it is associated with
significant pain, high-risk patients likely to require pacing should
receive a temporary pacemaker.

INDICATION FOR PACING IN INTRAVENTRICULAR CONDUCTION BLOCK

Guidelines for the placement of transcutaneous patches and external pacing and the use of temporary pacing after a myocardial infarction (Tables 24-3 and 24-4) (81) and implantation of cardiac pacemakers, have also been established by the ACC/AHA task force (Tables 24-5 through 24-7) (82). Although there are occasional cases that cannot be categorized according to these guidelines, they are, for the most part, all-encompassing and have been widely endorsed. Some indications for permanent pacing are relatively certain or unambiguous, whereas others require considerable expertise and judgment. The indications for pacemaker implantation have been divided into three specific groups:

Group I refers to conditions in which permanent pacing is definitely beneficial, useful, and effective.

Group II refers to conditions in which permanent pacing may be indicated, but there is conflicting evidence and/or divergence of opinion.

TABLE 24-4. RECOMMENDATIONS FOR TEMPORARY TRANSVENOUS PACING IN ACUTE MYOCARDIAL INFARCTION

Class I
  1. Asystole.
  2. Symptomatic bradycardia (includes sinus bradycardia with
     hypotension and type I second-degree AV block with
     hypotension not responsive to atropine).
  3. Bilateral BBB (alternating LBBB or RBBB with alternating
     LAFB/LPFB) (any age).
  4. New or indeterminate-age bifascicular block (RBBB with
     LAFB or LPFB, or LBBB) with first-degree AV block.
  5. Mobitz type II second-degree AV block.
Class IIa
  1. RBBB and LAFB or LPFB (new or indeterminate).
  2. RBBB with first-degree AV block.
  3. LBBB, new or indeterminate.
  4. Incessant ventricular tachycardia, for atrial or ventricular
     overdrive pacing.
  5. Recurrent sinus pauses (>3 s) not responsive to atropine.
Class IIb
  1. Bifascicular block of indeterminate age.
  2. New or age-indeterminate isolated RBBB.
Class III
  1. First-degree heart block.
  2. Type I second-degree AV block with normal
     hemodynamics.
  3. Accelerated idioventricular rhythm.
  4. BBB or fascicular block known to exist before acute
     myocardial infarction.

Note: In choosing an intravenous pacemaker system, patients with
substantially depressed ventricular performance, including right
ventricular infarction, may respond better to atrial/AV sequential
pacing than ventricular pacing. AV, atrioventricular; BBB, bundle
branch block; RBBB, right BBB; LAFB, left anterior fascicular block;
LPFB, left posterior fascicular block; LBBB, left BBB.

TABLE 24-5. INDICATIONS FOR PERMANENT PACING AFTER THE ACUTE PHASE OF MYOCARDIAL INFARCTION

Class I
1. Persistent second-degree atrioventricular (AV) block in the His-Purkinje system with bilateral bundle branch block or third-degree AV block within or below the His-Purkinje system after acute myocardial infarction.
2. Transient advanced (second- or third-degree) infranodal AV block and associated bundle branch block. If the site of block is uncertain, an electrophysiologic study may be necessary.
3. Persistent and symptomatic second- or third-degree AV block.

Class IIa
None.

Class IIb
Persistent second- or third-degree AV block at the AV nodal level.

Class III
1. Transient AV block in the absence of intraventricular conduction defects.
2. Transient AV block in the presence of isolated left anterior fascicular block.
3. Acquired left anterior fascicular block in the absence of AV block.
4. Persistent first-degree AV block in the presence of bundle branch block that is old or age indeterminate.

Group IIA refers to conditions in which the weight of evidence and opinion is in favor of usefulness and efficacy.

Group IIB refers to conditions in which the usefulness and efficacy is less well established by evidence/opinion.

Group III refers to conditions in which permanent pacing is not useful or effective and in some cases may be harmful.

TABLE 24-6. INDICATIONS FOR PERMANENT PACING IN CHRONIC BIFASCICULAR AND TRIFASCICULAR BLOCK

Class I
1. Intermittent third-degree atrioventricular (AV) block.
2. Type II second-degree AV block.

Class IIa
1. Syncope not proved to be caused by AV block when other likely causes have been excluded, specifically ventricular tachycardia.
2. Incidental finding at electrophysiologic study of markedly prolonged HV interval (≥100 ms) in asymptomatic patients.
3. Incidental finding at electrophysiologic study of pacing-induced infa-His block that is not physiologic.

Class IIb
None.

Class III
1. Fascicular block without AV block or symptoms.
2. Fascicular block with first-degree AV block without symptoms.

TABLE 24-7. INDICATIONS FOR PERMANENT PACING IN ACQUIRED ATRIOVENTRICULAR (AV) BLOCK IN ADULTS

Class I
1. Third-degree AV block at any anatomic level associated with any one of the following conditions:
   (a) Bradycardia with symptoms presumed to be caused by AV block.
   (b) Arrhythmias and other medical conditions that require drugs that result in symptomatic bradycardia.
   (c) Documented periods of asystole ≥3.0 s or any escape rate <40 bpm in awake, symptom-free patients.
   (d) After catheter ablation of the AV junction. There are no trials to assess outcome without pacing, and pacing is virtually always planned in this situation unless the operative procedure is AV junction modification.
   (e) Postoperative AV block that is not expected to resolve.
   (f) Neuromuscular diseases with AV block such as myotonic muscular dystrophy, Kearns-Sayre syndrome, Erb dystrophy (limb-girdle muscular dystrophy), and peroneal muscular atrophy.
2. Second-degree AV block regardless of type or site of block, with associated symptomatic bradycardia.

Class IIa
1. Asymptomatic third-degree AV block at any anatomic site with average awake ventricular rates of 40 bpm or faster.
2. Asymptomatic type II second-degree AV block.
3. Asymptomatic type I second-degree AV block at intra- or infra-His levels found incidentally at electrophysiologic study performed for other indications.
4. First-degree AV block with symptoms suggestive of pacemaker syndrome and documented alleviation of symptoms with temporary AV pacing.

Class IIb
1. Marked first-degree AV block (>0.30 second) in patients with left ventricular dysfunction and symptoms of congestive heart failure in whom a shorter AV interval results in hemodynamic improvement, presumably by decreasing left atrial filling pressure.

Class III
1. Asymptomatic first-degree AV block.
2. Asymptomatic type I second-degree AV block at the supra-His (AV node) level or not known to be intra- or infra-Hisian.
3. AV block expected to resolve and unlikely to recur (e.g., drug toxicity, Lyme disease).

REFERENCES

1. Wit AL. Cardiac arrhythmias: electrophysiologic mechanism. In: Reiser HJ, Horowitz LN, eds. *Mechanism and treatment of cardiac arrhythmias; relevance of basic studies to clinical management.* Baltimore, Munich: Urban & Schwarzenberg, 1985.
2. Schmitt FO, Erlanger J. Directional differences in the conduction of the impulse through the heart muscle and their possible relation to extrasystolic and fibrillary contractions. *Am J Physiol* 1928;87:326.
3. Lipsitz LA, Goldberger AL. Loss of complexity and aging. Potential application of fractals and chaos theory to senescence. *JAMA* 1992;267:1806.
4. Chialvo DR, Jalife J. On the non-linear equilibrium of the heart: locking behavior and chaos in Purkinje fibers. In: Zipes DP, Jal-

ife J, eds. *Cardiac electrophysiology. From cell to beside.* Philadelphia: WB Saunders, 1990.

5. Myerburg RJ, Gelband H, Hoffman BF. Functional characteristics of the gating mechanism in the canine A-V conduction system. *Circ Res* 1971;28:136.

6. Lazzara R, El Sherif N, Befeler B, Scherlag BJ. Regional refractoriness within the ventricular conduction system. An evaluation of the "gate" hypothesis. *Circ Res* 1976;39:254.

7. Spear JF, Moore EN. Supernormal excitability and conduction in the His-Purkinje system of the dog. *Circ Res* 1974;35:782.

8. Titus JL. Normal anatomy of the human cardiac conduction system. *Mayo Clin Proc* 1973;48:24.

9. Massing GK, James TN. Anatomical configuration of the His bundle and bundle branch in the human heart. *Circulation* 1976;53:609.

10. Demoulin JC, Kulbertus HE. Histopathological examination of the concept of left hemiblock. *Br Heart J* 1972;34:807.

11. Rosenbaum MB, Elizari MV, Lazzari JO. *The hemiblocks.* Oldsmar, FL: Tampa Tracings, 1970.

12. James TN. Anatomy of the coronary arteries in health and disease. *Circulation* 1965;32:1020.

12a. Cox J, Krajden M. Cardiovascular manifestations of Lyme disease. *Am Heart J* 1991;122:1449.

12b. Steere AC, Batsford WP, Weinberg M, et al. Lyme carditis: cardiac abnormalities of Lyme disease. *Ann Intern Med* 1980;93:8.

12c. Reznick JW, Braunstein DB, Walsh RL, et al. Lyme carditis: electrophysiologic and histopathologic study. *Am J Med* 1986; 81:923.

12d. van der Linde MR, Crijns HJGM, de Koning J, et al. Range of atrioventricular conduction disturbances in Lyme borreliosis: a report of four cases and review of other published reports. *Br Heart J* 1990;63:162.

13. Perloff JK. Cardiac involvement in heredofamilial neuromyopathic disease. *Cardiovasc Clin* 1972;4:333.

14. Arnett EN, Roberts WC. Active infective endocarditis. A clinicopathologic analysis of 137 necropsy patients. *Curr Probl Cardiol* 1976;7:1.

15. Lev M. Anatomical basis for atrioventricular block. *Am J Med* 1964;37:742.

16. Lenegre J. Etiology of bilateral bundle branch fibrosis in relation to complete heart block. *Prog Cardiovasc Dis* 1964;6:409.

17. Greenspahn BR, Denes P, Daniel W, Rosen KM. Chronic bifascicular block: evaluation of familial factors. *Ann Intern Med* 1976;84:521.

18. Davies MJ, Anderson RH, Becker AE. *The conduction system of the heart.* London: Butterworth-Heineman, 1983.

19. Rosen MR. Electrophysiology of the cardiac specialized conduction system. In: Narula OS, ed. *His bundle electrocardiography and clinical electrophysiology.* Philadelphia: FA Davis Co, 1975.

20. Cranefield PF, Klein HO, Hoffman BF. Conduction of the cardiac impulse. *Circ Res* 1971;28:199.

21. Gonzalez MD, Scherlag BJ, Mabo P, Lazzara R. Functional dissociation of cellular activation as a mechanism of Mobitz type II atrioventricular block. *Circulation* 1993;87:1389.

22. Dhingra, RC, Amat y Leon F, Pouget M, Rosen KM. Infranodal block. Diagnosis clinical significance and management. *Med Clin North Am* 1976;60:175.

23. Alpert MA, Flaker GC. Chronic fascicular block. Recognition, natural history and therapeutic implications. *Arch Intern Med* 1984;144:799.

23a. Eriksson P, Hansson P-O, Eriksson H, et al. Bundle-branch block in a general male population: the study of men born 1913. *Circulation* 1998;98:2494.

24. Schneider JF, Thomas HE, Kreger BE, et al. New acquired right bundle branch block. The Framingham Study. *Ann Intern Med* 1980;92:37.

25. Schneider JF, Thomas HE, Kreger BE, et al. New acquired left bundle branch block. The Framingham Study. *Ann Intern Med* 1979;90:303.

26. Rotman M, Triebwasser JH. A clinical and follow up study of right and left bundle branch. *Circulation* 1975;51:477.

27. Lasser RP, Haft JI, Friedberg CK. Relationship of right bundle branch block and marked left axis deviation (with left parietal or peri-infarction block) to complete heart block and syncope. *Circulation* 1968;37:429.

28. Scanlon PJ, Pryor R, Blount SG Jr. Right bundle branch block associated with left superior or inferior intraventricular block. Clinical setting, prognosis, and relation to complete heart block. *Circulation* 1970;43:1123.

29. DePasquale NP, Bruno MS. Natural history of combined right bundle branch block and left anterior hemiblock (bilateral bundle branch block). *Am J Med* 1973;54:297.

30. Pastore JO, Yurchak PM, Janis KM, et al. The risk of advanced heart block in surgical patients with right bundle branch block and left axis deviation. *Circulation* 1978;57:677.

30a. Grady TA, Chiu AC, Snader CE, et al. Prognostic significance of exercise-induced left bundle-branch block. *JAMA* 1998;279:153.

30b. Wagdy HM, Hodge D, Christian TF, et al. Prognostic value of vasodilator myocardial perfusion imaging in patients with left bundle-branch block. *Circulation* 1998;97:1563.

30c. Peteiro J, Monserrat L, Martinez D, Castro-Beiras A. Accuracy of exercise echocardiography to detect coronary artery disease in left bundle branch block unassociated with either acute or healed myocardial infarction. *Am J Cardiol* 2000;85:890.

31. Codini MA. Conduction disturbances in acute myocardial infarction: the use of pacemaker therapy. *Clin Prog Pacing Electrophysiol* 1983;2:142.

32. Lie KI, Wellens HJJ, Schuilenburg RM. Factors influencing prognosis of bundle branch block complicating acute anteroseptal infarction: the value of His bundle recording. *Circulation* 1974;50:935.

33. Hindman MC, Wagner GS, JaRo M, et al. The clinical significance of bundle branch block complicating acute myocardial infarction. 1. Clinical characteristics, hospital mortality, and one-year follow-up. *Circulation* 1978;58:679.

34. Hindman MC, Wagner GS, JaRo M, et al. The clinical significance of bundle branch block complicating acute myocardial infarction. 2. Indications for temporary and permanent pacemaker insertion. *Circulation* 1978;58:689.

35. Ginks WR, Sutton R, Ott W, et al. Long-term prognosis after acute anterior infarction with atrioventricular block. *Br Heart J* 1977;39:186.

36. Lie KI, Liem KL, Schuilenburg RM, et al. Early identification of patients developing late in-hospital ventricular fibrillation after discharge from the coronary care unit. A 52-year retrospective and prospective study of 1,897 patients. *Am J Cardiol* 1978; 41:674.

36a. Gruppo Italiano per lo Studio della Streptochinasi Nell'Infarto Miocardico. GISSI-2. A factorial randomised trial of alteplase versus streptokinase and heparin versus no heparin among 12,490 patients with acute myocardial infarction. *Lancet* 1990; 336:65.

36b. Grines C. A comparison of immediate angioplasty with thrombolytic therapy for acute myocardial infarction. *N Engl J Med* 1993;328:673.

36c. The GUSTO Investigators. An international randomized trial comparing four thrombolytic strategies for acute myocardial infarction. *N Engl J Med* 1993;329:673.

36d. Archbold RA, Sayer JW, Ray S, et al. Frequency and prognostic implications of conduction defects in acute myocardial infarction since the introduction of thrombolytic therapy. *Eur Heart J* 1998;19:893.

36e. Harpaz D, Behar S, Gottlieb S, et al, for the SPRINT Study Group and the Israeli Thrombolytic Survey Group. Complete atrioventricular block complicating acute myocardial infarction in the thrombolytic era. *J Am Coll Cardiol* 1999;34:1721.

36f. Newby KH, Pisano E, Krucoff MW, et al. Incidence and clinical relevance of the occurrence of bundle-branch block in patients treated with thrombolytic therapy. *Circulation* 1996;94:2424.

36g. Melgarejo-Moreno A, Galcera-Tomas J, Garcia-Alberola A, et al. Incidence, clinical characteristics, and prognostic significance of right bundle-branch block in acute myocardial infarction. A study in the thrombolytic era. *Circulation* 1997;96:1139.

36h. Haim M, Hod H, Kaplinsky E, et al, for the SPRINT Study Group. Frequency and prognostic significance of high-degree atrioventricular block in patients with a first non–Q wave acute myocardial infarction. *Am J Cardiol* 1997;79:674

37. Scherlag BJ, Lau SH, Helfant RG, et al. Catheter technique for recording His bundle activity in man. *Circulation* 1969;39:13.

38. Rosen KM. His bundle electrogram. *Circulation* 1972;46:831.

39. Kupersmith J, Kronsgrad E, Waldo AL. Conduction intervals and conduction velocity in the human cardiac conduction system. Studies during open heart surgery. *Circulation* 1973;47:776.

40. Dhingra RC, Rosen KM, Rahimtoola SH. Normal conduction intervals and responses in 61 patients using His bundle recording and atrial pacing. *Chest* 1973;64:55.

41. Dhingra RC, Wyndham C, Bauernfiend RA, et al. Significance of bundle block distal to the His bundle induced by atrial pacing in patients with chronic bifascicular block. *Circulation* 1979;60:1455.

42. Denes P, Wu D, Dhingra R, et al. The effects of cycle length on cardiac refractory periods in man. *Circulation* 1974;49:32.

43. Denker ST, Gilbert CG, Shenasa M, Akhtar M. An electrocardiographic-electrophysiologic correlation of aberrant ventricular conduction in man. *J Electrocardiol* 1983;16:269.

44. Elizari MV, Lazzari JO, Rosenbaum MB. Aberrant ventricular conduction: electrocardiographic manifestations and mechanism. In: Rosenbaum MB, Elizari MV, eds. *Frontiers of cardiac electrophysiology.* The Hague: Martinus Nijhoff, 1983.

45. Akhtar M, Gilbert C, Al-Nouri M, Denker S. Site of conduction delay during functional block in the His-Purkinje system in man. *Circulation* 1980;61:1239.

46. Damato AN, Lau SH, Helfant RH, et al. A study of heart block in man using His bundle recordings. *Circulation* 1969;39:297.

47. Rosen KM. The contribution of His bundle recordings to the understanding of cardiac conduction in man. *Circulation* 1971;43:961.

48. Narula OS, Scherlag BJ, Samet P, Javier RP. Atrioventricular block: localization and classification by His bundle recordings. *Am J Med* 1971;50:146.

49. Dhingra RC, Denes P, Wu D, et al. The significance of second degree atrioventricular block and bundle branch block. *Circulation* 1974;49:638.

50. Narula OS. Intraventricular conduction defects. In: Narula OS, ed. *His bundle electrocardiography.* Philadelphia: FA Davis Co, 1975.

51. Peuch P, Grolleau R, Guimond C. Incidence of different types of AV block and their localization by His bundle recording. In: Wellens HJJ, Lie KI, Janse MJ, eds. *The conduction system of the heart: structure, function, and clinical implications.* Philadelphia: Lea & Febiger, 1976.

52. Amat y Leon F, Dhingra R, Denes P, et al. The clinical spectrum of chronic His bundle block. *Chest* 1976;70:747.

53. McAnulty JH, Murphy E, Rahimtoola SH. A prospective evaluation of intra-Hisian delay. *Circulation* 1979;59:1035.

54. Rosen KM, Dhingra RC, Loeb HS, Rahimtoola SH. Chronic heart block in adults: clinical and electrocardiographic correlations. *Arch Intern Med* 1973;131:663.

55. Narula OS, Scherlag BJ, Javier RR. Analysis of the AV conduction defect in complete heart block utilizing His bundle electrograms. *Circulation* 1970;41:437.

56. Peters RW, Scheinman MM. Anatomic and electrophysiologic aspects of fascicular block. In: Levy S, Scheinman MM, eds. *Cardiac arrhythmias. From diagnosis to therapy.* Mount Kisco, NY: Futura Publishing, 1984.

57. Dhingra RC, Palileo E, Strasberg B, et al. Significance of HV interval in 517 patients with chronic bifascicular block. *Circulation* 1981;64:1265.

58. McAnulty J, Rahimtoola SH, Murphy E, et al. Natural history of "high risk" bundle branch block. Final report of a prospective study. *N Engl J Med* 1982;307:137.

59. Dhingra RC, Wyndham C, Amat y Leon F, et al. Incidence and site of atrioventricular block in patients with chronic bifascicular block. *Circulation* 1979;59:238.

60. Dhingra RC, Denes P, Wu D, et al. Prospective observations in patients with chronic bundle branch block and marked HV prolongation. *Circulation* 1976;53:600.

61. Denes P, Dhingra RC, Wu D, et al. Sudden death in patients with bifascicular block. *Arch Intern Med* 1977;137:1005.

62. Guerot C, Value PE, Lehner JR. Valeur predictive du test ajmaline dans le diagnostic des blocs auriculo-ventriculaires paroxystiques distaux. *Ann Med Interne* 1981;132:246.

63. Dhingra RC, Wyndham C, Bauernfiend R, et al. Significance of chronic bifascicular block without apparent organic heart disease. *Circulation* 1979;60:33.

64. Narula OS. Longitudinal dissociation in the His bundle: bundle branch block due to asynchronous conduction within the His bundle in man. *Circulation* 1977;56:996.

65. El-Sherif N, Amat y Leon F, Schonfield C, et al. Normalization of bundle branch block patterns by distal His bundle pacing. Clinical and experimental evidence of longitudinal dissociation in the pathologic His bundle. *Circulation* 1978;57:473.

66. Lazzara R, Yeh BK, Samet P. Functional transverse interconnections within the His bundle and the bundle branch. *Circ Res* 1973;32:509.

67. Denes P, Wu D, Dhingra RC, et al. Electrophysiological observations in patients with rate dependent bundle branch block. *Circulation* 1975;51:244.

68. Fisch C, Zipes DP, McHenry PL. Rate dependent aberrancy. *Circulation* 1973;48:714.

69. Rosenbaum MB, Lazzari JO, Elizari MV. The role of phase 3 and phase 4 block in clinical electrocardiography. In: Wellens HJJ, Lie KI, Janse MJ, eds. *The conduction system of the heart: structure, function, and clinical implications.* Philadelphia: Lea & Febiger, 1976.

70. Antzelevitch C, Jalife J, Moe GK. Frequency-dependent alterations of conduction in Purkinje fibers: a model of phase 4 facilitation and block. In: Rosenbaum MB, Elizari MV, eds. *Frontiers of cardiac electrophysiology.* The Hague: Martinus Nijhoff, 1983.

71. Halpern S, Chiale P, Nau GJ, et al. Effects of isoproterenol on abnormal intraventricular conduction. *Circulation* 1980;62:1357.

72. Denes P, Pick A, Miller RH, et al. A characteristic precordial T wave abnormality with intermittent left bundle branch block. *Ann Intern Med* 1978;89:55.

73. Chatterjee K, Harris AM, Davis JG, et al. T wave changes after artificial pacing. *Lancet* 1969;1:759.

74. Rosen KM, Gunnar R, Rahimtoola SH. Pseudo AV block secondary to premature nonpropagated His bundle depolarizations. *Circulation* 1970;42:367.

75. Akhtar M, Damato AN, Batsford WP, et al. Demonstration of reentry within the His-Purkinje system in man. *Circulation* 1974;50:1150.

76. Tchou P, Jazayeri M, Denker S, et al. Transcatheter electrical ablation of right bundle branch. A method of treating

macroreentrant ventricular tachycardia attributed to bundle branch reentry. *Circulation* 1988;78:246.

76a. Tchou P, Mehdirad AA. Bundle branch reentry ventricular tachycardia. *Pacing Clin Electrophysiol* 1995;18:1427.

77. Takagi T, Okada R. An electrocardiographic-pathologic correlative study on left axis deviation in hypertensive hearts. *Am Heart J* 1980;100:838.

78. Bharati S, Lev M. Histological and electrophysiological correlations in atrioventricular block and bundle branch block. In: Narula OS, ed. *Cardiac arrhythmias. Electrophysiology, diagnosis and management.* Baltimore: Williams & Wilkins, 1979.

79. Titus JL. Anatomy of the conduction system. *Circulation* 1973; 47:170.

80. Fisch C, DeSanctis RW, Dodge HT, et al. Guidelines for clinical intracardiac electrophysiologic studies. A report of the American College of Cardiology/American Heart Association Task Force on Assessment of Diagnostic and Therapeutic Cardiovascular Procedures. *Circulation* 1989;80:1925.

81. Ryan TJ, Antman EM, Brooks NH, et al. 1999 update: ACC/AHA guidelines for the management of patients with acute myocardial infarction: executive summary and recommendations. A report of the American College of Cardiology/American Heart Association Task force on Practice Guidelines (Committee on Management of Acute Myocardial Infarction). *Circulation* 1999;100:1016.

82. Gregoratos G, Cheitlin MD, Conill A, et al. ACC/AHA guidelines for implantation of cardiac pacemakers and antiarrhythmia devices: executive summary. A report of the American College of Cardiology/American Heart Association Task Force on Practice Guidelines (Committee on Pacemaker Implantation). *Circulation* 1998;97:1325.

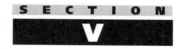

SECTION V

SPECIFIC SYNDROMES

25

ARRHYTHMIAS IN HYPERTROPHIC, DILATED, AND RIGHT VENTRICULAR CARDIOMYOPATHIES

WILLIAM J. MCKENNA
JOSEPH M. GALVIN
SHOAIB HAMID

The cardiomyopathies were originally defined as idiopathic and classified as dilated, hypertrophic, and restrictive based on anatomic and physiologic features. Improved understanding of the cause and pathogenesis led to revisions that maintain the established clinical definitions but recognize the evolution to a genetic or pathogenetic classification (1).

HYPERTROPHIC CARDIOMYOPATHY

Hypertrophic cardiomyopathy is a primary disorder of heart muscle that was first described more than 30 years ago (2,3). The condition is defined clinically by the presence of a hypertrophied and nondilated left ventricle in the absence of a cardiac or systemic cause (4,5). The prevalence, based on echocardiographic diagnostic criteria of disease in young adults, is approximately 1 in 500 (6). Symptoms result from abnormalities of diastolic function, elevated systolic left ventricular outflow tract gradients, ischemia, and arrhythmias. The condition carries an increased risk of sudden cardiac death and is the most common cause of sudden cardiac death among persons younger than 25 years of age (7–9).

Genetics

Hypertrophic cardiomyopathy has been described in Western, African, and Asian populations (10–13). Clinical genetic studies have established that hypertrophic cardiomyopathy has a familial pattern, with autosomal dominant transmission (14). Molecular genetic studies have identified eight different contractile protein gene abnor-

malities, thereby defining hypertrophic cardiomyopathy as a disease of the sarcomere (15,16). Mutations of the myocardial contractile protein genes include cardiac troponin T, cardiac troponin I, myosin regulatory light chain, cardiac myosin binding protein-C, essential light chain, β-cardiac myosin heavy chain, α-tropomyosin, cardiac troponin C, cardiac actin, and titin.

Pathology

The histopathologic hallmark of hypertrophic cardiomyopathy is myocardial disarray (17) (Fig. 25-1). Myocardial cells are invariably hypertrophied, and intercellular architecture is frequently bizarre. Areas of disarray are present in more than 95% of patients dying of hypertrophic cardiomyopathy. The extent and distribution of myocardial disarray is determined at postmortem examination; it cannot be readily assessed during life. It is probable that the disorganized architecture with abnormal myofiber and myofibrillar alignment provides a substrate for electrical instability and contributes to diastolic abnormalities. However, the precise relation of myocardial disarray with spontaneous arrhythmia and the threshold for ventricular fibrillation have not been established.

Hypertrophy of the interventricular septum, which may be a localized abnormality, and in some cases anterior displacement of the mitral valve causes resting or provocable left ventricular outflow tract obstruction in a subset of patients.

Mortality

Adults usually have a slow progression of symptoms over many years, and only a minority die of cardiac failure or require transplantation; however, there is a superimposed annual mortality rate from sudden cardiac death of 2% to 3% (18,19). In children and adolescents, sudden death is

W. J. McKenna, J. M. Galvin and S. Hamid: Department of Cardiac Medicine, St. Goerge's Hospital Medical School, London SW 17 ORE, United Kingdom.

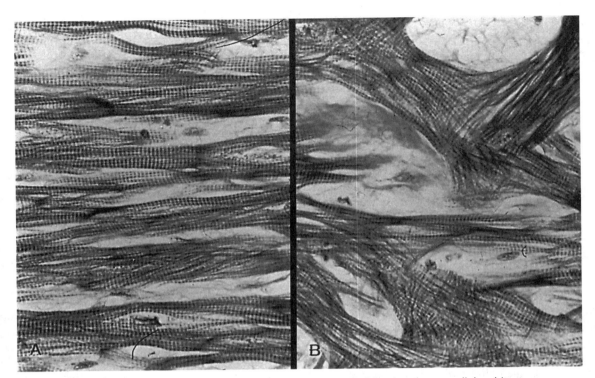

FIGURE 25-1. A: Normal myocardial cellular architecture. **B:** Disordered myocardial architecture demonstrates myocardial disarray, the histologic hallmark of hypertrophic cardiomyopathy. (Reproduced courtesy of Professor M. J. Davies, St. George's Hospital Medical School, London, UK.)

often the presenting feature of the disease (20). Numerous potential mechanisms of sudden cardiac death, in addition to an electrophysiologic predisposition to fatal arrhythmia, exist in these patients. Clinical arrhythmias are uncommon in children with the condition, and the identification of those children who are at high risk for sudden death is particularly difficult (21). In adults, arrhythmias are common, and the influence of ventricular arrhythmias on prognosis has been established (22,23).

Electrocardiogram

The 12-lead electrocardiogram (ECG) is normal for 5% of symptomatic patients and for 25% of asymptomatic patients, particularly those who are young (14,24). At the time of diagnosis, 5% to 10% of patients are in atrial fibrillation, 20% have left axis deviation, and 5% have right bundle branch block pattern (19,24). Most patients have an intraventricular conduction delay, but complete left bundle branch block (LBBB) is uncommon, although it may be seen after surgery and occasionally identified in the elderly. ST-segment depression and T-wave changes are the most common abnormalities and are usually associated with voltage changes of left ventricular hypertrophy or deep S waves in the anterior chest leads V_1 through V_3 (24). Repolarization changes are common, and occasionally, giant negative T waves are seen (12). Isolated voltage criteria for left ven-

tricular hypertrophy are unusual. Approximately 20% of patients have abnormal Q waves inferiorly (2, 3, and aVF) or less commonly in leads V_1 through V_3.

The distribution of the PR interval is similar to that in the normal population, but a short PR interval occasionally may be associated with a slurred upstroke to the QRS complex, similar to that seen in the Wolff-Parkinson-White syndrome. At electrophysiologic study, such changes are not usually associated with evidence of preexcitation, although patients with hypertrophic cardiomyopathy and accessory pathways have been described (25). P-wave abnormalities of left and right atrial overload are common, reflecting the difficulties faced by the atria in emptying their contents into poorly relaxing, stiff ventricles.

There are many electrocardiographic abnormalities, and therefore no ECG finding is typical of hypertrophic cardiomyopathy; a useful rule is to consider the diagnosis whenever the ECG is bizarre, particularly in younger patients in whom the manifestation of left ventricular hypertrophy on the ECG may precede its development documented by echocardiography (Fig. 25-2). Clinical and molecular genetic studies reveal that incomplete penetrance with abnormal electrocardiographic but normal echocardiographic left ventricular wall thickness may occur in up to 25% of gene carriers in some families (26,27). This finding led to the application of new diagnostic criteria in familial hypertrophic cardiomyopathy (28).

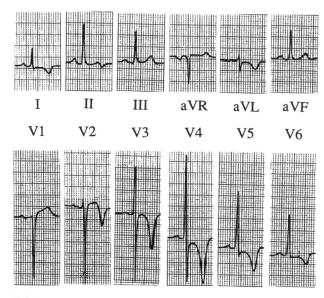

FIGURE 25-2. The 12-lead electrocardiogram from a patient with hypertrophic cardiomyopathy demonstrates marked left ventricular hypertrophy on voltage criteria, deeply inverted T waves, and slurring of the QRS complex.

Sinus and Atrioventricular Nodal Abnormalities

Holter monitoring of patients with hypertrophic cardiomyopathy does not suggest an increased incidence of sinoatrial disease or atrioventricular (AV) block compared with a normal population. Data from the largest series of patients undergoing detailed electrophysiologic evaluation (29) demonstrate abnormalities of sinus node function and disordered AV conduction in a significant number of subjects. Prolonged sinoatrial conduction time (≥120 ms) occurred in 66%, although only 6 (7%) patients demonstrated a prolonged sinus node recovery time (≥1,500 ms). The A-H interval was prolonged (≥120 ms) in 9 of 146, and H-V conduction was prolonged (H-V ≥55 ms) in 44 (30%) of 148. The prognostic significance of these abnormalities is uncertain, because the prevalence of such abnormalities is similar in asymptomatic patients and those with prior syncope and cardiac arrest.

Mechanism of Arrhythmia

Several factors predispose to the development of supraventricular tachycardias, particularly atrial fibrillation, including severe and diffuse hypertrophy, mitral, atrial dilatation, and restrictive left ventricular physiology (30,31). There are limited data on atrial pathology in hypertrophic cardiomyopathy, but some studies have shown extensive atrial fibrosis similar to that seen in patients with long-standing congestive heart failure (CHF) (32).

Factors predisposing to ventricular tachyarrhythmias in hypertrophic cardiomyopathy include myocardial hypertrophy, myocyte disarray (Fig. 25-1), myocardial fibrosis, myocardial ischemia, and autonomic disturbance. Sustained ventricular tachycardia is sometimes associated with apical left ventricular aneurysms in patients with long-standing midcavity obliteration has also been described as arising from the interventricular septum in patients with left ventricular outflow tract obstruction (33,34).

Supraventricular Arrhythmias

In adults with hypertrophic cardiomyopathy, supraventricular arrhythmias are common during 48-hour ambulatory electrocardiographic monitoring (22,35). Established atrial fibrillation is detected in 10% to 15% of consecutive patient populations; another 30% to 35% have episodes of paroxysmal atrial fibrillation or supraventricular tachycardia. Sustained atrial fibrillation lasting 30 seconds or longer may be poorly tolerated and carries an increased risk of embolism. When paroxysmal arrhythmias are sustained, important hemodynamic consequences may ensue. The acute onset of atrial fibrillation may be poorly tolerated hemodynamically with rapid deterioration to ventricular fibrillation or be tolerated with minimal hemodynamic embarrassment (36). This variable response to paroxysmal supraventricular arrhythmias depends on the ventricular heart rate response and the integrity of vascular responses (36–38).

In contrast, most children and adolescents are in sinus rhythm, and supraventricular arrhythmias during ambulatory electrocardiographic monitoring are uncommon (21). The increased incidence of supraventricular arrhythmias with age is not surprising, because the development of these arrhythmias is related to increased echocardiographic left atrial dimensions and increased left ventricular and end-diastolic pressure, both of which increase with age.

Atrial Fibrillation

Atrial fibrillation is the most common sustained arrhythmia seen in patients with hypertrophic cardiomyopathy, with a prevalence in most series of 15% to 20% (21,22,35). Establishment of atrial fibrillation was classically held to represent an important stage in the disease process with functional deterioration and risk of systemic emboli. One retrospective study of 52 patients found that the outcome of a cohort of patients with hypertrophic cardiomyopathy was not worsened by the presence of atrial fibrillation (37). However, the acute onset of atrial fibrillation led to symptomatic deterioration in 89%; restoration of sinus rhythm (63%) or control of ventricular rate with appropriate medical therapy (30%) led to restoration of original New York Heart Association (NYHA) functional class. Survival in the group with atrial fibrillation was compared with that of 122 patients who were matched for age, sex, known risk factors, and year of diagnosis and who remained in sinus rhythm during the same period. There were 19 deaths in the group with atrial fibrillation (six sudden, six from cardiac failure, two after myocardial infarction, two from stroke, and three from noncardiac causes); the 5-year mortality rate was 14%. Overall survival was similar for the patients who remained in sinus rhythm during the study period. None of the six patients with atrial fibrillation who were younger than 21 years at diagnosis died, compared with 11 (31%) of 35 patients of a similar age at diagnosis who did not develop atrial fibrillation. Among those 21 years or older at diagnosis, 22 (48%) of 46 patients with atrial fibrillation died, compared with 17 (20%) of 87 patients with sinus rhythm. This difference was not statistically different.

Symptomatic deterioration associated with the acute onset of atrial fibrillation may be seen in patients in whom the ventricular response is rapid, but most patients can be restored to their previous functional class by treatment, even if they remain in atrial fibrillation. The development of atrial fibrillation has not been shown to have an adverse effect on prognosis. A short duration of atrial fibrillation and amiodarone therapy were the most powerful predictors of a successful return to sinus rhythm. Patients with paroxysmal or established atrial fibrillation are at risk for emboli and should be administered anticoagulants (22,37).

Electrophysiologic Abnormalities

There is a limited amount of information about electrophysiologic assessment of supraventricular arrhythmias, and there is uncertainty over the significance of inducible atrial fibrillation in hypertrophic cardiomyopathy. Of 155 consecutive patients undergoing invasive electrophysiologic study at the National Institutes of Health (NIH), 145 of whom had one or more risk factors for sudden cardiac death, 9 patients (6%) had chronic atrial fibrillation (29). Sustained (≥30 seconds) atrial flutter or fibrillation could be induced in 15 (11%) of 136 patients who underwent the atrial stimulation protocol. Atrial fibrillation could be induced in 6 (55%) of the 11 patients who had paroxysmal atrial fibrillation on ambulatory monitoring but in only 9 (7%) of the 125 of patients without paroxysmal atrial fibrillation. Atrial tachycardia could be induced in 14 (10%) of 136 patients; in 4 (29%) of these, a similar arrhythmia had been detected spontaneously. Accessory AV pathways were present in 5%. Such pathways have been implicated in sudden cardiac death in patients with hypertrophic cardiomyopathy (25).

Ventricular Arrhythmias

Significance of Nonsustained Ventricular Tachycardia

Nonsustained ventricular tachycardia is seen on Holter monitoring in approximately 25% of adults with hypertrophic cardiomyopathy (22,23). Such arrhythmias appear to be clinically benign. The cause of nonsustained ventricular arrhythmias is unknown but may be associated with myocyte necrosis and myocardial fibrosis, which appear to be related to age. Episodes are almost invariably asymptomatic, occurring at night or during periods of predominant vagal tone. The ventricular rate is usually relatively slow (e.g., mean heart rate of 140 bpm in one series of 400 episodes in 52 patients). Analysis of different episodes in the same patient shows multiple morphologies, suggesting multiple origins in keeping with the diffuse nature of the disease.

Ventricular arrhythmias have marked biologic variability; at initial evaluation of a patient, 5 days of electrocardiographic monitoring is necessary to ensure at least a 75% chance of not missing nonsustained ventricular tachycardia (39). The recommendation of 48-hour taping represents a pragmatic compromise, which is unlikely to give rise to an important sampling error (39,40).

Although asymptomatic, the presence of nonsustained ventricular tachycardia on Holter monitoring carries a twofold to sevenfold increased risk of sudden cardiac death, depending on the patient population studied. The presence of such arrhythmias is the best single marker of increased risk of sudden cardiac death among adults 25 years of age or older. The negative predictive accuracy is high (97%), but the positive predictive accuracy is low (23%), reflecting the fact that most patients with nonsustained ventricular tachycardia on Holter do not die during short-term follow-up. There is a need for additional stratification in this high-risk cohort of adults.

Holter monitoring provides a sensitive marker for high-risk adults 25 years of age or older. They are, however, the survivors, and it is adolescents and young adults (<25 years) who are at greatest risk. Paradoxically, Holter-identified arrhythmias are less common in the young, and unlike in the adult, a negative Holter finding does not permit reassurance in relation to sudden death risk (21). In contrast to adults, the finding of nonsustained ventricular tachycardia in the young is relatively specific, and preliminary data suggest this is sufficient to consider prophylactic treatment (41).

Sustained Ventricular Tachycardia

Sustained monomorphic ventricular tachycardia in a clinical setting is uncommon in patients with hypertrophic cardiomyopathy. In one series of more than 250 patients with hypertrophic cardiomyopathy, of whom 51 had nonsustained ventricular tachycardia on Holter monitoring, only two patients had spontaneous episodes of sustained monomorphic ventricular tachycardia, with one patient presenting with hypotension and the other with syncope (42). Both had apical aneurysms demonstrated by angiography and phase analysis of technetium-99m radionuclide ventriculograms. In one, the focus of the tachycardia was mapped to the edge of the aneurysm. Sustained monomorphic ventricular tachycardia may also be seen in some cases of end-stage hypertrophic cardiomyopathy in which chamber dimensions tend to show relative chamber dilation that is often associated with a reduction in systolic function.

Exercise Hemodynamics and Autonomic Function

A significant proportion of sudden deaths in hypertrophic cardiomyopathy occur during or immediately after a period of exertion—hence the recommendation to avoid competitive sport and intense physical exertion (7–9,43). Such sudden deaths may not be associated with arrhythmias. Exertional syncope is an important symptom and carries an increased risk of sudden cardiac death (19,20). Classically, exertional syncope in hypertrophic cardiomyopathy was thought to be caused by true obstruction to left ventricular outflow. The occurrence of exertional syncope in patients without gradients, even with pharmacologic provocation and the finding of exercise hypotension despite a normal increase in cardiac output, has forced a revision of opinion.

. Approximately 30% of patients have a flat or hypotensive blood pressure response during upright exercise (44,45). In more than 90%, this is caused by an inappropriate decrease in systemic vascular resistance, rather than a failure to increase cardiac output (44,45). Such changes may also occur at rest and during normal daily activities (46). It is unclear whether inappropriate vascular responses are an important cause of syncopal episodes. Prospective evaluation, however, reveals that an abnormal exercise blood pressure response is associated with sudden death in the young, providing a sensitive marker of the high-risk young patient (47,48).

It is postulated that the ventricular baroreceptor reflex is activated, leading to withdrawal of peripheral sympathetic tone, and that this is explained by abnormally high left ventricular wall stress consequent on increased wall thickness, reduced cavity size, and increased sympathetic drive. Such abnormalities would be magnified in patients with the smallest left ventricular cavity dimensions. The importance of such abnormal reflexes has been established in patients recovering from myocardial infarction where unopposed sympathetic activity is a risk factor for recurrent arrhythmias and sudden cardiac death (49).

Identification of Patients at High Risk for Sudden Death

Previous reports have identified a number of clinical features that are associated with increased risk of sudden death. These include evidence of arrhythmic or hemodynamic instability, markers of ischemia, and adverse familial or genetic background (43–52). Specific β-myosin heavy chain mutations (e.g., Arg403Glu) and mutations in cardiac troponin T appear to be particularly lethal (15,16). Current clinical practice does not include genotyping, and the utility of a DNA diagnosis in risk stratification needs to be assessed in much larger cohorts. Previous risk stratification studies have been limited by the number of markers that could be appropriately included in multivariate analysis. One study revealed severe left ventricular hypertrophy

(>30 mm) to be an independent risk marker compared with other echocardiographic features (53). Seventy percent of patients who die suddenly, however, do not have severe left ventricular hypertrophy (43).

Preliminary data suggest that repolarization (T-wave) alternans (RPA) may predict arrhythmic events in patients with hypertrophic cardiomyopathy. In one series of 14 patients and 9 control subjects, RPA was present in 71% of those at high-risk for an arrhythmia (i.e., prior ventricular tachycardia, nonsustained ventricular tachycardia, abnormal paced electrograms or a family history); none of the low risk patients or control subjects had RPA (54). All patients with sustained ventricular tachycardia or abnormal ventricular electrograms exhibited RPA.

The presence of RPA may be related to the gene mutation and may be significantly abnormal in those mutations associated with the poorest prognosis. As an example, one study found a greater degree of RPA in 36 patients with a β-cardiac myosin heavy chain gene mutation compared with matched controls (55). RPA was particularly abnormal in patients with the Arg403Gln mutation who are at greatest risk for sudden death. Additional studies are required to verify and extend these data.

In a prospective study, we selected five markers derived from the history and simple noninvasive evaluation (e.g., exercise test, two-dimensional echocardiography/Doppler, Holter monitoring) that the literature suggested would be most useful in predicting sudden death risk in individual patients (56,57) (Table 25-1). The presence in isolation of each risk factor was associated with a relative risk of approximately 2 and an annual sudden death mortality of 1% or less. When two or more risk factors were present, relative risk was 6% to 8%, and annual sudden death rates increased to 2% to 6%, depending on the number and combination of risk factors. About 50% of patients, however, had no risk factors, and in the absence of markers of ischemia or coexistent coronary artery disease, there was no sudden death mortality at 6 years. This simple risk factor stratification algorithm provides the clinician with guidelines that at the extremes (i.e., no risk factors versus two or more) permit appropriate reassurance or the recommendation for prophylactic treatment.

Role of Programmed Ventricular Stimulation

The role of programmed electrical stimulation in hypertrophic cardiomyopathy has been controversial. The first

TABLE 25-1. RISK FACTORS FOR SUDDEN DEATH

Family history of hypertrophic cardiomyopathy with ≥2 sudden deaths (<40 years)
Syncope (within 1 year)
Abnormal exercise blood pressure response
Nonsustained ventricular tachycardia on Holter
Severe left ventricular hypertrophy (>30 mm)

issue is whether the commonly stimulated arrhythmias, ventricular fibrillation, polymorphic ventricular tachycardia, or ventricular flutter in any way mimic the clinical arrhythmias that cause the patient's death and therefore increase understanding of the mechanism of arrhythmogenesis. The second issue is the specificity of programmed stimulation in identifying high-risk patients. It is likely that, as a group, patients with hypertrophic cardiomyopathy are more likely to develop arrhythmias with programmed stimulation than are patients with normal ventricles and that high-risk patients, as a group, are more fragile than low-risk patients. Aggressive stimulation is required to produce an arrhythmia in patients who have survived ventricular fibrillation. However, the same protocol can induce an arrhythmia in a large number of patients and controls who do not die suddenly. This lack of discrimination makes programmed stimulation unhelpful in the management of patients unless other stratification methods are employed to refine the high-risk group.

In one series of 155 patients with hypertrophic cardiomyopathy undergoing electrophysiologic study, a variety of responses to programmed ventricular stimulation were observed (29). Nonsustained ventricular tachycardia was induced in 22 patients (14%); sustained arrhythmias (defined in this study as 3 to more than 30 consecutive ventricular beats at 120 bpm or greater, terminating spontaneously or requiring termination because of hemodynamic embarrassment) were induced in 66 (43%), among whom monomorphic ventricular tachycardia was seen in 16, polymorphic ventricular tachycardia in 48, and ventricular fibrillation in 2. Induction of sustained arrhythmias required two extrastimuli in 19 patients and three extrastimuli in 47. A left ventricular site for extrastimulation was required in 15 patients. Sixteen of 17 survivors of out-of-hospital ventricular fibrillation required three extrastimuli to produce sustained arrhythmia. It was claimed that the induction of sustained ventricular arrhythmia (polymorphic ventricular tachycardia in most of the study patients) was an abnormal finding in hypertrophic cardiomyopathy that might provide a useful guide to therapy, although the study also concluded that programmed ventricular stimulation using fewer than three extrastimuli induced ventricular tachycardia in only a small percentage of patients with hypertrophic cardiomyopathy. The usefulness of such induced arrhythmias remains uncertain, and a comparison with patients at low risk would help place these results in perspective.

The combined European experience, largely unpublished, is in general agreement with the incidence of induced ventricular arrhythmias in relation to the aggressiveness of the stimulation protocol. What is different is that the patients with inducible polymorphic ventricular tachycardia have not experienced the adverse outcome that the NIH study would have predicted for them (58,59).

Sudden cardiac death of patients with hypertrophic cardiomyopathy presents an unusual electrophysiologic prob-lem. There are reports of patients with monomorphic ventricular tachycardia preceding ventricular fibrillation (60). Patients who have monomorphic ventricular tachycardia as a precursor to ventricular fibrillation, however, usually do not have the clinical tachycardia induced by programmed ventricular stimulation. Polymorphic ventricular tachycardia or ventricular fibrillation, which is the usual result of programmed stimulation, is difficult to interpret in terms of clinical arrhythmias because these arrhythmias may be a nonspecific response to aggressive stimulation rather than a tachycardia that will occur in the patient and lead to sudden death.

This situation raises three problems in the investigation of hypertrophic cardiomyopathy. First, because they cannot be induced, the mechanisms of lethal arrhythmias cannot be studied using classic electrophysiologic methods such as observation of tachycardia initiation, activation sequence, and maneuvers such as entrainment and resetting. Second, in the absence of inducible tachycardias, the effects of drugs on arrhythmogenesis cannot be investigated except by controlled trials of their effect on survival. The detection of an arrhythmia substrate in patients who may be at risk for sudden cardiac death is frustrated because the arrhythmia itself cannot be studied to identify its substrate.

There is the paradox of assessing an arrhythmia that cannot be induced and studied directly but that may be lethal the first time that it occurs. Novel approaches to this problem that involve the detection of a putative arrhythmia substrate without induction of an arrhythmia are under investigation (61,62).

Therapeutic Approach to Arrhythmias

Atrial Fibrillation

Short episodes of paroxysmal atrial fibrillation or other supraventricular tachycardias do not warrant treatment, because patients are usually unaware of them and because their prognostic significance is uncertain. In established atrial fibrillation, digoxin is usually an appropriate agent for the control of the ventricular rate, but it is not very useful for the control of the heart rate in paroxysmal atrial fibrillation. Although digoxin may be contraindicated in the presence of hyperdynamic systolic function and a left ventricular outflow tract gradient, most patients in atrial fibrillation have impaired systolic function without a gradient and do not suffer any deleterious hemodynamic consequences from its use. Class I agents, particularly disopyramide and propafenone, have been used to prevent atrial fibrillation and to facilitate cardioversion. Their role in maintaining sinus rhythm has not been systematically assessed.

Amiodarone is also a useful drug in the treatment of established and paroxysmal atrial fibrillation. Amiodarone is effective in preventing the episodes and in attenuating the ventricular rate response if breakthrough does occur. Its use in high doses is associated with a significant incidence of side effects, including those that are relatively trivial (e.g., corneal deposits), troublesome (e.g., sleep disturbance, photosensitization, thyroid abnormalities), and life threatening (e.g., pulmonary fibrosis, hepatic failure). These adverse effects are generally seen with plasma amiodarone concentrations in excess of 2 mg/L (63), but suppression of supraventricular arrhythmias can usually be obtained with plasma concentrations of 0.5 to 1.0 mg/L (64). Significant adverse effects are seldom seen at these levels. In the study of the influence of atrial fibrillation on natural history, amiodarone therapy was associated with the maintenance of sinus rhythm, fewer alterations in drug therapy, fewer embolic episodes, and fewer attempts at direct current cardioversion (37).

Prevention of Sudden Death

Conventional noninvasive risk factor stratification identifies a cohort of patients who are at increased risk for sudden cardiac death. In approximately 30% of this group, a probable initiating mechanism that is amenable to specific therapy can be identified. A common initiating mechanism is paroxysmal atrial fibrillation, which can be effectively prevented with amiodarone. Sustained monomorphic ventricular tachycardia can be treated with drugs with or without an automatic implantable cardioverter-defibrillator (ICD); conduction disease, with a pacemaker; rapid AV conduction, through an accessory pathway by radiofrequency catheter ablation; ischemia, and autonomic disturbance with high-dose verapamil or a β blocker (Fig. 25-3); and left ventricular outflow tract obstruction by dual-chamber pacing (65), myectomy (66), or ethanol ablation (67). In the approximately 70% remaining, the patient is recognized to be at increased risk,

but there are multiple potential triggers or no identifiable triggers that can be targeted. Such patients include those who have been resuscitated from out-of-hospital ventricular fibrillation and those with two or more risk factors (Table 25-1). In such patients, implantation of an ICD is warranted and likely to be effective. Data from a retrospective registry indicates annual discharge rates for primary prevention of 2% to 3 %, whereas the risk of sudden death of those who have experienced out-of-hospital ventricular fibrillation is marginally greater (4%) (60,68,69). These discharge rates are less than those for high-risk coronary artery disease or dilated cardiomyopathy patients, and this finding has led some to question the utility of the ICD in treating hypertrophic cardiomyopathy (70). Long-term outcome remains to be determined, but it is anticipated that a single appropriate discharge may permit long-term survival in contrast to dilated cardiomyopathy and advanced coronary artery disease, for which the prognosis is likely to limit survival. Despite major advances in ICD technology, defibrillator use in the young with hypertrophic cardiomyopathy is associated with problems, including psychosocial adjustment, lead fracture or dislodgment, and inappropriate discharges, which appear to be more common than in older ICD patients (71).

A subset of high-risk hypertrophic cardiomyopathy patients also have clinical arrhythmias (mainly supraventricular) that may require concomitant use of amiodarone along with an ICD. Though amiodarone has been used successfully for sudden death prevention, its role in the ICD era is predominantly as additional therapy or use in those in whom an ICD is not acceptable or tolerated (72).

Effect of Atrioventricular Nodal Blocking Agents

Although β-blocking agents and calcium antagonists have been shown to provide symptomatic benefit, there is no evidence to suggest improved survival (19,73). The use of verapamil can be associated with serious complications (74). It can suppress impulse formation in the sinus node and adversely affect conduction through the AV node. It has been associated with the development of complete heart block in patients with preexisting but unsuspected conduction disease. The combination of conduction disturbance, negative inotropism, and vasodilator properties has caused pulmonary edema and death in some patients (74). Similarly, alcohol septal reduction and surgical myectomy are useful in the relief of symptoms and left ventricular outflow tract obstruction, but these procedures do not appear to prevent sudden death (66,67).

DILATED CARDIOMYOPATHY

Dilated cardiomyopathy (DCM) is a syndrome characterized by dilatation and impaired contraction of the left ven-

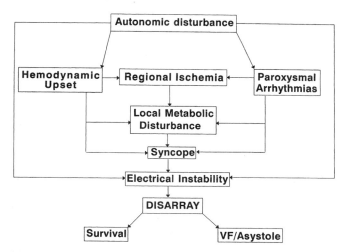

FIGURE 25-3. The schematic diagram illustrates the associations among autonomic dysfunction, hemodynamic upset, paroxysmal arrhythmias, and the arrhythmogenic substrate in the pathogenesis of sudden death in hypertrophic cardiomyopathy.

tricle or of both ventricles. It may be idiopathic, familial or genetic, viral or immunologic, alcoholic or toxic, or related to pregnancy (75). Some 20% to 30% of patients with unexplained DCM have familial disease. A common feature of DCM, regardless of the underlying cause, is a propensity to atrial and ventricular arrhythmias and an increased risk of sudden death.

Epidemiology

The incidence of DCM varies with geographic location, case ascertainment, and diagnostic criteria. The overall age-adjusted annual incidence rate from 1975 through 1984 in Olmsted County, Minnesota, was 6.0 cases per 100,000 persons, and the prevalence in 1985 was 36.5 cases per 100,000 persons, translating to about 100,000 affected individuals in the United States (76). More than 10,000 deaths in the United States are attributed to DCM each year.

Survival in DCM is principally determined by the source of referral and the duration of illness in the cohort being examined, varying from 46% at 1 year in a group of symptomatic patients refused transplantation (77) to 95% at 1 year in a population-based analysis (78) (Fig. 25-4). When ischemic and nonischemic cardiomyopathies are considered collectively, survival rates range from 48% to 76% at 1 year and from 19% to 66% at 2 years (77–80a).

Mechanisms of Arrhythmia

Multiple mechanisms for the loss of myocardial function have been demonstrated or postulated in DCM, including genetic abnormalities of the cardiac myocyte cytoskeleton (81–84) and infectious- (85) and immune-mediated (86) cardiomyocyte necrosis and apoptosis (87). Irrespective of the mechanism of loss of function, myocyte loss and replacement by fibrous tissue is common in DCM, creating a milieu for anisotropic conduction and reentrant arrhyth-

mias. At autopsy, extensive subendocardial scarring in the left ventricle has been described in 33% of patients and multiple patchy areas of replacement fibrosis in 57% of patients with DCM (88) (Fig. 25-5). The degree of left atrial fibrosis among patients with DCM in another autopsy series was almost four times that of controls who had died with a known prior myocardial infarction (13.1±6.1% versus 3.8±1.1%) (89).

In addition to structural changes, ion channel behavior and intracellular ion concentrations, particularly Ca^{2+}, can be altered. Li and colleagues found decreases in I_{to}, L-type I_{Ca}, and I_{Ks} activity and an increase in Na^{+}-Ca^{2+} exchange activity in atrial myocytes in dogs with ventricular pacing-induced heart failure (90). Ventricular I_{to} is decreased in dogs with pacing-induced CHF (91) and in cardiomyopathic Syrian hamsters (92). Ventricular I_{K1} is reduced in experimental (91,92) and clinical (93) CHF. Ventricular Na^{+}-Ca^{2+} exchange activity is increased in experimental CHF, resulting in prolongation of the action potential duration (94). Miyamoto and associates found that the abnormal decrease in systolic cytosol Ca^{2+} and increase in diastolic Ca^{2+} observed in failing myocardium may be reversed by overexpression of sarcoplasmic reticulum Ca^{2+} ATPase induced by adenoviral gene transfer, supporting the pivotal role of underexpression of this gene in loss of inotropy and arrhythmogenesis in failing myocardium (95). Other mechanical, hemodynamic, and neurohumoral factors play important roles in arrhythmia triggering and maintenance (Table 25-2).

Atrial Arrhythmias

The prevalence of atrial arrhythmias in DCM varies from 5% to 40% and increases with the severity of left ventricular dysfunction and the presence of symptoms of CHF (96,97). Atrial arrhythmias are a frequent consequence of and an infrequent precipitant of DCM. Occasionally, minimally

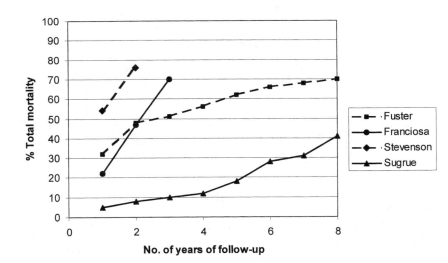

FIGURE 25-4. Survival curves from longitudinal studies of dilated cardiomyopathy (DCM) demonstrate how survival can vary depending on the population being examined. Stevenson and colleagues (77) examined survival in a group of patients with DCM and severe left ventricular dysfunction who were refused cardiac transplantation because of inadequate symptoms, and Sugrue and associates (78) analyzed a population-based cohort. Also included are data from Fuster (80) and Franciosa (80a).

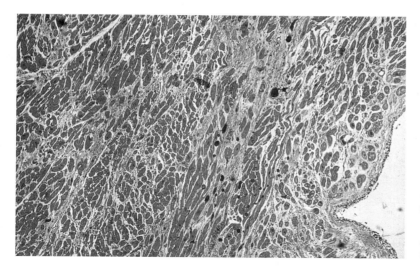

FIGURE 25-5. Hematoxylin-eosin stain of ventricular subendocardium demonstrates patchy fibrous tissue replacement of the myocardium in a case of idiopathic dilated cardiomyopathy (magnification ×370). (Courtesy of Dr. T Aretz, Department of Pathology, Massachusetts General Hospital, Boston, MA.)

symptomatic atrial tachycardia or atrial fibrillation is associated with a heart rate rapid enough to result in a gradual deterioration in left ventricular systolic function and DCM (98,99). Systolic function frequently returns to normal after termination and prevention of recurrence of the arrhythmia.

The most common arrhythmia in DCM is atrial fibrillation. Although single or dual focal sources of atrial fibrillation are not infrequent in the absence of structural heart disease (100), their incidence in DCM and amenability to catheter ablation are unknown. Development of atrial fibrillation in DCM is associated with a higher mortality rate (101,102) although some investigators disagree (96). In the largest study, 19% of 390 patients with advanced heart failure, including 191 patients with DCM, developed paroxysmal or chronic atrial fibrillation (101). The 1-year actuarial survival rates for patients with atrial fibrillation and for patients in sinus rhythm were 52% and 71% ($p = 0.001$),

respectively. However, this finding did not remain significant when corrected for an elevated pulmonary wedge pressure. The poor survival of patients with atrial fibrillation may not be cause and effect; rather, atrial fibrillation may merely be a marker of severe left ventricular dysfunction. Although atrial tachycardia, flutter, and other mechanisms of supraventricular tachycardia also occur, they are less common than atrial fibrillation, but the proportion of fibrillation initiated by these mechanisms remains unknown.

Ventricular Arrhythmias

Multiform premature ventricular contractions (PVCs), ventricular pairs, and nonsustained ventricular tachycardia are present in 80% to 95% of patients with DCM (103,104). In one study using 24-hour Holter monitoring, 53% of patients had more than 500 PVCs, 54% had ventricular pairs, and 31% experienced episodes of nonsustained ventricular tachycardia (105). In those with CHF, ventricular arrhythmias become more frequent and more complex as left ventricular function deteriorates (106). The prevalence of nonsustained ventricular tachycardia has been shown to increase from 15% to 20% in patients with class I or II CHF to 50% to 70% in patients with class IV CHF (97). Ventricular arrhythmias have been reported as independent predictors of total cardiac mortality (100) or sudden cardiac death by some but not by others (103). Although ventricular tachycardia usually arises in the myocardium, bundle branch reentry ventricular tachycardia (BBRVT) may be the mechanism responsible for ventricular tachycardia, and in one selected series, it was seen in 41% of patients with DCM (107). Bundle branch reentry produces ventricular tachycardia through a macroreentrant circuit involving the His-Purkinje system, usually with antegrade conduction over the right bundle branch and retrograde conduction over the left bundle branch. BBRVT is usually rapid, with a mean cycle length of 280 ms (108,109). It may be distinguished from myocardial ventricular tachy-

TABLE 25-2. FACTORS THAT CONTRIBUTE TO ARRHYTHMOGENESIS IN DILATED CARDIOMYOPATHY

Hypokalemia, hypomagnesemia (often related to diuretic use)
Sustained stretch-induced shortening of refractoriness and action potential duration predisposing to reentry
Short, pulsatile, stretch-induced arrhythmia after depolarizations
Diastolic calcium overload due to decreased sacrcoplasmic reticulum Ca^{2+} ATPase pump
Afterdepolarizations induced by increased Na^+-Ca^{2+} exchanger activity
Increased circulating catecholamines
Increased sympathetic tone
Myocardial fibrosis or scar
His-Purkinje system conduction delay
Increased endocardial surface area in dilated atrium or ventricle
Drugs (e.g., antiarrhythmics, digoxin, sympathomimetics, phosphodiesterase inhibitors)

cardia by the presence of a His or right bundle branch potential that precedes each QRS (110). The H-V interval in BBRVT equals or exceeds the value in sinus rhythm. Bundle branch reentrant tachycardia is an important arrhythmia to recognize because catheter ablation of the right or left bundle branch is almost always curative (111–113). DCM has been infrequently reported as a consequence of incessant ventricular tachycardia and rarely is caused by PVCs (114,115).

Predictors of Arrhythmia and Mortality

Clinical Predictors

The severity of left ventricular dysfunction is the most powerful predictor of mortality in patients with DCM and CHF (102,115–117). As CHF symptoms worsen, the risks of total mortality, sudden death, and CHF death increase (118,119), but the ratio of sudden death to CHF death decreases (118) (Fig. 25-6). When patients develop NYHA class IV symptoms, the ejection fraction is less valuable in predicting mortality (120). Syncope is a strong predictor of

death in general and sudden death in particular in patients with DCM (121). In one study, 1-year sudden death rates for patients with DCM increased from 12% to 45% when syncope was present (122).

Electrophysiologic Predictors

Electrocardiogram
First- and second-degree AV block (123) and the degree of QRS prolongation have all been associated with increased mortality (124) (Fig. 25-7).

Electrophysiologic Study
In most patients with nonischemic cardiomyopathy, programmed ventricular stimulation is unreliable in the induction of sustained monomorphic ventricular tachycardia. Polymorphic ventricular arrhythmias can be induced in up to 30% of patients with DCM, but these are nonspecific end points that are not useful for serial drug testing and are without prognostic significance (125–128). The poor positive and negative predictive value of programmed stimula-

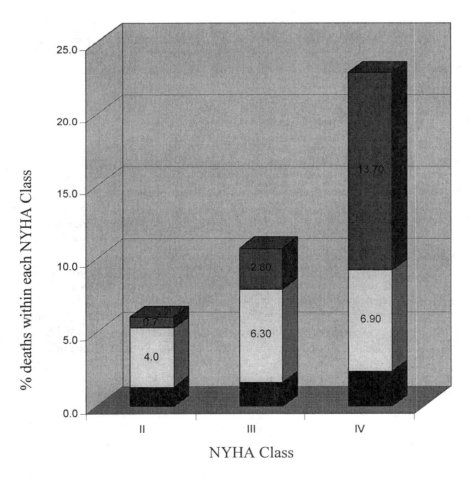

FIGURE 25-6. Death rates and mode of death according to New York Heart Association (NYHA) class in the Metoprolol CR/XL Randomized Intervention Trial in Congestive Heart Failure (MERIT-HF) (118). Rates are calculated as an average of death rates in the metoprolol and placebo groups in each NYHA class.

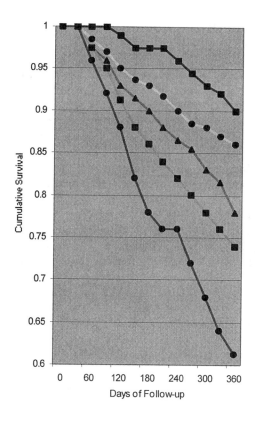

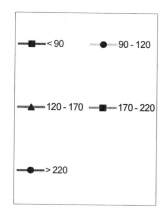

FIGURE 25-7. Survival among patients in the vesnarinone trial (VEST) as a function of QRS duration (in milliseconds) on baseline 12-lead electrocardiogram.

tion in the setting of DCM and nonsustained ventricular tachycardia preclude its routine use for risk stratification in this group (129–133) (Table 25-3).

Signal-Averaged Electrocardiogram

The sensitivity and specificity of the signal-averaged ECG in predicting ventricular tachycardia and sudden death in patients with nonischemic cardiomyopathy have varied from 22% to 100% and 45% to 96%, respectively

(134–135). The signal-averaged ECG has not been clearly demonstrated to have additional clinical benefit beyond assessment of systolic function and the frequent occurrence of bundle branch block in DCM limits its use.

Heart Rate Variability

Only a small number of studies of heart rate variability (HRV) in patients with DCM have been performed. In one study, Hoffmann and colleagues (139) examined 24-hour

TABLE 25-3. PROGRAMMED STIMULATION IN PATIENTS WITH DILATED CARDIOMYOPATHY AND NO HISTORY OF SUSTAINED VENTRICULAR ARRHYTHMIAS

		Inducible arrhythmia in Follow-up			Arrhythmic Events in Follow-up				Noninducible Patients	
Study	Year	Patients (n)	VES (n)	NSVT (%)	MMVT (%)	PMVT/VF (%)	Follow-up (mo)	Ind Patients	MMVT	PMVT/VF
Meinertz et al. (125)	1985	42	1–2	35%	0 (0%)	1 (2%)	16 ± 7	0 (0%)	0 (0%)	2 (5%)
Stamato (126)	1986	15	1–2	93%	0 (0%)	0 (0%)	19 ± 4	0 (0%)	0 (0%)	2 (13%)
Poll (127)	1986	20	1–3	100%	2 (10%)	4 (20%)	17 ± 14	0 (0%)	2 (50%)	5 (36%)
Das (128)	1986	24	1–3	NA	1 (4%)	4 (17%)	12 ± 6	1 (100%)	1 (25%)	2 (11%)
Gossinger (129)	1990	32	1–3	100%	4 (13%)	0 (0%)	21	1 (25%)	0 (0%)	2 (7%)
Brembilla (130)	1991	92	1–3	46%	3 (3%)	5 (5%)	24 ± 8	2 (67%)	2 (40%)	3 (4%)
Kadish (131)	1993	43	1–3	100%	6 (14%)	NA	20 ± 14	1 (17%)	NA	6 (16%)
Turrito (132)	1994	80	1–3	100%	10 (13%)	7 (9%)	22 ± 26	3 (30%)	0 (0%)	6 (10%)
Grimm (133)	1997	34	1–3	100%	3 (9%)	10 (29%)	24 ± 13	1 (33%)	3 (30%)	5 (24%)

Ind, inducible; MMVT, monomorphic ventricular tachycardia; NA, not available; Noninducible, no sustained ventricular arrhythmia inducible; NSVT, nonsustained ventricular tachycardia at baseline; PMVT/VF, polymorphic ventricular tachycardia or ventricular fibrillation, VES, ventricular extrastimuli used.
From Grimm W, Hoffmann J, Menz V, et al. Programmed ventricular stimulation for arrhythmia risk prediction in patients with idiopathic dilated cardiomyopathy and nonsustained ventricular tachycardia. *J Am Coll Cardiol* 1998;739–745, with permission.

HRV recordings, performing time and frequency domain analysis of 71 patients with DCM, 10 of whom developed ventricular tachycardia, ventricular fibrillation, or sudden death during 15 months of follow-up. A trend toward reduced HRV in time domain analysis but no differences between the two groups in frequency domain analysis were observed. A much larger group of 433 outpatients with CHF was evaluated in the United Kingdom Heart Failure Evaluation and Assessment of Risk Trial (UK-HEART) (140). After a follow-up of 482 days, HRV in the time domain was found to be an independent predictor of all-cause mortality and the most powerful predictor of death from progressive heart failure; the annual mortality rates for those with a standard deviation of the -R intervals of more than 100 ms (HRV present), 50 to 100 ms (intermediate HRV), and less than 50 ms (HRV absent) were 5.5%, 12.7%, and 51.4%, respectively.

QT Dispersion

Relatively few data exist on the predictive accuracy of QT dispersion in DCM. In the largest study, Grimm and colleagues found significantly longer QT, corrected QT (QTc), and adjusted (divided by the square root of the number of leads measured) QTc interval dispersions among 107 patients with DCM compared with healthy age- and sex-matched controls. QT dispersion was significantly longer (76 ± 17 versus 60 ± 26 ms, $p < 0.03$) among the 12 of 107 patients who developed sustained ventricular tachycardia, ventricular fibrillation, or sudden death during the 13-month follow-up period (141).

T wave Alternans

Results of studies for defining the role of RPA in patients with clinical CHF are emerging. In one prospective study of 81 patients with heart failure, no recent myocardial infarction, nor prior arrhythmias, the presence of RPA was associated with lower event-free survival at 2 years (80% versus 100% if RPA was absent) (142).

The presence of RPA is predictive of an arrhythmic event in patients with ischemic cardiomyopathy. As an example, one study of 87 patients with ischemic cardiomyopathy who received an implantable defibrillator for prior arrhythmia found RPA in 74% (143). The sensitivity, specificity, and negative and positive values for RPA predicting an arrhythmic event in this population were 86%, 52%, 76%, and 65%, respectively.

RPA is also a useful technique for identifying patients with nonischemic DCM who have ventricular tachycardia. As an example, one study of 58 patients with nonischemic DCM found that the percentage of patients with ventricular tachycardia on ambulatory monitoring was greater among those with RPA during bicycle exercise testing (61% versus 8% for those without RPA); the sensitivity, specificity, and predictive accuracy of RPA for ventricular tachycardia were 88%, 72%, and 77%, respectively (144).

Therapy for Arrhythmias

β-Adrenergic Blockers

Catecholamine excess in patients with DCM can result in several maladaptive responses, including downregulation of β-adrenergic receptors, inappropriate sinus tachycardia, increased transmural dispersion of refractoriness, and enhanced automaticity of atrial and ventricular ectopic foci. These responses may further reduce cardiac output while at the same time increasing the risk of atrial and ventricular arrhythmias. Three large, prospective, randomized trials redefined the role of β blockade in the treatment of patients with DCM and CHF (145–147). All three studies demonstrated a substantial reduction in sudden death rates and in total mortality, heart failure mortality, and hospitalization rates for heart failure (Table 25-4). The effects of β blockers on total mortality were marginally more marked in the ischemic than in the nonischemic patients in both studies that examined this question (147,148), although not significantly so, and it should not be presumed that the benefit is any less marked in patients with DCM. These studies have underlined the importance of β blockers and their role as one of the first-line drug therapies for patients with DCM and symptomatic but compensated heart failure.

Antiarrhythmic Drug Therapy

The use of class I antiarrhythmic drugs in the absence of an ICD has decreased in patients with heart failure or significant ventricular dysfunction because of an increased risk of death, specifically sudden death, demonstrated prospectively (148) and retrospectively (149–153). The increased mortality is almost certainly caused by ventricular proarrhythmia, although other mechanisms, including bradyarrhythmia and worsening of heart failure, may play a role. The use of serial drug testing does not decrease this risk in a coronary disease population (154). Although each of these trials was performed primarily in patients with ischemic heart disease, the results have been extrapolated by many to all patients with heart disease, including those with a nonischemic cardiomyopathy. How much of a role ischemia plays in the development of proarrhythmia and whether patients with DCM are at less of an increased risk than their ischemic counterparts are unclear, although proarrhythmia has been clearly documented previously in the setting of DCM and in the absence of structural heart disease (155,156). The risk of proarrhythmia is related to the degree of left ventricular dysfunction (156). In the Cardiac Arrhythmia Suppression Trial (CAST), major proarrhythmic effects were more common in patients with ejection fractions less than 0.30 compared with patients with ejection fractions greater than 0.30 (148). In the Stroke Prevention in Atrial fibrillation (SPAF) study, patients with atrial fibrillation and heart failure treated with antiarrhyth-

TABLE 25-4. RESULTS OF THE THREE LARGEST PROSPECTIVE, RANDOMIZED TRIALS OF BETA BLOCKERS IN TREATING CONGESTIVE HEART FAILURE

Trial	Number of Patients	DCM	Inclusion	Drug and Dosage	Relative Risk Reduction		
					TD	SD	CHFD
Carvedilol HFSG (145)	1,094	570 (52%)	NYHA II–IV, EF ≤ 0.35	Carvedilol 3.125–50 mg bid	65%	55%	79%
CIBIS II (146)	2,647	317 (12%)	NYHA III–IV, EF ≤ 0.35	Bisoprolol 1.25–10 mg/d	34%	44%	26%
MERIT-HF (147)	3,991	1,385 (35%)	NYHA II–IV, EF ≤ 0.4	Metoprolol CR/XL12.5–25 mg/d	34%	41%	49%

Carvedilol HFSG, Carvedilol Heart Failure Study Group; CIBIS II, Cardiac Insufficiency Bisoprolol Study II; MERIT-HF, Metoprolol CR/XL Randomized Intervention Trial in Congestive Heart Failure; DCM, Dilated Cardiomyopathy; NYHA, New York Heart Association Class; EF, Ejection Fraction; TD, Total Death; SD, Sudden Death; CHFD, Congestive Heart Failure Death.

mic drugs were at a 4.7-fold risk of cardiac death and 3.7-fold risk of sudden death compared with those who were not treated with antiarrhythmic drugs (150). In patients with no CHF, there was no increased risk associated with antiarrhythmic drug therapy.

Among the class III agents, two have been shown not to increase overall mortality in patients with heart failure. In the Danish Investigations of Arrhythmia and Mortality-congestive Heart Failure (DIAMOND-CHF), 1,518 patients with a history of heart failure and an ejection fraction of less than 0.35 were randomized to dofetilide (0.5 mg, given twice daily) or placebo, with no difference found in mortality at 3 years (157). Patients had in-hospital drug initiation, dose adjustment for creatinine clearance, and QTc measurements 2 to 3 hours after each of the first five doses. In addition to the lack of difference in mortality with dofetilide compared with placebo, the patients receiving dofetilide had a 12-fold increased likelihood of restoration of sinus rhythm if they were in atrial fibrillation (12% versus 1%) and a 65% reduction in further episodes of atrial fibrillation. The overall risk of torsade de pointes was 3.3% with dofetilide and 0% with placebo, with two fatalities among 762 patients in the treatment group. Female gender and NYHA class III or IV (versus class I or II) symptoms carried a 3.2- and 3.9-fold increased risk, respectively.

Sotalol is effective in the prevention of atrial and ventricular arrhythmias, although few data exist on the safety of sotalol in the setting of DCM or CHF. Proarrhythmia with sotalol and dofetilide is potentiated by renal insufficiency (i.e., both drugs are solely excreted by the kidney) and by diuretic-induced hypokalemia, necessitating caution when they are used in this population.

Amiodarone appears to be the most effective agent available for the prevention of atrial and ventricular arrhythmias and the least likely to result in proarrhythmia, although its use is limited by its side-effect profile. Two trials have demonstrated its lack of proarrhythmia in CHF populations. The first is the Congestive Heart Failure-Survival Trial of Antiarrhythmic Therapy (CHF-STAT), which randomly assigned 674 patients with symptomatic heart failure, fewer than nine PVCs per hour, and an ejection fraction less than 0.4 to

receive 300 mg of amiodarone daily or placebo (158). There were no differences between the two groups with respect to total mortality or sudden death. However, among the 193 patients (29%) with nonischemic cardiomyopathy, there was a trend toward a reduction in overall mortality ($p = 0.07$). The second is the Grupo de Estudio de la Sobrevida en la Insuficencia Cardiaca en Argentina (GESICA) trial, which randomized 516 patients with symptomatic CHF, 62% of whom had a nonischemic cause, and an ejection fraction of 0.35 on triple-drug therapy to amiodarone (300/day) or placebo and demonstrated a 28% reduction in overall mortality ($p = 0.024$) and a 27% reduction in sudden death ($p = 0.16$) among the amiodarone-treated patients (159).

Amiodarone, with appropriate close monitoring for potential side effects, should be considered as a first-choice drug in the treatment of atrial and ventricular arrhythmias in the setting of DCM, particularly in older patients with severe left ventricular dysfunction for whom life expectancy and therefore the long-term risk of pulmonary fibrosis is less than in younger patients.

Radiofrequency Ablation

Because of the risk of proarrhythmia with most antiarrhythmic drugs in patients with DCM, radiofrequency ablation provides an attractive alternative for the management of organized atrial arrhythmias such as ectopic atrial tachycardia and atrial flutter. Success rates of catheter ablation for ventricular tachycardia in the setting of DCM, however, have been less than those for ventricular tachycardia in the setting of coronary artery disease (160).

Angiotensin-Converting Enzyme Inhibition

Angiotensin-converting enzyme (ACE) inhibitors, in contrast to other vasodilators, may be unique in reducing sudden death in patients with heart failure (161). In Vasodilator Heart Failure Trial (VHeFT-II), the reduction in mortality (18% versus 28%) with enalapril was attributed to a reduction in the incidence of sudden death (37% versus 46%) in the enalapril group (162). Ventricular tachycardia was less frequent at 3 months and fewer new cases of ventricular tachycardia developed at 1 year and 2 years in the enalapril group (163). In contrast, the Cooperative North Scandinavian Enalapril Survival Study (CONSENSUS) and Studies of Left Ventricular Dysfunction (SOLVD) investigators failed to show a reduction in sudden death in 253 patients with NYHA class IV heart failure and 2,569 patients with left ventricular ejection fractions less than 0.35 respectively randomized to enalapril or placebo (164,165).

The superiority of the angiotensin II (AT1) receptor antagonist losartan to captopril in the prevention of sudden death in the Evaluation of Losartan in the Eldery (ELITE) trial (166) did not remain significant when subjected to the larger, adequately powered ELITE II study (167). Nonetheless, in patients unable to tolerate ACE inhibition because of cough or other side effects, the AT1 antagonists are a reasonable alternative.

Permanent Pacemakers

Severe bradycardia or electromechanical dissociation has been identified as the terminal rhythm among patients with CHF, severe left ventricular dysfunction, and class IV heart failure undergoing transplant evaluation (168). Beyond the role of preventing spontaneous or drug-induced symptomatic bradycardia or asystole, permanent pacing can correct two important intracardiac conduction abnormalities.

In the first case, prolongation of the PR interval, typically caused by AV nodal disease, has several deleterious effects on left ventricular hemodynamics, including a reduction in diastolic ventricular filling time and the development of end-diastolic tricuspid and mitral regurgitation. Correction of PR prolongation with short AV-delay, dual-chamber pacing has been shown to increase stroke volume (169) and blood pressure (170) and decrease mitral regurgitation (171) significantly, particularly when the baseline PR interval is more than 220 ms (172). In addition to improving hemodynamics directly, the increase in heart rate and blood pressure may cause secondary benefit by permitting a higher dose of β blocker and ACE inhibitor.

In the second case, much attention has been directed to the deleterious effect in CHF of intraventricular conduction delay in general and LBBB in particular. The resulting dyssynchronous contraction of the left ventricular free wall and interventricular septum and the late activation of the anterolateral papillary muscle may result in a decrease in effective left ventricular ejection and ejection fraction and an increase in functional mitral regurgitation, respectively (173). Both problems are potentially correctible by left ventricular free wall (or biventricular) pacing (174). Initially done epicardially, this can now be accomplished effectively and safely with specialized leads through the coronary sinus (175).

Early anecdotal reports of dramatic improvements in symptoms translated into significant improvements in NYHA class, 6-minute walk distance, quality of life, and ejection fraction in one nonrandomized trial (176) and in Vo2max and O2 consumption at anaerobic threshold in one randomized crossover trial (177). The clinical applicability of this technique will be decided by ongoing studies such as the Comparison of Medical Therapy, Pacing and Defibrillation in Chronic Heart Failure (COMPANION) and Multicenter InSync Randomized Clinical Evaluation (MIRACLE) trials. Because patients with DCM are at high risk for bradyarrhythmias and tachyarrhythmias, it is likely that the use of implantable defibrillators with demand pacing capability will prove to be more useful than either form of electrical therapy alone.

Implantable Cardioverter-Defibrillators in Heart Failure Patients with a Sustained Ventricular Tachyarrhythmia

The completed randomized trials of ICDs have concentrated primarily on patients with CAD. Only the Antiarrhythmics Versus Implantable Defibrillators (AVID) (178), Cardiac Arrest Study Hamburg (CASH) (179), and Canadian Implantable Defibrillator Study (CIDS) (180) trials included patients with DCM. Of the 162 patients without CAD in the AVID study (not all of whom had DCM), 77 received conventional drug therapy, and 75 received ICDs for cardiac arrest or sustained ventricular tachycardia that was felt to be life threatening on the basis of hemodynamic instability or depressed left ventricular function. The overall mortality was reduced among patients who were randomized to ICD therapy (9% versus 12% at 1 year, 11% versus 18% at 2 years, and 14% versus 38% at 3 years) (181). However, the outcome with an ICD was related to left ventricular ejection fraction; in those with a value between 0.20 and 0.34, survival was significantly better with the ICD, whereas in patients with a left ventricular ejection fraction of less than 0.20, survival tended to be better with the ICD than with drugs, but the difference was not statistically significant (182).

The CIDS trial analyzed the outcome of high-risk patients to establish whether some subsets of patients might benefit from the ICD (183). A multivariate risk model identified age, left ventricular ejection fraction, and NYHA class as independent predictors of risk, and based on these parameters, quartiles of risk were constructed. Patients in the highest-risk quartile, who had at least two risk factors (i.e., age ≥70 years, left ventricular ejection fraction ≤0.35, and NYHA class III or IV), had a significant reduction of death from the ICD compared with amiodarone (14.4% versus 30%); there was no benefit seen among patients in the other three quartiles.

Prophylactic Use of the Implantable Cardioverter-Defibrillator

Although previous myocardial infarction was an entry requirement for the Multicenter Automatic Defibrillator

Implantation Trial (MADIT) and Multicenter Unsustained Tachycardia Trial (MUSTT) (154,184), it has been suggested that patients with DCM who have the same characteristics of patients enrolled in MADIT (i.e., ejection fraction < 0.35%, nonsustained ventricular tachycardia [>3 beats], and inducible but nonsuppressible ventricular tachycardia) or MUSTT (i.e., asymptomatic nonsustained ventricular tachycardia, left ventricular ejection fraction ≤ 0.40, and inducible sustained ventricular tachycardia) may also benefit from a prophylactic ICD implant. However, the unreliability of programmed ventricular stimulation makes it difficult to fully extrapolate MADIT and MUSTT results to this population. The role of ICDs in the primary prevention of sudden death in patients with DCM will be defined over the next 3 years in a series of ongoing prospective, randomized trials: Defibrillators in Non-Ischemic Cardiomyopathy Treatment Evaluation (DEFINITE) (185), (AMIOVIRT), (DEBUT), Primary Implantation Cardioverter-Defibrillator (PRIDE), (CAT), and Sudden Cardiac Death–Heart Failure Trial (SCD-HeFT) (186).

ARRHYTHMOGENIC RIGHT VENTRICULAR CARDIOMYOPATHY

Arrhythmogenic right ventricular cardiomyopathy (ARVC), which has also been called arrhythmogenic right ventricular dysplasia, has been incorporated in the reclassification of the cardiomyopathies (187). Originally, it was described as a disease of the right ventricle, characterized by fibrofatty replacement of cardiomyocytes and extracellular matrix. Subsequent studies demonstrated that left ventricular involvement is common (188). The pathologic substrate may lead to the electrical instability and progressive ventricular dysfunction that is characteristic of the disease. ARVC may manifest with ventricular arrhythmias, heart failure, or sudden death. It probably represents a wide spectrum of disease, with clinicians seeing the more extreme cases (189,190).

Etiology

The cause and pathogenesis of ARVC are unknown, but proposed theories include apoptosis because programmed cell death has been observed in the right ventricular myocardium of patients with ARVC (191,192). An abnormality of a gene specific for cardiac muscle leading to a "myocardial dystrophy" has also been proposed (193). The inflammatory theory proposes that fibrofatty replacement of the right ventricle is the consequence of a continuous process of cell injury and repair in the setting of a chronic myocarditis (194–196). Support for this idea comes from the demonstration of inflammatory infiltrates at necropsy or endomyocardial biopsy. A genetic predisposition to

infections eliciting an immune reaction could account for the family history. Whether the myocarditis is a primary event or a reactive process secondary to the spontaneous myocyte death remains to be elucidated. The term *dysplasia* has been used to describe this disease, but the evidence does not support the concept of a congenital absence of myocardium.

Genetics

Familial disease appears to be common, affecting up to 50% of kindreds (197–202). In these families, segregation studies are most consistent with an autosomal dominant pattern of mendelian inheritance with variable penetrance. Six chromosomal loci have subsequently been published for the dominant form of the disease, although no gene has been identified: 14q23-q24 (203), 1q42-q43 (204), 14q12-q22 (205), 2q32 (206), 3p23 (207), and 10p12-p14 (208). An autosomal recessive form of ARVC (i.e., Naxos disease) has been reported exclusively in people on the Greek island of Naxos in whom there is cosegregation of cardiac, skin (nonepidermolytic palmoplantar keratoderma), and hair abnormalities (209). This distinctive phenotype allows for more accurate diagnosis of ARVC, which has offered a robust model for genetic studies. This variant of ARVC was mapped to the keratin 9 *(KRT9)* gene locus on chromosome 17q21, and a mutation of plakoglobin has been identified as the causative gene (210,211). Plakoglobin is a key protein in cell-cell adhesive junctions, such as the intercalated disc of the heart and the dermal-epidermal junctions of the epidermis (212). A 2-base pair deletion (Pk2157del2) caused a frame shift and premature termination at the 3′ end of the plakoglobin gene in affected individuals. This deletion was not identified in 43 autosomal dominant ARVC probands, suggesting that this form of the disease could be caused by mutations in other regions of the plakoglobin molecule or other functionally related proteins. *In vitro* studies and a plakoglobin-null mouse model reveal altered integrity at the cell-cell junction that, in conjunction with mechanical stress, leads to myocyte death (213).

Gross Pathology

ARVC is characterized pathologically by a fibrofatty replacement of the right ventricular free wall that may be segmental or diffuse (Fig. 25-8) and can affect the full thickness of the myocardium (214). Right ventricular aneurysms have been reported in up to 50% of postmortem cases (194) and are most commonly located in the apical, infundibular and subtricuspid areas, named the *triangle of dysplasia* (215).

Histology

Two histologic variants of ARVC have been described. The first is the so-called fatty pattern that predominantly

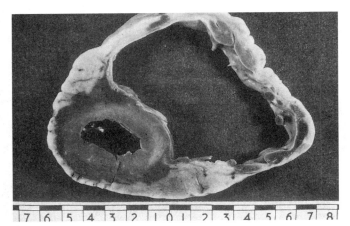

FIGURE 25-8. Cross-sectional, two-chamber view of a myocardium of a 25-year-old man who died suddenly from arrhythmogenic right ventricular cardiomyopathy. This specimen demonstrates gross dilatation of the right ventricle with diffuse fatty replacement. (Courtesy of Professor M. J. Davies, St. George's Hospital Medical School, London, UK.)

involves the apical and infundibular regions with sparing of the intraventricular septum and left ventricle (Fig. 25-9). There can be almost transmural replacement of the myocardium by fatty tissue, without any reduction in wall thickness. There is usually an absence of fibrous tissue and inflammatory infiltrates. The fibrofatty pattern is characterized by severe atrophy and scarring of the myocardium, with fibrous and fatty infiltration. The right ventricular wall thickness can be significantly reduced with aneurysmal dilatation. Inflow aneurysms appear to have a particular predilection for the diaphragmatic wall underneath the posterior leaflet of the tricuspid valve, and these are considered to be a diagnostic feature. Inflammatory infiltrates are pre-

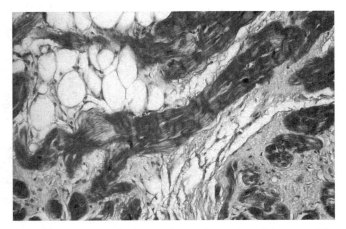

FIGURE 25-9. Histologic specimen from the right ventricle demonstrates replacement of myocytes *(black)* with fatty tissue *(white)* and interstitial fibrosis *(gray)*. (Courtesy of Professor M. J. Davies, St. George's Hospital Medical School, London, UK.)

sent, and the left ventricle can be involved. Electron microscopy of cardiac tissue from ARVC patients shows abnormal intercalated discs in right and left ventricles. The discs are attenuated and flattened with decreased Z band material (216).

The replacement of myocytes with fibrofatty tissue provides the histopathologic substrate for the genesis of ventricular arrhythmias. The disruption of normal cardiac fibers predisposes to fragmentation of ventricular depolarization and reentrant circuits.

Clinical Presentation

ARVC predominantly manifests in adolescents or young adults and appears to affect males more than females (217). Epidemiologic data are limited, but estimates of prevalence vary from 1 case in 10,000 to 1,000 persons (218). In certain geographic areas, such as the Veneto region of Italy, ARVC has been found to be the leading cause of sudden death in the young and in athletes (219). It appears to be a progressive disease with a variable clinical course, even within a single family. There are higher than expected rates of structural, functional, and ECG abnormalities in family members of persons with ARVC, which may be insufficient to fulfill the current diagnostic criteria but may represent early disease.

The information with regard to the natural history of ARVC, even in overt cases, is limited, but four stages of disease progression have been suggested (220). The first is an early "concealed" phase, with or without arrhythmias, during which sudden death may be the first manifestation of the disease (221). This can be followed by an "overt electrical disorder" phase, characterized by symptomatic arrhythmias that may lead to cardiac arrest. The patient may present with a spectrum of ventricular arrhythmias of left bundle branch morphology, suggesting a focus in the right ventricle. Progression of the underlying pathologic process can then lead to "right ventricular failure" with eventual left ventricular involvement leading to "biventricular pump failure." The true underlying diagnosis may be missed in these latter cases, with the patient diagnosed with idiopathic DCM (211).

Diagnosis

Compared with hypertrophic and dilated cardiomyopathies, for which a diagnosis can usually be based on the phenotypic features of the disease, a diagnosis of ARVC can be more difficult to establish. Clinical investigations such as electrocardiography may demonstrate nonspecific abnormalities, and structural and functional assessment of the right ventricle may be difficult. ARVC must be considered in the differential diagnosis when a patient presents with a

TABLE 25-5. CRITERIA FOR THE DIAGNOSIS OF ARRHYTHMOGENIC RIGHT VENTRICULAR CARDIOMYOPATHY DETECTED BY ECHOCARDIOGRAPHY, ANGIOGRAPHY, MAGNETIC RESONANCE IMAGING, OR RADIONUCLIDE SCINTIGRAPHY

1. Family history
   Major
     Familial disease confirmed at necropsy or surgery
   Minor
     Family history of premature sudden death (<35 years) caused by suspected arrhythmogenic right ventricular cardiomyopathy
     Family history (clinical diagnosis based on present criteria)
2. Electrocardiographic depolarization or conduction abnormalities
   Major
     Epsilon waves or localized prolongation (>110 ms) of the QRS complex in the right precordial leads (V_1 through V_3)
   Minor
     Late potentials seen on signal-averaged electrocardiogram
3. Repolarization abnormalities
   Minor
     Inverted T waves in right precordial leads (V_2 and V_3) in people >12 years and in the absence of right bundle branch block
4. Tissue characterization of walls
   Major
     Fibrofatty replacement of myocardium on endomyocardial biopsy
5. Global or regional dysfunction and structural alterations
   Major
     Severe dilatation and reduction of right ventricular ejection fraction with no (or only mild) left ventricular impairment
     Localized right ventricular aneurysms (akinetic or dyskinetic areas with diastolic bulging)
     Severe segmental dilatation of the right ventricle
   Minor
     Mild global right ventricular dilatation and/or ejection fraction reduction with normal left ventricle
     Mild segmental dilatation of the right ventricle
     Regional right ventricular hypokinesia
6. Arrhythmias
   Minor
     Left bundle branch block type ventricular tachycardia (sustained or nonsustained) documented on the electrocardiogram, Holter monitoring, or during exercise testing
     Frequent ventricular extrasystoles (more than 1,000/24 hours) on Holter monitoring

From McKenna WJ, Thiene G, Nava A, et al. Diagnosis of arrhythmogenic right ventricular dysplasia/cardiomyopathy. Task Force of the Working Group Myocardial and Pericardial Disease of the European Society of Cardiology and of the Scientific Council on Cardiomyopathies of the International Society and Federation of Cardiology. *Br Heart J* 1994;71:215–218, with permission.

ventricular arrhythmia of LBBB morphology and what may appear to be a structurally normal heart.

Definitive diagnosis of ARVC requires histologic confirmation of transmural fibrofatty replacement of the right ventricle at postmortem or surgery. This is not feasible in most cases, and a tissue diagnosis cannot always be obtained because of the segmental nature of the disease. A study group has proposed diagnostic criteria based on family history and on structural, functional, and electrocardiographic abnormalities (223) (Table 25-5). This diagnostic framework is being prospectively evaluated, but it is likely that less severe forms of the disease may not be encompassed by these criteria, and a genetic diagnosis can prove invaluable in improving diagnostic accuracy.

The differential diagnosis has to take account of Uhl's anomaly, which also involves the right ventricle and manifests at a younger age, characteristically with heart failure. In contrast to ARVC, histology in the Uhl anomaly is characterized by a complete absence of myocardial cells with apposition of epicardium and endocardium.

Evaluation

Electrocardiogram

The ECG in sinus rhythm demonstrates an abnormality in most long-standing cases but can initially appear normal. In a study of 74 patients with ARVC, 40% had a normal ECG 1-year after presenting with a ventricular arrhythmia (224). This number fell to 8% after 5 years, and no normal ECGs were seen after 6 years, demonstrating the progressive nature of this disease. T-wave inversion in the precordial leads V_1 through V_3 is the most common abnormality seen in at least 50% of cases (225,226), and extension throughout the precordial leads correlates with left ventricular involvement (188). Because these repolarization abnormalities of leads V_2 and V_3 are nonspecific, they are deemed to be minor criteria for the diagnosis of ARVC.

Various abnormalities of depolarization can occur in patients with ARVC. Incomplete right bundle branch block is more frequently observed than a complete block. A more specific finding is prolongation of the QRS complex to more than 110 ms in lead V_1, V_2, or V_3 (227). Epsilon waves occur in up to 30% of selected series and are ventricular postexcitation waves. They appear as small-amplitude potentials after the QRS complex and at the beginning of the ST segment (228). Epsilon waves can present with an atypical appearance, and their identification can be enhanced by the use of high-resolution electrocardiography or by a specific arrangement of the leads (229). These electrocardiographic changes are thought to reflect a parietal block rather than a defect in the conduction tissue of the bundle branches (230). The presence of epsilon waves or QRS prolongation in V_1 through V_3 is considered to be major diagnostic criteria for ARVC.

Signal-Averaged Electrocardiogram

Another minor diagnostic criterion is the presence of late potentials demonstrated by the signal-averaged ECG. They are thought to reflect areas of slow intraventricular conduction. The prevalence of late potentials varies in studies from 47% to 81% (231,232). The presence of late potentials in patients being assessed for ventricular arrhythmias favors an underlying myocardial disorder (231) and has been correlated with subsequent abnormal cardiac biopsy findings (233). An abnormal signal-averaged ECG has also been correlated with increased myocardial fibrosis and a reduction in the right ventricular ejection fraction, with a subsequent increased risk of sustained ventricular arrhythmias (232). However, one study demonstrated a closer relationship between the extent of the disease than with the presence of ventricular arrhythmias. QT dispersion has been shown to be increased in ARVC subjects, but it was not a predictive marker for life-threatening arrhythmias (234).

Echocardiography

Transthoracic echocardiography can be used to assess the structure and function of the right ventricle (235) and for excluding other cardiac disorders that may cause anatomic distortion of the right ventricle with associated arrhythmias. These include Ebstein's anomaly, atrial septal defects, tricuspid and pulmonary valve abnormalities, right ventricular infarction, partial anomalous pulmonary venous return, and congenital absence of the right hemipericardium (236). Structural abnormalities may include bulgings or sacculations in the apical and infero-posterior regions of the right ventricle, localized akinesia or dyskinesia, a prominent moderator band, and trabecular disarray (225,237,238). Formal quantification of right and left ventricular dimensions may reveal an increased ratio, with a right-to-left ventricular end-diastolic diameter greater than 0.5 having an 86% sensitivity, 93% sensitivity, and a negative predictive value of 93% for the diagnosis of ARVC (239). Structural and functional abnormalities in milder forms of the disease may be difficult to detect.

Echocardiography has also been a useful, noninvasive tool for screening asymptomatic relatives of ARVC subjects (240). Transesophageal echocardiography has been shown to be more accurate than transthoracic echocardiography in identifying subtle wall motion abnormalities (241).

Nuclear Ventricular Scintigraphy

Nuclear ventricular scintigraphy can be used to demonstrate ventricular size and contractility. By using ^{123}I–*meta*-iodobenzylguanidine scintigraphy, regional abnormalities of sympathetic myocardial innervation have been demonstrated in ARVC patients (242). Further study has demonstrated a significant reduction of postsynaptic β-adrenergic receptor density (243). It is hypothesized that increased sympathetic activity with abnormal adrenergic stimulation of the myocardium may result from increased noradrenaline concentrations in the synaptic cleft, which may be modulated by physical exertion. This condition may lead to fluctuations of cellular cAMP and protein phosphorylation, which can affect cellular calcium concentrations and a subsequent increase in the dispersion of repolarization. This may result in an increased propensity for arrhythmogenesis, with frequent stimulation of the β-adrenergic receptors leading to downregulation in their density. Consistent with this idea is the efficacy of β blockers as adjunctive therapy in the treatment of ventricular tachyarrhythmias.

Magnetic Resonance Imaging

Magnetic resonance imaging (MRI) is another imaging modality that enables detection of structural and functional abnormalities of the right ventricle. Cine-MRI allows detailed visualization of abnormal contraction patterns (244). MRI also allows tissue characterization, with adipose replacement represented by hyperintense signal on T1-weighted spin echo images (Fig. 25-10).However, the sensitivity of this technique for the diagnosis of ARVC varies from 22% to 100% (245,246). A study comparing patients who underwent MRI and endomyocardial biopsy found the invasive procedure to be more sensitive (89% versus 56%) (247). In most studies, spin echo MRI has a very high specificity for the diagnosis of ARVC. Fibrous tissue does not appear detectable on MRI. Technical problems, patient motion, or cardiac arrhythmias may lead to poor-quality cardiac-gated images during image acquisition. Another difficulty is the large discrepancy between observers in distinguishing adipose replacement from the presence of normal fatty tissue that occurs as part of the normal aging process and in assessing the degree of right ventricular free wall thinning. These aspects of MRI will improve with superior technology, and it is likely that MRI findings will be incorporated into any review of the current diagnostic criteria.

Contrast Ventriculography

Right ventricular angiography is considered by some to be the gold standard technique for the diagnosis of ARVC, and

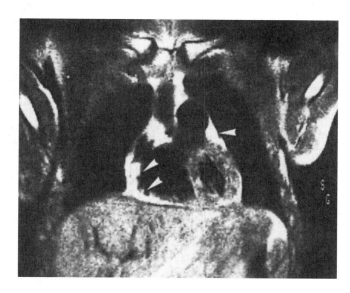

FIGURE 25-10. MR imaging of a case of dysplasia showing a *bright signal* suggesting fatty tissue infiltration. Superior to the left ventricle there is a *bright signal* that represents fat in the AV groove. This is a normal finding. The right ventricle is obviously dilated and demonstrates bright signals *(double arrows)* in the middle of the free wall. Some fatty tissue may be a normal component of the right ventricular free wall but the amount seen here is excessive.

because of the complex anatomy of the right ventricle, it is suggested that specific views be acquired during the study (229). Evidence of akinetic or dyskinetic bulges localized in the triangle of dysplasia have been shown to have a diagnostic specificity of more than 90% (248). However, insufficient information regarding this method of diagnosis and considerable interobserver variability in right ventricular wall motion abnormalities has been reported (249,250).

Endomyocardial Biopsy

Definitive diagnosis of ARVC in a patient undergoing investigations can be provided by transvenous endomyocardial biopsy. This technique has been shown to have a sensitivity of up to 89% (247). The samples are usually taken from the right ventricular septum, an area that is not commonly involved by the disease. The increased risk of perforation and cardiac tamponade precludes the sampling of the right ventricular free wall, which can be thin and atrophic, where the diagnostic yield may be higher. In view of the risk factors, an endomyocardial biopsy is recommended only if the noninvasive tests are inconclusive.

Arrhythmias

Supraventricular Tachyarrhythmias

Supraventricular tachyarrhythmias can be a feature of ARVC. In a series of 72 patients referred for management of ventricular arrhythmias, routine investigations (i.e., 12-lead electrocardiography and Holter monitoring) demonstrated atrial tachyarrhythmias in 24% of patients (251). There was no relationship between the type of ventricular arrhythmia and the presence or absence of supraventricular tachyarrhythmias.

Ventricular Tachyarrhythmias

Ventricular arrhythmias that may occur in ARVC include isolated ventricular premature ectopic beats, sustained monomorphic ventricular tachycardia, and ventricular fibrillation leading to cardiac arrest. During ventricular tachycardia, the QRS morphology is of a LBBB morphology, representing a focus in the right ventricle. Closer inspection of the 12-lead ECG during an episode of ventricular tachycardia may allow more precise anatomic location. The QRS axis is normal or displaced to the right when the tachycardia originates in the pulmonary infundibulum. Extreme left axis deviation represents a focus arising in the diaphragmatic wall or near the right ventricular apex (215).

During long-term follow-up, the various morphologies of ventricular tachycardia observed in a patient represent progression of the disease process. Familial effort-induced polymorphic ventricular tachycardia, linked to chromosome 1q42-43, has been reported in two families with a high number of young persons dying during exercise (252).

Patients presenting with ventricular tachyarrhythmias of a LBBB morphology with what may appear to be a structurally normal myocardium may be misdiagnosed with right ventricular outflow tract (RVOT) tachycardias, which generally have an excellent prognosis. The implications for family members who may then miss out on the potential benefits of screening can be potentially catastrophic. There is no family history of arrhythmias, and the baseline ECG is usually normal in RVOT tachycardias. From a treatment point of view, RVOT tachycardias can be definitively treated with radiofrequency ablation, whereas this treatment modality is not curative in ARVC. To add to the diagnostic confusion, focal structural abnormalities have been identified on MRIs in patients diagnosed with RVOT tachycardias (253). Whether RVOT tachycardias represent a minor form of ARVC is unknown.

Management

The treatment options for ARVC involve pharmacologic intervention for the prevention of arrhythmias and management of heart failure, catheter ablation, ICD, and in selected cases, surgical management. Because there is no standardized treatment algorithm, management is tailored to the individual symptoms. Patients diagnosed with ARVC should be advised to abstain from competitive sporting activity. Screening of first-degree family members should be undertaken with a 12-lead ECG, a signal-averaged ECG, transthoracic echocardiography, and exercise stress testing.

Risk Stratification

There is limited information on the risk factors for sudden arrhythmic death in ARVC. The predictive markers for those most at risk for arrhythmic death have yet to be defined by large, prospective, controlled studies. Retrospective analysis suggests that clinical markers that may be important in risk assessment include a history of syncope (254,255), family history and a young age (256), competitive sporting activity (219,257), diffuse right ventricular dilatation, and with left ventricular involvement (188,258).

Pharmacologic Treatment of Arrhythmias

Initial suggested therapy for patients with hemodynamically stable, non–life-threatening arrhythmias are β blockers and class I and III antiarrhythmic drugs, alone or in combination (259). Less empirical treatment, particularly for those with sustained ventricular tachycardia or ventricular fibrillation, can be derived from serial programmed stimulation (260).

Using such a management strategy, one study found doses of sotalol ranging from 320 to 480 mg/day to be the most efficacious antiarrhythmic therapy using invasive electrophysiologic and noninvasive methods (i.e., Holter monitoring and exercise testing) for evaluation of arrhythmia suppression; sotalol was effective in 68% and 83% of cases, respectively. A lack of response to sotalol predicted a similar response to amiodarone as evaluated by programmed ventricular stimulation. Each of the class I agents was effective in only a minority of the patients. In the group with inducible ventricular tachycardia, verapamil was the next most effective agent (50%) for suppressing arrhythmias, followed by β blockers (29%) and amiodarone (25%). In the group with arrhythmia inducible in baseline, the recurrence rate of nonfatal ventricular tachycardia during a 34-month follow-up period was 10%, with a 12% occurrence after an average of 14 months for the noninducible group. No patients discharged on antiarrhythmic therapy had a sudden cardiac death. However, there are limitations to this study in that the treatment allocation was not randomized or blinded.

Another study reported that combination antiarrhythmic drug therapy was effective in patients who did not respond to monotherapy. Six patients insufficiently treated by class I agents, β blockers, amiodarone or by combinations of class I agents with β blockers or amiodarone were successfully treated with a combination of β blockers and amiodarone (248).

Catheter Ablation

Catheter ablation has had success rates of about 90% in the short term, with no ventricular arrhythmias inducible on electrophysiologic testing 2 weeks after the procedure (261). However, during longer follow-up of 8 to 20 months, one half of the patients with an initially successful ablation demonstrated recurrence of ventricular tachycardia of a different morphology. This most likely represents progression of the underlying disease process and formation of new arrhythmogenic foci. This procedure should be considered in specific situations such as patients with drug-refractory, recurrent ventricular tachycardia and in patients experiencing severe side effects of drug therapy. Patients with focal disease who do not have ventricular tachycardia induced or those in whom pharmacologic therapy fails to suppress arrhythmia can also be considered for ablation.

Implantable Cardioverter-Defibrillator

ICDs are the treatment of choice for patients resuscitated from hemodynamically compromising ventricular tachycardia or ventricular fibrillation. Their benefit in survivors of cardiac arrest in whom the malignant arrhythmias cannot be reproduced during electrophysiologic studies has been demonstrated, although longer-term follow-up results are awaited (261–263). Because the primary arrhythmia in ARVC is ventricular tachycardia, antitachycardia pacing would be the main use on an ICD device. The administration of inappropriate therapy because of supraventricular tachycardias can be reduced by the implantation of a dual-chamber ICD.

As risk stratification in ARVC is further defined, indications for primary prevention of sudden death may evolve to include those with a strong family history of sudden cardiac death and poor tolerance of arrhythmias because of severe impairment of right and left ventricular function.

The potential complications of ICD insertion, which are more specific to ARVC, pertain to its distinct pathology. There is a potential risk of perforating the thin, atrophic, right ventricular free wall during the insertion of a transvenous lead. Pacing thresholds may be found to be higher and R-wave amplitudes lower during the time of device insertion. As the pathologic process progresses, problems with undersensing or pacing exit block may occur.

Surgical Treatment

Surgical management in patients with refractory ventricular tachycardia has involved simple ventriculotomy to interrupt macroreentry circuits (228) or complete disarticulation of the right ventricle, which prevents propagation of the abnormal electrical activity to the left ventricle (264). However, the long-term results of the former procedure have demonstrated a high recurrence rate of ventricular tachycardia, and the latter procedure is associated with adverse hemodynamic effects. A combination of myocardial resection and cryocoagulation has been reported as a safe and effective method when the origin of the recurrent ventricular tachycardia has been well defined on the basis of epicardial mapping (265). Cardiac transplantation may be the final treatment option for those with refractory congestive cardiac failure or cardiac arrhythmias.

Ongoing Challenges

ARVC is being recognized with increasing frequency, but there are many questions that need to be answered. The diagnosis should be considered when presented with a ventricular tachycardia of LBBB morphology or in the case of sudden death in a young person. A positive diagnosis is important for the affected person and may have implications for family members. The pathogenesis of this disease remains unknown. Further work is necessary to prospectively evaluate the current diagnostic criteria and the natural history of the disease in symptomatic probands and asymptomatic relatives who may be subsequently diagnosed. Identification of genetic markers will aid the diagnosis of more subtle cases of disease and provide a gold standard by which the clinical diagnostic criteria can be compared. Risk stratification needs to be defined for identifying those who are most at risk for life-threatening ventricular arrhythmias.

Other issues that should be addressed are the long-term clinical management of symptomatic and asymptomatic subjects. Management issues that need to be clarified include the long-term efficacy of empirical and electrophysiologically guided therapy, the benefit for asymptomatic relatives diagnosed with the disease of commencing prophylactic antiarrhythmic therapy, and the indications for nonpharmacologic therapy. It is hoped that the answers to these questions will be provided by collaboration in establishing an international registry to follow-up patients with this fascinating disease (266).

REFERENCES

1. Richardson P, McKenna W, Bristow M, et al. Report of the 1995 World Health Organization/International Society and Federation of Cardiology Task Force on the definition and classification of cardiomyopathies [Editorial]. *Circulation* 1996;93: 841–842
2. Brock R. Functional obstruction of the left ventricle (acquired aortic subvalvular stenosis). *Guys Hosp Rep* 1957;106:221–238.
3. Teare RD. Asymmetrical hypertrophy of the heart in young adults. *Br Heart J* 1958;20:1–8.
4. Maron BJ, Epstein SE. Hypertrophic cardiomyopathy: a discussion of nomenclature. *Am J Cardiol* 1979;43:1242–1244.
5. Goodwin JF. The frontiers of cardiomyopathy. *Br Heart J* 1982; 48:1–18.
6. Maron BJ, Gardin JM, Flack JM, et al. Prevalence of hypertrophic cardiomyopathy in a general population of young adults: echocardiographic analysis of 4111 subjects in the CARDIA study. Coronary Artery Risk Development in (Young) Adults. *Circulation* 1995;92:785–789.
7. Maron BJ, Bonow RO, Cannon RO, et al. Hypertrophic cardiomyopathy: interrelations of clinical manifestations, pathophysiology, and therapy (1). *N Engl J Med* 1987;316:780–789.
8. Maron BJ, Bonow RO, Cannon RO, et al. Hypertrophic cardiomyopathy: interrelations of clinical manifestations, pathophysiology, and therapy (2). *N Engl J Med* 1987;316:844–852.
9. Maron BJ, Roberts WC, McAllister HA, et al. Sudden death in young athletes. *Circulation* 1980;62:218–229.
10. Steingo L, Dansky R, Pocock WA, Barlow JB. Apical hypertrophic nonobstructive cardiomyopathy. *Am Heart J* 1982;104: 635–637.
11. Seftel HC. Cardiomyopathies in Johannesburg Bantu. *S Afr Med J* 1973;47:321–324.
12. Yamaguchi H, Ishimura T, Nishiyama S, et al. Hypertrophic nonobstructive cardiomyopathy with giant negative T waves (apical hypertrophy): ventriculographic and echocardiographic features in 30 patients. *Am J Cardiol* 1979;44:401–412.
13. Kawai C. Studies on cardiomyopathy in Japan. In: Sekiguchi M, Olsen EGJ, eds. *Clinical, pathological and theoretical aspects of cardiomyopathy.* Tokyo: University of Tokyo Press, 1980:3–10.
14. Braunwald E, Lambrew CT, Rockoff SD, et al. Idiopathic hypertrophic subaortic stenosis. I. A description of the disease based upon an analysis of 64 patients. *Circulation* 1964;29, 30[Suppl IV]:3–213.
15. Redwood CS, Moolman-Smook JC, Watkins H. Properties of mutant contractile proteins that cause hypertrophic cardiomyopathy. *Cardiovasc Res* 1999;44:20–36.
16. Bonne G, Carrier L, Richard P, et al. Familial hypertrophic cardiomyopathy: from mutations to functional defects. *Circ Res* 1998;83:580–593.
17. Davies MJ. The current status of myocardial disarray in hypertrophic cardiomyopathy. *Br Heart J* 1984;51:361–363.
18. McKenna WJ, Goodwin JF. The natural history of hypertrophic cardiomyopathy. *Curr Probl Cardiol* 1981;6:1–26.
19. McKenna W, Deanfield J, Faruqui A, et al. Prognosis in hypertrophic cardiomyopathy: role of age and clinical, electrocardiographic and hemodynamic features. *Am J Cardiol* 1981;47: 532–538.
20. McKenna WJ, Deanfield JE. Hypertrophic cardiomyopathy: an important cause of sudden death. *Arch Dis Child* 1984;59: 971–975.
21. McKenna WJ, Franklin RC, Nihoyannopoulos P, et al. Arrhythmia and prognosis in infants, children and adolescents with hypertrophic cardiomyopathy. *J Am Coll Cardiol* 1988;11: 147–153.
22. McKenna WJ, England D, Doi YL, et al. Arrhythmia in hypertrophic cardiomyopathy. I: Influence on prognosis. *Br Heart J* 1981;46:168–172.
23. Maron BJ, Savage DD, Wolfson JK, Epstein SE. Prognostic significance of 24 hour ambulatory electrocardiographic monitoring in patients with hypertrophic cardiomyopathy: a prospective study. *Am J Cardiol* 1981;48:252–257.
24. Savage DD, Seides SF, Clark CE, et al. Electrocardiographic

findings in patients with obstructive and nonobstructive hypertrophic cardiomyopathy. *Circulation* 1978;58:402–408.

25. Krikler DM, Davies MJ, Rowland E, et al. Sudden death in hypertrophic cardiomyopathy: associated accessory atrioventricular pathways. *Br Heart J* 1980;43:245–251.

26. McKenna WJ, Stewart JT, Nihoyannopoulos P, et al. Hypertrophic cardiomyopathy without hypertrophy: two families with myocardial disarray in the absence of increased myocardial mass. *Br Heart J* 1990;63:287–290.

27. Watkins H, McKenna WJ, Thierfelder L, et al. Mutations in the genes for cardiac troponin T and α-tropomyosin in hypertrophic cardiomyopathy. *N Engl J Med* 1995;332:1058–1064.

28. McKenna WJ, Spirito P, Desnos M, et al. Experience from clinical genetics in hypertrophic cardiomyopathy: proposal for new diagnostic criteria in adult members of affected families. *Heart* 1997;77:130–132.

29. Fananapazir L, Tracy CM, Leon MB, et al. Electrophysiologic abnormalities in patients with hypertrophic cardiomyopathy: a consecutive analysis in 155 patients. *Circulation* 1989;80:1259–1268.

30. Robinson K, Frenneaux MP, Stockins B, et al. Atrial fibrillation in hypertrophic cardiomyopathy: a longitudinal study. *J Am Coll Cardiol* 1990;15:1279.

31. Wigle ED, Sasson Z, Henderson MA, et al. Hypertrophic cardiomyopathy: the importance of the site and extent of hypertrophy. A review. *Prog Cardiovasc Dis* 1985;28:1–83.

32. Ohtani K, Yutani C, Nagata S, et al. High prevalence of atrial fibrosis in patients with dilated cardiomyopathy. *J Am Coll Cardiol* 1995;25:1162–1169.

33. Alfonso F, Frenneaux MP, McKenna WJ. Clinical sustained uniform ventricular tachycardia in hypertrophic cardiomyopathy: association with left ventricular apical aneurysm. *Br Heart J* 1989;61:178–181.

34. Borggrefe M, Schwammenthal E, Block M, Shulte HD. Pre- and postoperative electrophysiological findings in survivors of cardiac arrest and hypertrophic obstructive cardiomyopathy undergoing myectomy. *Circulation* 1993;88[Suppl I]:1120(abst).

35. Savage DD, Seides SF, Maron BJ, et al. Prevalence of arrhythmias during 24-hour electrocardiographic monitoring and exercise testing in patients with obstructive and nonobstructive hypertrophic cardiomyopathy. *Circulation* 1979;59:866–875.

36. Stafford WJ, Trohman RG, Bilsker M, et al. Cardiac arrest in an adolescent with atrial fibrillation and hypertrophic cardiomyopathy. *J Am Coll Cardiol* 1986;7:701–704.

37. Robinson K, Frenneaux MP, Stockins B, et al. Atrial fibrillation in hypertrophic cardiomyopathy: a longitudinal study. *J Am Coll Cardiol* 1990;15:1279–1285.

38. Mark AL, Kioschos JM, Abboud FM, et al. Abnormal vascular responses to exercise in patients with aortic stenosis. *J Clin Invest* 1973;52:1138–1146.

39. Mulrow JP, Healy MJ, McKenna WJ. Variability of ventricular arrhythmias in hypertrophic cardiomyopathy and implications for treatment. *Am J Cardiol* 1986;58:615–618.

40. McKenna WJ. Sudden death in hypertrophic cardiomyopathy: identification of the "high risk" patient. In: Brugada P, Wellens HJJ, eds. *Cardiac arrhythmias: where to go from here?* Mount Kisco, NY: Futura Publishing, 1987:353–365.

41. Monserrat L, Elliott P, Prasad K, et al. Non-sustained ventricular tachycardia and sudden death in hypertrophic cardiomyopathy. *J Am Coll Cardiol* 1998;31:26A.

42. Alfonso F, Frenneaux MP, McKenna WJ. Clinical sustained uniform ventricular tachycardia in hypertrophic cardiomyopathy: association with left ventricular apical aneurysm. *Br Heart J* 1989;61:178–181.

43. Maron BJ, Lipson LC, Roberts WC, et al. "Malignant" hypertrophic cardiomyopathy: identification of a subgroup of families with unusually frequent premature death. *Am J Cardiol* 1978;41:1133–1140.

44. Frenneaux MP, Counihan PJ, Caforio AL, et al. Abnormal blood pressure response during exercise in hypertrophic cardiomyopathy. *Circulation* 1990;82:1995–2002.

45. Counihan PJ, Frenneaux MP, Webb DJ, McKenna WJ. Abnormal vascular responses to supine exercise in hypertrophic cardiomyopathy. *Circulation* 1991;84;686–696.

46. Prasad K, Sneddon JF, Gould M, McKenna WJ. Episodic hypotension during daily activity in hypertrophic cardiomyopathy and propensity to sudden death: utility of continuous ambulatory BP monitoring. *Circulation* 1997;96:I-463(abst).

47. Sadoul N, Prasad K, Elliott PM, et al. Prospective assessment of blood pressure response during exercise in patients with hypertrophic cardiomyopathy. *Circulation* 1997;96:2987–2991.

48. Olivotto J, Maron BJ, Montereggi A, et al. Prognostic value of systemic blood pressure response during exercise in a community-based patient population with hypertrophic cardiomyopathy. *J Am Coll Cardiol* 1999;33;2044–2051.

49. Farrell TG, Paul V, Cripps TR, et al. Baroreflex sensitivity and electrophysiological correlates in patients after acute myocardial infarction. *Circulation* 1991;83:945–952.

50. McKenna WJ, Camm AJ. Sudden death in hypertrophic cardiomyopathy: assessment of patients at high risk [Editorial]. *Circulation* 1989;80:1489–1494.

51. McKenna WJ, Sadoul N, Slade AK, Saumarez RC. The prognostic significance of nonsustained ventricular tachycardia in hypertrophic cardiomyopathy [Editorial]. *Circulation* 1994;90:3115–3117.

52. Dilsizian V, Bonow RO, Epstein SE, Fananapazir L. Myocardial ischemia detected by thallium scintigraphy is frequently related to cardiac arrest and syncope in young patients with hypertrophic cardiomyopathy. *J Am Coll Cardiol* 1993;22:796–804.

53. Spirito P, Bellone P, Harris KM, et al. Magnitude of left ventricular hypertrophy and risk of sudden death in hypertrophic cardiomyopathy. *N Engl J Med* 2000;342:1778–1785.

54. Momiyama Y, Hartikainen J, Nagayoshi H, et al. Exercise-induced T wave alternans as a marker of high risk in patients with hypertrophic cardiomyopathy. *Jpn Circ J* 1997;61:650–656.

55. Atiga WL, Fananapazir L, McAreavey D, et al. Temporal repolarization lability in hypertrophic cardiomyopathy caused by beta-myosin heavy-chain gene mutations. *Circulation* 2000;101:1237–1242.

56. Elliott PM, Poloniecki J, Dickie S, et al. Sudden death in hypertrophic cardiomyopathy: identification of high risk patients. *J Am Coll Cardiol* 2000;36(7):2212–2218 .

57. Elliott PM, Gimeno Blanes JR, Mahon NG, et al. Relation between severity of left ventricular hypertrophy and prognosis in patients with hypertrophic cardiomyopathy. *Lancet* 2001;357:420–424.

58. Kuck KH, Kunze KP, Schluter M, et al. Programmed electrical stimulation in hypertrophic cardiomyopathy: results in patients with and without cardiac arrest or syncope. *Eur Heart J* 1988;9:177–185.

59. Borgreffe M, Podczeck A, Breithardt G. Electrophysiological studies in hypertrophic cardiomyopathy. *Circulation* 1986;74[Suppl II]:1992(abst).

60. Maron BJ, Shen W-K, Link MS, et al. Efficacy of the implantable cardioverter-defibrillator for the prevention of sudden death in hypertrophic cardiomyopathy. *N Engl J Med* 2000;342:365–373.

61. Saumarez RC, Camm AJ, Panagos A, et al. Ventricular fibrillation in hypertrophic cardiomyopathy is associated with increased fractionation of paced right ventricular electrograms. *Circulation* 1992;86:467–474.

62. Saumarez RC, Slade AK, Grace AA, et al. The significance of

paced electrogram fractionation in hypertrophic cardiomyopathy: a prospective study. *Circulation* 1995;91:2762–2768.

63. Harris L, McKenna WJ, Rowland E, et al. Side effects of long-term amiodarone therapy. *Circulation* 1983;67:45–51.

64. McKenna WJ, Harris L, Rowland E, et al. Amiodarone for long-term management of patients with hypertrophic cardiomyopathy. *Am J Cardiol* 1984;54:802–810.

65. Jeanrenaud X, Goy JJ, Kappenberger L. Effects of dual-chamber pacing in hypertrophic obstructive cardiomyopathy. *Lancet* 1992;339:1318–1323.

66. McIntosh CL, Maron BJ. Current operative treatment of obstructive hypertrophic cardiomyopathy. *Circulation* 1988;78:487–495.

67. Seggewiss H, Gleichmann U, Faber L, et al. Percutaneous transluminal septal myocardial ablation in hypertrophic obstructive cardiomyopathy: acute results and 3-month follow-up in 25 patients. *J Am Coll Cardiol* 1998;31:252–258.

68. Elliott PM, Sharma S, Varnava A, et al. Survival after cardiac arrest or sustained ventricular tachycardia in patients with hypertrophic cardiomyopathy. *J Am Coll Cardiol* 1999;33:1596–1601.

69. Cecchi F, Maron BJ, Epstein SE. Long-term outcome of patients with hypertrophic cardiomyopathy successfully resuscitated after cardiac arrest. *J Am Coll Cardiol* 1989;13:1283–1288.

70. Primo J, Geelen P, Brugada J, et al. Hypertrophic cardiomyopathy: role of the implantable cardioverter-defibrillator. *J Am Coll Cardiol* 1998;31:1081–1085.

71. Kron J, Oliver RP, Norsted S, Silka MJ. The automatic implantable cardioverter-defibrillator in young patients. *J Am Coll Cardiol* 1990;16:896–902.

72. McKenna WJ, Oakley CM, Krikler DM, Goodwin JF. Improved survival with amiodarone in patients with hypertrophic cardiomyopathy and ventricular tachycardia. *Br Heart J* 1985;53:412–416.

73. Bonow RO, Rosing DR, Bacharach SL, et al. Effects of verapamil on left ventricular systolic function and diastolic filling in patients with hypertrophic cardiomyopathy. *Circulation* 1981;64:787–796.

74. Epstein SE, Rosing DR. Verapamil: its potential for causing serious complications in patients with hypertrophic cardiomyopathy. *Circulation* 1981;64:437–441.

75. Richardson P, McKenna W, Bristow M, et al. Report of the 1995 WHO/International Society and Federation of Cardiology Task Force on the definition and classification of cardiomyopathies. *Circulation* 1996;93:841–842.

76. Codd MB, Sugrue DD, Gersh BJ, Melton LJ. Epidemiology of idiopathic dilated and hypertrophic cardiomyopathy: a population-based study in Olmsted County, Minnesota, 1975–1984. *Circulation* 1989;80:564–572.

77. Stevenson LW, Fowler MB, Schroeder JS, et al. Poor survival of patients with idiopathic cardiomyopathy considered too well for transplantation. *Am J Med* 1987;83:871–876.

78. Sugrue DD, Rodeheffer RJ, Codd MB, et al. The clinical course of idiopathic dilated cardiomyopathy: a population based study. *Ann Intern Med* 1992;117:117–123.

79. Cohn JN, Rector TS. Prognosis of congestive heart failure and predictors of mortality. *Am J Cardiol* 1988;62:25A–30A.

80. Fuster V, Gersh BJ, Giuliani ER, et al. The natural history of idiopathic dilated cardiomyopathy. *Am J Cardiol* 1981;47:525–531.

80a. Franciosa JA, Wilen M, Ziesche S, et al. Survival in men with severe chronic left ventricular failure due to either coronary heart disease or idiopathic dialated cardiomyopathy. *Am J Cardiol* 1983;51(5):831–836.

81. Olson TM, Michels VV, Thibodeau SN, et al. Actin mutations in dilated cardiomyopathy, a heritable form of heart failure. *Science* 1998;280:750–752.

82. Muntoni F, Cau M, Ganau A, et al. Brief report: deletion of the dystrophin muscle-promoter region associated with X-linked dilated cardiomyopathy. *N Engl J Med* 1993 ;329:921–925.

83. Li D, Tapscroft T, Gonzalez O, et al. Desmin mutation responsible for idiopathic dilated cardiomyopathy. *Circulation* 1999;100:461–464.

84. Fatkin D, MacRae C, Sasaki T, et al. Missense mutations in the rod domain of the Lamin A/C gene as causes of dilated cardiomyopathy and conduction system disease. *N Engl J Med* 1999;341:1715–1724.

85. Rose NR, Neumann DA, Herskowitz A. Coxsackie virus myocarditis. In: Stollerman GH, LaMont JJ, Sipperstein MD, eds. *Advances in internal medicine.* St Louis: Mosby–Year Book, 1992:411–429.

86. Luppi P, Rudert W, Zanone M, et al. Idiopathic dilated cardiomyopathy, a superantigen-driven autoimmune disease. *Circulation* 1998;98:777–785.

87. James TN. Normal and abnormal consequences of apoptosis in the human heart: from postnatal morphogenesis to paroxysmal arrhythmias. *Circulation* 1994;90:556–573.

88. Roberts WC, Siegel RJ, McManus BM. Idiopathic dilated cardiomyopathy: analysis of 152 necropsy patients. *Am J Cardiol* 1987;60:1340–1355.

89. Ohtani K, Yutani C, Nagat S, et al. High prevalence of atrial fibrosis in patients with dilated cardiomyopathy. *J Am Coll Cardiol* 1995;25:1162–1169.

90. Li D, Melnyk P, Feng J, et al. Effects of experimental heart failure on atrial cellular and ionic electrophysiology. *Circulation* 2000;101:2631–2638.

91. Kääb S, Nuss HB, Chiamvimonvat N, et al. Ionic mechanism of action potential prolongation in ventricular myocytes from dogs with pacing-induced heart failure. *Circ Res* 1996;78:262–273.

92. Thuringer D, Deroubaix E, Coulombe A, et al. Ionic basis of the action potential prolongation in ventricular myocytes from Syrian hamsters with dilated cardiomyopathy. *Cardiovasc Res* 1996;31:747–757.

93. Beuckelmann DJ, Nabauer M, Erdmann E. Alterations of K^+ currents in isolated human ventricular myocytes from patients with terminal heart failure. *Circ Res* 1993;73:379–385.

94. O'Rourke B, Kass DA, Tomaselli GF, et al. Mechanisms of altered excitation-contraction coupling in canine tachycardia-induced heart failure, I: experimental studies. *Circ Res* 1999;84:562–570.

95. Miyamoto MI, del Monte F, Schmidt U, et al. Adenoviral gene transfer of SERCA2a improves left-ventricular function in aortic-banded rats in transition to heart failure. *Proc Natl Acad Sci U S A* 2000;97:793–798.

96. Brembilla-Perrot B, Terrier de la Chaise A. Lack of prognostic implications of spontaneously occurring or stimulation induced atrial tachyarrhythmias in patients with dilated cardiomyopathy. *Eur Heart J* 1992;13:473–477.

97. Carson PE, Johnson GR, Dunkman WB, et al. The influence of atrial fibrillation on prognosis in mild to moderate heart failure. *Circulation* 1993;87[Suppl VI]:VI-102–VI-110.

98. Bertil Olsson S, Blomstrom P, Sabel KG, William-Olsson G. Incessant ectopic atrial tachycardia: successful surgical treatment with regression of dilated cardiomyopathy picture. *Am J Cardiol* 1984;53:1465–1466.

99. Grogan M, Smith HC, Gersh BJ, Wood DL. Left ventricular dysfunction due to atrial fibrillation in patients initially believed to have idiopathic dilated cardiomyopathy. *Am J Cardiol* 1992;69:1570–1573.

100. Haissaguerre M, Jais P, Shah D, et al. Spontaneous initiation of atrial fibrillation by ectopic beats originating in the pulmonary veins. *N Engl J Med* 1998;339:659–666.

101. Middlekauff HR, Stevenson WG, Stevenson LW. Prognostic significance of atrial fibrillation in advanced heart failure: a study of 390 patients. *Circulation* 1991;84:40–48.

102. Hofmann T, Meinertz T, Kasper W, et al. Mode of death in idiopathic dilated cardiomyopathy: a multivariate analysis of prognostic determinants. *Am Heart J* 1988;116:1455–1463.

103. DeMaria R, Gavazzi A, Caroli A, et al. Ventricular arrhythmias in dilated cardiomyopathy as an independent prognostic hallmark. *Am J Cardiol* 1992;69:1451–1457.

104. Meinertz T, Hofmann T, Kasper W, et al. Significance of ventricular arrhythmias in idiopathic dilated cardiomyopathy. *Am J Cardiol* 1984;53:902–907.

105. Huang SK, Messer JV, Denes P. Significance of ventricular tachycardia in idiopathic dilated cardiomyopathy: observations in 35 patients. *Am J Cardiol* 1983;51:507–512.

106. Packer M. Lack of relation between ventricular arrhythmias and sudden death in patients with chronic heart failure. *Circulation* 1992;85[Suppl I]:50–56.

107. Blanck Z, Dhala A, Deshpande S, Akhtar M. Bundle Branch reentrant ventricular tachycardia: cumulative experience in 45 patients. *J Cardiovasc Electrophysiol* 1993;4:253–259.

108. Caceres J, Jazayeri M, McKinnie J, et al. Sustained bundle branch reentry as a mechanism of clinical tachycardia. *Circulation* 1989;79:256–270.

109. Tchou P, Blanck Z, McKinnie J, et al. Mechanism of inducible ventricular tachycardia in patients with idiopathic dilated cardiomyopathy. *Circulation* 1983;67:674(abst).

110. Chien WW, Scheinman MW, Cohen TJ, Lesh MD. Importance of recording of the right bundle branch deflection in the diagnosis of His-Purkinje reentrant tachycardia. *Pacing Clin Electrophysiol* 1992;15:1015–1024.

111. Tchou P, Jazayeri M, Denker S, et al. Transcatheter electrical ablation of right bundle branch: a method of treating macroreentrant ventricular tachycardia attributed to bundle branch reentry. *Circulation* 1988;78:246–257.

112. Cohen TJ, Chien WW, Lurie KG, et al. Radiofrequency catheter ablation for treatment of bundle branch reentrant ventricular tachycardia: results and long-term follow-up. *J Am Coll Cardiol* 1991;18:1767–1773.

113. Blanck Z, Deshpande S, Jazayeri M, Akhtar M. Catheter ablation of the left bundle branch for the treatment of sustained bundle branch reentrant ventricular tachycardia. *J Cardiovasc Electrophysiol* 1995;6:40–43.

114. Fyfe DA, Gillette PC, Crawford FJ, Kline CH. Resolution of dilated cardiomyopathy after surgical ablation of ventricular tachycardia in a child. *J Am Coll Cardiol* 1987;9:231–234.

115. Chugh SS, Shen WK, Luria DM, Smith HC. First evidence of premature ventricular complex-induced cardiomyopathy: a potentially reversible cause of heart failure. *J Cardiovasc Electrophysiol* 2000;11:328–329.

116. Diaz RA, Obasohan A, Oakley CM. Prediction of outcome in dilated cardiomyopathy. *Br Heart J* 1987;58:393–399.

117. Schwarz F, Mall G, Zebe H, et al. Determinants of survival in patients with congestive cardiomyopathy: quantitative morphologic findings and left ventricular hemodynamics. *Circulation* 1984;70:923–928.

118. MERIT-CHF Study Group. Effect of metoprolol CR/XL in chronic heart failure: Metoprolol CR/XL Randomized Intervention Trial in Congestive Heart Failure. *Lancet* 1999;353:2001–2007.

119. Singh SN, Fletcher RD, Gross Fisher S, et al. Amiodarone in patients with congestive heart failure and asymptomatic ventricular arrhythmia. *N Engl J Med* 1995;333:77–82.

120. Alla F, Briancon S, Juilliere Y, et al, for the EPICAL investigators. Differential clinical prognostic classifications in dilated and ischemic advanced heart failure: the EPICAL study. *Am Heart J* 2000;139:895–904.

121. Fruwald FM, Eber B, Schumacher M, et al. Syncope in dilated cardiomyopathy is a predictor of sudden cardiac death. *Cardiology* 1996;87:177–180.

122. Middlekauf HR, Stevenson WG, Stevenson LW, Saxon LA. Syncope in advanced heart failure: high risk of sudden death regardless of origin of syncope. *J Am Coll Cardiol* 1993;21:110–116.

123. Schoeller R, Andresen D, Bittner P, et al. First- or second-degree atrioventricular block as a risk factor in idiopathic dilated cardiomyopathy. *Am J Cardiol* 1993;71:720–726.

124. Gotappy V, Krellis S, Fei L, et al. The resting electrocardiogram provides a sensitive and inexpensive marker of prognosis in patients with chronic congestive heart failure. *J Am Coll Cardiol* 1999;33:145A.

125. Meinertz T, Treese N, Kasper W, et al. Determinants of prognosis in idiopathic dilated cardiomyopathy as determined by programmed ventricular stimulation. *Am J Cardiol* 1985;56:337–341.

126. Stamato NJ, O'Connell JB, Murdock DK, et al. The response of patients with complex ventricular arrhythmias secondary to dilated cardiomyopathy to programmed electrical stimulation. *Am Heart J* 1986;112:205–508.

127. Poll DS, Marchlinski FE, Buxton AE, Josephson ME. Usefulness of programmed electrical stimulation in idiopathic dilated cardiomyopathy. *Am J Cardiol* 1986;58:992–997.

128. Das SK, Morady F, DiCarlo L, et al. Prognostic usefulness of programmed ventricular stimulation in idiopathic dilated cardiomyopathy without symptomatic ventricular arrhythmias. *Am J Cardiol* 1986;58:998–1000.

129. Gossinger HD, Jung M, Wagner L, et al. Prognostic role of inducible ventricular tachycardia in patients with dilated cardiomyopathy and asymptomatic nonsustained ventricular tachycardia. *Int J Cardiol* 1990;29:215–220.

130. Brembilla-Perrot B, Donetti J, Terrier de la Chaise A, et al. Diagnostic value of ventricular stimulation in patients with idiopathic dilated cardiomyopathy. *Am Heart J* 1991;121:1124–1131.

131. Kadish A, Schmaltz S, Calkins H, Morady F. Management of nonsustained ventricular tachycardia guided by electrophysiologic testing. *Pacing Clin Electrophysiol* 1993;16:1037–1050.

132. Turrito G, Ahuaja RK, Caref EB, El-Sherif N. Risk stratification for arrhythmic events in patients with nonischemic dilated cardiomyopathy and nonsustained ventricular tachycardia: role of programmed ventricular stimulation and the signal averaged electrocardiogram. *J Am Coll Cardiol* 1994;24:1523–1528.

133. Grimm W, Hoffmann J, Menz V, et al. Programmed ventricular stimulation for arrhythmia risk prediction in patients with idiopathic dilated cardiomyopathy and nonsustained ventricular tachycardia. *J Am Coll Cardiol* 1998;739–745.

134. Mancini DM, Wong KL, Simson MB. Prognostic value of an abnormal signal averaged electrocardiogram in patients with nonischemic congestive cardiomyopathy. *Circulation* 1993;87:1083–1092.

135. Middlekauff HR, Stevenson WG, Woo MA, et al. Comparison of frequency of late potentials in idiopathic dilated cardiomyopathy and ischemic cardiomyopathy with advanced congestive heart failure and their usefulness in predicting sudden death. *Am J Cardiol* 1990;66:1113–1117.

136. Keeling PJ, Kulakowski P, Yi G, et al. Usefulness of signal-averaged electrocardiograms in idiopathic dilated cardiomyopathy for identifying patients with ventricular arrhythmias. *Am J Cardiol* 1993;72:78–84.

137. Poll DS, Marchlinski FE, Falcone RA, et al. Abnormal signal-averaged electrocardiograms in patients with nonischemic congestive cardiomyopathy: relationship to sustained ventricular tachyarrhythmias. *Circulation* 1985;72:1308–1313.

138. Gonska BD, Bethge KP, Figulla HR, Kreuzer H. Occurrence and clinical significance of endocardial late potentials and fractionations in idiopathic dilated cardiomyopathy. *Br Heart J* 1988;59:39–46.

139. Hoffmann J, Grimm W, Menz V, et al. Heart rate variability

and major arrhythmic events in patients with idiopathic dilated cardiomyopathy. *Pacing Clin Electrophysiol* 1996;19[Suppl II]:1841–1844.

140. Nolan J, Batin PD, Andrews R, et al. Prospective study of heart rate variability and mortality in chronic heart failure: results of the United Kingdom Heart Failure Evaluation and Assessment of Risk Trial (UK-Heart). *Circulation* 1998;98:1510–1516.

141. Grimm W, Steder U, Menz V, et al. Clinical significance of increased QT dispersion in the standard 12-lead ECG for arrhythmia prediction in dilated cardiomyopathy. *Pacing Clin Electrophysiol* 1996;19[Suppl II]:1886–1889.

142. Klingenheben T, Cohen RJ, Peetermans JA, Hohnloser SH. Predictive value of T wave alternans in patients with congestive heart failure. *Circulation* 1998;98:I-864(abst).

143. MacMurdy KS, Shorofsky SR, Peters RW, et al. The accuracy of T wave alternans to predict the inducibility of ventricular tachycardia in patients with ischemic cardiomyopathy. *Circulation* 1998;98:I-648 (abst).

144. Adachi K, Ohnishi Y, Shima T, et al. Determinant of microvolt-level T-wave alternans in patients with dilated cardiomyopathy. *J Am Coll Cardiol* 1999;34:374–380.

145. The U.S. Carvedilol Heart Failure Study Group. The effect of carvedilol on morbidity and mortality in patients with chronic heart failure. *N Engl J Med* 1996;334:1349–1355.

146. CIBIS II Investigators and Committees. The Cardiac Insufficiency Bisoprolol Study II (CIBIS-II): a randomized trial. *Lancet* 1999;353:9–13.

147. MERIT-CHF Study Group. Effect of metoprolol CR/XL in chronic heart failure: Metoprolol CR/XL Randomized Intervention Trial in Congestive Heart Failure. *Lancet* 1999;353:2001–2007.

148. Echt DS, Liebson PR, Mitchell LB, et al. Mortality and morbidity in patients receiving encainide, flecainide, or placebo. The Cardiac Arrhythmia Suppression Trial. *N Engl J Med* 1991;324:781–788.

149. Coplen SE, Antman FE, Berlin JA, et al. Efficacy and safety of quinidine therapy for maintenance of sinus rhythm after cardioversion: a meta-analysis of randomized control trials. *Circulation* 1990;82:1106–1116.

150. Flaker GC, Blackshear JL, McBride R, et al. Antiarrhythmic drug therapy and mortality in atrial fibrillation. *J Am Coll Cardiol* 1992;20:527–532.

151. Pratt CM, Eaton T, Francis M, et al. The inverse relationship between baseline left ventricular ejection fraction and outcome of antiarrhythmic therapy: a dangerous imbalance in the risk-benefit ratio. *Am Heart J* 1989;118:433–440.

152. Chakko CS, Gheorghiade M. Ventricular arrhythmias in severe heart failure: incidence, significance, and effectiveness of antiarrhythmic therapy. *Am Heart J* 1985;109:497–504.

153. Middlekauf HR, Stevenson WG, Stevenson LW, Saxon LA. Antiarrhythmic drug therapy in 367 heart failure patients: class I drugs but not amiodarone are associated with increased sudden death risk. *J Am Coll Cardiol* 1991;17:92A(abst).

154. Buxton AE, Lee KL, Fisher JD, et al. A randomized study of the prevention of sudden death in patients with coronary artery disease. Multicenter Unsustained Tachycardia Trial Investigators. *N Engl J Med* 1999;341:1882–1890.

155. Morganroth J. Risk factors for the development of proarrhythmic events. *Am J Cardiol* 1987;59:32E–37E.

156. Podrid PJ, Lampert S, Graboys TB, et al. Aggravation of arrhythmia by antiarrhythmic drugs: incidence and predictors. *Am J Cardiol* 1987;59:38E–44E.

157. Torp-Pedersen C, Moller M, Bloch-Thomsen PE, et al. Dofetilide in patients with congestive heart failure and left ventricular dysfunction. Danish Investigations of Arrhythmia and Mortality on Dofetilide Study Group. *N Engl J Med* 1999;341:857–65.

158. Singh SN, Fletcher RD, Gross Fisher S, et al. Amiodarone in patients with congestive heart failure and asymptomatic ventricular arrhythmia. *N Engl J Med* 1995;333:77–82.

159. The GESICA Study Group. Grupo de estudio de la sobrevida en la insuficencia cardiaca en Argentina. *Lancet* 1994;344:493–498.

160. Kottkamp H, Hindricks G, Chen X, et al. Radiofrequency catheter ablation of sustained ventricular tachycardia in idiopathic dilated cardiomyopathy. *Circulation* 1995;92:1159–1168.

161. Cohn JN, Archibald DG, Ziesche S, et al. Effect of vasodilator therapy on mortality in patients with congestive heart failure: results of a Veterans' Administration cooperative study. *N Engl J Med* 1986;314:1547–1552.

162. Fletcher R, Cintron G, Johnson G, Cohn JN. Enalapril decreases ventricular tachycardia in heart failure: V-HeFT II. *Circulation* 1991;84:II-310(abst).

163. Fonarow G, Chelimsky-Fallick C, Stevenson LW, et al. Impact of vasodilator regimen on sudden death in advanced heart failure: a randomized trial of angiotensin-converting-enzyme inhibition and direct vasodilatation. *J Am Coll Cardiol* 1991;17:92A(abst).

164. The CONSENSUS Trial Study Group. Effects of enalapril on mortality in severe congestive heart failure: results of the Cooperative North Scandinavian Enalapril Survival Study (CONSENSUS). *N Engl J Med* 1987;316:1429–1435.

165. The SOLVD Investigators. Effect of enalapril on survival in patients with reduced left ventricular ejection fractions and congestive heart failure. *N Engl J Med* 1991;325:293–302.

166. Pitt B, Segal R, Martinez FA, et al, for The ELITE Investigators Randomised trial of losartan versus captopril in patients over 65 with heart failure (Evaluation of Losartan in the Elderly Study, ELITE). *Lancet* 1997;349:747–752.

167. Pitt B, Poole-Wilson PA, Segal R, et al. Effect of losartan compared with captopril on mortality in patients with symptomatic heart failure: randomised trial—the Losartan Heart Failure Survival Study ELITE II. *Lancet* 2000;355:1582–1587.

168. Luu M, Stevenson WG, Stevenson LW, et al. Diverse mechanisms of unexpected cardiac arrest in advanced heart failure. *Circulation* 1989;80:1675–1680.

169. Nishimura R, Holmes DR. Mechanism of hemodynamic improvement by dual chamber pacing for severe left ventricular dysfunction: an acute Doppler and catheterization hemodynamic study. *J Am Coll Cardiol* 1995;25:281–288.

170. Auricchio A, Salo RW. Acute hemodynamic improvement by pacing in patients with severe congestive heart failure. *Pacing Clin Electrophysiol* 1997;20[Suppl I]:313–324.

171. Rossi R, Muia N, Turco V, et al. Short Atrioventricular delay reduces the degree of mitral regurgitation in patients with a sequential dual chamber pacemaker. *Am J Cardiol* 1997;80:901–905.

172. Vardas PE, Simantirakis EN, Parthenakis FI, et al. AAIR versus DDDR pacing in patients with impaired sinus node chronotropy: an echocardiographic and cardiopulmonary study. *Pacing Clin Electrophysiol* 1997;20:1762–1768.

173. Askenazi J, Alexander JH, Koenigsberg DI, et al. Alteration of left ventricular performance by left bundle branch block simulated with atrioventricular sequential pacing. *Am J Cardiol* 1984;53:99–104.

174. Kass DA, Chen CH, Curry C, et al. Improved left ventricular mechanics from acute VDD pacing in patients with dilated cardiomyopathy and ventricular conduction delay. *Circulation* 1999;99:1567–1573.

175. Daubert J, Ritter P, Le Breton H, et al. Permanent left ventricular pacing with transvenous leads placed in the coronary sinus. *Pacing Clin Electrophysiol* 1998;21[Suppl II]:239–245.

176. Gras D, Mabo P, Tang T, et al. Multisite pacing as a supplemental treatment of congestive heart failure: preliminary results of the Medtronic Inc. InSync Study. *Pacing Clin Electrophysiol* 1998;21[Pt 2]:2249–2255.

177. Auricchio A, Stellbrink C, Sack S, et al. The Pacing Therapies for Congestive Heart Failure (PATH-CHF) study: rationale, design, and end points of a prospective randomized multicenter study. *Am J Cardiol* 1999;83:130D–135D.

178. Zipes DP, Wyse DG, Friedman PL, et al, on behalf of the AVID investigators. A comparison of antiarrhythmic drug therapy with implantable defibrillators in patients resuscitated from near-fatal ventricular arrhythmias. *N Engl J Med* 1997;337:1576–1583.

179. Kuck KH, Cappato R, Siebels J, Ruppel R, for the CASH Investigators. Randomized comparison of antiarrhythmic drug therapy with implantable defibrillators in patients resuscitated from cardiac arrest. The Cardiac Arrest Study Hamburg (CASH). *Circulation* 2000;102:748–754.

180. Connolly SJ, Gent M, Roberts RS, et al. Canadian implantable defibrillator study (CIDS): a randomized trial of the implantable cardioverter defibrillator against amiodarone. *Circulation* 2000;101:1297–1302.

181. Steinberg JS, Ehlert FA, Cannon DS, et al. Dilated cardiomyopathy versus coronary artery disease in patients with VT/VF: differences in presentation and outcome in the antiarrhythmics versus implantable defibrillators (AVID) registry. *Circulation* 1997;96:I-715A.

182. Domanski MJ, Saksena S, Epstein AE, et al. Relative effectiveness of the implantable cardioverter-defibrillator and antiarrhythmic drugs in patients with varying degrees of left ventricular dysfunction who have survived malignant ventricular arrhythmias. *J Am Coll Cardiol* 1999;34:1090–1095.

183. Sheldon R, Connolly S, Krahn A, et al. Identification of patients most likely to benefit from implantable cardioverter-defibrillator therapy: the Canadian Implantable Defibrillator Study. *Circulation* 2000;101:1660–1664.

184. Moss AJ, Hall J, Cannom DS, et al. Improved survival with an implanted defibrillator in patients with coronary disease at high risk for ventricular arrhythmia—Multicenter Automatic defibrillator implantation Trial (MADIT). *N Engl J Med* 1996;335:1933–1940.

185. Kadish A, Quigg R, Schaechter A, et al. Defibrillators in nonischemic cardiomyopathy treatment evaluation. *Pacing Clin Electrophysiol* 2000;23:338–343.

186. Klein H, Auricchio A, Reek S, Geller C. New primary prevention trials of sudden cardiac death in patients with left ventricular dysfunction: SCD-HEFT and MADIT-II [Review]. *Am J Cardiol* 1999;83[Suppl 5B]:91D–97D.

187. Richardson P, McKenna W, Bristow M, et al. Report of the 1995 World Health Organization/International Society and Federation of Cardiology Task Force on the Definition and Classification of cardiomyopathies. *Circulation* 1996;93:841–842.

188. Corrado D, Basso C, Thiene G, et al. Spectrum of clinicopathologic manifestations of arrhythmogenic right ventricular cardiomyopathy/dysplasia: a multicenter study. *J Am Coll Cardiol* 1997;30:1512–1520.

189. Fontaine G, Fontaliran F, Frank R. Arrhythmogenic right ventricular cardiomyopathies: clinical forms and main differential diagnoses. *Circulation* 1998;97:1532–1535.

190. Corrado D, Basso C, Thiene G. Arrhythmogenic right ventricular cardiomyopathy: diagnosis, prognosis, and treatment. *Heart* 2000;83:588–595.

191. Mallat Z, Tedgui A, Fontaliran F, et al. Evidence of apoptosis in arrhythmogenic right ventricular dysplasia. *N Engl J Med* 1996;335:1190–1196.

192. James TN. Normal and abnormal consequences of apoptosis in the human heart: from postnatal morphogenesis to paroxysmal arrhythmias. *Circulation* 1994;90:556–573.

193. Ahn AH, Kunkel LM. The structural and functional diversity of dystrophin. *Nat Genet* 1993;3:283–291.

194. Basso C, Thiene G, Corrado D, et al. Arrhythmogenic right ventricular cardiomyopathy: dysplasia, dystrophy, or myocarditis? *Circulation* 1996;94:983–991.

195. McFalls EO, van Suylen RJ. Myocarditis as a cause of primary right ventricular failure. *Chest* 1993;103:1607–1608.

196. Hofmann R, Trappe HJ, Klein H, Kemnitz J. Chronic (or healed) myocarditis mimicking arrhythmogenic right ventricular dysplasia. *Eur Heart J* 1993;14:717–720.

197. Canciani B, Nava A, Toso V, et al. A casual spontaneous mutation as possible cause of the familial form of arrhythmogenic right ventricular cardiomyopathy (arrhythmogenic right ventricular dysplasia). *Clin Cardiol* 1992;15:217–219.

198. Nava A, Thiene G, Canciani B, et al. Clinical profile of concealed form of arrhythmogenic right ventricular cardiomyopathy presenting with apparently idiopathic ventricular arrhythmias. *Int J Cardiol* 1992;35:195–206.

199. Ruder MA, Winston SA, Davis JC, et al. Arrhythmogenic right ventricular dysplasia in a family. *Am J Cardiol* 1985;56:799–800.

200. Zanardi F, Occari G, Cavazzini L, et al. [Familial arrhythmogenic dysplasia of the right ventricle: observation of 3 cases.] *G Ital Cardiol* 1986;16:4–14.

201. Nakanishi T, Shiroyama T, Inoue D, et al. [A family study of the two cases with arrhythmogenic right ventricular dysplasia with reference to genetic aspects.] *Kokyubyo To Junkan* 1986;34:1009–1014.

202. Laurent M, Descaves C, Biron Y, et al. Familial form of arrhythmogenic right ventricular dysplasia. *Am Heart J* 1987;113:827–829.

203. Rampazzo A, Nava A, Danieli GA, et al. The gene for arrhythmogenic right ventricular cardiomyopathy maps to chromosome 14q23-q24. *Hum Mol Genet* 1994;3:959–962.

204. Rampazzo A, Nava A, Erne P, et al. A new locus for arrhythmogenic right ventricular cardiomyopathy (ARVD2) maps to chromosome 1q42-q43. *Hum Mol Genet* 1995;4:2151–2154.

205. Severini GM, Krajinovic M, Pinamonti B, et al. A new locus for arrhythmogenic right ventricular dysplasia on the long arm of chromosome 14. *Genomics* 1996;31:193–200.

206. Rampazzo A, Nava A, Miorin M, et al. ARVD4, a new locus for arrhythmogenic right ventricular cardiomyopathy, maps to chromosome 2 long arm. *Genomics* 1997;45:259–263.

207. Ahmad F, Li D, Karibe A, et al. Localization of a gene responsible for arrhythmogenic right ventricular dysplasia to chromosome 3p23. *Circulation* 1998;98:2791–2795.

208. Li D, Ahmad F, Gardner MJ, et al. The locus of a novel gene responsible for arrhythmogenic right-ventricular dysplasia characterized by early onset and high penetrance maps to chromosome 10p12-p14. *Am J Hum Genet* 2000;66:148–156.

209. Protonotarios N, Tsatsopoulou A, Patsourakos P, et al. Cardiac abnormalities in familial palmoplantar keratosis. *Br Heart J* 1986;56:321–326.

210. Coonar AS, Protonotarios N, Tsatsopoulou A, et al. Gene for arrhythmogenic right ventricular cardiomyopathy with diffuse nonepidermolytic palmoplantar keratoderma and woolly hair (Naxos disease) maps to 17q21. *Circulation* 1998;97:2049–2058.

211. McKoy G, Protonotarios N, Crosby A, et al. Identification of a deletion in plakoglobin in arrhythmogenic right ventricular cardiomyopathy with palmoplantar keratoderma and woolly hair (Naxos disease). *Lancet* 2000;355:2119–2124.

212. Hertig CM, Butz S, Koch S, et al. N-cadherin in adult rat cardiomyocytes in culture. II. Spatio-temporal appearance of proteins involved in cell-cell contact and communication: forma-

tion of two distinct N-cadherin/catenin complexes. *J Cell Sci* 1996;109:11–20.

213. Ruiz P, Brinkmann V, Ledermann B, et al. Targeted mutation of plakoglobin in mice reveals essential functions of desmosomes in the embryonic heart. *J Cell Biol* 1996;135: 215–225.

214. Lobo FV, Heggtveit HA, Butany J, et al. Right ventricular dysplasia: morphological findings in 13 cases. *Can J Cardiol* 1992; 8:261–268.

215. Marcus FI, Fontaine GH, Guiraudon G, et al. Right ventricular dysplasia: a report of 24 adult cases. *Circulation* 1982;65: 384–398.

216. Guiraudon CM. Histological diagnosis of right ventricular dysplasia: a role for electron microscopy? *Eur Heart J* 1989;10 [Suppl D]:95–96.

217. Lascault G, Laplaud O, Frank R. Ventricular tachycardia features in right ventricular dysplasia. *Circulation* 1988;78:300(abst).

218. Fontaine G. Arrhythmogenic right ventricular dysplasia. *Curr Opin Cardiol* 1995;10:16–20.

219. Corrado D, Thiene G, Nava A, et al. Sudden death in young competitive athletes: clinicopathologic correlations in 22 cases. *Am J Med* 1990;89:588–596.

220. Nava A, Rossi L, Thiene G. *Arrhythmogenic right ventricular cardiomyopathy/dysplasia.* New York; Elsevier Science, 1997.

221. Furlanello F, Bertoldi A, Dallago M, et al. Cardiac arrest and sudden death in competitive athletes with arrhythmogenic right ventricular dysplasia. *Pacing Clin Electrophysiol* 1998;21: 331–335.

222. Nemec J, Edwards BS, Osborn MJ, Edwards WD. Arrhythmogenic right ventricular dysplasia masquerading as dilated cardiomyopathy. *Am J Cardiol* 1999;84:237–239, A9.

223. McKenna WJ, Thiene G, Nava A, et al. Diagnosis of arrhythmogenic right ventricular dysplasia/cardiomyopathy. Task Force of the Working Group Myocardial and Pericardial Disease of the European Society of Cardiology and of the Scientific Council on Cardiomyopathies of the International Society and Federation of Cardiology. *Br Heart J* 1994;71:215–218.

224. Abou-Jaoude S, Leclercq JF, Coumel P. Progressive ECG changes in arrhythmogenic right ventricular disease. *Eur Heart J* 1996;17: 1717–1722.

225. Metzger JT, de Chillou C, Cheriex E, et al. Value of the 12-lead electrocardiogram in arrhythmogenic right ventricular dysplasia, and absence of correlation with echocardiographic findings. *Am J Cardiol* 1993;72:964–967.

226. Canu G, Atallah G, Claudel JP, et al. [Prognosis and long-term development of arrhythmogenic dysplasia of the right ventricle.] *Arch Mal Coeur Vaiss* 1993;86:41–48.

227. Fontaine G, Sohal PS, Piot O, et al. Parietal block superimposed on right bundle branch block: a new ECG marker of right ventricular dysplasia. *J Am Coll Cardiol* 1997;29:110A(abst).

228. Fontaine G, Guiraudon G, Frank R, et al. Stimulation studies and epicardial mapping in VT: study of mechanisms and selection for surgery. In: Kulbertus HE, ed. *Re-entrant arrhythmias.* Lancaster, UK: MTP Publishers, 1977:334–350.

229. Fontaine G, Fontaliran F, Hebert JL, et al. Arrhythmogenic right ventricular dysplasia. *Annu Rev Med* 1999;50:17–35.

230. Fontaine G, Frank R, Guiraudon G, et al. [Significance of intraventricular conduction disorders observed in arrhythmogenic right ventricular dysplasia.] *Arch Mal Coeur Vaiss* 1984;77: 872–879.

231. Turrini P, Angelini A, Thiene G, et al. Late potentials and ventricular arrhythmias in arrhythmogenic right ventricular cardiomyopathy. *Am J Cardiol* 1999;83:1214–1219.

232. Blomstrom-Lundqvist C, Hirsch I, Olsson SB, Edvardsson N. Quantitative analysis of the signal-averaged QRS in patients with arrhythmogenic right ventricular dysplasia. *Eur Heart J* 1988;9:301–312.

233. Mehta D, Goldman M, David O, Gomes JA. Value of quantitative measurement of signal-averaged electrocardiographic variables in arrhythmogenic right ventricular dysplasia: correlation with echocardiographic right ventricular cavity dimensions. *J Am Coll Cardiol* 1996;28:713–719.

234. Benn M, Hansen PS, Pedersen AK. QT dispersion in patients with arrhythmogenic right ventricular dysplasia. *Eur Heart J* 1999;20:764–770.

235. Foale R, Nihoyannopoulos P, McKenna W, et al. Echocardiographic measurement of the normal adult right ventricle. *Br Heart J* 1986;56:33–44.

236. Kisslo JA. Two-dimensional echocardiography in arrhythmogenic right ventricular dysplasia. *Eur Heart J* 1989;10[Suppl D]:22–26.

237. Blomstrom-Lundqvist C, Beckman-Suurkula M, Wallentin I, et al. Ventricular dimensions and wall motion assessed by echocardiography in patients with arrhythmogenic right ventricular dysplasia. *Eur Heart J* 1988;9:1291–1302.

238. Pinamonti B, Sinagra G, Salvi A, et al. Left ventricular involvement in right ventricular dysplasia. *Am Heart J* 1992;123: 711–724.

239. Manyari DE, Duff HJ, Kostuk WJ, et al. Usefulness of noninvasive studies for diagnosis of right ventricular dysplasia. *Am J Cardiol* 1986;57:1147–1153.

240. Scognamiglio R, Fasoli G, Nava A, et al. Relevance of subtle echocardiographic findings in the early diagnosis of the concealed form of right ventricular dysplasia. *Eur Heart J* 1989; 10[Suppl D]:27–28.

241. De Piccoli B, Rigo F, Caprioglio F, et al. [The usefulness of transesophageal echocardiography in the diagnosis of arrhythmogenic cardiomyopathy of the right ventricle.] *G Ital Cardiol* 1993;23:247–259.

242. Wichter T, Hindricks G, Lerch H, et al. Regional myocardial sympathetic dysinnervation in arrhythmogenic right ventricular cardiomyopathy: an analysis using I-123-meta-iodobenzylguanidine scintigraphy. *Circulation* 1994;89:667–683.

243. Wichter T, Schafers M, Rhodes CG, et al. Abnormalities of cardiac sympathetic innervation in arrhythmogenic right ventricular cardiomyopathy: quantitative assessment of presynaptic norepinephrine reuptake and postsynaptic beta-adrenergic receptor density with positron emission tomography. *Circulation* 2000; 101:1552–1558.

244. Roul G, Germain P, Coulbois PM, et al. [MRI semeiology of segmental contraction abnormalities in arrhythmogenic dysplasia of the right ventricle.] *J Radiol* 1998;79:541–547.

245. Molinari G, Sardanelli F, Gaita F, et al. Right ventricular dysplasia as a generalized cardiomyopathy? findings on magnetic resonance imaging. *Eur Heart J* 1995;16:1619–1624.

246. Auffermann W, Wichter T, Breithardt G, et al. Arrhythmogenic right ventricular disease: MR imaging vs angiography. *Am J Roentgenol* 1993;161:549–555.

247. Menghetti L, Basso C, Nava A, et al. Spin-echo nuclear magnetic resonance for tissue characterisation in arrhythmogenic right ventricular cardiomyopathy. *Heart* 1996;76:467–470.

248. Daliento L, Rizzoli G, Thiene G, et al. Diagnostic accuracy of right ventriculography in arrhythmogenic right ventricular cardiomyopathy. *Am J Cardiol* 1990;66:741–745.

249. Le Guludec D, Slama MS, Frank R, et al. Evaluation of radionuclide angiography in diagnosis of arrhythmogenic right ventricular cardiomyopathy. *J Am Coll Cardiol* 1995;26:1476–1483.

250. Blomstrom-Lundqvist C, Selin K, Jonsson R, et al. Cardioangiographic findings in patients with arrhythmogenic right ventricular dysplasia. *Br Heart J* 1988;59:556–563.

251. Tonet JL, Castro-Miranda R, Iwa T, et al. Frequency of supraventricular tachyarrhythmias in arrhythmogenic right ventricular dysplasia. *Am J Cardiol* 1991;67:1153.

252. Bauce B, Nava A, Rampazzo A, et al. Familial effort polymor-

phic ventricular arrhythmias in arrhythmogenic right ventricular cardiomyopathy map to chromosome 1q42-43. *Am J Cardiol* 2000;85: 573–579.

253. Carlson MD, White RD, Trohman RG, et al. Right ventricular outflow tract ventricular tachycardia: detection of previously unrecognized anatomic abnormalities using cine magnetic resonance imaging. *J Am Coll Cardiol* 1994;24:720–727.

254. Blomstrom-Lundqvist C, Sabel KG, Olsson SB. A long term follow up of 15 patients with arrhythmogenic right ventricular dysplasia. *Br Heart J* 1987;58:477–488.

255. Marcus FI, Fontaine GH, Frank R, et al. Long-term follow-up in patients with arrhythmogenic right ventricular disease. *Eur Heart J* 1989;10[Suppl D]:68–73.

256. Nava A, Canciani B, Daliento L, et al. Juvenile sudden death and effort ventricular tachycardias in a family with right ventricular cardiomyopathy. *Int J Cardiol* 1988;21:111–126.

257. Thiene G, Nava A, Corrado D, et al. Right ventricular cardiomyopathy and sudden death in young people. *N Engl J Med* 1988;318:129–133.

258. Peters S, Peters H, Thierfelder L. Risk stratification of sudden cardiac death and malignant ventricular arrhythmias in right ventricular dysplasia-cardiomyopathy. *Int J Cardiol* 1999;71: 243–250.

259. Leclercq JF, Coumel P. Characteristics, prognosis and treatment of the ventricular arrhythmias of right ventricular dysplasia. *Eur Heart J* 1989;10[Suppl D]:61–67.

260. Wichter T, Martinez-Rubio A, Kottkamp H, et al. Reproducibility of programmed ventricular stimulation in arrhyth-mogenic right ventricular dysplasia/ cardiomyopathy. *Circulation* 1996;94[Suppl I]: 626(abst).

261. Shoda M, Kasanuki H, Ohnishi S, Umemura J. Recurrence of new ventricular tachycardia after successful catheter ablation in arrhythmogenic right ventricular dysplasia. *Circulation* 1992;86 [Suppl]:580(abst).

262. Breithardt G, Wichter T, Haverkamp W, et al. Implantable cardioverter defibrillator therapy in patients with arrhythmogenic right ventricular cardiomyopathy, long QT syndrome, or no structural heart disease. *Am Heart J* 1994;127: 1151–1158.

263. Link MS, Wang PJ, Haugh CJ, et al. Arrhythmogenic right ventricular dysplasia: clinical results with implantable cardioverter defibrillators. *J Interv Card Electrophysiol* 1997;1:41–48.

264. Guiraudon GM, Klein GJ, Gulamhusein SS, et al. Total disconnection of the right ventricular free wall: surgical treatment of right ventricular tachycardia associated with right ventricular dysplasia. *Circulation* 1983;67:463–470.

265. Misaki T, Watanabe G, Iwa T, et al. Surgical treatment of arrhythmogenic right ventricular dysplasia: long-term outcome. *Ann Thorac Surg* 1994;58:1380–1385.

266. Corrado D, Fontaine G, Marcus FI, et al. Arrhythmogenic right ventricular dysplasia/cardiomyopathy: need for an international registry. Study Group on Arrhythmogenic Right Ventricular Dysplasia/Cardiomyopathy of the Working Groups on Myocardial and Pericardial Disease and Arrhythmias of the European Society of Cardiology and of the Scientific Council on Cardiomyopathies of the World Heart Federation. *Circulation* 2000;101: E101–E106

26

ARRHYTHMIAS IN CONGENITAL HEART DISEASE

RONALD J. KANTER
ARTHUR GARSON

Cardiac rhythm abnormalities related to congenital heart defects may occur in response to hemodynamic influences on chamber dimensions, muscle mass, and the specialized conduction system; result from metabolic effects on myocardial tissue; or be caused by coexisting congenital abnormalities of the specialized conduction system. This chapter reviews the clinical arrhythmias associated with unoperated congenital heart defects, arrhythmias of clinical importance that occur immediately after congenital heart surgery, and arrhythmias that occur long after surgery for congenital heart defects. Management issues are emphasized in the sections regarding postoperative arrhythmias, with emphasis on newer treatment modalities.

ARRHYTHMIAS ASSOCIATED WITH UNOPERATED CONGENITAL HEART DEFECTS

Rhythm abnormalities in children with congenital heart defects before surgical intervention may be directly related to the malformation complex or result from progressive alterations caused by the defects. Table 26-1 summarizes the incidences of arrhythmias in the more common unoperated congenital heart defects.

Atrial Septal Defect

In ostium secundum and sinus venosus atrial septal defects (ASDs), chronic left-to-right shunting results in dilatation of the right atrium and right ventricle. Compared with patients having other types of congenital heart defects,

R. J. Kanter: Department of Cardiac Medicine and Electrophysiology, Division of Pediatrics, Duke University Medical Center, Durham, North Carolina 27710.

A. Garson: Department of Pediatric Cardiology, Division of Pediatrics, Baylor College of Medicine, Houston, Texas 88030.

those with ASDs had longer PR (154 versus 135 ms) and P-wave to atrial (P-A) (52 versus 29 ms) intervals, but atrial to His (A-H) and His to ventricular (H-V) intervals were not significantly different (1). The dilated right atrium in those with ASDs was thought to result in slowed intraatrial conduction. Typically, the electrocardiograms (ECGs) of patients with ASD also show right ventricular hypertrophy, manifested as an RSR' in lead V_1 and an RS in leads I and V_6 (Fig. 26-1).

Clark and Kugler evaluated 15 children (16 months to 18 years old) preoperatively with 24-hour ambulatory ECG monitoring and intracardiac electrophysiologic testing (2). Ten had prolonged corrected sinus node recovery times, and five had evidence of atrioventricular (AV) nodal dysfunction (i.e., prolonged A-H interval or abnormally slow AV nodal Wenckebach periodicity), but only two had ectopic atrial rhythms during ambulatory monitoring. Those having evidence of sinoatrial node dysfunction (SAND) tended to be older and to have a greater pulmonary to systemic flow ratio (Qp/Qs). Clark and colleagues compared the incidence of preoperative SAND in 28 patients with sinus venosus ASDs with the incidence among 68 patients having ostium secundum ASDs (3) and it occurred in 18% of the sinus venosus group and only 4% of the secundum group. Yabek and Jarmakani, in a review of SAND as an entity in children and young adults, identified 30 such individuals, 22 of whom had congenital heart defects (4). Only one was a preoperative case with a secundum ASD. Kyger and associates reported the clinical courses of 109 patients (age range, 1 to 72 years; median age, 14 years) with sinus venosus ASDs (5). Fourteen percent had preoperative arrhythmias, including four who were 10 years of age or younger; three had low atrial rhythms, and one had a junctional rhythm. Tachyarrhythmias were identified only in the older patients (>40 years old). These reports suggest that the subgroup of patients with sinus venosus ASDs may have as an additional predisposing factor for SAND the anatomic location of the defect with respect to the sinoatrial node.

TABLE 26-1. PREOPERATIVE INCIDENCE OF ARRHYTHMIAS IN PATIENTS WITH RELATED CONGENITAL HEART DEFECTS

Heart Defect	Atrial Fibrillation/ Flutter	Paroxysmal Supraventricular Tachycardia	Ventricular Tachycardia	Sudden Death	Sinus Bradycardial/ Junctional Rhythm	Atrioventricular Block
Second-degree and sinus venosus ASD	+–+++[a]				+–++	0–+
Ebstein's anomaly	+–++[a]	++		[b]		
VSD			+	+		
PDA	0–++++[a]					
Tetralogy of Fallot			0–+++[a]			
Aortic valve stenosis				[b]		
l-TGA		++			[b]	
Eisenmenger physiology			++	++		
"Polysplenia"		++			+–++++[a]	++
"Asplenia"	+			[b]		+

+, up to 10% incidence; ++, 10% to 40% incidence; +++, 40% to 60% incidence; ++++, 60% to 90% incidence; ASD, atrial septal defect; l-TGA, levo-transposition of the great arteries; PDA, patent ductus arteriosus; VSD, ventricular septal defect.
[a]Incidence increases with age.
[b]Incidence increases with lesion severity or associated defects.

More data are available on adults having ASDs. Sealy and coworkers reported their findings from 108 patients (3 to 63 years old) with ostium secundum ASDs (6). Thirty-two (29%) had arrhythmias, with an incidence of 8% to 24% in the group of patients 30 years of age and younger, 56% of those 31 to 50 years old, and 67% of those 51 to 63 years old. The predominant arrhythmias were atrial fibrillation and flutter. The researchers found no correlation between pulmonary artery pressure and incidence of arrhythmia, but 38% of those having a Qp/Qs of 3 : 1 or more, compared with only 11% of those with a Qp/Qs of 2 : 1 or less, had arrhythmias. Benedini and colleagues reported preoperative sinus node function in 26 adults (17 to 56 years old) having secundum ASDs (7). Ambulatory ECG monitoring and intracardiac electrophysiologic measurements were used to identify SAND, but all 17 patients who were described as having SAND had only prolonged sinoatrial conduction times or sinus node recovery times. The Holter evaluations

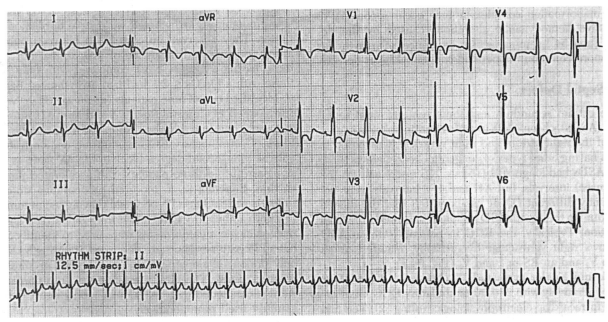

FIGURE 26-1. Electrocardiogram from a 3-year-old child with an ostium secundum atrial septal defect shows normal frontal plane QRS axis and typical rsR′ in V₁ (full standard chest leads; paper speed of 25 mm/sec).

were normal. The investigators concluded that SAND was "concealed" and could manifest postoperatively.

In a large report of 384 patients (16 to 72 years old) by Hamilton and associates, 8% had atrial fibrillation or flutter on routine ECG, 1% had third-degree AV block, 8% had minor conduction abnormalities, and 82% were in sinus rhythm (8). Eighty-eight percent had an incomplete right bundle branch block pattern identified in lead V_1. Although 44% complained of palpitations, only 20% had documented arrhythmias, with only eight patients having atrial fibrillation or flutter. Unlike Sealy's study, this group reported a correlation of atrial fibrillation or flutter with elevated pulmonary arteriolar resistance (Rp). The arrhythmia was present in 22% of those having an Rp $\geq$ 2 Wood units but in only 7% with an Rp $\leq$ 2 Wood units.

The relation of age to incidence of atrial fibrillation or flutter in adults with secundum ASD was investigated in five additional studies. Gatzoulis and coworkers described 213 adult patients with ASDs (9). Forty patients (19%) had preoperative atrial flutter or fibrillation. These patients tended to be older (59 versus 37 years) and to have higher mean pulmonary artery pressures (25 versus 20 mm Hg) than those not having preoperative arrhythmias. Rokseth reported that only 3 (4%) of 84 persons 20 to 40 years old, but 17 (28%) of 61 years of age or older, had atrial fibrillation or flutter (10). Paolillo and colleagues reviewed data from 49 persons 50 to 79 years old (11). Overall, 51% had documented atrial fibrillation or flutter or paroxysmal supraventricular tachycardia; however, among the small subgroup 77 to 79 years old, 80% had established arrhythmias. Forfang and associates in their experience found a similar incidence of atrial arrhythmia in their middle age population (12). Barbosa et al also reports a significant incidence of atrial fibrillation in patients with an ASD and with an atrial septal aneurysm, even if the shunt was small (13). In summary, preoperatively, ASDs are more frequently associated with atrial tachyarrhythmias in older persons, in those having the highest pulmonary blood flow, and perhaps in those with elevated Rp values. Although measurements of sinus node and atrial muscle automaticity or conduction may be abnormal in children, clinically important arrhythmias are uncommon.

Ebstein's Anomaly of the Tricuspid Valve

Ebstein's anomaly of the tricuspid valve is an abnormality in which there was separation of the right atrium from the right ventricle, with downward displacement of the tricuspid valve leaflets into the right ventricle. This configuration produced an "atrialized" portion of the right ventricle, often resulting in significant tricuspid regurgitation. In moderate or severe cases, it is associated with chronic cyanosis, with severe volume overload of both atria, and sometimes with right ventricular outflow tract obstruction. Dysplasia of part of the right ventricle and accessory AV connections are

intrinsic malformations that are variably present. This combination of physiologic and anatomic abnormalities results in a patient group with a high incidence of arrhythmias, even from early childhood. The ECGs of moderately or severely affected patients show marked right atrial enlargement and right ventricular conduction delay (Fig. 26-2).

Kumar and coworkers reviewed the natural history of 55 patients having Ebstein's anomaly (14). During follow-up, 12 patients had paroxysmal supraventricular tachycardia (PSVT), which was recurrent in 7. The Wolff-Parkinson-White (WPW) syndrome affected 5 of the 12 with PSVT and 3 others not having PSVT. Overall, 8 (15%) of 55 had WPW syndrome. Three patients not having WPW syndrome had multiple documented arrhythmias, including PSVT, atrial fibrillation, and nodal rhythm. At long-term follow-up (mean, 10 years), 22 (40%) had died, 2 suddenly. In a large collaborative study reported by Watson (15), data from 505 patients were reviewed; 438 were younger than 25 years of age. In the total group, 28% had reported paroxysmal arrhythmias, and 10% had WPW syndrome. Of 363 who underwent cardiac catheterization, 90 (25%) had arrhythmias during the procedure, including 46 (13%) with PSVT, 11 (3%) with atrial fibrillation or flutter, 10 (3%) with ventricular tachycardia, 23 (6%) with more than one tachyarrhythmia, and 1% each with complete AV block or severe bradycardia. During catheterization, 13 patients (3.6%) died, and 6 additional patients (1.7%) survived after cardiopulmonary resuscitation; all events were related to arrhythmias. Neither the presence of WPW syndrome nor a history of paroxysmal arrhythmias were predictive of arrhythmias or death at cardiac catheterization or of subsequent sudden cardiac death.

In several natural history studies, the incidence of arrhythmia increases with age at presentation (16–18), although in the Celermajer's report of 220 cases of Ebstein's anomaly, arrhythmia was the most common presenting symptom (42%) in the adolescent and adult age groups only (16). Actuarial survival was only 59% at 10 years, but among 58 deaths, only 8 were sudden. Although arrhythmias were the major contributor to morbidity, they rarely were fatal. Oh and colleagues reviewed 52 consecutive patients with Ebstein's anomaly at the Mayo clinic (18). Forty-one patients (79%) had documented arrhythmias (i.e., 18 with PSVT, 10 with atrial flutter or fibrillation, 13 with nonsustained ventricular arrhythmias, and 3 with high-grade AV block or a history of palpitations, syncope, or presyncope). Six patients (12%) had WPW syndrome. Those having proven or presumed arrhythmias were older than those not having symptomatic or proven arrhythmias (21 versus 9 years, $p \leq 0.01$).

Gentles and associates retrospectively analyzed predictors of long-term survival in 48 patients, 10 (21%) of whom had WPW syndrome (19). Seventeen patients presented in the first week of life. Seven (41%) died by 5 months, none of whom had WPW syndrome. Of the 41 older patients, there were 28 long-term survivors (68%) who were followed for a

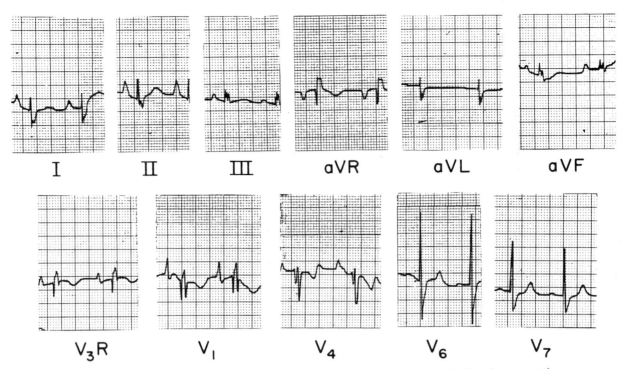

FIGURE 26-2. On the electrocardiogram for an 11-year-old patient with Ebstein's anomaly, notice the large P waves in leads II, V$_1$, and V$_3$ and the relatively low-voltage QRS. There is marked right ventricular conduction delay and first-degree atrioventricular block (full standard chest leads; paper speed of 25 mm/sec). (From Van Mierop LHS, Scheibler GL, Victorica BE. Ebstein's anomaly. In: Adams FH, Emmanouilides GC, eds. *Heart disease in infants, children, and adolescents.* Baltimore: Williams & Wilkins, 1979, with permission.)

mean of 11 years. PSVT was present in 43% of survivors and in 31% of those who had died (p = ns); WPW syndrome was present in 34% of survivors but in none who died (p = 0.05). Atrial fibrillation was not present in any of the survivors, and all who had developed atrial fibrillation were dead within 5 years (p = 0.03). For eight older patients who experienced sudden cardiac death, ventricular fibrillation related to severe cardiomegaly was thought to be the cause.

Most supraventricular tachycardias associated with accessory pathways can be treated nonpharmacologically. However, because of the abnormal anatomy and complex electrophysiology, radiofrequency catheter ablation of supraventricular tachycardia substrates has been especially challenging. Data from 65 Ebstein's patients were analyzed and reported by Reich and coworkers (20). There were 82 nondecremental accessory pathways (i.e., 62% right free wall, 34% right septal, and 4% left sided) and 17 other supraventricular tachycardias (i.e., one atrial ectopic tachycardia, seven AV node reentry tachycardias, five Mahaim fiber–related tachycardias, and four intraatrial reentry tachycardias). Catheter ablation success rates ranged from 75% for those not involving accessory pathways to 89% for septal accessory pathways. The overall recurrence rate was 30%. Smaller patient size and lesser degrees of tricuspid regurgitation predicted better short-term and long-term success rates.

Pulmonary Valve Stenosis

Patients born with valvar pulmonic stenosis develop right ventricular hypertrophy relative to the severity of outflow tract obstruction (Fig. 26-3). Surgical or balloon valvuloplasty may result in pulmonary valve regurgitation with subsequent right ventricular volume overload. In their report of the Second Joint Study on the Natural History of Congenital Heart Defects (NHS-2), Wolfe and colleagues reviewed arrhythmias from 182 patients with pulmonic stenosis (21). Twenty-two percent of those patients had premature supraventricular beats (PSVBs) at a rate exceeding 0.5 per hour (i.e., upper limits of normal).

Ventricular Septal Defect

A ventricular septal defect (VSD) is the most common congenital heart defect. Although defects occur in all portions of the interventricular septum, their effects on the cardiac conduction system and the risk of arrhythmia in unoperated patients probably result mostly from their hemodynamic effects and not their locations. Most moderate or large defects are associated with ECG findings of right and left ventricular hypertrophy and left atrial enlargement. Even when a VSD is an isolated abnormality, associated arrhythmias are common in children and adults. In NHS-

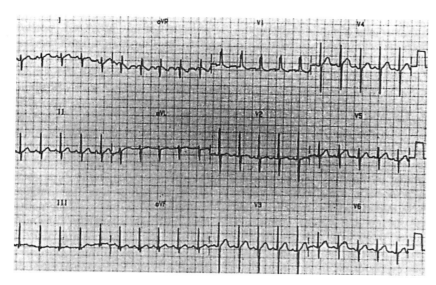

FIGURE 26-3. The electrocardiogram for a 4-year-old girl with moderate pulmonary valve stenosis indicates right axis deviation (QRS axis of 120 degrees) and right ventricular hypertrophy. An R wave in V_1 of less than 20 mm with an R : S ratio greater than 4 : 1 is typical (full standard chest leads; paper speed of 25 mm/sec).

2, Wolfe and associates reviewed 24-hour ECG data from 439 patients having VSDs (21). Among the younger group (<40 years), 58 (15.3%) had more PSVBs than the others, and 22 (10.6%) had more premature ventricular beats (PVBs) than the control population. Ventricular couplets (17.3%) and multiform PVBs (26.3%) were more prevalent than expected among patients younger than 50 years of age, and 5.7% of all patients had at least one episode of ventricular tachycardia ($p < 0.0001$ versus controls). In this group of patients who had not had surgery, the best independent predictors for having serious arrhythmias were the mean pulmonary artery pressure at the time of entry into the NHS-1 and age at the NHS-2.

In a separate study of 109 Norwegian adults 16 to 65 years old (52 were younger than 25 years) having VSD, atrial fibrillation was documented in only one patient with a large defect (22). An additional 37 patients had complaints of "palpitations and atypical chest pain." This experience may have underestimated the incidence of atrial fibrillation, because a later report of 188 young adults (mean age, 29.2 years), all of whom had small VSDs (23), documented age-related symptomatic tachycardias, mostly atrial fibrillation, in 8.5%.

Atrioventricular Septal Defect

In all forms of atrioventricular septal defect (AVSD), there are common abnormalities of the course of the conduction system. As emphasized by Anderson and Ho, the AV node maintains its position between the insertion of the inlet ventricular septum and the atrial septum (24). In an AVSD, this results in posteroinferior displacement of the AV node and left bundle branch (25), a longer than normal penetrating bundle (24), and relative hypoplasia of the anterior portion of the left bundle branch (25). This configuration produces the familiar left axis deviation of the QRS complex with the

superior counterclockwise vector loop in the frontal plane. Chamber enlargement, as reflected on the ECG, depends on the resultant hemodynamics. In most instances of complete AVSDs, the ECG shows biventricular hypertrophy and biatrial enlargement (Fig. 26-4). In patients with an ostium primum ASD or with a complete AVSD but a small VSD, the ECG resembles that from a patient with an ostium secundum ASD plus the QRS axis shift. In older children or adults with unoperated AVSDs, Eisenmenger physiology often has supervened, resulting in marked right ventricular hypertrophy. Fournier and coworkers performed preoperative electrophysiology studies in 18 children (median age, 3 years) with AVSDs and identified first-degree AV block in five because of a prolonged P-A interval in one, prolonged A-H intervals in two, and normal intervals in two, prolonged P-A intervals with normal PR intervals in four, and sinus node dysfunction in one (26). The investigators concluded that electrophysiologic abnormalities were rare preoperatively in patients with AVSDs.

Accessory AV connections and PSVT may be associated with this congenital defect. In our experience, accessory pathways tend to be posteroseptally located.

Patent Ductus Arteriosus

Like the VSD, a patent ductus arteriosus (PDA) that has a persistent left-to-right shunt results in volume loading of the left atrium and the left ventricle. Arrhythmias in general and atrial tachyarrhythmias in particular are most unusual in the infant, child, or teenager with an isolated PDA. Marquis and colleagues (27) reported 37 patients who survived beyond 50 years from among 804 with PDAs who were seen in Edinburgh from 1940 to 1979; 32 had exclusive left-to-right shunts, and 15 of those underwent surgical ligation. Five of the 15 had atrial fibrillation preoperatively, and three of those could be maintained in sinus rhythm

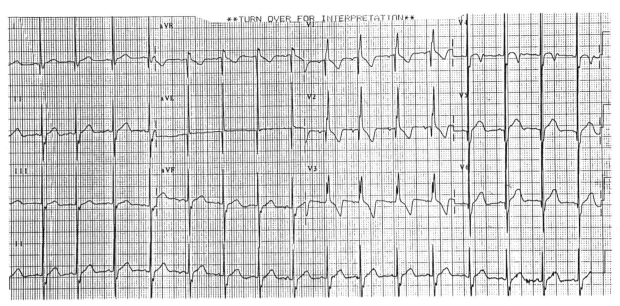

FIGURE 26-4. The electrocardiogram for a 4-month-old child with unoperated complete atrioventricular septal defect shows a left axis deviation (QRS axis of –30 degrees) with a counterclockwise QRS vector loop in frontal plane, biventricular hypertrophy, and left atrial enlargement (full standard chest leads; paper speed of 25 mm/sec).

postoperatively. The investigators observed that atrial fibrillation accompanies congestive heart failure by the fifth or sixth decades of life inexorably among those not undergoing surgical repair. Other arrhythmias are uncommon. These findings were corroborated by McManus' report of 46 adults with PDAs (28). When ECGs were available, 18 of 21 patients were found to have persistent or intermittent atrial fibrillation.

Tetralogy of Fallot

Tetralogy of Fallot is a common cardiac entity in which there is hypoplasia and anterior malalignment of the infundibular septum, infundibular and often valvar pulmonic stenosis, overriding aorta, and perimembranous-to-outlet VSD. The hemodynamic findings in patients preoperatively with tetralogy of Fallot include right ventricular hypertension with associated hypertrophy, normal pulmonary arteriolar resistance, and systemic arterial desaturation with secondary polycythemia. The preoperative ECG usually shows right ventricular hypertrophy and right axis deviation (Fig. 26-5). There is an age-related increase in ventricular arrhythmia in these patients. Deanfield and associates investigated 60 patients (3 months to 63 years old) who had not undergone surgical repair; 20% had significant ventricular ectopy (Lown grade II or higher). (29). Ventricular ectopy was not present in those 8 years old or younger. One of five children 8 to 16 years old had a 5-beat run of ventricular tachycardia, and 58% of those 16 years and older were affected, including four (21%) with 3- to 12-beat runs. Similarly, supraven-

tricular arrhythmias were found in only three children, all of whom were older than 8 years. Only four children of the entire group of 60 were symptomatic.

The incidence of spontaneous ventricular ectopy has also been compared preoperatively and postoperatively in 50 patients with tetralogy of Fallot (30). None of the younger patients (<7 years) had ectopy preoperatively that was greater than Lown grade I, and 44% of 18 patients 30 to 43 years old had a higher assessment than Lown grade II. At a mean of 44 months postoperatively, 29% of the younger group had Lown grade II or III ectopy compared with 33% of the older group. The investigators concluded that the high frequency of ventricular ectopy in patients with tetralogy of Fallot was not attributable to the operation alone but was also related to the preoperative milieu, including age at repair.

Defects Causing Left Ventricular Outflow Tract Obstruction

Congenital heart defects causing left ventricular outflow tract obstruction include subvalvar, valvar, and supravalvar aortic stenosis and coarctation of the aorta. Increased left ventricular wall stress and development of secondary hypertrophy are related to the severity of obstruction. Bush and coworkers performed electrophysiologic evaluations on right atrial tissue obtained at the time of aortic valve surgery from 58 children and adults having valvar aortic stenosis (31). Only 18% of those younger than 20 years but 67% of those older than 40 years of age had postoperative supraventricular arrhythmias. The younger group had equal dis-

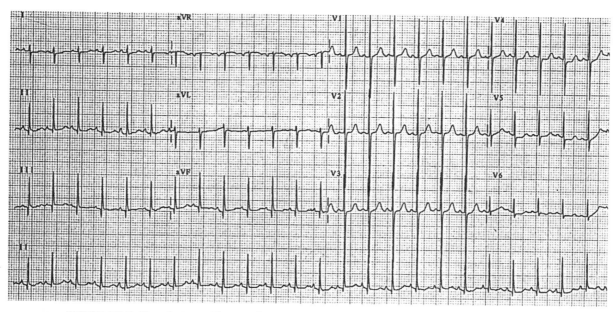

FIGURE 26-5. The electrocardiogram for a 3-month-old infant with unoperated tetralogy of Fallot shows right ventricular hypertrophy with positive T waves in leads V_1 and V_2 (full standard chest leads; paper speed of 25 mm/sec).

tribution of atrial fibrillation or flutter, premature atrial beats, junctional tachycardia (JT), and PSVT, but atrial fibrillation or flutter was the predominant arrhythmia in the older group. Diffuse phase 4 depolarizations and local conduction abnormalities were present in right atrial tissue from the older but not the younger patients. The investigators also found that these abnormalities were not present in the atria of older persons who did not have aortic stenosis, suggesting progressive influence on the electrophysiologic milieu of the right atrium by the long-standing hemodynamic effects of aortic stenosis.

Aortic stenosis in children is only occasionally associated with arrhythmias. Bisset and colleagues found no conduction defects or arrhythmias in 15 children about to undergo aortic valve replacement (32). In a study by Bricker and associates of 2,761 children and young adults who had undergone exercise testing at Baylor University, only 6 patients had developed exercise-related bundle branch block; 2 had subvalvar aortic stenosis, and 1 had valvar aortic stenosis (33). These three patients represented a relatively significant percentage (0.5%) of the total population of patients having aortic stenosis.

Among adults with unoperated aortic stenosis and without coronary artery disease, Klein demonstrated high-grade ventricular ectopy by ambulatory ECG monitoring in 34% of patients, compared with only 6% of controls (34). Von Olshausen and coworkers (35) and Santinga and colleagues (36) confirmed the high incidence of complex ventricular ectopy in patients with aortic stenosis. They further showed that its occurrence correlated with a lower left ventricular ejection fraction, higher wall stress, and no magnitude of

peak systolic ejection gradient across the aortic valve. Possible mechanisms for sudden death of patients with this lesion are paroxysmal ischemic changes, AV dissociation, electrical standstill, ventricular tachycardia, and nonsustained ventricular flutter.

Wolfe and associates reviewed 24-hour ECG monitor data from 134 patients with aortic stenosis as part of the ongoing NHS-2 investigation (21). PSVBs occurred with greater than normal frequency in this patient group than in controls. However, the prevalence of PVBs was not greater than expected.

Conduction abnormalities may complicate native aortic valve infective endocarditis. In a report by DiNubile and coworkers, 9% of 211 patients with infective endocarditis developed conduction abnormalities (37). This was more likely to occur in those having aortic valve disease than in those having other valve involvement, especially if the infection had spread beyond the valve anulus. Increasing severity of the AV block, including isolated bundle branch or hemiblock, first-degree or second-degree AV block with or without bundle branch or hemiblock, or third-degree AV block, was an independent predictor of death. The investigators concluded that valve replacement was indicated in those with bacterial endocarditis in the presence of unstable AV conduction; this was especially the case when the aortic valve was involved.

In patients having unrepaired coarctation of the aorta, there usually is discrete narrowing of the aorta just distal to the takeoff of the left subclavian artery. This results in hypertension of the proximal aorta and left ventricle, manifested as left ventricular hypertrophy on the ECG (Fig. 26-6).

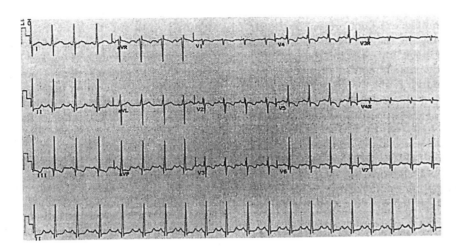

FIGURE 26-6. The electrocardiogram for a 9-month-old child with severe coarctation of the aorta demonstrates left ventricular hypertrophy and "strain" (one-half standard chest leads; paper speed of 25 mm/sec).

Coarctation of the aorta has been reported in a case of congenital AV block (38) and in another with WPW syndrome (39). Two additional cases of sudden death have been reported, one in a 31-year-old patient who had a history of Stokes-Adams attacks occurring over several years and associated with progressive AV block (40) and the other in a 20-year-old patient with recurrent episodes of atrial fibrillation 9 years after surgical repair of coarctation of the aorta (41). Although subarachnoid hemorrhage and ruptured aorta are the most frequently considered causes of sudden death of persons with coarctation of the aorta, both of these patients had marked histologic abnormalities of the AV conduction system identified at postmortem examination.

Sudden death has also been reported for a child with supravalvar aortic stenosis, pulmonary artery stenosis, and hypoplasia of the left anterior descending coronary artery as part of William's syndrome (42). The cause of death was myocardial infarction.

d-Transposition of the Great Arteries

Babies born with d-transposition of the great arteries (d-TGA) have ventriculoarterial discordance, with an anterior aorta arising from the right ventricular outflow tract and a pulmonary artery arising posteriorly from the left ventricle. As long as the right ventricle remains the systemic ventricle (as it must before or after an atrial redirection operation), the ECG maintains a pattern of right ventricular hypertrophy in these patients (Fig. 26-7). Because the normal newborn's right ventricle is already at systemic pressure, the newborn with d-TGA usually has a normal ECG for age.

The high incidence of rhythm disturbances after atrial redirection procedures for simple d-TGA prompted two large investigations enrolling preoperative patients with this malformation. Southall and colleagues reviewed the rhythms from 120 consecutive patients with d-TGA who were admitted over a 6-year period (43); 80% had undergone balloon atrial septostomy, 2.5% had atrial septectomy, and 17.5%

had neither. One of the 120 had first-degree AV block, and a second acquired a first-degree AV block during cardiac catheterization; both had complete AV block postoperatively. Twenty-four-hour ambulatory ECG monitoring was performed preoperatively and postoperatively in 19 children. Preoperatively, there were periods of second-degree and complete sinoatrial block in 10 of the 19; one patient also had premature atrial beats, and six had periods of junctional rhythm. Two other patients had only premature atrial beats at less than 12 per hour, and periods of junctional rhythm were observed in only one additional patient. The lowest heart rate observed was 50 bpm in all but two children. In comparing the results of 134 healthy newborns and 92 healthy juveniles, the investigators concluded that the electrocardiographic patterns in these 19 children were normal.

Martin and associates reported preoperative findings from 92 survivors of the Mustard operation performed in 115 patients over a 10-year period (44). Eighty-three percent of children were in normal sinus rhythm, 12.2% had Lown grade I ventricular ectopy, and there was one child each with frequent premature atrial beats, atrial fibrillation, and Lown grade V ventricular ectopy. The Southall and Martin groups concluded that the preoperative rhythm in children with d-TGA was not different from that of normal children.

l-Transposition of the Great Arteries

In patients with "corrected" transposition of the great arteries (l-TGA or "ventricular inversion"), there is AV and ventriculoarterial discordance, and desaturated systemic venous return therefore enters the pulmonary arteries, and fully saturated pulmonary venous return is directed to the aorta as it should be. The aorta arises from a left-sided right ventricular outflow tract, leftward and anterior to the pulmonary artery. In this condition, the ventricles are said to be l (levo) looped rather than having the normal ventricular d (dextro) looping. Associated congenital heart defects include VSD or pulmonic stenosis in most patients and insufficiency of the tricuspid

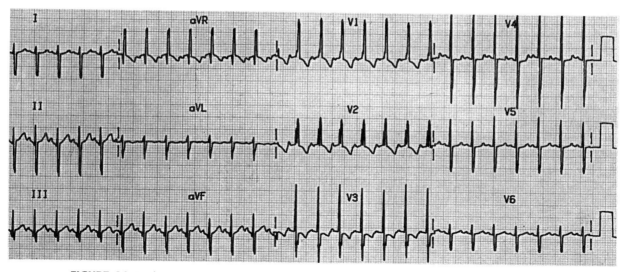

FIGURE 26-7. Electrocardiogram for a 6-month-old infant with d-transposition of the great arteries before a Senning operation. He received a balloon atrial septostomy shortly after birth. Notice the right ventricular hypertrophy and right axis deviation (QRS axis of 180 degrees in the frontal plane). This patient would have undergone an arterial switch operation in the first week of life in the modern surgical era (full standard chest leads; paper speed of 25 mm/sec).

valve, which is the left AV valve that functions as the systemic AV valve, in up to one third of patients (45).

Conduction Abnormalities

The specialized AV conduction system is structurally different, usually giving a QS or qR pattern in V_1 and an rS or RS pattern in V_6 on a standard ECG (Fig. 26-8). The specialized conduction systems in 11 patients with l-TGA were dissected and described by Anderson and coworkers (46). In all cases, the connecting AV node was located anteriorly in the right atrium at the mitral-pulmonary junction, with an anteriorly positioned His bundle that encircled the anterolateral region of the pulmonary valve. The His bundle bifurcated

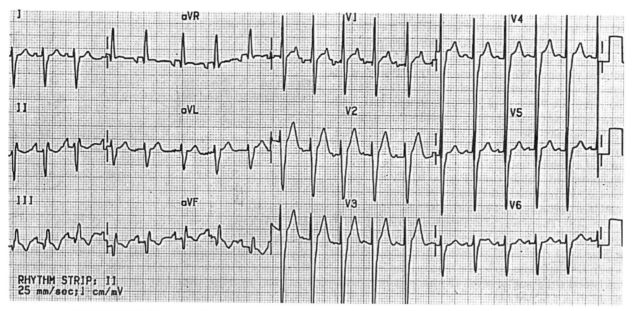

FIGURE 26-8. Electrocardiogram for a 2-year-old child with l-transposition of the great arteries and moderately severe dysplasia of the left-sided tricuspid valve with tricuspid insufficiency. He had already undergone patch closure of a ventricular septal defect. Notice the qR in V_1 and the rS in V_6, representing initial right-to-left ventricular septal activation and right-sided ventricular hypertrophy (full standard chest leads; paper speed of 25 mm/sec).

on the anterior ventricular septum. Of eight cases in which there was a coexisting VSD, the bundle bordered the anterior quadrant of the defect in all. In most cases, a hypoplastic posterior AV node just anterior to the coronary sinus was also present, but only in one did it connect with the ventricular mass through a posterior penetrating bundle. In specimens from older patients, the elongated encircling bundles were infiltrated with fibrous tissue or completely disrupted. Five patients had had ECG evidence of complete AV block, and the investigators postulated that the anterior encircling AV bundle was predisposed to fibrous degeneration because of its increased length and perhaps position. Congenital AV block due to a lack of continuity between the atria and specialized conduction system in patients with l-TGA has also been reported (46).

Further clinical correlation with these pathologic findings is provided in two noteworthy reports. Daliento and colleagues described the rhythm and conduction disturbances in 17 patients with l-TGA and no coexisting defects (47). Two patients had had episodes of palpitations most of their lives, and the remainder were asymptomatic. Ten patients had a normal PR interval, two had first-degree AV block (12%), and five had complete AV block (29%). Complete AV block was present in all five patients at a mean age of 15.8 years and was known to have been preceded by first- or second-degree AV block in two. The escape rhythm was junctional in four and idioventricular in one. The level of block was supra-Hisian in two patients and intra-Hisian in one patient. Lown grade IVa ventricular ectopy on Holter monitoring was present in each of the four patients with AV block, whereas among the 11 patients not having complete AV block, two patients had Lown grade III, and two had Lown grade Ia. One patient with complete AV block died suddenly, many years after developing block, from ventricular tachycardia

that degenerated into ventricular fibrillation. Histologic examination of this woman's conduction system demonstrated fibrosis and disruption of the proximal penetrating bundle. The investigators recommended elective pacemaker placement in patients with l-TGA, complete AV block, and high-grade ventricular ectopy. Of the two patients with palpitations, electrophysiologic studies suggested that one had AV node reentry tachycardia and showed that the other had a retrograde-only left lateral accessory AV connection.

Huhta and associates reviewed the data on 107 patients with l-TGA who were between 2 and 76 years of age at follow-up (45). Coexisting cardiac defects were present in most patients; four (3.7%) had congenital complete AV block, and 19 others developed complete AV block between the ages of 4 months and 52 years (mean, 18.1 years). Twenty-two percent of this patient group had complete AV block. Data analysis showed a risk of developing AV block after diagnosis of approximately 2% per year. The risk was higher for those not having a VSD, and the risk was not increased after VSD closure if intraoperative AV block did not occur. The only death in this series was a 28-year-old patient who died suddenly during exercise 4 years after the onset of AV block. The investigators concluded that prophylactic pacemaker placement was unnecessary in children as long as their heart rates were higher than 50 bpm.

Arrhythmia

Cases of PSVT have been reported in series of young patients having l-TGA (47,48), although the incidence is not established. Most cases are AV reentry tachycardia, using an accessory AV connection associated with the tricuspid valve; when the patient has situs solitus, the pathway usually is in the left free wall or septum, and multiple path-

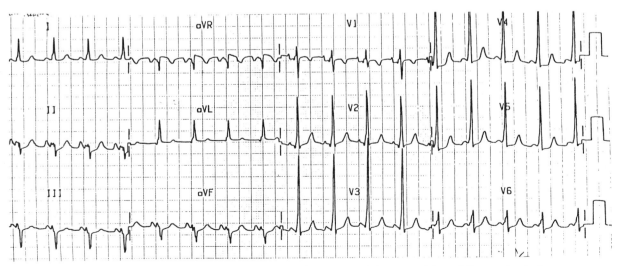

FIGURE 26-9. Electrocardiogram for an 11-year-old girl with l-transposition of the great arteries and mild pulmonic stenosis. She also had Wolff-Parkinson-White syndrome and recurrent episodes of paroxysmal supraventricular tachycardia.

ways may exist (48) (Fig. 26-9). Because of the high prevalence of tricuspid valve abnormalities in this condition, tricuspid regurgitation may be associated with atrial tachyarrhythmias or may necessitate valve replacement. The risk of postoperative complete AV block is substantial in this subgroup of patients.

Symptomatic ventricular tachycardia has been reported in unoperated older patients having l-TGA (49,50), and atrial tachycardias seem to be ubiquitous in these patients, starting in the fifth decade (50). In Prieto's report of 40 patients with l-TGA (51), the 20-year survival rates for unoperated patients were 60% for those having and 100% for those not having significant tricuspid regurgitation (i.e., systemic AV valve); not all deaths were arrhythmic, however.

Cardiac Defects Associated with the Heterotaxy Syndromes

The heterotaxy syndromes refer to patterns of malformation thought to occur after failure of lateralization of thoracic and abdominal viscera into situs solitus or situs inversus. They frequently involve the cardiovascular system, often with severe congenital malformations. Although they are usually categorized as right (RAI) or left atrial isomerism (LAI), there is great variability within each group. The cardiac conduction system is usually structurally abnormal, and congenital or acquired AV block is the most important clinical conduction defect.

Electrocardiographic Abnormalities

Histopathologic studies have demonstrated bilateral sinus node–like structures in patients with RAI, each at the superior vena caval–right atrial junction when bilateral cavae are present (52,53). This is consistent with the observed P-wave

axes of 0 to 90 degrees in 64% and 90 to 180 degrees in 34% of serial ECGs obtained for 59 patients with RAI and reported by Wren and coworkers (54). Momma and colleagues reported an inferior P-wave axis in almost all of the 50 patients with RAI they reviewed (55). In that series, the sinus rate remained stable over time in all but two patients. We have observed two P-wave axes at different times in each of two patients with RAI (Fig. 26-10).

In the report by Wren and associates, 67 patients had LAI, and the P-wave axis was 0 to −90 degrees in 8%, −90 to −180 degrees in 41%, 0 to 90 degrees in 37%, and 90 to 180 degrees in 14% of the ECGs reviewed (54). Among 14 patients who had 24-hour ECG monitoring, only four had a stable "sinus" P-wave axis, and almost one third demonstrated subsequent P-wave shifts of 90 degrees or more. Momma and coworkers also reported a dominance of superior P-wave axes in children (mean age, 7.4 years) with LAI, with 70% being −30 to −90 degrees (55). There was a tendency toward atrial rate slowing over time. By age 15 years, two thirds had slow atrial or junctional rhythms. Dickinson and colleagues showed that patients with LAI had sinus node–like tissue, often hypoplastic, occurring in the lateral atrial wall of seven of nine patients but entirely absent in two (53).

Conduction Abnormalities

Complete AV block, congenital or acquired, is common in patients with LAI. In the series by Rand and associates, 15% had AV block at presentation (54), and Garcia and coworkers reported six such patients, four of whom had congenital blocks and all of whom died (56). Case reports also exist for congenital AV block in persons with RAI (52), and cases of unexplained sudden death of patients with "asplenia" (RAI) have been reported (57). We know of one case of acquired

continuous

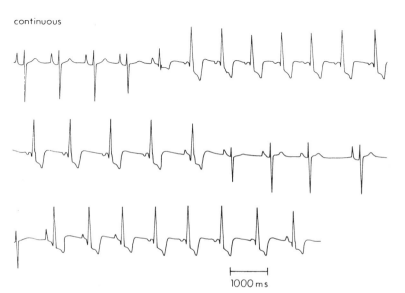

1000 ms

FIGURE 26-10. Rhythm strip from a 16-year-old boy with right atrial isomerism with cardiac defects, including left-sided inferior vena cava, right-sided superior vena cava, total anomalous pulmonary venous return, complete atrioventricular septal defect, ventricular l-looping, hypoplastic morphologically right ventricle, double-outlet right ventricle, and pulmonary valve atresia. Two atrial pacemakers are manifested as two P-wave morphologies. Every P-wave change is followed within two beats by changes in the PR interval and QRS morphology, suggesting two junctional and infrajunctional systems.

complete AV block in a patient with RAI and a single ventricle. However, the incidence appears to be lower among patients with RAI than those with LAI. In the report by Dickenson and colleagues, a detailed analysis of the histopathology of the AV conduction system of 13 patients with LAI or RAI may explain this clinical observation (53). All four patients with RAI had anterior and posterior AV nodes and penetrating bundles. In only one was there discontinuity between the anterior AV node and corresponding bundle. However, of nine with LAI, two had discontinuity between anterior and posterior AV nodes and their bundles. All three patients with LAI, ventricular d-looping, and two ventricles had a normal (single posterior) AV node and continuous His bundle, meaning that among the six patients with LAI and a single ventricle, ventricular l-looping, or both conditions, two had complete AV block. A connecting sling of conduction tissue between the anterior and posterior penetrating bundles was identified in all patients in whom both penetrating bundles existed. Its clinical relevance is unknown. One patient with LAI had an accessory AV connection and WPW syndrome identified on the ECG.

Arrhythmia

Clinically important tachycardias are less common than AV block. When WPW syndrome is present, AV reentry tachycardia may occur. Atrial flutter (54) may be related to atrial stretch from volume loading due to AV valve regurgitation, left atrial enlargement from left-to-right shunting in the presence of a VSD, or chronic changes caused by chronic tissue hypoxemia and polycythemia.

The clinical relevance of all arrhythmias in this group of patients is heightened by the associated hemodynamic abnormalities imposed by the structural defects. Tachycardia suppression and support of unduly slow rate with artificial pacing are of great importance.

Tricuspid Atresia

Tricuspid atresia is a congenital abnormality of alignment in which there is absence of the AV connection to the morphologically right ventricle (58). The ventricular septum maintains its early developmental position; therefore, the AV node is located in the normal location or posterolateral to the blind-ending dimple in the floor of the right atrium. It is related normally to the tendon of Todaro and coronary sinus (24).

Electrocardiographic Abnormalities

The surface ECG demonstrates right atrial enlargement in almost all patients with tricuspid atresia, left axis deviation in about three fourths (59), a short PR interval (<0.10 second) in up to 12% (60), and the WPW syndrome in 0.29% to 0.51% (60,61) (Fig. 26-11). When Zellers and associates

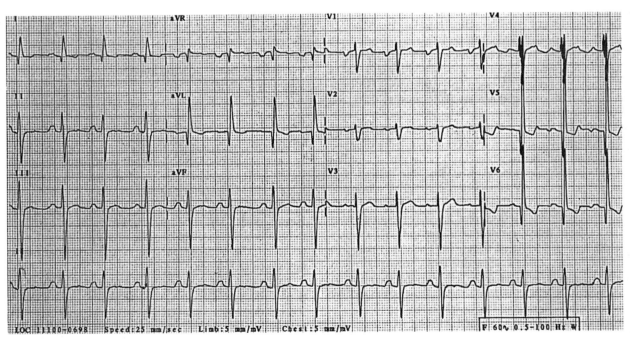

FIGURE 26-11. Electrocardiogram for a 15-year-old adolescent with tricuspid atresia who had undergone Potts' anastomosis (i.e., descending aorta to left pulmonary artery) as a young child. Salient features include biatrial enlargement, left axis deviation with counterclockwise QRS vector loop in the frontal plane (−55 degrees), and left ventricular hypertrophy with "strain" (one-half standard chest leads; paper speed of 25 mm/sec).

systematically evaluated 183 patients with tricuspid atresia, they found that only one of nine fulfilling ECG criteria for WPW syndrome had an accessory pathway; the remainder of the patients had an ECG abnormality called *pseudo-pre-excitation,* in which AV nodal conduction was normal or enhanced. It was postulated that impaired conduction in a portion of the left bundle branch accounted for the slurred QRS upstroke. Of those nine patients, five had had clinical PSVT. Dick and coworkers reported a case of tricuspid atresia and WPW syndrome in a teenager who had recurrent PSVT using a single right posterior accessory pathway (61).

Arrhythmia

Patients with tricuspid atresia appear to be prone to arrhythmias during cardiac catheterization. Dick and colleagues, in a series of 101 patients, found that four suffered arrhythmias during cardiac catheterization: one had asystole, one had fatal ventricular fibrillation, and two developed atrial fibrillation or flutter (60). Three other teenage patients had chronic atrial fibrillation, presumably from volume overloading of the atria by long-standing systemic-to-pulmonary artery shunts.

Hypoplastic Left Heart Syndrome

Hypoplastic left heart syndrome (HLHS) is a group of congenital defects that includes abnormalities ranging from mitral and aortic atresia with no demonstrable left ventricular chamber to a uselessly small left ventricle with mitral or aortic valve hypoplasia. It is the most common form of functional single ventricle and is uniformly lethal without surgical intervention. Before improvements in surgical technique and perioperative management, interest in arrhythmias in these patients was academic. The specialized conduction system in HLHS usually is normal, but there seems to be a higher than expected incidence of coexistent atrial ectopic tachycardia, especially in cases of familial HLHS (62).

Single Ventricle

This section considers other congenital heart defects in which there is only one functional ventricle. This group of complex congenital heart defects usually has abnormalities of the specialized conduction system. It is useful to consider single-ventricle morphologies according to whether there is left ventricular dominance or right ventricular dominance and according to whether there is ventricular d-looping or l-looping. When the ventricle is l-looped, there may be two AV nodes, one posteriorly located and the other along the anterolateral margin of the right AV orifice. All of these considerations influence the course of the conduction system and potential for natural or surgical AV block.

In the case of double-inlet left ventricle, there is connection of the right atrium to the left ventricle, and neither atrium connects with a vestigial right ventricular outlet chamber. This defect complex may exist as d- or l-looping of the ventricle. In either case, the ventricular septum does not extend to the crux but contacts the AV ring anteriorly. The primary ring of conduction tissue forms to the right of the interatrial septum, placing the AV node at the right margin of the inner heart tube, anterior and lateral to the atrial septum to connect to the trabecular septum (24). Besides the difference in location of the penetrating bundle to the persistent bulboventricular foramen (i.e., functional VSD) in l- versus d-looped hearts (24) and in double-inlet left ventricle, its elongated course in l-looped hearts makes it prone to fibrous degeneration and complete AV block, just as in hearts with two ventricles and l-TGA. If, in the case of an l-looped double-inlet left ventricle, there are two AV nodes, the posterior one usually does not make contact with the ventricular septum. Atresia of the right AV orifice may also occur and results in a single anterolateral or posterolateral AV node, similar to that found in classic tricuspid atresia (63).

When there is a dominant right ventricle, the ventricular septum generally contacts the crux of the heart, permitting a normally located AV node to descend into the ventricular septum. In a few patients with double-inlet right ventricle or straddling of the right AV valve plus ventricular l-looping, there may be an additional "sling" of conduction tissue (63). In the presence of ventricular d-looping and a dominant right ventricle, the AV node is normally positioned with respect to atrial landmarks, and the penetrating bundle directly enters the ventricular septum (64).

Eisenmenger Syndrome

Eisenmenger syndrome is irreversible elevation of pulmonary vascular resistance that develops in certain congenital heart defects as a result of pulmonary artery blood flow and pulmonary artery pressure, which are initially increased. With the elevation in pulmonary arteriolar resistance and increased right-sided pressures, patients begin to develop right-to-left shunting, which results in chronic hypoxemia and development of polycythemia and myocardial hypoxia. Despite what should be an excellent substrate for arrhythmias, early reports described only rare cases of primarily supraventricular arrhythmias (65,66). However, sudden unexpected death occurred in 12% to 18% of patients (65,66). Supraventricular tachyarrhythmias were an independent predictor of mortality in a group of 109 affected adults (67).

As part of the group of patients with VSDs in the NHS-2 report (21), Wolfe and associates included 20 patients with Eisenmenger's syndrome. During 24-hour ECG monitoring, 80% had a frequency of PVBs exceeding that of a normal population, 72.2% had ventricular couplets, 88.9% had multiform PVBs, and 20% had more than one ventricular tachycardia episode. The prevalence of ventricular arrhythmia far exceeded that from all other patient groups with VSDs, aortic stenosis, or pulmonic stenosis. However, the relation of these findings to risk of sudden, unexpected death is unproved. We have observed sudden, severe bradycardia at the moment of demise in a few patients. It is possible that a sudden additional rise in pulmonary vascular resistance could have been the cause of sudden death in these patients.

Persistent Left Superior Vena Cava

This hemodynamically benign defect occurs in about 0.5% of the general population and results from persistence of the left anterior cardinal vein. This structure usually courses across the posterolateral wall of the left atrium approximately where the oblique vein of Marshall exists, where it enters the right atrium by way of the great cardiac vein and coronary sinus. It may exist as a discrete defect or may accompany other congenital heart defects. When it accompanies a sinus venosus–type ASD, a low atrial rhythm, also known as a *coronary sinus rhythm* with a superior P-wave axis, may be expected (68). Impaired sinus node function may occur when there is a persistent left and no right superior vena cava. In one report, this combination plus abnormal AV node function was thought to cause fatal bradycardia in two children (69).

If transvenous pacemaker implantation is required because of intrinsic or postsurgical AV conduction system disease, there are special considerations. In patients with a coexisting right superior vena cava, that approach is preferable. Otherwise, a right ventricular lead placed from the left subclavian vein is usually best passed into the coronary sinus, because the innominate vein often is small and may even be lacking. It must then be looped in the right atrium so that it may enter the right ventricle. Prior knowledge of the existence of a left superior vena cava should permit safe and reliable placement of an active fixation system using biplane imaging (Fig. 26-12). Reported complications have included atrial perforation and thrombosis of the coronary sinus (70,71).

Congenital Abnormalities of the Coronary Arteries

Congenital abnormalities of the origin and course of the coronary arteries are rare but disproportionately important defects, because they may be associated with sudden myocardial ischemia, ventricular fibrillation, and death. When the left coronary artery arises from the pulmonary artery, symptoms almost always occur, usually in early infancy, but if collateral coronary blood supply from the right coronary artery is adequate, symptoms may occur as late as adolescence (72).

In another group of defects, the left main coronary artery may arise from the right sinus of Valsalva (73–76), or less frequently, the right may arise from the left sinus (77,78). In either instance, the aberrantly arising coronary artery tends to have a partially intramural course, may have a narrowed origin, and may be prone to compression between the ascending aorta and pulmonary artery during exercise.

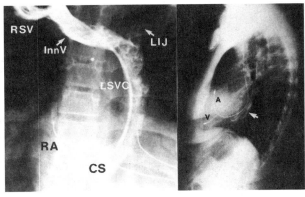

FIGURE 26-12. A: Posteroanterior venogram of a 12-year-old patient having absent right superior vena cava and mirror-image venous return to a left superior vena cava (LSVC) that enters the right atrium (RA) by means of the coronary sinus (CS). His rhythm was low atrial and junctional. **B:** Lateral chest radiograph of an adult with similar anatomy illustrates the posterior and inferior location *(arrowhead)* of atrial (A) and ventricular (V) pacing leads as they enter the right atrium. The ventricular lead must then loop almost 180 degrees before entering the tricuspid valve and right ventricle. (From Van Nooten G, Verbeet T, Deuvaert FE. Atrial perforation by a screw-in electrode via a left superior vena cava. *Am Heart J* 1990;119:1439–1440, with permission.)

Symptoms of exercise-induced syncope preceded sudden death in approximately 50% of affected individuals. In series reporting sudden unexplained death of patients ranging in age from children to middle-aged adults by Waller and coworkers (79), Topaz and Edwards (80), Maron and colleagues (81), and Driscoll and Edwards (82), 5% to 35% of autopsy cases had one of these anomalies. In another autopsy series by Barth and Roberts, 61% of 38 patients having the left main coronary artery arising from the right sinus had died by 20 years of age (76). The risk of arrhythmia and death for all persons having one of these anomalies is unknown, although thought to be high. However, Berdoff and associates demonstrated an incidence of 5.6 cases of anomalous right coronary artery form the left sinus per 1,000 patients, and most had had a benign clinical course (83).

Myocardial overbridging of the left anterior descending coronary artery in association with hypoplasia or absence of the posterior descending coronary artery and septal fibrosis has been found in otherwise healthy teenagers or young adults dying during strenuous exercise (83). Myocardial overbridges have been identified in 0.5% to 2.7% of otherwise normal coronary angiograms (84), making those with associated hypoplasia of coronary arteries a small subset of overbridging or a different disease altogether.

Ventricular Aneurysms and Diverticula and Left Ventricular False Tendons

Congenital ventricular diverticula may be muscular and arise from the apex in association with midline abnormalities in other parts of the body or may be fibrous and arise from the apex or left ventricular base (85). Although these patients most commonly present with congestive heart failure, valvular insufficiency, or embolic events, nonsustained and sustained ventricular tachycardia and sudden death have been reported (85,86). These rare lesions may manifest at any age, and reports of successful abolition of ventricular tachycardia after surgical repair exist (85). Even less common are right ventricular diverticula.

Left ventricular false tendons are chordal strands that connect the ventricular septum to other left ventricular structures. They are present in more than 50% of healthy persons, and there is an unexpectedly high prevalence of coexisting ventricular ectopy (87). Suwa and colleagues reported 40 such patients, 11 of whom had high-grade ventricular ectopy (87). In a separate report, Suwa and coworkers reported surgical correction of paroxysmal sustained ventricular tachycardia in a 31-year-old man by resecting one such false tendon (88). The mechanism for tachycardia was not proved, but the false tendon did contain Purkinje fibers, prompting speculation that postural and other volume changes might have caused traction on this structure with resultant ectopic beats.

Primary Cardiac Tumors in Children

Primary cardiac tumors in infants and children are rare, accounting for only 0.0017% (89), 0.027% (90), and 0.08% (91) of cases in three autopsy series. Tumor types most frequently observed to be associated with cardiac rhythm disturbances are rhabdomyomas, fibromas, histiocytoid tumors, and less commonly, hemangiomas, teratomas, and primary malignant cardiac tumors.

Rhabdomyomas tend to be multiple and usually involve the ventricular septum, but they may occur in the ventricular free wall, papillary muscles, and atrial wall (92). More than two thirds of children with rhabdomyomas present when younger than 2 years of age, and rhabdomyomas therefore are considered true congenital lesions. Although their hemodynamic effects are emphasized in most reports, ventricular tachycardia is common (89,92), and complete AV block (92) and WPW syndrome with PSVT (92,93) have also been reported. We managed a case of tachycardia-induced cardiomyopathy in a patient having atrial ectopic tachycardia originating from an atrial septal rhabdomyoma. The management difficulties of such arrhythmias are highlighted in a report by Case and associates of an infant who died despite tumor cryoablation, pacemaker implantation, and aggressive antiarrhythmic drug therapy (93). This infant had monomorphic ventricular tachycardia, polymorphic ventricular tachycardia, and antidromic reciprocating tachycardia.

A benign cardiac tumor of early infancy is the fibroma. The fibroma tends to be single, occurs most commonly in the left ventricular free wall or ventricular septum, and has

been associated with PSVT, ventricular tachycardia, and sudden death (92).

Incessant and frequently fatal ventricular tachycardia may occur in patients who at autopsy or surgery are found to have single or multiple small, flat, pale, tan-colored lesions variously described as localized histiocytoid cardiomyopathy, Purkinje cell tumors, or myocardial hamartomas. Ferrans and colleagues reported 14 infants with this disease, 2 to 24 months old, 12 of whom were female and all of whom died (94). Although nine infants were thought to have PSVT, it is likely that they had ventricular tachycardia. Garson reported 21 infants with incessant ventricular tachycardia and cardiac tumors, ranging in age from birth to 30 months (mean age, 10.5 months) (95). The clinical presentation was cardiac arrest in 11 and congestive heart failure in six; three patients had coexisting WPW syndrome. Electrophysiologic studies localized the ventricular tachycardia focus to the left ventricle in 17 and the right ventricle in four patients. Because antiarrhythmic drugs failed to eliminate incessant ventricular tachycardia, all patients underwent surgery. Myocardial hamartoma was the diagnosis for 15 patients, and resection, cryoablation, or both procedures successfully eliminated ventricular tachycardia in these 15 patients.

Myxosarcoma, hemangiosarcoma, and malignant teratomas are rare malignant childhood cardiac tumors. They have been associated with right ventricular conduction delay, right bundle branch block, left bundle branch block, short PR interval, and complete AV block (92).

Tachycardia-Induced Cardiomyopathy

Although not a structural congenital heart defect, tachycardia-induced cardiomyopathy often manifests in early childhood and results from an incessant congenital tachyarrhythmia. Some understanding of the pathogenesis of cardiomyopathy and, after termination of pacing, of cardiomyopathy recovery comes from chronically paced animals that serve as a model of this disease. This type of cardiomyopathy is almost always recoverable (96–98) after the heart rate is controlled, emphasizing the importance of an accurate diagnosis and expeditious treatment. The incessant tachyarrhythmias in children that have a congenital basis include congenital JT, the permanent form of junctional reciprocating tachycardia (PJRT), some cases of atrial ectopic tachycardia (AET), and rare cases of ventricular tachycardia such as those associated with a cardiac tumor.

Mechanisms of Cardiomyopathy

Chronic supraventricular and ventricular tachycardias produce left ventricular dilatation (98–100), diminished left ventricular systolic function (98–100), but no left ventricular hypertrophy (98,100). Using a chronically atrially paced pig model, Tomita and coworkers demonstrated systolic and diastolic dysfunction (101). As observed clinically, these animals have reduced left ventricular ejection fractions, elevated left ventricular end-systolic and diastolic volumes, and elevated left ventricular end-diastolic pressures. The investigators also observed increased systolic wall stress, impaired rate of left ventricular relaxation, reduced rate of early diastolic filling, and increased indices of wall stiffness. Four weeks after normalization of heart rhythm, the pigs developed left ventricular hypertrophy, normalized left ventricular wall stress, improved systolic function, and reduced left ventricular end-systolic and diastolic volumes. Their end-diastolic pressures remained elevated with reduced rate of relaxation. These findings are consistent with the clinical observations of reduced left ventricular volume, increased ejection fraction, and improvement in clinical symptoms in humans in whom supraventricular or ventricular tachycardia has been eliminated (97–100, 102).

In a follow-up study, Spinale and associates used the same model and demonstrated reduced myocardial blood flow and reduced myofibrillar content during the tachycardia phase of the study (103). Four weeks after tachycardia resolution, myocardial blood flow normalized at rest, but during cardiovascular stress (i.e., rapid pacing), it was still reduced when compared with control animals. This reduced flow was thought to be caused by persistent elevation of left ventricular pressure and reduced transmural coronary perfusion pressure, exacerbated by rapid pacing.

In animal models of tachycardia-induced cardiomyopathy, histologic changes include reduced mitochondrial density, interstitial fibrosis, and myocyte injury (104). Chronic ventricular tachycardia is associated with elevated catecholamine levels and reduction in myocardial high-energy phosphate levels (98).

The time course of improvement in left ventricular systolic function is related to the duration of the chronic tachycardia; the longer the period of tachycardia, the longer is the required period of recovery.

Congenital Junctional Tachycardia

Congenital JT is an automatic rhythm that manifests in the first 6 months of life. In the review by Villain and colleagues (105), most of the 26 affected babies presented with an average ventricular rate of 230 bpm and congestive heart failure. In three patients, JT may have been present *in utero*. About 50% of these patients had a positive family history of tachycardia.

The surface ECG shows a narrow QRS tachycardia. If there is AV dissociation, the atrial rate is slower than the ventricular rate, and there may be sinus capture beats. Ventriculoatrial conduction may be present, in which case the tachycardia is of the short RP variety and is regular. This rhythm may be transiently overdrive suppressed by rapid atrial or ventricular pacing but cannot be truly interrupted by any pacing maneuvers or by electrical cardioversion.

In Villain's series, the mortality rate was higher than 30%. Initial treatment consists of cardiovascular stabilization, aimed at lowering the ventricular rate. Standard therapy for congestive heart failure is appropriate, including diuretics and digoxin. Exogenous catecholamines may accelerate the rate and should be avoided, if possible. Amiodarone is the safest and most efficacious agent for more immediate treatment (105). Class Ia and Ic antiarrhythmic drugs may reach therapeutic levels more rapidly but do not have as desirable a risk-benefit profile. Ongoing trials of intravenous amiodarone probably will show this route of administration to be the therapy of choice for initial control of JT.

Once stable, chronic therapy with amiodarone is the most effective approach, although successful rhythm control using propafenone, quinidine, and sotalol has also been reported (106–108). Combination drug therapy may be necessary. Sudden death and pathologic abnormalities of the His bundle and AV node have been reported in a few cases of congenital JT (109,110), raising speculation that backup permanent pacing should be mandatory adjunctive therapy.

Selective radiofrequency catheter ablation of the focus of JT with preservation of AV conduction has been reported (111–113). The technique requires identification of the earliest atrial activation during JT, if possible, and targeting that location, usually just superoposterior to the compact AV node.

Atrial Ectopic Tachycardia

AET represents about 10% of all supraventricular tachycardias in children (114). AET may appear at any age, and there may be differences in the natural history of AET according to the age at presentation. It has been our anecdotal experience that AET in neonates may be a self-limited condition in a large proportion of cases (Fig. 26-13). Control of rate and treatment of congestive heart failure by medical means for about 1 year may be sufficient until sinus rhythm supervenes. An unusual variety of incessant atrial tachycardia in neonates known as *chaotic atrial tachycardia*, in which there are a variety of atrial pacemakers, usually converts to AET or "burns itself out"` altogether. Ventricular rate control is frequently sufficient therapy for this tachycardia, although there is anecdotal evidence that propafenone is especially effective in providing complete suppression. AET in older children is more likely to be permanent, although it may be reasonable to attempt rhythm control with drugs for a finite period before going to ablative therapy, even in this group.

AET may emanate from a single focus or multiple foci. The most commonly mapped locations responsible for AET are at the ostia or within the pulmonary veins, especially the upper pulmonary veins; along the crista terminalis onto the eustachian valve and into the coronary sinus; and along the AV valve annuli. However, they may occur anywhere in the atria, including the apex of the triangle of

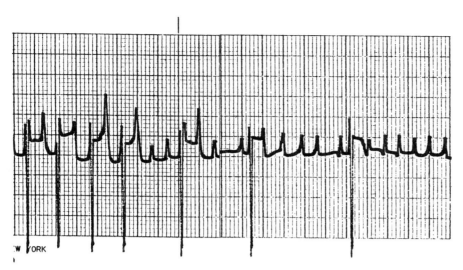

FIGURE 26-13. Electrocardiogram for a newborn with atrial ectopic tachycardia and an atrial rate of almost 500 bpm. An acceptable ventricular rate response was attained with digoxin. The ventricular systolic function remained normal, and the patient converted to sinus rhythm at 2 months of age (full standard chest leads; paper speed of 25 mm/sec).

Koch, into the proximal superior vena cava, and in the atrial appendages.

AET is one mechanism for a long RP tachycardia, and the P-wave morphology suggests the focus location. This may be very difficult to determine from the ECG, especially in the cases of foci located in the interatrial septum and in the presence of multiple foci. The mechanism is most commonly enhanced automaticity, although this is not always the case. The differential diagnosis includes sinus tachycardia, PJRT, and atypical AV node reentry (aAVNRT). If there is an apparent high right atrial focus, the P-wave axis may be normal in the frontal plane, and discrimination from sinus tachycardia secondary to primary dilated cardiomyopathy may be difficult. In AET, the rate is faster, the P-wave axis is more posterior (i.e., negative P-wave in leads V_1 and V_2), and there are more likely to be periods of second-degree AV block (115). If the P-wave morphology suggests a low septal focus, AET must be differentiated from PJRT and from aAVNRT. In AET, maneuvers causing transient AV block (e.g., intravenous adenosine) may permit persistence of the tachycardia, manifested as at least two consecutive P waves without an intervening QRS complex, proving that this is not PJRT. If the tachycardia incessantly stops and starts, there may be cycle-length alternation at the onset of PJRT or aAVNRT but usually not in AET. A ventricular premature beat placed when the His bundle is refractory may preexcite or postexcite the next atrial electrogram in PJRT but not in AET. If a premature beat placed any time in diastole postexcites the next atrial electrogram, it cannot be AET. The atrial activation sequence during ventricular pacing maneuvers may not be helpful in discriminating these tachycardias.

Pharmacologic therapy for congestive heart failure is indicated for all affected patients, and the resultant reduction in intrinsic catecholamine levels by improvement in ventricular function after treatment with digoxin may slow the AET rate slightly. However, digoxin does not usually suppress the focus. Similarly, calcium channel and β-blocking drugs may reduce the ventricular response to AET but do not control the AET itself. Class Ia drugs are also not very effective (116). Moricizine (117), class Ic agents (i.e., flecainide and propafenone) (118), and class III drugs (i.e., amiodarone and sotalol) (119), used alone or in combination, have been successful. If drug therapy fails or drug side effects become problematic, catheter ablation using radiofrequency energy is highly efficacious for curing children with a single AET focus, with success rates at medium-term follow-up of at least 90%. Multiple foci may be more difficult, and surgical methods for abolition of foci, including cryoablation, surgical extirpation, and surgical exclusion (120,121), may be necessary. Precise mapping of the foci before surgery is highly desirable, because one or more of the foci may become suppressed by general anesthesia, making intraoperative mapping difficult.

Permanent Form of Junctional Reciprocating Tachycardia

PJRT, an uncommon arrhythmia, is a form of orthodromic reciprocating tachycardia in which the ventriculoatrial limb of the reentry circuit is a decrementally conducting concealed accessory AV pathway. The retrograde pathway has a slow conduction time, giving a long RP appearance to the ECG. Typically, the tachycardia is incessant. Even when incessant, it may have frequent terminations in the accessory pathway (i.e., block after the QRS), followed after one or more sinus beats by reinitiation (Fig. 26-14). The pathway usually has a posteroseptal location. This tachycardia may begin any time from fetal life to early adulthood. Pharmacologic therapy in children may be very difficult, and drugs whose actions are limited to the AV node are generally useless when used alone. Class Ic and class III agents are of greatest value. Catheter ablation methods are highly successful for curing this arrhythmia.

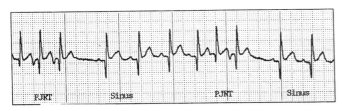

FIGURE 26-14. Rhythm strip for a 15-year-old boy with a permanent form of junctional reciprocating tachycardia (PJRT) alternating with periods of sinus rhythm (full standard chest leads; paper speed of 25 mm/sec).

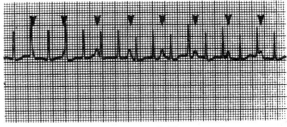

Lead II

FIGURE 26-15. On the rhythm strip for junctional tachycardia, atrioventricular dissociation is evident, with P waves marked by arrowheads (full standard chest leads; paper speed of 25 mm/sec).

ARRHYTHMIAS IMMEDIATELY AFTER CONGENITAL HEART SURGERY

In the immediate postoperative period, children with congenital heart defects develop tachyarrhythmias associated with changes in cardiac chamber dimension resulting from impaired ventricular contractility, subendocardial ischemia, effects of residual defects, localized injury to the specialized conduction system, metabolic imbalances, or central nervous system injury. Rarely, postoperative endocarditis manifests with new-onset ventricular or atrial ectopy.

Junctional Tachycardia

JT, also called junctional ectopic or His bundle tachycardia, generally occurs within 24 hours of congenital heart operations. It has been reported to occur in up to 8% of open-heart operations (122). Cardiac procedures most frequently associated with JT are tetralogy of Fallot repair, Mustard operation for d-TGA, VSD closure, AVSD repair, repair of total anomalous pulmonary venous return, and after the Fontan operation (122–124).

Procedures involving suture lines near the penetrating bundle of His may result in a transient period of injury and edema of the bundle. However, procedures remote from this structure may also cause JT, probably from stretch on the bundle, as may occur with postoperative pulmonary artery hypertension. JT has had a reported mortality rate of up to 50%, caused by the adverse effects of rate-related reduction in ventricular filling and AV asynchrony.

Similar to congenital JT, postoperative JT is a regular tachycardia with a rate usually greater than 200 bpm and a QRS morphology identical to that seen during sinus rhythm. There is usually ventriculoatrial dissociation, with a ventricular rate faster than the atrial rate and with occasional sinus capture beats (Fig. 26-15). This condition can be best demonstrated by epicardial wire electrograms. Occasionally, there is ventriculoatrial conduction, with negative P waves in the inferior leads. In those instances, JT may be confused with atrial ectopic tachycardia and first-degree AV block. JT appears to result from an automatic mechanism and cannot be terminated by introduction of atrial or ventricular extrastimuli or overdrive pacing, or by

direct current cardioversion. These maneuvers may result in overdrive suppression, which may last a few seconds before a gradual "warm up" to the previous rate (125). Garson and Gillette demonstrated a normal H-V interval in four children with nonsurgical JT (125).

If the patient's hemodynamic status can be improved, given time, JT generally resolves. Unfortunately, the agents used to improve inotropic function tend to increase the rate of JT. The goals of therapy are to reduce the ventricular rate to less than 180 bpm in infants and less than 150 bpm in older children. Successful reduction in rate has been reported in small series of patients using a variety of antiarrhythmic agents, including digoxin (122), flecainide (124), propafenone (125), moricizine (126), and amiodarone (127). Hypotension, especially during the intravenous administration of intravenous propafenone (128) or amiodarone (127) is a definite risk. Walsh and coworkers used a more systematic approach in evaluating treatment options in 71 consecutive children having postoperative JT (129). They were listed in the following order: reduction in exogenous catecholamines, correction of fever, atrial pacing, digoxin, phenytoin or propranolol or verapamil, procainamide or hypothermia, and procainamide plus hypothermia. Only correction of fever and combined procainamide plus hypothermia appeared to be efficacious. Amiodarone was not used in this study. Moderate hypothermia (32°C to 34°C) (130) usually requires pharmacologic paralysis and may result in metabolic acidosis.

In patients in whom AV asynchrony is thought to be deleterious and in those whose heart rates have been reduced by drugs or hypothermia, atrial pacing may be employed to achieve AV association. This may be accomplished with atrial pacing at a rate faster than that of the JT or by coupling atrial paced events to the prior ventricular sensed event (124). Till and associates used moderate hypothermia and atrial pacing to successfully treat 8 of 11 patients (124). Success seemed to be related to early intervention, generally within 1 hour of tachycardia onset. Survivors returned to sinus rhythm 1 to 10 days after therapy.

Patients refractory to all measures may be considered for transcatheter or surgical His bundle ablation and dual-chamber pacemaker implantation (111–113,131).

Other Arrhythmias in the Immediate Postoperative Period

Virtually any arrhythmia may occur immediately postoperatively, depending on hemodynamic or metabolic alterations. In general, onset of new tachyarrhythmias in the early postoperative period warrants investigation of the cause. Correction of the hemodynamic, mechanical, or metabolic problem should be attempted first. The decision to use pharmacologic therapy must weigh the risks of coexisting hemodynamic deterioration caused by the arrhythmia or potential for worse arrhythmias against adverse effects from the drugs themselves.

An unusual but recognized cause for sudden hypotension and bradycardia in the immediate postoperative period was identified in four infants within 18 hours of completion of intracardiac surgery (132). Their responses to intravenous atropine boluses and infusions suggested to the investigators that a hypervagotonic response to myocardial stretch (i.e., Bezold-Jarisch reflex) was the cause. If other causes of sudden hypotension and bradycardia (e.g., airway obstruction, pericardial tamponade) have been excluded, this cause should be considered and treated with atropine.

EVALUATION AND MANAGEMENT OF PATIENTS WITH CHRONIC ARRHYTHMIAS AFTER SURGERY FOR CONGENITAL HEART DISEASE

Table 26-2 summarizes the rates of arrhythmias after the more commonly performed congenital heart operations.

Chronic Arrhythmias after Operations on the Atria

The greatest experience with arrhythmias after atrial surgery is with the Mustard and Senning operations for d-TGA. Creation of an intraatrial baffle with prosthetic material or pericardium (i.e., Mustard operation) or atrial wall itself (i.e., Senning operation) results in damage to the sinus node, perinodal structures, and their blood supplies (133) and to pacemaker tissue throughout the atrium. Symptomatic bradycardia manifests as exercise intolerance, fatigue, early morning headaches, or rarely as presyncope and syncope. Intraatrial reentry tachycardia or flutter also occurs and, in certain rare circumstances, may predispose to sudden death.

All variations of the Fontan operation are designed to direct systemic venous return to the pulmonary arteries in patients with a single ventricle. These operations usually result in all or part of the right atrium having a chronically elevated mean pressure. Hence, hemodynamic factors in addition to surgical scars likely account for the atrial tachycardias observed in these patients.

After repair of ostium secundum or sinus venosus ASDs or of partial or total anomalous pulmonary venous return, sick sinus syndrome may also occur (Fig. 26-16).

Incidence and Natural History

After the Mustard operation, there is a progressive decrease in the percentage of patients having sinus rhythm. When evaluated by routine ECG or 24-hour Holter 5 to 10 years postoperatively, 20% to 40% are in sinus rhythm (134–137), 7% to 35% are in junctional rhythm (134,136,137), up to 40% are in a slow ectopic atrial rhythm (137), and 10% have atrial reentry tachycardia or flutter (134,136,138,139). In their series of 249 patients, Gewillig and colleagues reported a 2.4% per year loss of sinus rhythm, and the presence of junctional rhythm carried a 2.1-fold increased risk of developing atrial flutter ($p < 0.05$) (136). In a multiple-institution report

TABLE 26-2. INCIDENCE OF ARRHYTHMIAS AND RELATED PROBLEMS IN PATIENTS AFTER SELECTED OPERATIONS FOR CONGENITAL HEART DEFECTS

Operation	Atrial Fibrillation/ Flutter	Ventricular Tachycardia	Sudden Death	Sinus or Junctional Bradycardia	Atrioventricular Block	Pacemaker Requirement
Mustard/Senning operation	++–+++	+++[a]	++–++++[a]	+++–++++[b]	+–++	+++
Fontan operation	+++++	+++[a]	++[a]	++++	++[a]	+++
Tetralogy of Fallot repair	+–++	+–++++[a]	++[a]		++	+–++
ASD closure	+–+++++[c]			+–++	+	+–++
VSD closure		+–+++++[a]	+–++[a]			0–+++[a]
Pulmonic stenosis repair	0–+++[b]		+			
Aortic stenosis repair		+++–++++[a]	++–+++[a]			

+, 0% to 1% incidence; ++, 1% to 5% incidence; +++, 5% to 10% incidence; ++++, 10% to 20% incidence; +++++, 20 to 60% incidence; ASD, atrial septal defect; VSD, ventricular septal defect.
[a]Increased with worse hemodynamic status or associated defects.
[b]Related to increased time since surgery.
[c]Increased with older age at time of surgery.

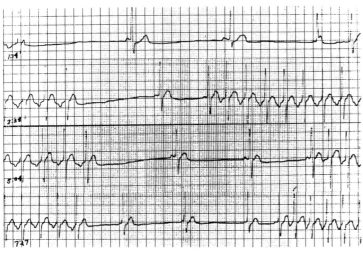

24 Hr Ambulatory ECG – Lead II

FIGURE 26-16. Bradyarrhythmias and tachyarrhythmias recorded in a patient who had undergone closure of an atrial septal defect. Periods of sinus or junctional bradycardia alternate with runs of atrial reentry tachycardia (paper speed of 25 mm/sec).

of 182 patients, there was also a progressive loss of sinus rhythm over time, but the prevalence of atrial tachyarrhythmias was relatively constant at 2.1% to 7.1% over a mean follow-up period of 4.5 to 8.3 years (139). Between 5% and 11% of patients had received pacemakers (140,141), usually for unacceptably low heart rates, syncope, or as adjunctive therapy to antiarrhythmic drugs other than digoxin. An even longer-duration follow-up for smaller groups of patients has been reported by Puley and coworkers (142); at a median follow-up of 23 years for 86 adults who had undergone the Mustard operation, 48% experienced supraventricular tachycardia (mostly atrial flutter), and 22% had pacemakers (142). Risk factors for supraventricular tachycardia included pulmonary hypertension, right ventricular dysfunction, and junctional rhythm. Helbing compared the long-term outcomes (median follow-up, 16 years) of 60 Mustard with 62 Senning patients (143). SAND was significantly more likely in the Mustard group.

Sudden death occurs late after these operations and affects 3% to 15% of patients (134,136,142,144). In the report by Lucet and associates on 123 patients after Mustard or Senning operations, four sudden deaths occurred, and three of those patients had severe right ventricular dysfunction (145). In Gewilleg's report, right ventricular dysfunction was present in 38% of those who later developed atrial flutter ($p < 0.01$), and the presence of atrial flutter increased the risk of sudden death 4.7-fold ($p < 0.01$) (136). This point was also emphasized in a large collaborative study of 380 children with atrial flutter (138). The most frequent diagnosis was "postoperative Mustard operation," and the 6-year mortality rate in this subgroup was 21%. The risk of sudden death among those whose atrial flutter could not be eliminated was fourfold that of those who had had no recurrences. The mechanism of sudden death was thought to be 1:1 AV conduction during atrial flutter directly causing ventricular fibrillation, or followed by

marked overdrive suppression of all subsidiary pacemakers with resultant asystole (Fig. 26-17). It is probable that another cause of sudden death in this group of patients is ventricular tachycardia, especially in those patients who have depressed right ventricular function or in those who have had additional ventricular surgery for VSDs or left ventricular outflow tract obstruction.

In their report of 30 individuals undergoing the Fontan operation, Weber and colleagues documented one late arrhythmic death and a gradual increase in supraventricular arrhythmias during a 10.7-year follow-up among survivors (146). Of 23 who had been in sinus rhythm preoperatively, 11 (48%) developed late arrhythmias, five of whom required pacemaker implantation and eight of whom were receiving multiple antiarrhythmic drugs. They further identified a prolonged P-wave duration and deeply negative P wave in lead V_1 on preoperative ECG as predictors of long-term postoperative PSVT. Driscoll and coworkers found 20% of 352 patients required antiarrhythmic drugs, pacemaker implantation, or both at 5 to 15 years of follow-up (147). They identified right atrial stretch, impaired ventricular function, and AV valve insufficiency as potential causes for the tachycardia-bradycardia syndrome, although postoperative AV block occurred in several instances, and ventricular tachycardia occurred in 6% of patients. Gewillig and associates found an 18% incidence of arrhythmias at 8-year follow-up assessment of 78 long-term survivors of the modified Fontan operation (148). Multivariate analysis disclosed older age, increased right atrial size, and elevated pulmonary artery pressures as risk factors for arrhythmia development ($p < 0.001$). In another report, among 32 patients undergoing the modified Fontan operation for tricuspid atresia, 15% of survivors had developed recurrent atrial tachyarrhythmias at a mean follow-up of 8.9 years (149). The most sobering report comes from the National Heart Hospital in London, England, where the actuarial arrhyth-

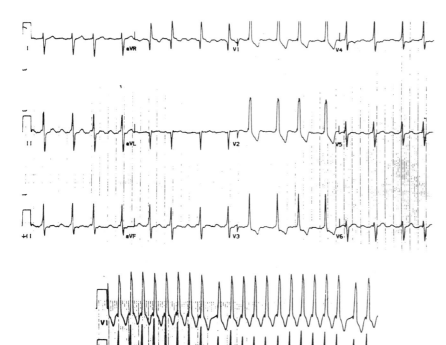

FIGURE 26-17. Top: Electrocardiogram for a 30-year-old man who had undergone the Mustard operation for d- transposition of the great arteries. He has chronic atrial flutter and presyncope during exercise. Notice the right ventricular hypertrophy and right axis deviation (QRS axis of 150 degrees). **Bottom:** Three-channel rhythm strip for the same patient during stage IV of a treadmill test using a Bruce protocol. The patient became presyncopal, requiring termination of the test (full standard chest leads; paper speed of 25 mm/sec).

mia-free survival rate for hospital survivors was only 60% at 10 years (150). These patients tended to have higher mean right atrial pressures and lower ejection fractions.

Cavopulmonary procedures of several types are known to render patients susceptible to a wide range of arrhythmias (151–157). An interesting postoperative tachycardia described in occasional patients who had undergone the Bjork-type Fontan operation (i.e., right atrial appendage directly anastomosed to the right ventricular outflow tract) is orthodromic AV reciprocating tachycardia involving spontaneous establishment of conduction across the suture line (158). We have even had a case of late postoperative onset of WPW syndrome having a right anteroseptal ECG pattern and requiring complete electrical dissociation of that suture line by catheter ablation.

Pacemakers are required in 5% to 15% of patients after the modified Fontan operation (146,147,159). The indications for pacing include tachycardia-bradycardia syndrome, congenital AV block, or postoperative AV block. The reported incidence of late arrhythmic death overall is 2% to 3% (146,147,160). These data are influenced by newer surgical techniques. There is early evidence that the staged approach involving a bidirectional Glenn operation or the hemi-Fontan procedure before the total cavopulmonary connection may increase the likelihood of developing SAND (161).

Reports of small numbers of patients after total anomalous pulmonary venous connection (162) or ostium primum ASD (163) repairs have shown a high incidence of conduction abnormalities, including sinus, ectopic atrial or junctional bradycardia, and atrial flutter or fibrillation. Complete AV block may occur after ostium primum repair. Murphy and colleagues described the natural history of 123 patients who had undergone repair of ostium secundum or sinus venosus ASDs at the Mayo Clinic (164). Late follow-up (27 to 32 years) revealed that the incidence of atrial flutter or fibrillation increased directly with age at repair; it was 4% if the patient was 11 years of age or younger at the time of surgery, 17% for those between 12 and 24 years, 41% for those between 25 and 41 years, and 59% for patients older than 41 years. The incidence of pacemaker requirement was low for all groups (4% of total, including two with AV block). These findings were corroborated by a later report in which late postoperative atrial flutter or fibrillation was predicted by older age at surgery (>40 years), the presence of preoperative atrial flutter or fibrillation, or the occurrence of immediate postoperative atrial flutter or fibrillation or junctional rhythm (13).

Most babies born today with simple d-TGA undergo the arterial switch operation instead of the Mustard or Senning procedure. Midterm follow-up (24 to 29 months) after the arterial switch operation at two centers failed to demonstrate significant rhythm disturbances by 24-hour ECG monitoring of 250 infants (165,166). Electrophysiologic testing of 158 patients undergoing the arterial switch operation at Children's Hospital, Boston, revealed normal corrected sinus node recovery times and A-H intervals in 97% of patients but a high incidence of simple atrial ectopy (167). At a mean follow-up period of 2.1 years, the incidence was 5% for supraventricular tachycardia and less than 1% for ventricular tachycardia.

Noninvasive Evaluation

After the Mustard, Senning, or Fontan operations, we obtain a 24-hour ECG before discharge from the hospital. If there are signs of sinus node dysfunction at this point, more aggressive patient surveillance than usual is indicated. Otherwise, 24-hour ambulatory ECGs are sufficient every 2 to 5 years. In patients having chronic fatigue and in those having syncope or dizziness at rest or with exercise, a 24-hour ECG and exercise test should be performed. Hesslein and coworkers performed treadmill tests on 25 children at an average age of 10.2 years after the Mustard operation (168). Using a modified Bruce protocol, patients exercised to exhaustion in 90% of tests. In 70.4% of tests, the maximum attained heart rates were more than two standard deviations below predicted values ($p < 0.001$), and in 59.3% of tests, heart rates 5 minutes after exercise were more than two standard deviations below predicted values ($p < 0.001$). This relatively sudden drop in heart rate immediately after exercise may correlate with the frequently observed fatigue and dizziness that many patients experience immediately after exercise. Forty-seven percent of the patients tested had abnormally low exercise capacity. For patients having less frequent paroxysmal episodes of syncope, dizziness, or palpitations, newer ambulatory electrocardiographic monitoring systems, such as transtelephonic monitoring and implantable recorders may prove valuable.

Electrophysiologic Testing

After the Mustard operation, electrophysiologic abnormalities found during invasive electrophysiologic testing have included prolongation of the sinus node or pacemaker recovery times in more than 50% of patients and prolongation of the sinoatrial conduction time in more than 33% (169,170) (Fig. 26-18). Vetter and associates also demonstrated intraatrial conduction delay in 90% and increased atrial effective refractory period in 41% of patients tested. Sustained atrial reentry tachycardia was inducible in 51% of patients, 48% of whom later developed spontaneous atrial flutter (137). AV conduction is usually normal.

For 30 patients who underwent the modified Fontan operation, Kurer and colleagues performed invasive electrophysiologic testing at a mean of 1.9 years postoperatively

(171). Fifty percent had prolongation of the corrected sinus node or pacemaker recovery times. Seventy percent were in sinus rhythm, but only one half of those had normal sinoatrial conduction times. The remaining 30% had ectopic atrial or junctional rhythms. Atrial electrical function was also abnormal; there was a prolonged atrial refractory period in 43%, intraatrial conduction delays in 76%, and inducible sustained atrial reentry tachycardia in 27% of patients. There were AV conduction abnormalities in 10% of patients.

We recommend electrophysiologic study after atrial surgery in any patient who has developed syncope, presyncope, or palpitations suggesting a sustained tachyarrhythmia or who has documented tachycardia other than atrial flutter. Even if noninvasive monitoring shows bradycardia as the source for syncope, cardiac catheterization and electrophysiologic study are indicated before pacemaker implantation to evaluate AV nodal function for identification and possible ablation of tachyarrhythmias that may be contributing to symptoms and to demonstrate anatomic patency of venous and atrial structures pertinent to permanent lead implantation.

Management

The recommendations of the American Heart Association and the American College of Cardiology Joint Committee on Pacing (172) as they relate to patients who have undergone atrial surgery are to insert a pacemaker in any patient with: "symptomatic" bradycardia, defined as dizziness, lightheadedness, and near or frank syncope, marked exercise intolerance, or congestive heart failure (class I indication), or with the tachycardia-bradycardia syndrome and a tachyarrhythmia requiring treatment with an antiarrhythmic drug other than digitalis that could suppress the sinus node (e.g., β-blocking drugs, verapamil, quinidine, procainamide, disopyramide, flecainide, propafenone, sotalol, amiodarone) (i.e., class II indication).

If symptoms are convincing but cannot be reproduced by ambulatory monitoring, tachyarrhythmias are not inducible, and if there is moderate bradycardia while awake (<60 bpm in an infant younger than 2 years, 50 bpm in children 2 to 10 years old, or 40 bpm in patients older than 10 years), we recommend pacemaker implantation.

The second indication is reasonable in view of most clinicians' observations that progressive bradycardia and AV conduction abnormalities may occur in patients treated with many of these drugs. Implanting a pacemaker in such a patient may also protect against the severe bradycardia that may result after an episode of atrial flutter.

Absent from these recommendations is an asymptomatic "extreme" bradycardia, defined as a resting but awake heart rate less than 50 bpm in an infant younger than 1 year of age, less than 40 bpm in children 1 to 10 years of age, and less than 30 bpm in children older than 10 years of age who have undergone atrial surgery. Although most such patients

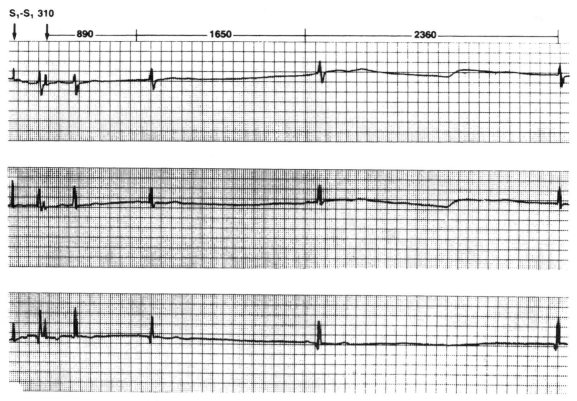

FIGURE 26-18. Using standard electrocardiography, the surface electrocardiogram (leads I, II, and III, *top to bottom*) was recorded at bedside from a 4-year-old girl who had undergone repair of sinus venosus atrial septal defect 3 days earlier. After 30 seconds of pacing (S₁-S₁) by means of the right atrial epicardial wires at a 310-ms cycle length, the sinus node recovered 890 ms later. The resting sinus cycle length was 640 ms; therefore, the corrected sinus node recovery time was 250 ms. Secondary pauses of 1,650 and 2,360 ms suggested the presence of sinus node entrance block during the atrial pacing (paper speed of 50 mm/sec).

have accompanying episodes of tachycardia or symptoms related to the bradycardia, some patients have no other symptoms. There probably are heart rates below which patients are at risk of life-threatening events, but there are scant data to support this idea. Based on the study by Lucet that related the coexistence of tachyarrhythmias and bradyarrhythmias in these patients (145), we would consider placing a pacemaker in such a patient in hope of preventing tachyarrhythmias.

Several investigators have described favorable experiences with atrial pacing, including antitachycardia pacing, after Mustard, Senning, or Fontan operations (173–175). In some cases, novel approaches to lead placement may be required. Advances in interventional catheterization have benefited some patients when superior vena caval baffle obstruction is present. Catheter-delivered stents can relieve untoward hemodynamic abnormalities and may permit placement of intravenous pacing systems. If AV conduction is also inadequate, dual-chamber pacing is necessary. AV synchrony is especially important in Fontan patients, and ventricular pacing alone, even with rate adaptiveness, may not be acceptable (176). Dual-chamber epicardial lead sys-

tems or transvenous atrial and epicardial ventricular lead systems are required in these instances.

Management of tachyarrhythmia after the Senning or Mustard operations may be controversial because many patients remain asymptomatic despite the presence of atrial flutter with 2 : 1 AV conduction. We generally recommend prophylactic digoxin in patients after these operations, hoping to reduce the risk of 1 : 1 AV conduction if atrial flutter develops. In the presence of adequate ventricular function, calcium channel or β-blocking agents can serve the same purpose and are more likely than digoxin to control the ventricular rate during exercise. Patients who present with atrial flutter (with or without symptoms) should undergo transvenous or transesophageal overdrive pacing termination or direct current cardioversion. If they do not have a therapeutic blood concentration of digoxin or they have not been on any medications, we attempt chronic treatment with digoxin alone for a first episode. Failing this, several options are available: antitachycardia pacing (with digoxin therapy), class Ia (with digoxin and bradycardia pacing) or class III agents (with bradycardia pacing), or radiofrequency catheter ablation. Implantation of an antitachycardia pacemaker may obviate the need for second-line drugs, but the efficacy of this modality must be demonstrated by electrophysiologic testing in the drug-free state.

Because sudden death in Mustard and Senning patients is most likely linked to tachyarrhythmias, complete arrhythmia suppression is the goal of therapy. Radiofrequency ablation of atrial reentrant tachycardia can be performed with success rates at medium-term follow-up of 70% to 80% (177,178). This has become our preferred approach in patients with recurrent intraatrial reentry tachycardia (Fig. 26-19).

After the modified Fontan operation, medical suppression of tachyarrhythmias may be difficult. The requirements for AV synchrony and adequate diastolic filling time makes arrhythmia control especially crucial (179). For these challenging patients, combinations of antiarrhythmic drugs, often including amiodarone, are sometimes necessary. Antitachycardia pacing is sometimes possible (175), but it may result in acceleration of one atrial tachycardia to another. Radiofrequency catheter ablation of intraatrial reentry tachycardia substrates is being performed in these patients with increasing success rates. Standard techniques to identify areas critical to common atrial flutter circuits in the normal heart are being successfully applied, including recognition of presystolic and split potentials and entrainment with concealed conduction and a short postpacing interval. Successful ablation of more than 70% of these circuits is being achieved (180–182). Even better results can be expected with the advent of electroanatomic mapping techniques (183) and chilled-tip ablation catheters.

In a group of 14 patients, a more radical approach involving surgical conversion to total cavopulmonary connection–type Fontan with concomitant intraoperative mapping and cryoablation of intraatrial reentry tachycardia circuits has been reported by Mavroudis and coworkers (184). These patients experienced improvement in hemodynamic status and in arrhythmia control. The inferomedial right atrium, superior rim of the old ASD patch, and the lateral right atrium usually were the regions requiring cryoablation lesions. Only 2 of 12 patients undergoing cryoablation still required antiarrhythmic drugs at a median follow-up period of 25 months (185).

Chronic Arrhythmias after Operation on the Ventricles

Most studies of chronic arrhythmias occurring after operation on the ventricles have been of patients with tetralogy of Fallot (186–191). In general, the less serious the defect, the less serious is the outcome. For example, late sudden death occurs in approximately 4% of patients who have had VSD repair (26,192), 0% to 5% of those who have had tetralogy of Fallot repair (186,191), 18% of those who have had double-outlet right ventricle repair (193), and 18% of those who have had surgery for truncus arteriosus with a single pulmonary artery (194).

The surgical repair of tetralogy of Fallot always involves patch closure of the VSD and resection of some infundibular muscle, usually through a right infundibulotomy. Pulmonary regurgitation always results if the right ventricular

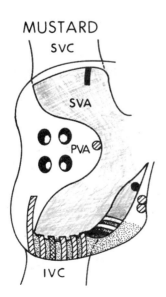

FIGURE 26-19. Successful and unsuccessful ablation sites of substrates for supraventricular tachycardia after the Mustard and Senning operations for d- transposition of the great arteries in 11 patients using radiofrequency catheter ablation. Linear lesions were placed for intraatrial reentry tachycardia (i.e., atypical atrial flutter), and focal lesions were placed for focal atrial tachycardia or for the typical variety of atrioventricular node reentry tachycardia. IVC, inferior vena cava; MV, mitral valve; PVA, pulmonary venous atrium; SVA (shaded gray in Mustard figure), systemic venous atrium; SVC, superior vena cava; TV, tricuspid valve; stippled area in Mustard figure, isthmus between inferior vena cava and tricuspid valve. (From Kanter RJ, Papagiannis J, Carboni MP, et al. Radiofrequency catheter ablation of supraventricular tachycardia substrates after Mustard and Senning operations for d-transposition of the great arteries. *J Am Coll Cardiol* 2000;35:428–441, with permission.)

outflow tract enlargement must extend across the pulmonary valve anulus.

Conduction Disturbance

Incidence

After repair of tetralogy of Fallot, approximately 80% of patients have complete right bundle branch block, an additional 11% have the combination of right bundle branch block with left axis deviation, and 3% have the combination of right bundle branch block, left axis deviation, and first-degree AV block (186) (Fig. 26-20). Early studies of these patients suggested that the combination of right bundle branch block with left axis deviation (195) or with additional first-degree AV block (196) predicted late sudden death. Later experience found that late sudden death is not often caused by conduction disturbances.

Clinical Significance

Among patients having syncope after ventricular repair of congenital heart defects, electrophysiologic findings of prolonged H-V interval or abnormally slow rate of AV Wenckebach block may help guide clinical decision making. However, the very common finding of right bundle branch block is more difficult to interpret. The ECG finding of right bundle branch block may result from proximal damage to the bundle itself or from the right ventriculotomy, interrupting the distal Purkinje fibers in the right ventricular free wall.

Irrespective of the site of conduction delay, the finding of right bundle branch block after right ventriculotomy appears to carry a benign early and midterm prognosis. It only obscures the ECG with regard to interpretation of ventricular dilatation or hypertrophy. Perhaps more importantly, in patients with "true" proximal right bundle branch block, the development of left bundle branch block, which occasionally accompanies atherosclerotic heart disease later in life, places these patients at risk for complete AV block.

Evaluation

On follow-up ECGs, the patterns of right bundle branch block, right bundle branch block–left axis deviation, and right bundle branch block–left axis deviation–first-degree AV block all have inconstant intracardiac correlates. Friedli and Bolens associated a normal Q wave with right ventricular apex activation times in most patients having ECG criteria for *bifascicular block* (i.e., right bundle block plus left axis deviation) and normal H-V intervals in three of five patients having ECG criteria for *trifascicular block* (i.e., right bundle branch block, left axis deviation, and first-degree AV block) (197). The recommendation was therefore made that these terms not be used to describe the ECG, unless there is an intracardiac correlate (i.e., prolonged Q-wave to right ventricular apex activation time for bifascicular block and additional H-V interval prolongation for trifascicular block).

Even if intracardiac conduction intervals support the diagnosis of "true" bifascicular or trifascicular block, we become concerned primarily if there is type II second-degree AV block; complete AV block; marked H-V interval prolongation (>100 ms), even in the absence of symptoms; syncope with any H-V interval prolongation and no inducible tachyarrhythmias; or block below the His bundle at atrial-paced rates below 120 bpm. In the presence of transient postoperative type II second-degree AV block or complete AV block lasting less than 7 days postoperatively,

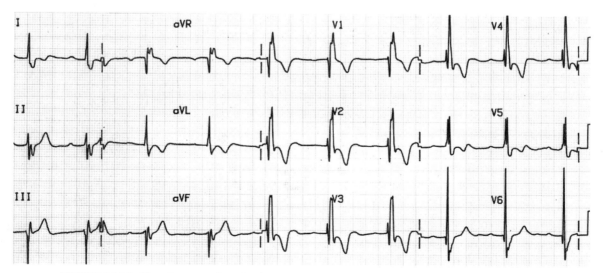

FIGURE 26-20. The electrocardiogram for an 11-year-old girl 6 years after repair of tetralogy of Fallot indicates a first-degree atrioventricular block, left-axis deviation, and right bundle branch block. She remains asymptomatic (full standard chest leads; paper speed of 25 mm/sec).

24-hour ECG monitoring should be performed before discharge and then regularly. All patients after ventricular surgery involving the ventricular septum should have 24-hour ECG monitoring every 2 to 5 years. Exercise testing may be of value to evaluate the maximum conducted sinus rate. If it is less than 120 bpm, closer surveillance of their rhythm and symptoms may be warranted, although type I second-degree AV block is acceptable in the absence of symptoms.

In the patient who has had an operation on the ventricles and had a negative noninvasive evaluation but has syncope or presyncope, electrophysiology study is indicated. The cause of syncope could be AV block, ventricular arrhythmias, or occasionally atrial flutter with rapid AV conduction.

Garson and associates reported their findings from electrophysiologic studies from 27 patients after tetralogy repair (198). Forty-one percent had an abnormal corrected sinus node recovery time, 15% had a prolonged A-H interval, 41% had an abnormally slow AV Wenckebach rate, and 22% had a prolonged H-V interval. Similarly, Friedli and Bolens demonstrated conduction disturbances in 10 of 52 patients (197). Three patients developed block below the His bundle with atrial pacing rates below 120 bpm, and two of them developed complete AV block within 5 years. Based on these limited data, we would consider electrophysiologic testing for a patient with AV Wenckebach rates less than 120 bpm during exercise testing to assess the level of block. Otherwise, routine electrophysiologic testing in an asymptomatic patient is not indicated.

Management

A pacemaker should be implanted in any child with type II second-degree or complete AV block lasting more than 7 days after heart surgery. A pacemaker should also be implanted in the patient with syncope or presyncope and a prolonged H-V interval or AV block below the His at atrial paced rates below the 120 bpm. If ventricular tachycardia is also inducible, therapy must be individualized and ambulatory ECG event recording may be useful. Asymptomatic patients with prolonged H-V interval or AV block below the His at atrial-paced rates below 120 bpm should be followed closely with 24-hour ECG monitoring and exercise testing every 6 months. However, the value of exercise testing to determine the maximum conducted sinus rate in these patients is unproved.

Some patients undergo pacemaker insertion in the postoperative period but regain AV conduction shortly thereafter; data are not available to predict their risk of recurring AV block. This issue is usually of importance after their pulse generator reaches depletion parameters and elective replacement is required. In such instances, we use stringent criteria from 24-hour ECG monitoring and electrophysiologic testing (i.e., normal AV Wenckebach rate and normal H-V interval) before considering discontinuation of pacing.

Ventricular Tachyarrhythmias

Incidence

During long-term follow-up of repair of tetralogy of Fallot, ventricular arrhythmias were evident in approximately 5% to 10% of patients on routine electrocardiogram (186, 198,199), 20% to 40% on treadmill exercise testing (186,198,199), and 40% to 60% by 24-hour ECG monitoring (186,191,198,199). The mean age at the time of repair in these studies was 5 to 10 years. The presence and severity (i.e., Lown grade) of ventricular ectopy was most frequently reported to be related to older age at repair (191,200,201), elevation of right ventricular systolic pressure (usually ≥60 mm Hg) (186,191,198,201), and longer periods of follow-up after surgery (191,198,201). Depressed right ventricular ejection fraction (201), elevation of right ventricular end-diastolic pressure (198), duration of cardiopulmonary bypass during repair, and presence of a Potts anastomosis (200) also correlated with the incidence of ventricular arrhythmia in single reports. Walsh and colleagues found different results for 220 patients, all of whom had had tetralogy of Fallot repair before 18 months of age (189). Among 184 late survivors, followed for a mean of 60 months, there were no late deaths caused by arrhythmias, and only one patient required a pacemaker (for sinoatrial node disease). Among 41 patients who had 24-hour ECG data, only one patient had greater than Lown grade I ventricular ectopy. The investigators postulated that the earlier age of repair (compared with most other series) may protect the heart from deleterious changes accrued from long-standing right ventricular hypertension, left ventricular volume overloading, and systemic desaturation.

In an early report by Quattlebaum and coworkers, sudden death in three patients after ventricular surgery was thought to be related to conduction disturbance (196), but virtually all later reports suggest that ventricular arrhythmias are the cause (186,191,196,198,200). The overall incidence of late sudden cardiac death after repair of tetralogy of Fallot ranges from 1.5% to 5% (186,191,196,200–205).

Evaluation

The main goal of routine evaluation of patients after ventricular surgery is to identify individuals who are at risk for symptoms or death from ventricular arrhythmias. Unfortunately, there is no one diagnostic test that represents the gold standard for determining such risk. The 12-lead ECG, chest radiograph, 24-hour ECG, treadmill exercise test, and echocardiogram all have roles in outpatient surveillance. Follow-up is stricter for those with poor hemodynamics than for those with excellent hemodynamics. Equivocal or minor symptoms may be evaluated with event recorders, but paroxysmal palpitations, syncope, or presyncope merits invasive electrophysiologic testing.

Based on study results, the 12-lead ECG may prove to be the most valuable screen for patients at risk for dangerous ventricular arrhythmias (i.e., ventricular tachycardia and sudden death). An increased QRS duration appears to be sensitive (206) and perhaps specific (207) for such risk, with a cutoff value of at least 180 ms providing the greatest accuracy. The coexistence of increased JT interval dispersion may enhance the predictive value, suggesting that both repolarization and depolarization abnormalities are important. The British study also found a correlation between an increased cardiothoracic ratio by chest radiograph with QRS prolongation (206).

The finding of complex ventricular arrhythmias (i.e., couplets, multiform PVBs, or ventricular tachycardia) on 24-hour ECG monitoring reliably identifies patients who subsequently have inducible ventricular tachycardia by electrophysiologic testing (191), but the relationship of such ectopy to clinical events is still unproved. Garson's report of 488 patients showed that 33% of 21 patients having high-grade ventricular ectopy confirmed by Holter monitoring later died, compared with no deaths among the 421 without ventricular ectopy (208). Harrison and associates corroborated those findings and found that ventricular ectopy was of prognostic importance, especially when it coexisted with poor ventricular function or residual structural defects (209). However, the value of Holter monitoring has been called into question by Cullen's report of 47 patients prospectively followed for 12 years after an original postoperative Holter assessment (210). Those originally having high-grade ventricular ectopy (including seven with nonsustained ventricular tachycardia) were no more likely to later have clinical ventricular tachycardia or to die suddenly than those not originally having ventricular ectopy. Importantly, the hemodynamic status was similar in patients of both groups. In conclusion, the presence of high-grade ventricular arrhythmias determined by ambulatory monitoring in one of these patients with poor ventricular function or the presence of a QRS duration of 180 ms or longer appeared to identify a patient at high risk for clinical ventricular tachycardia or sudden death.

The value of exercise testing is less clear for detecting patients at risk for symptomatic ventricular arrhythmias after right ventricular surgery. Garson and colleagues found that, among 104 patients who had undergone treadmill testing after tetralogy repair, those who had exercise-induced ventricular arrhythmias were older and had higher right ventricular systolic and diastolic pressures than those with no ectopic beats (198).

Signal averaging of the QRS complex to detect late potentials has been investigated in patients after tetralogy of Fallot repair. Although the QRS_d cannot be used to detect late potentials in the presence of right bundle branch block, an increased low-amplitude signal plus a decreased root mean square voltage correctly identified four of nine patients who had serious ventricular arrhythmias; no episodes of clinically relevant ventricular arrhythmias occurred in any patient not having late potentials by these criteria (211). Continued investigation in this area is needed.

We recommend invasive electrophysiologic testing after ventricular surgery in patients having sustained palpitations, syncope, or presyncope. The demonstration of symptomatic sustained monomorphic ventricular tachycardia by noninvasive means is an indication for electrophysiologic testing as a guide for antiarrhythmic drug selection (190). In the absence of symptoms, we would also consider ventricular programmed stimulation if a patient had echocardiographic or catheterization-proven impairment of hemodynamics, as well as Lown grade III or higher-grade ectopy by 24-hour ECG or high-grade ventricular ectopy during exercise testing.

Garson and coworkers used a pacing protocol consisting of paired ventricular extrastimuli and burst pacing at the right ventricular apex at one cycle length in 26 patients after tetralogy repair (198). They induced nonsustained ventricular tachycardia in 26% and sustained ventricular tachycardia in 7% of patients (Fig. 26-21). Of the 33% with any inducible ventricular tachycardia, 44% had had syncope, 67% had high-grade ventricular ectopy demonstrated by Holter monitoring, 56% had elevated right ventricular systolic pressures, and 45% had reduced right ventricular ejection fractions, whereas none of these abnormalities was present in the patients without inducible tachycardias. In a multicenter study, Chandar and associates observed that ventricular tachycardia was not inducible in the setting of a negative 24-hour ambulatory ECG recording and normal right ventricular systolic pressure, but that it was inducible in 45% of patients having syncope, in 27% of those having high-grade ventricular ectopy, and in 47% of those having ventricular tachycardia demonstrated by Holter monitoring (191). Of five late deaths, none had inducible ventricular tachycardia with double extrastimuli, but all had at least one risk factor as defined previously. Alexander and coworkers applied sophisticated statistical methods to a group of 130 patients who underwent programmed ventricular stimulation; 33% had tetralogy of Fallot, 25% had d-TGA, and 12% had left ventricular outflow tract obstructive lesions (212). By univariate analysis, a positive study result was associated with a sixfold increased risk of decreased survival, yielding an 87% sensitivity in predicting mortality. However, there was a 33% false-negative rate for 21 patients having documented clinical ventricular tachycardia, and the positive predictive value of sudden cardiac death was only 20%. This group of patients had a 3% annual mortality and event risk, much higher than any previous reports. The subjective decision to perform ventricular programmed stimulation identified a group with a high prevalence of poor outcome.

It is becoming evident that a search is indicated for supraventricular tachycardias in symptomatic patients after ventricular surgery (212,213). For 53 tetralogy patients with a median age of 23 years, Roos-Hesselink and colleagues demonstrated atrial flutter or fibrillation in 23% and other supraventricular tachycardias in 11% (213). We ablated AV node reentry in four postoperative tetralogy patients.

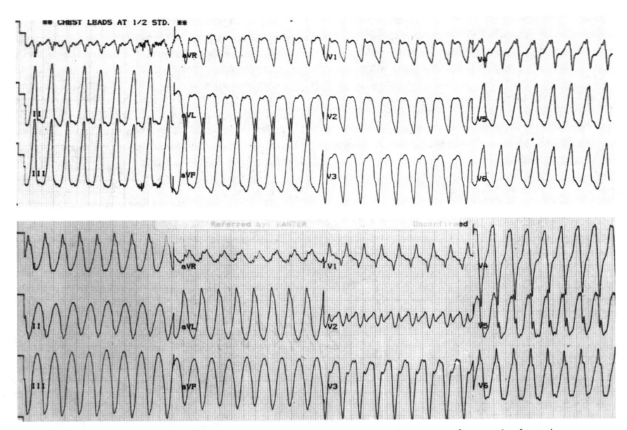

FIGURE 26-21. Two electrocardiograms for a 25-year-old man many years after repair of tetralogy of Fallot who suffered from recurrent near-syncope. These tracings were obtained during programmed ventricular stimulation and represent macroreentry ventricular tachycardia from around the right ventricular outflow tract patch *(top)* and from around the VSD patch *(bottom)*. Precise intraoperative mapping confirmed the location of the tachycardia circuits. He has been free of arrhythmia for 8.5 years after intraoperative argon photoablation of the reentry circuits (one-half standard chest leads; paper speed of 25 mm/sec).

Supraventricular tachycardias tend to be more poorly tolerated by these patients than by patients with normal hearts.

Management

When considering treatment for ventricular arrhythmias after ventricular surgery, the two major concerns are patient selection and standards for efficacy. Symptomatic ventricular tachycardia requires treatment. The diagnosis is established by noninvasive ambulatory ECG event recording or induction of sustained ventricular tachycardia by ventricular programmed stimulation in a syncopal or presyncopal patient. In separate reports by Kugler and coworkers (214) and Deal and associates (190), serial electrophysiology studies identified antiarrhythmic drugs (mostly phenytoin and propranolol) that effectively suppressed ventricular tachycardia reinducibility. In follow-up, no patient had clinical ventricular tachycardia. The positive predictive value of serial drug testing using ventricular programmed stimulation is less well established. We have found that quinidine and procainamide are not very useful drugs for sustained ventricular

tachycardia in these patients and that class Ic agents may be especially proarrhythmic (215). Anecdotal experience has shown the value of amiodarone or sotalol in some patients.

Because of potential drug side effects, nonpharmacologic therapy has become more attractive in recent years. After complete tachycardia circuit mapping in the electrophysiology laboratory, surgical resection, cryoablation (216), and argon photoablation have all met with variable success. Radiofrequency catheter ablation has been used to successfully interrupt macroreentry ventricular tachycardia circuits in several patients (217,218), even when there are multiple ventricular tachycardia circuits and when ventricular tachycardia is poorly hemodynamically tolerated (218). Implantable cardioverter-defibrillators may provide antitachycardia pacing as well as the safety net of cardioversion or defibrillation, if necessary (219).

Less clear are the indications for treating asymptomatic patients with high-grade ventricular ectopy by 24-hour ECG monitoring or exercise testing. If their hemodynamics are acceptable, we follow these patients closely, without any therapy. In those with poor hemodynamics, we consider ventricular programmed stimulation to help identify patients with inducible sustained tachycardia and to help guide medical therapy. Until there are randomized clinical trials involving treatment and nontreatment of such patients with induced ventricular tachycardia, we recommend treatment with antiarrhythmic drugs. Drugs with low proarrhythmic risk (i.e., β blocker, phenytoin, mexiletine, and perhaps sotalol) are emphasized for these patients.

For patients who have undergone ventricular surgery, we recommend consideration of treatment for those in the following categories: asymptomatic patients with poor hemodynamics and high-grade ventricular ectopy by 24-hour ECG monitoring; asymptomatic patients with poor hemodynamics and inducible ventricular tachycardia during electrophysiologic testing; and any patients with clinical sustained ventricular tachycardia.

Arrhythmias after Repair of Other Congenital Heart Defects

Ebstein's Anomaly of the Tricuspid Valve

In the report by Oh and colleagues, for 52 patients with Ebstein's anomaly who underwent surgical repair, the procedure included accessory pathway interruption in six with WPW syndrome, and five no longer had PSVT at follow-up (18). Of 18 patients with preoperative PSVT, four (22%) continued to have episodes at a mean follow-up of 40 months. Similarly, 3 (30%) of 10 with atrial fibrillation or flutter had recurrences at 36 months. Of seven postoperative deaths, two were early (ventricular fibrillation), three late (1, 5, and 27 months), and two were not associated with arrhythmias. Those having late arrhythmic deaths had had ventricular tachycardia (2 patients) or severe bradycardia (1 patient) perioperatively. Of the 11 patients without preoperative arrhythmias, none were found to have died or developed arrhythmias at late follow-up.

The effect of Ebstein's anomaly on outcome of surgical ablation of accessory pathway was evaluated by Pressley and coworkers (220). Thirty-eight patients with WPW syndrome and Ebstein's anomaly were compared with 384 patients having only WPW syndrome. In the Ebstein group, the postoperative 10-year survival rate (92.4%), freedom from significant arrhythmias (82%), incidence of atrial fibrillation (9%), and incidence of becoming disabled (9.4%) were no different from the values for the control group. The investigators concluded that Ebstein's anomaly should not preclude accessory pathway ablation. The acceptance of transcatheter ablation of accessory pathways makes this option even more attractive and may make future congenital surgery less risky in this disease.

Newer surgical techniques for improving tricuspid valve and right heart function, as introduced by Carpentier, have been shown to reduce or eliminate atrial tachycardias at 58 months median follow-up (221).

Pulmonary Valve Stenosis

In the NHS-2, Wolfe and associates followed 182 patients with pulmonary valve stenosis, and 92.8% had undergone surgical valvotomy (21). Among patients younger than 40 years of age, 18.7% had PSVBs at a rate exceeding 0.5 per hour (i.e., upper limits of normal). Three of the 16 patients older than 40 years who had undergone surgery had more than 4.0 PSVBs per hour (i.e., upper limits of normal). These rates were all significantly greater than for the control population.

For all ages, 11.2% of the surgically managed group ($p < 0.001$ versus control) had PVBs at a rate exceeding the upper limits of normal. Of all patients younger than 50 years of age who were treated medically or surgically, 14.3% had at least one ventricular couplet ($p < 0.001$ versus control). Similarly, 26.3% of patients younger than 50 years had multiform PVBs ($p < 0.001$ versus controls), also occurring in greater than expected frequency in medically and surgically treated groups. Of the 169 surgically treated patients, six (8.3%) had ventricular tachycardia. At least one serious arrhythmia was present in 28% of the surgically treated group. Age on admission was the only independent predictor of occurrence of a serious arrhythmia. Presence of cardiomyopathy, age at NHS-2 enrollment, and functional class at NHS-2 admission were marginally significant. The investigators concluded that the prevalence of arrhythmias was higher for these patients than for the control population but that serious arrhythmias were less commonly observed than in patients with aortic valve stenosis or VSD. The occurrence of sudden, unexpected death (0.05%) was significantly lower than in patients with either of the other defects ($p < 0.0001$).

Evidence from medium-term follow-up evaluation shows that balloon valvotomy may be associated with less ventricular ectopy than observed after surgical valvotomy (222), perhaps because there is less pulmonary insufficiency after balloon valvotomy. Whether reduction in pulmonary insufficiency by homograft valve insertion is associated with a reduction in ventricular ectopy is unclear (223).

Ventricular Septal Defect

The most extensive data from patients after surgical closure of VSD come from the NHS-2 (18). Serious arrhythmias, excluding patients with Eisenmenger physiology, were present in 36.8% of patients. Of those having undergone surgery, the risk of having serious arrhythmias was increased in those functioning below New York Heart Association class I or in those having cardiomegaly. At the time of final status, the occurrence of sudden, unexpected death was 4.2%.

Atrioventricular Septal Defect

In the report by Fournier and colleagues, 14 patients with an AVSD underwent postoperative electrophysiologic studies (26). There was first-degree AV block in nine (i.e., A-H interval prolongation in two, H-V interval prolongation in one, and combined "upper normal intervals" in three), sinus node dysfunction in three, AV nodal dysfunction in four, and right bundle branch block in 13. Postoperative complete AV block is now uncommon after repair of this lesion because of modification of the surgical technique.

Noninvasive evaluation by Holter monitoring has also been performed. Daliento and coworkers demonstrated a 33% incidence of ventricular and 10% incidence of atrial arrhythmias in 106 patients after AVSD repair (224). Ectopy was more likely in larger (and therefore older) patients if they had a higher postoperative right ventricular end-diastolic dimension or a larger VSD or if there was postoperative right bundle branch block. The type of AVSD did not correlate with the presence of arrhythmia. These investigators reported no episodes of sudden death.

Left Ventricular Outflow Tract Obstructive Lesions

Wolfe described 61 patients younger than 40 years of age with left outflow tract obstruction due to aortic stenosis after surgical aortic valvulotomy or valve replacement (21). The prevalences of PSVBs and PVBs were higher than a control population. Ventricular tachycardia occurred in 10.1% of the valvotomy and 13.9% of the valve replacement groups; this incidence was significantly greater than that in the general population ($p < 0.0001$). Likewise, 21.6% of all patients had at least one ventricular couplet, and 41% had multiform PVBs. Serious arrhythmias occurred in 44.8% of patients and were significantly more likely to be present in surgically treated patients ($p = 0.0056$). Using a multivariate logistic model, the odds of experiencing a serious arrhythmia were increased by an elevated left ventricular end-diastolic pressure, coexistence of aortic insufficiency, and male gender. Of greatest concern, the occurrence of sudden, unexpected death at last follow-up was 5.4%, significantly higher than for the group with pulmonic stenosis. The failure of surgical relief of obstructive left ventricular outflow tract lesions to prevent life-threatening arrhythmias has also been reported by Silka and associates (225). They demonstrated incremental risk of sudden death 20 years after repair of aortic stenosis or coarctation of the aorta.

REFERENCES

1. Anderson PAW, Rogers MC, Canent RV, et al. Atrioventricular conduction in secundum atrial septal defects. *Circulation* 1973; 48:27–31.

2. Clark EB, Kugler JD. Preoperative secundum atrial septal defect with coexisting sinus node and atrioventricular node dysfunction. *Circulation* 1982;65:976–980.

3. Clark EB, Roland JMA, Varghese PJ, et al. Should the sinus venosus type ASD be closed? A review of the atrial conduction defects and surgical results in twenty eight children. *Am J Cardiol* 1975;35:127–134.

4. Yabek SM, Jarmakani JM. Sinus node dysfunction in children, adolescents, and young adults. *Pediatrics* 1978;61:593–598.

5. Kyger ER, Frazier H, Cooley DA, et al. Sinus venosus atrial septal defect: early and late results following closure in 109 patients. *Ann Thorac Surg* 1978;25:44–50.

6. Sealy WC, Farmer JC, Young G, et al. Atrial dysfunction and atrial secundum defects. *J Thorac Cardiovasc Surg* 1969;57: 245–250.

7. Benedini G, Affatato A, Bellandi M, et al. Pre-operative sinus node function in adult patients with atrial septal defect (ostium secundum type). *Eur Heart J* 1985;6:261–265.

8. Hamilton WT, Haffajee CI, Dalen JE, et al. Atrial septal defect secundum: clinical profile with physiologic correlates in children and adults. *Cardiovasc Clin* 1979;10:267–277.

9. Gatzoulis MA, Freeman MA, Siu SC, et al. Atrial arrhythmia after surgical closure of atrial septal defects in adults. *N Engl J Med* 1999;340:839–846.

10. Rokseth R. Congenital heart disease in middle-aged adults. *Acta Med Scand* 1968;183:131–138.

11. Paolillo V, Dawkins KD, Miller GAH. Atrial septal defect in patients over the age of 50. *Int J Cardiol* 1985;9:139–147.

12. Forfang K, Simonsen S, Andersen A, Efskind L. Atrial septal defect in the middle aged. *Am Heart J* 1977;94:44–54.

13. Barbosa MM, Pena JL, Motta MM, et al. Aneurysms of the atrial septum diagnosed by echocardiography and their associated cardiac abnormalities. *Int J Cardiol* 1990;29:71–78.

14. Kumar AE, Fyler DC, Miettinen OS, Nadas AS. Ebstein's anomaly: clinical profile and natural history. *Am J Cardiol* 1971; 28:84–95.

15. Watson H. Natural history of Ebstein's anomaly of tricuspid valve in childhood and adolescence. *Br Heart J* 1974;36:417–427.

16. Celermajer DS, Bull C, Cullen S, et al. Ebstein's anomaly: presentation and outcome from fetus to adult. *J Am Coll Cardiol* 1994;23:170–176.

17. Radford DJ, Graff RF, Neilson GH. Diagnosis and natural history of Ebstein's anomaly. *Br Heart J* 1985;54: 517–522.

18. Oh JK, Holmes DR, Hayes DL, et al. Cardiac arrhythmias in patients with surgical repair of Ebstein's anomaly. *J Am Coll Cardiol* 1985;6:1351–1357.

19. Gentles TL, Calder AL, Clarkson PM, Neutze JM. Predictors of long-term survival with Ebstein's anomaly of the tricuspid valve. *Am J Cardiol* 1992;69:377–381.

20. Reich JD, Auld D, Hulse E, et al. The Pediatric Radiofrequency Ablation Registry's experience with Ebstein's anomaly. *J Cardiovasc Electrophysiol* 1998;9:1370–1377.

21. Wolfe RR, Driscoll DJ, Gersony WM, et al. Arrhythmias in patients with valvar aortic stenosis, valvar pulmonary stenosis, and ventricular septal defect. *Circulation* 1993;87[Suppl I]: 89–101.

22. Otterstad JE, Nitter-Hauge S, Myhre E. Isolated ventricular septal defect in adults. *Br Heart J* 1983;50:343–348.

23. Neumayer U, Stone S, Somerville J. Small ventricular septal defects in adults. *Eur Heart J* 1998;19:1573–1582.

24. Anderson RH, Ho SY. The morphologic substrates for pediatric arrhythmias. *Cardiol Young* 1991;1:159–176.

25. Feldt RH, DuShane JW, Titus JL. The atrioventricular conduction system in persistent common atrioventricular canal defect. *Circulation* 1970;42:437–444.

26. Fournier A, Young M-L, Garcia OL, et al. Electrophysiologic

cardiac function before and after surgery in children with AV canal. *Am J Cardiol* 1986;57:1137–1141.

27. Marquis RM, Miller HC, McCormack RJM, et al. Persistence of ductus arteriosus with left to right shunt in the older patient. *Br Heart J* 1982;48:469–484.

28. McManus BM. Patent ductus arteriosus. In: Robertson C, ed. *Adult congenital heart disease.* Philadelphia: FA Davis, 1987: 455–476.

29. Deanfield JE, McKenna WJ, Presbitero P, et al. Ventricular arrhythmia in unrepaired and repaired tetralogy of Fallot. *Br Heart J* 1984;52:77–81.

30. Sullivan ID, Presbitero P, Gooch VM, et al. Is ventricular arrhythmia in repaired tetralogy of Fallot an effect of operation or a consequence of the course of the disease? *Br Heart J* 1987; 58:40–44.

31. Bush HL, Gelband H, Hoffman BF, et al. Electrophysiological basis for supraventricular arrhythmias following surgical procedures for aortic stenosis. *Arch Surg* 1971;103: 620–625.

32. Bisset GS, Meyer RA, Hirschfeld SS, et al. Aortic valve replacement in childhood: evaluation of left ventricular function by electrocardiography, echocardiography and graded exercise testing. *Am J Cardiol* 1983;52:568–572.

33. Bricker JT, Traweek MS, Danford DA, et al. Exercise related bundle branch block in children. *Am J Cardiol* 1985;56:796–797.

34. Klein RC. Ventricular arrhythmias in aortic valve disease: analysis of 102 patients. *Am J Cardiol* 1984;53:1079–1083.

35. von Olshausen K, Schwarz F, Appelbach J, et al. Determinants of the incidence and severity of ventricular arrhythmias in aortic valve disease. *Am J Cardiol* 1983;51:1103–1109.

36. Santinga JT, Kirsh MM, Brady TJ, et al. Left ventricular function in patients with ventricular arrhythmias and aortic valve disease. *Ann Thorac Surg* 1983;35:152–155.

37. DiNubile MJ, Calderwood SB, Steinhaus DM, et al. Cardiac conduction abnormalities complicating native valve active infective endocarditis. *Am J Cardiol* 1986;58:1213–1217.

38. Lev M, Silverman J, Fitzmaurice FM, et al. Lack of connection between the atria and the more peripheral conduction system in congenital atrioventricular block. *Am J Cardiol* 1971;27:481–490.

39. Bodlander JW. The Wolff-Parkinson-White syndrome in association with congenital heart disease: coarctation of the aorta. *Am Heart J* 1946;31:785–793.

40. Clark RJ, Firminger HI. Coarctation of the aorta associated with Adams-Stokes syndrome, complete heart block and bicuspid calcareous aortic valve. *N Engl J Med* 1949;240:710–714.

41. James TN, Jackson DA. De subitaneis mortibus: XXVII. Histological abnormalities in the sinus node, atrioventricular node and His bundle associated with coarctation of the aorta. *Circulation* 1977;56:1094–1102.

42. Terhune PE, Buchino JJ, Rees AH. Myocardial infarction associated with supravalvular aortic stenosis. *J Pediatr* 1985;106: 251–254.

43. Southall DP, Keeton BR, Leanage R, et al. Cardiac rhythm and conduction before and after Mustard's operation for complete transposition of the great arteries. *Br Heart J* 1980;43:21–30.

44. Martin RP, Radley-Smith R, Yocoub MH. Arrhythmias before and after anatomic correction of transposition of the great arteries. *J Am Coll Cardiol* 1987;10:200–204.

45. Huhta JC, Maloney JD, Ritter DG, et al. Complete atrioventricular block in patients with atrioventricular discordance. *Circulation* 1983;67:1374–1377.

46. Anderson RH, Becker AE, Arnold R, et al. The conducting tissues in congenitally corrected transposition. *Circulation* 1974; 50:911–923.

47. Daliento L, Corrado D, Buja G, et al. Rhythm and conduction disturbances in isolated, congenitally corrected transposition of the great arteries. *Am J Cardiol* 1986;58:314–318.

48. Kanter RJ, Pressley JC, Packer DL, et al. Impact of coexisting heart disease on outcome of surgery for the Wolff-Parkinson-White syndrome in children. *J Am Coll Cardiol* 1989;13:138A.

49. Fontaine JM, Kamal BM, Sokil AB, et al. Ventricular tachycardia: a life-threatening arrhythmia in a patient with congenitally corrected transposition of the great arteries. *J Cardiovasc Electrophysiol* 1998;9:517–522.

50. Presbitero P, Somerville J, Rabajoli F, et al. Corrected transposition of the great arteries without associated defects in adult patients: clinical profile and follow up. *Br Heart J* 1995;74: 57–59.

51. Prieto LR, Hordof AJ, Secic M, et al. Progressive tricuspid valve disease in patients with congenitally corrected transposition of the great arteries. *Circulation* 1998;98:997–1005.

52. Rossi L, Montella S, Frescura C, et al. Congenital atrioventricular block in right atrial isomerism (asplenia). *Chest* 1984;85: 578–580.

53. Dickinson DF, Wilkinson JL, Anderson KR, et al. The cardiac conduction system in situs ambiguus. *Circulation* 1979;59: 879–886.

54. Wren C, MacCartney FJ, Deanfield JE. Cardiorhythm in atrial isomerism. *Am J Cardiol* 1987;59:1156–1158.

55. Momma K, Takao A, Shibata T. Characteristics and natural history of abnormal atrial rhythms in left isomerism. *Am J Cardiol* 1990;65:231–236.

56. Garcia OL, Mehta AV, Pichoff AS, et al. Left isomerism and complete atrioventricular block: a report of six cases. *Am J Cardiol* 1981;48:1103–1107.

57. Kotcher AL. Familial asplenia, other malformations, and sudden death. *Pediatrics* 1980;65: 633–635.

58. Rao PS. *Tricuspid atresia.* Mt. Kisco, NY: Futura Publishing, 1992.

59. Dick M, Fyler DC, Nadas AS. Tricuspid atresia: clinical course in 101 patients. *Am J Cardiol* 1975;36:327–337.

60. Zellers TM, Porter C, Driscoll DJ. Pseudo-preexcitation in tricuspid atresia. *Tex Heart Inst J* 1991;18:124–126.

61. Dick M, Behrendt DM, Byrum CJ, et al. Tricuspid atresia and the Wolff-Parkinson-White syndrome: evaluation methodology and successful surgical treatment of the combined disorders. *Am Heart J* 101;1981:496–500.

62. Hajdu J, Marton T, Toth-Pal E, et al. Familial association of congenital left heart abnormalities and sustained fetal arrhythmia. *Pediatr Cardiol* 1999;20:368–370.

63. Becker AE, Wilkinson JL, Anderson RH. Atrioventricular conduction tissues: a guide in understanding the morphogenesis of the univentricular heart. In: Van Praagh R, Takao A, eds. *Etiology and morphogenesis of congenital heart disease.* Mount Kisco, NY: Futura Publishing, 1980.

64. Wilkinson JL, Dickinson D, Smith A, et al. Conducting tissues in univentricular heart of right ventricular type with double or common inlet. *J Thorac Cardiovasc Surg* 1979;77:691–698.

65. Clarkson PM, Frye RL, DuShane JW, et al. Prognosis for patients with ventricular septal defect and severe pulmonary vascular obstructive disease. *Circulation* 1968;38:129–135.

66. Young D, Mark H. Fate of the patient with the Eisenmenger syndrome. *Am J Cardiol* 1971;28:658–669.

67. Cantor WJ, Harrison DA, Moussadji JS, et al. Determinants of survival and length of survival in adults with Eisenmenger syndrome. *Am J Cardiol* 1999;84:677–681.

68. Hancock EW. Coronary sinus rhythm in sinus venosus defect and persistent left superior vena cava. *J Am Coll Cardiol* 1964; 14:608–615.

69. James TN, Marshall TK, Edwards JE. De subitaneis mortibus: XX. Cardiac electrical instability in the presence of a left superior vena cava. *Circulation* 1976;54:689–697.

70. Van Nooten G, Verbeet T, Deuvaert FE. Atrial perforation by a

screw-in electrode via a left superior vena cava. *Am Heart J* 1990;119:1439–1440.

71. Chaithiraphan S, Goldberg E, Wolff W, et al. Massive thrombosis of the coronary sinus as an unusual complication of transvenous pacemaker insertion in a patient with persistent left, and no right superior vena cava. *J Am Geriatr Soc* 1974;22:70–85.

72. Virmani R, Robinowitz M, Clark MA, et al. Sudden death and partial absence of the right ventricular myocardium: a report of three cases and a review of the literature. *Arch Pathol Lab Med* 1982;106:163–167.

73. Liberthson RR, Dinsmore RE, Bharati S, et al. Aberrant coronary artery origin from the aorta: diagnosis and clinical significance. *Circulation* 1974;50:774–779.

74. Cheitlin MD, DeCastro CM, McAllister HA. Sudden death as a complication of anomalous left coronary origin from the anterior sinus of Valsalva: a not-so-minor congenital anomaly. *Circulation* 1979;50:780–787.

75. Liberthson RR, Zaman L, Weyman A, et al. Aberrant origin of the left coronary artery from the proximal right coronary artery: diagnostic features and pre-and post-operative course. *Clin Cardiol* 1982;5:377–381.

76. Barth CW III, Roberts WC. Left main coronary artery originating from the right sinus of Valsalva and coursing between the aorta and pulmonary trunk. *J Am Coll Cardiol* 1986;7:366–373.

77. Roberts WC, Siegel RJ, Zipes DP. Origin of the right coronary artery from the left sinus of Valsalva and its functional consequences: analysis of 10 necropsy patients. *Am J Cardiol* 1982;49:363–368.

78. Liberthson RR, Gang DL, Custer J. Sudden death in an infant with aberrant origin of the right coronary artery from the left sinus of Valsalva of the aorta: case report and review of the literature. *Pediatr Cardiol* 1983;4:45–48.

79. Waller BF. Exercise-related sudden death in young (age ≤30 years) and old (age ≥30 years) conditioned subjects. *Cardiovasc Clin* 1985;15:9–73.

80. Topaz O, Edwards JE. Pathologic features of sudden death in children, adolescents, and young adults. *Chest* 1985;87:476–482.

81. Maron BJ, Roberts WC, McAllister HA, et al. Sudden death in young adults. *Arch Intern Med* 1988;148:303–308.

82. Driscoll DJ, Edwards WD. Sudden unexplained death in children and adolescents. *J Am Coll Cardiol* 1985;5:118B–121B.

83. Berdoff R, Haimowitz A, Kupersmith J. Anomalous origin of the right coronary artery from the left sinus of Valsalva. *Am J Cardiol* 1986;58:656–657.

84. Morales AR, Romanelli R, Boucek RJ. The mural left anterior descending coronary artery, strenuous exercise, and sudden death. *Circulation* 1980;62:230–237.

85. Shen EN, Fukuyama O, Herre JM, et al Ventricular tachycardia with congenital ventricular diverticulum. *Chest* 1991;100:283–285.

86. Fellows CL, Bardy GH, Ivey TD, et al. Ventricular dysrhythmias associated with congenital left ventricular aneurysms. *Am J Cardiol* 1986;57:997–999.

87. Suwa M, Hirota Y, Kaku K, et al. Prevalence of the coexistence of left ventricular false tendons and premature ventricular complexes in apparently healthy subjects. *J Am Coll Cardiol* 1988;12:910–914.

88. Suwa M, Yoneda Y, Nagao H, et al. Surgical correction of idiopathic paroxysmal ventricular tachycardia possibly related to left ventricular false tendon. *Am J Cardiol* 1989;64:1217–1220.

89. Garson A, Gillette PC, Titus JL, et al. Surgical treatment of ventricular tachycardia in infants. *N Engl J Med* 1984;310:1443–1445.

90. Nadas AS, Ellison RC. Cardiac tumors in infancy. *Am J Cardiol* 1968;21:363–366.

91. Simcha A, Wells BG, Tynan MJ, et al. Primary cardiac tumors in childhood. *Arch Dis Child* 1971;46:508–514.

92. Arcinegus E, Hakimi M, Farooki ZQ, et al. Primary cardiac tumors in children. *J Thorac Cardiovasc Surg* 1980;79:582–591.

93. Case CL, Gillette PC, Crawford FA. Cardiac rhabdomyoma causing supraventricular and lethal ventricular arrhythmias in an infant. *Am Heart J* 1991;122:1484–1486.

94. Ferrans VJ, McAllister HA, Haese WH. Infantile cardiomyopathy with histiocytoid change in cardiac muscle cells. *Circulation* 1976;53:708–719.

95. Garson A, Smith RT, Moak JP, et al. Incessant ventricular tachycardia in infants: myocardial hamartomas and surgical cure. *J Am Coll Cardiol* 1987;10:619–626.

96. Packer DL, Bardy GH, Worley SJ, et al. Tachycardia-induced cardiomyopathy: a reversible form of left ventricular dysfunction. *Am J Cardiol* 1986;57:563–570.

97. Gillette PC, Smith RT, Garson A, et al. Chronic supraventricular tachycardia: a curable cause of congestive cardiomyopathy. *JAMA* 1985;253:391–392.

98. Coleman HN, Taylor RR, Pool PE, et al. Congestive heart failure following chronic tachycardia. *Am Heart J* 1971;81:790–798.

99. Gillette PC, Wampler DG, Garson A, et al. Treatment of atrial automatic tachycardia by ablation procedures. *J Am Coll Cardiol* 1985;6:405–409.

100. McLaran CJ, Bersh BJ, Sugrue DD, et al. Tachycardia-induced myocardial dysfunction—a reversible phenomenon? *Br Heart J* 1985;53:323–327.

101. Tomita M, Spinale FG, Crawford FA, et al. Changes in left ventricular volume, mass, and function during the development and regression of supraventricular tachycardia-induced cardiomyopathy. *Circulation* 1991;83:635–644.

102. Garson A, Gillette PC, Titus JL, et al. Surgical treatment of ventricular tachycardia in infants. *Med Intelligence* 1984;310:1443–1449.

103. Spinale FG, Tanaka R, Crawford FA, et al. Changes in myocardial blood flow during development of and recovery from tachycardia-induced cardiomyopathy. *Circulation* 1992;85:717–729.

104. Spinale FG, Hendrick DA, Crawford FA, et al. Chronic supraventricular tachycardia causes ventricular dysfunction and subendocardial injury in swine. *Am J Physiol* 1990;259:H218–H229.

105. Villain E, Vetter VL, Garcia JM, et al. Evolving concepts in the management of congenital junctional tachycardia: a multicenter study. *Circulation* 1990;81:1544–1549.

106. Reimer A, Paul T, Kallfelz H-C. Efficacy and safety of intravenous and oral propafenone in pediatric cardiac dysrhythmias. *Am J Cardiol* 1991;68:741–744.

107. Bolens M, Friedli B. Junctional ectopic tachycardia with a benign course in a premature infant. *Pediatr Cardiol* 1990;11:216–218.

108. Maragnes P, Fournier A, Davignon A. Usefulness of oral sotalol for the treatment of junctional ectopic tachycardia. *Int J Cardiol* 1992;35:165–167.

109. Brechenmacher C, Coumel P, James TM. De subitaneis mortibus: XVI. Intractable tachycardia in infancy. *Circulation* 1976;53:377–381.

110. Bharati S, Moskowitz WB, Scheinman M. Junctional tachycardias: anatomic substrate and its significance in ablative procedures. *J Am Coll Cardiol* 1991;18:179–186.

111. Hamdan M, Van Hare GF, Fisher W, et al. Selective catheter ablation of the tachycardia focus in patients with nonreentrant junctional tachycardia. *Am J Cardiol* 1996;78:1292–1297.

112. Ehlert FA, Goldberger JJ, Deal BJ, et al. Successful radiofrequency energy ablation of automatic junctional tachycardia preserving normal atrioventricular nodal conduction. *Pacing Clin Electrophysiol* 1993;16:54–61.

113. Van Hare GF, Velvis H, Langberg JJ. Successful transcatheter ablation of congenital junctional ectopic tachycardia in a ten-month-old infant using radiofrequency energy. *Pacing Clin Electrophysiol* 1990;13:730–735.

114. Garson A. Supraventricular tachycardia. In: Gillette PC, Garson A, eds. *Pediatric cardiac dysrhythmias.* New York: Grune & Stratton, 1981:177–253.

115. Gelb BD, Garson A. Noninvasive discrimination of right atrial ectopic tachycardia from sinus tachycardia in "dilated cardiomyopathy." *Am Heart J* 1990;120:886–891.

116. Mehta AV, Sanchez GR, Sacks EJ, et al. Ectopic automatic atrial tachycardia in children: clinical characteristics, management, and follow-up. *J Am Coll Cardiol* 1988;11:379–385.

117. Evans VL, Garson A, Smith RT, et al. Ethmozine (moricizine HCl): a promising drug for "automatic" atrial ectopic tachycardia. *Am J Cardiol* 1987;60:83F–86F.

118. Kunze K-P, Kuck K-H, Schluter M, et al. Effect of encainide and flecainide on chronic ectopic atrial tachycardia. *J Am Coll Cardiol* 1986;7:1121–1126.

119. Colloridi V, Perri C, Ventriglia F, et al. Oral sotalol in pediatric atrial ectopic tachycardia. *Am Heart J* 1992;123:254–256.

120. Lawrie GM, Lin H-T. Wyndham CRC, et al. Surgical treatment of supraventricular tachycardia arrhythmias. *Ann Surg* 1987; 205:700–711.

121. Gillette PC, Wampler DG, Garson A, et al. Treatment of atrial automatic tachycardia by ablation procedures. *J Am Coll Cardiol* 1985;6:405–409.

122. Grant JW, Serwer GA, Armstrong BE, et al. Junctional tachycardia in infants and children after open heart surgery for congenital heart disease. *Am J Cardiol* 1987;59:1216–1218.

123. Bach SE, Shah JJ, Albers WH, et al. Hypothermia for the treatment of postsurgical greatly accelerated junctional ectopic tachycardia. *J Am Coll Cardiol* 1987;10:1095–1099.

124. Till JA, Rowland E. Atrial pacing as an adjunct to the management of post-surgical His bundle tachycardia. *Br Heart J* 1991; 66:225–229.

125. Garson A, Gillette PC. Junctional ectopic tachycardia in children: electrocardiography, electrophysiology, and pharmacologic response. *Am J Cardiol* 1979;44: 298–302.

126. Mehta AV, Subrahmanyam AB, Long JB, et al. Experience with moricizine HCl in children with supraventricular tachycardia. *Int J Cardiol* 1996;57:31–35.

127. Perry JC, Fenrich AL, Hulse JE, et al. Pediatric use of intravenous amiodarone: efficacy and safety in critically ill patients from a multicenter protocol. *J Am Coll Cardiol* 1996;27: 1246–1250.

128. Vignati G, Mauri L, Figini A. The use of propafenone in the treatment of tachyarrhythmias in children. *Eur Heart J* 1993; 14:546–550.

129. Walsh EP, Saul JP, Sholler GF, et al. Evaluation of a staged treatment protocol for rapid automatic junctional tachycardia after operation for congenital heart disease. *J Am Coll Cardiol* 1997; 29:1046–1053.

130. Pfammatter JP, Paul T, Ziemer G, et al. Successful management of junctional tachycardia by hypothermia after cardiac operations in infants. 1995;60:556–560.

131. Gillette PC, Garson A, Porter CJ, et al. Junctional automatic ectopic tachycardia: new proposed treatment by transcatheter His bundle ablation. *Am Heart J* 1983;106:619–623.

132. Fullerton DA, St Cyr JA, Clarke DR, et al. Bezold- Jarisch reflex in postoperative pediatric cardiac surgical patients. *Ann Thorac Surg* 1991;52:534–536.

133. Martin TC, Smith L, Hernandez A, et al. Dysrhythmias following the Senning operation for dextro-transposition of the great arteries. *J Thorac Cardiovasc Surg* 1983;85:928–932.

134. Hayes CJ, Gersony WM. Arrhythmias after the Mustard oper-

ation for transposition of the great arteries: a long-term study. *J Am Coll Cardiol* 1986;7:133–137.

135. Warnes CA, Somerville J. Transposition of the great arteries: late results in adolescents and adults after the Mustard procedure. *Br Heart J* 1987;58:148–155.

136. Gewillig M, Cullen S, Mertens B, et al. Risk factors for arrhythmia and death after Mustard operation for simple transposition of the great arteries. *Circulation* 1991;84[Suppl III]:187–192.

137. Vetter VL, Tanner CS, Horowitz LN. Electrophysiologic consequences of the Mustard repair of d-transposition of the great arteries. *J Am Coll Cardiol* 1987;10:1265–1273.

138. Garson A, Bink-Boelkens M, Hesslein PS, et al. Atrial flutter in the young: a collaborative study of 380 cases. *J Am Coll Cardiol* 1985;6:871–878.

139. Flinn CJ, Wolff GS, Campbell RM, et al. Natural history of supraventricular rhythms in 182 children following the Mustard operation. *J Am Coll Cardiol* 1983;1:613–618.

140. Turina M, Siebenmann R, Nussbaumer P, et al. Long-term outlook after atrial correction of transposition of great arteries. *J Thorac Cardiovasc Surg* 1988;95:828–835.

141. Turley K, Hanley FL, Verrier ED, et al. The Mustard procedure in infants (less than 100 days of age): ten year follow-up. *J Thorac Cardiovasc Surg* 1988;96:849–853.

142. Puley G, Siu S, Connelly M, et al. Arrhythmia and survival in patients >18 years of age after the Mustard procedure for complete transposition of the great arteries. *Am J Cardiol* 1999;83: 1080–1084.

143. Helbing WA, Hansen B, Ottenkamp J, et al. Long-term results of atrial correction for transposition of the great arteries. *J Thorac Cardiovasc Surg* 1994;108:363–372.

144. Vetter VL, Tanner CS, Horowitz LN. Inducible atrial flutter after the Mustard repair of complete transposition of the great arteries. *Am J Cardiol* 1988;61:428–435.

145. Lucet V, Batisse A, Nyoc DD, et al. Troubles du rhythme apres corrections atriales des transpositions des gros vaisseaux. *Arch Mal Coeur* 1986;79:640–647.

146. Weber HS, Hellenbrand WE, Kleinman CS, et al. Predictors of rhythm disturbances and subsequent morbidity after the Fontan operation. *Am J Cardiol* 1989;64:762–767.

147. Driscoll DJ, Offord KP, Feldt RH, et al. Five- to fifteen-year follow-up after Fontan operation. *Circulation* 1992;85:469–496.

148. Gewillig M, Wyse RK, DeLeval MR, et al. Early and late arrhythmias after the Fontan operation: predisposing factors and clinical consequences. *Br Heart J* 1992;67:72–79.

149. Girod DA, Fontan F, Deville C, et al. Long-term results after the Fontan operation for tricuspid atresia. *Circulation* 1987;75:605–610.

150. Peters NS, Somerville J. Arrhythmias after the Fontan procedure. *Br Heart J* 1992;68:199–204.

151. Rodefeld MD, Bromberg BI, Schuessler RB, et al. Atrial flutter after lateral tunnel construction in the modified Fontan procedure: a canine model. *J Thorac Cardiovasc Surg* 1996;111: 514–526.

152. Gardiner HM, Dhillon R, Bull C, et al. Prospective study of the incidence and determinants of arrhythmia after total cavopulmonary connection. *Circulation* 1996;94[Suppl II]:17–21.

153. Viullo DA, DeLeon SY, Berry TE, et al. Clinical improvement after revision in Fontan patients. *Ann Thorac Surg* 1996;61: 1797–1804.

154. Hashimoto K, Kurosawa H, Tanaka A, et al. Total cavopulmonary connection without the use of prosthetic material: technical considerations and hemodynamic consequences. *J Thorac Cardiovasc Surg* 1995;110:625–632.

155. Pearl JM, Laks H, Stein DG, et al. Total cavopulmonary anastomosis versus conventional modified Fontan procedure. *Ann Thorac Surg* 1991;52:189–196.

156. Amodeo A, Galletti L, Marianeschi S, et al. Extracardiac Fontan operation for complex cardiac anomalies: seven years' experience. *J Thorac Cardiovasc Surg* 1997;114:1020–1030.

157. Weber HS, Gleason MM, Myers JL, et al. The Fontan operation in infants less than 2 years of age. *J Am Coll Cardiol* 1992;19:828–833.

158. Rosenthal E, Bostock J, Gill J. Iatrogenic atrioventricular bypass tract following a Fontan operation for tricuspid atresia. *Heart* 1997;77:283–285.

159. Mair DD, Hagler DJ, Julsrud PR, et al. Early and late results of the modified Fontan procedure for double-inlet left ventricle: the Mayo Clinic experience. *J Am Coll Cardiol* 1991;18:1727–1732.

160. Taliercio CP, Vlietstra RE, McGoon MD, et al. Permanent cardiac pacing after the Fontan procedure. *J Thorac Cardiovasc Surg* 1985;90:414–419.

161. Manning PB, Mayer JE Jr, Wernovsky G, et al. Staged operation to Fontan increases the incidence of sinoatrial node dysfunction. *J Thorac Cardiovasc Surg* 1996;111:833–839.

162. Davis JT, Ehrlich R, Hennessey JR, et al. Long-term follow-up of cardiac rhythm in repaired total anomalous pulmonary venous drainage. *Thorac Cardiovasc Surg* 1986;34:172–175.

163. Portman MA, Beder SD, Cohen MH, et al. Conduction abnormalities detected by electrophysiologic testing following repair of ostium primum atrioventricular septal defect. *Int J Cardiol* 1986;11:111–119.

164. Murphy JG, Gersh BJ, McGoon MD, et al. Long-term outcome after surgical repair of isolated atrial septal defect. *N Engl J Med* 1990;323:1645–1650.

165. Wernovsky G, Hougen TJ, Walsh EP, et al. Midterm results after the arterial switch operation for transposition of the great arteries with intact ventricular septum: clinical, hemodynamic, echocardiographic, and electrophysiologic data. *Circulation* 1988;77:1333–1344.

166. Kramer H-H, Rammos S, Krogmann O, et al. Cardiac rhythm after Mustard repair and after arterial switch operation for complete transposition. *Int J Cardiol* 1991;32:5–12.

167. Rhodes LA, Wernovsky G, Keane JF, et al. Arrhythmias and intracardiac conduction after the arterial switch operation. *J Thorac Cardiovasc Surg* 1995;109:303–310.

168. Hesslein PS, Gutgesell HP, Gillette PC. Exercise assessment of sinoatrial node function in children after Mustard's operation. *Pediatr Res* 1980;14:445–451.

169. Saalouke MG, Rios J, Perry LW, et al. Electrophysiologic studies after Mustard's operation for d-transposition of the great vessels. *Am J Cardiol* 1978;41:1104–1109.

170. Gillette PC, Kugler JD, Garson A, et al. Mechanisms of cardiac arrhythmias after the Mustard operation for transposition of the great arteries. *Am J Cardiol* 1980;45:1225–1230.

171. Kurer CC, Tanner CS, Vetter VL. Electrophysiologic findings after Fontan repair of functional single ventricle. *J Am Coll Cardiol* 1991;17:174–181.

172. Dreifus LS. Guidelines for implantation of cardiac pacemaker and antiarrhythmia devices. *J Am Coll Cardiol* 1991;18:1–13.

173. Gillette PC, Wampler DG, Shannon C, et al. Use of cardiac pacing after the Mustard operation for transposition of the great arteries. *J Am Coll Cardiol* 1986;7:138–141.

174. Gillette PC, Zeigler V, Case CL, et al. Atrial antitachycardia pacing in children and young adults. *Am Heart J* 1991;122:844–849.

175. Porter CJ, Fukushige J, Hayes DL, et al. Permanent antitachycardia pacing for chronic atrial tachyarrhythmias in post-operative pediatric patients. *Pacing Clin Electrophysiol* 1991;14:2056–2057.

176. Karpawich PP, Paridon SM, Pinsky WW. Failure of rate-responsive ventricular pairing to improve physiological performance in the univentricular heart. *Pacing Clin Electrophysiol* 1991;14:2058–2061.

177. Van Hare GF, Lesh MD, Ross BA, et al. Mapping and radiofrequency ablation of intraatrial reentrant tachycardia after the Senning or Mustard procedures for transposition of the great arteries. *Am J Cardiol* 1996;77:985–991.

178. Kanter RJ, Papagiannis J, Carboni MP, et al. Radiofrequency catheter ablation of supraventricular tachycardia substrates after Mustard and Senning operations for d-transposition of the great arteries. *J Am Coll Cardiol* 2000;35:428–441.

179. Fishberger SB, Wernovsky G, Gentles TL, et al. Long-term outcome in patients with pacemakers following the Fontan operation. *Am J Cardiol* 1996;77:887–889.

180. Kalman JM, Van Hare GF, Olgin JE, et al. Ablation of 'incisional' reentrant atrial tachycardia complicating surgery for congenital heart disease: use of entrainment to define critical isthmus of conduction. *Circulation* 1996;93:502–512.

181. Triedman JK, Saul JP, Weindling SN, et al. Radiofrequency ablation of intra-atrial reentrant tachycardia after surgical palliation of congenital heart disease. *Circulation* 1995;91:707–714.

182. Baker BM, Lindsay BD, Bromberg BI, et al. Catheter ablation of clinical intraatrial reentrant tachycardias resulting from previous atrial surgery: localizing and transecting the critical isthmus. *J Am Coll Cardiol* 1996;28:411–417.

183. Dorostkar PC, Cheng J, Scheinman MM. Electroanatomical mapping and ablation of the substrate supporting intraatrial reentrant tachycardia after palliation for complex congenital heart disease. *Pacing Clin Electrophysiol* 1998;21:1810–1819.

184. Mavroudis C, Backer CL, Deal BJ, et al. Fontan conversion to cavopulmonary connection and arrhythmia circuit cryoablation. *J Thorac Cardiovasc Surg* 1998;115:547–556.

185. Deal BJ, Mavroudis C, Backer CL, et al. Impact of arrhythmia circuit cryoablation during Fontan conversion for refractory atrial tachycardia. *Am J Cardiol* 1999;83:563–568.

186. Garson A, Nihill MR, McNamara DG, et al. Status of the adult and adolescent after repair of tetralogy of Fallot. *Circulation* 1979;59:1232–1240.

187. Kavey RE, Blackman MS, Londheimer HM. Incidence and severity of chronic ventricular dysrhythmias after repair of tetralogy of Fallot. *Am Heart J* 1982;103:342–350.

188. Fuster V, McGoon DC, Kennedy MA. Long-term evaluation (12–22 years) of open heart surgery for tetralogy of Fallot. *Am J Cardiol* 1980;46:635–640.

189. Walsh EP, Rockenmacher S, Keane JF, et al. Late results in patients with tetralogy of Fallot repaired during infancy. *Circulation* 1988;77:1062–1067.

190. Deal BJ, Scagliotti D, Miller SM, et al. Electrophysiologic drug testing in symptomatic ventricular arrhythmias after repair of tetralogy of Fallot. *Am J Cardiol* 1987;59:1380–1385.

191. Chandar JS, Wolff GS, Garson A, et al. Ventricular arrhythmias in postoperative tetralogy of Fallot. *Am J Cardiol* 1990;65:655–661.

192. Moller JH, Patton C, Varco RL, et al. Postoperative ventricular septal defect: 24–30 years' follow-up of 232 patients. In: *Proceedings of the Second World Congress of Pediatric Cardiology.* New York: Springer-Verlag, 1985:20.

193. Shen W-K, Holmes DR, Porter CJ, et al. Sudden death after repair of double-outlet right ventricle. *Circulation* 1990;81:128–136.

194. Fyfe DA, Driscoll DJ, DiDonato RM, et al. Truncus arteriosus with single pulmonary artery: influence of pulmonary vascular obstructive disease on early and late operative results. *J Am Coll Cardiol* 1985;5:1168–1172.

195. Wolff GS, Rowland TW, Ellison RC. Surgically induced right bundle branch block with left anterior hemiblock. *Circulation* 1972;45:587–593.

196. Quattlebaum TG, Varghese PJ, Neill CA, et al. Sudden death

among postoperative patients with tetralogy of Fallot: a follow-up study of 243 patients for an average of twelve years. *Circulation* 1975;54:289–293.

197. Friedli B, Bolens M. Intraventricular conduction disturbances after correction of tetralogy of Fallot: can bifascicular and trifascicular block be diagnosed from the surface ECG. *Pediatr Cardiol* 1985;6:133–136.

198. Garson A Jr, Gillette PC, Gutgesell HP, et al. Stress-induced ventricular arrhythmia after repair of tetralogy of Fallot. *Am J Cardiol* 1980;46:1006–1012.

199. Deanfield JE, McKenna WJ, Hallidie-Smith KA. Detection of late arrhythmia and conduction disturbance after correction of tetralogy of Fallot. *Br Heart J* 1980;44:248–253.

200. Katz NM, Blackstone EH, Kirklin JW, et al. Late survival and symptoms after repair of tetralogy of Fallot. *Circulation* 1982;65:403–410.

201. Kobayashi J, Hirose H, Nakano S, et al. Ambulatory electrocardiographic study of the frequency and cause of ventricular arrhythmia after correction of tetralogy of Fallot. *Am J Cardiol* 1984;54:1310–1313.

202. Horowitz LN, Vetter VL, Harken AH, et al. Electrophysiologic characteristics of sustained ventricular tachycardia occurring after repair of tetralogy of Fallot. *Am J Cardiol* 1980;46:446–452.

203. Silka MJ, Cutler JE, Kron J. Catecholamine-dependent ventricular tachycardia following repair of tetralogy of Fallot. *Am Heart J* 1991;122:586–587.

204. Garson A. Ventricular arrhythmias after congenital heart surgery: a canine model. *Pediatr Res* 1984;18:1112–1120.

205. Erickson CC, Sprague K, Garson A. Pulmonary insufficiency: a risk factor for ventricular arrhythmias in animals with right ventriculotomy. *J Am Coll Cardiol* 1991;17:153A.

206. Gatzoulis MA, Till JA, Somerville J, et al. Mechanoelectrical interaction in tetralogy of Fallot: QRS prolongation relates to right ventricular size and predicts malignant ventricular arrhythmias and sudden death. *Circulation* 1995;92:231–237.

207. Berul CI, Hill SL, Geggel RL, et al. Electrocardiographic markers of late sudden death risk in postoperative tetralogy of Fallot children. *J Cardiovasc Electrophysiol* 1997;8:1349–1356.

208. Garson A, Randall DC, Gillette PC, et al. Prevention of sudden death after repair of tetralogy of Fallot: treatment of ventricular arrhythmias. *J Am Coll Cardiol* 1985;6:221–227.

209. Harrsion DA, Harris L, Siu SC, et al. Sustained ventricular tachycardia in adult patients late after repair of tetralogy of Fallot. *J Am Coll Cardiol* 1997;30:1368–1373.

210. Cullen S, Celermajer DS, Franklin RCG, et al. Prognostic significance of ventricular arrhythmia after repair of tetralogy of Fallot: A 12-year prospective study. *J Am Coll Cardiol* 1994;23:1151–1155.

211. Rovamo L, Makijarvi M, Pesonen E, et al. Late potentials on signal-averaged electrocardiograms in children after right ventriculotomy. *Pediatr Cardiol* 1995;16:114–119.

212. Alexander ME, Walsh EP, Saul JP, et al. Value of programmed ventricular stimulation in patients with congenital heart disease. *J Cardiovasc Electrophysiol* 1999;10:1033–1044.

213. Roos-Hesselink J, Perlroth MG, McGhie J, et al. Atrial arrhythmias in adults after repair of tetralogy of Fallot. Correlations with clinical, exercise, and echocardiographic findings. *Circulation* 1995;91:2214–2219.

214. Kugler JD, Cheatham JP, Gumbiner CH, et al. Results of phenytoin and propranolol drug electrophysiology studies for ventricular tachycardia in patients having repaired lesions with tetralogy of Fallot physiology. *Circulation* 1985;72:III-341.

215. Reimer A, Paul T, Kallfelz HC. Efficacy and safety of intravenous and oral propafenone in pediatric cardiac dysrhythmias. *Am J Cardiol* 1991;68:741–744.

216. Downar E, Harris L, Kimber S, et al. Ventricular tachycardia after surgical repair of tetralogy of Fallot: results of intraoperative mapping studies. *J Am Coll Cardiol* 1992;20:648–655.

217. Horton RP, Canby RC, Kessler DJ, et al. Ablation of ventricular tachycardia associated with tetralogy of Fallot: demonstration of bidirectional block. *J Cardiovasc Electrophysiol* 1997;8:432–435.

218. Papagiannis J, Kanter RJ, Wharton JM. Radiofrequency catheter ablation of multiple haemodynamically unstable ventricular tachycardias in a patient with surgically repaired tetralogy of Fallot. *Cardiol Young* 1998;8:379–382.

219. Silka MJ, Kron J, Dunnigan A, et al. Sudden cardiac death and the use of implantable cardioverter-defibrillators in pediatric patients. *Circulation* 1993;87:800–807.

220. Pressley JC, Wharton JM, Tang ASL, et al. Effect of Ebstein's anomaly on short- and long-term outcome of surgically treated patients with Wolff-Parkinson-White syndrome. *Circulation* 1992;86:1147–1155.

221. Senni M, Chauvaud S, Crupi G, et al. Early and intermediate results of Carpentier's repair for Ebstein's anomaly. *Giorn Ital Cardiol* 1996;26:1415–1420.

222. O'Connor BK, Beekman RH, Lindauer A, et al. Intermediate-term outcome after pulmonary balloon valvuloplasty: comparison with a matched surgical control group. *J Am Coll Cardiol* 1992;20:169–173.

223. Hokken RB, Bogers AJ, Spitaels SE, et al. Pulmonary homograft insertion after repair of pulmonary stenosis. *J Heart Valve Dis* 1995;4:182–186.

224. Daliento L, Rizzoli G, Marchiori MC, et al. Electrical instability in patients undergoing surgery for atrioventricular septal defect. *Int J Cardiol* 1991;30:15–21.

225. Silka MJ, Hardy BG, Menashe VD, et al. A population-based prospective evaluation of risk of sudden cardiac death after operation for common congenital heart defects. *J Am Coll Cardiol* 1998;32:245–251.

27

ARRHYTHMIAS AND CONDUCTION DISTURBANCES ASSOCIATED WITH PREGNANCY

SAMER R. DIBS
LESLIE A. SAXON

The arrhythmias and conduction disturbances associated with pregnancy can originate in the mother's gravida or her fetus. This chapter focuses on the spectrum of rhythm and conduction disturbances and their diagnosis and treatment in the setting of normal cardiac structure and function and in the setting of acquired or congenital malformations of the heart and circulation (1). The arrhythmias or conduction defects per se or any given therapeutic strategy potentially affect the mother and the fetus (1–12).

EPIDEMIOLOGY OF HEART DISEASE AND PREGNANCY

Epidemiologic information must consider the population under study, particularly comparisons between populations in developed and underdeveloped countries. In Western Europe and North America, maternal mortality from all causes has been steadily decreasing for decades. Advances in cardiovascular medicine, obstetrics, anesthesiology, and reproductive biology have resulted in a substantial improvement in safety for the mother and the fetus. The frequency of pregnancy complicated by heart disease does not appear to have changed significantly during the past several decades, ranging from 0.4% to just more than 4% (13,14). The major changes have been the steady decline in maternal mortality rates and changes in the relative incidence of the various types of cardiac disorders in pregnant women. In the 1950s, cardiac disease was the second leading cause of maternal death, reflecting a high incidence of rheumatic fever in childhood and rheumatic heart disease in adults. In

North America and Europe, there has been a dramatic decrease in the incidence of rheumatic fever, as well as a decline in its severity and in the incidence of subsequent rheumatic heart disease. The decrease in frequency of rheumatic heart disease in pregnancy has coincided with an increase in maternal congenital heart disease. Although the rate of occurrence of congenital heart disease remains relatively constant at 0.6% to 0.8% of live births (14–16), advances in diagnostic techniques and in the surgical and medical care of women with congenital malformations of the heart and circulation permit an increasing number of women with disorders that were previously fatal in early life to reach reproductive age (17,18).

HEMODYNAMIC AND ELECTROCARDIOGRAPHIC CHANGES IN NORMAL PREGNANCY

New-onset, or latent, arrhythmias may become manifest during pregnancy partly because of the altered hemodynamic state (19,20) and partly because of hormonal (21) and autonomic (22) changes. Alternatively, the arrhythmias may reflect worsening of preexisting structural heart disease or newly acquired cardiac or metabolic disorders (23–43).

Knowledge of the circulatory adjustments that accompany gestation, labor, delivery, and the puerperium is basic to an understanding of the diagnosis and management of arrhythmias and conduction disturbances in the gravid patient (19,44,45). Hormonally mediated decreases in systemic vascular resistance and increases in blood volume and cardiac output of 30% to 50%, compared with pregestational levels, provide for the needs of the developing fetus (19,46). Cardiac output is increased by 5 weeks after the last menstrual period and increases until 24 weeks, after which time, it does not change significantly until term.

S. R. Dibs: Department of EP/Cardiology, Northwestern University, Chicago, Illinois 60611.

L. A. Saxon: Department of Medicine, University of California, San Francisco, California 94143.

TABLE 27-1. HEMODYNAMIC CHANGES DURING PREGNANCY

Parameter	Precon	5 wk	8 wk	12 wk	24 wk	36 wk	38 wk	SE
HR (bpm)	75	79	80	83	84	88	87	1
SV (mL)	65.8	68.6	76.9	82.8	86.5	84.0	83.6	1.3
CO (L/min)	4.88	5.40	6.12	6.72	7.21	7.34	7.22	0.11
SVR (dyn/s.cm^5)	1,326	1,213	1,052	943	902	966	966	22
SBP (mm Hg)	108	109	107	106	108	114	114	2
DBP (mm Hg)	67	66	63	64	65	71	72	1

Note: Values quoted are means preconception (precon) and at specified weeks of gestation; standard error (SE) determined by analysis of variance. HR, heart rate; SV, aortic stroke volume; CO, aortic cardiac output; SVR, systemic vascular resistance; SBP, systolic blood pressure; DBP, diastolic blood pressure.
(From Robson SC, Hunter S, Boys R, et al. Serial study of factors influencing changes in cardiac output during human pregnancy. *Am J Physiol* 1989;256:H1060–H1065, with permission.)

Heart rate and stroke volume contribute to cardiac output increases. Heart rate is increased by 5 weeks of gestation and continues to increase until 32 weeks, after which time, it does not significantly change until term; 10% of pregnant women will have sinus tachycardia (20). Stroke volume starts increasing between 5 and 8 weeks and reaches a maximum level at 20 weeks, after which time, it does not change significantly until the last month when it may decrease slightly (Table 27-1) (19).

The surface electrocardiogram (ECG) may exhibit subtle changes during normal pregnancy. QT-interval shortening and slight PR interval shortening may accompany increases in heart rate (46,47). Frontal lead QRS axis changes are minor despite significant elevation of the diaphragm (47). Nonspecific abnormalities of the ST segments and T waves may be seen in pregnancy (48). Horizontal or downsloping ST depression with exercise was observed in 20% to 25% of healthy pregnant women, not significantly different from age-matched healthy nonpregnant women (48).

Heart rate variability data from Holter monitor recordings have been analyzed in healthy (and preeclamptic) pregnant women, to evaluate cardiac autonomic modulation changes (49–54). Total heart rate variability is reduced in normal pregnancy, and some studies suggest a shift of sympathovagal balance toward vagal withdrawal and sympathetic dominance (49,51).

PREGNANCY IN THE PRESENCE OF STRUCTURAL HEART DISEASE

The clinical and hemodynamic consequences of arrhythmias and conduction defects during pregnancy largely depend on the underlying heart disease (46). Poor maternal functional class or cyanosis, myocardial dysfunction, left heart obstruction, prior arrhythmia, and prior cardiac events (heart failure, transient ischemic attack, or stroke) not resulting from a cardiac intervention are predictive of maternal cardiac complications, including new-onset heart failure, symptomatic tachyarrhythmia or bradyarrhythmia,

stroke or transient ischemic attack of cardiac origin, and cardiac death. Poor maternal functional class or cyanosis is also predictive of neonatal events, defined as prematurity, "small for gestational age" birth weight, respiratory distress syndrome, intraventricular hemorrhage after birth, neonatal death, or still birth (23).

Acquired heart disease is present in a small proportion of pregnant women (10). Loss of atrial contribution to ventricular filling, as occurs in atrial fibrillation, may cause hemodynamic and clinical deterioration in severe aortic or mitral stenosis and regurgitation, hypertrophic cardiomyopathy, or hypertensive heart disease. Tachycardia in patients with coronary artery disease may precipitate ischemia. Also, tachycardia may have adverse effects on left ventricular filling and output in severe mitral stenosis and in conditions associated with left ventricular diastolic dysfunction. Bradycardia, on the other hand, may be detrimental in patients with chronic severe aortic regurgitation (55).

Congenital heart disease may complicate pregnancy (Table 27-2) (14,24–27,56–58). In patients with cyanotic congenital heart disease, tachycardia may precipitate hypercyanotic episodes as a result of increased right-to-left shunting (58). Pharmacologic or electrical conversion to normal sinus rhythm serves to improve symptoms and cardiac performance (59).

ASYMPTOMATIC ARRHYTHMIAS AND CONDUCTION DEFECTS

The incidence of asymptomatic atrial and ventricular premature complexes at various stages of pregnancy is unknown. Data from 24-hour Holter monitoring demonstrate that isolated atrial and ventricular premature beats occur in 58% and 40% respectively, in pregnant women who have no symptom of arrhythmia, which is not significantly different from their incidence in pregnant women with complaints of palpitations, dizziness, presyncope, or syncope who are otherwise healthy. Whereas only a small minority of either group of patients had frequent atrial premature beats (10 or more per

TABLE 27-2. SIGNIFICANT ARRHYTHMIAS AND CONDUCTION DISTURBANCES IN CONGENITAL HEART DISEASE (CHD)

CHD	Preoperative Arrhythmias	Postoperative Arrhythmias	Pregnancy Issues
ASD	Ectopic atrial rhythm (SV) AFL/AF (OS, OP) PR prolongation (OS, OP) Advanced AV block (OP)	Sinus node dysfunction (SV, OS, OP) Ectopic atrial rhythm (SV) AFL/AF (OS, OP) Advanced/complete AV block (OP)	Pregnancy generally well tolerated Preop: large ASD: heart failure may develop Preop: SVT may cause RV failure, risk of deep venous thrombosis, paradoxical embolism
VSD	AV block (membranous VSD) VT/VF	PR prolongation RBBB, RBBB/LAFB, Complete AV block	Pregnancy usually well tolerated Preop: nonrestrictive VSD with Eisenmenger reaction: decreased systemic arterial resistance and increased systemic venous return increase right-to-left shunt and decrease PaO_2
TOF	VPCs, VT/VF	Sinus node dysfunction AT/AFL/AF PR prolongation RBBB, RBBB/LAFB, Advanced/complete AV block VPCs, VT	Preop: decreased systemic arterial resistance and increased systemic venous return cause increase in right-to-left shunt and hypoxemia; increased blood volume may cause heart failure
EATV	PR prolongation AFL/AF Ventricular fib Junctional tachycardia AV reciprocating tachycardia RBBB Bundle branch reentrant tachycardia Atrialized RV tachycardia/ fibrillation (inducible)	AFL/AF Advanced AV block Ventricular fibrillation	Preop: right-to-left shunt via PFO/ASD may occur AV reciprocating tachycardia may occur more frequently

TGA	Sinus node dysfunction
	Atrial tachyarrhythmias
		Mustard and Senning operations:
		  Sinus node dysfunction
		  Ectopic atrial/junctional rhythms
		  AT/AFL/AF
		  Junctional tachycardia, AVNRT
		  Advanced/complete AV block
		Jatene operation:
		  APCs
			Postop: pregnancy not advisable if there is severe RV dysfunction or pulmonary hypertension

CTGA	Atrial tachyarrhythmias AV reciprocating tachycardia ('L Ebstein') PR prolongation 2 : 1 AV block; complete AV block with narrow QRS escape rhythm	Atrial tachyarrhythmias Complete AV block	Preop: systemic RV vulnerable to hemodynamic overload

TA	AF	Fontan procedure:
		  Sinus node dysfunction
		  AT/AFL/AF
		  Junctional tachycardia
		  Complete AV block
		  VT/VF
			Postop: pregnancy with increased risk of miscarriage

SV	Complete AV block (LV with inverted outlet chamber) Ventricular tachyarrhythmias	Fontan procedure: similar to TA	Postop: similar to TA

ASD, atrial septal defect; SV, sinus venosus; OS, ostium secundum; OP, ostium primum; VSD, ventricular septal defect; TOF, tetralogy of Fallot; EATV, Ebstein anomaly of tricuspid valve; TGA, complete transposition of great arteries; CTGA, congenitally corrected transposition of great arteries; TA, tricuspid atresia; VT, ventricular tachycardia; VF, ventricular fibrillation; AFL, atrial flutter; AF, atrial fibrillation; RBBB, right bundle branch block; VPC, ventricular premature contraction; RV, right ventricular; AV, atrioventricular; LAFB, left anterior fascicular block; AT, atrial tachycardia; AVNRT, atrioventricular nodal reentrant tachycardia; LV, left ventricle; SVT, supraventricular tachycardia; PFO, patent foramen ovale.

hour), frequent ventricular premature beats (10 or more per hour) occurred in a significantly larger proportion of symptomatic patients (20%), compared with asymptomatic patients (2%). Nevertheless, there was no correlation between the incidence of arrhythmias and occurrence of symptoms; only 10% of symptomatic episodes were accompanied by the presence of arrhythmia, suggesting that physiologic changes during pregnancy may contribute to those symptoms (20).

The incidence of atrial and ventricular premature beats is greater during pregnancy than during the postpartum period, suggesting that the "hyperdynamic" state of pregnancy may itself be arrhythmogenic in selected patients (20). However, these data should be interpreted cautiously because the incidence of atrial and ventricular premature beats detected by Holter monitoring in asymptomatic and symptomatic individuals without clinically apparent structural heart disease is high (60). Moreover, there is marked day-to-day variability of ectopic beats which may be as great as 23% (61). In any event, in the absence of structural heart disease, the presence of asymptomatic or mildly symptomatic premature atrial and ventricular ectopic beats or sinus bradycardia is prognostically benign and does not warrant therapeutic intervention (13,60,62).

The incidence of asymptomatic premature beats is high in patients with structural heart disease, and in the absence of clinical signs of cardiac decompensation, they are associated with the underlying cardiac disease in the pregnant patient (58,62). In the rare instance of a pregnant patient with coronary artery disease and prior infarction, the presence of asymptomatic premature ventricular complexes represents a threefold increase in risk of sudden cardiac death (63). However, antiarrhythmic therapy has not been shown to prevent sudden death in this setting, and empiric treatment with antiarrhythmic agents may be hazardous (64).

SUPRAVENTRICULAR TACHYCARDIAS

Mechanisms and Classification

Supraventricular tachycardias may be caused by disorders of impulse formation or impulse conduction (65,66). Disorders of impulse formation are attributable to abnormal automaticity or triggered activity (afterdepolarizations). Disorders of impulse conduction may result in reentrant tachycardias, which constitute the largest group of sustained tachyarrhythmias encountered in pregnant patients with or without heart disease (67).

Natural History

It is not clear whether pregnancy is associated with an increased risk of new-onset paroxysmal supraventricular tachycardia, particularly because the childbearing years are a time when supraventricular tachycardia often occurs for the first time. Nevertheless, there is evidence of exacerba-

tion of symptoms during tachycardia as well as an increase in the frequency of preexisting tachycardia during pregnancy (68–70). This may be a result of hemodynamic and autonomic alterations influencing the electrophysiologic substrate during pregnancy (69). A close correlation between occurrence of supraventricular tachycardic episodes and plasma concentrations of ovarian hormones at various stages of the menstrual cycle has been demonstrated (21); hormonal changes may also play a role in pregnancy-related changes in supraventricular tachycardia occurrence.

Atrial Tachycardias

In the general population, atrial tachycardias are the least common supraventricular tachycardia and are often associated with cardiac or pulmonary disease. The atrial rate ranges between 150 and 250 beats per minute (bpm) (71). Digitalis intoxication and metabolic derangements such as hyperthyroidism or alcohol ingestion may be causal (71). Atrial tachycardia mechanism may be automatic, reentrant, or triggered (71). Atrial tachycardias can be recognized on the surface ECG by a P-wave morphology that differs from the sinus P wave and first-degree atrioventricular (AV) block that does not affect the rate of the atrial tachycardia (66,71). Atrial tachycardias have been reported in pregnant patients without structural heart disease, and preexisting paroxysmal atrial tachycardia may become incessant during gestation. With appropriate therapy, these tachyarrhythmias rarely result in serious compromise to maternal or fetal health (13,72).

Atrial reentrant tachycardias are commonly observed in patients with congenital heart disease as sequelae of extensive intraatrial surgery (59,73).

AV Nodal Reentrant Tachycardia

AV nodal reentry is the most commonly encountered supraventricular tachycardia in the healthy gravid and the nongravid patient and has no predilection for associated structural heart disease (66). Tachycardia rates range from 150 to 250 bpm (71). Reentry is thought to occur within the AV nodal and atrial perinodal structures as a result of functional or anatomic dissociation of the AV node into slow and rapid conducting pathways (71). Tachycardia is initiated by conduction delay and unidirectional block, which can occur with a properly timed atrial premature beat (Fig. 27-1). In most cases, retrograde P waves are not observed on the surface ECG, because the retrograde limb is the fast pathway of the circuit in typical AV nodal reentrant tachycardia, which conducts rapidly, resulting in simultaneous atrial and ventricular depolarization (71).

AV Reciprocating Tachycardia

AV reciprocating tachycardias, associated with an accessory pathway, are second in frequency to AV nodal reentry and

A

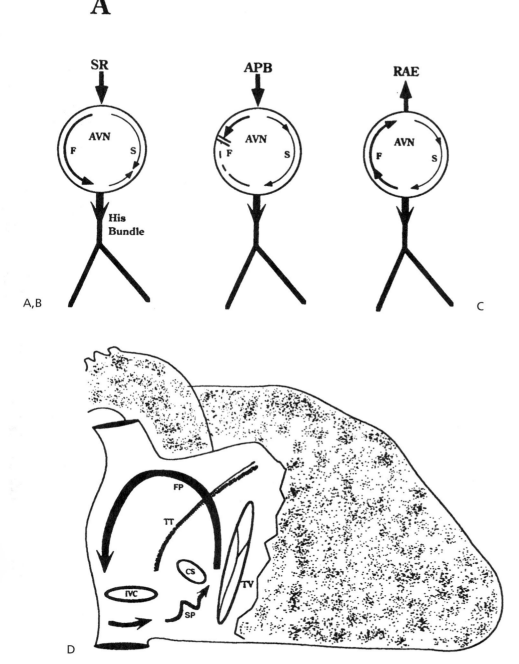

D

FIGURE 27-1. Atrioventricular (AV) nodal reentry. **A:** Atrial impulse is conducted antegradely in fast pathway *(F)* of AV node *(AVN)* during sinus rhythm *(SR)*. Antegrade wavefront in slow pathway *(S)* and returning retrograde wavefront from fast pathway collide and terminate in slow pathway. **B:** Atrial premature beat (APB) is conducted antegradely in slow pathway and is blocked antegradely in fast pathway because of its longer refractory period. Returning retrograde wavefront is also blocked in fast pathway. **C:** Timing of atrial impulse and AV pathway characteristics are such that APB is conducted antegradely in slow pathway and returns retrogradely in fast pathway where it is conducted back to the right atrium as an echo beat *(RAE)*. This may be the initiating beat of typical AVN reentrant tachycardia, in which antegrade conduction by way of slow pathway and retrograde conduction by way of fast pathway form the reentry circuit. **D:** A schematic diagram illustrating AVN reentry in the context of AV nodal and perinodal structures. (SP, slow pathway; FP, fast pathway; CS, coronary sinus; TT, tendon of Todaro; IVC, inferior vena cava; TV, tricuspid valve.)

are caused by the presence of an accessory pathway (74,75). There are two types of reciprocating tachycardias, depending on whether the accessory pathway is the antegrade or the retrograde limb of the tachycardia circuit. Orthodromic tachycardia, which is more frequent, uses the AV node as the antegrade limb and the accessory pathway as the retrograde limb of the tachycardia circuit. Tachycardia rates range from 150 to 250 bpm (Fig. 27-2) (71). Antidromic tachycardia uses the accessory pathway as the antegrade limb and the AV node as the retrograde limb. These tachy-

cardias may be quite rapid and are generally wide complex, resulting from ventricular depolarization occurring over the accessory pathway. It may be difficult to differentiate antidromic tachycardia from ventricular tachycardia on the surface ECG (76,77).

Ventricular preexcitation is present on the surface ECG in up to 25% of patients with Ebstein's anomaly of the tricuspid valve (58). Approximately one third of those patients with preexcitation have more than one accessory pathway (58). Symptomatic supraventricular tachycardias are com-

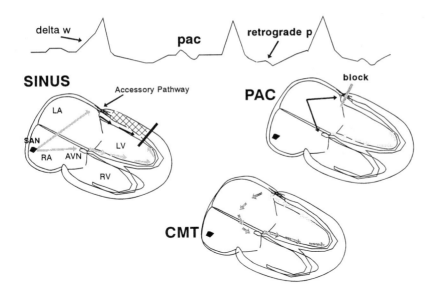

FIGURE 27-2. Atrioventricular (AV) reciprocating tachycardia or circus movement tachycardia using an accessory pathway. In the schematic electrocardiogram **(top)**, the first complex is a preexcited QRS electrogram caused by simultaneous ventricular depolarization from the AV node and left-sided accessory pathway. Next, a premature atrial complex *(PAC)* blocks in the accessory pathway, and ventricular depolarization is only from the AV nodal-His bundle pathway. However, retrograde atrial activation occurs as a result of the recovery of accessory pathway conduction, and circus movement tachycardia is initiated. (SAN, sinoatrial node; RA, right atrium; LA, left atrium; AVN, atrioventricular node; RV, right ventricle; LV, left ventricle.)

mon, may occur during pregnancy, and can result in serious hemodynamic deterioration (58).

Atrial Flutter

In typical atrial flutter, the atrial rate is 250 to 350 bpm (71); flutter is most often observed in pregnancy associated with structural cardiac disease or a metabolic derangement such as Graves disease (13,71).

Atrial flutter, or more aptly *incisional atrial tachycardia,* is not infrequent in patients who have had or who have not had surgery for congenital heart disease (58,73) and is caused by reentry around abnormal anatomic structures or surgical incision scars. These patients—including the nonsurgical group with atrial septal defects, those with Ebstein's anomaly with or without an accessory pathway, and particularly those who have undergone the Mustard or Senning procedure for transposition of the great arteries—are particularly susceptible to hemodynamic deterioration with the onset of atrial flutter (57,58).

Atrial Fibrillation

Atrial fibrillation is characterized by a chaotic atrial rhythm with atrial rates of 400 to 600 bpm (71). The ventricular response is typically between 100 and 160 bpm (71) but in the presence of an antegradely conducting accessory pathway may exceed 300 bpm with risk of inducing ventricular fibrillation (71,78). In the absence of structural heart disease, atrial fibrillation is rare in pregnancy unless associated with thyrotoxicosis (13,79).

In patients with rheumatic mitral stenosis, atrial fibrillation can have grave consequences for mother and fetus (13). In one large series of pregnant patients with rheumatic heart disease, atrial fibrillation was present before pregnancy in

4.1% of all pregnancies (79). On the other hand, atrial fibrillation developed during pregnancy in 2.5% of all pregnancies. Heart failure complicated 26% of pregnancies with preexistent atrial fibrillation. In comparison, heart failure occurred in 72% of pregnancies with new-onset atrial fibrillation. One third of the heart failure occurrences in the latter group preceded onset of atrial fibrillation (79). The outcome of pregnancy in women with artificial heart valves has also been studied. The incidences of maternal atrial fibrillation and heart failure were 5.8% and 2.9%, respectively (34).

Atrial fibrillation is also encountered in patients with congenital heart disease and may be present in surgical and nonsurgical patients with atrial septal defects, Ebstein's anomaly, or after Fontan, Mustard, or Senning repairs (58). In the patient with a rapidly conducting antegrade accessory pathway, including those with Ebstein's anomaly, atrial fibrillation may have serious hemodynamic consequences (58).

VENTRICULAR TACHYCARDIA

Definition

Ventricular tachycardia is defined as a rhythm of ventricular origin, arising distal to the bundle of His with rates ranging between 110 and 250 bpm (71). QRS complexes are broad (exceeding 0.12 seconds), and in up to 75% of cases, AV dissociation is present (71,80).

Idiopathic Ventricular Tachycardia

Ventricular tachycardia is uncommon in pregnancy and relatively rare in patients without heart disease. However, new-onset ventricular tachycardia or worsening of nonsustained ventricular tachycardia may become manifest in otherwise healthy pregnant women (81). In that setting, the ventricular tachycardia is considered to be idiopathic and may originate in the right or left ventricle (82–84). In most reported cases of idiopathic ventricular tachycardia complicating pregnancy, the tachycardias have originated in the right ventricle and appear to be exacerbated by exercise, emotional stress, or other provocative stimuli. Despite the rapid rate or associated syncope, these tachycardias are generally brought under control with medical therapy and when properly treated have a very benign prognosis (85).

Ventricular Tachycardia Resulting from Metabolic Derangement

Paroxysmal ventricular tachycardia has been described in association with thyrotoxicosis and hyperemesis and with hypomagnesemia. Ventricular tachycardia resolved with correction of the metabolic derangements (86). Ventricular tachycardia in association with pheochromocytoma not causing hypertension has also been reported (87).

Ventricular Tachycardia Resulting from Adverse Effects of Medication

Premature atrial and ventricular beats were rarely noted in a large obstetric population receiving subcutaneous terbutaline infusion for treatment of preterm labor (88). At least one case of sudden death in pregnancy has been attributed to terbutaline use (89). Also, any over-the-counter preparations containing a sympathomimetic agent may cause hypertension and symptomatic ventricular arrhythmias (90) and should be avoided.

Ventricular Tachycardia in Mitral Valve Prolapse

Ventricular tachycardia may rarely occur in pregnant patients with mitral valve prolapse, even in the absence of significant mitral regurgitation (91,92).

Ventricular Tachycardia in Congenital Long QT Syndrome

Ventricular tachycardia resulting from congenital long QT syndrome may occur in pregnancy (93–96). Appropriate pharmacologic or device therapy should be administered (97). Although pregnancy is not associated with an increase in cardiac events in patients with long QT syndrome, the postpartum interval is a time of increased risk for sudden death, aborted cardiac arrest, and syncope. Treatment with β blockers results in a significant decrease in the risk for cardiac events during pregnancy and postpartum (96).

Ventricular Tachycardia in Hypertension

Nonsustained ventricular tachycardia has been observed in up to 70% of pregnant subjects with hypertensive crises and correlates with the severity of the hypertension (40). In these cases, ventricular irritability may be caused by increased catecholamine levels or myocardial ischemia. Successful treatment of hypertension results in resolution of arrhythmias (38,39).

Ventricular Tachycardia with Myocardial Infarction

Myocardial infarction is rare in pregnancy and may be caused by coronary artery spasm, hypercoagulability, atherosclerosis (premature coronary artery disease resulting from the usual risk factors), or coronary artery dissection (42,43). Hemodynamically unstable ventricular tachycardia or fibrillation may occur during or after acute myocardial infarction (98).

Ventricular Tachycardia in Cardiomyopathy

Sustained or nonsustained ventricular tachycardia may be the initial manifestation of peripartum cardiomyopathy. A thorough evaluation of the pregnant patient in her third trimester with new-onset ventricular tachycardia is therefore essential (35,36). Patients with hypertrophic obstructive cardiomyopathy generally tolerate pregnancy satisfactorily, with a maternal and fetal mortality rate reported from the world literature of only 1.8% (37). However, ventricular arrhythmias may worsen during pregnancy, and fatal sustained ventricular tachycardia has been reported in a mother at 36 weeks of gestation (99).

Ventricular Tachycardia in Congenital Heart Disease

Ventricular tachycardia may occur in the setting of nonsurgical and surgical patients with congenital heart disease, particularly after repaired tetralogy of Fallot (18,23). The general risk (irrespective of pregnancy) of late sudden cardiac death for patients surviving operations for common congenital heart defects is 25 to 100 times more than age-matched controls and is increased primarily after the second postoperative decade (18). This increased risk is mainly represented by patients with obstructive left heart lesions or cyanotic lesions, i.e., aortic stenosis, coarctation of the aorta, tetralogy of Fallot, and transposition of the great arteries (18). Three quarters of the sudden deaths are arrhythmic in origin, with the documented arrhythmias being more commonly ventricular tachycardia or fibrillation and less commonly advanced AV block (18). Nevertheless, the absolute risk of sudden cardiac death is only 1 of 454 patient-years in high-risk patients (18), suggesting a small total risk for the duration of pregnancy. Furthermore, large studies of women who have undergone surgery for congenital heart disease do not suggest an increase in significant ventricular arrhythmias during pregnancy (24,26).

AV CONDUCTION DISTURBANCES

AV conduction disturbances exist when an atrial impulse is not conducted or is conducted with delay to the ventricle at a time when the AV junction is not physiologically refractory to stimulation (71,100,101).

First-Degree AV Block

First-degree AV block is defined as prolongation of the PR interval beyond 0.2 seconds. Each atrial impulse is conducted to the ventricles. First-degree block is rarely observed in pregnancy in the absence of rheumatic heart disease or congenital heart disease, particularly congenitally corrected transposition of the great arteries and Ebstein's anomaly of the tricuspid valve (13,58). The site of AV delay is usually located above the bundle of His and does not progress to advanced heart block, and the block itself is not associated with maternal or fetal risk.

Second-Degree AV Block

Second-degree AV block may occur at any level of the ventricular conduction system and is present when some atrial impulses fail to reach the ventricle.

Type I (Wenckebach) second-degree AV block refers to progressive delay in AV conduction time before AV block, and unlike type II second-degree AV block, the block is typically above the bundle of His and progression to complete heart block is rare (101,102).

Type II second-degree AV block is recognized when two or more atrial beats are conducted to the ventricles with identical PR intervals before AV block. This form of AV block is reported in less than 0.2% of pregnancies, and most cases have been found in association with organic heart disease or in the presence of digitalis therapy (13).

In patients with congenital heart disease, second-degree AV block most commonly occurs in repaired tetralogy of Fallot and less commonly after repair of ventricular septal defects (58).

Most cases of second-degree AV block in pregnancy are Wenckebach block and are not associated with symptomatic bradycardia. In the absence of symptoms or marked bradycardia, removal of potentially aggravating causes is all that is indicated.

Complete Heart Block

Complete heart block (third-degree AV block) can be acquired or congenital and is present when no atrial impulses reach the ventricle by way of the AV node. Acquired complete heart block is most commonly infra-Hisian, whereas congenital complete heart block is usually above the His bundle (71).

Acquired complete heart block is rare in gravidas, and in one series of more than 92,000 pregnancies, it occurred in only 0.02% (13). Stokes-Adams attacks were observed in 10% of cases, with maternal death in 20% of cases, directly related to the severity of the coexisting heart disease. Postoperative complete heart block may occur after tetralogy of Fallot repair, ventricular septal defect or ostium primum atrial septal defect repair, atrial switch (Mustard or Senning), or Fontan operation (58).

Maternal and fetal outcomes are favorable in gravidas with isolated congenital complete heart block, particularly when the QRS complex is narrow, which is usually the case (13,103). In the absence of symptomatic bradycardia, a wide QRS escape rhythm, or ventricular dysfunction, pacing support for congenital complete heart block is not necessary (101).

FETAL ARRHYTHMIAS

Fetal heart rate can be monitored externally using maternal abdominal ECG or fetal echocardiography or internally using fetal scalp electrode recordings (104–107). Fetal scalp recordings are technically superior but require rupture of the membranes (107). Sustained trends in fetal heart rate and heart rate variability are as important as absolute heart rate in diagnosing fetal distress (108,109). Maternal abdominal ECG recordings show maternal and fetal (ventricular) cardiac electrical activity. Fetal scalp ECG recordings show fetal cardiac electrical activity in a single lead and require rupture of the membranes. Available ECG methods are, therefore, limited in discriminating fetal arrhythmias (107). Fetal real-time echocardiography with Doppler provides information on heart rate and AV conduction and has emerged as a valuable tool for diagnosing *in utero* fetal tachyarrhythmias and bradyarrhythmias and high-degree heart block and for evaluating the effects of therapy (107,110–112). In addition to the previously mentioned ECG and echocardiographic methods, fetal magnetocardiography, which registers the magnetic field generated by the fetal heart, may hold some advantage for external monitoring of fetal heart rate and rhythm, particularly after the 20th week of gestation (Fig. 27-3) (113,114).

The fetal conduction system is fully developed by the 16th week of gestation (10,106,107). Fetal heart rate normally falls between 120 and 160 bpm during the second and third trimesters (106,107) and normally demonstrates pronounced variability (108,109). Significant fetal tachycardia is present when the heart rate exceeds 180 bpm (Table 27-3). A fetal ECG or fetal echocardiogram should be obtained to differentiate sinus from supraventricular tachycardia. Most cases of fetal sinus tachycardia are secondary to potentially treatable causes (107). Significant fetal bradycardia may indicate fetal distress and is diagnosed when the heart rate falls below 100 bpm and is sustained for more than 1 minute (Table 27-4) (107,115,116). This may represent fetal sinus bradycardia, which has several possible causes. Alternatively, this may represent sinoatrial or AV

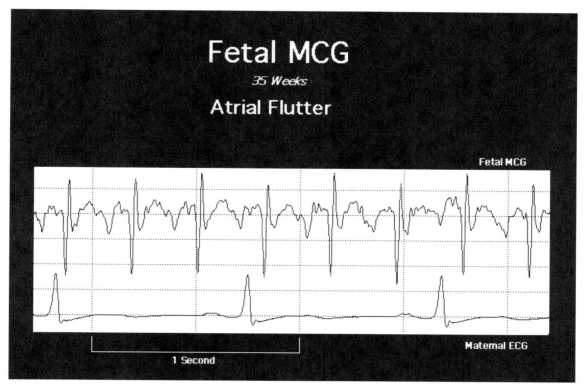

FIGURE 27-3. A sample fetal magnetocardiogram obtained at 35 weeks of gestation. Fetal rhythm is atrial flutter with 2 : 1 atrioventricular conduction **(top tracing)**. There is no significant interference from maternal rhythm, which is in normal sinus rhythm as displayed **(bottom tracing)**. (Courtesy of Paul R. Steiner, M.D., University of California, San Francisco.)

block. The former, a sign of umbilical cord or occasionally head compression, may be difficult to discern on fetal ECG without adequate P-wave recording. Although the association of congenital complete AV block and congenital heart disease is well known (117), there has been increasing attention to the association between congenital heart block and maternal autoimmune disease (systemic lupus erythematosus, anti-Ro and anti-La autoantibodies) (118–120). The prognosis of intrauterine complete heart block is largely related to the coexisting cardiac disease (103). In fetuses

with congenital complete heart block and structurally normal hearts, a single heart (ventricular) rate does not accurately predict the outcome *in utero* or the need for postnatal pacing (121).

Atrial premature beats and bigeminy and trigeminy are detected by intrapartum fetal ECG in at least 1% of monitored births and are associated with a benign course (122). Paroxysmal supraventricular tachycardia is the most common serious tachyarrhythmic disorder detected *in utero* and is accompanied by congenital heart disease in approximately 5% to 10% of cases (117,123). Persistent supraventricular tachycardia can lead to fetal hydrops. Atrial fibrilla-

TABLE 27-3. CAUSES OF FETAL TACHYCARDIA

Sinus tachycardia
   Amnionitis
   Cytomegalovirus disease
   Drugs, e.g., atropine
   Maternal fever
   Early fetal hypoxia
   Maternal anxiety
   Electrolyte imbalance
   Thyrotoxicosis
   Meconium aspiration
   Circulatory collapse
Supraventricular tachycardia
Ventricular tachycardia (rare)

TABLE 27-4. CAUSES OF FETAL BRADYCARDIA

Sinus bradycardia
   Fetal head and umbilical cord compression
   Maternal hypotension
   Maternal seizures
   Maternal voiding
   Paracervical block anesthesia
   Drugs, e.g., β blockers
   Long QT syndrome
Sino-Atrial Block:
   Umbilical cord or head compression
Atrio ventricular block

tion or flutter is a less common but nonetheless important cause of fetal tachycardia (124–126). Supraventricular tachyarrhythmias have a favorable prognosis if recognized *in utero,* are properly treated, and if they occur in the absence of congenital heart disease (123,127). Ventricular tachycardia is very rare in the healthy fetal heart and is usually found in conjunction with complex congenital heart disease or long QT syndrome or severe metabolic abnormalities (107, 115,117,122,128,129).

Therapy of fetal arrhythmias usually involves maternal administration of antiarrhythmic agents (transplacental therapy) (130–132). Direct fetal antiarrhythmic therapy has occasionally been used for treatment of supraventricular tachycardia (130,132–135). Additionally, fetal ventricular pacing for hemodynamically compromising complete congenital heart block has been reported (130,136).

PHARMACOLOGIC THERAPY OF ARRHYTHMIAS

General Considerations

Conservative therapy may be appropriate in some pregnant patients with arrhythmia. Avoidance of exertion and cardiac stimulants may be helpful in reducing frequency

of paroxysmal tachycardias sensitive to adrenergic tone (65,71). Vagal measures such as Valsalva maneuver may acutely terminate paroxysmal reentrant supraventricular tachycardias using the AV node as part of the reentry circuit (137,138).

All antiarrhythmic agents have potential adverse effects during pregnancy, and the risk extends to mother and fetus (2–9,138–142). Accordingly, judicious use of these agents in treating arrhythmias in the mother or the fetus is obligatory. Table 27-5 lists commonly used antiarrhythmic agents, their indications, and potential adverse effects for mother and fetus. Table 27-6 lists antiarrhythmic agents considered to be compatible with breast feeding (142).

Adjustments in antiarrhythmic drug dosing may be required during pregnancy, given pregnancy-related changes in gastrointestinal absorption, intravascular volume, plasma protein concentration, hepatic metabolism, and renal clearance (2).

Adenosine

Adenosine is a ubiquitous endogenous nucleoside capable of causing AV nodal block (143–145). Intravenous adenosine transiently suppresses sinus node automaticity and depresses AV nodal conduction (141). The drug does not

TABLE 27-5. ANTIARRHYTHMIC DRUGS IN PREGNANCY: CLINICAL USE AND ADVERSE EFFECTS

Drug	Applications	Adverse Effects on Fetus and Labor	
		Definite Association	**Possible Association**
Adenosine	Maternal SVT (acute termination)		
Digoxin	Maternal or fetal SVT		Premature labor
	Maternal or fetal heart failure		Low birth weight
β-adrenoreceptor blockers	Maternal or fetal SVT	Fetal bradycardia	Prolonged labor (propranolol)
	Selected VTs	Fetal apnea	Fetal polycythemia
	Maternal hypertension	Fetal growth retardation	Fetal hypoglycemia
	Maternal thyrotoxicosis		Fetal hyperbilirubinemia
Calcium channel blockers	Maternal or fetal SVT	Fetal bradycardia/heart block	Congenital malformation
	Selected VTs	Fetal hypotension/depression of cardiac contractility	
	Maternal hypertension		
	Premature labor		
Class Ia antiarrhythmics	Maternal or fetal SVT or VT		Fetal thrombocytopenia (quinidine)
	Maternal malaria (quinidine)		Fetal eighth cranial nerve injury (quinidine)
	Labor induction (disopyramide)		Premature labor (quinidine)
Class Ib antiarrhythmics	VT	Fetal bradycardia	Fetal hypoglycemia (mexiletine)
		Fetal CNS depression (IV lidocaine)	Congenital malformation (phenytoin)
Class Ic antiarrhythmics	Maternal or fetal SVT		
	Selected VTs		
Class III antiarrhythmics	Maternal or fetal SVT or VT	Fetal bradycardia	Spontaneous abortion
		Fetal QT prolongation	Fetal growth retardation
		Fetal hypo- or hyperthyroidism (amiodarone)	Premature labor (amiodarone)
			Congenital malformation

SVT, supraventricular tachycardia; VT, ventricular tachycardia; CNS, central nervous system.

TABLE 27-6. ANTIARRHYTHMIC DRUGS USUALLY COMPATIBLE WITH BREASTFEEDING

Digoxin
Propranolol
Metoprolol
Labetalol
Verapamil
Diltiazem
Quinidine
Procainamide
Disopyramide
Lidocaine
Mexiletine
Flecainide
Sotalol

From American Academy of Pediatrics Committee on Drugs. *The transfer of drugs and other chemicals into human breastmilk. Pediatrics* 1994;93:137–150, with permission.

significantly depress conduction in most accessory pathways (146). Adenosine is indicated for the acute termination of supraventricular tachycardias such as AV nodal reentrant tachycardia and AV reciprocating tachycardia and has an efficacy of more than 90%. Adenosine can transiently slow the ventricular response rate of atrial fibrillation or flutter by causing AV nodal block, but it does not slow atrial activity. The duration of the drug effect is less than 20 seconds after an intravenous bolus of 6 or 12 mg. Side effects are usually mild and nonsustained; they include flushing, chest pain, and dyspnea (138). Adenosine terminates supraventricular tachycardia more rapidly than intravenous verapamil and is much less apt to result in drug-induced hypotension (147). Adenosine's AV nodal effect is antagonized by theophylline and enhanced by dipyridamole. Adenosine should be used with caution in patients with chronic obstructive pulmonary disease unassociated with bronchospasm and should be avoided in asthmatic patients, because of risk of bronchoconstriction (141,144). Adenosine may cause transient sinus arrest or complete AV block and may induce atrial fibrillation (138).

Use of adenosine in pregnancy for termination of supraventricular tachycardia has been reported without adverse maternal or fetal effects (148,149). Fetal AV block has not been reported after maternal adenosine administration. Adenosine, however, causes dose-dependent contraction of human placental vessels *in vitro*; if similar contraction results *in vivo,* an adverse effect on the fetus may occur if adenosine is administered to pregnant women at term or during labor (150).

Digitalis

Digitalis glycosides exert inotropic effects by inhibition of Na,K-ATPase (141). The predominant cardiac antiarrhythmic action is on the atria and proximal AV nodal tissues mediated by the vagus nerve. In the atrium, digitalis enhances conduction and shortens the refractory period whereas the drug slows AV nodal conduction by lengthening refractory period and decreasing conduction velocity. The drug may be used for the treatment of maternal and fetal supraventricular arrhythmias including AV nodal reentrant tachycardias and for control of ventricular response to atrial fibrillation or flutter (151–153), but its effects are greatest in the presence of vagal tone. Digoxin readily crosses the placenta, and in the latter half of gestation, fetal blood levels approximate maternal blood levels after maternal digitalization (151). Sera of pregnant women and fetuses contain digoxin-like immunoreactive factors, which may interfere with serum level of digoxin. Ultrafiltration of the serum sample before analysis appears to minimize this interference (154). Although digoxin is secreted in breast milk, infant blood levels are below therapeutic digoxin concentrations, so use of the drug is considered safe in lactating mothers (142).

There is a potential but unproven association between digoxin use in pregnancy and premature labor or low-birth-weight infants (155). However, the safe use of digoxin for maternal and fetal arrhythmias has been borne out in large numbers of patients (10).

β-Adrenoreceptor Antagonists

β-Adrenoreceptor antagonists act by blocking β_1, β_2, or both receptors. Cardiac effects are mediated through β_1 receptors (138). β_2 Drug effects are predominantly on the bronchi and blood vessels. In pregnancy, myometrial relaxation is a β_2-receptor–mediated process, and β blockers with both β_1 and β_2 activity may counteract the effect of β_2 stimulation (156). β Blockers with nonselective β_1 and β_2 activity include propranolol, labetalol (which also has α-blocking properties), nadolol, and timolol. Selective β_1 antagonists include atenolol, metoprolol, betaxolol, and esmolol (available only as intravenous infusion). Selective β_1 antagonists with intrinsic sympathetic activity include oxprenolol, acebutolol, and pindolol. β Antagonists are predominantly used in pregnancy to treat hypertension and thyrotoxicosis (10). However, the use of these agents, particularly propranolol, which has seen the largest use in pregnancy, is somewhat controversial because of individual reports of fetal apnea, growth retardation, bradycardia, premature labor, and fetal metabolic abnormalities (156–158). The relative safety of selective versus nonselective agents in pregnancy has not been established (10,11). Although the safety of all of these agents in pregnancy has not been established definitively, they have been used widely to treat maternal and fetal supraventricular arrhythmias, as well as certain forms of maternal ventricular tachycardia (82,93,94).

Propranolol, labetalol, atenolol, nadolol, and metoprolol are known to be excreted in breast milk (10,142); no significant adverse effects on infants from breast feeding have been reported (142).

Calcium Channel Antagonists

The calcium channel antagonists are a group of agents that exert antiarrhythmic effects by inhibiting the slow inward calcium current, resulting in lengthening of AV nodal refractory periods and slowing of AV nodal conduction (138). These agents also have vasodilatory activity by blocking calcium entry into vascular smooth muscle cells. Verapamil, diltiazem, nifedipine, isradipine, nicardipine, felodipine, and nimodipine are calcium antagonists that have been investigated in pregnancy. Their primary use in pregnancy has been in the treatment of gestational hypertension and for suppression of preterm labor.

The calcium blockers that have the most selective myocardial or heart rate slowing effects are verapamil and diltiazem, which are effective in the treatment of supraventricular reentrant tachycardias and for control of ventricular response to atrial fibrillation or flutter (138). These drugs have no direct effect on conduction in accessory pathways (138). Calcium blockers have also proved efficacious in the treatment of selected idiopathic ventricular tachycardias (82).

Acute or chronic maternal use does not appear to affect uteroplacental blood flow or fetal heart rate even if transient maternal hypotension from drug administration does occur (159). However, *in vitro* studies of the effects of various calcium channel blockers including verapamil and diltiazem on growth and morphologic differentiation of rat embryos show dose-dependent and reversible reductions of embryonic heart rate, as well as developmental abnormalities (160,161). Verapamil is detected in breast milk, but not in infant plasma; the hazard to the suckling infant, therefore, appears to be small (162).

Class I Antiarrhythmics

Class I agents act by blocking sodium channels. They are further subdivided into types a, b, and c, depending on their differential effects on V_{max} (rate of depolarization in phase 0) and action potential duration (138).

Ia Agents

Class Ia drugs include quinidine, procainamide, and disopyramide, which reduce V_{max} and prolong action potential duration. These agents have been used in the treatment of ventricular and supraventricular arrhythmias, including those involving an accessory pathway (138). They are also useful for the termination of atrial fibrillation or flutter after the ventricular rate has been slowed (138). For the therapy of atrial flutter, they should be used in conjunction with an AV nodal blocking agent, as they are capable of slowing the rate of atrial flutter, and as a result of a decrease in concealed AV nodal conduction, there may be an increase in ventricular rate (138).

In addition to the previously mentioned indications, use of these agents in pregnancy has included fetal supraventricular and ventricular arrhythmias, induction of labor (disopyramide), and maternal malaria (quinidine) (134,163).

Care must be taken when administering this class of drugs because adverse reactions, which are exacerbated by electrolyte abnormalities, are potentially fatal and include polymorphic ventricular tachycardia caused by early afterdepolarizations resulting from drug-induced QT-interval prolongation (138).

Quinidine has been used safely in pregnancy for more than 50 years (81,164). Quinidine is excreted in breast milk and may accumulate in the newborn liver (142). Case reports of adverse fetal effects include thrombocytopenia, premature labor, and eighth nerve toxicity (165).

Procainamide has no known teratogenic effects and, like quinidine, is a useful agent in treating various maternal and fetal arrhythmias (131). However, concern regarding chronic use in pregnancy is warranted because of the known autoimmune response to long-term therapy (138).

Disopyramide has been less widely used as an antiarrhythmic agent in pregnancy because of concerns regarding the initiation of premature labor. In a placebo-controlled study, disopyramide has proven to be an effective agent for the induction of uterine contractions when used in patients requiring labor induction (163). The drug is excreted in breast milk, and disopyramide and its metabolite are detected in the infant's urine (166).

Ib Agents

Class Ib drugs include lidocaine, which is available only in intravenous form, and mexiletine and tocainide, which are oral preparations. These agents do not significantly reduce V_{max}, but they shorten action potential duration. Class Ib agents are indicated in the treatment of ventricular tachycardia or fibrillation (intravenous lidocaine) (138).

Lidocaine appears to be well tolerated in pregnancy and is widely used, primarily as a local or epidural anesthetic, but also as an intravenous antiarrhythmic agent (10). Lidocaine and its metabolites can be detected in fetal blood; fetal metabolism of lidocaine is impaired by fetal acidosis (167–169). In animals, central nervous system and cardiovascular toxic manifestations of lidocaine do not appear to be exacerbated in pregnancy (170).

Mexiletine has had limited usage in pregnancy, with no adverse fetal effects, except for newborn hypoglycemia (92). Mexiletine is found in fetal blood and breast milk, but deleterious effects on the breast-fed infant have not been reported (142).

There is no published experience with tocainide in pregnancy.

Ic Agents

Flecainide and propafenone are class Ic agents, whose primary action is to reduce V_{max} with little effect on action potential duration (138). Propafenone also has weak β-adrenergic and calcium channel-blocking activity. These agents are indicated in the treatment of ventricular arrhythmias and supraventricular tachycardias, including those involving an accessory pathway. Flecainide should not be used in the treatment of ventricular tachycardia that occurs in the setting of a recent myocardial infarction in light of the results of the Cardiac Arrhythmia Suppression Trial, demonstrating increased mortality in postinfarction patients treated with flecainide versus placebo for ventricular premature beats (64). Propafenone is approved for the treatment of ventricular tachycardia, but cautious use is prudent in patients with depressed left ventricular function or an acute myocardial infarction because of antiarrhythmic activity similar to that associated with flecainide (138). In the treatment of atrial fibrillation or flutter, as with class Ia agents, class Ic agents should be used with an AV nodal blocking drug to avoid rapid ventricular rates (138).

Flecainide has been used in the treatment of refractory maternal atrial tachycardia (72,171). Moreover, flecainide has been an effective agent in the treatment of refractory fetal supraventricular tachycardia, particularly in association with fetal hydrops (172,173). Transplacental passage occurs, and the drug is detected in fetal serum and breast milk (174), but other than sporadic cases (175), no adverse fetal or infant effects have been reported.

Propafenone use in pregnancy is extremely limited (139). It has reported efficacy in the treatment of new-onset ventricular tachycardia during pregnancy in the setting of normal cardiac function. Drug concentrations are found in fetal plasma and breast milk (142).

Class III Antiarrhythmics

Class III drugs block potassium channels and prolong repolarization and refractoriness. They include amiodarone, sotalol, bretylium, ibutilide, and dofetilide (138,141). Amiodarone, available for oral and intravenous use, is a highly effective drug for treating maternal and fetal ventricular and supraventricular tachycardias, including those using an accessory pathway. Amiodarone also exerts α- and β-adrenergic blocking effects. Sotalol is approved for treatment of ventricular tachycardia and has been used for treatment of supraventricular tachycardias. It is available as an oral agent. Sotalol, only available in oral form, also has β-adrenergic blocking properties. Cautious use is prudent in patients with depressed left ventricular function. Bretylium is an intravenous agent indicated for the treatment of drug refractory or life-threatening ventricular tachycardias. Ibutilide is available in intravenous form and is indicated for acute conversion of atrial fibrillation and flutter (176). Dofetilide is a novel class III agent with potential usefulness in acute conversion of atrial flutter and fibrillation as well as chronic rhythm management of heart failure patients with atrial fibrillation (177,178).

Amiodarone has unique characteristics that mandate guarded use in pregnancy. The drug is highly protein and lipid bound, resulting in a large body store and a mean plasma elimination half-life of 2 months (141). Each 200-mg amiodarone tablet contains 75 mg of iodine; thus, amiodarone has direct action on the thyroid gland (141). These effects may result in hypothyroidism or hyperthyroidism in the mother or fetus (179–181). Fetal bradycardia, fetal QT-interval prolongation, premature labor, and low-birth-weight infants have also been reported in association with maternal amiodarone therapy (179). Concern about fetal neurotoxicity has also been raised (182). Amiodarone is found in fetal tissue and breast milk, but other than hypothyroidism, no adverse effects on the breast-fed infant have been reported (142). In addition to treatment of serious maternal arrhythmias, amiodarone has been an effective agent in the treatment of life-threatening fetal tachycardia and hydrops fetalis by direct injection into the umbilical vein (183). Use of amiodarone in pregnancy should be reserved for those maternal and fetal arrhythmias not responding to agents with known safety.

Sotalol use during pregnancy has been reported in the treatment of refractory maternal and fetal supraventricular tachycardias and maternal ventricular tachycardia (174). Drug is found in fetal serum and breast milk (142,174). Congenital malformations and fetal death, as well as behavioral abnormalities in offspring, have been reported after administration of d-sotalol in rat experiments (184–186).

There is no experience with the use of intravenous bretylium in pregnancy (187), so its use cannot be recommended except in instances of life-threatening maternal or fetal ventricular tachycardia. Moreover, available animal data on ibutilide and dofetilide suggest possible teratogenic and embryotoxic effects (184,185,188).

NONPHARMACOLOGIC THERAPIES OF ARRHYTHMIAS

Cardiopulmonary Resuscitation

Resuscitation from cardiopulmonary arrest in a pregnant patient should be done in accord with standard protocols (189,190). To minimize the effect of the gravid uterus on systemic venous return and cardiac output, the uterus should be displaced to the side manually or by using a wedge (e.g., multiple pillows) or by positioning the pregnant patient's back on the kneeling rescuer's thighs (human wedge) (189–191).

The decision to perform a "perimortem" cesarean section is difficult but should be made quickly. Cesarean section within 5 minutes of arrest may improve outcome for the mother and the fetus (189,190,192,193).

Direct Current Cardioversion

External cardioversion is indicated for maternal ventricular or supraventricular tachyarrhythmia associated with adverse hemodynamic consequences. Electrical cardioversion has been used in pregnancy and is well tolerated (98,194,195). Fetal monitoring is recommended immediately after cardioversion (196), although risk of induction of fetal arrhythmia appears to be minimal, perhaps because of low electrical energy reaching the fetus or high defibrillation threshold of the fetal heart (2).

Cardiac Arrhythmia Surgery

Cardiac sympathectomy involves selective removal of the left sympathetic innervation to the heart. Sympathetic overactivity is thought to be involved in ventricular tachycardia occurring in the setting of idiopathic long QT syndrome (97,197). Ventricular tachycardia in association with myocardial ischemia may also be neurally mediated (198). Uncomplicated pregnancy has been reported in a patient with congenital long QT syndrome who had undergone left stellectomy (199).

Operations for treatment of supraventricular tachycardias have been largely replaced by radiofrequency catheter ablation (138). Direct surgical treatment of ventricular arrhythmias is not widely applied (138). There are no published reports on the effect of cardiac arrhythmia surgery on human pregnancy.

Radiofrequency Catheter Ablation

Radiofrequency ablation is a transvenous catheter technique that offers potential permanent cure of most supraventricular tachycardias, including AV reciprocating tachycardia (involving accessory pathway), AV nodal reentrant tachycardia, atrial flutter, and ectopic atrial tachycardia (200,201). Radiofrequency energy destroys a segment of an accessory pathway, a critical component of a reentrant circuit, or an arrhythmia focus. Tissue damage is achieved by thermal heating. This technique is also effective in the treatment of selected ventricular tachycardias (202).

Catheter position for radiofrequency ablation requires the use of fluoroscopy, generally excluding its use during pregnancy. Nevertheless, radiofrequency ablation was performed without complication for a right posteroseptal accessory pathway, which had been causing recurrent hemodynamically compromising episodes of orthodromic supraventricular tachycardia that were refractory to medical treatment (194). Echocardiographic guidance to electrophysiologic testing has been proposed as an alternative to fluoroscopy (203). More importantly, however, radiofrequency therapy is attractive for the patient who is on antiarrhythmic therapy, who is contemplating pregnancy, and who seeks definitive arrhythmia control to remove fetal risk associated with drug therapy.

Cardiac Pacemaker

Temporary or permanent cardiac pacing may be indicated in a pregnant woman for sinus node dysfunction, advanced AV block, congenital long QT syndrome, or neurocardiogenic syncope (101,204,205). Transthoracic and transesophageal echocardiography have been used to guide pacemaker lead positioning in lieu of fluoroscopy (206–208).

Implantable Cardioverter-Defibrillator

Implantable cardioverter-defibrillators are a highly effective form of therapy for the prevention of sudden death in patients with a history of or high risk for sustained ventricular tachycardia or fibrillation (101). A multicenter retrospective analysis of women with implantable cardioverter-defibrillators implanted before conception did not show an increased risk of major implantable cardioverter-defibrillator–related complications or an increased number of implantable cardioverter-defibrillator–related discharges (209). Specifically, there were no adverse sequelae of implantable cardioverter-defibrillator discharges on fetal outcome (209,210).

REFERENCES

1. Saxon LA, Perloff JK. Arrhythmias and conduction disturbances associated with pregnancy. In: Podrid PJ, Kowey PR, eds. *Cardiac arrhythmia: mechanisms, diagnosis and management.* Baltimore: Williams & Wilkins, 1995:1161–1174.
2. Page RL. Treatment of arrhythmias during pregnancy. *Am Heart J* 1995;130:871–876.
3. Chow T, Galvin J, McGovern B. Antiarrhythmic drug therapy in pregnancy and lactation. *Am J Cardiol* 1998;82:58I–62I.
4. Joglar JA, Page RL. Treatment of cardiac arrhythmias during pregnancy: safety considerations. *Drug Safety* 1999;20:85–94.
5. Cox JL, Gardner MJ. Treatment of cardiac arrhythmias during pregnancy. *Prog Cardiovasc Dis* 1993;36:137–178
6. Thilaen U, Olsson SB. Pregnancy and heart disease: a review. *Eur J Obstet Gynecol Reprod Biol* 1997;75:43–50.
7. Meijboom EJ, van Engelen AD, van de Beek EW, et al. Fetal arrhythmias. *Curr Opinion Cardiol* 1994;9:97–102.
8. Ito S, Magee L, Smallhorn J. Drug therapy for fetal arrhythmias. *Clin Perinatol* 1994;21:543–572.
9. Ward RM. Drug therapy of the fetus. *J Clin Pharmacol* 1993; 33:780–789.
10. Elkayam U, Gleicher N. *Cardiac problems in pregnancy: diagnosis and management of maternal and fetal disease.* New York: Wiley-Liss, 1998.
11. Gleicher N. *Principles and practice of medical therapy in pregnancy.* Stamford, CT: Appleton & Lange, 1998.
12. Hamilton B, Thomson KJ. *The heart in pregnancy and the childbearing age.* Boston: Little, Brown and Co, 1941.
13. Mendelson CL. Disorders of the heartbeat during pregnancy. *Am J Obstet Gynecol* 1956;72:1268–1301.
14. Perloff JK. Pregnancy and congenital heart disease. *J Am Coll Cardiol* 1991;18:340–342.
15. Stumpflen I, Stumpflen I, Wimmer M, et al. Effect of detailed fetal echocardiography as part of routine prenatal ultrasonographic screening on detection of congenital heart disease. *Lancet* 1996;348:854–857.
16. Montana E, Khoury MJ, Cragan JD, et al. Trends and outcomes after prenatal diagnosis of congenital cardiac malformations by fetal echocardiography in a well defined birth population, Atlanta, Georgia, 1990–1994. *J Am Coll Cardiol* 1996;28:1805–1809.
17. Connelly MS, Webb GD, Somerville J, et al. Canadian consen-

sus conference on adult congenital heart disease 1996. *Can J Cardiol* 1998;395–452.

18. Silka MJ, Hardy BG, Menashe VD, Morris CD. A population-based prospective evaluation of risk of sudden cardiac death after operation for common congenital heart defects. *J Am Coll Cardiol* 1998;32:245–251.

19. Hunter S, Robson SC. Adaptation of maternal heart in pregnancy. *Br Heart J* 1992;68:540–543.

20. Shotan A, Ostrzega E, Mehra A, et al. Incidence of arrhythmias in normal pregnancy and relation to palpitations, dizziness, and syncope. *Am J Cardiol* 1997;79:1061–1064.

21. Rosano GMC, Leonardo F, Sarrel PM, et al. Cyclical variation in paroxysmal supraventricular tachycardia in women. *Lancet* 1996;347:786–788.

22. Ekholm EM, Piha SF, Erkkola RU, et al. Autonomic cardiovascular reflexes in pregnancy. A longitudinal study. *Clin Auton Res* 1994;4:161–165.

23. Siu SC, Sermer M, Harrison DA, et al. Risk and predictors for pregnancy-related complications in women with heart disease. *Circulation* 1997;96:2789–2794.

24. Zuber M, Gautschi N, Oechslin E, et al. Outcome of pregnancy in women with congenital shunt lesions. *Heart* 1999;81: 271–275.

25. Siu S, Chitayat D, Webb G. Pregnancy in women with congential heart defects: what are the risks? *Heart* 1999;81:225–226.

26. Presbitero P, Somerville J, Stone S, et al. Pregnancy in cyanotic congenital heart disease. Outcome of mother and fetus. *Circulation* 1994;89:2673–2676.

27. Schmaltz AA, Neudorf U, Winkler UH. Outcome of pregnancy in women with congenital heart disease. *Cardiol Young* 1999;1: 88–96.

28. Canobbio MM, Mair DD, van der Velde M, et al. Pregnancy outcomes after Fontan repair. *J Am Coll Cardiol* 1996;28: 763–767.

29. Lao TT, Sermer M, Colman JM. Pregnancy following surgical correction for transposition of the great arteries. *Obstet Gynecol* 1994;83:665–668.

30. Lynch-Salamon DI, Maze SS, Combs CA. Pregnancy after Mustard repair for transposition of the great arteries. *Obstet Gynecol* 1993;82:676–679.

31. Megerian G, Bell JG, Huhta JC, et al. Pregnancy outcome following Mustard procedure for transposition of the great arteries: a report of five cases and review of the literature. *Obstet Gynecol* 1994;83:512–516.

32. Genoni M, Jenni R, Hoerstrup SP, et al. Pregnancy after atrial repair for transposition of the great arteries. *Heart* 1999;81: 276–277.

33. Weiss BM, von Segesser LK, Alon E, et al. Outcome of cardiovascular surgery and pregnancy: a systematic review of the period 1984–1996. *Am J Obstet Gynecol* 1998;179:1643–1653.

34. Suri V, Sawhney H, Vasishta K, et al. Pregnancy following cardiac valve replacement surgery. *Int J Gynaecol Obstet* 1999;64: 239–246.

35. Brown CS, Bertolet BD. Peripartum cardiomyopathy: a comprehensive review. *Am J Obstet Gynecol* 1998;178:409–414.

36. Lampert MB, Lang RM. Peripartum cardiomyopathy. *Am Heart J* 1995;130:860–870.

37. Piacenza JM, Kirkorian G, Andra PH, et al. Hypertrophic cardiomyopathy and pregnancy. *Eur J Obstet Gynecol Reprod Biol* 1998;80:17–23.

38. Magee LA, Ornstein MP, von Dadelszen P. Fortnightly review: management of hypertension in pregnancy. *BMJ (Clin Res Ed)* 1999;318:1332–1336.

39. Sibai BM. Treatment of hypertension in pregnant women. *N Engl J Med* 1996;335:257–265.

40. Naidoo DP, Bhorat I, Moodley J, et al. Continuous electrocardiographic monitoring in hypertensive crises in pregnancy. *Am J Obstet Gynecol* 1991;164:530–533.

41. Weiss BM, Zemp L, Seifert B, et al. Outcome of pulmonary vascular disease in pregnancy: a systematic overview from 1978 through 1996. *J Am Coll Cardiol* 1998;31:1650–1657.

42. Roth A, Elkayam U. Acute myocardial infarction associated with pregnancy. *Ann Intern Med* 1996;125:751–762.

43. Badui E, Enciso R. Acute myocardial infarction during pregnancy and puerperium: A review. *Angiology* 1996;47:739–756.

44. Robson SC, Hunter S, Boys R, et al. Serial study of factors influencing changes in cardiac output during human pregnancy. *Am J Physiol* 1989;256:H1060–H1065.

45. Clapp JF 3rd, Capeless E. Cardiovascular function before, during, and after the first and subsequent pregnancies. *Am J Cardiol* 1997;80:1469–1473.

46. Elkayam U. Pregnancy and cardiovascular disease. In: Braunwald E, ed. *Heart disease: a textbook of cardiovascular medicine.* Philadelphia: WB Saunders, 1997:1843–1864.

47. Carruth JE, Mirvis SB, Brogan DR, et al. The electrocardiogram in normal pregnancy. *Am Heart J* 1981;102:1075–1078.

48. Veille JC, Kitzman DW, Bacevice AE. Effects of pregnancy on the electrocardiogram in healthy subjects during strenuous exercise. *Am J Obstet Gynecol* 1996;175:1360–1364.

49. Ekholm EM, Hartiala J, Huikuri HV. Circadian rhythm of frequency-domain measures of heart rate variability in pregnancy. *Br J Obstet Gynecol* 1997;104:825–828.

50. Stein PK, Hagley MT, Cole PL, et al. Changes in 24-hour heart rate variability during normal pregnancy. *Am J Obstet Gynecol* 1999;180:978–985.

51. Chen GY, Kuo CD, Yang MJ, et al. Comparison of supine and upright positions on autonomic nervous activity in late pregnancy: the role of aortocaval compression. *Anaesthesia* 1999;54: 215–219.

52. Speranza G, Verlato G, Albiero A. Autonomic changes during pregnancy: assessment by spectral heart rate variability analysis. *J Electrocardiol* 1998;31:101–109.

53. Eneroth E, Storck N. Preeclampsia and maternal heart rate variability. *Gynecol Obstet Invest* 1998;45:170–173.

54. Lewinsky RM, Riskin-Mashiah S. Autonomic imbalance in preeclampsia: evidence for increased sympathetic tone in response to the supine-suppressor test. *Obstet Gynecol* 1998; 91:935–939.

55. Braunwald E, ed. *Heart disease: a textbook of cardiovascular medicine.* Philadelphia: WB Saunders, 1997.

56. Perloff JK. *The clinical recognition of congenital heart disease.* Philadelphia: WB Saunders, 1994.

57. Perloff JK, Koos B. Pregnancy and congenital heart disease: The mother and the fetus. In: Perloff JK, Child JS, eds. *Congenital heart disease in adults.* Philadelphia: WB Saunders, 1998: 144–164.

58. Natterson PD, Perloff JK, Klitzner TS, et al. Electrophysiologic abnormalities: unoperated occurrence and postoperative residua and sequelae. In: Perloff JK, Child JS, eds. *Congenital heart disease in adults.* Philadelphia: WB Saunders, 1998:316–345.

59. Wessel HU, Benson DW Jr, Braunlin EA, et al. Exercise response before and after termination of atrial tachycardia after congenital heart disease surgery. *Circulation* 1989;80:106–111.

60 Kennedy HL, Whitlock JA, Sprague MK, et al. Long term follow-up of asymptomatic healthy subjects with frequent and complex ventricular ectopy. *N Engl J Med* 1985;312:193–197.

61. Morganroth J, Michelson EL, Horowitz LN, et al. Limitations of routine long-term electrocardiographic monitoring to assess ventricular ectopic frequency. *Circulation* 1978;58:408–414.

62. Moss AJ. Clinical significance of ventricular arrhythmias in patients with and without coronary artery disease. *Prog Cardiovasc Dis* 1980;23:33–52.

63. Ruberman W, Weinblatt E, Goldberg JD, et al. Ventricular premature beats and mortality after myocardial infarction. *N Engl J Med* 1977;297:750–757.

64. Echt DS, Liebson PR, Mitchell B, et al, for the CAST Investigators. Mortality and morbidity in patients receiving encainide, flecainide, or placebo. *N Engl J Med* 1991;324:781–788.

65. Zipes DP. Genesis of cardiac arrhythmias: electrophysiological considerations. In: Braunwald E, ed. *Heart disease: a textbook of cardiovascular medicine.* Philadelphia: WB Saunders, 1997: 548–592.

66. Josephson ME. *Clinical cardiac electrophysiology: techniques and interpretations.* Philadelphia: Lea & Febiger, 1993.

67. Rotmensch HH, Rotmensch S, Elkayam U. Management of cardiac arrhythmias during pregnancy: current concepts. *Drugs* 1987;33:623–633.

68. Tawam M, Levine I, Mendelson M, et al. Effect of pregnancy on paroxysmal supraventricular tachycardia. *Am J Cardiol* 1993; 72:838–840.

69. Lee SH, Chen SA, Wu TJ, et al. Effects of pregnancy on first onset and symptoms of paroxysmal supraventricular tachycardia. *Am J Cardiol* 1995;76:675–678.

70. Kounis NG, Zavras GM, Papdaki PJ, et al. Pregnancy-induced increase of supraventricular arrhythmias in Wolff-Parkinson-White syndrome. *Clin Cardiol* 1995;18:137–140.

71. Zipes DP. Specific arrhythmias: diagnosis and treatment. In: Braunwald E, ed. *Heart disease: a textbook of cardiovascular medicine.* Philadelphia: WB Saunders, 1997:640–704.

72. Treakle K, Kostic B, Hulkower S. Supraventricular tachycardia resistant to treatment in a pregnant woman. *J Fam Pract* 1992; 35:581–584.

73. Flinn CJ, Wolff GS, MacDonald D II, et al. Cardiac rhythm after the Mustard operation for complete transposition of the great arteries. *N Engl J Med* 1984;310:1635–1638.

74. Al-Khatib SM, Pritchett EL. Clinical features of Wolff-Parkinson-White syndrome. *Am Heart J* 1999;138:403–413.

75. Obel OA, Camm AH. Accessory pathway reciprocating tachycardia. *Eur Heart J* 1998;19[Suppl E]:E13–24,E50–51.

76. Sager PT, Bhandari AK. Wide complex tachycardias. Differential diagnosis and management. *Cardiol Clin* 1991;9:595–618.

77. Steurer G, Gursoy S, Frey B, et al. The differential diagnosis on the electrocardiogram between ventricular tachycardia and pre-excited tachycardia. *Clin Cardiol* 1994;17:306–308.

78. Mozo de Rosales F, Moreno J, Bodegas A, et al. Conversion of atrial fibrillation with ajmaline in a pregnant woman with Wolff-Parkinson-White syndrome. *Eur J Obstet Gynecol Reprod Biol* 1994;56:63–66.

79. Szekely P, Snaith L. Atrial fibrillation and pregnancy. *Br Med J* 1961;1:1407–1410.

80. Brugada P, Brugada J, Mont L, et al. A new approach to the differential diagnosis of a regular tachycardia with a wide QRS complex. *Circulation* 1991;83:1649–1659.

81. McMillan TM, Bellet S. Ventricular paroxysmal tachycardia: report of case in pregnant girl of 16 years with apparently normal heart. *Am Heart J* 1931;7:70–71.

82. Altemose GT, Buxton AE. Idiopathic ventricular tachycardia. *Annu Rev Med* 1999;50:159–177.

83. Lerman BB, Stein KM, Markowitz SM. Idiopathic right ventricular outflow tract tachycardia: a clinical approach. *Pace* 1996;19:2120–2137.

84. Lerman BB, Stein KM, Markowitz SM. Mechanisms of idiopathic left ventricular tachycardia. *J Cardiovasc Electrophysiol* 1997;8:571–583.

85. Chandra NC, Gates EA, Thamer M. Conservative treatment of paroxysmal ventricular tachycardia during pregnancy. *Clin Cardiol* 1991;14:347–350.

86. Varon ME, Sherer DM, Abramowicz JS, et al. Maternal ventricular tachycardia associated with hypomagnesemia. *Am J Obstet Gynecol* 1992;167:1352–1355.

87. Bassoon-Zaltzman C, Sermer M, Lao TT, et al. Bladder pheochromocytoma in pregnancy without hypertension. A case report. *J Reprod Med* 1995;40:149–150.

88. Perry KG Jr, Morrison JC, Rust OA, et al. Incidence of adverse cardiopulmonary effects with low-dose continuous terbutaline infusion. *Am J Obstet Gynecol* 1995;173:1273–1277.

89. Hudgens DR, Conradi SE. Sudden death associated with terbutaline sulfate administration. *Am J Obstet Gynecol* 1993;169: 120–121.

90. Onuigbo M, Alikhan M. Over-the-counter sympathomimetics: a risk factor for cardiac arrhythmias in pregnancy. *South Med J* 1998;91:1153–1155.

91. Braverman AC, Bromley BS, Rutherford JD. New onset ventricular tachycardia during pregnancy. *Int J Cardiol* 1991; 409–412.

92. Gregg AR, Tomich PG. Mexiletine use in pregnancy. *J Perinatol* 1988;8:33–35.

93. Ledwich JR, Fay JE. Idiopathic recurrent ventricular fibrillation. *Am J Cardiol* 1969;24:255–258.

94. O'Callaghan AC, Normandale JP, Morgan M. The prolonged QT syndrome: a review with anaesthetic implications and a report of two cases. *Anaesth Intensive Care* 1982;10:50–55.

95. McCurdy CM Jr, Rutherford SE, Coddington CC. Syncope and sudden arrhythmic death complicating pregnancy. A case report of Romano-Ward syndrome. *J Reprod Med* 1993;38:233–234.

96. Rashba EJ, Zareba W, Moss AJ, et al. Influence of pregnancy on the risk for cardiac events in patients with hereditary long QT syndrome. *Circulation* 1998;97:451–456.

97. Schwartz PJ. The long QT syndrome. *Curr Probl Cardiol* 1997; 22:297–351.

98. Garry D, Leikin E, Fleisher AG, et al. Acute myocardial infarction in pregnancy with subsequent medical and surgical management. *Obstet Gynecol* 1996;87:802–804.

99. Shah DM, Sunderji SG. Hypertrophic cardiomyopathy and pregnancy: report of a maternal mortality and review of literature. *Obstet Gynecol Surv* 1985;40:444–448.

100. Wagner GS. *Marriott's practical electrocardiography.* Baltimore: Williams & Wilkins, 1994.

101. Gregoratos G, Cheitlin MD, Conill A, et al. ACC/AHA guidelines for implantation of cardiac pacemakers and antiarrhythmia devices: a report of the American College of Cardiology/American Heart Association Task Force on Practice Guidelines (Committee on Pacemaker Implantation). *J Am Coll Cardiol* 1998;31: 1175–1209.

102. Copeland GD, Stern TN. Wenckebach periods in pregnancy and puerperium. *Am Heart J* 1958;56:291–298.

103. Pinsky WW, Gillette PC, Garson A Jr, et al. Diagnosis, management, and long-term results of patients with congenital complete atrioventricular block. *Pediatrics* 1982;69:728–733.

104. Brumund MR, Lutin WA. Advances in antenatal diagnosis and management of the fetus with a heart problem. *Pediatr Ann* 1998;27:486–490.

105. Ferrer PL. Fetal arrhythmias. In: Deal BJ, Wolff GS, Gelband H, eds. *Current concepts in diagnosis and management of arrhythmias in infants and children.* Armonk, NY: Futura Publishing, 1998:17–63.

106. Case CL, Fyfe DA. Fetal dysrhythmias. In: Gilette PC, Garson A Jr, eds. *Pediatric arrhythmias: electrophysiology and pacing.* Philadelphia: WB Saunders, 1990:637–647.

107. Buttino L Jr, Cusick W, Gleicher N. Fetal heart rate and rhythm disorders. In: Elkayam U, Gleicher N, eds. *Cardiac problems in pregnancy: diagnosis and management of maternal and fetal disease.* New York: Wiley-Liss, 1998:583–602.

108 Hon EH. The electronic evaluation of the fetal heart rate. Pre-

liminary report. 1958 [Classical article]. *Am J Obstet Gynecol* 1996;175:747–748.

109. Hon EH. *An atlas of fetal heart rate patterns.* New Haven, CT: Harty Press, 1968.

110. Fyfe DA, Meyer KB, Case CL. Sonographic assessment of fetal cardiac arrhythmias. *Semin Ultrasound Comput Tomogr Magn Reson* 1993;14:286–297.

111. DeVore GR, Siassi B, Platt LD. Fetal echocardiography. III. The diagnosis of cardiac arrhythmias using real-time directed M-mode ultrasound. *Am J Obstet Gynecol* 1983;146:792–799.

112. Kleinman CS, Donnerstein RL, Jaffe CC, et al. Fetal echocardiography: a tool for evaluation of in utero cardiac arrhythmias and monitoring of *in utero* therapy: analysis of 71 patients. *Am J Cardiol* 1983;51:237–243.

113. Hukkinen K, Kariniemi V, Katila TE, et al. Instantaneous fetal heart rate monitoring by electromagnetic methods. *Am J Obstet Gynecol* 1976;125:1115–1120.

114. Menaendez T, Achenbach S, Moshage W, et al. Prenatal recording of fetal heart action with magnetocardiography. *Zeitschrift Kardiologie* 1998;87:111–118.

115. Hofbeck M, Ulmer H, Beinder E, et al. Prenatal findings in patients with prolonged QT interval in the neonatal period. *Heart* 1997;77:198–204.

116. Vigliani M. Romano-Ward syndrome diagnosed as moderate fetal bradycardia. A case report. *J Reprod Med* 1995;40:725–728.

117. Shenker L. Fetal cardiac arrhythmias. *Obstet Gynecol Surv* 1979; 34:561–572.

118. Smeenk RJ. Immunological aspects of congenital atrioventricular block. *Pace* 1997;20:2093–2097.

119. Olah KS, Gee H. Antibody mediated complete congenital heart block in the fetus. *Pace* 1993;16:1872–1879.

120. Press J, Uziel Y, Laxer RM, et al. Long-term outcome of mothers of children with complete congenital heart block. *Am J Med* 1996;100:328–332.

121. Groves AM, Allan LD, Rosenthal E. Outcome of isolated congenital complete heart block diagnosed *in utero. Heart* 1996;75: 190–194.

122. Young BK, Klein SA, Katz M. Intrapartum fetal cardiac arrhythmias. *Obstet Gynecol* 1979;54:427–432.

123. Klapholz H, Schifrin BS, Rivo E. Paroxysmal supraventricular tachycardia in the fetus. *Obstet Gynecol* 1974;43:718–721.

124. Jaeggi E, Fouron JC, Drblik SP. Fetal atrial flutter: diagnosis, clinical features, treatment, and outcome. *J Pediatr* 1998;132: 335–339.

125. Soyeur DJ. Atrial flutter in the human fetus: diagnosis, hemodynamic consequences, and therapy. *J Cardiovasc Electrophysiol* 1996;7:989–998.

126. Hourvitz A, Achiron R, Abraham A, et al. Induced cardioversion of fetal flutter by artificial rupture of membranes at term. *J Perinat Med* 1995;23:403–407.

127. Van der Horst RL. Congenital atrial flutter and cardiac failure presenting as hydrops foetalis at birth. *S Afr Med J* 1970;44: 1037–1039.

128. Yamada M, Nakazawa M, Momma K. Fetal ventricular tachycardia in long QT syndrome. *Cardiol Young* 1998;8:119–122.

129. Lopes LM, Cha SC, Scanavacca MI, et al. Fetal idiopathic ventricular tachycardia with nonimmune hydrops: benign course. *Pediatr Cardiol* 1996;17:192–193.

130. Cusick W, Buttino L Jr, Gleicher N. Intrauterine therapy of rhythm and rate disorders and heart failure. In: Elkayam U, Gleicher N, eds. *Cardiac problems in pregnancy: diagnosis and management of maternal and fetal disease.* New York: Wiley-Liss, 1998:603–613.

131. Kleinman CS, Copel JA, Weinstein EM, et al. Treatment of fetal supraventricular tachyarrhythmias. *J Clin Ultrasound* 1985;13:265–273.

132. Simpson JM, Sharland GK. Fetal tachycardias: management and outcome of 127 consecutive cases. *Heart* 1998;79: 576–581.

133. Parilla BV, Strasburger FJ, Socol ML. Fetal supraventricular tachycardia complicated by hydrops fetalis: a role for direct fetal intramuscular therapy. *Am J Perinatol* 1996;13:483–486.

134. Hallak M, Neerhof MG, Perry R, et al. Fetal supraventricular tachycardia and hydrops fetalis: combined intensive, direct, and transplacental therapy. *Obstet Gynecol* 1991;78:523–525.

135. Weiner CP, Thompson MI. Direct treatment of fetal supraventricular tachycardia after failed transplacental therapy. *Am J Obstet Gynecol* 1988;158:570–573.

136. Carpenter RJ Jr, Strasburger JR, Garson A Jr, et al. Fetal ventricular pacing for hydrops secondary to complete atrioventricular block. *J Am Coll Cardiol* 1986;8:1434–1436.

137. Souma ML, Cabaniss CD, Nataraj A, et al. The Valsalva maneuver: a test of autonomic nervous system function in pregnancy. *Am J Obstet Gynecol* 1983;145:274–278.

138. Zipes DP. Management of cardiac arrhythmias: pharmacological, electrical, and surgical techniques. In: Braunwald E, ed. *Heart disease: a textbook of cardiovascular medicine.* Philadelphia: WB Saunders, 1997:593–639.

139. Rosen MR, Strauss HC, Janse MJ. The classification of antiarrhythmic drugs. In: Zipes DP, Jalife J, eds. *Cardiac electrophysiology: from cell to bedside.* Philadelphia: WB Saunders, 1995: 1277–1286.

140. Koren G, Pastuszak A, Ito S. Drugs in pregnancy. *N Engl J Med* 1998;338:1128–1137.

141. *Physicians' Desk Reference 1999.* Montvale, NJ: Medical Economics Company, 1999.

142. American Academy of Pediatrics Committee on Drugs. The transfer of drugs and other chemicals into human breast milk. *Pediatrics* 1994;93:137–150.

143. Wilbur SL, Marchlinski FE. Adenosine as an antiarrhythmic agent. *Am J Cardiol* 1997;79:30–37.

144. Camm AJ, Garratt C. Adenosine and supraventricular tachycardia. *N Engl J Med* 1991;325:1621–1629.

145. Cohen TJ, Tucker KJ, Abbott JA, et al. Usefulness of adenosine in augmenting ventricular preexcitation for noninvasive localization of accessory pathways. *Am J Cardiol* 1992;69:1178–1185.

146. Chen SA, Tai CT, Chiang CE, et al. Electrophysiologic characteristics, electropharmacologic responses and radiofrequency ablation in patients with decremental accessory pathway. *J Am Coll Cardiol* 1996;28:732–737.

147. Sellers TD, Kirchhoffer JB, Modesto TA. Adenosine: a clinical experience and comparison with verapamil for the termination of supraventricular tachycardias. *Prog Clin Biol Res* 1987;230: 283–299.

148. Merson N. Adenosine treatment of supraventricular tachycardia following epidural test dose: a case study. *AANA J* 1993;61: 521–523.

149. Kanai M, Shimizu M, Shiozawa T, et al. Use of intravenous adenosine triphosphate (ATP) to terminate supraventricular tachycardia in a pregnant woman with Wolff-Parkinson-White syndrome. *J Obstet Gynaecol Res* 1996;22:95–99.

150. Omar HA, Rhodes LA, Ramirez R, et al. Alteration of human placental vascular tone by antiarrhythmic medications in vitro. *J Cardiovasc Electrophysiol* 1996;7:1197–1203.

151. Rogers MC, Willerson JT, Goldblatt A, et al. Serum digoxin concentrations in the human fetus, neonate, and infant. *N Engl J Med* 1972;287:1010–1013.

152. Luxford AME, Kellaway GSM. Pharmacokinetics of digoxin in pregnancy. *Eur J Clin Pharmacol* 1983;25:117–121.

153. Okita GT, Plotz EJ, Davis ME. Placental transfer of radioactive digitoxin in pregnant women and its fetal distribution. *Circ Res* 1956;4:376–380.

154. Schlebusch H, von Mende S, Grunn U, et al. Determination of digoxin in the blood of pregnant women, fetuses and neonates before and during antiarrhythmic therapy using four immuno-chemical methods. *Eur J Clin Chem Clin Biochem* 1991;29:57–66.

155. Weaver JB, Pearson JF. Influence of digitalis on time of onset and duration of labour in women with cardiac disease. *Br Med J* 1973;3:519–520.

156. Barden TP, Stander RW. Effects of adrenergic blocking agents and catecholamines in human pregnancy. *Am J Obstet Gynecol* 1968;102:226–235.

157. Paran E, Holzberg G, Mazor M, et al. Beta-adrenergic blocking agents in the treatment of pregnancy-induced hypertension. *Int J Clin Pharmacol Ther* 1995;33:119–123.

158. Kaaja R, Hiilesmaa V, Holma K, et al. Maternal antihypertensive therapy with beta-blockers associated with poor outcome in very-low birthweight infants. *Int J Gynecol Obstet* 1992;38:195–199.

159. Byerly W, Hartmann A, Tannenbaum A. Verapamil in the treatment of maternal paroxysmal supraventricular tachycardia. *Ann Emerg Med* 1991;20:552–554.

160. Ban Y, Nakatsuka T, Matsumoto H. Effects of calcium channel blockers on cultured rat embryos. *J Appl Toxicol* 1996;16:147–151.

161. Stein G, Srivastava MK, Marker HJ, et al. Effects of calcium channel blockers on the development of early rat postimplantation embryos in culture. *Arch Toxicol* 1990;64:623–638.

162. Miller MR, Withers R, Bhamra R, Holt DW. Verapamil and breast feeding. *Eur J Clin Pharmacol* 1986;30:125–126.

163. Tadmor OP, Keren A, Rosenak D, et al. The effect of disopyramide on uterine contractions during pregnancy. *Am J Obstet Gynecol* 1990;162:482–486.

164. Meyer J, Lackner JE, Schochet SS. Paroxysmal tachycardia in pregnancy. *JAMA* 1930;94:1901–1904.

165. Mauer AM, Devaux LO, Lahey ME. Neonatal and maternal thrombocytopenic purpura due to quinidine. *Pediatrics* 1957;19:84–87.

166. Ellsworth AJ, Horn JR, Raisys VA, et al. Disopyramide and N-monodesalkyl disopyramide in serum and breast milk. *Drug Intell Clin Pharm* 1989;23:56–57.

167. Kuhnert BR, Knapp DR, Kuhnert PM, et al. Maternal, fetal and neonatal metabolism of lidocaine. *Clin Pharmacol Ther* 1979;26:213–220.

168. Brown WU Jr, Bell GC, Alper MH. Acidosis, local anesthetics, and the newborn. *Obstet Gynecol* 1976;48:27–30.

169. Banzai M, Sato S, Tezuka N, et al. Placental transfer of lidocaine hydrochloride after prolonged continuous maternal intravenous administration. *Can J Anaesth* 1995;42:338–340.

170. Morishima HO, Finster M, Arthur GR, et al. Pregnancy does not alter lidocaine toxicity. *Am J Obstet Gynecol* 1990;162:1320–1324.

171. Ahmed K, Issawi I, Peddireddy R. Use of flecainide for refractory atrial tachycardia of pregnancy. *Am J Crit Care* 1996;5:306–308.

172. Polak PE, Stewart PA, Hess J. Complete atrioventricular dissociation and His bundle tachycardia in a new born: problems in prenatal diagnosis and post natal management. *Int J Cardiol* 1989;22:269–271.

173. Frohn-Mulder IM, Stewart PA, Witsenburg M, et al. The efficacy of flecainide versus digoxin in the management of fetal supraventricular tachycardia. *Prenat Diag* 1995;15:1297–1302.

174. Wagner X, Jouglard J, Moulin M, et al. Coadministration of flecainide acetate and sotalol during pregnancy: lack of teratogenic effects, passage across the placenta, and excretion in human breast milk. *Am Heart J* 1990;119:700–702.

175. Vanderhalt AL, Cocjin J, Santulli TV, et al. Conjugated hyper-bilirubinemia in a newborn infant after maternal (transplacen-

tal) treatment with flecainide acetate for fetal tachycardia and fetal hydrops. *J Pediatr* 1995;126:988–990.

176. Murray KT. Ibutilide. *Circulation* 1998;97:493–497.

177. Falk RH, Pollak A, Singh SN, Friedrich T. Intravenous Dofetilide Investigators. Intravenous dofetilide, a class III antiarrhythmic agent, for the termination of sustained atrial fibrillation or flutter. *J Am Coll Cardiol* 1997;29:385–390.

178. Torp-Pedersen C, Moller M, Bloch-Thomsen PE, et al. Danish Investigations of Arrhythmia and Mortality on Dofetilide Study Group. Dofetilide in patients with congestive heart failure and left ventricular dysfunction. *N Engl J Med* 1999;341:857–865.

179. Widerhorn J, Bhandari AK, Bughi S, et al. Fetal and neonatal adverse effects profile of amiodarone treatment during pregnancy. *Am Heart J* 1991;122:1162–1166.

180. Magee LA, Downar E, Sermer M, et al. Pregnancy outcome after gestational exposure to amiodarone in Canada. *Am J Obstet Gynecol* 1995;172:1307–1311.

181. Matsumura LK, Born D, Kunii IS, et al. Outcome of thyroid function in newborns from mothers treated with amiodarone. *Thyroid* 1992;2:279–281.

182. Magee LA, Nulman I, Rovet JF, et al. Neurodevelopment after in utero amiodarone exposure. *Neurotoxicol Teratol* 1999;21:261–265.

183. Gembruch U, Manz M, Bald R, et al. Repeated intravascular treatment with amiodarone in a fetus with refractory supraventricular tachycardia and hydrops fetalis. *Am Heart J* 1989;118:1335–1338.

184. Webster WS, Brown-Woodman PD, Snow MD, et al. Teratogenic potential of almokalant, dofetilide, and d-sotalol: drugs with potassium channel blocking activity. *Teratology* 1996;53:168–175.

185. Abrahamsson C, Palmer M, Ljung B, et al. Induction of rhythm abnormalities in the fetal rat heart. A tentative mechanism for the embryotoxic effect of the class III antiarrhythmic agent almokalant. *Cardiovasc Res* 1994;28:337–344.

186. Speiser Z, Gordon I, Rehavi M, et al. Behavioral and biochemical studies in rats following prenatal treatment with beta-adrenoceptor antagonists. *Eur J Pharmacol* 1991;195:75–83.

187. Gutgesell M, Overholt E, Boyle R. Oral bretylium tosylate use during pregnancy and subsequent breast feeding: a case report. *Am J Perinatol* 1990;7:144–145.

188. Marks TA, Terry RD. Developmental toxicity of ibutilide fumarate in rats after oral administration. *Teratology* 1996;54:157–164.

189. Emergency Cardiac Care Committee and Subcommittees, American Heart Association. Guidelines for cardiopulmonary resuscitation and emergency cardiac care. IV: special resuscitation situations. *JAMA* 1992;268:2242–2250.

190. Kloeck W, Cummins RO, Chamberlain D, et al. Special resuscitation situations: an advisory statement from the International Liaison Committee on Resuscitation. *Circulation* 1997;95:2196–2210.

191. Goodwin AP, Pearce AJ. The human wedge: a manoeuvre to relieve aortocaval compression in resuscitation during late pregnancy. *Anaesthesia* 1992;47:433–434.

192. Katz VL, Dotters DJ, Droegemueller W. Perimortem cesarean delivery. *Obstet Gynecol* 1986;68:571.

193. Perkins V. CPR during pregnancy. *Am Heart J* 1996;132:1319.

194. Domainguez A, Iturralde P, Hermosillo AG, et al. Successful radiofrequency ablation of an accessory pathway during pregnancy. *Pace* 1999;22:131–134.

195. Meitus ML. Fetal electrocardiography and cardioversion with direct current countershock. Report of a case. *Dis Chest* 1965;48:324–325.

196. Rosemond RL. Cardioversion during pregnancy. *JAMA* 1993;269:3167.

197. Schwartz PJ, Locati EH, Moss AJ, et al. Left cardiac sympathetic denervation in the therapy of congenital long QT syndrome: a worldwide report. *Circulation* 1991;84:503–511.

198. Stevenson WG. Surgical sympathectomy to prevent sudden death. *J Cardiovasc Electrophysiol* 1992;3:17–20.

199. Bruner JP, Barry MJ, Elliott JP. Pregnancy in a patient with idiopathic long QT syndrome. *Am J Obstet Gynecol* 1984;149: 690–691.

200. Jackman WM, Wang X, Friday KJ, et al. Catheter ablation of accessory atrioventricular pathways (Wolff-Parkinson-White syndrome) by radiofrequency current. *N Engl J Med* 1991;324: 1605–1611.

201. Calkins H, Sousa J, El-Atassi R, et al. Diagnosis and cure of the Wolff-Parkinson-White syndrome or paroxysmal supraventricular tachycardias during a single electrophysiologic test. *N Engl J Med* 1991;324:1612–1618.

202. Coggins DL, Lee RJ, Sweeney J, et al. Radiofrequency catheter ablation as a cure for idiopathic tachycardia of both left and right ventricular origin. *J Am Coll Cardiol* 1994;23:1333–1341.

203. Lee MS, Evans SJ, Blumberg S, et al. Echocardiographically guided electrophysiologic testing in pregnancy. *J Am Soc Echocardiogr* 1994;7:182–186.

204. Schonbrun M, Rowland W, Quiroz AC. Complete heart block in pregnancy. Successful use of an intravenous pacemaker in 2 patients during labor. *Obstet Gynecol* 1966;27:243–246.

205. Berestka SA, Spellacy WN. Complete heart block associated with pregnancy and treated with an internal pacemaker. *Lancet* 1967;87:461–463.

206. Geudal M, Kervancioglu C, Oral D, et al. Permanent pacemaker implantation in a pregnant woman with the guidance of ECG and two-dimensional echocardiography. *Pace* 1987;10: 543–545.

207. Jordaens LJ, Vandenbogaerde JF, Van de Bruaene P, et al. Transesophageal echocardiography for insertion of a physiological pacemaker in early pregnancy. *Pace* 1990;13:955–957.

208. Antonelli D, Block L, Rosenfeld T. Implantation of permanent dual chamber pacemaker in a pregnant woman by transesophageal echocardiographic guidance. *Pace* 1999;22:534–535.

209. Natale A, Davidson T, Geiger MJ, et al. Implantable cardioverter-defibrillators and pregnancy: a safe combination? *Circulation* 1997;96:2808–2812.

210. Piper JM, Berkus M, Ridgway LE III. Pregnancy complicated by chronic cardiomyopathy and an automatic implantable cardioverter defibrillator. *Am J Obstet Gynecol* 1992;167:506–507.

28

ARRHYTHMIA IN ATHLETES

MICHAEL A. BRODSKY
CYRIL Y. LEUNG

INTRODUCTION

Cardiovascular disease has been the leading cause of death in the industrialized world since the middle of the 20th century. One possible cause of this problem was a change in the work environment from a physical to a nonphysical labor force as subsequent research has shown physical inactivity to be a risk factor for the development of cardiovascular disease (1). Data from the United States aerobics center longitudinal study have suggested that the level of cardiorespiratory fitness is directly correlated to cardiovascular disease and all-cause mortality rate (2). This relationship has been confirmed in various other populations by metaanalysis of multiple studies (3). Physical fitness has also been associated with other benefits related to cardiovascular risk factors such as improved lipid profile, better glucose metabolism, lower blood pressure and body weight, and nonsmoking (2).

Coincidentally, revival of the Olympics in 1896 helped arouse an international focus on sports. The results of the games were interpreted as criteria on which to judge the local culture. In this way, organized sports became an important part of a community's identity. Eventually the best athletes became icons of their society. Thus, modern society placed great value on athleticism and attention to fitness.

This attitude toward athleticism has resulted in a mass movement toward exercise, particularly in the United States; however, questions have been raised about the risks and benefits of exercise, as athletic training with regular exercise can have a definite effect on cardiovascular structure and function, as well as the heart rhythm (4,5). Although exercise is generally beneficial for the heart, it has been implicated in cardiovascular disease and in rare circumstances can be associated with serious fatal events (4). Of the myriad opinions on this subject, most authors agree that arrhythmia, exercise, athleticism, and sudden cardiac death (SCD) are important interconnected concepts that need to be understood (4–6). The purpose of this chapter is to review the physiologic and morphologic changes the heart undergoes as a result of exercise. We review the current data about arrhythmias and the pathophysiology of SCD in this population. In addition, recommendations for preathletic participation evaluation screening, diagnosis, and management are considered.

PHYSIOLOGIC CHANGES WITH EXERCISE

The cardiovascular effects of both acute and chronic exertion are complex and require a basic understanding of exercise physiology. Exercise is often classified as either dynamic/isotonic or static/isometric. Dynamic activities include those with active change in muscle length, such as running, cycling, rowing, or swimming. Static activities, which increase the resistance against which muscles work, include weight lifting, wrestling, and shot putting. Few activities are purely either dynamic or static; they usually have components of both.

The parameter most frequently used in assessing the level of training or the intensity of an exercise is oxygen uptake, which equals the product of cardiac output and arterial-venous O_2 difference (7,8). In dynamic exercise, there are increases in heart rate, stroke volume, and mean blood pressure, and there is a decrease in total peripheral resistance (9). The rise in heart rate seen with initiation of exercise is primarily a result of withdrawal of parasympathetic tone (10); however, heart rate increases to more than 130 beats per minute (bpm) are usually a result of elevated levels of circulating catecholamines (8,11). Stroke volume increases with acute dynamic exercise because of an increased myocardial contractility resulting from catecholamines and the Frank-Starling mechanism, and because dynamic exercise causes an increased venous return that results in a cardiovascular volume load and hence an increase in contractility (12). With initiation of exercise, intrathoracic pressures fall to a greater negative value, and this, combined with enhanced venous return secondary to the milking effect of muscular contraction, causes greater inflow into the right and left ventricles with a concomitant

M. A. Brodsky and C. Y. Leung: Department of Cardiology, University of California, Irvine Medical Center, Orange, California 92868.

increase in ventricular diameter and subsequent invocation of the Frank-Starling mechanism (13). Circulating catecholamines cause enhanced myocardial contractility and improvement in left ventricular (LV) ejection fraction as documented with echocardiography (14).

Static exercise, on the other hand, causes a smaller increase in oxygen consumption, cardiac output, and heart rate, and no significant increase in stroke volume (15). Although end-diastolic ventricular volume may increase because of increased venous return and greater negative intrathoracic pressures, the end-systolic volume may also increase, reflecting exaggerated afterload, resulting in no net increase in stroke volume. There is also a marked increase in mean arterial blood pressure but no appreciable change in total peripheral resistance. Thus, dynamic exercise primarily causes a volume load on the LV, whereas static exercise causes a pressure overload on the cardiovascular system. In real life, the combination of these effects results in adaptive physiologic and morphologic cardiovascular changes.

Morphologic Cardiac Changes

There are specific morphologic cardiac changes associated with exercise. Echocardiographic analysis has suggested that isometrically trained athletes have an increase in LV wall thickness without concomitant increase in cavity size, whereas endurance training results in an increase in LV cavity size and LV wall thickness (16). Studies comparing the differences in cardiac dimensions between athletes and nonathletes have shown that the athletic group had significant increases in ventricular septal thickness, posterior free wall thickness, LV end-diastolic dimension, LV mass, and right ventricular (RV) transverse diameter; however, these parameters are usually within normal limits in the healthy, nontrained population (17,18). LV hypertrophy criteria are frequently met in endurance and statically trained individuals, reflecting larger cavity size and wall thickness, respectively (19) (Fig. 28-1). Despite these changes in wall thickness and size, the LV shape is not altered (20). Douglas and colleagues (21) noted that the RV and LV had different responses to exercise; echocardiographic images obtained immediately after prolonged exercise showed that RV size increased significantly, whereas the LV size was reduced. Pelliccia and colleagues (22) reviewed echocardiographic data in 947 elite athletes (78% men) looking for the upper limit of physiologic cardiac hypertrophy. They noted that less than 2% of athletes had a LV wall thickness of more than or equal to 13 mm. The thickest LV sizes were noted in rowers, canoeists, and a cyclist, each of whom additionally had an enlarged LV cavity (22). Henriksen and colleagues (23) also noted similar findings in 127 male elite endurance athletes. In their analysis, 13% had a LV wall thickness of more than 13 mm, but none had a wall thickness of more than 15 mm. These data help differentiate

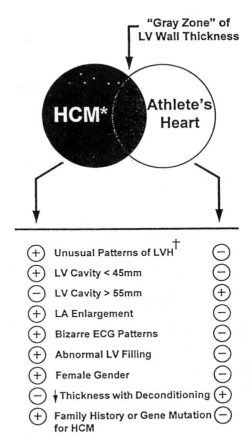

FIGURE 28-1. Flow chart showing criteria used to distinguish hypertrophic cardiomyopathy (HCM) from athlete's heart when the left ventricular (LV) wall thickness is within the shaded area of overlap, consistent with both diagnoses. (* Assumed to be the nonobstructive form of HCM, as the presence of substantial mitral valve systolic motion would confirm the diagnosis of HCM in an athlete. † May involve various morphologic abnormalities including heterogeneous distribution of left ventricular hypertrophy in which the asymmetry is prominent—adjacent regions may differ in thickness, with sharp transitions evident between segments; and patterns in which the anterior ventricular septum is spared from the hypertrophic process and the region of predominant thickening may be in the posterior portion of the septum or the anterolateral or posterior free wall.) LA, left atrial. (From Maron BJ, Pelliccia A, Spirito P. Cardiac disease in young trained athletes: insights into methods for distinguishing athlete's heart from structural heart disease, with particular emphasis on hypertrophic cardiomyopathy. *Circulation* 1995;91:1596–1601, with permission of American Heart Association.)

"physiologic" hypertrophy from hypertrophy seen in hypertrophic cardiomyopathy (HCM).

The myocardial hypertrophy seen in athletes is usually symmetric, as opposed to that seen in individuals with HCM, which is most often asymmetric, involving predominantly the interventricular septum (24). There are many other distinctive morphologic and echocardiographic differences between athletic LV hypertrophy and HCM (25,26) (Fig. 28-1). HCM, usually an autosomally dominant transmitted genetic disease, is characterized by a hypertrophic nondilated LV, which is present in the absence of an obvious cause of hypertrophy such as hypertension and aortic stenosis and is often associated with an exaggerated interventricular septum to posterior wall ratio (more than 1.3 : 1) and bizarre cellular architecture with an increased number of abnormal-appearing intramural coronary arteries with thickened walls and compromised lumina (27). This distinction is particularly important in determining the difference between a physiologic adaptation and a pathologic, often life-threatening, condition.

Henriksen and colleagues (23) found that the RV inflow tract diameter and right and left atrial measurements were significantly greater in endurance athletes compared with those of normal subjects (23); in addition, the RV free wall was slightly thicker than what was seen in normal active subjects but the differences were small. These data suggest that cardiac enlargement occurs symmetrically in right and left cavities, probably reflecting greater hemodynamic loading, a mechanism by which athletes sustain a high cardiac output during exercise.

Most of the aforementioned data have been obtained in young male athletes. Specific studies of women found that female resistance and endurance-trained athletes exhibited a lesser degree of LV changes than male athletes (28,29). LV cavity size exceeding normal limits was evident in a minority (8%) of women athletes and was rarely (1% of athletes) within the range of dilated cardiomyopathy (29). Elderly athletes have also been noted to have a lesser degree of LV changes than their youthful counterparts (30). Many, if not all, of these physiologic changes in men and women resolve with deconditioning usually within 3 months (31).

INCIDENCE OF SPECIFIC TYPES OF ARRHYTHMIAS AND CONDUCTION DISTURBANCES

Cardiac electrophysiology changes in response to exercise in much the same way as the aforementioned cardiac structure evolves. In general, most of the electrical phenomena are likely the results of physiologic hypertrophy and increased parasympathetic tone. Analysis of beat-to-beat variations in the R-R intervals of athletes has shown increased heart rate variability in all spectral bands reflecting changing autonomic tone (32–34). Puig and colleagues (33) suggested that the bradycardia and heart rate variability seen in athletes indicated an increase in parasympathetic activity without reduction in sympathetic tone. Significant electrocardiographic (ECG) changes begin to occur within 11 weeks of training and disappear soon after cessation of exercise (19). To understand the athlete's cardiac electrical phenomena, one must comprehend the normal cardiac electrophysiology.

The most comprehensive study of electrophysiology in a normal population was published by Hiss and Lamb (35) in 1962 and was based on a standard 12-lead ECG, which

recorded 1 minute of information per subject, obtained in 122,043 Air Force recruits aged 16 and older. Subsequently, dynamic (Holter) ECG was developed, which allowed for further evaluation of the heart's rhythm. This information allowed approximately 24 hours of two- or three-lead ECG typically during a wide range of behavior including the activity of daily living and exercise. Throughout the last three decades, there have been numerous Holter studies of the heart rhythm of controls and athletes. To analyze data from controls and athletes, we selected four control Holter studies, four athlete Holter studies, and six studies directly comparing athletes with controls (34,36–48). In these reports, the subjects varied by age, trained athletic activity, and geography, although most of the subjects were men (Tables 28-1 and 28-2).

Sinus Node Function

Analysis of the ECGs in Air Force recruits found that 24% had sinus bradycardia, 3% had sinus tachycardia, and 2% had sinus arrhythmia (35). The control Holter studies found an average heart rate of 68 to 82 bpm in the different populations (34,36–39,48) (Tables 28-1 and 28-2). Sinus bradycardia and tachycardia were transiently found in all 50 of the male medical students and a heart rate of less than 40 bpm was noted in 24%, most often occurring during sleep. Marked bradycardia was slightly less common in women; the minimum heart rate was 33 bpm in men and 40 bpm in women (37). In the elderly population, the men also had a slower heart rate than women (38). Control data from the study of 100 teenage boys was consistent with the adult data. The minimum sinus heart rate noted was 35 bpm (39). As expected, bradycardia was even more common in athletes than in controls. The athlete's average heart rate ranged from 50 to 66 bpm and the minimum heart rate averaged in the 30s. Sinus arrhythmia was noted in all individuals, although there were more episodes of marked R-R–interval changes in athletes, and more in men than in women with few exceptions. The longest pause was only slightly longer than 2 seconds in the controls but often longer than 2.5 seconds in the athletes. In the direct comparison studies, athletes had slower average and minimum heart rate and longer pauses than controls, regardless of age.

Although resting bradycardia is a commonly encountered phenomenon in athletes, several studies have confirmed that circadian heart rate variation in this group of individuals is maintained and normal (42,49,50). Although speculation exists regarding the mechanism of bradycardia in this group, the exact cause remains unclear. Potential explanations include alterations of autonomic nervous system activity, changes in sinus node sensitivity to cholinergic influences, and a secondary effect of increased stroke volume (8,32–34,51). The mechanism of prolonged pauses in the athletic population is likely due to the same reasons as bradycardia. These long sinus pauses can be disconcerting but are unlikely to be of clinical significance. Ogawa and

TABLE 28-1. AMBULATORY ELECTROCARDIOGRAPHY IN CONTROLS AND ATHLETES

Author/Year	N	Age	% Male	Time (h)	Sport	Avg HR	Min HR	Long Sinus Pause	1st AVB	2nd AVB I	2nd AVB II 3rd AVB	APD (%)	SVT/AF (%)	VPD (%)	Complex VPD (%)	VT (%)
Controls																
Brodsky, 1977 (36)	50	25	100	24	C	73	33	2.06	8	6	0	56	2	50	18	2
Sobotka, 1981 (37)	50	25	0	24	C	82	40	1.92	12	4	0	64	2	54	14	2
Fleg, 1982 (38)	98	60–85	70	24	C	72	34	1.88	6	1	0	88	28	80	11	4
Dickinson, 1984 (39)	100	15	100	48	C	—	23	4.5	12	11	1	44	0	41	16	3
Athletes																
Hanne-Paparo, 1981 (40)	32	24	100	12	V	—	36	1.68	3	3	0	9	3	6	0	0
Talan, 1982 (42)	20	21	100	24	R	61	31	2.81	45	40	0	100	10	70	20	0
Zeppilli, 1983 (43)	20	39	100	24	R	53	24	2.96	10	5	0	65	5	40	10	0
Pilcher, 1983 (44)	80	31	65	24	R	50	35	—	0	0	0	41	0	50	4	1

Avg HR, average heart rate in bpm; APD, atrial premature depolarization; C, control; Long pause, duration of longest R-R interval in seconds; Min HR, minimum heart rate in bpm; N, no. of subjects; R, running; SVT/AF, supraventricular tachycardia/atrial fibrillation; V, various (cycling, running); VPD, ventricular premature depolarization; VT, ventricular tachycardia; AV, atrioventricular; 1st AVB, first-degree AV block; 2nd AVB, second-degree AV block; 3rd AVB, third-degree AV block.

TABLE 28-2. AMBULATORY ELECTROCARDIOGRAPHY IN CONTROLS AND ATHLETES: DIRECT COMPARATIVE STUDIES

Author/Year	N	Age	% Male	Time (h)	Sport	Avg HR	Min HR	Long Sinus Pause	1st AVB	2nd AVB I	2nd AVB II 3rd AVB	APD (%)	SVT/AF (%)	VPD (%)	Complex VPD (%)	VT (%)
Viitasato, 1982 (41)	35	23	100	16	C	68	33	2.60	14	6	0	—	—	42	3	6
Viitasato, 1982 (41)	35	23	100	16	V	60	24	2.76	37	23	9	—	—	32	0	0
Viitasato, 1984 (45)	35	15	100	24	C	72	38	2.02	11	3	0	—	—	57	3	0
Viitasato, 1984 (45)	35	15	100	24	V	66	31	2.42	23	17	6	—	—	60	0	3
Palatini, 1985 (46)	40	19	100	24	C	79	52	—	5	3	0	63	3	55	0	0
Palatini, 1985 (46)	40	20	100	24	V	66	45	—	28	15	0	72	0	70	3	8
Northcote, 1989 (47)	20	56	100	48	C	74	47	—	0	0	0	—	—	90	5	10
Northcote, 1989 (47)	20	56	100	48	R	59	37	15	30	20	15	—	—	75	10	0
Jensen-Urstad, 1997 (34)	13	25	—	48	C	71	46	2.28	—	15	0	—	—	—	—	0
Jensen-Urstad, 1997 (34)	16	25	100	48	R	55	31	3.06	44	19	7	25	—	82	—	13
Jensen-Urstad, 1998 (48)	12	74	100	48	C	69	48	2.3	0	8	0	33	25	100	41	17
Jensen-Urstad, 1998 (48)	11	73	100	48	V	60	40	2.6	9	22	0	82	18	100	82	9

Avg HR, average heart rate in bpm; APD, atrial premature depolarization; C, control; Long pause, duration of longest R-R interval in seconds; Min HR, minimum heart rate in bpm; N, no. of subjects; R, running; SVT/AF, supraventricular tachycardia/atrial fibrillation; V, various (cycling, running); VPD, ventricular premature depolarization; VT, ventricular tachycardia; AV, atrioventricular; 1st AVB, first-degree AV block; 2nd AVB I, type I second-degree AV block; 2nd AVB II, type II second-degree AV block; 3rd AVB, type I third-degree AV block.

colleagues (52) reported that there was no long-term sequelae from this type of finding in athletes.

AV Conduction

In the Air Force recruits studied by Hiss and Lamb, the
incidence of first-degree atrioventricular (AV) block was
0.7% (35). Among the control subjects undergoing Holter
monitoring, first-degree AV block occurred in 0% to 14%
of the population with no difference between gender or
age. In athletes, the frequency of first-degree AV block
ranged from 9% to 45% (35–43). Conducting PR intervals as long as 0.52 seconds have been reported (53). These
findings reflect the fact that the AV node, which accounts
for most of AV conduction time, is highly sensitive to sympathetic and parasympathetic tone, and the overriding
parasympathetic state present in athletes is felt to account
for the PR prolongation. Although numerous studies confirm either no change or a shortening of the PR interval

after exercise, Hunt reported that in champion swimmers
who had a normal PR interval at rest, the PR interval
increased by as much as 0.04 seconds or more in 12 of 20
of these swimmers after a 110-yard sprint (54–57) (Fig.
28-2A, B).

In their study of 122,043 ECGs, Hiss and Lamb (35)
recorded only four cases of Wenckebach and four other
cases of second-degree AV block, for an incidence of 0.06
per 1,000. Holter monitoring control data noted second-
degree AV block type I ranging from 0% to 11% with no
trend regarding age or gender. The athletes had a higher frequency of second-degree AV block type I, noted in up to
40%. This distinction is most striking in the comparison
studies in which athletes averaged 18% and controls averaged only a 6% incidence. As with first-degree AV block,
type I second-degree AV block (Wenckebach) appears to
occur with an increased frequency in the athletic population, seems to be related to training intensity, and is functionally associated with hypervagotonia (58–60). Zeppilli

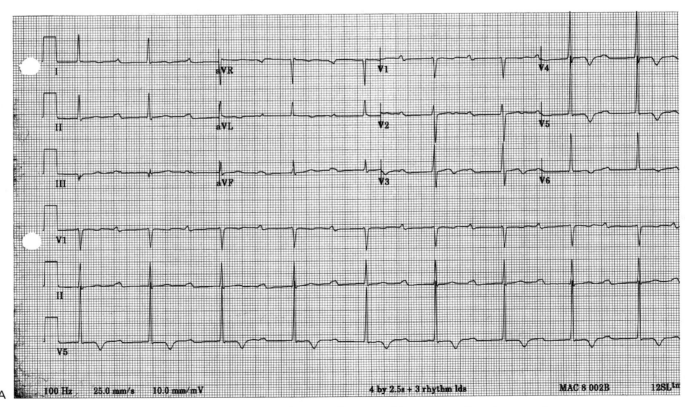

FIGURE 28-2. A: Baseline electrocardiogram of 55-year-old asymptomatic male runner (averaging 40 miles per week for more than 20 years). Note first-degree atrioventricular block and pattern of left ventricular hypertrophy with strain. **B:** Individual developed paroxysmal atrial fibrillation with exercise testing at peak exercise and at a second test at early recovery. Note relatively
slow ventricular response at 65 beats per minute even though this was at 2 minutes of recovery
from exercise test. Echocardiogram was consistent with athletic heart. Left ventricular hypertrophy was not evident. Cardiac catheterization revealed normal coronaries.

and colleagues (61) reported normalization of second-degree AV block in 9 of 10 athletes by exercise and/or intravenous isoproterenol administration and in all after 0.6 mg of intravenous atropine. Meytes and colleagues (58) studied 126 athletes and found three cases of type I second-degree AV block, all of which disappeared after a change in position from lying to sitting, or standing, or after discontinuation of exercise.

In the Air Force data, the incidence of type II second-degree AV block or third-degree AV block was 0.02 per 1,000 (35). During 24-hour Holter monitoring in control populations, these abnormalities were extremely rare, found in only 1 out of more than 450 subjects. This conduction abnormality was found more frequently in athletes, noted in 9 out of more than 300 subjects. Thus, type II second-degree AV block or third-degree AV block is exceedingly

rare in normals, and although it is more frequently seen in a healthy athlete, it is still an uncommon event (32–43). Most of those reports are anecdotal and do not completely exclude organic heart disease with certainty. Northcote and colleagues (47) reviewed ECG, Holter, and treadmill data on 20 veteran male endurance runners older than 45 years and found three athletes who had intermittent third-degree AV block. One of these individuals had 846 long pauses during the 24-hour monitoring period, with the longest pause lasting 15 seconds. Although asymptomatic, this man had a dual-chamber pacemaker implanted and reportedly felt "more energetic" after its insertion. In a separate account, Northcote and colleagues reported on a 52-year-old former professional boxer who ran 11 km daily and complained of recurrent syncope (62). He had documented intermittent ventricular standstill or asystole lasting up to

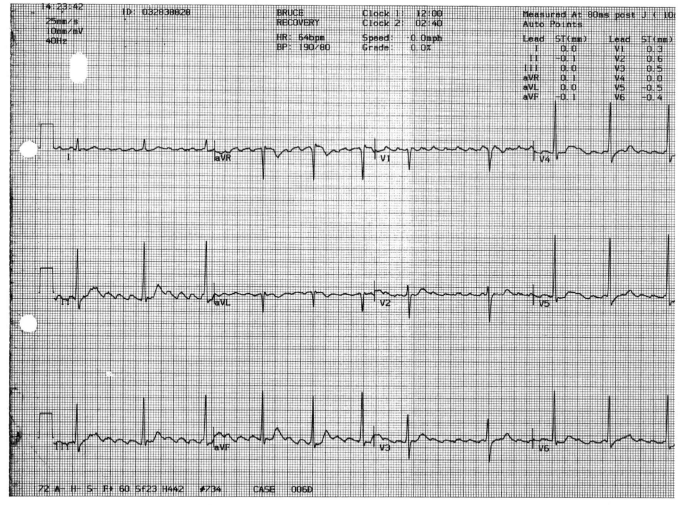

FIGURE 28-2. *(continued)*

B

30 seconds, and after permanent pacemaker implantation, he had resolution of his symptoms. Cooper and colleagues (63) described two cases of young, well-conditioned individuals who had third-degree AV block and syncope. One of the subjects stopped vigorous exercise, and subsequently AV block and syncope disappeared. The other individual, a 19-year-old woman with intermittent first-, second-, and third-degree AV block underwent an electrophysiology study and was found to have a prolonged A-H interval of 200 ms and type I and II second-degree AV block during atrial pacing at rates of 110 bpm. The HV interval was normal. The A-H interval normalized after administration of atropine. After stopping exercise, the woman's symptoms and ECG abnormalities resolved. After returning to a vigorous exercise program, however, she experienced five additional syncopal episodes in a 6-month period. Follow-up Holter monitoring studies again showed all types of AV block.

Intraventricular Conduction

The QRS complex of the athlete tends to be of normal duration, but of exaggerated voltage (19). The QRS configuration of precordial lead V_1 is often noted to have an rSr' configuration, consistent with incomplete right bundle branch block (49,54–56). Lichtman and colleagues (64) analyzed 10 separate studies involving ECGs obtained on 527 athletes and found a 16% incidence of incomplete right bundle branch block.

In contrast, the incidence of a complete right or left bundle branch block is much lower. In the healthy population, Hiss and Lamb (35) noted complete right bundle branch block in 0.18% of subjects and complete left bundle branch block in even fewer. They found that none of the 44,231 recruits younger than 25 years had a left bundle branch block, perhaps because individuals with this degree of block would likely have a structural heart disorder and not enter the Air Force.

Supraventricular and Ventricular Arrhythmias

On 24-hour Holter monitoring, the control subjects had a great variation of ectopic atrial activity, with most of the subjects with arrhythmia having primarily isolated atrial premature depolarizations. The range of supraventricular arrhythmia was from 33% to 88% with no clear trend regarding age or gender. There was a slight trend of more frequent supraventricular arrhythmia in athletes compared with normals, but the percentages were not significant. Supraventricular tachycardia and atrial fibrillation were rarely seen in the control or the athletic population. Pantano and Oriel (65) evaluated 24-hour ECG monitors and treadmill testing in 60 runners (75% men; mean age, 32)

and found similar results. Supraventricular arrhythmia was noted in 40% of the subjects including three with tachycardia and one with atrial fibrillation. Holter monitoring in part during running was more revealing than a standard symptom-limited exercise test (65).

The most common mechanisms of supraventricular tachycardias are AV nodal reentrant tachycardia (most often resulting from a second AV nodal pathway), and AV reciprocating tachycardia (resulting from an accessory pathway and often associated with ECG evidence of a preexcitation syndrome such as Wolff-Parkinson-White [WPW]). Early reports suggested an increased incidence of WPW syndrome in athletes; however, this has not been borne out in subsequent studies (19). Although ventricular preexcitation may be more evident because of slower antegrade conduction over the AV node secondary to enhanced vagal tone in the athlete with WPW syndrome, there is no reason *a priori* for these individuals to have a higher incidence of this anomaly or of the associated arrhythmia. No increase has been reported in AV nodal reentrant tachycardia in athletes.

During 24-hour Holter monitoring of young healthy subjects or athletes, atrial fibrillation or atrial flutter were rarely noted. Hiss and Lamb noted an incidence of atrial fibrillation of 0.004% on a baseline resting ECG (35). Abdon and colleagues (66) from Sweden noted atrial fibrillation along with sinus bradycardia in a number of middle-aged athletes who presented with dizziness, syncope, or stroke. Zehender and colleagues (19) suggested that atrial fibrillation was more common in athletes than in the general population, but the frequency was still low at 0.06%. There was no apparent age dependence of this arrhythmia in their study, in contrast to what has been observed in the general population. One could postulate, however, that the milieu for atrial fibrillation is frequently present in athletes given their increase in vagal tone and the resultant dispersion of atrial refractoriness and left atrial dilation resulting from LV hypertrophy. Italian investigators reported their evaluation of 13 elite athletes with atrial fibrillation (67). They noted a 6% incidence of atrial fibrillation among all arrhythmias in their special referral population. There was a substrate for arrhythmias in five athletes (three with WPW syndrome, one with RV dysplasia, and one with healed myocarditis), whereas eight had lone atrial fibrillation. Former athletes, particularly as they become older, may also have the appropriate electrophysiologic conditions for atrial fibrillation (Figs. 28-2B and 28-3).

In the control population, the incidence of ventricular arrhythmia on 24 hour Holter monitoring was remarkably similar to that of supraventricular arrhythmia with a wide variation ranging from 41% to 100% of subjects. In this group, there was a tendency of older subjects to have more arrhythmia. However, complex ventricular arrhythmia,

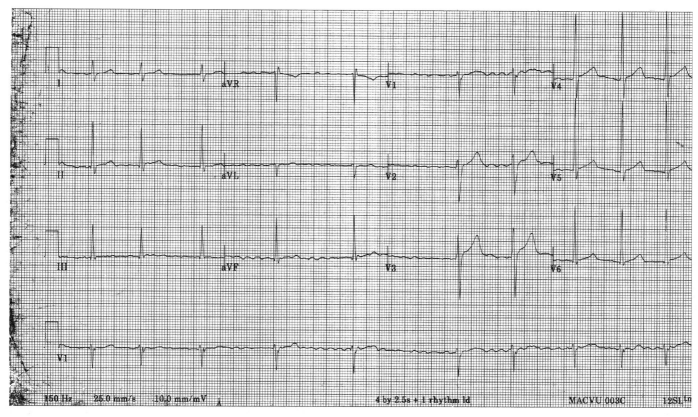

FIGURE 28-3. Electrocardiogram from a 30-year-old professional hockey player with paroxysmal lone atrial fibrillation. He was taking no cardiac therapy. Arrhythmia developed with exercise. Cardioversion was uneventful. Within 2 weeks of procedure, he was traded.

including ventricular couplets, R-on-T phenomenon or multiformed ventricular premature depolarizations, and ventricular tachycardia, occurred infrequently in all of these studies. The rare episodes of ventricular tachycardia were of short duration and of slow rate. There was no significantly greater incidence of ventricular premature depolarizations and complex ventricular arrhythmia in the group of athletes than in the control population. Pantano and Oriel (65) noted that 60% of their subjects had ventricular arrhythmia, but none had tachycardia. As with supraventricular arrhythmia, Holter monitoring exposed more arrhythmia than exercise testing. In an attempt to determine the significance of ventricular arrhythmia in this population, Biffi and colleagues (68) reported on 71 athletes referred with frequent and complex ventricular arrhythmia noted on Holter monitoring. During a follow-up of 8.3 ± 3.5 years, the only death noted occurred in a 24-year-old who was told not to exercise because of RV dysplasia and participated in ice hockey against medical advice. The authors concluded that complex arrhythmia may be associated with structural heart disease. They fur-

ther suggested that complex ventricular arrhythmia alone did not have an associated adverse clinical significance (68) (Fig. 28-4A, B).

Repolarization

It is common for an athlete to demonstrate ECG variations from normal repolarization. Unusual ST segments have included elevation (often labeled *early repolarization*) and depression (suggested to be pseudoischemia). Marked T-wave abnormalities have often been seen commensurate with the ST changes. Much of the literature on this subject has concluded that these repolarization changes are benign based on several facts (19,49,50,54–57,64,69–72). Firstly, ECG abnormalities usually normalize with exercise. Secondly, stress testing results with nuclear imaging are usually normal. Thirdly, the subjects are almost always completely asymptomatic. Fourthly, the long-term outcome has been excellent. Fifthly, repolarization abnormalities resolve with deconditioning. Pelliccia and colleagues compared ECG patterns with cardiac morphology in 1,005 Italian athletes

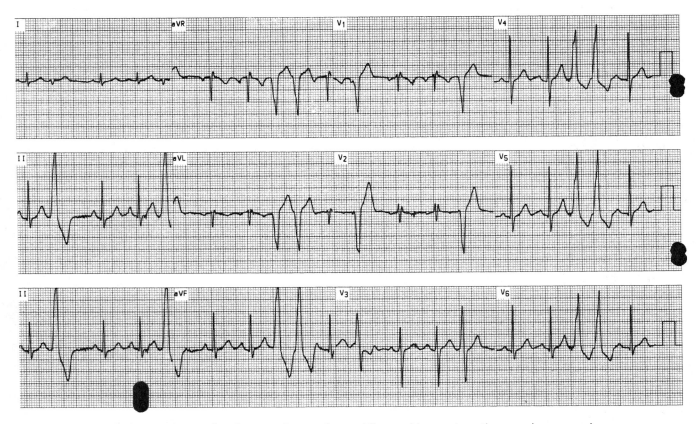

FIGURE 28-4. Exercise electrocardiogram from a 54-year-old asymptomatic man who engaged in various athletic pursuits including running, bicycling, hiking, and weight lifting. He typically exercised 10 hours weekly. An irregular rhythm was noted on routine physical examination. Note sinus tachycardia, incomplete right bundle branch block, T-wave inversion in leads V_1 through V_2, and frequent and repetitive ventricular extrasystoles. The ventricular arrhythmia has a left bundle branch block, rightward axis configuration. Echocardiography results were normal, as was the results of magnetic resonance imaging.

competing in 38 sporting disciplines. They noted that abnormal ECG findings were mostly associated with young men participating in endurance sports. These unusual ECG findings were often noted in subjects with larger than normal size hearts, but were not necessarily indicative of pathology (72).

In summary, the cardiovascular electrophysiologic system undergoes specific definable changes in response to athletic training. Electrical impulses traverse the heart of an athlete typically in a slower fashion including slower activation of the sinus node and mild prolongation of AV conduction. The normal respiratory phasic and diurnal variations are usually maintained. There is usually no significant difference in the frequency of supraventricular or ventricular ectopic activity or tachycardia comparing athletes with a control population. In comparing the normal control population with the athlete, there is a significant overlap of these electrophysiologic findings partly because of the high frequency of bradycardia and AV conduction "abnormalities" in normal subjects. The mechanism of most of the changes is likely an increased parasympathetic tone in athletes. There exists a milieu for pathologic transformation after prolonged training in certain situations. Some athletes may be at risk for syncope or stroke resulting from sick sinus node syndrome with severe sinus bradycardia, prolonged pauses from sinus arrest, high-grade AV block, or even atrial fibrillation. Many of these electrophysiologic changes may resolve after cessation of exercise for 3 months.

SUDDEN DEATH IN ATHLETES

SCD most often affects middle-aged and older individuals with significant underlying cardiac disease. SCD in a young athletic person is an unusual event, often making news. In Orange County, California, an area of 2.5 million people, there has been approximately 1 death per year throughout the last decade in athletic participants younger than 20 years (age range, 7 to 19 years). The sports involved were basketball (3), water polo (2), soccer (2), football (1), gymnastics (1), track (1), and volleyball (1). This phenomenon has also been noted internationally (73–83). After the reporting of these data, there has been an outcry for information. The most prominent response to this call has been the two Bethesda conferences, the 16th in 1985 and the 26th in 1994 (84,85).

Calculating the incidence of SCD in athletes is difficult for several reasons. First, the definition of an athlete is extremely broad and encompassing (86). Strictly defined, an athlete is a competitor in the physical exercises—such as running, leaping, boxing, wrestling—that formed part of the public games in ancient Greece and Rome. Additionally, it is one who by special training and exercise has acquired great physical strength (86). Therefore, some may suggest that anyone going to a school in which exercise and games are mandatory, including senior citizens occasionally engaging in community jogging, may be considered an athlete. The aforementioned Bethesda conferences, which were designed to provide guidelines for cardiovascular screening of competitive athletes in high school and college, defined a competitive athlete as one who participates in an organized team or individual sport that requires regular competition against others as a central component, places a high premium on excellence and achievement, and requires vigorous and intense training in a systematic fashion (87). This latter definition, however, ignores the many individuals who participate in school athletics or recreational sports and it is not clear whether the definition of an athlete should include an arbitrary cutoff for performance, training, exercise duration, or age. An additional concern is the problem that SCD may be caused by errors in judgment rather than an underlying cardiac disorder—for example, SCD resulting from situations like heat stroke or exercising while ill. Lastly, an important consideration may be matching the activity to the age of the participant. Each year, a significant number of people older than 35 years die suddenly during exercise and often they are engaging in extreme sports like long-distance marathon running, which may be too physically demanding. For others with perhaps significant underlying cardiac disease, even a brisk walk may be too stressful.

Definition of Sudden Cardiac Death

Although the definition of SCD has been variable through the years, the precise definition has significant implications for communication and preparticipation screening.

Currently SCD is most commonly defined as nontraumatic, nonviolent, unexpected death resulting from cardiac causes within 6 hours of the onset of symptoms. Some important causes of death associated with athletics, such as commotio cordis or cardiac concussion, which are caused by collision (trauma) with another player or with a projectile and lead to lethal arrhythmia, will not be discussed here (88).

Prevalence of Sudden Cardiac Death in Athletes

The overall incidence of SCD varies and depends on the age of the population and the type of exercise; however, regardless of the type of exercise and age, it is fortunately an uncommon event. Some of the reported frequencies are 1 incidence in 13,000 hours of cross-country skiing, 1 in 215,000 hours of marathon running, and 1 in 396,000 hours of jogging (89–91). Calculations based on individuals show that yearly frequencies are 1 of 15,240 joggers per year, and 1 of 20,000 exercisers per year (89,92). In Minnesota, the calculated risk for SCD in men was 1 death per 300,000 sports participants annually (93). In France, there are between 1,200 and 1,500 episodes of SCD related to sports annually (83). Its occurrence, nonetheless, is unexpected in an individual who is thought to be not only healthy, but in peak physical condition. Ironically, most cases of SCD occur in individuals with significant underlying structural heart disease.

Electrophysiologic Basis of Sudden Cardiac Death in Athletes

Data on athletes with life-threatening arrhythmia symptoms have provided insight into this SCD syndrome (94,95). This information confirms that certain arrhythmias create symptoms and are potentially dangerous despite the presence or absence of other clinical pathologies. These arrhythmias are generally associated with a very rapid or very slow heart rate that compromises hemodynamic function.

Italian investigators reported data on 16 athletes who were resuscitated from cardiac arrest (94). The electrophysiologic events included eight with ventricular tachycardia developing into ventricular fibrillation, five with WPW syndrome and rapid preexcited atrial fibrillation, two with long QT syndrome associated torsade de pointes then ventricular fibrillation, and one with high-grade AV block and atrial fibrillation. Significant structural heart disease was present in only those patients presenting with ventricular tachycardia. Coelho and colleagues (95), from Chicago, Illinois, performed extensive electrophysiologic testing on eight athletes with a history of symptomatic ventricular tachycardia (95). The most complex structural heart disease reported was mitral valve prolapse. In seven of the eight athletes, the ventricular tachycardia had been provoked during exercise. The arrhythmia was reproducible during exercise testing in four of eight, during isoproterenol infusion in four of seven, and during programmed stimulation in four of eight.

The final common pathway for SCD in athletes, as in nonathletes, is most often ventricular fibrillation. This complex rhythm disturbance has been extensively studied in animal preparations, yet many questions regarding its nature remain unanswered. Surawicz (96) described the factors that may enhance vulnerability to ventricular fibrillation including increased automaticity of Purkinje fibers, slow conduction, prolonged action potential, and increased nonuniformity of refractoriness (96). Clinically, many factors may occur in athletes that can enhance the potential for ventricular fibrillation, such as bradycardia (increasing the duration of the relative refractory period), cardiac hypertrophy, hypokalemia (resulting in increased automaticity of Purkinje fibers), acidosis, sympathetic stimulation, and emotional factors. Sympathetic nervous system activity during exercise has been investigated but remains incompletely described (11,97–101). There are many hormonal responses to exercise and physical training including an effort-dependent increase in epinephrine and norepinephrine levels. There is a continued increase in their concentrations after exercise, with a 10-fold rise over baseline for norepinephrine and a threefold rise for epinephrine, which may help explain the phenomenon of SCD immediately after exercise (98). Asystole may alternatively be a mechanism for SCD. Asystole with a duration as long as 8 minutes after exercise and associated with syncope has been reported by Osswald and colleagues (99) and was thought to be caused by neurocardiogenic reflexes.

Pathophysiologic Basis of Sudden Cardiac Death in Athletes

Many factors influence the risk of SCD in athletes (Table 28-3). Although the most important is underlying structural heart disease, a combination of adverse conditions usually predispose individuals to SCD. Those with underlying structural heart disease will usually require the addition of a significant transient stress to precipitate the life-threatening event. For a situation of SCD to occur, there is commonly a

TABLE 28-3. FACTORS FOR SUDDEN CARDIAC DEATH IN ATHLETES

1. Cardiovascular structural disease
2. Primary electrophysiologic conditions
3. Personal characteristics and general medical status
4. The environment
5. Exposure to toxins
6. Preparation for or performance in an event

factor whose threshold is exceeded. Among the various factors, cardiovascular structure is the most well studied.

Cardiovascular Structural Disease

During the last 20 years, there have been several reports of cardiovascular pathologic abnormalities in athletic victims of SCD (73–83) (Table 28-4). Upon review of these data, one finds several readily apparent trends. First, age is the most important variable when predicting the presence of an underlying cardiovascular structural disorder associated with SCD. Of the victims of SCD who are younger than 30 years, most have some type of structural, nonatherosclerotic heart disease, whereas those older than 30 years typically have underlying coronary atherosclerosis. Second, among those younger than 30 years who died suddenly, the most common cardiac pathology found was HCM, followed by coronary artery anomalies, and then a potpourri of disorders. Third, geographic location, particularly country of origin, is also an important variable when considering the cardiac cause of death. In Italy, several investigators have noted arrhythmogenic RV dysplasia to be an important cause of SCD, although this is a rare finding in North America (102,103). Fourth, there appears to be great variation in pathologic diagnosis, even after adjusting for location and date of report.

Hypertrophic Cardiomyopathy

HCM is the most common underlying cardiovascular abnormality in young athletic victims of SCD (73–83). HCM is an uncommon primary cardiac disease with a prevalence of about 0.2% (104). It is usually genetically transmitted and is characterized by a hypertrophic, nondilated LV in the absence of another cardiac or systemic disease that may produce LV hypertrophy. Although the inheritance pattern and hemodynamic effects of HCM, including diminished LV compliance, reduced LV filling, and in severe cases, LV outflow tract obstruction, have been well established, the mechanism of SCD in these patients is not clear (105,106). Studies have shown that HCM is a common cause of SCD in the young population and particularly among black men, and that HCM usually occurs in patients without previous symptoms (27,107). HCM as a cause of SCD in athletes is not limited to the young. Noakes and colleagues (108) reported SCD in a 42-year-old experienced male ultramarathoner during a standard 26.2-mile marathon. Despite ischemic symptoms in prior races, this individual was found to have normal coronary arteries at autopsy; however, the LV wall was 2.4 cm thick with myofiber disarray. Several potential mechanisms by which SCD occurs in HCM have been described (109–118). Although most athletes who die with HCM appear to have the nonobstructive form, the hemodynamic effects of LV outflow tract obstruction have never been disproved as a cause of death. Ventricular fibrillation may occur in these patients as a primary event related to cellular disar-

TABLE 28-4. CARDIOVASCULAR DISORDERS IN ATHLETIC VICTIMS OF SUDDEN CARDIAC DEATH

Study/Year	Location	Age (Y)	Cardiovascular Condition (N)									
			Total	HCM	CAA	LVH	RVD	VHD	ASHD	M	EP/UNK	OTH
<30 y old												
Maron, 1980 (73)	United States	19 (13–30)	29	14	4	5	0	0	3	0	1	2
Tsung, 1982 (74)	Indiana	17 (14–18)	4	1	2	0	0	0	0	0	1	0
Waller, 1984 (76)	Indiana	20 (13–29)	17	4	2	6	0	3	0	0	2	0
Kennedy, 1984 (77)	Missouri	<30	4	2	1	0	0	0	0	0	1	0
Corrado, 1990 (79)	Northern Italy	23 (11–35)	22	0	2	0	6	2	4	0	3	5
Burke, 1991 (80)	Maryland	26 (14–34)	34	8	4	3	1	0	9	2	6	0
Van Camp, 1995 (81)	United States	17 (13–24)	136	56	16	0	1	9	3	7	1	43
Maron, 1996 (82)	United States	17 (12–40)	134	48	25	14	4	8	3	5	3	24
Tabib, 1999 (83)	France	<30	27	8	4	0	7	2	1	0	1	4
>30 y old												
Virmani, 1982 (75)	United States	36 (18–57)	30	0	0	0	0	1	22	0	7	0
Waller, 1984 (76)	Indiana	48 (37–65)	10	0	0	0	0	0	10	0	0	0
Kennedy, 1984 (77)	Missouri	>30	7	0	0	0	0	0	7	0	0	0
Northcote, 1986 (78)	United Kingdom	46 (22–66)	60	1	0	0	0	4	51	0	2	2
Tabib, 1999 (83)	France	>30	53	10	1	0	2	0	26	0	4	10

N, no. of subjects; HCM, hypertrophic cardiomyopathy; CAA, coronary artery anomalies; LVH, left ventricular hypertrophy; RVD, right ventricular dysplasia; VHD, valvular heart disease; ASHD, atherosclerotic heart disease; M, myocarditis; EP, primary electrophysiologic abnormality; UNK, unknown; OTH, other; includes dilated cardiomyopathy as the most common disorder.

ray, in response to ischemia associated with increased LV mass and diminished coronary supply, or secondary to a preceding rhythm disturbance such as extreme bradycardia, supraventricular tachycardia, atrial fibrillation, or ventricular tachycardia. There have been few clinical variables that are reliable for predicting a high-risk group of individuals with HCM, including SCD in a first-degree relative, presence of ventricular tachycardia on 24-hour Holter monitoring, syncope, and an abnormal blood pressure response to exercise (109–116). Although SCD in nonathletic patients with HCM shows a predilection for the early morning hours (similar to that described in coronary artery disease with acute myocardial infarction and angina), trained competitive athletes with HCM usually die in the late afternoon and early evening hours, which is associated with their peak periods of exertion during practice or games. These relationships underline the trigger effect of exercise in provoking the mechanism for SCD in competitive athletes with HCM (117).

Congenital Coronary Artery Anomalies

The second most common cardiovascular pathologic finding associated with SCD in the young athlete is anomalous coronary arteries (73–83). Origin of the left main coronary artery from the right sinus of Valsalva represents the most common clinically relevant anomaly, and as reported by Burke and colleagues, is associated with a 46% incidence of SCD (118,119). The abrupt angular takeoff of the slitlike left coronary ostium in this case is felt to be further compromised by exercise as the engorged aorta and pulmonary artery further compress the coronary artery, resulting in ischemia-mediated ventricular fibrillation. Coronary malformation is rarely diagnosed during life but is usually identified for the first time at autopsy. However, a substantial proportion of these individuals experience prodromal symptoms, most commonly syncope or angina (114). Therefore, a high index of suspicion is necessary to identify individuals with an anomalous left main coronary artery during life. Unfortunately, conventional echocardiography and stress testing have not been consistently helpful in uncovering this problem (120–122). Origin of the right coronary artery from the left sinus of Valsalva is a less common anomaly and is associated with a far lower reported incidence of SCD of 17% (110).

Idiopathic Left Ventricular Hypertrophy

Idiopathic LV hypertrophy has been found in some pathology series of young athletes who experienced SCD (67,76,82,118). It is a symmetric, concentric hypertrophy in which the LV mass exceeds that of physiologic hypertrophy. It is not associated with genetic transmission or hypertension, and there is no cellular disarray microscopically, as is seen with HCM. This has also been noted to be more common in blacks and may represent a variant of HCM.

Arrhythmogenic Right Ventricular Dysplasia

Arrhythmogenic RV dysplasia is a myopathic process characterized by segmental fatty infiltration and fibrosis of the RV; the septum and LV are typically spared. RV aneurysms are reported to occur over the anterior surface of the pulmonary infundibulum, at the apex of the RV, and along the inferior RV segment (123). Arrhythmogenic RV dysplasia may be associated with recurrent or intractable ventricular arrhythmias and may have a familial occurrence (79,123, 124). It is the most common cause of SCD in young competitive athletes in the Veneto region of northern Italy (103,125). Corrado and colleagues reviewed the causes of death in 22 athletes aged 11 to 35 years who had died suddenly; of the 14 cases in which ventricular fibrillation was felt to be the cause of death, RV dysplasia accounted for 6 deaths (79). This geographical finding is thought also to correlate with a presumed genetic basis of arrhythmogenic RV dysplasia. Although familial clustering has been seen in northern Italy, arrhythmogenic RV dysplasia is a relatively uncommon entity in North America. Goodin and colleagues (126) reported this entity as the cause of SCD in 3 cases of 547 cardiac deaths in the state of Maryland from 1983 to 1989. This geographical discrepancy may partly be because of the systematic Italian national screening in which athletes with HCM would be selectively disqualified (127).

ECG findings in patients with arrhythmogenic RV dysplasia usually include T-wave inversion in the precordial leads (V_1 through V_3) and isolated premature contractions with left bundle branch block morphology (128). Two-dimensional echocardiography may rarely show abnormalities of the RV such as fatty infiltration, but magnetic resonance imaging appears to be more sensitive in diagnosing this condition (129). In an attempt to determine risk factors for SCD in arrhythmogenic RV dysplasia, Peters and Reil (130) analyzed 60 patients, 40 of whom had clinical sustained ventricular tachycardia or cardiac arrest. They suggested that RV size, RV ejection fraction, number of RV wall motion abnormalities, and results of electrophysiologic testing were all predictive of this condition. The data are consistent with those of previous studies of VT in the setting of normal LV function (131).

Valvular Heart Disease

Mitral valve prolapse affects up to 3% to 5% of the population and is therefore occasionally associated with malignant arrhythmias and SCD. Of the subjects with mitral valve prolapse, those particularly with severe leaflet thickening and redundancy or with moderate to severe mitral regurgitation may be the ones most at risk for SCD (132–135). Although early studies revealed no significant increase in malignant arrhythmias in these individuals, more recent investigations have shown malignant ventricular ectopy before a fatal event (132–135). Nevertheless, mitral valve prolapse as the sole cause of SCD in competitive athletes is very rare, and there is no evidence that these arrhythmic complications are exercise-related. A permissive attitude toward participation in sports has been advocated, unless the subject with mitral valve prolapse has a history of syncope, disabling chest pain, complex ventricular arrhythmias, significant mitral regurgitation, prolonged QT interval, Marfan syndrome, or a family history of SCD (114,132).

Aortic stenosis has been noted in autopsy studies in athletic victims of SCD (81,82). This seems surprising because these individuals should be identified antemortem before engaging in exercise with a preparticipant history (syncope) or physical (heart murmur) (114). Of note, all reported deaths occurred in men, a group more likely to deny or ignore prodromal symptoms.

Atherosclerotic Coronary Artery Disease

Atherosclerotic coronary artery disease is a relatively uncommon cause of SCD in young athletes, and if it does occur, it appears to affect individuals who have marked hyperlipidemia (114,119). Despite Bassler's claim that marathon running would invoke an immunity from or resolution of atherosclerosis in the athlete, subsequent reports have proven this untrue (136). In athletes older than 30 years, atherosclerotic coronary artery disease is the leading cause of SCD (75–78,83). It accounted for 100% of the cases of those older than 40 years who died suddenly while running, as reported by Waller and Roberts (137). Coronary atherosclerosis in these older individuals is often recognized before death, as these individuals often have a knowledge of risk factors and symptoms of angina (138–140). Katzel and colleagues (141) further documented that trained athletes older than 50 years had a 16% incidence of exercise-induced silent ischemia, a figure comparable to that of nonathletes. Several studies have described risk factors for atherosclerosis associated SCD such as family history of premature atherosclerosis or a personal history of hyperlipidemia, smoking, hypertension, prodromal symptoms of chest pain, or fatigue (138–140).

The mechanism of athletic death in patients with coronary artery disease is not entirely clear. It is thought that the chronic fixed coronary lesion may not be responsible for the cause of death. Although not proven, observational studies have suggested that exercise may induce plaque rupture and thrombus formation and coronary spasm leading to a terminal arrhythmic event (142,143).

Myocarditis

Myocarditis from any cause (e.g., viral, fungal, bacterial, atypical bacterial, and collagen vascular disease) may result in SCD (114). It is infrequently cited as a cause of SCD in this population, although there appears to be an increased incidence of myocarditis-associated SCD in Swedish athletes (144–147). Myocarditis can cause arrhythmias ranging from isolated extrasystoles, which are most common, to

atrial fibrillation or life-threatening ventricular arrhythmias, which are uncommon (144). Although not proven, it has been suggested that healed myocarditis with interstitial fibrosis may provide an arrhythmogenic substrate, and SCD is felt to result from ventricular arrhythmia. Of 19 SCDs in screened Air Force recruits reported by Philips and colleagues, myocarditis was thought to be the underlying cause in 6 and represented the most common underlying cardiovascular disorder (148).

Other

Dilated cardiomyopathy has been reported as a cause of SCD in athletes (81–83). This disorder is often seen as a consequence of hypertension or viral illness. It can be identified by signs or symptoms of an enlarged poorly contracting LV. These individuals often develop serious ventricular arrhythmia.

Myocardial bridging is a condition in which a coronary artery can be compressed by an unusually thickened, adversely located myocardium. Consequences of the disorder also known as *mural tunneled vessels* are most pronounced at times of increased myocardial contractility such as during exertion. Morales and colleagues (149) and later Agirbasli and colleagues (150) described ischemia, infarction, and SCD in athletes with myocardial bridging as their only cardiovascular abnormality (149,150). Yetman and colleagues (151) noted correlation of bridging with HCM. Those who had both conditions were at a markedly increased risk of death.

Marfan syndrome is a heritable connective tissue abnormality that principally affects the heart but also affects the eyes and musculoskeletal system (114). The cardiovascular complications of this disorder include mitral valve prolapse (more than 50%), aortic valve regurgitation, and aortic dissection. The life expectancy of individuals affected is often significantly reduced. Individuals may be at risk for SCD as a consequence of aortic dissection or rupture (152).

Kawasaki disease is a disorder of coronary arteries caused by vasculitis and the subsequent healing process. It usually affects children and results in segmental narrowing alternating with aneurysmal dilation of the arteries (114). This disorder has been associated with infarction and SCD with exercise (80,83).

Coronary vasospasm is a transient, abrupt reduction, and often complete cessation, in coronary blood flow that can have life-threatening consequences. Often, potentially affected individuals have a normal response to cardiovascular stress, except in unusual circumstances. Exercise, particularly in the cold weather, is one of the many potential triggers for coronary vasospasm and SCD (153).

Scarred myocardial bruising is a term coined by Tabib and colleagues (83) to reflect a pathologic finding at autopsy. In two cases of SCD during athletic competition, middle-aged men had scarring of the posterior wall of the LV. Microscopic analysis suggested previous hemorrhage. Historically, both cases had frontal sternal thoracic shock or trauma.

Sarcoidosis has also been noted, albeit rarely, in reports of SCD in athletes (82). This disorder has a predilection for blacks and is associated with bradyarrhythmias and tachyarrhythmias (154).

Primary Electrophysiologic Conditions

The most common primary electrophysiologic abnormalities found in athletes without structural heart disease who die suddenly include WPW syndrome, long QT syndrome, and idiopathic ventricular fibrillation (114,155–157). There are no data, however, to suggest that these disorders occur more frequently in athletes than in the general population (19). Thiene and colleagues (158) reported on the pathologic analysis of three young athletes who succumbed suddenly during athletic endeavors; each of these patients had an accessory pathway. Wiedermann and colleagues (159) described the case of an 18-year-old football player with overt ventricular preexcitation caused by a posteroseptal pathway. The victim had been empirically placed on antiarrhythmic drug therapy after an episode of atrial fibrillation with ventricular rates ranging from 214 to 380 bpm. He died suddenly 10 days after discharge while engaged in ordinary daily activities, presumably from atrial fibrillation–related ventricular fibrillation. Electrophysiologic testing had not been carried out before death.

Primary conduction abnormalities causing SCD are difficult to detect even on postmortem examination. Subtle findings in otherwise unexplainable SCD have included narrowed or sclerotic sinus node arteries as a result of hyperplasia and intimal proliferation, sinoatrial and AV nodal fibrotic scarring, or congenital anomalies of the conduction system (160–162).

Personal Characteristics and General Medical Status

Age and gender are known risk factors for SCD during exercise. It has been observed that the risk of SCD during exercise is 5 to 14 times greater in men than women (81,89, 163). There are many potential explanations for this gender difference, including general attitude, prevalence and risk factors for coronary artery disease, and type and style of exercise (75). However, there are no differences in overall number of men (versus women) who exercise or time spent in exercise activity. Age is an inconsistent factor for SCD with exercise. In Finland, the incidence of SCD was greatest among older men, whereas in Washington State, those younger than 45 years were at a greater risk (89,163).

Reports of SCD in military populations (younger than 35 years) have been inconsistent with the usual pathology data from young athletes. Lynch (164) evaluated SCD during or soon after exertion or sport in young British soldiers and noted that more than half had significant atherosclerotic coronary artery disease. Among typical cardiovascular risk factors, only hyperlipidemia has been noted to be a factor for SCD with exercise (138–141,165). Sickle cell trait has been associated with death during exercise (81,82). In some cases, death is sudden, but in others, rhabdomyolysis may develop, as noted in military recruits (166,167). Pulmonary disease has been an occasional factor in causing athletic death. Individuals may suddenly develop an unstable asthmatic condition (or exercise-induced anaphylaxis) or an individual may exercise while ill and gradually have respiratory distress. Van Camp and colleagues (81) noted that respiratory illness played a role in the deaths of five high school or collegiate athletes. Others have also reported SCD during exercise in athletes with pulmonary disease (168,169).

The Environment

Many athletic endeavors occur in less than ideal weather conditions. Some athletes may train in adverse conditions attempting to build character; unfortunately, this may occasionally result in serious consequences for the participants. Van Camp and colleagues noted over a 10-year period that 15 men died in organized high school and college athletics from weather-related conditions, including hyperthermia (81). Takada and colleagues (170) noted a correlation between meteorological conditions, physical activities, and the risk of SCD in 76 pediatric cases. They suggested that SCDs during competitive sports were somehow associated with particular weather patterns.

Exposure to Toxins

In 1967 a British cyclist competing in the Tour de France died and tested positive for amphetamines (171). Partly as a result of this event, the International Olympic Committee began drug testing the year after (172). During the last 30 years, these tests have shown that athletes are willing to employ various dangerous substances to possibly improve their performance. Included among the items found and later banned by the Olympic Organization are stimulants, narcotics, anabolic agents, antiasthma drugs, diuretics, hormones, alcohol, and marijuana. Some of these agents may create unfair advantage for the user for the short-term athletic event. Serious cardiovascular problems have been reported after the use of some of these therapies. Adgey and colleagues (173) noted that of the more than 120 deaths annually in the United Kingdom associated with substance abuse, some occur during athletic activity. When evaluating any possible cardiovascular problem in athletes, the physician should be aware of the potential for abusing these myriad substances.

Stimulants such as amphetamines and cocaine are the most common substances associated with athletic SCD (174,175). Amphetamines are sympathomimetic agents that have effects similar to those of norepinephrine; cocaine blocks the reuptake of noradrenaline, thereby producing an excess of neurotransmitter in the synapse and increased receptor stimulation. The increase in noradrenaline produces tachycardia, vasoconstriction, acute increase in blood pressure, and ventricular arrhythmias. Anabolic agents have been thought to cause cardiovascular disorders by increasing the risk of atherosclerosis, thrombosis, vasospasm, and direct myocardial injury (176,177).

Preparation for and Performance of Event

Siscovick and colleagues (92) showed that the level of habitual exercise (training) was an important factor for the risk of SCD. Among sedentary men, the transient increase in risk of SCD during exercise was large compared with the risk of regular exercisers. Tabib and colleagues (83) suggested that recreational sports activity may be dangerous and that individuals may experience SCD after sport for which they had been inadequately trained.

In considering organized high school or collegiate athletics, there was no significant risk of SCD for one sporting event over another (81). High school and collegiate football and basketball were reported to be the sports with the highest number of SCD fatalities, but these failed to reach statistical significance because of the high number of participants and small number of SCD events.

In summary, many potential factors must be considered regarding SCD in athletes. There is a small but persistent prevalence of SCD in active people. The mechanism of death is most commonly ventricular fibrillation. Structural cardiac disease is the most important of the myriad of risk factors for fatal arrhythmia. Younger athletic victims are more likely to have HCM, coronary artery anomalies, or a mixed bag of cardiac disorders (114). Those older than 30 years are more likely to have typical atherosclerotic coronary artery disease. Additional important factors include the individual's general medical status, personal habits, and preparation for exercise along with the environment. Despite attention to these details, some athletes are still at risk for SCD. The next challenge is to determine whether we can predict those at risk by screening.

PREPARTICIPATION SCREENING

Cardiovascular deaths in competitive athletes often occur in the setting of previously unsuspected cardiovascular disease. The sudden occurrence of these events is often perceived by the public as a catastrophe and reinvigorates the debate over preparticipation screening. The purpose of screening in competitive sports through routine and systematic evaluations is to identify clinically relevant and preexisting cardiovascular abnormalities and thereby reduce the risk associated with organized sports. Some suggest that given the significant percentage of recognizable disease accounting for SCD, it seems logical that identification of these conditions with preparticipation screening should drastically

reduce the incidence of exercise-related SCD (178–180). On the other hand, some regard this exercise as futile (181).

Consideration of Various Studies in Preparticipation Screening

The American Heart Association published a position paper to guide health professionals on evaluating prospective athletes. This opinion was supported by the American Academy of Pediatrics Section on Cardiology and endorsed by the Board of Trustees of the American College of Cardiology (6).

The American Heart Association recommended that "some form of preparticipation cardiovascular screening for high school and collegiate athletes is justifiable and compelling, based on ethical, legal, and medical grounds." They concluded that a complete and careful personal and family history and physical examination designed to identify (or raise suspicion of) those cardiovascular lesions known to cause sudden death or disease progression in young athletes is the best available and most practical approach to screening populations of competitive sports participants, regardless of age. Such cardiovascular screening is an obtainable objective and should be mandatory for all athletes. They recommended that both a history and physical examination be performed before participation in organized high school (grades 9 through 12) and collegiate sports. They strongly recommended that athletic screening be performed by a health care worker with the requisite training, medical skills, and background to reliably obtain a detailed cardiovascular history, perform a physical examination, and recognize heart disease. Specifically, athletic screening evaluations should include a complete medical history, emphasizing prior occurrence of exertional chest pain or discomfort, syncope or near syncope, palpitations suggesting tachycardia, excessive or unexplained dyspnea or fatigue associated with exertion, past detection of a heart murmur or hypertension, and family history of premature SCD or cardiovascular disease in close relatives younger than 50 years. The physical examination should include brachial artery blood pressure measurement, precordial auscultation in both the supine and the standing position to identify murmurs consistent with dynamic LV outflow obstruction, assessment of femoral pulses to exclude coarctation of the aorta, and recognition of physical stigmata of Marfan syndrome. Screening should then be repeated every 2 years. In intervening years, an interim history should be obtained. They recommended developing a national standard for preparticipation medical evaluations.

In athletes older than 35 years, despite the limitation of the history and physical examination in detecting coronary heart disease, a personal history of coronary risk factors or family history of premature atherosclerosis may be useful for identifying disease; therefore, it should be performed before initiating competitive exercise. Additionally, selective medically supervised exercise stress testing in men older than 40 and women older than 50 who wish to engage in regular physical training and competitive sports would be useful, particularly for those with two or more coronary risk factors.

This opinion paper was designed to allow for a risk reduction for athletic participation. In considering this position, the authors evaluated the likely causes of SCD and the cost efficiency of various tests for mass screening. As a public policy, there is often an important focus on financial consideration. Supporting that notion, the American Heart Association published an addendum 2 years after the initial report to reduce the frequency of the evaluations to every 3 to 4 years for collegiate athletes (182). The American Heart Association suggested that the previous requirement for testing every 2 years placed a "considerable burden" on the National Collegiate Athletic Association. This report commented on the "economic restraints and the availability of facilities, personnel, and time." Despite these official recommendations, there has been only a limited response by organized school programs. Glover and Maron (183) reviewed cardiovascular screening by high schools and found only 40% followed at least 70% of the American Heart Association recommendations. Pfister and colleagues surveyed collegiate screening programs and noted that only 26% adhered to 75% of the recommendation. Furthermore, examinations were commonly done by orthopedic surgeons, athletic trainers, or nurse practitioners. Cardiologists were included as examiners in only 5% of schools (184).

Epstein and Maron suggested that because SCD in athletes is an infrequent event, the cost efficiency of in-depth large-scale screening was prohibitively impractical (178). They concluded that to prospectively identify the one young athlete who will die suddenly, 200,000 athletes would have to be screened. Of these 200,000, 0.5% (or 1,000) would have congenital heart disease, of which 1% (or 10) would have disease capable of causing SCD. Of this group, 10% (or 1) might go on to die suddenly.

There are many possible tests available for screening potential participants. It has been generally agreed on that the medical history interview has been ineffective in uncovering worthwhile data in the young athlete (6). This changes, however, once participants are older than 30, as the history will likely uncover more worthwhile data. This difference is probably because of a number of factors including the likely underlying cardiovascular disorder and a willingness of the participant to admit to symptoms or risk factors that might curtail his or her activity.

The standard physical examination has been even more disappointing in detecting significant cardiovascular risk (6). Most of the common causes of significant cardiovascular disease do not exhibit prominent physical findings. Many individuals will have heart murmurs, most of which are innocent. Even a focused cardiovascular examination with maneuvers designed to enhance pathologic findings are rarely helpful. This is partly because these procedures are not often appropriately accomplished.

ECG has been considered a possible tool in the screening process. The 12-lead ECG findings are abnormal in most patients with significant disorders such as HCM. However, recent data indicate that a certain proportion of genetically affected individuals with long QT syndrome may have little or no phenotypic expression on the ECG (156). ECG also has a relatively low specificity as a screening test in the athletic populations because of the high frequency of ECG alterations that are associated with the normal "athlete's heart" (19). One study, however, suggested ECG may be worthwhile. Fuller and colleagues studied 5,615 high school athletes during a 3-year period in northern Nevada and noted outcome measures in 22 student athletes (185). ECG was the most effective screening tool, with value in 1 of 350 athletes. In contrast to these data, Maron and colleagues (186) found no athlete with definitive evidence of cardiovascular disease of major clinical consequence in 501 athletes screened with personal and family histories and 12-lead ECGs. Ninety of these athletes went on to have echocardiography because of positive findings and 75 of these athletes had no evidence for cardiovascular disease. In a study by LaCorte and colleagues (187), personal and family histories and 12-lead ECGs obtained from 1,424 student athletes, aged 12 to 18 years, resulted in further evaluation in 11%. Cardiovascular abnormalities were not identified on more intensive evaluation in young athletes (188).

Signal-average ECG results have been disappointing when evaluated as a screening tool for potentially uncovering risk for SCD. Moroe and colleagues (189) used this technique to prospectively evaluate 796 athletes. Abnormal results were noted in 8.5% of subjects. There were neither serious ventricular arrhythmias nor SCD during an average follow-up of 20 months. Biffi and colleagues (190) used signal averaging in 60 top-level athletes, 60% without arrhythmia and 40% with frequent and complex ventricular arrhythmia. Ventricular late potentials were found in 20% of the athletes with arrhythmia and 0% of the athletes without arrhythmia. These results did not correlate with any anatomic abnormality. Sustained VT was not induced in any subject, although nonsustained VT was provoked more commonly in those with late potentials (190). These data are not surprising, given the relatively low yield of the signal-averaged ECG in subjects with no significant coronary artery disease (191,192).

Holter monitoring has often been used as a diagnostic tool for screening, but there are no data supporting its usefulness. Part of the problem with prolonged ECG monitoring, as well as other screening tests, is finding unusual, not necessarily abnormal, results that may cause needless anxiety. For most situations, this test has a low yield for finding significant problems and is costly and inconvenient. One possible role for screening ambulatory monitoring is in older subjects at risk for coronary disease (104).

Although echocardiography can detect structural heart disease such as valvular heart disease, aortic root dilation, LV dysfunction, and most forms of HCM, it may lack the sensitivity to detect coronary artery anomalies and arrhythmogenic RV dysplasia. Assuming the occurrence of HCM in a young athletic population is 1 of 500, at a cost of $500 per echocardiogram, it would theoretically cost $250,000 to detect one previously undiagnosed case (97).

Furthermore, two-dimensional echocardiography has the potential for false-positive or false-negative results. False-positive results may arise from the difficulty in differentiating the athletic heart from pathologic conditions such as HCM; this can generate unnecessary anxiety and medical workup and expenses. False-negative results may occur because phenotypic expression of HCM may not be evident or complete until adolescence.

Comprehensive screening has been reported to be of value in special circumstances, however. Corrado and colleagues (193) used history, physical examination, ECG, and limited exercise testing as preliminary screening tests for athletes in northern Italy. If positive findings were encountered, additional testing was performed including echocardiography, Holter monitoring, and more vigorous exercise testing. They suggested that their approach successfully identified individuals at risk. There was no comment regarding cost.

ELIGIBILITY FOR PARTICIPATION AND RECOMMENDATIONS FOR SPECIFIC ARRHYTHMIAS

All athletic individuals should be evaluated by at least a history and physical examination before participation. This includes competitors from school age to the elderly. Clearance for athletic participation should be based on the individual's scheduled activity and medical status. The latter involves a cardiovascular history (risk factors, symptoms) and focused examination of cardiovascular structure and function, including the heart rhythm. If a significant abnormality is detected, the athlete's activity should be restricted until further analysis is done. Consideration of participation should be based on the type of activity (specific classification of the sport) and cardiovascular structure and function.

The 16th and later 26th Bethesda conferences made specific recommendations for athletic participation for individuals with many different types of cardiovascular conditions. Task forces reviewed the important considerations regarding congenital heart disease, acquired valvular heart disease, mitral valve prolapse, HCM, myocarditis, and other myopericardial diseases (194–196). Additionally, there were data on systemic hypertension, coronary artery disease, and arrhythmia (197–199). The section on arrhythmia included information on ectopic beats, bradyarrhythmia (sinus node function, AV conduction), supraventricular and ventricular tachyarrhythmia, preexcitation, long QT syndrome, and syncope (199). As listed in Tables 28-5 through 28-7, most documented and suspected conditions required further evaluation in the form of noninvasive tests,

TABLE 28-5. BRADYARRHYTHMIAS

	Noninvasive Workup[a]		Comments and Treatment Options	Competitive Sports Participation Recommendations[b,c]
Arrhythmias	No Symptoms	Symptoms		
Sinus nodal dysfunction	No	Yes	No treatment if asymptomatic; pacemaker may be necessary if pauses are >3 s and secondarily symptomatic	FP if heart rate increases appropriately or arrhythmias appropriately treated without recurrence for 3–6 mo
1st-degree AV block	No[d]	Yes	None	FP if no symptoms and/or no worsening of AV block with exercise
2nd-degree AV block Mobitz type I	No[e]	Yes	None if no symptoms; for associated symptoms, consider pacemaker	FP if no significant worsening of AV block with exercise; LP if AV block worsens with exercise[f]
2nd-degree Mobitz type II, acquired or congenital 3rd-degree AV block	Yes	Yes	Pacemaker unless asymptomatic with normal heart and heart rate of >40 at rest and no other arrhythmia	LP if pacemaker necessary[g]
Complete RBBB	Yes	Yes	None if no symptoms	FP if no symptoms
Complete LBBB	Yes	Yes	EPS likely necessary; pacemaker if HV interval is >90 ms in the setting of LBBB	FP if no symptoms; LP if pacemaker is needed[g]

AV, atrioventricular; RBBB, right bundle branch block; LBBB, left bundle branch block; EPS, electrophysiologic study; FP, full participation; LP, limited participation.
[a]Full noninvasive workup includes 12-lead electrocardiogram (ECG), echocardiogram, exercise stress test, and 24-h ambulatory ECG (Holter) monitoring, the latter in part during sports activity.
[b]Based on reference no. 176.
[c]Degree of participation of athletes with structural heart disease depends on the limitation of the underlying disease.
[d]Unless PR interval >0.3 or if QRS is abnormal.
[e]Unless QRS is abnormal or block occurs with exercise.
[f]EPS may be necessary in some patients.
[g]Athletes on anticoagulants or with pacemaker and defibrillator systems should not participate in sports with danger of bodily collision.

TABLE 28-6. SUPRAVENTRICULAR ARRHYTHMIAS

Arrhythmias	Diagnostic Approach	Comments and Treatment Options	Sports Participation Recommendations[a,b,c]
APD, JPD	None if no symptoms	None, β blocker	FP. β Blockers are banned by Olympics in some sports
AF, AFL	NI[d] EPS likely for AFL	AV blockade, AAD, RFA, AC	FP as long as rate controlled during physical activity
AT, SNRT, NPJT	NI[d] EP likely for most patients	RFA, AV blockade	FP as long as rate controlled during physical activity
PSVT	NI[d] EPS for most patients	RFA, digoxin, β blocker, CCB, AAD	Curative RFA or drug therapy; if after successful medical therapy, FP participation after 6 mo if no recurrence of arrhythmias
WPW	EPS for risk stratification with or without symptoms	If asymptomatic and low risk, no therapy; if high risk, RFA	RFA is recommended for all individuals who have hemodynamically compromised symptoms before FP; FP if >30 y old if asymptomatic FP after curative RFA with no recurrence of symptoms or arrhythmia for 6 mo

APD, atrial premature depolarizations; JPD, junctional premature depolarizations; AF, atrial fibrillation; AFL, atrial flutter; AT, atrial tachycardia; SNRT, sinus nodal reentrant tachycardia; NPJT, nonparoxysmal junctional tachycardia; PSVT, paroxysmal supraventricular tachycardia; WPW, Wolff-Parkinson-White syndrome; AV, atrioventricular; AAD, antiarrhythmic drugs; RFA, radiofrequency ablation; AC, anticoagulation; CCB, calcium channel blocker; FP, full participation; NI, noninvasive; EPS, electrophysiologic study.
[a]Based on reference no. 176.
[b]Degree of participation of athletes with structural heart disease depends on the limitation of the underlying disease.
[c]Athletes on anticoagulants or with pacemaker and defibrillators should not participate in sports with danger of bodily collision.
[d]Full NI workup includes 12-lead electrocardiogram (ECG), echocardiogram, exercise stress test and 24-h ambulatory ECG (Holter) monitoring, the latter in part during sports activity.

TABLE 28-7. VENTRICULAR ARRHYTHMIAS, OTHER

Arrhythmias	Diagnostic Approach	Comment and Treatment Options	Sports Participation Recommendations[a,b]
VPD	NI[c]	Reassurance, BB Treat SHD if indicated	FP if no SHD; if SHD present, LP with or without treatment
VT	NI[c] Cardiac catheterization and EPS strongly recommended with sustained symptomatic arrhythmia	**No SHD:** BB, AAD or RFA **SHD:** BB, AAD, or ICD	**No SHD:** Restriction from sport participation for 6 mo or longer depending on results of treatment; if no more VT after treatment, FP permitted; if asymptomatic NSVT and no worsening during sport activity, FP permitted **SHD:** LP[b]
VF	NI[c] EPS and cardiac catheterization	ICD and BB, and/or AAD	LP only after adequate treatment and no recurrence for 6 mo regardless of SHD
Long QT syndrome	Family history, NI[c]	BB and/or ICD	Restricted from all competitive sports
Syncope	NI[c], TTM, tilt, EPS may be necessary	Depends on diagnosis	Depends on SHD and control of symptoms

VPD, ventricular premature depolarization; VT, ventricular tachycardia; VF, ventricular fibrillation; NI, noninvasive; EPS, electrophysiologic study; TTM, transtelephonic monitor; BB, β blocker; SHD, structural heart disease; AAD, antiarrhythmic drugs; RFA, radiofrequency ablation; ICD, implantable cardiometer-defibrillator; FP, full participation; LP, limited participation; NSVT, nonsustained ventricular tachycardia;
[a]Based on reference no. 176.
[b]Degree of participation of athletes with SHD depends on limitations of the underlying disease.
[c]Full NI workup includes 12-lead electrocardiogram (ECG), echocardiogram, exercise stress test, and 24-h ambulatory ECG (Holter) monitoring, the latter in part during sports activity.

to define the cardiovascular structure and extent of the arrhythmia.

The general initial workup for significant symptoms (syncope, presyncope, or palpitations suggesting tachycardia) and most documented arrhythmias should start with an ECG, echocardiogram, 24-hour Holter recording, and symptom-limited exercise test. If symptoms develop during sports activity, the individual should ideally be evaluated during his activity using Holter monitoring. Some individuals will require a more extensive workup such as blood analysis, tilt test, cardiac catheterization, and invasive electrophysiologic testing. Occasionally, subjects will require therapy (drug, ablation, device). Rarely, someone will be precluded from participation and may even seek legal intervention (200). More often, however, prospective athletes will require delay in participation in the sport until the specialist can review the test results and certify the safety of exercise. One extreme example of restriction is up to a 3-month rest to allow for deconditioning. This may allow for a distinction between a physiologic athletic heart versus a pathologic condition such as HCM. If therapy is necessary, close monitoring is essential. This may require blood analysis, second noninvasive testing, or even invasive testing. Athletes will need to be constantly encouraged to adhere to their therapy, even if it restricts them.

Athletes with syncope present a special diagnostic dilemma. This complaint is relatively common in a young healthy population and therefore is often written off as a benign condition (201). However, syncope may be the presenting complaint of a life-threatening cardiovascular condition such as HCM, coronary artery disorder, or ventricular tachycardia and therefore must be taken seriously (114,201). A focused history and physical examination should suggest the diagnosis in most cases. Often, despite a suspected diagnosis, the physician should perform a further workup to confirm the diagnosis. Sometimes an athlete may have more than one possible mechanism for syncope such as HCM and neurally mediated syncope. After the standard noninvasive evaluation, tilt testing has a high yield in these patients (202,203). Oftentimes, continuous loop recorders and invasive electrophysiologic studies are necessary to make the definitive diagnosis. Most athletes can return to active participation, because those with neurally mediated syncope can be treated effectively.

Levy, in a National Institutes of Health pamphlet, suggested that individuals can begin a sensible exercise program on their own, without seeing a physician first, if they have neither a history of cardiovascular symptoms nor risk factors for cardiovascular disease (204). On the other hand, Chung (205) suggests that a stress test is appropriate for screening for any man older than 40 years before starting an exercise program. When presented with an individual who wishes to begin or continue athletic training, the physician must be cognizant of the fact that neither superior fitness nor habitual exercise guarantees protection against an exercise-related death (206). Athletes will often run and exercise through pain that in a nonathletic setting could cause them to seek medical attention. It thus seems prudent to fully evaluate any individual engaged in or about to become involved with athletics who presents with a symptom that may represent a cardiac source. The issue of large-scale screening of apparently healthy athletes with all its ramifications remains unresolved.

REFERENCES

1. Powell KE, Thompson PD, Caspersen CJ, Kendrick JS. Physical activity and the incidence of coronary heart disease. *Annu Rev Public Health* 1987;8:253–287.
2. Blair SN, Kampert JB, Kohl HW III, et al. Influences of cardiorespiratory fitness and other precursors on cardiovascular disease and all-cause mortality in men and women. *JAMA* 1996;276:205–210.
3. Berlin JA, Colditz GA. A meta-analysis of physical activity in the prevention of coronary heart disease. *Am J Epidemiol* 1990;132:612–628.
4. Thompson PD. The cardiovascular complications of vigorous physical activity. *Arch Intern Med* 1996;156:2297–2302.
5. Wight JN, Salen D. Sudden cardiac death and the athlete's heart. *Arch Intern Med* 1995;155:1473–1480.
6. Maron BJ, Thompson PD, Puffer JC, et al. Cardiovascular preparticipation screening of competitive athletes. *Circulation* 1996;94:850–856.
7. Scheuer J, Tipton C. Cardiovascular adaptations to physical training. *Annu Rev Physiol* 1977;39:221–251.
8. Blomquist CG, Saltin B. Cardiovascular adaptations to physical training. *Annu Rev Physiol* 1983;45:169–189.
9. Mitchell JH, Haskell WL, Raven PB. Classification of sports. *J Am Coll Cardiol* 1994;24:864–866.
10. Robinson BF, Epstein SF, Beiser GD, Braunwald E. Control of heart rate by the autonomic nervous system: studies in man on the interrelation between baroreceptor mechanisms and exercise. *Circ Res* 1966;19:400–411.
11. Christensen NJ, Galbo H. Sympathetic nervous activity during exercise. *Annu Rev Physiol* 1983;45:139–153.
12. Park RC, Crawford MH. Heart of the athlete. *Curr Probl Cardiol* 1985;10:1–73.
13. Crawford MH. Physiologic consequences of systematic training. *Cardiol Clin* 1992;10:209–218.
14. Poliner LR, Dehmer GJ, Lewis SE, et al. Left ventricular performance in normal subjects: a comparison of the responses to exercise in the upright and supine positions. *Circulation* 1980;62:528–534.
15. Crawford MH, White DH, Amon KW. Echocardiographic evaluation of left ventricular size and performance during hand grip and supine and upright bicycle exercise. *Circulation* 1979;59:1158–1196.
16. Morganroth J, Maron BJ, Henry WL, Epstein SL. Comparative left ventricular dimensions in trained athletes. *Ann Intern Med* 1975;82:521–524.
17. Maron BJ. Structural features of the athlete heart as defined by echocardiography. *J Am Coll Cardiol* 1986;7:190–203.
18. Shapiro LM. Morphologic consequences of systematic training. *Cardiol Clin* 1992;10:219–226.
19. Zehender M, Meinertz T, Keul J, Just H. ECG variants and cardiac arrhythmias in athletes: clinical relevance and prognostic importance. *Am Heart J* 1990;119:1378–1391.
20. Pelliccia A, Avelar E, DeCastro S, Pandian N. Global left ventricular shape is not altered as a consequence of physiologic remodeling in highly trained athletes. *Am J Cardiol* 2000;86:700–702.

21. Douglas PS, O'Toole ML, Hiller WDB, Reichek N. Different effects of prolonged exercise on the right and left ventricles. *J Am Coll Cardiol* 1990;15:64–69.

22. Pelliccia A, Maron BJ, Spataro A, et al. The upper limit of physiologic cardiac hypertrophy in highly trained elite athletes. *N Engl J Med* 1991;324:295–301.

23. Henriksen E, Landeliust J, Wesslen L, et al. Echocardiographic right and left ventricular measurements in male elite endurance athletes. *Eur Heart J* 1996;17:1121–1128.

24. Shapiro LM, Kleinebenne A, McKenna WJ. The distribution of left ventricular hypertrophy in hypertrophic cardiomyopathy: comparison to athletes and hypertensives. *Eur Heart J* 1985;6:967–974.

25. Maron BJ, Pelliccia A, Spirito P. Cardiac disease in young trained athletes: insights into methods for distinguishing athlete's heart from structural heart disease, with particular emphasis on hypertrophic cardiomyopathy. *Circulation* 1995;91:1596–1601.

26. Maron BJ, Pelliccia A, Spataro A, Granata M. Reduction in left ventricular wall thickness after deconditioning in highly trained Olympic athletes. *Br Heart J* 1993;69:125–128.

27. Maron BJ, Bonow RO, Cannon RO III, et al. Hypertrophic cardiomyopathy: interrelation of clinical manifestations, pathophysiology, and therapy. *N Engl J Med* 1987;316:780–789,844–852.

28. George KP, Wolfe LA, Burggraf GW, Norman R. Electrocardiographic and echocardiographic characteristics of female athletes. *Med Sci Sports Exerc* 1995;27:1362–1370.

29. Pelliccia A, Maron BJ, Culasso F, et al. Athletes heart in women: echocardiographic characterization of highly trained elite female athletes. *JAMA* 1996;276:211–215.

30. Fleg JL, Shapiro EP, O'Connor F, et al. Left ventricular diastolic filling performance in older male athletes. *JAMA* 1995;273:1371–1376.

31. Ehsani AA, Hagberg JM, Hickson RC. Rapid changes in left ventricular dimensions and mass in response to physical conditioning and deconditioning. *Am J Cardiol* 1978;42:52–56.

32. DeMeersman RE. Heart rate variability and aerobic fitness. *Am Heart J* 1993;125:726–731.

33. Puig J, Freitas J, Carvalho MJ, et al. Spectral analysis of heart rate variability in athletes. *J Sports Med Phys Fitness* 1993;33:44–48.

34. Jensen-Urstad K, Saltin B, Ericson M, et al. Pronounced resting bradycardia in male elite runners is associated with high heart rate variability. *Scand J Med Sci Sports* 1997;7:274–278.

35. Hiss RG, Lamb LE. Electrocardiographic findings in 122,043 individuals. *Circulation* 1962;25:947–961.

36. Brodsky M, Wu D, Kanakis C, Rosen KM. Arrhythmias documented by 24 hour continuous electrocardiographic monitoring in 50 male medical students without apparent heart disease. *Am J Cardiol* 1977;39:390–395.

37. Sobotka PA, Mayer JH, Bauernfeind RA, et al. Arrhythmias documented by 24 hour continuous ambulatory electrocardiographic monitoring in young women without apparent heart disease. *Am Heart J* 1981;101:753–759.

38. Fleg JL, Kennedy HL. Cardiac arrhythmias in a healthy elderly population. *Chest* 1982;81:302–307.

39. Dickinson DF, Scott O. Ambulatory electrocardiographic monitoring in 100 healthy teenage boys. *Br Heart J* 1984;51:179–183.

40. Hanne-Paparo N, Kellermann JJ. Long-term Holter ECG monitoring of athletes. *Med Sci Sports Exerc* 1981;13:294–298.

41. Viitasalo MT, Kala R, Eisalo A. Ambulatory electrocardiographic recording in endurance athletes. *Br Heart J* 1982;47:213–220.

42. Talan DA, Bauernfeind RA, Ashley WW, et al. Twenty-four hour continuous ECG recordings in long-distance runners. *Chest* 1982;82:19–24.

43. Zeppilli P. High-grade arrhythmias in well-trained runners. *Am Heart J* 1983;4:775–777.

44. Pilcher GF, Cook J, Johnston BL, Fletcher GF. Twenty-four hour continuous electrocardiography during exercise and free activity in 80 apparently healthy runners. *Am J Cardiol* 1983;52:859–861.

45. Viitasalo MT, Kala R, Eisalo A. Ambulatory electrocardiographic findings in young athletes between 14 and 16 years of age. *Eur Heart J* 1984;5:2–6.

46. Palatini P, Maraglino G, Sperti G, et al. Prevalence and possible mechanisms of ventricular arrhythmias in athletes. *Am Heart J* 1985;110:560–567.

47. Northcote RJ, Canning GP, Ballantyne D. Electrocardiographic findings in male veteran endurance athletes. *Br Heart J* 1989;61:155–160.

48. Jensen-Urstad K, Bouvier F, Saltin B, Jensen-Urstad M. High prevalence of arrhythmias in elderly male athletes with a lifelong history of regular strenuous exercise. *Heart* 1998;79:161–164.

49. VanGanse W, Versee L, Eylenbosch W, Vuylsteek K. The electrocardiogram of athletes. *Br Heart J* 1970;32:160–164.

50. Balady GJ, Cadigan JB, Ryan TJ. Electrocardiogram of the athlete: an analysis of 289 professional football players. *Am J Cardiol* 1984;53:1339–1343.

51. Lewis SF, Nylander E, Gad P, Areskoy NH. Non-autonomic component in bradycardia of endurance trained men at rest and during exercise. *Acta Physiol Scand* 1980;109:297–305.

52. Ogawa S, Tabata H, Ohishi S, et al. Prognostic significance of long ventricular pauses in athletes. *Jpn Circ J* 1991;55:761–766

53. Hansen EO. Intermittent partial heart block in a well trained top sportsman. *Nord Med* 1959;62:1386–1388.

54. Gibbons LW, Cooper KH, Martin RP, Pollock ML. Medical examination and electrocardiographic analysis of elite distance runners. *Ann N Y Acad Sci* 1977;301:283–396.

55. Smith WG, Cullen KJ, Thorburn IO. Electrocardiograms of marathon runners in 1962 Commonwealth Games. *Br Heart J* 1964;26:469–476.

56. Nakamoto K. Electrocardiograms of 25 marathon runners before and after 100 meter dash. *Jpn Circ J* 1969;33:105–128.

57. Hunt EA. Electrocardiographic study of 20 champion swimmers before and after 110 yard sprint swimming competition. *Can Med Assoc J* 1963;88:1251–1253.

58. Meytes I, Kaplinsky E, Yahini J, et al. Wenckebach AV block: a frequent feature following heavy physical training. *Am Heart J* 1990;90:426–430.

59. Cullen KJ, Collin R. Daily running causing Wenckebach heart block. *Lancet* 1964;1:729–730.

60. Sargin O, Alp C, Tansi C, Karaca L. Wenckebach phenomenon with nodal and ventricular escape in marathon runners. *Chest* 1970;57:102–105.

61. Zeppilli P, Fenici R, Sassara M, et al. Wenckebach seconddegree AB block in top-ranking athletes: an old problem revisited. *Am Heart J* 1980;100:281–294.

62. Northcote R, Rankin A, Scullion R, Logan W. Is severe bradycardia in veteran athletes an indication for a permanent pacemaker? *Br Med J* 1989;298:213–232.

63. Cooper JP, Fraser AG, Penny WJ. Reversibility and benign recurrence of complete heart blocking athletes. *Int J Cardiol* 1992;35:118–120.

64. Lichtman J, O'Rourke RA, Klein A, Karliner J. Electrocardiogram of the athlete. *Arch Intern Med* 1973;132:763–770.

65. Pantano JA, Oriel RJ. Prevalence and nature of cardiac arrhythmias in apparently normal well-trained runners. *Am Heart J* 1982;104:762–768.

66. Abdon NJ, Landin K, Johansson BW. Athlete's bradycardia as an embolising disorder? *Br Heart J* 1984;52:660–666.

67. Furlanello F, Bertoldi A, Dallago M, et al. Atrial fibrillation in elite athletes. *J Cardiovasc Electrophysiol* 1998;9:S63–S68.

68. Biffi A, Verdile L, Pelliccia A, et al. Long-term significance of

apparently life-threatening ventricular tachyarrhythmias in trained athletes. *Circulation* 2000;102:2550.

69. Zeppilli P, Pirrami MM, Sassara M, Fenici R. T wave abnormalities in top-ranking athletes: effects of isoproterenol, atropine, and physical exercise. *Am Heart J* 1980;100:213–222.

70. Serra Grimma JS, Carrio I, Estorch M, et al. ECG alterations in the athlete type "pseudoischemia." *J Sports Cardiol* 1986;3:9–16.

71. Serra Grima R, Estorch M, Carrio I, et al. Marked ventricular repolarization abnormalities in highly trained athletes' electrocardiograms: clinical and prognostic implications. *J Am Coll Cardiol* 2000;36:1310–1316.

72. Pelliccia A, Maron BJ, Culasso F, et al. Clinical significance of abnormal electrocardiographic patterns in trained athletes. *Circulation* 2000;102:278–284.

73. Maron BJ, Roberts WC, McAllister HA, et al. Sudden death in young athletes. *Circulation* 1980;62:218–229.

74. Tsung SH, Huang TY, Chang HH. Sudden death in young athletes. *Arch Pathol Lab Med* 1982;106:168–170.

75. Virmani R, Robinowitz M, McAllister HA. Nontraumatic death in joggers: a series of 30 patients at autopsy. *Am J Med* 1982;72:874–881.

76. Waller BF, Newhouse P, Pless J, et al. Exercise-related sudden death in 27 conditioned subjects aged ≥30 years: coronary artery abnormalities are the culprit. *J Am Coll Cardiol* 1984;3:621(abst).

77. Kennedy HL, Whitlock JA. Sports related sudden death in young persons. *J Am Coll Cardiol* 1984;3:622(abst).

78. Northcote RJ, Flannigan C, Ballantyne D. Sudden death and vigorous exercise—a study of 60 deaths associated with squash. *Br Heart J* 1986;55:198–203.

79. Corrado D, Thiene G, Nava A, et al. Sudden death in young competitive athletes: clinicopathologic correlations in 22 cases. *Am J Med* 1990;89:588–596.

80. Burke AP, Farb A, Virmani R, et al. Sports-related and non-sports related sudden cardiac death in young adults. *Am Heart J* 1991;121:568–575.

81. Van Camp SP, Bloor CM, Mueller FO, et al. Nontraumatic sports death in high school and college athletes. *Med Sci Sports Exerc* 1995;27:641–647.

82. Maron BJ, Shirani J, Poliac LC, et al. Sudden death in young competitive athletes. *JAMA* 1996;276:199–204.

83. Tabib A, Miras A, Taniere P, Loire R. Undetected cardiac lesions cause unexpected sudden cardiac death during occasional sport activity. *Eur Heart J* 1999;20:900–903.

84. Mitchell JH, Maron BJ, Epstein SE. 16th Bethesda Conference: cardiovascular abnormalities in the athlete: recommendations regarding eligibility for competition. *J Am Coll Cardiol* 1985;6:1186–1232.

85. Maron BJ, Mitchell JH. 26th Bethesda Conference: revised eligibility recommendations for competitive athletes with cardiovascular abnormalities. *J Am Coll Cardiol* 1994;24:845–899.

86. *Oxford English Dictionary.* Oxford: Oxford University Press, 1971:533.

87. Maron BJ, Mitchell JH. Revised eligibility recommendations for competitive athletes with cardiovascular abnormalities. *J Am Coll Cardiol* 1994;24:848–850.

88. Maron BJ, Poliac LC, Kaplan JA, Mueller FO. Blunt impact to the chest leading to sudden death from cardiac arrest during sports activities. *N Engl J Med* 1995;333:337–342.

89. Thompson PD, Funk EJ, Carleton RA, Sturner NQ. Incidence of death during jogging in Rhode Island from 1975 through 1980. *JAMA* 1982;63:287–304.

90. Vuori I. Sudden death and physical activity. *Cardiology* 1978;63:287–304.

91. Maron BJ, Poliac LC, Roberts WO. Risk for sudden cardiac death associated with marathon running. *J Am Coll Cardiol* 1996;28:428–431.

92. Siscovick DS, Weiss NS, Fletcher RH, Lasky T. The incidence of primary cardiac arrest during vigorous exercise. *N Engl J Med* 1984;311:874–877.

93. Maron BJ, Gohman TE, Aeppli D. Prevalence of sudden cardiac death during competitive sports activities in Minnesota high school athletes. *J Am Coll Cardiol* 1998;32:1881–1884.

94. Furlanello F, Bertoldi A, Bettini R, et al. Life threatening arrhythmias in athletes. *Pace* 1992;15:1403–1411.

95. Coelho A, Palileo E, Ashley W, et al. Tachyrrhythmias in young athletes. *J Am Coll Cardiol* 1986;7:237–243.

96. Surawicz B. Ventricular fibrillation. *J Am Coll Cardiol* 1985;5:43B–54B.

97. Hartley LH, Mason JW, Hogan RP, et al. Multiple hormonal responses to prolonged exercise in relation to physical training. *J Appl Physiol* 1972;33:607–610.

98. Dimsdale JE, Moss J. Plasma catecholamines in stress and exercise. *JAMA* 1980;243:340–342.

99. Osswald S, Brooks R, O'Nunain SS, et al. Asystole after exercise in healthy persons. *Ann Intern Med* 1994;120:630–632.

100. Dimsdale JE, Hartley LH, Gainey T, et al. Post-exercise period plasma catecholamines and exercise. *JAMA* 1984;251:630–632.

101. Waller BF. What causes sudden cardiac death in athletes? *Cardiovasc Rev Rep* 1988;1:39–44.

102. Nava A, Thiene G, Canciani B, et al. Familial occurrence of right ventricular dysplasia: a study involving nine families. *J Am Coll Cardiol* 1988;12:1222–1228.

103. Thiene G, Nava A, Corrado D. et al. Right ventricular cardiomyopathy and sudden death in young people. *N Engl J Med* 1988;318:129–133.

104. Maron BJ, Gardin JM, Flack JM, et al. Prevalence of hypertrophic cardiomyopathy in a general population of young adults. *Circulation* 1995;92:785–789.

105. Maron BJ, Nichols PF, Pickle LW, et al. Patterns of inheritance in hypertrophic cardiomyopathy: assessment of M-mode and two-dimensional echocardiography. *Am J Cardiol* 1984;53:1087–1094.

106. Lardani H, Serrano JA, Villanul RJ. Hemodynamics and coronary angiography in idiopathic hypertrophic subaortic stenosis. *Am J Cardiol* 1978;41:476–481.

107. Hardarson T, De la Calzada CS, Curiel R, Goodwin JF. Prognosis and mortality of hypertrophic cardiomyopathy. *Lancet* 1973;2:1462–1467.

108. Noakes TD, Rose AG, Opie LH. Hypertrophic cardiomyopathy associated with sudden death during marathon racing. *Br Heart J* 1979;41:624–627.

109. Goodwin JF, Krikles DM. Arrhythmias as a cause of sudden death in hypertrophic cardiomyopathy. *Lancet* 1976;2:937–940.

110. Maron BJ, Lipson LC, Roberts WC, et al. "Malignant" hypertrophic cardiomyopathy: identification of a subgroup of families with unusually frequent premature death. *Am J Cardiol* 1978;41:1133–1140.

111. Maron BJ, Savage DD, Wolfson J, Epstein SE. Prognostic significance of 24 hour ambulatory electrocardiographic monitoring in patients with hypertrophic cardiomyopathy: a prospective study. *Am J Cardiol* 1981;48:252–254.

112. Maron BJ, Roberts WC, Epstein SE. Sudden death in hypertrophic cardiomyopathy: a profile of 78 patients. *Circulation* 1982;65:1388–1394.

113. Frennaux MP, Counihan PJ, Caforio ALP, et al. Abnormal blood pressure response during exercise in hypertrophic cardiomyopathy. *Circulation* 1990;82:1995–2002.

114. McCaffrey FM, Braconier DS, Strong WB. Sudden cardiac death in young athletes. *Am J Dis Child* 1991;145:177–183.

115. Sadoul N, Prasad K, Elliott PM, et al. Prospective prognostic assessment of blood pressure response during exercise in

patients with hypertrophic cardiomyopathy. *Circulation* 1997; 96:2987–2991.

116. Maki S, Ikeda H, Muro A, et al. Predictors of sudden cardiac death in hypertrophic cardiomyopathy. *Am J Cardiol* 1998;82: 774–778.

117. Maron BJ, Kogan J, Proschan MA, et al. Circadian variability in the occurrence of sudden cardiac death in patients with hypertrophic cardiomyopathy. *J Am Coll Cardiol* 1994;23:1405–1409.

118. Virmani R, Rogan K, Cheitlin MD. Congenital coronary artery anomalies: pathologic aspects. In: Virmani R, Forman MB, eds. *Nonatherosclerotic ischemic heart disease*. New York: Raven Press, 1989:153–183.

119. Burke AP, Farb A, Virmani R. Causes of sudden death in athletes. *Cardiol Clin* 1992;10:303–317.

120. Maron BJ, Leon MB, Swain JA, et al. Prospective identification by two-dimensional echocardiography of anomalous origin of the left main coronary artery from the right sinus of Valsalva. *Am J Cardiol* 1991;68:140–142.

121. Zeppilli P, Dello Russo A, Santini C, et al. *In vivo* detection of coronary artery anomalies in asymptomatic athletes by echocardiographic screening. *Chest* 1998;114:89–93.

122. Basso C, Maron BJ, Corrado D, Thiene G. Clinical profile of congenital coronary artery anomalies with origin from the wrong aortic sinus leading to sudden death in young competitive athletes. *J Am Coll Cardiol* 2000;35:1493–1501.

123. Marcus F, Fontaine G, Guirandon G, et al. Right ventricular dysplasia: a report of 24 adult cases. *Circulation* 1982;65:384–398.

124. Nava A, Thiene G, Canciani B, et al. Familial occurrence of right ventricular dysplasia: a study involving nine families. *J Am Coll Cardiol* 1988;12:1222–1223.

125. Furlanello F, Bertoldi A, Dallago M, et al. Cardiac arrest and sudden death in competitive athletes with arrhythmogenic right ventricular dysplasia. *Pace* 1998;21:331–335.

126. Goodin JC, Farb A, Smialek JE, et al. Right ventricular dysplasia associated with sudden death in young adults. *Modern Pathol* 1991;4:702–706.

127. Pelliccia A, Maron BG. Preparticipation cardiovascular evaluation of the competitive athlete: perspectives from the 30-year Italian experience. *Am J Cardiol* 1995;75:827–829.

128. Metzger JT, De Chillou C, Cheriex E, et al. Values of the 12-lead electrocardiogram in arrhythmogenic right ventricular dysplasia, and absence of correlation with echocardiographic findings. *Am J Cardiol* 1993;72:964–967.

129. Ricci C, Longo R, Pagnan L, et al. Magnetic resonance imaging in right ventricular dysplasia. *Am J Cardiol* 1992;70:1589–1595.

130. Peters S, Reil GH. Risk factors of cardiac arrest in arrhythmogenic right ventricular dysplasia. *Eur Heart J* 1995;16:77–80.

131. Brodsky MA, Orlov MV, Winters RJ, Allen BJ. Determinants of inducible ventricular tachycardia in patients with clinical ventricular tachycardia and no apparent structural heart disease. *Am Heart J* 1993;126:1113–1120.

132. Jeresaty RM. Sudden death in mitral valve prolapse syndrome. *Am J Cardiol* 1976;37:317–318.

133. Savage DD, Garrison RJ, Devereux RB, et al. Mitral valve prolapse in the general population. Epidemiologic features: the Framingham Study. *Am Heart J* 1983;106:571–576.

134. Kligfield P, Tochreiter C, Kramer H, et al. Complex arrhythmias in mitral regurgitation with and without mitral valve prolapse: contrast to arrhythmias in mitral valve prolapse without mitral regurgitation. *Am J Cardiol* 1985;55:1545–1549.

135. Vohra J, Sathe S, Warren R, et al. Malignant ventricular arrhythmias with mitral valve prolapse and mild mitral regurgitation. *Pace* 1993;16:387–393.

136. Bassler TJ. Marathon running and immunity to atherosclerosis. *Ann N Y Acad Sci* 1977;301:579–592.

137. Waller BF, Roberts WC. Sudden death while running in conditioned runners aged 40 years or over. *Am J Cardiol* 1980;45: 1292–1300.

138. Thompson PD, Stern MP, Williams P, et al. Death during jogging or running. *JAMA* 1979;242:1265–1267.

139. Northcote RJ, Ballantyne D. Sudden cardiac death in sport. *Br Med J* 1983;287:1357–1359.

140. Jackson RT, Beaglehole R, Sharpe N. Sudden death in runners. *N Z Med J* 1983;96:289–292.

141. Katzel LI, Fleg JL, Busby-Whitehead J, et al. Exercise-induced silent myocardial ischemia in master athletes. *Am J Cardiol* 1998;81;261–265.

142. Black A, Black MM, Gensini G. Exertion and acute coronary artery injury. *Angiology* 1975;26:759–783.

143. Davies MJ, Thomas A. Thrombosis and acute coronary lesions in sudden cardiac ischemic death. *N Engl J Med* 1984;310: 1137–1140.

144. Viquola PH, Honumi K, Swage PS, et al. Lymphocytic myocarditis presenting as unexplained ventricular arrhythmias: diagnosis with endomyocardial biopsy and response to immunosuppression. *J Am Coll Cardiol* 1984;4:812–819.

145. Neuspiel DR. Sudden death from myocarditis in young athletes [Letter]. *Mayo Clin Proc* 1986;61:226–227.

146. Wesslen L, Pahlson C, Lindquist O, et al. An increase in sudden unexpected cardiac deaths among Swedish orienteers during 1979–1992. *Eur Heart J* 1996;17:902–910.

147. Friman G, Wesslen L, Fohlman J, et al. The epidemiology of infectious myocarditis, lymphocytic myocarditis and dilated cardiomyopathy. *Eur Heart J* 1995;16:36–41.

148. Phillips M, Robinowitz M, Higgins J, et al. Sudden cardiac death in Air Force recruits. A 20-year review. *JAMA* 1986;256: 2696–2699.

149. Morales AR, Romanelli R, Boucek JB. The mural left anterior descending coronary artery, strenuous exercise and sudden death. *Circulation* 1980;62:230–237.

150. Agirbasli M, Martin GS, Stolt JB, et al. Myocardial bridge as a cause of thrombus formation and myocardial infarction in a young athlete. *Clin Cardiol* 1997;20:1032–1036.

151. Yetman AT, McCrindle BW, MacDonald C, et al. Myocardial bridging in children with hypertrophic cardiomyopathy—a risk factor for sudden death. *N Engl J Med* 1998;339:1201–1209.

152. Bain M, Zumwalt R, van der Bel-Kahn J. Marfan syndrome presenting as aortic rupture in a young athlete: sudden unexpected death? *Am J Forensic Med Pathol* 1987;8:334–337.

153. Gordon JB, Ganz P, Nabel EG, et al. Atherosclerosis influences the vasomotor response of epicardial coronary arteries to exercise. *J Clin Invest* 1989;83:1946–1952.

154. Roberts WC, McAllister HJ, Ferrans VJ. Sarcoidosis of the heart: a clinicopathologic study of 35 necropsy patients and review of 78 previously described necropsy patients. *Am J Med* 1977;63:86–106.

155. Munger TM, Packer DL, Hammil SC, et al. A population study of the natural history of Wolff-Parkinson-White syndrome in Olmsted County, Minnesota, 1953–1989. *Circulation* 1993;87: 866–873.

156. Jackman WM, Friday KJ, Anderson JL, et al. The long QT syndromes: a critical review, new clinical observations and unifying hypothesis. *Prog Cardiovasc Dis* 1988;31:115–172.

157. Benson DW Jr, Benditt DG, Anderson RW, et al. Cardiac arrest in young, ostensibly healthy patients: clinical, hemodynamic, and electrophysiologic findings. *Am J Cardiol* 1983;52:65–69.

158. Thiene G, Pennelli N, Rossi L. Cardiac conduction system abnormalities as a possible cause of sudden death in young athletes. *Hum Pathol* 1983;14:705–709.

159. Wiedermann CJ, Becker AE, Hopferwieser T, et al. Sudden death in a young competitive athlete with Wolff-Parkinson-White syndrome. *Eur Heart J* 1987;8:651–655.

160. James TN, Froggett P, Marshall TK. Sudden death in young athletes. *Ann Intern Med* 1967;67:1013–1021.

161. Bharati S, Cantor GH, Leach JB III, et al. The conduction system in sudden death in Alaskan sled dogs during the Iditarod race and/or during training. *Pace* 1997;20:654–666.

162. Bharati S, Lev M. *The cardiac conduction system in unexplained sudden death*. Mt. Kisco, NY: Futura Publishing, 1990.

163. Siscovick DS. Exercise and its role in sudden cardiac death. *Cardiol Clin* 1997;15:467–470.

164. Lynch P. Soldiers, sport, and sudden death. *Lancet* 1980;1: 1235–1237.

165. Siscovick DS, Ekelund LG, Johnson JL, et al. Sensitivity of exercise electrocardiography for acute cardiac events during moderate and strenuous physical activity. *Arch Intern Med* 1991;151:325–330.

166. Kark JA, Posey DM, Schumacher HR, Ruehle CJ. Sickle cell trait as a risk factor for sudden death in physical training. *N Engl J Med* 1987;317:781–787.

167. Kerle KK, Nishimura KD. Exertional collapse and sudden death associated with sickle cell trait. *Am Fam Physician* 1996; 54:237–240.

168. Willems S. Sudden cardiac death in young athletes: orienteering on *Chlamydia pneumoniae*? *Eur Heart J* 1996;17:810–812.

169. Sedivy R, Bankl HC, Stimpfl T, et al. Sudden, unexpected death of a young marathon runner as a result of bronchial malformation. *Modern Pathol* 1997;10:247–251.

170. Takada K, Nagashima M, Takada H, et al. Sudden death in school children: role of physical activities and meteorological conditions. *Pediatr Int* 1999;41:151–156.

171. Beckett AH, Cowan DA. Misuse of drugs in sport. *Br J Sports Med* 1979;12:185–194.

172. Catlin DH, Murray TH. Performance-enhanced drugs, fair competition, and olympic sport. *JAMA* 1996;276:231–237.

173. Adgey AAJ, Johnston PW, McMechan S. Sudden cardiac death and substance abuse. *Resuscitation* 1995;29:219–221.

174. Cregler LL. Cocaine as a risk factor for cardiovascular disease. *Clin Cardiol* 1991;14:450–455.

175. Isner JM, Estes NAM III, Thompson PD, et al. Acute cardiac events temporally related to cocaine abuse. *N Engl J Med* 1986;315:1438–1443.

176. Melchert RB, Welder AA. Cardiovascular effects of androgenic-anabolic steroids. *Med Sci Sports Exerc* 1995;27:1252–1262.

177. Luke JL, Farb A, Virmani R, Sample RH. Sudden cardiac death during exercise in a weight lifter using anabolic androgenic steroids: pathological and toxicological findings. *J Forensic Sci* 1990;35:144–147.

178. Epstein SE, Maron BJ. Sudden death and the competitive athlete: perspectives on preparticipation screening studies. *J Am Coll Cardiol* 1986;7:220–230.

179. Sharma S, Whyte G, McKenna WJ. Sudden death from cardiovascular disease in young athletes: fact or fiction? *Br J Sports Med* 1997;31:269–276.

180. Franklin BA, Fletcher GF, Gordon NF, et al. Cardiovascular evaluation of the athlete. *Sports Med* 1997;2:97–119.

181. Shephard RJ. The athlete's heart: is big beautiful? *Br J Sports Med* 1996;30:5–10.

182. Maron BJ, Thompson PD, Puffer JC, et al. Cardiovascular preparticipation screening of competitive athletes: addendum. *Circulation* 1998;97:2294.

183. Glover DW, Maron BJ. Profile of preparticipation cardiovascular screening for high school athletes. *JAMA* 1998;279:1817–1819.

184. Pfister GC, Puffer JC, Maron BJ. Preparticipation cardiovascular screening for US collegiate student-athletes. *JAMA* 2000; 283:1597–1599.

185. Fuller CM, McNulty CM, Spring DA, et al. Prospective screening of 5,615 high school athletes for risk of sudden cardiac death. *Med Sci Sports Exerc* 1997;29:1131–1138.

186. Maron BJ, Bodison SA, Wesley YE, et al. Results of screening a large group of intercollegiate competitive athletes for cardiovascular disease. *J Am Coll Cardiol* 1987;10:1214–1221.

187. LaCorte MA, Boxer RA, Gottesfeld IB, et al. EKG screening program for school athletes. *Clin Cardiol* 1989;12:42–44.

188. Pelliccia A, Maron BJ, Culasso F, et al. Clinical significance of abnormal electrocardiographic patterns in trained athletes. *Circulation* 2000;102:278–284.

189. Moroe K, Kimoto K, Inoue T, et al. Evaluation of abnormal signal-averaged electrocardiograms in young athletes. *Jpn Circ J* 1995;59:247–256.

190. Biffi A, Ansalone G, Verdile L, et al. Ventricular arrhythmias and athlete's heart: role of signal-averaged electrocardiography. *Eur Heart J* 1996;17: 557–563.

191. Orlov YSK, Brodsky MA, Orlov MV, et al. Is the time domain signal-averaged electrocardiogram helpful in patients with ventricular tachycardia without apparent structural heart disease? *Clin Cardiol* 1995;18:568–572.

192. Northcote RJ, MacFarlane P, Ballantyne D. Ambulatory electrocardiography in squash players. *Br Heart J* 1983;50:372–377.

193. Corrado D, Basso C, Schiavon M, Thine G. Screening for hypertrophic cardiomyopathy in young athletes. *N Engl J Med* 1998;339:364–369.

194. Graham TP Jr, Bricker JT, James FW, Strong WB. Task force 1: congenital heart disease. *J Am Coll Cardiol* 1994;24:867–873.

195. Cheitlin MD, Douglas PS, Parmley WW. Task force 2: acquired valvular heart disease. *J Am Coll Cardiol* 1994;24:874–880.

196. Maron BJ, Isner JM, McKenna WJ. Task force 3: hypertrophic cardiomyopathy, myocarditis and other myopericardial diseases and mitral valve prolapse. *J Am Coll Cardiol* 1994;24:880–885.

197. Kaplan NM, Deveraux RB, Miller HS. Task force 4: systemic hypertension. *J Am Coll Cardiol* 1994;24:885–888.

198. Thompson PD, Klocke FJ, Levine BD, VanCamp SP. Task force 5: coronary artery disease. *J Am Coll Cardiol* 1994;24:888–892.

199. Zipes DP, Garson A. Task force 6: arrhythmias. *J Am Coll Cardiol* 1994;24:892–899.

200. Maron BJ, Mitten MJ, Quandt EF, Zipes DP. Competitive athletes with cardiovascular disease—the case of Nicholas Knapp. *N Engl J Med* 1998;339:1632–1635.

201. Driscoll DJ, Jacobsen SJ, Porter CJ, Wollan PC. Syncope in children and adolescents. *J Am Coll Cardiol* 1997;29:1039–1045.

202. Calkins H, Seifert M, Morady F. Clinical presentation and long-term follow-up of athletes with exercise-induced vasodepressor syncope. *Am Heart J* 1995;129:1159–1164.

203. Sakaguchi S, Shultz JJ, Remole SC, et al. Syncope associated with exercise, a manifestation of neurally mediated syncope. *Am J Cardiol* 1995;75:476–481.

204. Levy RI. *Exercise and your heart* [Pamphlet]. Washington: US Dept of Health and Human Services; 1981; NIH publication no 81-1677.

205. Chung EK. Exercise ECG testing: is it indicated for asymptomatic individuals before engaging in any exercise program? *Arch Intern Med* 1980;140: 895–896.

206. Zeppilli P. High grade arrhythmias in well-trained runners. *Am Heart J* 1983;106:775–778.

29

ARRHTHMIAS AFTER CARDIAC AND NONCARDIAC SURGERY

MINA K. CHUNG
CRAIG R. ASHER
DAVID YAMADA
KIM A. EAGLE

Arrhythmias rank among the most common postoperative complications of cardiac surgery. Atrial tachyarrhythmias, in particular atrial fibrillation, are the most frequent type of significant arrhythmia (Table 29-1) (1–5). Although ventricular ectopy is common, serious, sustained ventricular tachyarrhythmias are distinctly uncommon after most types of cardiac surgery (6–10). Bradyarrhythmias are frequent but usually transient, and given the nearly routine use of epicardial pacing wires, are less frequently of long-term clinical significance. This chapter addressed the epidemiology, pathogenesis, diagnosis, treatment, prevention, and complications of arrhythmias after surgery, particularly after cardiac surgery.

SUPRAVENTRICULAR ARRHYTHMIAS

Atrial Arrhythmias

Epidemiology

Although occurrence rates are greatest after cardiac surgery, major noncardiac surgery carries a risk of supraventricular arrhythmias on the order of 3% to 4% (11,12). The requirement of thoracotomy for noncardiac surgical procedures increases the risk to 12% to 46% (13–16). Higher incidences are reported after total compared with partial pneumonectomy (14,16). Other factors that correlated with atrial fibrillation after lung surgery included history of ischemic heart disease, congestive heart failure, intraoperative cardiac arrest, and need for repeat thoracotomy.

After cardiac surgery, atrial tachyarrhythmias, particularly atrial fibrillation, are the most common significant arrhythmia. Atrial arrhythmias have been reported to occur in 5% to 100% of patients after coronary artery bypass graft (CABG) (1) with recent studies still reporting incidences of 17% to 40% after CABG (1–5,17). Incidences are even higher after valvular surgery and range from 37% to 64% (2,18,19).

The clinical impact of atrial fibrillation after surgery is significant, because it can prolong hospital stay and escalate expenses. Atrial arrhythmias after cardiac surgery usually occur with a peak incidence on postoperative days 2 to 3. One analysis of 1,666 patients showed that 4.7% of supraventricular arrhythmias developed on the day of surgery, with peak incidence of 43.1% occurring on day 2 and only 0.4% occurring 9 or more days after surgery (5). However, hospital length of stay after CABG can be extended by 2 to 3 days with additional costs of several thousand dollars incurred per patient (2,17,20,21). Higher risks of stroke after cardiac surgery (2,22–24) and mortality after cardiac and major noncardiothoracic surgery (24,25) have been associated with postoperative atrial fibrillation.

Pathogenesis

Factors that may contribute to the development of atrial fibrillation after cardiac surgery include surgically induced

M. K. Chung, C. R. Asher and D. Yamada: Department of Cardiology, Cleveland Clinic Foundation, Cleveland, Ohio 44195.

K. A. Eagle: Department of Internal Medicine, University of Michigan Medical Center, Ann Arbor, Michigan 48109.

TABLE 29-1. INCIDENCE OF ARRHYTHMIAS AFTER CARDIAC SURGERY

Type of Arrhythmia	Incidence (%)
Atrial fibrillation[a]	5–40%
Nonsustained ventricular ectopy	36%
Sustained ventricular tachycardia or fibrillation	0.4–1.5%
Sinus node dysfunction	0.8–21%
Bundle branch or fascicular block	17–45%
Complete atrioventricular block	≤4%

[a]Includes atrial flutter and supraventricular tachycardia.

acute atrial enlargement, hypertension or stretch; atrial ischemia or infarction from inadequate atrial protection from cardioplegia during bypass; trauma from cannulation; electrolyte abnormalities, such as hypomagnesemia; inflammation resulting from pericarditis; and β-blocker withdrawal (26–36). Increasing age, the most consistent clinical predictor of postoperative atrial fibrillation, may also decrease the threshold for atrial fibrillation.

Intrinsic predisposition to postoperative atrial fibrillation is suggested to be associated with age-related changes in electrophysiologic properties of the atria (37), preoperative prolongation of P-wave duration (38,39), and inducibility of atrial fibrillation before cardiopulmonary bypass (40). In patients undergoing surgery for aortic stenosis, Bush and colleagues (37) reported that patients older than 40 years had a 67% incidence of postoperative supraventricular arrhythmias, compared with an 18% incidence in patients younger than 20 years. Right atrial tissue from older patients displayed diffuse spontaneous phase 4 depolarization, local conduction disturbances, decrease in the resting membrane potential with slower V_{max} of the action potential, and shorter action potential duration. Kecskemeti and colleagues (41) also studied right atrial appendage cells from patients undergoing cardiac surgery. Postoperative atrial fibrillation occurred in 1 of 10 patients with normal action potentials, compared with 8 of 10 patients with abnormal action potentials, characterized by depolarized resting membrane potential, slowed upstroke that could cause slowed conduction, reduced amplitude, and prolonged refractoriness. Lowe and colleagues (40) predicted postoperative atrial fibrillation by the intraoperative inducibility of atrial fibrillation using alternating current applied to the right atrium before the initiation of cardiopulmonary bypass with a sensitivity of 94%, though only modest specificity of 41%.

Excessive sympathetic or decreased parasympathetic activity may precede the onset of postoperative atrial fibrillation in some patients. Hogue and colleagues (42) reported that among 36 patients undergoing CABG, those who developed atrial fibrillation had reduced heart rate complexity, higher heart rates, and more frequent atrial ectopy before the onset of the atrial arrhythmia. However, in this study, R-R–interval heart rate variability could be lower or higher before the onset of arrhythmias, suggesting that heightened sympathetic or vagal activation might promote atrial fibrillation in individual patients. Dimmer and colleagues (43) reported that the onset of atrial fibrillation after CABG was preceded by an increase in the number of atrial premature contractions, as well as increase in standard deviation of R-R intervals (SDNN) and an initial lower than higher low frequency–high frequency ratio, interpreted as consistent with a loss of vagal tone and moderate increase in sympathetic tone before the onset of atrial fibrillation. Pichlmaier and colleagues (44) recorded monophasic action potentials continuously after surgery and observed that in

seven of nine episodes of atrial fibrillation, monophasic action potential duration decreased, and in the two patients in whom the mean arterial pressure increased, beat-to-beat variability of cycle length increased; suggesting that in some patients, fluctuation in autonomic tone may be contributory. Tittelbach and colleagues (45) also reported involvement of the adrenergic system by demonstrating changes in guanine nucleotide–binding protein (G protein) expression after CABG. On average, ratios of G(s alpha)/G (i alpha) mRNA and protein expression increased after CABG in patients who developed atrial fibrillation and decreased in patients without atrial fibrillation.

Intraoperative atrial ischemia resulting from inadequate cold cardioplegic arrest has also been associated with slowed atrial conduction in animal models (28,29). Sato and colleagues (28) reported no significant effect of augmented atrial hypothermia on atrial refractory periods and inducibility of atrial arrhythmias in the canine heart, but atrial conduction times were significantly prolonged during the first 2 hours after bypass. Atrial fibrillation that was inducible by extrastimulation was associated with increased dispersion of refractoriness and a prolongation of conduction time. Smith and colleagues (30) noted that in humans and dogs, there exists a disparity in the ability to cool the atrial and ventricular septa, as well as a more rapid increase in atrial septal temperature after cessation of infusion of cardioplegia. They postulated that ischemic injury resulting from inadequate atrial hypothermia may be related to postoperative rhythm disturbances. Using a bipolar atrial electrogram, Tchervenkov and colleagues (46) monitored atrial activity from the time of administration of cardioplegia until removal of the aortic cross-clamp. Among patients who developed postoperative supraventricular tachyarrhythmias, the mean duration of atrial activity was markedly longer than that of arrhythmia-free patients (46 ± 4.7 versus 22.6 ± 4.0 minutes; $p < 0.001$).

The contribution of inflammatory mechanisms to postoperative atrial arrhythmias is supported by the observation that postoperative atrial fibrillation is most prevalent 2 to 3 days after surgery. Atrial injury from direct ischemia or trauma might be expected to provoke atrial fibrillation earlier in the postoperative period. Pericardial effusions, likely mediated by inflammation after cardiac surgery, have been correlated with postoperative supraventricular arrhythmias (47).

Shortening of action potential duration may be contributory to postoperative atrial fibrillation, as has been seen in non-postoperative atrial fibrillation. Studies by Pichlmaier and colleagues (44) showed monophasic action potential shortening in the 60 minutes before seven of nine episodes of postoperative atrial fibrillation.

Cellular mechanisms underlying electrical remodeling and susceptibility to postoperative atrial fibrillation have been elucidated by Van Wagoner and colleagues (48,49). This group showed that in contrast to expectation, the shortening of action potential duration was not caused by an increase in outward K⁺ currents but resulted from a reduction in density of l-type Ca²⁺ channels. Reduced densities of the transient and the sustained outward K^+ currents with decreased expression of Kv1.5 K^+ channels were found in atrial myocytes derived from patients with chronic atrial fibrillation undergoing cardiac surgery (48). This group also studied voltage-dependent l-type calcium currents in atrial myocytes isolated from 42 patients in sinus rhythm at the time of cardiac surgery and 11 patients with chronic atrial fibrillation (49). Of the patients in sinus rhythm, 50% developed postoperative atrial fibrillation. In contrast to chronic atrial fibrillation, which was characterized by reduced I_{Ca}, patients with the greatest I_{Ca} had an increased incidence of postoperative atrial fibrillation, independent of age. This finding was consistent with the concept that calcium overload may be important in the initiation of atrial fibrillation. The subsequent development of reduced I_{Ca} density once atrial fibrillation becomes established and persistent may be an adaptive response to atrial fibrillation–induced calcium overload. Thus, patients at highest risk for postoperative atrial fibrillation may be more easily susceptible to atrial calcium overload occurring in response to high sympathetic tone, atrial injury, or inflammation in the postoperative state, whereas patients with lower basal I_{Ca} may be at a lower risk for the afterdepolarizations that might trigger premature atrial contractions or activation of latent atrial pacemakers. These studies provide a rationale for the effectiveness of β blockers in preventing postoperative atrial fibrillation and suggest that β blockers or calcium channel blockers may be a more logical therapy than digoxin, which might further exacerbate calcium overload (49).

Risk Factors

The most commonly reported preoperative, intraoperative, and postoperative risk factors for supraventricular arrhythmias after cardiac surgery are listed in Table 29-2.

Preoperative Factors

The most consistent clinical predictor of postoperative atrial fibrillation after CABG has been advanced age (2,3,5,17, 20,21,50,51). In a multivariate analysis of 1,666 patients, Fuller and colleagues (5) demonstrated that age was the leading correlate of postoperative atrial fibrillation ($p = 0.0001$). In a review of 5,807 CABG patients, Leitch and colleagues (3) found that the risk of a postoperative supraventricular arrhythmia was 27.7% for patients 70 years or older, compared with only 3.7% for patients younger than 40 years. Advanced age was the strongest independent predictor of postoperative atrial fibrillation or flutter ($p < 0.001$). Likewise, Curtis and colleagues (16) reported that after pulmonary resection, the average age of patients was older among those with postoperative supraventricular arrhythmias than in those without. Age-related changes in electrophysiologic properties may lower the threshold for atrial fibrillation in the elderly (36,52).

TABLE 29-2. REPORTED RISK FACTORS FOR ATRIAL FIBRILLATION AFTER CARDIAC SURGERY

	Strength of association
Preoperative factors	
Age (older)	+++
Valvular disease	++
Prior atrial fibrillation	+
Left atrial enlargement	+
Congestive heart failure	+
Surface P-wave duration	+
Male gender	+/–
Preoperative digoxin	+/–
Preoperative β blockers	+/–
Chronic obstructive lung disease	+/–
Right coronary artery stenosis	+/–
Intraoperative factors	
Hypomagnesemia	+
Hypokalemia	+
Prolonged Aortic cross-clamp and cardiopulmonary bypass times	+/–
Type of cardioplegia	+/–
Method of cannulation	+/–
Inadequate atrial protection	+/–
Internal mammary artery graft	+/–
Postoperative factors	
Postoperative β blocker use (protective)	+++
Postoperative β blocker withdrawal	+/–
Pericarditis or pericardial effusion	+/–

+/–, Unclear evidence or conflicting studies; +, some supporting evidence; ++, moderate supporting evidence; +++, strong supporting evidence.
Source: Asher CR, Chung MK, Eagle KA, Lauer MS. Atrial fibrillation following cardiac surgery. In: Falk R, Podrid P, eds. Atrial fibrillation: mechanisms and management, 2nd ed. New York: Lippincott–Raven Publishers, 1997, with permission.

Other reported preoperative risk factors for postoperative atrial fibrillation have included prior atrial fibrillation (21,53), male gender (17,21), cardiomegaly (51), history of congestive heart failure (21), left atrial enlargement (51), right coronary artery stenosis (54–56), sinoatrial nodal and atrioventricular (AV) nodal artery disease (57), and sleep-disordered breathing (58). In a prospective review of 104 patients with proximal or mid right coronary artery stenosis, 45 (43%) had postoperative atrial fibrillation, compared with 12 (19%) of 64 patients without more than 70% lumen narrowing of the right coronary artery ($p = 0.001$) (54). Pehkonen and colleagues (55) reported that retrograde cardioplegia and right coronary artery stenosis were associated with atrial fibrillation. The authors proposed that with stenosis of the right coronary artery, this type of cardioplegia offers poorer atrial myocardial protection. A higher incidence of postoperative atrial arrhythmias has also been reported in patients undergoing CABG with concomitant right coronary endarterectomy (59). However, a large recent study by Mathew and colleagues (21) reported no association with 75% stenosis of the right coronary artery. Noncardiac diseases, such as chronic obstructive pulmonary disease (2,3) and chronic renal failure (3), have been associated with postoperative atrial fibrillation in some studies (21).

Preoperative use of digoxin (2,5) has been studied retrospectively, but results are not consistent. Creswell and colleagues (2) studied 2,833 patients undergoing CABG and reported that preoperative digoxin was an independent predictor of postoperative atrial arrhythmias (incidence, 44.7% versus 32.4%; $p < 0.001$). Fuller and colleagues (5), however, reported that preoperative digoxin use was a univariate but not an independent predictor of postoperative atrial arrhythmias. Morrison and Killip (60) and Rose and colleagues (61) failed to find a correlation between digoxin levels and atrial arrhythmias.

Studies of preoperative use of β blockers (2,3,5) have also yielded inconsistent results. Leitch and colleagues (3) reported preoperative β blockers to be an independent predictor of arrhythmias (incidence, 17.9% versus 14.9%; $p = 0.011$). However, other large studies have not found this association (2,5). A large prospective observational study of 2,417 patients undergoing CABG with or without concurrent valvular surgery by Mathew and colleagues (21) reported a lower incidence of atrial fibrillation in patients receiving β-blocking agents in the preoperative period. As β blockers are frequently used in the treatment of coronary artery disease, many patients have received chronic beta blockade before surgery, and Weightman and colleagues (62) reported an association with preoperative β-blocker use and improved in-hospital mortality rate after coronary artery surgery.

Electrophysiologic parameters have been examined to preoperatively identify patients at risk for developing supraventricular arrhythmias. These include preoperative P-wave duration by standard electrocardiogram (ECG) (38,63) or signal-average ECG (39,64–69). In a study of preoperative P-wave prolongation in 99 patients undergoing CABG, Buxton and colleagues (38) reported that the mean P-wave duration was 126 ms in patients developing atrial fibrillation or flutter, compared with 116 ms in patients remaining in sinus rhythm ($p < 0.001$). An intraatrial conduction defect (single standard-lead P-wave duration of more than 116 ms) had a sensitivity of 83% and a specificity of 43% in the prediction of postoperative atrial arrhythmias. Chang and colleagues (63) also reported a 2.9-fold greater risk of postoperative atrial fibrillation with a P-wave duration of 100 or more ms in lead II. Stafford and colleagues (67) showed signal-averaged P-wave duration to be a better predictor than standard ECG or echocardiographic criteria for left atrial enlargement. Zaman and colleagues (66) reported that the combination of signal-averaged P-wave duration and low serum magnesium on the first postoperative day could identify most patients with postoperative atrial fibrillation. Tamis and Steinberg (39) reported that the combined use of abnormal P-wave signal-average ECG and low left ventricular ejection fraction could identify a group with 50% risk for atrial fibrillation after cardiac surgery, which was nine times higher than patients with normal test results. However, signal-averaged P-wave duration was not a predictor of postoperative atrial fibrillation after noncardiac thoracic surgery in a study by Amar and colleagues (70) and in one study by Frost and colleagues (71) after CABG when controlled for effects of increasing age and body weight. Overall, these methods have moderate sensitivity and specificity but are not currently in widespread use.

Intraoperative Factors
Intraoperative factors that may contribute to the development of atrial fibrillation after cardiac surgery (Table 29-2) include inadequate atrial myocardial protection with ischemia or infarction, acute atrial enlargement, trauma from cannulation, hypomagnesemia, long cardiopulmonary bypass and cross-clamp times, and pulmonary vein venting (2,21,27,30,31).

Atrial ischemia has been proposed to trigger atrial fibrillation in patients with underlying vulnerability to this arrhythmia (72). Higher rates of postoperative atrial fibrillation have been reported after longer aortic cross-clamp or total pump time (2,73,74), although not consistently (4,5,51,75). Lower atrial fibrillation incidence has been reported after minimally invasive CABG (76) or valvular (77,78) surgery or without cardiopulmonary bypass, although again not universally (78,79).

Conventional hypothermic cardioplegia may not adequately cool the atria or produce complete electrical arrest in the atria (36,72). Mullen and colleagues (80) found that cold hyperkalemic cardioplegic solution was associated with the highest incidence of postoperative supraventricular arrhythmias compared with blood and diltiazem-containing cardioplegic solutions (63%, 40%, 47%, respectively; $p < 0.05$). Although crystalloid cardioplegia cooled the right atrium, it did not arrest the atrium and resulted in the most perioperative ischemic injury. The duration of atrial activity monitored by atrial electrograms during cardioplegic arrest has been associated with an increased incidence of supraventricular arrhythmias postoperatively in some studies (30,46,80).

Nevertheless, the incidence of atrial fibrillation has not been reduced by various methods of cardioplegia. Although Rousou and colleagues (27) reported that warm blood cardioplegia was associated with a lower incidence of postoperative supraventricular arrhythmias when compared with cold cardioplegia, other studies have not shown different rates and with various methods (59,75,81–83). One large retrospective review by Arom and colleagues (84) reported higher postoperative atrial fibrillation in 4,224 patients who underwent retrograde cardioplegia when compared with 2,808 patients who received anterograde/retrograde cardioplegia. However, both approaches appeared to provide good myocardial protection with no difference in operative mortality rates, and anterograde/retrograde approaches may be associated with longer pump times. No difference in arrhythmias with high-volume versus low-volume crystalloid solutions has also been reported (27).

Studies of bicaval cannulation versus atrial cannulation have shown variable results in the CABG population, although bicaval anastomosis does appear to reduce atrial arrhythmias after orthotopic heart transplantation. Hearse and colleagues (36) reported that double-caval cannulation and intracavitary cooling during aortic valve replacement reduced the incidence of atrial fibrillation from 50% to 13% when compared with single atrial cannulation, which allowed right atrial and septal rewarming by systemic venous return. However, a retrospective analysis found the choice of a single atriocaval cannula versus bicaval cannulation had no effect on the incidence of conduction disturbances or atrial arrhythmias in patients receiving low-volume crystalloid cardioplegic solution for coronary bypass procedures (27). One randomized trial in 78 patients of augmented right heart cooling with bicaval cannulation did not demonstrate a decrease in postoperative atrial arrhythmias when compared with a standard system of single venous cannulation, although technical difficulties associated with multiple cannulation and longer cardiopulmonary bypass times complicated this analysis (85). Mathew and colleagues (21) reported a higher incidence of postoperative atrial fibrillation with bicaval cannulation, as well as pulmonary vein venting. However, after heart transplantation, Brandt and colleagues (86) and others report that the atrial fibrillation incidence is lower after bicaval anastomoses compared with right atrial anastomoses (4% versus 40%; $p < 0.001$).

Early studies suggested that the use of internal mammary artery conduits may increase the risk of postoperative atrial fibrillation. A small study of 80 patients compared postoperative atrial fibrillation in groups receiving internal mammary artery grafts in addition to saphenous vein grafts versus saphenous vein grafts alone and showed a 31% versus 24% incidence, respectively, of atrial fibrillation (32). Patients with the arterial grafts had a 16% higher rate of postoperative pericarditis. However, the study by Mathew and colleagues (21) reported a lower incidence of atrial fibrillation in patients receiving an internal mammary artery graft.

The role of electrolyte disturbances, including magnesium and potassium, in the generation of supraventricular arrhythmias, remains controversial. Jensen and colleagues [(87) showed that patients who developed postoperative atrial fibrillation had lower skeletal muscle potassium concentration before CABG and higher sodium levels. In addition, during CABG, potassium levels fell and sodium increased in right atrial and skeletal muscle. Postoperatively, magnesium levels in right atrial or skeletal muscle did not change, although serum levels decreased. This fall in magnesium levels after cardiac surgery has been reported by other groups (88), and low serum levels may correlate with episodes of postoperative arrhythmias (31). However, administration of magnesium decreased the incidence of supraventricular arrhythmias in only two of four studies of magnesium after CABG or noncardiac thoracic surgery

(Table 29-8) (31,89–91). Wahr and colleagues (92) reported that hypokalemia ($K^+ < 3.5$ mmol/L) was associated with higher risk for perioperative serious arrhythmia, need for cardiopulmonary resuscitation, intraoperative arrhythmia, and postoperative atrial fibrillation or flutter. The authors reinforced the importance of potassium repletion before surgery.

Inducibility of atrial fibrillation before bypass surgery has also been studied. Lowe and colleagues (40) attempted to predict postoperative atrial fibrillation by determining the intraoperative inducibility of atrial fibrillation using alternating current applied to the right atrium before the initiation of cardiopulmonary bypass in 50 patients. Inducibility of atrial fibrillation identified patients at risk for postoperative atrial fibrillation with a sensitivity of 94%, specificity of 41%, negative predictive value of 93%, and positive predictive value of 47%. However, this method has not achieved widespread clinical use and may be limited by limited specificity and practical issues with preoperative atrial fibrillation induction.

Postoperative Factors

Circulating endogenous or exogenous catecholamines can be elevated in the postoperative period, but no consistent correlation with postoperative atrial fibrillation has been demonstrated. Engelman and colleagues (93) demonstrated elevations in serum norepinephrine and epinephrine in the first 3 postoperative days but found no correlation between atrial fibrillation and no protection by β-blocker use after surgery. Mohr and colleagues (94) reported no additional risk of supraventricular tachyarrhythmias among the groups receiving exogenous catecholamines in a population given intravenous norepinephrine on a routine basis.

The β-adrenergic blocker withdrawal syndrome has been implicated as a possible mechanism predisposing to atrial arrhythmias after cardiac surgery. As β blockers are frequently used in the treatment of coronary artery disease and heart failure, many patients have received chronic beta blockade before surgery. The heightened catecholamine sensitivity resulting from higher density of β-adrenergic receptors induced by chronic β-blocker use, along with the increase in perioperative catecholamine levels, may lead to the β-blocker withdrawal syndrome if preoperative β blockers are not continued in the postoperative period. β Blockers are commonly discontinued for fear of perioperative hemodynamic effects. Such withdrawal may play a role in the pathogenesis of a number of adverse cardiac events, including atrial arrhythmias (33–35,95,96). In a small study of β-blocker prophylaxis for atrial fibrillation, Daudon and colleagues (97) reported that in the control group that was not treated with postoperative β blockers, 18 of 39 patients (46%) who received β blockers preoperatively developed atrial arrhythmias, compared with 2 of 11 patients (18%) who did not receive preoperative β blockers. These differences did not reach statistical significance.

Pericarditis and pericardial effusions have been studied as factors associated with atrial fibrillation. Pericardial effusions are common after cardiac surgery, and Weitzman and colleagues (98) reported that in 122 patients, 85% had effusions, with most being first apparent on postoperative day 2. Although prospective analyses of patients after CABG have shown no consistent correlation between postoperative pericarditis and supraventricular arrhythmias (4,51,99), this may be a result of the inaccuracy of detecting pericarditis because of the absence of sensitive and specific clinical criteria (e.g., pericardial rubs, ECG changes, pleuritic chest pain). Although the pericardial effusions did not correlate with clinical signs of pericarditis, such as pericardial rub, pain, or fever, Angelini and colleagues (47) reported that 22 of 35 (63%) patients with pericardial effusions detected by echocardiography within 3 to 5 days after CABG and valvular surgery had supraventricular arrhythmias, compared with 9 of 79 patients (11%) without effusions ($p < 0.001$).

A number of factors have been found not to correlate well with the occurrence of postoperative atrial tachyarrhythmias. These have included hypertension, previous myocardial infarction, unstable angina, left ventricular function, extent of coronary artery disease, lipid profiles, and arterial blood gas values. Although some authors have reported that more advanced coronary artery disease or more preoperative infarcts predispose to atrial fibrillation (55), in general, coronary artery disease risk factors, severity of coronary artery disease, and preoperative hemodynamic parameters have not been consistently shown to predict postoperative atrial fibrillation (2,3,53,73,99–102).

In summary, atrial fibrillation is a common arrhythmia after cardiac surgery. With the exceptions of advanced age, β-blocker use, and pericardial effusions, a number of

reviews evaluating many clinical correlates have failed to demonstrate clearly reproducible preoperative, intraoperative, and postoperative correlates of atrial fibrillation. This may be because several potentially independent causes of arrhythmias are operating simultaneously. In addition, sample sizes in several of the studies are too small to allow meaningful evaluation of many independent and interrelated arrhythmogenic factors.

Prophylaxis

The prevention of postoperative atrial arrhythmias has been studied using multiple agents, although most studies have used randomized open-label designs and relatively few patients. The studies of digoxin have shown mixed results, and metaanalyses have shown no benefit (103,104). In contrast, β-adrenergic blockers have produced the most consistent benefit in preventing postoperative atrial arrhythmias in multiple randomized studies. Other pharmacologic agents, such as verapamil, diltiazem, and magnesium, have yielded variable, negative, or inconclusive results. Recent studies of sotalol and amiodarone show some promise in prophylaxis of postoperative atrial fibrillation.

Digoxin

Prospective nonrandomized and randomized studies of prophylactic digoxin have yielded mixed results (Tables 29-3 through 29-5) (100,105–109). Table 29-3 summarizes the six major digoxin prophylaxis trials. Although two nonrandomized trials suggested a benefit to digoxin, two of the four randomized trials failed to show a benefit, and one study showed an increase in atrial fibrillation with digoxin use. Table 29-4 summarizes trials that used a combination of β blockers and digoxin. Two metaanalyses of digoxin

TABLE 29-3. DIGOXIN PROPHYLAXIS TRIALS

Author	Year	Patients (N)	Design	Digoxin Regimen	Control	Digoxin	p value
					SVA		
Johnson and colleagues (107)	1976	120	R	1–1.5 mg PO 2–3 d before surgery; 0.25 mg qd (pod 1)	26.0%	5.5%	<0.01
Tyras and colleagues (108)	1978	140	R	1–1.5 mg PO 1 d before surgery; 0.25 qd (pod 1)	11.4%	27.8%	<0.05
Parker and colleagues (109)	1983	120	R	1–1.5 mg PO 1 d before surgery; 0.25 qd (pod 1)	21.4%	3.1%	<0.005
Weiner and colleagues (105)	1986	98	R	0.75–1.0 mg IV (dos); 0.25 PO qd	16%	15%	NS
Chee and colleagues (100)	1982	182	NR	0.75 mg 1 d before surgery; 0.25 mg qd (dos)	72% 95%	5%	<0.01 <0.01
Csicsko and colleagues (106)	1981	407 (270 historic controls)	NR	1 mg IV (dos); 0.25 mg qd	15%	2%	<0.01

N, number of patients; R, randomized; NR, nonrandomized; SVA, supraventricular arrhythmias; pod, postoperative day; dos, day of surgery; ICU, intensive care unit; NS, not significant; monitoring period, period of continuous telemetry or Holter monitoring; ECGs, electrocardiograms.
Source: Asher CR, Chung MK, Eagle KA, Lauer MS. Atrial fibrillation following cardiac surgery. In: Falk R, Podrid P, eds. Atrial fibrillation: mechanisms and management, 2nd ed. New York: Lippincott–Raven Publishers, 1997, with permission.

TABLE 29-4. COMBINATION β-BLOCKER PROPHYLAXIS TRIALS (PROSPECTIVE RANDOMIZED, CONTROLLED TRIALS WITH ≥100 PATIENTS)

Author	Year	N	Design	Monitoring Period/ ECGs	Control	Treatment	SVA Control	SVA Treatment	p value
Mills and colleagues (118)	1983	179	R	7 d	No treatment	Digoxin 1 mg IV (dos), 0.25 mg PO (pod 1) propranolol 10 mg PO q6h (dos)	30.0%	3.4%	<0.001 +
Rubin and colleagues (99)	1987	123	R	4 d	No treatment	Propranolol 20 mg PO q6h (pod 1)	37.5%	16.2%	<0.03
						Digoxin 0.5 mg (pod 1), 0.25 mg PO qd		32.6%	NS
Roffman and colleagues (102)	1981	172	NR	7 d	No treatment	Digoxin 1 mg IV (dos); 0.25 mg PO (pod 1)	28.2%	28.9%	NS
						Digoxin 1 mg IV (dos); 0.25 mg PO (pod 1) + propranolol 20 mg PO tid (pod 2)		2.2%	<0.005
Kowey and colleagues (119)	1997	157	R,DB	7 d	Digoxin 1 mg IV/PO over 24 hr, then 0.125–0.25 mg qd	Digoxin IV/PO 1 mg over 24 h, 0.125–0.25 mg qd + acebutolol 200 mg PO/NGT q12h	32%	24%	0.11

N, number of patients; R, randomized; NR, nonrandomized; monitoring period, period of continuous telemetry or Holter monitoring; ECGs, electrocardiograms; pod, postoperative day; dos, day of surgery; SVA, supraventricular arrhythmias.
Source: Asher CR, Chung MK, Eagle KA, Lauer MS. Atrial fibrillation following cardiac surgery. In: Falk R, Podrid P, eds. Atrial fibrillation: mechanisms and management, 2nd ed. New York: Lippincott–Raven Publishers, 1997, with permission.

prophylaxis trials showed no significant advantage of digoxin in preventing supraventricular arrhythmias after CABG (Table 29-5) (103,104). However, there has not been a placebo-controlled, double-blind trial of digoxin use for this purpose.

β-Adrenergic Blockers

Multiple randomized studies of postoperative β blockers have found them to be almost uniformly beneficial in preventing postoperative atrial fibrillation. Among the agents

shown to be of benefit are propanolol, timolol, metoprolol, nadolol, and acebutolol (1,35,94,96,97,99,101,110–116). Table 29-6 summarizes 10 randomized prospective trials of β-blocker prophylaxis for postoperative supraventricular arrhythmias; only two of these trials were double-blind, placebo-controlled. Two metaanalyses have also shown overall significant 50% to 74% reductions in postoperative supraventricular arrhythmias with β blockers (103,104). Jakobsen and colleagues (117) also showed that perioperative metoprolol could reduce the frequency of atrial fibrilla-

TABLE 29-5. METAANALYSES OF TRIALS FOR THE PROPHYLAXIS OF SUPRAVENTRICULAR ARRHYTHMIAS AFTER CABG

Author	Date	Treatment	Total patients (N)	SVA Control	SVA Drug	p value
Andrews and colleagues (104)	1991	β Blocker	1,549	34.0%	8.7%	<0.0001
		Digoxin	507	17.6%	14.2%	0.88
		Verapamil	432	18.2%	18.2%	0.69
Kowey and colleagues (103)	1992	β Blocker	1,418	20.2%	9.8%	<0.001
		Digoxin	875	19.1%	15.4%	NS
		Digoxin + β blocker	292	29.4%	2.2%	<0.001

SVA, supraventricular arrhythmias; CABG, coronary artery bypass graft.
Source: Asher CR, Chung MK, Eagle KA, Lauer MS. Atrial fibrillation following cardiac surgery. In: Falk R, Podrid P, eds. Atrial fibrillation: mechanisms and management, 2nd ed. New York: Lippincott–Raven Publishers, 1997, with permission.

TABLE 29-6. β BLOCKER PROPHYLAXIS TRIALS (PROSPECTIVE RANDOMIZED, CONTROLLED TRIALS WITH ≥100 PATIENTS)

Author	Year	N	Design	Regimen	SVA Control	SVA Drug	p value	Comments
Vecht and colleagues (1)	1986	132	R, DB, P	Timolol 5 mg PO q12h (dos), 10 mg PO bid (pod 1)	19.7%	7.5%	<0.05	Most on β-blockers preoperatively
Silverman and colleagues (101)	1982	100	R, NB	Propanolol 10 mg PO q6h (pod 1)	28.0%	6.0%	<0.01	All on preoperative β blockers; included patients with LV dysfunction
Ivey and colleagues (240)	1983	109	R, DB, P	Propanolol 20 mg PO q6h (pod 1)	16.1%	13.2%	>0.10	All on propanolol preoperatively
Daudon (97)	1986	100	R, NB	Acebutolol 200 mg PO bid, start dose 36 h post-operatively	40%	0%	p < 0.001	Some on preoperative β blockers
Matangi and colleagues (110)	1985	164	R, NB	Propanolol 5 mg PO q6h (dos)	23.0%	9.8%	0.02	All on preoperative β blockers
Stephenson and colleagues (112)	1980	223	R, NB	Propanolol 10 mg PO q6h on transfer from ICU	18%	8%	NS	Many on preoperative β blockers
Khuri and colleagues (113)	1987	141	R, DB, P	Nadolol 40 mg qd, start dose (pod 1)	42%	9%	<0.001	Most on preoperative β blockers
Abel and colleagues (115)	1983	100	R, NB	Propanolol IV 1 mg × 2 pre-operatively at CPB; 2 mg q4h (dos) until able to take PO, then 10 mg PO q6h × 24 h, then 20 mg PO q6h to pod 6, then 10 mg PO q6h × 3 d	38%	17%	<0.05	All taking preoperative propanolol. No benefit to using postoperative propranolol in patients taking propranolol ≥320 mg preoperatively
Mohr and colleagues (94)	1981	103	R, NB	Propanolol preoperative, 5–10 mg PO 6 h post-operative (dos)		5%		Included patients with LV dysfunction
				Propanolol preoperative, none postoperative	40%		<0.001	
				No propranolol preoperative, treated postoperative		27%	<0.01	
Ali and colleagues (241)	1997	210	R	Postoperative resumption of preoperative β blocker	38%	17%	<0.02	All on preoperative β blockers; not resumed in control group

N, number of patients; R, randomized; DB, double-blind; NB, nonblind; P, placebo-controlled; monitoring period, period of continuous telemetry or Holter monitoring; ECGs, electrocardiograms; dos, day of surgery; pod, postoperative day; CPB, cardiopulmonary bypass; SVA, supraventricular arrhythmias; LV, left ventricular; ICU, intensive care unit; NS, not significant.
Source: Asher CR, Chung MK, Eagle KA, Lauer MS. Atrial fibrillation following cardiac surgery. In: Falk R, Podrid P, eds. Atrial fibrillation: mechanisms and management, 2nd ed. New York: Lippincott–Raven Publishers, 1997, with permission.

tion after thoracotomy for lung resection from 40% in a placebo group to 6.7% in a group treated with 100 mg of metoprolol daily preoperatively and postoperatively.

Despite evidence supporting the efficacy of β blockers in preventing postoperative atrial arrhythmias, these agents have been used in a limited manner for prophylaxis, presumably because of apprehension over potential hemodynamic or pulmonary intolerance. β Blockers have been demonstrated to be safe when used in postoperative trials, although most studies excluded patients with contraindications, including impaired left ventricular function, AV block greater than first degree, and significant obstructive lung disease.

Combined β-Blocker and Digoxin Prophylaxis

Four trials have studied combined use of β blockers and digoxin (Table 29-4). Roffman and Feldman (102) in a non-randomized controlled study compared postoperative administration of digoxin plus propranolol and digoxin alone with a control group. Control patients and those given

digoxin had only a 22% incidence of supraventricular arrhythmias, compared with only 2.1% in the combined digoxin-propranolol group. It appeared that the β blocker played a major role in preventing postoperative arrhythmias. Mills and colleagues (118) also showed a beneficial effect of digoxin plus propranolol for preventing supraventricular and ventricular arrhythmias. In the Kowey and colleagues metaanalysis (103) of these two studies (Table 29-5), the combination of β blockers and digoxin caused a larger reduction than β blockers or digoxin alone, from 29.4% to 2.2%, suggesting a possible synergistic effect. This group subsequently performed a randomized, double-blind trial of digoxin with acebutolol versus digoxin and placebo in 157 patients with randomization stratified by preoperative β-blocker use (119). There was a trend toward lower incidence of atrial fibrillation and flutter among patients in the digoxin-acebutolol group (24%) compared with patients treated with digoxin alone (32%; $p = 0.11$), with the incidence being 17% versus 32%, respectively, in an analysis of patients that could complete the study ($p = 0.048$).

Calcium Channel Blockers

Two studies have shown oral verapamil to be ineffective in preventing atrial fibrillation after CABG. (120,121). However, when atrial fibrillation did occur in patients on verapamil, ventricular rates were slower. In the study by Davison and colleagues (120), hypotension and pulmonary edema occurred more frequently in the verapamil-treated group.

After lung operations, verapamil had only modest efficacy for prophylaxis of postoperative atrial fibrillation. Van Mieghem and colleagues (122) randomized 199 patients undergoing pneumonectomy or lobectomy to placebo or verapamil 10 mg intravenously over 2 minutes followed by a 30-minute infusion of 0.375 mg per minute, then 0.125 mg per minute for 3 days. Atrial fibrillation occurred in 15% of the placebo patients, compared with 8% of patients on verapamil (not significant), and side effects required discontinuation of verapamil in 9% because of bradycardia and in 14% because of hypotension.

Intravenous diltiazem may be better tolerated hemodynamically than verapamil. Intravenous diltiazem has been compared with nitroglycerin by two groups. In a randomized study of 120 patients undergoing CABG by Seitelberger and colleagues (123), a 24-hour infusion of intravenous diltiazem (0.1 mg per hour) reduced postoperative atrial fibrillation from 18% to 5% (p = 0.05), premature ventricular beats per hour, and ventricular runs per hour compared with nitroglycerin. El-Sadek and Krause (124) also reported less supraventricular tachyarrhythmias and Lown class 4 ventricular arrhythmias with diltiazem after CABG in a study of 40 patients randomized to treatment with diltiazem or nitroglycerin.

Antiarrhythmic Agents

Trials studying the effect of class I or III antiarrhythmic drugs in the prevention of postoperative atrial fibrillation are reviewed in Table 29-7.

Class Ia Antiarrhythmic Agents. *Procainamide* has shown some efficacy in the prevention of postoperative atrial fibrillation after CABG. In a double-blind, randomized, placebo-controlled pilot trial of procainamide used for prevention of atrial fibrillation after CABG in 46 patients, Laub and colleagues (125) reported that procainamide reduced the number of atrial fibrillation episodes per hour. Gold and colleagues (126) showed a nonsignificant reduction in incidence of atrial fibrillation, although number of patient days in atrial fibrillation was significantly lower, as was the incidence of ventricular tachycardia (2% versus 20%; p < 0.01). In addition, the incidence of atrial fibrillation was significantly reduced in patients achieving therapeutic procainamide serum levels, supporting the importance of achieving therapeutic levels for efficacy with procainamide. Nausea was a significant side effect of therapy.

Quinidine has not been studied well for prophylaxis after surgery and its use remains appropriately limited in view of its proarrhythmic potential, particularly in the setting of hypokalemia, which may occur commonly with diuresis after surgery. Quinidine has been shown in one study to be ineffective in preventing atrial fibrillation after mitral valvotomy (127).

Class Ic Antiarrhythmic Agents. The use of class Ic drugs is usually limited to patients without significant ventricular dysfunction or coronary artery disease because of results of the Cardiac Arrhythmia Suppression Trial (CAST), which showed a higher mortality rate in postinfarction patients treated with flecainide and encainide. However, flecainide may be useful in patients with valvular disease, and short-term propafenone has been used by many clinicians after even CABG. *Propafenone* has been reported in one study to be of similar efficacy to atenolol (128). *Flecainide* given intravenously reduced atrial fibrillation or flutter when compared with digoxin used after thoracic surgery (129).

Class III Antiarrhythmic Agents. *Sotalol,* a class III antiarrhythmic agent with β-blocker activity, has been effective in reducing postoperative supraventricular arrhythmias (130–134). Sotalol appears to be more effective than β blockers without class III activity.

Sotalol's potent β-blocking activity requires vigilance for beta-blockade–associated hemodynamic and bradycardia side effects. A small study showed hemodynamically significant adverse effects requiring discontinuation of the drug in 6 of 25 patients (24%) given an intravenous load followed by oral sotalol (135). Nystrom and colleagues (132) reported that 11 of 50 (22%) patients required reduction or discontinuation of sotalol dosed at 160 mg twice daily because of bradycardia, with two also discontinued because of hypotension. This dose may be excessive for some patients, particularly if other β blockers or negatively chronotropic drugs are continued. Gomes and colleagues (131) demonstrated that oral sotalol begun 2 days before cardiac surgery at 80 to 120 mg twice daily and continued for 4 days after surgery reduced atrial fibrillation with good hemodynamic tolerance. Temporary pacing using temporary epicardial pacing leads from surgery was used as necessary for bradycardia. Suttorp and colleagues (136) also reported that low-dose sotalol (40 mg q8h) was better tolerated than high-dose (80 mg q8h) sotalol. Only rare proarrhythmia has been reported (133). Thus, sotalol appears effective, but caution is indicated to avoid the hemodynamic adverse effects associated with its β-adrenergic blocking activity.

Amiodarone has also been studied for prophylaxis of postoperative atrial fibrillation, although the most cost-effective and practical dosing regimen has not been established (Table 29-7) (137–141). Effective regimens have included a total intravenous dose of 4.5 g over the first 4 postoperative days (137); 15 mg/kg delivered after removal of the aortic cross-clamp for 24 hours followed by 600 mg orally in three divided doses for 5 days (138); preoperative oral amiodarone

TABLE 29-7. CLASS I AND III ANTIARRHYTHMIC DRUG PROPHYLAXIS TRIALS

Author	Year	N	Design	Control	Drug Regimen	SVA Control	Drug	p value	Comments
Laub and colleagues (125)	1993	46	R, DB, P	Placebo	Procainamide 12 mg/kg IV load, 2 mg/min, then weight-adjusted PO (dos-pod 5)	38%	18%	0.2	
Gold and colleagues (126)	1996	100	R, DB, P	Placebo	Procainamide po adjusted by weight × 4 d	38%	26%	NS	38 → 13% reduction in patients with therapeutic levels (p < 0.05)
Merrick and colleagues (128)	1995	207	R, DB	Atenolol 50 mg qd	Propafenone 300 mg bid	10.8%	12.4%	0.89	
Borgeat and colleagues (129)	1991	30	R	Digoxin 10 μg/kg × 12 h, then 0.24 mg/ 24 h	Flecainide 2 mg/kg IV load, then 0.15 mg/g/h	47%	7%	<0.05	Thoracic surgery patients
Suttorp and colleagues (136)	1990	429	R	Propranolol 10 mg q6h	Sotalol 40 mg q8h	18.8%	13.9%	NS	Trend toward less SVA in sotalol groups; fewer adverse effects in low-dose groups
				Propranolol 20 mg q6h	Sotalol 80 mg q8h	13.7%	10.9%		
Suttorp and colleagues (130)	1991	300	R, DB, P	Placebo	Sotalol 40 mg PO q6h (dos-pod 6)	33%	16%	<0.005	
Janssen (242)	1986	130	R	Control	Sotalol IV dos (0.3 mg/kg), 80 mg PO tid (pod 1)	36.0%	2.4%	<0.01	
					Metoprolol IV (dos) 0.1 mg/kg, 50 mg PO tid (pod 1)		15.3%	<0.05	
Nystrom and colleagues (132)	1993	101	R	β blockers	Sotalol 160 mg PO bid	29%	10%	0.028	Dose reduction or discontinuation: 22% sotalol
Parikka and colleagues (134)	1998	191	R	Metoprolol 75 mg/d	Sotalol 120 mg/d	32%	16%	<0.01	QT longer on sotalol
Jacquet and colleagues (135)	1994	42	R	Control	Sotalol IV 1 mg/kg over 2 h, 0.15 mg/kg/h × 24 h, then 80 mg PO q8–12h	29%	16%	NS	
Gomes and colleagues (131)	1999	85	R, DB, P	Placebo	Sotalol 80–120 mg bid begun 2 d preoperatively, continued 4 d postoperative	38%	12.5%	0.008	2/40 (5%) hypotension, bradycardia on sotalol
Pfisterer and colleagues (133)	1997	255	R, DB, P	Placebo	Sotalol 80 mg bid begun 2 h preoperatively × 3 mo	46%	26%	0.0012	1 proarrhythmia; >90% AF within 9 d; 70% of sotalol SEs after 9 d
Hohnloser and colleagues (137)	1991	77	R, P	Placebo	Amiodarone IV 300 mg over 2 h, 1,200 mg/d × 2 d, then 900 mg/d × 2 d	21%	5%	<0.05	NSVT, HR reduced, JT prolonged by amiodarone; discontinued in 2 for QT
Butler and colleagues (138)	1993	120	R, DB, P	Placebo	Amiodarone 15 mg/kg IV over 24 h, 200 mg PO × 5 d	20%	8%	0.07	Reduced total treated SVA, V arrhythmias, p = 0.05, more bradycardia with drug
Daoud and colleagues (139)	1997	124	R, DB, P	Placebo	Amiodarone PO 600 mg qd min. 7 d preoperative then 200 mg qd until discharge	53%	25%	0.003	Hospitalization costs reduced in amiodarone group
Redle and colleagues (140)	1999	143	R, DB, P	Placebo	Amiodarone PO 2 g, divided 1–4 d preoperatively; 400 mg qd × 7 d postoperative	33%	25%	0.30	Hospital cost no different
Guarnier and colleagues (141)	1999	300	R, DB, P	Placebo	Amiodarone IV 1 g/d × 2 d	47%	35%	0.01	Hospital stay not reduced

N, number of patients; R, randomized; DB, double-blind; P, placebo-controlled; dos, day of surgery; pod, postoperative day; SVA, supraventricular arrhythmias; NSVT, nonsustained ventricular tachycardia; V, ventricular; NS, not significant; HR, heart rate; AF, atrial fibrillation.

given for a minimum of 7 days (mean dose of 4.6 g) followed by 200 mg per day until discharge (139); and 2 g of intravenous amiodarone given over the first 2 postoperative days (141). Another study of oral amiodarone using 2 g of amiodarone in divided doses given 1 to 4 days before surgery and 400 mg daily for 7 days postoperatively also showed a trend toward reduction of atrial fibrillation (140).

Magnesium

Hypomagnesemia is common after cardiopulmonary bypass (31,142,143), and a number of groups have demonstrated reductions in atrial arrhythmias with magnesium (Table 29-8). The effectiveness of magnesium administration in preventing arrhythmias may depend on the achievement of adequate magnesium blood levels (31,144,145).

TABLE 29-8. MAGNESIUM PROPHYLAXIS TRIALS

Author	Year	N	Design	Control	Drug Regimen	SVA Control	Mg	p value	Comments
Nurozler and colleagues (90)	1996	50	R, P, DB	Placebo	MgSO$_4$ IV 100 mEq pod 1, then 25 mEq/d × 4 d	20%	4%	0.02	All on β blockers
Fanning and colleagues (143)	1991	99	R, P, DB	Placebo	MgSO$_4$ 40 mEq/L + KCL 20 mEq/L in D5W at 100 mL/h × 24 h, then 25 mL/h for h 25–96	28%	14.3%	<0.02	
Terzi and colleagues (91)	1996	194	R	No treatment or digoxin 0.5 mg	MgSO$_4$ 2 g (16 mEq) intraoperative and in 6 h	26.7%	10.7%	0.008	Noncardiac thoracic surgery
Katholi and colleagues (144)	1990	128	R, P, DB	Placebo	MgCl$_2$ 48 mEq IV, then 15 mEq PO qd	14%			No reduction in nonresponders
					Responders: Mg ≥ 2 mEq/L		7%	<0.05	
					Nonresponders: Mg < 2 mEq/L		14%	NS	
England and colleagues (31)	1992	100	R, P, DB	Placebo	MgCl$_2$ 2 g intraoperative after CPB termination	34%	20%	0.11	Decreased postoperative ventricular arrhythmias (34% vs. 16%, $p < 0.04$)
Casthely and colleagues (145)	1994	140		No Mg	MgSO$_4$ 10 mg/kg IV Pre-CPB Post-CPB Pre- and post-CPB	11.4%	11.4% 2.9% 0%	NS	Lowest arrhythmias and higher Mg levels in pre- and post-CPB Mg group
Jensen and colleagues (89)	1997	57	R, P	Placebo	MgSO$_4$ 10 mmol q8h × 4 d	35.7%	34.5%	NS	Reduced duration of AF
Parikka and colleagues (146)	1993	140	R, P	Placebo	MgSO$_4$ 70 mmol IV over 1st 48 h	26%	29%	NS	Mg level did not correlate with AF reduction
Wistbacka and colleagues (147)	1995	81	R, DB	MgSO$_4$ and MgCl$_2$ low-dose regimen	MgSO$_4$ and MgCl$_2$ high-dose regimen, intraoperative—pod 2	45%	24.3%	0.063	

N, number of patients; R, randomized; DB, double-blind; P, placebo-controlled; CPB, cardiopulmonary bypass; dos, day of surgery; pod, postoperative day; SVA, supraventricular arrhythmias; NSVT, nonsustained ventricular tachycardia; V, ventricular; NS, not significant; AF, atrial fibrillation; MgSO$_4$, magnesium sulfate.

However, other trials have shown negative or borderline results using magnesium supplementation despite an increase in magnesium levels (89,146,147).

Atrial Pacing

Right atrial or biatrial overdrive pacing has shown variable effectiveness in preventing postoperative atrial fibrillation (Table 29-9) (21,148–152). In a large prospective observational study of 2,417 patients undergoing CABG with or without valve surgery, Mathew and colleagues (21) identified atrial pacing, but not AV pacing, as an independent predictor of postoperative atrial fibrillation. Chung and colleagues (150) reported that atrial pacing in the AAI mode did not reduce the incidence of atrial fibrillation and was associated with an increase in, instead of suppression of, frequent atrial premature depolarizations. A substantial proportion of paced patients were found to have atrial undersensing, loss of capture, and sinus rhythm overriding the AAI pacing, producing competitive atrial pacing and premature beats. These results suggest that this mode of pacing is not beneficial in suppressing postoperative atrial fibrillation. Preliminary results of a follow-up study using an automatic atrial overdrive pacing algorithm likewise showed no reduction in atrial fibrillation. No additional benefit to right atrial pacing by alternative site or biatrial pacing has been consistently shown

(148,149,151). A study by Gerstenfeld and colleagues (148) of no atrial, right atrial, or biatrial pacing also showed no significant reduction in atrial fibrillation after CABG. Kurz and colleagues (149) studied biatrial synchronous AAI pacing in a randomized study after heart surgery. The study was prematurely aborted after 21 patients out of a planned 200 patients because of a proarrhythmic effect of the pacing. Sensing failure developed in 6 of 12 paced patients, provoking atrial fibrillation in 5 of these patients, compared with 2 of 9 patients developing atrial fibrillation in the control group. However, atrial pacing may be more effective in patients treated with β blockers (148,151). Greenberg and colleagues (151) reported a reduction in atrial fibrillation using atrial pacing concomitantly with β-blocker therapy. In the Gerstenfeld and colleagues study (148), a reduction in atrial fibrillation was observed in the paced patients treated with concomitant β blockers (no atrial pacing, 38%; right atrial pacing, 15%; biatrial pacing, 0%; $p < 0.05$). Blommaert and colleagues (152) also reported a reduction in atrial fibrillation on postoperative day 2 with atrial pacing. Approximately 60% of these patients were using β blockers. We do not advocate the use of routine AAI atrial overdrive pacing to suppress atrial arrhythmias after cardiac surgery, but concomitant use with β blockers particularly with improved consistent overdrive pacing algorithms might be beneficial.

TABLE 29-9. PROSPECTIVE RANDOMIZED TEMPORARY PACING STUDIES FOR PREVENTION OF ATRIAL ARRHYTHMIAS AFTER CARDIAC SURGERY

Author	Year	N	Atrium Paced	Pacing regimen	SVA Control	SVA Paced	p value	Comments
Gerstenfeld and colleagues (148)	1999	61	RA, RA + LA	100 bpm	33%	29% 37%	> 0.7	AF induced by A pacing during A repolarization in 3 pts. In PATs on β blockers, trend toward less AF in paced groups
Kurz and colleagues (149)	1999	21	RA + LA	AAI 10 bpm above underlying max 110 bpm × 3 days	22%	42%	NS	Study stopped due to proarrhythmia: 6/12 paced had sensing failure → AF in 5. No AF in 3 that completed the pacing protocol
Chung and colleagues (150)	2000	100	RA	AAI 10 bpm above underlying, max 110 bpm × 4 d	28.6%	25.5%	0.90	Increase in atrial ectopy with A pacing; frequent undersensing, loss of capture
Blommaert and colleagues (152)	2000	96	RA	Dynamic AAI overdrive lower rate 80 bpm × 24 h on pod 2	27%	10%	0.036	59% on β blockers; pacing and end points on pod 2
Greenberg and colleagues (151)	2000	154	RA, LA, RA + LA	AAI 100–110 bpm × 72 h	37.5%	8% 20% 26%	0.002 0.14 0.40	Overall paced 17% AF, p < 0.005

RA, right atrium; LA, left atrium; AF, atrial fibrillation; A, atrial; pod, postoperative day; bpm, beats per minute.

Other Prophylactic Strategies

Miscellaneous other methods have been tested for prophylaxis of atrial fibrillation after surgery. Other pharmacologic prophylactic regimens studied have included steroids and thyroid supplementation. Triiodothyronine (T_3) supplementation (153) was tested in a placebo-controlled, randomized study of 142 patients with depressed left ventricular function undergoing CABG. Patients randomized to T_3 0.8 μg/kg intravenous bolus at the time of aortic cross-clamp removal followed by 0.113 μg/kg per hour for 6 hours had a lower incidence of atrial fibrillation (24% versus 46%; p = 0.009). Methylprednisolone studied for its effects on extubation times incidentally produced no reduction in postoperative atrial fibrillation in one prospective, randomized, double-blind, placebo-controlled study of 60 patients who underwent CABG (154).

Intraoperative strategies have included use of heparin coating of cardiopulmonary bypass circuits, intraoperative glucose-insulin-potassium solutions, and posterior pericardiotomy. There is one report of reduced atrial fibrillation after the use of completely heparin-coated cardiopulmonary bypass circuits (155). Intraoperative glucose-insulin-potassium solutions have been promoted to ensure adequate metabolic substrates during surgery but have produced variable results for the reduction of postoperative arrhythmias (156,157). Lazar and colleagues (156) randomized 30 patients undergoing CABG for unstable angina to 30% dextrose, 80 mEq per liter of potassium, and 50 U regular insulin versus 5% dextrose and reported higher cardiac indices, shorter ventilator support time, and lower incidence of atrial fibrillation (13.3% versus 53.3%; p = 0.02) In contrast, Wistbacka and colleagues (157) randomized 32 CABG patients to glucose 0.6 g/kg per hour, insulin 0.12 U/kg per hour, and potassium chloride 0.12 mmol/kg per hour from induction of anesthesia to start of cardiopulmonary bypass versus Ringer's acetate only and found no differences in myocardial injury, hemodynamics, or arrhythmia frequency.

Posterior pericardiotomy during cardiac surgery has also been advocated to reduce postoperative atrial fibrillation (158,159). Kuralay and colleagues (158) randomized 200 patients undergoing CABG to posterior pericardiotomy using a longitudinal incision parallel and posterior to the left phrenic nerve extending from the left inferior pulmonary vein to the diaphragm versus no posterior pericardiotomy. The incidence of atrial fibrillation was 6% in the pericardiotomy group, compared with 34% in the no pericardiotomy group (p < 0.001). This result has yet to be confirmed by other studies.

Summary

A strategy that we have used at the Cleveland Clinic Foundation for prophylaxis of atrial fibrillation after cardiac surgery is shown in Figure 29-1. Patients who are eligible for β-blocker prophylaxis are begun on metoprolol for 5 days, monitored for occurrence of supraventricular tachyarrhythmias or side effects, and then tapered off over 3 days.

Diagnosis and Treatment

The diagnosis of postoperative atrial fibrillation is often easily made from surface ECGs. The diagnosis of atrial fibrillation, flutter, or other forms of supraventricular or ventricular tachycardia can also be made with the aid of atrial electrograms obtained from temporary atrial epicardial pacing wires that are often placed routinely at the time of cardiac surgery.

Onset of atrial fibrillation in the postoperative period is likely to be symptomatic because it is often associated with rapid ventricular rates. Although postoperative atrial fibrillation generally is self-limited, symptoms, hemodynamic compromise, and concern over risk of thromboembolism usually justify intervention. Treatment of postoperative atrial fibrillation differs little from treatment of this

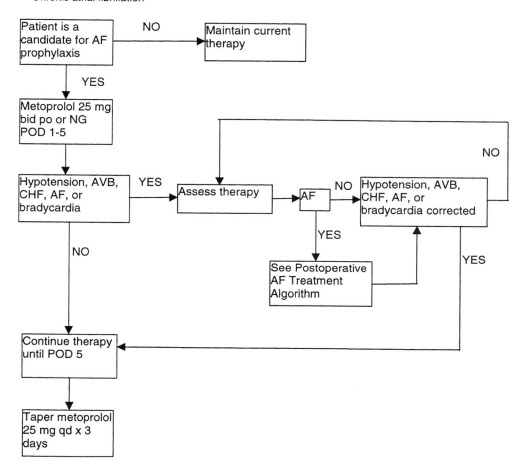

FIGURE 29-1. Algorithm for prevention of atrial fibrillation (AF) after cardiac surgery. AV, atrioventricular; AVB, AV block; CHF, congestive heart failure; CABG, coronary artery bypass grafting; LV, left ventricle; LVEF, LV ejection fraction; NG, nasogastric tube; POD, postoperative day.

arrhythmia in other situations. A general approach to postoperative atrial fibrillation and algorithms for treatment can be found in Figure 29-2.

Clinical instability manifested by hypotension, ischemia, or congestive heart failure should prompt immediate electrical cardioversion, usually beginning with 200 J of synchronized energy. Atrial overdrive pacing can be attempted if atrial flutter is the dominant rhythm.

In the absence of the need for urgent cardioversion, control of the ventricular rate becomes the primary concern during the first 24 hours. The goal is to achieve a heart rate of 70 to 100 beats per minute at rest. The choice of pharmacologic

agent depends on the clinical profile of the patient and physician preference. Commonly used agents include digoxin, β blockers, and calcium channel blockers (Table 29-10). Intravenous and oral forms of each agent can be used, although intravenous dosing is preferred to accelerate the onset of action. High postoperative sympathetic tone makes rate control with digoxin alone frequently ineffective. Tisdale and colleagues (160) compared ventricular rate control with diltiazem versus digoxin for atrial fibrillation after CABG. Diltiazem achieved rate control earlier than digoxin, and after 6 hours, response rates were higher with diltiazem (85% versus 45%; *p* = 0.02). After 24 hours, response rates were similar

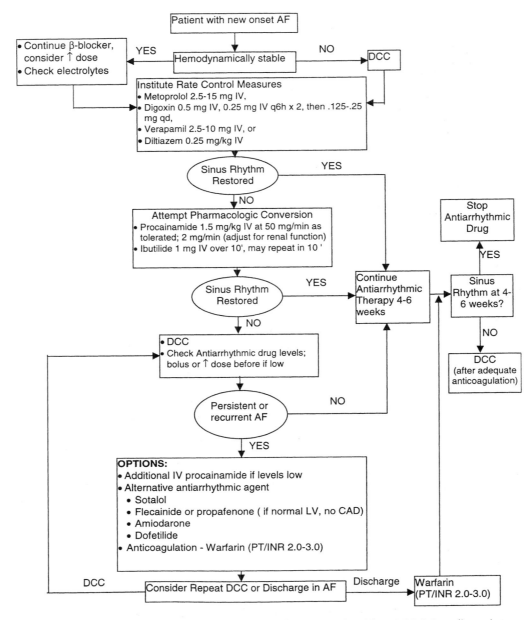

FIGURE 29-2. Postoperative atrial fibrillation (AF) treatment algorithm. DCC, DC cardioversion; LV, left ventricle; CAD, coronary artery disease; PT, prothrombin time; INR, international normalized ratio.

and conversion occurred in 55% of patients on diltiazem and 65% patients on digoxin (*p* = 0.75). Monitoring for hypotension and possibly negative inotropic effects is advised for β blockers or calcium channel blockers.

In patients without a prior history of atrial fibrillation, spontaneous conversion to sinus rhythm frequently occurs without the need for further therapy (161,162). Myers and colleagues (162) evaluated a rate-control approach to 59 patients after CABG. The use of digoxin with or without verapamil was associated with spontaneous conversion to sinus rhythm in 55 patients. Two to 4 weeks later, two of

the four patients with continued atrial fibrillation were in sinus rhythm and two others in sinus rhythm had reverted to atrial fibrillation. Thus, even with this rate-control approach, more than 90% of patients were in sinus rhythm 2 to 4 weeks after the onset. Solomon and colleagues (163) reported that 12 of 67 patients with postoperative atrial fibrillation who were discharged in atrial fibrillation had shorter length of stay with no repeated hospitalizations, bleeding complications, or thromboembolic events.

Nevertheless, in patients whose atrial arrhythmia persists for more than 24 hours or even earlier despite adequate rate

TABLE 29-10. RATE CONTROL FOR POSTOPERATIVE ATRIAL ARRHYTHMIAS

Agent	Loading Dose	Maintenance Dose	Side Effects/Toxicity	Comments
Digoxin	0.25–0.5 mg IV or PO, then 0.25 mg q 4–6 h to 1 mg in 1st 24 h	0.125–0.25 mg PO or IV qd	Anorexia, nausea; AV block; ventricular arrhythmias; accumulates in renal failure	Used in CHF; vagotonic effects on the AVN; delayed onset of action; narrow therapeutic window; less effective in postop, paroxysmal AF with high adrenergic states
β Blockers			Bronchospasm; CHF; low BP	Effective in heart rate control; rapid onset of action
Propranolol	1 mg IV q 2–5 h to 0.1–0.2 mg/kg	10–80 mg PO tid-qid		
Metoprolol	5 mg IV q5 h to 15 mg	25–100 mg PO bid-tid		
Esmolol	500 ug/kg IV over 1 h	50 µg/kg IV for 4 h; repeat load prn and ↑ maintenance 20–50 µg/kg/min q5–10 h		Esmolol shortacting
Calcium channel blockers			Low BP, CHF	Rapid onset, can be used safely in COPD and DM
Verapamil	2.5–10 mg IV over 2 h	5–10 mg IV q30–60 h or 40–160 mg PO tid or 120–480 mg/d, sustained release	High digoxin level	
Diltiazem	0.25 mg/kg over 2 h, repeat prn p 15 h at 0.35 mg/kg	5–15 mg/h IV or 30–90 mg PO qid or 120–360 mg sustained-release qd		Often well tolerated with low LVEF pts

CHF, congestive heart failure; BP, blood pressure; AVN, atrioventricular node; AF, atrial fibrillation; COPD, chronic obstructive pulmonary disease; DM, diabetes mellitus; LVEF, left ventricular ejection fraction; AV, atrioventricular.

control, pharmacologic or electrical cardioversion can generally be attempted. Trials testing the efficacy of class I or III antiarrhythmic drugs in the treatment of postoperative atrial fibrillation are summarized in Table 29-11. Pharmacologic conversion can be attempted using intravenous or oral regimens. The reported efficacy and dosing regimens of antiarrhythmic agents used for the acute conversion of atrial fibrillation after cardiac surgery are summarized in Table 29-12. The agents with intravenous forms are most commonly used after surgery. These include procainamide, ibutilide, and amiodarone. The use of quinidine is limited by proarrhythmia concerns, particularly in the postoperative setting in which electrolyte depletion resulting from diuresis might be more common. Disopyramide use has also been limited by side effects, including urinary retention. Oral flecainide and propafenone have been usually reserved for patients with no coronary artery disease and with normal ventricular function but may be of use in patients who have undergone valve surgery and who fit these criteria. Oral sotalol can be used in patients who can tolerate beta blockade, but close attention to QT intervals and electrolyte balance is important because of the risk of proarrhythmia.

Availability of intravenous and oral forms makes procainamide a typical first-line choice after rate control has been achieved. A loading dose of 10 to 15 mg/kg intravenously at less than or equal to 50 mg per minute is followed by a continuous infusion at 1 to 2 mg per minute. Oral sustained-release preparations can subsequently be used, typically at 2 to 4 g per day in two to four divided doses, depending on the preparation. Doses should be adjusted according to serum levels, which should be checked daily while on intravenous dosing. Levels of *N*-acetylprocainamide, an active metabolite of procainamide, can accumulate to toxic levels with renal dysfunction. Potential side effects include hypotension, QRS widening, and proarrhythmia, including QT prolongation and torsade de pointes. Hemodynamic effects may be seen in patients with severe left ventricular dysfunction. Gastrointestinal problems can also be a limiting factor, and procainamide can be a cause of postoperative fever (164). If the drug is continued long-term, arthralgias and a lupus-like syndrome may develop. However, if used only for postoperative atrial arrhythmias, procainamide often can be stopped by 4 to 6 weeks after surgery.

Intravenous ibutilide, a class III potassium channel blocker, can also acutely convert atrial arrhythmias after cardiac surgery with success rates of up to 57% (165). One study showed ibutilide to be more efficacious than procainamide in conversion of short-term atrial fibrillation or flutter (166). Another study reported higher success rates for termination of atrial flutter using rapid atrial pacing with less acceleration to atrial fibrillation when using ibu-

TABLE 29-11. CLASS I OR III ANTIARRHYTHMIC DRUG TRIALS FOR THE TREATMENT OF POSTOPERATIVE ATRIAL ARRHYTHMIAS

Author	Year	N	Design	Drug Regimen 1	Drug Regimen 2	% Conversion Drug 1	% Conversion Drug 2	p value	Comments
Gavaghan and colleagues (243)	1985	156	NR	Disopyramide IV 2 mg/kg, then 0.4 mg/kg/h or PO 600 mg qd		48			93% converted by discharge; 19% with side effects
Hjelms and colleagues (244)	1992	30	R	Procainamide IV 25 mg/min, max 15 mg/kg	Digoxin IV 0.75–1 mg	87	60	0.05	
McAlister and colleagues (245)	1990	80	R, P	Quinidine PO 400 mg, then 400 mg in 4 h prn	Amiodarone IV 5 mg/kg × 20 h	64	41	0.04	More side effects with quinidine
Gentili and colleagues (170)	1992	50	NR	Propafenone IV 2 mg/kg × 10 h		70			
Connolly and colleagues (171)	1987	14	R, DB, P	Propafenone 2 mg/kg over 10 min	Control	43	0	<0.001	Decreased VR, BP with propafenone
Geelen and colleagues (246)	1999	62	R, DB	Propafenone IV 2 mg/kg × 10 h	Procainamide IV 20 mg/kg @ 30 mg/min to 1,000 mg	76	61	NS	Propafenone better at 15 h; procainamide ↑, propafenone ↓ VR
Di Biasi and colleagues (247)	1995	84	R, DB	Propafenone IV 2 mg/kg × 15 h, then 10 mg/kg × 24 h prn	Amiodarone IV 5 mg/kg × 15 h, then 15 mg/kg × 24 h prn	68.4	82.6	NS	↓ VR with both; Propafenone better in 1st h
Larbuisson and colleagues (248)	1996	40	R	Propafenone IV 1–2 mg/kg × 10 h, then 420 mg/24 h	Amiodarone IV 2.5–5.0 mg/kg × 10 h, then 900 mg × 24 h	67	77	NS	Propafenone effective earlier
Wafa and colleagues (249)	1989	29	R	Flecainide IV 1 mg/kg × 10 h, 1.5 mg/kg/h × 1 h, 0.25 mg/kg/h × 23 h	Digoxin 0.5 mg, then 0.25 mg q6h × 2 doses	60	0	< 0.01	
Gavaghan and colleagues (250)	1988	56	R	Flecainide IV 2 mg/kg × 2 h, 0.2 mg/kg/h × 12 h, then PO	Digoxin 0.75 mg IV, then after 2 h disopyramide 2 mg/kg IV, 0.4 mg/kg/h × 10 h	86	89	NS	Time to conversion shorter with flecainide; 1 death, intractable ventricular arrhythmia in patient with toxic flecainide, poor ventricular and hepatic function d 5
Campbell and colleagues (251)	1985	40	R	Sotalol IV 1 mg/kg, then 0.2 mg/kg × 12 h	Digoxin 0.75 mg IV, 2 h later disopyramide 2 mg/kg IV, then 0.4 mg/kg/h × 10 h	85	85	NS	Drug 1 effective earlier; acute urinary retention with drug 2
Installe and colleagues (252)	1981	90	NR	Amiodarone IV 2.5–5.0 mg/kg IV		61			Hypotension in 18%, transient unless ↓ LV
Cochrane and colleagues (253)	1994	30	R, P	Amiodarone IV 5 mg/kg to 400 mg max over 30 h, then after 30 h 25 mg/h adjusted to 40 mg/h if HR > 120 bpm until 24 h after conversion to SR	Digoxin 0.5 mg IV × 30 h, 0.25 mg IV after 2 h, 0.125 mg IV after 5 and 9 h, then weight/renal adjusted PO after 12 h	93	80	NS	Crossover to ½ dose alternate arm if in AF at 24 h; 24-h end point listed; 15/15 (100%) converted on amiodarone, 2 recurred, then converted on digoxin; 13/15 converted on digoxin, 3 recurred transiently
Frost (169)	1997	98	R, DB, P	Dofetilide IV × 15 h 4 µg/kg to 8 µg/kg	Placebo	36 / 44	24	0.27 / 0.11	Short runs aberrancy, VT: 9% at 8 µg/kg

N, number of patients; R, randomized; DB, double-blind; P, placebo-controlled; BP, blood pressure; VR, ventricular rate; VT, ventricular tachycardia; LV, left ventricle; HR, heart rate; SR, sinus rhythm; NS, not significant.

TABLE 29-12. REGIMENS FOR PHARMACOLOGIC CONVERSION OF POSTOPERATIVE ATRIAL ARRHYTHMIAS

Drug	Route	Dose	Success Rate	Adverse Effects/Comments
Quinidine	PO	400 mg, then 400 mg in 4 h	64%	TdP, PMVT; GI; hypotension; enhanced AVN conduction; usually avoided postoperatively because of risk of proarrhythmia with diuresis/electrolyte imbalances
Disopyramide	IV	2 mg/kg, then 0.4 mg/kg/h	48–85%	Urinary retention; enhanced AVN conduction; AFL 1 : 1; VT; hypotension, TdP
	PO	600 mg qd		
Procainamide	IV	1–1.5 g at 25–50 mg/min	61–87%[a]	Fever; enhanced AVN conduction; accumulates in renal failure, TdP, PMVT
Propafenone	PO	600 mg	55–87%	?Avoid in CAD, LV dysfunction
	IV	2 mg/kg over 10 min	43–76%	
Flecainide	PO	300 mg	90%[a]	Avoid in CAD, LV dysfunction
	IV	2 mg/kg over 10 min	65–90%[a]	
	IV	1 mg/kg × 10 h, 1.5 mg/kg/h × 1 h, 0.25 mg/kg/h × 23 h	60%	
	IV	2 mg/kg × 2 h, 0.2 mg/kg/h × 12 h	86%	
Amiodarone	IV	2.5–5.0 mg/kg IV over 20 min, 15 mg/kg over 24 h; or 1.2 g over 24 h	41–93%	Hypotension
Sotalol	PO	80–160 mg, then 160–360 mg/d	52%[a]	Bradycardia; hypotension; CHF; TdP
	IV	1 mg/kg, then 0.2 mg/kg × 12 h	85%	
Dofetilide	IV	4–8 µg/kg over 15 h	36–44%	TdP; VT; must adjust dose for renal function
	PO	125–500 µg bid	29–32%[a]	
Ibutilide	IV	1 mg over 10 min, repeat in 10 h if no conversion	57%	TdP; PMVT

TdP, torsade de pointes; PMVT, polymorphic ventricular tachycardia; GI, gastrointestinal; AVN, atrioventricular node; AFL, atrial flutter; VT, ventricular tachycardia; CAD, coronary artery disease; LV, left ventricular
[a]Nonsurgical atrial arrhythmia studies.

tilide or procainamide (167). Patients should be monitored for QT prolongation and torsade de pointes.

Intravenous amiodarone has been advocated in postoperative patients, but cost can be limiting. Intravenous amiodarone is not frequently required for atrial arrhythmias in the postoperative patient but may be helpful in hemodynamically unstable patients, recurrent atrial fibrillation despite cardioversion or other antiarrhythmic drugs, rate control refractory to conventional AV nodal blocking drugs, or intolerance to standard antiarrhythmic or rate-controlling drugs because of negative inotropic effects. Rapid oral loading, however, can usually be achieved in patients with intact gastrointestinal function (168).

Dofetilide, a new class III antiarrhythmic agent, has been studied for termination of atrial fibrillation or flutter after CABG. In a double-blind, placebo-controlled, randomized trial of 98 patients, dofetilide (4 to 8 µg/kg intravenously) converted 36% and 44% of patients to sinus rhythm within 3 hours, compared with 24% on placebo (169). In this study, dofetilide was well tolerated and no torsade de pointes was reported, although short episodes of aberrancy and ventricular tachycardia occurred in three patients. The dose of dofetilide should be reduced if renal dysfunction is present.

Intravenous propafenone has been studied for postoperative atrial arrhythmias, although it is not available in this form in this country (170,171). Earlier times to conversion compared with intravenous amiodarone or procainamide and contribution to ventricular rate control have been reported.

Patients remaining in atrial fibrillation after approximately a 24-hour trial of drug therapy typically undergo electrical cardioversion. A short-acting anesthetic, such as etomidate or methohexital, is administered before cardioversion. An R-wave synchronized shock is delivered usually at initial energies of 200 J for atrial fibrillation, 50 to 100 J for atrial flutter, or 25 to 50 J if using a biphasic waveform. Anteroposterior patch positions (e.g., right parasternal–left paraspinal) are more optimal for atrial defibrillation than the anterior-anterior positions (e.g., right parasternal–left apical) that are often used for ventricular defibrillation. Low-energy internal defibrillation has also been reported to be successful using epicardial wire defibrillation electrodes placed during open-heart surgery (172–174).

Rates of recurrence after successful conversion to sinus rhythm are not well established. One study documented recurrence in 62% of patients after electrical cardioversion, despite concurrent treatment with procainamide (175). However, persistence of the arrhythmia to hospital discharge is infrequent, particularly with treatment, and even less frequently does it persist to the 6-week follow-up visit (161,162,176). A study by Yilmaz and colleagues (176) reported that in 120 patients who were converted to and maintained in sinus rhythm with pharmacologic therapy or direct current (DC) cardioversion, the rate of recurrent atrial fibrillation was low (3.3% to 6.7%) after discharge from the hospital.

Nevertheless, recurrence of atrial fibrillation is often problematic, because underlying conditions, such as inflammation, injury, and high sympathetic tone, are ongoing. Recurrent atrial fibrillation may be treated with a trial of a different antiarrhythmic drug, such as sotalol or amiodarone, or in the absence of coronary artery disease or ventricular dysfunction, propafenone or flecainide, followed by repeated electrical cardioversion. Alternatively, if the arrhythmia is well tolerated, the patient may be discharged on anticoagulation and followed up for another attempt at cardioversion after recovery from surgery, often at 4 to 6 weeks. Patients who maintain sinus rhythm with the aid of an antiarrhythmic drug may be discharged on that medication, which may be discontinued at the 4- to 6-week follow-up visit if there is no evidence of recurrence.

The management of postoperative atrial flutter presents special challenges because medical treatment is often ineffective. However, electrical cardioversion or rapid atrial pacing by way of transthoracic epicardial wires has been successfully employed (177,178). For recurrent typical atrial flutter, catheter ablation of the posterior right atrial isthmus between the tricuspid annulus and inferior vena cava has been successful in long-term management (179).

Patients with valvular disease may be more difficult to maintain in sinus rhythm. One early study suggested that success is limited when the duration of atrial fibrillation is more than 3 years or the left atrial size is more than 5.2 cm (180). However, achievement and maintenance of sinus rhythm can often be done with a reasonable expectation of success after valve surgery (181).

As in nonsurgical atrial fibrillation, anticoagulation is an important consideration for patients with postoperative trial fibrillation, particularly those in whom atrial fibrillation persists for more than 48 hours or continues to recur after cardioversion. Atrial fibrillation is known to increase the risk of stroke in nonsurgical settings, as well as in the postoperative state (2,22,23). The available evidence favors anticoagulation if atrial fibrillation persists for more than 48 hours, particularly if cardioversion is anticipated after this time (182,183). Heparin may be used but may not be feasible in the immediate postoperative period. During the subacute period after surgery, initiation of oral warfarin (target international normalized ratio of 2.0 to 3.0) without intravenous heparin may be preferred by some surgeons. However, data supporting the benefits over risks of anticoagulation in the postoperative period remain lacking.

Prognosis and Complications

Although usually benign, adverse clinical consequences of postoperative supraventricular arrhythmias may occur, and in a few patients, these may result in significant adverse clinical consequences. Potential complications include embolism, particularly cerebrovascular accidents; hemodynamic compromise, sustained atrial fibrillation; and increased resource use, including increased length of hospital stay.

Mortality

With notable exceptions, most large studies of postoperative atrial fibrillation have not reported an associated increase in mortality rate. Aranki and colleagues (17) in a study of 570 patients undergoing CABG, overall operative mortality rate was 1.8% in patients maintaining sinus rhythm and 3.9% in patients who developed atrial fibrillation ($p = 0.15$). However, Brathwaite and Weissman (25) reported that among 462 patients who underwent noncardiothoracic surgery, 10.2% of patients with new-onset atrial arrhythmias had higher mortality rate (23.4%), as did the 13% of patients with a prior history of atrial arrhythmias (mortality rate of 8.6%), when compared with patients without atrial arrhythmias (mortality rate of 4.3%) ($p < 0.02$), although most of the deaths were noncardiac and resulted from sepsis or cancer. In a Department of Veteran Affairs study of 3,855 patients undergoing open cardiac surgery, postoperative atrial fibrillation was associated with a higher hospital mortality rate (5.9% atrial fibrillation versus 2.47% no atrial fibrillation), as well as 6-month mortality rate (9.36% versus 4.17%) ($p < 0.001$) (24).

Atrial Thrombus Formation and Systemic Emboli

Stroke is an infrequent, yet serious, consequence of CABG (184). Evidence for an association between postoperative stroke and atrial fibrillation has been reported by several groups. Taylor and colleagues (22) prospectively evaluated 453 consecutive patients undergoing CABG for neurologic complications. Stroke or transient ischemic attack (TIA) occurred in 10 patients (2.2%). Postoperative atrial fibrillation occurred in 6 of these 10 patients (60%), compared with its occurrence in 80 of 443 patients (18%) who did not have stroke or TIA ($p < 0.005$). Other clinical correlates of post-CABG stroke or TIA included a prior history of stroke or TIA and presence of a carotid bruit. A history of stroke or TIA and postoperative atrial fibrillation was identified as an independent predictor of post-CABG neurologic events. These findings are further supported by a case-control study by Reed and colleagues (23) from the Massachusetts General Hospital. Postoperative atrial fibrillation occurred in 29 of 54 (54%) cases of postoperative stroke or TIA after CABG but in only 15 of 54 (28%) of the controls; the odds ratio for stroke with postoperative atrial fibrillation was 3.0 (95% confidence interval, 1.4–6.7). Mathew and colleagues (21) also reported that patients with major and minor neurologic injury had higher incidences of atrial fibrillation (major, 7% AF versus 2% no AF; minor, 6% versus 2%; $p < 0.01$). Almassi and colleagues (24) reported in a study of 3,855 Veterans Administration patients undergoing open cardiac surgery that the stroke rate was 5.26% in patients with postoperative atrial fibrillation, compared with 2.95% in patients without atrial fibrillation ($p < 0.001$). Aranki and colleagues (17) reported that the stroke incidence was 4 of 381 (1%) in patients remaining in sinus rhythm after CABG, compared with 7 of 189 (3.7%) in patients who developed postoperative atrial fibrillation ($p = 0.025$). D'Agostino and colleagues (185) also reported postoperative atrial fibrillation to be an independent predictor of postoperative neurologic events ($p = 0.0014$) among 1,279 patients who underwent CABG and who had undergone noninvasive carotid artery screening. In contrast, Hogue and colleagues (186) studied risk factors for early or delayed stroke after cardiac surgery among 2,972 patients and reported that atrial fibrillation had no impact on postoperative stroke rate unless it was accompanied by low cardiac output syndrome. Although these and other data do not conclusively show a cause-effect relationship between brief paroxysms of atrial fibrillation and clinically significant systemic emboli, they heighten the concern for such an association.

Hemodynamic Deterioration

An important potential complication of post-CABG atrial fibrillation is hemodynamic deterioration—either hypotension, congestive heart failure, or both—as a consequence of the arrhythmia or its treatment. How well atrial fibrillation is tolerated often depends on three major factors: (a) the ventricular rate, (b) the status of the patient's underlying ventricular function, and (c) the duration of the arrhythmia. In addition, the loss of atrial systole may contribute to hemodynamic deterioration. Gentili and colleagues (170) reported an increase in cardiac index from 2.7 ± 0.4 to 3.4 ± 0.1 L per minute ($p < 0.05$) after conversion of postoperative atrial fibrillation to sinus rhythm by propafenone. Mathew and colleagues (21) reported a greater incidence of postoperative congestive heart failure, duration of intubation, and renal insufficiency in patients who developed postoperative atrial fibrillation. Almassi and colleagues (24) also reported higher incidences of intensive care unit readmission (13% versus 3.9%, AF versus no AF), perioperative myocardial infarction (7.41% versus 3.36%), persistent congestive heart failure (4.57% versus 1.4%), and reintubation (10.59% versus 2.47%). Aranki and colleagues (17) reported that atrial fibrillation was also associated with higher rates of reoperation, ventilator requirement for more than 24 hours, reintubation, ventricular arrhythmias, cardiac arrest, renal failure, infection, and pacemaker requirement, although this may at least in part reflect a sicker population.

In the post-CABG patient, atrial fibrillation does not commonly result in hypotension severe enough to require the use of sympathomimetic pressors or other therapy. Davison and colleagues (120) observed only one clinically significant episode of hypotension in the 23 patients of a control group that developed atrial fibrillation. Rubin and colleagues (99) reported that 2 of 36 patients with postoperative atrial fibrillation experienced syncope, compared with 4 of 87 patients without atrial fibrillation ($p = NS$). No patients required DC cardioversion.

However, hemodynamic compromise, including congestive heart failure or significant bradyarrhythmias, might also occur as a result of therapy but generally is not common even with β blocker, calcium channel blocker, sotalol, or other antiarrhythmic drug therapy. Proarrhythmia from antiarrhythmic drug therapy for postoperative atrial fibrillation is fortunately rare but can occur (187). Because 90% of the incidence of atrial fibrillation occurred within 9 days of surgery and side effects from prophylactic antiarrhythmic therapy were greatest after 9 days, Pfisterer and colleagues (133) suggest that limitation of prophylactic therapy (sotalol in this case) to less than 9 days might be most efficacious and safe.

Although hemodynamic decompensation from postoperative atrial fibrillation is a concern, its occurrence in clinical practice appears to be unusual. Episodes of postoperative atrial fibrillation are usually of short duration. The bypass procedure itself reduces the ischemic jeopardy imposed by the arrhythmia. Finally, patients with very poor left ventricular function are less commonly subjected to cardiac surgery. Nonetheless, in occasional patients, atrial fibrillation can precipitate serious hemodynamic deterioration. For these individuals, the urgent termination of the arrhythmia and its further prevention are of paramount importance.

Prolonged Atrial Fibrillation

New-onset atrial fibrillation occurring after surgery usually is transient. In one European study (188) of 19 of 100 consecutive patients (19%) undergoing CABG who developed atrial fibrillation, one quarter of these patients were still in atrial fibrillation at the time of hospital discharge. Landymore and Howell (161) reported data on ambulatory ECG monitoring in 43 patients who developed post-CABG atrial fibrillation and 15 who did not. Despite frequent episodes of asymptomatic atrial fibrillation immediately before hospital discharge, at 3 and 6 weeks after surgery, atrial fibrillation almost never occurred. Most studies of patients previously free of atrial tachyarrhythmias (35,94,96,97,100–102,106–108,110,120,176) suggest this arrhythmia rarely persists for longer than a few days, even though it is often recurrent when it develops. Yilmaz and colleagues (176,189) showed a low rate of recurrent atrial fibrillation (3.3% to 10%) in patients discharged from the hospital with or without antiarrhythmic drugs. Thus, chronic atrial fibrillation developing *de novo* post–cardiac surgery appears to be unusual and long-term drug treatment for atrial fibrillation prevention is generally unnecessary.

Resource Utilization

Multiple studies have shown that postoperative atrial fibrillation is associated with prolonged hospital lengths of stay. Angelini and colleagues (95) noted that after surgery for coronary heart disease, postoperative atrial fibrillation significantly increased length of hospital stay from 9.9 to 11.4 days. Similarly, Rubin and colleagues (99) in a study of 123 patients noted that atrial fibrillation occurrence was associated with a 2-day increase in length of stay (14.4 ± 6 days versus 12.4 ± 4 days; $p < 0.02$). Lowe and colleagues (40) in a study of 50 patients undergoing CABG with or without other cardiac procedures found that postoperative atrial fibrillation was associated with a longer length of stay in the intensive care unit (3.6 versus 1.9 days; $p = 0.02$). Paone and colleagues (190) reported that increased length of stay in elderly patients aged 70 years or older was largely attributable to an increased incidence of atrial fibrillation. Other recent studies have confirmed a 2- to 5-day increase in length of stay and increases in hospital costs of several thousand dollars per patient associated with postoperative atrial fibrillation (2,17,20,21,103).

Valvular Disease

Postoperative arrhythmias after valvular surgery have been less well studied than arrhythmias after CABG. In a prospective study of 50 consecutive patients undergoing cardiac valve replacement, Smith and colleagues (191) found that atrial fibrillation was the most common postoperative arrhythmia, occurring in 21 of 66 arrhythmic episodes (32%). Supraventricular arrhythmias were more common after mitral valve replacement than after aortic valve replacement (73% versus 43%; $p < 0.05$). In a study of 70 patients undergoing cardiac surgery, atrial fibrillation occurred in 9 of 15 patients (60%), whereas it occurred in only 19 of 50 patients (38%) undergoing CABG (p = NS) (19). The reported incidence of postoperative atrial fibrillation after valve surgery ranges from 37% to 64% (2,18,19), and many valve patients have persistent atrial fibrillation before surgery.

As with CABG, among patients undergoing valvular surgery, age also appears to be an important independent predictor of postoperative atrial fibrillation. Douglas and colleagues, in reviewing 118 patients undergoing surgery for aortic stenosis, noted that the strongest independent predictor of postoperative atrial fibrillation was age (192). Creswell and colleagues (2) reported highest postoperative atrial arrhythmia incidences after a combination of CABG with carotid endarterectomy (60.0%), aortic valve replacement (60.1%), mitral valve repair (62.2%), or mitral valve replacement (63.6%). In a study of 915 patients undergoing valvular surgery, Asher and colleagues (18) identified

older age, mitral stenosis, left atrial enlargement, use of systemic hypothermia, and prior surgery as predictors of postoperative atrial fibrillation. Advanced age, mitral stenosis, and left atrial enlargement were confirmed as independent risk factors in a validation cohort.

Asher and colleagues (77) also reported a trend toward a decrease in the incidence of atrial fibrillation after minimally invasive valve surgery, compared with conventional mitral valve surgery (26.3% minimally invasive versus 38.0% midline sternotomy; $p = 0.08$). Tambeur and colleagues (193) reported no difference in the incidence of atrial fibrillation after left atrial versus extended transseptal approaches to mitral valve surgery. Age again was an independent predictor of atrial fibrillation or flutter after mitral valve surgery.

An additional issue in valvular heart disease patients is whether it is worthwhile to attempt to restore sinus rhythm after valve replacement or repair in patients with chronic persistent atrial fibrillation preoperatively. Flugelman and colleagues (180) studied 40 patients with pure mitral stenosis and chronic atrial fibrillation who underwent mitral valve replacement or commissurotomy. Cardioversion with DC shock and quinidine or disopyramide was performed in all patients less than 6 months after the procedure. Twenty-four patients (60%) remained in sinus rhythm for more than 3 months after cardioversion and were therefore considered successes. Patients who were "successes" were younger (38 versus 47 years; $p < 0.05$), had symptoms for a shorter period of time (3.0 versus 6.4 years; $p < 0.02$), and by echocardiography had a smaller preoperative left atrial size (4.9 versus 5.5 cm; $p < 0.03$). Following multivariate analysis, the authors concluded that for patients with preoperative left atrial sizes of more than 5.2 cm and symptoms for more than 3 years, the likelihood of successful cardioversion was too low to justify any attempt. In a more recent study, Obadia and colleagues (194) reported that the probability of return to sinus rhythm after mitral valve repair was 94% when sinus rhythm was present preoperatively, 80% when atrial fibrillation was intermittent or when the duration of atrial fibrillation was less than 1 year, but markedly lower for durations of more than 1 year. Postoperative return to sinus rhythm was associated with better 1- and 4-year survival rates, compared with postoperative atrial fibrillation.

Late recurrence of atrial fibrillation after mitral valve repair was studied by Vogt and colleagues (195). In this study of 189 patients, 72 with preoperative chronic or paroxysmal atrial fibrillation, followed for 12.2 ± 10 years, predictors of late atrial fibrillation included older age, preoperative atrial fibrillation, preoperative antiarrhythmic drug treatment, and elevated pulmonary artery pressure, heart rate, and left ventricular ejection fraction. The authors suggested that patients with these risk factors might be candidates for combined mitral valve repair and surgery for atrial fibrillation.

Conclusions

Atrial fibrillation is a frequent complication of CABG and other types of cardiac surgery, occurring in 20% to 40% of patients, and is particularly common in elderly patients. Despite a wealth of data, its specific pathogenesis or precipitants are incompletely understood. Although it occurs commonly, it is most often a benign, self-limited arrhythmia with adverse effects primarily limited to increases in length of hospital stay, need for antiarrhythmic therapies, and postoperative stroke. Treatment primarily consists of rate control using β-adrenergic blocking agents, calcium channel blockers, and digoxin. In some cases, there may be a need for additional antiarrhythmic agents. Electrical cardioversion may be required in some patients, particularly if the arrhythmia is associated with hemodynamic instability or symptoms. The most effective prophylactic strategies include low-dose β-adrenergic blocking drugs, avoidance of β-blocker withdrawal, and targeting of these strategies to patients at higher risk for atrial fibrillation.

Ventricular Arrhythmias

Compared with atrial fibrillation and other supraventricular tachyarrhythmias, serious ventricular arrhythmias are much less common as complications of cardiac surgery. However, sustained ventricular tachycardia and ventricular fibrillation do represent life-threatening events and in some postoperative cardiac arrest cases may have long-term treatment implications.

Epidemiology and Incidence

New isolated premature ventricular complexes (PVCs) or nonsustained ventricular arrhythmias are fairly common with an incidence of up to 36%, often associated with electrolyte or other metabolic imbalances. However, sustained ventricular arrhythmias have decreased and are quite uncommon with reported incidences after cardiac surgery ranging from 0.41% to 1.4% (7–10) after initial reports of a 6% incidence of postoperative ventricular fibrillation (196). Abedin and colleagues (197) reported that among 1,599 patients undergoing CABG, only 7 had sustained ventricular tachycardia and 11 had ventricular fibrillation (total of 1.2%); 12 of these events occurred on the first postoperative day. Only one of these patients had a perioperative myocardial infarction. After 30 months of follow-up, only two patients died (one of myocardial infarction and one of noncardiac causes), and no patients had recurrent symptomatic ventricular arrhythmias. Michelson and colleagues (19) monitored 70 patients with CABG 1 and 5 days after discharge from the intensive care unit. Whereas 18 of 50 had some ventricular ectopy, only 4 had ventricular tachycardia, defined as at least three consecutive ventricular premature depolarizations.

Among patients undergoing valvular surgery, Michelson and colleagues (19) reported that 3 of 15 patients had ventricular premature depolarizations of Holter monitoring, but none had ventricular tachycardia or ventricular fibrillation. Hoie and Forfang (198) followed 44 patients who underwent aortic valve replacement. Only two had ventricular premature depolarizations "requiring" treatment. There were no episodes of sustained ventricular tachycardia and only one episode of ventricular fibrillation, which in retrospect was caused by acute hypoxemia from ventilator failure.

Recognizable Antecedent Causes

A number of conditions predispose to postoperative ventricular arrhythmias, including preoperative ventricular tachycardia or fibrillation; electrolyte or metabolic abnormalities such as hypokalemia or hypomagnesemia; hypoxemia or acidosis; drugs, including inotropic sympathomimetics, digoxin, or antiarrhythmic agents used for treatment of other arrhythmias such as atrial fibrillation; perioperative myocardial infarction or ischemia; hemodynamic instability; low cardiac output states; or reperfusion after cessation of cardiopulmonary bypass (9,31,142,143,199–202).

Unexpected De Novo Ventricular Arrhythmias

In 1984 Kron and colleagues (8) reported that 18 of 1,251 (1.4%) patients undergoing open-heart surgery had experienced unanticipated sustained ventricular tachycardia or fibrillation during the first 6 weeks after cardiac surgery. In 13 patients, the event occurred during the first 48 hours after surgery. Of the 10 patients who had the arrhythmia in the surgical intensive care unit, 8 were hemodynamically stable. Only 3 of the 18 patients had an intraoperative myocardial infarction. For five of the patients, the ventricular arrhythmia was fatal; three more patients died of recurrent ventricular arrhythmias, for an overall early mortality rate of 44%.

Topol and colleagues (7) reported that 12 of 1,675 patients undergoing CABG had new-onset sustained ventricular tachycardia and/or ventricular fibrillation after surgery. None of these patients had evidence of intraoperative or perioperative myocardial infarctions, syncope, or palpitations preoperatively greater than Lown class 2 preoperative ventricular ectopy, or hemodynamic compromise or electrolyte abnormality preceding the arrhythmia. Ten of the 12 patients had prior myocardial infarctions. Graft closure was documented in three patients. The arrhythmia occurred a mean of 27 days after surgery with a range of 2 days to 5 months. At 11 ± 4 months of follow-up, two patients died and four had implantable cardioverter-defibrillators (ICDs). Tam and colleagues (9) noted unexpected, sustained ventricular tachyarrhythmias in 16 of 2,364 patients (0.68%) undergoing open-heart surgery. Most of the arrhythmias occurred during the first 7 postoperative days. All the patients had significant preoperative left ventricular dysfunction. All 16 patients were successfully resuscitated, but 12 had recurrent ventricular arrhythmias with 3 deaths. Saipin and colleagues (10) reported on 19 patients who had unexpected ventricular tachycardia or ventricular fibrillation within 7 days of cardiac surgery. Most had left ventricular systolic dysfunction. Six of the 19 patients had recurrent arrhythmia. There were no arrhythmic deaths during the follow-up, and three received ICDs after electrophysiologic study.

Mechanisms of Unexpected Ventricular Arrhythmias

Structural or functional abnormalities may underlie ventricular arrhythmias after surgery (203). Structural abnormalities include myocardial infarction, hypertrophy, and primary myopathic processes such as dilation and fibrosis. Functional abnormalities include transient myocardial ischemia and reperfusion, systemic factors such as hypoxemia and metabolic imbalance, and drug toxicities. Because there are very few patients with serious *de novo* ventricular arrhythmias after cardiac surgery, no systematic data defining specific mechanisms exist. Reperfusion and release of endogenous catecholamines after stresses of surgery may contribute (7). Kron and colleagues (8) noted that four of six patients with initial ventricular fibrillation had an acute ischemic event. Thus, postoperative ventricular tachycardia and ventricular fibrillation may represent different pathophysiologic entities. Ventricular fibrillation may more likely result from acute ischemia from graft spasm or thrombosis, whereas ventricular tachycardia may be more related to nonischemic mechanisms, such as reperfusion and altered metabolism, conduction, or repolarization abnormalities in the border region of myocardial scar (204).

Prognosis

Prognosis of ventricular arrhythmias is correlated with the type of ventricular arrhythmia and degree of structural heart disease. Patients with simple PVCs postoperatively have not been shown to exhibit increased risk for developing malignant ventricular arrhythmias, and their long-term prognosis is not impaired (200,205). Complex ventricular arrhythmias, including frequent PVCs (more than 30 PVCs per hour) and nonsustained ventricular tachycardia, have no impact on short-term outcome (200). Regarding long-term outcome, Pinto and colleagues (206) studied 185 patients with postoperative frequent PVCs and nonsustained ventricular tachycardia and reported an incidence of death at average follow-up of 36 months of 8%, compared with 5% for matched controls, although the differences were not statistically significant and left ventricular ejection fraction was not reported. Huikuri and colleagues (205) studied 126 patients with postoperative complex ventricular ectopy and reported that patients with a left ventricular ejection fraction of 0.40 or less had a 75% mortality rate and 33% incidence of sudden death at an average follow-up of 15 months, whereas none of the patients with normal left ventricular function had sudden death. Thus, long-term outcome after complex ventricular arrhythmias occurring postoperatively appears to be related to the degree of ventricular dysfunction.

Patients with sustained ventricular arrhythmias have poorer short-term and long-term prognoses. A hospital mortality rate of up to 50% has been reported in patients with sustained ventricular arrhythmias after surgery; of initial survivors, up to 40% will have a recurrence. Up to 20% will die a cardiac death within 24 months (7–10). Aggressive management, potentially with an ICD and possibly an electrophysiologic study, is often indicated, particularly if no reversible cause, including ischemia or infarction, is found.

Diagnosis

The diagnosis of ventricular tachycardia or ventricular fibrillation can usually be made from the surface ECG results, but occasionally the possibility of supraventricular tachycardia with aberrant conduction needs to be considered. Temporary epicardial atrial electrodes can be used to record an atrial electrogram simultaneously with a surface ECG. This should facilitate detection of AV association or dissociation.

Management of Ventricular Arrhythmias

Because unexpected severe ventricular arrhythmias in post–cardiac surgical patients are uncommon, there are little systematic data to help define optimal management of this situation compared with serious ventricular arrhythmias in the nonoperative patient.

Acute Treatment

Premature ventricular depolarizations and even short runs of nonsustained ventricular tachycardia usually do not need routine treatment if they are not hemodynamically significant or symptomatic, because little evidence suggests the risk of acute progression to more serious arrhythmias. Correction of any reversible causes of ventricular arrhythmias, as listed previously, should be routine. For hemodynamically significant or symptomatic PVCs or nonsustained ventricular tachycardia, lidocaine has been used successfully, although no benefits in morbidity or mortality have been demonstrated (7,207,208). Overdrive pacing, using atrial or AV sequential pacing, has been advocated by some, although evidence of efficacy has been lacking (209).

Sustained ventricular tachycardia, if hemodynamically stable, may be treated initially with intravenous antiarrhythmic medication. Lidocaine is generally the first drug of choice and is given first in a loading dose of 1 to 1.5 mg/kg, up to a total dosage of 2 to 3 mg/kg as needed in two divided doses spaced over approximately 10 to 15 minutes. An intravenous continuous infusion of 2 to 4 mg per minute may be started if the loading dose terminates the arrhythmia. Lidocaine dose may need to be modified in patients who are elderly, who have congestive heart failure, or who have hepatic dysfunction. Procainamide is often the second-line drug, given as an infusion at 20 to 50 mg per minute for a total loading dose of 15 mg/kg and then at a rate of 1 to 4 mg per minute if the drug appears to be successful. The loading dose should be stopped early if the QRS complex widens by more than 50% or if hypotension develops. Procainamide is renally excreted and dose modifications or even avoidance may be required in the presence of renal insufficiency. The metabolite *N*-acetylprocainamide may accumulate to toxic levels with renal failure. Bretylium is probably less effective than the first two agents in treating ventricular tachycardia but may be given as a 5- to 10-mg/kg loading dose over 10 minutes, followed by 1- to 2-mg per minute intravenous infusion. A common side effect is postural hypotension. Intravenous amiodarone has also been used as a first-line treatment for ventricular arrhythmias. A bolus of 150 mg is given intravenously over 10 minutes, followed by the initial infusion at 0.5 to 1 mg per minute with tapering after loading. Additional 150-mg intravenous boluses may be given over the first few hours for recurrent hemodynamically significant ventricular tachycardia or fibrillation. If possible, however, frequent boluses during the first 24 hours should be limited preferably to keep the total dose to less than 2,000 mg over the first 24 hours because of the risk of hepatic toxicity. Hypotension is a potential side effect that may require dose reduction or slowing of the infusion or bolus rates. High-dose oral amiodarone loading can also be effective if a patient is able to take medication orally or through a nasogastric tube. In this method, doses up to approximately 2,400 mg could be administered in divided doses over the first 24-hour loading period. In patients with left ventricular dysfunction, amiodarone is often better tolerated than other antiarrhythmic agents.

In patients with slower tachycardias and ventricular epicardial wires still in place, overdrive ventricular pacing may be attempted by pacing the ventricle at rates that exceed the tachycardia rate for a short burst. Because this procedure may accelerate the tachycardia to ventricular fibrillation, means for electrical cardioversion or defibrillation should be in place before the attempt.

For ventricular fibrillation or hemodynamically compromising ventricular tachycardia, unsynchronized DC electrical defibrillation or cardioversion should be performed. Electrical cardioversion should also be performed for sustained ventricular tachycardias that do not respond to antiarrhythmic medication. Energy levels generally required range from 200 to 360 J. Awake patients should be anesthetized with a short-acting agent, such as midazolam, etomidate, or methohexital, ideally in a fasting state. Intravenous access and personnel skilled in airway management

should be present. Depending on the urgency of the clinical situation, some of these measures may not be possible to implement. As noted previously, because ventricular fibrillation may be more indicative of acute ischemia, the possibility of acute graft spasm or thrombosis should be considered. Acute treatment may also include use of antiarrhythmic agents such as lidocaine, procainamide, bretylium, or amiodarone.

For patients who do not respond to conventional resuscitative measures, intraaortic balloon counterpulsation or initiation of emergency cardiopulmonary bypass in the surgical intensive care unit could be considered. Roussou and colleagues reported a 56% long-term survival rate for patients undergoing this procedure with no resultant mediastinitis and a 22% incidence of soft tissue infections (210).

Long-Term Management

Because long-term prognosis of patients with ventricular arrhythmias after cardiac surgery has not been studied in large numbers (7–10), decisions can be difficult regarding device implantation and permanent drug therapy. Postarrhythmia evaluation includes risk stratification by assessment of left ventricular function and exercise-induced ventricular arrhythmias, as well as selective use of electrophysiologic studies. Because of many acute exogenous and endogenous metabolic disturbances in the early postoperative period, some studies suggest that electrophysiologic study should be performed at least 1 week after surgery (6,211). Otherwise, long-term management differs little from that of non–postoperative ventricular arrhythmias and is discussed in other chapters.

Applicability of many of the multicenter studies to nonsustained ventricular tachycardia detected in the immediate postoperative period after cardiac surgery is unknown. Patients with recent (within 2 months) cardiac surgery were excluded from the trials. In addition, the CABG Patch trial, which randomized patients with low ejection fraction and a positive signal-average ECG to ICD versus no ICD implantation at the time of CABG surgery, showed that the population was at a high risk for death, but no difference in mortality rate was seen in the treatment groups (212). The reasons for the discrepancy between the results of this trial and those of the Multicenter Automatic Defibrillator Implantation Trial and the Multicenter Unsustained Tachycardia Trial may include a removal of risk from bypass surgery that relieved ischemia-provoked arrhythmias and/or the limitation of benefits in mortality because of a higher operative mortality rate from undergoing ICD implantation at the time of the thoracotomy. The mortality risk from ICD implantation has improved with the modern use of nonthoracotomy implantation methods.

Finally, regarding the prevention of postoperative ventricular arrhythmias, almost all available data are on nonsustained arrhythmias and thus of unclear value. Such studies with magnesium demonstrated a reduction in the frequency and severity of nonsustained arrhythmias (31). To the extent that surges in catecholamines postoperatively represent a predisposing factor, use of β-blocking drugs may also reduce the incidence of ventricular arrhythmias.

BRADYARRHYTHMIAS

Considerations by Type of Surgery

Noncardiac Surgery

Bradycardia may occur during or after noncardiac surgery but usually is precipitated by the use of pharmacologic agents that exacerbate preexisting bradycardia. It can often be managed with atropine and chronotropic agents such as isoproterenol. Situations that may warrant a temporary pacemaker include marked vasovagal cardioinhibitory responses, asymptomatic but marked bradycardia, or advanced conduction system disease. In addition, right heart catheterization in the setting of left bundle branch block may warrant placement of a prophylactic temporary pacemaker. Transcutaneous pacing can be an alternative and acceptable method of providing temporary pacing support until a temporary or permanent pacing device can be placed.

Cardiac Surgery

In cardiac surgery, bradyarrhythmias are common at least transiently but have not had an adverse impact on overall survival. Treatment has been facilitated by the practice of implanting temporary epicardial atrial and ventricular pacing wires at the time of surgery (213). The clinical challenge remains in postoperative patients to determine for an individual how long to allow for recovery of AV conduction or sinus node dysfunction before committing them to permanent pacing. It has been common practice to implant permanent pacemakers if symptomatic complete heart block or severe sinus node dysfunction persists past 5 to 7 days postoperatively, or even earlier depending on the presence or absence of underlying intrinsic rhythm or failure of temporary pacing leads. However, recovery is frequent with long-term follow-up. Reported pacemaker requirements after CABG, valve surgery, and orthotopic heart transplantation are summarized in Figure 29-3. The management of bradyarrhythmias after cardiac transplantation is discussed in Chapter 32.

CABG

Bradyarrhythmias after CABG requiring at least temporary pacing is common. AV conduction disturbances and sinus node dysfunction can occur. Most bradycardias are transient. New conduction disturbances are reported to occur in 22.5% to 45% of patients after CABG (214–216). Most conduction disturbances or bradycardias requiring temporary pacing recover within the first 6 hours after surgery (217), with a mean recovery time from temporary pacing requirement

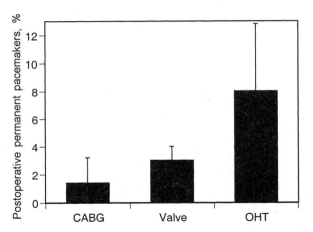

FIGURE 29-3. Postoperative permanent pacemaker requirements. Pacemaker implantation rates in the perioperative period after coronary artery bypass graft (CABG), valve, and orthotopic heart transplant (OHT) surgery, summarized from published literature from two CABG (n = 2,081), three valve (2,941), 25 OHT (n = 4,583) studies. Mean plus standard deviation is graphed.

reported to be 66 minutes in one study (216). In a study by Caspi and colleagues (217) of the 56 of 348 patients (16%) with AV block after CABG, block resolved in less than 6 hours in 32 and persisted after this point in 24 patients. Persistent AV block lasting more than 6 hours was associated with perioperative myocardial infarction and low cardiac output. Baerman and colleagues (215) reported that in the 46 of 93 patients (49%) with a new bundle branch, fascicular, or complete heart block, the block resolved partially or completely in 54% by hospital discharge. Bundle branch block was frequent, but the resolution rate was high and progression to complete AV block was rare if not present by postoperative day 1. Although in this study complete heart block resolved by postoperative day 2 in one patient and all three patients receiving a pacemaker with complete heart block were in sinus rhythm with 1 : 1 AV conduction 2 months later, resolution of complete AV block could be transient, and monitoring for several days before discharge was recommended, if a pacemaker was not implanted.

Persistent conduction disturbances occur in 5.5% to 34% of patients (218,219). Permanent pacing has been required in 0.3% to 3.4% of patients undergoing CABG because of sinus node dysfunction or AV conduction disturbances (215,218,220,221). Tuczu and colleagues (218) reported that the incidence of new postoperative conduction disturbances that persisted to hospital discharge among 2,000 consecutive patients undergoing CABG was 5.5% (111 patients), although only 6 (0.3%) required permanent pacing, and long-term prognosis was not affected.

Long-term recovery of AV conduction or sinus node dysfunction can occur within the first few days to weeks after surgery. In a 3-year follow-up study of 26 patients requiring pacemakers for complete heart block and 10 patients for sinus node dysfunction, only 30% of patients with sinus node dysfunction remained pacemaker-dependent, although 65% of patients with complete heart block remained dependent (222). Emlein and colleagues (220) reported that 11 of 13 patients demonstrated persistent AV conduction or sinus node dysfunction requiring continuous pacing on follow-up. All eight patients with complete heart block and two of five patients with sick sinus syndrome had no recovery or only partial recovery. Severe or complete AV block appears less likely than sinus node dysfunction to recover with long-term observation.

Factors that have been associated with bradyarrhythmias requiring temporary pacing after CABG include older age, preoperative bradycardia, preoperative left bundle branch block, preoperative use of β-adrenergic blockers and calcium channel blockers, number of vessels grafted, higher potassium levels, duration of aortic cross-clamp times, and excessively low myocardial temperatures during cardioplegia (216,219,220). Multivessel coronary disease, including left main trunk disease with occluded dominant right coronary anatomy and nongraftable or endarterectomy of the right coronary artery, were associated with AV block (217). Factors that have been associated with the need for permanent pacemakers after CABG include older age, preoperative left bundle branch block, left ventricular aneurysmectomy, left main coronary artery stenosis, number of bypassed arteries, cardiopulmonary bypass time, aortic cross-clamp time, and blood instead of crystalloid cardioplegia (215,219–221).

Valvular Surgery

Bradycardia after valve operations usually is caused by complete or high-degree AV block, presumably resulting from surgery near the AV conduction system, and occurs particularly after mitral or aortic valve procedures. Transient AV block has been reported in 17.6% of patients undergoing aortic valve replacement and 13% of patients undergoing mitral valve replacement (223). Moore and Wilkoff (224) reported that 4% of patients undergoing aortic valve replacement and 1% of patients undergoing mitral valve replacement develop complete heart block. Permanent pacing is required in approximately 2% to 4% of patients after valve surgery (223,225–227), although the requirement can be much higher with some types of procedures. Pacemakers have been implanted in up to 24% of patients after surgery for calcific aortic stenosis (228) and 22% after tricuspid valve replacement (229). Mitral valve repair and replacement have been associated with equal frequencies of clinically important second- or third-degree AV block, with an incidence of new conduction disturbances of 30.6%, and complete heart block in 1.5% (226). The right lateral atriotomy that is necessary with minimally invasive mitral valve operations or other transseptal superior approaches to the mitral valve may transect the sinus node artery (230). Sinus node dysfunction with persistent symptomatic sinus bradycardia requiring permanent pacing is not infrequent in

these patients. Pacemaker requirement is also higher after repeated valve surgeries (7.7% versus 2.0% after initial valve surgery) with preoperative PR-interval prolongation and preexisting infective endocarditis increasing the risk of needing postoperative permanent pacing (225).

Significant perivalvular calcification appears to predispose to AV block after surgery requiring pacing. Nair and colleagues (228) reported that in 76 patients undergoing aortic valve replacement for calcific aortic stenosis, 15 of 45 (33%) patients with mitral annulus calcification required a permanent pacemaker, compared with 3 of 31 (10%) without mitral annulus calcification. Gaillard and colleagues (227) noted that after aortic valve surgery, calcific aortic stenosis was the main pathology in all patients paced.

Other significant risk factors include older age, preoperative left bundle branch block, left ventricular aneurysmectomy, left main coronary artery stenosis, number of bypassed arteries, and cardiopulmonary bypass time. The incidence of AV block may be reduced by decreasing the concentration of potassium in the reinfusion cardioplegia solution (231).

Technical Aspects of Epicardial Temporary Pacing

The ability to maintain effective pacing in the postoperative period decreases with time from intraoperative temporary epicardial electrode placement. Optimization of electrode positioning can enhance sensing and pacing thresholds (232,233). In one small study, sites at the inferolateral caudal right atrial free wall and above the sinus node produced the best pacing thresholds and resistance (233). Complications that may occur with temporary epicardial pacing leads include the potential for local or mediastinal infection and laceration with bleeding and cardiac tamponade on lead removal (234). Patients on anticoagulants are probably at higher risk for the latter complication, and if possible, anticoagulation is usually held around the time of wire removal or not begun until after removal and assurance of hemodynamic stability.

Treatment

There is usually no need to consider temporary pacing measures before cardiac surgery, because it is standard surgical practice to implant temporary epicardial atrial and ventricular pacing wires at the time of surgery. The difficulty lies in determining the amount of time to allow for recovery of AV conduction or sinus node after surgery before committing the patient to permanent pacing, as recovery is not uncommon with long-term follow-up. Even among patients deemed suitable for permanent pacing, only 30% to 40% of patients with sinus node dysfunction remain pacemaker-dependent. Among patients with complete heart block, 65% to 100% remain dependent. The usual practice is to implant a permanent pacemaker if symptomatic complete heart block or severe sinus node dysfunction persists for more than 5 to 7 days postoperatively. If underlying intrinsic rhythm is absent or temporary pacing leads fail, permanent pacing may be warranted even sooner.

Chronotropic medications, such as theophylline or aminophylline, are used occasionally for sinus bradycardia after transplantation to improve sinus node dysfunction (235) or high-grade AV block (236). Use of these medications has been postulated to decrease the need for permanent pacing (237,238).

Pacing in the postoperative state after cardiac surgery is sometimes used to improve hemodynamics by shortening the AV delay. This maneuver may improve cardiac index in patients with impaired ejection fraction and prolonged native AV intervals of 200 ms or more (239). However, concurrent hemodynamic monitoring is recommended to individualize treatment, as the optimal timing for a given patient must be empiric and cannot be predicted.

SUMMARY

Arrhythmias are common after surgery, particularly after cardiac surgery. Atrial fibrillation is the most common arrhythmia encountered postoperatively, although ventricular arrhythmias and conduction disturbances can occur. Prompt and proper recognition, assessment of hemodynamic stability, acute treatment, and assessment of long-term treatment strategies are similar to those of nonsurgically associated arrhythmias but are critical to appropriate management of these arrhythmias.

REFERENCES

1. Vecht RJ, Nicolaides EP, Ikweuke JK, et al. Incidence and prevention of supraventricular tachyarrhythmias after coronary bypass surgery. *Int J Cardiol* 1986;13:125–134.
2. Creswell LL, Schuessler RB, Rosenbloom M, Cox JL. Hazards of postoperative atrial arrhythmias. *Ann Thoracic Surg* 1993;56:539–549.
3. Leitch JW, Thomson D, Baird DK, Harris PJ. The importance of age as a predictor of atrial fibrillation and flutter after coronary artery bypass grafting. *J Thorac Cardiovasc Surg* 1990;100:338–342.
4. Crosby LH, Pifalo WB, Woll KR, Burkholder JA. Risk factors for atrial fibrillation after coronary artery bypass grafting. *Am J Cardiol* 1990;66:1520–1522.
5. Fuller JA, Adams GG, Buxton B. Atrial fibrillation after coronary artery bypass grafting. Is it a disorder of the elderly? *J Thorac Cardiovasc Surg* 1989;97:821–825.
6. Carlson MD, Biblo LA, Waldo AL. Post open heart surgery ventricular arrhythmias. *Cardiovasc Clin* 1992;22:241–253.
7. Topol EJBK, Platia EV, Griffith LSC. De novo refractory ventricular tachyarrhythmias after coronary revascularization. *Am J Cardiol* 1986;1986:57–59.
8. Kron IL DJ, Crosby IK, Mentzer RM, et al. Unanticipated postoperative ventricular tachyarrhythmias. *Ann Thoracic Surg* 1984;38:317–322.
9. Tam SKC MJ, Edmunds LH. Unexpected, sustained ventricular tachyarrhythmia after cardiac operations. *J Thorac Cardiovasc Surg* 1991;102.
10. Saipin PM WA, Foster JR. Unexpected ventricular tachyarrhythmias soon after cardiac surgery. *Am J Cardiol* 1991;68:1099–1100.
11. Goldman L. Supraventricular tachyarrhythmias in hospitalized adults after surgery. Clinical correlates in patients over 40 years of age after major noncardiac surgery. *Chest* 1978;73:450–454.
12. Johnston K. Multicenter prospective study of nonruptured abdominal aortic aneurysm. *J Vasc Surg* 1989;9:437–447.
13. Nielsen J, Sorensen H, Alstrup P. Atrial fibrillation following thoracotomy for non-cardiac diseases, in particular cancer of the lung. *Acta Med Scand* 1973;193:425–429.
14. Dyszkiewicz W, Skrzypczak M. Atrial fibrillation after surgery of the lung: clinical analysis of risk factors. *Eur J Cardiothorac Surg* 1998;13:625–628.
15. Krowka MJ, Pairolero PC, Trastek VF, et al. Cardiac dysrhythmia following pneumonectomy. Clinical correlates and prognostic significance. *Chest* 1987;91:490–495.
16. Curtis JJ, Parker BM, McKenney CA, et al. Incidence and predictors of supraventricular dysrhythmias after pulmonary resection. *Ann Thorac Surg* 1998;66:1766–1771.
17. Aranki SF, Shaw DP, Adams DH, et al. Predictors of atrial fibrillation after coronary artery surgery. Current trends and impact on hospital resources. *Circulation* 1996;94:390–397.
18. Asher CR, Miller DP, Grimm RA, et al. Analysis of risk factors for development of atrial fibrillation early after cardiac valvular surgery. *Am J Cardiol* 1998;82:892–895.
19. Michelson EMJ, MacVaugh H. Postoperative arrhythmias after coronary artery and cardiac valvular surgery detected by long-term electrocardiographic monitoring. *Am Heart J* 1979;97:442–448.
20. Borzak S, Tisdale JE, Amin NB, et al. Atrial fibrillation after bypass surgery: does the arrhythmia or the characteristics of the patients prolong hospital stay? *Chest* 1998;113:1489–1491.
21. Mathew JP, Parks R, Savino JS, et al. Atrial fibrillation following coronary artery bypass graft surgery: predictors, outcomes, and resource utilization. MultiCenter Study of Perioperative Ischemia Research Group. *JAMA* 1996;276:300–306.
22. Taylor GJ, Malik SA, Colliver JA, et al. Usefulness of atrial fibrillation as a predictor of stroke after isolated coronary artery bypass grafting. *Am J Cardiol* 1987;60:905–907.
23. Reed GLD, Singer DE, Picard EH, DeSanctis RW. Stroke following coronary-artery bypass surgery. A case-control estimate of the risk from carotid bruits. *N Engl J Med* 1988;319:1246–1250.
24. Almassi GH, Schowalter T, Nicolosi AC, et al. Atrial fibrillation after cardiac surgery: a major morbid event? *Ann Surg* 1997;226:501–513.
25. Brathwaite D, Weissman C. The new onset of atrial arrhythmias following major noncardiothoracic surgery is associated with increased mortality. *Chest* 1998;114:462–468.
26. Boyden PA, Hoffman BF. The effects on atrial electrophysiology and structure of surgically induced right atrial enlargement in dogs. *Circ Res* 1981;49:1319–1331.
27. Rousou JA, Meeran MK, Engelman RM, et al. Does the type of venous drainage or cardioplegia affect postoperative conduction and atrial arrhythmias? *Circulation* 1985;72:II259–II263.
28. Sato S, Yamauchi S, Schuessler RB, et al. The effect of augmented atrial hypothermia on atrial refractory period, conduction, and atrial flutter/fibrillation in the canine heart. *J Thorac Cardiovasc Surg* 1992;104:297–306.
29. Chen XZ, Newman M, Rosenfeldt FL. Internal cardiac cooling improves atrial preservation: electrophysiological and biochemical assessment. *Ann Thorac Surg* 1988;46:406–411.
30. Smith PK, Buhrman WC, Levett JM, et al. Supraventricular conduction abnormalities following cardiac operations. A com-

plication of inadequate atrial preservation. *J Thorac Cardiovasc Surg* 1983;85:105–115.

31. England MR, Gordon G, Salem M, Chernow B. Magnesium administration and dysrhythmias after cardiac surgery. A placebo-controlled, double-blind, randomized trial. *JAMA* 1992;268:2395–2402.

32. Salem BI, Chaudhry A, Haikal M, et al. Sustained supraventricular tachyarrhythmias following coronary artery bypass surgery comparing mammary versus saphenous vein grafts. *Angiology* 1991;42:441–446.

33. Oka Y, Frishman W, Becker RM, et al. Clinical pharmacology of the new beta-adrenergic blocking drugs. Part 10. Beta-adrenoceptor blockade and coronary artery surgery. *Am Heart J* 1980;99:255–269.

34. Hammon JW Jr, Wood AJ, Prager RL, et al. Perioperative beta blockade with propranolol: reduction in myocardial oxygen demands and incidence of atrial and ventricular arrhythmias. *Ann Thorac Surg* 1984;38:363–367.

35. Salazar C, Frishman W, Friedman S, et al. Beta-blockade therapy for supraventricular tachyarrhythmias after coronary surgery: a propranolol withdrawal syndrome? *Angiology* 1979; 30:816–819.

36. Hearse D, Braimbridge M, Jynge P. *Protection of the ischemic myocardium: cardioplegia.* New York: Raven Press, 1981.

37. Bush HL Jr, Gelband H, Hoffman BF, Malm JR. Electrophysiological basis for supraventricular arrhythmias: following surgical procedures for aortic stenosis. *Arch Surg* 1971;103:620–625.

38. Buxton AE, Josephson ME. The role of P wave duration as a predictor of postoperative atrial arrhythmias. *Chest* 1981;80:68–73.

39. Tamis JE, Steinberg JS. Value of the signal-averaged P wave analysis in predicting atrial fibrillation after cardiac surgery. *J Electrocardiol* 1998;30:36–43.

40. Lowe JE, Hendry PJ, Hendrickson SC, Wells R. Intraoperative identification of cardiac patients at risk to develop postoperative atrial fibrillation. *Ann Surg* 1991;213:388–392.

41. Kecskemeti V, Kelemen K, Solti F, Szabo Z. Physiological and pharmacological analysis of transmembrane action potentials of human atrial fibers. *Adv Myocardiol* 1985;6:37–47.

42. Hogue CW Jr, Domitrovich PP, Stein PK, et al. RR interval dynamics before atrial fibrillation in patients after coronary artery bypass graft surgery. *Circulation* 1998;98:429–434.

43. Dimmer C, Tavernier R, Gjorgov N, et al. Variations of autonomic tone preceding onset of atrial fibrillation after coronary artery bypass grafting. *Am J Cardiol* 1998;82:22–25.

44. Pichlmaier AM, Lang V, Harringer W, et al. Prediction of the onset of atrial fibrillation after cardiac surgery using the monophasic action potential. *Heart* 1998;80:467–472.

45. Tittelbach V, Schwab M, Volff JN, et al. Atrial fibrillation after coronary artery bypass surgery: association with changes in G protein levels in mononuclear leukocytes. *Naunyn Schmiedebergs Arch Pharmacol* 1999;359:204–211.

46. Tchervenkov CI, Wynands JE, Symes JF, et al. Persistent atrial activity during cardioplegic arrest: a possible factor in the etiology of postoperative supraventricular tachyarrhythmias. *Ann Thorac Surg* 1983;36:437–443.

47. Angelini GD, Penny WJ, el-Ghamary F, et al. The incidence and significance of early pericardial effusion after open heart surgery. *Eur J Cardiothorac Surg* 1987;1:165–168.

48. Van Wagoner DR, Pond AL, McCarthy PM, et al. Outward K$^+$ current densities and Kv1.5 expression are reduced in chronic human atrial fibrillation. *Circ Res* 1997;80:772–781.

49. Van Wagoner DR, Pond AL, Lamorgese M, et al. Atrial L-type Ca^{2+} currents and human atrial fibrillation. *Circ Res* 1999; 85:428–436.

50. Frost L, Molgaard H, Christiansen EH, et al. Atrial fibrillation and flutter after coronary artery bypass surgery: epidemiology, risk factors and preventive trials. *Int J Cardiol* 1992;36:253–261.

51. Dixon FE, Genton E, Vacek JL, et al. Factors predisposing to supraventricular tachyarrhythmias after coronary artery bypass grafting. *Am J Cardiol* 1986;58:476–478.

52. Kitzman DW, Edwards WD. Age-related changes in the anatomy of the normal human heart. *J Gerontol* 1990;45:M33–M39.

53. Hashimoto K, Ilstrup DM, Schaff HV. Influence of clinical and hemodynamic variables on risk of supraventricular tachycardia after coronary artery bypass. *J Thorac Cardiovasc Surg* 1991;101: 56–65.

54. Mendes LA, Connelly GP, McKenney PA, et al. Right coronary artery stenosis: an independent predictor of atrial fibrillation after coronary artery bypass surgery. *J Am Coll Cardiol* 1995; 25:198–202.

55. Pehkonen E, Honkonen E, Makynen P, et al. Stenosis of the right coronary artery and retrograde cardioplegia predispose patients to atrial fibrillation after coronary artery bypass grafting. *Thorac Cardiovasc Surg* 1998;46:115–120.

56. Terada Y, Mitsui T, Matsushita S, et al. Atrial fibrillation after coronary artery bypass grafting. An increase in high-frequency atrial activity in patients with right coronary artery revascularization. *Jpn J Thorac Cardiovasc Surg* 1999;47:6–13.

57. Kolvekar S, D'Souza A, Akhtar P, et al. Role of atrial ischaemia in development of atrial fibrillation following coronary artery bypass surgery. *Eur J Cardiothorac Surg* 1997;11:70–75.

58. Mooe T, Gullsby S, Rabben T, Eriksson P. Sleep-disordered breathing: a novel predictor of atrial fibrillation after coronary artery bypass surgery. *Coron Artery Dis* 1996;7:475–478.

59. Pattison CW, Dimitri WR, Williams BT. Dysrhythmias following coronary artery surgery. A comparison between cold cardioplegic and intermittent ischaemic arrest (32 degrees C) with the effect of right coronary endarterectomy. *J Cardiovasc Surg (Torino)* 1988;29:601–605.

60. Morrison J, Killip T. Serum digitalis and arrhythmia in patients undergoing cardiopulmonary bypass. *Circulation* 1973;47: 341–352.

61. Rose MR, Glassman E, Spencer FC. Arrhythmias following cardiac surgery: relation to serum digoxin levels. *Am Heart J* 1975;89:288–294.

62. Weightman WM, Gibbs NM, Sheminant MR, et al. Drug therapy before coronary artery surgery: nitrates are independent predictors of mortality and beta-adrenergic blockers predict survival. *Anesth Analg* 1999;88:286–291.

63. Chang CM, Lee SH, Lu MJ, et al. The role of P wave in prediction of atrial fibrillation after coronary artery surgery. *Int J Cardiol* 1999;68:303–308.

64. Steinberg JS, Zelenkofske S, Wong SC, et al. Value of the P-wave signal-averaged ECG for predicting atrial fibrillation after cardiac surgery. *Circulation* 1993;88:2618–2622.

65. Klein M, Evans SJ, Blumberg S, et al. Use of P-wave–triggered, P-wave signal-averaged electrocardiogram to predict atrial fibrillation after coronary artery bypass surgery. *Am Heart J* 1995; 129:895–901.

66. Zaman AG, Alamgir F, Richens T, et al. The role of signal averaged P wave duration and serum magnesium as a combined predictor of atrial fibrillation after elective coronary artery bypass surgery. *Heart* 1997;77:527–531.

67. Stafford PJ, Kolvekar S, Cooper J, et al. Signal averaged P wave compared with standard electrocardiography or echocardiography for prediction of atrial fibrillation after coronary bypass grafting. *Heart* 1997;77:417–422.

68. Dimmer C, Jordaens L, Gorgov N, et al. Analysis of the P wave with signal averaging to assess the risk of atrial fibrillation after coronary artery bypass surgery. *Cardiology* 1998;89:19–24.

69. Aytemir K, Aksoyek S, Ozer N, et al. Atrial fibrillation after

coronary artery bypass surgery: P wave signal averaged ECG, clinical and angiographic variables in risk assessment. *Int J Cardiol* 1999;69:49–56.

70. Amar D, Roistacher N, Zhang H, et al. Signal-averaged P-wave duration does not predict atrial fibrillation after thoracic surgery. *Anesthesiology* 1999;91:16–23.

71. Frost L, Lund B, Pilegaard H, Christiansen EH. Re-evaluation of the role of P-wave duration and morphology as predictors of atrial fibrillation and flutter after coronary artery bypass surgery. *Eur Heart J* 1996;17:1065–1071.

72. Cox JL. A perspective of postoperative atrial fibrillation in cardiac operations. *Ann Thorac Surg* 1993;56:405–409.

73. Ormerod OJ, McGregor CG, Stone DL, et al. Arrhythmias after coronary bypass surgery. *Br Heart J* 1984;51:618–621.

74. Caretta Q, Mercanti CA, De Nardo D, et al. Ventricular conduction defects and atrial fibrillation after coronary artery bypass grafting. Multivariate analysis of preoperative, intraoperative and postoperative variables. *Eur Heart J* 1991;12:1107–1111.

75. Butler J, Chong JL, Rocker GM, et al. Atrial fibrillation after coronary artery bypass grafting: a comparison of cardioplegia versus intermittent aortic cross-clamping. *Eur J Cardiothorac Surg* 1993;7:23–25.

76. Abreu JE, Reilly J, Salzano RP, et al. Comparison of frequencies of atrial fibrillation after coronary artery bypass grafting with and without the use of cardiopulmonary bypass. *Am J Cardiol* 1999;83:775–776,A9.

77. Asher CR, DiMengo JM, Arheart KL, et al. Atrial fibrillation early postoperatively following minimally invasive cardiac valvular surgery. *Am J Cardiol* 1999;84:744–747,A9.

78. Cohn LH, Adams DH, Couper GS, et al. Minimally invasive cardiac valve surgery improves patient satisfaction while reducing costs of cardiac valve replacement and repair. *Ann Surg* 1997;226:421–428.

79. Saatvedt K, Fiane AE, Sellevold O, Nordstrand K. Is atrial fibrillation caused by extracorporeal circulation? *Ann Thorac Surg* 1999;68:931–933.

80. Mullen JC, Khan N, Weisel RD, et al. Atrial activity during cardioplegia and postoperative arrhythmias. *J Thorac Cardiovasc Surg* 1987;94:558–565.

81. Investigators TWH. Randomised trial of normothermic versus hypothermic coronary bypass surgery. The Warm Heart Investigators. *Lancet* 1994;343:559–563.

82. Fontan F, Madonna F, Naftel DC, et al. Modifying myocardial management in cardiac surgery: a randomized trial. *Eur J Cardiothorac Surg* 1992;6:127–136.

83. Pehkonen EJ, Honkonen EL, Makynen PJ, et al. Conduction disturbances after different blood cardioplegia modes in coronary artery bypass grafting. Including comparison with an earlier patient series. *Scand J Thorac Cardiovasc Surg* 1996;30:149–155.

84. Arom KV, Emery RW, Petersen RJ, Bero JW. Evaluation of 7,000+ patients with two different routes of cardioplegia. *Ann Thorac Surg* 1997;63:1619–1624.

85. Cheung EH, Arcidi JM Jr, Jackson ER, et al. Intracavitary right heart cooling during coronary bypass surgery. A prospective randomized trial. *Circulation* 1988;78:III173–III179.

86. Brandt M, Harringer W, Hirt SW, et al. Influence of bicaval anastomoses on late occurrence of atrial arrhythmia after heart transplantation. *Ann Thorac Surg* 1997;64:70–72.

87. Jensen BM, Alstrup P, Klitgard NA. Postoperative arrhythmias and myocardial electrolytes in patients undergoing coronary artery bypass grafting. *Scand J Thorac Cardiovasc Surg* 1996; 30:133–140.

88. Aglio LS, Stanford GG, Maddi R, et al. Hypomagnesemia is common following cardiac surgery. *J Cardiothorac Vasc Anesth* 1991;5:201–208.

89. Jensen BM, Alstrup P, Klitgard NA. Magnesium substitution and postoperative arrhythmias in patients undergoing coronary artery bypass grafting. *Scand Cardiovasc J* 1997;31:265–269.

90. Nurozler F, Tokgozoglu L, Pasaoglu I, et al. Atrial fibrillation after coronary artery bypass surgery: predictors and the role of MgSO4 replacement. *J Cardiac Surg* 1996;11:421–427.

91. Terzi A, Furlan G, Chiavacci P, et al. Prevention of atrial tachyarrhythmias after non-cardiac thoracic surgery by infusion of magnesium sulfate. *Thorac Cardiovasc Surg* 1996;44:300–303.

92. Wahr JA, Parks R, Boisvert D, et al. Preoperative serum potassium levels and perioperative outcomes in cardiac surgery patients. Multicenter Study of Perioperative Ischemia Research Group. *JAMA* 1999;281:2203–2210.

93. Engelman RM, Haag B, Lemeshow S, et al. Mechanism of plasma catecholamine increases during coronary artery bypass and valve procedures. *J Thorac Cardiovasc Surg* 1983;86:608–615.

94. Mohr R, Smolinsky A, Goor DA. Prevention of supraventricular tachyarrhythmia with low-dose propranolol after coronary bypass. *J Thorac Cardiovasc Surg* 1981;81:840–845.

95. Angelini P, Feldman MI, Lufschanowski R, Leachman RD. Cardiac arrhythmias during and after heart surgery: diagnosis and management. *Prog Cardiovasc Dis* 1974;16:469–495.

96. White HD, Antman EM, Glynn MA, et al. Efficacy and safety of timolol for prevention of supraventricular tachyarrhythmias after coronary artery bypass surgery. *Circulation* 1984;70:479–484.

97. Daudon P, Corcos T, Gandjbakhch I, et al. Prevention of atrial fibrillation or flutter by acebutolol after coronary bypass grafting. *Am J Cardiol* 1986;58:933–936.

98. Weitzman LB, Tinker WP, Kronzon I, et al. The incidence and natural history of pericardial effusion after cardiac surgery—an echocardiographic study. *Circulation* 1984;69:506–511.

99. Rubin DA, Nieminski KE, Reed GE, Herman MV. Predictors, prevention, and long-term prognosis of atrial fibrillation after coronary artery bypass graft operations. *J Thorac Cardiovasc Surg* 1987;94:331–335.

100. Chee TP, Prakash NS, Desser KB, Benchimol A. Postoperative supraventricular arrhythmias and the role of prophylactic digoxin in cardiac surgery. *Am Heart J* 1982;104:974–977.

101. Silverman NA, Wright R, Levitsky S. Efficacy of low-dose propranolol in preventing postoperative supraventricular tachyarrhythmias: a prospective, randomized study. *Ann Surg* 1982; 196:194–197.

102. Roffman JA, Fieldman A. Digoxin and propranolol in the prophylaxis of supraventricular tachydysrhythmias after coronary artery bypass surgery. *Ann Thorac Surg* 1981;31:496–501.

103. Kowey PR, Taylor JE, Rials SJ, Marinchak RA. Meta-analysis of the effectiveness of prophylactic drug therapy in preventing supraventricular arrhythmia early after coronary artery bypass grafting. *Am J Cardiol* 1992;69:963–965.

104. Andrews TC, Reimold SC, Berlin JA, Antman EM. Prevention of supraventricular arrhythmias after coronary artery bypass surgery. A meta-analysis of randomized control trials. *Circulation* 1991;84:III236–III244.

105. Weiner B, Rheinlander HF, Decker EL, Cleveland RJ. Digoxin prophylaxis following coronary artery bypass surgery. *Clin Pharm* 1986;5:55–58.

106. Csicsko JF, Schatzlein MH, King RD. Immediate postoperative digitalization in the prophylaxis of supraventricular arrhythmias following coronary artery bypass. *J Thorac Cardiovasc Surg* 1981;81:419–422.

107. Johnson LW, Dickstein RA, Fruehan CT, et al. Prophylactic digitalization for coronary artery bypass surgery. *Circulation* 1976;53:819–822.

108. Tyras DH, Stothert JC Jr, Kaiser GC, et al. Supraventricular tachyarrhythmias after myocardial revascularization: a randomized trial of prophylactic digitalization. *J Thorac Cardiovasc Surg* 1979;77:310–314.

109. Parker FB Jr, Greiner-Hayes C, Bove EL, et al. Supraventricular arrhythmias following coronary artery bypass. The effect of preoperative digitalis. *J Thorac Cardiovasc Surg* 1983;86:594–600.

110. Matangi MF, Neutze JM, Graham KJ, et al. Arrhythmia prophylaxis after aorta-coronary bypass. The effect of minidose propranolol. *J Thorac Cardiovasc Surg* 1985;89:439–443.

111. Martinussen HJ, Lolk A, Szczepanski C, Alstrup P. Supraventricular tachyarrhythmias after coronary bypass surgery—a double blind randomized trial of prophylactic low dose propranolol. *Thorac Cardiovasc Surg* 1988;36:206–207.

112. Stephenson LW, MacVaugh HD, Tomasello DN, Josephson ME. Propranolol for prevention of postoperative cardiac arrhythmias: a randomized study. *Ann Thorac Surg* 1980;29:113–116.

113. Khuri SF, Okike ON, Josa M, et al. Efficacy of nadolol in preventing supraventricular tachycardia after coronary artery bypass grafting. *Am J Cardiol* 1987;60:51D–58D.

114. Boudoulas H, Snyder GL, Lewis RP, et al. Safety and rationale for continuation of propranolol therapy during coronary bypass operation. *Ann Thorac Surg* 1978;26:222–227.

115. Abel RM, van Gelder HM, Pores IH, et al. Continued propranolol administration following coronary bypass surgery. Antiarrhythmic effects. *Arch Surg* 1983;118:727–731.

116. Shafei H, Nashef SA, Turner MA, Bain WH. Does low-dose propranolol reduce the incidence of supraventricular tachyarrhythmias following myocardial revascularisation? A clinical study. *Thorac Cardiovasc Surg* 1988;36:202–205.

117. Jakobsen CJ, Bille S, Ahlburg P, et al. Perioperative metoprolol reduces the frequency of atrial fibrillation after thoracotomy for lung resection. *J Cardiothorac Vasc Anesth* 1997;11:746–751.

118. Mills SA, Poole GV Jr, Breyer RH, et al. Digoxin and propranolol in the prophylaxis of dysrhythmias after coronary artery bypass grafting. *Circulation* 1983;68:II222–II225.

119. Kowey PR, Dalessandro DA, Herbertson R, et al. Effectiveness of digitalis with or without acebutolol in preventing atrial arrhythmias after cardiac surgery. *Am J Cardiol* 1997;79:1114–1117.

120. Davison R, Hartz R, Kaplan K, et al. Prophylaxis of supraventricular tachyarrhythmia after coronary bypass surgery with oral verapamil: a randomized, double-blind trial. *Ann Thorac Surg* 1985;39:336–339.

121. Smith EE, Shore DF, Monro JL, Ross JK. Oral verapamil fails to prevent supraventricular tachycardia following coronary artery surgery. *Int J Cardiol* 1985;9:37–44.

122. Van Mieghem W, Tits G, Demuynck K, et al. Verapamil as prophylactic treatment for atrial fibrillation after lung operations. *Ann Thorac Surg* 1996;61:1083–1086.

123. Seitelberger R, Hannes W, Gleichauf M, et al. Effects of diltiazem on perioperative ischemia, arrhythmias, and myocardial function in patients undergoing elective coronary bypass grafting. *J Thorac Cardiovasc Surg* 1994;107:811–821.

124. el-Sadek M, Krause E. Postoperative antiarrhythmic effects of diltiazem in patients undergoing coronary bypass grafting. *Cardiology* 1994;85:290–297.

125. Laub GW, Janeira L, Muralidharan S, et al. Prophylactic procainamide for prevention of atrial fibrillation after coronary artery bypass grafting: a prospective, double-blind, randomized, placebo-controlled pilot study. *Crit Care Med* 1993;21:1474–1478.

126. Gold MR, O'Gara PT, Buckley MJ, DeSanctis RW. Efficacy and safety of procainamide in preventing arrhythmias after coronary artery bypass surgery. *Am J Cardiol* 1996;78:975–979.

127. McCarty RJ, Jahnke EJ, Walker WJ. Ineffectiveness of quinidine in preventing atrial fibrillation following mitral valvotomy. *Circulation* 1966;34:792–794.

128. Merrick AF, Odom NJ, Keenan DJ, Grotte GJ. Comparison of propafenone to atenolol for the prophylaxis of postcardiotomy supraventricular tachyarrhythmias: a prospective trial. *Eur J Cardiothorac Surg* 1995;9:146–149.

129. Borgeat A, Petropoulos P, Cavin R, et al. Prevention of arrhythmias after noncardiac thoracic operations: flecainide versus digoxin. *Ann Thorac Surg* 1991;51:964–968.

130. Suttorp MJ, Kingma JH, Peels HO, et al. Effectiveness of sotalol in preventing supraventricular tachyarrhythmias shortly after coronary artery bypass grafting. *Am J Cardiol* 1991;68:1163–1169.

131. Gomes JA, Ip J, Santoni-Rugiu F, et al. Oral d,l-sotalol reduces the incidence of postoperative atrial fibrillation in coronary artery bypass surgery patients: a randomized, double-blind, placebo-controlled study. *J Am Coll Cardiol* 1999;34:334–339.

132. Nystrom U, Edvardsson N, Berggren H, et al. Oral sotalol reduces the incidence of atrial fibrillation after coronary artery bypass surgery. *Thorac Cardiovasc Surg* 1993;41:34–37.

133. Pfisterer ME, Kloter-Weber UC, Huber M, et al. Prevention of supraventricular tachyarrhythmias after open heart operation by low-dose sotalol: a prospective, double-blind, randomized, placebo-controlled study. *Ann Thorac Surg* 1997;64:1113–1119.

134. Parikka H, Toivonen L, Heikkila L, et al. Comparison of sotalol and metoprolol in the prevention of atrial fibrillation after coronary artery bypass surgery. *J Cardiovasc Pharmacol* 1998;31:67–73.

135. Jacquet L, Evenepoel M, Marenne F, et al. Hemodynamic effects and safety of sotalol in the prevention of supraventricular arrhythmias after coronary artery bypass surgery. *J Cardiothorac Vasc Anesth* 1994;8:431–436.

136. Suttorp MJ, Kingma JH, Tjon Joe Gin RM, et al. Efficacy and safety of low- and high-dose sotalol versus propranolol in the prevention of supraventricular tachyarrhythmias early after coronary artery bypass operations. *J Thorac Cardiovasc Surg* 1990;100:921–926.

137. Hohnloser SH, Meinertz T, Dammbacher T, et al. Electrocardiographic and antiarrhythmic effects of intravenous amiodarone: results of a prospective, placebo-controlled study. *Am Heart J* 1991;121:89–95.

138. Butler J, Harriss DR, Sinclair M, Westaby S. Amiodarone prophylaxis for tachycardias after coronary artery surgery: a randomised, double blind, placebo controlled trial. *Br Heart J* 1993;70:56–60.

139. Daoud EG, Strickberger SA, Man KC, et al. Preoperative amiodarone as prophylaxis against atrial fibrillation after heart surgery. *N Engl J Med* 1997;337:1785–1791.

140. Redle JD, Khurana S, Marzan R, et al. Prophylactic oral amiodarone compared with placebo for prevention of atrial fibrillation after coronary artery bypass surgery. *Am Heart J* 1999;138:144–150.

141. Guarnieri T, Nolan S, Gottlieb SO, et al. Intravenous amiodarone for the prevention of atrial fibrillation after open heart surgery: the Amiodarone Reduction in Coronary Heart (ARCH) trial. *J Am Coll Cardiol* 1999;34:343–347.

142. Khan RM, Hodge JS, Bassett HF. Magnesium in open-heart surgery. *J Thorac Cardiovasc Surg* 1973;66:185–191.

143. Fanning WJ, Thomas CS Jr, Roach A, et al. Prophylaxis of atrial fibrillation with magnesium sulfate after coronary artery bypass grafting. *Ann Thorac Surg* 1991;52:529–533.

144. Katholi R, Taylor G, Woods W, et al. MgCl2 replacement after bypass surgery to prevent atrial fibrillation: a double blind, randomized trial. *Circulation* 1990;82[Suppl III]:III58.

145. Casthely PA, Yoganathan T, Komer C, Kelly M. Magnesium and arrhythmias after coronary artery bypass surgery. *J Cardiothorac Vasc Anesth* 1994;8:188–191.

146. Parikka H, Toivonen L, Pellinen T, et al. The influence of intravenous magnesium sulphate on the occurrence of atrial fibrilla-

tion after coronary artery by-pass operation. *Eur Heart J* 1993; 14:251–258.

147. Wistbacka JO, Koistinen J, Karlqvist KE, et al. Magnesium substitution in elective coronary artery surgery: a double-blind clinical study. *J Cardiothorac Vasc Anesth* 1995;9:140–146.

148. Gerstenfeld EP, Hill MR, French SN, et al. Evaluation of right atrial and biatrial temporary pacing for the prevention of atrial fibrillation after coronary artery bypass surgery. *J Am Coll Cardiol* 1999;33:1981–1988.

149. Kurz DJ, Naegeli B, Kunz M, et al. Epicardial, biatrial synchronous pacing for prevention of atrial fibrillation after cardiac surgery. *Pacing Clin Electrophysiol* 1999;22:721–726.

150. Chung M, Augostini R, Asher C, et al. Ineffectiveness and potential proarrhythmia of atrial pacing for the prevention of atrial fibrillation after coronary artery bypass surgery. *Ann Thorac Surg* 2000 *(in press)*.

151. Greenberg MD, Katz NM, Iuliano S, et al. Atrial pacing for the prevention of atrial fibrillation after cardiovascular surgery [Comments]. *J Am Coll Cardiol* 2000;35:1416–1422.

152. Blommaert D, Gonzalez M, Mucumbitsi J, et al. Effective prevention of atrial fibrillation by continuous atrial overdrive pacing after coronary artery bypass surgery [see comments]. *J Am Coll Cardiol* 2000;35:1411–1415.

153. Klemperer JD, Klein IL, Ojamaa K, et al. Triiodothyronine therapy lowers the incidence of atrial fibrillation after cardiac operations. *Ann Thorac Surg* 1996;61:1323–1329.

154. Chaney MA, Nikolov MP, Blakeman B, et al. Pulmonary effects of methylprednisolone in patients undergoing coronary artery bypass grafting and early tracheal extubation. *Anesth Analg* 1998;87:27–33.

155. Ovrum E, Am Holen E, Tangen G, Ringdal MA. Heparinized cardiopulmonary bypass and full heparin dose marginally improve clinical performance. *Ann Thorac Surg* 1996;62: 1128–1133.

156. Lazar HL, Philippides G, Fitzgerald C, et al. Glucose-insulin-potassium solutions enhance recovery after urgent coronary artery bypass grafting. *J Thorac Cardiovasc Surg* 1997;113: 354–362.

157. Wistbacka JO, Kaukoranta PK, Nuutinen LS. Prebypass glucose-insulin-potassium infusion in elective nondiabetic coronary artery surgery patients. *J Cardiothorac Vasc Anesth* 1992;6:521–527.

158. Kuralay E, Ozal E, Demirkili U, Tatar H. Effect of posterior pericardiotomy on postoperative supraventricular arrhythmias and late pericardial effusion (posterior pericardiotomy). *J Thorac Cardiovasc Surg* 1999;118:492–495.

159. Asimakopoulos G, Della Santa R, Taggart DP. Effects of posterior pericardiotomy on the incidence of atrial fibrillation and chest drainage after coronary revascularization: a prospective randomized trial. *J Thorac Cardiovasc Surg* 1997;113:797–799.

160. Tisdale JE, Padhi ID, Goldberg AD, et al. A randomized, double-blind comparison of intravenous diltiazem and digoxin for atrial fibrillation after coronary artery bypass surgery. *Am Heart J* 1998;135:739–747.

161. Landymore RW, Howell F. Recurrent atrial arrhythmias following treatment for postoperative atrial fibrillation after coronary bypass operations. *Eur J Cardiothorac Surg* 1991;5:436–439.

162. Myers MG, Alnemri K. Rate control therapy for atrial fibrillation following coronary artery bypass surgery. *Can J Cardiol* 1998;14:1363–1366.

163. Solomon AJ, Kouretas PC, Hopkins RA, et al. Early discharge of patients with new-onset atrial fibrillation after cardiovascular surgery. *Am Heart J* 1998;135:557–563.

164. Murray KD, Vlasnik JJ. Procainamide-induced postoperative pyrexia. *Ann Thorac Surg* 1999;68:1072–1074.

165. VanderLugt JT, Mattioni T, Denker S, et al. Efficacy and safety of ibutilide fumarate for the conversion of atrial arrhythmias after cardiac surgery. *Circulation* 1999;100:369–375.

166. Volgman AS, Carberry PA, Stambler B, et al. Conversion efficacy and safety of intravenous ibutilide compared with intravenous procainamide in patients with atrial flutter or fibrillation. *J Am Coll Cardiol* 1998;31:1414–1419.

167. Stambler BS, Wood MA, Ellenbogen KA. Comparative efficacy of intravenous ibutilide versus procainamide for enhancing termination of atrial flutter by atrial overdrive pacing. *Am J Cardiol* 1996;77:960–966.

168. Mostow ND, Vrobel TR, Noon D, Rakita L. Rapid control of refractory atrial tachyarrhythmias with high-dose oral amiodarone. *Am Heart J* 1990;120:1356–1363.

169. Frost L, Mortensen PE, Tingleff J, et al. Efficacy and safety of dofetilide, a new class III antiarrhythmic agent, in acute termination of atrial fibrillation or flutter after coronary artery bypass surgery. Dofetilide Post-CABG Study Group. *Int J Cardiol* 1997;58:135–140.

170. Gentili C, Giordano F, Alois A, et al. Efficacy of intravenous propafenone in acute atrial fibrillation complicating open-heart surgery. *Am Heart J* 1992;123:1225–1228.

171. Connolly SJ, Mulji AS, Hoffert DL, et al. Randomized placebo-controlled trial of propafenone for treatment of atrial tachyarrhythmias after cardiac surgery. *J Am Coll Cardiol* 1987;10: 1145–1148.

172. Liebold A, Haisch G, Rosada B, Kleine P. Internal atrial defibrillation—a new treatment of postoperative atrial fibrillation. *Thorac Cardiovasc Surg* 1998;46:323–326.

173. Kleine P, Blommaert D, van Nooten G, et al. Multicenter results of TADpole heart wire system used to treat postoperative atrial fibrillation. *Eur J Cardiothorac Surg* 1999;15:525–527.

174. Liebold A, Rodig G, Birnbaum DE. Performance of temporary epicardial stainless steel wire electrodes used to treat atrial fibrillation: a study in patients following open heart surgery. *Pacing Clin Electrophysiol* 1999;22:315–319.

175. Raitt M, Dolack G, Kino K, et al. Procainamide has limited effectiveness for the treatment of atrial fibrillation after open heart surgery. *Circulation* 1994;90:I376.

176. Yilmaz AT, Demirkilic U, Arslan M, et al. Long-term prevention of atrial fibrillation after coronary artery bypass surgery: comparison of quinidine, verapamil, and amiodarone in maintaining sinus rhythm. *J Cardiac Surg* 1996;11:61–64.

177. Waldo AL, MacLean WA, Cooper TB, et al. Use of temporarily placed epicardial atrial wire electrodes for the diagnosis and treatment of cardiac arrhythmias following open-heart surgery. *J Thorac Cardiovasc Surg* 1978;76:500–505.

178. Malcolm ID, Cherry DA, Morin JE. The use of temporary atrial electrodes to improve diagnostic capabilities with Holter monitoring after cardiac surgery. *Ann Thorac Surg* 1986;41:103–105.

179. Feld GK, Fleck RP, Chen PS, et al. Radiofrequency catheter ablation for the treatment of human type 1 atrial flutter. Identification of a critical zone in the reentrant circuit by endocardial mapping techniques. *Circulation* 1992;86:1233–1240.

180. Flugelman MY, Hasin Y, Katznelson N, et al. Restoration and maintenance of sinus rhythm after mitral valve surgery for mitral stenosis. *Am J Cardiol* 1984;54:617–619.

181. Skoularigis J, Rothlisberger C, Skudicky D, et al. Effectiveness of amiodarone and electrical cardioversion for chronic rheumatic atrial fibrillation after mitral valve surgery. *Am J Cardiol* 1993;72:423–427.

182. Laupacis A, Albers G, Dalen J, et al. Antithrombotic therapy in atrial fibrillation. *Chest* 1998;114:579S–589S.

183. Arnold AZ, Mick MJ, Mazurek RP, et al. Role of prophylactic anticoagulation for direct current cardioversion in patients with atrial fibrillation or atrial flutter. *J Am Coll Cardiol* 1992;19: 851–855.

184. Gardner TJ, Horneffer PJ, Manolio TA, et al. Stroke following coronary artery bypass grafting: a ten-year study. *Ann Thorac Surg* 1985;40:574–581.

185. D'Agostino RS, Svensson LG, Neumann DJ, et al. Screening carotid ultrasonography and risk factors for stroke in coronary artery surgery patients. *Ann Thorac Surg* 1996;62:1714–1723.

186. Hogue CW Jr, Murphy SF, Schechtman KB, Davila-Roman VG. Risk factors for early or delayed stroke after cardiac surgery. *Circulation* 1999;100:642–647.

187. Humphries JO. Unexpected instant death following successful coronary artery bypass graft surgery (and other clinical settings): atrial fibrillation, quinidine, procainamide, et cetera, and instant death. *Clin Cardiol* 1998;21:711–718.

188. Yousif H, Davies G, Oakley CM. Peri-operative supraventricular arrhythmias in coronary bypass surgery. *Int J Cardiol* 1990;26:313–318.

189. Yilmaz AT, Demirkilic U, Kuralay E, et al. Long-term prevention of atrial fibrillation after coronary artery surgery. *Panminerva Med* 1997;39:103–105.

190. Paone G, Higgins RS, Havstad SL, Silverman NA. Does age limit the effectiveness of clinical pathways after coronary artery bypass graft surgery? *Circulation* 1998;98:II41–II45.

191. Smith R, Grossman W, Johnson L, et al. Arrhythmias following cardiac valve replacement. *Circulation* 1972;45:1018–1023.

192. Douglas PS, Hirshfeld JW Jr, Edmunds LH Jr. Clinical correlates of atrial tachyarrhythmias after valve replacement for aortic stenosis. *Circulation* 1985;72:II159–II163.

193. Tambeur L, Meyns B, Flameng W, Daenen W. Rhythm disturbances after mitral valve surgery: comparison between left atrial and extended trans-septal approach. *Cardiovasc Surg* 1996;4:820–824.

194. Obadia JF, el Farra M, Bastien OH, et al. Outcome of atrial fibrillation after mitral valve repair. *J Thorac Cardiovasc Surg* 1997;114:179–185.

195. Vogt PR, Brunner-LaRocca HP, Rist M, et al. Preoperative predictors of recurrent atrial fibrillation late after successful mitral valve reconstruction. *Eur J Cardiothorac Surg* 1998;13:619–624.

196. Favaloro RG, Effler DB, Groves LK, et al. Direct myocardial revascularization with saphenous vein autograft. Clinical experience in 100 cases. *Dis Chest* 1969;56:279–283.

197. Abedin Z, Soares J, Phillips DF, Sheldon WC. Ventricular tachyarrhythmias following surgery for myocardial revascularization. A follow-up study. *Chest* 1977;72:426–428.

198. Hoie J, Forfang K. Arrhythmias and conduction disturbances following aortic valve implantation. *Scand J Thorac Cardiovasc Surg* 1980;14:177–183.

199. Johnson RG, Shafique T, Sirois C, et al. Potassium concentrations and ventricular ectopy: a prospective, observational study in post–cardiac surgery patients. *Crit Care Med* 1999;27:2430–2434.

200. Smith RC KF, Merrick S, Mangano DT. Ventricular dysrhythmias in patients undergoing coronary artery bypass graft surgery: incidence, characteristics, and prognostic importance. *Am Heart J* 1992;123:73–81.

201. Tchervenkov CI, Wynands JE, Symes JF, et al. Electrical behavior of the heart following high-potassium cardioplegia. *Ann Thorac Surg* 1983;36:314–319.

202. Surawicz B. Is hypomagnesemia or magnesium deficiency arrhythmogenic? *J Am Coll Cardiol* 1989;14:1093–1096.

203. Myerburg RJ, Kessler KM, Bassett AL, Castellanos A. A biological approach to sudden cardiac death: structure, function and cause. *Am J Cardiol* 1989;63:1512–1516.

204. Moran JM. Postoperative ventricular arrhythmia. *Ann Thorac Surg* 1984;38:312–313.

205. Huikuri HVKU, Ikaheimo MJ, Takkunen JT. Prevalence and prognostic significance of complex ventricular arrhythmias after coronary arterial bypass graft surgery. *Int J Cardiol* 1990;27:333–339.

206. Pinto RPNW, Scheir JJ, Surawicz B. Prognosis of patients with frequent premature ventricular complexes and nonsustained ventricular tachycardia after coronary artery bypass graft surgery. *Clin Cardiol* 1996;19:321–324.

207. King FGAA, Peters SD. Prophylactic lidocaine for the postoperative coronary artery bypass patient: a double-blind, randomized trial. *Can J Anesthesiol* 1990;37:363–368.

208. Landow LWJ. An improved lidocaine infusion protocol for cardiac surgical patients. *J Cardiothorac Vasc Anesth* 1991;5.

209. Shigemitsu OHT, Takasami H, Shirabe J, Ito M. Analysis of perioperative ventricular arrhythmias in valvular heart diseases by Holter ECG recording. *Jpn Circ J* 1991;55:951–961.

210. Rousou JA, Engelman RM, Flack JE 3rd, et al. Emergency cardiopulmonary bypass in the cardiac surgical unit can be a life-saving measure in postoperative cardiac arrest. *Circulation* 1994;90:II280–II284.

211. Bhandari AK, Au PK, Rose JS, et al. Decline in inducibility of sustained ventricular tachycardia from two to twenty weeks after acute myocardial infarction. *Am J Cardiol* 1987;59:284–290.

212. Bigger JT Jr, and the CABG Patch Trial Investigators. Prophylactic use of implanted cardiac defibrillators in patients at high risk for ventricular arrhythmias after coronary-artery bypass graft surgery. Coronary Artery Bypass Graft (CABG) Patch Trial Investigators. *N Engl J Med* 1997;337:1569–1575.

213. Takeda M, Furuse A, Kotsuka Y. Use of temporary atrial pacing in management of patients after cardiac surgery. *Cardiovasc Surg* 1996;4:623–627.

214. Wexelman W, Lichstein E, Cunningham JN, et al. Etiology and clinical significance of new fascicular conduction defects following coronary bypass surgery. *Am Heart J* 1986;111:923–927.

215. Baerman JM, Kirsh MM, de Buitleir M, et al. Natural history and determinants of conduction defects following coronary artery bypass surgery. *Ann Thorac Surg* 1987;44:150–153.

216. Baraka AS, Taha SK, Yazbeck VK, et al. Transient atrioventricular block after release of aortic cross-clamp. *Anesth Analg* 1995;80:54–57.

217. Caspi J, Amar R, Elami A, et al. Frequency and significance of complete atrioventricular block after coronary artery bypass grafting. *Am J Cardiol* 1989;63:526–529.

218. Tuzcu EM, Emre A, Goormastic M, et al. Incidence and prognostic significance of intraventricular conduction abnormalities after coronary bypass surgery. *J Am Coll Cardiol* 1990;16:607–610.

219. Hippelainen M, Mustonen P, Manninen H, Rehnberg S. Predictors of conduction disturbances after coronary bypass grafting [Comments]. *Ann Thorac Surg* 1994;57:1284–1287.

220. Emlein G, Huang SK, Pires LA, et al. Prolonged bradyarrhythmias after isolated coronary artery bypass graft surgery. *Am Heart J* 1993;126:1084–1090.

221. Gundry SR, Sequeira A, TR C, McLaughlin JS. Postoperative conduction disturbances: a comparison of blood and crystalloid cardioplegia. *Ann Thorac Surg* 1989;47:384–390.

222. Feldman S, Glikson M, Kaplinsky E. Pacemaker dependency after coronary artery bypass. *Pacing Clin Electrophysiol* 1992;15:2037–2040.

223. Keefe DL, Griffin JC, Harrison DC, Stinson EB. Atrioventricular conduction abnormalities in patients undergoing isolated aortic or mitral valve replacement. *Pacing Clin Electrophysiol* 1985;8:393–398.

224. Moore SL, Wilkoff BL. Rhythm disturbances after cardiac surgery. *Semin Thorac Cardiovasc Surg* 1991;3:24–28.

225. Jaeger FJ, Trohman RG, Brener S, Loop F. Permanent pacing following repeat cardiac valve surgery. *Am J Cardiol* 1994;74:505–507.

226. Brodell GK, Cosgrove D, Schiavone W, et al. Cardiac rhythm and conduction disturbances in patients undergoing mitral valve surgery. *Cleve Clin J Med* 1991;58:397–399.

227. Gaillard D, Lespinasse P, Vanetti A. Cardiac pacing and valvular surgery. *Pacing Clin Electrophysiol* 1988;11:2142–2148.

228. Nair CK, Sketch MH, Ahmed I, et al. Calcific valvular aortic stenosis with and without mitral anular calcium. *Am J Cardiol* 1987;60:865–870.

229. Cooper JP, Jayawickreme SR, Swanton RH. Permanent pacing in patients with tricuspid valve replacements. *Br Heart J* 1995;73:169–172.

230. Takeshita M, Furuse A, Kotsuka Y, Kubota H. Sinus node function after mitral valve surgery via the transseptal superior approach. *Eur J Cardiothorac Surg* 1997;12:341–344.

231. Ellis RJ, Mavroudis C, Gardner C, et al. Relationship between atrioventricular arrhythmias and the concentration of K+ ion in cardioplegic solution. *J Thorac Cardiovasc Surg* 1980;80:517–526.

232. Ferguson TB Jr, Cox JL. Temporary external DDD pacing after cardiac operations. *Ann Thorac Surg* 1991;51:723–732.

233. Almassi GH, Wetherbee JN, Hoffmann RG, Olinger GN. Optimal lead positioning for postoperative atrial pacing. *Chest* 1992;101:1194–1196.

234. Del Nido P, Goldman BS. Temporary epicardial pacing after open heart surgery: complications and prevention. *J Cardiac Surg* 1989;4:99–103.

235. Heinz G, Kratochwill C, Buxbaum P, et al. Immediate normalization of profound sinus node dysfunction by aminophylline after cardiac transplantation. *Am J Cardiol* 1993;71:346–349.

236. Haught WH, Bertolet BD, Conti JB, et al. Theophylline reverses high-grade atrioventricular block resulting from cardiac transplant rejection. *Am Heart J* 1994;128:1255–1257.

237. Bertolet BD, Eagle DA, Conti JB, et al. Bradycardia after heart transplantation: reversal with theophylline. *J Am Coll Cardiol* 1996;28:396–399.

238. Raghavan C, Maloney JD, Nitta J, et al. Long-term follow-up of heart transplant recipients requiring permanent pacemakers. *J Heart Lung Transplantation* 1995;14:1081–1089.

239. Broka SM, Ducart AR, Collard EL, et al. Hemodynamic benefit of optimizing atrioventricular delay after cardiopulmonary bypass. *J Cardiothorac Vasc Anesth* 1997;11:723–728.

240. Ivey MF, Ivey TD, Bailey WW, et al. Influence of propranolol on supraventricular tachycardia early after coronary artery revascularization. A randomized trial. *J Thorac Cardiovasc Surg* 1983;85:214–218.

241. Ali IM, Sanalla AA, Clark V. Beta-blocker effects on postoperative atrial fibrillation. *Eur J Cardiothorac Surg* 1997;11:1154–1157.

242. Janssen J, Loomans L, Harink J, et al. Prevention and treatment of supraventricular tachycardia shortly after coronary artery bypass grafting: a randomized open trial. *Angiology* 1986;37:601–609.

243. Gavaghan TP, Feneley MP, Campbell TJ, Morgan JJ. Atrial tachyarrhythmias after cardiac surgery: results of disopyramide therapy. *Aust N Z J Med* 1985;15:27–32.

244. Hjelms E. Procainamide conversion of acute atrial fibrillation after open-heart surgery compared with digoxin treatment. *Scand J Thorac Cardiovasc Surg* 1992;26:193–196.

245. McAlister HF, Luke RA, Whitlock RM, Smith WM. Intravenous amiodarone bolus versus oral quinidine for atrial flutter and fibrillation after cardiac operations. *J Thorac Cardiovasc Surg* 1990;99:911–918.

246. Geelen P, O'Hara GE, Roy N, et al. Comparison of propafenone versus procainamide for the acute treatment of atrial fibrillation after cardiac surgery. *Am J Cardiol* 1999;84:345–347, A8—A9.

247. Di Biasi P, Scrofani R, Paje A, et al. Intravenous amiodarone vs propafenone for atrial fibrillation and flutter after cardiac operation. *Eur J Cardiothorac Surg* 1995;9:587–591.

248. Larbuisson R, Venneman I, Stiels B. The efficacy and safety of intravenous propafenone versus intravenous amiodarone in the conversion of atrial fibrillation or flutter after cardiac surgery. *J Cardiothorac Vasc Anesth* 1996;10:229–234.

249. Wafa SS, Ward DE, Parker DJ, Camm AJ. Efficacy of flecainide acetate for atrial arrhythmias following coronary artery bypass grafting. *Am J Cardiol* 1989;63:1058–1064.

250. Gavaghan TP, Koegh AM, Kelly RP, et al. Flecainide compared with a combination of digoxin and disopyramide for acute atrial arrhythmias after cardiopulmonary bypass. *Br Heart J* 1988;60:497–501.

251. Campbell TJ, Gavaghan TP, Morgan JJ. Intravenous sotalol for the treatment of atrial fibrillation and flutter after cardiopulmonary bypass. Comparison with disopyramide and digoxin in a randomised trial. *Br Heart J* 1985;54:86–90.

252. Installe E, Schoevaerdts JC, Gadisseux P, et al. Intravenous amiodarone in the treatment of various arrhythmias following cardiac operations. *J Thorac Cardiovasc Surg* 1981;81:302–308.

253. Cochrane AD, Siddins M, Rosenfeldt FL, et al. A comparison of amiodarone and digoxin for treatment of supraventricular arrhythmias after cardiac surgery. *Eur J Cardiothorac Surg* 1994;8:194–198.

30

PERIINFARCTION ARRHYTHMIAS

AZAD V. GHURAN
A. JOHN CAMM

More than 300,000 people die suddenly in the United States each year of coronary artery disease, with the development of ventricular tachyarrhythmias after myocardial infarction being the most common cause (1,2). Sixty percent of deaths associated with acute myocardial infarction occur within the first hour (3) and are attributable to arrhythmias, particularly ventricular fibrillation.

Numerous experimental laboratory studies and clinical observations have furthered our understanding of the pathophysiologic mechanisms underlying malignant arrhythmias in the acute phase of myocardial infarction. Improvements in arrhythmia detection and treatment have had a major impact on the management of primary arrhythmias (i.e., those resulting from ischemia), such that the in-hospital mortality rate for arrhythmias has decreased significantly, and most deaths are now caused by the complications of left ventricular failure occurring 3 to 4 days after infarction (3–5).

VENTRICULAR ARRHYTHMIAS

The correlation between ischemic heart disease and arrhythmias is well established. Angina was linked to sudden death in the 18th century by Heberden (6), and the connection between acute coronary obstruction and ventricular arrhythmias was made in 1840 by Erichsen, who demonstrated that ligation of a coronary artery in dogs resulted in cessation of ventricular action with a "a slight tremulous motion alone continuing" (7).

Life-threatening ventricular arrhythmias most commonly occur in the setting of ischemic heart disease (8,9), and abnormal ventricular rhythms, stable and unstable, are a common occurrence in the periinfarction period. The reported incidence of periinfarction ventricular arrhythmia varies considerably, with ventricular premature contractions occurring in 10% to 93%, ventricular tachycardia in 3% to 39%, and ventricular fibrillation in 4% to 36% (10,11). The occurrence of life-threatening ventricular arrhythmias is almost certainly underestimated in view of the proportion of patients for whom sudden death is the first presenting feature of their myocardial infarction (12,13).

Lethal periinfarction ventricular arrhythmias are caused by an interplay between three basic components: substrate, such as the presence of potential reentry circuits within the infarcted area; trigger, such as premature ventricular contractions (PVCs), variations in cycle length, and heart rate; and modulating factors, such as ischemia-induced electrolyte imbalance, dysfunction of the autonomic nervous system, and impaired left ventricular function, which may act on substrate and trigger to induce arrhythmia. Investigation of these components has led to the development of a large number of animal models. Clinical observations have also played an important role (14).

Cellular Effects of Acute Ischemia

Myocardial ischemia has rapid and profound effects on the electrophysiologic characteristics of the myocyte. Changes in the resting membrane potential and the inward and outward ionic fluxes during the action potential lead to alterations in conduction, refractoriness, and automaticity of cardiac muscle cells, all of which contribute to the occurrence of ventricular arrhythmias (15).

Resting Membrane Potential

Experimental coronary artery occlusion causes myocardial cells to depolarize (16). The fall in resting potential is associated with an alteration in transmembrane potassium distribution and an increase in extracellular potassium concentration from 4 to 14.7 mM within 15 minutes of coronary occlusion in guinea pig hearts (17). Potassium accumulation occurs in two phases. The first is amenable to reversibility with reperfusion (provided this occurs within

A. V. Ghuran: Department of Cardiology, Houston Medical School, Houston, Texas 77030.

A. J. Camm: Department of Cardiological Science, St. George's Medical School, London SW 17 ORE, United Kingdom.

15 minutes), and the second phase is irreversible, representing permanent cellular damage (18–20).

Alterations of potassium distribution caused by acute ischemia reflect an imbalance between potassium influx and efflux. Studies from rabbit hearts have demonstrated that the primary component of ischemia-induced extracellular potassium rise is excess potassium efflux compared with influx (20). Further animal experiments have shown that in the early stages of ischemia (<10 minutes) the sodium-potassium pump is only mildly depressed (15). It has been suggested that potassium loss results from increased permeability of the cell membrane to anions, such as inorganic phosphate and lactate (21). The development of intracellular acidosis has also been implicated in potassium loss from myocardial cells (17).

Among other products accumulating in ischemic myocardium, a group of compounds known as lysophosphoglycerides (LPGs) have been implicated in mediating adverse electrophysiologic changes. Of these, lysophosphatidylcholine and lysophosphatidylethanolamine are the most important (22). When LPG is added to the superfusate of isolated normal myocardium and Purkinje fibers, electrical changes are produced that are similar to those of ischemic myocardium: depolarization of resting membrane potential, separation of the action potential upstroke into two components, and postrepolarization refractoriness (23–25). Small amounts of LPG augment the effect of hypoxia and elevated potassium, and this phenomenon is intensified by the influence of acidosis (26). High concentrations of LPG cause disruption of the cell membrane, contributing to massive calcium entry and eventually to cell death (27,28).

Changes in the Action Potential

The action potential is also significantly affected by acute ischemia. The changes that occur include a reduction in amplitude, upstroke velocity, and duration. The alterations seen are not merely a result of changes in the resting membrane potential; action potentials with similar properties may be produced by coronary perfusion with solutions containing no substrate, very low Po_2, and high potassium levels, and a low pH.

In the central ischemic zone, postrepolarization refractoriness results in lengthening of the refractory period, whereas in the areas bordering the main area of infarction, refractory periods shorten. This inhomogeneity is partly caused by diffusion of potassium from the ischemic areas of the myocardium toward more normal myocardium. This situation, together with catecholamine-induced stimulation of the sodium-potassium pump, allows previously inexcitable cells to regain their excitability, and after 10 to 20 minutes of ischemia, extracellular potassium levels begin to return to normal (15).

Changes in action potential upstroke characteristics cause a reduction in conduction velocity by approximately 50% during the first 5 to 10 minutes of ischemia; thereafter, coupling resistance increases rapidly, indicating irreversible injury (15). As heart rate increases, there is a further reduction in conduction velocity brought about by rate-dependent changes in intracellular sodium and calcium ion concentrations (29,30). This rate-dependent conduction slowing is an important mechanism in the origin of reentry arrhythmias.

Mechanisms of Periinfarction Ventricular Arrhythmia

When considering the mechanisms responsible for periinfarction ventricular arrhythmias, a distinction must be made between the acute phase of myocardial ischemia (i.e., first 30 minutes) and the subacute or delayed phase (i.e., 6 to 72 hours after infarction). This distinction is necessary because of variations in clinical arrhythmia type, cellular mechanisms, and immediate prognostic implications.

Acute-Phase Ischemia

During experimental coronary artery occlusion, arrhythmias occurring within the first 30 minutes demonstrate a bimodal distribution. Arrhythmias occurring after 2 to 10 minutes of ischemia are known as "immediate" or phase 1a ventricular arrhythmias, having a peak incidence after 5 to 6 minutes of ischemia. Delayed or phase 1b arrhythmias occur after approximately 12 to 30 minutes of coronary artery occlusion (31).

Experimental evidence suggests that phase 1a and 1b arrhythmias have different mechanisms. Phase 1a arrhythmias occur when there is marked conduction slowing and delayed activation in the subepicardial muscle, which is coincident with highly abnormal subepicardial electrograms due to membrane depolarization and the consequent decrease in membrane action potential amplitude (10). As a result of these changes, some electrograms are altered from smooth, high-amplitude deflections to fractionated electrograms, and there is evidence to suggest that these are a result of inhomogeneous conduction (32).

One phenomenon of the fractionated electrogram is diastolic bridging, which often precedes ventricular ectopic activity. Diastolic bridging is most easily recorded on a composite electrode, which is an electrode with multiple recording poles covering a large area of the epicardial surface (33). On the basis of these electrocardiographic findings, it was proposed and later confirmed that reentry is a dominant mechanism of phase 1a arrhythmias (32,34–36).

Reentry, or circus movement, is a major cause of ventricular tachyarrhythmias. It requires an area with abnormally slow conduction and an adjacent pathway exhibiting unidirectional block. Sufficiently slow conduction to allow recovery of excitability in the blocked pathway is necessary to permit retrograde conduction over this route to complete the circuit. The characteristic slow and inhomogeneous activation of the ischemic myocardium coupled with the association between fractionated electrograms and early postinfarction arrhythmias supports reentry as a likely mechanism. More concrete evidence for reentry in this context has been derived from mapping experiments, in which circus movements with a diameter of 1 to 2 cm were found to be the mechanism of ventricular tachycardia, occurring 2 to 10 minutes after coronary occlusion in porcine and canine hearts (37). During ventricular fibrillation, multiple reentrant wavelets are present, which travel independently around multiple islets of temporary conduction block (10). It has also been suggested that during phase 1a, a nonreentry mechanism initiates ventricular premature depolarizations, which may precipitate reentrant arrhythmias. The possible origin for this series of events is triggered activity resulting from afterdepolarizations and abnormal automaticity (i.e., spontaneous impulse formation based on phase 4 depolarization in cells with reduced maximum diastolic potential) (38).

The mechanism that gives rise to phase 1b arrhythmias has not been fully elucidated. They possibly arise as a result of abnormal automaticity because of the increased catecholamine release that occurs after 15 to 20 minutes of ischemia (39–41). Subepicardial electrograms recorded during phase 1b are not as abnormal as those recorded during phase 1a, and there may be less spatial inhomogeneity of subepicardial activation. In animal experiments, phase 1b arrhythmias are always preceded by spontaneous improvement in action potential amplitude and by shortening of the refractory period, (15) but these changes are absent when the hearts are pretreated with propranolol.

Delayed Ventricular Arrhythmias

The delayed events generally occur 3 to 6 hours into the evolving myocardial infarction, but this phase of arrhythmias may last up to 3 days. The most frequently observed ventricular arrhythmias during the delayed phase of acute infarction are ventricular ectopic beats (i.e., single or in runs of two or three beats), ventricular tachycardia, and accelerated idioventricular rhythm (42,43). In studies in which electrocardiographic monitoring was initiated within 8 hours after infarction, a 47% incidence of ventricular tachycardia or slow ventricular rhythms was reported (44).

The exact mechanism leading to the genesis of delayed periinfarction arrhythmias in humans remains virtually unknown. In the canine model, myocardial necrosis after coronary artery occlusion begins several millimeters from the endocardial surface and progresses as a wavefront toward the epicardium, and in full-thickness infarcts, it stops short of the epicardium by 1 to 30 muscle fiber widths (45–47). The progressing infarction also causes attrition of the endocardial layers until, by 14 hours, only scattered islands of irreversibly damaged myocardial cells remain. Most of the subendocar-

dial surface is then taken up with surviving Purkinje cells, and it is these cells that are thought to be the initiators of most delayed postinfarction arrhythmias (45,48); the probable dominant mechanism is abnormal automaticity in surviving Purkinje fibers (15), although there is some evidence that enhanced normal automaticity may also play a role (49). Surviving Purkinje cells have an increased sensitivity to catecholamines, and delayed arrhythmias can be provoked by stimulation of the sympathetic nervous system. Some arrhythmias may be caused by a combination of focal activity and reentry in Purkinje cells, because prolongation of the action potential in these cells produces unidirectional block, which enables reentry to occur.

Role of the Autonomic Nervous System

Relative excess in sympathetic over vagal activity may result in increased arrhythmogenesis resulting from alteration of the sodium-potassium pump or potassium conductance of the myocardial cell membrane, leading to hyperpolarization of the membrane (50).

In animal experiments, impaired vagal competence and a relative excess in sympathetic activity, when associated with acute ischemia, result in an increased incidence of ventricular arrhythmias and sudden death (51). Further experiments have suggested that decreased vagal activity may result from tonic sympathetic restraint caused by increased activity in sympathetically innervated myocardial stretch receptors (52). In clinical studies, a greater reduction in baroreflex sensitivity has been seen in inferior than in anterior infarction (53), suggesting a greater decrease in vagal activity; it has been proposed that this results from excess damage to afferent parasympathetic neurons, which have their greatest concentration in the posteroinferior portion of the heart. Conversely, stimulation of these parasympathetic afferent neurons can cause a reflex bradycardia, vasodilatation, and hypotension (i.e., Benzold-Jarisch reflex) (54). This transient increase in vagal activity is one of the factors involved in the development of bradyarrhythmias during inferior myocardial infarctions.

In the late postinfarction period, impaired parasympathetic tone, as documented by decreased baroreflex sensitivity and heart rate variability (HRV), has been associated with increased inducibility of sustained monomorphic ventricular tachycardia and with sudden death (55–57).

Clinical Features of Ventricular Arrhythmias

Premature Ventricular Contractions

PVCs are common after acute myocardial infarction; the reported incidence is as high as 93% (10). Patients are usually asymptomatic, and physical findings are limited to irregularities in the pulse and occasional cannon waves in the jugular venous pulse. Before the widespread use of thrombolysis, aspirin, and β-blocker therapy, it was felt that the frequency, multiformity, and coupling intervals of PVCs were harbingers for the development of ventricular arrhythmias. It is now clear that PVCs in the early periinfarction period (in contrast to the late infarction period) are not correlated with mortality or the development of ventricular tachyarrhythmias (58,59).

Ventricular Tachycardia

Accelerated idioventricular rhythm (60) has a rate between 50 and 120 bpm. It occurs commonly in the setting of acute myocardial infarction (up to 50% of cases) and has been associated with reperfusion of the myocardium after thrombolytic therapy (61). It is caused by an abnormal ventricular focus, which takes over as the dominant pacemaker during periods of depressed sinoatrial or atrioventricular (AV) nodal automaticity. It can also occur during periods of high vagal tone.

Ventricular tachycardia is defined as three or more consecutive beats arising below the AV node, with an R-R interval of less than 500 ms (>120 bpm). It can be described as sustained or nonsustained and as monomorphic, multiple monomorphic, or polymorphic.

In the setting of acute myocardial infarction, polymorphic ventricular tachycardia (PVT) (Fig. 30-1) has an overall incidence of 2% (62) and is not consistently related to QT interval prolongation, sinus bradycardia, sinus pauses, or electrolyte abnormalities. When present, it is most often associated with symptoms or signs of recurrent myocardial ischemia.

The manifestations of ventricular tachycardia during acute myocardial infarction depend on the characteristics of the tachycardia and on left ventricular function. Significant hemodynamic compromise may occur if the tachycardia is sustained and rapid or left ventricular function is poor. Dyspnea, palpitations, or chest pain may occur if a paroxysm is short lived or left ventricular function has been maintained. In both situations, ventricular tachycardia increases myocardial oxygen demand, which may result in exacerbation of ischemia and possible infarct extension. Occasionally, ventricular tachycardia is the presenting feature of an otherwise silent myocardial infarction.

In the setting of acute myocardial infarction, the initial priority is to obtain electrocardiographic documentation of the cardiac rhythm. At first, this can be done with a bedside monitor, but if the situation allows, a 12-lead electrocardiogram (ECG) should be obtained when the patient has a sustained arrhythmia. The main differential diagnosis to be considered is supraventricular tachycardia with aberrant (e.g., bundle branch block) or preexcited AV conduction. This distinction is important, because it has immediate implications with respect to management. Misdiagnosis and inappropriate treatment at this stage can have severe consequences (63,64). Intravenous adenosine (to a dose of 0.25 mg/kg), because of its short-lived dromotropic effect on the AV node, can terminate or reveal most supraventricular tachycardias, but it has no effect on ventricular arrhythmias and is therefore useful and safe for diagnosis. Given the clinical context of acute ischemia, if there is any doubt, the tachycardia should be treated as ventricular in origin until there is irrefutable evidence to the contrary.

Ventricular Fibrillation

Ventricular fibrillation is a rapid, disorganized ventricular arrhythmia associated with unrecordable blood pressure and no cardiac output. Untreated, the arrhythmia is almost universally lethal, with very few recorded spontaneous reversions to sinus rhythm. During ventricular fibrillation, the ECG shows rapid (150 to 400 bpm), irregular, shapeless QRST undulations of variable amplitude. Some examples of apparent asystole may be low-amplitude or fine ventricular fibrillation (65). Ventricular fibrillation peaks in the early hours of infarction and subsequently declines as the myocardial electrophysiologic environment stabilizes. Approximately 60% of episodes occur within 4 hours and 80% within 12 hours (42). It is the most common cause of out-of-hospital cardiac arrest, accounting for approximately three-fourths of cases, although less than one half of these patients seem to have had an acute myocardial infarction. For reasons not entirely known, the incidence of periinfarction ventricular fibrillation has been declining over the past decade (66). This decline may be related to strategies ensuring early coronary reperfusion with thrombolysis or intervention and with the use of aspirin and β blockers. Periinfarction ventricular fibrillation associated with cardiogenic shock has a poor prognosis, with a mortality rate of 40% to 60% (67).

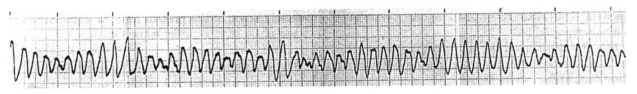

FIGURE 30-1. Polymorphic ventricular tachycardia.

Treatment of Periinfarction Ventricular Arrhythmias

Premature Ventricular Contractions

PVCs are almost universal in the setting of acute myocardial infarction (10). Frequent and complex PVCs are present in the same proportion of patients who develop ventricular fibrillation as those who do not (58). Numerous randomized trials have compared routine antiarrhythmic drugs with placebo. Although a reduction in PVC frequency has been observed, none of the agents administered (with the exception of β blockers) has conclusively reduced arrhythmia, and all cause death (68–70). PVCs are treated conservatively with correction of any ongoing cardiac ischaemia or electrolyte and metabolic disturbances. The β blockers should be administered as early as possible to avoid the proarrhythmic effect of sympathetic stimulation. If periinfarction PVCs are occurring frequently enough to cause hemodynamic compromise and treatment is required, lidocaine (71) is the drug of choice (Table 30-1). It is given as a slow intravenous bolus, followed by an infusion of 1 to 4 mg/min.

Ventricular Tachycardia

Accelerated idioventricular rhythm does not appear to have an adverse effect on mortality, and there is no evidence that its presence increases the incidence of ventricular fibrillation. Most episodes are transient, benign, and require no treatment. However, if the rhythm is causing hemodynamic compromise, such as because of loss of AV synchrony, increasing the sinus node rate with atropine or atrial pacing is indicated.

Rapid treatment of ventricular tachycardia in the periinfarction period is mandatory because of the deleterious effect on cardiac output, the exacerbation of myocardial ischemia, and the risk of deterioration into ventricular fibrillation. The American Heart Association and the American College of Cardiology (ACC/AHA) has published guidelines for the treatment of ventricular tachycardia in the setting of acute myocardial infarction (72) (Table 30-2). Direct current (DC) countershock using 100 to 200 J should be used immediately if there is hemodynamic compromise. After this, an intravenous bolus of lidocaine should be given, and a lidocaine infusion is commenced. Provided that the patient is hemodynamically stable, a trial of drug treatment using intravenous lidocaine, amiodarone, or procainamide should be considered (Table 30-1). Recurrent arrhythmias may be a reflection of continuing ischemia or uncorrected electrolyte imbalance; hypokalemia and hypomagnesemia increase the risk of ventricular arrhythmias (73), and the serum potassium and magnesium levels should be kept above 4.0 and 2 mmol/L, respectively. For recurrent arrhythmias, bretylium can be considered (74). Bretylium results in an initial catecholamine release followed by a reduction and can be particularly effective in suppressing resistant ventricular tachycardia (74). However, a delay of 30 minutes can occur before bretylium exerts its antiarrhythmic effect, and it may be associated with hypotension. Of the available drug therapies, high-dose intravenous amiodarone has been shown to be effective in controlling recalcitrant destabilizing ventricular arrhythmias when other agents such as lidocaine, procainamide, and bretylium had failed (75–77).

Overdrive pacing can also be used to treat persistent recalcitrant ventricular tachycardia, particularly when it is monomorphic (78). It may provide a means of terminating the arrhythmia until the precipitating factors have been controlled or until drug treatment has become effective. Over-

TABLE 30-1. DRUGS USED IN THE TREATMENT OF VENTRICULAR ARRHYTHMIAS DURING MYOCARDIAL INFARCTION

Antiarrhythmic Drugs	Loading Dose	Maintenance	Comments
Lidocaine	1–1.5 mg/kg	1–4 mg/min; reduce after 24 hours to 1–2 mg/min	Additional boluses of 0.5–0.75 mg/kg every 5–10 minutes as needed, to a maximum of 3 mg/kg
Procainamide	10–15 mg/kg over 30–60 min	1–4 mg/min	Caution in patients with renal insufficiency
Amiodarone	150 mg over 10 min	Early infusion of 1 mg/min for 6 hours followed by 0.5 mg/min	Additional infusions of 150 mg frequently needed
Bretylium	5 mg/kg over 10 min	1–2 mg/min	For resistant ventricular fibrillation, repeated dose of 10 mg/kg can be given at 5-minute intervals to a maximum dose of 30–35 mg/kg. A delay of 30 minutes can occur before bretylium exerts its antiarrhythmic effects.

Adapted from Ryan TJ, Antman EM, Brooks NH, et al. 1999 Update: ACC/AHA guidelines for the management of patients with acute myocardial infarction: Executive summary and recommendations. A report of the American College of Cardiology/American Heart Association Task Force on Practice Guidelines (Committee on Management of Acute Myocardial Infarction). *Circulation* 1999;100:1016–1030, with permission.

TABLE 30-2. RECOMMENDATIONS FOR TREATING VENTRICULAR TACHYCARDIA OR VENTRICULAR FIBRILLATION IN ACUTE MYOCARDIAL INFARCTION

Class I

1. Ventricular fibrillation (VF) should be treated with an unsynchronized electric shock with an initial energy of 200 J; if unsuccessful, a second shock of 200 to 300 J should be given, and if necessary, a third shock of 360 J should be given.
2. Sustained (>30 seconds or causing hemodynamic collapse) polymorphic ventricular tachycardia (VT) should be treated with an unsynchronized electric shock using an initial energy of 200 J; if unsuccessful, a second shock of 200 to 300 J should be given, and if necessary, a third shock of 360 J should be given.
3. Episodes of sustained monomorphic VT associated with angina, pulmonary edema, or hypotension (blood pressure <90 mm Hg) should be treated with a synchronized electric shock of 100 J initial energy. Increasing energies may be used if not initially successful.
4. Sustained monomorphic VT not associated with angina, pulmonary edema, or hypotension (blood pressure <90 mm Hg) should be treated with one of the following regimens:
   a. Lidocaine: bolus 1.0 to 1.5 mg/kg. Supplemental boluses of 0.5 to 0.75 mg/kg every 5 to 10 minutes to a maximum of 3 mg/kg total loading dose may be given as needed. Loading is followed by infusion of 2 to 4 mg/min (30 to 50 μg/kg per minute).
   b. Procainamide: 20 to 30 mg/min loading infusion, up to 12 to 17 mg/kg. This may be followed by an infusion of 1 to 4 mg/min.
   c. Amiodarone: 150 mg infused over 10 minutes followed by a constant infusion of 1.0 mg/min for 6 hours and then a maintenance infusion of 0.5 mg/min.
   d. Synchronized electrical cardioversion starting at 50 J (brief anesthesia is necessary).
   Comment: Knowledge of the pharmacokinetics of these agents is important because dosing varies considerably, depending on age, weight, and hepatic and renal function.

Class IIa

1. Infusions of antiarrhythmic drugs may be used after an episode of VT/VF but should be discontinued after 6 to 24 hours and the need for further arrhythmia management assessed.
2. Electrolyte and acid-base disturbances should be corrected to prevent recurrent episodes of VF when an initial episode of VF has been treated.

Class IIb

1. Drug-refractory polymorphic VT should be managed by aggressive attempts to reduce myocardial ischemia, including therapies such as β-adrenoceptor blockade, intraaortic balloon pumping, and emergency angioplasty or bypass surgery. Amiodarone, 150 mg infused over 10 minutes followed by a constant infusion of 1.0 mg/min for up to 6 hours and then a maintenance infusion at 0.5 mg/min, may also be helpful.

Class III

1. Treatment of isolated ventricular premature beats, couplets, runs of accelerated idioventricular rhythm, and nonsustained VT.
2. Prophylactic administration of antiarrhythmic therapy when using thrombolytic agents.

Adapted from Ryan TJ, Antman EM, Brooks NH, et al. *Circulation* 1999;100:1016–1030, with permission.

drive pacing is performed using a transvenous temporary pacing wire positioned in the right ventricle; a burst of 20 to 50 beats, introduced at a rate 10 to 20 bpm faster than the tachycardia, terminates 80% of ventricular tachycardias. However, there is a risk that pacing can result in acceleration of the tachycardia followed by deterioration into ventricular fibrillation. Atrial or ventricular pacing at rates higher than the intrinsic heart rate can help prevent the onset of bradycardic related ventricular tachyarrhythmias.

Distinction between monomorphic ventricular tachycardia and PVT is important and has therapeutic implications. PVT is uncommon and more likely to be associated with ongoing cardiac ischemia. PVT can degenerate into ventricular fibrillation and should be treated as unstable ventricular tachycardia with urgent DC cardioversion. It has a variable response to class 1 agents and may be suppressed by intravenous amiodarone therapy (62). Bretylium may also be more effective for PVT compared with its limited benefit for monomorphic ventricular tachycardia. Intravenous magnesium and overdrive pacing may not be effective in suppressing recurrences. Early nonpharmacologic intervention such as coronary angioplasty or bypass surgery may sometimes be effective (62). Recommendations for the duration of antiarrhythmic drug therapy are discussed in the next section.

Ventricular Fibrillation

The ACC/AHA has published guidelines for the treatment of ventricular fibrillation in the setting of an acute myocardial infarction (72) (Table 30-2). Defibrillation with a DC shock is the definitive treatment for ventricular fibrillation. Defibrillation should be performed as soon as the diagnosis of ventricular fibrillation is considered with an initial shock of 200 J, followed by further shocks of 200 J and 360 J if a stabilized rhythm has not been achieved (79). The likelihood of survival decreases 10% for each minute of time after the onset of uncorrected ventricular fibrillation. According to standard international resuscitation guidelines (79), after three rapid shocks delivered in a row, the patient should be intubated and intravenous access obtained. Epinephrine (1 mg, given intravenously) should be administered and followed by defibrillation at 360 J within 30 to 60 seconds. Epinephrine is given principally as a vasoconstrictor (i.e., α-agonist effect) to increase the efficiency of basic life support, not as an adjuvant to defibrillation, and it should be repeated every 3 minutes. If ventricular fibrillation persists, an antifibrillatory agent such as lidocaine, amiodarone, procainamide, or bretylium can be administered (72) and followed within 30 to 60 seconds by another 360-J shock. There are few data to support lidocaine for the treatment of shock-resistant ventricular fibrillation; rather, the opposite is true, because lidocaine is known to increase the defibrillation threshold. Results from a randomized study of out-of-hospital cardiac arrest suggest that early use of intravenous amiodarone leads to an increase in the proportion resuscitated (80).

There are no definitive data about when to discontinue intravenous antiarrhythmic drug infusions. It is common clinical practice to continue the infusion for a minimum of 48 hours to several days and to discontinue the infusion provided there is no arrhythmia recurrence. For patients with refractory ventricular arrhythmias, high-dose β blockade coupled with atrial or dual-chamber pacemaker therapy, and light anesthesia together with muscle relaxation and artificial ventilation may be lifesaving. Urgent referral for coronary revascularization, implantable cardioverter-defibrillator insertion, or both procedures should be considered for patients who develop ventricular arrhythmias more than 48 hours after the index myocardial infarction or in whom the arrhythmias persist beyond this period.

ATRIAL ARRHYTHMIAS

Sinus Bradycardia

Sinus bradycardia (<60 bpm) is common, occurring in 25% to 40 % of patients within the first hour after a myocardial infarction and decreasing to 15% to 20% after 4 hours (58). This arrhythmia is less common in patients with infarctions involving the left coronary system (81). It often results from hypervagotonia and responds well to intravenous atropine (0.6 to 1 mg) in most cases (82). The ACC/AHA has published guidelines for the use of atropine in the setting of an acute myocardial infarction (72) (Table 30-3). Death as a result of periinfarction sinus bradycardia is rare (83), but its significance is related to the effect of decreasing myocardial efficiency, thereby exacerbating ischemia and the possible development of a more sinister escape rhythm (84).

Treatment of sinus bradycardia is necessary only if the patient is symptomatic or has evidence of hemodynamic compromise. Persistent bradycardia despite intravenous atropine warrants consideration of temporary cardiac pacing (82); atrial or sequential AV pacing is superior to ventricular pacing particularly in right ventricular infarction (84). The ACC/AHA has published guidelines for use of transvenous or transcutaneous pacing in the setting of an acute myocardial infarction (72) (Table 30-4).

Sinus Tachycardia

Sinus tachycardia occurs in approximately 30% of acute myocardial infarctions (11,85). Sinus tachycardia can result in an increase in myocardial oxygen consumption and a reduction in diastolic coronary artery perfusion, thereby augmenting myocardial ischemia. Persistent sinus tachycardia may signify pump failure, and under these circumstances, it is a poor prognostic sign that is associated with an increase in mortality. Sinus tachycardia can also occur as

TABLE 30-3. RECOMMENDATIONS FOR ATROPINE

From Early After Onset of Acute Myocardial Infarction to 6 to 8 Hours Afterward

Class I
1. Sinus bradycardia with evidence of low cardiac output and peripheral hypoperfusion or frequent premature ventricular complexes at onset of symptoms of acute myocardial infarction (AMI)
2. Acute inferior infarction with type I second- or third-degree atrioventricular (AV) block associated with symptoms of hypotension, ischemic discomfort, or ventricular arrhythmias
3. Sustained bradycardia and hypotension after administration of nitroglycerin
4. For nausea and vomiting associated with administration of morphine
5. Ventricular asystole

Class IIa
1. Symptomatic patients with inferior infarction and type I second- or third-degree heart block at the level of the AV node (i.e., with narrow QRS complex or with known existing bundle branch block)

Class IIb
1. Administration concomitant with (before or after) administration of morphine in the presence of sinus bradycardia
2. Asymptomatic patients with inferior infarction and type I second-degree heart block or third-degree heart block at the level of the AV node
3. Second- or third-degree AV block of uncertain mechanism when pacing is not available

Class III
1. Sinus bradycardia greater than 40 bpm without signs or symptoms of hypoperfusion or frequent premature ventricular contractions
2. Type II AV block and third-degree AV block with new wide QRS complex presumed to be caused by AMI

More Than 8 Hours After Presentation

Class I
1. Symptomatic sinus bradycardia (generally, heart rate less than 50 bpm associated with hypotension, ischemia, or escape ventricular arrhythmia)
2. Ventricular asystole
3. Symptomatic atrioventricular (AV) block occurring at the AV nodal level (second-degree type I or third-degree with a narrow-complex escape rhythm)

Class II
None

Class III
1. AV block occurring at an infranodal level (usually associated with anterior myocardial infarction with a wide-complex escape rhythm)
2. Asymptomatic sinus bradycardia

Adapted from Ryan TJ, Antman EM, Brooks NH, et al. *Circulation* 1999;100:1016–1030, with permission.

a result of sympathetic overactivity, anxiety, ongoing chest pain, pyrexia, and hypovolemia. Management is aimed at treating the underlying cause. Patients with left ventricular dysfunction should be treated with an angiotensin-converting enzyme (ACE) inhibitor and diuretics. A β blocker can then be added cautiously after the condition is stabilized.

TABLE 30-4. INDICATIONS FOR TRANSCUTANEOUS OR TRANSVENOUS TEMPORARY PACING

Disturbances	Strength of Indication
Rate Disturbances	
Sinus bradycardia without hypotension, ventricular ectopic activity, angina, left ventricular failure or syncope	Class III
Sinus bradycardia with any of the above, despite atropine	Class I
Accelerated idioventricular rhythm	Class III
Idioventricular rhythm with bradycardia and hypotension or rate less than 45 bpm	Class I
Recurrent sinus pauses (>3 seconds) not responsive to atropine	Class IIa
Incessant ventricular tachycardia (atrial or ventricular overdrive pacing)	Class IIa
Asystole	Class I
Conduction Disturbances	
First-degree atrioventricular (AV) block	Class III
Second-degree AV block	
Mobitz I with normal hemodynamics	Class III
Mobitz I with bradycardia or hypotension	Class I
Mobitz II	Class I
Third-degree heart block	Class I
Preexisting bundle branch block or fascicular block	Class III
New left bundle branch block or bifasicular block	Class IIA
Right bundle branch block with first-degree AV block	Class IIA
New, isolated right bundle branch block	Class IIb
New bifasicular block or left bundle branch block with first-degree AV block (trifascicular block)	Class I
Alternating bundle branch block or right bundle branch block with alternating anterior or posterior fasicular block	Class I

Class I, conditions for which there is evidence and/or general agreement that pacing is beneficial, useful, and effective; class II, conditions for which there is conflicting evidence or a divergence of opinion about the usefulness or efficacy of pacing (class IIa: weight of evidence or opinion is in favor of pacing; class IIb, usefulness or efficacy is less well established by evidence or opinion); class III, there is no evidence or general agreement that pacing is useful or effective and may be harmful. Because transcutaneous pacing is uncomfortable, a transvenous system should be inserted, if a prolonged period of pacing is required.
Adapted from Ryan, TJ, Antman, EM, Brooks, NH, et al. 1999 Update: ACC/AHA guidelines for the management of patients with acute myocardial infarction: executive summary and recommendations. A report of the American College of Cardiology/American Heart Association Task Force on Practice Guidelines (Committee on Management of Acute Myocardial Infarction). *Circulation* 1999;100:1016–1030, with permission.

The β-blocking drugs have reduced all-cause and arrhythmic mortality rates for patients with heart failure (86,87). When sinus tachycardia is thought to be inappropriately fast, given the physiologic state of the patient, slowing of the heart rate with β blockade, particularly if the patient has ongoing chest pain, is helpful. For continuing chest pain, adequate analgesia and a nitrate infusion followed by cardiac catheterization are warranted. Anxious patients should be adequately sedated.

Atrial Tachyarrhythmias: Atrial Fibrillation and Flutter

Incidence and Pathogenesis

The overall incidence of atrial tachyarrhythmias during the periinfarction period is between 10% and 20% (83,85,88). Atrial fibrillation (Fig. 30-2) is the most common atrial tachyarrhythmia, occurring in 10% to 15% of patients with acute myocardial infarction (89–92). Atrial flutter in the periinfarction period is often transient and occurs in less than 5% of patients (93). Although atrial flutter is less common, its clinical significance and management are similar to atrial fibrillation.

Atrial fibrillation and flutter occur predominantly within the first 72 hours after an infarction (88), with only 3% arising in the very early phase (<3 hours) (94). Increased ventricular rates and loss of atrial systole to left ventricular filling result in a significant reduction in cardiac output and an increase in cardiac ischemia.

Several factors are associated with periinfarction atrial fibrillation. These include atrial infarction or ischemia, sinus node dysfunction, age (90,92), metabolic abnormalities (i.e., ischemic atrial tissue can release endogenous adenosine, which can shorten the atrial refractory period) (95), pericarditis (96), pericardial infusion (96), right ventricular infarction (90), congestive heart failure and left ventricular dysfunction (90,92), higher peak creatinine kinase level (92), increased heart rate (92), diabetes mellitus (92), history of hypertension (92), and iatrogenic causes such as the use of inotropic drugs.

Most studies of atrial fibrillation during acute myocardial infarction have been relatively small, were performed in the prethrombolytic era, and gave conflicting results. Moreover, patients who developed atrial fibrillation were thought

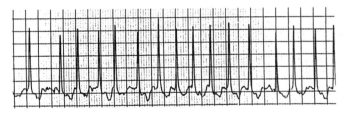

FIGURE 30-2. Atrial fibrillation with a fast ventricular response.

to represent a higher-risk population, and atrial fibrillation was considered to be a nonindependent factor for in-hospital and long-term mortality. Data from Sakata and colleagues (90) and the Global Utilization of Streptokinase and t-PA (tissue-type plasminogen activator, alteplase) for Occluded Coronary Arteries (GUSTO-1) trial (92) have shown an independent association of atrial fibrillation with in-hospital and long-term mortality, reinfarction rates, ventricular arrhythmias, advanced AV conduction disturbances, asystole, cardiogenic shock, and ischemic strokes. Atrial fibrillation is more likely to be associated with more extensive coronary artery disease and poorer reperfusion of the infarct-related artery (92).

The location of the infarct-related coronary artery lesion and the onset time of atrial fibrillation remain controversial. Hod and associates (94) demonstrated that in patients who developed atrial fibrillation within 6 hours of the onset of chest pain, all had inferior infarcts with proximal occlusion of the circumflex artery before the left atrial branch. All patients with atrial fibrillation had compromised blood flow down the AV branch of the right coronary artery. Atrial fibrillation did not occur if the occlusion was in the distal circumflex artery or if there was no concomitant involvement of the AV nodal artery. Atrial fibrillation also did not occur in lone occlusions of a dominant right coronary artery (i.e., supplying the sinoatrial and AV nodes), where there was no involvement of the proximal circumflex artery. The investigators concluded that, because these arteries supplied the left atrial muscle and the sinoatrial and AV nodes, left atrial dysfunction is an important factor in the development of periinfarction atrial fibrillation. In contrast, Sakata and coworkers (90) demonstrated that the incidence of occlusion of the right proximal coronary artery causing the infarct was significantly higher in patients who developed atrial fibrillation in less than 24 hours. They suggested that atrial and sinus node ischemia or right atrial overload due to right ventricular dysfunction were possible causes for the development of atrial fibrillation. They also showed that patients who developed atrial fibrillation 24 hours or longer after an acute infarction tended to have anterior myocardial infarction with increased pulmonary capillary wedge pressure, left ventricular dilation, and reduced ejection fraction. The true situation almost certainly lies within a combination of left atrial dysfunction, nodal artery involvement, and other factors, such as pericardial irritation, electrolyte imbalance, and biventricular failure.

Treatment of Atrial Tachyarrhythmias

The management of periinfarction supraventricular tachyarrhythmias is important, because any tachycardia may increase myocardial oxygen demand and thereby exacerbate ischemia and decrease cardiac output. The initial management of atrial fibrillation or flutter depends on the clinical situation and associated symptoms.

If the patient is compromised by the ventricular rate or by loss of the atrial contribution to cardiac output, synchronized DC cardioversion should be performed, initially using 25 to 50 J for atrial flutter and 100 to 200 J for atrial fibrillation, with gradual increases up to 360 J for unsuccessful shocks. In patients who are hemodynamically stable, attention should be focused on ensuring an adequate ventricular rate control of less than 100 bpm. Provided there are no contraindications (Table 30-5), a β blocker (Table 30-6) is the best agent for rate control. Esmolol, a short-acting β blocker, can be used intravenously if there are concerns regarding the use of a β blocker. Alternative agents such as intravenous diltiazem or intravenous verapamil can also be used, but because of their negative inotropic effects, caution is needed when one of these drugs is administered. Intravenous digoxin is useful, especially if atrial fibrillation is associated with congestive cardiac failure. However, it may take up to 2 hours to be effective (97). Its principal mechanism of action, an increase in vagal tone with consequent prolongation of AV conduction, is easily reversed by sympathetic overactivity, which is often seen in the early periinfarction period. Patients with persistent atrial fibrillation should be considered for DC or pharmacologic cardioversion while in the hospital or at a later date. If permanent atrial fibrillation must be accepted (i.e., resistant to pharmacologic or electrical cardioversion), adequate rate control must be ensured. Agents such as procainamide (58) or amiodarone (98) can be used for the pharmacologic cardioversion of atrial fibrillation. If long-term therapy is needed to aid elective DC cardioversion or control paroxysms of atrial fibrillation, class 1 agents should be avoided in view of their proarrhythmic effects and the increased mortality associated with these agents (99–101). Amiodarone (102–103) or sotalol (104) are alternative drugs that are safe and have the advantage of slowing the ventricular rate if atrial fibrillation recurs. Although newer class 3

TABLE 30-5. RELATIVE CONTRAINDICATION TO β BLOCKERS DURING THE PERIINFARCTION PERIOD

- Heart rate less than 60 bpm
- Systolic arterial pressure less than 100 mm Hg
- Moderate or severe left ventricular failure
- Signs of peripheral hypotension
- PR interval of 0.24 seconds
- Second- or third-degree AV block
- Severe chronic obstructive pulmonary disease
- History of asthma
- Severe peripheral vascular disease
- Insulin-dependent diabetes mellitus

Adapted from Ryan TJ, Antman EM, Brooks NH, et al. 1999 Update: ACC/AHA guidelines for the management of patients with acute myocardial infarction: executive summary and recommendations. A report of the American College of Cardiology/American Heart Association Task Force on Practice Guidelines (Committee on Management of Acute Myocardial Infarction). *Circulation* 1999;100:1016–1030, with permission.

TABLE 30-6. DRUGS USED FOR VENTRICULAR RATE CONTROL DURING ATRIAL FIBRILLATION

Drug	Loading dose	Maintenance	Comments
Metoprolol	IV: 2.5 mg over 2–4 minutes, may repeat every 5 minutes up to 15 mg	IV: 5–10 mg every 6 hours. Orally: 50 mg every 6 hours for 48 hours, then 100 mg twice daily	Hypotension, bronchospasm, negative inotrope and chronotrope. Acts synergistically with digoxin
Propranolol	IV: 0.5–1 mg every 5 minutes to a maximum 0.15–0.2 mg/kg	Orally: 40–240 mg/d in 3–4 divided doses	As for metoprolol
Atenolol	IV: 5–10 mg	Orally: 100 mg/d	As for metoprolol
Esmolol	IV: 0.5 mg/kg/min	IV: 0.05 mg–0.2 mg/kg/min	Very short half-life, as for metoprolol
Digoxin	IV/orally: 0.25–0.5 mg every 6–8 hours up to 1 mg/24 hours	IV/orally: 0.125–0.5 mg/d	Peak effects may take up to 2 hours
Verapamil	IV: 2.5–10 mg over 2 minutes; can repeat dose after 30 minutes	IV: 0.125 mg/min. Orally: 160–180 mg/d in divided doses	Acts synergistically with digoxin, increase digoxin levels, hypotension, bradycardia, negative inotrope
Diltiazem	IV: 0.25–0.35 mg/kg over 2 minutes	IV: 5–15 mg/h. Orally: 90–240 mg/d in divided doses	As for verapamil

Kowey PR, Marinchak RA, Rials SJ et al. Acute Treatment of Atrial Fibrillation. *Am J Cardiol* 1998;81[Suppl 5A]:16C–22C, with permission.

agents such as ibutilide (105) and dofetilide (106) have been successful in terminating acute episodes of atrial fibrillation, their efficacy and safety in the periinfarction period are limited and are being evaluated (107).

Because of the increased risk of thromboembolism in patients with atrial fibrillation, provided there are no clinical contraindications, all patients should be heparinized and considered for oral anticoagulation if atrial fibrillation persists or is paroxysmal. Patients who develop atrial fibrillation transiently or persistently in the periinfarction period are more likely to have multiple coronary artery vessel disease, poorer coronary artery reperfusion and left ventricular dysfunction. These patients probably can benefit from early cardiac catheterization and interventional strategies.

CONDUCTION DISTURBANCES

Acute myocardial ischemia can produce a wide range of conduction disturbances involving the AV node and infranodal structures. These arrhythmias have various degrees of clinical significance, from benign to potentially lethal, and they can reflect the degree of myocardial damage. Although in the current thrombolytic era early reperfusion can shorten the duration of AV block and reduce the need for temporary pacing, it has not reduced the incidence of complete AV block, which has remained relatively constant.

Atrioventricular Block

First-Degree Heart Block

The electrocardiographic finding of first-degree heart block (Fig. 30-3) occurs for up to 14% of patients with acute myocardial infarction admitted to coronary care units and is more common for those with inferior infarction. Most often, the block occurs within the AV node (108). First-

degree heart block that is below the His bundle is more commonly associated with anterior myocardial infarcts and has a worse prognosis. First-degree heart block may also be a manifestation of hypervagotonia, bradycardia, and drugs such as digoxin, β blockers, and calcium antagonists.

Second-Degree Heart Block

Mobitz Type I or Wenckebach Heart Block
Mobitz type I heart block (Fig. 30-4A) is present in 4% to 10% of patients with acute myocardial infarction and accounts for about 90% of patients with second-degree heart block. This rhythm is usually transient (seldom persisting beyond 72 hours) and is more common after inferior infarctions. It is caused by conduction delay within the AV node and is most commonly associated with AV nodal ischemia resulting from occlusion of the right coronary artery (109,110).

Mobitz Type II Heart Block
Mobitz type II heart block is rare in the context of acute myocardial infarction, with an overall incidence of less than 1% (58). It most often occurs with anterior infarction indicating damage to the AV junction or His bundle. The QRS

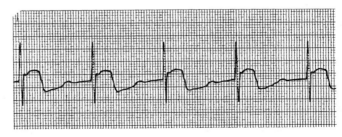

FIGURE 30-3. First-degree heart block (PR interval of 440 ms).

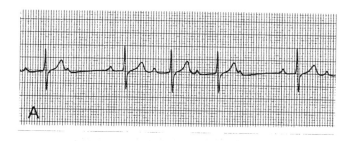

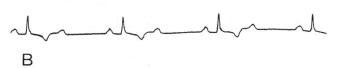

FIGURE 30-4. Second-degree heart block: **A:** Mobitz type I. **B:** A 2 : 1 second-degree heart block.

complexes are usually narrow, but when widened, they reflect distal fascicular disease and a high risk of sudden progression to complete heart block (111). Advanced heart block such as 2 : 1 second-degree heart block (Fig. 30-4B) may be caused by block within the AV node (Mobitz type I) or more distal block within the His-Purkinje system (Mobitz type II). A 3 : 1 (or higher) AV block is usually caused by intra-Hisian or infra-Hisian disease.

Third-Degree or Complete Heart Block

The blood supply to the AV node is derived from two sources, the AV branch of the right coronary artery and a small proportion from a septal perforating branch of the left anterior descending artery. This dual blood supply is thought to account for the increased overall mortality of patients with acute myocardial infarction who develop complete heart block (Fig. 30-5), because it suggests more extensive coronary artery disease (106). Complete heart block in an anterior infarction is also considered to be a

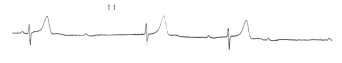

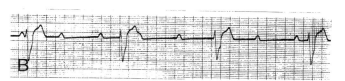

FIGURE 30-5. Third-degree (complete) heart block. **A:** Narrow QRS complex escape rhythm. **B:** Wide QRS complex escape rhythm.

reflection of extensive myocardial necrosis with damage below the AV node and accounts for the difference in presentation and prognosis.

Complete AV block has an incidence of about 6 % (111, 112). It is twice as common with inferoposterior infarcts compared with anterior infarction (7.7% versus 3.9%) (111), with most occurring within the first 72 hours (112,113). The development of advanced forms of AV block complicating myocardial infarctions appears more complex and multifactorial, involving ischemic damage and other metabolic and electrolyte changes that alter cardiac conduction (112).

There are few studies concerning the incidence of complete heart block after thrombolysis. Moreover, most of the data are limited to patients presenting with inferior myocardial infarction. Data from the second Thrombolysis in Myocardial Infarction (TIMI II) trial (114) suggest that 5.7% of patients presenting with an inferior myocardial infarction develop second- or third-degree heart block within 24 hours of receiving a thrombolytic agent; these patients were older and a greater proportion had cardiogenic shock. Other features that may be associated with complete heart block include female gender, β-blocker therapy, increased infarct size, heart failure, diabetes mellitus, chemical and interventional reperfusion (angioplasty), and reocclusion (112).

In general, complete heart block associated with inferior infarction is thought to be caused by block above the bundle of His (111), and it often occurs after progression from first-degree or Mobitz type I second-degree heart block. The consequent escape rhythm is usually stable and often junctional, with narrow QRS complexes and a rate exceeding 40 bpm, but slower rates with broad QRS complexes (>120 ms) may also be seen. In the setting of inferior myocardial infarction, complete heart block is often self-limiting, resolving within 1 week. In contrast, patients with anterior infarction may develop complete heart block suddenly 12 to 24 hours after the onset of acute ischemia. It is usually preceded by intraventricular conduction abnormalities (e.g., left or right bundle branch block, bifascicular or trifascicular block) or Mobitz type II heart block. In this setting, the escape rhythm is often unstable (<40 bpm) with broad QRS complexes and may progress suddenly to asystole.

The in-hospital mortality rates for anterior and inferior infarctions are increased by the occurrence of complete heart block, even when other confounding variables have been accounted for. Anterior infarction has a significantly higher in-hospital mortality rate (63%) than inferior infarction (41.9%) in this context (111,113,115). The time of appearance of advanced AV block has no effect on mortality (116).

Intraventricular Conduction Disturbances

Conduction disturbances involving the left and right bundle branches of the His-Purkinje system occur in 10% to 24% of patients with acute myocardial infarction (109,117). The right bundle and the left posterior fascicle have a dual blood supply derived from the right coronary artery and the left anterior descending artery (58). The blood supply to the anterior fascicle of the left bundle is derived from the septal perforator branches of the left anterior descending artery. Although thrombolytic therapy reduces the overall mortality rate associated with persistent bundle branch block (117), the mortality for patients with persistent bundle branch block is significantly higher than those without (8.7% versus 3.5%) (117). Persistent bundle branch block is an independent marker for mortality (118,119). In contrast, for patients with transient disturbances who recover normal conduction during hospitalization, the prognosis is similar to patients who never develop this complication (118,119).

Left Anterior Hemiblock

Left anterior hemiblock involves conduction block or delay in the left anterior fascicle and appears on the surface ECG as a left axis deviation (Fig. 30-6). It occurs in 3% to 5% of people with acute myocardial infarction (120), and the mortality rate is slightly increased for these patients.

Left Posterior Hemiblock

Left posterior hemiblock represents conduction block of the left posterior fascicle and manifests as right axis deviation on the ECG. This conduction disturbance occurs in 1% to 2% of patients with acute myocardial infarction. The posterior fascicle is larger than the anterior fascicle, and posterior hemi-

block usually reflects more severe damage than anterior hemiblock and has a higher associated mortality rate (113).

Right Bundle Branch Block

New right bundle branch block has an incidence of 2% in patients with acute myocardial infarction and is frequently associated with anteroseptal infarcts and complete AV block (58,118). Its onset often reflects significant myocardial damage and is therefore associated with a higher mortality rate (112).

Bifascicular Block

Bifascicular block describes a conduction block of two of the three major divisions of the His-Purkinje system and may appear as a new feature on the ECG after a myocardial infarction. The electrocardiographic appearances consist of right bundle branch block in association with left or right axis deviation (reflecting left anterior or left posterior hemiblock, respectively) or complete left bundle branch block.

When associated with myocardial infarction, bifascicular block is associated with an increased incidence of progression to complete heart block (113); coexisting first-degree heart block (i.e., trifascicular block) further increases this risk. Mortality is also increased as a result of the extensive myocardial damage that occurs to bring about such widespread conduction abnormalities and is more common in cases of anterior than inferior infarction. Such damage puts these patients at higher risk for cardiogenic shock, asystole,

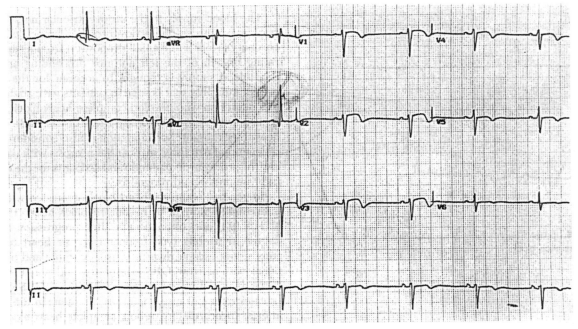

FIGURE 30-6. Left axis deviation with acute anterior infarction.

and ventricular arrhythmias (121). In one study, Sgarbossa and colleagues (118) showed that the conduction defects associated with most deaths were right bundle branch block plus left anterior fascicular block (23%, $p < 0.001$, odds ratio = 2.5) and isolated right bundle branch block (21%, p = 0.003, odds ratio = 2.17). The mortality rate for patients with right bundle branch block plus left posterior fascicular block or with left bundle branch block was only 10%.

Treatment of Periinfarction Conduction Disturbances

Atrioventricular Conduction Disturbances

Noninvasive external temporary cardiac pacing is widely available and is acceptable to most patients, although not well tolerated for long periods. It is virtually free of complications and has a role in patients awaiting insertion of temporary transvenous pacing wires who are at high risk for bleeding or at relatively low risk for progression to complete heart block. Because transcutaneous pacing can be uncomfortable and painful, a transvenous system should be inserted as soon as possible if a prolonged period of pacing is required. Indications for the use of transvenous or transcutaneous pacing have been published by the ACC/AHA (72) (Table 30-4).

First-degree heart block in itself does not require any specific treatment unless there is evidence of progression to higher degrees of conduction block. Similarly, Mobitz type I second-degree heart block does not require specific treatment provided that the ventricular rate is adequate; if this conduction disturbance causes hemodynamic compromise, temporary cardiac pacing is indicated. Because patients with Mobitz type II second-degree heart block have a significant risk of progression to complete heart block, the introduction of a temporary pacemaker is appropriate. Complete heart block occurring within 6 hours of the onset of ischemia probably is caused in part by hypervagotonia, especially if the QRS complexes are narrow, and it can be successfully treated with atropine; complete heart block occurring after this time probably requires temporary cardiac pacing (122).

Although AV block and bundle branch block carry independent risks for mortality and in-hospital complications, perhaps related to infarct size, the use of pacing during this period does not alter mortality (112). However, temporary cardiac pacing can protect against transient hypotension and consequent exacerbation of ischemia and may also prevent malignant ventricular escape rhythms. In cases of anterior infarction, there is a significant risk of asystole in patients with complete AV block, and pacing has obvious benefits in this clinical situation. The indications for the insertion of a permanent pacemaker after conduction disturbances, as recommended by the ACC/AHA, are summarized in Table 30-7 (72). The decision regarding the placement of a permanent pacemaker in patients with inferior myocardial infarctions should be delayed for 14 to 16 days (123).

TABLE 30-7. ACC/AHA GUIDELINES FOR THE INSERTION OF A PERMANENT PACEMAKER AFTER MYOCARDIAL INFARCTION

Class I
1. Persistent second-degree atrioventricular (AV) block in the His-Purkinje system with bilateral bundle branch block or complete heart block within or below the His-Purkinje system after an acute myocardial infarction
2. Transient advanced (second- or third-degree) infranodal AV block and associated bundle branch block. If the site of block is uncertain, an electrophysiological study may be necessary.
3. Persistent and symptomatic second- or third-degree AV block

Class IIA
None

Class IIB
1. Persistent second- or third-degree AV block at the AV node level

Class 3
1. Transient AV block in the absence of intraventricular conduction defects
2. Transient AV block in the presence of isolated left anterior fascicular block
3. Acquired left anterior fascicular block in the absence of AV block
4. Persistent first-degree AV block in the presence of bundle branch block that is old or age indeterminate

Adapted from Ryan TJ, Antman EM, Brooks NH, et al. 1999 Update: ACC/AHA guidelines for the management of patients with acute myocardial infarction: executive summary and recommendations. A report of the American College of Cardiology/American Heart Association Task Force on Practice Guidelines (Committee on Management of Acute Myocardial Infarction). *Circulation* 1999;100:1016–1030, with permission.

Intraventricular Conduction Disturbance

In view of the risk of progression to complete AV block, patients with new alternating bundle branch or trifascicular block should be temporarily paced. With other forms of intraventricular conduction disturbances, such as isolated left or right bundle branch block and bifascicular block, the development of higher degrees of block or asystole is greater, and left ventricular function is likely to be impaired and less able to compensate if complete heart block develops. Some authorities recommend prophylactic pacing in this group, but this form of management is controversial.

REPERFUSION ARRHYTHMIAS

With the increasing use of intravenous thrombolytics for acute myocardial infarction, reperfusion arrhythmias may become a more significant aspect of acute coronary care. These arrhythmias consist of ventricular ectopic beats, accelerated idioventricular rhythm, ventricular tachycardia, and ventricular fibrillation.

Reperfusion arrhythmias are one manifestation of a spectrum of reperfusion injury, which also comprises vascular damage (i.e., no reflow phenomenon), myocardial stunning, accelerated necrosis of reversibly damaged cells, and cell swelling and accelerated necrosis of irreversibly damaged myocytes (124,125). Reperfusion injury is thought to be mediated by three main mechanisms: the calcium paradox, the oxygen paradox, and the production of oxygen free radicals.

The calcium paradox occurs when calcium is restored to the extracellular space after having been depleted by ischemia. Instead of homeostasis being restored, severe cell damage results with muscle contracture and cell death (126). This phenomenon is thought to arise because of depletion of mitochondrial energy resulting from excess intracellular calcium, which causes damage to the respiratory chain and decreases ATP production (129). The oxygen paradox is closely linked to the calcium paradox, because oxygen mediates the uptake of calcium by the mitochondria (128). During reperfusion, oxygen also leads to cell damage by the formation of oxygen free radicals (129).

With the marked fluxes in calcium occurring during reperfusion, the situation lends itself to calcium recycling when ATP is restored, with possible adverse electrophysiologic effects, particularly the development of calcium-dependent arrhythmias (129,130). Animal experiments have demonstrated that excess calcium oscillations in the reoxygenation phase of reperfusion coincide with ventricular arrhythmias in a papillary muscle model (131).

The role of free radicals in the genesis of reperfusion arrhythmias is uncertain. Free radical scavengers have reduced the occurrence of reperfusion ventricular fibrillation (132). However, free radical-induced membrane damage occurs 5 to 10 minutes after reperfusion (133), making this unlikely to be the sole cause of reperfusion arrhythmias, which usually occur within seconds of abrupt restoration of blood flow (134). Several studies have shown no protective effect by free radical scavengers on early reperfusion arrhythmias (130).

The incidence of reperfusion arrhythmias is influenced by the severity and duration of ischemia. No arrhythmias are seen to arise from dead cells, which supports the concept that reperfusion arrhythmias are energy dependent. The occurrence of arrhythmias follows a bell-shaped curve; as the duration of ischemia increases, so do reperfusion arrhythmias, with the peak incidence occurring at 5 to 10 minutes after the onset of ischemia, presumably as ATP stores become depleted (127,128).

Several lines of evidence suggest that reperfusion arrhythmias are related to the severity of ischemia. First, calcium-dependent reperfusion arrhythmias can develop after the metabolic changes induced by ischemia, such as the accumulation of cyclic AMP, which predispose to calcium oscillations (135,136). Second, the fatty acid metabolite palmityl carnitine accumulates during ischemia, facilitating the opening of calcium channels (134). Third, the greater the degree of hypoperfusion, the greater is the rate of formation of oxygen free radicals in the myocardium on reperfusion (136).

Fourth, increased heart rate increases the severity of ischemic injury and the incidence of reperfusion arrhythmias (137). This disruption on a cellular level is thought to be translated into the clinical picture of reperfusion arrhythmias by effects on delayed afterdepolarizations (causing triggered activity) and ventricular automaticity (128,136).

There are, however, some important differences between experimental models and the clinical situation. Reperfusion arrhythmias in animal models occur after 5- to 15-minute periods of coronary artery occlusion not associated with infarction (138); in these models, if the duration of ischemia is extended to 1 to 3 hours, arrhythmias occur during the period of ischemia; however, reperfusion is not associated with a dramatic increase in arrhythmia (139).

A pooled analysis (139) of intracoronary thrombolytic trials suggested that these life-threatening arrhythmias were more likely to occur when the interval between the onset of infarction and thrombolytic therapy was short (analogous to experimental models). The rate of lysis may also be important. Serious arrhythmias are more common when thrombolytic agents are given into the coronary artery and lysis is rapid (similar to the animal model). They are less frequent when intravenous thrombolytic agents are used.

In humans, thrombolytic therapy is usually given more than 2 to 4 hours after the onset of coronary occlusion, when significant myocardial infarction is already present. It seems likely that ischemia, rather than reperfusion, is responsible for most arrhythmias seen in patients with myocardial infarction. This idea is supported by the observation that trials of intravenous thrombolytic therapy have not demonstrated any increase in life-threatening arrhythmias that could be attributed to reperfusion (140,141).

Reperfusion arrhythmias should be managed in an identical fashion to arrhythmias occurring in a different context. Unfortunately, animal data suggest that antiarrhythmic drugs are less effective for reperfusion arrhythmia. No prophylactic therapeutic maneuvers have been proven to reduce the incidence of these events, but interest is being shown in calcium channel blocking agents (e.g., adenosine, dipyridamole) and free radical scavengers (e.g., superoxide dismutase). Yoshida and associates demonstrated the antiarrhythmic effect of dipyridamole in the treatment of reperfusion arrhythmias generated during primary angioplasty for myocardial infarction (142). Dipyridamole, an inhibitor of cellular uptake of adenosine, may prevent or terminate reperfusion arrhythmias by decreasing cyclic AMP-mediated intracellular calcium overload and hence a reduction in triggered activity.

RISK STRATIFICATION

There has been considerable interest in identifying patients at increased risk for ventricular tachyarrhythmias and arrhythmic death after myocardial infarction who have been treated optimally for residual ischemia. This is important because

TABLE 30-8. INCIDENCE OF SUSTAINED VENTRICULAR ARRHYTHMIAS OR SUDDEN CARDIAC DEATH IN PATIENTS AFTER MYOCARDIAL INFARCTION

Test	Adverse Outcome (%)	
	For Normal Test Results	For Abnormal Test Results
Signal-averaged electrocardiogram	1–3	17–29
Ejection fraction	5–6	16–24
Holter monitor	7–9	14–23
Heart rate variability	1–23	16–17
Programmed stimulation	0–4	12–32

Adapted from Cain ME, Anderson JL, Arnsdorf MF, et al. Signal-averaged electrocardiography: ACC expert consensus document. *J Am Coll Cardiol* 1996;27:238, with permission.

most antiarrhythmic agents have the unwelcome adverse effect of proarrhythmia, and implantable cardioverter-defibrillators (ICDs) are expensive. The selection of patients most at risk is therefore crucial to ensure that the prophylactic treatment of sudden cardiac death is safe and cost-effective.

Two limitations confound the proper identification and therapy of patients at increased risk for serious arrhythmias after a myocardial infarction. First, no one factor alone is highly predictive of a fatal arrhythmia. Second, no form of therapy has been shown to improve the outcome for high-risk patients. Despite these caveats, many different clinical features have been evaluated as possible risk factors for the development of a fatal arrhythmia after an acute myocardial infarction (143) (Table 30-8).

In view of the widely held belief that frequent or complex PVCs in the recovery period after a myocardial infarction are an independent marker of sudden cardiac death, more than 50 placebo-controlled trials have been performed using class I antiarrhythmic agents in the setting of acute myocardial infarction (144) in an attempt to suppress PVCs and reduce the triggering mechanism of ventricular tachycardia and ventricular fibrillation. Overall, no beneficial effect on mortality was shown, with an odds ratio of 1.17 (range, 1.03 to 1.31), indicating a potential harmful effect on mortality (Table 30-9).

The Cardiac Arrhythmia Suppression Trial (CAST) was the largest placebo-controlled trial designed to investigate whether suppression of asymptomatic PVCs with class I agents could reduce the risk of death from arrhythmias after myocardial infarction (99,100). More than 1,400 patients in whom antiarrhythmic treatment produced significant suppression of single or repetitive PVCs were randomized to encainide, flecainide, moricizine, or placebo and followed for a mean period of 10 months. Despite suppression of more than 80% of single PVCs and more than 90% of runs of ventricular tachycardia, the mortality rate was significantly higher for patients treated with antiarrhythmic drugs compared with patients in the placebo arm (Fig. 30-7). d-Sotalol, an isomer of d,l-sotalol that is devoid of β-blocking activity but has only class III antiarrhythmic effects, was evaluated in a postinfarction study known as Survival with Oral d-Sotalol (SWORD) (145). This trial randomized patients with a reduced left ventricular ejection fraction (LVEF) and a recent myocardial infarction or symptomatic heart failure and a remote myocardial infarction to d-sotalol or placebo. The trial was stopped after less than one half of the planned 6,400 patients were enrolled because of an increased incidence of death (5.0% versus 3.1%, *p* = 0.006) among patients treated with d-sotalol primarily because of presumed arrhythmic deaths (3.6% versus 2.0%, *p* = 0.008) (Fig. 30-8).

The only antiarrhythmic agent that has been shown to reduce the incidence of cardiac arrhythmias and mortality after myocardial infarction is a β blocker; the ACC/AHA have published recommendations for the use of a β blocker after a myocardial infarction (72) (Table 30-10). Although amiodarone has been shown to significantly reduce arrhythmic mortality, there is no significant reduction in all-cause mortality (102,103) (Fig. 30-9). However, subset analysis of patients in the European Myocardial Infarct Amiodarone Trial (EMIAT) showed that amiodarone reduced total mor-

TABLE 30-9. PROPHYLACTIC ANTIARRHYTHMIC DRUG THERAPY IN ASYMPTOMATIC POSTMYOCARDIAL INFARCTION PATIENTS

Class of AA	Number of Trials	Total Number of Patients	Placebo Mortality (%)	Active Mortality (%)	Odds Ratio (95% CI)
I	57	21,780	5.2	6.0	1.17 (1.03–1.31)
Ia	17	5,229	8.2	9.7	1.22 (1.00–1.47)
Ib	32	14,013	4.0	4.3	1.06 (0.89–1.26)
Ic	8	2,538	6.0	7.4	1.42 (0.95–1.95)
II	55	53,268	6.6	5.4	0.81 (0.75–0.87)
III	7	1,293	14.2	10.3	0.66 (0.47–0.93)
IV	24	20,342	9.3	9.7	1.04 (0.95–1.14)

AA, antiarrhythmic drug (Vaughan-Williams classification); CI, confidence interval.
Adapted from Teo K, Yusuf C, Furberg C. Effect of prophylactic antiarrhythmic drug therapy on post-myocardial infarction mortality. *Eur Heart J* 1992;13:224, with permission.

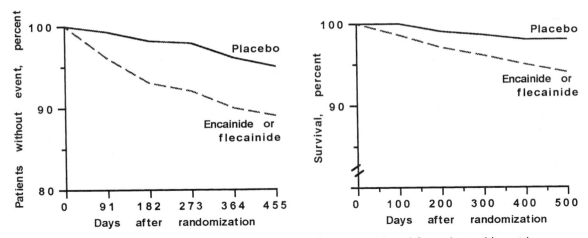

FIGURE 30-7. Results of the Cardiac Arrhythmia Suppression Trial (CAST) for patients with ventricular premature beats after myocardial infarction. Compared with those receiving placebo, patients receiving encainide or flecainide had a significantly lower rate of avoiding a cardiac event (i.e., death or resuscitated cardiac arrest) (*left*, p = 0.001) and a lower overall survival (*right*, p = 0.0006). The cause of death was arrhythmia or cardiac arrest. (Adapted from Echt DS, Liebson PR, Mitchell B, et al. Mortality and morbidity in patients receiving encainide, flecainide or placebo: the Cardiac Arrhythmia Suppression Trial. *N Engl J Med* 1991;324:781–788, with permission.).

tality rates for patients with an ejection fraction of less than 0.30, with premature ventricular beats on the initial Holter assessment, or with concurrent β blocker therapy (146,147) (Fig. 30-10). Amiodarone reduced total mortality (18% versus 23% for placebo) for patients with reduced HRV, defined as a HRV index of 20 U or less (148). In contrast, there was a trend toward increased total mortality for patients without these features. The safety and efficacy of newer class III agents such as azimilide (149) and dofetilide (107) in the postinfarction period are being evaluated.

Left ventricular function is a powerful predictor of sudden death after myocardial infarction (150,151); however, the predictive value of resting LVEF alone is low, and assessment of myocardial function during exercise may be more useful (152) (Table 30-8). The predictive value of LVEF for sudden arrhythmic death can be increased by combining other risk factors such as the signal-averaged ECG, HRV, or baroreflex sensitivity.

Late potentials demonstrated on the signal-averaged ECG identify patients at risk for sustained ventricular

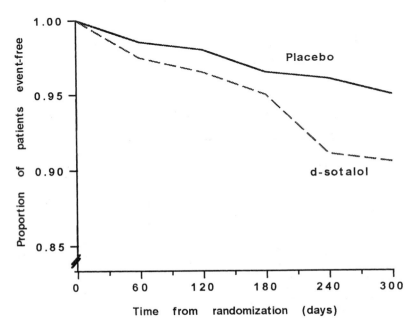

FIGURE 30-8. Results from the Survival with Oral d-Sotalol (SWORD) trial. The administration of d-sotalol to patients with an ejection fraction ≤ 0.35 after recent myocardial infarction (MI) or after symptomatic heart failure with a remote (> 42 days) MI was associated with increased mortality compared with placebo (5% versus 3.1%). The excess number of deaths was presumed to result primarily from arrhythmias. (Adapted from Waldo A, Camm J, de Ruyter H, et al. Effect of d-sotalol on mortality in patients with left ventricular dysfunction after recent and remote myocardial infarction. *Lancet* 1996;348:7, with permission.)

TABLE 30-10. β-ADRENOCEPTOR BLOCKING AGENTS IN MYOCARDIAL INFARCTION

Recommendations for Early Therapy

Class I
1. Patients without a contraindication (see Table 30-5) to β-adrenoceptor blocker therapy who can be treated within 12 hours of onset of infarction, irrespective of administration of concomitant thrombolytic therapy or performance of primary angioplasty
2. Patients with continuing or recurrent ischemic pain
3. Patients with tachyarrhythmias, such as atrial fibrillation with a rapid ventricular response
4. Patients with non-ST elevation myocardial infarction

Class IIb
1. Patients with moderate left ventricular (LV) failure (the presence of bibasilar rales without evidence of low cardiac output) or other relative contraindications (see Table 30-5) to β-adrenoceptor blocker therapy, provided they can be monitored closely

Class III
1. Patients with severe LV failure

Recommendations for Long-Term Therapy

Class I
1. All but low-risk patients without a clear contraindication to β-adrenoceptor blocker therapy. Treatment should begin within a few days of the event (if not initiated acutely) and continue indefinitely.

Class IIa
1. Low-risk patients without a clear contraindication to β-adrenoceptor blocker therapy
2. Survivors of non-ST elevation myocardial infarction

Class IIb
1. Patients with moderate or severe left ventricular failure or other relative contraindications to β-adrenoceptor blocker therapy, provided they can be clearly monitored

Class III
None

Adapted from Ryan TJ, Antman EM, Brooks NH, et al. *Circulation* 1999;100:1016–1030, with permission.

tachycardia or sudden death (153,154). However, like LVEF, the predictive value of signal-averaged ECG alone is low (143) (Table 30-8).

HRV is defined as the periodic variation of heart rate over time. A number of studies have shown a reduction in HRV to be associated with an increased risk of all-cause and arrhythmic mortality after a myocardial infarction (55–57,155). Moreover, the predictive value is independent of other risk predictors such as PVC frequency, signal-averaged ECG, and LVEF (55,155) (Table 30-8).

Baroreflex sensitivity is a quantitative assessment of the integrity of the autonomic nervous system (primarily vagal reflexes) to respond to abrupt changes in arterial pressure. A prospective study showed that a reduction in baroreflex sensitivity was an independent predictor of mortality after myocardial infarction (57).

Although electrophysiologic testing has been used to predict the risk of sudden death in patients with recent myocardial infarction, only 6.2% to 35% of patients have

inducible tachyarrhythmias (145–147,156). Of these patients with inducible, sustained tachyarrhythmias, arrhythmic events have occurred in 14% to 36% over 1 to 2 years (157,158). The wide variation between studies reflect the heterogeneity of the populations investigated, and varying numbers of patients, left ventricular function, stimulation protocols, and administration of thrombolytic therapy. The role of electrophysiologic testing for risk stratification in the postinfarction period remains debatable (Table 30-8). Moreover, it is an invasive procedure and therefore not ideally suited as a screening test for a large number of patients; it may be more appropriately applied to preselected patients with positive noninvasive test results (159,160).

T-wave alternans (TWA) is characterized by the alternation on a beat-to-beat basis of the amplitude (microvolt level) and morphology of T waves on the surface ECG. Experimental studies suggest a temporal correlation among rate, ischemia-induced alternans, dispersion of repolarization, and susceptibility to ventricular arrhythmias (161,162). However, multivariate prospective data using TWA as a risk stratifier in the postinfarction period are lacking.

QT dispersion is a measure of interlead variations of QT interval duration on the surface 12-lead ECG and is believed to reflect regional differences in repolarization heterogeneity and may provide an indirect marker of arrhythmogenicity. The comprehensive study by Zabel and coworkers (163) casts doubt on the value of QT dispersion as a risk predictor in patients after myocardial infarction.

Heart rate turbulence describes a pattern acceleration and later deceleration of the succeeding sinus rhythm after a single premature beat (164). Patients at low risk after myocardial infarction appear to have this characteristic pattern. In contrast, this phenomena was not seen in high-risk patients and was an independent predictor of mortality when compared with age, previous myocardial infarction, left ventricular dysfunction, arrhythmias on Holter monitoring, and HRV.

A combination of variables may provide more clinically applicable information. Farrell and colleagues have shown that the combination of impaired HRV and late potentials had a sensitivity of 58%, with a positive predictive accuracy of 33% for arrhythmic events (165). By selecting patients with a high risk of arrhythmic death (using decreased HRV) and deselecting patients with a high risk of non-arrhythmic death (using low ejection fractions), Hartikanen and associates (166) were able to identify a group of patients in which 75% of deaths were arrhythmic. Similarly, by selecting patients with the lowest ejection fraction and omitting patients with the lowest HRV, they were able to identify a group of patients in which 75% of deaths were nonarrhythmic. The combined use of noninvasive and electrophysiologic testing has been studied by Pedretti and coworkers (160). They demonstrated that the combination of two or more variables among LVEF less than 0.40, posi-

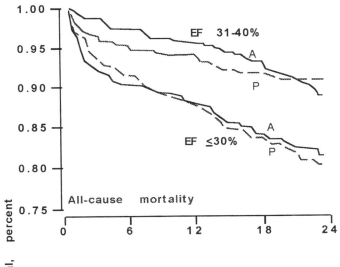

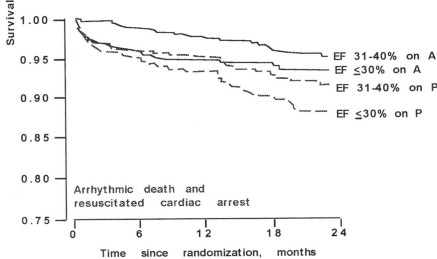

FIGURE 30-9. Effect of amiodarone in 1,486 postmyocardial patients who were randomized to amiodarone (A) or placebo (P) in the European Myocardial Infarct Amiodarone Trial (EMIAT). When analyzed by baseline ejection fraction (EF), amiodarone had no effect on all-cause mortality *(top)* but reduced the incidence of arrhythmic death or resuscitated cardiac arrest *(bottom)*. The benefit was greatest in patients with an EF ≤ 0.30 *(dashed lines)*. (Adapted from Julian DG, Camm AJ, Frangin G, et al, for the European Myocardial Infarct Amiodarone Trial Investigators. Randomized trial of effect of amiodarone on mortality in patients with left-ventricular dysfunction after recent myocardial infarction: EMIAT. *Lancet* 1997; 349:675–682, with permission.)

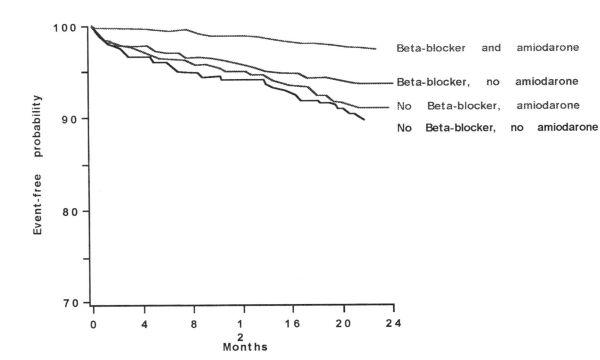

tive late potentials, repetitive ventricular premature complexes, and a subsequent positive programmed stimulation test identified a group of post–myocardial infarction patients with a 65% risk of arrhythmic events. The combined use of noninvasive tests and programmed stimulation tests revealed a sensitivity of 81%, specificity of 97%, positive predictive accuracy of 65%, and a negative predictive accuracy of 99%.

MANAGEMENT OF THE HIGH-RISK POST–MYOCARDIAL INFARCTION PATIENT

More than 50% of deaths of patients who survive acute myocardial infarction are caused by lethal ventricular tachyarrhythmias and are likely to occur within the first year. Before thrombolytic therapy, about 5% to 10% of patients suffered sudden cardiac death within the first year after acute myocardial infarction. In the current thrombolytic era, this figure has decreased to probably 1% to 2% within the first year (167). High-risk post–myocardial infarction patients can be categorized as follows:

1. Asymptomatic, high-risk individuals, based on the results of invasive and noninvasive testing
2. Those with episodes of nonsustained ventricular tachycardia remote from the index infarction (>48 hours)
3. Those with late episodes of sustained ventricular tachycardia and fibrillation

The first group has already been discussed, and although some of these tests may be sensitive, they all have a low positive predictive accuracy. Management strategies for this group of patients have not been fully defined, and the standard antiarrhythmic drugs (with the exception of β blockers and amiodarone) could be potentially proarrhythmic. It is imperative, when appropriate, that all patients are discharged on a β blocker, an ACE inhibitor (if there is associated left ventricular dysfunction), aspirin, and a lipid-lowering drug (if the cholesterol level is raised). There is no evidence to support the routine administration of prophylactic amiodarone therapy. Several ongoing studies are investigating the prophylactic insertion of ICDs in this high-risk group:

1. The Multicenter Automatic Defibrillator Implantation Trial II (MADIT II) investigates survival of patients with high-risk coronary artery disease and with a low ejection fraction (<0.35) who are randomized to ICD or non-ICD therapy.
2. The Defibrillator in Acute Myocardial Infarction Trial (DINAMIT) investigates high-risk patients with a reduced ejection fraction (<0.35) and a depressed HRV or an elevated heart rate (mean R-R interval ≤750 ms) on 24-hour Holter monitoring.
3. The Beta-Blocker Strategy plus Implantable Cardioverter-Defibrillator Trial (BEST-ICD) compares electrophysiologically guided therapy (drug or ICD) with conventional therapy in patients with a recent myocardial infarction, an ejection fraction less than 0.36, and at least one other risk factor: 10 or more ventricular premature complexes per hour, reduced HRV, or late ventricular potentials (168).

The results of the Multicenter Unsustained Tachycardia Trial (MUSTT) (158) and MADIT (169) studies suggest that in patients with coronary artery disease, asymptomatic nonsustained ventricular tachyarrhythmias, a reduced LVEF (<0.40), and nonsuppressibility of sustained ventricular tachycardia on electrophysiologic testing are significantly protected with an ICD (Figs. 30-11 and 30-12).

In the past, survivors of sustained ventricular arrhythmia or cardiac arrest who had been optimally treated for any residual cardiac ischemia underwent electrophysiologic testing. In this patient population, ventricular arrhythmias were inducible in 60% to 80% (170–172). In patients with inducible ventricular arrhythmias, electrophysiologically guided therapy was successful in reducing the recurrence of further events. For instance, Wilber and colleagues (172), demonstrated that during a median follow-up period of 21 months, cardiac arrest recurred in 12% in whom inducible arrhythmias had been suppressed, 33% in whom inducible arrhythmias persisted, and 17% in whom arrhythmias could not be induced. The widely accepted strategy during the 1980s and early 1990s for the treatment of life-threatening ventricular arrhythmias was serial electrophysiologically guided antiarrhythmic drug therapy using mainly class I agents.

FIGURE 30-10. A pooled analysis of patients in the European Myocardial Infarct Amiodarone Trial (EMIAT) and Canadian Amiodarone Myocardial Infarction Arrhythmia Trial (CAMIAT) shows that all-cause mortality after a myocardial infarction is lower with a combination of amiodarone and a β blocker compared with a β blocker alone or no β blocker with or without amiodarone. (Adapted from Boutitie F, Boissel JP, Connnolly SJ, et al, and the EMIAT and CAMIAT Investigators. Amiodarone Interaction with β-blockers: analysis of the merged EMIAT [European Myocardial Infarct Amiodarone Trial] and CAMIAT [Canadian Amiodarone Myocardial Infarction Trial] databases. *Circulation* 1999;99:2268, with permission.)

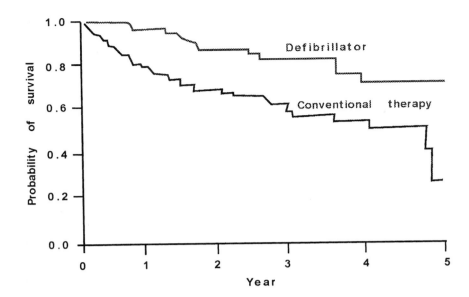

FIGURE 30-11. Kaplan-Meier cumulative survival curves in the Multicenter Automatic Defibrillator Implantation Trial (MADIT) show that selected high-risk patients (i.e., prior infarction, left ventricular ejection fraction ≤ 0.35, nonsustained ventricular tachycardia, and an inducible sustained ventricular tachyarrhythmia not suppressible with procainamide) have a better survival rate with an implantable defibrillator compared with conventional therapy with antiarrhythmic drugs (*p* = 0.009). (Adapted from Moss AJ, Hall WJ, Cannom DS, et al, for the Multicenter Automatic Defibrillator Implantation Trial Investigators. Improved survival with an implanted defibrillator in patients with coronary disease at high risk for ventricular arrhythmias. *N Engl J Med* 1996;335:1933, with permission.)

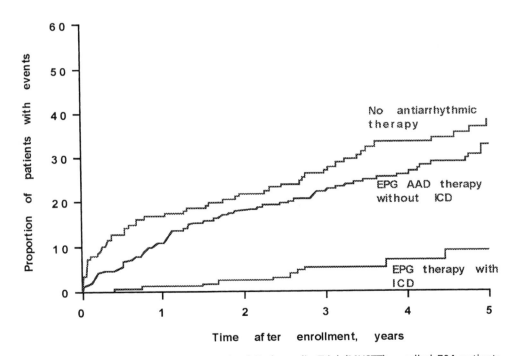

FIGURE 30-12. The Multicenter Unsustained Tachycardia Trial (MUSTT) enrolled 704 patients with coronary artery disease, nonsustained ventricular tachycardia, and a left ventricular tachycardia (VT) induced during electrophysiologic (EP) study. Kaplan-Meier estimates show that the incidence of cardiac arrest or death from arrhythmia is significantly lower among those receiving an implantable cardioverter-defibrillator (ICD) compared with those receiving no therapy or those with EP-guided (EPG) antiarrhythmic drug (AAD) therapy (9% versus 32% and 25%, respectively; *p* < 0.001 for ICD versus no ICD and for ICD versus no antiarrhythmic therapy.) (Data from Buxton AE, Lee KL, Fisher JD, et al. A randomized study of the prevention of sudden death in patients with coronary artery disease. *N Engl J Med* 1999;341:1882, with permission.)

The management strategies of patients with major arrhythmic events have changed significantly during the past decade. The increasing use of aspirin, thrombolytic therapy, β blockers, and ACE inhibitors has resulted in a significant reduction in mortality and may have altered the vulnerable myocardial substrate responsible for arrhythmogenesis. As a result, the initial benefits seen with class I agents in the 1980s and 1990s have changed, with a shift toward an adverse outcome for patients given these agents (70,99–101,144). This is also reflected in the findings of the Cardiac Arrest in Seattle: Conventional versus Amiodarone Drug Evaluation (CASCADE) study, which demonstrated that empiric amiodarone therapy was more effective than electrophysiologically guided treatment with class I agents (173).

There is substantial evidence that demonstrates the superiority of ICDs over antiarrhythmic drug therapy in reducing total mortality in this high-risk patient population (174–177) (Fig. 30-13). Consequently, patients with sustained ventricular tachycardia and survivors of cardiac arrest are considered to have a class I indication (as recommended by the ACC/AHA) for ICD insertion (178).

CONCLUSIONS

Arrhythmias such as ventricular and atrial tachyarrhythmias and conduction disturbances are frequently encountered during the periinfarction period. These arrhythmias arise because of a complex interaction between ionic, metabolic, and neurohormonal changes, with consequent electrophysiologic instability. The arrhythmias generated contribute significantly to the morbidity and mortality seen in the periinfarction period. The past decades have seen improvements in the diagnosis and management of these arrhythmias and consequently a decrease in mortality in the early postinfarction period (3).

A large number of laboratory and clinical experiments have enabled us to understand many of the mechanisms leading to these arrhythmias, particularly the influence of the autonomic nervous system, but there are still areas that require further investigation, such as the mechanism, treatment, and prevention of reperfusion arrhythmias and the development of strategies to identify patients at high risk for sudden arrhythmic death, thereby allowing targeted therapy. Despite advances in nonpharmacologic management of high-risk patients such as the use of ICDs, pharmacologic management has remained disappointing, and further studies are needed to provide effective treatment for resistant periinfarction arrhythmias, especially ventricular fibrillation.

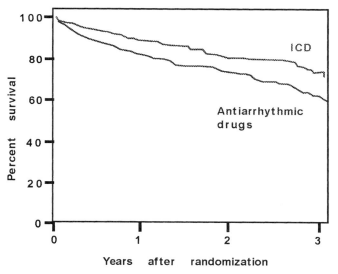

FIGURE 30-13. The Antiarrhythmic Versus Implantable Defibrillators (AVID) trial randomized 1,016 patients with a history of ventricular fibrillation, ventricular tachycardia, or syncope thought to result from arrhythmia to an implantable cardioverter-defibrillator (ICD) or antiarrhythmic therapy (i.e., sotalol or amiodarone). After a 3-year follow-up period, survival was significantly better in the ICD group (*p* < 0.02), but the improvement in mean survival was only 2.6 months. (Adapted from The Antiarrythmics Versus Implantable Defibrillator [AVID] Investigators. A comparison of antiarrhythmic drug therapy with implantable defibrillators in patients resuscitated from near fatal ventricular arrhythmia *N Engl J Med* 1997;337:1576, with permission.)

REFERENCES

1. Lown B. Sudden cardiac death: the major challenge confronting contemporary cardiology. *Am J Cardiol* 1979;43:313–329.
2. Myerburg RJ, Kessler KM, Castellanos A. Sudden cardiac death: structure, function and time-dependence of risk. *Circulation* 1992;85[Suppl 1]:2–10.
3. Rosamond WD, Chambless LE, Folsom AR, et al. Trends in the incidence of myocardial infarction and in mortality due to coronary heart disease. *N Engl J Med* 1998;339:861–867.
4. Yusuf S, Wittes J, Friedman L. Overview of results of randomized clinical trials in heart disease: 1. Treatments following myocardial infarction. *JAMA* 1988;260:2088–2093.
5. Ong L, Green S, Reiser P, Morrison J. Early prediction of mortality in patients with acute myocardial infarction: a prospective study of clinical and radionuclide risk factors. *Am J Cardiol* 1986;57:33–38.
6. Snellen HA. History of cardiology. Rotterdam, The Netherlands: Donker Academic, 1984.
7. Erichsen F. On the influence of the coronary circulation on the action of the heart. *Lond Med Gazette* 1841–1842;2:561.
8. Davies MF. Pathological view of sudden cardiac death. *Br Heart J* 1981;45:88.
9. Goldstein S, Landis JR, Leighton R, et al. Characteristics of resuscitated out-of-hospital cardiac arrest victims with coronary artery disease. *Circulation* 1981;64:977–984.
10. Bigger JT, Dresdale RT, Heissenbattel RH, et al. Ventricular arrhythmias in ischemic heart disease: mechanism, prevalence, significance and management. *Prog Cardiovasc Dis* 1977;19:255–300.
11. O'Doherty M, Taylor DI, Quinn E, et al. Five hundred patients

with myocardial infarction monitored within one hour of symptoms. *Br Med J* 1983;286:1405.

12. Pisa Z. Sudden death: a worldwide problem. In: Kulbertus H, Wellens HJ, eds. *Sudden death.* The Hague: Martinus Nijhoff, 1980.

13. Kannel WB, Doyle JT, McNamara PM, et al. Precursors of sudden coronary death: factors related to the incidence of sudden death. *Circulation* 1975;51:606.

14. Coumel P. The management of clinical arrhythmias: an overview on invasive versus non-invasive electrophysiology. *Eur Heart J* 1987;8:92–99.

15. Janse MJ, Wit AL. Electrophysiological mechanisms of ventricular arrhythmias resulting from myocardial ischaemia and infarction. *Physiol Rev* 1989;69:1049—1069.

16. Downer E, Janse AL, Durrer D. The effect of acute coronary occlusion on subepicardial transmembrane potentials in the intact porcine heart. *Circulation* 1977;56:217.

17. Kleber AG. Resting membrane potential, extracellular potassium activity and intracellular sodium activity during global ischemia in isolated perfused guinea-pig hearts. *Circ Res* 1983; 52:442–450.

18. Hill JL, Gettes LS. Effects of acute coronary artery occlusion on local myocardial and extracellular potassium activity in swine. *Circulation* 1980;61:768—778.

19. Hirche HJ, Franz C, Bos L, et al. Myocardial extracellular potassium and hydrogen increase and noradrenaline release as a possible cause of early arrhythmias following acute coronary occlusion in pigs. *J Mol Cell Cardiol* 1980;12:579.

20. Guarnieri T, Strauss H. Intracellular potassium activity in guinea-pig papillary muscle during prolonged hypoxia. *J Clin Invest* 1982;69:435–442.

21. Rau EE, Shine KL, Langer GA. Potassium exchange and mechanical performance in anoxic mammalian myocardium. *Am J Physiol* 1977;232:H85–H94.

22. Sobel BE, Corr PB, Robinson AK, et al. Accumulation of lysophosphoglycerides with arrhythmogenic properties in ischemic myocardium. *J Clin Invest* 1978;62:546–553.

23. Clarkson CW, Sawicki G. The effects of lysophosphatidylcholine, a toxic metabolite of ischemia, on the components of cardiac excitability in sheep Purkinje fibers. *Circ Res* 1981;49:16.

24. Clarkson CW, Ten Eick RE. On the mechanism of lysophosphatidylcholine-induced depolarization of cat ventricular myocardium. *Circ Res* 1983;52:543–556.

25. Corr PB, Cain ME, Witkowski FX, et al. Potential arrhythmogenic electrophysiological derangements in canine Purkinje fibres induced by lysophosphoglycerides. *Circ Res* 1979;44: 822–832.

26. Basset AL, Gelband H, Nilsson K, et al. Electrophysiology following healed experimental myocardial infarction. In: Kulbertus HE, ed. *Reentrant arrhythmias-mechanisms and treatment.* Lancaster, UK: MTP Press, 1979:242.

27. Corr PB, Yamada KA, Creer MH, et al. Lysophosphoglycerides and ventricular fibrillation early after the onset of ischaemia. *J Mol Cell Cardiol* 1987;19[Suppl V]:45–53.

28. Katz AM. Membrane-derived lipids and the pathogenesis of ischemic myocardial damage. *J Mol Cell Cardiol* 1982;14: 627–632.

29. Cohen CJ, Fozzard HA, Sheu SS. Increase in intracellular sodium ion activity during stimulation in mammalian cardiac muscle. *Circ Res* 1982;50:651–662.

30. Lado MG, Sheu SS, Fozzard HA. Changes in intracellular calcium activity with stimulation in sheep cardiac Purkinje strands. *Am J Physiol* 1982;243:133–137.

31. Harris AS. Delayed development of ventricular ectopic rhythms following experimental coronary artery occlusion. *Circulation* 1950;1:1318.

32. Boineau J, Cox JL. Slow ventricular activation in acute myocardial infarction: a source of re-entrant premature contraction. *Circulation* 1973;48:703–713.

33. El-Sherif NR, Hope R, Scherlag BJ, Lazzara R. Reentrant ventricular arrhythmias in the late myocardial infarction period: I. Conduction characteristics in the infarction zone. *Circulation* 1977;55:686.

34. Kaplinsky E, Ogawa S, Balke C, Dreifus LS. Two periods of early ventricular arrhythmias in the canine acute infarction model. *Circulation* 1979;60:397–403.

35. Sherlag BJ, Helfant LA, Haft JI, Damato AN. Electrophysiology underlying ventricular arrhythmias due to coronary ligation. *Am J Physiol* 1970;219:1665.

36. Waldo AL, Kaiser GA. A study of ventricular arrhythmias associated with acute myocardial infarction in the canine heart. *Circulation* 1970;47:1222.

37. Janse MJ, Van Capelle FJ, Morsink H, et al. Flow "injury" currents and patterns of excitation during early ventricular arrhythmias in regional myocardial ischemia in isolated porcine and canine hearts: evidence for 2 different mechanisms. *Circ Res* 1980;47:151.

38. Hoffman B, Singer DH. Appraisal of the effects of catecholamines on cardiac electrical activity. *Circ Res* 1981;49:1.

39. Carlsson L. Mechanisms of local noradrenaline release in acute myocardial infarction. *Acta Physiol Scand* 1978;129[Suppl]:7.

40. Schomig A, Dart AM, Dietz R, et al. Release of endogenous catecholamines in the ischemic myocardium of the rat. *Circ Res* 1984;55:689.

41. Penny WJ. The deleterious effects of myocardial catecholamines on cellular electrophysiology and arrhythmias during ischemia and reperfusion. *Eur Heart J* 1984;5:960.

42. Campbell RW, Murray A, Julian DG. Ventricular arrhythmias in the first 12 hours of acute myocardial infarction. *Br Heart J* 1981;46:351.

43. Northover BJ. Ventricular tachycardia during the first 72 hours after acute myocardial infarction. *Cardiology* 1982;69:149.

44. Spann JF, Moellering RC, Haber E, Wheeler EO. Arrhythmias in acute myocardial infarction. *N Engl J Med* 1964;271:427.

45. Fengoli JJ, Karaquezian HS, Freidman P, et al. Time course of infarct growth toward the endocardium after coronary occlusion. *Am J Physiol* 1979;236:H356.

46. Lowe JE, Cummings RG, Adams DH, Hull-Ryde EA. Evidence that cell death begins in the endocardium independent of variations in collateral flow or wall tension. *Circulation* 1983; 68:190.

47. Reimer KA, Jennings RB. The wavefront phenomenon of myocardial ischemic cell death. II. Transmural progression of necrosis within the framework of ischemic bed size (myocardium at risk) and collateral flow. *Lab Invest* 1979;40:633.

48. Fenoglia JJ, Albala A, Silva FC, et al. Structural basis of ventricular arrhythmias in human myocardial infarction: a hypothesis. *Hum Pathol* 1976;7:547.

49. Sugi K, Karagueuzian HS, Fishbein MC, et al. Spontaneous ventricular tachycardia associated with isolated right ventricular infarction one day after right coronary occlusion in the dog: studies on the site of origin and mechanism. *Am Heart J* 1985;109:232.

50. Bryden PA, Cranefield PF, Gadsby DC. Noradrenaline hyperpolarizes cells of the canine coronary sinus by increasing their permeability to potassium ions. *J Physiol Lond* 1983;339:185.

51. Schwartz PJ. The autonomic nervous system and sudden death. *Eur Heart J* 1998;19:F72–F80.

52. Cerati D, Schwartz PJ. Single cardiac nerve fiber activity, acute myocardial infarction and sudden death. *Circ Res* 1991;69: 1389.

53. La Rovere MT, Specchia G, Mortara A, Schwartz PJ. Baroreflex

sensitivity, clinical correlates and cardiovascular mortality among patients with first myocardial infarction. *Circulation* 1988;78:816.

54. Feigl D. Early and late atrioventricular block in acute inferior myocardial infarction. *J Am Coll Cardiol* 1984;4:35.

55. Cripps TR, Malik M, Farrell TG, Camm AJ. Prognostic value of reduced heart rate variability after myocardial infarction: clinical evaluation of a new analysis method. *Br Heart J* 1991; 65:14.

56. Lanza GA, Guido V, Galeazzi M, et al. Prognostic role of heart rate variability in patients with a recent myocardial infarction. *Am J Cardiol* 1998;82:1323–1328.

57. La Rovere MT, Bigger JT, Marcus FI, et al, for the ATRAMI investigators. Baroreflex sensitivity and heart rate variability in prediction of total cardiac mortality after myocardial infarction. *Lancet* 1998;351:478–484.

58. Antman EM, Braunwald E. Acute myocardial infarction. In: Braunwald E, ed. *Heart disease,* 5th ed. Philadelphia: WB Saunders, 1997:1245–1254.

59. Maggioni AP, Zuanetti G, Franzosi MG, et al. Prevalence and prognostic significance of ventricular arrhythmias after myocardial infarction in the fibrinolytic era: GISSI-2 results. *Circulation* 1993;87:312–322.

60. Rothfeld EL, Zucker IR, Parsonnet V, Alinsonorin CA. Idioventricular rhythm in acute myocardial infarction. *Circulation* 1968;37:203–209.

61. Gorgels APM, Vos MA, Letsch IS, Verschuuren EA, et al. Usefulness of the accelerated idioventricular rhythm as a marker for myocardial necrosis and reperfusion during thrombolytic therapy in acute myocardial infarction. *Am J Cardiol* 1988;61:231–235.

62. Wolfe CL, Nibley C, Bhandari A, et al. Polymorphous ventricular tachycardia associated with acute myocardial infarction. *Circulation* 1991;84:1543–1551.

63. Stewart RB, Bardy GH, Greene HL. Wide complex tachycardias: misdiagnosis and outcome after emergent therapy. *Ann Intern Med* 1986;104:766.

64. Dancy M, Camm AJ, Ward D. Misdiagnosis of chronic recurrent ventricular tachycardia. *Lancet* 1985;2:320–323.

65. Ewy GA. Ventricular fibrillation masquerading as asystole. *Ann Emerg Med* 1984;14:11.

66. Antman EM, Berlin JA. Declining incidence of ventricular fibrillation in myocardial infarction. *Circulation* 1992;86:1033–1035.

67. Behar S, Reccher-Ress H, Schechter M, et al. Frequency and prognostic significance of secondary ventricular fibrillation complicating acute myocardial infarction. *Circulation* 1985; 72:623.

68. May GS, Furberg CD, Eberlein KA, Geraci BJ. Secondary prevention after myocardial infarction: a review of short-term acute phase trials. *Prog Cardiovasc Dis* 1983;25:335.

69. Hine LK, Laird N, Hewitt P, Chalmers TC. Meta-analytic evidence against prophylactic use of lidocaine in acute myocardial infarction. *Arch Intern Med* 1989;149:2694.

70. Naccarelli GV, Wolbrette DL, dell'Orfano JT. A decade of clinical trial developments in postmyocardial infarction, congestive heart failure, and sustained ventricular tachyarrhythmia patients: from CAST to AVID and Beyond. *J Cardiovasc Electrophysiol* 1998;9:864–891.

71. Lie KI, Wellens HJ, Van Capelle FJ, Durrer D. Lidocaine in the prevention of primary ventricular fibrillation. *N Engl J Med* 1974;291:324.

72. Ryan TJ, Antman EM, Brooks NH, et al. 1999 Update: ACC/AHA guidelines for the management of patients with acute myocardial infarction: executive summary and recommendations. A report of the American College of Cardiology/American Heart Association Task Force on Practice Guidelines (Committee on Management of Acute Myocardial Infarction). *Circulation* 1999;100:1016–1030.

73. Nordehaug JE, Johannessen KA, von der Lippe G. Serum potassium as a risk factor for ventricular arrhythmias early in acute myocardial infarction. *Circulation* 1985;71:645.

74. Heissenbuttel RH, Bigger JT Jr. Bretylium tosylate: a newly available antiarrhythmic drug for ventricular arrhythmias. *Ann Intern Med* 1979;91:229–238.

75. Kowey PR, Bharucha DB, Rials SJ, et al. Intravenous antiarrhythmic therapy for high-risk patients. *Eur Heart J* 1999;1: C36–C40.

76. Scheinman MM, Levine JH, Cannom DS, et al. Dose-ranging study of intravenous amiodarone in patients with life-threatening ventricular tachyarrhythmias. *Circulation* 1995;92:3264.

77. Kowey PR, Levine JH, Herre JM, et al. Randomized, double-blind comparison of intravenous amiodarone and bretylium in the treatment of patients with recurrent, hemodynamically destabilizing ventricular tachycardia or fibrillation. The Intravenous Amiodarone Multicenter Investigators Group. *Circulation* 1995;92:3255.

78. Cook JR, Kirchhoffer JB, Fitzgerald TF, Lajzer DA. Comparison of decremental and burst overdrive pacing as treatment for ventricular tachycardia associated with coronary artery disease. *Am J Cardiol* 1992;70:311–315.

79. Advanced Life Support Working Group of the European Resuscitation Council. The 1998 European resuscitation guidelines for adult advanced life support. *Br Med J* 1998;316:1863–1869.

80. Kudenchuk PJ, Cobb LA, Copass MK, et al. Amiodarone for resuscitation after out-of-hospital cardiac arrest due to ventricular fibrillation. *N Engl J Med* 1999;341:871–878.

81. George M, Greenwood TW. Relationship between bradycardia and the site of myocardial infarction. *Lancet* 1967;1:739.

82. Zipes DP. The clinical significance of bradycardic arrhythmias in acute myocardial infarction. *Am J Cardiol* 1969;24:814.

83. Liberthson RR, Salisbury KW, Hutter AH, DeSanctis RW. Atrial tachyarrhythmias in acute myocardial infarction. *Am J Med* 1976;60:956–960.

84. Topol EJ, Goldschlager N, Ports TA, et al. Hemodynamic benefit of atrial pacing in right ventricular myocardial infarction. *Ann Intern Med* 1982;96:594.

85. Jewitt DE, Raftery EB, Balcon R, Oram S. Incidence and management of supraventricular arrhythmias after acute myocardial infarction. *Am Heart J* 1976;60:956–960.

86. CIBIS-II Investigators and Committees. The Cardiac Insufficiency Bisoprolol Study II (CIBIS-II): a randomised trial. *Lancet* 1999;353:9–13.

87. MERIT-HF Study Group. Effect of metoprolol CR/XL in chronic heart failure: Metoprolol CR/XL Randomized Intervention Trial in Congestive Heart failure (MERIT-HF). *Lancet* 1999;353:2001–2007.

88. James TN. Myocardial infarction and atrial arrhythmias. *Circulation* 1961;24:761.

89. Behar S, Zahavi Z, Goldbourt U, Reicher-Reiss H. Long-term prognosis of patients with paroxysmal atrial fibrillation complicating acute myocardial infarction: SPRINT study group. *Eur Heart J* 1992;13:45–50.

90. Sakata K, Kurihara H, Iwamori K, et al. Clinical and prognostic significance of atrial fibrillation in acute myocardial infarction. *Am J Cardiol* 1997;80:1522–1527.

91. Madias JE, Patel DC, Singh D. Atrial fibrillation in acute myocardial infarction: a prospective study based on data from a conservative series of patients admitted to the coronary care unit. *Clin Cardiol* 1996;19:180.

92. Crenshaw BS, Ward SR, Granger CB, et al. Atrial fibrillation in the setting of acute myocardial infarction: the GUSTO-1 experience. *J Am Coll Cardiol* 1997;30:406–413.

93. Berisso MZ, Carratino L, Ferroni A, et al. Frequency characteristics and significance of supraventricular tachyarrhythmias detected by 24-hour electrocardiographic recordings in the late hospital phase of acute myocardial infarction. *Am J Cardiol* 1990;65:1064.

94. Hod H, Lew AS, Keltae M, et al. Early atrial fibrillation during evolving myocardial infarction. *Circulation* 1987;75:146.

95. Bertolet BD, Hill JA, Kerensky RA, et al. Myocardial infarction related atrial fibrillation: role of endogenous adenosine. *Heart* 1997;78:88–90.

96. Nagahama Y, Sugiura T, Takehana K, et al. The role of infarction associated pericarditis on the occurrence of atrial fibrillation. *Eur Heart J* 1998;19:287–292.

97. Kowey PR, Marinchak RA, Rials SJ, et al. Acute treatment of atrial fibrillation. *Am J Cardiol* 1998;81[Suppl 5A]:16C–22C.

98. Cowan JC, Gardiner P, Reid DS, et al. Amiodarone in the management of atrial fibrillation complicating myocardial infarction. *Br J Clin Pract* 1986;40:155–161.

99. Echt DS, Liebson PR, Mitchell LB, et al. Mortality and morbidity in patients receiving encainide, flecainide or placebo: the Cardiac Arrhythmia Suppression Trial. *N Engl J Med* 1991;324:781–788.

100. The Cardiac Arrest Suppression Trial II Investigators. Effect of the antiarrhythmic agent moricizine on survival after myocardial infarction. *N Engl J Med* 1992;327:227–233.

101. Impact research Group. International mexiletine and placebo antiarrhythmic coronary trial: I. Report on arrhythmia and other findings. *J Am Coll Cardiol* 1984;4:1148–1163.

102. Julian DG, Camm AJ, Franglin G, et al, for the European Myocardial Infarct Amiodarone Trial Investigators. Randomized trial of effect of amiodarone on mortality in patients with left-ventricular dysfunction after recent myocardial infarction: EMIAT. *Lancet* 1997;349:675–682.

103. Cairns JA, Connolly SJ, Roberts R, et al, for the Canadian Amiodarone Myocardial Infarction Arrhythmia Trial Investigators. Randomized trial of outcome after myocardial infarction in patients with frequent or repetitive ventricular premature depolarizations: CAMIAT. *Lancet* 1997;349:675–682.

104. Julian DG, Prescott RJ, Jackson FS, et al. Controlled trial of sotalol for one year after myocardial infarction. *Lancet* 1982;1:1142–1147.

105. Abi-Mansour P, Carberry PA, McCowan RJ, et al. Conversion efficacy and safety of repeated doses of ibutilide in patients with atrial flutter and atrial fibrillation. *Am Heart J* 1998;136:632–642.

106. Norgaard BL, Wachtell K, Christensen PD, et al. Efficacy and safety of intravenously administered dofetilide in acute termination of atrial fibrillation and flutter: a multicenter, randomized, double-blind, placebo-controlled trial. Danish Dofetilide in Atrial Fibrillation and Flutter Study Group. *Am Heart J* 1999;137:1062–1069.

107. Danish Investigations of Arrhythmias and Mortality on Dofetilide. Dofetilide in patients with left ventricular dysfunction and either heart failure or acute myocardial infarction: rationale, design, and patient characteristics of the DIAMOND studies. *Clin Cardiol* 1997;20:704–710.

108. Damato AN, Lau SH. Clinical value of the electrogram of the conducting system. *Prog Cardiovasc Dis* 1970;13:119.

109. Feigl D, Aschenazy J, Kishon Y. Early and late atrioventricular block in acute inferior myocardial infarction. *J Am Coll Cardiol* 1984;4:35–38.

110. Kyriakidis M, Barbetseas J, Antonoloulos A, et al. Early atrial arrhythmias in acute myocardial infarction. *Chest* 1992;101:944.

111. Goldberg RJ, Zeravallos JC, Yarzebski J, et al. Prognosis of acute myocardial infarction complicated by complete heart block (the Worcester Heart Attack Study). *Am J Cardiol* 1992;69:1135.

112. Simons GR, Sgarbosa E, Wagner G, et al. Atrioventricular and intraventricular conduction disorders in acute myocardial infarction: a reappraisal in the thrombolytic era. *Pacing Clin Electrophysiol* 1998;21:2651–2663.

113. Clemenson P, Bates ER, Califf RM, et al, for the TAMI Study Group. Complete atrioventricular block complicating acute inferior myocardial infarction treated with reperfusion therapy. *Am J Cardiol* 1991;67:225.

114. Berger PR, Roucco NA Jr, Ryan TJ, et al. Incidence and prognostic implications of heart block complicating inferior myocardial infarction treated with thrombolytic therapy: results from TIMI II. *J Am Coll Cardiol* 1992;20:533–540.

115. Nicod P, Gilpin E, Dittrich H, et al. Long-term outcome in patients with inferior myocardial infarction and complete atrioventricular block. *J Am Coll Cardiol* 1988;12:589–594.

116. Altun A, Ozkan B, Gurcagan A, et al. Early and late atrioventricular block in acute inferior myocardial infarction. *Coron Artery Dis* 1998;9:1–4.

117. Newby KH, Pisano E, Krucoff MW, et al. Incidence and clinical relevance of the occurrence of bundle branch block in patients with thrombolytic therapy. *Circulation* 1996;94:2424–2428.

118. Sgarbossa EB, Pinski SL, Topol EJ, et al, for the GUSTO Investigators. Acute myocardial infarction and complete bundle branch block at hospital admission: clinical characteristics and outcome in the thrombolytic era. Global Utilization of Streptokinase and t-PA (tissue-type plasminogen activator) for Occluded Coronary Arteries. *J Am Coll Cardiol* 1998;31:105–110.

119. Melgarejo-Moreno A, Galcera-Tomas J, Garcia-Alberola A. Incidence, clinical characteristics and prognostic significance of right bundle branch block in acute myocardial infarction: a study in the thrombolytic era. *Circulation* 1997;96:1139–1144.

120. Klein RC, Vera Z, Mason DT. Intraventricular conduction defects in acute myocardial infarction: incidence, prognosis and therapy. *Am Heart J* 1984:1007–1013.

121. Goodman MJ, Lassers BW, Julian DG. Complete bundle branch block complicating acute myocardial infarction. *N Engl J Med* 1970;282:237.

122. Norris RM, Mercer CJ. Significance of idioventricular rhythms in acute myocardial infarction. *Prog Cardiovasc Dis* 1974;16:445.

123. Barold SS. American College of Cardiology/American Heart Association guidelines for pacemaker implantation after acute myocardial infarction: what is persistent advanced block at the atrioventricular node? *Am J Cardiol* 1997;80:770–774.

124. Zimmerman ANE, Hulsman WC. Paradoxical influences of calcium on the permeability of the isolated rat heart. *Nature* 1960;211:646.

125. Hearse DJ, Humphrey SM, Bullock GR. The oxygen paradox and the calcium paradox: two facets of the same problem? *J Mol Cell Cardiol* 1978;10:641.

126. Opie LH. Reperfusion injury and its pharmacologic modification. *Circulation* 1989;80:1049.

127. Opie LH, Coetzee WA. Role of calcium ions in reperfusion arrhythmias: relevance to pharmacologic intervention. *Cardiovasc Drugs Ther* 1988;2:623.

128. Coetzee WA, Opie LH. Effects of components of ischemia and metabolic inhibition on delayed afterdepolarizations in guinea pig papillary muscle. *Circ Res* 1987;61:157.

129. Allen DG, Lee JA, Smith GL. The effects of simulated ischaemia on intracellular calcium and tension in ferret ventricular muscle. *J Physiol (Lond)* 1988;401:81P.

130. Hearse DJ, Tosaki A. Free radicals and calcium: simultaneous interacting triggers as determinants of vulnerability to reperfusion-induced arrhythmias in the rat heart. *J Mol Cell Cardiol* 1988;20:213.

131. Pallandi RT, Perry MA, Campbell TJ. Proarrhythmic effects of an oxygen-derived free radical generating system on cation potentials recorded from guinea pig ventricular myocardium: a possible cause of reperfusion induced arrhythmias. *Circ Res* 1987;60:50.

132. Ambrosio G, Weisfeldt ML, Jacobus WE, et al. Evidence for a reversible oxygen mediated component of reperfusion injury: reduction by recombinant human superoxide dismutase administered at the time of reflow. *Circulation* 1987;75:282.

133. Saman S, Gaetzee WA, Opie LH. Inhibition by simulated ischaemia or hypoxia of delayed afterdepolarizations provoked by cyclic AMP: significance for ischaemia and reperfusion arrhythmias. *J Mol Cell Cardiol* 1988;20:91.

134. Spedding M, Mir AK. Direct activation of calcium channels by palmityl carnitive, a putative endogenous ligand. *Br J Pharmacol* 1987;92:457.

135. Ledermen SN, Wenger TL, Harrell FE, et al. Effects of different paced heart rates on canine coronary artery occlusion and reperfusion arrhythmias. *Am Heart J* 1987;113:1365.

136. Naylor WG, Elz JS. Reperfusion injury: laboratory artefact or clinical dilemma? *Circulation* 1986;74:215.

137. Jennings RB, Reiner KA, Steenbergen C. Myocardial ischemia revisited: the osmolar load, membrane damage and reperfusion. *J Mol Cell Cardiol* 1986;18:769.

138. Manning AS, Hearse DJ. Reperfusion-induced arrhythmias: mechanisms and prevention. *J Mol Cell Cardiol* 1984;16:497; 518.

139. Hagar JM, Kloner RA. Reperfusion arrhythmias: experimental and clinical aspects. *Age Reperfusion* 1990;2:1–5.

140. ISIS-2 (Second International Study of Infarct Survival) Collaborative Group. Randomised trial of intravenous streptokinase, oral aspirin, both, or neither among 17,187 cases of suspected acute myocardial infarction: ISIS-2. *Lancet* 1988;2:349–360.

141. Gruppo Italiano per lo Studio della Streptochinasi nell' infarto miocardico (GISSI). Effectiveness of intravenous thrombocytic treatment in acute myocardial infarction. *Lancet* 1986; 1:397–402.

142. Yoshida Y, Hirai M, Yamada T, et al. Antiarrhythmic efficacy of dipyridamole in treatment of reperfusion arrhythmias: evidence for cAMP-mediated triggered activity as a mechanism responsible for reperfusion arrhythmias. *Circulation* 2000;101:624–630.

143. Cain ME, Anderson JL, Arnsdorf MF, et al. Signal-averaged electrocardiography: ACC expert consensus document. *J Am Coll Cardiol* 1996;27:238.

144. Teo K, Yusuf S, Furberg C. Effect of prophylactic antiarrhythmic drug therapy on post-myocardial infarction mortality. *JAMA* 1993;270:1589–1595.

145. Waldo A, Camm J, de Ruyter H, et al. Effect of d-sotalol on mortality in patients with left ventricular dysfunction after recent and remote myocardial infarction. *Lancet* 1996;348:7.

146. Malik M, Camm AJ, Janse MJ, et al, on behalf of the EMIAT Investigators. Depressed heart rate variability identifies postinfarction patients who might benefit from prophylactic treatment with amiodarone: a substudy of EMIAT (the European Myocardial Infarct Amiodarone Trial). *J Am Coll Cardiol* 2000;35:1263.

147. Boutitie F, Boissel J-P, Connolly SJ, et al, and the EMIAT and CAMIAT Investigators. Amiodarone Interaction with β-blockers: analysis of the merged EMIAT (European Myocardial Infarct Amiodarone Trial) and CAMIAT (Canadian Amiodarone Myocardial Infarction Trial) databases. *Circulation* 1999;99:2268.

148. Janse MJ, Malik M, Camm AJ, et al, on behalf of the EMIAT Investigators. Identification of post–acute myocardial infarction patients with potential benefit from prophylactic treatment with amiodarone: a substudy of EMIAT (the European Myocardial Infarct Amiodarone Trial). *Eur Heart J* 1998;19:85.

149. Camm AJ, Karam R, Pratt CM. The Azimilide Post-Infarct Survival Evaluation (ALIVE) trial. *Am J Cardiol* 1998;81[Suppl 6A]:35D–39D.

150. Nicod P, Gilpin E, Dittrich H, et al. Influence on prognosis and mortality of left ventricular ejection fraction with and without signs of left ventricular failure after acute myocardial infarction. *Am J Cardiol* 1988;61:1165–1171.

151. The Multicenter Postinfarction Research Group. Risk stratification and survival after myocardial infarction. *N Engl J Med* 1983;309:331–336.

152. Hung J, Goris ML, Nash E, et al. Comparative value of maximal treadmill testing, exercise thallium myocardial perfusion scintigraphy and exercise radionuclide ventriculography for distinguishing high- and low-risk patients after acute myocardial infarction. *Am J Cardiol* 1984;53:1221–1227.

153. Gomes JA, Winters SL, Stewart D, et al. A new noninvasive index to predict sustained ventricular tachycardia and sudden death in the first year after myocardial infarction: based on signal-averaged electrocardiogram, radionuclide ejection fraction and Holter monitoring. *J Am Coll Cardiol* 1987;10:349–357.

154. Steinberg JS, Regan A, Sciacca RR, et al. Predicting arrhythmic events after acute myocardial infarction using the signal-averaged electrocardiogram. *Am J Cardiol* 1992;69:13–21.

155. Kleiger RE, Miller JP, Bigger JT Jr, et al. Decreased heart rate variability and its association with increased mortality after acute myocardial infarction. *Am J Cardiol* 1987;59:256–262.

156. Denniss RA, Richards DA, Cody DV, et al. Prognostic significance of ventricular tachycardia and fibrillation induced at programmed stimulation and delayed potentials detected on the signal-averaged electrocardiograms of survivors of acute myocardial infarction. *Circulation* 1986;74:731–745.

157. Bourke JP, Richards DA, Ross DL. Routine programmed stimulation in survivors of acute myocardial infarction for prediction of spontaneous ventricular tachyarrhythmias during follow-up: results optimal stimulation protocol and cost effective screening. *J Am College Cardiol* 1991;18:780–788.

158. Buxton AE, Lee KL, Fisher JD, et al. A randomized study of the prevention of sudden death in patients with coronary artery disease. *N Engl J Med* 1999;341:1882–1890.

159. Zoni-Berisso M, Molini D, Mel GS, et al. Value of programmed ventricular stimulation in predicting sudden death and sustained ventricular tachycardia in survivors of acute myocardial infarction. *Am J Cardiol* 1996;77:673.

160. Pedretti R, Etro MD, Laporta A, et al. Prediction of late arrhythmic events after acute myocardial infarction from combined use of non-invasive prognostic variables and inducibility of sustained monomorphic ventricular tachycardia. *Am J Cardiol* 1993;71:1131–1141.

161. Murdah M, Mckenna WJ, Camm AJ. Repolarization alternans: techniques, mechanisms, and cardiac vulnerability. *Pacing Clin Electrophysiol* 1997;20[Pt II]:2641–2657.

162. Nearing BD, Oesterle SN, Verrier RL. Quantification of ischaemia induced vulnerability by precordial T wave alternans analysis in dog and human. *Pacing Clin Electrophysiol* 1994;28: 1440–1449.

163. Zabel M, Klingenheben ZM, Franz MR, et al. Assessment of QT dispersion for prediction of mortality or arrhythmic events after myocardial infarction: results of a prospective, long term follow-up study. *Circulation* 1998;97:2543–2550.

164. Schmidt G, Malik M, Barthel P, et al. Heart-rate turbulence after ventricular premature beats as a predictor of mortality after acute myocardial infarction. *Lancet* 1999;353:1390–1396.

165. Farrell TG, Bashir Y, Cripps T, et al. Risk stratification for arrhythmic events in postinfarction patients based on heart rate variability, ambulatory electrocardiographic variables and the signal-averaged electrocardiogram. *J Am Coll Cardiol* 1991;18: 687–697.

166. Hartikanen JE, Malik M, Staunton A, et al. Distinction between arrhythmic and nonarrhythmic death after acute myocardial infarction based on heart rate variability, signal-averaged electrocardiogram, ventricular arrhythmias and left ventricular ejection fraction. *J Am Coll Cardiol* 1996;28: 296–304.

167. Andresen D, Steinbeck G, Bruggemann T, et al. Risk stratification following myocardial infarction in the thrombolytic era: a two-step strategy using non-invasive and invasive methods. *J Am Coll Cardiol* 1999;33:131–138.

168. Schron EB. Friedman LM, Greene HL. Future clinical trials. In: Woosley RL, Singh SN, eds. *Arrhythmia treatment and therapy: evaluation of clinical trial evidence.* New York: Marcel Dekker, 2000;351–360.

169. Moss AJ, Hall WJ, Cannom DS, et al, for The Multicenter Automatic Defibrillator Implantation Trial Investigators. Improved survival with an implanted defibrillator in patients with coronary disease at high risk for ventricular arrhythmias. *N Engl J Med* 1996;335:1933–1940.

170. Ruskin JN, DiMarco JP, Garan H. Out of hospital cardiac arrest: electrophysiologic observations and selection of long term antiarrhythmic therapy. *N Engl J Med* 1980;303:607–612.

171. Roy D, Waxman HL, Kienzle MG, et al. Clinical characteristics and long term follow-up in 119 survivors of cardiac arrest: relation to inducibility at electrophysiologic testing. *Am J Cardiol* 1983;52:969–974.

172. Wilber DJ, Garan H, Finkelstein D, et al. Out of hospital cardiac arrest: role of electrophysiologic testing in prediction of long term outcome. *N Engl J Med* 1988;318:19–24.

173. The CASCADE Investigators. Randomised antiarrhythmic drug therapy in survivors of cardiac arrest (the CASCADE study). *Am J Cardiol* 1993;72:280–287.

174. The Antiarrhythmic Versus Implantable Defibrillators (AVID) Investigators. A comparison of antiarrhythmic drug therapy with implantable defibrillators in patients resuscitated from near fatal ventricular arrhythmias. *N Engl J Med* 1997;337:1576–1583.

175. Connolly SJ, Gent M, Roberts RS, et al. Canadian Implantable Defibrillator Study (CIDS): a randomised trial of the implantable cardioverter defibrillator against amiodarone. *Circulation* 2000;101:1297–1302.

176. Wever EF, Hauer RN, van Capelle FL, et al. Randomized study of implantable defibrillator as first-choice therapy versus conventional strategy in postinfarct sudden death survivors. *Circulation* 1995;91:2195–203.

177. Newman D, Sauve MJ, Herre J, et al. Randomized study of implantable defibrillator as first-choice therapy versus conventional strategy in postinfarct sudden death survivors. *Circulation* 1992;69:899–903.

178. Gregoratos G, Cheitlin MD, Conill A, et al. ACC/AHA Practice Guidelines. ACC/AHA guidelines for the implantation of cardiac pacemakers antiarrhythmia devices: a report of the American College of Cardiology and the American Heart Association Task Force on Practice Guidelines (Committee on Pacemaker Implantation). *J Am Coll Cardiol* 1998;31:1175–1209.

31

ARRHTHMIAS IN MITRAL VALVE DISEASE

PAUL KLIGFIELD
RICHARD B. DEVEREUX

Symptomatic and asymptomatic arrhythmia are common features of mitral valve disease. The development of atrial fibrillation in patients with rheumatic mitral stenosis has long been an important transitional event between a less symptomatic early phase of the disease and a period of progressive dyspnea and fatigue with higher risk of embolization (1,2). Atrial fibrillation and a range of ventricular arrhythmias are prominent features of rheumatic mitral regurgitation. Although rheumatic heart disease remains an important worldwide health problem, its prevalence in developed countries has decreased dramatically during the past half century. Throughout the last 30 years, mitral valve prolapse (MVP) has emerged as the most commonly diagnosed abnormality of the heart valves. As a consequence, MVP has emerged as the most frequent cause of hemodynamically important nonischemic, nonmyopathic mitral regurgitation in the United States. During this period, the clinical features and significance of arrhythmias in many patients with MVP uncomplicated by mitral regurgitation have remained controversial.

Early studies of MVP emphasized the prevalence of palpitation in affected subjects, and incorporation of atrial and ventricular arrhythmias within a combined clinical, auscultatory, electrocardiographic (ECG), and echocardiographic syndrome unified previously unexplained symptoms and physical findings in many patients (3–9). Occasional reports of unexpected sudden death in subjects with MVP (5,10–14) focused on the prevalence, prognostic value, and treatment of arrhythmias associated with this disorder (15–25). However, it has become increasingly evident that MVP is most often a rather benign clinical finding with only a small incidence of serious complications (9,26–28). The management challenge in this population is to predict and prevent these complications while providing reassur-

ance for the many people in whom isolated, uncomplicated MVP has no important risk.

This chapter examines arrhythmias in patients with mitral valve disease, with particular focus on the general features, arrhythmic profile, and arrhythmic complications of MVP, with and without hemodynamically important mitral regurgitation (29–40). Arrhythmias in patients with significant mitral regurgitation, with and without underlying MVP, are separately compared. We review the effect of selection bias on arrhythmias found in populations with MVP, and we suggest that arrhythmia complexity in MVP is predominantly determined by the presence of associated severe mitral regurgitation. Evidence for an association of MVP with arrhythmic sudden death is examined, and incidence rates of sudden death are estimated for patients with MVP with and without hemodynamically important mitral regurgitation. We discuss data bearing on mechanisms of arrhythmogenesis in mitral valve disease and recommendations for treatment of patients with MVP. Recent reviews address the biology, clinical characteristics, natural history, and complications of MVP in supplementary detail (9,27,28, 37–45).

MITRAL VALVE PROLAPSE
Prevalence

Depending on the echocardiographic criteria used for ascertainment, the prevalence of MVP ranges from about 2.4% to 5.0% in the general adult population (8,9,27,43,46,47), making it one of the most common structural cardiac abnormalities seen in clinical practice. MVP is most often a benign disorder, and recognized complications are fortunately rare (9,27,28). However, as a consequence of the many prevalent cases, even the occurrence of complications with very low incidence, such as complex arrhythmia and arrhythmic death, can affect a substantial number of patients (32,35).

P. Kligfield and R. B. Devereux: Department of Medicine, Weill Medical College of Cornell University, New York, New York 10021.

Echocardiographic Features

Recognition of MVP evolved from bedside detection of mid-systolic clicks and late systolic apical murmurs that have been shown to arise from the mitral apparatus (3,48). Because auscultatory features of MVP vary between examinations, echocardiography has become a primary method of detection and diagnostic confirmation (41,42). As revealed by these methods, the anatomic abnormalities of MVP include mitral leaflet enlargement, thickening, and connective tissue and chordal disruption leading to systolic protrusion of a leaflet or leaflets across the plane of the mitral anulus. The diagnosis of MVP can be made with high specificity by M-mode recordings when there is at least 2 mm of systolic posterior leaflet displacement behind the C-D line. Diagnosis is made by two-dimensional methods when there is systolic protrusion of a leaflet across the anular plane in the parasternal long-axis view. When 2 mm of protrusion in this view is required for definition of MVP (27,28), its prevalence in screened populations will be lower than when lesser protrusion is used for diagnosis. Specificity is unacceptably low if the apical four-chamber view is used alone for diagnosis (42), because of geometric distortions caused by the saddle shape of the mitral anulus.

Clinical Features

Family studies demonstrate that the condition may be inherited in a classic, autosomal dominant pattern with variable age- and sex-dependent expression more likely in women (41,49). Only preliminary evidence has been obtained for linkage between MVP and a chromosome region that might code for one or more connective tissue proteins (50). Family studies also demonstrate that MVP is associated with minor thoracic skeletal abnormalities, such as pectus excavatum, scoliosis, and straight back, with reduced body weight and reduced blood pressure (41,46,49,51,52), with occasional orthostatic hypotension (53), and with symptomatic palpitation and syncope (52). Even so, as discussed in this chapter, associations between MVP and complex atrial and ventricular arrhythmias are less strong than has been generally inferred from early reports.

Case-control family studies do not support a true association between MVP and clinical features of atypical chest pain, dyspnea, panic or anxiety attacks, or ECG repolarization abnormalities (9,52); these findings are also more common in women than in men in the absence of MVP. Chest pain, dyspnea, syncope, heart failure, cerebrovascular disease, and atrial fibrillation were found with similarly low prevalence among people with and without MVP in the Framingham offspring cohort (27,28). In population-based studies, individuals with MVP have had lower body weight and blood pressure, as well as lower prevalence of diabetes and overt coronary heart disease than individuals without this condition (28,47). The prevalence, severity, and signif-

icance of autonomic dysfunction in MVP have been subject to selection bias and have been incompletely studied (9). The extent to which orthostatic hypotension, sinus tachycardia, or even marked sinus arrhythmias might result in perception of symptomatic palpitation or dizziness in MVP has important implications for the interpretation and management of arrhythmia in these patients. However, no clear link has been established between autonomic dysfunction and arrhythmia in MVP.

NONARRHYTHMIC COMPLICATIONS

Major complications of MVP include the development of infective endocarditis, progressive mitral regurgitation, occasional cases of cerebral embolization, and as discussed in detail later in this chapter, sudden death (54–68). Among patients with MVP, the risks of endocarditis and of progressive severe mitral regurgitation are strongly concentrated in men, rather than in women, and in people older than 45 years (54,56,57). The risk of endocarditis is increased in patients with MVP with demonstrable mitral regurgitation (56–58). Age appears to be an important factor in the subsequent development of complications in prospectively studied MVP populations. Thus, for example, Bisset and colleagues (64) found no progression of mitral regurgitation, one case each of infective endocarditis and cerebrovascular accident, and no sudden death among 119 children, whose mean age at entry was 10 years, over a mean follow-up of 7 years. In contrast, Duren and colleagues (63) found substantially higher incidences of infective endocarditis, progressive mitral regurgitation, and cerebrovascular accidents during a mean 6-year follow-up of adults with MVP, a number of whom had varying amounts of mitral regurgitation at study entry and whose mean age was 42 years.

Overall, it has been estimated that MVP is associated with a 25-fold increased risk of severe mitral regurgitation (54), with cumulative lifetime risk of hemodynamically important regurgitation for individuals reaching about 1% to 2% for women and about 5% for men (9,55,57). Even when mitral regurgitation is not overt, increased heart size by standard criteria (69) has been a common finding among subjects with MVP examined at autopsy (66–68). Although more than 1,000 cases of infective endocarditis occur among patients with MVP in the United States alone each year, because of the high prevalence of MVP in the general population, individual risk is quite low, perhaps 1 in 5,000 per year (9). This risk appears to be concentrated in the subset of patients with MVP with apical systolic murmurs and significant mitral regurgitation, in whom antibiotic prophylaxis for procedures is indicated (56,58,59).

Morphology of the mitral leaflet may be related to subsequent complications. Nishimura and colleagues (61) have shown that the risk of important mitral regurgitation, infective endocarditis, and cerebral embolic events, as well as sudden death, are concentrated in patients with MVP who have thickened, redundant mitral valve leaflets demonstrated by echocardiography. Marks and colleagues (62) found that complications of endocarditis, progression to moderate to severe mitral regurgitation, and referral for mitral valve replacement, but not of stroke, are significantly more frequent in patients with MVP who have leaflet thickening than in patients without this finding. However, a study of patients with MVP with a low prevalence of severe regurgitation failed to find an association between thickened mitral leaflets and the subsequent risk of major complications (70), and other studies have shown thickening of mitral leaflets in 60% or more of individuals with uncomplicated MVP (71,72).

ARRHYTHMIAS IN MITRAL PROLAPSE, MITRAL REGURGITATION, AND MITRAL STENOSIS

Arrhythmias in Heterogeneous MVP Populations

A wide range of arrhythmias have been detected by ambulatory ECG in patients with MVP. During recording periods of varying duration in variously selected populations, atrial premature contractions (APCs) have been recorded in 35% to 90% and atrial tachycardia has been documented in 6% to 32% of patients (18–20,23,24,29–40). Ventricular premature contractions (VPCs) have been found in 58% to 89% of MVP study groups. Complex ventricular arrhythmias have been reported in 30% to 59% of adult patients with MVP, but definitions of arrhythmia complexity within these studies have included frequent and multiform VPCs (19,23) or occasionally multiform single VPCs alone (20,24) as complex forms. Other definitions of complexity have been limited to repetitive forms alone, to include only VPC couplets, salvos, or nonsustained ventricular tachycardia (18). Even with comparable definitions, the prevalence of repetitive ventricular arrhythmias in MVP has been highly variable. Within these heterogeneous study populations, the reported prevalence of VPC couplets has ranged from 6% to 50% and that for VPC salvos or nonsustained ventricular tachycardia has ranged from 5% to 21%.

Although some cases of block within and below the level of the atrioventricular (AV) node have been reported (73,74), conduction defects beyond modest prolongation of the PR interval or occasional Wenckebach periods are uncommon in general populations of subjects with MVP (23,24). On the other hand, among highly symptomatic patients referred for electrophysiologic study, abnormal sinus node function, A-H interval prolongation, prolongation of the HV interval and spontaneous second- or even third-degree AV block, and chronic bundle branch block have been found, each in 10% to 20% of cases (33,34,75).

Reasons for the highly variable prevalence of arrhythmias in MVP found in different reports include significant selection bias when highly symptomatic patients are concentrated in a study group (76). This bias limits our ability to extrapolate data obtained from electrophysiologic studies in symptomatic referred patients to the general MVP population. Further, patient populations often differ in symptoms and in clinical severity of disease, as do normal controls. It is now well appreciated that atrial and ventricular ectopy also occur commonly in clinically healthy subjects (77–83). Thus, by way of example, Brodsky and colleagues (78) found APCs in 56% and VPCs in 50% of clinically healthy young men, whereas Sobotka and colleagues (79) found APCs in 64% and VPCs in 54% of healthy young women. Thus, evaluation of potential excess prevalence of arrhythmias attributable to MVP requires selection of both representative patients and suitable control populations.

Selection bias results when symptomatic patients with MVP are inadvertently compared with asymptomatic healthy subjects or volunteers. To reduce this bias, Kramer and colleagues (24) compared ambulatory arrhythmias in patients with uncomplicated MVP with control subjects who had similar prevalences of palpitation, chest pain, dyspnea, and dizziness. Indeed, many of the control patients in this study were originally referred with a tentative diagnosis of MVP, based on symptoms alone, which was ultimately disproved by subsequent auscultatory and echocardiographic examination. Selection bias also was avoided in the study of Savage and colleagues (23), in which subjects with MVP and randomly chosen controls were identified independent of symptom status, from participants in a systematic evaluation of offspring of the original cohort of the Framingham Study.

Regarding atrial arrhythmias, Kramer and colleagues (24) found that patients with MVP had modest trends toward more APC couplets (30%) and more brief runs of supraventricular tachycardia (32%) than similarly symptomatic controls, but these differences did not reach statistical significance (Fig. 31-1). A similar trend toward more supraventricular tachycardia (24%) among randomly selected subjects with MVP than among controls was also found in the Framingham Study (23). Combining these two studies, which used similar echocardiographic and ambulatory ECG methods, suggests a higher prevalence of supraventricular tachycardia, predominantly brief three- to eight-beat runs of sequential APCs, in MVP than in similarly selected controls (28% versus 17%; $p < 0.02$) (Fig. 31-2).

Regarding ventricular arrhythmias, Kramer and colleagues (24) found no significant differences in the prevalence of frequent VPCs (3%), multiform VPCs (43%), ventricular couplets (6%), or ventricular salvos and nonsustained ventricular tachycardia (5%) in patients with MVP compared with similarly selected control subjects (Fig. 31-3). Interestingly, both MVP and randomly selected control groups in the Framingham Study had equal prevalences of VPC couplets or brief

Group Prevalence (%)

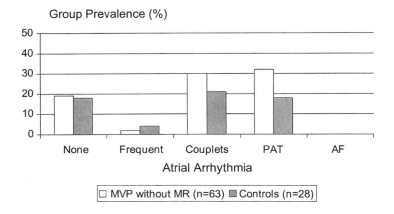

Atrial Arrhythmia

FIGURE 31-1. Atrial arrhythmias in patients with mitral valve prolapse, with no important mitral regurgitation, and in similarly symptomatic control subjects. Prevalences (in percentages) of no atrial premature contractions (APCs), frequent APCs (>10 per 1,000 total beats), APC couplets, brief paroxysmal atrial tachycardia (PAT), and atrial fibrillation (AF) are shown on the vertical axis. Patients with mitral valve prolapse have trends toward more APC couplets and PAT, but these differences do not reach significance. (From Kramer HM, Kligfield P, Devereux RB, et al. Arrhythmias in mitral valve prolapse: effect of selection bias. *Arch Intern Med* 1984;144:2360–2364, with permission.)

Group Prevalence of Atrial Tachycardia (%)

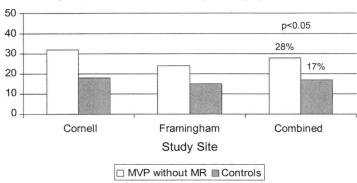

Study Site

FIGURE 31-2. Differences in group prevalence of paroxysmal atrial tachycardia (PAT) between subjects with mitral valve prolapse, without important mitral regurgitation, and similarly selected control subjects reach significance when data are pooled from the Cornell and the Framingham studies. (From Kramer HM, Kligfield P, Devereux RB, et al. Arrhythmias in mitral valve prolapse: effect of selection bias. *Arch Intern Med* 1984;144:2360-2364, and Savage DD, Levy D, Garrison RJ, et al. Mitral valve prolapse in the general population. *Am Heart J* 1983;106:582–586, with permission.)

Group Prevalence (%)

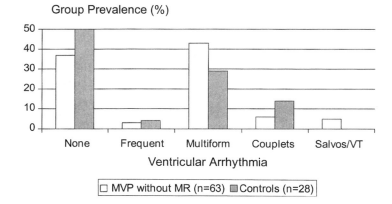

Ventricular Arrhythmia

FIGURE 31-3. Ventricular arrhythmias in patients with mitral valve prolapse, with no important mitral regurgitation, and in similarly symptomatic control subjects. Prevalences (in percentages) of frequent ventricular premature contractions (VPCs) (>10 per 1,000 total beats), multiform VPCs, VPC couplets, VPC salvos or ventricular tachycardia (more than three sequential VPCs at a rate of >100 beats per minute), and early-cycle forms. No differences reach significance. (From Kramer HM, Kligfield P, Devereux RB, et al. Arrhythmias in mitral valve prolapse: effect of selection bias. *Arch Intern Med* 1984;144:2360–2364, with permission.)

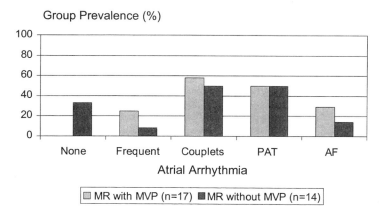

FIGURE 31-4. Atrial arrhythmias in patients with mitral regurgitation, with and without mitral valve prolapse. Prevalences (in percentages) of no atrial premature contractions (APCs), frequent APCs (>10 per 1,000 total beats), APC couplets, brief paroxysmal atrial tachycardia, and atrial fibrillation are shown on the vertical axis. Note similar profile of arrhythmias in patients with mitral regurgitation, independent of origin. (From Kligfield P, Hochreiter C, Kramer H, et al. Complex arrhythmias in mitral regurgitation with and without mitral valve prolapse: contrast to arrhythmias in mitral valve prolapse with and without mitral regurgitation. *Am J Cardiol* 1985;55:1545–1549, with permission.)

runs of ventricular tachycardia (15%) (23). Thus, when ambulatory MVP populations are compared with comparably symptomatic or comparably asymptomatic control subjects, it is not apparent that there is a higher group prevalence of frequent or complex arrhythmia, other than brief supraventricular tachycardia, in patients with MVP who do not have mitral regurgitation.

Arrhythmias in Severe Mitral Regurgitation, with and without MVP

It has long been recognized that atrial and ventricular arrhythmias are common among patients with pure mitral regurgitation (84,85). Chronic atrial fibrillation is common, and repetitive atrial arrhythmias and brief bursts of atrial tachycardia in patients in sinus rhythm can be found in half of such patients by ambulatory ECG. Repetitive ventricular arrhythmias are also commonly detected by ambulatory recording, with VPC couplets found in more than half, and VPC salvos or brief bursts of nonsustained ventricular tachycardia found in about one third of patients (87). Similar prevalences of complex arrhythmias have been demonstrated in patients with comparable severity of mitral regurgitation resulting from MVP or other causes (87), as

shown in Figures 31-4 and 31-5. These findings suggest that arrhythmias found in populations with MVP are strongly influenced by the degree of mitral regurgitation.

Effect of Mitral Regurgitation on Arrhythmias in Mitral Prolapse

The development of significant mitral regurgitation is an uncommon but well-established complication of MVP in adults (47,54,55,57,60–64). Indeed, because MVP is so common, it is now emerging as the most common cause of hemodynamically important mitral regurgitation in industrialized countries (54,57,86,87). The relationship between valvular regurgitation and the arrhythmias observed in patients with MVP (87,88) is particularly relevant to the problem of sudden death.

The effect of hemodynamically important mitral regurgitation on the group prevalence of atrial arrhythmias in MVP is summarized from the data of Kligfield and colleagues (87) in Table 31-1 and Figure 31-6. Atrial arrhythmias were more frequent and more complex in patients with MVP with associated clinically severe mitral regurgitation. All patients with mitral regurgitation had some atrial arrhythmia, nearly one third were in sustained atrial fibrillation (29%), and very frequent APCs (more than 10 per 1,000 beats) in patients in

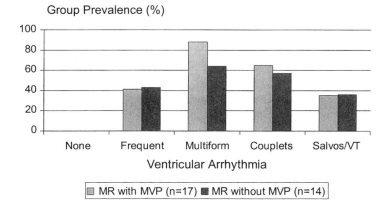

FIGURE 31-5. Ventricular arrhythmias in patients with mitral regurgitation, with and without mitral valve prolapse. Prevalences (in percentages) of frequent ventricular premature contractions (VPCs) (>10 per 1,000 total beats), multiform VPCs, VPC couplets, and VPC salvos or ventricular tachycardia (more than three sequential VPCs at a rate of >100 beats per minute). No differences reach significance. (From Kligfield P, Hochreiter C, Kramer H, et al. Complex arrhythmias in mitral regurgitation with and without mitral valve prolapse: contrast to arrhythmias in mitral valve prolapse with and without mitral regurgitation. *Am J Cardiol* 1985;55:1545–1549, with permission.)

TABLE 31-1. PREVALENCE OF ARRHYTHMIAS DETECTED BY AMBULATORY ELECTROCARDIOGRAPHY IN ADULT POPULATIONS WITH MITRAL VALVE PROLAPSE

		Arrhythmia Prevalence (%)				
	N	Any APCs	SVT	Any VPCs	Complex VPCs[a]	Repetitive VPCs[b]
Kramer et al. (24)	63	81	32	63	43	8
Savage et al. (23)	61	90	24	89	56	15
DeMaria et al. (19)	31	35	6	58	52	
Campbell et al. (20)	20		10	80	50	30
Winkle et al. (18)	24	63	29	75	50	50

Source: Kramer HM, Kligfield P, Devereux RB, et al. *Arrhythmias in mitral valve prolapse: effect of selection bias.* Arch Intern Med 1984;144:2360–2364, with permission.
SVT, supraventricular tachycardia; VPCs, ventricular premature complexes.
[a]Definitions of complex VPCs vary among studies, and generally include multiform VPCs.
[b]Repetitive VPCs include pairs, salvos, and ventricular tachycardia.

sinus rhythm were common (25%). In contrast, none of the patients with MVP without mitral regurgitation had atrial fibrillation, and frequent APCs were rare (2%). Patients with MVP and mitral regurgitation also had trends toward more prevalent APC couplets (58%) and episodes of brief supraventricular tachycardia (50%) than were found in patients with uncomplicated MVP alone, but these differences did not reach statistical significance.

The effect of important mitral regurgitation on ventricular arrhythmias in MVP (73) is also shown in Table 31-1 and Figure 31-7. Similar to the findings for atrial arrhythmias, ventricular arrhythmias are more frequent and more complex when mitral regurgitation complicates MVP. All patients with mitral regurgitation had ventricular ectopy, and more than 41% had very frequent VPCs (more than 10 per 1,000 beats). In contrast, frequent VPCs were present in only 3% of patients with MVP without mitral regurgitation. Further, patients with MVP with severe mitral regurgitation had markedly increased prevalences of multiform VPCs (88%), VPC couplets (65%), and nonsustained ventricular tachycardia (35%), with peak Lown grades of 4A or 4B in nearly two thirds (59%) of this subset. Babuty and colleagues (39) have more recently demonstrated a significant concentration of multiform and repetitive VPCs in patients with MVP with

mitral regurgitation, even when the grade of regurgitation was only mild to moderate. These findings indicate that patients with MVP with hemodynamically important mitral regurgitation are likely to have more frequent and more complex atrial and ventricular arrhythmias than patients without mitral regurgitation. Accordingly, the prevalence of complex arrhythmia within different MVP populations will vary with the proportion of patients who have underlying important mitral regurgitation in the group.

Arrhythmias in Mitral Stenosis

Atrial arrhythmias, including atrial fibrillation, are common in patients with rheumatic mitral stenosis. Selzer and Cohn (2) considered atrial fibrillation to be the most common complication of mitral stenosis and the factor most responsible for the transition from compensation to disability in these people. In the large series reported by Wood (1) in 1954, chronic atrial fibrillation was present in approximately 40% and paroxysmal atrial fibrillation was recognized in an additional 6% of patients.

In patients with mitral stenosis who were in sinus rhythm, 24-hour ambulatory monitoring by Ramsdale and

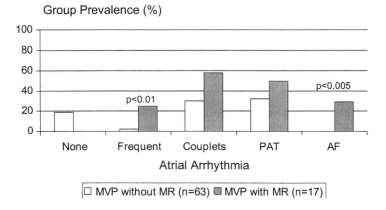

FIGURE 31-6. Atrial arrhythmias in patients with mitral valve prolapse, with and without hemodynamically important mitral regurgitation. Patients with mitral regurgitation have a higher prevalence of frequent atrial premature contractions (APCs) and atrial fibrillation, whereas trends toward more APC couplets and paroxysmal atrial tachycardia do not reach statistical significance. (From Kligfield P, Hochreiter C, Kramer H, et al. Complex arrhythmias in mitral regurgitation with and without mitral valve prolapse: contrast to arrhythmias in mitral valve prolapse with and without mitral regurgitation. *Am J Cardiol* 1985;55:1545–1549, with permission.)

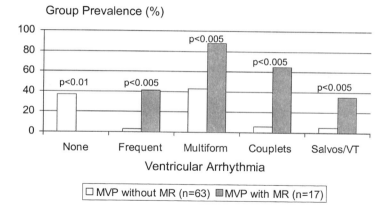

Group Prevalence (%)

FIGURE 31-7. Ventricular arrhythmias in patients with mitral valve prolapse, with and without hemodynamically important mitral regurgitation. Patients with mitral regurgitation have a higher prevalence of ventricular premature contractions (VPCs), frequent VPCs, multiform VPCs, VPC couplets, and VPC salvos or ventricular tachycardia. (From Kligfield P, Hochreiter C, Kramer H, et al. Complex arrhythmias in mitral regurgitation with and without mitral valve prolapse: contrast to arrhythmias in mitral valve prolapse with and without mitral regurgitation. *Am J Cardiol* 1985;55:1545–1549, with permission.)

colleagues (89) revealed one or more transient and generally asymptomatic supraventricular tachyarrhythmia in 55%. In this population, 40% had paroxysmal atrial tachycardia, 22% had paroxysmal atrial fibrillation, 13% had multifocal atrial tachycardia, and 8% had transient atrial flutter. Nearly all patients had single APCs, 64% had APC couplets or triplets, and arrhythmias were more common in older patients.

PROGNOSTIC SIGNIFICANCE OF ARRHYTHMIA

Sudden Death and Complex Arrhythmias in MVP

Rare cases of sudden death have been associated with MVP since its early recognition (5,8,10), and it has become generally accepted that a small but important subset of patients with MVP has complex arrhythmias that are potentially lethal (11–14,32). A link between arrhythmic death and MVP is supported by demonstration of MVP as the only autopsy finding in some cases of sudden death (13,14, 66–68, 90), as the only abnormality in survivors of cardiac arrest (65), and as the only clinical finding in patients referred for management of refractory, symptomatic complex ventricular arrhythmias (11,22,88). Although it is presumed that the basis for sudden death in MVP is arrhythmic, it is clear that the number of patients with MVP with complex arrhythmias greatly exceeds the number who die suddenly. Further, it is far from established that complex arrhythmias that might indicate a high level of risk are indeed present before the fatal event in those patients with MVP suffering sudden death (32).

The incidence of sudden death during prospective follow-up of selected patient groups has ranged from 0% to 0.5% yearly (26,27,61–64). However, inferences from these longitudinal data are limited by symptomatic and clinical heterogeneity of study populations, by varied referral patterns, by inconstant reporting of associated findings such as mitral regurgitation, and by lack of absolute autopsy con-

firmation that MVP was the sole cause of death, particularly in older patients.

Among prospectively followed cohorts, with variable selection characteristics, Nishimura and colleagues (61) found 6 cases of sudden death among 237 minimally symptomatic patients with MVP followed for an average of 6 years. This prevalence corresponds to an annual mortality rate of approximately 0.4% to 0.5%, which is twice the incidence of sudden death expected in the general adult population (91,92). Other studies have found lower risk. Duren and colleagues (63) reported three cases of sudden death during a 6-year evaluation of 300 adults with MVP, and Zuppiroli and colleagues (28) reported three instances of sudden death among 312 patients with MVP followed for a mean of 8.5 years. In these populations, the arrhythmic death rate is approximately 0.1% to 0.2%. All patients with sudden death in the report by Nishimura and colleagues (61) had echocardiographic evidence of mitral leaflet redundancy (thickening), but the mortality rate was not independently found to be associated with severe mitral regurgitation. However, two thirds of the cases of sudden death occurred in men older than 55 years, and autopsy evidence was not available in these patients to exclude occult ischemic disease that might explain this mortality rate (92). Only one of three patients with sudden death reported by Zuppiroli and colleagues (28) was younger than 70 years.

Interestingly, two of the three cases of sudden death reported by Duren and colleagues (63) also occurred in patients older than 50 years, but in partial contrast, both had evidence of hemodynamically important mitral regurgitation. This is quite similar to the forensic necropsy finding of significant mitral regurgitation in 9 of the 13 cases of sudden death attributed to MVP by Davies and colleagues (14). Two younger patients followed by Duren and colleagues (63), including the third case of sudden death, were successfully resuscitated from ventricular fibrillation at least once. This is consistent with observations of MVP as the only clinical abnormality in a significant proportion of survivors of potentially fatal arrhythmia

(11,22,65,88). For example, Wei and colleagues (22) found 10 patients with MVP and a similar number with no detectable heart disease among 60 consecutive patients referred for management of refractory complex ventricular arrhythmias. Somberg and colleagues found 15 patients with MVP among 87 patients without significant coronary artery disease, cardiomyopathy, or other major conditions in a group of more than 900 patients referred for electrophysiologic study after successful resuscitation from cardiac arrest or with sustained ventricular tachycardia. La Vecchia and colleagues (88) found MVP in 7 of 28 patients with documented ventricular tachycardia and no other evidence of heart disease. If no selection bias governed referral to these groups with complex arrhythmias but without otherwise detectable disease, the 16% to 25% prevalence of MVP is approximately four to six times the number that would be expected from random inclusion of the estimated 3% to 4% of the general population with MVP. Thus, important arrhythmias may be significantly concentrated in some subgroups of the general MVP population.

Sudden Death and Complex Arrhythmias in Mitral Regurgitation

Sudden death in patients with nonischemic mitral regurgitation is increased in subgroups with poor ventricular function and complex ventricular arrhythmias (84,93), and some patients with primary valvular disease have been found in series of survivors of out-of-hospital cardiac arrest (91,94). However, arrhythmic death in these studies, during a number of years, does not appear to be common in patients with important mitral regurgitation and complex ventricular arrhythmias when right and left ventricular function are preserved (84). The potential role of standard electrophysiologic investigation in these patients remains to be established.

Findings during ambulatory ECG monitoring, other than repetitive ventricular arrhythmias, have been found to have prognostic value for mortality risk in patients with hemodynamically severe mitral regurgitation (95–97). Clustering of VPCs by fractal analysis, independent of arrhythmia frequency or complexity, was found to concentrate risk of death in patients with nonischemic mitral regurgitation of mixed causes (95). Similar concentration of risk was also found in the subgroup of patients in sinus rhythm who had reduced statistical measures of heart rate variability (96). Interestingly, reduced variability of heart rate also was prognostically useful in patients with mitral regurgitation who were in atrial fibrillation (97). In these patients, outcome appeared more closely related to cardiac rhythm than to the specific cause of mitral regurgitation. If mitral regurgitation, rather than its causes, is separately a factor in arrhythmia complexity and in sudden death, its role in the natural history of MVP requires careful analysis.

Risk of Sudden Death in MVP Populations

Some approximation of the relative risk and incidence of sudden death in patients with MVP can be formulated from available observations. Estimates of sudden death are derived from forensic necropsy data from Davies and colleagues (14), differences in arrhythmia profile in patients with MVP with and without mitral regurgitation (87), limited natural history data in small groups of patients with valvular heart disease (84,92), and approximations of the risk of development of important mitral regurgitation (54). From these data, we have estimated the annual risk of sudden death to be extremely small in general populations with uncomplicated MVP (32,35). In contrast, mortality risk appears to be highly concentrated in the small subgroup of patients with MVP with hemodynamically severe mitral regurgitation. However, it must be reemphasized that even an event with low incidence can have major cumulative consequences within large populations.

Based on a 3% to 4% estimated prevalence (9,46,54) of echocardiographically documented MVP among adults in the United States, approximately 7 million of the 200 million adults in this country are affected. From the first available data, the annual risk of sudden death attributable to MVP alone has been estimated at approximately 2 per 10,000 patients with MVP who do not have mitral regurgitation, or 0.02% yearly (32,35). The risk caused by MVP is actually lower than the annual risk of sudden death from all causes, which has been estimated at 22 per 10,000 for the adult U.S. population (91). This risk is also lower than the 7 per 10,000 annual risk for sudden death found in subjects 45 to 54 years old without antecedent clinical evidence of coronary disease in the combined Albany-Framingham study (92).

Accordingly, sudden death in patients with MVP who do not have mitral regurgitation or coronary disease should be uncommon enough to be rarely encountered in any unselected study population. This is entirely consistent with the generally innocent prognosis of patients with this condition (9,26,27), and it might even be argued from these data that sudden death in patients with MVP without mitral regurgitation may be independent of MVP itself. However, even a very low incidence of sudden death among the approximately 7 million adults with MVP in the United States who do not have important mitral regurgitation would be associated with enough events to be detected in highly selected series of patients who have been autopsied (66–68) or resuscitated (65).

Although the strength of the association between sudden death and MVP in patients without mitral regurgitation remains uncertain, sudden death does appear to be a major risk in patients with MVP who have hemodynamically important mitral regurgitation. Early implication of this association is found in the data of Davies and colleagues (14), in which 12 cases of unexpected death associated with isolated primary MVP occurred during a 5-year period among forensic necropsies that were specifically screened for prolapse. During this period, approximately 1,250 sudden deaths were caused by ischemic heart disease in the population at risk. As previously noted, two thirds of the autopsy cases of patients with MVP had evidence of significant mitral regurgitation caused by ruptured chordae; in only four cases, three of which were young women, were no important structural changes consistent with valve regurgitation noted (14). We have previously used these observations, with estimates of the prevalence of clinically significant mitral regurgitation in the general MVP population, to calculate an annual mortality rate in this subgroup of 94 to 188 per 10,000, or 0.9% to 1.9% yearly (32,35), which is 50- to 100-fold greater than the risk calculated in patients with MVP who do not have mitral regurgitation. These estimates can be adjusted in context of several recent additional observations.

A similar preponderance of underlying important mitral regurgitation is also seen among the few cases of sudden death in the large clinical series reported by Duren and colleagues (63), but other clinical and autopsy reports (61,65–68) suggest a smaller proportion of severe regurgitation among patients with MVP with actual or potentially fatal events. Demonstrated severe mitral regurgitation in these reports ranges from 0% to 67%, but the overall proportion with evidence of mitral regurgitation or with otherwise unexplained evidence of cardiac enlargement or hypertrophy (69,90) ranges from about 28% to about 50%. Based on an estimate that 2% to 4% of the general MVP population has clinically significant mitral regurgitation (55,57), the relative risk of sudden death in patients with MVP can be calculated to be within the range of 9- to 49-fold higher when important mitral regurgitation is present.

This revised estimate confirms that the risk of sudden death in patients with MVP is strongly concentrated in those with mitral regurgitation. It is consistent with observations that complex ventricular arrhythmias are significantly more prevalent in patients with MVP when mitral regurgitation is present (87). The magnitude of mitral regurgitation associated with increased risk has not yet been quantified. Patients with MVP with regurgitation who had a high prevalence of complex arrhythmias in the report by Kligfield and colleagues (87) had holosystolic murmurs and large left atrial and left ventricular dimensions. However, complex ventricular arrhythmias were also concentrated in patients with MVP with lesser degrees of mitral regurgitation in the study of Babuty and colleagues (39). The mortality rate reported by Hochreiter and colleagues (84) in patients with documented severe mitral regurgitation was strongly concentrated in those with reduced right and left ventricular ejection fractions at rest. These findings suggest that patients with MVP at greatest risk for sudden death have hemodynamically severe mitral regurgitation. Whether this risk develops discretely with hemodynamic compromise or is continuous with progressively important mitral regurgitation still requires systematic evaluation.

MECHANISM OF ARRHYTHMIA

Arrhythmogenesis in MVP and Mitral Regurgitation

Potential sources of arrhythmia in MVP exist in the prolapsing valve and in the valve support apparatus, the conduction system, and the atrial and ventricular endocardium. Mechanical stretch and distortion of the prolapsing mitral valve or its papillary muscle support might initiate arrhythmias. For example, Wit and colleagues (98) found that atrial depolarization could be propagated into the mitral valve leaflet in an experimental canine preparation, and that under some experimental conditions of stretch and catecholamine stimulation, muscle fibers found within the mitral leaflet could demonstrate spontaneous diastolic depolarization. Wit and Cranefield (99) also reported that simian mitral valve fibers could initiate slow response potentials leading to triggered activity. Nonvalvular sites of potential arrhythmogenic abnormality have also been observed within the atrium. In several cases examined by Chesler and colleagues (13), platelet and fibrin aggregates were found in the angle between the posterior mitral leaflet and the left atrial wall, and a hemorrhagic lesion in this angle was also reported by Pocock and colleagues (100).

Bharati and colleagues (73) suggested that alternative arrhythmogenic sites might reside in areas of fatty infiltration around the sinoatrial and AV nodes, and additional conduction disorders within or below the level of the AV node were also reported by Chandraratna and colleagues (74). Complex atrial arrhythmias might be related to sudden death in MVP if accessory pathways found in some symptomatic patients with MVP (8,75,101) predisposed to unstable and rapid ventricular response rates during atrial flutter or fibrillation. Dual AV nodal pathways have been found in a significantly higher proportion of symptomatic patients with MVP than in similarly symptomatic patients without MVP (75), and these observations support a reentrant mechanism for the excess prevalence of supraventricular tachyarrhythmias found in some populations with MVP.

Intracardiac mapping in patients with MVP has suggested that a left ventricular myocardial origin of ectopic activation regularly occurs in areas adjacent to the papillary muscle (102). In contrast, Chesler and colleagues (13) found left ventricular mural friction lesions in the endocardial tissue of a high proportion of patients with MVP in an early review of sudden death with adequate autopsy data. These friction lesions, also noted by Pocock and colleagues (100), suggest a possible substrate for arrhythmogenesis as a consequence of mechanical irritation and localized scarring of the ventricular endocardium by thickened chordae. La Vecchia and colleagues (88) found increased fibrosis on endocardial biopsy in patients with MVP with ventricular tachycardia, and Morales and colleagues (67) reported extensive fibrosis adjacent to conduction tissue in patients with MVP who died suddenly. Association and coincidence are difficult to separate in other studies. Martini and colleagues (103) found evidence of coexisting arrhythmogenic right ventricular dysplasia in a patient with nonsustained ventricular fibrillation and MVP. Coincidence of unassociated events may explain this observation, as well as the inducible monomorphic right ventricular tachycardia found in a patient with MVP and possible right ventricular dysplasia by Kosmas and colleagues (104).

Arrhythmia and Substrate in MVP Sudden Death

In addition to complex ventricular arrhythmias and important mitral regurgitation, a number of other clinical findings have been associated with sudden death in patients with MVP, including the presence of thickened redundant mitral leaflets, prolonged QT intervals, and abnormal repolarization on the resting ECG. However, no single finding or combination of findings has been consistently associated with sudden death in patients with MVP, and risk stratification is further complicated by the paucity of evidence concerning the occurrence of suspected risk factors before sudden death (32).

Although it is clear that the mechanism of sudden death is usually arrhythmic, detection of complex arrhythmias in patients with MVP who have survived cardiac arrest does not prove that complex arrhythmias regularly precede sudden death in less highly selected patients. Thus, in six patients who died suddenly during a prospective study of the natural history of MVP, Nishimura and colleagues (61) found redundant (thickened) mitral leaflets by echocardiography in all six, but detected antecedent complex ventricular arrhythmias in only three. This suggests that in addition to low specificity and extremely poor predictive value for sudden death, complex ventricular arrhythmias detected by routine ambulatory monitoring may also suffer from low sensitivity for subsequent sudden death in the general MVP population.

Even so, sudden death in patients with MVP is likely to result from more complex factors than the mere presence of complex or repetitive arrhythmias per se, because these occur commonly in patients with MVP and in healthy subjects, with generally benign consequences (105). Additional neurohumoral factors may play an important role, and it is possible that arrhythmic mortality risk in patients with MVP results from a cluster of pathophysiologic circumstances that might not be present during routine monitoring of rhythm before the fatal event. This consideration is important in the management of arrhythmias in patients with MVP who are otherwise asymptomatic and free of additional risk factors.

In patients with MVP with significant mitral regurgitation, the risk of sudden death and the prevalence of complex ventricular arrhythmias appear to be greater than in the general prolapse population (14,87). Because patients with mitral regurgitation who have poor ventricular function

have been found to have detectable complex arrhythmias before death (84,93), it is possible that the combination of arrhythmias and ventricular dysfunction may identify a subgroup of patients with MVP at particularly high risk of sudden death. If the proportion of patients with sudden death caused by MVP who have evidence of coincident important mitral regurgitation remains in the range estimated previously, it could be concluded that one quarter to one half of cases of sudden death caused by MVP may be concentrated within a high-risk subgroup comprising the 2% to 4% of the entire MVP population who have severe valvular regurgitation (32,35). Other studies suggest that ventricular hypertrophy may be an additional risk factor for sudden death in patients with MVP (69,90). These small subgroups clearly deserve attention and further study. However, important mitral regurgitation has not been frequently noted among MVP survivors of potentially fatal arrhythmia (11,22,65,91,94). This might be explained by a weaker association between mitral regurgitation and sudden death in MVP than has been suggested, or alternatively, by a lower prevalence of successful resuscitation or spontaneous reversion to normal rhythm when mitral regurgitation or ventricular hypertrophy is present.

Abnormalities of repolarization, including ST depression, T-wave flattening and inversion, and prolongation of the QT interval, have been linked to arrhythmogenesis and to sudden death in patients with MVP (5,8,10,22,106,107), but these associations have been inconstant (11,13,65). Although the relationships between the congenital QT syndromes, autonomic dysfunction, and sudden death are well known (108), the prevalence of QT prolongation in MVP appears to be the same, or not much greater, as that found in the general population (109). It is also clear that circulating catecholamines can affect the QT interval (110), but it remains speculative whether these factors, together with observed catecholamine-sensitive automaticity and triggered activity in abnormal mitral valve tissue (99), might provide a contributory mechanism for arrhythmogenesis in MVP. In addition to intrinsic prolongation of the QT interval, nonspecific repolarization changes have been associated with potentially malignant arrhythmias in patients with MVP, and the potential arrhythmogenic role of electrolyte abnormalities and drug effects on the duration of repolarization in patients with MVP requires further study (11,12,111,112). QT dispersion measured from the surface ECG has been associated with ventricular arrhythmias in patients with MVP (40,113), but the prognostic value of this observation remains to be examined.

Because of the much residual uncertainty regarding the predictive value of suspected risk factors for sudden death in patients with MVP who have no mitral regurgitation, additional data are necessary to identify patients at concentrated risk. Prevalence and incidence estimates would be strengthened by careful autopsy examination for MVP as the only cardiac abnormality in cases of sudden death; a centralized registry might be useful to coordinate these otherwise isolated reports. To more accurately quantify the occurrence of sudden death in patients with MVP, a cooperative study might be established to pool prospective observations in patients with MVP with potential markers of risk. These markers might include repetitive ventricular arrhythmias, QT prolongation, resting repolarization abnormalities, and echocardiographic features such as redundant mitral leaflets. Uniform acquisition of clinical and laboratory profiles of such patients, based on standardized diagnostic criteria, would lead to more accurate assessment of arrhythmic mortality rates in patients with MVP and would improve our ability to identify and study interventions in the small subset of patients with MVP who are at risk of sudden death.

Arrhythmogenesis in Mitral Stenosis

Direct rheumatic involvement of the atrium is not required for initiation of atrial arrhythmias (1,114). Although mitral valve area alone may not be the major determinant of atrial size in patients with mitral stenosis and marked atrial dilation may more often be the result of, rather than the cause of, atrial fibrillation (114), atrial arrhythmias in patients with mitral stenosis generally can be related to age and atrial size and pressure (1,2,89). Whether these factors promote sensitivity to stretch or catecholamines (98) or whether other causes of heterogeneity of action potential properties in response to a wide range of atrial abnormalities lead to arrhythmia in this population is not clear.

METHODS FOR EVALUATION OF ARRHYTHMIA IN MITRAL VALVE DISEASE
Rest, Exercise, and Ambulatory ECG

Arrhythmias in subjects with mitral valve disease may be symptomatic or asymptomatic, and symptomatic palpitation may or may not be coincident with disordered rhythm in some patients. Although the prevalence of ambulatory arrhythmias in patients with MVP is underestimated by the limited period of recording of routine ECGs (29), exercise testing and ambulatory ECG recording lead to increased detection of arrhythmias (15–21). Although exercise may markedly exacerbate arrhythmias in patients with MVP, several studies of adults with MVP demonstrate that the sensitivity of 24-hour ambulatory ECG for the detection of arrhythmias exceeds that of stress testing (18,19,23). Similar findings were reported in children with MVP by Kavey and colleagues (25). The role of QT dispersion and other measures of subtle repolarization abnormality in prognosis requires evaluation, as does the role of heart rate variability.

Electrophysiologic Studies of MVP

In early studies, accessory pathways were reported in 10% to 25% of symptomatic patients with MVP (74,101), but

this is clearly an overestimate of the prevalence of bypass tracts in the general prolapse population. Levy and Savage (43) found no cases of classic Wolff-Parkinson-White conduction among nearly 300 subjects with MVP who were identified by echocardiographic findings in the Framingham Study. Even the rare occurrence of preexcitation in patients with MVP has important implications for arrhythmogenesis and drug therapy, because acceleration of conduction in accessory tissue, particularly in the setting of atrial flutter or fibrillation, is a recognized danger. Although Josephson and colleagues (101) found a high prevalence of left-sided accessory pathways in patients with MVP with documented supraventricular tachycardia, antidromic conduction was rare in this group. Of the 10% of symptomatic patients with MVP with accessory pathways detected by Ware and colleagues (75) during electrophysiologic study, half were concealed and half were manifest, a proportion similar to that reported by Schaal (34). A higher prevalence of atrial fibrillation in patients with MVP with mitral regurgitation might predispose to sudden death in the presence of accessory pathways. In this context, the relatively low prevalence of atrial flutter and fibrillation in patients with MVP without mitral regurgitation is reassuring.

Electrophysiologic studies do support a reentrant mechanism for the modest excess prevalence of supraventricular tachycardia found in patients with MVP. Ware and colleagues (75) demonstrated dual AV nodal pathways in 40% of patients with MVP with symptomatic palpitation or syncope, a prevalence that was nearly twice that found in similarly selected symptomatic patients without MVP. Among patients with MVP with spontaneous sustained supraventricular tachycardia whose arrhythmia was reproduced during electrophysiologic study, AV nodal reentry was the mechanism in two thirds of the cases; and accessory pathway reentry, the mechanism in one third. The same distribution of underlying mechanism was also found by Schaal in a larger, symptomatic referral population (34).

The role of electrophysiologic assessment of ventricular arrhythmias in patients with MVP remains controversial (115–118). Although highly symptomatic patients with MVP may often have arrhythmias that are inducible in the laboratory (34,115–117), the prognostic and therapeutic use of these findings remain uncertain (116,117). Patients with MVP without syncope or presyncope who are not able to have arrhythmias induced by standard, or even aggressive, stimulation protocols have a benign short-term natural history even when complex ventricular arrhythmias are detected by ambulatory ECG, consistent with the extremely low incidence of sudden death in these patients. Of course, these observations do not mean that electrophysiologic study might not be a sensitive method for the identification of asymptomatic patients at risk of arrhythmic death, but because of the low event rate, the predictive value would be quite low and many asymptomatic patients would need to be studied to detect one case at actual risk of sudden death.

Among symptomatic patients with frequent or complex ventricular ectopy studied by Morady and colleagues (116), recurrent syncope was infrequent and was similar in groups who were treated empirically or whose therapy was guided by electrophysiologic testing. However, electrophysiologically guided drug therapy may provide a benefit for some highly symptomatic patients with inducible sustained tachycardias and in some patients with documented sustained ventricular tachycardia who have nonsustained inducible rhythms, but this possibility requires clinical evaluation in a large series.

THERAPEUTIC MODALITIES AND THEIR OUTCOME

Pharmacologic Therapy in MVP

It is difficult to synthesize these often discordant observations into a useful plan for the management of arrhythmias in patients with MVP, and it is evident that any treatment algorithm must remain flexible as further information becomes available. Clearly, most patients with MVP require no treatment, either for the control of symptoms or for the prevention of arrhythmic death (32,35). On the other hand, the higher prevalence of sudden death found in patients with MVP with important mitral regurgitation, particularly in the presence of ventricular dysfunction and in the context of their significantly increased prevalence of complex arrhythmias (84,87,93), suggests that these patients require more intensive study of therapeutic intervention than lower risk patients without regurgitation.

No data exist regarding the role of electrophysiologic testing for drug selection or the efficacy of antiarrhythmic therapy in patients with MVP who have hemodynamically important mitral regurgitation. Whether β blockers (when tolerated), other antiarrhythmic drugs, implantable cardioverter-defibrillator devices, or even valve repair or replacement (when indicated) can reverse this risk is unknown, and these approaches require prospective study. β-Blocking drugs seem preferable to alternative antiarrhythmic drugs when ventricular performance permits, with ambulatory monitoring follow-up.

Standard ECG should be used to identify patients who have evidence of preexcitation or other anomalous pathways and prolongation of the rate-corrected QT interval. Because each of these subgroups may be at increased risk of sudden death, such patients should be separated from the general MVP population for more intensive evaluation. Asymptomatic patients with prolonged QT intervals might be considered for a prospective trial of beta blockade, particularly when ventricular arrhythmias are present by ambulatory monitoring. If the QT shortens or the arrhythmias decrease without a serious side effect, medication might be continued on a prophylactic basis, with mortality rate examined in comparison with that of similar patients. Drugs that prolong the QT interval should be avoided.

Although this is rational (107,108), no data yet support the presumptive efficacy of this approach in patients with MVP.

Asymptomatic patients with none of these findings on clinical evaluation need not be routinely required to undergo ambulatory monitoring, because the documented risk of mortality, even when complex ventricular arrhythmias are detected, is markedly less than the expected incidence of serious complication or proarrhythmic effects of administering antiarrhythmic drugs to large populations. Even if antiarrhythmic therapy were effective and risk free in patients with MVP without mitral regurgitation, the 40% to 50% prevalence of complex ventricular arrhythmias among 7 million adult patients with MVP suggests that approximately 2,000 patients with multiform VPCs or repetitive forms would require effective treatment for a year in an attempt to prevent one unexpected MVP death.

If treatment were restricted to the 8% to 9% of adults with ambulatory MVP without mitral regurgitation who had either VPC pairs or ventricular tachycardia by ambulatory ECG (23,24), at least 300 patients would need to be effectively treated for a year to prevent each sudden arrhythmic death. Of course, these estimates assume that the proposed therapy is completely effective to prevent sudden death, that therapy produces no offsetting proarrhythmic or other adverse consequences in large populations among whom no benefit can be expected, and that the presence of complex or repetitive arrhythmias is sensitive for the identification of patients with MVP at risk of subsequent sudden death. Because each of these limiting assumptions can be seriously questioned, these patients should not be treated pharmacologically in the absence of additional risk, further data, or prospective therapeutic trial.

In patients with MVP who are symptomatic with palpitation, pharmacologic treatment of detected arrhythmias may be necessary for alleviation of discomfort or for protection against sudden death. However, it must be appreciated that palpitation is exceedingly common in patients with MVP and not all patients require therapy. It has not been shown that symptomatic palpitation is a useful marker for complex arrhythmias. Ambulatory monitoring should be performed in this subgroup to identify patients with VPC couplets or nonsustained ventricular tachycardia. A therapeutic trial of β-blocking therapy (119) might be instituted in this subgroup, with follow-up evaluation by repeated ambulatory recording. At present, because of the high incidence of symptomatic intolerance, problems with compliance, untoward side effects, and potential proarrhythmic effects of other antiarrhythmic agents, their risk must be weighed against their potential symptomatic benefits in this setting. Hemodynamically uncompromised patients with nonsustained ventricular arrhythmias who do not respond to β blockers are probably best left untreated, unless control of palpitation per se is the therapeutic goal or until more accurate predictors of concentrated risk for sudden death are available.

A substantial subset of patients with symptomatic palpitations will be found to have brief bursts of nonsustained supraventricular arrhythmias. Patients with transient atrial fibrillation are uncommon, and when this is present, the possibility of coincident mitral regurgitation should be considered. Patients with atrial flutter or fibrillation should be carefully screened by repeated resting ECG recordings for evidence of preexcitation. When present, this combination in a patient with MVP probably warrants electrophysiologic study. The mildly symptomatic patient with brief supraventricular tachycardia may require only explanation and reassurance, with reduction of caffeine, nicotine, and alcohol when appropriate. When symptoms remain limiting, a trial of beta blockade may be considered. The efficacy of β-blocking drugs should be assessed by serial ambulatory recording and perhaps with additional exercise testing. Because electrophysiologic study does not clearly improve patient management and does not clearly define drug efficacy in this subgroup (115–118), pending further study, it should be reserved for symptomatic patients who do not respond to β blockers in whom potentially life-threatening proarrhythmic drug effects must be avoided (112). Alternatively, when there is no risk of rapid preexcitation, digitalis or a calcium channel-blocking drug may be effective for symptom control. Refractory symptomatic cases may benefit from electrophysiologic study to document and potentially ablate underlying dual AV nodal pathways or contributory accessory pathways.

Patients with dizziness, presyncope, or syncope who have evidence of VPC couplets, VPC salvos, or nonsustained ventricular tachycardia require therapy, certainly for symptoms if not for survival. Orthostatic hypotension should be excluded as a cause of syncope or presyncope, as this may cause these symptoms in patients with MVP (53) independently of arrhythmias and this might be exacerbated by some forms of antiarrhythmic treatment. One could reasonably suggest that implantable cardioverter-defibrillators be considered for patients with MVP with symptomatic ventricular tachycardia and survivors of out-of-hospital cardiac arrest.

Electrophysiologic and Surgical Intervention in MVP

To the extent that symptomatic supraventricular tachycardia in patients with MVP can be related to underlying dual AV nodal pathways, accessory pathways, or localized trigger sites, radiofrequency ablation may be preferable to chronic pharmacologic therapy (120,121). Refractory ventricular tachycardia has been treated by overdrive pacing in at least one instance of mitral prolapse (122), and mitral valve anuloplasty has been reported to provide relief of palpitation and syncope in some patients with malignant arrhythmia associated with MVP (123–125). As an example, Reece and colleagues (124) reported on two patients with preoperatively documented ventricular fibrillation and syncope who remained well up to 4 years after mitral valve surgery. Kay

and colleagues (125) reported on six patients with severe prolapse but without mitral regurgitation who underwent mitral valve repair for debilitating symptoms; there was a subsequent reduction, but not elimination, of arrhythmia.

A survival advantage with implantable defibrillators for patients with mitral regurgitation and reduced ejection fraction (126) is a reasonable but unproved extrapolation from ongoing trials in ischemic and myopathic patients with complex arrhythmias and reduced left ventricular function. Similarly, the effect of high-risk surgical correction on survival in patients with mitral regurgitation who have severely depressed ejection fractions requires clarification.

Rate and Rhythm Control in Mitral Stenosis

Reduction of resting and exercise heart rate can have an important effect on the effort tolerance of patients with mitral stenosis, even when in sinus rhythm. Klein and colleagues (127) found a significant increase in exercise time with atenolol in patients in sinus rhythm. Similarly, Ahuja and colleagues (128) demonstrated improvement in exercise capacity during sinus rhythm that was considerably more marked with treatment with metoprolol or with verapamil than with digoxin. Although atrial fibrillation can reduce the cardiac output in mitral stenosis independent of heart rate (1,129), stroke volume and pulmonary venous pressure are strongly dependent on the duration of diastole when mitral stenosis is severe (1,2,130). Rate control, particularly during exercise, is therefore particularly important in patients with mitral stenosis and atrial fibrillation. For patients with atrial fibrillation, Ahuja and colleagues (128) also found improvement in exercise capacity to be greater with metoprolol or with verapamil than with digoxin alone, an effect attributed to different degrees of resting and peak effort rate control with the different drugs.

Cardioversion of atrial fibrillation to sinus rhythm can reduce atrial volume in patients with mitral valve disease, including those with rheumatic mitral stenosis (131). Restoration of effective atrial contraction after cardioversion and after valve surgery is occasionally problematic in patients with mitral stenosis and with mitral regurgitation, particularly when atrial size is very large. Recent reports have suggested that the atrial maze procedure performed in conjunction with valve replacement or repair may facilitate return to sinus rhythm with effective contraction (132, 133), but further study is needed to evaluate the long-term consequences of these techniques.

REFERENCES

1. Wood P. An appreciation of mitral stenosis. *Br Med J* 1954; I:1051–1063.
2. Selzer A, Cohn KE. Natural history of mitral stenosis: a review. *Circulation* 1972;45:878–890.

3. Barlow JB, Pocock WA, Marchand P, Denny M. The significance of late systolic murmurs. *Am Heart J* 1963;66:443–452.

4. Criley JM, Lewis KB, Humphries JO, Ross RS. Prolapse of the mitral valve: clinical and angiographic findings. *Br Heart J* 1966;28:488–496.

5. Hancock EW, Cohn K. The syndrome associated with midsystolic click and late systolic murmur. *Am J Med* 1966;41:183–196.

6. Pocock WA, Barlow JB. Etiology and electrocardiographic features of the billowing posterior mitral leaflet syndrome. *Am J Med* 1971;51:731–738.

7. Wooley CF. Where are the diseases of yesteryear? DaCosta's syndrome, soldier's heart, the effort syndrome, neurocirculatory asthenia, and the mitral valve prolapse syndrome [Editorial]. *Circulation* 1976;53:749–751.

8. Devereux RB, Perloff JK, Reichek N, Josephson ME. Mitral valve prolapse. *Circulation* 1976;54:3–14.

9. Devereux RB, Kramer-Fox R, Kligfield P. Mitral valve prolapse: causes, clinical manifestations, and management. *Ann Intern Med* 1989;111:305–317.

10. Shappell SD, Marshall CE, Brown RE, Bruce TA. Sudden death and the familial occurrence of mid-systolic click, late systolic murmur syndrome. *Circulation* 1973;48:1128–1134.

11. Winkle RA, Lopes MG, Popp RL, Hancock EW. Life-threatening arrhythmias in the mitral valve prolapse syndrome. *Am J Med* 1976;60:961–967.

12. Jeresaty RM. Sudden death in the mitral valve prolapse-click syndrome [Editorial]. *Am J Cardiol* 1976;37:317–318.

13. Chesler E, King RA, Edwards JE. The myxomatous mitral valve and sudden death. *Circulation* 1983;67:632–639.

14. Davies MJ, Moore BP, Braimbridge MV. The floppy mitral valve: study of incidence, pathology, and complications in surgical, necropsy, and forensic material. *Br Heart J* 1978;40:468–481.

15. Pocock WA, Barlow JB. Postexercise arrhythmias in the billowing posterior mitral leaflet syndrome. *Am Heart J* 1970;80:740–745.

16. Gooch AS, Vicencio F, Maranhao V, Goldberg H. Arrhythmias and left ventricular asynergy in the prolapsing mitral leaflet syndrome. *Am J Cardiol* 1972;29:611–620.

17. Sloman G, Wong M, Walker J. Arrhythmias on exercise in patients with abnormalities of the posterior leaflet of the mitral valve. *Am Heart J* 1972;83:312–317.

18. Winkle RA, Lopes MG, Fitzgerald JW, et al. Arrhythmias in patients with mitral valve prolapse. *Circulation* 1975;52:73–81.

19. DeMaria AN, Amsterdam EA, Vismara LA, et al. Arrhythmias in the mitral valve prolapse syndrome: prevalence, nature, and frequency. *Ann Intern Med* 1976;84:656–660.

20. Campbell RWF, Godman MG, Fiddler GI, et al. Ventricular arrhythmias in syndrome of balloon deformity of mitral valve: definition of possible high risk group. *Br Heart J* 1976;38:1053–1057.

21. Malcolm AD, Ahuja SP. The electrocardiographic response to exercise in 44 patients with mitral leaflet prolapse. *Eur J Cardiol* 1978;8:359–370.

22. Wei JY, Bulkley BH, Schaeffer AH, et al. Mitral-valve prolapse syndrome and recurrent ventricular tachyarrhythmias: a malignant variant refractory to conventional drug therapy. *Ann Intern Med* 1978;89:6–9.

23. Savage DD, Levy D, Garrison RJ, et al. Mitral valve prolapse in the general population. *Am Heart J* 1983;106:582–586.

24. Kramer HM, Kligfield P, Devereux RB, et al. Arrhythmias in mitral valve prolapse: effect of selection bias. *Arch Intern Med* 1984;144:2360–2364.

25. Webb Kavey R-E, Blackman MS, Sondheimer HM, Byrum CJ. Ventricular arrhythmias and mitral valve prolapse in childhood. *J Pediatr* 1984;105:885–890.

26. Allen H, Harris A, Leatham A. Significance and prognosis of an isolated late systolic murmur. *Br Heart J* 1974;36:525–532.

27. Freed LA, Levy D, Levine RA, et al. Prevalence and clinical outcome of mitral-valve prolapse. *N Engl J Med* 1999;341:1–7.

28. Zuppiroli A, Rinaldi M, Kramer-Fox R, et al. Natural history of mitral valve prolapse. *Am J Cardiol* 1995;75:1028–1032.

29. Swartz MH, Teichholz LE, Donoso E. Mitral valve prolapse: a review of associated arrhythmias. *Am J Med* 1977;62:377–389.

30. Mason DT, Lee G, Chan MC, DeMaria AN. Arrhythmias in patients with mitral valve prolapse. Types, evaluation, and therapy. *Med Clin North Am* 1984;68:1039–1049.

31. Kligfield P, Devereux RB. Arrhythmias in mitral valve prolapse. *Clin Prog Electrophysiol Pacing* 1985;3:403–418.

32. Kligfield P, Levy D, Devereux RB, Savage DD. Arrhythmias and sudden death in mitral valve prolapse. *Am Heart J* 1987;113:1298–1307.

33. Levy S. Arrhythmias in the mitral valve prolapse syndrome: clinical significance and management. *Pace* 1992;15:1080–1088.

34. Schaal SF. Mitral valve prolapse: cardiac arrhythmias and electrophysiological correlates. In: Boudoulas H, Wooley GF, eds. *Mitral valve prolapse and the mitral valve prolapse syndrome.* Mount Kisco, NY: Futura Publishing, 1988:567–590.

35. Kligfield P, Devereux RB. Is the patient with mitral valve prolapse at high risk for sudden death identifiable? In: Cheitlin MD, ed. *Dilemmas in clinical cardiology. Cardiovascular clinics.* Philadelphia: FA Davis Co, 1990:143–157.

36. Yabek SM. Ventricular arrhythmias in children with an apparently normal heart. *J Pediatr* 1991;119:1–11.

37. Boudoulas H, Wooley CF. Mitral valve prolapse and the mitral valve prolapse syndrome. *Prog Cardiovasc Dis* 1986;14:275–309.

38. Zuppiroli A, Mori F, Favilli S, et al. Arrhythmias in mitral valve prolapse: relation to anterior mitral leaflet thickening, clinical variables, and color Doppler echocardiographic variables. *Am Heart J* 1994;128:919–927.

39. Babuty D, Cosnay P, Breuillac JC, et al. Ventricular arrhythmia factors in mitral valve prolapse. *Pacing Clin Electrophysiol* 1994;17:1090–1099.

40. Kulan K, Komsuoglu B, Tuncer C, Kulan C. Significance of QT dispersion on ventricular arrhythmias in mitral valve prolapse. *Int J Cardiol* 1996;54:251–257.

41. Devereux RB, Kramer-Fox R, Shear MK, et al. Diagnosis and classification of severity of mitral valve prolapse: methodologic, biologic and prognostic considerations. *Am Heart J* 1987;113:1265–1280.

42. Levine RA, Triulzi MO, Harrigan P, Weyman AE. The relationship of mitral annular shape to the diagnosis of mitral valve prolapse. *Circulation* 1987;75:756–767.

43. Levy D, Savage D. Prevalence and clinical features of mitral valve prolapse. *Am Heart J* 1987;113:1281–1290.

44. Retchin SM, Fletcher RH, Earp J, et al. Mitral valve prolapse. Disease or illness? *Arch Intern Med* 1986;146:1081–1084.

45. Devereux RB, Kligfield P. Mitral valve prolapse. In: Rakel RE, ed. *Current therapy 1992.* Philadelphia: WB Saunders, 1992:237–242.

46. Savage DD, Garrison RJ, Devereux RB, et al. Mitral valve prolapse in the general population. *Am Heart J* 1983;106:571–578.

47. Devereux RB, Jones EC, Lee ET, et al. Prevalence and correlates of mitral valve prolapse in a general population sample: the Strong Heart Study. *Circulation* 1999;100[Suppl I]:I212(abst).

48. Fontana ME, Wooley CF, Leighton RF, Lewis RP. Postural changes in left ventricular and mitral valvular dynamics in the systolic click–late systolic murmur syndrome. *Circulation* 1975;51:165–173.

49. Devereux RB, Brown WT, Kramer-Fox R, Sachs I. Inheritance of mitral valve prolapse. Effect of age and sex on gene expression. *Ann Intern Med* 1982;97:826–832.

50. Disse S, Abergel E, Berrebi A, et al. Mapping of a first locus for autosomal dominant myxomatous mitral valve prolapse to

chromosome 16p11.2-p12.1. *Am J Hum Genetics* 1999;65: 1242–1251.

51. Devereux RB, Brown WT, Lutas EM, et al. Association of mitral valve prolapse with low body-weight and low blood pressures. *Lancet* 1982;2:792–795.

52. Devereux RB, Kramer-Fox R, Brown WT, et al. Relation between clinical features of the mitral prolapse syndrome and echocardiographically documented mitral valve prolapse. *J Am Coll Cardiol* 1986;8:763–772.

53. Santos AD, Mathew PK, Hilal A, Wallace WA. Orthostatic hypotension: a commonly unrecognized cause of symptoms in mitral valve prolapse. *Am J Med* 1981;71:746–750.

54. Devereux RB, Hawkins I, Kramer-Fox R, et al. Complications of mitral valve prolapse: disproportionate occurrence in men and older patients. *Am J Med* 1986;81:751–756.

55. Wilcken DE, Hickey AJ. Lifetime risk for patients with mitral prolapse of developing severe valve regurgitation requiring surgery. *Circulation* 1988;78:10–14.

56. MacMahon SW, Roberts JK, Kramer-Fox R, et al. Mitral valve prolapse and infective endocarditis. *Am Heart J* 1987;113: 1291–1298.

57. Singh RG, Cappucci R, Kramer-Fox R, et al. Severe mitral regurgitation due to mitral valve prolapse: risk factors for development, progression and need for mitral valve surgery. *Am J Cardiol*, in press.

58. Danchin A, Voiriot P, Briancon S, et al. Mitral valve prolapse as a risk factor for infective endocarditis. *Lancet* 1989;1:743–745.

59. Devereux RB, Frary CJ, Kramer-Fox R, et al. Cost effectiveness of infective endocarditis for mitral valve prolapse with or without a mitral regurgitant murmur. *Am J Cardiol* 1994;74: 1024–1029.

60. Kolibash AJ Jr, Kilman JW, Bush CA, et al. Evidence for progression from mild to severe mitral regurgitation in mitral valve prolapse. *Am J Cardiol* 1986;58:762–767.

61. Nishimura RA, McGoon MD, Shub C, et al. Echocardiographically documented mitral-valve prolapse. *N Engl J Med* 1985; 313:1305–1309.

62. Marks AR, Choong CY, Sanfilippo AJ, et al. Identification of high-risk and low-risk subgroups of patients with mitral-valve prolapse. *N Engl J Med* 1989;320:1031–1036.

63. Duren DR, Becker AE, Dunning AJ. Long-term follow-up of idiopathic mitral valve prolapse in 300 patients: a prospective study. *J Am Coll Cardiol* 1988;11:42–47.

64. Bisset GS, Schwartz DC, Meyer RA, et al. Clinical spectrum and long term follow-up of isolated mitral valve prolapse in 119 children. *Circulation* 1980;62:423–429.

65. Boudoulas H, Schaal SF, Stang JM, et al. Mitral valve prolapse: cardiac arrest with long term survival. *Int J Cardiol* 1990;26: 37–44.

66. Dollar AL, Roberts WC. Morphologic comparison of patients with mitral valve prolapse who died suddenly with patients who died from severe valvular dysfunction or other conditions. *J Am Coll Cardiol* 1991;17:921–931.

67. Morales AR, Remanelli R, Boncek RJ, et al. Myxoid heart disease: an assessment of extraordinary cardiac pathology in severe mitral valve prolapse. *Hum Pathol* 1992;23:129–137.

68. Farb A, Tang AL, Atkinson JB, et al. Comparison of cardiac findings in patients with mitral valve prolapse who die suddenly to those who have congestive heart failure from mitral regurgitation and those with fatal noncardiac conditions. *Am J Cardiol* 1992;70:234–239.

69. Roberts WC. The hypertensive diseases: evidence that systemic hypertension is a greater risk factor to the development of other cardiovascular diseases than previously suspected. *Am J Med* 1975;591:523–532.

70. Zuppiroli A, Roman MJ, O'Grady M, Devereux RB. A family

study of anterior mitral leaflet thickness and mitral valve prolapse. *Am J Cardiol* 1998;82:823–826.

71. Weissman NJ, Pini R, Roman MJ, et al. *In vivo* mitral valve morphology and motion in mitral valve prolapse. *Am J Cardiol* 1994;73:1080–1088.

72. Malkowski MJ, Boudoulas H, Wooley CF, et al. Spectrum of structural abnormalities in floppy mitral valve: echocardiographic evaluation. *Am Heart J* 1996;132:145–151.

73. Bharati S, Granston AS, Liebson PR, et al. The conduction system in mitral valve prolapse syndrome with sudden death. *Am Heart J* 1981;101:667–670.

74. Chandraratna PAN, Ribas-Meneclier C, Littman BB, Samet P. Conduction disturbances in patients with mitral valve prolapse. *J Electrocardiol* 1977;10:233–236.

75. Ware JA, Magro SA, Luck JC, et al. Conduction system abnormalities in symptomatic mitral valve prolapse: an electrophysiologic analysis of 60 patients. *Am J Cardiol* 1984;53:1075–1078.

76. Motulsky AG. Biased ascertainment and the natural history of diseases. *N Engl J Med* 1978;298:1196–1197.

77. Southall DP, Johnston F, Shinebourne EA, Johnston PGB. 24-hour electrocardiographic study of heart rate and rhythm patterns in population of healthy children. *Br Heart J* 1981;45: 281–291.

78. Brodsky M, Wu D, Denes P, et al. Arrhythmias documented by 24 hour continuous electrocardiographic monitoring in 50 male medical students with apparent heart disease. *Am J Cardiol* 1977;39:390–395.

79. Sobotka PA, Mayer JH, Bauernfeind RA, et al. Arrhythmias documented by 24-hour continuous ambulatory electrocardiographic monitoring in young women without apparent heart disease. *Am Heart J* 1981;101:753–758.

80. Hinkle LE, Carver ST, Stevens M. The frequency of asymptomatic disturbances of cardiac rhythm and conduction in middle-aged men. *Am J Cardiol* 1969;24:629–650.

81. Clarke JM, Shelton JR, Hamer J, et al. The rhythm of the normal human heart. *Lancet* 1976;2:508–512.

82. Glasser SP, Clark PI, Applebaum HJ. Occurrence of frequent complex arrhythmias detected by ambulatory monitoring: findings in an apparently healthy asymptomatic elderly population. *Chest* 1979;75:565–568.

83. Camm AJ, Evans KE, Ward ED, Martin A. The rhythm of the heart in active elderly subjects. *Am Heart J* 1980;99:598–603.

84. Brigden W, Leatham A. Mitral incompetence. *Br Heart J* 1953; 15:55–73.

85. Kligfield P, Hochreiter C, Kramer H, et al. Complex arrhythmias in mitral regurgitation with and without mitral valve prolapse: contrast to arrhythmias in mitral valve prolapse without mitral regurgitation. *Am J Cardiol* 1985;55:1545–1549.

86. Hochreiter C, Niles N, Devereux RB, et al. Mitral regurgitation: relationship of non-invasive right and left ventricular performance descriptors to clinical and hemodynamic findings and to prognosis in medically and surgically treated patients. *Circulation* 1986;73:900–912.

87. Waller BF, Morrow AG, Maron BJ, et al. Etiology of clinically isolated severe, chronic, pure mitral regurgitation: analysis of 97 patients over 30 years of age having mitral valve replacement. *Am Heart J* 1982;104:276–288.

88. La Vecchia L, Ometto R, Centofante P, et al. Arrhythmic profile, ventricular function, and histomorphometric findings in patients with idiopathic ventricular tachycardia and mitral valve prolapse: clinical and prognostic evaluation. *Clin Cardiol* 1998; 21:731–735.

89. Ramsdale DR, Arumugam N, Singh SS, et al. Holter monitoring in patients with mitral stenosis and sinus rhythm. *Eur Heart J* 1987;8:164–170.

90. Carrado D, Basso C, Nara A, et al. Sudden death in young peo-

ple with apparently isolated mitral valve prolapse. *G Ital Cardiol* 1997;27:1097–1105.

91. Ruskin JN, DiMarco JP, Garan H. Out-of-hospital cardiac arrest. Electrophysiologic observations and selection of long-term antiarrhythmic therapy. *N Engl J Med* 1980;303:607–613.

92. Kannel WB, Doyle JT, McNamara PM, et al. Precursors of sudden coronary death: factors related to the incidence of sudden death. *Circulation* 1975;51:606–613.

93. Kligfield P, Hochreiter C, Niles N, et al. Relation of sudden death in pure mitral regurgitation, with and without mitral valve prolapse, to repetitive ventricular arrhythmias and right and left ventricular ejection fractions. *Am J Cardiol* 1987;60: 397–399.

94. Myerburg RJ, Conde CA, Sung RJ, et al. Clinical, electrophysiologic and hemodynamic profile of patients resuscitated from prehospital cardiac arrest. *Am J Med* 1980;68:568–576.

95. Stein KM, Borer JS, Hochreiter C, Kligfield P: Fractal clustering of ventricular ectopy and sudden death in mitral regurgitation. *J Electrocardiol* 1993;25[Suppl]:178–181.

96. Stein KM, Borer JS, Hochreiter C, et al. Prognostic value and physiologic correlates of heart rate variability in chronic severe mitral regurgitation. *Circulation* 1993;88:127–135.

97. Stein K, Borer JS, Hochreiter C, Herrold EM, Kligfield P: Variability of the ventricular response in atrial fibrillation and prognosis in chronic non-ischemic mitral regurgitation. *Am J Cardiol* 1994;74:906–911.

98. Wit AL, Fenoglio JJ, Wagner BM, Bassett AL. Electrophysiological properties of cardiac muscle in the anterior mitral valve leaflet and the adjacent atrium in the dog: possible implications for the genesis of atrial dysrhythmias. *Circ Res* 1973;32: 731–745.

99. Wit AL, Cranefield PF. Triggered activity in cardiac muscle fibers of the simian mitral valve. *Circ Res* 1976;38:85–98.

100. Pocock WA, Bosman CK, Chesler E, et al. Sudden death in primary mitral valve prolapse. *Am Heart J* 1984;107:378–382.

101. Josephson ME, Horowitz LN, Kastor JA. Paroxysmal supraventricular tachycardia in patients with mitral valve prolapse. *Circulation* 1977;57:111–115.

102. Muilwijk SLC, SippensGroenewegen A, van Hernel NM, et al. Ventricular arrhythmias in patients with mitral valve prolapse: identification of the site of origin using body surface mapping. *Circulation* 1992;86[suppl I]:I584.

103. Martini B, Basso C, Thiene G. Sudden death in mitral valve prolapse with Holter monitoring-documented ventricular fibrillation: evidence of coexisting arrhythmogenic right ventricular cardiomyopathy. *Int J Cardiol* 1995;49:274–278.

104. Kosmas CE, Dalessandro DA, Langieri G, et al. Monomorphic right ventricular tachycardia in a patient with mitral valve prolapse. *Pacing Clin Electrophysiol* 1996;19:509–513.

105. Kennedy HL, Whitlock JA, Sprague MK, et al. Long-term follow-up of asymptomatic healthy subjects with frequent and complex ventricular ectopy. *N Engl J Med* 1985;312:193–197.

106. Bekheit SG, Ali AA, Deglin SM, Jain AC. Analysis of QT interval in patients with idiopathic mitral valve prolapse. *Chest* 982;81:620–625.

107. Puddu PE, Pasternac A, Tubau JF, et al. QT interval prolongation and increased plasma catecholamine levels in patients with mitral valve prolapse. *Am Heart J* 1983;105:422–428.

108. Moss AJ, Schwartz PJ, Crampton RS, et al. The long Q-T syndrome: prospective longitudinal study of 328 families. *Circulation* 1991;84:1136–1144.

109. Cowan MD, Fye WB. Prevalence of QTc prolongation in women with mitral valve prolapse. *Am J Cardiol* 1989;63: 133–134.

110. Abildskov JA. Adrenergic effects on the QT interval of the electrocardiogram. *Am Heart J* 1976;92:210–216.

111. Salmela PI, Ikaheimo M, Juustila H. Fatal ventricular fibrillation after treatment with digoxin in a 27-year-old man with mitral leaflet prolapse syndrome. *Br Heart J* 1981;46:338–341.

112. Velebit V, Podrid P, Lown B, et al. Aggravation and provocation of ventricular arrhythmias by antiarrhythmic drugs. *Circulation* 1982;65:886–893.

113. Tieleman RG, Crijns HJ, Wiesfeld AC, et al. Increased dispersion of refractoriness in the absence of QT prolongation in patients with mitral valve prolapse and ventricular arrhythmias. *Br Heart J* 1995;73:37–40.

114. Probst P, Goldschlager N, Selzer A. Left atrial size and atrial fibrillation in mitral stenosis: factors influencing their relationship. *Circulation* 1973;48:1282–1287.

115. Engel TR, Meister SG, Frankl WS. Ventricular extrastimulation in the mitral valve prolapse syndrome. Evidence for ventricular reentry. *J Electrocardiol* 1978;11:137–142.

116. Morady F, Shen E, Bhandari A, et al. Programmed ventricular stimulation in mitral valve prolapse: analysis of 36 patients. *Am J Cardiol* 1984;53:135–138.

117. Rosenthal ME, Hamer A, Gang ES, et al. The yield of programmed ventricular stimulation in mitral valve prolapse patients with ventricular arrhythmias. *Am Heart J* 1985;110: 970–976.

118. Naccarelli GV, Prystowsky EN, Jackman WM, et al. Role of electrophysiologic testing in managing patients who have ventricular tachycardia unrelated to coronary artery disease. *Am J Cardiol* 1982;50:165–171.

119. Winkle RA, Lopes MG, Goodman DJ, et al. Propranolol for patients with mitral valve prolapse. *Am Heart J* 1977;93: 422–427.

120. Wu D, Yeh S-N, Wang C-C, et al. Nature of dual atrioventricular node pathways and the tachycardia circuit as defined by radiofrequency ablation technique. *J Am Coll Cardiol* 1992;20: 884–895.

121. Jackman WM, Wang X, Friday KJ, et al. Catheter ablation of accessory atrioventricular pathways (Wolff-Parkinson-White syndrome) by radiofrequency current. *N Engl J Med* 1991;324: 1605–1611.

122. Ritchie JL, Hammermeister KE, Kennedy JW. Refractory ventricular tachycardia and fibrillation in a patient with the prolapsing mitral leaflet syndrome: successful control with overdrive pacing. *Am J Cardiol* 1976;37:314–316.

123. Pocock WA, Barlow JB, Marcus RH, Barlow CW. Mitral valvuloplasty for life-threatening ventricular arrhythmias in mitral valve prolapse. *Am Heart J* 1990;121:199–202.

124. Reece JJ, Cooley DA, Painvin GA, et al. Surgical treatment of mitral systolic click syndrome: results in 37 patients. *Ann Thorac Surg* 1985;39:155–158.

125. Kay JH, Krohn BG, Zubiate P, Hoffman RL. Surgical correction of severe mitral prolapse without mitral insufficiency but with pronounced cardiac arrhythmias. *J Thorac Cardiovasc Surg* 1979;78:259–268.

126. Fogoros RN, Elson JJ, Bonnet CA, et al. Efficacy of the automatic implantable cardioverter-defibrillator in prolonging survival in patients with severe underlying cardiac disease. *J Am Coll Cardiol* 1990;16:381–386.

127. Klein HO, Sareli P, Schamroth CL, et al. Effects of atenolol on exercise capacity in patients with mitral stenosis with sinus rhythm. *Am J Cardiol* 1985;56:598–601.

128. Ahuja RC, Sinha N, Saran RK, et al. Digoxin or verapamil or metoprolol for heart rate control in patients with mitral stenosis: a randomised cross-over study. *Int J Cardiol* 1989;25:325–331.

129. Koide T, Nakanishi A, Ito I, et al. Hemodynamic and clinical significances of atrial fibrillation, pulmonary vascular resistance and left ventricular function in rheumatic mitral stenosis. *Jpn Heart J* 1975;16:122–142.

130. Kligfield P. Systolic time intervals in atrial fibrillation and mitral stenosis. *Br Heart J* 1974;36:798–805.
131. Gosselink AT, Crijns HJ, Hamer HP, et al. Changes in left and right atrial size after cardioversion of atrial fibrillation: role of mitral valve disease. *J Am Coll Cardiol* 1993;22:1666–1672.
132. Kosakai U, Kawaguchi AT, Isobe F, et al. Cox maze procedure for chronic atrial fibrillation associated with mitral valve disease. *J Thorac Cardiovasc Surg* 1994;108:1049–1054.
133. Yuda S, Nakatani S, Isobe F, et al. Comparative efficacy of the maze procedure for restoration of atrial contraction in patients with and without giant left atrium associated with mitral valve disease. *J Am Coll Cardiol* 1998;31:1097–1102.

32

ARRHYTHMIAS IN CARDIAC TRANSPLANTATION

STEVEN A. ROTHMAN
JOYCE WALD
HOWARD J. EISEN

Cardiac transplantation is widely accepted as definitive therapy for end-stage congestive heart failure for which there are no alternative therapies. The transplanted heart presents a unique electrophysiologic milieu in that the heart is denervated and is subject to immunologic assaults not found in other cardiovascular diseases. Despite this, arrhythmias and conduction system disease are fairly common and range in significance from atrial premature depolarizations (APDs) to sustained and potentially lethal arrhythmias. The causes of these arrhythmias are quite varied and include situations unique to cardiac transplantation, such as acute allograft rejection and ischemia from the transplantation surgery or from transplant vasculopathy.

ELECTROPHYSIOLOGIC FEATURES OF THE TRANSPLANTED HEART

Effect of Denervation

The most striking feature of the transplanted heart is the increase in the resting sinus rate because of the lack of parasympathetic innervation. The heart rate is usually greater than 80 bpm and, in the absence of sinus node dysfunction, varies inversely with the donor's age (1,2). Although not affected by parasympathetic or sympathetic innervation early after transplantation, the donor heart appears to have an increased susceptibility to circulating catecholamines. It has been demonstrated that isoproterenol has a greater effect on heart rate in the trans-

S. A. Rothman: Department of Medicine, Division of Clinical Electrophysiology, Temple University School of Medicine, Philadelphia, Pennsylvania 19140.

J. Wald: Department of Medicine, Temple University School of Medicine, Philadelphia, Pennsylvania 19140.

H. J. Eisen: Department of Medicine, Division of Heart Transplantation, Cardiology Section, Temple University School of Medicine, Philadelphia, Pennsylvania 19140.

planted heart when directly compared with the innervated recipient heart, increasing the sinus rate by 40 bpm in the donor atria and 18 bpm in the recipient atria (3). Similar results have been obtained when comparing the chronotropic response to an infusion of isoprenaline in denervated orthotopic and heterotopic hearts with innervated heterotopic recipient hearts and with hearts of normal volunteers (4). After β blockade, these heart rate responses were attenuated to the same extent in all hearts, suggesting a "supersensitivity" of the β receptor. Other mechanisms, however, may also play a role in the increased effectiveness of circulating catecholamines. In a study evaluating the effects of norepinephrine and epinephrine on cardiac transplant recipients and hypertensive controls, the cardiac transplant recipients showed a greater response to these agents and had a twofold to threefold increase in plasma concentrations of these agents, suggesting a diminished systemic clearance (5). Lurie and colleagues (6) demonstrated in rabbit isografts that a twofold increase in postsynaptic β-receptor density may be the cause of a marked increase in isoproterenol-stimulated adenylate cyclase activity.

An increased sensitivity to adenosine has also been demonstrated in the denervated heart. Ellenbogen and colleagues (7) studied the effects of adenosine in the donor and recipient atria of transplanted hearts, as well as in normal controls. Adenosine was found to cause a threefold to fourfold greater change in the sinus cycle length in transplanted donor hearts when compared with the recipient atria and with controls. A similar increase was observed in the PR interval change. This response was thought to result from an exaggerated sensitivity at the presynaptic or postreceptor level. Clinically, this effect has resulted in an increased risk of heart block during adenosine pharmacologic stress testing (8) and in the need for smaller doses of the drug when used to induce transient atrioventricular (AV) block for diagnostic or therapeutic purposes.

Reinnervation

Historically, the transplanted heart has been thought of as a denervated organ that would remain so over time. The observations of heart rate variability and heart rate changes during exercise, however, have suggested that reinnervation does occur to some extent (9,10). A variety of techniques have since been used to demonstrate sympathetic reinnervation. Studies using tracers taken up by intact sympathetic neurons, such as *meta*-iodobenzylguanidine scintigraphy and positron emission tomography with ^{11}C-hydroxyephedrine, have shown partial sympathetic reinnervation to occur late after transplantation (11,12). Intracoronary injections of tyramine, which cause release of norepinephrine from intact presynaptic sympathetic nerve terminals, have also demonstrated heterogeneous sympathetic reinnervation to occur at least 1 year after transplantation (13,14). When sympathetic reinnervation affects the sinus node, an improved heart rate response can be seen during exercise and the recovery period (15). In a study assessing the effect of sympathetic reinnervation on heart rate variability, Lord and associates (16) found a significant relationship between the low-frequency component of the spectrum and the response to tyramine, demonstrating that sympathetic reinnervation increases heart rate variability. Neither the low-frequency nor high-frequency components of the heart rate variability spectrum were affected by atropine in cardiac transplant recipients.

Although evidence for sympathetic reinnervation accumulates, parasympathetic reinnervation remains controversial. In a study of 10 orthotopic heart transplant recipients who underwent tilt-table testing, Fitzpatrick and coworkers (17) observed a vasovagal response in seven patients. All seven of these had a vasodepressor effect, but three also had a concomitant decrease in donor heart rate by a mean of 23 bpm. This latter effect was thought to result from parasympathetic reinnervation. In a report by Morgan-Hughes and colleagues (18), tilt-table testing, Valsalva maneuvers, and heart rate responses to tyramine and exercise were studied in seven heart transplant recipients. Four of the seven patients had a vasodepressor response to tilt-table testing, and two of the four also had a marked decrease in donor heart rate. Evidence of sympathetic reinnervation was present only in the two patients with associated donor bradycardia, suggesting that the bradycardic response of the donor heart may have been caused by sympathetic withdrawal rather than parasympathetic reinnervation.

Arrowood and colleagues (19) demonstrated an absence of parasympathetic reinnervation by using a trigeminal nerve reflex and an arterial baroreflex in two groups of cardiac transplant recipients, one early (<24 months) and one late (>45 months) after transplantation. Both reflexes caused marked changes in recipient sinus heart rates but no significant change in the donor sinus rate. By using external neck suction to induce a carotid baroreceptor reflex, Bernardi et al (20) observed only a low-frequency compo-

nent in the heart rate variability spectrum that was not abolished by atropine. In a later study, however, this group compared the baroreceptor response in transplant recipients that underwent an atrial or a bicaval surgical anastomosis (21). In 4 of 10 patients who underwent bicaval anastomosis, a high-frequency component in the R-R interval spectrum was recorded, suggesting parasympathetic reinnervation, and it was abolished after the administration of atropine. In contrast, this high-frequency component in the heart rate variability spectrum was only seen in 2 of 79 atrial anastomosis patients. Because most parasympathetic fibers may be left intact (i.e., most end at the level of the atria) when using an atrial anastomosis, the severing of all parasympathetic fibers when performing a bicaval anastomosis was thought to provide a greater stimulus for nerve fiber regeneration.

Pharmacologic Therapy

The absence of autonomic innervation in the transplanted heart can also alter the effects of many other antiarrhythmic and cardioactive agents. The intravenous administration of digoxin has had little effect on the transplanted heart, causing no change in AV nodal conduction because its actions are predominantly mediated by the vagus nerve (22). For the same reason, atropine has also been shown to be ineffective in the transplanted heart (23), although a paradoxical parasympathomimetic effect has been reported. Brunner-La Rocca et al (24) reported three cases of high-grade AV block after atropine administration in cardiac transplant recipients, a response similar to that seen with low doses of atropine in normal patients. Although the mechanism for this is not clear, they postulated that at least partial parasympathetic reinnervation had occurred in those patients. Others have suggested that this effect may be caused by a central site of action (23).

Because of the transplanted heart's dependence on circulating catecholamines, β-blocking agents can have a significant effect on the heart's chronotropic and inotropic function, particularly during exercise. An early study of transplant recipients by Bexton and associates (25) demonstrated a marked decrease in exercise capacity from 6.8 minutes to 4.5 minutes after the administration of intravenous propranolol. In this study, the resting heart rate decreased from 109 ± 28 to 83 ± 16 bpm, and the peak heart rate was markedly reduced from 138 ± 34 bpm in the baseline test to only 96 ± 18 bpm after the administration of propranolol. Subsequent studies have shown a similar effect (26), and in a study by Verani and coworkers (27), β blockade caused a greater decrease in the resting ejection fraction of transplant recipients compared with normal controls (−16% ± 12.6% versus −5.4% ± 2.6%) and a 42% decrease in the peak cardiac index. In a study of heterotopic and orthotopic transplant recipients, Yusuf and colleagues (28) observed a 15% decrease in exercise duration, a 34% reduction in systolic blood pressure increase, and a 40% attenuation in heart rate increase after β blockade. In the heterotopic recipients, β blockade produced similar effects on heart rate in the denervated donor hearts and the innervated recipient hearts during and after mild exercise, but during peak exercise β blockade attenuated the rate to a greater extent in the donor hearts. In a study comparing a β_1-selective β blocker and a nonselective β blocker, the systolic blood pressure increase during exercise was totally blocked by both agents, but the heart rate increase was blunted 50% more by the nonselective agent, suggesting that nonselective β blockade may be less well tolerated in cardiac transplant patients than β_1-selective blockade (29).

A marked potentiation of the negative chronotropic and dromotropic effects of calcium antagonists has also been demonstrated in denervated hearts. Qi and associates (30) compared the effects of intravenous verapamil in dogs, after pharmacologic autonomic blockade and orthotopic transplantation, with a control group of normal dogs. An initial decrease in the sinus cycle length that was seen in the control group was absent in both groups of animals with denervated hearts. A subsequent increase in the sinus cycle length occurred promptly in the denervated hearts and was more pronounced than that seen in innervated hearts. Effects on AV nodal conduction were also more pronounced in the denervated groups. In a study of heterotopic heart transplanted dogs, the effects of verapamil, diltiazem, and nifedipine were compared in the recipient and donor hearts. Sinus automaticity and AV nodal conduction were depressed to a greater degree in the transplanted hearts, with the greatest effect on automaticity caused by verapamil (31). These effects may result from the absence of adrenergic reflexes mediated by the autonomic nervous system.

The effects of several antiarrhythmic agents are also different in orthotopic heart transplant recipients. Without its autonomically mediated anticholinergic effect, disopyramide causes a decrease in heart rate and prolongs the conduction time in the AV node and in the His-Purkinje system (32). Quinidine can increase the sinus cycle length and AV nodal conduction times in the donor heart while significantly decreasing the recipient sinus node cycle length (33). Procainamide and mexiletine have lesser effects on donor hearts

compared with recipient heterotopic hearts in dogs (34). Amiodarone, however, can cause a marked depression of the sinus node, and its long half-life (34) and widespread use in cardiomyopathy patients can cause significant bradycardia in the early posttransplantation period (35). Nanas and coworkers (36) studied the pharmakinetics of amiodarone in transplant recipients who had been taking oral amiodarone up until the time of their transplantation. Plasma concentrations of amiodarone decreased steadily but remained detectable up to the third month after transplantation. Myocardial concentrations of the agent, however, increased in the early postoperative period, with a peak concentration about 2 weeks after transplantation. The sinus-slowing effects of amiodarone may therefore worsen in the early posttransplantation period and can persist for up to several months.

Drug Interactions

A final consideration in the use of cardioactive agents is their potential interaction with the immunosuppressive agents used to prevent rejection of the transplanted heart (Table 32-1). Several drugs have been shown to increase the serum level of cyclosporine, potentially causing toxicity. Diltiazem has been the most widely studied agent, and its effect on cyclosporine concentrations has been used to decrease the total dosage of cyclosporine, resulting in substantial savings (37). Amiodarone and propafenone have also been shown to cause a substantial increase in cyclosporine levels (38–40). Proarrhythmic effects have been reported with another immunosuppressive agent, tacrolimus. This agent is a macrolide antibiotic and can cause prolongation of the QT interval. Torsade de pointes has been reported during therapy with this agent (41,42). The concomitant use of other QT prolonging agents or drugs that may increase its plasma concentration must be avoided or done with caution. The same is true for rapamycin, another macrolide antibiotic.

Arrhythmogenic Substrate

The transplanted heart is susceptible to several mechanisms of arrhythmogenesis. Surgical trauma to the sinoatrial and

TABLE 32-1. COMMON IMMUNOSUPPRESSIVE AGENTS AND POSSIBLE INTERACTIONS WITH ANTIARRHYTHMIC DRUGS

Immunosuppressive Agent	Antiarrhythmic	Effect
Cyclosporine	Diltiazem, verapamil, propafenone, amiodarone	Increase cyclosporine levels by inhibition of hepatic enzymes (cytochrome P450)
	Digoxin	Possible increase in digoxin level by decreasing digoxin clearance
Tacrolimus (Prograf, FK506) (prolongs the QT interval)	Amiodarone, diltiazem, lidocaine, propafenone, quinidine, verapamil	Increase plasma levels of tacrolimus by inhibition of hepatic enzymes (cytochrome P450)
Mycophenolate (CellCept)	None	No known interactions
Azathioprine (Imuran)	None	No known interactions

AV nodes, ischemia during preservation, surgical suture lines, rejection, and accelerated atherosclerosis all play a part in the formation of an arrhythmogenic substrate. The denervated donor heart has increased sensitivity to sympathetic amines and adenosine, and various degrees of reinnervation may occur. During rejection, an increase in the atrial and ventricular effective refractory periods has been observed, as well as an increase in the functional refractory period of the AV node (43). In an animal model, increases in the refractory period of the conduction system have directly correlated with the degree of rejection (44). Other electrophysiologic changes caused by rejection have been observed on the cellular level and include a significant reduction in the resting membrane potential, the action potential amplitude, and the maximum upstroke velocity of phase zero (45). All of these factors may contribute to the cardiac rhythm disturbances seen in the orthotopic heart transplant recipient. Given the multiple changes that occur over time, it is likely that early postoperative arrhythmias probably arise from different mechanisms from those occurring later.

Modifications in the surgical technique of cardiac transplantation have led to a decreased incidence of some arrhythmias. The standard orthotopic heart transplantation technique, initially described by Lower and Shumway, (46) involves an atrial anastomosis in which the donor atria are sutured directly to a remnant cuff of recipient right and left atria that includes the vena cavae, a portion of the atrial septum, and the pulmonary veins. Many centers are performing a bicaval anastomosis procedure in which the inferior and superior vena cavae are directly sutured to the recipient vena cavae (47,48) (Fig. 32-1). The left atria is attached with a small remnant of recipient atrial tissue that includes only the pulmonary veins. In addition to a decreased incidence of bradyarrhythmias (49–51) and some atrial dysrhythmias (52,53), improvements in atrial function and hemodynamics have been observed (54–56).

BRADYARRHYTHMIAS AND CONDUCTION DISTURBANCES

Sinus Node Dysfunction

The normal resting sinus rate of the denervated heart is usually greater than 80 bpm and may exceed 100 bpm in hearts transplanted from young donors. Sinus node dysfunction, which may be manifested by a "relative" bradycardia, has historically been the most common arrhythmia seen after orthotopic heart transplantation, occurring in up to 40% to 50% of patients in the first several weeks after transplantation (57–59). This dysrhythmia may result in significant patient morbidity, and as many as 16% of orthotopic heart transplant recipients require permanent pacing (59). Long-term mortality rates for these patients, however, do not appear to be different from those for other heart transplant recipients (60).

A variety of definitions for sinus node dysfunction have been used, ranging from the need for permanent pacing to formal programmed stimulation techniques with corrected sinus node recovery times longer than 520 ms (Fig. 32-2). The use of such overdrive suppression techniques in the intact human heart has been insensitive and poorly reproducible. This, however, does not hold true for the denervated transplanted heart. Mason (61) compared the sinus node response with overdrive suppression in the recipient and donor nodes of orthotopic heart transplant recipients and control subjects. Curves describing the relationship between the corrected sinus node recovery time and the cycle length of overdrive pacing were smooth and predictable for 72% of the donor atria compared with only 17% of the recipient atria and 20% of the control atria (Fig. 32-3). Similar results were found by Bexton and colleagues (1), who also observed a close correlation in the calculated sinoatrial conduction time when assessed by the methods of Strauss et al (62) or Narula and colleagues (63).

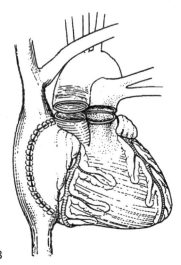 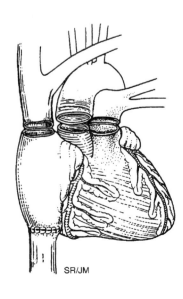

A,B

SR/JM

FIGURE 32-1. Surgical technique of orthotopic heart transplantation. Right anterior oblique projections of the donor heart are shown during implantation using a standard atrial anastomosis technique **(A)** and a bicaval anastomosis technique **(B)**.

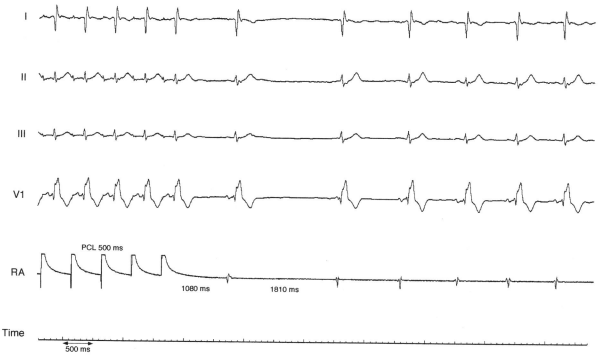

FIGURE 32-2. Abnormal sinus node function in an orthotopic heart transplant recipient. Simultaneous surface electrocardiographic recordings for leads I, II, III, and V₁ are shown along with an intracardiac recording from the donor right atrium (RA). Although pacing at a cycle length of 500 ms in the donor atria results in a normal primary pause of 1,080 ms (corrected sinus node recovery time, 280 ms), abnormal sinus node function is manifested by the prolonged secondary pause of 1,810 ms.

Potential causes of sinus node dysfunction have included ischemia during hypothermic preservation, immunologic processes, rejection, and surgical trauma to the sinus node, perinodal atrium, or sinoatrial artery (59,64). During the past two decades, changes in explantation techniques and storage solutions have allowed harvesting from greater dis-

tances, resulting in longer ischemic times of the donor heart. Heinz and colleagues (35) found no correlation between abnormal sinus node function and two cardioplegias commonly used at that time. Although a study comparing the University of Wisconsin and Stanford solutions showed an earlier restoration of normal sinus rhythm using

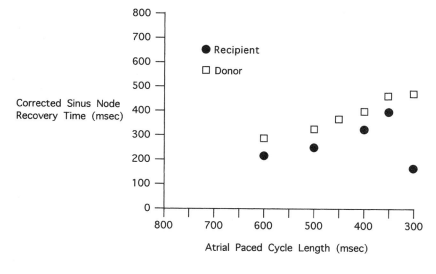

FIGURE 32-3. Sinus node recovery times in the recipient and donor atria of an orthotopic heart transplant recipient with normal sinus node function. A prolongation of the donor atria's corrected sinus node recovery time is seen at subsequently shorter paced cycle lengths. In the recipient atria, a discontinuous curve results when the corrected sinus node recovery time abruptly decreases at the shortest paced cycle length.

the University of Wisconsin solution, there was no significant difference by the third postoperative day (65). Several studies have demonstrated a correlation between the donor ischemic time and abnormal sinus node function (58,66). A similar correlation was found in a study assessing sinus node function in the early postoperative period, but this did not hold true for orthotopic heart transplant recipients with persistent sinus node dysfunction (62). Similarly, one large, retrospective series demonstrated no difference in the donor ischemic time for 41 of 556 orthotopic heart transplant recipients who required implantation of a permanent pacemaker (67).

Marked bradyarrhythmias due to severe cellular or humoral rejection have been reported (68,69), and for such patients, the prognosis is extremely poor. Blanche and colleagues (70) reviewed the clinical course and outcome of 15 patients who required a permanent pacemaker for bradyarrhythmias: six associated with acute or chronic rejection and nine not associated with rejection. The overall mortality rate was 100% for the rejection group, compared with only 1 (11%) of 9 patients in the nonrejection group. Several of the deaths in the rejection group occurred early after implantation of the pacemaker. For most patients with abnormal sinus node function, however, rejection is probably not a significant cause. Dibiase and colleagues at Stanford (67) described 41 of 556 orthotopic heart transplant recipients who required implantation of a permanent pacemaker. Only 24% of the pacemaker group had concomitant rejection requiring treatment, an incidence similar to those not requiring permanent pacemaker implantation. Miyamoto and colleagues (66) also showed no association between rejection and early postoperative bradyarrhythmias, but three of six patients requiring implantation of permanent pacemaker late after transplantation did have significant rejection. In a series of 50 consecutive orthotopic heart transplant recipients who underwent overdrive pacing to assess sinus node function, there was no difference between groups in the frequency of moderate to severe rejection (68). This study also failed to show an association with the pretransplantation disease state, donor age, or recipient age.

In the series reported by DiBiase and associates (67), patients who required permanent pacemakers had a significantly higher prevalence of abnormal sinoatrial nodal arteries compared with a control group of heart transplant recipients with normal sinus node function. Surgical trauma to the sinoatrial node or its blood supply has also been implicated by other groups as a possible cause of sinus node dysfunction (71–73). Such trauma can be avoided by performing a bicaval anastomosis rather than the standard atrial anastomosis (47,48), and several centers have since reported a decreased need for temporary and permanent pacing using this technique (50,51). In a prospective series of 70 orthotopic heart transplant recipients, we found the incidence of sinus node dysfunction, as determined by atrial pacing techniques, to decrease from 44% in those undergoing standard atrial anastomosis to 5% in the bicaval anastomosis group (49). When patients treated with amiodarone preoperatively were excluded, those requiring treatment of their bradycardia decreased from 35% in the atrial anastomosis group to 3% in the bicaval anastomosis group.

Normalization of posttransplantation sinus node dysfunction and bradyarrhythmias can occur in up to 55% of patients during the first 3 postoperative months (57). In patients who have received a permanent pacemaker early after transplantation, only 38% continue to pace at 3 months, and less than 20% are pacer dependent at 1 year (74). Holt and colleagues reviewed a policy change whereby pacemaker implantation in heart transplant recipients was delayed for at least 3 weeks after transplantation. Although this resulted in a decrease in the incidence of permanent pacemaker implantation from 11% to 8% (75), hospitalization was increased from a mean of 14 days to 24 days (76). To avoid implantation of a permanent pacemaker during this period, the use of theophylline (69,77,78) or terbutaline (79) has been advocated to increase the sinus rate.

Theophylline's effect most likely results from its action as an adenosine receptor antagonist. It is not clear whether posttransplantation sinus node dysfunction is an adenosine-mediated disease, but the effects of theophylline appear to be specific for donor hearts with abnormal sinus node function (80,81). In our study evaluating the acute effects of aminophylline, the corrected sinus node recovery time decreased by 33% in donor hearts with abnormal sinus node function, compared with a decrease of only 4% in normal donor hearts (80). Tables 32-2 and 32-3 show the acute effects of aminophylline (6 mg/kg, given intravenously) and terbutaline (0.25 mg, given subcutaneously), respectively, in 10 consecutive heart transplant recipients with sinus node dysfunction and 10 heart transplant recipients with normal sinus node function (82). Both agents show a marked decrease in the corrected sinus node recovery time of heart transplant recipients with sinus node dysfunction, but terbutaline significantly decreased the sinus node recovery time of normal recipients as well. Nonetheless, these agents have only a modest effect on the sinus node cycle length and recovery time, with incomplete correction of the underlying sinus node abnormality. In the latter study of 10 patients, only four patients had complete normalization of their sinus node abnormalities with either agent. These agents are probably best reserved for patients with only mild or moderate sinus node dysfunction or those with postoperative bradycardia due to prior amiodarone use.

Conduction Disturbances

The most common conduction abnormality after orthotopic heart transplantation is the occurrence of a new right bundle branch delay when compared with the donor electrocardiogram. This can occur in up to 70% of patients in the early postoperative period and usually manifests as an

TABLE 32-2. ELECTROPHYSIOLOGIC EFFECTS OF AMINOPHYLLINE IN ORTHOTOPIC HEART TRANSPLANT RECIPIENTS WITH AND WITHOUT SINUS NODE DYSFUNCTION

Sinus Node Function	Before Aminophylline (ms)	After Aminophylline (ms)	% Change	p Value
Normal				
SCL	731 ± 97	661 ± 90	9 ± 5	< 0.05
CSNRT	336 ± 111	286 ± 88	7 ± 22	NS
SACT	146 ± 35	136 ± 33	1 ± 22	NS
Abnormal				
SCL	798 ± 140	718 ± 101	10 ± 4	< 0.05
CSNRT	570 ± 312	428 ± 273	16 ± 5	< 0.05
SACT	172 ± 49	162 ± 38	4 ± 13	NS

CSNRT, corrected sinus node recovery time; SACT, sinoatrial conduction time; SCL, sinus cycle length; SN, sinus node.

incomplete right bundle branch block (83). The conduction abnormality may persist, and in one study (84) it was associated with a prolonged donor ischemic time and multiple episodes of rejection. Other studies, however, have failed to show any association with coronary artery disease, rejection, or ischemic time (83,85). Mechanical or thermal injury to the right bundle branch has also been postulated, whereas increased pulmonary artery pressures or changes in heart orientation have not been found to have a significant correlation (83,86).

Other common electrocardiographic changes that can be seen after orthotopic heart transplantation include changes in the QRS axis, a decrease in precordial lead voltages and shortening of the QT interval. The observance of a new left bundle branch block is uncommon, seen in less than 4% of orthotopic heart transplant recipients (84). In patients in whom large remnants of the recipient atria are left intact, intraatrial dissociation may occur and can sometimes lead to a false diagnosis (Fig. 32-4). In this situation, there is evidence of atrial activity (P wave) from the donor and recipient. The donor P-wave rate is faster than that of the recipient because of vagal denervation of the donor sinus node.

High-grade AV block is an uncommon finding after heart transplantation, particularly in the early postoperative period (58). Although AV block accounts for less than 10% of pacemaker implantations early after transplantation,

(67,87) it is a more common cause for permanent pacing more than 1 year after heart transplantation (73). The cause of late AV block is probably multifactorial. Rejection may play a role because of lymphocytic infiltration and hemorrhage within the His-Purkinje system (88,89); although this cause has been reported (66), it remains uncommon. Severe graft coronary disease has also been reported as a cause for the late development of heart block (73). Of greatest concern is the increased mortality associated with the late development of heart block (86,90). An extensive evaluation for coronary artery disease and rejection is warranted for such patients.

Pacing in the Transplanted Heart

For the orthotopic heart transplant recipient who requires permanent pacing for sinus node dysfunction or AV block, atrial-ventricular synchronization is the optimal approach. Hemodynamic studies comparing atrial and ventricular pacing have demonstrated significant increases in cardiac output with AV synchrony. Midei and colleagues (91) evaluated the effects of AAI and VVI pacing in nine consecutive orthotopic heart transplant recipients. A markedly higher cardiac output was observed with AAI pacing compared with VVI pacing (5.5 ± 1.4 L/min versus 4.6 ± 1.5 L/min), as well as an increased systemic arterial pressure. Parry and coworkers (92)

TABLE 32-3. ELECTROPHYSIOLOGIC EFFECTS OF TERBUTALINE IN ORTHOTOPIC HEART TRANSPLANT RECIPIENTS WITH AND WITHOUT SINUS NODE DYSFUNCTION

Sinus Node Function	Before Terbutaline (ms)	After Terbutaline (ms)	% Change	p Value
Normal				
SCL	714 ± 95	625 ± 86	12 ± 5	< 0.05
CSNRT	310 ± 101	210 ± 67	30 ± 18	< 0.05
SACT	120 ± 25	101 ± 31	16 ± 18	NS
Abnormal				
SCL	712 ± 139	616 ± 73	13 ± 7	< 0.05
CSNRT	504 ± 244	378 ± 157	21 ± 16	NS
SACT	192 ± 44	200 ± 38	6 ± 7	NS

CSNRT, corrected sinus node recovery time; SACT, sinoatrial conduction time; SCL, sinus cycle length; SN, sinus node.

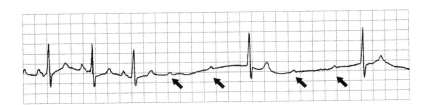

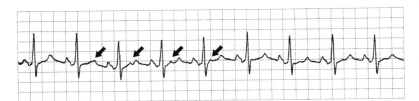

FIGURE 32-4. Pseudo-heart block in an orthotopic heart transplant recipient. **A:** Recipient atrial activity *(arrow)* gives the appearance of complete heart block during a sinus pause and junctional escape rhythm in the donor atria, which is driving the ventricle. **B:** After the return of donor atrial activity, atrial dissociation of the donor and recipient P waves *(arrows)* is evident. The donor P waves are associated with the QRS.

demonstrated similar results with an 11% and 8% improvement in cardiac output during AAI and DDD pacing compared with VVI pacing. In a study comparing the effects of AV synchrony in patients with a bicaval or atrial anastomosis, the improvement in cardiac output with AAI pacing was even greater in the bicaval group (55). No studies have compared these pacing modes in patients with symptomatic bradyarrhythmias, and it is not clear whether maintaining AV synchrony in such patients would result in long-term symptomatic improvement.

For patients with sinus node dysfunction but normal AV conduction, AAI pacing is probably adequate. Long-term follow-up of such patients has not revealed any latent AV block, although the number of reported patients is low (71,93). Some centers, however, take a more cautious approach, using a single ventricular lead with VVI pacing (66,67). Lead dislodgment during endomyocardial biopsy is a potential problem when using ventricular leads and can occur in up to 10% of patients (67). Fluoroscopic guidance and an active fixation permanent pacing lead are used at our institution to help minimize this problem.

Another approach for pacing heart transplant recipients has been to synchronize the recipient and donor atria, allowing the recipient atria with intact innervation to control the heart rate and provide better hemodynamic support. Nagele and colleagues (94) reported 21 patients with donor sinus node disease and normal recipient sinus rhythm. Each patient had a dual-chamber pacemaker with a bipolar pacing wire to each atria, whereby the donor atria was paced after a sensed recipient atrial beat (i.e., atrial synchronization), or a single-chamber pacemaker with a unipolar lead to each atria connected by a Y adapter that allowed sensing and triggered pacing of both atria. When compared with other age- and sex-matched heart transplant recipients, those with atrial synchronization showed a greater increase in heart rate response to exercise, improved cardiac index at rest and exercise, and decreased pulmonary pressures. In a study by Parry and coworkers (92), synchronization of the recipient and

donor atria did not improve resting hemodynamics beyond that achieved with donor atrial pacing alone.

Technically, placement of an atrial lead may be more difficult in the heart transplant recipient, and the rate of lead dislodgment has been reported to be higher than that in nontransplantation patients (95). The atria should be carefully mapped to find the optimal pacing and sensing site, and active-fixation leads should be used. Care must be taken to avoid sensing the recipient atria, which may inhibit pacing in an AAI system or trigger rapid ventricular pacing in a DDD system. Woodard reported a case of an AAI pacemaker sensing recipient atrial flutter and causing inhibition of atrial pacing with symptomatic bradycardia (96). Rate-responsive pacing should be considered in all orthotopic heart transplant recipients, but the optimal sensor probably depends on the activity level of the individual patient. Most patients with bradycardia early after transplantation do improve, but up to 40% of those who do require permanent pacing continue to pace during long-term follow-up (75).

SUPRAVENTRICULAR TACHYARRHYTHMIAS

Atrial Premature Depolarizations

Isolated APDs and nonsustained atrial dysrhythmias are common in the early postoperative transplantation period, occurring in 55% to 76% of patients (58,97,98). The prevalence is lower at long-term follow-up, decreasing from 55% in the early postoperative period to 30% at a mean of 24 months after transplantation in one study (97). Although several studies have shown no significant difference in the incidence of APDs during rejection, others have reported that their frequency may be increased (98,99).

Atrial Fibrillation and Flutter

Atrial fibrillation and flutter have been reported to occur in as many as 18% to 50% of orthotopic heart transplant recipients (52,98,100), with an even higher incidence in the era before cyclosporine (97). Changes in surgical technique have decreased the incidence even further. The use of a bicaval anastomosis decreased the incidence of atrial flutter and fibrillation in one series from 40% of patients with a standard atrial anastomosis to 4% of patients who underwent a bicaval anastomosis (52,53). Acute allograft rejection needs to be excluded in patients presenting with these dysrhythmias, because they may occur in the setting of rejection. MacDonald (101) described nine patients with 16 episodes of atrial flutter over a 2-year period. Twelve of these episodes were associated with rejection that was moderate to severe in nine of the episodes. Other investigators have not demonstrated as strong a correlation, and in a study by Pavri and associates (100), only 16% of atrial dysrhythmias were associated with moderate to severe rejection. This study did show an increased risk of death in cardiac transplant recipients who had a history of atrial fibrillation. The investigators speculated that atrial fibrillation may have been a marker for more extensive myocardial disease or facilitated by an abnormal hormonal milieu caused by an underlying infection or multiple-organ failure.

The cause of atrial dysrhythmias during rejection is unknown, but the patchy nature of rejection may result in an heterogeneous impairment of atrial conduction and refractoriness, allowing the formation of multiple microreentrant circuits. Atrial hemodynamics may be altered by the reduced ventricular function and compliance that occurs during rejection. Treatment of these arrhythmias includes control of the ventricular response rate and additional immunosuppressive therapy if concurrent rejection is found. The β blockers and calcium antagonists may be used for rate control, but no studies show either agent to be more efficacious. Many orthotopic heart transplant recipients are treated with diltiazem for hypertension and prevention of cardiac transplant vasculopathy (102), and in these patients, the addition of a β-adrenergic blocker would be warranted if further rate control is needed. There is no role for digoxin because its effects on AV nodal conduction are predominantly mediated by the vagus nerve (9).

Acute termination of atrial fibrillation and flutter can be performed pharmacologically, electrically, or by pacing techniques. Ibutilide has been reported to be efficacious in one case report (103), and other antiarrhythmic agents, such as procainamide, can also be considered. Because of its simplicity and high efficacy, we prefer electrical cardioversion for atrial fibrillation if the rhythm does not terminate spontaneously. For atrial flutter, overdrive pacing can be performed at the time of the myocardial biopsy with a more than 90% success rate for terminating the arrhythmia (101).

Several factors should be considered when using antiarrhythmic agents for the treatment of recurrent atrial arrhythmias. First, many antiarrhythmic agents, including propafenone, amiodarone, and quinidine, may interfere with the metabolism of immunosuppressive agents, and

drug levels need to be monitored closely. Second, the prevalence of cardiac transplant vasculopathy is as high as 15% at 1 year and 50% at 5 years (104), and patients with an acute event often present silently or with atypical symptoms (105). The use of type Ic agents should therefore be avoided or used cautiously. QT-prolonging agents should be avoided in heart transplant recipients who are being treated with the immunosuppressive agent tacrolimus because of the risk of torsade de pointes. Recurrent atrial flutter may be amenable to radiofrequency catheter ablation, avoiding antiarrhythmic side effects and drug interactions. Mapping of atrial flutter in the orthotopic heart transplant recipient demonstrates a macroreentrant circuit around the tricuspid annulus (106), and radiofrequency ablation of the flutter circuit can be performed by creating bidirectional conduction block between the tricuspid annulus and the atrial anastomosis suture line, proximal to the inferior vena cava (107–110).

Other Supraventricular Tachycardias

A variety of supraventricular arrhythmias have been described in orthotopic heart transplant recipients, including several reports of AV reentrant tachycardia involving a concealed or overt AV bypass tract (111–113), Wolff-Parkinson-White syndrome (114,115), AV nodal reentrant tachycardia (116), and sustained atrial tachycardias (100, 117,118). Radiofrequency catheter ablation has been performed in many of these of patients, and success rates similar to those for patients not receiving transplants can probably be expected, along with a low complication rate. At our center, radiofrequency catheter ablation has been used successfully in 11 orthotopic heart transplant recipients without complication: three patients had an atrial tachycardia, five patients had AV nodal reentrant tachycardia, two patients had Wolff-Parkinson-White syndrome, and one patient had a concealed AV bypass tract.

One arrhythmia unique to the orthotopic heart transplant recipient is caused by interatrial conduction from the recipient to donor atria. Bexton and colleagues (119) initially described a case of donor and recipient atrial synchronization that persisted while pacing either atrium, and two cases of unidirectional interatrial conduction were later described by Anselme et al (120). Postulated mechanisms for these arrhythmias included mechanical coupling, electrotonic transmission, and electrical conduction. In one patient with an atrial tachycardia caused by 1 : 1 and 2 : 1 conduction from a recipient atrial tachycardia (Fig. 32-5), termination of the donor arrhythmia was achieved by radiofrequency catheter ablation along the right atrial suture line (121), making direct interatrial impulse propagation or electrotonic influences the most likely mechanism for this phenomenon. During the past several years, there have been several more case reports of this type of dysrhythmia (122–124). In all of the reported cases, orthotopic heart transplantation was performed using a standard atrial

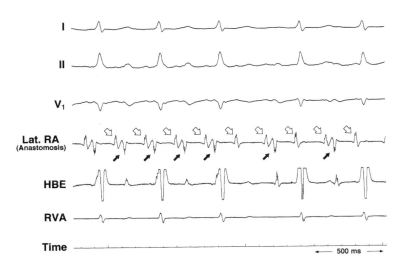

FIGURE 32-5. Intracardiac electrogram demonstrates recipient atrial tachycardia *(open arrows)* with 1 : 1 and 2 : 1 conduction to the donor atria *(solid arrows)*. Shown are surface electrocardiographic recordings I, II, and V₁ and intracardiac recordings from the right atrial anastomosis (Lat. RA), the His bundle electrogram (HBE), and the right ventricular apex (RVA).

anastomosis, and most patients presented with this dysrhythmia several years after transplantation. In an attempt to determine the prevalence of this dysrhythmia, Lefroy and colleagues (125) evaluated the rest and exercise electrocardiograms of 50 patients more than 5 years after transplantation. Frequent APDs with variable coupling to the preceding sinus beats or changes in P-wave morphology during exercise were found in five subjects, with both features present in one subject. Based on these results, they concluded that at least intermittent recipient to donor atrial conduction may occur in up to 10% of patients more than 5 years after orthotopic heart transplantation.

VENTRICULAR DYSRHYTHMIAS

Premature Ventricular Complexes and Nonsustained Ventricular Tachycardia

Premature ventricular complexes (PVCs) are common in the early posttransplantation period, occurring in up to 100% of patients (58,98). Nonsustained ventricular tachycardia and accelerated idioventricular rhythms are also frequent in the early posttransplantation period and may in part result from an increased sensitivity to circulating catecholamines (4) or rejection (58). Supporting the role of rejection, Little and coworkers (97) observed a trend toward a decreased prevalence of ventricular arrhythmias in transplant recipients treated with cyclosporine compared with azathioprine. After the early postoperative period, the prevalence of PVCs and nonsustained ventricular arrhythmias decreased significantly (97–99). Complex ventricular ectopy (i.e., multifocal PVCs and couplets) and nonsustained ventricular arrhythmias that occur late after transplantation, however, have been associated with an increased presence of coronary artery disease (99,126). Treatment of ventricular ectopy and nonsustained ventricular tachycardia is rarely warranted, but an evaluation for secondary causes

should be pursued. The predictive value of electrophysiologic testing in heart transplant recipients with nonsustained ventricular tachycardia, left ventricular dysfunction, and coronary arteriopathy is not clear.

Sustained Ventricular Arrhythmias

Sustained ventricular arrhythmias are uncommon in the donor heart (127) and, when they occur, are usually associated with severe atherosclerosis or allograft rejection. Two cases of sustained ventricular tachycardia not associated with rejection have been reported. Scott and associates (98) described a patient with sustained ventricular tachycardia who had been treated with flecainide for atrial dysrhythmias. This was treated successfully with direct current (DC) cardioversion, and after discontinuation of the antiarrhythmic agent, there were no further recurrences. A biopsy at the time showed no rejection. In the case reported by Clarke and colleagues (128), hemodynamically stable ventricular tachycardia occurred in an orthotopic heart transplant recipient 5 weeks after transplantation. The tachycardia had a right bundle branch block morphology with a left axis deviation, and although an initial biopsy showed moderate focal rejection, the tachycardia continued to recur after treatment. Multiple antiarrhythmic agents were tried empirically without success until the diagnosis of a fascicular tachycardia was entertained, and the arrhythmia was terminated with intravenous verapamil. The patient was ultimately cured with radiofrequency catheter ablation. Sustained or symptomatic nonsustained ventricular arrhythmias arising from the right ventricular outflow tract have not been reported.

Documented episodes of polymorphic ventricular tachycardia or ventricular fibrillation have almost exclusively been associated with severe rejection (Fig. 32-6). Berke and colleagues (129) described two patients who developed ventricular fibrillation while undergoing intensive in-hospital treatment for severe acute rejection. Both patients were initially

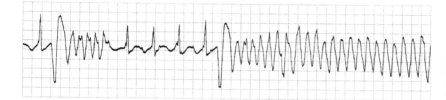

FIGURE 32-6. Polymorphic ventricular tachycardia and the onset of ventricular fibrillation are shown in an orthotopic heart transplant recipient with a grade 3B/4 cellular rejection.

resuscitated with DC cardioversion, but one subsequently died of unremitting rejection. In a case described by de Jonge (130), ventricular fibrillation occurred repeatedly in a patient undergoing antirejection therapy and was initially treated with procainamide after lidocaine failed to suppress recurrences. This patient had a subsequent episode of ventricular fibrillation several days later and was changed to flecainide for the remainder of his treatment course. Ventricular fibrillation has also been reported as a complication of endomyocardial biopsy in a patient with moderate acute rejection (131).

CLINICAL SYNDROMES

Sudden Cardiac Death

Sudden cardiac death is a frequent cause of mortality among orthotopic heart transplant recipients. Patel and colleagues from the Texas Heart Institute (132) reviewed the records of 257 recipient deaths and found 25 patients who had sudden cardiac deaths (9.7%). Eighty percent of the episodes occurred more than 1 year after transplantation and 20% after more than 5 years. Endomyocardial biopsies performed a mean of 3.8 months before death showed no evidence of rejection in 95% of the subjects. Of the five patients who died within 1 year of transplantation, three had severe coronary artery disease on autopsy, and one had severe rejection; no autopsy was performed on the fifth patient. Among the patients who died more than 1 year after transplantation, 16 had coronary artery disease. Overall, of the subjects for whom autopsy or angiographic data were available, 95% had evidence of severe coronary disease. This high prevalence of severe coronary atherosclerosis or recent myocardial infarction has been demonstrated in other autopsy studies of patients with sudden cardiac death (86,129,133). Although ventricular tachyarrhythmias are thought to be the mode of sudden cardiac death, severe bradycardic events may also occur in the setting of advanced atherosclerosis (59,134). Whereas most heart transplant recipients with significant allograft rejection present with symptoms of congestive heart failure, the lack of anginal symptoms in the denervated heart may play a role in the development of severe, asymptomatic coronary artery disease.

Syncope

Syncope can occur in the orthotopic heart transplant recipient and can be caused by a variety of mechanisms.

Sick sinus syndrome can manifest initially with syncope (67), and heart block can occur late after transplantation. Weinfeld and colleagues at Brigham and Woman's Hospital in Boston (73) described their experience with 11 patients with bradyarrhythmias later after transplantation. Five of these patients presented with syncope, and the remainder all had near syncope. The most common arrhythmia was AV block, occurring in seven patients. In one patient, the AV block resulted from coronary spasm. Sinus node dysfunction occurred in four patients. All patients in this study were treated with pacemakers, except for the patient with coronary spasm, who was successfully treated medically.

Tachyarrhythmias are also potential causes of syncope in this patient population. The orthotopic heart transplant recipient is at risk for a variety of supraventricular arrhythmias. Zhu reported one patient with recurrent syncope who was found to have poorly tolerated AV nodal reentrant tachycardia on electrophysiologic study. After radiofrequency catheter modification of the AV node, the patient had no further episodes of syncope (116). Of more concern, however, are life-threatening arrhythmias that initially present as syncope. In Patel's study of 25 heart transplant recipients who died of sudden cardiac death, four patients had a history of syncope (132). All four patients also had evidence of coronary vasculopathy on autopsy.

Neurocardiogenic mechanisms may also cause syncope in orthotopic heart transplant recipients. Scherrer et al initially described the occurrence of vasovagal symptoms in a cardiac transplant recipient who was participating in a study designed to assess arterial baroreceptor control of sympathetic outflow (135). While recording peripheral sympathetic nerve activity, the patient was given an intravenous infusion of nitroprusside, causing a drop in systolic blood pressure from 131 to 116 mm Hg. After an initial increase in sympathetic nerve activity, the patient began to yawn and complain of nausea. Sympathetic nerve activity was then almost completely inhibited, and the patient became pale and hypotensive; recovery occurred after the infusion of saline and phenylephrine. During this episode there was no change in the donor heart rate, except for a slight increase at the end of the episode, probably because of an increase in circulating catecholamines. Several spontaneous cases of vasovagal syncope have since been reported (136,137), and in one case, decreases in the donor heart rate and blood pressure were observed.

Neurocardiogenic syncope has also been induced in asymptomatic heart transplant recipients undergoing head-upright tilt-table testing. Fitzpatrick (17) reported the outcome of tilt-table testing on 10 subjects at a mean of 22 months after heart transplantation. Surprisingly, 7 of the 10 patients had vasovagal reactions manifested by a mean decrease in blood pressure of 55 mm Hg and a mean decrease in recipient heart rate by 25 bpm. The donor heart rate remained unchanged in four patients, but in three patients, there was a mean decrease of 23 bpm. In a study by Lord and coworkers (138), head-upright tilt-table testing was compared for 17 asymptomatic orthotopic heart transplant recipients and 12 normal controls. Syncope or presyncope was induced in 7 of 17 heart transplant recipients and in 11 of 12 controls using an aggressive protocol. For patients with a positive result, the time to tilt-induced symptoms was markedly greater in the heart transplant recipients than in the normal controls (28.7 ± 18.8 versus 12.5 ± 10.2 minutes). In this study, there was no significant change in the donor heart rate during symptoms.

At our institution, 23 orthotopic heart transplant recipients presented with a syncopal or severe near-syncopal event. The causes of syncope in this group are listed in Table 32-4. The most common cause was bradycardia, including five patients who presented with new-onset AV block. This dysrhythmia was associated with severe posttransplantation coronary arteriopathy in four patients and severe cellular rejection in a fifth. Tachyarrhythmias were found in three patients. One patient had an exercise-induced ventricular tachycardia that was treated successfully with medical therapy. Polymorphic ventricular tachycardia was inducible in another patient who subsequently underwent implantation of a cardioverter-defibrillator. A third patient who presented with AV nodal reentry was successfully treated with radiofrequency catheter ablation. A cause for syncope could not be determined in 26% of orthotopic heart transplant recipients. Workup of these patients included a negative electrophysiology study, normal tilt-table study, normal left and right heart catheterization, and normal right ventricular biopsy. All of these patients have had no recurrent events without treatment.

TABLE 32-4. CAUSES OF SYNCOPE IN 23 ORTHOTOPIC HEART TRANSPLANT RECIPIENTS

Cause of Syncope	Number of Patients (%)
Sinus node dysfunction	6 (26)
Atrioventricular (AV) block	5 (22)
Neurocardiogenic syncope	2 (9)
Ventricular tachycardia	2 (9)
Carotid sinus hypersensitivity	1 (4)
Supraventricular tachycardia (AV nodal reentry)	1 (4)
Unknown	6 (26)

Treatment

Orthotopic heart transplant recipients who present with sustained ventricular arrhythmias, cardiac arrest, or syncope due to ventricular arrhythmias should be aggressively evaluated for rejection and coronary arteriopathy. Treatment for these patients should be directed toward the underlying cause, and if no reversible cause is found, implantation of a cardioverter-defibrillator is warranted. AV block and bradyarrhythmias are probably best treated with a pacemaker, and most patients with recurrent vasovagal syncope can be treated with conservative measures, such as hydration and support stockings. Because most heart transplant recipients with neurocardiogenic syncope present with a predominant vasodepressor effect, centrally acting agents or peripheral vasoconstrictors can be expected to have the most efficacy. Patients who present with syncope of an unknown cause and have no evidence of coronary artery disease or rejection probably do not require further treatment. We are not aware of any therapeutic trials for the treatment of these syndromes in heart transplant recipients, and therefore more definitive recommendations cannot be made.

DETECTION OF TRANSPLANT REJECTION WITH PACEMAKERS

One of the major causes of morbidity and mortality after cardiac transplantation is acute cellular allograft rejection, a process in which the allograft is damaged by infiltrating host T lymphocytes. The mainstay for diagnosing allograft rejection is endomyocardial biopsy, an invasive procedure associated with a some morbidity and mortality (139). Questions have been raised about the reliability of endomyocardial biopsy (140,141). The development of noninvasive or less invasive diagnostic approaches for the detection of cardiac transplant rejection is desirable.

Alterations in QRS voltages on electrocardiograms as a result of transplant rejection have been observed since the early era of cardiac transplantation (142). Intramyocardial electrograms (IMEGs) have been studied prospectively using pacemakers implanted at the time of transplantation (143). In a prospective study of 32 cardiac transplant patients, IMEG amplitudes were recorded by a dual-chamber pacemaker implanted at the time of transplant. A loss of 8% or more of the IMEG voltage below the individual patient range of variability from overnight recordings was thought to indicate rejection. Endomyocardial biopsies were performed concurrently in this patient cohort. Of 27 episodes of acute rejection occurring during the study, 22 were accurately identified by IMEG, and five could only be identified by biopsy because the IMEG results were inconclusive. IMEG and endomyocardial biopsy were positive in 16 cases and negative in 228. The negative predictive value for the treatment of rejection for IMEG was 100%, with a sensitivity of 100% and a specificity of 97%. This single-center study showed that IMEG analysis from an implanted pacemaker could be used as a screen for endomyocardial biopsies and could be used to replace many of the endomyocardial biopsies performed.

An alternative approach to the noninvasive detection of rejection in heart transplant recipients using pacemakers implanted at the time of transplantation was to study changes in ventricular-evoked response amplitudes (VERAs) acquired during short periods of ventricular pacing (144). In the initial single-center study using this approach, 17 patients were enrolled and had VVI pacemakers placed at the time of transplantation. One-minute sequences of ventricular pacing at 100 bpm were obtained, and the data were compared with endomyocardial biopsy results using International Society of Heart and Lung Transplantation (ISHLT) grades. Grade 2 or higher is considered significant. The VERA was found to have a sensitivity and specificity of 84% and 81%, respectively, for an ISHLT grade 2 or higher-grade rejection. A subsequent single-center study of 29 patients showed that changes in VERAs could detect 89 ISHLT grade 1B or higher rejection episodes, with reversal of the VERA changes after reversal of the rejections using corticosteroids (145,146).

A rejection-sensitive parameter (RSP) was identified in the subsequent studies. The RSP was defined as the maximum slope of the descending side of the T wave (i.e., T-slew rate) of the ventricular-evoked response. Comparison of the T-slew rates from 239 recordings obtained when there was no biopsy evidence of rejection with nine recordings obtained at the time of biopsy-proved rejection showed a significant difference in the RSP (p = 0.0031). The sensitivity and specificity for the detection of ISHLT grade 2 or higher-grade rejection were 71% and 76%, respectively, with positive and negative predictive values of 11% and 98%, respectively. A multicenter study of 30 transplant patients at five transplantation centers in the United States further investigated the utility of this pacemaker-guided analysis of the RSP, T-slew, for the noninvasive detection of cardiac transplant rejection (147). Pacemaker data obtained from 1-minute periods of VVI pacing at 100 bpm were compared with the results of endomyocardial biopsy. During 850 follow-up evaluations, 3,515 epimyocardial electrograms were recorded, and 307 endomyocardial biopsies were obtained. The sensitivity and specificity of T-slew for detecting rejection were 69% and 75%, respectively. The negative and positive predictive values were 96% and 23%, respectively. The epimyocardial electrogram parameters measured at the time of rejection were significantly lower than those obtained when no rejection was present (87% versus 99%, p < 0.001). Using this approach, 71% of endomyocardial biopsies could potentially have been eliminated if the epimyocardial electrogram parameter values had been used as a screen to determine whether rejection was present.

The ultimate utility of these pacemaker-guided approaches for the detection of rejection may be as a screen for determining if more invasive diagnostic techniques, such as endomyocardial biopsy, are warranted, sparing patients the cost and expense of many of the biopsies that are now performed. Further work in larger studies will be required to define the role of pacemaker-guided monitoring of rejection in cardiac transplant recipients.

CONCLUSIONS

Although most arrhythmias after orthotopic heart transplantation are benign, the occurrence of several types of arrhythmias should alert the physician to exclude serious underlying causes. Sustained atrial flutter and fibrillation may be associated with allograft rejection, and complex ventricular ectopy or AV block may be caused by acute rejection or severe coronary atherosclerosis. Early postoperative bradyarrhythmias due to sinus node dysfunction are probably caused by surgical trauma to the sinoatrial node or its blood supply and can be avoided using a bicaval anastomosis technique.

REFERENCES

1. Bexton RS, Nathan AW, Hellestrand KJ, et al. Sinoatrial function after cardiac transplantation. *J Am Coll Cardiol* 1984;3:712–723.
2. Strobel JS, Epstein AE, Bourge RC, et al. Nonpharmacologic validation of the intrinsic heart rate in cardiac transplant recipients. *J Interv Card Electrophysiol* 1999;3:15–18.
3. Cannom DS, Rider AK, Stinson EB, Harrison DC. Electrophysiologic studies in the denervated transplanted human heart. II. Response to norepinephrine, isoproterenol and propranolol. *Am J Cardiol* 1975;36:859–866.
4. Yusuf S, Theodoropoulos S, Mathias CJ, et al. Increased sensitivity of the denervated transplanted human heart to isoprenaline both before and after beta-adrenergic blockade. *Circulation* 1987;75:696–704.
5. Leenen FH, Davies RA, Fourney A. Catecholamines and heart function in heart transplant patients: effects of beta₁- versus nonselective beta-blockade. *Clin Pharmacol Ther* 1998;64:522–535.
6. Lurie KG, Bristow MR, Reitz BA. Increased beta-adrenergic receptor density in an experimental model of cardiac transplantation. *J Thorac Cardiovasc Surg* 1983;86:195–201.
7. Ellenbogen KA, Thames MD, DiMarco JP, et al. Electrophysiological effects of adenosine in the transplanted human heart: evidence of supersensitivity. *Circulation* 1990;81:821–828.
8. Toft J, Mortensen J, Hesse B. Risk of atrioventricular block during adenosine pharmacologic stress testing in heart transplant recipients. *Am J Cardiol* 1998;82:696–697.
9. Fallen EL, Kamath MV, Ghista DN, Fitchett D. Spectral analysis of heart rate variability following human heart transplantation: evidence for functional reinnervation. *J Auton Nerv Syst* 1988;23:199–206.
10. Rudas L, Pflugfelder PW, Menkis AH, et al. Evolution of heart rate responsiveness after orthotopic cardiac transplantation. *Am J Cardiol* 1991;68:232–236.
11. De Marco T, Dae M, Yuen-Green MS, et al. Iodine-123 metaiodobenzylguanidine scintigraphic assessment of the transplanted human heart: evidence for late reinnervation. *J Am Coll Cardiol* 1995;25:927–931.

12. Schwaiger M, Hutchins GD, Kalff V, et al. Evidence for regional catecholamine uptake and storage sites in the transplanted human heart by positron emission tomography. *J Clin Invest* 1991;87:1681–1690.

13. Wilson RF, Christensen BV, Olivari MT, et al. Evidence for structural sympathetic reinnervation after orthotopic cardiac transplantation in humans. *Circulation* 1991;83:1210–1220.

14. Wilson RF, Laxson DD, Christensen BV, et al. Regional differences in sympathetic reinnervation after human orthotopic cardiac transplantation. *Circulation* 1993;88:165–171.

15. Lord SW, Brady S, Holt ND, et al. Exercise response after cardiac transplantation: correlation with sympathetic reinnervation. *Heart* 1996;75:40–43.

16. Lord SW, Clayton RH, Mitchell L, et al. Sympathetic reinnervation and heart rate variability after cardiac transplantation. *Heart* 1997;77:532–538.

17. Fitzpatrick AP, Banner N, Cheng A, et al. Vasovagal reactions may occur after orthotopic heart transplantation [See comments]. *J Am Coll Cardiol* 1993;21:1132–1137.

18. Morgan-Hughes NJ, Kenny RA, Scott CD, et al. Vasodepressor reactions after orthotopic cardiac transplantation: relationship to reinnervation status. *Clin Auton Res* 1994;4:125–129.

19. Arrowood JA, Minisi AJ, Goudreau E, et al. Absence of parasympathetic control of heart rate after human orthotopic cardiac transplantation. *Circulation* 1997;96:3492–3498.

20. Bernardi L, Bianchini B, Spadacini G, et al. Demonstrable cardiac reinnervation after human heart transplantation by carotid baroreflex modulation of RR interval. *Circulation* 1995;92:2895–2903.

21. Bernardi L, Valenti C, Wdowczyck-Szulc J, et al. Influence of type of surgery on the occurrence of parasympathetic reinnervation after cardiac transplantation. *Circulation* 1998;97:1368–1374.

22. Goodman DJ, Rossen RM, Cannom DS, et al. Effect of digoxin on atrioventricular conduction. studies in patients with and without cardiac autonomic innervation. *Circulation* 1975;51:251–256.

23. Epstein AE, Hirschowitz BI, Kirklin JK, et al. Evidence for a central site of action to explain the negative chronotropic effect of atropine: studies on the human transplanted heart. *J Am Coll Cardiol* 1990;15:1610–1617.

24. Brunner-La Rocca HP, Kiowski W, Bracht C, et al. Atrioventricular block after administration of atropine in patients following cardiac transplantation. *Transplantation* 1997;63:1838–1839.

25. Bexton RS, Milne JR, Cory-Pearce R, et al. Effect of beta blockade on exercise response after cardiac transplantation. *Br Heart J* 1983;49:584–588.

26. Kushwaha SS, Banner NR, Patel N, et al. Effect of beta blockade on the neurohumoral and cardiopulmonary response to dynamic exercise in cardiac transplant recipients. *Br Heart J* 1994;71:431–436.

27. Verani MS, Nishimura S, Mahmarian JJ, et al. Cardiac function after orthotopic heart transplantation: response to postural changes, exercise, and beta-adrenergic blockade. *J Heart Lung Transplant* 1994;13:181–193.

28. Yusuf S, Theodoropoulos S, Dhalla N, et al. Influence of beta blockade on exercise capacity and heart rate response after human orthotopic and heterotopic cardiac transplantation. *Am J Cardiol* 1989;64:636–641.

29. Leenen FH, Davies RA, Fourney A. Role of cardiac beta 2-receptors in cardiac responses to exercise in cardiac transplant patients. *Circulation* 1995;91:685–690.

30. Qi AZ, Tuna IC, Gornick CC, et al. Potentiation of cardiac electrophysiologic effects of verapamil after autonomic blockade or cardiac transplantation. *Circulation* 1987;75:888–893.

31. Alvarez L, Escudero C, Torralba A, Millan I. Electrophysiologic assessment of calcium channel blockers in transplanted hearts: an experimental study. *J Electrocardiol* 1998;31:51–56.

32. Bexton RS, Hellestrand KJ, Cory-Pearce R, et al. The direct electrophysiologic effects of disopyramide phosphate in the transplanted human heart. *Circulation* 1983;67:38–45.

33. Mason JW, Winkle RA, Rider AK, et al. The electrophysiologic effects of quinidine in the transplanted human heart. *J Clin Invest* 1977;59:481–489.

34. Alvarez L, Escudero C, Torralba A, Millan I. Electrophysiologic effects of procainamide, mexiletine, and amiodarone on the transplanted heart: experimental study. *J Thorac Cardiovasc Surg* 1995;109:899–904.

35. Heinz G, Ohner T, Laufer G, et al. Demographic and perioperative factors associated with initial and prolonged sinus node dysfunction after orthotopic heart transplantation: the impact of ischemic time. *Transplantation* 1991;51:1217–1224.

36. Nanas JN, Anastasiou-Nana MI, Margari ZJ, et al. Redistribution of amiodarone in heart transplant recipients treated with the drug before operation. *J Heart Lung Transplant* 1997;16:387–389.

37. Valantine H, Keogh A, McIntosh N, et al. Cost containment: coadministration of diltiazem with cyclosporine after heart transplantation. *J Heart Lung Transplant* 1992;11:1–7; discussion 7–8.

38. Mamprin F, Mullins P, Graham T, et al. Amiodarone-cyclosporine interaction in cardiac transplantation [Letter, comment]. *Am Heart J* 1992;123:1725–1726.

39. Nicolau DP, Uber WE, Crumbley AJ, Strange C. Amiodarone-cyclosporine interaction in a heart transplant patient. *J Heart Lung Transplant* 1992;11:564–568.

40. Spes CH, Angermann CE, Horn K, et al. Ciclosporin-propafenone interaction. *Klin Wochenschr* 1990;68:872.

41. Hodak SP, Moubarak JB, Rodriguez I, et al. QT prolongation and near fatal cardiac arrhythmia after intravenous tacrolimus administration: a case report. *Transplantation* 1998;66:535–537.

42. Johnson MC, So S, Marsh JW, Murphy AM. QT prolongation and torsades de pointes after administration of FK506. *Transplantation* 1992;53:929–930.

43. Wnuk-Wojnar AM, Zembala M, Religa Z, et al. Electrophysiologic properties of transplanted human heart with and without rejection. *J Heart Lung Transplant* 1992;11:435–441.

44. Kitamura M, Berry GJ, Billingham ME, et al. Assessment of cardiac allograft rejection with electrophysiology of the conduction system and histopathology of the ventricle. *J Heart Lung Transplant* 1992;11:280–288.

45. Binah O, Zhang HL, Oluwole SF, et al. Mechanical and electrophysiologic changes in rat cardiac allografts during immunologic rejection. *Transplantation* 1991;52:508–512.

46. Lower RR, Stofen RR Shumway NE. Homovital transplantation of the heart. *J Thorac Cardiovasc Surg* 1961;41:196–201.

47. Dreyfus G, Jebara V, Mihaileanu S, Carpentier AF. Total orthotopic heart transplantation: an alternative to the standard technique [See comments]. *Ann Thorac Surg* 1991;52:1181–1184.

48. Sarsam MA, Campbell CS, Yonan NA, et al. An alternative surgical technique in orthotopic cardiac transplantation [See comments]. *J Card Surg* 1993;8:344–349.

49. Rothman SA, Jeevanandam V, Combs WG, et al. Eliminating bradyarrhythmias after orthotopic heart transplantation. *Circulation* 1996;94[Suppl II]:278–282.

50. Deleuze PH, Benvenuti C, Mazzucotelli JP, et al. Orthotopic cardiac transplantation with direct caval anastomosis: is it the optimal procedure? *J Thorac Cardiovasc Surg* 1995;109:731–737.

51. el Gamel A, Yonan NA, Grant S, et al. Orthotopic cardiac transplantation: a comparison of standard and bicaval Wythenshawe techniques. *J Thorac Cardiovasc Surg* 1995;109:721–729.

52. Brandt M, Harringer W, Hirt SW, et al. Influence of bicaval anastomoses on late occurrence of atrial arrhythmia after heart transplantation. *Ann Thorac Surg* 1997;64:70–72.

53. Forni A, Faggian G, Luciani GB, et al. Reduced incidence of

cardiac arrhythmias after orthotopic heart transplantation with direct bicaval anastomosis. *Transplant Proc* 1996;28:289–292.

54. Aleksic I, Freimark D, Blanche C, et al. Resting hemodynamics after total versus standard orthotopic heart transplantation in patients with high preoperative pulmonary vascular resistance. *Eur J Card Thorac Surg* 1997;11:1037–1044.

55. el-Gamel A, Deiraniya AK, Rahman AN, et al. Orthotopic heart transplantation hemodynamics: does atrial preservation improve cardiac output after transplantation? *J Heart Lung Transplant* 1996;15:564–571.

56. Leyh RG, Jahnke AW, Kraatz EG, Sievers HH. Cardiovascular dynamics and dimensions after bicaval and standard cardiac transplantation. *Ann Thorac Surg* 1995;59:1495–1500.

57. Heinz G, Hirschl M, Buxbaum P, et al. Sinus node dysfunction after orthotopic cardiac transplantation: postoperative incidence and long-term implications. *Pacing Clin Electrophysiol* 1992;15:731–737.

58. Jacquet L, Ziady G, Stein K, et al. Cardiac rhythm disturbances early after orthotopic heart transplantation: prevalence and clinical importance of the observed arrhythmias. *J Am Coll Cardiol* 1990;16:832–837.

59. Mackintosh AF, Carmichael DJ, Wren C, et al. Sinus node dysfunction in the first three weeks after cardiac transplantation. *Br Heart J* 1982;48:584–588.

60. Heinz G, Kratochwill C, Koller-Strametz J, et al. Benign prognosis of early sinus node dysfunction after orthotopic cardiac transplantation. *Pacing Clin Electrophysiol* 1998;21:422–429.

61. Mason JW. Overdrive Suppression of the transplanted heart: effect of the autonomic nervous system on human sinus node recovery. *Circulation* 1980;62:688–696.

62. Strauss HC, Bigger JT, Saroff AL, Giardina EGV. Electrophysiologic evaluation of sinus node function in patients with sinus node dysfunction. *Circulation* 1976;53:763–776.

63. Narula OS, Shantha N, Vasquez M, et al. A new method for measurement of sinoatrial conduction time. *Circulation* 1978; 58:706–714.

64. Ellenbogen KA, Stanbler BS, Wood MA. Cardiac transplantation. In: Podrid P, Kowey P, eds. *Cardiac Arrhythmia: Mechanisms, Diagnosis, and Management.* Baltimore: Williams & Wilkins, 1995.

65. Stein DG, Drinkwater DC Jr, Laks H, et al. Cardiac preservation in patients undergoing transplantation. a clinical trial comparing University of Wisconsin solution and Stanford solution. *J Thorac Cardiovasc Surg* 1991;102:657–665.

66. Miyamoto Y, Curtiss EI, Kormos RL, et al. Bradyarrhythmia after heart transplantation: incidence, time course, and outcome. *Circulation* 1990;82[Suppl IV]:313–317.

67. DiBiase A, Tse TM, Schnittger I, et al. Frequency and mechanism of bradycardia in cardiac transplant recipients and need for pacemakers. *Am J Cardiol* 1991;67:1385–1389.

68. Blanche C, Czer LS, Trento A, et al. Bradyarrhythmias requiring pacemaker implantation after orthotopic heart transplantation: association with rejection [See comments]. *J Heart Lung Transplant* 1992;11:446–452.

69. Ellenbogen KA, Szentpetery S, Katz MR. Reversibility of prolonged chronotropic dysfunction with theophylline following orthotopic cardiac transplantation. *Am Heart J* 1988;116:202–206.

70. Blanche C, Czer LS, Fishbein MC, et al. Permanent pacemaker for rejection episodes after heart transplantation: a poor prognostic sign. *Ann Thorac Surg* 1995;60:1263–1266.

71. Payne ME, Murray KD, Watson KM, et al. Permanent pacing in heart transplant recipients: underlying causes and long-term results. *J Heart Lung Transplant* 1991;10:738–742.

72. Kratochwill C, Schmid S, Koller-Strametz J, et al. Decrease in pacemaker incidence after orthotopic heart transplantation. *Am J Cardiol* 1996;77:779–783.

73. Weinfeld MS, Kartashov A, Piana R, Hauptman PJ. Bradycardia: a late complication following cardiac transplantation. *Am J Cardiol* 1996;78:969–971.

74. Scott CD, Omar I, McComb JM, et al. Long-term pacing in heart transplant recipients is usually unnecessary. *Pacing Clin Electrophysiol* 1991;14:1792–1796.

75. Holt ND, Tynan MM, Scott CD, et al. Permanent pacemaker use after cardiac transplantation: completing the audit cycle. *Heart* 1996;76:435–438.

76. Holt ND, Parry G, Tynan MM, et al. Permanent pacemaker implantation after cardiac transplantation: extra cost of a conservative policy. *Heart* 1996;76:439–441.

77. Redmond JM, Zehr KJ, Gillinov MA, et al. Use of theophylline for treatment of prolonged sinus node dysfunction in human orthotopic heart transplantation. *J Heart Lung Transplant* 1993; 12:133–138.

78. Bertolet BD, Eagle DA, Conti JB, et al. Bradycardia after heart transplantation: reversal with theophylline. *J Am Coll Cardiol* 1996;28:396–399.

79. Cook LS, Will KR, Moran J. Treatment of junctional rhythm after heart transplantation with terbutaline. *J Heart Transplant* 1989;8:342–344.

80. Rothman SA, Jeevanandam V, Seeber CP, et al. Electrophysiologic effects of intravenous aminophylline in heart transplant recipients with sinus node dysfunction. *J Heart Lung Transplant* 1995;14:429–435.

81. Conti JB, Bertolet B, Belardinelli L, et al. Sinus bradycardia in transplant patients is not associated with elevated endogenous adenosine concentrations. *Circulation* 1995;92:I-334(abst).

82. Rothman SA, Jeevanandam V, Hsia H, et al. A comparison of the electrophysiologic effects of aminophylline and terbutaline in heart transplant recipients with sinus node dysfunction. *Circulation* 1995;92:I-334(abst).

83. Villa AE, de Marchena EJ, Myerburg RJ, Castellanos A. Comparisons of paired orthotopic cardiac transplant donor and recipient electrocardiograms. *Am Heart J* 1994;127:70–74.

84. Leonelli FM, Pacifico A, Young JB. Frequency and significance of conduction defects early after orthotopic heart transplantation. *Am J Cardiol* 1994;73:175–179.

85. Golshayan D, Seydoux C, Berguer DG, et al. Incidence and prognostic value of electrocardiographic abnormalities after heart transplantation. *Clin Cardiol* 1998;21:680–684.

86. Leonelli FM, Dunn K, Young JB, Pacifico A. Natural history, determinants, and clinical relevance of conduction abnormalities following orthotopic heart transplantation. *Am J Cardiol* 1996;77:47–51.

87. Markewitz A, Schmoeckel M, Nollert G, et al. Long-term results of pacemaker therapy after orthotopic heart transplantation. *J Card Surg* 1993;8:411–416.

88. Bieber CP, Stinson EB, Shumway NE. Pathology of the conduction system in cardiac rejection. *Circulation* 1969;39:567–575.

89. Stovin PGI, Hewitt S. Conduction tissue in the transplanted human heart. *J Pathol* 1986;149:183–189.

90. Rubin S, Hsia H, Mather P, et al. Etiology and prognostic implications of post-transplant conduction system disease. *J Heart Lung Transplant* 1996;15:S60(abst).

91. Midei MG, Baughman KL, Achuff SC, et al. Is atrial activation beneficial in heart transplant recipients? *J Am Coll Cardiol* 1990;16:1201–1204.

92. Parry G, Malbut K, Dark JH, Bexton RS. Optimal pacing modes after cardiac transplantation: is synchronisation of recipient and donor atria beneficial? *Br Heart J* 1992;68:195–198.

93. Heinz G, Kratochwill C, Buxbaum P, et al. Long-term intrinsic pacemaker function in patients paced for sinus node deficiency after cardiac transplantation. *Pacing Clin Electrophysiol* 1992;15: 2061–2067.

94. Nagele H, Doring V, Kalmar P, et al. Long-term hemodynamic benefit of atrial synchronization with A2A2D or A2A2T pacing in sinus node syndrome after orthotopic heart transplantation. *J Heart Lung Transplant* 1998;17:906–912.

95. Woodard DA, Conti JB, Mills RMJ, et al. Permanent atrial pacing in cardiac transplant patients. *Pacing Clin Electrophysiol* 1997;20:2398–2404.

96. Woodard DA, Conti JB, Curtis AB. Oversensing of atrial flutter in the recipient atrium of a heart transplant patient with a permanent atrial pacemaker. *Clin Cardiol* 1996;19:597–598.

97. Little RE, Kay GN, Epstein AE, et al. Arrhythmias after orthotopic cardiac transplantation: prevalence and determinants during initial hospitalization and late follow-up. *Circulation* 1989; 80[Suppl III]:140–146.

98. Scott CD, Dark JH, McComb JM. Arrhythmias after cardiac transplantation. *Am J Cardiol* 1992;70:1061–1063.

99. Romhilt DW, Doyle M, Sagar KB, et al. Prevalence and significance of arrhythmias in long-term survivors of cardiac transplantation. *Circulation* 1982;66[Suppl I]:219–222.

100. Pavri BB, O'Nunain SS, Newell JB, et al. Prevalence and prognostic significance of atrial arrhythmias after orthotopic cardiac transplantation. *J Am Coll Cardiol* 1995;25:1673–1680.

101. Macdonald P, Hackworthy R, Keogh A, et al. Atrial overdrive pacing for reversion of atrial flutter after heart transplantation. *J Heart Lung Transplant* 1991;10:731–737.

102. Schroeder JS, Gao SZ, Alderman EL, et al. A preliminary study of diltiazem in the prevention of coronary artery disease in heart-transplant recipients. *N Engl J Med* 1993;328:164–170.

103. Kaufman LJ, Kofalvi AE, Hong RA, et al. Cardioversion of atrial fibrillation with ibutilide in an orthotopic heart transplant patient [Review]. *J Heart Lung Transplant* 1999;18:1018–1020.

104. Gao SZ, Schroeder JS, Alderman EL, et al. Prevalence of accelerated coronary artery disease in heart transplant survivors: comparison of cyclosporine and azathioprine regimens. *Circulation* 1989;80[Suppl II]:100–105.

105. Gao SZ, Schroeder JS, Hunt SA, et al. Acute myocardial infarction in cardiac transplant recipients. *Am J Cardiol* 1989;64: 1093–1097.

106. Arenal A, Almendral J, Munoz R, et al. Mechanism and location of atrial flutter in transplanted hearts: observations during transient entrainment from distant sites. *J Am Coll Cardiol* 1997;30:539–546.

107. Li YG, Gronefeld G, Hohnloser SH. Radiofrequency catheter ablation of atrial flutter after orthotopic heart transplantation. *J Cardiovasc Electrophysiol* 1996;7:1086–1090.

108. Pitt MP, Bonser RS, Griffith MJ. Radiofrequency catheter ablation for atrial flutter following orthotopic heart transplantation. *Heart* 1998;79:412–413.

109. Pinski SL, Bredikis AJ, Winkel E, Trohman RG. Radiofrequency catheter ablation of atrial flutter after orthotopic heart transplantation: insights into the redefined critical isthmus. *J Heart Lung Transplant* 1999;18:292–296.

110. Delacretaz E, Stevenson WG, Winters GL, Friedman PL. Radiofrequency ablation of atrial flutter. *Circulation* 1999;99:E1–E2.

111. Goy JJ, Kappenberger L, Turina M. Wolff-Parkinson-White syndrome after transplantation of the heart. *Br Heart J* 1989;61: 368–371.

112. Gallay P, Albat B, Thevenet A, Grolleau R. Direct current catheter ablation of an accessory pathway in a recipient with refractory reciprocal tachycardia. *J Heart Lung Transplant* 1992; 11:442–445.

113. Neuzner J, Friedl A, Pitschner HF. Radiofrequency catheter ablation of a concealed accessory atrioventricular pathway after heart transplantation. *Pacing Clin Electrophysiol* 1994;17:1778–1781.

114. Thompson E, Steinhaus D, Long N, Borkon AM. Preexcitation syndrome in a donor heart. *J Heart Transplant* 1989;8:177–180.

115. Rothman SA, Hsia HH, Bove AA, et al. Radiofrequency ablation of Wolff-Parkinson-White syndrome in a donor heart after orthotopic heart transplantation. *J Heart Lung Transplant* 1994; 13:905–909.

116. Zhu DW, Sun H. Case report: radiofrequency catheter ablation of atrioventricular nodal reentrant tachycardia in a patient with heart transplantation. *J Interv Card Electrophysiol* 1998;2:87–89.

117. Ott P, Kelly PA, Mann DE, et al. Tachycardia-induced cardiomyopathy in a cardiac transplant recipient: treatment with radiofrequency catheter ablation. *J Cardiovasc Electrophysiol* 1995;6:391–395.

118. Hoffmann E, Reithmann C, Nimmermann P, et al. Atrial reentrant tachycardia after heart transplantation. *Circulation* 1999; 99:326–327.

119. Bexton RS, Hellestrand KJ, Cory-Pearce R, et al. Unusual atrial potentials in a cardiac transplant recipient: possible synchronization between donor and recipient atria. *J Electrocardiol* 1983;16:313–321.

120. Anselme F, Saoudi N, Redonnet M, Letac B. Atrioatrial conduction after orthotopic heart transplantation. *J Am Coll Cardiol* 1994;24:185–189.

121. Rothman SA, Miller JM, Hsia HH, Buxton AE. Radiofrequency ablation of a supraventricular tachycardia due to interatrial conduction from the recipient to donor atria in an orthotopic heart transplant recipient. *J Cardiovasc Electrophysiol* 1995;6:544–550.

122. Saoudi N, Redonnet M, Anselme F, et al. Catheter ablation of atrioatrial conduction as a cure for atrial arrhythmia after orthotopic heart transplantation. *J Am Coll Cardiol* 1998;32: 1048–1055.

123. Gasparini M, Mantica M, Lunati M, et al. Congestive heart failure induced by recipient atrial tachycardia conducted to the donor atrium after orthotopic heart transplantation: complete regression after successful radiofrequency ablation. *J Cardiovasc Electrophysiol* 1999;10:399–404.

124. Lai W, Kao A, Silka MJ, et al. Recipient to donor conduction of atrial tachycardia following orthotopic heart transplantation. *Pacing Clin Electrophysiol* 1998;21:1331–1335.

125. Lefroy DC, Fang JC, Stevenson LW, et al. Recipient-to-donor atrioatrial conduction after orthotopic heart transplantation: surface electrocardiographic features and estimated prevalence. *Am J Cardiol* 1998;82:444–450.

126. Park JK, Hsu DT, Hordof AJ, Addonizio LJ. Arrhythmias in pediatric heart transplant recipients: prevalence and association with death, coronary artery disease, and rejection. *J Heart Lung Transplant* 1993;12:956–964.

127. Alexopoulos D, Yusuf S, Bostock J, et al. Ventricular arrhythmias in long term survivors of orthotopic and heterotopic cardiac transplantation. *Br Heart J* 1988;59:648–652.

128. Clarke N, Mason M, Paul V. Radiofrequency ablation of a fascicular tachycardia after orthotopic cardiac transplantation. *Heart* 1998;79:414–416.

129. Berke DK, Graham AF, Schroeder JS, Harrison DC. Arrhythmias in the denervated transplanted human heart. *Circulation* 1973;48:113–115.

130. de Jonge N, Jambroes G, Lahpor JR, Woolley SR. Ventricular fibrillation during acute rejection after heart transplantation. *J Heart Lung Transplant* 1992;11:797–798.

131. Oldham N, Ott RA, Allen BA, et al. Ventricular fibrillation complicating endomyocardial biopsy of a cardiac allograft. *Cathet Cardiovasc Diagn* 1991;23:300–301.

132. Patel VS, Lim M, Massin EK, et al. Sudden cardiac death in cardiac transplant recipients. *Circulation* 1996;94[Suppl II]: 273–277.

133. Uretsky BF, Kormos RL, Zerbe TR, et al. Cardiac events after heart transplantation: incidence of and predictive value of coronary arteriography. *J Heart Lung Transplant* 1992;11:S45–51.

134. Grinstead WC, Smart FW, Pratt CM, et al. Sudden death caused by bradycardia and asystole in a heart transplant patient with coronary arteriography. *J Heart Lung Transplant* 1991;10:931–936.

135. Scherrer U, Vissing S, Morgan BJ, et al. Vasovagal syncope after infusion of a vasodilator in a heart-transplant recipient [See comments]. *N Engl J Med* 1990;322:602–604.

136. Rudas L, Pflugfelder PW, Kostuk WJ. Vasodepressor syncope in a cardiac transplant recipient: a case of vagal re-innervation? *Can J Cardiol* 1992;8:403–405.

137. Montebugnoli L, Montanari G. Vasovagal syncope in heart transplant patients during dental surgery. *Oral Surg Oral Med Oral Pathol Oral Radiol Endod* 1999;87:666–669.

138. Lord SW, Brady S, Baylis PH, et al. Vasopressin release during orthostatic hypotension after cardiac transplantation. *Clin Auton Res* 1996;6:351–357.

139. Billingham ME, Cary NRB, Hammond ME, et al, for the Internal Society for Heart Transplantation. A working formulation for the standardization of nomenclature in the diagnosis of heart and lung rejection: Heart Rejection Study group. *J Heart Lung Transplant* 1990;9:587–593.

140. Nealson H, Soerensen FB, Neilsen B. Reproducibility of acute rejection diagnosis in human cardiac allograft: the Stanford Classification of the International Grading System. *J Heart Lung Transplant* 1993;12:239–243.

141. Nakhleh RE, Jones J, Goswitz JJ. Correlation of endomyocardial biopsy findings with autopsy findings in human cardiac allografts. *J Heart Lung Transplant* 1992;11:479–485.

142. Oyer PE, Stinson EB, Bieber CP, et al. Diagnosis and treatment of acute cardiac allograft rejection. *Transplant Proc* 1979;11:296–303.

143. Warnecke H, Muller J, Cohnert T, et al. Clinical heart transplantation without routine endomyocardial biopsy. *J Heart Lung Transplant* 1992;11:1093–1102.

144. Auer T, Schreier G, Hutten H, et al. Paced epimyocardial electrograms for noninvasive rejection monitoring after heart transplantation. *J Heart Lung Transplant* 1996;15:993–998.

145. Iberer F, Grasser B, Schreier G, et al. Introducing a new clinical method for noninvasive rejection monitoring after heart transplantation to clinical practice analysis of intramyocardial electrograms. *Transplant Proc* 1998;30:895–899.

146. Grasser B, Schreier G, Iberer F, et al. Noninvasive monitoring of rejection therapy based intramyocardial electrograms after orthotopic heart transplantation. *Transplant Proc* 1996;28:3276–3277.

147. Eisen HJ, Bourge R, Hershberger R, et al. Noninvasive rejection monitoring of heart transplants using high resolution pacemaker telemetry-initial us multicenter results. *Pacing Clin Electrophysiol* 1998;21:814.

33

SYNCOPE: PATHOPHYSIOLOGY, EVALUATION, AND TREATMENT

DAVID G. BENDITT

Syncope is best considered as a syndrome, the principal features of which are relatively abrupt loss of consciousness and postural tone with subsequent spontaneous recovery. Presyncope or near syncope are conditions in which the individual experiences a sense that true syncope is imminent, but it does not fully materialize. In these latter instances, patients may describe their symptoms using nonspecific terms such as *lightheaded spells* or *dizziness*. As a rule, syncope and presyncope are alarming symptoms for patients, and they often trigger a request for medical consultation.

The causes of syncope and presyncopal symptoms are numerous and in many individuals are multifactorial. Recently, considerable attention has been focused on improving understanding of the pathophysiology of syncope, identifying contributing factors, and developing an organized approach to its diagnostic evaluation and treatment. This chapter summarizes the progress made in these areas.

EPIDEMIOLOGY AND PROGNOSIS

Syncope is an important cause of morbidity in almost all age groups. The Framingham Study data, based on 26 years of follow-up in 2,336 men and 2,873 women, suggests that approximately 3% of the population experience syncope during their lifetime (1). The incidence may even be higher, reportedly up to 37%, if a young population of individuals is examined (2). Additionally, in the same Framingham Study, syncope in the absence of evident cardiac or neurologic findings (so-called *isolated syncope*) accounted for 79% and 88% of episodes in men and women, respectively. The

latter finding suggests that in a general population, the neurally mediated reflex syncopal syndromes (particularly the vasovagal faint) and disturbances of orthostatic blood pressure control (including idiopathic orthostatic hypotension and drug-induced orthostasis) are probably the predominant causes of syncope. Further, given an initial syncopal event, recurrence of symptoms can be expected in about 30% of cases (1–5).

Studies examining the impact of syncope on the health care system are generally in need of updating. Nevertheless, it has been estimated that syncope accounts for approximately 3% of emergency department visits and from 1% to 6% of general hospital admissions in the United States (6–8). In the case of patients admitted to the hospital, most probably have or are suspected of having clinically significant underlying structural heart or cardiovascular disease. However, in a broader population of individuals in the community, this is not the case. As noted earlier, isolated syncope (i.e., syncope without cardiac or neurologic findings) accounted for most fainting episodes in the Framingham Study (1). Among these individuals, the first syncope occurred at an average age of 52 years (range, 17 to 78 years) for men and 50 years (range, 13 to 87 years) for women. Further, the prevalence of isolated syncope increased with advancing age; the range increased from 8 per 1,000 person examinations in the 35- to 44-year-old age group to approximately 40 per 1,000 person examinations in the older than 75 years age group (Fig. 33-1). Among elderly patients confined to long-term care institutions, the annual incidence may be as high as 6%, with 30% recurrence rates (9,10).

Recently, there has been increased interest in the possibility that syncope may account for an important fraction of unexplained falls, particularly in older individuals. In particular, in this setting, syncope may result in physical injury, loss of employment or avocation, loss of driving privilege, and possibly a need for premature placement in a long-term care institution. In the end, older syncope patients are at considerable risk of loss of an independent lifestyle.

D. G. Benditt: Cardiovascular Division, Department of Medicine, University of Minnesota Medical School, Minneapolis, Minnesota 55455.

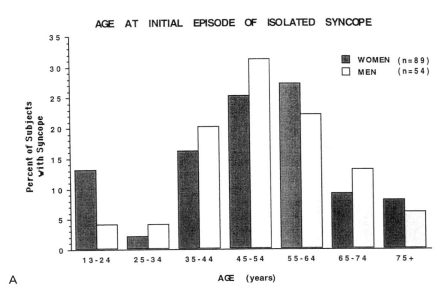

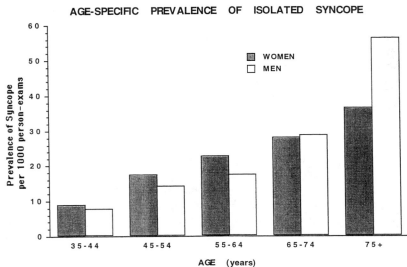

FIGURE 33-1. Graph depicting the age at initial episode **(A)** and age-specific prevalence of isolated syncopal events. These findings, obtained after 26 years of follow-up in the Framingham Study, illustrate that syncope in the absence of overt structural or neurologic disease occurs in all **(A)** age groups, although there is a particular predilection in **(B)** older individuals (From Savage DD, Corwin L, McGee DL, et al. Epidemiologic features of isolated syncope: the Framingham Study. *Stroke* 1985;16:626–629, with permission.)

Assessment of the origins of syncope based on early clinical reports (including primarily history, physical examination, and basic laboratory studies) is problematic given the often limited capabilities available for substantiating suspected diagnoses. The subsequent evolution of tools for identifying structural or functional cardiovascular disease and for obtaining correlation between such findings (e.g., valvular disease and arrhythmias) and the occurrence of symptoms has been particularly valuable in the evaluation of the syncope patient. Nonetheless, in one of the earliest clinical reports, which was a retrospective review of medical records, Wayne (11) determined that in approximately one half of cases (about 500 of the 1,000

cases reviewed), no specific diagnosis could be made. Of the cases in which a diagnosis was made, vasovagal syncope accounted for almost 60% (or about 30% of all cases if one includes the "no diagnosis" group). In subsequent reports (3,5,7,8,12,13), emanating from various hospital services (emergency rooms, intensive care units, inpatients), the proportion of diagnoses has differed widely, probably reflecting the nature of the patient population examined. Thus, for example, the incidence of cardiac disease and cardiac arrhythmias as a suspected cause of syncope has varied from approximately 1% to as high as 40% in these reports (Table 33-1). On the other hand, common threads include the observations that the neurally

TABLE 33-1. CAUSES OF SYNCOPE: BASIC CLINICAL EVALUATION

Cause	Pooled (1980s)	Kapoo (1990) (6)	Wayne (1961) (11)
Neurally Mediated			
VVS	8–37	16	30
CSS	0–4	1.2	1.5
Other	1–8	0	3
Orthostatic/dysautonomic			
Orthostatic	4–10	10	28
Drugs	1–7	2	0
Cardiac			
Arrhythmia	4–38	11	2.5
Organic heart disease	1–8	0	1.8
Cerbrovascular	0	2	2.6
Psychologic/Neurologic			
Psychologic	1–7	0	.04
Neurologic	3–32	1.5	2.8
Unknown	13–41 (34)	1	51

VVS, vasovagal syncope; CSS, carotid sinus syndrome.

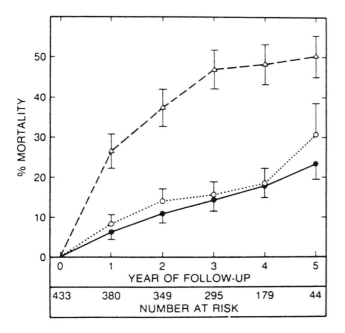

FIGURE 33-2. Graph depicting actuarial mortality rates of patients with cardiac cause of syncope (*triangles*), noncardiac cause of syncope (*unfilled circles*), and syncope of unknown cause (*filled circles*). The mortality rate in patients with a cardiac cause of syncope was significantly higher than that in patients with a noncardiac cause or patients with syncope of unknown cause. (From Kapoor W. Evaluation and outcome of patients with syncope. *Medicine* 1990;69:160–175, with permission.)

mediated faints have tended to be the most frequent causes of syncope, and "no diagnosis" has tended to remain in the range of 30% to 50% of cases.

The prognosis associated with a syncopal spell correlates primarily with the nature and severity of the underlying disease processes, particularly in terms of heart disease. In a relatively early examination of this issue, Kapoor and colleagues (3) noted that the poor outcome in patients with syncope of presumed cardiovascular origin, compared with noncardiovascular causes, was directly related to the presence of underlying structural heart and vascular disease. In a more recent update, Kapoor (6) reported a 5-year mortality rate of 50.5% among patients with a presumed cardiac cause of syncope, compared with 30% in patients believed to have a noncardiac cause and 24% among patients in whom the basis of syncope remained unknown (Fig. 33-2). The corresponding sudden death percentages were 33%, 5%, and 8.5%. The critical importance of identifying the basis of syncope in patients with symptoms of cardiac origin is evidenced by the fact that many of the arrhythmias observed are now treatable with drugs or devices. Thus, among the 43 patients who died suddenly during follow-up, 28 were in the group in which syncope was of cardiac origin: ventricular tachycardia (VT), 16; other conduction system disease, 7; pulmonary events, 2; myocardial infarction, 2; and aortic dissection, 1. These observations suggest a more benign prognosis for patients with syncope in whom a structural cardiovascular cause is excluded. Nonetheless, a 5% first-year mortality rate remains a concern and has been a relatively consistent observation in the literature (14). Further, mortality aside, such patients continue to be at risk for physical injury and may encounter employment- and recreation-related restrictions, as well as life and disability insurance dilemmas.

Invasive electrophysiologic testing currently plays an important role in evaluating the basis for syncope evaluation and in clarifying prognostic issues. Regarding the former, the greatest use of electrophysiologic testing lies in identifying arrhythmic disturbances in individuals having cardiac disease (e.g., ischemic heart disease and cardiomyopathy) or structural anomalies (e.g., accessory connections). In these settings, presumably because of the preponderance of structural heart disease in syncope patients with diagnostic electrophysiologic tests, there is a higher propensity for sudden death and total mortality than in syncope patients with nondiagnostic electrophysiologic studies (Fig. 33-3) (5). On the other hand, syncope recurrence rates are roughly comparable in both groups (Fig. 33-3) (5). Consequently, aggressive pursuit of an etiologic diagnosis is warranted in all patients presenting with syncope, in an attempt to evaluate and potentially reduce mortality risk and to prevent morbidity associated with recurrent episodes.

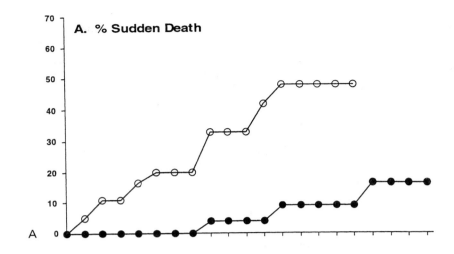

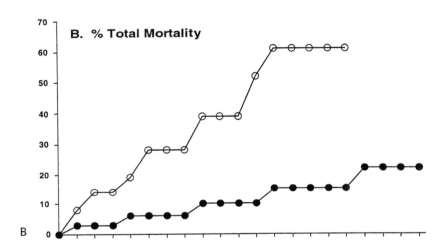

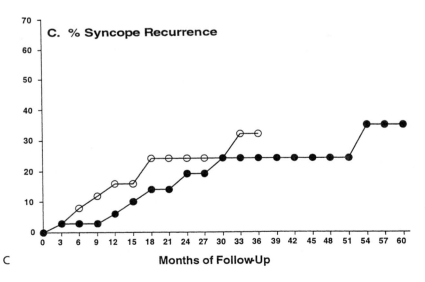

Months of Follow-Up

FIGURE 33-3. Graphs adapted from Bass and colleagues (5) depicting clinical events during follow-up in patients referred for conventional electrophysiologic (EP) study of syncope. Unfilled circles represent the subgroup of patients in whom EP testing provided a basis for syncope (EP positive), whereas filled circles represent the subgroup of patients in whom EP testing failed to provide a basis for syncope (EP negative). The percentages of patients in each subgroup exhibiting **(A)** sudden death, **(B)** total mortality, and **(C)** syncope recurrence are indicated on the ordinate, and months of follow-up are indicated on the abscissa. See text for further discussion. (Adapted from Bass EB, Elson JJ, Fogoros RN, et al. Long-term prognosis of patients undergoing electrophysiology, with permission.)

PATHOPHYSIOLOGY: GENERAL PRINCIPLES

The specific factors resulting in syncope vary from patient to patient depending on the cause of the symptoms. These factors will be discussed in conjunction with the diagnostic classification provided later in this chapter. However, a number of general principles are relevant to the development of syncope.

It has been estimated that maintenance of consciousness requires cerebral oxygen (O_2) delivery of at least 3.5 mL of O_2 per 100 g of tissue each minute (15,16). As a rule, in the healthy younger to middle-aged individual, with cerebral blood flow in the range of 50 to 60 mL per minute per 100 g of tissue, O_2 requirements are usually easily achieved. However, the integrity of a number of important cerebrovascular circulatory control mechanisms is crucial for maintaining adequate cerebral nutrient delivery, including the following:

1. "autoregulatory" features permit cerebral blood flow to be maintained over a relatively wide range of perfusion pressures (16);
2. chemoresponsiveness permits cerebral vasodilation to occur in the presence of either diminished P_{O_2} or elevated P_{CO_2};
3. baroreceptor-induced adjustments of heart rate and systemic vascular resistance, which allow changes in systemic circulatory dynamics in an attempt to protect cerebral flow;
4. vascular volume regulation in which renal and hormonal influences help to maintain central volume and venous return to the heart, thereby diminishing syncope risk.

Transient failure of protective mechanisms or the intervention of other factors (e.g., drugs and hemorrhage) that reduce central systemic pressure below the autoregulatory range for 8 to 10 seconds or longer may induce a syncopal episode. In this setting, syncope risk is even greater in older or ill patients in whom crucial compensatory mechanisms may be compromised. Aging alone has been associated with substantial diminution of cerebral blood flow (17,18). At the same time, neural mechanisms needed to trigger compensatory mechanisms may be less effective in the older patient. For instance, in elderly individuals, carotid baroreceptor responsiveness may be functionally less reliable (19–21). Thus, compensatory heart rate and vascular changes may be inadequate to adjust for even transient hemodynamic disturbances such as abrupt postural change, cough, straining, or dehydration. Additionally, certain common disease states may diminish protection usually accorded cerebral blood flow. For example, hypertension has been associated with a shift of the autoregulatory range to higher pressures (22), whereas diabetes alters the chemoresponsiveness of the cerebrovascular bed (23). Similarly, other chronic disease states such as congestive heart failure, peripheral or cerebrovascular disease, or venous insufficiency may substantially increase the risk of syncope. These and other concomitant disease conditions are common among older syncope patients (9,10,12,24).

DIFFERENTIAL DIAGNOSTIC CONSIDERATIONS

A number of studies have delineated the multiple potential causes of syncope in various settings (Table 33-2). However, application of these findings to medical practice is limited by the nature of the environment in which patients were enrolled and the variable manner in which symptoms were evaluated. In one report from an important ongoing study of syncope patients, Kapoor (6) summarized observations in 433 syncope patients initially enrolled between April 1981 and February 1984. Evaluation of these patients included history, physical, and neurologic examination, hematologic and biochemical studies, 12-lead electrocar-

TABLE 33-2. LOSS OF CONCIOUSNESS: DIAGNOSTIC CLASSIFICATION

Neurally mediated (neurocardiogenic) reflex syncopal syndromes
  Vasovagal faint
  Carotid sinus syncope
  Cough syncope and related disorders
  Gastrointestinal, pelvic, or urologic origin
Orthostatic, dysautonomic, and drug-induced
  Blood/plasma loss (hemorrhage, diarrhea, Addison disease, pheochromocytoma)
  Idiopathic orthostatic hypotension
  Primary autonomic failure syndromes (acute pure dysautonomia, pure autonomic failure, multiple system atrophy, Parkinson disease with autonomic failure)
  Secondary autonomic failure syndromes (diabetic neuropathy, amyloid neuropathy)
  Drug-induced orthostasis
Primary cardiac arrhythmias
  Sinus node dysfunction (including bradycardia-tachycardia syndrome)
  Atrioventricular conduction system disease
  Paroxysmal supraventricular and ventricular tachycardias
  Implanted device (pacemaker, implantable cardioverter-defibrillator) malfunction
Structural cardiac or cardiopulmonary disease
  Cardiac valvular disease/ischemia
  Acute myocardial infarction
  Obstructive cardiomyopathy
  Pericardial disease/tamponade
  Pulmonary embolus
  Pulmonary hypertension
Cerebrovascular, neurologic
  Vascular steal syndromes (including "subclavian steal" syndrome)
  Seizure disorders
Miscellaneous syncope-like conditions
  Psychiatric disturbances
    Panic attacks
    Hysteria
    Somatization
    Generalized anxiety
  Metabolic and others
    Hyperventilation (hypocapnia)
    Hypoglycemia
    Hypoxemia

diogram (ECG), and a minimum of 24 hours of ambulatory ECG monitoring. Further studies, including angiography, electroencephalogram, and computer tomographic scans, were obtained when clinically warranted. Electrophysiologic testing was only used for a portion of the time encompassed by this report and was performed in relatively few patients. Head-up tilt testing was not available.

Among the patients reported by Kapoor (6), a cause of syncope was assigned in 254 of 433 patients, with a cardiovascular cause being responsible in most cases. The most common causes of syncope were neurally mediated (vasodepressor) syncopal syndromes (71 patients), VT (49 patients), orthostatic hypotension (43 patients), and drug-induced syncope (9 patients). Carotid sinus syncope was identified in only 5 of 254 patients (2%) and seizure disorders only in 7 of 254 patients (3%). Vascular disease compromising cerebral blood flow accounted for 10 cases of 254 (4%), of whom, 2 patients were diagnosed as having subclavian steal syndrome.

History and physical examination were considered the most useful means for assessing a "cause" of syncope (140 of 254 patients, or 55%), whereas the ECG and ECG monitoring (30 and 54 patients, respectively) were the next most valuable tools (Fig. 33-4). Of importance, neurologic studies were of diagnostic use in only 4 of 254 patients, whereas computed tomographic scans were not reported to be of diagnostic use in any patient.

Important limitations of Kapoor's analysis include the fact that the specificity of a diagnosis based solely on the history and physical examination is uncertain at best. Further, even in experienced hands, there was a disturbing inability to characterize a basis for syncope in a substantial percentage of patients (179 of 433, or 41%). This latter finding is consistent with that of many other reports (Table 33-1). Consequently, although history and physical examination are crucial steps in the syncope evaluation, judicious but directed and aggressive use of available laboratory testing techniques (particularly tilt table tests and electrophysiologic studies) is essential (Fig. 33-4). The ultimate goal is to optimize chances of obtaining a sufficiently certain diagnosis to permit a confident statement regarding prognosis and appropriate therapy.

The findings reported by Kapoor (6) are consistent with what should be expected in general patient populations. Consequently, given the previously noted caveats, these observations are important for physicians in emergency rooms and general medical and cardiology practice. By contrast, syncope patients reported from electrophysiology laboratories are more highly selected and usually comprise a high proportion of older patients with structural cardiovascular disease, who in turn tend to exhibit a higher incidence of conduction system disease and ventricular and supraventricular arrhythmias as the cause of syncope. This selection bias is particularly relevant to the interpretation of reports in which electrophysiologic testing was conducted without benefit of tilt table study.

In older patients, the predominant referral population for conventional electrophysiologic testing, VT has been the most commonly identified basis for syncope, although supraventricular tachyarrhythmias (SVTs), conduction sys-

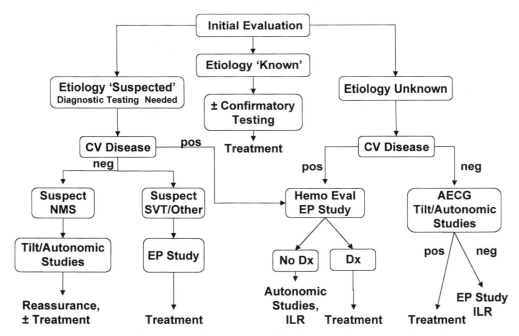

FIGURE 33-4. Schematic depicting a strategy for evaluation of patients presenting with syncope. The initial evaluation includes a detailed medical history, physical examination, 12-lead electrocardiogram, and an echocardiogram if deemed appropriate.

tem disease, and sinoatrial dysfunction are also reported (5,25–33). Nonetheless, more recent studies suggest that within this patient population, and in the younger patient, neurally mediated syncope represents an important diagnostic consideration (24,34). As a rule, the syncope patient with evident structural cardiac disease should undergo a conventional electrophysiologic study first, and if the finding are not diagnostic, then a tilt table test and related studies of autonomic nervous system function (e.g., carotid sinus massage and baroreceptor sensitivity) are warranted (Fig. 33-4). The reverse strategy would be appropriate in the individual with no evidence of structural cardiovascular disease.

CLASSIFICATION OF THE CAUSES OF SYNCOPE AND THEIR EVALUATION

Classifications of the causes of syncope have often focused on two broad categories: cardiovascular and noncardiovascular disorders (with the cardiovascular category sometimes including the neurally mediated syncope disorders, but not always). Unfortunately, however, the use of such a simple classification system is diminished because most syncope episodes fall into the cardiovascular class. Further, within such a broad cardiovascular category, there is a wide range of pathophysiologies and prognoses. For example, current concepts suggest that syncope associated with valvular aortic stenosis is not only the result of reduced forward flow (i.e., diminished cardiac output), but perhaps more importantly a reflection of neural reflex effects (particularly inappropriate vasodilation in the setting of a restricted ability to increase forward flow) (35–37). Finally, the conditions encompassed within such a broad class have quite different implications. The prognosis associated with aortic stenosis and syncope is much more worrisome than that of most other forms of neurally mediated syncope.

In an attempt to avoid some of the liabilities associated with the conventional clinical classification of syncope, clinical conditions associated with syncope are here divided into six major diagnostic categories:

1. neurally mediated reflex disturbances of blood pressure control
2. orthostatic and dysautonomic disturbances of blood pressure control
3. primary cardiac arrhythmias
4. structural cardiovascular and cardiopulmonary disease
5. cerebrovascular and neurologic origin
6. noncardiovascular disorders

Neurally Mediated Reflex Disturbances of Blood Pressure Control

Pathophysiology

Neurally mediated disturbances of blood pressure control (Table 33-2), particularly the vasovagal faint, are the most

common causes of syncope (38–41). From a pathophysiologic perspective, the various conditions within this group exhibit a number of common features. Differences are primarily the result of the "trigger factors" associated with each of the specific conditions and possibly the manner in which the central nervous system receives and processes afferent (incoming) neural signals generated by these triggers (Fig. 33-5). In general, the afferent neural signals, which initiate these forms of syncope, may originate directly from the central nervous system or may be derived from various peripheral "receptors" that respond to mechanical or chemical stimuli, pain, or possibly even temperature change. The former is exemplified by faints after exposure to noxious smells, unpleasant sights or thoughts, or pain. The latter encompasses syncope associated with venipuncture, prolonged exposure to upright posture, heat, dehydration, and physical exertion. Other peripheral triggers include carotid sinus stimulation, gastrointestinal or genitourinary stimulation, coughing, sneezing, and other forms of airway irritation (40,41). Emotional state and hydration status may play important contributory roles in determining susceptibility to fainting at a given point in time.

In the case of carotid sinus syndrome, carotid artery mechanoreceptors (baroreceptors) have been presumed to be the principal origin of the afferent neural signals triggering the event (40–45). However, recent research suggests that the problem is more complex, with discordance of afferent signals from the carotid baroreceptors and nearby neck muscle proprioceptor sites being the source of the problem in many cases. Potentially, discordance of afferent signals from multiple origins may be important in other forms of neurally mediated syncope.

In certain forms of neurally mediated syncope, cardiac receptor sites of various types are believed to be responsible for triggering the faint. For example, mechanoreceptors and to some extent chemoreceptors located in atrial and ventricular myocardium normally provide an important stream of afferent neural signals that play a crucial role in central nervous system regulation of heart rate and vascular tone. However, at certain times and in certain as yet poorly understood situations, the efferent responses to these afferent signals are seemingly inappropriate, possibly resulting in undesirable consequences. Thus, in aortic stenosis, severe hemorrhage or dehydration, or myocardial ischemia, the central nervous system efferent response may initiate hemodynamic instability resulting from excessive bradycardia and vasodilation. Possibly other factors, such as the status of other central nervous system activity or discordance of signals from multiple peripheral sites, are required to set the stage for symptomatic hypotension.

Cardiac receptor sites are not the sole source of afferent signals capable of provoking vasodepressor syncope in subjects susceptible to the "emotional" or "vasovagal" faint. Evidence for this comes from the observation that vasovagal syncope can occur in heart transplant patients in whom

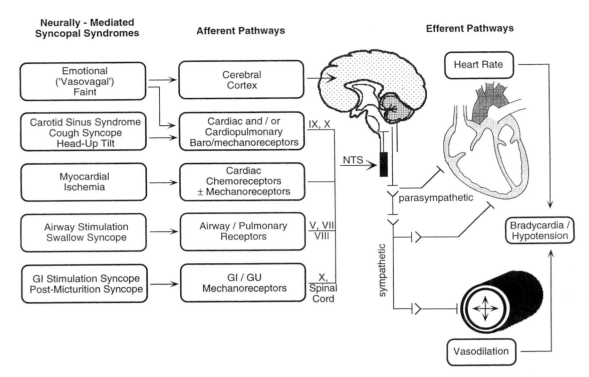

FIGURE 33-5. Schematic illustration depicting present concepts regarding the mechanisms of the neurally mediated syncopal syndromes. The principal neurally mediated syncopal syndromes are indicated at left. Currently suspected peripheral receptors ("triggers") and afferent neural pathways are also depicted. Efferent neural pathways are at the right. (NTS, nucleus tractus solitarius.) See text for discussion.

ventricular and atrial mechanoreceptors were presumably decentralized (46). It now seems clear that peripheral receptors of multiple types in various organ systems may participate in initiating symptomatic episodes.

The ultimate cause of loss of consciousness in most cases of neurally mediated syncope is transient diminution of cerebrovascular perfusion pressure, resulting in inadequacy of global cerebral nutrient supply. However, the electrophysiologic and hemodynamic picture responsible for this disturbance varies considerably from individual to individual. Certain fainters exhibit a predominantly cardioinhibitory picture, in which severe bradycardia, or even asystole, is the proximate cause of the faint. A few fainters exhibit a pure vasodepressor syndrome. Most, however, present a mixed vasodepressor and cardioinhibitory response (47–49) (Table 33-3), but it is the vasodepressor element that is generally the more crucial in these cases. The bradycardia is primarily of parasympathetic origin, and even if reversed by atropine (or pacing), substantial hypotension persists. The vasodepressor element, on the other hand, is thought to be predominantly the result of abrupt peripheral sympathetic neural withdrawal with consequent inappropriate peripheral vascular dilation (50,51). Potentially, excess β-adrenergic influence on vascular tone also contributes to the vasodepressor phenomenon. Markedly ele-

TABLE 33-3. HEART RATE AND HEMODYNAMIC RESPONSES TO HEAD-UP TILT-TABLE TESTING[a]

Type 1: Mixed
  Heart rate rises initially then falls, but the ventricular rate does not fall to less than 40 bpm or falls to 40 bpm for less than 10 s with or without asystole for less than 3 s.
  Blood pressure rises initially then falls before heart rate falls.
Type 2A: Cardioinhibitory
  Heart rate rises initially then falls to a ventricular rate of less than 40 bpm for more than 10 s or asystole occurs for more than 3 s.
  Blood pressure rises initially then falls before heart rate falls.
Type 2B: Cardioinhibitory
  Heart rate rises initially then falls to a ventricular rate less than 40 bpm for more than 10 s or asystole occurs for more than 3 s.
  Blood pressure rises initially and only falls to hypertensive levels of less than 80 mm Hg systolic at or after onset of rapid and severe heart rate fall.
Type 3: Pure Vasodepressor
  Heart rate rises progressively and does not fall more than 10% from peak at time of syncope.
  Blood pressure falls to cause syncope.

[a]Based on initial proposal of a recently formed international study group (VASIS, VasoVagal International Study). Exceptions proposed by the study group are not incorporated into this Table. Future modifications to this classification should be expected. (From Sutton R, Petersen M, Brignole M, et al. Proposed classification for tilt induced vasovagal syncope. *Eur J Cardiac Pacing Electrophysiol* 1992;2:180–183, with permission.)

vated circulating epinephrine levels are well known to occur during the evolution of certain types of neurally mediated syncope, particularly the vasovagal faint. Conceivably, altered epinephrine-norepinephrine balance may undermine vascular control (52,53). Finally, failure of baroreceptor feedback to compensate for the evolving hypotension is an important but poorly understood aspect of the neurally mediated hypotensive episode.

As noted earlier, the cerebral hypoperfusion associated with vasovagal episodes is believed to be primarily the result of marked central vascular hypotension. However, other factors may contribute and perhaps even be crucial in some individuals. Thus, transcranial Doppler study has raised the interesting possibility that paradoxical cerebrovascular arterial vasoconstriction may account for some faints (54). Further study of this phenomenon is needed.

Diagnostic Evaluation

The diagnosis of most forms of the neurally mediated faint relies on carefully taking medical history, particularly information provided by witnesses. Thus, recognition that symptoms occurred in conjunction with cough (so-called cough syncope), after voiding (postmicturition syncope), or during gastrointestinal or genitourinary instrumentation is usually sufficient for making a diagnosis. Similarly, in the case of carotid sinus syndrome or vasovagal faint, a classic history in an otherwise well individual is often enough to be confident of the diagnosis. However, in many instances, the history is not clear and further testing is needed.

In the case of carotid sinus syndrome, demonstration of an asystolic pause of more than 5 seconds when the carotid sinus is subjected to moderate pressure, linear massage is usually considered diagnostic. However, the validity of this diagnostic criterion alone is uncertain. Reproduction of symptoms, such as by undertaking carotid massage with the patient in the upright posture secured to a tilt table while monitoring both the ECG and the arterial blood pressure, is desirable. In regard to vasovagal syncope, head-up tilt testing has evolved into a valuable laboratory diagnostic tool (41,45,49,55–61). In addition (a) the patient obtains confidence that the physician has witnessed the symptoms and is thereby better equipped to provide prognostic and treatment advice, (b) the patient may learn to recognize warning symptoms to take evasive action in the future, and (c) although somewhat controversial, tilt table testing may be helpful in assessing effectiveness of therapy.

As a diagnostic tool, tilt table testing discriminates well between symptomatic vasovagal syncope patients and asymptomatic control subjects. Most studies suggest that tilt table testing at angles of 60 to 70 degrees, in the absence of pharmacologic provocation, exhibits a specificity of approximately 90%. In the presence of pharmacologic provocation, test specificity may be reduced, but the magnitude of this reduction seems to be small, particularly in the case of low-

dose isoproterenol infusion (61). Other provocative agents (e.g., nitroglycerin, edrophonium, and adenosine) have yet to be thoroughly studied in this regard (61a,61b). Tilt testing sensitivity is more difficult to quantitate than its specificity given the absence of an alternative gold standard for comparison. Nonetheless, tilt table testing appears to be useful for identifying a subset of patients with syncope with apparent susceptibility to neurally mediated syncope.

As is true of many evolving procedures in medicine, the methodology of tilt table testing has exhibited substantial variations from report to report. However, recently an Expert Consensus Report from the American College of Cardiology summarized a desirable tilt table testing methodology for practitioners (62). In essence, the laboratory should be quiet and comfortable, the patient should rest in the supine position for 30 to 45 minutes before beginning the test, and care should be taken to provide fluid replenishment in patients who have been fasting overnight. Three or more simultaneous ECG leads should be recorded continuously, and beat-to-beat blood pressure recordings using the least intrusive method possible should also be recorded. The patient should be gently secured to prevent falling, and footboard support should be provided. Tilt angles in the 70-degree range are recommended with a maximum tilt test duration of 45 minutes. Pharmacologic provocation (e.g., isoproterenol, edrophonium, nitroglycerin) remains a secondary step to be used for eliciting susceptibility to hypotension bradycardia during head-up tilt testing when the baseline drug-free tilt has been nondiagnostic.

Orthostatic and Dysautonomic Disturbances of Vascular Control (Including Drug Effects)

Pathophysiology

Presyncopal or syncopal symptoms associated with abrupt assumption of upright posture are extremely common. All age groups appear to exhibit susceptibility to this phenomenon. However, the elderly, less physically fit, or otherwise dehydrated or volume-depleted individual is at greatest risk for frank syncope in this setting. Iatrogenic factors such as excessive diuresis or overly aggressive use of certain antihypertensive agents are important contributors.

In the older or infirm patient, environmental factors (e.g., excessive heat), impaired mobility, and a reduced appetite may aggravate susceptibility to orthostatic hypotension by reducing circulating fluid volume and diminishing fitness level. The latter, in particular, has an adverse impact on ability to vasoconstrict and venoconstrict promptly in the setting of gravitational stress. Additionally, chronotropic incompetence may contribute to the problem by preventing appropriate compensatory heart rate changes with upright posture. Furthermore, in some cases, abrupt diminution of central volume with upright posture may trigger neural reflexes comparable to those described for neurally mediated syncope. The consequent vasodilation and relative bradycardia may then additionally complicate the pathophysiology of the orthostatic syncopal event. In certain cases, the coincidence of neurally mediated and intrinsic electrophysiologic disturbances (e.g., sinus node dysfunction) appear to have been implicated in syncope occurrences (58,63).

Primary autonomic nervous system dysfunction, such as multiple system atrophy (formerly Shy-Drager syndrome) may lead to disturbances of vascular control (40,55,64). These are, however, relatively rare. More commonly, disturbances of autonomic vascular control are secondary in nature (e.g., neuropathies of alcohol or diabetic origin, spinal cord lesions, or paraneoplastic syndromes). Additionally, and even more frequently, a wide range of commonly used vasoactive drugs or sedatives may impair normal neural reflex compensation and increase susceptibility to symptomatic orthostasis. For example, angiotensin-converting enzyme inhibitors and other vasodilators may prevent adequate vasoconstriction in the setting of movement to upright posture. β-Adrenergic blocking drugs or other sympatholytic antihypertensive agents may preclude appropriate heart rate response to gravitational stress.

Diagnostic Evaluation

Medical history, with particular emphasis on concomitant diseases and drug therapy, remains the principal diagnostic tool. However, with increasing recognition of primary autonomic dysfunction as a cause for syncope, autonomic system evaluation (including but not restricted to tilt table testing) becomes an important element in the diagnosis. Expert neurologic consultation may be needed in such cases.

Primary Cardiac Arrhythmias

Pathophysiology

Primary cardiac arrhythmias encompass those rhythm disturbances associated with intrinsic cardiac disease, accessory conduction pathways, or other structural abnormalities (e.g. postoperative disturbances). Intrinsic sinus node dysfunction (bradyarrhythmias and tachyarrhythmias), atrioventricular (AV) conduction system disturbances, and SVTs and VTs are included; VT is a more common cause than SVT.

The basis of syncope in the setting of a cardiac arrhythmia may seem evident in some cases, such as in conjunction with an extended asystolic spell or a very rapid nonsustained ventricular tachyarrhythmia. However, in many other instances, it is less clear-cut. Thus, certain patients may faint in association with onset of paroxysmal SVT or atrial fibrillation whereas others do not. Heart rate and ventricular function do not necessarily distinguish the fainter and the nonfainter. In this regard, the speed and effectiveness of autonomically mediated vasoconstriction appears to be an important contributing factor (58,63).

Diagnostic Evaluation

In general, among patients with clinically significant structural heart disease, primary cardiac arrhythmias are probably the most common cause of syncope. Thus, a careful physical examination and use of selected studies (particularly echocardiography and occasionally radionuclide scanning) is an important first step in determining the likelihood of a primary arrhythmic cause for syncope. Subsequently, other studies may be appropriately selected in an attempt to ascertain a basis for symptoms. These studies may include ambulatory ECG (including Holter-type monitors, external event recorders, and implantable loop recorders), exercise testing, signal-average ECG (SAECG), electrophysiology testing, and tilt table testing.

Ambulatory Electrocardiography

The use of conventional 24- to 48-hour ambulatory ECG monitors or patient-activated ECG recorders has limited effectiveness in the syncope evaluation. Clearly, if symptoms occur during such a recording session, the arrhythmic basis may be unequivocally documented. However, the pathophysiology of the arrhythmia may remain unclear (e.g., sinus bradycardia caused by intrinsic sinoatrial disease versus a neurally mediated reflex phenomenon). Furthermore, clinical experience suggests that the productivity of this approach is marginal. For example, Gibson and Heitzman (65) reported a diagnostic finding in only 2% of more than 1,500 24-hour ambulatory ECG recordings in patients being assessed for syncope. In Kapoor's assessment of his experience (6), conventional Holter-type ECG monitoring was carried out in 249 patients in whom an initial tentative basis for syncope was not available. Of these patients, only seven developed syncope during monitoring and two of these had normal sinus rhythm at the time; the other diagnoses included VT, sinus pause, and heart block—each in one patient and sinus bradycardia in two patients. Although 54 other patients were interpreted to have had a diagnostic finding, the specificity of these observations remains arguable. Consequently, the overall use of conventional Holter-type monitoring in this setting was only 7 of 249 (3%).

For many years, it has been recognized that symptomatic periods do not occur during ambulatory ECG recordings, and even when symptoms do occur, there is often no clear-cut associated abnormal rhythm (66,67). Recently, an American College of Cardiology and the American Health Association Guidelines Committee reviewed findings in 2,612 patients with syncope in whom ambulatory ECG was used as part of the diagnostic evaluation (67). Symptoms occurred during monitoring in 19% of cases, but only 112 of 2,612 (4%) had a documented arrhythmia. Conversely, although 79% of patients were asymptomatic during the recording period, 369 of the 2,612 (14%) exhibited arrhythmias. Consequently, from a cost-effectiveness perspective, conventional Holter-type ambulatory ECG has limited use in the syncope evaluation. However, the economics can be improved by only reviewing tapes associated with symptomatic episodes. Ambulatory ECG tapes unassociated with symptoms are simply recycled without review.

Event recorders have become of increasing importance in the syncope evaluation. These devices can be made available to the patient for longer periods of time than can a conventional Holter recorder (67b). When appropriate, they can be used in a continuous loop mode to record transient symptomatic arrhythmias.

The most recent innovation in ambulatory ECG is the development of a small implantable electronic ECG recording device (implantable loop recorder; Reveal, Medtronic, Inc, Minneapolis, MN) with memory and telemetry capability (68). The current device is about the size of a small rectangular box of matches and has two sensing electrodes spaced approximately 32 mm apart on its shell. Battery capacity permits the patient to make intermittent symptom recordings for approximately 18 months. Currently, an external patient-operated module is used to trigger the implantable loop recorder to save a symptomatic episode in memory. The device can be programmed to retain for later review an extended period of recording time before the trigger event, thereby possibly recording onset of the symptom episode. Records are accessed by conventional telemetry techniques, comparable to those used by standard pacemakers. The next generation of this device is in clinical trials and incorporates certain automatic recording triggers (for tachycardias and bradycardias), as well as using the external patient-trigger module.

Results from centers specializing in the evaluation of syncope suggest that the implantable loop recorder is applicable in about 5% to 10% of a selected referred syncope population (68,69). These individuals have generally undergone detailed evaluation for syncope, but a satisfactory diagnosis has not been obtained. Preliminary findings suggest that arrhythmias (bradycardias and tachycardias) are ultimately identified in about 40% of cases, whereas another 40% are found to have nonarrhythmic syncope and 20% have no documented syncope recurrences.

Apart from difficulty obtaining a diagnostic finding during ambulatory ECG monitoring, the patient remains exposed to the hazards of recurrent symptoms. Further, nonspecific findings (e.g., sinus rhythm during syncope) are common because of the absence of corroborative data such as blood pressure recording. Ultimately, easy-to-use monitors, capable of monitoring multiple hemodynamic parameters simultaneously, will need to be developed.

Exercise Testing

In the evaluation of patients with syncope, exercise testing is largely restricted to those cases in which history suggests that exertion is associated with spontaneous symptoms. Apart from the potential for identification of underlying ischemic heart disease (with hypotension secondary to ischemia or aggravation of left ventricular dysfunction), such testing may detect chronotropic incompetence, rate-dependent AV block, or the exertional variant of neurally mediated syncope (41,70–72). On certain occasions, exercise may induce tachyarrhythmias, thereby providing a basis for syncope.

Exercise testing is not particularly cost-effective in assessment of syncope. Among the 433 patient evaluations reported by Kapoor (6), stress tests were only useful in 2 cases (1 SVT and 1 nonsustained VT).

Signal-Average Electrocardiogram

In patients referred for electrophysiologic testing for syncope, the SAECG has been used to assess susceptibility to inducible VT. The correlation of positive SAECG results with inducible VT has been high in ischemic heart disease settings, but more variable in other conditions (73–75). For example, among 136 patients with syncope, Kuchar and colleagues (73) found positive SAECG results in 29 (21%), and 22 of 29 patients had inducible VT in the laboratory. The reported sensitivity of the test was 73%, with a specificity of 89%. Overall, the positive predictive accuracy of the SAECG is inadequate in syncope. However, the negative predictive accuracy is quite high. Consequently, normal SAECG results may be useful in diminishing the priority accorded electrophysiologic testing for VT in a given patient.

Specific Arrhythmic Conditions and Clinical Electrophysiologic Testing

Intrinsic sinus node dysfunction is most common in older patients but may be observed in younger individuals. However, even when present, its role in causing syncope may not be easily proven. Furthermore, because symptoms associated with sinus node dysfunction may be caused by tachyarrhythmias or bradyarrhythmias, a thorough evaluation of each patient is essential before embarking on a course of treatment (76). Currently, ECG documentation of a symptomatic event remains the only definitive way of invoking sinus node dysfunction as a cause of syncope. However, this is rarely accomplished. A somewhat lower level of diagnostic certainty is achievable with documentation of spontaneous pauses lasting more than 3.5 seconds. Nonetheless, this finding remains arguable (77,78). Conventional electrophysiologic testing of sinus node function is a relatively unreliable tool for attempting to correlate symptoms with evidence of abnormal sinoatrial function. Although abnormalities of sinus node recovery after periods of rapid atrial pacing, or disturbances of sinoatrial conduction time or refractory periods, may tend to support a diagnosis of sinus node dysfunction, the relationship to syncope must still be substantiated more directly. In this regard, Gann and colleagues (79) were able to show a correlation between symptoms that ultimately required a pacemaker implantation and a prolonged sinus node recovery time. Nonetheless, the findings did not exhibit a sufficiently strong positive predictive value to permit making an immediate treatment decision.

As in the case of sinus node dysfunction, establishing a causal role of AV conduction system disease in precipitating syncope may be difficult except in the most overt cases of high-grade AV block. Because cardiac conduction system disease is relatively common, particularly in the setting of underlying structural heart disease, its presence may be a nonspecific finding with respect to syncope. Consequently, in the absence of documented second- or third-degree AV block, the role of conduction system disease in the patient with syncope requires careful assessment, often including invasive electrophysiologic study. Additionally, conduction system disease tends to coexist with regional or generalized myocardial disease. Thus, these patients share the physical substrate for other arrhythmias (particularly ventricular tachyarrhythmias). Frequently ventricular tachyarrhythmias, rather than AV block, account for the syncopal symptoms (80–82).

In general, SVTs are less often implicated as causes of syncope than VTs. Nonetheless, syncope can be associated with SVT, particularly in those patients who exhibit susceptibility to neurally mediated syncope (63). In a survey of published studies incorporating patients of all ages, Camm and Lau (39) concluded that SVT accounted for only 8% of diagnoses; the ventricular tachyarrhythmias accounted for 20%.

Table 33-4 summarizes findings of several studies in which electrophysiologic testing has been employed to evaluate the basis of syncope. The close association of underlying structural heart disease with a positive diagnostic finding is evident. Other studies further confirm this impression. For example, in a retrospective analysis of the evaluation of 201 patients with syncope of unknown origin, Haissaguerre and colleagues (83) detected a probable etiologic diagnosis in 50 patients (25%). Factors associated with a positive (presumably diagnostic) electrophysiologic test included male gender, presence of underlying heart disease, evidence of underlying bundle branch block, and injury associated with the syncopal event. Similar conclusions can be derived from the report by Gossinger and colleagues (84), which incorporated findings from 108 patients undergoing electrophysiologic study for assessment of syncope. Positive findings correlated with asymptomatic runs of SVT on ambulatory ECG recordings, older age, more frequent episodes of syncope, organic heart disease, and male gender. Camm and Lau (39) suggest that electrophysiologic testing provides a diagnosis in 56% of all patients. However, the testing is clearly more successful in patients with (71%) than in those without (36%) evident structural cardiac disease.

It seems clear that evidence of underlying heart disease and conduction system abnormalities is associated with a greater probability that conventional electrophysiologic study will elicit an abnormal finding in the patient with syncope. However, the specificity of the finding must be carefully evaluated. For example, among 21 patients with syncope in whom documented intermittent AV block or sinus pauses were associated with symptoms, Fujimura and colleagues (85) undertook electrophysiologic testing at a time when the heart rhythm had returned to normal. Only three of eight patients with documented sinus pauses and two patients with documented AV block were found to exhibit appropriate abnormalities during electrophysiologic testing. On the other hand, other abnormalities not known to have occurred spontaneously in these individuals were often induced during study. Consequently, not only may a negative electrophysiologic study overlook an arrhythmic cause of syncope, but induction of unrelated rhythm disturbances may occur and lead to inappropriate selection of treatment. Therefore, findings during electrophysiologic studies in patients with syncope must be interpreted carefully.

Structural Cardiovascular or Cardiopulmonary Disease

Pathophysiology

Syncopal episodes resulting directly from structural abnormalities of the heart or blood vessels (excluding arrhythmias) are relatively infrequent causes of syncope, and when they do occur, the basis for the faint is often multifactorial. Thus, probably the most common cause of syncope seemingly

TABLE 33-4. ELECTROPHYSIOLOGIC TESTING IN SYNCOPE OF UNKNOWN ORIGIN

Reference	No. of patients	No. with heart disease	Overall EP positive	EP positive with heart disease	EP positive without heart disease
Akhtar and colleagues (1983) (27)	30	18	16 (53%)	15 (83%)	1 (8%)
Morady and colleagues (1983) (28)	53	38	30 (57%)	27 (71%)	3 (20%)
Teichmann and colleagues (1985) (30)	150	75	112 (75%)	64 (85%)	48 (64%)
Crozier and colleagues (1986) (32)	94	42	26 (28%)	16 (38%)	10 (20%)
Sra and colleagues (1991) (33)	86	31	29 (34%)	22 (71%)	7 (13%)
Total	413	204	213 (52%)	144 (71%)	69 (33%)

EP positive, patients in whom conventional electrophysiologic (EP) testing provided a plausible diagnostic basis for syncope.

attributable directly to left ventricular disease is that which occurs in conjunction with acute myocardial ischemia or infarction (86,87). However, in this case, the origin of syncope is complex, including not only transient reduction of cardiac output but also important neural reflex effects (including the Bezold-Jarisch reflex) and cardiac arrhythmias.

Syncope associated with aortic stenosis or hypertrophic obstructive cardiomyopathy is also relatively rare but important to recognize because of the reportedly poor prognosis (particularly in valvular aortic stenosis) if untreated. The basis for the faint is often attributed to inadequate blood flow resulting from mechanical obstruction, cardiac arrhythmias, or both. However, ventricular mechanoreceptor-mediated bradycardia and vasodilation (comparable to that alluded to previously in the section on neurally mediated syncope) is thought to play an important role (35–37). In the case of hypertrophic obstructive cardiomyopathy, neural reflex mechanisms may also play a role, but syncope may be more often related to diminished cardiac output in conjunction with abrupt onset of atrial tachyarrhythmias (particularly atrial fibrillation) or VT. McKenna and colleagues (88) reported syncope to be an important predictor of sudden death in these patients, a finding yet to be confirmed by others (89).

Other even less common conditions that may be associated with syncope include left ventricular inflow obstruction such as in patients with mitral stenosis or atrial myxoma, right ventricular outflow obstruction, right-to-left shunting secondary to pulmonic stenosis or pulmonary hypertension. In the latter case (i.e., pulmonary hypertension), neural reflex effects may contribute to symptoms.

Diagnostic Evaluation

Echocardiography rarely provides a definitive basis for syncope. Nonetheless, the echocardiogram is invaluable given the importance of identifying underlying structural heart disease in patients with syncope. Further, in some cases, the echocardiogram may provide direct clues to the cause if, for example, hypertrophic obstructive cardiomyopathy, severe valvular aortic stenosis, intracardiac tumor (e.g., myxoma), or anomalous origin of one or coronary arteries are detected. Ultrasound techniques also are appropriately employed to assess vascular disturbances detected on physical examination. Thus, assessment of the carotid and/or subclavian system may be an appropriate step in selected individuals. Other imaging modalities, such as radionuclide imaging, are reserved for specific clinical indications.

The combination of tilt table testing and invasive electrophysiologic testing has substantially enhanced diagnostic capabilities in patients with syncope. Sra and colleagues (33) reported results of electrophysiologic testing in conjunction with head-up tilt testing in 86 consecutive patients referred for evaluation of unexplained syncope. Electrophysiologic testing results were abnormal in 29 (34%) patients, with most of these (21 patients) being inducible sustained monomorphic VT. Among the remaining patients, head-up tilt testing proved positive in 34 (40%) cases, and 23 patients (26%) remained undiagnosed. In general, patients exhibiting positive electrophysiologic findings were older, were more frequently men, and exhibited lower ventricular ejection fractions and higher frequency of evident heart disease than was the case in patients with positive head-up tilt test results or patients in whom no diagnosis was determined.

In a further evaluation of the combined use of electrophysiologic testing and head-up tilt testing in assessment of syncope, Fitzpatrick and colleagues (56) analyzed findings in 322 syncope patients. Conventional electrophysiologic testing provided a basis for syncope in 229 of 322 cases (71%), with 93 patients having normal electrophysiologic study findings. Among the patients with abnormal electrophysiologic findings, AV conduction disease was diagnosed in 34%, sinus node dysfunction in 21%, carotid sinus syndrome in 10%, and an inducible sustained tachyarrhythmia in 6%. In the 93 patients with normal electrophysiologic study findings, tilt table testing was undertaken in 71 cases and reproduced syncope, consistent with a vasovagal faint, in 53 (75%) patients.

Syncope Caused by Cerebrovascular or Neurologic Disturbances

Pathophysiology

Cerebrovascular disease and vascular "steal" syndromes are rare causes of true syncope. However, transient ischemic attacks caused by vertebrobasilar disease may mimic syncope (only rarely is carotid vessel–mediated ischemia associated with syncope, such as in the patient with an extremely compromised cerebral circulation). In such cases, there are usually associated neurologic findings to lead the physician toward the correct diagnosis. Thus, vertebrobasilar disease is usually accompanied by at least some of the following symptoms: vertiginous complaints, ocular disturbances, or speech problems.

In subclavian steal syndrome, narrowing of the subclavian artery at its origin, results in syncope or dizziness in conjunction with ipsilateral upper extremity exercise as blood is shunted from the brain to the exercising limb by way of the vertebral artery system. Usually a bruit can be detected over the affected subclavian artery, along with diminution of brachial artery pressure on the affected side (40). Rarely, extrinsic disturbances of the cerebrovascular supply may be at fault. Thus, syncope or dizziness associated with neck extension or rotation may be caused by vertebral artery compression by cervical spondylosis, cervical osteoarthritis, or a cervical rib.

It has been estimated that 3% of the U.S. population is susceptible to seizures. For many of these cases, epilepsy is the etiologic diagnosis, and differentiation from true syncope may be made based on careful history and appropriate neurologic assessment. On the other hand, seizure-like activity may occur in conjunction with cerebral hypoperfusion of any cause. Recently, there has been increased interest in the possibility that unsuspected arrhythmias or neurally mediated faints may be responsible for symptoms in certain treatment refractory seizure patients.

In some patients, temporal lobe seizures may mimic (or induce) neurally mediated reflex bradycardia and hypotension. Differentiation of such events from true syncope may be difficult. However, seizures tend to be independent of position, are usually associated with immediate convulsive activity and loss of bowel or urinary continence, and are typically followed by a confusional state. On the other hand, apparent seizure-like motor activity may also accompany transient cerebral hypoperfusion of any cause (including neurally mediated reflex syncope). However, in the latter case, the abnormal motor activity tends to be relatively brief and unassociated with bladder or bowel incontinence.

Diagnostic Evaluation

Imaging techniques (magnetic resonance imaging, echo, and angiography) are only infrequently undertaken with the express purpose of identifying a cerebrovascular basis for syncope. Consequently, the reported clinical experience is too small to make any judgment. Nonetheless, in those few cases where vascular disease is believed to be the basis of syncope, noninvasive imaging provides very safe and accurate methods for defining the extent of disease.

Overall, conventional neurologic laboratory studies (electroencephalogram, head computed tomographic imaging, and magnetic resonance imaging) have had a relatively low yield in unselected syncope patients. Among the 433 syncope evaluations reviewed by Kapoor (4), an electroencephalogram was helpful in only 3 cases. As a rule, neurologic consultation and these types of laboratory studies should be reserved for situations in which clinical observations (history or physical findings) suggest organic nervous system disease. On the other hand, given the importance of orthostatic and dysautonomic causes of syncope, tilt table testing and other tests of autonomic function have an increasingly important role to play. Specifically, various orthostatic intolerance disorders are now being recognized by virtue of tilt table testing and autonomic studies. These include postural orthostatic tachycardia syndrome, orthostatic hypotension (of various causes), inappropriate sinus tachycardia, chronic fatigue syndrome, and the neurally mediated faints. Syncope has been associated with each of these disorders, although the mechanism of the faint is often unclear.

A few recent case studies have pointed to the potential value of implantable loop recorder monitoring in seizure patients unresponsive to conventional treatments; some of these individuals have been found to have previously undocumented arrhythmias as the cause of their symptoms. Alternatively, a similar subset of treatment refractory patients have been reported to have positive tilt test results, suggesting that the diagnosis may have been neurally mediated hypotension bradycardia rather than a true seizure (94).

Syncope of Noncardiovascular Origin and Miscellaneous

Metabolic or endocrine disturbances rarely cause true syncope (40,41). More often, they result in confusion or behavioral disturbances. Hyperventilation episodes with marked reductions of P_{CO_2}, presumably leading to vasoconstriction and reduced cerebral blood flow, may be one of the more frequent causes of transient loss of consciousness in this category.

Syncope may be mimicked by anxiety attacks, hysteria, or other psychiatric disturbances (92–94). In this regard, Linzer and colleagues (92) indicated that panic disorder and major depression were common findings in their syncope patients and attributed approximately 25% to 30% of events to such causes. Similarly, Kapoor and colleagues (93) reported a psychiatric diagnosis in 24% (major depression, 12%; others, 12%), whereas Grubb and colleagues (94) also concluded that a psychogenic origin can be expected in approximately 25% of cases. However, except in cases in which loss of consciousness is witnessed and demonstrated to be associated with a normotensive state, such a diagnosis should be considered only once other causes have been clearly excluded.

Persistent Dizziness

The problem of persistent dizziness is often lumped with syncope. It has been estimated that dizziness accounts for about 8 million outpatient medical visits per year (95) and is probably one of the most common and refractory of all health-related complaints. In an evaluation of the problem, Kroenke and colleagues (96) found vertigo of various forms to be the most common primary or contributory cause (54%), with psychiatric disturbances being second in frequency (16%). Others (97–99) have observed a similar breakdown of diagnoses (Table 33-5). In perhaps more than 50% of instances, however, dizziness is multifactorial (96), and the establishment of an etiologic diagnosis requires substantial persistence on the part of the physician.

TABLE 33-5. CAUSES OF PERSISTENT DIZZINESS[a]

Study	Kroenke and colleagues (96)	Drachman and Hunt (97)	Nedzeiski and colleagues (98)	Herr and colleagues (99)
No. of points	100	102	2222	125
Cause (%)				
Vertigo	54	46	45	50
Benign positional	(16)	(12)	(17)	NA
Ménière	(4)	(4)	(10)	(1)
Nonspecific vertigo	(10)	(10)	NA	NA
Psychiatric disorder	16	9	21	11
Presyncope	6	4	NA	14
Dysequilibrium	2	16	NA	1
Hyperventilation	1	23	NA	5
Multicausal[b]	13	12	NA	NA
Unknown	8	9	19	10

NA, Not assigned or not available.

[a]In some studies, percentages may exceed 100% if multiple etiologies were assigned. Note that the principal subcategories under vertigo are noted, but these do no add up to the total because of omission of less frequent categories.

[b]Multicausal: one or more primary causes as listed above were identified, but no single one predominated. Six of these patients had 2 causes, and 7 patients had 3 causes.

Source: Kroenke K, Lucas CA, Risenberg ML, et al. Causes of persistent dizziness: A perspective study of 100 patients in ambulatory care. Ann Intern Med 1992;117:989–904, with permission.

TREATMENT

The key requirement for effective treatment of the patient with syncope is an accurate etiologic diagnosis. Thereafter, a wide range of pharmacologic and device therapies can be considered.

In most cases, the treatment of syncope focuses on secondary prevention of syncope recurrences in individuals who have already experienced (or are suspected of having experienced) a syncopal spell. Primary prevention in patients considered to be at high risk is, however, encountered in selected situations. Examples include currently asymptomatic patients in whom severe cardiac conduction system disease has been identified, or individuals known to have long QT syndrome or Brugada syndrome.

Neurally Mediated Syncope

In the case of neurally mediated syncope, treatment strategies should whenever possible address apparent trigger factors (e.g., avoiding rapid neck movement or tight collars in carotid sinus syndrome, suppressing the cause of cough in cough syncope). However, often such an approach is not feasible or is not sufficient. Thus, for patients with susceptibility to symptomatic bradycardia resulting from vagally induced sinus arrest or paroxysmal AV block, a cardiac pacemaker may be necessary. In patients with a prominent vasodepressor component accounting for hypotension, aggressive attention to volume maintenance along with the use of vasoconstrictor agents becomes the treatment focus. In some patients, treatment with fludrocortisone, amino-phylline, theophylline, support stockings, or ephedrine may also be helpful. The serotonin uptake inhibitors have been helpful for patients with syncope caused by carotid sinus hypersensitivity in several small series (99a,99b).

Vasovagal syncope is the most frequently encountered of all the neurally mediated syncopes, and its treatment has been the subject of considerable interest. For most patients, no specific treatment is needed. Education related to recognizing triggering events or situations and maintenance of hydration (possibly including fludrocortisone, salt tablets, sport drinks) and avoidance of extended periods of upright posture, along with reassurance, are usually sufficient. However, in cases in which recurrent or severe symptoms demand a more aggressive approach, several pharmacologic strategies have been proposed. β-Adrenergic blocking drugs, serotonin reuptake inhibitors, disopyramide, and vasoconstrictor agents (e.g., midodrine) have been the agents of principal interest; other agents that may be effective include scopolamine, theophylline, aminophylline, and ephedrine. However, for any of these agents, only a small amount of experience currently exists and large controlled treatment trials are lacking (100–104).

Many young patients with neurocardiogenic syncope respond poorly to medical therapy. Orthostatic training may be an effective approach in this group; patients undergo a series of five in-hospital upright tilt table studies; the duration of the study is 10 minutes initially and is increased by 10 minutes each day up to 50 minutes. This training program is continued at home, under the supervision of a family member, by standing against a wall for up to 40 minutes twice a day. In one study of 47 refractory patients followed for mean of 18 months, none of the trained patients had spontaneous recurrent syncope, whereas 57% of controls experienced a recurrent episode (104a).

Cardiac pacing has proved highly successful in carotid sinus syndrome and is considered the treatment of choice when bradycardia has been documented (105–108). In contrast, until recently, experience with pacing in vasovagal syncope and other forms of neurally mediated syncope has been limited. In this regard, the North American Vasovagal Pacing Study (109), a prospective randomized controlled multicenter trial, found an annual actuarial rate of recurrent syncope of approximately 19% for paced patients and 60% in control subjects. The Vasovagal International Study in Europe, recently submitted for publication, obtained essentially the same outcome (110). Consequently, for very symptomatic vasovagal syncope patients, cardiac pacing now becomes an important consideration. Regarding pacing, Sheldon and colleagues (111) reported outcomes, including quality-of-life indices, in 12 difficult-to-treat vasovagal syncope patients provided pacemaker therapy and followed for an average of 1 year. Compared with symptom status before pacemaker implantation, pacing was associated not only with fewer symptoms, but also with a substantial increase in quality-of-life scores.

Orthostasis and Dysautonomias

The treatment of patients with syncope resulting from orthostasis or dysautonomias, after elimination of drug-induced hypotension, relies heavily on physical maneuvers (e.g., support stockings, elevation of the head of the bed at night, and tilt training) (112,113). The mainstay of pharmacologic treatment has been attempts at chronic expansion of central circulating volume (e.g., fludrocortisone, salt tablets, and sport drinks). Additional benefit may be achieved with the use of erythropoietin, which acts to increase circulating blood volume. A second element in the strategy is reduction of the tendency for central volume to be displaced to the lower extremities with upright posture. To this end, vasoconstrictors have been employed, although with limited success because of the tendency for tachyphylaxis to develop. Of greatest current interest is midodrine, an agent that has prominent venoconstriction properties and good overall tolerance (114–116). Physical rehabilitation (gentle progressive increments of exercise), with enforced periods of increasing exposure to upright posture (so-called *tilt training*) is also advisable. Cardiac pacing at relatively rapid rates may prove valuable in certain very difficult cases but is not widely accepted. Tolerance to persistent rapid pacing rates and long-term adverse effects on left ventricular function are a concern.

Primary Cardiac Arrhythmias

In the treatment of syncope resulting from primary cardiac bradyarrhythmias, cardiac pacemaker therapy is clearly effective, whether the arrhythmia is caused by sinus node dysfunc-tion or AV conduction disturbances. In the case of syncope associated with paroxysmal SVTs, the efficacy of conventional antiarrhythmic drug treatment is not well studied but is likely to be quite good if the drugs are tolerated and compliance is maintained. However, such patients are more often considered for curative transcatheter ablation techniques.

In the case of paroxysmal atrial fibrillation, syncope may occur as a result of the tachyarrhythmia itself (i.e., excessively rapid rate or possibly reduced cardiac output resulting from loss of atrial contribution) or prolonged bradycardia at the termination of a tachycardia episode. Treatment may focus on abolishing the atrial fibrillation events, but given the difficulty of accomplishing this goal, backup pacing is often needed. In terms of curative ablation, preliminary results have been encouraging, but the procedure is not yet widely available and may not be warranted for most patients. Currently, many symptomatic paroxysmal atrial fibrillation patients, and particularly those who have experienced syncope as a consequence of the tachyarrhythmia, are being treated with long-term amiodarone therapy. Other drugs such as flecainide and propafenone are also very effective in selected individuals with symptomatic atrial fibrillation, although in patients with demonstrable structural heart disease, there are generally greater safety concerns with these agents than there are with amiodarone. In the future, implantable low-energy atrial cardioverters may prove beneficial in some of the most difficult to control cases of atrial fibrillation (117,118).

In the case of syncope caused by VT, underlying left ventricular dysfunction is often present. In such settings, the proarrhythmic risk associated with antiarrhythmic drug therapy is markedly increased. The risk has been reported to range from 5% to 15% with class I agents (e.g., quinidine and disopyramide). Pharmacologic therapeutic strategies in this setting often involve early introduction of class III agents (particularly amiodarone). However, several recent large studies suggest that even amiodarone may not provide optimal prophylaxis against sudden death, particularly in the setting of poor left ventricular systolic function (i.e., an ejection fraction of less than 0.30) (119–123). Consequently, implantable pacemaker cardioverter-defibrillators are increasingly recommended for high-risk patients. Cardiac ablation techniques for mapping and elimination of VT are evolving. This approach is a first-choice therapy only in right ventricular outflow tract tachycardia and bundle branch reentrant tachycardia. However, as technology advances, transcatheter ablation may find a greater role in the control of ventricular tachyarrhythmias (124).

Structural Cardiovascular or Cardiopulmonary Disease

In patients in whom structural cardiovascular or cardiopulmonary disease is the cause of syncope, treatment must be directed at the specific structural lesion or its consequences.

Thus, in syncope associated with myocardial ischemia, pharmacologic therapy or revascularization is clearly the appropriate strategy in most cases. Similarly, when syncope is closely associated with surgically addressable lesions (e.g., valvular aortic stenosis, pericardial disease, atrial myxoma, and congenital cardiac anomaly), a direct corrective approach is often feasible. On the other hand, when syncope is caused by certain difficult-to-treat conditions such as primary pulmonary hypertension or restrictive cardiomyopathy, it is often impossible to ameliorate the underlying problem adequately. Even modifying outflow gradients in hypertrophic obstructive cardiomyopathy is not readily achieved surgically. Recent success with cardiac pacing techniques may offer promise for certain very symptomatic individuals, but this approach remains quite controversial (125–127).

SUMMARY

Syncope is a common symptom with many possible causes. Establishing the cause is the principal task faced by the physician. It is often said that the combination of a detailed medical history and a thorough physical examination may provide a working diagnosis in approximately 60% of syncope episodes. However, confirming a diagnostic suspicion is crucial to establish a degree of certainty sufficient to permit arriving at a confident assessment of prognosis and establishing an effective treatment program. To this end, patient and persistent efforts are usually needed.

The careful assessment of the diagnostic possibilities, along with careful use of noninvasive and invasive testing, should result in defining a basis for symptoms in approximately 75% to 80% of syncope episodes. The principal initial diagnostic step is differentiation of those patients with normal cardiovascular status from those with evident structural heart disease. In the former individuals, autonomic testing (particularly tilt table testing) is probably the most cost-effective first diagnostic step. In the latter group, a functional assessment of the suspected structural disturbance (i.e., hemodynamic, angiographic, and electrophysiologic studies as appropriate) is crucial. In all cases, the ultimate objective is to obtain a sufficiently strong correlation between the symptoms and the detected abnormalities to permit effective and confident treatment decisions.

ACKNOWLEDGMENT

The authors thank Wendy Markuson and Barry L. S. Detloff for assistance in preparation of the manuscript.

REFERENCES

1. Savage DD, Corwin L, McGee DL, et al. Epidemiologic features of isolated syncope: the Framingham Study. *Stroke* 1985;16:626–629.
2. Dermksian G, Lamb LE. Syncope in a population of healthy young adults. *JAMA* 1958;1200–1207.
3. Kapoor WN, Karpf M, Wieand S, et al. A prospective evaluation and follow-up of patients with syncope. *N Engl J Med* 1983;309:197–204.
4. Kapoor WN, Peterson J, Wieand HS, et al. Diagnostic and prognostic implications of recurrences in patients with syncope. *Am J Med* 1987;83:700–708.
5. Bass EB, Elson JJ, Fogoros RN, et al. Long-term prognosis of patients undergoing electrophysiologic studies for syncope of unknown origin. *Am J Cardiol* 1988;62:1186–1191.
6. Kapoor W. Evaluation and outcome of patients with syncope. *Medicine* 1990;69:160–175.
7. Day SC, Cook EF, Funkenstein H, Goldman L. Evaluation and outcome of emergency room patients with transient loss of consciousness. *Medicine* 1982;72:15–23.
8. Gendelman HE, Linzer M, Gabelman M, Smoller J. Syncope in a general hospital population. *N Y State J Med* 1983;83:116–165.
9. Lipsitz LA, Wei JY, Rowe JW. Syncope in an elderly, institutionalized population: prevalence, incidence, and associated risk. *Q J Med* 1985;55:45–55.
10. Lipsitz, LA, Pluching FC, Wei JY, Rowe JW. Syncope in institutionalized elderly: the impact of multiple pathological conditions and situational stress. *J Chronic Dis* 1986;39:619–630.
11. Wayne HH. Syncope: physiological considerations and an analysis of the clinical characteristics in 510 patients. *Am J Med* 1961;30:418–438.
12. Silverstein MD, Singer DE, Mulley AG, et al. Patients with syncope admitted to medical intensive care units. *JAMA* 1982;248:1185–1189.
13. Martin GJ, Adams SL, Martin HG, et al. Prospective evaluation of syncope. *Ann Emerg Med* 1984;13:499–504.
14. Mahoney CB, Benditt DG. Syncope: a meta-analysis examining causes and outcomes in tertiary health care environments with particular emphasis on the effects of cardiac pacing. *Pace* 1999;22:168(abst).
15. Gibson GE, Pulsinelli W, Blass JP, et al. Brain dysfunction in mild to moderate hypoxia. *Am J Med* 1981;70:1247–1254.
16. Rowell LB. *Human circulation. Regulation during physical stress.* New York: Oxford University Press, 1986.
17. Scheinberg P, Blackburn I, Rich M, et al. Effects of aging on cerebral circulation and metabolism. *Arch Neurol Psychol* 1953;70:77–85.
18. Cook P, James I. Cerebral vasodilators. *N Engl J Med* 1981;305:1508–1513.
19. Heidorn GH, McNamara AP. Effect of carotid sinus stimulation on the electrocardiograms of clinically normal individuals. *Circulation* 1956;14:1104–1113.
20. Lown B, Levine JA. The carotid sinus. Clinical value of its stimulation. *Circulation* 1961;23:766–789.
21. Brown KA, Maloney JD, Smith HC, et al. Carotid sinus reflex in patients undergoing coronary angiography: relationship of degree and location of coronary artery disease to response to carotid sinus massage. *Circulation* 1980;62:697–703.
22. Scheinberg P, Blackburn I, Rich M, Saslaw M. Effects of aging on cerebral circulation and metabolism. *Arch Neurol Psychol* 1953;70:77–85.
23. Dandona P, James IM, Newbury PA, et al. Cerebral blood flow in diabetes mellitus: evidence of abnormal cerebral vascular reactivity. *Br Med J* 1978;2:325–326.
24. Grubb BP, Wolfe D, Samoil D, et al. Recurrent unexplained syncope in the elderly: the use of head-upright tilt table testing in evaluation and management. *J Am Geriatr Soc* 1992;40:1123–1128.
25. DiMarco JP. Electrophysiologic studies in patients with unexplained syncope. *Circulation* 1987;75[Supp III]:140–143.

26. Hess DS, Morady F, Scheinman MM. Electrophysiologic testing in the evaluation of patients with syncope of undetermined origin. *Am J Cardiol* 1982;50:1309–1315.

27. Akhtar M, Shenasa M, Denker S, et al. Role of cardiac electrophysiologic studies in patients with unexplained recurrent syncope. *Pace* 1983;6:192–201.

28. Morady F, Shen E, Schwartz A, et al. Long-term follow-up of patients with recurrent unexplained syncope evaluated by electrophysiologic testing. *J Am Coll Cardiol* 1983;2:1053–1059.

29. Olshansky B, Mazuz M, Martins JB. Significance of inducible tachycardia in patients with syncope of unknown origin: a long-term follow-up. *J Am Coll Cardiol* 1983;5:216–223.

30. Teichman SL, Felder SD, Matos JA, et al. The value of electrophysiologic studies in syncope of undetermined origin: report of 150 cases. *Am Heart J* 1985;110:469–479.

31. Denes P, Ezri MD. The role of electrophysiologic studies in the management of patients with unexplained syncope. *Pace* 1985; 8:424–435.

32. Crozier I, Low CJS, Dow LJ, Ikram H. Cardiac electrophysiological assessment and the natural history of unexplained syncope. *N Z Med J* 1988;101:106–108.

33. Sra JS, Anderson AJ, Sheikh SH, et al. Unexplained syncope evaluated by electrophysiologic studies and head-up tilt testing. *Ann Intern Med* 1991;114:1013–1019.

34. Lipsitz LA, Micrus I, Mosely GB, Goldberger A. Spectral characteristics of heart rate variability before and during postural tilt: relation to aging and risk of syncope. *Circulation* 1990;81: 1803–1810.

35. Lombard JT, Selzer A. Valvular aortic stenosis. *Ann Intern Med* 1987;106:292–298.

36. Atwood JE, Kawanishi S, Myers J, et al. Exercise testing in patients with aortic stenosis. *Chest* 1988;93:1083–1087.

37. Johnson AM. Aortic stenosis, sudden death, and the left ventricular baroreceptors. *Br Heart J* 1971;33:1–5.

38. Kudenchuk PJ, McAnulty JH. Syncope: evaluation and treatment. *Mod Conc Cardiovasc Dis* 1985;54:25–29.

39. Camm AJ, Lau CP. Syncope of undetermined origin: diagnosis and management. *Prog Cardiol* 1988;1:139–156

40. Ross RT. *Syncope.* London: WB Saunders, 1988.

41. Benditt DG. Syncope. In: Evans RW, ed. *Diagnostic testing in neurology.* Philadelphia: WB Saunders, 1999:391–404.

42. Weiss S, Baker JP. The carotid sinus reflex in health and disease. Its role in the causation of fainting and convulsions. *Medicine* 1933;12:297–354.

43. Nathanson MH. Hyperactive cardioinhibitory carotid sinus reflex. *Arch Intern Med* 1946;77:491–502.

44. Thomas JE. Hyperactive carotid sinus reflex and carotid sinus syncope. *Mayo Clin Proc* 1969;44:127–139.

45. Almquist A, Goldenberg IF, Milstein S, et al. Provocation of bradycardia and hypotension by isoproterenol and upright posture in patients with unexplained syncope. *N Engl J Med* 1989; 320:346–351.

46. Scherrer U, Vissing S, Morgan BJ, et al. Vasovagal syncope after infusion of a vasodilator in a heart-transplant recipient. *N Engl J Med* 1990;332:602–604.

47. Almquist A, Gornick CC, Benson DW Jr, et al. Carotid sinus hypersensitivity: evaluation of the vasodepressor component. *Circulation* 1985;67:927–936.

48. Chen M-Y, Goldenberg IF, Milstein S, et al. Cardiac electrophysiologic and hemodynamic correlates of neurally mediated syncope. *Am J Cardiol* 1989;63:66–72.

49. Sutton R, Petersen M, Brignole M, et al. Proposed classification for tilt induced vasovagal syncope. *Eur J Cardiac Pacing Electrophysiol* 1992;2:180–183.

50. Wallin BG, Sundlof G. Sympathetic outflow in muscles during vasovagal syncope. *J Auton Nerv Syst* 1982;6:287–291.

51. Ziegler MG, Echon C, Wilner KD, et al. Sympathetic nervous withdrawal in the vasodepressor (vasovagal) reaction. *J Auton Nerv Syst* 1986;17:273–278.

52. Chosy JJ, Graham DT. Catecholamines in vasovagal fainting. *J Psychosom Res* 1965;9:189–194.

53. Fitzpatrick A, Williams T, Ahmed R, et al. Echocardiographic and endocrine changes during vasovagal syncope induced by prolonged head-up tilt. *Eur J Cardiac Pacing Electrophysiol* 1992;2:121–128.

54. Grubb BP, Gerard G, Roush K, et al., Cerebral vasoconstriction during head-up tilt-induced vasovagal syncope. A paradoxic and unexpected response. *Circulation* 1991;84:1157–1164.

55. Abi-Samra F, Maloney JD, Fouad-Tarazi FM, et al. The usefulness of head-up tilt testing and hemodynamic investigations in the workup of syncope of unknown origin. *Pace* 1988;11: 1202–1214.

56. Fitzpatrick A, Sutton R. Tilting towards a diagnosis in unexplained syncope. *Lancet* 1989;1:658–660.

57. Raviele A, Gasparini G, Di Pede F, et al. Usefulness of head-up tilt test in evaluating patients with syncope of unknown origin and negative electrophysiologic study. *Am J Cardiol* 1990;65: 1322–1327.

58. Brignole M, Menozzi C, Gianfranchi L, et al. Neurally mediated syncope detected by carotid sinus massage and head-up tilt test in sick sinus syndrome. *Am J Cardiol* 1991;68:1032–1036.

59. Grubb BP, Temesy-Armos P, Hahn H, et al. Utility of upright tilt table testing in the evaluation and management of syncope of unknown origin. *Am J Med* 1991;90:6–10.

60. Grubb BP, Gerard G, Roush K, et al. Differentiation of convulsive syncope and epilepsy with head-up tilt testing. *Ann Intern Med* 1991;115:871–876.

61. Natale A, Akhtar M, Jazayeri M, et al. Provocation of hypotension during head-up tilt testing in subjects with no history of syncope or presyncope. *Circulation* 1995;92:54–58.

61a. Mittal S, Stein KM, Markowitz SM, et al. Induction of neurally mediated syncope with adenosine. *Circulation* 1999;99: 1318–1324.

61b. Zeng C, Zhu Z, Hu W, et al. Value of sublingual isosorbide dinitrate before isoproterenol tilt test for diagnosis of neurally mediated syncope. *Am J Cardiol* 1999;83:1059–1063.

62. Benditt DG, Ferguson DW, Grubb BP, et al. Tilt-table testing for assessing syncope. An American College of Cardiology expert consensus document. *J Am Coll Cardiol* 1996;28(1): 263–275.

63. Leitch JW, Klein GJ, Yee R, et al. Syncope associated with supraventricular tachycardia. An expression of tachycardia rate or vasomotor response. *Circulation* 1992;85(3):1064–1071.

64. Bannister RF, Mathias CJ, eds. *Autonomic failure,* 3rd ed. New York: Oxford University Press, 1992:1–953.

65. Gibson JC, Heitzman MR. Diagnostic efficacy of 24 hour electrocardiographic monitoring for syncope. *Am J Cardiol* 1984; 53:1013–1017.

66. Clark PI, Glasser SP, Spoto E. Arrhythmias detected by ambulatory monitoring. Lack of correlation with symptoms of dizziness and syncope. *Chest* 1980;77:722–725.

67. Awford et al. ACC/AHA Guidelines for Ambulatory Electrocardiography. J Am Coll Cardiol 1999;34:912–948

67a. Zimetbaum PJ, Josephson ME. The evolving role of ambulatory arrhythmia monitoring in general clinical practice. *Ann Intern Med* 1999;130:848–856.

68. Krahn AD, Klein GJ, Yee R, et al, and the Reveal Investigators. Use of an extended monitoring strategy in patients with problematic syncope. *Circulation* 1999;99(3):406–410.

69. Zaidi A, Fitzpatrick A. Outcomes from a syncope clinic: role of the insertable loop recorder. *Arch Mal Coeur* 1998;91[Suppl III]:138(abst).

70. Hirata T, Yano K, Okoi T, et al. Asystole with syncope following strenuous exercise in a man without organic heart disease. *J Electrocardiol* 1987;20:280–283.

71. Edward C, Hyucke MD, Harold G, et al. Post-exertional cardiac asystole in a young man without organic heart disease. *Ann Intern Med* 1987;106:844–845.

72. Grubb BP, Temesy-Armos PN, Samoil D, et al. Tilt table testing in the evaluation and management of athletes with recurrent exercise-induced syncope. *Med Sci Sports Exerc.* 1993;25:24–28.

73. Kuchar DL, Thorburn CW, Sammel NL. Signal-averaged electrocardiogram for evaluation of recurrent syncope. *Am J Cardiol* 1986;58:949–953.

74. Gang ES, Peter T, Rosenthal ME, et al. Detection of late potentials on the surface electrocardiogram in unexplained syncope. *Am J Cardiol* 1986;58:1014–1020.

75. Winters SL, Steward D, Gomes JA. Signal averaging of the surface QRS complex predicts inducibility of ventricular tachycardia in patients with syncope of unknown origin: a prospective study. *J Am Coll Cardiol* 1987;10:775–781.

76. Benditt DG, Milstein S, Goldstein M, et al. Sinus node dysfunction: pathophysiology, clinical features, evaluation and treatment. In: Zipes DP, Jalife J, eds. *Cardiac electrophysiology: from cell to bedside.* Philadelphia: WB Saunders, 1990:708–734.

77. Ector H, Rolies L, DeGeest H. Dynamic electrocardiography and ventricular pauses of 3 seconds and more etiology and therapeutic implications. *Pace* 1983;6:548–551.

78. Hilgard J, Ezri MD, Denes P. Significance of ventricular pauses of three seconds or more detected on twenty-four hour Holter recordings. *Am J Cardiol* 1985;55:1005–1008.

79. Gann D, Tolentino R, Samet P. Electrophysiologic evaluation of elderly patients with sinus bradycardia. *Ann Intern Med* 1979;90:242–249.

80. Dhingra RC, Denes P, Wu D, et al. Syncope in patients with chronic bifascicular block. Significance, causative mechanisms, and clinical implications. *Ann Intern Med* 1974;81:302–306.

81. Ezri M, Lerman BB, Marchilinski FE, et al. Electrophysiologic evaluation of syncope with bifascicular block. *Am Heart J* 1983; 106:693–697.

82. Morady F, Higgins J, Peters RW, et al. Electrophysiologic testing in bundle branch block and unexplained syncope. *Am J Cardiol* 1984;54:587–591.

83. Haissaguerre M, Commenges D, Maio JO, et al. Etude electrophysiologique des syncopes: prevision du resultat. *Presse Med* 1989;5:212–220.

84. Gossinger HD, Siostrozonek P, Jong M, et al. Prediction of electrophysiological abnormality in patients with otherwise unexplained syncope. *J Cardiovasc Electrophysiol* 1991;2:2–8.

85. Fujimura O, Yee R, Klein GJ, et al. The diagnostic sensitivity of electrophysiologic testing in patients with syncope caused by transient bradycardia. *N Engl J Med* 1989;321:1703–1707.

86. Pathy MS. Clinical presentation of myocardial infarction in the elderly. *Br Heart J* 1967;29:190–199.

87. Dixon MS, Thomas P, Sheridon DJ. Syncope is the presentation of unstable angina. *Int J Cardiol* 1988;19:125–129.

88. McKenna WJ, Deanfield J, Faruqui A, et al. Prognosis in hypertrophic cardiomyopathy: role of age and clinical electrocardiographic and hemodynamic features. *Am J Cardiol* 1981;47: 532–538.

89. Maron BJ, Roberts WC, Epstein SE. Sudden death in hypertrophic cardiomyopathy: a profile of 78 patients. *Circulation* 1982;65(7):1388–1394.

90. Duthie EH, Gambert SR, Tresch D. Evaluation of the systolic murmur in the elderly. *J Am Geriatr Soc* 1981;29:498–502.

91. Krasnow, Stein RA. Hypertrophic cardiomyopathy in the aged. *Am Heart J* 1978;96:326–336.

92. Linzer M, Varia I, Pontinen M, et al. Medically unexplained syncope: relationship to psychiatric illness. *Am J Med* 1992;92: 18–25.

93. Kapoor WN, Fortunato M, Sefcik T, Schulberg H. Psychiatric illness in patients with syncope. *Clin Res* 1989;37:316(abst).

94. Grubb BP, Gerard G, Wolfe DA, et al. Syncope and seizures of psychogenic origin: Identification with head-up tilt table testing. *Clin Cardiol* 1992;15:839–842.

95. Sloane PD. Dizziness in primary care: results from the National Ambulatory Medical Care Survey. *J Fam Pract* 1989;29:33–38.

96. Kroenke K, Lucas CA, Rosenberg ML, et al. Causes of persistent dizziness. A perspective study of 100 patients in ambulatory care. *Ann Intern Med* 1992;117:989–904.

97. Drachman DA, Hart CW. An approach to the dizzy patient. *Neurology* 1972;22:323–334.

98. Nedzeiski JM, Barben HO, McIlmoyl L. Diagnoses in a dizziness unit. *J Otolaryngol* 1986;15:101–104.

99. Herr RD, Zun L, Mathews JJ. A directed approach to the dizzy patient. *Ann Emerg Med* 1989;18:664–672.

99a. Grubb BP, Samoil D, Kosinski D, et al. The use of serotonin reuptake inhibitors in the treatment of recurrent syncope due to carotid sinus hypersensitivity unresponsive to dual chamber cardiac pacing. *Pacing Clin Electrophysiol* 1994;17:1434–1436.

99b. Dan S, Grubb BP, Mouhaffel AH, et al. Use of serotonin reuptake inhibitors as primary therapy for carotid sinus hypersensitivity. *Pacing Clin Electrophysiol* 1997;20:1633–1635.

100. Fitzpatrick AP, Ahmed R, Williams S, et al. A randomized trial of medical therapy in malignant vasovagal syndrome or neurally-mediated bradycardia/hypotension syndrome. *Eur J Cardiac Pacing Electrophysiol* 1991;1:991–202.

101. Brignole M, Menozzi C, Gianfranchi L, et al. A controlled trial of acute and long-term medical therapy in tilt-induced neurally mediated syncope. *Am J Cardiol* 1992;70:339–342.

102. Morillo CA, Leitch JW, Yee R, et al. A placebo-controlled trial of intravenous and oral disopyramide for prevention of neurally mediated syncope induced by head-up tilt. *J Am Coll Cardiol* 1993;22:1843–1848.

103. Moya A, Permanyer-Miralda G, Sagrista-Sauleda J, et al. Limitations of head-up tilt test for evaluating the efficacy of therapeutic interventions in patients with vasovagal syncope: Results of a controlled study of etilefrine versus placebo. *J Am Coll Cardiol* 1995;25:65–69.

104. Mahanonda N, Bhuripanyo K, Kangkagate C, et al. Randomized double-blind placebo-controlled trial of oral atenolol in patients with unexplained syncope and positive upright tilt table results. *Am Heart J* 1995;130:1250–1253.

104a. Di Girolamo E, Di Iorio C, Leonzio L, et al. Usefulness of a tilt training program for the prevention of refractory neurocardiogenic syncope in adolescents: a controlled study. *Circulation* 1999;100:1798–1801.

105. Morley CA, Perrins EJ, Grant P, et al. Carotid sinus syncope treated by pacing. Analysis of persistent symptoms and role of atrioventricular sequential pacing. *Br Heart J* 1982;47:411–418.

106. Brignole M, Sartore B, Barra M, et al. Ventricular and dual chamber pacing for treatment of carotid sinus syndrome. *Pace* 1989;12:582–590.

107. Deschamps D, Richard A, Citron B, et al. Hypersensibilite sino-carotidienne. Evolution a moyen et a long terme des patients traites par stimulation ventriculaire. *Arch Mal Coeur* 1990;83:63–67.

108. Cardiac pacing for carotid sinus syndrome and vasovagal syncope. In: Barold S, Mugica J, eds. *New perspectives in cardiac pacing,* 3rd ed. Mount Kisco, NY: Futura Publishing, 1993:15–28.

109. Sheldon RS, Gent M, Roberts RS, Connolly SJ, for the NAV-PAC Investigators. North American Vasovagal Pacemaker Study: study design and organization. *Pace* 1997;20:844–848.

110. Sutton R, Brignole M, Menozzi C, et al, for the VASIS Investi-

gators. Dual-chamber pacing in the treatment of neurally-mediated tilt-positive cardioinhibitory syncope. Pacemaker versus no therapy: a multicentre randomized study. *Circulation* 2000; 102:294–299.

111. Sheldon R, Koshman ML, Wilson W, et al. Effect of dual-chamber pacing with automatic rate-drop sensing on recurrent neurally-mediated syncope. *Am J Cardiol* 1998;81:158–162.

112. Ten Harkel ADJ, van Lieshout JJ, Wieling W. Treatment of orthostatic hypotension with sleeping in the head-up position, alone and in combination with fludrocortisone. *J Intern Med* 1992;232:139–145.

113. Ector H, Reybrouck T, Heidbuchel H, et al. Tilt training: a new treatment for recurrent neurocardiogenic syncope or severe orthostatic intolerance. *Pace* 1998;21:193–196.

114. Jankovic J, Gilden JL, Hiner BC, et al. Neurogenic orthostatic hypotension: a double-blind placebo-controlled study with midodrine. *Am J Med* 1993;95:38–48

115. Sra J, Maglio C, Biehl M, et al. Efficacy of midodrine hydrochloride in neurocardiogenic syncope refractory to standard therapy. *J Cardiovasc Electrophysiol* 1997;8:42–46..

116. Benditt DG, Wilbert L, Fahy G, et al. In: Raviele A, ed. Midodrine for treatment of vasovagal syncope. *Cardiac arrhythmias 1999*, vol 1. Milan, Italy: Springer-Verlag Italia, 2000.

117. Murgatroyd FD, Johnson EE, Cooper RAS, et al. Safety of low-energy transvenous atrial defibrillation—world experience. *Circulation* 1994;90;I14.

118. Ayers GM. Internal atrial defibrillation and implantable atrial defibrillators. In: Ali Oto M, ed. *Practice and progress in cardiac pacing and electrophysiology.* Dordecht, The Netherlands, Kluwer Academic Publishers, 1996:309–316.

119. Middelkauff HR, Stevenson WG, Stevenson LW, Saxon LA. Syncope in advanced heart failure: high risk of sudden death regardless of origin of syncope. *J Am Coll Cardiol* 1993;21:110–116.

120. Middelkauff HR, Stevenson WG, Saxon LA. Prognosis after syncope: impact of left ventricular function. *Am Heart J* 1993; 125:121–127.

121. Moss AJ, Hall WJ, Cannom DS, et al. Improved survival with an implanted defibrillator in patients with coronary disease at high risk for ventricular arrhythmia. *N Engl J Med* 1996;335: 1933–1940.

122. The Antiarrhythmics versus Implantable Defibrillators (AVID) Investigators. A comparison of antiarrhythmic drug therapy with implantable defibrillators in patients resuscitated from near-fatal ventricular arrhythmias. *N Engl J Med* 1997;337: 1576–1583.

123. Bigger JT Jr, for the CABG Patch Trial Investigators. Prophylactic use of implanted cardiac defibrillators in patients at high risk for ventricular arrhythmias after coronary-artery bypass graft surgery. *N Engl J Med* 1997;337:1569–1575.

124. Benditt DG, Adler SW, Beatty G, et al. Advances in transcatheter endocardial mapping and radiofrequency ablation of ventricular arrhythmias. In: Oto MA, ed. *Practice and progress in cardiac pacing and electrophysiology.* Dordrecht, The Netherlands: Kluwer Academic Publishers, 1996:277–287.

125. .McKenna W, Deanfield J, Faruqui A, et al. Prognosis in hypertrophic cardiomyopathy: role of age and clinical electrocardiographic and hemodynamic features. *Am J Cardiol* 1981;47(3): 532–538.

126. McAreavey D, Epstein ND, Fananapazir L. Dual chamber pacing is effective therapy for hypertrophic cardiomyopathy patients with provocable LV outflow tract obstruction and symptoms refractory to medical therapy. *J Am Coll Cardiol* 1994;23:11(abst).

127. Maron BJ, Nishimura RA, McKenna WJ, et al. Assessment of permanent dual-chamber pacing as a treatment for drug-refractory symptomatic patients with obstructive hypertrophic cardiomyopathy. A randomized, double-blind, crossover study (M-PATHY). *Circulation* 1999;99(22):2927–2933.

INDEX

Page numbers followed by "f" denote figures. Page numbers followed by "t" denote tables.

A

AAVRT. See Antidromic atrioventricular reentrant tachycardia
Ablation therapy, for Wolff-Parkinson-White syndrome, 542–543, 543f. See also Catheter ablation; Cryoablation; Radiofrequency catheter ablation
ACC. See American College of Cardiology
Accelerated idioventricular rhythm, 573
Accessory atrioventricular connection, in the retrograde refractory period, 15t
Accessory pathways, pathogenesis and preexcitation, 517–521, 518f, 519f, 520f, 521f
ACE. See Angiotensin-converting enzyme inhibitors
Acebutolol. See also Clinical studies
Acebutolol et Prevention Secondaire de l'Infarctus (APSI) Trial, 113–114
Acebutolol (Sectral)
    adverse effects, 282
    for arrhythmias in pregnancy, 795
    dosing, 282
    drug classification, 273t
    efficacy, 282
    electrophysiology, 282
    pharmacokinetics, 282
    prophylaxis trials, 838t
Acetylprocainamide, postoperative atrial arrhythmias and, 845
Actin-related autosomal dominant dilated cardiomyopathy, 89–90
Action potential (AP)
    atrial myocyte, 40
    atrioventricular nodal cells, 39–40
    changes in, 864
    chloride channels, 48
    configuration, 42t
    definition, 37
    in disease states, 48–49
    duration, 213–214, 266–267
    effective refractory period, 38
    His-Purkinje system, 40–41
    hyperpolarization-activated, 48
    membrane current underlying, 42–48, 43f, 44f, 45t, 46f, 46t, 47f
    membrane responsiveness curve, 38
    potassium channels and, 46–48, 46t, 47f
        molecular basis of, 46–47, 47f
        β subunits, 47–48
    sinoatrial nodal cells, 39–40

sodium current and, 42–45, 43f
    auxiliary β-subunit modulation, 43–44
    calcium channels, 45, 45t
    sodium channel regulation by second messengers, 44
supernormal period, 38
transmural variation of the action potential in the ventricle and atrium, 41, 41f, 42t
vagal stimulation, 40
variation, 38f
ventricular myocyte, 37–39, 37f, 38f
Activation sequence mapping, 254–256, 256f, 390–391, 390f
Acute ischemia, cardiac action potential in, 48
Acute myocardial infarction (AMI)
    etiology and predisposing factors, 460–461
    indications for temporary cardiac pacing, 328–329, 330t
    intraventricular block from, 702–703, 708–711, 709f, 710f
    risk for nocturnal cardiac events, 119t
    treatment and indications for pacing, 689
Adenocard. See Adenosine
Adenosine (Adenocard)
    adverse effects, 293
    for antidromic atrioventricular reentrant tachycardia in WPW syndrome, 541
    for arrhythmias in pregnancy, 794–795
    for atrial tachycardia, 419
    for atrioventricular nodal reentry tachycardia, 448
    clinical use and adverse effects in pregnancy, 794t
    dosing, 293
    drug classification, 273t
    effect during preexcited atrial fibrillation, 473f
    efficacy, 293
    electrophysiology, 292–293
    for orthodromic atrioventricular reentrant tachycardia in WPW syndrome, 540
    pharmacokinetics, 293
    for reperfusion arrhythmias, 876
Advanced Cardiac Life Support guidelines, 631
AET. See Atrial ectopic tachycardia
AFFIRM. See Atrial Fibrillation Follow-up Investigation of Rhythm Management Trial

Afterdepolarizations
    delayed (DAD), 70–72
    early (EAD), 68–70
    triggered activity and, 68–72, 69f, 71f
Age. See also Children; Elderly
    atrial fibrillation and, 458, 458t, 459f
    exercise testing and, 181
    preparticipation screening for athletes and, 821–822
    prevalence of nonsustained ventricular tachycardia in asymptomatic subjects, 554, 554t
    relation to incidence of atrial fibrillation/flutter, 751
    syncope and, 925, 926f
AHA. See American Heart Association
Alcohol, as predisposing factor to atrial fibrillation, 462
Algorithm 1, 158f, 159–161, 159f, 160f, 161f
Algorithm 2, 161–163, 161f, 162f
Allele, definition, 100
α helix, definition, 100
α-methyldopa, for sinus node dysfunction induction or worsening, 659t
α-tropomyosin gene mutations, 88
Alternative splicing, definition, 100
Ambasilide
    frequency dependence, 268
    for Torsade de Pointes, 609
Ambulatory monitoring. See Holter monitoring
American College of Cardiology (ACC)
    guidelines for implantation of ICDs, 364
    guidelines for insertion of a permanent pacemaker after myocardial infarction, 875t
    guidelines for placement of transcutaneous patches and external pacing, 713, 713t, 714t
    guidelines for the use of temporary pacing, 329
    guidelines for treatment of ventricular tachycardia and ventricular fibrillation in the setting of acute myocardial infarction, 867, 868t
    recommendations for the use of electrophysiologic testing, 712, 712t, 713t
    tilt-table testing methodology, 933

American Heart Association (AHA), 631
  guidelines for amiodarone as therapy for
    hemodynamically stable ventricular
    tachycardia, 588
  guidelines for implantation of ICDs, 364
  guidelines for insertion of a permanent
    pacemaker after myocardial
    infarction, 875t
  guidelines for placement of
    transcutaneous patches and external
    pacing, 713, 713t, 714t
  guidelines for the use of temporary
    pacing, 329
  guidelines for treatment of ventricular
    tachycardia and ventricular
    fibrillation in the setting of acute
    myocardial infarction, 867, 868t
  recommendations for preparticipation
    screening for athletes, 821–822
  recommendations for the use of
    electrophysiologic testing, 712,
    712t, 713t
AMI. *See* Acute myocardial infarction
Amino acids, 44f
Amino acid sequence, definition, 100
Aminophylline, 413
  cardiac transplantation and, 912, 913t
  electrophysiologic effects of, 913t
Amiodarone (Cordarone). *See also* Clinical
    studies
  adverse effects, 285
  for antidromic atrioventricular reentrant
    tachycardia in WPW syndrome, 541
  for arrhythmias, 740
    assessment, 167
    in pregnancy, 797
    prevention, 482
    termination of atrial fibrillation,
      478–479
  for atrial fibrillation, 726–727, 727
    in WPW syndrome, 541
  for atrial flutter, 512
  for atrial tachyarrhythmias, 871
  for atrial tachycardia, 422
    multifocal, 413
  cardiac transplantation and, 909, 915
  for congestive heart failure, 765
  for dilated cardiomyopathy, 733
  dosing, 283
  drug classification, 273t
  drug trials for treatment of postoperative
    atrial arrhythmias, 846t
  effect of catecholamine infusion on
    efficacy of, 186t
  effect on defibrillation threshold, 376t
  effect on postmyocardial patients, 880f
  effect on ventricular tachycardia rate,
    376t
  efficacy, 283–285, 284t, 285t
  electrophysiology, 283
  frequency dependence, 268–269
  for heart rate control in atrial fibrillation,
    474
  hemodynamic effects, 271
  versus ICD therapy, 364
  ICD trials, 283–284, 284t

interaction with immunosuppressive
    agents, 909t
  for long-term therapy of the sudden
    cardiac death survivor, 634, 634f
  metabolism, 266
  for nonsustained ventricular tachycardia,
    561
  for orthodromic atrioventricular reentrant
    tachycardia in WPW syndrome, 540
  pharmacokinetics, 283, 283t
  for postoperative atrial arrhythmias, 847
  for pretreatment for cardioversion, 476
  for prevention of postoperative atrial
    fibrillation, 839–840, 840t
  for prevention of rejection of the
    transplanted heart, 909
  regimen for postoperative atrial
    arrhythmias, 847t
  as repolarization-prolonging drug, 273t
  for sinoatrial nodal atrial tachycardia, 425
  for sinus node dysfunction induction or
    worsening, 659t
  for sudden cardiac death, 642–643, 645f
  for sustained monomorphic ventricular
    tachycardia, 577, 588
  for Torsade de Pointes, 609, 610
  for treatment of ventricular arrhythmias
    during myocardial infarction, 867t
  for ventricular arrhythmias, 853
  for ventricular premature depolarizations,
    561
  for ventricular tachycardia or ventricular
    fibrillation in acute myocardial
    infarction, 868t
AMIOVIRT, 735
Amphetamines, sudden cardiac death in
    athletes and, 820–821
Amyloidosis, as a cause of sinus node
    dysfunction, 659
Anger
  behavioral studies and risk of cardiac
    events, 118t
  ventricular arrhythmias and, 116, 116f
Angina, risk for nocturnal cardiac events,
    119t
Angioplasty, for ventricular tachycardia or
    ventricular fibrillation in acute
    myocardial infarction, 868t
Angiotensin-converting enzyme (ACE)
    inhibitors
  for dilated cardiomyopathy, 733–734
  for sudden cardiac death, 632
Anterograde conduction
  atrioventricular conduction pathways, 17
  refractoriness and patterns of conduction,
    14–21, 14t, 15f, 15t, 16f
Anterograde periods, definition, 14, 14t
Anthopleurin-A (AP-A), 606
Antiarrhythmic agents, 177, 178f, 185,
    185f, 186t, 263–301. *See also* Clinical
    studies; individual drug names
  absorption, 265
  for arrhythmias, 732–733
  for atrial flutter, 508
  for atrial tachycardia, 422
  bioavailability, 265–266

cardiac transplantation and, 909
  classification, 272–294, 273t
  class III drugs under development, 273t,
    290–291
  clinical use and adverse effects in
    pregnancy, 794t
  combination therapy, 272–294
  dilated cardiomyopathy and, 729t
  drug-receptor mechanism for channel
    blockade, 267, 267f
  elimination, 266
  for fetal arrhythmias, 794
  frequency dependence, 268–269, 268f,
    269f, 270f
  for heart rate control, 473–474
    in atrial fibrillation, 473–474
  hemodynamic effects, 271
  implantable cardioverter-defibrillator
    interactions, 375–377, 376t
  for long-term therapy of the sudden
    cardiac death survivor, 634
  metabolism, 266
  pacing for drug-induced
    bradyarrhythmias, 329–330
  pharmacokinetic and pharmacodynamic
    principles of, 265–266
  pretreatment for cardioversion, 476
  for prevention of postoperative atrial
    fibrillation, 839–840, 840t
  for prevention of sudden cardiac death,
    642, 643f, 644f
  proarrhythmic effects of, 269–271
    atrial proarrhythmia, 271
    monomorphic ventricular tachycardia,
      270
    Torsade de pointes, 270–271
    ventricular proarrhythmia, 269–271
  prophylactic use
    in congentive heart failure, 561–562,
      561f, 562f
    in coronary artery disease, 563–567,
      563f, 564f, 565f, 566f
    in myocardial infarction, 563–567,
      563f, 564f, 565f, 566f
  receptor physiology, 266–271
  for sinus node dysfunction, 659
    induction or worsening, 659t
  for sinus node reentrant tachycardia, 656
  for sudden cardiac death, 631–632
  for sustained monomorphic ventricular
    tachycardia, 588
  for Torsade de Pointes, 609–611
  as trigger for sudden cardiac death, 626
  for Wolff-Parkinson-White syndrome,
    539–541
Antiarrhythmic Drugs Versus Implantable
    Defibrillator (AVID) trial, 241, 245,
    283–284, 284t, 364–366, 576–577,
    637, 638f, 639f, 734, 883, 883f
Anticoagulation
  in atrial fibrillation, 487
  for atrial flutter, 512
  heart rate control versus rhythm control,
    482–483
  for postoperative atrial arrhythmias,
    848

recommendations before cardioversion, 489

Antidepressants, for sinus node dysfunction induction or worsening, 659t

Antidromic atrioventricular reentrant tachycardia (AAVRT)
  as cause of wide QRS complex tachycardia, 150t
  pharmacologic therapy, 541
  Wolff-Parkinson-White syndrome and, 524, 524f, 534–535, 536f, 537f

Antihistamines
  for sinus node dysfunction or worsening, 659t
  Torsade de Pointes and, 611

Antihypertensive therapy
  for prevention of sudden cardiac death, 641
  for sinus node dysfunction or worsening, 659t

Antitachycardia devices, for Wolff-Parkinson-White syndrome, 541–542, 542f

Anxiety, behavioral studies and risk of cardiac events, 118t

Aortic dissection, as complication of invasive cardiac electrophysiologic studies, 235t

Aortic stenosis, incidence of arrhythmias after repair of, 767t

AP. *See* Action Potential

AP-A. *See* Anthopleurin-A

APDs. *See* Atrial premature depolarizations

APSI. *See* Acebutolol et Prevention Secondaire de l'Infarctus

ARREST trial, 631, 631f, 868–869

Arrhythmias
  abnormal impulse formation, 66–72
    abnormal automaticity, 67, 67f
    afterdepolarizations and triggered activity, 68–72, 69f, 71f
    automaticity as a mechanism of cardiac arrhythmias, 67
    normal automaticity, 66–67
    parasystole and modulated parasystole, 67–68, 68f, 69f
  adrenergically-induced cardiac vulnerability, 112–115, 112f, 113f, 114f
  after cardiac and noncardiac surgery, 831–862
  after heart surgery, 766–767
  anatomic substrates associated with development of, 8t
  α_1- and α_2-adrenergic receptor blockade in preventing ischemia-induced vulnerability, 113–115
  arrhythmogenesis mechanisms, 112–113, 114f
  arrhythmogenic anatomy, 7–9, 7f, 8t, 9f
  associated with congenital heart disease, 749–783
  in athletes, 805–829
  autonomic factors and behavioral state on, 109–123

behavioral stress and arrhythmogenesis
    experimental studies, 115–118, 115f, 116f, 117f, 118f, 118t
    clinical evidence, 116–118, 117f, 118f, 118t
  β-adrenergic blocking agents and, 732, 733t, 740
  calcium channel blockers and, 479, 796
  cardiac action potential in, 48
  in cardiomyopathies, 721–748
  chronic, after operation on the ventricles, 772–777
  classification, 51, 52f
  and conduction disturbances in pregnancy, 787t
  ECG for assessment of, 167
  electrocardiogram in the diagnosis of, 127–164. *See also* Electrocardiogram
  evaluation of sudden cardiac death, 633
  exercise testing for assessment and management, 165–194. *See also* Exercise testing
  fetal, 792–794, 793f, 793t
  genetics of, 81–107
  Holter monitoring for assessment and management, 165–194. *See also* Holter monitoring
  incidence during exercise, 180–182
  inheritance patterns, 81–83, 82f, 83f
  inherited electrical disorders and, 93–97
  limitations in electrocardiographic interpretation of, 127
  mechanism of, 897–899
    arrhythmia and substrate in mitral valve prolapse sudden death, 898–899
    arrhythmogenesis in mitral stenosis, 899
    arrhythmogenesis in mitral valve prolapse and mitral regurgitation, 897–898
  mechanisms of, 8t, 51–79, 127–139, 128f, 129f
  in mitral valve disease, 889–905
  multiple risk factors, 202f, 224–225
  periinfarction, 863–888
  pharmacologic treatment, 476–479, 740
  physiologic basis for assessment, 195–196
  predictive value in, 202, 202f
  pregnancy and, 785–803
  preoperative incidence in patients with related congenital heart defects, 750t
  primary cardiac and syncope, 934–936
  prognostic significance of, 895–897
  reentry, 51–66
    circus movement, 51–56, 52f, 53f, 54f, 55f
    phase 2, 58
    reflection, 56–58, 56f, 57f
    role of heterogeneity, 58–65, 58f–59f, 60f, 62f, 63f, 64f, 65f
    slow or delayed conduction, 65–66
  reperfusion, 875–876
  reproducibility of exercise-induced, 184
  risk for nocturnal cardiac events, 119t
  sleep-related cardiac risk, 119–120, 119t

sudden cardiac death and, 621–623, 622f
  surgery for sudden cardiac death, 635
  surgical therapy for, 383–386
  sympathetic-parasympathetic nerve interactions, 112, 113f
  syncope, 925–944
  therapeutic options for termination of, 475–479
  therapy for prevention of, 480–485
  therapy for Wolff-Parkinson-White syndrome and, 539–543
  treatment of syncope, 940
  T-wave alternans and, 111t, 110–112, 110f, 111f
  types of, 8t
  variability, 556t

Arrhythmogenesis, mechanisms of, 112–113, 114f

Arrhythmogenic right ventricular cardiomyopathy (ARVC), 85t, 735–741. *See also* Arrhythmogenic right ventricular dysplasia
  clinical presentation, 736
  diagnosis, 736–737, 737t
  etiology, 735
  evaluation, 737–738
  genetics, 735
  gross pathology, 735, 736f
  histology, 735–736, 736f
  management, 740–741
    catheter ablation, 740
    implantable cardioverter-defibrillator, 740
    pharmacologic treatment, 740
    risk stratification, 740
    surgical treatment, 741
  supraventricular tachyarrhythmias and, 738–739
  ventricular tachyarrhythmias and, 739–740

Arrhythmogenic right ventricular dysplasia (ARVD), 241, 591–592, 592f
  diagnosis, 591, 592f
  imaging techniques, 592

ARVC. *See* Arrhythmogenic right ventricular cardiomyopathy

ARVD. *See* Arrhythmogenic right ventricular dysplasia

ASDs. *See* Atrial septal defects

Ashman phenomenon, 704–705

Asp, 451

Aspirin, for prevention of thromboembolism, 486–487

Atenolol
  for arrhythmias in pregnancy, 795
  combination therapy for rate control of atrial fibrillation, 471–472, 472f
  for ventricular rate control during atrial fibrillation, 872t

Athletes, 805–829. *See also* Exercise
  atrioventricular conduction in, 810, 811f
  cardiovascular disorders in, 817t
  eligibility for participation and recommendations for specific arrhythmias, 823–825, 823t, 824t

Athletes (*contd.*)
  incidence of arrhythmias and conduction
    disturbances in, 807–815, 808t,
    809t
  intraventricular conduction in, 810
  morphlogic cardiac changes with exercise,
    806–807, 806f
  physiologic changes with exercise,
    805–807
  preparticipation screening, 821–823
  repolarization in, 813–815
  sinus node function in, 807, 810
  sudden death in, 815–821
    arrhythmogenic right ventricular
      dysplasia and, 818
    atherosclerotic coronary artery disease
      and, 819
    cardiovascular structural disease and,
      816–820, 817t
    congenital coronary artery anomalies
      and, 818
    definition, 815
    electrophysiologic basis, 815–816
    environment and, 820
    exposure to toxins, 820–821
    hypertrophic cardiomyopathy and,
      816, 818
    idiopathic left ventricular hypertrophy
      and, 818
    myocarditis and, 819
    pathophysiologic basis, 816–821,
      816t
    personal characteristics and general
      medical status, 820
    preparation for and performance of
      event, 821
    prevalence in athletes, 815
    primary electrophysiologic conditions,
      820
    valvular heart disease and, 818–819
  supraventricular and ventricular
    arrhythmias in, 810–813, 811f,
    812f–813f, 814f
ATRAMI. *See* Autonomic Tone and Reflexes
  After Myocardial Infarction
Atrial activation, 129–144
  absence of, 129–137, 136f, 137f, 138f
  of the conduction system, 16, 16f
  long RP–short PR relationships in
    tachycardias, 139, 141f, 142f–143f
  P-wave morphology and axis, 141–144,
    144f
  short RP–long PR relationships in
    tachycardias, 136f, 139, 139f, 140f
Atrial arrhythmias
  after cardiac and noncardiac surgery,
    831–851
    diagnosis and treatment, 842–848
    epidemiology, 831
    pathogenesis, 831–833
    prognosis and complications, 848–850
    prophylaxis, 836–842
    risk factors, 833–836, 833t
      intraoperative factors, 834–835
      postoperative factors, 835–836
      preoperative factors, 833–834

  valvular disease and, 850–851
  atrial pacing for prevention of
    postoperative atrial fibrillation, 841,
    842t
  atrial tachyarrhythmias, 870–872, 870f,
    871t, 872t
  drug prophylaxis, 836–842
  rate control for postoperative, 845t
  sinus bradycardia, 869, 869t, 870t
  sinus tachycardia, 869–870
Atrial cannulation, 835
Atrial ectopic tachycardia (AET), 764–765,
  765f
Atrial fibrillation, 98, 457–500. *See also*
  Clinical studies
  acute drug therapy, 541
  after cardiac surgery, 462, 836
  age- and gender-specific prevalence, 458,
    458t, 459f
  anticoagulation in, 487
  approach to the patient with new-onset,
    470–471
  atrial ischemia and, 834
  atrial pacing for prevention of
    postoperative, 841, 842t
  calcium channel blockers and, 479
  cardiac action potential in, 48–49
  cardiac transplantation and, 914–915
  cardiovascular and noncardiovascular
    precipitants of, 460t
  catheter ablation and, 484–485
  causes of hemodynamic impairment in,
    469t
  chronic drug therapy, 541
  classification, 457–458
  as complication of invasive cardiac
    electrophysiologic studies, 235t
  definition, 457
  diagnosis and treatment of postoperative,
    842–848, 844f, 845t, 846t, 847t
  drugs for ventricular rate control during,
    872t
  electrical remodeling of the atrium,
    466–467, 467f
  electrocardiographic manifestations of,
    464
  electrophysiology, 464–468, 465f
    cellular, and ionic basis of electrical
      remodeling, 467, 468f
  epidemiology, 458
  etiology and predisposing factors,
    458–463, 459t
  exercise testing
    for management of, 188, 188f
    in the treatment of, 182, 183f
  external cardioversion for arrhythmia
    termination, 475–476
  familial, 85t
  focal, 468
  hemodynamics, 469–470, 469t, 470f
  in hypertrophic cardiomyopathy,
    723–724
  implantable atrial defibrillator for
    arrhythmia termination, 479
  indications, use, and outcomes of catheter
    ablation, 395–396, 396f

  inducibility before CABG patch surgery,
    835
  internal electrical cardioversion for
    arrhythmia termination, 476
  lone. *See* Lone atrial fibrillation
  morphologic changes in the atrium
    predisposing to, 464
  multiple-wavelet hypothesis, 465–466
  pacemakers and, 485
  3-P classification, 457
  pharmacologic therapy for arrhythmia
    termination, 476–479
  postoperative treatment algorithm, 844f
  in pregnancy, 790
  preoperative incidence of arrhythmias in
    patients with related congenital
    heart defects, 750t
  prognostic implications, 463–464
  prolonged, 849–850
  prophylaxis after cardiac surgery, 842,
    843f
  recurrence, 848
  risk for nocturnal cardiac events, 119t
  role of antiarrhythmic drugs for heart rate
    control, 473–474
  role of cardioversion and defibrillation in,
    314–315, 315t
  role of the autonomic nervous system in,
    468–469
    sympathetic atrial fibrillation, 469
    parasympathetic nervous system, 468
    sympathetic nervous system, 469
    vagal atrial fibrillation, 468–469
  surgical treatment of, 384–385, 384f,
    484
  therapeutic approach to, 726–727
  therapeutic options for arrhythmia
    termination, 475–479
  therapy for arrhythmia prevention,
    480–485
    catheter ablation, 484–485
    pacemakers, 485
    pharmacologic, 480–482
    rate control and anticoagulation versus
      rhythm control, 482–483
    surgical therapy, 484
  therapy to control ventricular rate,
    471–475
  thromboembolism and role of
    anticoagulation, 485–489
    antithrombotic therapy before
      cardioversion, 487–489
    risk factors in chronic atrial fibrillation,
      485–486
    therapy for prevention of stroke in
      chronic atrial fibrillation, 486–487
    treatment recommendations in chronic
      atrial fibrillation, 487
    transesophageal echocardiography and,
      488–489
  wavelength and, 465–466, 465f, 466f
  in Wolff-Parkinson-White syndrome,
    535–538, 537f, 538f, 539f
Atrial Fibrillation Follow-up Investigation of
  Rhythm Management (AFFIRM) Trial,
  314, 483

Atrial flutter, 501–516
  anticoagulant therapy, 512
  with atrioventricular block, 507f
  atypical, 502
  calcium channel blockers and, 508
  cardiac mapping, 253, 254f
  cardiac transplantation and, 914–915
  catheter ablation for treatment of,
    511–512
  clinical electrophysiology, 508
  clinical significance, 502–503
  diagnosis, 505–508
    electrocardiographic manifestations
      and diagnostic features, 506–507,
      506f, 507f
    physical examination, 505–506
    of suspected, 507–508
  direct current cardioversion to convert to
    sinus rhythm, 511
  "drug-induced," 512
  drug therapy for, 512
  hemodynamic effects, 505
  history, 501–502, 501f, 502f
  implanted antitachycardia pacemaker,
    512
  incidence and clinical setting, 502
  incisional atrial reentry, 502
  indications, use, and outcomes of catheter
    ablation, 393–395, 393f, 394f
  left, 502
  management, 508–513
    acute treatment, 508–511, 509f, 510f
    chronic treatment, 511–513
    of postoperative, 848
  mapping studies, 503
  mechanisms, 503–505, 504f
  pacing to interrupt, 509–510, 509f, 510f
  in pregnancy, 790
  preoperative incidence of arrhythmias in
    patients with related congenital
    heart defects, 750t
  QRS complex and, 507
  reverse typical, 502, 502f
  role of cardioversion and defibrillation in,
    315
  surgical treatment of, 384, 513
  symptoms, 505
  typical, 502, 502f
  in Wolff-Parkinson-White syndrome,
    535–538, 537f, 538f, 539f
Atrial implantable cardioverter-defibrillators,
  378–379
Atrial ischemia, atrial fibrillation and, 834
Atrial mapping, for evaluation of atrial
  tachycardias, 422
Atrial pacing, 327–328. *See also* Clinical
  studies
  atrioventricular bypass tract function
    during, 525–528, 526f, 527f, 528f,
    529f
  decremental atrioventricular nodal
    conduction and, 17–20, 18f, 19f
  for postoperative atrial fibrillation, 841,
    842t
Atrial premature depolarizations (APDs),
  cardiac transplantation and, 914

Atrial proarrhythmia, antiarrhythmic agents
    and, 271
Atrial septal defects (ASDs), 753, 754f
Atrial tachyarrhythmias
  atrial arrhythmias and, 871t, 870–872,
    870f, 872t
  postoperative, 836
Atrial tachycardias, 413–423
  automatic, 142f–143f
  β-adrenergic blocking agents and, 419,
    422
  calcium channel blockers and, 422
  cardiac mapping, 252–253, 253f
  circuits in intracardiac electrograms, 137f
  definition, 413–414, 414f, 415f
  ECG characteristics, 416, 417f
  electrophysiologic mechanisms, 417–419
    effect of pharmacologic agents, 419
    incessant atrial tachycardia, 418
    paroxysmal atrial tachycardia with
      block, 418
    paroxysmal sustained atrial tachycardia,
      417–418, 418f
    short bursts, 417
  etiology, 416
    automatic ectopic atrial tachycardia,
      416
    paroxysmal atrial tachycardia with
      block, 416
    short bursts, 416
    sustained reentrant atrial tachycardia,
      416
  evaluation methods, 419–422
    atrial mapping, 422
    atrial tachycardia
      caused by abnormal automaticity,
        419
      caused by reentry, 420, 420f, 421f
      caused by triggered automaticity,
        422
  incidence/prevalence, 414–416
    incessant atrial tachycardia, 415
    paroxysmal atrial tachycardia with
      block, 415–416
    paroxysmal sustained atrial tachycardia,
      415
    short bursts, 414–415
  indications, use, and outcomes of catheter
    ablation, 392–393, 392f
  physical examination, 419
  in pregnancy, 788
  prognostic/clinical significance, 419
  recipient, cardiac transplantation and,
    915, 916f
  symptoms and presentation, 419
  therapy, 422–423
    digoxin toxicity, 423
    pharmacologic therapy, 422
    surgical or catheter ablation, 422–423
Atrial thrombus formation, postoperative
  atrial arrhythmias and, 848
Atrionodal bundles, 5
Atrioventricular block, 872–873
  2:1, 146–147, 677
  with atrial flutter, 507f
  β-adrenergic blocking agents and, 680

  bradyarrhythmias and, 236–237
  electrophysiologic manifestations of His-
    Purkinje disease and, 705–707, 706f
  electrophysiology, 673–674
    in acquired, 712t
  etiology, 679–682
  first-degree. *See* First-degree
    atrioventricular block
  incidence and prevalence, 676f, 677, 678f
  indications for permanent cardiac pacing,
    335–337, 335t, 336t
  preoperative incidence of arrhythmias in
    patients with related congenital
    heart defects, 750t
  second-degree. *See* Second-degree
    atrioventricular block
  during supraventricular tachyarrhythmia,
    146–147
  terminology of, 674–675, 674f, 675f,
    676f
  third-degree. *See* Third-degree
    atrioventricular block
  variable, 147
Atrioventricular conduction, 128f. *See also*
    Clinical studies
  accessory connections, 20–21, 20f, 22f
  anterograde pathways, 17
  in athletes, 810, 811f
  disturbances in pregnancy, 792
  treatment of periinfarction disturbances,
    875, 875t
Atrioventricular dissociation, 147, 147f,
    157–158
  electrophysiology, 673–674
Atrioventricular fusion, 157–158
Atrioventricular junction, indications, use,
  and outcomes of catheter ablation,
  399–400
Atrioventricular nodal ablation
  indications, use, and outcomes of catheter
    ablation, 400
  indications for permanent cardiac pacing
    after, 341
Atrioventricular nodal blocking agents,
  effect of, 727
Atrioventricular nodal reentrant tachycardia
  (AVNRT), 433–456
  β-adrenergic blocking agents and,
    447–448
  cardiac mapping, 252, 252f
  cardiac transplantation and, 915
  clinical aspects and diagnosis, 437–445
    differential diagnosis, 440–445, 444f,
      445f, 446f, 447f
    electrocardiographic and
      electrophysiologic considerations,
      438–440, 439f, 440f, 441f, 442f
  common type, 136f, 138f
  indications, use, and outcomes of catheter
    ablation, 398–399, 399f
  management, 445–453
    approach to therapy, 453
    autonomic influences, 445–447
    nonpharmacologic therapy, 448–451,
      449f, 450f, 452f, 453f
    pharmacologic therapy, 447–448

Atrioventricular nodal reentrant tachycardia (*contd.*)
    radiofrequency ablation, 451, 453
    nodal anatomy, 433–434, 433f, 434f
    nodal physiology, 434–435
    in pregnancy, 788, 789f
    studies of atrioventricular node reentry, 435–437
        basic, 435–436, 436f
        clinical, 436–437
Atrioventricular node, 671–692. *See also* Clinical studies
    anatomy, 433–434, 433f, 434f, 671
    cells, 39–40
    ECG manifestations, 682–684
        first-degree AV block, 682
        second-degree AV block, 682–683
        third-degree AV dissociation block and, 683–684
    electrophysiologic mechanisms, 684–686
        first-degree AV block, 684–685
        second-degree AV block, 685–686, 685f, 686f
        third-degree AV dissociation and block, 686
    electrophysiology, 672–677, 672f, 673f
        atrioventricular dissociation block and, 673–674
        bradyarrhythmias, 675–677
        concealed conduction, 673
        tachyarrhythmias, 675–677
        terminology of atrioventricular block, 674–675, 674f, 675f, 676f
    etiology of atrioventricular block, 679–682
        cardiomyopathies and infiltrative processes, 681
        congenital heart disease, 681–682
        drugs, 679–680, 680f
        electrolyte imbalance, 681
        fibrosis and sclerosis, 679
        increased vagal tone, 680–681
        infective endocarditis, 681
        ischemic heart disease, 679
        myocarditis, 681
        trauma, 681
        valvular disease, 681
    with fast and slow pathways, 19f
    history, 671
    incidence and prevalence of atrioventricular block, 676f, 677, 678f
        first-degree AV block, 677
        second-degree AV block, 677
        third-degree (complete) AV block, 676f, 677, 678f
    indication for and evaluation with electrophysiologic studies, 687–688
    physical examination, 686
    physiology, 434–435
    prognostic implications in different disease states, 686–687
    retrograde refractory period, 15t
    symptoms, 686
    treatment and indications for pacing, 688–689

        first-degree AV block, 688–689
        high-degree heart block associated with an acute myocardial infarction, 689
        second-degree AV block, 689
        third-degree AV block, 689
Atrioventricular reciprocating tachycardia, in pregnancy, 788–790, 790f
Atrioventricular reentrant tachycardia (AVRT), Wolff-Parkinson-White syndrome and, 523–524, 523f, 524f
Atrioventricular septal defect (AVSD), 753, 754f
    arrhythmias after repair of, 778
Atrioventricular tachycardias, circuits in intracardiac electrograms, 137f
Atrium
    chronic arrhythmias after, 767–772, 768f, 769f
    electrical remodeling of, 466–467, 467f
    morphologic changes predisposing to atrial fibrillation, 464
    transmural variation of the action potential in, 41, 41f
    vulnerability of, 16, 17f
Atropine
    ACC/AHA recommendations for, 869, 869t
    for atrioventricular nodal reentry tachycardia, 445
    cardiac transplantation and, 908
    sinus bradycardia and, 655
    for sinus node dysfunction, 664
ATXII. *See* Sea anemone toxin
Atypical atrial flutter, 502
Automatic ectopic atrial tachycardia, etiology of, 416
Automaticity
    abnormal, 67, 67f
        evaluation of atrial tachycardias, 419
    definition, 66
    as a mechanism of cardiac arrhythmias, 67
    normal, 66–67
    triggered, evaluation of atrial tachycardia caused by, 422
Autonomic nervous system
    innervation and control, 6–7
    parasympathetic, 468
    role in atrial fibrillation, 468–469
    sympathetic, 469
        sustained monomorphic ventricular tachycardia and, 576–577
    vagal atrial fibrillation and, 468–469
    ventricular arrhythmias and, 865
Autonomic Tone and Reflexes After Myocardial Infarction (ATRAMI), 203, 203f
Autosomal dominant
    definition, 81, 83f
    dilated cardiomyopathy and, 85t
Autosomal recessive, definition, 81, 83f
Autosome, definition, 100
AVID. *See* Antiarrhythmics Versus Implantable Defibrillator trial
AVNRT. *See* Atrioventricular nodal reentrant tachycardia

AVRT. *See* Atrioventricular reentrant tachycardia
ASD. *See* Atrial septal defect
Azathioprine (Imuran), interaction with antiarrhythmic agents, 909t
Azimilide, 290–291
    frequency dependence, 268
    as repolarization-prolonging drug, 273t
    for Torsade de Pointes, 609

B

Band designation, definition, 100
Barth syndrome, 85t
    Tafazzin-related, 91–92
Base pair, definition, 100
Base pair substitution, definition, 100
Base pairs, DNA, definition, 100
BBB. *See* Bundle branch block
BBRT. *See* Bundle branch reentrant tachycardia
Belladonna alkaloids, for sinus node dysfunction, 664
BEST-ICD. *See* Beta-Blocker Strategy plus Implantable Cardioverter-Defibrillator Trial
β-adrenergic blocking agents. *See also* Clinical studies
    for acute control of heart rate, 472, 473f, 473t
    for antidromic atrioventricular reentrant tachycardia in WPW syndrome, 541
    for arrhythmias, 732, 733t, 740
    for atrial tachycardia, 419, 422
    atrioventricular block and, 680
    for atrioventricular nodal reentry tachycardia, 447–448
    cardiac transplantation and, 908–909
    contraindications, 871, 871t
    for heart rate control in atrial fibrillation, 474, 474t
    interaction with ICDs, 376
    for Long QT syndrome, 94
    for mitral valve prolapse, 900–901
    for multifocal atrial tachycardia, 413
    for orthodromic atrioventricular reentrant tachycardia in WPW syndrome, 540
    preoperative use, 834
    prophylaxis trials, 837–838, 838t
    prophylaxis with digoxin, 838
    randomized trials, 733t
    rate control for postoperative atrial arrhythmias, 845t
    for rate control of atrial fibrillation, 471, 472f
    for sinoatrial nodal atrial tachycardia, 425
    for sinus node
        dysfunction, 659
        worsening, 659t
        reentrant tachycardia, 656
    for sudden cardiac death, 632
    for sustained monomorphic ventricular tachycardia, 588
    withdrawal syndrome after cardiac surgery, 835
β-adrenergic receptor blockade
    central effects, 114–115

hemodynamic effects, 271
peripheral sites of action, 114
β-adrenoreceptor blockers
for arrhythmias in pregnancy, 795
clinical use and adverse effects in
pregnancy, 794t
Beta-Blocker Heart Attack Trial, 113
Beta-Blocker Strategy plus Implantable
Cardioverter-Defibrillator Trial (BEST-
ICD), 881
β-myosin
dilated cardiomyopathy, 90
heavy chain mutations, 87–88
Betapace. *See* Sotalol
Betaxolol, for arrhythmias in pregnancy,
795
Bicarbonate, for sudden cardiac death, 631
Bicaval cannulation, 835
Bifascicular block, 696, 697f, 874–875
indications for permanent cardiac pacing,
337, 337t
Biochemicals, changes during exercise, 179
Biopsy, endomyocardial. *See*
Endomyocardial biopsy
Bisoprolol. *See* Clinical studies
Blanking period, 324
Bleeding
with anticoagulants, 487
as complication of invasive cardiac
electrophysiologic studies, 235t
Blood pressure
neurally mediated reflex disturbances and
syncope, 931–933
Blood supply of the His bundle, 694
Bradyarrhythmias
after cardiac surgery, 854–856
after noncardiac surgery, 854
athletes and, 823, 823t
atrioventricular block and conduction
disturbances evaluation, 236–237
cardiac transplantation and, 910–914,
911f, 913t, 914f
as a complication of defibrillation and
cardioversion, 316–317
coronary artery bypass graft surgery and,
854–855
drug-induced, indications for temporary
cardiac pacing, 329–330
electrophysiology, 675–677
diagnosis and management, 236–237
epicardial temporary pacing for, 855–856
sinus node dysfunction evaluation, 236
Torsade de pointes and, 612
valvular surgery and, 855
Bradycardia, causes of fetal, 793t
Bradycardia-tachycardia syndrome, 461,
507, 656, 657f, 658f
Bradytachycardia syndrome, 561
Bretylium (Bretylol)
adverse effects, 287
antiadrenergic effects, 286
for arrhythmias in pregnancy, 797
dosing, 286
drug classification, 273t
effect on defibrillator threshold, 376t
efficacy, 286–287

electrophysiology, 286
hemodynamic effects, 271
pharmacokinetics, 286
for sudden cardiac death, 631
for sustained monomorphic ventricular
tachycardia, 588
for treatment of ventricular arrhythmias
during myocardial infarction, 867t
Bretylol. *See* Bretylium
Brevibloc. *See* Esmolol hydrochloride
Brockenbrough effect, 553, 554f
Brugada syndrome, 60–61, 62f
genetics and, 85t, 96–97
sudden cardiac death and, 624
syncope and, 939
Bundle branch block (BBB)
change in SVT rate and, 150
as complication of invasive cardiac
electrophysiologic studies, 235t
intermittent, 709–711, 709f, 710f
from longitudinal dissociation in the His
bundle, 708
Bundle branch reentrant tachycardia
(BBRT)
electrophysiologic manifestations of His-
Purkinje disease and, 711
indications, use, and outcomes of catheter
ablation, 401
sustained monomorphic ventricular
tachycardia and, 583, 590–591,
590f

C

CABG Patch. *See* Coronary Artery Bypass
Graft Patch trial
Caffeine, effect on reuptake of calcium, 72
Calan. *See* Verapamil
Calcium, for multifocal atrial tachycardia,
413
Calcium channel blockers, 45, 45t
for antidromic atrioventricular reentrant
tachycardia in WPW syndrome, 541
for arrhythmias in pregnancy, 796
for arrhythmia termination in atrial
fibrillation, 479
for atrial flutter, 508
for atrial tachycardia, 422
cardiac transplantation and, 909
clinical use and adverse effects in
pregnancy, 794t
for heart rate control in atrial fibrillation,
474
metabolism, 266
for orthodromic atrioventricular reentrant
tachycardia in WPW syndrome, 540
for pretreatment for cardioversion, 476
prophylaxis for atrial fibrillation after
CABG, 839
rate control for postoperative atrial
arrhythmias, 845t
for rate control of atrial fibrillation, 471,
472f
for sinoatrial nodal atrial tachycardia,
425
for sinus node dysfunction or worsening,
659t

Calcium current, comparison in cardiac
muscle, 45t
CAMIAT. *See* Canadian Amiodarone
Myocardial Infarction Arrhythmia Trial
Canadian Amiodarone Myocardial
Infarction Arrhythmia Trial
(CAMIAT), 167, 272, 284, 284t,
285t, 564, 564f, 565f, 642, 644f
Canadian Implantable Defibrillator Study
(CIDS), 241, 283–284, 284t,
366–367, 637, 639f, 734
Cannulation
atrial, 835
bicaval, 835
CAPS. *See* Cardiac Arrhythmia Pilot Study
Capture beats, 157–158
Cardiac arrest
cardiopulmonary resuscitation and, 312,
313f
risk for nocturnal cardiac events, 119t
role of cardioversion and defibrillation in,
312–313, 313f
Cardiac Arrest in Seattle: Conventional
versus Amiodarone Drug Evaluation
(CASCADE) trials, 231, 241, 284,
284t, 588, 634, 634f
Cardiac Arrest Study Hamburg (CASH),
241, 283–284, 284t, 367, 734
Cardiac Arrhythmia Pilot Study (CAPS),
204
Cardiac Arrhythmia Suppression Trial
(CAST), 113, 177, 178f, 211, 211f,
272, 512, 588, 626, 732–733, 839,
877, 877t, 878f
Cardiac Arrhythmia Suppression Trial
(CAST II), 564
Cardiac catheterization, indications for
temporary cardiac pacing during, 330
Cardiac disease, electrophysiology in
nonischemic, 243–244
Cardiac electrophysiology, definition, 3
Cardiac failure, risk of development of atrial
fibrillation, 459t
Cardiac Insufficiency Bisoprolol Study II
(CIBIS II), 732, 733t
Cardiac mapping
activation sequence mapping, 254–256,
256f
of atrioventricular nodal reentrant
tachycardia, 252, 252f
definition, 246–247
electrophysiologic testing and, 231–262
entrainment mapping, 256, 257f
limitations of endocardial mapping,
256–257
methodology, 248–249
noncontact endocardial activation
mapping, 249, 250f
nonfluoroscopic electroanatomic
mapping, 248–249
single-catheter, 248
noncontact endocardial activation, 249,
250f
nonfluoroscopic electroanatomic,
248–249
pace mapping, 254, 255f

Cardiac mapping (*contd.*)
single-catheter, 248
of specific tachyarrhythmias, 249–256
atrial flutter, 253, 254f
atrial tachycardia, 252–253, 253f
atrioventricular nodal reentry, 252, 252f
preexcitation syndromes, 249–252, 250f, 251f
ventricular tachycardia, 253–256, 255f, 256f, 257f
surgical ablation and, 389–392
voltage mapping, 253, 256
Cardiac pacing. *See* Pacemakers; Pacing
Cardiac Pathways Cooled RF Ablation clinical trial, 402
Cardiac resuscitation
active compression-decompression, 630–631
adjunctive drug therapy, 631–632, 631f
in sudden cardiac death, 630–632, 631f
Cardiac surgery. *See also* Cardiac transplantation
arrhythmias after, 766–767, 831–862
repair of congenital heart defects, 777–778
atrial arrhythmias after, 831–851
diagnosis and treatment, 842–848
epidemiology, 831
pathogenesis, 831–833
prognosis and complications, 848–850
prophylaxis, 836–842
risk factors, 833–836, 833t
intraoperative factors, 834–835
postoperative factors, 835–836
preoperative factors, 833–834
valvular disease and, 850–851
atrial fibrillation after, 462
bradyarrhythmias after, 854–856
as a cause of sinus node dysfunction, 659
incidence of arrhythmias after, 767t, 831t
in pregnancy, 798
risk factors for atrial fibrillation after, 833t
supraventricular arrhythmias after, 831–854
ventricular arrhythmias after, 851–854
Cardiac tamponade, as a complication of invasive cardiac electrophysiologic studies, 235t
Cardiac transplantation. *See also* Cardiac surgery
arrhythmogenic substrate, 909–910, 910f
β-adrenergic blocking agents and, 908–909
bradyarrhythmias and conduction disturbances, 910–914
conduction disturbances, 912–913, 914f
sinus node dysfunction, 910–912, 911f, 913t
calcium channel blockers and, 909
causes of syncope in orthotopic recipients, 918t
detection of transplant rejection with pacemakers, 918–919
drug interactions, 909, 909t
electrophysiologic features of the transplanted heart, 907–910
effect of denervation, 907
reinnervation, 908
indications for permanent cardiac pacing after, 341, 341t
orthotopic surgical technique, 910, 910f
pacing in the transplanted heart, 913–914
pharmacologic therapy, 908–909
pseudo-heart block in an orthotopic heart transplant recipient, 914, 915f
sudden cardiac death and, 917
supraventricular tachyarrhythmias and, 914–916
atrial fibrillation and flutter, 914–915
atrial premature depolarizations, 914
recipient atrial tachycardia, 915, 916f
syncope and, 917–918, 918t
theophylline for sinus bradycardia after, 856
vasculopathy and, 915
ventricular dysrhythmias, 916–917
premature ventricular complexes and nonsustained ventricular tachycardia, 916
sustained ventricular arrhythmias, 916–917, 917f
Cardiac tumors, in children, 763
Cardioactive drugs
sudden cardiac death and, 632
that may induce or worsen sinus node dysfunction, 659, 659t
Cardiogenic shock, as complication of invasive cardiac electrophysiologic studies, 235t
Cardiomyopathies. *See also* Clinical studies
arrhythmias in, 721–748
arrhythmogenic right ventricular. *See* Arrhythmogenic right ventricular cardiomyopathy
autosomal dominant dilated, 85t
definition, 721
dilated. *See* Dilated cardiomyopathies
ECG for risk assessment of, 176, 176f
etiology and predisposing factors, 461, 681
familial hypertrophic, 85t
hypertrophic. *See* Hypertrophic cardiomyopathy
hypertrophic/obstructive, 86–88
indications for permanent cardiac pacing, 340, 340t
identification of patients at high risk for sudden death, 725–726, 725t
indications, use, and outcomes of catheter ablation in nonischemic, 402
mechanisms of, 763–764
in pregnancy, 791
prevalence of nonsustained ventricular tachycardia and, 555, 555t
right ventricular, 92–93
role of programmed electrical stimulation in patients with nonsustained ventricular tachycardia, 559
role of programmed ventricular stimulation, 725–726
tachycardia-induced, 763–765
tachycardia-mediated, 502–503
therapeutic approach to arrhythmias, 726–727
atrial fibrillation, 726–727
effect of atrioventricular nodal blocking agents, 727
prevention of sudden death, 727, 727f
X-linked, 85t
Cardiopulmonary bypass, for ventricular arrhythmias, 853
Cardiopulmonary disease, syncope and, 936–937
Cardiopulmonary resuscitation (CPR). *See also* Resuscitation
during defibrillation, 312, 313f
in pregnancy, 797
Cardioquin. *See* Quinidine
Cardiovascular disease (CD)
in athletes, 816–820, 817t
risk of development of atrial fibrillation, 459t
syncope and, 936–937
treatment, 940–941
Cardioversion, 303–322. *See also* Clinical studies
calcium channel blockers and, 476
clinical considerations, 312
complications, 316–318
direct current, for atrial tachycardia, 422
electrophysiology, 303–308, 304f, 305f, 306f, 307f, 308f
external, for arrhythmia termination in atrial fibrillation, 475, 476
internal, 316
for arrhythmia termination in atrial fibrillation, 476
low-energy, 364
recommendations for anticoagulation before, 489
role in specific arrhythmias, 312–316
for ventricular arrhythmias, 853
for ventricular tachycardia or ventricular fibrillation in acute myocardial infarction, 868t
Cardizem. *See* Diltiazem
Carotid sinus syndrome, syncope and, 931, 932f
Carvedilol Heart Failure Study Group (Carvedilol HFSG), 732, 733t
Carvedilol HFSG. *See* Carvedilol Heart Failure Study Group
CASCADE. *See* Cardiac Arrest in Seattle: Conventional versus Amiodarone Drug Evaluation trials
CASH. *See* Cardiac Arrest Study Hamburg
CAST II. *See* Cardiac Arrhythmia Suppression Trial
Catecholaminergic polymorphic ventricular tachycardia (CPVT), 85t, 97
Catecholamines
exercise testing and, 185, 185f, 186t
to improve conduction, 711

Catheter ablation, 386–403. *See also*
Ablation; Cryoablation;
Radiofrequency catheter ablation
for arrhythmias, 740
atrial fibrillation and, 484–485
for atrial tachycardias, 422–423
biophysics of radiofrequency catheter
ablation, 387–388, 388f, 389f
complications, 402–403
hardware, 388–389
indications, use, and outcomes of,
392–402
mapping, 389–392
activation, 390–391, 390f
entrainment, 391, 391f
pace, 391
overview, 386
for permanent form of junctional
reciprocating tachycardia, 765
for prevention of arrhythmias in atrial
fibrillation, 484–485
principles of, 386–387, 387f
radiofrequency, 388f
for sinoatrial nodal atrial tachycardia, 426
sudden cardiac death, 635–636, 636f
for treatment of atrial flutter, 511–512
Catheterization, complications of invasive
cardiac electrophysiologic studies and,
235t
CAT trial, 735
CD. *See* Cardiovascular disease
CellCept. *See* Mycophenolate
Cellular telephones, pacemakers and, 353
Centimorgans (cM), definition, 100
Cerebrovascular diseases
syncope caused by, 937–938
Torsade de pointes and, 612
Channel block, drug-receptor mechanism
for, 267, 267f
Chaotic atrial tachycardia. *See* Multifocal
atrial tachycardia
CHD. *See* Coronary heart disease
CHF. *See* Congestive heart failure
CHF-STAT. *See* Congestive Heart
Failure–Survival Trial of
Antiarrhythmic Therapy; Veterans
Administration Heart Failure Trial
Children. *See also* Congenital heart
disease
diagnosis of atrioventricular nodal
reentrant tachycardia in, 437–438
primary cardiac tumors in, 763
primary conduction disease in, 695
Chloride channels, action potentials and, 48
Chromatin, definition, 100
Chromosome, definition, 101
Chromosome bands, definition, 101
Chronic intraventricular block
electrophysiologic manifestations of His-
Purkinje disease and, 707–708
electrophysiologic studies, 713t
exercise testing and left bundle branch
block, 701–702
His-Purkinje disease and, 701–702
natural history of conduction
abnormalities, 701

prevalence, 701
significance, 701
Chronotropic incompetence, 654–655
CIBIS II. *See* Cardiac Insufficiency
Bisoprolol Study II
CIDS. *See* Canadian Implantable
Defibrillator Study
Cimetidine, 266
metabolism, 266
for sinus node dysfunction induction or
worsening, 659t
Circus movement reentry, 51–56, 52f, 53f,
54f, 55f
definition, 51
figure-of-eight model, 54, 54f
leading circle model, 53–54, 53f
ring model, 51–53, 52f
spiral waves and rotors, 54–56, 55f
Cisapride, Torsade de Pointes and, 611
Clinical studies
Acebutolol et Prevention Secondaire de
l'Infarctus (APSI) Trial, 113–114
β-adrenergic blockers, 837–838, 838t
AMIOVIRT, 735
antiarrhythmic drug prophylaxis trials,
840t
antiarrhythmic drug trials for treatment
of postoperative atrial arrhythmias,
846t
Antiarrhythmics Versus Implantable
Defibrillator (AVID) trial, 241, 245,
283–284, 284t, 364–366, 576–577,
637, 638f, 639f, 734, 883, 883f
ARREST trial, 631, 631f, 868–869
Atrial Fibrillation Follow-up Investigation
of Rhythm Management (AFFIRM)
Trial, 314, 483
atrial pacing for postoperative atrial
fibrillation, 841, 842t
of atrioventricular node reentry, 435–436
Autonomic Tone and Reflexes After
Myocardial Infarction (ATRAMI),
203, 203f
of AV conduction in athletes, 810
of behavioral stress and arrhythmogenesis,
115–118, 115f, 116f, 117f, 118f,
118t
Beta-Blocker Heart Attack Trial, 113
Beta-Blocker Strategy plus Implantable
Cardioverter-Defibrillator Trial
(BEST-ICD), 881
Canadian Amiodarone Myocardial
Infarction Arrhythmia Trial
(CAMIAT), 167, 272, 284, 284t,
285t, 564, 564f, 565f, 642, 644f
Canadian Implantable Defibrillator Study
(CIDS), 241, 283–284, 284t,
366–367, 637, 639f, 734
Cardiac Arrest in Seattle: Conventional
versus Amiodarone Drug Evaluation
(CASCADE) trials, 231, 241, 284,
284t, 588, 634, 634f
Cardiac Arrest Study Hamburg (CASH),
241, 283–284, 284t, 367, 734
Cardiac Arrhythmia Pilot Study (CAPS),
204

Cardiac Arrhythmia Suppression Trial
(CAST), 113, 177, 178f, 211, 211f,
272, 512, 588, 626, 732–733, 839,
877, 877t, 878f
Cardiac Arrhythmia Suppression Trial
(CAST II), 564
Cardiac Insufficiency Bisoprolol Study II
(CIBIS II), 732, 733t
Cardiac Pathways Cooled RF Ablation
clinical trial, 402
Carvedilol Heart Failure Study Group
(Carvedilol HFSG), 732, 733t
CAT trial, 735
COMPANION, 734
Congestive Heart Failure–Survival Trial of
Antiarrhythmic Therapy (CHF-
STAT), 206, 284, 284t, 642–643,
645f, 733
Cooperative North Scandinavian
Enalapril Survival Study
(CONSENSUS), 734
Coronary Artery Bypass Graft Patch
(CABG Patch) trial, 212, 368, 646,
646f, 853
Coronary Drug Project, 175
Danish Investigations of Arrhythmia and
Mortality on Dofetilide-Myocardial
Infarction (DIAMOND) study, 201,
733
DEBUT, 735
Defibrillator in Acute Myocardial
Infarction Trial (DINAMIT), 207,
881
Defibrillators in Non-Ischemic
Cardiomyopathy Treatment
Evaluation (DEFINITE), 246,
735
digoxin prophylaxis trials, 836–837,
836t, 837t
electrophysiologic, 724
electrophysiologic methodology of,
232–234
Electrophysiologic Study Versus
Electrocardiographic Monitoring
(ESVEM), 166–167, 167f, 231,
241, 272, 583, 583f
ELITE trial, 734
European Myocardial Infarction
Amiodarone Trial (EMIAT), 167,
206, 272, 285t, 564, 642, 643f,
877–878, 880f–881f
German Pharmacological Intervention in
Atrial Fibrillation (PIAF) study, 483
GESICA, 176, 176f, 562
GISSI-2, 559
Global Utilization of Streptokinase and t-
PA for Occluded Coronary Arteries
(GUSTO-1) trial, 460–461, 703,
871
Goteborg Metoprolol Trial, 113, 114
Grupo de Estudio de la Sobrevida en la
Insuficiencia Cardiac en Argentina
(GESICA) trial, 284, 284t,
642–643, 645f, 733
HV interval significance, 707–708
indications for, 232–234

Clinical studies (*contd.*)
  Left Ventricular Dysfunction Prevention and Treatment Trials, 463
  magnesium prophylaxis trials, 840–841, 841t
  Metoprolol CR/XL Randomized Intervention Trial in Congestive Heart Failure (MERIT-HF), 730, 730f, 732, 733t
  Multicenter Automatic Defibrillator Implantation Trial (MADIT I), 231, 245, 367–368, 565–567, 566f, 643, 646, 646f, 734–735
  Multicenter Automatic Defibrillator Implantation Trial (MADIT II), 881
  Multicenter InSync Randomized Clinical Evaluation (MIRACLE), 734
  Multicenter Pacing Therapy for Hypertrophic Cardiomyopathy (M-PATHY) trial, 340
  Multicenter Post Infarction Trial, 176
  Multicenter Unsustained Tachycardia Trial (MUSTT), 212, 231, 245, 284, 368–369, 559–560, 646–647, 647f, 734–735, 881, 882f
  North American Vasovagal Pacemaker Study, 338
  Pacing in Cardiomyopathy (PIC) study, 340
  Pacing Therapies for Congestive Heart Failure (PATH-CHF) study, 341
  Primary Implantation Cardioverter-Defibrillator (PRIDE) trial, 735
  Rate Control versus Electrical cardioversion (RACE) study, 483
  SPRINT study group, 703
  Stroke Prevention in Atrial Fibrillation (SPAF) study, 732–733
  Studies of Left Ventricular Dysfunction (SOLVD), 734
  Sudden Cardiac Death–Heart Failure Trial (SCD-HeFT), 246, 368, 735
  Survival With Oral d-Sotalol (SWORD) Trial, 177, 178f, 877, 878f
  TAMI 9 trial, 703
  Thrombolysis in Myocardial Infarction (TIMI II) trial, 873
  Trandolapril Cardiac Evaluation (TRACE) study, 461
  of T-wave alternans, 222
  on T-wave alternans in high-risk patients, 111t
  United Kingdom Heart Failure Evaluation and Assessment of Risk Trial (UK-HEART), 205–207, 206f, 732
  Vasovagal Syncope International Study (VASIS), 338
  VEST trial, 730, 731f
  Veterans Administration Heart Failure Trial (CHF-STAT), 561–562
Clofilium, for prolonged repolarization, 72
Clone, definition, 101
Clonidine
  intravenous, for acute control of heart rate, 472–473
    for sinus node dysfunction induction or worsening, 659t
Cloning, definition, 101
cM. *See* Centimorgans
Cocaine, sudden cardiac death in athletes and, 820–821
"Cocktail" treatment, 543
Coding region, definition, 101
Codon, definition, 101
Commotio cordis, sudden cardiac death and, 624
COMPANION study, 734
Complete heart block
  as complication of invasive cardiac electrophysiologic studies, 235t
  electrophysiological criteria and His-Purkinje disease, 707
  in pregnancy, 792
Concealed conduction, 17f, 28–30, 29f
  electrophysiology, 673
Concealed entrainment, 584, 585f
Concealed pathways, indications, use, and outcomes of catheter ablation, 396–398, 397f
Conduction system
  abnormalities
    heterotaxy syndromes, 759–760
    His-Purkinje disease, 693–717
    natural history of, 701
    sudden cardiac death, 624–625
    l-transposition of the great arteries, 757–758, 757f
  accessory atrioventricular connections, 20–21, 20f, 22f
  acute conduction blocks in the prethrombolytic era, 702–703
  acute conduction blocks with thrombolytic therapy, 703
  advanced disease in the His bundle, 234f
  anatomy, 3–7, 4f, 5f, 6f
  anterograde
    atrioventricular conduction pathways, 17
    refractoriness and patterns of conduction, 14–21, 14t, 15f, 15t, 16f
  arrhythmogenic anatomy, 7–9, 7f, 8t, 9f
  asymptomatic arrhythmias in pregnancy and, 786, 787
  atrial pacing and decremental atrioventricular nodal conduction, 17–20, 18f, 19f
  atrial vulnerability, 16, 17f
  atrioventricular block, 872–873
    first-degree heart block, 872, 872f
    second-degree heart block, 872–873, 873f
    third-degree heart block, 873, 873f
  atrioventricular block evaluation, 236–237
  autonomic innervation and nervous control, 6–7
  autosomal dominant defects, 91
  baseline conduction intervals, 12–13, 12f
  cardiac transplantation and, 912–913, 914f
    concealed, 17f, 28–30, 29f
    disease in the elderly, 695
    electrophysiology, 9–31
    gap phenomenon, 30, 30t
    incidence in athletes, 807–815, 808t, 809t
    intraatrial, 16, 16f
    and atrial activation, 16, 16f
    intracardiac electrograms, 9–10, 10f
    intraventricular defects, 696–701, 696f, 697f, 698f, 699f, 700f
    intraventricular disturbances, 873–875
      bifascicular block, 874–875
      left anterior hemiblock, 874, 874f
      left posterior hemiblock, 874
      right bundle branch block, 874
    intraventricular in athletes, 810
    junction, 694
    normal, 3–4, 4f
    pacing protocols and programmed electrical stimulation, 10–12, 11f, 12t
    parietal block, 696
    preexcitation and, 20–21
    pseudo-supernormal, 30–31, 31f
    retrograde
      refractoriness assessment, 21–28
      using accessory ventriculoatrial connections, 27–28, 27f, 28f
    retrograde ventriculoatrial, 22–26, 23f, 24f, 25f, 26f, 27f
    sinoatrial node function evaluation, 13, 13f
    slow or delayed, 65–66
    supernormal, 30–31, 31f
    treatment of periinfarction disturbances, 875, 875t
      atrioventricular conduction disturbances, 875, 875t
      intraventricular conduction disturbances, 875
    use of exercise testing to expose abnormalities, 186f
    vascular supply, 6
Congenital, definition, 101
Congenital heart disease, 749–783. *See also* Children
  arrhythmias
    after heart surgery, 766–767
    after repair of other congenital heart defects, 777–778
    associated with unoperated, 749–765
    and conduction disturbances in pregnancy, 787t
    immediately after congenital heart surgery
      in the immediate postoperative period, 767
    junctional tachycardia, 766–767, 766f
  in athletes, 818
  atrial septal defects, 749–751, 750f
  atrioventricular septal defect, 753, 754f
  chronic arrhythmias after operation on the ventricles, 772–777

congenital abnormalities of the coronary
arteries, 762
defects causing left ventricular outflow
tract obstruction, 754–756, 756f
Ebstein's anomaly of the tricuspid valve,
751–752, 752f
Eisenmenger syndrome, 761–762
etiology, 681–682
evaluation and management
of chronic arrhythmias after surgery
for, 767–778
of patients with chronic arrhythmias
afer surgery for congenital heart
disease
chronic arrhythmias after operations
on the atria, 767–772
incidence, 767t
heterotaxy syndromes, 759–760
arrhythmia, 760
conduction abnormalities, 759–760
electrocardiographic abnormalities,
759, 759f
hypoplastic left heart syndrome, 761
patent ductus arteriosus, 753–754
persistent left superior vena cava, 762,
762f
in pregnancy, 791
primary cardiac tumors in children,
763
pulmonary valve stenosis, 752, 753f
single ventricle, 761
tachycardia-induced cardiomyopathy,
763–765
atrial ectopic tachycardia, 764–765,
765f
congenital junctional tachycardia,
764–765
mechanisms of cardiomyopathy,
763–764
permanent form of junctional
reciprocating tachycardia, 765,
766f
tetralogy of Fallot, 754, 755f
l-transposition of the great arteries,
756–759
arrhythmia, 758–759, 758f
conduction abnormalities, 757–758,
757f
d-transposition of the great arteries, 756,
757f
tricuspid atresia, 760–761
arrhythmia, 761
electrocardiographic abnormalities,
760–761, 760f
ventricular aneurysms and diverticula and
left ventricular false tendons,
762–763
ventricular septal defect, 752–753
Congenital junctional tachycardia, 764–765
Congestive heart failure (CHF). *See also*
Clinical studies
amiodarone for prevention of, 642–643,
645f
atrial fibrillation and, 463
as complication of invasive cardiac
electrophysiologic studies, 235t

predictive value of QT dispersion, 216
prophylactic use of antiarrhythmic agents,
561–562, 561f, 562f
Congestive Heart Failure–Survival Trial of
Antiarrhythmic Therapy (CHF-STAT),
206, 284, 284t, 642–643, 645f, 733
Connecticut Peer Review Organization,
487
Consciousness, diagnostic classification of
loss of, 929, 929t
CONSENSUS. *See* Cooperative North
Scandinavian Enalapril Survival Study
Contrast ventriculography, for evaluation of
arrhythmogenic right ventricular
cardiomyopathy, 738
Convulsive incoordination, 303
Cooperative North Scandinavian Enalapril
Survival Study (CONSENSUS), 734
Cordarone. *See* Amiodarone
Coronary arteries, congenital abnormalities
of, 762
Coronary artery bypass graft patch (CABG
patch) surgery. *See also* Clinical studies
bradyarrhythmias and, 854–855
hemodynamic deterioration following,
849
inducibility of atrial fibrillation before,
835
for long-term management of ventricular
arrhythmias, 853
postoperative atrial fibrillation, 849
prolonged atrial fibrillation following,
849–850
Coronary Artery Bypass Graft Patch (CABG
Patch) trial, 212, 368, 646, 646f,
853
Coronary artery disease
with polymorphous ventricular
tachycardia, 616f
prophylactic use of antiarrhythmic agents,
563–567, 563f, 564f, 565f, 566f
role of programmed electrical stimulation
and, 559–560
sudden cardiac death in athletes and,
819
Coronary Drug Project, 175
Coronary heart disease (CHD)
ECG for risk assessment of, 175–176
risk of development of atrial fibrillation,
459t
Coronary sinus, perforation as complication
of invasive cardiac electrophysiologic
studies, 235t
Coronary sinus rhythm. *See* Persistent left
superior vena cava
Coronary stenosis, as complication of
invasive cardiac electrophysiologic
studies, 235t
Coronary vasospasm, sudden cardiac death
in athletes and, 819
Corvert. *See* Ibutilide
Cough syncope, 933
CPR. *See* Cardiopulmonary resuscitation
CPVT. *See* Catecholaminergic polymorphic
ventricular tachycardia
Crosstalk, 349f

Cryoablation, for atrial flutter, 513. *See also*
Ablation therapy; Catheter ablation;
Radiofrequency catheter ablation
Crystodigin. *See* Digitoxin
Cyclosporine, 266
interaction with antiarrhythmic agents,
909t
CYP. *See* Cytochrome P450 enzymes
Cytochrome P450 enzymes (CYP),
metabolism, 266
Cytogenetic map, definition, 101
Cytoskeleton
definition, 101
dilated cardiomyopathy and, 89

D

DADs. *See* Delayed afterdepolarizations
Danish Investigations of Arrhythmia and
Mortality on Dofetilide-Myocardial
Infarction (DIAMOND) study, 201,
733
DCM. *See* Dilated cardiomyopathy
DEBUT, 735
Defibrillation, 303–322
atrial fibrillation, 303
clinical considerations, 312
complications, 316–318
convulsive incoordination, 303
electrode polarity, 311
electrode position, 311
electrophysiology, 303–308, 304f, 305f,
306f, 307f, 308f
implantable
for arrhythmia termination in atrial
fibrillation, 479
atrial, 479
internal, 316
role in specific arrhythmias, 312–316
success factors, 308–312
transthoracic impedance, 311, 311t
undulatory stage, 303
waveforms and, 308–310, 309f, 310f,
359
Defibrillator in Acute Myocardial Infarction
Trial (DINAMIT), 207, 881
Defibrillators in Non-Ischemic
Cardiomyopathy Treatment Evaluation
(DEFINITE), 246, 735
DEFINITE. *See* Defibrillators in Non-
Ischemic Cardiomyopathy Treatment
Evaluation
Delayed afterdepolarizations (DADs),
70–72
as cause of arrhythmia, 72
causes and origin of, 71–72, 71f
ionic mechanisms underlying, 72
triggered activity and, 70–71
Deletion, definition, 101
Delta wave, 517, 518f
Deoxyribonucleic acid (DNA)
bases of, definition, 100
definition, 101
Depression, behavioral studies and risk of
cardiac events, 118t
Desmin-related autosomal dominant dilated
cardiomyopathy, 90

DIAMOND. *See* Danish Investigations of Arrhythmia and Mortality on Dofetilide-Myocardial Infarction study
Diastolic bridging, 864
Digitalis
  for arrhythmias in pregnancy, 795
  for atrial flutter, 508
  for atrial tachycardia, 422
  for chronic arrhythmias, 770
  excess, 680, 680f
  induced delayed afterdepolarizations, 71, 71f
  intoxication, 418
  for sinus node
    dysfunction, 659
    dysfunction induction or worsening, 659t
    reentrant tachycardia, 656
Digitoxin (Crystodigin)
  adverse effects, 294
  dosing, 293–294
  drug classification, 273t
  efficacy, 294
  electrophysiology, 294
  pharmacokinetics, 294
Digoxin (Lanoxin, Lanoxicaps). *See also* Clinical studies
  adverse effects, 294
  for antidromic atrioventricular reentrant tachycardia in WPW syndrome, 541
  for arrhythmia prevention, 480
  for arrhythmia termination in atrial fibrillation, 479
  for atrial fibrillation in WPW syndrome, 541
  for atrial flutter, 508
  for atrial tachyarrhythmias, 871
  for atrial tachycardia, 422
  atrioventricular block and, 680
  for atrioventricular nodal reentry tachycardia, 446, 447–448
  clinical use and adverse effects in pregnancy, 794t
  combination therapy for rate control of atrial fibrillation, 471–472, 472f
  for congestive heart failure, 765
  dilated cardiomyopathy and, 729t
  dosing, 293–294
  drug classification, 273t
  efficacy, 294
  electrophysiology, 293
  for heart rate control in atrial fibrillation, 474, 474t
  interaction with immunosuppressive agents, 909t
  for orthodromic atrioventricular reentrant tachycardia in WPW syndrome, 540
  pharmacokinetics, 293
  preoperative use, 834
  prophylaxis
    with β-adrenergic blocking agents, 838
    trials, 836–837, 836t, 837t
  for rate control
    of atrial fibrillation, 471, 872t

    of postoperative atrial arrhythmias, 845t
  for slowing ventricular response rates during atrial fibrillation, 473t
  for sudden cardiac death, 632
  toxicity in atrial tachycardias, 423
  for ventricular rate control during atrial fibrillation, 872t
Dilated cardiomyopathy (DCM), 88–92, 727–735
  actin-related autosomal dominant, 89–90
  arrhythmia mechanisms, 728, 729f, 729t
  arrhythmia therapy, 732–735
    β-adrenergic blockers, 732, 733t
    angiotensin-converting enzyme inhibition, 733–734
    antiarrhythmic drug therapy, 732–733
    implantable cardioverter-defibrillators in heart failure patients with a sustained ventricular tachycardia, 734
    permanent pacemakers, 734
    prophylactic use of the implantable cardioverter-defibrillator, 734–735
    radiofrequency ablation, 733
  atrial arrhythmias in, 728–729
  autosomal dominant
    with conduction defects, 91
    Emery-Dreifuss muscular dystrophy, 91
  with defects of proteins of the nuclear lamina and nuclear envelope, 90–91
  with defects of the cytoskeletal proteins, 89
  desmin-related autosomal dominant, 90
  epidemiology, 728, 728f
  indications for permanent cardiac pacing, 340–341, 340t
  loci associated with, 92
  mitochondrial, 92
  α-myosin heavy chain and Troponin-T related, 90
  predictors of arrhythmia and mortality, 730–732
    clinical predictors, 730, 730f
    electrophysiologic predictors, 730–732, 731f, 731t
  sudden cardiac death in athletes and, 819
  Tafazzin-related Barth syndrome, 91–92
  ventricular arrhythmias in, 729–730
  X-linked, 85
    dystrophin, 89
    Emery-Dreifuss muscular dystrophy, 90–91
Diltiazem (Cardizem)
  adverse effects, 292
  for arrhythmias in pregnancy, 796
  for atrial flutter, 508
  for atrial tachyarrhythmias, 871
  cardiac transplantation and, 915
  as cause of atrioventricular block, 679
  dosing, 292
  drug classification, 273t
  efficacy, 292
  electrophysiology, 292

  for heart rate control in atrial fibrillation, 474t
  interaction with immunosuppressive agents, 909t
  for postoperative atrial fibrillation, 843–844
  for prevention of cardiac transplant vasculopathy, 915
  for prevention of rejection of the transplanted heart, 909
  prophylaxis for atrial fibrillation after CABG, 839
  rate control for postoperative atrial arrhythmias, 845t
  for sinus node
    dysfunction, 659
    induction or worsening, 659t
    reentrant tachycardia, 656
  for slowing ventricular response rates during atrial fibrillation, 473t
  for ventricular rate control during atrial fibrillation, 872t
DINAMIT. *See* Defibrillator in Acute Myocardial Infarction Trial
Dipyridamole, for reperfusion arrhythmias, 876
Direct current cardioversion
  for atrial tachycardia, 422
  to convert atrial flutter to sinus rhythm, 511
  in pregnancy, 797–798
Direct current countershock, for ventricular tachycardia, 867
Disopyramide (Norpace, Norpace CR)
  adverse effects, 276
  for arrhythmias
    in pregnancy, 796
    prevention, 481
  for atrial fibrillation, 726–727
  for atrial flutter, 508, 512
  atrioventricular block and, 680
  for atrioventricular nodal reentry tachycardia, 448
  cardiac transplantation and, 909
  dosing, 276
  drug classification, 273t
  drug trials for treatment of postoperative atrial arrhythmias, 846t
  effect on defibrillator threshold, 376t
  effect on ventricular tachycardia rate, 376t
  efficacy, 276
  electrophysiology, 276
  hemodynamic effects, 271
  pharmacokinetics, 274t, 276
  regimen for postoperative atrial arrhythmias, 847t
  side effects, 845
  for sinus node dysfunction or worsening, 659t
Dissociation
  by default, 684
  incomplete AV, 684
  interference, 683
  isorhythmic, 683
  by usurpation, 684

Diuretics, for sudden cardiac death, 632
Dizziness, syncope and, 938, 939t
DNA. *See* Deoxyribonucleic acid
Dofetilide (Tikosyn). *See also* Clinical
  studies
  adverse effects, 290
  for arrhythmias
    in pregnancy, 797
    prevention, 482
    termination in atrial fibrillation, 478
  for atrial fibrillation in WPW syndrome,
    541
  for atrial flutter, 512
  dosing, 289–290
  drug classification, 273t
  drug trials for treatment of postoperative
    atrial arrhythmias, 846t
  efficacy, 290
  electrophysiology, 289
  frequency dependence, 268
  hemodynamic effects, 271
  pharmacokinetics, 289, 289t
  for postoperative atrial arrhythmias, 847
  regimen for postoperative atrial
    arrhythmias, 847t
  as repolarization-prolonging drug, 273t
  for sustained monomorphic ventricular
    tachycardia, 588
  for Torsade de Pointes, 609, 610–611
Dominant inheritance, definition, 101
Dopamine, for sudden cardiac death, 631
Dressler beat (ventricular capture), 684
Dronedarone, 291
  as repolarization-prolonging drug, 273t
Drugs. *See also* Antiarrhythmic drugs;
  individual drug names
  adverse reactions as complication of
    invasive cardiac electrophysiologic
    studies, 235t
  cardioactive. *See* Cardioactive drugs
  classification of antiarrhythmic drugs,
    272–273, 273t
  toxicity and exercise testing, 185–187,
    186f, 187t
  as trigger for sudden cardiac death,
    626–627
  use dependency, 185
Dry erosion, 352
Dual-chamber pacing, 327–328, 334f, 335f,
  342, 344, 344f, 345f
Duchenne dystrophy, as a cause of sinus
  node dysfunction, 659
Dysautonomias, syncope and, 940
Dysplasia, arrhythmogenic right ventricular,
  591–592, 592f
Dystrophin
  dilated cardiomyopathy and, 89
  X-linked dilated cardiomyopathy, 89

E

EADs. *See* Early afterdepolarizations
Early afterdepolarizations (EADs), 68–70
  as cause of arrhythmia, 70
  characteristics, 68–70
  ionic mechanisms underlying, 70
  origin of, 70

Ebstein's anomaly, 738
  arrhythmias after repair of, 777
  congenital heart disease and, 751–752,
    752f
ECGs. *See* Electrocardiograms
Echocardiography
  for evaluation of syncope, 937
  preparticipation screening for athletes
    and, 822
  transthoracic. *See* Transthoracic
    echocardiography
Effective refractory period (ERP), 38
Eisenmenger syndrome, 761–762
Elderly, primary conduction disease in, 695
Electrical remodeling, 466
Electroanatomic mapping, 248–249
Electrocardiograms (ECGs). *See also* Holter
  monitoring and electrocardiography
  analysis, 152–155, 153f, 154f, 155f, 156f
  for arrhythmia diagnosis, 173–175
  atrial fibrillation and, 464
  atrial tachycardia characteristics of, 416,
    417f
  of atrioventricular node, 682–684
  diagnostic features of atrial flutter,
    506–507, 506f, 507f
  for hypertrophic cardiomyopathy, 722,
    723f
  multifocal atrial tachycardia
    characteristics, 412
  rate and regularity on, 149–150
  for risk assessment, 175–177
  signal-averaged. *See* Signal-averaged
    electrocardiogram
  sinoatrial tachycardia characteristics, 424
  for sustained monomorphic ventricular
    tachycardia, 579–581, 579f, 580f,
    581t
  in Wolff-Parkinson-White syndrome,
    525–539
Electrocardiographic system, 168–169,
  168f, 169f, 170f
  solid-state ECG recording, 169, 171,
    171f
Electrocardiography
  in athletes, 808t, 809t
  atrial activity and, 129–144
    absence of, 129–137, 136f, 137f, 138f
    long RP–short PR relationships in
      tachycardias, 139, 141f,
      142f–143f
    P-wave morphology and axis,
      141–144, 144f
    short RP–long PR relationships in
      tachycardias, 136f, 139, 139f,
      140f
  atrioventricular block during
    supraventricular tachyarrhythmia,
    146–147
    2:1 atrioventricular block, 146–147
    atrioventricular dissociation, 147,
      147f
    variable atrioventricular block, 147
  diagnosis and evaluation of a wide QRS
    complex tachycardia, 150–163
    causes, 150, 150t

  clinical approach to, 150–155, 151t,
    154f, 155f
    criteria for distinguishing between
      tachyarrhythmias, 155–158, 157f
    stepwise approach to, 158f, 159–163,
      159f, 160f, 161f, 162f
  diagnostic interventions, 149, 149f
  for evaluation of syncope, 934–935
  initiation/termination of supraventricular
    tachyarrhythmia, 147–149
    arrhythmia initiation, 147–149, 148f
    termination of the arrhythmia, 149
  limitations, 127, 158
  mechanisms of arrhythmias and,
    127–129, 128f, 129f
  narrow-complex tachycardias and,
    129–150
  QRS morphology, 144–145
    bundle branch block and
      atrioventricular reentrant
      tachycardia, 145, 145f
    bundle branch block and
      supraventricular tachyarrhythmia,
      144
    pseudo-alterations in the QRS
      complex, 144
    QRS alternans, 144
    wide QRS complex not related to
      bundle branch block, 145, 146f
  rate and regularity on the
    electrocardiogram, 149–150
Electrodes
  pacemaker, 324–325
  polarity, 311
  position in defibrillation, 311
Electrograms
  intracardiac, 9–10, 10f
  recording of His-Purkinje disease and,
    703–705, 704f, 705f
Electrolyte disturbances
  etiology, 681
  as trigger for sudden cardiac death,
    626
Electromagnetic interference, pacemakers
  and, 352–353
Electronic surveillance systems, pacemakers
  and, 353
Electrophysiologic Study Versus
  Electrocardiographic Monitoring
  (ESVEM), 166–167, 167f, 231, 241,
  272, 583, 583f
Electrophysiology. *See also* Clinical studies
  action potential and, 37–50
  in athletes, 815–816
  of atrial fibrillation, 464–468, 468f
  of atrioventricular node, 672–677, 672f,
    673f
  cardiac mapping and, 231–262
  of cardioversion and defibrillation,
    303–308, 304f, 305f, 306f, 307f,
    308f
  changes during exercise, 180
  components of basic diagnostic study,
    12t
  of the conduction system, 9–31
  definition, 3

Electrophysiology (*contd.*)
in diagnosis and management of
bradyarrhythmias, 236–237
atrioventricular block and conduction
disturbances evaluation, 236–237
sinus node dysfunction evaluation, 236
in diagnosis and management of
tachyarrhythmias, 237–241
narrow QRS complex tachycardia,
237–240, 238f, 239f, 240f
wide-complex tachycardia, 240–241
equipment, 387f
in evaluating the high-risk patient,
245–246, 246f
of His-Purkinje disease, 703–711, 704f,
705f, 706f, 709f, 710f
indication for and evaluation of
atrioventricular node, 687–688
indications for cardiac studies, 231, 231t
indications for testing His-Purkinje
disease, 712, 712t, 713t
"jump," 673
in management of ventricular
tachyarrhythmias, 241–243
application and protocols, 241–242
ventricular tachycardia in ischemic
heart disease, 242–243
mechanisms of sinoatrial tachycardias,
424–425, 425f
methodology of cardiac studies, 232–234
approach to the patient, 232
baseline cardiac recordings and
analysis, 232–233, 233f, 234f,
234t
equipment and personnel, 232
polymorphous ventricular tachycardia
induced during testing, 613
safety issues in invasive studies, 234, 235t
in syncope of unknown origin, 244–245
testing
in asymptomatic individuals, 528–529
in syncope of unknown origin, 936t
of the transplanted heart, 907–910
for ventricular tachyarrhythmias in
nonischemic cardiac disease,
243–244
ELITE trial, 734
Embolism, as a complication of
defibrillation and cardioversion, 317
Emery-Dreifuss muscular dystrophy
autosomal dominant dilated
cardiomyopathy and, 91
X-linked, 90–91
EMIAT. *See* European Myocardial Infarction
Amiodarone Trial
Enalapril, 734
Encainide
for atrial tachycardia, 422
effect of catecholamine infusion on
efficacy of, 186t
effect on ventricular tachycardia rate,
376t
as trigger for sudden cardiac death, 626
Endless-loop tachycardia, 351, 351f
Endocardial mapping
limitations of, 256–257

noncontact, 249, 250f
Endomyocardial biopsy, for evaluation of
arrhythmogenic right ventricular
cardiomyopathy, 738
Entrainment mapping, 256, 257f, 391, 391f
Environment, sudden cardiac death in
athletes and, 820
Epicardial pacing, 327
bradyarrhythmias and, 855–856
Epinephrine, for sudden cardiac death, 631
ERP. *See* Effective refractory period
Ersentilide, 291
as repolarization-prolonging drug, 273t
Erythromycin, 266
Torsade de Pointes and, 611
Esmolol hydrochloride (Brevibloc)
adverse effects, 282
for arrhythmias in pregnancy, 795
for atrial flutter, 508
for atrial tachyarrhythmias, 871
dosing, 282
drug classification, 273t
efficacy, 282
electrophysiology, 282
for multifocal atrial tachycardia, 413
for orthodromic atrioventricular reentrant
tachycardia in WPW syndrome, 540
pharmacokinetics, 282
rate control for postoperative atrial
arrhythmias, 845t
for slowing ventricular response rates
during atrial fibrillation, 473t
for ventricular rate control during atrial
fibrillation, 872t
ESVEM. *See* Electrophysiologic Study
Versus Electrocardiographic
Monitoring
Ethmozine. *See* Moricizine
European Myocardial Infarction
Amiodarone Trial (EMIAT), 167, 206,
272, 285t, 564, 642, 643f, 877–878,
880f–881f
Excitable gap, 338
Exercise. *See also* Athletes
cardiac transplantation and, 908
hemodynamics and autonomic function in
hypertrophic cardiomyopathy, 725
mitral valve disease and, 899
morphologic cardiac changes with,
806–807, 806f
physiologic changes with, 805–807
as trigger for sudden cardiac death, 627
Exercise testing
for assessment and management of
arrhythmias, 165–194, 179t
chronic intraventricular block and,
701–702
for detection of ventricular
tachyarrhythmias, 775
for evaluation
of QT syndrome, 188
of syncope, 935
of Wolff-Parkinson-White syndrome,
188
incidence of arrhythmia during exercise,
180–182

supraventricular arrhythmia, 182,
182t, 183f
ventricular arrhythmia, 180–182, 180t,
181f
left bundle branch block and, 701–702
for management
of atrial fibrillation, 188, 188f
of supraventricular arrhythmia,
187–188, 188f
of ventricular arrhythmia, 184–187,
184f
catecholamines and antiarrhythmic
drugs, 185, 185f, 186t
exposure of drug-related toxicity
and, 185–187, 186f, 187f
physiologic effects of exercise, 179–180,
179f
biochemical changes, 179
electrophysiologic effects, 180
hemodynamic changes, 180
mechanical effects, 179–180
prognostic significance of ventricular
arrhythmia during, 182–184, 183t
reproducibility of exercise-induced
arrhythmia, 184
role in arrhythmia management,
179–189
safety, 188–189
for sustained monomorphic ventricular
tachycardia, 581, 581f
Exhaustion, behavioral studies and risk of
cardiac events, 118t
Exons, definition, 101
External pacing, 326, 326f, 327f, 328f
Extrastimulation, atrioventricular bypass
tract function during, 525–528, 526f,
527f, 528f, 529f

F
Familial atrial fibrillation, 85t
Familial hypertrophic cardiomyopathy, 85t
Family history
for diagnosis of arrhythmogenic right
ventricular cardiomyopathy, 737t
identification of patients at high risk for
sudden cardiac death, 725, 725t
sudden cardiac death and, 642
Fascicular disease, indications for permanent
cardiac pacing, 337, 337t
FDA. *See* Food and Drug Administration
Felodipine, for arrhythmias in pregnancy,
796
Fetus. *See also* Pregnancy
arrhythmias in, 792–794, 793f, 793t
causes of bradycardia, 793t
causes of tachycardia, 793t
Fibrillation, atrial, 303
Fibroma, 763
Fibrosis, etiology, 679
Figure-of-eight model of reentry, 51–53, 52f
First-degree atrioventricular block, 872,
872f
ECG manifestations, 682
electrophysiological criteria and His-
Purkinje disease, 705–706, 706f
electrophysiologic mechanisms, 684–685

incidence and prevalence, 677
treatment and indications for pacing, 688–689
Flecainide (Tambocor)
adverse effects, 279
for arrhythmias
in pregnancy, 796–797
prevention, 481
termination in atrial fibrillation, 478
for atrial fibrillation in WPW syndrome, 541
for atrial flutter, 512
for atrial tachycardia, 422
for atrioventricular nodal reentry tachycardia, 448
for congestive heart failure, 765
dosing, 278
drug classification, 273t
drug trials for treatment of postoperative atrial arrhythmias, 846t
effect of catecholamine infusion on efficacy of, 186t
effect on defibrillation threshold, 376t
effect on ventricular tachycardia rate, 376t
efficacy, 278–279
electrophysiology, 278
exercise testing and, 187f
frequency dependence, 269
hemodynamic effects, 271
for multifocal atrial tachycardia, 413
for orthodromic atrioventricular reentrant tachycardia in WPW syndrome, 540
pharmacokinetics, 278, 279t
for postoperative atrial arrhythmias, 845
for prevention of postoperative atrial fibrillation, 839, 840t
regimen for postoperative atrial arrhythmias, 847t
for sinus node dysfunction induction or worsening, 659t
as trigger for sudden cardiac death, 626
Fluoxetine (Prozac), metabolism and, 266
Fontan operation
antitachycardia pacing after, 771
incidence of arrhythmias after, 767t
Food and Drug Administration (FDA), approval of implantable cardioverter-defibrillators, 357
Frame (reading frame), definition, 101
Frame shift, definition, 101
Frank-Starling mechanism, 805
Frequency domain, survival curves, 201f
Friedreich's ataxia, as a cause of sinus node dysfunction, 659

G

Gap phenomenon, 30, 30t
classification, 30t
Gate phenomenon, 693
Gender. *See also* Men; Women
atrial fibrillation and, 458, 458t, 459f
exercise testing and, 181
Gene, definition, 101
Gene maps, 92
Genetic linkage

definition, 101
to hypertrophic cardiomyopathy, 721
Genetics
in acquired long QT syndrome, 612
of arrhythmogenic disorders, 81–107
of arrhythmogenic right ventricular cardiomyopathy, 735
in diagnosing, 99–100
electrical disorders associated with ventricular arrhythmias, 93–97
inherited structural abnormalities of the heart, 86–93
Mendelian patterns of inheritance, 81–83, 82f, 83f
molecular, 86–87
nomenclature for genes and chromosomes, 83–85, 84f, 85t
supraventricular arrhythmias and, 98–99
testing, 84f, 99–100
Genomic DNA, definition, 101
Genotype, definition, 101
Genotype-phenotype correlation
hypertrophic cardiomyopathy and, 87–88
of Long QT syndrome, 95
German Pharmacological Intervention in Atrial Fibrillation (PIAF) study, 483
GESICA trial, 176, 176f, 562. *See* Grupo de Estudio de la Sobrevida en la Insuficiencia Cardiac en Argentina trial
GISSI-2 trial, 559
Glasgow program, 215
Global Utilization of Streptokinase and t-PA for Occluded Coronary Arteries (GUSTO-1) trial, 460–461, 703, 871
Glucose-insulin-potassium, for postoperative atrial fibrillation, 842
Goteborg Metoprolol Trial, 113, 114
G protein, 40
Graves disease, as a cause of sinus node dysfunction, 659
Grupo de Estudio de la Sobrevida en la Insuficiencia Cardiac en Argentina (GESICA) trial, 284, 284t, 642–643, 645f, 733
Guanabenz, for sinus node dysfunction induction or worsening, 659t
GUSTO-1. *See* Global Utilization of Streptokinase and t-PA for Occluded Coronary Arteries trial

H

Haloperidol, causing Torsade de Pointes, 611
Heart
anatomy, 384f
of left heart, 522f
comparison of calcium currents in cardiac muscle, 45t
inherited structural abnormalities, 86–93
normal, 574
normal conduction system, 3–4, 4f
structurally abnormal, 574
Heart defects, preoperative incidence of arrhythmias in patients with related congenital heart defects, 750t
Heart disease
congenital, etiology, 681–682

ECG for risk assessment in healthy persons, 176–177
epidemiology in pregnancy, 785
ischemic, electrophysiologic management of, 242–243
predictive value in, 199–203
structural, in pregnancy, 786, 787t
sudden cardiac death and, 624–625
prevention, 642–647
Heart failure. *See also* Clinical studies
risk for nocturnal cardiac events, 119t
sudden cardiac death and, 623
as trigger for sudden cardiac death, 626
Heart rate
acceleration, 614
antiarrhythmic drugs for control of, 473–474
β-adrenergic blocking agents and, 472, 473f, 473t
calcium channel blockers and, 474
cardiac action potential in, 48–49
control with anticoagulation versus rhythm control, 482–483
Heart rate variability. *See* R-R interval variability
Heart surgery. *See* Cardiac surgery
Hemangiosarcoma, 763
Hematoma, as complication of invasive cardiac electrophysiologic studies, 235t
Hemochromatosis, as a cause of sinus node dysfunction, 659
Hemodynamics
changes during exercise, 180
as a complication of defibrillation and cardioversion, 317
Hemopericardium, as complication of invasive cardiac electrophysiologic studies, 235t
Heparin
for atrial tachyarrhythmias, 872
for postoperative atrial fibrillation, 842
for thromboembolic prophylaxis, 487
Heterogeneity, reentry and, 58–65, 58f–59f, 60f, 62f, 63f, 64f, 65f
Heterotaxy syndromes, 759–760
arrhythmia, 760
conduction abnormalities, 759–760
electrocardiographic abnormalities, 759, 759f
His bundle
advanced conduction disease in, 234f
blood supply, 694
branching portion, 694
recording, 704f
His-Purkinje disease
chronic intraventricular block, 701–702
exercise testing and left bundle branch block, 701–702
natural history of conduction abnormalities, 701
prevalence, 701
significance, 701
clinical electrophysiologic manifestations and diagnosis, 703–711
atrioventricular blocks, 705–707, 706f

His-Purkinje disease, (*contd.*) (clinical electrophysiologic manifestations and diagnosis
  bundle branch reentrant sustained ventricular tachycardia, 711
  chronic intraventricular blocks, 707–708
  electrogram recording, 703–705, 704f, 705f
  intraventricular block from acute myocardial infarction, 708–711, 709f, 710f
  pseudoatrioventricular block, 711
  ECG manifestations and diagnosis of intraventricular conduction defects, 696–701, 696f, 697f, 698f, 699f, 700f
  etiology, 694–695
    acute reversible causes, 695
    structural, 694–695
  histologic and electrophysiologic correlation, 712
  indications for electrophysiologic testing, 712, 712t, 713t
  indications for pacing in intraventricular conduction block, 713–714, 713t, 714t
  intraventricular blocks from acute myocardial infarction, 702–703
    acute conduction blocks in the prethrombolytic era, 702–703
    acute conduction blocks with thrombolytic therapy, 703
    non–Q-wave myocardial infarction, 703
  mechanism of, 695–696
His-Purkinje system
  action potentials and, 40–41
  anatomy of the conduction system, 694
  blood supply, 694
  disease of, 693–717
  electrophysiologic properties, 693–694
  retrograde refractory period, 15t
HLHS. *See* Hypoplastic left heart syndrome
Hodgkin-Huxley model, 42
Holiday heart syndrome, 462
Holter monitoring. *See also* Electrocardiograms
  for assessment and management of arrhythmias, 165–194
  ECG for arrhythmia diagnosis, 173–175
  ECG for risk assessment, 175–177
    in cardiomyopathy, 176, 176f
    in coronary heart disease, 175–176
    in healthy persons without heart disease, 176–177
    in symptomatic ventricular tachycardia or ventricular fibrillation, 177
  information derived from, 167–168
    role for arrhythmia assessment, 167
    role for assessment of late potentials, 168
    role for assessment of ST-segment and QT-interval changes, 167–168
  methodology and technology, 168–173

conventional ambulatory electrocardiographic system, 168–169, 168f, 169f, 170f
  implantable loop recorders, 172–173
  in-hospital telemetry, 171
  solid-state ECG recording systems, 169, 171, 171f
  transtelephonic recording devices, 171–172, 173f, 174t
  pathophysiology of cardiac arrhythmias and, 165–167, 166f, 167f
  preparticipation screening for athletes and, 822
  role of, 165–179
  for sustained monomorphic ventricular tachycardia, 581–582
  therapeutic intervention, 177–179
    with antiarrhythmic drug therapy, 177, 178f
    pacemaker evaluation, 177–179
Hot spot, definition, 101
Hydralazine, for sinus node dysfunction, 664
Hyperpolarization-activated action potential, 48
Hypersensitive carotid syndrome, indications for permanent cardiac pacing, 337, 338t
Hypertension, in pregnancy, 791
Hypertrophic cardiomyopathy, 86–88
  arrhythmia mechanism, 723
  cardiac Troponin T, 88
  as a cause of sinus node dysfunction, 659
  clinical characteristics and clinical diagnosis, 86
  clinical management, 86
  electrocardiogram, 722, 723f
  etiology and predisposing factors, 461
  genetics, 721
  genotype-phenotype correlation, 87–88
  molecular genetics, 86–87
  mortality and, 721–722
  myosin-binding protein C mutations, 88
  α-myosin heavy chain mutations, 87–88
  pathology, 721, 722f
  prevalence and inheritance, 86
  prophylactic use of antiarrhythmic agents, 562
  role of programmed electrical stimulation and, 559
  sinus and atrioventricular nodal abnormalities, 723
  sudden cardiac death in athletes and, 816, 818
  supraventricular arrhythmias, 723–724
    atrial fibrillation, 723–724
    electrophysiologic abnormalities, 724
  α-tropomyosin gene mutations, 88
  ventricular arrhythmias, 724–725
    exercise hemodynamics and autonomic function, 725
    significance of nonsustained ventricular tachycardia, 724
    sustained ventricular tachycardia, 724

Hypertrophic obstructive cardiomyopathy, indications for permanent cardiac pacing, 340, 340t
Hypokalemia, dilated cardiomyopathy and, 729
Hypomagnesemia, dilated cardiomyopathy and, 729t
Hypoplastic left heart syndrome (HLHS), 761
Hypothermic cardioplegia, 834
Hysteresis, 350, 350f

I

Ibutilide (Corvert)
  adverse effects, 289
  for arrhythmias
    in pregnancy, 797
    termination in atrial fibrillation, 478
  for atrial flutter, 508
  cardiac transplantation and, 915
  to convert atrial flutter to sinus rhythm, 511
  dosing, 289
  drug classification, 273t
  efficacy, 289
  electrophysiology, 288
  frequency dependence, 269
  pharmacokinetics, 288–289, 289t
  for postoperative atrial arrhythmias, 845, 847
  for pretreatment for cardioversion, 476
  regimen for postoperative atrial arrhythmias, 847t
  as repolarization-prolonging drug, 273t
  for sustained monomorphic ventricular tachycardia, 588
  for Torsade de Pointes, 610
ICDs. *See* Implantable cardioverter-defibrillators
IDCM. *See* Idiopathic dilated cardiomyopathy
Idiopathic dilated cardiomyopathy (IDCM), 243
  prognostic significance of nonsustained ventricular tachycardia and, 557, 557t
  prognostic significance of signal-averaged electrocardiogram and, 560
  sustained monomorphic ventricular tachycardia and, 593–594, 594f
Idiopathic left ventricular hypertrophy, sudden cardiac death in athletes and, 818
Idiopathic ventricular fibrillation, 97, 128f
  sudden cardiac death and, 624
Idiopathic ventricular tachyarrhythmias, 72
Idiopathic ventricular tachycardia, 97, 592–594
  indications, use, and outcomes of catheter ablation, 400–401, 401f
  left posterior fascicular, 593–594, 594f
  in pregnancy, 790–791
  right ventricular outflow tract, 592–593, 593f
Idioventricular rhythms, 72
  accelerated, 573
IMEGs. *See* Intramyocardial electrograms

Impedance mismatch, 521
Implantable atrial defibrillator, 479
    atrial, 378–379
    for sudden cardiac death, 636–640, 638f,
        639f
    for ventricular arrhythmias, 851–852
Implantable cardioverter-defibrillators
    (ICDs), 357–382. *See also* Clinical
    studies
    versus amiodarone, 364
    antiarrhythmic drug interactions,
        375–377, 376t
    antitachycardia pacing, 363–364
    for arrhythmias, 740
    β-adrenergic blocking agents and, 376
    in conditions associated with ventricular
        tachyarrhythmias, 369
    defibrillation waveforms, 359
    detection enhancements, 359–362, 360f,
        361f
    diagnostic storage capabilities, 362–363,
        363t
    dual-chamber devices, 377–378, 377f,
        378f
    features, 358t
    follow-up, 374–375
    future developments, 379
    hardware components, 358–363
    in heart failure patients with a sustained
        ventricular tachyarrhythmia, 734
    in high-risk patients, 367–369
    history of, 357
    implantation techniques and testing of
        ICD function, 370–373, 370f, 371f,
        372f
    indications, use, and outcomes of catheter
        ablation and, 402
    indications for implantation, 364–370,
        365t
    low-energy cardioversion, 364
    manufacturers, 358t
    nonthoracotomy lead (NTL) systems,
        359
    outcome after implantation for secondary
        prevention, 364–367
    pacemaker interactions, 373–375, 373t
    in pregnancy, 798
    for prevention of sudden cardiac death in
        high-risk patients, 643, 646–647,
        646f, 647f
    prophylactic use of, 734–735
    role of cardioversion and defibrillation in,
        314
    for sustained monomorphic ventricular
        tachycardia, 588–589, 589f
    for syncope, 940
    tachycardia termination improvement,
        363–364
Impulse formation
    abnormal automaticity, 67, 67f
    abnormal formation, 66–72
    afterdepolarizations and triggered activity,
        68–72, 69f, 71f
    automaticity as a mechanism of cardiac
        arrhythmias, 67
    normal automaticity, 66–67

parasystole and modulated parasystole,
    67–68, 68f, 69f
Imuran. *See* Azathioprine
Inappropriate sinus tachycardia (IST),
    indications, use, and outcomes of
    catheter ablation, 393
Incessant atrial tachycardia
    electrophysiologic mechanisms, 418
    incidence/prevalence, 415
Incisional atrial reentry, 502
Incisional atrial tachycardia. *See* Atrial
    flutter
Incomplete AV dissociation, 684
Incomplete dominance, definition, 101
Inderal. *See* Propranolol
Inderal-LA. *See* Propranolol
Infections
    as complication of invasive cardiac
        electrophysiologic studies, 235t
    with implantable cardioverter-
        defibrillators, 373
    pacemaker, 351–352
    Staphylococcus aureus, 351
    Staphylococcus epidermis, 351, 373
Infective endocarditis, etiology, 681
Infra-Hisian block, 704, 705f
Insertion, definition, 101
Interference dissociation, 683
International Liaison Committee on
    Resuscitation, recommendations for
    amiodarone as therapy for
    hemodynamically stable ventricular
    tachycardia, 588
International normalized ratio (INR),
    512
International Society of Heart and Lung
    Transplantation (ISHLT), 919
Intraaortic balloon counterpulsation, for
    ventricular arrhythmias, 853
Intraatrial conduction, 16, 16f
Intracardiac pacing, 326
Intracranial hypertension, as a cause of sinus
    node dysfunction, 659
Intramyocardial electrograms (IMEGs), for
    detection of transplant rejection with
    pacemakers, 918–919
Intraventricular block
    acute myocardial infarction and,
        702–703, 708–711, 709f, 710f
Intron-exon boundaries, definition, 101
Ischemia
    acute-phase, 48, 864–865
    α$_1$- and α$_2$-adrenergic receptor blockade
        in preventing, 113–115
    clinical stress testing and, 117–118, 118f,
        118t
    risk for nocturnal cardiac events, 119t
    sustained monomorphic ventricular
        tachycardia and, 576
Ischemic heart disease
    electrophysiologic management of,
        242–243
    etiology, 679
    indications, use, and outcomes of catheter
        ablation for ventricular tachycardia
        in, 401–402

polymorphous ventricular tachycardia
    and, 613
    ventricular arrhythmias and, 863–869
ISHLT. *See* International Society of Heart
    and Lung Transplantation
Isoproterenol
    for atrioventricular nodal reentry
        tachycardia, 445
    for programmed cardiac stimulation,
        234t
Isoptin. *See* Verapamil
Isorhythmic dissociation, 683
Isradipine, for arrhythmias in pregnancy,
    796
IST. *See* Inappropriate sinus tachycardia

J
Jaundice, as a cause of sinus node
    dysfunction, 659
Jervell and Lange-Nielsen syndrome, 85t,
    608
JRT. *See* Junctional reciprocating tachycardia
Junctional escape rhythm, 683
    preoperative incidence of arrhythmias in
        patients with related congenital
        heart defects, 750t
Junctional reciprocating tachycardia (JRT),
    763
Junctional tachycardia
    congenital heart disease and, 764–765,
        766–767, 766f
    permanent form of reciprocating, 765,
        766f

K
Kawasaki disease, sudden cardiac death in
    athletes and, 819
Ketoconazole, 266
    Torsade de Pointes and, 611
Knoten, 433

L
Labetalol, for arrhythmias in pregnancy,
    795
LAFB. *See* Left anterior fascicular block
LAI. *See* Left atrial isomerism
Lange-Nielson syndrome, 185–186
Lanoxicaps. *See* Digoxin
Lanoxin. *See* Digoxin
Late potentials, ECG for assessment of, 168
Lead electrodes, 324–325
    removal, 350, 350t
    system failure, 349–350
Leading circle model of reentry, 53–54,
    53f
Left anterior fascicular block (LAFB), 696,
    697f
Left anterior hemiblock, 874, 874f
Left atrial flutter, 502
Left atrial isomerism (LAI), 759
Left heart syndrome, hypoplastic, 761
Left posterior fascicular block (LPFB),
    696
Left posterior hemiblock, 874
Left superior vena cava, persistent, 762,
    762f

Left ventricular dysfunction. *See also*
Clinical studies
risk stratification of SAECG after,
212–213
in sudden cardiac death, 632
Left Ventricular Dysfunction Prevention
and Treatment Trials (SOLUD), 463
Left ventricular outflow tract obstruction
arrhythmias after repair of, 778
congenital heart defects causing,
754–756, 756f
Lenègre-Lev disease (progressive cardiac
conduction defect), 98–99, 695
Lev disease, 695
Lidocaine hydrochloride (Xylocaine)
adverse effects, 277
for arrhythmias in pregnancy, 796
dosing, 277
drug classification, 273t
effect on defibrillator threshold, 376t
efficacy, 277
electrophysiology, 276
hemodynamic effects, 271
interaction with immunosuppressive
agents, 909t
metabolism, 266
pharmacokinetics, 276–277
for sinus node dysfunction induction or
worsening, 659t
for sudden cardiac death, 631
for sustained monomorphic ventricular
tachycardia, 588
for tachycardia, 152
for treatment of ventricular arrhythmias
during myocardial infarction, 867t
for ventricular arrhythmias, 852–853
for ventricular tachycardia or ventricular
fibrillation in acute myocardial
infarction, 868t
Lifestyle, modification for prevention of
sudden cardiac death, 641–642
Lipid lowering, for prevention of sudden
cardiac death, 641
Lithium, for sinus node dysfunction
induction or worsening, 659t
Locus
associated with dilated cardiomyopathy,
92
definition, 101
Lod (logarithm of odds) score, definition,
101
Lone atrial fibrillation, etiology and
predisposing factors, 460
Long QT syndrome, 61–65, 63f, 64f, 65f,
85t
acquired, 608–612, 609t
β-adrenergic blocking agents and, 94
clinical management, 94
clinical manifestations, 93–94
congenital, 607–608
genetic factors, 607, 607t
in pregnancy, 791
prevalence and clinical presentation,
607–608
sudden cardiac death and, 624–625
drug-induced, 83

genetics
basis of, 94–95
considerations, 612
-specific therapy, 95–96
genotype-phenotype correlation, 95
Jervell and Lange-Nielsen type, 85t
QT dispersion to assess prognosis, 217
quinidine-induced, 552, 553f
risk factors for drug-induced, 611, 611t
risk for nocturnal cardiac events, 119t
Romano-Ward type, 85t
Loop recorders, implantable, 172–173, 174t
Low-molecular-weight heparin, for
thromboembolic prophylaxis, 487
LPFB. *See* Left posterior fascicular block
LPGs. *See* Lysophosphoglycerides
Lupus erythematosus, as a cause of sinus
node dysfunction, 659
Lysophosphoglycerides (LPGs), 864

M

Macrolide antibiotics, for Torsade de
Pointes, 611
MADIT. *See* Multicenter Automatic
Defibrillator Implantation Trial
Magnesium sulfate. *See also* Clinical studies
for polymorphous ventricular tachycardia,
614
for prevention of postoperative atrial
arrhythmias, 840–841, 841t
for sudden cardiac death, 631
Magnetic resonance imaging (MRI)
for evaluation of arrhythmogenic right
ventricular cardiomyopathy, 738,
739f
pacemakers and, 353
Mahaim fiber tachycardia, 145, 146f
Malignant teratomas, 763
Manifest accessory connection, 20
Mapping
activation, 390–391, 390f
atrial
for evaluation of atrial tachycardias,
422
studies, 503
entrainment, 391, 391f
intracardiac, in patients with mitral valve
prolapse, 897–898
pace, 254, 255f, 391
sustained monomorphic ventricular
tachycardia, 584, 586–587, 586f,
587f
Marfan syndrome
preparticipation screening for athletes
and, 821–822
sudden cardiac death in athletes and, 819
Marker, definition, 101
MAT. *See* Multifocal atrial tachycardia
MEANS. *See* Modular ECG analysis system
Mechanical effects, changes during exercise,
179–180
Membrane responsiveness curve, 38
Men. *See also* Gender
risk of development of atrial fibrillation,
459t
sudden cardiac death in athletes and, 820

MERIT-HF. *See* Metoprolol CR/XL
Randomized Intervention Trial in
Congestive Heart Failure
Meta-iodobenzylguanidine scintigraphy, 908
Methylprednisolone, for postoperative atrial
fibrillation, 842
Metoprolol. *See also* Clinical studies
for acute myocardial infarction, 113
for arrhythmias in pregnancy, 795
for congestive heart failure, 114
death rates and mode of death with, 730,
730f
for multifocal atrial tachycardia, 413
for orthodromic atrioventricular reentrant
tachycardia in WPW syndrome, 540
rate control for postoperative atrial
arrhythmias, 845t
for ventricular rate control during atrial
fibrillation, 872t
Metoprolol CR/XL Randomized
Intervention Trial in Congestive Heart
Failure (MERIT-HF), 730, 730f, 732,
733t
Mexiletine (Mexitil)
adverse effects, 278
for arrhythmias in pregnancy, 796
cardiac transplantation and, 909
dosing, 278
drug classification, 273t
effect on defibrillator threshold, 376t
effect on ventricular tachycardia rate,
376t
efficacy, 278
electrophysiology, 278
hemodynamic effects, 271
metabolism, 266
pharmacokinetics, 277t, 278
for sinus node dysfunction induction or
worsening, 659t
Mexitil. *See* Mexiletine
MIRACLE. *See* Multicenter InSync
Randomized Clinical Evaluation
Missense mutation, definition, 101
Mitral stenosis
arrhythmias in, 894–895
arrhythmogenesis in, 899
rate and rhythm control in, 901
Mitral valve disease
arrhythmias in, 889–905
evaluation methods, 899–900
ambulatory ECG, 899
electrophysiologic studies of mitral
valve prolapse, 899–900
exercise, 899
rest, 899
mitral stenosis, 894–895
mitral valve prolapse. *See* Mitral valve
prolapse
mitral valve regurgitation, 893–894,
894f, 894t, 895f
therapeutic modalities and outcome,
900–901
Mitral valve prolapse (MVP), 93, 414–415
arrhythmias
in heterogeneous populations,
891–893, 892f

and substrate in sudden cardiac death, 898–899

arrhythmogenesis and mitral regurgitation, 894f, 897–898

β-adrenergic blocking agents and, 900–901

as a cause of sinus node dysfunction, 659

clinical features, 890

echocardiographic features, 890

effect of mitral valve regurgitation on arrhythmias in, 893–894, 894f, 894t, 895f

electrophysiologic and surgical intervention in, 901

electrophysologic studies of, 899–900

nonarrhythmic complications, 890–891

pharmacologic therapy, 900–901

in pregnancy, 791

prevalence, 889

risk of sudden cardiac death and, 896–897

sudden cardiac death and, 895–896

Mitral valve regurgitation

arrhythmias in, 893, 893f

arrhythmogenesis in mitral valve prolapse and, 897–898

effect on arrhythmias in mitral prolapse, 893–894, 894f, 894t, 895f

sudden cardiac death and, 896

Mobitz type I atrioventricular block, 674f, 677, 699f, 872, 873f

ECG manifestations, 682–683

electrophysiologic mechanisms, 685, 685f

prognostic implications, 687

symptoms, 686

Mobitz type II atrioventricular block, 675f, 677, 700f, 872–873, 873f

ECG manifestations, 683

electrophysiologic mechanisms, 685–686, 686f

prognostic implications, 687

symptoms, 686

Modeling

of action potentials, 40

Hodgkin-Huxley, 42

Modular ECG analysis system (MEANS), 215, 217

Molecular genetics, 86–87

diagnosis in clinically affected individuals, 99

diagnosis in clinically unaffected individuals, 99–100

Molecular structure, of potassium channels, 46–47, 47f

Moricizine (Ethmozine)

adverse effects, 281

for atrial tachycardia, 422

for atrioventricular nodal reentry tachycardia, 448

for congestive heart failure, 765

dosing, 280

drug classification, 273t

effect on defibrillation threshold, 376t

effect on ventricular tachycardia rate, 376t

efficacy, 280–281

electrophysiology, 280

for nonsustained ventricular tachycardia, 561

pharmacokinetics, 279t, 280

for sinus node dysfunction or worsening, 659t

for ventricular premature depolarizations, 561

Mortality

after thrombolysis, 202–203

for anterior and inferior infarctions, 873

causes of in-hospital, 629, 629f

with combined risk factors, 202f

of hypertrophic cardiomyopathy, 721–722

postoperative atrial arrhythmias and, 848

risk factors for sudden cardiac death, 629, 630t

M-PATHY. *See* Multicenter Pacing Therapy for Hypertrophic Cardiomyopathy

MRI. *See* Magnetic resonance imaging

Multicenter Automatic Defibrillator Implantation Trial (MADIT I), 231, 245, 367–368, 565–567, 566f, 643, 646, 646f, 734–735

Multicenter Automatic Defibrillator Implantation Trial (MADIT II), 881

Multicenter InSync Randomized Clinical Evaluation (MIRACLE), 734

Multicenter Pacing Therapy for Hypertrophic Cardiomyopathy (M-PATHY) trial, 340

Multicenter Post Infarction Trial, 176

Multicenter Unsustained Tachycardia Trial (MUSTT), 212, 231, 245, 284, 368–369, 559–560, 646–647, 647f, 734–735, 881, 882f

Multifocal atrial tachycardia (MAT), 411–413, 764

β-adrenergic blocking agents and, 413

definition, 411, 411f

ECG characteristics, 412, 412f

electrophysiologic mechanisms, 412

etiology, 411–412

evaluation methods, 413

incidence/prevalence, 411

physical examination, 412–413

prognostic/clinical significance, 413

symptoms and presentation, 412–413

therapy, 413

Multiple system atrophy, 934

Multiple-wavelet hypothesis, 465–466

Mural tunneled vessels, sudden cardiac death in athletes and, 819

Mustard procedure, 769

antitachycardia pacing after, 771

as a cause of sinus node dysfunction, 659

electrophysiologic testing after, 770, 771f

incidence of arrhythmias after, 767t

sudden cardiac death after, 772

MUSTT. *See* Multicenter Unsustained Tachycardia Trial

MVP. *See* Mitral valve prolapse

Mycophenolate (CellCept), interaction with antiarrhythmic agents, 909t

Myocardial bridging, sudden cardiac death in athletes and, 819

Myocardial dysfunction, as a complication of defibrillation and cardioversion, 318

Myocardial infarction. *See also* Clinical studies

ACC/AHA guidelines for insertion of a permanent pacemaker after myocardial infarction, 875t

acute. *See* Acute myocardial infarction

α-adrenoreceptor blocking agents in, 879t

antiarrhythmic agents for prevention of sudden cardiac death, 642, 643f, 644f

baroreceptor sensitivity and effect on, 203–207

early recovery, 204

late recovery, 204

predictive value, 204–205, 204t, 205f

prognosis assessment, 204t, 205–207, 205f

as complication of invasive cardiac electrophysiologic studies, 235t

controlled behavioral studies of behavioral stress and, 117, 117f

incidence of sustained ventricular arrhythmias or sudden cardiac death after, 877t

management of the high-risk post-infarction patient, 881–883, 882f, 883f

non–Q-wave, 703

predictive value of prognosis after, 199–201, 200f

in pregnancy, 791

prevalence of nonsustained ventricular tachycardia in the late hospital phase, 554, 555t

prognostic significance of signal-averaged electrocardiogram and survivors of, 560

prophylactic use of antiarrhythmic agents, 563–567, 563f, 564f, 565f, 566f

QT dispersion for prognoses, 216–217

risk for nocturnal cardiac events, 119t

risk stratification of SAECG after, 210–211

sudden cardiac death and, 623

Myocardial ischemia

as complication of invasive cardiac electrophysiologic studies, 235t

sudden cardiac death and, 623

syncope and, 932f

as trigger for sudden cardiac death, 626

Myocardial necrosis

as a complication of defibrillation and cardioversion, 318

as complication of invasive cardiac electrophysiologic studies, 235t

Myocarditis

as a cause of sinus node dysfunction, 659

etiology, 681

sudden cardiac death in athletes and, 819

Myocardium, abnormalities and sudden cardiac death, 623–624

Myocytes
atrial, 40
ventricular, 37–39, 37f, 38f
Myosin-binding protein C mutations, 88
Myotonic dystrophy, as a cause of sinus
node dysfunction, 659
Myxedema, as a cause of sinus node
dysfunction, 659
Myxosarcoma, 763

N

Nacetylprocainamide, effect on defibrillator
threshold, 376t
Nadolol
for arrhythmias in pregnancy, 795
prophylaxis trials, 838t
NASPE. *See* North American Society of
Pacing and Electrophysiology
National Institutes of Health (NIH),
electrophysiologic studies, 724
Naxos disease, 92
Neurally mediated syncope
indications for permanent cardiac pacing,
337–338
treatment, 939–940
Neurocardiogenic syncope, 918
Neurologic examination, in sudden cardiac
death, 633
Neurology, disturbances and syncope,
937–938
Nicardipine, for arrhythmias in pregnancy,
796
Nifedipine, for arrhythmias in pregnancy,
796
NIH. *See* National Institutes of Health
Nimodipine, for arrhythmias in pregnancy,
796
Nodal approaches, 5
Nodal conduction, atrial pacing and
decremental atrioventricular, 17–20,
18f, 19f
Nodal tachycardias, circuits in intracardiac
electrograms, 137f
Noncontact endocardial activation cardiac
mapping, 249, 250f
Nonfluoroscopic electroanatomic cardiac
mapping, 248–249
Nonischemic dilated cardiomyopathy, role
of programmed electrical stimulation
and, 559–560
Non–Q-wave infarction, 703
risk for nocturnal cardiac events, 119t
Nonsustained ventricular tachycardia
(NSVT), 549–571, 552f
clinical manifestations, 552–554, 554f
electrocardiographic characteristics,
549–552, 550f, 551f, 552f, 553f
mechanisms, 556–557
prevalence, 554–555, 554t, 555t, 556t
prognostic significance, 557–560
with coronary artery disease, 558–559,
559t
with hypertrohic cardiomyopathy, 557
with nonischemic dilated
cardiomyopathy, 557, 557t, 558f
in a normal population, 557

role of signal-averaged electrocardiogram,
560
role of programmed electrical stimulation
and, 559–560
treatment, 560–567
sudden cardiac death reduction,
561–567
symptom relief, 560–561
Nonthoracotomy lead (NTL) systems, 359
Norepinephrine, for sudden cardiac death,
631
Normal pathway, 17
Norpace. *See* Disopyramide
North American Society of Pacing and
Electrophysiology (NASPE), protocols
for programmed ventricular
stimulation, 241–242
North American Vasovagal Pacemaker
Study, 338
Naxos disease, 85t
NSVT. *See* Nonsustained ventricular
tachycardia
NTL. *See* Nonthoracotomy lead systems
Nuclear ventricular scintigraphy, for
evaluation of arrhythmogenic right
ventricular cardiomyopathy, 738

O

OAVRT. *See* Orthodromic atrioventricular
reentrant tachycardia
Opioid blockers, for sinus node dysfunction
induction or worsening, 659t
Orthodromic atrioventricular reentrant
tachycardia (OAVRT), 129, 130f,
529–533, 530f, 531f, 532f–533f, 534f
β-adrenergic blocking agents and, 540
calcium channel blockers and, 540
circuits in intracardiac electrograms, 137f
pharmacologic therapy for acute,
539–540
pharmacologic therapy for chronic, 540
schematic, 523f
Orthostasis, syncope and, 940
Ouabain, for sinoatrial nodal atrial
tachycardia, 425
Overdrive pacing, 339. *See also* Pacing
for ventricular arrhythmias, 853
for ventricular tachycardia, 867–868
Oxprenolol, for arrhythmias in pregnancy,
795

P

Pacemakers, 323–356. *See also* Clinical
studies
for arrhythmias in pregnancy, 798
for asymptomatic sinus node dysfunction,
659
atrial fibrillation and, 485
bradyarrhythmias and, 854, 854f
codes, 325–326, 325t
dependency, 345
detection of cardiac transplant rejection
with, 918–919
dry erosion and, 352
dysfunction as a complication of
defibrillation and cardioversion, 318

evaluation, 177–179
follow-up evaluation and function
assessment, 345–346, 346f
implantable cardioverter-defibrillator
interactions, 373–375, 373t
implanted antitachycardia for atrial
flutter, 512
lead electrodes for, 324–325
malfunction and complications, 346–350
failure to pace appropriately, 346–347,
346f, 347f, 348f
failure to sense appropriately, 347–349,
349f
lead removal, 350, 350t
lead system failure, 349–350
permanent insertion, 332–333, 333f,
334f, 335f
for prevention of arrhythmias in atrial
fibrillation, 485
"pseudocoupling," 683
pulse generators for, 323–324
for sinus node dysfunction, 664
system performance on follow-up
problems, 350–353
electromagnetic interference, 352–353
hysteresis, 350, 350f
mode switching frequency, 350–351
pacemaker syndrome, 351, 352f
pacemaker system infection, 351–352
proarrhythmic syndromes, 351, 351f
Pacemaker syndrome, 351, 352f
Pace mapping, 254, 255f, 391
Pacing. *See also* Clinical studies
ACC/AHA recommendations for
temporary, 870t
antitachycardia, 363–364
atrial
atrioventricular bypass tract function
during, 525–528, 526f, 527f,
528f, 529f
and decremental atrioventricular nodal
conduction, 17–20, 18f, 19f
decremental atrioventricular nodal
conduction and, 17–20, 18f, 19f
for postoperative atrial fibrillation,
841, 842t
atrioventricular bypass tract function
during, 525–528, 526f, 527f, 528f,
529f
changing ramp, 339
dual-chamber, 342, 344, 344f, 345f
epicardial, bradyarrhythmias and,
855–856
with extrastimuli, 11
fixed-cycle-length, 11, 11f
fixed-rate, 11, 11f
indications for, 688–689
in intraventricular conduction block,
713–714, 713t, 714t
to interrupt atrial flutter, 509–510, 509f,
510f
mode switching, 344–345
overdrive, 339
permanent
implantation, 332–353
indications for, 333–341

precipitation of inadvertent and deliberate atrial fibrillation, 510–511, 510f
for prevention of postoperative atrial fibrillation, 841, 842t
protocols and programmed electrical stimulation, 10–12, 11f, 12t
rate-adaptive, 344
resynchronization therapy, 340–341, 340t
single-chamber, 341–342, 343f
syncope and, 940
system selection, 341–345, 342f, 343f, 343t, 344f
temporary, 326–332
    atrial and dual-chamber, 327–328
    epicardial, 327
    external, 326, 326f, 327f, 328f
    indications for, 328–332
    intracardiac, 326
    for a reversible condition, 331–332
    transesophageal, 326–327, 329f
tiered therapy, 339
in the transplanted heart, 913–914
for ventricular arrhythmias, 853
for ventricular tachycardia, 867–868
Pacing in Cardiomyopathy (PIC) study, 340
Pacing Therapies for Congestive Heart Failure (PATH-CHF) study, 341
Pain, as complication of invasive cardiac electrophysiologic studies, 235t
Parasympathetic nervous system, atrial fibrillation and, 468
Parasystole
abnormal impulse formation and, 67–68, 68f, 69f
modulated, 68, 68f
Parietal block, 696
Paroxetine (Paxil), metabolism, 266
Paroxysmal atrial tachycardia with block
definition, 413–414
electrophysiologic mechanisms, 418
etiology, 416
incidence/prevalence, 415–416
Paroxysmal supraventricular tachycardia (PSVT), 433. *See also* Atrioventricular nodal reentrant tachycardia
preoperative incidence of arrhythmias in patients with related congenital heart defects, 750t
surgical treatment of, 385–386
Paroxysmal sustained atrial tachycardia
electrophysiologic mechanisms, 417–418, 418f
incidence/prevalence, 415
Patent ductus arteriosus (PDA), 753–754
PATH-CHF. *See* Pacing Therapies for Congestive Heart Failure
Pathlength, 52
Paxil. *See* Paroxetine
PDA. *See* Patent ductus arteriosus
Pealing back of refractoriness, 15–16
Penetrance, definition, 101
Perforation, as complication of invasive cardiac electrophysiologic studies, 235t
Pericarditis
after cardiac surgery, 836

as a cause of sinus node dysfunction, 659
as complication of invasive cardiac electrophysiologic studies, 235t
Periinfarction arrhythmias, 863–888
atrial arrhythmias, 869–872
conduction disturbances, 872–875
management of the high-risk post-myocardial infarction patient, 881–883
reperfusion arrhythmias, 875–876
risk stratification, 876–881
ventricular arrhythmias, 863–869
Permanent junctional reciprocating tachycardia (PJRT), 533–534, 535f
Persistent left superior vena cava, 762, 762f
PES. *See* Programmed electrical stimulation
PET. *See* Positron emission tomography
Pharmacologic agents
for atrial tachycardias, 422
effect on atrial tachycardias, 419
Phase 3 block, 711
Phase 4 block, 711
Phase 2 reentry, 58
Phenothiazines, for sinus node dysfunction or worsening, 659t
Phenotype, definition, 101
Phenytoin, 266
effect on defibrillator threshold, 376t
for sinus node dysfunction induction or worsening, 659t
Pheochromocytoma, as a cause of sinus node dysfunction, 659
Phobias, behavioral studies and risk of cardiac events, 118t
Phosphate, for sudden cardiac death, 631
Phosphodiesterase inhibitors, dilated cardiomyopathy and, 729t
Phrenic nerve, paralysis as complication of invasive cardiac electrophysiologic studies, 235t
PIC. *See* Pacing in Cardiomyopathy study
Pinacidil, effect on reuptake of calcium, 72
Pindolol
for arrhythmias in pregnancy, 795
for sinus node dysfunction, 659
PJRT. *See* Permanent junctional reciprocating tachycardia
PM. *See* Purkinje-myocardial junction
Point mutation, definition, 102
Polymerase chain reaction, definition, 102
Polymorphic ventricular tachycardia, 916–917, 917f
Polymorphism, definition, 102
Polymorphous ventricular tachycardia, 573, 603–619
definition, 603
electrocardiographic characteristics, 603–605, 604f
electrophysiologic mechanisms, 603
associated with prolonged repolarization, 605–607
induced during electrophysiologic testing, 613
induction of sustained, 615f
initiating sequences of Torsade de Pointes, 603–604, 604f

ionic mechanisms and, 605–606
rate-dependence of Torsade de Pointes, 603
sympathetic imbalance, 607
therapy, 613–614
with triple vessel coronary artery disease, 616f
T-wave alternans and, 604, 605f
Population-based studies, 217
Positron emission tomography (PET), 908
Posterior pericardiotomy, for postoperative atrial fibrillation, 842
Postural orthostatic tachycardia syndrome (POTS), 393
Potassium channel blocking agents, for Torsade de Pointes, 609
Potassium channels
action potentials and, 46–48–46t, 47f
characteristics of, 46f
comparison of properties of delayed rectifier currents, 46t
molecular basis of, 46–47, 47f
β subunits, 47–48
structure, 47f
POTS. *See* Postural orthostatic tachycardia syndrome
Preexcitation
cardiac mapping, 249–252, 250f, 251f
conduction system and, 20–21
epidemiology of, 522
Preexcitation syndromes, 98, 541
indications, use, and outcomes of catheter ablation, 396–398, 397f
Pregnancy. *See also* Fetus
arrhythmias and conduction disturbances associated with, 785–803
asymptomatic arrhythmias and conduction defects in, 786, 787
AV conduction disturbances, 792
complete heart block, 792
second-degree AV block, 792
calcium channel blockers and, 796
epidemiology of heart disease and, 785
fetal arrhythmias, 792–794, 793f, 793t
hemodynamic and electrocardiographic changes in normal, 785–786, 786t
nonpharmacologic therapy of arrhythmias, 797–798
cardiac arrhythmia surgery, 798
cardiopulmonary resuscitation, 797
direct current cardioversion, 797–798
implantable cardioverter-defibrillator, 798
radiofrequency catheter ablation, 798
pharmacologic therapy of arrhythmias, 794–797, 794t, 795t
adenosine, 794–795
α-adrenoreceptor antagonists, 795
calcium channel antagonists, 796
class I antiarrhythmic agents, 796–797
class III antiarrhythmic agents, 797
digitalis, 795
general considerations, 794, 794t, 795t
in the presence of structural heart disease, 786, 787t

Pregnancy (*contd.*)
  supraventricular tachycardias and,
      788–790
    atrial fibrillation, 790
    atrial flutter, 790
    atrial tachycardias, 788
    AV nodal reentrant tachycardia, 788,
        789f
    AV reciprocating tachycardia,
        788–790, 790f
    mechanisms and classification, 788
    natural history, 788
  ventricular tachycardias and, 790–791
    from adverse effects of medication, 791
    in cardiomyopathy, 791
    in congenital heart disease, 791
    in congenital long QT syndrome, 791
    definition, 790
    in hypertension, 791
    idiopathic, 790–791
    from metabolic derangement, 791
    in mitral valve prolapse, 791
    with myocardial infarction, 791
Premature ventricular complexes (PVCs), 851
    treatment, 867, 867t
    ventricular arrhythmias and, 865–866
Pressor agents, for sudden cardiac death,
    631
PRIDE. *See* Primary Implantation
    Cardioverter-Defibrillator trial
Primary electrical abnormality, as
    predisposing factor to atrial fibrillation,
    462–463
Primary electrical disease. *See* Idiopathic
    ventricular fibrillation
Primary Implantation Cardioverter-
    Defibrillator (PRIDE) trial, 735
Prinzmetal angina, risk for nocturnal cardiac
    events, 119t
Proarrhythmia, 269–271
    atrial, 271
    as complication of invasive cardiac
        electrophysiologic studies, 235t
    ventricular, 269–271
Proarrhythmic syndromes, 351, 351f
Procainamide (Procan-SR, Pronestyl-SR,
    Procanbid)
    adverse effects, 275–276
    for antidromic atrioventricular reentrant
        tachycardia in WPW syndrome, 541
    for arrhythmias
      in pregnancy, 796
      prevention, 481
      termination of atrial fibrillation, 478
    for atrial fibrillation in WPW syndrome,
        541
    for atrial flutter, 508, 512
    for atrial tachyarrhythmias, 871
    atrioventricular block and, 680
    for atrioventricular nodal reentry
        tachycardia, 448
    cardiac transplantation and, 909, 915
    dosing, 275
    drug classification, 273t
    drug trials for treatment of postoperative
        atrial arrhythmias, 846t

effect of catecholamine infusion on
    efficacy of, 186t
effect on defibrillator threshold, 376t
effect on ventricular tachycardia rate,
    376t
efficacy, 275
electrophysiology, 275
hemodynamic effects, 271
for orthodromic atrioventricular reentrant
    tachycardia in WPW syndrome, 540
pharmacokinetics, 274t, 275
for postoperative atrial arrhythmias, 845,
    847
for prevention of postoperative atrial
    fibrillation, 839, 840t
regimen for postoperative atrial
    arrhythmias, 847t
for sinus node dysfunction induction or
    worsening, 659t
for sudden cardiac death, 631
for sustained monomorphic ventricular
    tachycardia, 588
for treatment of ventricular arrhythmias
    during myocardial infarction, 867t
for ventricular tachycardia or ventricular
    fibrillation in acute myocardial
    infarction, 868t
Procanbid. *See* Procainamide
Procan-SR. *See* Procainamide
Prograf. *See* Tacrolimus
Programmed electrical stimulation (PES),
    10–12, 11f, 12t
    with nonsustained ventricular
        tachycardia, 559
    ventricular, 725–726
Progressive cardiac conduction defect
    (Lenègre-Lev disease), 98–99
Progressive familial heart block type I, 85t
Pronestyl-SR. *See* Procainamide
Propafenone (Rythmol)
    adverse effects, 280
    for arrhythmia
      prevention, 481
    for arrhythmias
      in pregnancy, 796–797
      termination in atrial fibrillation, 478
    for atrial fibrillation, 726–727
      in WPW syndrome, 541
    for atrial flutter, 512
    for atrioventricular nodal reentry
        tachycardia, 448
    cardiac transplantation and, 915
    for congestive heart failure, 765
    dosing, 280
    drug classification, 273t
    drug trials for treatment of postoperative
        atrial arrhythmias, 846t
    effect on defibrillation threshold, 376t
    effect on ventricular tachycardia rate,
        376t
    efficacy, 280
    electrophysiology, 279
    exercise testing and, 184, 184f
    frequency dependence, 269
    interaction with immunosuppressive
        agents, 909t

for orthodromic atrioventricular reentrant
    tachycardia in WPW syndrome, 540
pharmacokinetics, 279–280, 279t
for postoperative atrial arrhythmias, 845,
    847
for prevention of postoperative atrial
    fibrillation, 839, 840t
regimen for postoperative atrial
    arrhythmias, 847t
for sinus node dysfunction induction or
    worsening, 659t
Propranolol (Inderal, Inderal-LA)
    adverse effects, 281–282
    for arrhythmias in pregnancy, 795
    for atrioventricular nodal reentry
        tachycardia, 447
    cardiac transplantation and, 908
    dosing, 281
    drug classification, 273t
    effect on defibrillator threshold, 376t
    efficacy, 281
    electrophysiology, 281
    for orthodromic atrioventricular reentrant
        tachycardia in WPW syndrome, 540
    pharmacokinetics, 281
    prophylaxis trials, 837t, 838t
    rate control for postoperative atrial
        arrhythmias, 845t
    for ventricular rate control during atrial
        fibrillation, 872t
Proximal heart block, 687–688
Prozac. *See* Fluoxetine
Pseudoatrioventricular block, His-Purkinje
    disease and, 711
Pseudo-preexcitation, 761
Pseudo-supernormal conduction, 30–31,
    31f
PSVT. *See* Paroxysmal supraventricular
    tachycardia
Psychoactive drugs, for Torsade de Pointes,
    611
Psychosocial stress, as trigger for sudden
    cardiac death, 627–628
Pulmonary stenosis, incidence of
    arrhythmias after repair of, 767t
Pulmonary thromboembolism, as
    complication of invasive cardiac
    electrophysiologic studies, 235t
Pulmonary valve stenosis, 752, 753f
    arrhythmias after repair of, 777
Pulmonary vein stenosis, as complication of
    invasive cardiac electrophysiologic
    studies, 235t
Pulse generators, 323–324
Purkinje-myocardial (PM) junction, 40
PVCs. *See* Premature ventricular complexes
P-wave morphology, axis and, 141–144,
    144f

Q
QRS complex, 158
    atrial flutter and, 507
    electrophysiologic diagnosis and
        management, 237–240, 238f, 239f,
        240f
    tachycardia, 438, 439f

QRS morphology, 144–145
  bundle branch block and atrioventricular
    reentrant tachycardia, 145, 145f
  bundle branch block and supraventricular
    tachyarrhythmia, 144
  pseudo-alterations in the QRS complex,
    144
  QRS alternans, 144
  wide QRS complex not related to bundle
    branch block, 145, 146f
QRS tachycardia, wide complex
  causes, 150, 150t
  clinical approach to, 150–155, 151t,
    154f, 155f
  criteria for distinguishing between
    tachyarrhythmias, 155–158, 157f
  diagnosis and evaluation, 150–163
  stepwise approach to, 158f, 159–163,
    159f, 160f, 161f, 162f
QT dispersion, 213–218, 732
  to assess prognosis after myocardial
    infarction, 216–217
  automated software packages, 215
  long QT syndrome and, 217
  measurement methods, 214–216, 215f
  physiologic basis, 213–214
  predictive value of, 216
  to predict mortality in population-based
    studies, 217, 218f
QT Guard program, 215
QT-interval changes, ECG for assessment
  of, 167–168
QT syndrome
  exercise testing for evaluation of, 188
  syncope and, 939
Quality-of-life scores, in atrial fibrillation,
  475f
Quinaglute. *See* Quinidine
Quinidex. *See* Quinidine
Quinidine (Quinidex, Quinaglute,
    Cardioquin)
  adverse effects, 274–275
  for arrhythmias
    in pregnancy, 796
    prevention, 481
    termination in atrial fibrillation,
      477
  for atrial flutter, 512
  atrioventricular block and, 680
  for atrioventricular nodal reentry
    tachycardia, 448
  cardiac transplantation and, 909, 915
  dosing, 274
  drug classification, 273t
  drug trials for treatment of postoperative
    atrial arrhythmias, 846t
  effect of catecholamine infusion on
    efficacy of, 186t
  effect on defibrillator threshold, 376t
  effect on ventricular tachycardia rate,
    376t
  efficacy, 274
  electrophysiology, 273–274
  hemodynamic effects, 271
  induced long QT syndrome, 552,
    553f

interaction with immunosuppressive
    agents, 909t
  metabolism, 266
  pharmacokinetics, 274, 274t
  postoperative atrial arrhythmias and, 845
  for prevention of postoperative atrial
    fibrillation, 839
  for prolonged repolarization, 72
  regimen for postoperative atrial
    arrhythmias, 847t
  for sinus node dysfunction induction or
    worsening, 659t
  for Torsade de Pointes, 609
Quinidine syncope, 609

R
RACE. *See* Rate Control versus Electrical
    cardioversion study
Radiation skin burns, as complication of
    invasive cardiac electrophysiologic
    studies, 235t
Radiofrequency catheter ablation. *See also*
    Ablation therapy, Catheter ablation;
    Cryoablation
  for atrioventricular nodal reentry
    tachycardia, 451–453
  cardiac transplantation and, 915
  "cocktail" treatment, 543
  for dilated cardiomyopathy, 733
  in pregnancy, 798
  for sustained monomorphic ventricular
    tachycardia, 589–590, 589f
  for ventricular tachyarrhythmias,
    776–777
  for Wolff-Parkinson-White syndrome,
    542, 543f
RAI. *See* Right atrial isomerism
Rapamycin, for prevention of rejection of
    the transplanted heart, 909
Rate-adaptive pacing, 344
Rate Control versus Electrical cardioversion
    (RACE) study, 483
Reading frame, definition, 101
Receptor physiology, of antiarrhythmic
    agents, 266–271
Recording systems
  solid-state ECG, 169, 171, 171f
  transtelephonic, 171–172, 173f, 174t
Reentry, 51–66
  atrioventricular node, 148f
  as a cause of ventricular
    tachyarrhythmias, 864–865
  circuits in intracardiac electrograms, 137f
  circus movement, 51–56, 52f, 53f, 54f,
    55f
  evaluation of atrial tachycardia caused by,
    420, 420f, 421f
  fascicular tachycardia, 591
  incisional atrial, 502
  phase 2, 58
  reflection, 56–58, 56f, 57f
  role of heterogeneity, 58–65, 58f–59f,
    60f, 62f, 63f, 64f, 65f
  sinus node, 655–656, 656f, 657f
  slow or delayed conduction, 65–66
Reflection, reentry and, 56–58, 56f, 57f

Refractory periods, 14–16, 15f, 324
  definition, 15t
  effective, 14, 15f
  functional, 14–15, 15f
  peeling back, 15–16
  relative, 14
Regulatory sequence, definition, 102
Reperfusion, SAECG after, 211–212, 211f
Reperfusion arrhythmias, 875–876
Repolarization
  in athletes, 813–815
  reserve, 611
Reserpine, for sinus node dysfunction
    induction or worsening, 659t
Resting membrane potential, 863–864
Resuscitation. *See also* Cardiopulmonary
    resuscitation
  of noncardiac sudden death patients,
    628–629
  outcome in sudden cardiac death,
    628–629, 628t
Resynchronization therapy, 340–341, 340t
Retrograde conduction
  normal ventriculoatrial, 22–26, 23f, 24f,
    25f, 26f, 27f
  refractoriness assessment, 21–28
  using accessory ventriculoatrial
    connections, 27–28, 27f, 28f
Reverse typical atrial flutter, 502, 502f
Rhabdomyomas, 763
Rheumatic heart disease
  etiology and predisposing factors, 461
  risk of development of atrial fibrillation,
    459t
Rhythms, idioventricular, 72
Rifampin, 266
Right atrial isomerism (RAI), 759
Right bundle branch block, 874
Right ventricular cardiomyopathy, 92–93
Right ventricular dysplasia, in athletes, 818
Ring model of reentry, 51–53, 52f
RK506. *See* Tacrolimus
Romano-Ward syndrome, 85t, 93–96,
    185–186, 608
R on T phenomenon, 551, 551f
R-R interval variability, 195–207
  baroreceptor sensitivity and effect of
    myocardial infarction on, 203–207
    early recovery, 204
    late recovery, 204
    predictive value, 204–205, 204t, 205f
    prognosis assessment, 205–207, 206f,
      207f
  methodology, 196–199
    day-to-day reproducibility, 199
    physiologic sequence of standard
      frequency bands, 198–199, 199t
    spectral analysis, 197–198, 197f
    time domain analysis, 196–197, 196t
  physiologic basis for arrhythmia
    assessment, 195–196
  predictive value in heart disease,
    199–203
    of arrhythmic events, 202, 202f
    to assess prognosis after myocardial
      infarction, 199–201, 200f

R-R interval variability predictive value in heart disease (*contd.*)
of death and arrhythmic events after thrombolysis, 202–203
short-term measures, 201–202
survival curves, 200f
Ryanodine, effect on reuptake of calcium, 72
Rythmol. *See* Propafenone

S
SA. *See* Sinoatrial node
SACT. *See* Sinoatrial conduction time
SAECG. *See* Signal-averaged electrocardiogram
Sarcoidosis, sudden cardiac death in athletes and, 820
Scarred myocardial bruising, sudden cardiac death in athletes and, 819–820
SCD-HeFT. Sudden Cardiac Death–Heart Failure Trial. *See* Sudden cardiac death
Scintigraphy, meta-iodobenzylguanidine, 908
Sclerosis, etiology, 679
Scroll wave reentry, 55, 55f
Sea anemone toxin (ATXII), 606
Seattle Heart Watch program, 629
Second-degree atrioventricular block, 699f, 872–873, 873f
ECG manifestations, 682–683
electrophysiologic criteria and His-Purkinje disease, 706, 706f
electrophysiologic mechanisms, 685–686, 685f, 686f
incidence and prevalence, 677
in pregnancy, 792
treatment and indications for pacing, 689
Sectral. *See* Acebutolol
Sedative-hypnotic agents, for sustained monomorphic ventricular tachycardia, 588
Sematilide, frequency dependence, 268
Senning operation, 769
antitachycardia pacing after, 771
incidence of arrhythmias after, 767t
sudden cardiac death after, 772
Sensing threshold, 324, 345
Sepsis, as complication of invasive cardiac electrophysiologic studies, 235t
Serotonin uptake inhibitors, metabolism, 266
Short bursts of arrhythmia
electrophysiologic mechanisms, 417
etiology, 416
incidence/prevalence, 414–415
Shy-Drager syndrome, 934
Sicilian Gambit, 272
Sick sinus syndrome (SSS), 98, 656–664
diagnostic evaluation, 660–663, 661f, 662f, 663f
etiology and predisposing factors, 461, 659–660
indications for permanent pacing, 333
pathophysiology, 659–660
prevalence, 658

recognition, 656–658, 657f, 658f, 659f
significance, 658–659, 659t
therapy, 663–664
SIDS. *See* Sudden infant death syndrome
Signal-averaged electrocardiogram (SAECG), 208–213
for arrhythmogenic right ventricular cardiomyopathy, 737
clinical applications, 210–213
for evaluation of syncope, 935
interpretation and classification criteria, 208, 209, 209t
pathophysiology, 210, 210f
preparticipation screening for athletes and, 822
risk stratification
after myocardial infarction, 210–211
in patients with left ventricular dysfunction, 212–213
sustained monomorphic ventricular tachycardia, 581
technical aspects, 208–209, 208f
unexplained syncope, 213
use after reperfusion, 211–212, 211f
Single-catheter cardiac mapping, 248
Single-chamber pacing, 341–342, 343f
Sinoatrial conduction time (SACT), 13, 13f, 236, 662, 662f
Sinoatrial nodal tachycardia
βα-adrenergic blocking agents and, 425
calcium channel blockers and, 425
Sinoatrial node (SA)
cells, 39–40
functional evaluation, 13, 13f
Sinoatrial tachycardias, 423–426
definition, 423
ECG characteristics, 424
electrophysiologic mechanisms, 424–425, 425f
etiology, 424
evaluation methods, 425
physical examination, 425
prevalence, 423–424
prognostic/clinical significance, 425
symptoms and presentation, 425
therapy, 425–426, 426f
Sinus arrhythmia, 549–550, 550f, 653–654, 654f
Sinus bradycardia, 655
atrial arrhythmias and, 869, 869t, 870t
preoperative incidence of arrhythmias in patients with related congenital heart defects, 750t
theophylline after transplantation, 856
Sinus node
cardiac transplantation and, 910–912, 911f, 913t
dysfunction, 653–670
definitions, 910, 911f
evaluation, 236
electrophysiologic testing for evaluation of syncope, 935
function, 653–670
in athletes, 807, 810
indications for permanent cardiac pacing, 333, 335, 335t

reentry, 655–656, 656f, 657f
sick sinus syndrome, 656–664
diagnostic evaluation, 660–663, 661f, 662f, 663f
etiology and pathophysiology, 659–660
prevalence, 658
recognition, 656–658, 657f, 658f, 659f
significance, 658–659, 659t
therapy, 663–664
sinus rhythm, 653–655
normal, 653
sinus arrhythmia, 653–654, 654f
sinus bradycardia, 655
sinus tachycardia, 654–655
Sinus node recovery time (SNRT), 13, 13f, 236
Sinus rhythm
atrioventricular bypass tract function during, 525–528, 526f, 527f, 528f, 529f
normal, 653
Sinus tachycardia, 654–655
atrial arrhythmias and, 869–870
shock therapy for, 360, 360f
Sleep, cardiac risk and, 119–120, 119t
SNRT. *See* Sinus node recovery time
Sodium channel blocking agents
for atrioventricular nodal reentry tachycardia, 448
for Torsade de Pointes, 609
Sodium current
action potentials and, 42–45, 43f
auxiliary β-subunit modulation, 43–44
calcium channels and, 45, 45t
sodium channel regulation by second messengers, 44
SOLVD. *See* Studies of Left Ventricular Dysfunction
Sotalol (Betapace). *See also* Clinical studies
adverse effects, 288
for arrhythmias, 740
in pregnancy, 797
prevention, 481–482
termination of atrial fibrillation, 479
for atrial fibrillation in WPW syndrome, 541
for atrial flutter, 512
for congestive heart failure, 765
dosing, 288
drug classification, 273t
drug trials for treatment of postoperative atrial arrhythmias, 846t
effect on defibrillation threshold, 376t
effect on ventricular tachycardia rate, 376t
efficacy, 288
electrophysiology, 287–288
frequency dependence, 269
for heart rate control in atrial fibrillation, 474
hemodynamic effects, 271
interaction with ICDs, 376
for long-term therapy of the sudden cardiac death survivor, 634, 635f

pharmacokinetics, 287t, 288
for postoperative atrial arrhythmias,
845
for prevention of postoperative atrial
fibrillation, 839, 840t
regimen for postoperative atrial
arrhythmias, 847t
as repolarization-prolonging drug, 273t
for sinus node dysfunction or worsening,
659t
for sustained monomorphic ventricular
tachycardia, 588
for Torsade de Pointes, 609–610
SPAF. *See* Stroke Prevention in Atrial
Fibrillation study
Spiral wave reentry, 54–56, 55f
Sports. *See* Athletes
SPRINT study group, 703
SSS. *See* Sick sinus syndrome
Staphylococcus aureus, 351
Staphylococcus epidermis, 351, 373
Steroids, for postoperative atrial fibrillation,
842
Stimulation threshold, 324–325
Streptokinase, 460–461, 703, 871
Stress. *See also* Clinical studies
behavioral studies and risk of cardiac
events, 118t
as trigger for sudden cardiac death,
627–628
ventricular arrhythmias and, 115, 115f
Stroke. *See also* Clinical studies
atrial fibrillation and, 463–464
as complication of invasive cardiac
electrophysiologic studies, 235t
postoperative, 848–849
therapy for prevention of, 486–487
Stroke Prevention in Atrial Fibrillation
(SPAF) study, 732–733
Strong Heart Study, 217
ST-segment
changes as a complication of
defibrillation and cardioversion,
317, 317f
ECG for assessment of, 167–168
Studies of Left Ventricular Dysfunction
(SOLVD), 734
Sudden cardiac death. *See also* Clinical
studies
Sudden Cardiac Death–Heart Failure Trial
(SCD-HeFT), 246, 368, 735
Sudden cardiac death (SCD), 621–652
after the Mustard procedure, 772
after the Senning operation, 772
arrhythmia and substrate in mitral valve
prolapse and, 898–899
arrhythmic mechanism of, 621–623, 622f
arrhythmogenic right ventricular
dysplasia and, 818
atherosclerotic coronary artery disease
and, 819
in athletes, 815–821
cardiac transplantation and, 917
cardiovascular structural disease and,
816–820, 817t
causes, 623–625, 623t

absence of structural heart disease,
624–625
Brugada syndrome, 624
commotio cordis, 624
conduction system abnormalities,
624–625
congenital long QT syndrome,
624–625
heart failure, 623
myocardial abnormalities, 623–624
myocardial ischemia and infarction,
623
clinical risk factors for, 625–626, 625f
complex arrhythmias in mitral
regurgitation, 896
congenital heart disease in athletes and,
818
definitions, 621, 815
electrophysiologic basis, 815–816
environment and, 820
evaluation and management, 630–633,
630t
arrhythmia evaluation, 633
cardiac resuscitation, 630–632, 631f
patient evaluation, 632–633, 633f
exposure to toxins and, 820–821
familial form, 624
hypertrophic cardiomyopathy and, 816,
818
identification of patients at high risk for,
725–726, 725t
idiopathic left ventricular hypertrophy
and, 818
incidence, 621, 622f
of sustained ventricular arrhythmias or
sudden cardiac death after
myocardial infarction, 877t
long-term therapy of the survivor,
634–640
nonpharmacologic therapy, 635–640
arrhythmic surgery, 635
catheter ablation, 635–636, 636f
implantable defibrillator, 636–640,
638f, 639f
pharmacologic therapy, 634, 634f,
635f
myocarditis and, 819
pathophysiologic basis, 816–821, 816t
preoperative incidence of arrhythmias in
patients with related congenital
heart defects, 750t
prevalence in athletes, 815
prevention in patients with heart disease,
642–647, 727, 727f
amiodarone in congestive heart failure,
642–643, 645f
antiarrhythmic agents after myocardial
infarction, 642, 643f, 644f
prevention in the general population,
640–642, 640f
antihypertensive therapy, 641
family history and, 642
implantable cardioverter-defibrillators
in high-risk patients, 643,
646–647, 646f, 647f
lifestyle modification, 641–642

lipid lowering, 641
primary electrophysiologic conditions,
820
prognostic significance of arrhythmia in
mitral valve prolapse, 895–896
reduction in, 561–567
resuscitation outcome, 628–629, 628t
causes of in-hospital mortality, 629,
629f
factors related to, 629
of noncardiac sudden death,
628–629
risk factors for mortality, 629, 630t
risk in mitral valve prolapse populations,
896–897
syncope as risk factor for, 725t
triggers for, 626–628, 627f
drugs, 626–627
electrolyte disturbances, 626
exercise, 627
heart failure and myocardial ischemia,
626
psychosocial stress, 627–628
valvular heart disease and, 818–819
Sudden infant death syndrome (SIDS), risk
for nocturnal cardiac events, 119t
Sudden unexplained nocturnal death
(SUNDS), risk for nocturnal cardiac
events, 119t
SUNDS. *See* Sudden unexplained nocturnal
death
Supernormal conduction, 30–31, 31f
Supernormal period, 38
Superoxide dismutase, for reperfusion
arrhythmias, 876
Supraventricular arrhythmias, 98–99
in athletes, 810–813, 811f, 812f–813f,
814f, 824t
2:1 block, 143f
diagnostic value of tracings, 139f
exercise testing for management of,
187–188, 188f
incidence during exercise, 182, 182t,
183f
Supraventricular tachyarrhythmias
(SVTs)
arrhythmia
initiation, 147–149, 148f
termination, 149
cardiac transplantation and, 914–916
incessant, 150
premature ventricular contraction during,
150
rate, 149–150
relationship of P to QRS, 136f
termination, 142f
Supraventricular tachycardia, 10, 10f,
129f
as cause of wide QRS complex
tachycardia, 150t
electrocardiographic and mechanistic
characteristics, 135f
narrow complex, 131f, 131t
in pregnancy, 787–790
regularity, 149
role of cardioversion in, 315–316

Surgery
for arrhythmias, 383–386, 740
arrhythmias after cardiac and noncardiac, 831–862
for atrial fibrillation, 384–385, 384f
atrial fibrillation after, 462
for atrial flutter, 384, 513
for atrial tachycardias, 422–423
for mitral valve prolapse, 901
orthotopic technique of heart transplantation, 910, 910f
for paroxysmal supraventricular tachycardia, 385–386
for sudden cardiac death, 635
therapy for arrhythmia prevention, 484
for ventricular tachyarrhythmias, 386
Survival With Oral d-Sotalol (SWORD) Trial, 177, 178f, 877, 878f
Sustained monomorphic ventricular tachycardia, 573–601
arrhythmogenic right ventricular dysplasia and, 591–592, 592f
bundle branch reentrant tachycardia and, 590–591, 590f
clinical evaluation, 578–587
diagnostic evaluation, 579
electrocardiogram, 579–581, 579f, 580f, 581t
electrophysiologic studies, 582–584, 582f, 583f, 584t, 585f
exercise testing, 581, 581f
Holter and event monitoring, 581–582
mapping ventricular tachycardia, 584, 586–587, 586f, 587f
physical examination, 578–579
signal-averaged electrocardiogram, 581
clinical presentation, 577–578, 578f
definition, 573
idiopathic ventricular tachycardia and, 592–594
left posterior fascicular, 593–594, 594f
right ventricular outflow tract, 592–593, 593f
pathogenesis, 574–577, 575f, 576f, 577f
prevalence, 573–574
reentrant fascicular tachycardia and, 591
therapy, 587–590
acute, 587–588
chronic, 588–590
antiarrhythmic drugs, 588
implantable cardioverter-defibrillator, 588–589, 589f
radiofrequency catheter ablation, 589–590, 589f
Sustained reentrant atrial tachycardia, etiology, 416
SVTs. *See* Supraventricular tachyarrhythmias
SWORD. *See* Survival With Oral d-Sotalol Trial
Sympathetic nervous system, atrial fibrillation and, 469
Sympathetic-parasympathetic nervous system, interactions with arrhythmias, 112, 113f
Sympatholytic antihypertensives, for sinus node dysfunction or worsening, 659t

Sympathomimetics, dilated cardiomyopathy and, 729t
Symptomatic ventricular tachycardia, ECG for risk assessment of, 177
Syncope, 925–944. *See also* Clinical studies
cardiac transplantation and, 917–918, 918t
causes in orthotopic heart transplant recipients, 918t
classification and evaluation of the causes, 931–938
neurally mediated reflex disturbances of blood pressure control, 931–933
diagnostic evaluation, 933
pathophysiology, 931–933, 932f, 932t
orthostatic and dysautonomic disturbances of vascular control, 933–934
diagnostic evaluation, 934
pathophysiology, 933–934
persistent dizziness, 938, 939t
primary cardiac arrhythmias, 934–936
diagnostic evaluation, 934–936, 936t
pathophysiology, 934
structural cardiovascular or cardiopulmonary disease, 936–937
diagnostic evaluation, 937
pathophysiology, 936–937
syncope caused by cerebrovascular or neurologic disturbances, 937–938
diagnostic evaluation, 938
pathophysiology, 937–938
syncope of noncardiovascular origin, 938
differential diagnostic considerations, 929–931, 929t, 930f
electrophysiologic testing for unknown origin, 936t
epidemiology, 925–928, 926f, 927f, 927t, 928f
isolated, 925
mortality rates, 927, 927f
neurally mediated, indications for permanent cardiac pacing, 337–338
neurocardiogenic, 918
pathophysiology, 929
patient evaluation, 930f, 931
preparticipation screening for athletes and, 825
prognosis, 925–928, 926f, 927f, 927t, 928f
as risk factor for sudden cardiac death, 725t
SAECG in unexplained, 213
treatment, 939–941
of neurally mediated syncope, 939–940
orthostasis and dysautonomias, 940
of primary cardiac arrhythmias, 940
structural cardiovascular/cardiopulmonary disease, 940–941

of unknown origin, electrophysiologic management, 244–245
Systemic thromboembolism
as complication of invasive cardiac electrophysiologic studies, 235t

T
Tachyarrhythmias
cardiac mapping, 249–256
as a complication of defibrillation and cardioversion, 317
criteria for distinguishing between, 155–158, 157f
electrophysiology, 675–677
diagnosis and management, 237–241
idiopathic ventricular, 72
indications for permanent cardiac pacing, 332f, 338–340, 338t, 339f, 339t
narrow QRS complex tachycardia, 237–240, 238f, 239f, 240f
physical examination, 151–152
wide-complex tachycardia, 240–241
Tachycardia. *See also* Clinical studies
catecholaminergic polymorphic ventricular, 85t
causes of fetal, 793t
circuits in patients with Wolff-Parkinson-White syndrome, 130f
continuation, 149f
electrophysiologic significance, 140f
endless-loop, 351, 351f
indications for temporary cardiac pacing, 330–331, 331f, 332f
interventions and drugs, 152
junctional, 147f
long RP–short PR, 141f
relationships in, 139, 141f, 142f–143f
Mahaim fiber, 145, 146f
narrow-complex, 129–150
not requiring an atrioventricular bypass tract for initiation and maintenance of the arrhythmia, 524–525, 525f
pacing indications for prevention of, 338, 338t
pathophysiology associated with atrioventricular accessory pathways, 523–525, 523f, 524f, 525f
repetitive junctional, 128f
requiring an atrioventricular bypass tract for arrhythmia initiation and maintenance, 523–524, 523f, 524f
short RP–long PR relationships in, 136f, 139, 139f, 140f
sinoatrial reentrant, 144f
termination improvement with implantable cardioverter-defibrillators, 363–364
ventricular polymorphic, 64f, 65
V_1-negative wide QRS, 156–157, 157f
V_1-positive wide QRS, 156, 157f
wide complex
versus supraventricular, 151t
wide-complex, 153f, 240–241
in Wolff-Parkinson-White syndrome, 517–548

Tachycardia-bradycardia syndrome, 461, 507, 656, 657f, 658f
Tachycardia-mediated cardiomyopathy, 502–503
Tacrolimus (Prograf, RK506)
　interaction with antiarrhythmic agents, 909t
　for prevention of rejection of the transplanted heart, 909
　for Torsade de pointes, 909
Tafazzin-related Barth syndrome, 91–92
Tambocor. *See* Flecainide
TAMI 9 trial, 703
TdP. *See* Torsade de pointes
Tedisamil, 291
　as repolarization-prolonging drug, 273t
TEE. *See* Transesophageal echocardiography
Telemetry, in-hospital, 171
Terbutaline, electrophysiologic effects of, 913t
Terfenadine, 266
　Torsade de Pointes and, 611
Tetralogy of Fallot, 754, 755f
　incidence of arrhythmias after repair of, 767t
d-TGA. *See* d-Transposition of the great arteries
l-TGA. *See* l-Transposition of the great arteries
Theophylline, 413
　cardiac transplantation and, 912, 913t
　for sinus bradycardia after transplantation, 856
Third-degree atrioventricular block, 700f, 873, 873f
　ECG manifestations, 683–684
　electrophysiologic mechanisms, 686
　incidence and prevalence, 676f, 677, 678f
　treatment and indications for pacing, 689
Threshold current, 10
Thromboembolism
　antithrombotic therapy before cardioversion, 487–489
　risk factors in chronic atrial fibrillation, 485–486
　role of anticoagulation and, 485–489
　therapy for prevention of stroke in chronic atrial fibrillation, 486–487
　treatment recommendations in chronic atrial fibrillation, 487
Thrombolysis. *See also* Clinical studies
　predictive value in death and arrhythmic events after, 202–203
Thrombolysis in Myocardial Infarction (TIMI II) trial, 873
Thrombolytic therapy
　with acute conduction blocks, 703
　for coronary occlusion, 876
Thrombophlebitis, as complication of invasive cardiac electrophysiologic studies, 235t
Thyroid
　abnormalities as predisposing factor to atrial fibrillation, 462
　supplementation for postoperative atrial fibrillation, 842
TIA. *See* Transient Ischemic Attack

Tikosyn. *See* Dofetilide
Tilt-table testing
　for evaluation of syncope, 932, 932t, 937
　testing methodology, 933
Time domain analysis, 196–197, 196t
　definitions, 196t
TIMI II. *See* Thrombolysis in Myocardial Infarction trial
Timolol
　for arrhythmias in pregnancy, 795
　prophylaxis trials, 838t
Tocainide (Tonocard)
　adverse effects, 277
　dosing, 277
　drug classification, 273t
　effect on ventricular tachycardia rate, 376t
　efficacy, 277
　electrophysiology, 277
　hemodynamic effects, 271
　pharmacokinetics, 277, 277t
　for sinus node dysfunction or worsening, 659t
Tonocard. *See* Tocainide
Torsade de pointes (TdP), 65
　antiarrhythmic agents and, 270–271
　bradyarrhythmias and, 612
　cerebrovascular diseases and, 612
　clinical conditions associated with, 607–613
　　acquired long QT syndromes, 608–612
　　congenital long QT syndrome, 607–608
　　polymorphous ventricular tachycardia in the absence of prolonged cardiac repolarization, 612–613
　drug-induced, 83
　initiating sequences of, 603–604, 604f
　mapping, 70
　polymorphous ventricular tachycardia, 603, 604f
　Quinidine syncope and, 609
　rate-dependence, 603
　repolarization reserve, 611
　risk factors for drug-induced, 611, 611t
　short QT interval and, 612–613
　tacrolimus and, 909
　therapy, 613–614
Toxicity
　for chronic treatment of orthodromic atrioventricular reentrant tachycardia in WPW syndrome, 540
　drug-related and exercise testing, 185–187, 186f, 187t
Toxins, exposure to, 820–821
d-Transposition of the great arteries (d-TGA), 756–757f
l-Transposition of the great arteries (l-TGA), 756–759, 757f
Trandolapril Cardiac Evaluation study (TRACE), 461
Transcatheter ablation, complications of invasive cardiac electrophysiologic studies and, 235t

Transesophageal echocardiography (TEE), atrial fibrillation and, 488–489
Transesophageal pacing, 326–327, 329f
Transient ischemic attack (TIA), as complication of invasive cardiac electrophysiologic studies, 235t
Transplacental therapy, for fetal arrhythmias, 794
Transplantation. *See* Cardiac transplantation
Transthoracic echocardiography, for evaluation of arrhythmogenic right ventricular cardiomyopathy, 738
Transthoracic impedance, 311, 311t
　factors affecting, 311t
Trauma
　as a complication of defibrillation and cardioversion, 318
　etiology, 681
Trecetilide, 291
　repolarization-prolonging drug, 273t
Tremulous incoordination, 303
Triangle of Koch, 433, 433f
Tricuspid atresia, 760–761, 760f
Trifascicular disease, 237
　indications for permanent cardiac pacing, 337, 337t
Triiodothyronine (T₃), supplementation for postoperative atrial fibrillation, 842
Tromethamine, for sudden cardiac death, 631
Troponin T, hypertrophic cardiomyopathy and, 88
Tumors
　as a cause of sinus node dysfunction, 659
　primary cardiac, in children, 763
T-wave alternans, 218–225. *See also* Clinical studies
　arrhythmias and, 110–112, 110f, 111f, 111t
　cellular electrophysiologic mechanisms underlying, 218–219
　clinical studies, 222, 223f
　dependence on heart rate, 220
　ICD shock prediction, 224
　interpretation, 220–221, 221f
　measurement, 219–222, 219f
　polymorphous ventricular tachycardia and, 604, 605f
　risk stratification
　　after myocardial infarction, 222–223, 224f
　　in congestive heart failure, 223
　ventricular arrhythmias and, 219
Twiddler's syndrome, as a complication of implantable cardioverter-defibrillators, 374
Typical atrial flutter, 502, 502f

U

Uhl's anomaly, 737
UK-HEART. *See* United Kingdom Heart Failure Evaluation and Assessment of Risk Trial
ULV. *See* Upper limit of vulnerability
United Kingdom Heart Failure Evaluation and Assessment of Risk Trial (UK-HEART), 205–207, 206f, 732

Unstable angina, risk for nocturnal cardiac events, 119t
Upper limit of vulnerability (ULV), 304
Use dependency, 185

V
Vagal atrial fibrillation, autonomic nervous system and, 468–469
Vagal stimulation, action potential and, 40
Vagal tone, 680–681
Vagolytic agents, for atrioventricular nodal reentry tachycardia, 446–447
Valvular disease
  etiology, 681
  postoperative arrhythmias after surgery, 850
  sudden cardiac death in athletes and, 818–819
  surgery, bradyarrhythmias and, 855
Vascular supply, 6
  orthostatic and dysautonomic disturbances and syncope, 933–934
Vasculopathy, cardiac transplantation and, 915
VASIS. *See* Vasovagal Syncope International Study
Vasovagal Syncope International Study (VASIS), 338
Ventricle
  chronic arrhythmias after operation on, 772–777
    clinical significance, 773
    evaluation, 773–774
    incidence, 773, 773f
    management, 774
  retrograde refractory period, 15t
  transmural variation of the action potential in, 41, 41f
Ventricular arrhythmias
  after cardiac and noncardiac surgery, 851–854
    diagnosis, 852
    epidemiology and incidence, 851
    management, 852–854
    mechanisms of unexpected, 852
    prognosis, 852
    recognizable antecedent causes, 851
    unexpected de novo ventricular arrhythmias, 851–852
  antecedent causes, 851
  in athletes, 810–813, 811f, 812f–813f, 814f, 824t
  cardiac action potential in, 48
  cellular effects of acute ischemia, 863–864
    changes in the action potential, 864
    resting membrane potential, 863–864
  clinical features, 865–866
    premature ventricular contractions, 865–866
    ventricular fibrillation, 866
    ventricular tachycardia, 866, 866f
  delayed, 865
  diagnosis, 852
  drugs used during myocardial infarction, 867t

epidemiology and incidence, 851
exercise testing
  for management of, 184–187, 184f
  prognostic significance, 182–184, 183t
  in hypertrophic cardiomyopathy, 724–725
incidence
  during exercise, 180–182, 180t, 181f
  of sustained ventricular arrhythmias or sudden cardiac death after myocardial infarction, 877t
ischemic heart disease and, 863–869
management, 852
  acute treatment, 852–853
  long-term, 853–854
mechanisms of periinfarction, 864–865
  acute-phase ischemia, 864–865
  delayed ventricular arrhythmias, 865
  role of the autonomic nervous system, 865
prognosis, 852
psychological stress and, 115, 115f
significance of nonsustained ventricular tachycardia, 724
treatment of periinfarction, 867–869, 867t, 868t
unexpected de novo, 851–852
Ventricular bigeminy, 551, 551f
Ventricular capture (Dressler beat), 684
Ventricular dysrhythmias
  cardiac transplantation and, 916–917
  premature ventricular complexes and nonsustained ventricular tachycardia, 916
  sustained ventricular arrhythmias, 916–917, 917f
Ventricular-evoked response amplitudes (VERAs), for detection of transplant rejection with pacemakers, 919
Ventricular fibrillation
  as a complication of invasive cardiac electrophysiologic studies, 235t
  ECG for risk assessment of, 177
  idiopathic, 97
  recommendations in acute myocardial infarction, 868t
  termination by potassium chloride infusion, 305f
  treatment, 868–869
  ventricular arrhythmias and, 866
Ventricular flutter, 573
Ventricular parasystole, 550, 550f
Ventricular preexcitation, 8
Ventricular premature beats (VPBs)
  prognostic significance of exercise-induced, 182, 183f, 184
Ventricular premature contractions (VPCs), in mitral valve prolapse, 891–893, 892f
Ventricular premature depolarizations (VPDs), 549–571, 551f, 552f
  clinical manifestations, 552–554, 554f
  electrocardiographic characteristics, 549–552, 550f, 551f, 552f, 553f
  mechanisms, 556–557
  prevalence, 554–555, 554t, 555t, 556t

prognostic significance, 557–560
  with coronary artetry disease, 558–559, 559t
  with hypertrophic cardiomyopathy, 557
  with nonischemic dilated cardiomyopathy, 557, 557t, 558f
  in a normal population, 557
treatment, 560–567
  sudden cardiac death reduction, 561–567
  symptom relief, 560–561
Ventricular proarrhythmia, antiarrhythmic agents and, 269–271
Ventricular rate, therapy to control, 471–475
Ventricular septal defect (VSD), 752–753
  arrhythmias after repair of, 777
Ventricular tachyarrhythmias
  electrophysiologic management of, 241–243
    application and protocols, 241–242
    in ischemic heart disease, 242–243
  electrophysiology in nonischemic cardiac disease, 243–244
  evaluation, 774–776, 776f
  implantable cardioverter-defibrillators and, 359
  incidence, 774
  management, 776–777
  surgical treatment of, 386
Ventricular tachycardia (VT)
  with atrioventricular dissociation, 154f
  cardiac mapping, 253–256, 255f, 256f, 257f
  catecholaminergic polymorphic, 97
  as cause of wide QRS complex tachycardia, 150t
  changes in ST segments, 154f
  definition, 866
  determination of the mechanism of, 584, 584t
  effect of antiarrhythmic drugs on rate, 376t
  electrophysiologic study, 156f
  exercise-induced, 581, 581f
  idiopathic, 97
  indications, use, and outcomes of catheter ablation, 400–402
  mapping, 584–587, 586f, 587f
  monomorphic, antiarrhythmic agents and, 270
  prediction of inducible, 216
  in pregnancy, 790–791
  preoperative incidence of arrhythmias in patients with related congenital heart defects, 750t
  recommendations in acute myocardial infarction, 868t
  role of cardioversion and defibrillation in, 313–314, 314f
  significance of nonsustained, 724
  sustained, 724
  sustained monomorphic. *See* Sustained monomorphic ventricular tachycardia
  treatment, 867–868, 868t

with two morphologies, 154f
ventricular arrhythmias and, 866, 866f
Ventriculography, contrast. *See* Contrast ventriculography
Verapamil (Calan, Isoptin)
adverse effects, 292
for arrhythmias in pregnancy, 796
for atrial flutter, 508
for atrial tachyarrhythmias, 871
for atrial tachycardia, 419
for atrioventricular nodal reentry tachycardia, 448
as cause of atrioventricular block, 679
complications, 727
dosing, 291–292
drug classification, 273t
effect on defibrillator threshold, 376t
efficacy, 292
electrophysiology, 291
for heart rate control in atrial fibrillation, 474, 474t
interaction with immunosuppressive agents, 909t
for multifocal atrial tachycardia, 412, 413
for orthodromic atrioventricular reentrant tachycardia in WPW syndrome, 540
pharmacokinetics, 291
for pretreatment for cardioversion, 476
prophylaxis
for atrial fibrillation after CABG, 839
trials, 837t
for rate control
of atrial fibrillation, 471–472
of postoperative atrial arrhythmias, 845t
for sinoatrial nodal atrial tachycardia, 425
for sinus node
dysfunction, 659
dysfunction induction or worsening, 659t
reentrant tachycardia, 656
for slowing ventricular response rates during atrial fibrillation, 473t
for ventricular rate control during atrial fibrillation, 872t

VERAs. *See* Ventricular-evoked response amplitudes
VEST trial, 730, 731f
Veterans Administration Heart Failure Trial (CHF-STAT), 561–562
Voltage mapping, 253, 256
Voltage pulse, 324
VPBs. *See* Ventricular premature beats
VPCs. *See* Ventricular premature contractions
VPDs. *See* Ventricular premature depolarizations
VSD. *See* Ventricular septal defect
VT. *See* Ventricular tachycardia

W

Warfarin
for atrial flutter, 512
for postoperative atrial arrhythmias, 848
for prevention of thromboembolism, 486–487
Waveforms, defibrillation and, 308–310, 309f, 310f, 359
Wavelength, 52
atrial fibrillation and, 465–466, 465f, 466f
Wild type, definition, 102
Wolff-Parkinson-White (WPW) syndrome, 98
anatomic considerations, 521–522, 521f, 522f
antidromic atrioventricular reentrant tachycardia (AAVRT), 534–535, 536f, 537f
in athletes, 811–812
cardiac transplantation and, 915
as cause of wide QRS complex tachycardia, 150t
electrocardiographic and electrophysiologic manifestations, 525–539
electrophysiologic testing in asymptomatic individuals, 528–529
epidemiology of preexcitation, 522

etiology and predisposing factors, 461–462
exercise testing for evaluation of, 188
heart rate control in, 473, 473f
history, 517
orthodromic atrioventricular reentrant tachycardia and, 529–533, 530f, 531f, 532f–533f, 534f
pacemaker management of, 331, 332f
pathogenesis of accessory pathways and preexcitation, 517–521, 518f, 519f, 520f, 521f
pathophysiology of tachycardias associated with atrioventricular accessory pathways, 523–525, 523f, 524f, 525f
permanent junctional reciprocating tachycardia and, 533–534, 535f
surgery and, 385, 513
tachycardia circuits in patients with, 130f
tachycardias in, 517–548
therapy for arrhythmias associated with, 539–543
ablation therapy, 542–543, 543f
antitachycardia devices, 541–542, 542f
pharmacologic therapy, 539–541
Women. *See also* Gender
arrhythmias and conduction disturbances associated with pregnancy. *See* Pregnancy
risk of development of atrial fibrillation, 459t
sudden cardiac death in athletes and, 820
Worry, behavioral studies and risk of cardiac events, 118t
WPW. *See* Wolff-Parkinson-White syndrome

X

X-linked dominant, definition, 81, 83f
X-linked recessive, definition, 81, 83f
Xylocaine. *See* Lidocaine hydrochloride